CAMPBELL'S
UROLOGY

Edited by

Patrick C. Walsh, M.D.

David Hall McConnell Professor
The Johns Hopkins University School of Medicine
Urologist-in-Chief
Brady Urological Institute
The Johns Hopkins Hospital
Baltimore, Maryland

Alan B. Retik, M.D.

Professor of Surgery (Urology)
Harvard Medical School
Chief, Division of Urology
Children's Hospital
Boston, Massachusetts

Thomas A. Stamey, M.D.

Professor and Chairman
Department of Urology
Stanford University School of Medicine
Stanford, California

E. Darracott Vaughan, Jr., M.D.

James J. Colt Professor of Urology
Cornell University Medical College
Urologist-in-Chief
The New York Hospital–Cornell Medical Center
New York, New York

Sixth Edition

CAMPBELL'S UROLOGY

W. B. SAUNDERS COMPANY
A Division of Harcourt Brace & Company

Philadelphia   London   Toronto   Montreal   Sydney   Tokyo

W. B. SAUNDERS COMPANY

A Division of
Harcourt Brace & Company

The Curtis Center
Independence Square West
Philadelphia, PA 19106

Library of Congress Cataloging-in-Publication Data

Campbell's Urology—6th ed. / [edited by] Patrick C. Walsh
. . . [et al.]

     p.   cm.

Includes bibliographical references and index.

ISBN 0–7216–3059–6 (set)

1. Urology.   I. Campbell, Meredith F. (Meredith
Fairfax),   . II. Walsh, Patrick C.,   . III. Title:
Urology.
[DNLM: 1. Urologic Diseases.   WJ 100 C192]

RC871.C33 1992   616.6—dc20   90–9237
DNLM/DLC

Listed here are the latest translated editions of this book together with the language of the translation
and the publisher.

Italian (3rd Edition)   Casa Editrice Universo,
                      Rome, Italy

Portuguese (1st Edition) Editora Guanabara Koogan,
                      Rio de Janeiro, Brazil

Editor: W. B. Saunders Staff
Developmental Editor: Rosanne Hallowell
Designer: Maureen Sweeney
Production Manager: Carolyn Naylor
Manuscript Editors: Mary Anne Folcher, Carol Robins,
                  Mary Ellen Ford, and Terry Belanger
Illustration Coordinator: Walter Verbitski
Indexers: Angela Holt and Julie Figures
Cover Designer: Michelle Maloney

Volume 1 ISBN 0–7216–4048–6
Volume 2 ISBN 0–7216–4049–4
Volume 3 ISBN 0–7216–4050–8
Set ISBN 0–7216–3059–6

Campbell's Urology, 6th edition

Printed in the United States of America.

Last digit is the print number: 9   8   7   6   5   4   3

CONTRIBUTORS

Mark C. Adams, M.D.

Assistant Professor of Urology, Indiana University School of Medicine, Indianapolis, Indiana. Attending Physician, Department of Urology, James Whitcomb Riley Hospital for Children, Indianapolis.

> AUGMENTATION CYSTOPLASTY IMPLANTATION OF ARTIFICIAL URINARY SPHINCTER IN MEN AND WOMEN AND RECONSTRUCTION OF THE DYSFUNCTIONAL URINARY TRACT

John M. Barry, M.D.

Professor of Surgery, and Chairman, Division of Urology and Renal Transplantation, Oregon Health Sciences University, Portland, Oregon. Staff Surgeon, University Hospital; and Consultant, Veterans Hospital, Portland.

> RENAL TRANSPLANTATION

Stuart B. Bauer, M.D.

Associate Professor of Surgery (Urology), Harvard Medical School, Boston, Massachusetts. Associate in Surgery (Urology), Children's Hospital, Boston.

> ANOMALIES OF THE UPPER URINARY TRACT
> NEUROGENIC VESICAL DYSFUNCTION IN CHILDREN

Arie Belldegrun, M.D.

Associate Professor of Surgery/Urology, University of California School of Medicine, Los Angeles, California. Attending Physician, UCLA Medical Center; Chief, Division of Urology, Olive View/UCLA Medical Center; and Clinical Director, Adoptive Immunotherapy Core Laboratory, Jonsson Comprehensive Cancer Center, Los Angeles.

> RENAL TUMORS

Mitchell C. Benson, M.D.

Associate Professor of Clinical Urology, Columbia University College of Physicians and Surgeons, New York, New York. Director, Urologic Oncology, Columbia–Presbyterian Medical Center, New York.

> URINARY DIVERSION

Richard E. Berger, M.D.

Associate Professor of Urology, University of Washington, Seattle, Washington. Attending Physician, University of Washington Affiliated Hospitals, Seattle.

> SEXUALLY TRANSMITTED DISEASES: THE CLASSIC DISEASES

Jon David Blumenfeld, M.D.

Assistant Professor of Medicine, Cornell University Medical College, New York, New York. Assistant Attending Physician in Medicine, The New York Hospital, New York.

> THE ADRENALS

Charles B. Brendler, M.D.

Associate Professor of Urology, The Johns Hopkins University School of Medicine, Baltimore, Maryland. Attending Physician, The Johns Hopkins Hospital, Baltimore.

> EVALUATION OF THE UROLOGIC PATIENT: HISTORY, PHYSICAL EXAMINATION, AND URINALYSIS
> URETHRECTOMY
> PERIOPERATIVE CARE

Peter N. Burns, Ph.D.

Associate Professor of Medical Biophysics and Radiology, University of Toronto, Toronto, Ontario, Canada. Senior Scientist, Sunnybrook Health Science Centre, Toronto.

> IMAGING OF THE URINARY TRACT: ULTRASONOGRAPHY OF THE URINARY TRACT

H. Ballentine Carter, M.D.

Assistant Professor of Urology, The Johns Hopkins University School of Medicine, Baltimore, Maryland. Department of Urology, The Johns Hopkins Hospital and Francis Scott Key Hospital, Baltimore.

> EVALUATION OF THE UROLOGIC PATIENT: INSTRUMENTATION AND ENDOSCOPY

William J. Catalona, M.D.
Professor of Surgery/Urology, Washington University School of Medicine, St. Louis, Missouri. Attending Physician, Barnes Hospital, The Jewish Hospital of St. Louis, and St. Louis Children's Hospital, St. Louis.
UROTHELIAL TUMORS OF THE URINARY TRACT

Thomas S. K. Chang, Ph.D.
Associate Professor, Department of Urology, The Johns Hopkins School of Medicine, Baltimore, Maryland.
PHYSIOLOGY OF MALE REPRODUCTION: THE TESTIS, EPIDIDYMIS, AND DUCTUS DEFERENS

Robert L. Chevalier, M.D.
Professor and Vice-Chairman, Department of Pediatrics, University of Virginia School of Medicine, Charlottesville, Virginia. Attending Pediatrician, and Chief, Division of Pediatric Nephrology, University of Virginia Health Sciences Center, Charlottesville.
RENAL FUNCTION IN THE FETUS AND NEONATE

Robert J. Churchill, M.D.
Professor and Chairman of Radiology, University of Missouri School of Medicine, Columbia, Missouri. Chairman, Department of Radiology, University of Missouri Hospital and Clinics, Columbia.
IMAGING OF THE URINARY TRACT: COMPUTED TOMOGRAPHY OF THE URINARY TRACT

Ralph V. Clayman, M.D.
Professor of Urologic Surgery and Radiology, Washington University School of Medicine, St. Louis, Missouri. Attending Physician, Barnes Affiliated Hospitals, Barnes Hospital, Veterans Administration Hospital, The Jewish Hospital of St. Louis, and St. Louis Children's Hospital, St. Louis.
ENDOSURGICAL TECHNIQUES FOR THE DIAGNOSIS AND TREATMENT OF NONCALCULOUS DISEASE OF THE URETER AND KIDNEY

Donald S. Coffey, Ph.D.
Professor, The Johns Hopkins University School of Medicine, Baltimore, Maryland.
PHYSIOLOGY OF MALE REPRODUCTION: THE MOLECULAR BIOLOGY, ENDOCRINOLOGY, AND PHYSIOLOGY OF THE PROSTATE AND SEMINAL VESICLES

Giulio J. D'Angio, M.D.
Professor of Radiation Oncology, Radiology, and Pediatric Oncology, University of Pennsylvania School of Medicine, Philadelphia, Pennsylvania. Vice-Chairman, Department of Radiation Oncology, Hospital of the University of Pennsylvania, Philadelphia.
PEDIATRIC ONCOLOGY

Jean B. deKernion, M.D.
Professor of Surgery/Urology, and Chief, Division of Urology, University of California School of Medicine, Los Angeles, California. Professor of Surgery/Urology—UCLA School of Medicine, and Chief, Division of Urology, Los Angeles.
RENAL TUMORS

Francesco Del Greco, M.D.
Professor of Medicine, Northwestern University Medical School, Chicago, Illinois. Attending Physician and Medical Director, Dialysis Center, Northwestern Memorial Hospital, Chicago. Visiting Attending Physician, Veterans Administration Lakeside Hospital, Chicago.
OTHER RENAL DISEASES OF UROLOGIC SIGNIFICANCE

Charles J. Devine, Jr., M.D.
Professor of Urology, Eastern Virginia Medical School, Norfolk, Virginia. Attending Physician, The Devine Center for Genitourinary Reconstructive Surgery, Sentara Norfolk General Hospital, Sentara Leigh Memorial Hospital, and Children's Hospital of the King's Daughters, Norfolk.
SURGERY OF THE PENIS AND URETHRA

William C. DeWolf, M.D.
Associate Professor of Surgery, Harvard Medical School, Boston, Massachusetts. Urologist-in-Chief, Beth Israel Hospital, Boston.
GENETIC DETERMINANTS OF UROLOGIC DISEASE

George W. Drach, M.D.
Professor of Surgery, and Chief of Urology, University of Arizona, Tucson, Arizona. Attending Urologist, University Medical Center; and Consultant in Urology, Veterans Administration Medical Center, Tucson.
URINARY LITHIASIS: ETIOLOGY, DIAGNOSIS, AND MEDICAL MANAGEMENT

John W. Duckett, M.D.
Professor of Urology in Surgery, University of Pennsylvania School of Medicine, Philadelphia, Pennsylvania. Director, Division of Urology, Children's Hospital of Philadelphia, Philadelphia.
HYPOSPADIAS

J. S. Dunbar, M.D.
Professor Emeritus, Department of Radiology, University of Toronto, Toronto, Ontario, Canada. Consultant in Radiology, Hospital for Sick Children, Toronto.
IMAGING OF THE URINARY TRACT: EXCRETORY UROGRAPHY IN INFANTS AND CHILDREN

Jack S. Elder, M.D.
Associate Professor of Urology and Pediatrics, Case Western Reserve University School of Medicine, Cleveland, Ohio. Director of Pediatric Urology, Rainbow Babies and Children's Hospital and MetroHealth Hospital, Cleveland.
CONGENITAL ANOMALIES OF THE GENITALIA

Audrey E. Evans, M.D.
Professor of Pediatrics and Human Genetics, University of Pennsylvania School of Medicine, Philadelphia, Pennsylvania. Professor of Pediatric Oncology, Children's Hospital of Philadelphia, Philadelphia.
PEDIATRIC ONCOLOGY

William R. Fair, M.D.
Professor of Surgery/Urology, Cornell University Medical College, New York, New York; and Member, Sloan–Kettering Institute, New York. Chief, Urology Service, Memorial Sloan–Kettering Cancer Center; and Attending Surgeon, Memorial Hospital and New York Hospital, New York.
OVERVIEW OF CANCER BIOLOGY AND PRINCIPLES OF ONCOLOGY

Fuad S. Freiha, M.D.
Professor of Urology, Stanford University School of Medicine, Stanford, California. Chief, Urologic Oncology, Stanford University Medical Center, Stanford.
OPEN BLADDER SURGERY

Richard M. Friedenberg, M.D.
Professor and Chairman, Department of Radiological Sciences, University of California, Irvine, California. Chairman, Department of Radiological Sciences, University of California, Irvine Medical Center, Orange, California.
IMAGING OF THE URINARY TRACT: EXCRETORY UROGRAPHY IN THE ADULT

John P. Gearhart, M.D.
Associate Professor of Pediatric Urology and Pediatrics, The Johns Hopkins University School of Medicine, Baltimore, Maryland. Director of Pediatric Urology, The Johns Hopkins Hospital; and Consultant in Pediatric Urology, Francis Scott Key Hospital, The University of Maryland Hospital, and John F. Kennedy Hospital, Baltimore.
EXSTROPHY OF THE BLADDER, EPISPADIAS, AND OTHER BLADDER ANOMALIES

Fredrick W. George, Ph.D.
Assistant Professor of Internal Medicine, Department of Internal Medicine, University of Texas Southwestern Medical Center, Dallas, Texas.
EMBRYOLOGY OF THE GENITAL TRACT

Bruce R. Gilbert, M.D., Ph.D.
Clinical Instructor in Surgery (Urology), The New York Hospital–Cornell Medical Center, New York, New York. Assistant Attending Surgeon (Urology), The New York Hospital, New York.
NORMAL RENAL PHYSIOLOGY

Jay Y. Gillenwater, M.D.
Professor and Chairman of Urology, University of Virginia Medical School, Charlottesville, Virginia. Chairman of Urology, University of Virginia Hospital, Charlottesville.
THE PATHOPHYSIOLOGY OF URINARY TRACT OBSTRUCTION

Kenneth I. Glassberg, M.D.
Professor of Urology, State University of New York Health Science Center, Brooklyn, New York. Director, Division of Pediatric Urology, University Hospital of Brooklyn, Kings County Hospital Center, and Long Island College Hospital; Attending Physician in Urology at Maimonides Medical Center, Brooklyn.
RENAL DYSPLASIA AND CYSTIC DISEASE OF THE KIDNEY

Irwin Goldstein, M.D.
Professor of Urology, Boston University School of Medicine, Boston, Massachusetts. Visiting Surgeon, University Hospital, Boston.
DIAGNOSIS AND THERAPY OF ERECTILE DYSFUNCTION

Marc Goldstein, M.D.
Associate Professor of Surgery (Urology), Cornell University Medical College; and Staff Scientist, Center for Biomedical Research, The Population Council, New York, New York. Associate Attending Surgeon and Director, The Male Reproduction and Microsurgery Unit, The James Buchanan Brady Foundation, Department of Surgery, Division of Urology, The New York Hospital–Cornell Medical Center, New York.
SURGERY OF MALE INFERTILITY AND OTHER SCROTAL DISORDERS

Edmond T. Gonzales, Jr., M.D.
Professor of Urology, Scott Department of Urology, Baylor College of Medicine, Houston, Texas. Chief, Urology Service, and Head, Department of Surgery, Texas Children's Hospital, Houston.
POSTERIOR URETHRAL VALVES AND OTHER URETHRAL ANOMALIES

Rafael Gosalbez, M.D.
Fellow, Pediatric Urology, Emory University School of Medicine, Atlanta, Georgia.
NEONATAL AND PERINATAL EMERGENCIES

James G. Gow, M.D., Ch.M., F.R.C.S.
Former Clinical Lecturer, University of Liverpool, Liverpool, United Kingdom. Attending Physician, Lourdes Private Hospital, Liverpool.
GENITOURINARY TUBERCULOSIS

Damian R. Greene, M.B., F.R.C.S.I.
Post-Doctoral Research Fellow in Urologic Oncology, Baylor College of Medicine, Houston, Texas.
UROLOGIC ULTRASONOGRAPHY

Alexander Greenstein, M.D.
Assistant Professor of Urology, Department of Urology, Sourasky Medical Center, Ichilov Hospital, Tel-Aviv University, Tel-Aviv, Israel.
SURGERY OF THE URETER

James E. Griffin, M.D.
Professor of Internal Medicine, University of Texas Southwestern Medical Center, Dallas, Texas. Attending Physician, Parkland Memorial Hospital, Dallas.
DISORDERS OF SEXUAL DIFFERENTIATION

John Hale, Ph.D.
Professor Emeritus, Radiological Physics, University of Pennsylvania School of Medicine, Philadelphia, Pennsylvania.
IMAGING OF THE URINARY TRACT: RADIATION PROTECTION

W. Hardy Hendren, M.D.
Robert E. Gross Professor of Surgery, Harvard Medical School, Boston, Massachusetts. Chief of Surgery, Children's Hospital, and Visiting Surgeon, Massachusetts General Hospital, Boston.
CLOACAL MALFORMATIONS
URINARY UNDIVERSION: REFUNCTIONALIZATION OF THE PREVIOUSLY DIVERTED URINARY TRACT

Harry W. Herr, M.D.
Associate Professor of Surgery, Cornell University Medical College, New York, New York. Associate Attending Surgeon, Memorial Sloan–Kettering Cancer Center, New York.
SURGERY OF PENILE AND URETHRAL CARCINOMA

Marjorie Hertz, M.D.
Professor of Radiology and Head, Section of Imaging, Sackler Faculty of Medicine, Tel-Aviv University, Ramat Aviv, Israel. Senior Radiologist, Imaging Department, Sheba Medical Center, Tel-Hashomer, Israel.
IMAGING OF THE URINARY TRACT: CYSTOURETHROGRAPHY

Warren D. W. Heston, Ph.D.
Associate Member and Director of Urologic Oncology Research, Memorial Sloan–Kettering Cancer Center, New York, New York.
OVERVIEW OF CANCER BIOLOGY AND PRINCIPLES OF ONCOLOGY

Stuart S. Howards, M.D.
Professor of Urology and Physiology, University of Virginia Health Sciences Center, Charlottesville, Virginia. Staff Urologist, University of Virginia Hospital, Charlottesville.
MALE INFERTILITY
SURGERY OF THE SCROTUM AND TESTIS IN CHILDHOOD

Jeffry L. Huffman, M.D.
Associate Professor of Urology, University of Southern California School of Medicine, Los Angeles, California. Attending Physician, USC University Hospital, Los Angeles.
URETEROSCOPY

Robert D. Jeffs, M.D., F.R.C.S.(C.)
Professor of Pediatric Urology, The Johns Hopkins University School of Medicine, Baltimore, Maryland. Director Emeritus of Pediatric Urology, The Johns Hopkins Hospital; and Consultant in Pediatric Urology, Francis Scott Key Medical Center, University of Maryland Hospital, and John F. Kennedy Institute, Baltimore.
EXSTROPHY OF THE BLADDER, EPISPADIAS, AND OTHER BLADDER ANOMALIES

Gerald H. Jordon, M.D.
Associate Professor, Department of Urology, Eastern Virginia Medical School, Norfolk, Virginia. Attending Physician, Sentara Hospitals, Norfolk General and Leigh Memorial, The Children's Hospital of the King's Daughters, and DePaul Medical Center, Norfolk.
TUMORS OF THE PENIS
SURGERY OF THE PENIS AND URETHRA

Saad Juma, M.D.
Assistant Clinical Professor, Division of Urology, University of California School of Medicine, San Diego, California.
FEMALE UROLOGY

John N. Kabalin, M.D.
Assistant Professor of Urology, Stanford University School of Medicine, Stanford, California. Chief, Urology Section, Veterans Administration Medical Center, Palo Alto, California.
SURGICAL ANATOMY OF THE GENITOURINARY TRACT: ANATOMY OF THE RETROPERITONEUM AND KIDNEY

Louis R. Kavoussi, M.D.
Assistant Professor, Harvard Medical School, Boston, Massachusetts. Head, Section of Endourology, Division of Urologic Surgery, Brigham and Women's Hospital, Boston.
ENDOSURGICAL TECHNIQUES FOR THE DIAGNOSIS AND TREATMENT OF NONCALCULOUS DISEASE OF THE URETER AND KIDNEY

Lowell R. King, M.D.
Professor of Urology, Associate Professor of Pediatrics, and Head, Section on Pediatric Urology, Duke University, Durham, North Carolina. Attending Urologist, Duke University Medical Center, Durham.
VESICOURETERAL REFLUX, MEGAURETER, AND URETERAL REIMPLANTATION

Saulo Klahr, M.D.
John E. and Adaline Simon Professor of Medicine, Washington University School of Medicine, St. Louis, Missouri. Physician-in-Chief, The Jewish Hospital of St. Louis, and Physician, Barnes Hospital, St. Louis.
RENAL ENDOCRINOLOGY

Stephen A. Koff, M.D.
Professor of Surgery, Ohio State University College of Medicine, Columbus, Ohio. Chief, Division of Pediatric Urology, Children's Hospital, Columbus.
ENURESIS

Warren W. Koontz, Jr., M.D.
Professor and Chairman, Division of Urology, Medical College of Virginia, Virginia Commonwealth University, Richmond, Virginia.
SURGERY OF THE URETER

Robert J. Krane, M.D.
Professor and Chairman, Department of Urology, Boston University School of Medicine, Boston, Massachusetts.
DIAGNOSIS AND THERAPY OF ERECTILE DYSFUNCTION

Herbert Y. Kressel, M.D.
Professor of Radiology, University of Pennsylvania School of Medicine, Philadelphia, Pennsylvania. Chief of MRI, Hospital of the University of Pennsylvania, Philadelphia.
IMAGING OF THE URINARY TRACT: MAGNETIC RESONANCE IMAGING

John N. Krieger, M.D.
Associate Professor, Department of Urology, University of Washington School of Medicine, Seattle, Washington.
SEXUALLY TRANSMITTED DISEASES: THE ACQUIRED IMMUNODEFICIENCY SYNDROME AND RELATED CONDITIONS

Elroy D. Kursh, M.D.
Associate Professor of Urology, Case Western Reserve University School of Medicine, Cleveland, Ohio. Attending Urologist, University Hospitals of Cleveland, MetroHealth Medical Center, and Veterans Administration Medical Center, Cleveland.
EXTRINSIC OBSTRUCTION OF THE URETER

Elliott C. Lasser, M.D.
Professor, Department of Radiology, University of California, San Diego, California. Attending Physician, UCSD Medical Center, San Diego.
IMAGING OF THE URINARY TRACT: CONTRAST MEDIA FOR UROGRAPHY

Jay Stauffer Lehman, M.D.*
Formerly, Assistant Director, The Edna McConnell Clark Foundation, New York, New York.
PARASITIC DISEASES OF THE GENITOURINARY SYSTEM

Bruce R. Leslie, M.D.
Staff Physician, Division of Hypertensive Diseases, Ochsner Medical Institutions, New Orleans, Louisiana.
NORMAL RENAL PHYSIOLOGY

John A. Libertino, M.D.
Associate Clinical Professor of Surgery, Harvard Medical School, Boston, Massachusetts. Chief of Surgery, Lahey Clinic Medical Center, Burlington, Massachusetts.
RENOVASCULAR SURGERY

Nancy A. Little, M.D.
Assistant Clinical Professor, Division of Urology, University of Texas Health Science Center at San Antonio, Texas.
FEMALE UROLOGY

*Deceased.

Leon Love, M.D.
Professor of Radiology, and Acting Chairman, Loyola University Medical Center, Maywood, Illinois. Chairman, Department of Radiology, Cook County Hospital, Chicago.
IMAGING OF THE URINARY TRACT: COMPUTED TOMOGRAPHY OF THE URINARY TRACT

Franklin C. Lowe, M.D.
Assistant Professor of Clinical Urology, Columbia College of Physicians and Surgeons, New York, New York. Associate Director, Department of Urology, St. Luke's–Roosevelt Hospital Center, New York.
EVALUATION OF THE UROLOGIC PATIENT: HISTORY, PHYSICAL EXAMINATION, AND URINALYSIS

Tom F. Lue, M.D.
Associate Professor of Urology, University of California School of Medicine, San Francisco, California.
PHYSIOLOGY OF ERECTION AND PATHOPHYSIOLOGY OF IMPOTENCE

Peter J. Lynch, M.D.
Professor and Head, Department of Dermatology, University of Minnesota Medical School, Minneapolis, Minnesota. Attending Physician, University of Minnesota Hospital and Clinic, Minneapolis.
CUTANEOUS DISEASES OF THE EXTERNAL GENITALIA

Max Maizels, M.D.
Associate Professor of Urology, Northwestern University Medical School, Chicago, Illinois. Attending Physician, Children's Memorial Hospital and Northwestern Memorial Hospital, Chicago.
NORMAL DEVELOPMENT OF THE URINARY TRACT

James Mandell, M.D.
Associate Professor of Surgery, Harvard Medical School, Boston, Massachusetts. Associate in Surgery, Children's Hospital, Boston.
RENAL FUNCTION IN THE FETUS AND NEONATE
PRENATAL AND POSTNATAL DIAGNOSIS AND MANAGEMENT OF CONGENITAL ABNORMALITIES

David L. McCullough, M.D.
William H. Boyce Professor and Chairman, Department of Urology, Bowman Gray School of Medicine of Wake Forest University, Winston-Salem, North Carolina. Chairman, Department of Urology, North Carolina Baptist/Wake Forest University Medical Center, Winston-Salem.
EXTRACORPOREAL SHOCK WAVE LITHOTRIPSY

W. Scott McDougal, M.D.
Professor of Surgery (Urology), Harvard Medical School, Boston, Massachusetts. Chief, Department of Urology, Massachusetts General Hospital, Boston.
USE OF INTESTINAL SEGMENTS IN THE URINARY TRACT: BASIC PRINCIPLES

John E. McNeal, M.D.
Clinical Professor of Urology (Surgery), Stanford University School of Medicine, Stanford, California.
ADENOCARCINOMA OF THE PROSTATE

Edwin M. Meares, Jr., M.D.
Charles M. Whitney Professor and Chairman, Division of Urology, Tufts University School of Medicine, Boston, Massachusetts. Chairman, Department of Urology, New England Medical Center Hospitals, Boston.
PROSTATITIS AND RELATED DISORDERS

Winston K. Mebust, M.D.
Professor of Surgery/Urology, University of Kansas School of Medicine, Kansas City, Kansas. Professor and Chairman, Section of Urology, University of Kansas Medical Center, Kansas City.
TRANSURETHRAL SURGERY

Edward M. Messing, M.D.
Associate Professor of Surgery and Human Oncology, Division of Urology, University of Wisconsin School of Medicine, Madison, Wisconsin. Attending Urologist, University Hospital; and Consulting Urologist, Middleton Veterans Administration Hospital, Madison.
INTERSTITIAL CYSTITIS AND RELATED SYNDROMES

Michael E. Mitchell, M.D.
Professor of Urology, University of Washington School of Medicine, Seattle, Washington. Chief, Division of Pediatric Urology, Children's Hospital and Medical Center, Seattle.
AUGMENTATION CYSTOPLASTY IMPLANTATION OF ARTIFICIAL URINARY SPHINCTER IN MEN AND WOMEN AND RECONSTRUCTION OF THE DYSFUNCTIONAL URINARY TRACT

Andrew C. Novick, M.D.
Chairman, Department of Urology, Cleveland Clinic Foundation, Cleveland, Ohio.
SURGERY OF THE KIDNEY

Carl A. Olsson, M.D.
Professor and Chairman, Department of Urology, Columbia University College of Physicians and Surgeons, New York, New York. Chairman, Department of Urology, Columbia–Presbyterian Medical Center, New York.
URINARY DIVERSION

Olle Olsson, M.D.
Professor Emeritus, Consulting Radiologist, Department of Diagnostic Radiology, University Hospital, Lund, Sweden.
IMAGING OF THE URINARY TRACT: AN OVERVIEW OF URORADIOLOGY

David F. Paulson, M.D.
Professor of Surgery, Duke University School of Medicine, Durham, North Carolina. Chief of Urologic Surgery, Duke University Medical Center, Durham.
PERINEAL PROSTATECTOMY

Alan D. Perlmutter, M.D.
Professor of Urology, Wayne State University School of Medicine, Detroit, Michigan. Chief, Department of Pediatric Urology, Children's Hospital of Michigan, Detroit.
ANOMALIES OF THE UPPER URINARY TRACT
SURGICAL MANAGEMENT OF INTERSEXUALITY

Craig A. Peters, M.D.
Assistant Professor in Surgery, Harvard Medical School, Boston, Massachusetts. Assistant in Surgery, Children's Hospital, Boston.
PRENATAL AND POSTNATAL DIAGNOSIS AND MANAGEMENT OF CONGENITAL ABNORMALITIES
ECTOPIC URETER AND URETEROCELE

Paul C. Peters, M.D.
E.E. and Greer Garson Fogelson Distinguished Professor of Urology, The University of Texas Southwestern Medical School, Dallas, Texas. Chief of Service, Parkland Memorial Hospital; and Attending Physician, Dallas Veterans Administration Medical Center, Baylor University Medical Center, Children's Medical Center, Zale Lipshy University Hospital, Dallas, and John Peter Smith Hospital, Fort Worth.
GENITOURINARY TRAUMA

Howard M. Pollack, M.D.
Professor of Radiology and Urology, University of Pennsylvania School of Medicine, Philadelphia, Pennsylvania. Chief, Section of Uroradiology, Department of Radiology, Hospital of the University of Pennsylvania, Philadelphia.
IMAGING OF THE URINARY TRACT

Jacob Rajfer, M.D.
Professor of Surgery/Urology, University of California School of Medicine, Los Angeles, California. Chief, Division of Urology, Harbor–UCLA Medical Center, Los Angeles.
CONGENITAL ANOMALIES OF THE TESTIS

R. Beverly Raney, M.D.
Professor and Chairman, Department of Clinical Pediatrics, Non-Neuro Solid Tumor Section, M.D. Anderson Cancer Center, Houston, Texas. Deputy Head, Division of Pediatrics, M.D. Anderson Cancer Center, Houston.
PEDIATRIC ONCOLOGY

Shlomo Raz, M.D.
Professor of Surgery/Urology, Center for Health Sciences, University of California School of Medicine, Los Angeles, California.
FEMALE UROLOGY

Claude Reitelman, M.D.
Assistant Professor of Urology, Wayne State University School of Medicine, Detroit, Michigan. Associate Attending Physician, Department of Pediatric Urology, Children's Hospital of Michigan, Detroit.
SURGICAL MANAGEMENT OF INTERSEXUALITY

Martin I. Resnick, M.D.
Lester Persky Professor of Urology, Case Western Reserve University School of Medicine, Cleveland, Ohio. Director of Urology, University Hospitals of Cleveland; and Attending Urologist, Veterans Administration Medical Center, Cleveland.
EXTRINSIC OBSTRUCTION OF THE URETER

Neil M. Resnick, M.D.
Assistant Professor of Medicine, Harvard Medical School, Boston, Massachusetts. Chief of Geriatrics and Director of the Continence Center, Brigham and Women's Hospital; and Geriatric Research and Education Clinical Center, Brockton/West Roxbury Veterans Administration Medical Center, Boston.
EVALUATION AND MEDICAL MANAGEMENT OF
   URINARY INCONTINENCE

Alan B. Retik, M.D.
Professor of Surgery (Urology), Harvard Medical School, Boston, Massachusetts. Chief, Division of Urology, Children's Hospital, Boston.
ANOMALIES OF THE UPPER URINARY TRACT
PRENATAL AND POSTNATAL DIAGNOSIS AND
   MANAGEMENT OF CONGENITAL ABNORMALITIES
ECTOPIC URETER AND URETEROCELE

Jerome P. Richie, M.D.
Elliott C. Cutler Professor of Urologic Surgery, Harvard Medical School, Boston, Massachusetts. Chairman, Harvard Program in Urology (Longwood area); and Chief of Urology, Brigham and Women's Hospital, Boston.
NEOPLASMS OF THE TESTIS

Christopher M. Rigsby, M.D.
Attending Radiologist, Fairfax Hospital, Falls Church, Virginia.
IMAGING OF THE URINARY TRACT:
   ULTRASONOGRAPHY OF THE URINARY TRACT

Richard C. Rink, M.D.
Associate Professor of Urology, Indiana University School of Medicine, Indianapolis, Indiana. Chief, Pediatric Urology, James Whitcomb Riley Hospital for Children, Indianapolis.
AUGMENTATION CYSTOPLASTY IMPLANTATION OF
   ARTIFICIAL URINARY SPHINCTER IN MEN AND
   WOMEN AND RECONSTRUCTION OF THE
   DYSFUNCTIONAL URINARY TRACT

Roberto Romero, M.D.
Associate Professor, and Director of Perinatal Research, Department of Obstetrics and Gynecology, Yale University Medical School, New Haven, Connecticut.
IMAGING OF THE URINARY TRACT:
   ULTRASONOGRAPHY OF THE URINARY TRACT

Arthur T. Rosenfield, M.D.
Professor of Diagnostic Radiology and Surgery (Urology), Yale University School of Medicine, New Haven, Connecticut. Attending Radiologist, and Director of

Computed Tomography, Yale–New Haven Hospital, New Haven.
IMAGING OF THE URINARY TRACT:
   ULTRASONOGRAPHY OF THE URINARY TRACT

Daniel B. Rukstalis, M.D.
Instructor in Surgery, University of Chicago Medical School, and University of Chicago Hospital, Chicago, Illinois.
GENETIC DETERMINANTS OF UROLOGIC DISEASE

Arthur I. Sagalowsky, M.D.
Professor of Urology, University of Texas Southwestern Medical School, Dallas, Texas. Attending Physician, Parkland Memorial Hospital, Baylor University Medical Center, Veterans Administration Medical Center, and Zale Lipshy University Hospital, Dallas.
GENITOURINARY TRAUMA

Peter T. Scardino, M.D.
Russell and Mary Hugh Scott Professor and Chairman, Scott Department of Urology, Baylor College of Medicine, Houston, Texas. Chief of Urology Service, The Methodist Hospital and Harris County Hospital District, Houston.
UROLOGIC ULTRASONOGRAPHY

Anthony J. Schaeffer, M.D.
Professor and Chairman, Department of Urology, Northwestern University Medical School, Chicago, Illinois. Attending Physician, Northwestern Memorial Hospital, Children's Memorial Hospital, and Veterans Administration Lakeside Hospital, Chicago.
INFECTIONS OF THE URINARY TRACT
OTHER RENAL DISEASE OF UROLOGIC SIGNIFICANCE

Paul F. Schellhammer, M.D.
Professor and Chairman, Department of Urology, Eastern Virginia Medical School, Norfolk, Virginia. Attending Physician, Sentara Hospitals, Norfolk General and Leigh Memorial, The Children's Hospital of the King's Daughters, and DePaul Medical Center, Norfolk.
TUMORS OF THE PENIS

Peter N. Schlegel, M.D.
Assistant Professor of Surgery (Urology), Cornell University Medical College, New York, New York. Staff Scientist, The Population Council, Center for Biomedical Research, New York. Assistant Attending Surgeon, The New York Hospital, New York.
PHYSIOLOGY OF MALE REPRODUCTION: THE TESTIS,
   EPIDIDYMIS, AND DUCTUS DEFERENS

Steven M. Schlossberg, M.D.
Associate Professor, Departments of Urology and Anatomy, Eastern Virginia Medical School, Norfolk, Virginia. Attending Physician, Sentara Hospitals, Norfolk General and Leigh Memorial, The Children's Hospital of the King's Daughters, and DePaul Medical Center, Norfolk.
TUMORS OF THE PENIS
SURGERY OF THE PENIS AND URETHRA

Robert W. Schrier, M.D.
Professor and Chairman, Department of Medicine, University of Colorado School of Medicine, Denver, Colorado. Chief, Renal Division, University Hospital at the University of Colorado Health Sciences Center, Denver.
ETIOLOGY, PATHOGENESIS, AND MANAGEMENT OF RENAL FAILURE

Joseph W. Segura, M.D.
Carl Rosen Professor of Urology, Mayo Medical School, Mayo Clinic, Rochester, Minnesota. Staff Consultant, St. Mary's Hospital and Rochester Methodist Hospital, Rochester.
PERCUTANEOUS MANAGEMENT

Ridwan Shabsigh, M.D.
Assistant Professor of Urology, Department of Urology, Columbia University, New York, New York. Attending Physician, Columbia–Presbyterian Hospital, New York.
UROLOGIC ULTRASONOGRAPHY

Joseph I. Shapiro, M.D.
Assistant Professor of Medicine and Radiology, University of Colorado School of Medicine, Denver, Colorado. Co-Director, NMR Spectroscopy, and Director, Chronic Dialysis, University Hospital at the University of Colorado Health Sciences Center, Denver.
ETIOLOGY, PATHOGENESIS, AND MANAGEMENT OF RENAL FAILURE

Linda M. Dairiki Shortliffe, M.D.
Associate Professor of Urology, Stanford University School of Medicine, Stanford, California. Chief of Pediatric Urology, Lucile Salter Packard Children's Hospital at Stanford.
URINARY TRACT INFECTIONS IN INFANTS AND CHILDREN

Mark Sigman, M.D.
Assistant Professor of Urology, Division of Urology, Brown University, Providence, Rhode Island. Staff Urologist, Rhode Island Hospital and Veterans Administration Hospital, Providence.
MALE INFERTILITY

Donald G. Skinner, M.D.
Professor and Chairman, Department of Urology, University of Southern California, Los Angeles, California. Chief of Surgery and Urology, Kenneth Norris Jr. Cancer Hospital; and Chairman, Department of Urology, USC/LAC Medical Center, Los Angeles.
SURGERY OF TESTICULAR NEOPLASMS

Eila C. Skinner, M.D.
Assistant Professor of Urology, University of Southern California, Los Angeles, California. Provisional Staff Physician, Norris Cancer Hospital and Hospital of Good Samaritan, Los Angeles.
SURGERY OF TESTICULAR NEOPLASMS

Jerome Hazen Smith, M.D.
Professor of Pathology, University of Texas Medical Branch, Galveston, Texas. Attending Physician, University of Texas Medical Branch Hospitals, Galveston.
PARASITIC DISEASES OF THE GENITOURINARY SYSTEM

Joseph A. Smith, Jr., M.D.
Professor and Chairman, Department of Urology, Vanderbilt University, Nashville, Tennessee. Chief of Urologic Surgery, Vanderbilt University Hospital, Nashville.
UROLOGIC LASER SURGERY

M. J. Vernon Smith, M.D., Ph.D.
Professor of Urology, Medical College of Virginia, Virginia Commonwealth University, Richmond, Virginia.
SURGERY OF THE URETER

Howard M. Snyder III, M.D.
Associate Professor of Urology, Department of Surgery, University of Pennsylvania School of Medicine, Philadelphia, Pennsylvania. Associate Director, Division of Pediatric Urology, Children's Hospital of Philadelphia, Philadelphia.
PEDIATRIC ONCOLOGY

R. Ernest Sosa, M.D.
Assistant Professor of Surgery, Division of Urology, Cornell University Medical College, New York, New York. Assistant Attending Surgeon, New York Hospital–Cornell Medical Center, New York.
RENOVASCULAR HYPERTENSION

Thomas A. Stamey, M.D.
Professor and Chairman, Department of Urology, Stanford University School of Medicine, Stanford, California.
ADENOCARCINOMA OF THE PROSTATE
URINARY INCONTINENCE IN THE FEMALE: THE STAMEY ENDOSCOPIC SUSPENSION OF THE VESICAL NECK FOR STRESS URINARY INCONTINENCE

William D. Steers, M.D.
Assistant Professor of Urology, University of Virginia Health Science Center, Charlottesville, Virginia. Attending Physician, University of Virginia Hospital, Charlottesville.
PHYSIOLOGY OF THE URINARY BLADDER

Stevan B. Streem, M.D.
Head, Section of Stone Disease and Endourology, Department of Urology, Cleveland Clinic Foundation, Cleveland, Ohio.
SURGERY OF THE KIDNEY

Ray E. Stutzman, M.D.
Associate Professor of Urology, The Johns Hopkins University School of Medicine, Baltimore, Maryland.

Staff Physician, The Johns Hopkins Hospital; and Chief of Urology, Francis Scott Key Medical Center, Baltimore.
SUPRAPUBIC AND RETROPUBIC PROSTATECTOMY

Ronald S. Swerdloff, M.D.
Professor of Medicine, University of California School of Medicine, Los Angeles, California. Chief, Division of Endocrinology, Harbor–UCLA Medical Center, Los Angeles.
PHYSIOLOGY OF MALE REPRODUCTION:
   HYPOTHALAMIC-PITUITARY FUNCTION

Emil A. Tanagho, M.D.
Professor and Chairman, Department of Urology, University of California School of Medicine, San Francisco, California.
SURGICAL ANATOMY OF THE GENITOURINARY
   TRACT: ANATOMY OF THE LOWER URINARY TRACT

E. Darracott Vaughan, Jr., M.D.
James J. Colt Professor of Urology, Cornell University Medical College, New York, New York. Urologist-in-Chief, The New York Hospital–Cornell Medical Center, New York.
NORMAL RENAL PHYSIOLOGY
RENOVASCULAR HYPERTENSION
THE ADRENALS

Franz von Lichtenberg, M.D.
Professor of Pathology, Harvard Medical School, Boston, Massachusetts. Pathologist, Peter Bent Brigham Hospital, Boston.
PARASITIC DISEASES OF THE GENITOURINARY
   SYSTEM

Patrick C. Walsh, M.D.
David Hall McConnell Professor, The Johns Hopkins University School of Medicine, Baltimore, Maryland. Urologist-in-Chief, Brady Urological Institute, The Johns Hopkins Hospital, Baltimore.
BENIGN PROSTATIC HYPERPLASIA
SUPRAPUBIC AND RETROPUBIC PROSTATECTOMY
RADICAL RETROPUBIC PROSTATECTOMY

Christina Wang, M.D.
Professor of Medicine, University of California Medical Center, Los Angeles, California. Director of Andrology, Division of Endocrinology/Metabolism and Division of Reproductive Endocrinology/Infertility, Cedars–Sinai Medical Center, Los Angeles.
PHYSIOLOGY OF MALE REPRODUCTION:
   HYPOTHALAMIC-PITUITARY FUNCTION

Alan J. Wein, M.D.
Professor and Chairman, Division of Urology, University of Pennsylvania School of Medicine, Philadelphia, Pennsylvania. Chief of Urology, Hospital of the University of Pennsylvania, Philadelphia.
NEUROMUSCULAR DYSFUNCTION OF THE LOWER
   URINARY TRACT

Robert M. Weiss, M.D.
Professor and Chief, Section of Urology, Yale University School of Medicine, New Haven, Connecticut. Professor and Chief, Section of Urology, Yale–New Haven Hospital, New Haven.
PHYSIOLOGY AND PHARMACOLOGY OF THE RENAL
   PELVIS AND URETER

Richard D. Williams, M.D.
Professor and Head, Department of Urology, University of Iowa, Iowa City, Iowa. Chief of Urology, University of Iowa Hospitals and Clinics; and Consultant, Iowa City Veterans Affairs Medical Center, Iowa City.
SURGERY OF THE SEMINAL VESICLES

Jean D. Wilson, M.D.
Professor of Internal Medicine, University of Texas Southwestern Medical Center, Dallas, Texas. Attending Physician, Parkland Memorial Hospital, Dallas.
EMBRYOLOGY OF THE GENITAL TRACT
DISORDERS OF SEXUAL DIFFERENTIATION

Gilbert J. Wise, M.D.
Clinical Professor, Department of Urology, State University of New York Health Science Center, Brooklyn, New York. Director, Division of Urology, Maimonides Medical Center, Brooklyn.
FUNGAL INFECTIONS OF THE URINARY TRACT

John R. Woodard, M.D.
Clinical Professor of Surgery (Urology) and Director of Pediatric Urology, Emory University School of Medicine, Atlanta, Georgia. Chief, Urology Section, Egleston Hospital for Children at Emory University; Attending Physician, Scottish Rite Children's Medical Center, Atlanta.
NEONATAL AND PERINATAL EMERGENCIES
PRUNE-BELLY SYNDROME

Subbarao V. Yalla, M.D.
Associate Professor of Surgery (Urology), Harvard Medical School, Boston, Massachusetts. Chief of Urology, Brockton/West Roxbury Medical Center of Veterans Affairs; and Associate Surgeon, Brigham and Women's Hospital, Boston.
EVALUATION AND MEDICAL MANAGEMENT OF
   URINARY INCONTINENCE

PREFACE

In the six years that have elapsed since the last edition was published, the field of urology has undergone a major transformation. Today, advances in basic science, pharmacology, diagnostic imaging, instrumentation, and surgical technique have expanded the field and added to the complexity of patient management. In response to these changes, the Sixth Edition of *Campbell's Urology* has been expanded and rewritten. The authors of each chapter were challenged to take a scholarly, encyclopedic approach to each topic rather than provide merely a personal viewpoint. In doing so, we hope to maintain the reputation of this book as "the bible of urology." Also, to keep pace with these rapid advances in the future, an "Update" series is planned. These Updates will complement *Campbell's Urology* and will cover the latest advances in urology. This will enable the reader to maintain a contemporary grasp of the field until the next edition is published.

More than half of the three-volume Sixth Edition is new, with 22 new chapters and 27 new contributors. To provide a completely fresh approach to all topics, there are two new editors: Dr. Alan B. Retik, Professor and Chairman of Pediatric Urology, Boston Children's Hospital and Harvard Medical School; and Dr. E. Darracott Vaughan, Jr., Professor and Chairman of Urology, Cornell Medical Center, The New York Hospital.

The Sixth Edition begins with a new chapter, "Surgical Anatomy of the Genitourinary Tract," complete with full-page color illustrations of the gross anatomy correlated with cross-sections of whole body tomography. The topic of renal physiology has been expanded by the addition of two new chapters: "Renal Endocrinology" and "Renal Function in the Fetus and Neonate." Recognizing the importance of office ultrasound procedures, we have added a new chapter, "Urologic Ultrasonography." The coverage of male sexual dysfunction has been expanded by the development of two new chapters: "Physiology of Erection and Pathophysiology of Impotence" and "Diagnosis and Therapy of Erectile Dysfunction." These two chapters complement one another and provide a comprehensive approach to the understanding of male sexual dysfunction, its pathophysiology, and its management. Similarly, because of increased interest in female urology, we have also added two new chapters: "Evaluation and Medical Management of Urinary Incontinence" and "Female Urology."

The section on pediatric urology has been expanded to include "Prenatal and Postnatal Diagnosis and Management of Congenital Abnormalities," "Posterior Urethral Valves and Other Urethral Anomalies," "Congenital Anomalies of the Genitalia," and "Surgery of the Scrotum and Testis in Childhood." The topic of renal calculus disease and related disorders is described in separate chapters: "Extracorporeal Shock Wave Lithotripsy," "Percutaneous Management," "Ureteroscopy," and "Endosurgical Techniques for the Diagnosis and Treatment of Noncalculous Disease of the Ureter and Kidney."

Recognizing the expanded role of reconstruction of the lower urinary tract in urology, we have created three new complementary chapters: "Use of Intestinal Segments in the Urinary Tract: Basic Principles"; "Augmentation Cystoplasty Implantation of Artificial Sphincter in Men and Women and Reconstruction of the Dysfunctional Urinary Tract"; and "Urinary Diversion," with a major emphasis on continent urinary diversion. In addition, we have added new chapters on laser surgery and the surgery of male infertility.

We wish to thank the editors and authors of prior editions, since this new edition has been built upon the solid foundation they laid. Our gratitude is greatest for the contingent of contributing authors who collectively represent the best scientists and clinicians associated with the field of urology. A work of this scope and magnitude cannot be accomplished without the assistance of a great number of persons whose effort may not be specifically attributed within this book. Specifically, we wish to express our thanks to Martin J. Wonsiewicz, William J. Lamsback, Rosanne Hallowell, Carolyn Naylor, Carol Robins, Mary Anne Folcher, Walter Verbitski, Maureen Sweeney, and the staff of the W. B. Saunders Company for their patience and help in bringing this ambitious undertaking to publication.

PATRICK C. WALSH
For the Editors

CONTENTS

THE MOLECULAR BIOLOGY, ENDOCRINOLOGY, AND
PHYSIOLOGY OF THE PROSTATE AND SEMINAL
VESICLES, 221
Donald S. Coffey, Ph.D.

7

GENETIC DETERMINANTS OF UROLOGIC DISEASE

William C. DeWolf, M.D. and Daniel B. Rukstalis, M.D.

II

THE UROLOGIC EXAMINATION AND DIAGNOSTIC TECHNIQUES

8

EVALUATION OF THE UROLOGIC PATIENT

HISTORY, PHYSICAL EXAMINATION, AND URINALYSIS, 307
Franklin C. Lowe, M.D. and Charles B. Brendler, M.D.

INSTRUMENTATION AND ENDOSCOPY, 331
H. Ballentine Carter, M.D.

VI
SEXUAL FUNCTION

16
PHYSIOLOGY OF ERECTION AND PATHOPHYSIOLOGY OF IMPOTENCE

Tom F. Lue, M.D.

VII
INFECTIONS AND INFLAMMATION OF THE GENITOURINARY TRACT

17
INFECTIONS OF THE URINARY TRACT

Anthony J. Schaeffer, M.D.

21
PARASITIC DISEASES OF THE GENITOURINARY SYSTEM 883

Jerome Hazen Smith, M.D., Franz von Lichtenberg, M.D.
and Jay Stauffer Lehman, M.D.

22
FUNGAL INFECTIONS OF THE URINARY TRACT 928

Gilbert J. Wise, M.D.

23
GENITOURINARY TUBERCULOSIS 951

James G. Gow, M.D.

X

EMBRYOLOGY AND ANOMALIES OF THE GENITOURINARY TRACT

33

RENAL FUNCTION IN THE FETUS AND NEONATE 1344
Robert L. Chevalier, M.D. and James Mandell, M.D.

34

ANOMALIES OF THE UPPER URINARY TRACT 1357
Stuart B. Bauer, M.D., Alan D. Perlmutter, M.D. and Alan B. Retik, M.D.

35

RENAL DYSPLASIA AND CYSTIC DISEASE OF THE KIDNEY 1443
Kenneth I. Glassberg, M.D.

Volume 3

XIII

62
ENDOSURGICAL TECHNIQUES FOR THE DIAGNOSIS AND TREATMENT OF NONCALCULOUS DISEASE OF THE URETER AND KIDNEY

Ralph V. Clayman, M.D. and Louis R. Kavoussi, M.D.

XIV
UROLOGIC SURGERY

63
PERIOPERATIVE CARE

Charles B. Brendler, M.D.

64
THE ADRENALS 2360
E. Darracott Vaughan, Jr., M.D. and Jon David Blumenfeld, M.D.

65
SURGERY OF THE KIDNEY 2413
Andrew C. Novick, M.D. and Stevan B. Streem, M.D.

66
RENAL TRANSPLANTATION 2501
John M. Barry, M.D.

73

URINARY UNDIVERSION: REFUNCTIONALIZATION OF THE PREVIOUSLY DIVERTED URINARY TRACT
W. Hardy Hendren, M.D.

74

OPEN BLADDER SURGERY
Fuad S. Freiha, M.D.

82
SURGERY OF THE SEMINAL VESICLES

Richard D. Williams, M.D.

83
SURGERY OF THE PENIS AND URETHRA

Charles J. Devine, Jr., M.D., Gerald H. Jordan, M.D. and Steven M. Schlossberg, M.D.

XIII
URINARY LITHIASIS

58
URINARY LITHIASIS: ETIOLOGY, DIAGNOSIS, AND MEDICAL MANAGEMENT

George W. Drach, M.D.

Anthropologic history provides evidence that urinary calculi existed as long as 7000 years ago and perhaps longer. The "specialty" of urologic surgery was even recognized by Hippocrates, who, in his famous oath for the physician, stated, "I will not cut, even for the stone, but leave such procedures to the practitioners of the craft" (Clendening, 1942). The recognition of different varieties of urinary calculi also resulted in more varieties of medical treatment, most of which failed. Now, however, many major advances have greatly improved our understanding of the causes of stone disease. Although not all patients with urinary calculi can be cured, patients with one of the five major types of urinary calculi now have at least an 80 per cent chance of cure or control with medical therapy alone. Procedural therapy continues to be important as an aspect of management of urinary calculi, but it is only one step in the total plan for patients with urinary lithiasis.

Considerable selection, through May 1990, has been exercised in choosing the literature for the references for this chapter. Also, several research symposia in urinary lithiasis have been conducted within the past 2 decades. These have resulted in authoritative volumes with valuable information about worldwide research on urinary lithiasis. A separate list of the proceedings of these research symposia has also been included.

This chapter first summarizes the history and theories necessary for the understanding and care of patients with urinary calculi. A discussion of treatment of the acute stone episode follows. The problem of renal damage caused by stones is surveyed in a discussion of the pathophysiology of obstruction due to urinary calculi, nephrocalcinosis, and urinary tract epithelial changes related to urinary lithiasis. For each stone type, a brief historical review is followed by epidemiologic factors concerning the incidence of urolithiasis, such as heredity, age, sex, geography, environment, occupation, or economic level. Next, the aspects of etiology are discussed in general terms with reference to both clinical and laboratory findings.

Having progressed through the etiologic and diagnostic aspects of urinary lithiasis, we classify the individual patient with regard to the type of stone and the degree of activity of the disease. Based on this classification, we discuss specific treatments available for each type of stone disease. Some practical aspects of management of stones that have passed out of the kidney into the ureter or have formed in other specific anatomic locations are presented. These include stones of the bladder, prostate, and urethra. We also summarize observations on stone disease in children.

Urinary lithiasis management represents a realm of sharing between the urologist and his or her medical colleagues. In some instances, medical specialists with training in endocrinologic disease perform evaluation and treatment of urinary stone disease. In many locales, however, this is not possible or feasible. Decisions about evaluation and treatment of patients with urinary lithiasis often rest with the urologist. Urologists must therefore understand all aspects of the etiology, diagnosis, and surgical and procedural treatment of urinary lithiasis.

HISTORY

Humans of ancient times were undoubtedly afflicted with stone disease just as humans are now. Riches (1968)

This chapter is dedicated to the memory of Birdwell Finlayson, M.D., of Gainesville, Florida, who died on July 22, 1988. Birdwell contributed immensely to our understanding of urinary stones, especially those physicochemical aspects that are so difficult for most of us to comprehend. More importantly, he was a sounding board for all of us who studied this disease of human lithiasis. He served us quietly as a sharpening stone to help hone our thoughts and theories to a razor's edge. For these contributions, in the community of those who study stone disease, Birdwell has gained immortality.

refers to the stone that was found in the pelvis, presumably in the bladder, of an Egyptian skeleton estimated to be over 7000 years old. Perhaps because of the admonition of Hippocrates, surgical treatment of bladder calculi was for centuries traditionally left to numbers of traveling lithotomists.

By the 17th and 18th centuries many of them had become famous. Wangensteen and co-workers, (1969) referred to some of the more famous lithotomists of that time. They included Colot, Friar Jacques, Rau, Friar Come, and others. Soon, however, surgeons trained in anatomy and other aspects of medical practice recognized that traveling lithotomists were not as adept at their calling as might be desired. Many of these well-trained individuals, whom Wangensteen classified as "professionals," began to take an interest in urinary lithiasis. Most of their interest centered on improvement of techniques for removal of bladder calculi. As an example, Dupuytren, who is famous in many areas of medicine and surgery, developed a new type of perineal instrument for removal of bladder calculi (Drach, 1974a).

Celsius, Franco, and Cheselden were other great contributors to the development of improved lithotomy techniques. Civiale and Bigelow, although separated in time by half a century, were instrumental in the development of practical lithotrity and litholapaxy techniques that are still used.

Sir Henry Thompson became famous for his interest in medical therapy of bladder stone and suggested the possibility of treatment of bladder stone by dissolution (Thompson, 1873, cited by Thorwald, 1956). Only after this period of improvement in surgery did a significant amount of attention turn to the medical treatment of urolithiasis, although naturopaths had tried unsuccessfully to treat "disease of the stone" for centuries. Galen, for example, treated stone disease with wine and honey, parsley and caraway seed; Howship recommended administration of alkalis or acids to arrest calculi, as did Sir Astley Cooper (cited by Wesson, 1935).

As Europeans moved to America, they brought with them their predisposition to form bladder calculi. Wangensteen and associates (1969) summarized several reviews of lithotomy practice in America during the years 1810 to 1853. Vogel (1970) noted that in America, urinary calculous disease was isolated preponderantly to immigrant Europeans. For instance, he reviews the statement that "Savages were unacquainted with a great many diseases that afflict the Europeans, such as the gout, dropsy, gravel." Citing another reference, he notes that North Carolina Indians were " . . . never troubled by scurvy, dropsy, or stone." In 1559, an Inca reportedly stated that he thought that corn was the factor that prevented the occurrence of urinary calculi in native American Indians (cited by Vogel). Many Indian herbal treatments were adapted to the treatments of urinary calculus or gravel. Thus, Vogel mentions the use of haw or hawthorn tree, persimmon, sarsaparilla, and decoctions of multiple other leaves and twigs as remedies for stone.

In contrast, Beck and Mulvaney (1966) reported two urinary calculi associated with the bony remains of two Indians buried in Fulton County, Illinois, and Marion County, Indiana. Both stones were preponderantly carbonate apatite, although one contained a small amount of struvite. Dating of these archeologic sites placed one inhabitant at 1500 B.C. and the other at 1500 A.D. Because, as we shall learn, pure apatitic calculi usually accompany metabolic disease, it seems possible that these calculi were caused by such a disease and that, indeed, idiopathic urinary stone disease rarely afflicted native American Indians.

Whether or not stone disease of early centuries was governed more by heredity or by environment, there is no doubt that bladder calculi were an endemic part of life prior to the 20th century (Ellis, 1969; Ostergaard, 1973). King (1971) and Prien (1971) noted the historical trend away from bladder calculi toward upper urinary tract calculi whenever a country becomes more industrialized and diet becomes more nutritious. When agrarian and primitive pursuits remain the primary way of life for a population, the incidence of bladder stone disease continues to be high, as it is in Thailand (Lonsdale, 1968b; Suvachittanont et al., 1973). By the early 1900s, observers had already begun to notice an increased occurrence of renal and ureteral calculi and a decreased occurrence of bladder calculi in Europe, the British Isles, and America. This change seemed to parallel the change toward industrialization.

Investigators began to report some significant physiologic observations that were associated with the production of urinary calculi. These included the importance of diet, especially in association with uric acid bladder calculi (Gutman and Yu, 1968). Hypercalciuria was clearly defined as one factor contributing to the formation of calcium calculi (Flocks, 1939). Hypercalciuria due to hyperparathyroidism was identified and distinguished from idiopathic hypercalciuria (Albright and Reifenstein, 1948; Flocks, 1940).

The importance of nucleation of stones in the kidney was studied intensively by Randall (1937), who described the famous "Randall's plaques." Urinary crystals and colloid were described, and the "crystalloid" and "colloid" composition of all stones was determined (Wesson, 1935). The effects of infections on stone formation were noted to be different from the effects of excessive excretion of crystalloids in the absence of infection. Much groundwork was laid for the worldwide resurgence of research into the etiology and prophylaxis of urolithiasis that followed World War II. The remainder of this chapter is concerned mostly with the immense amount of information about urinary stone disease gained since 1950.

The history of stone disease implies that many diverse factors might be involved in its causation: heredity, environment, age, sex, urinary infection, metabolic diseases, and dietary excesses or deficiencies. Review of epidemiologic aspects of urinary calculi begins our survey of urolithiasis.

EPIDEMIOLOGIC ASPECTS

Andersen (1973) presents an interesting, multifaceted theory of epidemiology of urinary calculi. He notes that the incidence of upper tract urinary calculi varies greatly with age, anatomic site, and geographic distribution and that unexplained increases during different periods of history have occurred. He believes, therefore, that at least two separate epidemiologic factors are involved in the genesis of urinary calculi. The first of these may be considered intrinsic. Intrinsic factors are related to the inherited biochemical or anatomic makeup of the individual. For example, African Bantu natives and the related North American blacks tend to have very few urinary calculi (Modlin, 1967; Pantanowitz et al., 1973).

A subcategory of this racial or ethnic factor includes any familial tendency toward generation of calculi. Familial inheritance of calcium stone disease has been reported by Resnick and colleagues (1968) and by McGeown (1960) and reviewed by Finlayson (1974). No true sex-linked inheritance of urinary lithiasis has been defined, but Transbol and Frydendal (1973) have reported that male relatives of patients with hypercalciuric stone disease were more often affected than female relatives.

Intrinsic factors of urolithiasis, therefore, include ethnic, racial, and familial background and any inherited physiologic or anatomic predisposition to urinary calculi. Most of these factors are discussed further in the sections on specific types of calculi, although the effects of heredity, age, and sex on incidence of calculi are discussed in this section.

Superimposed on these apparent intrinsic factors are those that Andersen (1973) terms extrinsic. Another term for these might be "environmental factors." These include climate, drinking water, dietary patterns of populations and of households of individuals, presence or absence of trace elements in foodstuffs and drinking water, and occupations. Some of these extrinsic factors are definitely related to the occurrence of urinary calculi, but first several intrinsic factors are reviewed.

Intrinsic Factors

Heredity

Underlying all epidemiologic concepts of causation of urinary calculi is the role of heredity. Numerous workers have noted that urinary calculi are relatively rare in the North American Indian, the blacks of Africa and America, and the native-born Israeli. It would appear that resistance to urinary stone disease has been part of the natural selection of individuals for persistence of their race in areas that have relatively hot climates. Conversely, the incidence of stone disease is known to be highest in some of the colder temperate areas of the world populated primarily by Eurasians and whites. Although the incidence of bladder stones seems to be related primarily to dietary habits and malnutrition in underdeveloped and primitive countries, dietary improvement over the years has probably resulted only in a change of the site of occurrence of urinary calculi from bladder to kidney (Sutor, 1972).

The hereditary capability of forming stones persists while the anatomic site has changed. We find evidence in studies of this nature by Gram (1932) and by Goldstein (1951). As noted earlier, genetic studies have been performed by Resnick and co-workers (1968) and by McGeown (1960). These investigators concluded that urolithiasis requires a polygenic defect (more than one gene is involved). In addition, genetic predisposition to urinary lithiasis has partial penetrance, so that the severity of stone disease may differ from generation to generation even though the individual has the gene defects necessary for urinary lithiasis.

However, White and colleagues (1969) caution against accepting familial or hereditary theories of stone formation too readily. They studied patients who were stone formers and their spouses and similar pairs of individuals who were not stone formers. These workers noted that urinary calcium excretion was significantly higher in spouses of patients who were stone formers than in the control persons of the same sex in households of persons who did not form stones. Hence, household diet as well as familial tendencies must be considered in theories of etiology of urinary lithiasis.

Renal tubular acidosis (RTA) is one hereditary disease that has certainly been associated with frequent episodes of urinary lithiasis. Nephrolithiasis and nephrocalcinosis have been reported to occur in almost 73 per cent of patients with this disease (Dretler et al., 1969; Marquardt, 1973; Giugliani, et al., 1985). Incomplete RTA also appears to be transmitted as a hereditary trait that results in urinary lithiasis.

Cystinuria is a prime example of familial transmission of a type of urinary lithiasis that is definitely hereditary. Cystinuria is known to be expressed when two recessive genes for cystinuria are present—it is a homozygous recessive disease (Crawhall and Watts, 1968). The genetic defect is that of excessive excretion of cystine, ornithine, lysine, and arginine (COLA). Only cystine becomes insoluble in urine. Interestingly, some patients with cystinuria do not develop urinary calculi (Giugliani, et al., 1985; King, 1967, 1971). It therefore appears that at least two gene defects (polygenic) are required to predispose some cystinuric patients toward formation of cystine urinary calculi. Hence, only stone-forming cystinuric patients carry the additional gene defect that causes formation of urinary calculi of cystine.

Age and Sex

Figure 58–1 shows the typical age and sex distributions of incidence of urinary calculi in a group of 119 patients. Note that the peak age incidence of urinary calculi occurs in the 3rd to 5th decades. About three males are afflicted for every female. These observations are generally confirmed by most studies of age and sex incidence of urinary calculi (Blacklock, 1969; Fetter and Zimskind, 1961; Inada et al., 1958; Pak, 1987).

Several investigators have pointed out that the maximum incidence of urinary lithiasis appears to occur in the 30- to 50-year-old age group (Bailey et al., 1974; Burkland and Rosenberg, 1955; Fetter and Zimskind, 1961; Frank et al., 1959; Prince and Scardino, 1960). But when does urolithiasis begin? If we determine the age of patients depicted in Figure 58–1 at the onset of disease, we obtain the results shown in Figure 58–2. The majority of patients report onset of disease in the 2nd decade of life, with decreasing onset through the

3rd, 4th, and 5th decades. If we combine this fact with the apparent observation in Figure 58–1 that the maximum incidence of disease occurs in the 5th decade, we recognize that urinary calculous disease has a tendency to persist over a long period of an individual's life.

Blacklock (1969), in a long-term study of individuals in military service, found that the chance of having one or more recurrences of urinary calculous disease during a period of many years was 67 per cent for the male patient with idiopathic urinary lithiasis. Sutherland and colleagues (1985) reported peak risk of recurrence of calculi at 1½ and 8 years. Figures 58–1 and 58–2 also show that in this group of patients, females constitute about one third the total number. This is the same proportion reported in most other studies of incidence of urinary calculi by sex. However, Lonsdale (1968b) observed that incidence of upper urinary tract calcification is approximately equal in males and females at the time of autopsy. For some reason, therefore, the symptomatic appearance of urinary calculous disease is more prevalent in males. In females, most upper urinary tract calculous disease is caused by chronic urinary tract infections or metabolic defects, such as cystinuria or hyperparathyroidism. Most upper urinary tract lithiasis throughout the world is accounted for by recurrent idiopathic calcific or uric acid calculi in males.

Several investigators have commented on the apparently equal tendency toward urinary lithiasis in males and females during childhood (Malek and Kelalis, 1975; Prince and Scardino, 1960). This observation, coupled with reports that increased serum testosterone levels resulted in increased endogenous oxalate production by the liver (Liao and Richardson, 1972), led Finlayson (1974) to postulate that lower serum testosterone levels may contribute to some of the protection women and children have against oxalate stone disease. Yet, van Aswegen and associates (1989) found that the urinary testosterone concentration of patients who were stone formers was lower than that of controls.

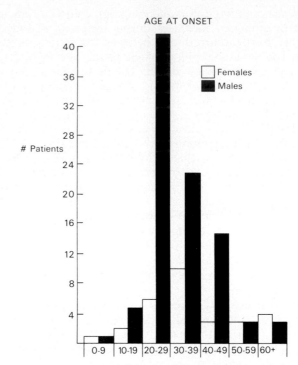

Figure 58–2. Age and sex distribution of 119 patients at the time of first episode of proven renal lithiasis. Only 6 per cent of males had onset after age 50, but 25 per cent of females had onset after age 50. As noted in the text, this later onset of some stone disease in females was correlated with renal infection or metabolic diseases, especially hyperparathyroidism.

Welshman and McGeown (1975) have demonstrated increased urinary citrate concentrations in the urine of females. These workers postulate that this finding may aid in protecting females from calcium urolithiasis.

Extrinsic Factors

Geography

Given the fact that heredity, age, and sex must have important effects on the incidence of urinary lithiasis, numerous other studies attempt to relate high or low incidence to the geographic distribution of this disease. For example, there is a noticeable increase in urinary calculi in those who live in mountainous, desert, and tropical areas. Boyce and co-workers (1956) performed an extensive study of the incidence of calculous disease in the United States. Their results were updated by Sierakowski and associates (1978) (Fig. 58–3). A similar survey of the United States had been conducted earlier by Burkland and Rosenberg (1955) and had shown essentially the same results. Whereas Boyce and colleagues tended to emphasize reports of stone disease on the East Coast, Burkland and Rosenberg emphasized disease in the western United States. Results shown in Figure 58–3 summarize those for the entire United States.

All investigative groups agreed that the areas of highest incidence of urolithiasis in the United States are

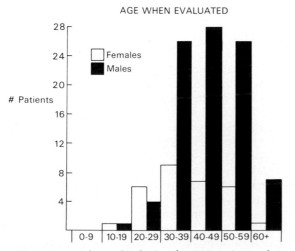

Figure 58–1. Age and sex distribution for 119 patients who were evaluated completely for recurrent renal lithiasis. A male-to-female ratio of 3:1 is evident. Compare with Figure 58–2.

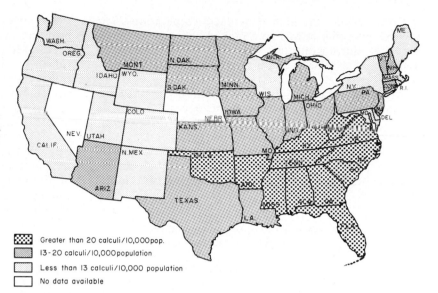

Figure 58–3. Geographic distribution of urinary lithiasis in the United States in 1974, based on a hospital discharge survey. (From Sierakowski, R., Finlayson, B., and Landes, R.: Urol. Res., 1:157, 1978.)

Greater than 20 calculi/10,000 pop.

13-20 calculi/10,000 population

Less than 13 calculi/10,000 population

No data available

the northwest, the southeast, and the arid southwest. Finlayson (1974) reviewed several worldwide geographic surveys and stated that the United States is relatively high in the incidence of urinary calculous disease for its population. Other high-incidence areas are the British Isles, Scandinavian countries, Mediterranean countries, northern India and Pakistan, northern Australia, Central Europe, portions of the Malayan peninsula, and China.

In certain other areas of the world, a relatively low occurrence of idiopathic urinary lithiasis is found. Low-incidence areas include Central and South America, most of Africa, and those areas of Australia populated by aborigines. Many of the areas with a low incidence of stone disease have large populations of native inhabitants. One wonders whether the processes of natural selection have previously eliminated those individuals with genetic tendencies toward development of urinary lithiasis.

In addition to the various incidences for all urinary calculi combined, differences are noted in the types of urinary stone disease in various areas of the world. Lonsdale (1968 a and b) and Sutor and Wooley (1970, 1971, 1974a) have reported extensive geographic surveys of types of urinary calculi. They have noted, for example, that stones from Great Britain, Scotland, and Sudan are similar and are composed primarily of mixed calcium oxalate and calcium phosphate. Sutor and colleagues (1974a) reported that many oxalate but few struvite calculi were found in the stone collections of the Royal Navy. Sharma and colleagues (1989) noted the same low incidence of struvite stones in India. Hence, it seems to confirm that struvite stones are associated primarily with upper urinary tract infections in females or in patients with neurogenic bladders and chronic urinary infections (Griffith, 1979). Sexual differences in the type and incidence of stones affect the geographic and occupational distribution of urolithiasis.

Upper urinary tract calculi composed of uric acid tend to be more common in Czechoslovakia and Israel (Herbstein et al., 1974), and possibly Chicago (Gutman and Yu, 1968). Conversely, Hazarika and colleagues (1974) and Sharma and colleagues (1989) noted that upper urinary tract calculi analyzed in India contained mostly calcium oxalate or calcium phosphate (apatite). Uric acid or ammonium urate calculi were rarely encountered. Pantanowitz and co-workers (1973) reported that calcium oxalate and phosphate were found in 53 per cent of 256 South African stones analyzed by them. Most of the remaining stones in this series contained "triple phosphates (struvite)."

In summary, geography influences the incidence of urinary calculi and the types of calculi that occur within a given area. However, the capability of individuals to transport the intrinsic genetic tendencies toward urinary stone formation from area to area makes it likely that the major tendencies contributing to urinary lithiasis reside in the individual. The effects of geography represent just one aspect of the environment superimposed on the intrinsic factors. Andersen (1973) further stated in his stone formation hypothesis presented previously that, given an intrinsic predisposition toward urinary lithiasis "Dietary structure provides the baseline of stone incidence in all countries or regions." He points out that certain types of geography tend to establish dietary patterns. Geography has an effect in terms of temperature and humidity, which also seem to influence the incidence of human urinary calculi.

Climatic and Seasonal Factors

It is difficult to find direct evidence for the influence of climate on the occurrence of urinary lithiasis. Several workers, however, have attempted to show a relationship between higher environmental temperature and higher seasonal incidence of urinary stone disease. For example, Prince and associates (1956) related their observations on seasonal variation in incidence of urinary calculi to high summer temperatures in the southeastern United States. Figure 58–4A is derived from data presented in their article. Peak incidence of lithiasis occurred in July, August, and September, which are also the months with the highest average temperatures. The relative humidity in this area ranged between 70 and 80 per cent throughout the year and therefore did not appear to be related to the peak incidence of urinary stone disease.

Prince and Scardino (1960) followed this study with a prospective analysis of 922 occurrences of ureteral stones. Once again, the peak incidence occurred in July, August, and September. In examining their later report, one notes that the highest incidence of urinary calculi appears to occur 1 to 2 months following the achievement of the maximum mean annual temperature in the study area.

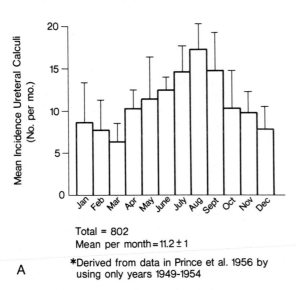

Seasonal Incidence of Ureteral Calculi*
(Southeastern U.S.A.)

Total = 802
Mean per month = 11.2 ± 1

A   *Derived from data in Prince et al. 1956 by using only years 1949-1954

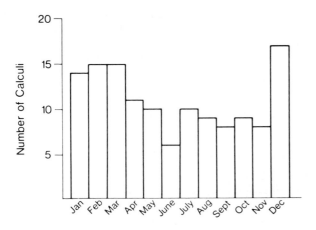

Monthly Incidence of Free (Ureteral) Urinary Calculi*
(Perth, Western Australia)

B   *Derived from data in Bateson, 1973

Figure 58–4. Comparison of occurrence of ureteral stones in southeastern United States *(A)* and Western Australia *(B)*. Highest incidences are in summer months. (Derived from data in Prince, C. L., Scardino, P. L., and Wolan, T. C.: The effect of temperature, humidity, and dehydration on the formation of renal calculi. J. Urol., 75:209, 1956, [using only years 1949–1954]; and from data in Bateson, E. M.: Renal tract calculi and climate. Med. J. Aust., 2:111, 1973.)

An interesting contrast to the studies by Prince and Scardino is found in the communication by Bateson (1973). He reported the incidence of upper urinary tract calculi in the area surrounding Perth in Western Australia. Figure 58–4*B* also shows the incidence of calculi per month in 188 of his patients. The peak incidence of urinary calculi occurs in December through March. This finding coincides with the peak maximum summer temperatures in that geographic area. A comparison indicates that in both areas, increased mean environmental temperatures seem to be related to increased incidence of urinary calculi. Summer in Perth, Western Australia, usually includes the months of December through March, while summer in Savannah, Georgia, includes May through September. Mean temperatures in Perth for the summer months are near 83.2°F, whereas mean temperatures in summer in Savannah are about 79.2°F. Bateson stated that the dry climate of Perth contributes to the formation of stones. In contrast, the relative humidity for the Savannah area is near 75 per cent.

Rivera (1973) studied the seasonal incidence of urinary calculi in the area surrounding San Juan, Puerto Rico. Maximum incidence of urolithiasis in this Northern Hemisphere region occurred in July through October in most years. Highest average monthly temperatures in the area occurred in the months of August and September. During the study, some unusual seasonal changes occurred, including unusual coolness during periods when relatively high temperatures would be expected. A decrease in the number of calculi during these unexpected cool periods was noted. Rivera concluded that urinary calculi follow a recurrent annual cycle with increased occurrence during the hot months. Peak incidence immediately followed periods of higher temperature, increased humidity, increased precipitation, and slower winds. Al-Dabbagh and Fahadi (1977) drew similar conclusions.

In contrast, Elliott (1975) concluded from a 10-year study of seasonal variations in urolithiasis that peak stone incidence occurred during periods of above average temperature and below average rainfall. In view of the conflicting data accumulated from humid or dry regions, it appears that mean temperature remains the most critical factor.

Parry and Lister (1975) presented an alternative viewpoint that implicates increased exposure to sunlight as a cause of increased urinary calcium excretion. This occurrence may lead to a higher incidence of urolithiasis. However, Blacklock (1969) reported a higher incidence of urinary calculi in naval personnel who worked below deck in a hot environment (cooks, boiler stokers) than in personnel above deck who supposedly receive more sunlight. The sunlight theory requires much more prospective study to prove its value (Varghese et al., 1989).

Elevated environmental temperature seems, therefore, to be related to a greater risk of stone disease in those populations capable of forming stones. High temperatures increase perspiration, which may result in a higher concentration of urine. This hyperconcentration could contribute to stone formation in many ways. For example, if the individual has, as noted previously, an inborn tendency toward formation of calculi, dehydration would result in decreased urine volume and increased urinary concentration of these molecules as well as excessive urinary acidity (Toor et al., 1964). These changes could promote crystallization of the respective molecules. Hallson and Rose (1977) have shown increased crystalluria in patients who form stones during summer months. Yet, Caduff and co-workers (1988) found no difference in summer or winter urinary osmolality between urology clinic patients who form stones and patients who do not form stones. Hence, the "dehydration/hyperconcentration" theory requires more investigation.

Patients with a tendency toward formation of uric acid or cystine calculi would have an additional risk. Acid urine holds much less uric acid or cystine in solution. One admonition to patients who form stones, as derived from these studies, might be to "keep cool."

Water Intake

Two factors involved in the relationship between water intake and urolithiasis are (1) the volume of water ingested as opposed to that lost by perspiration and respiration and (2) the mineral or trace element content of the water supply of the region. One of the prevailing assumptions in the literature concerning urolithiasis is that increased water intake and increased urinary output decrease the incidence of urinary calculi in those patients who are predisposed to the disease.

In their survey of urolithiasis in the United States, Burkland and Rosenberg (1955) questioned urologists about their opinions of methods of preventing recurrence of urinary stone disease. "Forcing water" received the highest total number of positive responses, along with elimination of infection and elimination of urinary obstruction. This opinion is reaffirmed in reviews by Drach (1976a), Smith and Boyce (1969), Finlayson (1974), Thomas (1975), and Seftel and Resnick (1990). Finlayson pointed out the theoretical criticism that urine dilution by increased water intake may actually increase ion activity coefficients and, hence, crystallization of the elements in urine. But water diuresis does reduce the average time of residence of free crystal particles in urine and dilutes absolutely the components of urine that may crystallize. Finlayson concluded that the dilutional effects of water diuresis probably outweigh the changes in ion activity and therefore do help to prevent stone formation. For example, in patients who form urinary calculi of calcium oxalate, Finlayson (1974) demonstrated that a higher urine flow causes a reduction in urine oxalate concentration. However, to be effective, a urine output of more than 3600 ml/day would be theoretically necessary. Few patients ingest enough water to create such a high urinary output unless they are educated to do so.

Environment, family education, heredity, and other factors are associated with various habits of ingestion of fluids, especially water. Lonsdale (1968b) pointed out that the habitual low levels of water intake may have been related to the high incidence of uric acid stones of British adults in earlier times.

A revealing series of studies of water drinking habits were reported by Frank and co-workers (1959, 1966). They first investigated the epidemiologic aspects of occurrence of urinary lithiasis in native and immigrant groups populating Israeli communities. They noted that the areas of highest incidence of urolithiasis were the warmer desert regions as opposed to the cooler mountain regions. Within desert areas, the incidence of calculi formation was highest in immigrants from Europe, lower in those from East and North Africa, and lowest in the native-born population of Israel. Overall incidence of calculi rose markedly after age 18.

These investigators selected one factor as the most important in increasing risk of stone disease—low urinary output in an area of high environmental temperatures. They also believed that low urinary output was secondary to the low intake drinking habits brought to Israel by the immigrants. To further test this hypothesis, they selected one village and attempted to increase the consumption of water by the population by emphasizing that water drinking would decrease the incidence of urinary calculi. In a second village, no attempt was made to increase water drinking or to educate the people about calculous disease, but observations on water drinking and on incidence of calculous disease were continued. Without giving any further explanations to the second village, these workers conducted surveys of average daily urinary output in both villages. Their educational program on water drinking appeared to be effective. Between 1962 and 1965, a consistent difference in the average urinary output of individuals in the two villages was evident. Those in the "educated" village produced an average of 200 to 300 ml more urine per day than those in the control village.

These investigators reported an interesting incidental observation. In the control village, there was little difference between the average summer urinary output (1041 ml/day) and the average winter output (1060 ml/day). The posteducation incidence of urinary calculi was 0.07 per cent in the village with high urinary output and 1.80 per cent in the village with low urinary output, a highly significant difference. This well-performed study implies that low daily urinary volume is a very important factor in the causation of urolithiasis.

In support of this theory, Blacklock (1969) reported that by increasing urinary output from approximately 800 to 1200 ml/day, incidence of urinary calculi in sailors decreased by 86 per cent. Those clinicians who treat patients with urinary lithiasis with medications need to remember these reports of the effectiveness of increased urinary output alone.

Although volume of water drinking and subsequent urinary output play a part in causing urolithiasis, other investigators have suggested that the mineral content of water may contribute to the causation of stone disease. Data are conflicting, however (Churchill et al., 1980; Shuster et al., 1982). Some state that excessive water hardness (e.g., calcium sulfate) contributes to calculi (Rose and Westbury, 1975), whereas others state that excessive softness (e.g., sodium carbonate) causes a greater incidence of stone disease (Juuti and Heinonen, 1980; Sierakowski et al., 1976; Sierakowski et al., 1978). Additionally, the presence or absence of certain trace elements in water has been implicated in the formation of urinary calculi. For example, zinc is an inhibitor of calcium crystallization (Elliot and Eusebio, 1967), and low urinary levels of zinc could therefore further a tendency toward stone formation. Yet, Yendt and Cohanim (1973) reported improvement in their patients who form stones after treatment with thiazide, even though urinary zinc concentrations in most of these patients declined. Proof that water hardness or softness or trace element content is critical to stone formation requires a well-constructed prospective study similar to that conducted on water drinking by Frank and associates (1959, 1966).

Diet

Little doubt can exist that dietary intake of various foods and fluids, which result in the greater urinary excretion of substances that produce stones, has a significant effect on the incidence of urinary calculi. Ingestion of excessive amounts of purines (uric acid) (Hodgkinson, 1976), oxalates (Thomas, 1975), calcium, phosphate, and other elements often results in excessive excretion of these components in urine. Effects of diet in relation to specific types of urinary calculi are reviewed in later sections of this chapter.

One must be very cautious about assuming that the dietary patterns of an individual are the same as those of the community in which he or she lives. Lonsdale (1968b) points out that patients who form stones may have exceptional dietary patterns because of previous habits, or because they cannot assimilate the normal diet. Peculiar dietary excesses may also occur, such as the following: use of large amounts of Worcestershire sauce with its high oxalate content (Finlayson, personal communication; Holmes, 1971), a vegetarian diet associated with childhood urolithiasis, and the habitual excessive ingestion of milk products in the form of cheese or ice cream.

Not only the diet but also its source may be important. Identical vegetables grown in various parts of Thailand contain amounts of oxalate that differ by 50 per cent or more (Suvachittanont et al., 1973). Practical problems associated with analysis of the total diet for a large group of people make such studies highly suspect. In addition, the most important diet is that of the individual patient who forms stones. A careful dietary history is critical to the evaluation of every individual who forms stones.

Occupation

Lonsdale (1968b) indicated that urinary calculi are much more likely to be found in individuals who have sedentary occupations. Blacklock (1969) reported that the incidence of urinary calculi was higher in administrative and sedentary personnel of the Royal Navy than in manual workers. The highest incidences were found in cooks and engineering room personnel, and, as discussed previously, these were probably associated with work conditions that included a hot environment. The rate of stone formation was lowest in the "active" group of Royal Marines.

Mates (1969) performed an extensive survey of regional differences in the occurrence of stone disease in Czechoslovakia. He reported that of all epidemiologic factors studied, the occupation of the individual was of greatest importance. The lowest incidence of stone disease in this country was found in agricultural and border populations. The highest incidence was found in industrial areas. Within these areas, incidence was especially high among sedentary workers and among civil service employees.

Mates then described an interesting method for prevention of stone disease based on his epidemiologic studies: "A large consumption of beer and butter is associated with minimal stone disease." Andersen (1973) emphasized that the relationship between diet and heredity is the major determinant for urolithiasis but that occupation is also important. He postulated that the economic level of living, related to occupation, and the diet predicated by this level are as likely to be involved in the genesis of upper urinary tract calculi as they have been in the genesis of endemic stones of the bladder.

Sutor and Wooley (1974a) correlated occupation with incidence of urinary calculi in 856 patients. Professional and managerial groups had a much higher than expected incidence of calculi, whereas skilled and partly skilled groups had the expected frequency. Unskilled laborers had a slightly lower than expected incidence. Manual workers had a much lower than expected frequency of urinary calculi. Occupation also tends to determine exposure to other factors, such as high environmental temperature, which may increase a tendency toward formation of urinary calculi.

Robertson and colleagues (1979 a and b) performed extensive studies of the relationship between occupation, social class, and risk of stone formation. They confirmed that the risk of formation of calcium urinary calculi was increased in the most affluent countries, regions, societies, and individuals. These persons have more disposable income to spend on animal protein, which leads to increased urinary concentrations of calcium, oxalate, and uric acid (Robertson et al., 1979 a and b). In fact, these investigators have gone so far as to suggest an alternative to high-protein ("rich-man's") diets in their paper, *Should Recurrent Calcium Oxalate Stone-Formers Become Vegetarians?* (Robertson et al., 1979c). Hence, it becomes difficult to assess whether occupation itself is a primary factor in stone disease or whether it merely establishes other aspects of environment such as diet, heat exposure, and water drinking. Alterations in these factors may be the actual instigators of urolithiasis.

In summary, this review of the epidemiology of urinary lithiasis leads us to conclude that the following factors all play some part in the genesis of urinary calculi: heredity, age, sex, geographic location, environmental temperature, water intake, diet, social class, and occupation of the individual. Given the fact that for urolithiasis to occur, the individual must have the capability of forming urinary calculi, we now discuss the physical and chemical factors that have a role in the formation of urinary calculi.

THEORETICAL BASIS OF ETIOLOGY

Modern concepts of etiology of urinary calculous disease may be separated conveniently into four major theories (Table 58–1): (1) supersaturation/crystallization theory; (2) matrix nucleation theory; (3) inhibitor absence theory; and (4) epitaxy (Coe et al., 1980; Elliot, 1973b; Finlayson, 1974, 1978; Malek and Boyce, 1973; Pak, 1987; Resnick and Boyce, 1978; Scott, 1975; Vermeulen and Lyon, 1968; Williams, 1974a).

Robertson and associates (1976) developed a combined theory of saturation of urine with crystallizable agents versus inhibition by certain proteins. In 1981, they presented an extended combined theory, in which the major factors contributing to, for example, calcium crystallization, were evaluated by discriminate analysis (Robertson and Peacock, 1983). They showed that risk of calcium oxalate crystallization was related to the following factors (in order of importance): calcium oxalate crystallization increased as urinary concentrations of oxalate, uric acid, pH, and calcium increased; it decreased as urinary concentrations of protein inhibitors and total volume increased.

To understand the present theories of the causation of stone disease, it is necessary first to explain some of the basic processes involved in crystallization in biologic systems. Some aspects of renal anatomy that are critical to the application of these crystallization processes to urinary lithiasis are discussed. Urinary excretion patterns of some substances that are critical in the formation of specific types of calculi are examined. Specific discussions of each type of calculus follow this general introduction to etiology.

Processes of Crystallization

As Finlayson (1974) emphasized, it is impossible to discuss present-day concepts of stone disease without becoming acquainted with the vocabulary of biologic crystallization. Therefore, some descriptions and examples of crystallization processes are introduced, so that the use of these words in discussing the diagnosis and treatment of urolithiasis is clear. Terms to be reviewed include saturation and saturation concentration, supersaturation, solubility product, formation product or formation saturation, metastable region of supersaturation, crystal nucleation, crystal growth, crystal aggregation, epitaxy, and zeta potential.

Saturation

If the increasing amounts of substances capable of crystallizing are added to pure water at a given pH and temperature, eventually a high enough concentration is reached for crystals to form. When crystals begin to form, the solution has become saturated with the substance. A specific limit to the amount of solids or solute that can be held in solution exists. Crystallization of a single substance, such as cystine or uric acid, will occur when enough of the substance is added to water at given pH and temperature to saturate the solution (saturation concentration). When two or more substances are combined to form the crystal, as is the case with table salt (sodium chloride) or calcium oxalate, the level of saturation is governed by the product of the concentrations of the two or more substances. The point at which saturation is reached and crystallization begins is referred to as the solubility product (SP), which is defined as the product of the molar concentrations of the two substances at the point of saturation.

Note that pH and temperature are always specified for any crystallization process. Alteration in either factor may greatly change the amount of substance or solute that may be held in solution. Perhaps the best known illustration of the effects of temperature on solubility is the increased solubility of sugar in hot water. For all practical purposes, there need be no concern about temperature in our discussion of urolithiasis because it must occur at body temperature, near 37°C. One must be cautious in analyzing the results of some in vitro studies of stone crystallization, however, because many such studies are performed at room temperature rather than at body temperature (Finlayson, 1974). Because urine varies widely in pH, this factor must be considered in any explanation of urolithiasis.

Saturation and solubility product in water are simple to define, but urine is a much more complex solution. In urine, when the concentration of a substance reaches the point at which saturation would occur in water, crystallization does not occur as expected. Urine has the ability to hold more solute in solution than does pure water. Although all elements and molecules in urine are suspended in water, the mixture of many electrically active ions in urine causes interactions that change the solubility of their elements. Such a solution is called polyionic, and the definition of saturation or solubility product of a given substance in this type of solution becomes very complex and difficult. In addition, many organic molecules such as urea, uric acid, citrate, and complex mucoproteins of urine all mutually affect the solubility of other substances. For example, citrate is known to combine with calcium to form a soluble complex. It therefore prevents some calcium from combining with oxalate or phosphate and becoming crystalline. As a corollary to this statement, Finlayson (1974), Elliot (1973a), Welshman and McGeown (1975), Nicar and co-workers (1983), Menon and Mahle (1983), and Schwille and co-workers (1982) have reported that deficiency in urinary citrate is one of many factors found in the urine of patients who form stones.

Electrical attraction or repulsion of ions in biologic solutions is also involved in the stone-forming crystallization process. Rollins and Finlayson (1973) studied electrical fields of urine-like solutions and the effects of various additives on the electrical attraction of urinary

Table 58–1. MODERN THEORIES OF ETIOLOGY OF CALCIUM STONE DISEASE

Supersaturation/crystallization
Matrix initiation
Inhibitor lack
Epitaxy
Combinations of above

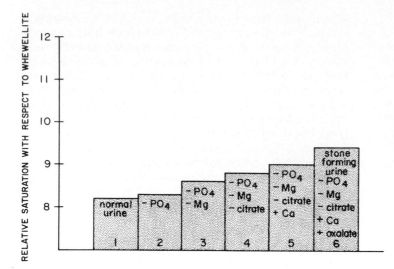

Figure 58–5. Effect of certain urinary components on degree of saturation of urine with whewellite (calcium oxalate monohydrate). Removal of some (PO_4, magnesium, citrate) or addition of others (calcium, oxalate) results in increased saturation and increased risk of precipitation of stone crystals. (Used with permission of Birdwell Finlayson, M.D.)

substances. This type of biologic, electrical activity is called zeta potential (Gardner, 1969; Scurr and Robertson, 1986).

In an attempt to simplify the study of urinary stone disease, many investigators have tried to eliminate urinary components that they believe do not contribute to or detract from a tendency to form urinary calculi. The most elemental of these solutions requires, for calcium oxalate crystals, the presence of calcium, oxalate, sodium, and chloride ions (Finlayson and Roth, 1973). But even this simple solution does not adequately reproduce all the ionic activity present in urine, nor does it reproduce other ionic effects on stone formation. A further discussion of ionic activity and its relationship to urolithiasis is beyond the scope of this chapter. The interested reader is referred to the works of Finlayson (1978), Robertson and colleagues (1968 and 1972a), Nordin and colleagues (1979), and Isaacson (1968) for further information. However, the presence of such a large number of ionically active substances does change the solubility of any given element or substance in urine.

Supersaturation

The most significant and beneficial effect of these ionic and protein-element interactions is to raise the solubility of various substances that otherwise might crystallize at the concentrations present in urine (Fig. 58–5). Hence, if a given amount of calcium and oxalate that would crystallize when placed in a solution of water at given pH and temperature is placed in urine, it will be held in solution. If the amount of calcium and oxalate is increased progressively in the same volume of urine at constant pH and temperature, the calcium and oxalate will remain in solution even though the solubility product has been exceeded. In doing this, we are actually creating supersaturation. This area of supersaturation is called the metastable region or zone and is illustrated in Figure 58–6. The amount of substance in urine can be increased to a point at which urine will no longer hold it in solution. Spontaneous nucleation of the crystals then begins. The area of supersaturation between

the solubility product and spontaneous urinary crystallization is the metastable zone for a given substance.

The point at which spontaneous nucleation of crystals occurs is known as the formation product (FP) for urine. Although urine contains multiple and complex solubilizing factors for that particular crystal, the amount of substance in urine may eventually become so great that it is capable of crystallizing in spite of the solubilizers and inhibitors that are present (Breslau and Pak, 1980; Chang-Ti et al., 1987; Dyer and Nordin, 1967; Finlayson, 1974; Fleisch, 1965; Hodgkinson and Nordin, 1971; Lonsdale, 1968 a and b; Mullin, 1972; Thomas, 1974; Walton, 1965, 1967; Williams, 1974 a and b).

Crystal Nucleation

Nucleation of crystals occurs when active ions and molecules in a solution no longer flow randomly in a completely dissociated fashion but cluster together closely enough to form the earliest crystal structure that

PROCESSES OF CRYSTALLIZATION RELATED TO STONE FORMATION

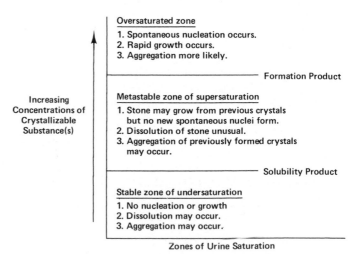

Figure 58–6. Concepts of crystallization in urine summarized. (See text for full discussion of various zones.)

TRIGGER OR LIMIT CONCEPT OF CALCULUS FORMATION

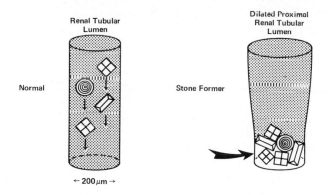

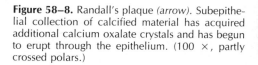

← 200 μm →

Figure 58–7. "Triggering" of urolithiasis may occur when many crystals or spherules aggregate to occlude a urinary tubule *(arrow)*, or a single crystal may become lodged in the tubule and grow larger, as urine in the metastable zone of saturation flows by.

will not dissolve. This structure has the form of a lattice that is characteristic of that crystal. If this process occurs spontaneously in a pure solution, such as sodium plus chloride in distilled deionized water, the process is called homogeneous nucleation. But pure solutions are difficult to create. Dust particles, glass chips, and other contaminants may enter the solution and serve as nuclei. The analogy is that of a chemical catalyst: Other particles that start nucleation "catalyze" the process. This type of secondary nucleation is most probable in urine and is referred to as heterogeneous nucleation.

No matter what type of nucleation occurs, it requires energy to "push" the crystal nucleus together (Uhlmann and Chalmers, 1965). The energy required for nucleation is higher than that required for simple crystal growth and is provided when the amount of supersaturation is high enough in the oversaturated zone to cause nucleation. According to Walton (1965), the physical factors that tend to control nucleation are those of interfacial energy, temperature, and frequency of collision. Frequency of collision increases as supersaturation increases; therefore, enough energy is ultimately created to allow nucleation.

These two concepts of nucleation may be further separated into the free particle theory and the fixed particle theory (Finlayson and Reid, 1978) In free particle nucleation, multiple crystals are formed simultaneously in the upper urinary system when the formation product of a substance is exceeded. One concept of free particle nucleation also allows for the fact that urine probably contains multiple, previously formed microliths in the kidney papillae. These are subsequently excreted and may then serve as nuclei for other ions. To conform to this theory, however, these particles must float freely in urine and must serve as nuclei for further growth or aggregation of crystals. In the theory of fixed particle nucleation, it is suggested that because of excessive concentration of certain ions in certain areas of kidney, precipitation of crystals or spherules may occur in the renal papillae either within the tubular lumina or beneath the surface of the papillae (Drach and Boyce, 1972; Finlayson and Reid, 1978; Hautmann et al., 1980; Malek and Boyce, 1973; Randall, 1937; Resnick and Boyce, 1978; Resnick and Boyce, 1978; Vermeulen and Lyon, 1968) (Figs. 58–7 and 58–8). These particles remain "fixed" and serve as nuclei for further growth.

Crystal Growth

Once nucleation has occurred in the complex solution known as urine, certain nuclei may continue to grow if the urine remains supersaturated. Not only will such nuclei continue to grow in the zone above the formation product (the zone that permits spontaneous nucleation), they will continue to grow even if the saturation of urine falls into the metastable zone between solubility product

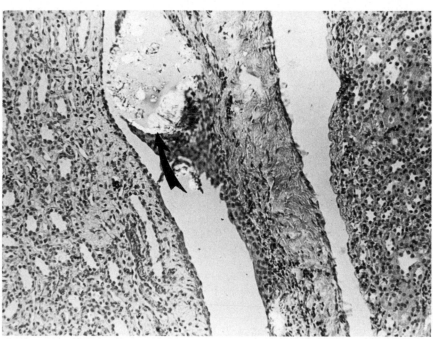

Figure 58–8. Randall's plaque *(arrow)*. Subepithelial collection of calcified material has acquired additional calcium oxalate crystals and has begun to erupt through the epithelium. (100 ×, partly crossed polars.)

and formation product (see Fig. 58–6). The concept of increasing the urine concentration to the level in which the formation product is exceeded is important to certain theories of urinary stone formation in which homogeneous nucleation is a critical event. In other theories, however, saturation is required only to the range of metastable supersaturation. It is postulated that adequate heterogeneous nuclei are already created by biologic processes in the kidney (Carr, 1969; Drach and Boyce, 1972; Malek and Boyce, 1973; Randall, 1937). Stones then grow on these preformed nuclei.

Crystal Aggregation

Another concept is necessary to promote our understanding of the probable genesis of urinary calculi. This concept is that of aggregation. If multiple nuclei and crystals are formed spontaneously and float freely, these nuclei become active kinetically and bounce about in the urine. If they remain small, free, and independent within the solution, they will pass through the urinary tract within a given amount of time and will be voided. Under certain conditions, however, these nuclei can grow and may come close enough to each other to be bound together by various chemical forces. Therefore, nuclei or larger growing crystals may aggregate and form larger crystal masses (Baumann and Wacker, 1979; Sallis, 1987).

Epitaxy

One other aspect of crystallization that has received considerable attention is epitaxy (Hench, 1972; Lonsdale, 1968 a and b; Seifert, 1967). If a crystal has a pattern or organization of ions that is regular and predictable, this structure is called a lattice. This surface lattice may resemble very closely that of a second but different type of crystal. Depending on the closeness of resemblance, the second type of crystal may actually be able to grow on the surface of the first. Calcium oxalate and uric acid do have crystal lattices that are similar enough to permit this process of epitaxy, or the deposit of one type of crystal upon the surface of another. In some situations, the degree of mismatch between the surface lattices of two crystals is so great that epitaxy is not likely to occur. It is for this reason that cystine crystals rarely deposit on the surface of a previously formed nucleus of uric acid or calcium oxalate. The mismatch in surface lattices is too great.

Epitaxy requires oriented overgrowth of one crystal on the surface of another. Because of this requirement, the opportunity exists to modify crystal surfaces to prohibit epitactic overgrowth and to interfere with stone formation and growth. In some concepts of inhibition of stone formation, this theory is the basis of attempts to "poison" growing surfaces of crystals. At the present time, however, no known method of interfering with stone growth includes epitaxy or inhibition of epitaxy as its primary mechanism of action (Finlayson, 1974; Lonsdale, 1968a).

Relationship Between Time Allowed for Crystal Growth and Size of Passages

In a simple water solution the growth of a crystal occurs over a period of time. For a given crystal, this growth may be estimated by measuring the increase in size or weight per unit of time. In a static solution such as that in a test tube in a laboratory, this is a relatively simple procedure. One can take a portion of the mixture, weigh and count the crystals in this portion, and estimate the total mass of crystals present in the container. The crystals will continue to grow as long as additional solutes are added to the solution to promote supersaturation. If solutes are not added, however, the growth will continue only until the level of crystallizable solute in the supernatant has dropped below the solubility product. At this point, we say that supersaturation has been relieved, and growth ceases.

But normal urine is not a static solution. It flows continuously, and new solutes are continuously excreted. Therefore, crystals may form best at the point of greatest supersaturation of urine, usually the renal papillae (see Fig. 58–7) (Hautmann et al., 1980; Jordan et al., 1978; Vermeulen and Lyon, 1968). As soon as these crystals form, they can flow within 3 to 5 minutes into the renal pelvis, down the ureter, and into the bladder, where they remain for a period of approximately 3 to 6 hours. Transit time of urine from the normal kidney to the normal bladder is estimated to be from 5 to 10 minutes.

The lumen of the nephron is smallest at the level of the collecting duct, where its diameter is 50 to 200 μm. Anatomically, this portion occurs in the renal papilla (Finlayson, 1974). If the crystal does not have time to grow large enough to obstruct any renal tubule, it passes into the ureter, where the minimum diameter that can cause obstruction within 10 minutes is approximately 2 mm. This statement is a clinical observation based on the fact that the majority of urinary calculi that cause symptoms are greater than 2 mm in diameter (Lehtonen, 1973; Sutor and Wooley, 1975; and many others). After the crystal has reached the bladder, it may still grow and may achieve a size that exceeds 6 mm in diameter. Such a crystal could still be voided through the urethra without difficulty.

To summarize this theory, urinary crystals form in the small lumen of the renal tubule and progress through the renal pelvis to the ureter, into the bladder, and out the urethra. Even if crystals grow as they progress through the urinary tract, they are able to pass because the conduits become progressively larger as they progress toward the outside. The urinary tract is anatomically constructed like an inverted cone. The diameters are smallest in the renal tubule and become progressively larger in the ureter, the bladder, and the urethra.

Teleologically, it's a good system that allows passage of any possible small particles. But if a particular crystal becomes lodged, growth can continue for long periods whenever urinary supersaturation or aggregation of new crystals occurs. Hence, if the crystal mass becomes lodged in the renal papilla or tubule it is no longer able to move through the system (see Figs. 58–7 and 58–8). The crystal remains at that point and continues to grow in supersaturated urine. Intermittent layered growth of stones has been reviewed by Lonsdale (1968a). If the crystal breaks off or breaks away from the renal papilla when it is too small to obstruct the ureter, it will pass through the system without causing symptoms. But if the crystal attains a diameter of greater than approximately 2 mm, it may pass into the ureter and create urinary obstruction, becoming a symptomatic urinary calculus.

What about bladder calculi? A calculus of 2 to 3 mm may pass through the ureter and into the bladder with relatively few symptoms. But let us suppose it enters a bladder in which there is obstruction of the urinary outlet. This problem occurs especially often in males. Bladder calculi are extremely rare in females. If, because of prostatic obstruction or a narrow bladder neck, the stone cannot enter the urethra but remains in the base of the bladder or in a diverticulum, it can continue to grow whenever the urine is supersaturated with the substances that created the stone. Such stones may achieve enormous size (Fig. 58–9), the largest reported weighing over 1 kg (Becher et al., 1978). Urinary stasis in the bladder also allows growth of stones on the distal ends of stents, whereas the upper portions remain relatively free of crystals (Fig. 58–10).

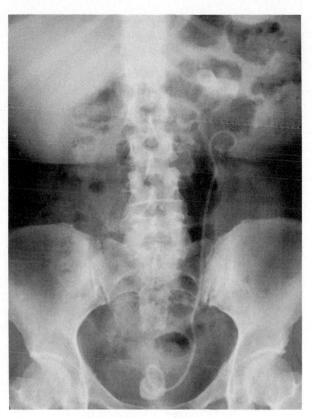

Figure 58–10. Encrustation of the bladder portion of a ureteral stent in a patient with recurrent urinary lithiasis.

Matrix

A noncrystalline protein-like matrix of urinary calculi was first described by Anton von Heyde in 1684 (cited

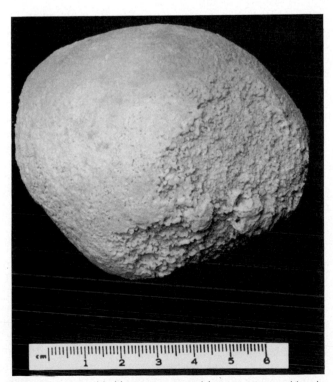

Figure 58–9. Large bladder stone removed from an 87-year-old male.

by King, 1967). The exact influence of matrix on formation and crystallization of urinary calculi has been forcefully debated for years. Boyce and colleagues (1969) have pursued the role of matrix in stone formation since their earliest report in 1954. Extensive investigations have characterized matrix as a derivative of several of the mucoproteins of urine and serum (Sugimoto et al., 1985; Rahman et al., 1986). Matrix content of a given stone varies, but most solid urinary calculi have a matrix content of about 3 per cent by weight (Boyce and King, 1959). Alternatively, matrix calculi, composed of an average of 65 per cent of matrix by weight, may occur, especially in association with urinary infection (Allen and Spence, 1966; Mall et al., 1975). The matrix content of some calculi may be very small—uric acid calculi, for example, may have a matrix content of less than 2 per cent.

Chemical analysis of stone matrix reveals it to be about 65 per cent hexosamine and 10 per cent bound water (Boyce, 1968). Uromucoid, the major mucoid component of urine, is very similar in composition to matrix, except that it also contains about 3.5 per cent sialic acid, whereas matrix has none. Malek and Boyce (1973) have postulated that this distinctive lack of sialic acid may be due to cleavage of the acid from uromucoid molecules by the renal enzyme sialidase.

Whether matrix truly initiates stone formation or plays a part in causation of stone disease continues to be uncertain. Several investigations (Finlayson et al., 1961; Vermeulen and Lyon, 1968) have indicated that matrix may be only an adventitious coprecipitate with the crystals that form stones. Sutor and O'Flynn (1973) demonstrated that matrix crept into a previously crystallized mass placed by a patient into her bladder.

However, as Finlayson (1974) concludes, simple coprecipitation cannot explain all the interactions observed between stone crystals and matrix. For example, polymerization of matrix must occur in order to form the matrix stone. Watanabe (1972) and Lanzalaco and coworkers (1988) believe that matrix participates in the formation of stone crystals. Matrix must originate in the renal tubules, probably in the proximal tubule (Herrman, 1963; Keutel, 1965; Malek and Boyce, 1973). Malek and Boyce demonstrated that kidneys of patients with idiopathic calcium lithiasis show a large number of intranephronic calculi in the renal tubules. These microliths are laminated structures of matrix and crystals that mimic the structures of larger stones. Such microliths were not found in kidneys of patients who formed struvite, uric acid, or cystine stones. Therefore, matrix-related growth or aggregation of these small intranephronic stones may be one primary event in the causation of calcigerous lithiasis.

Boyce and associates (1962) described one component that is immunologically unique to stone matrix and is different from any of the other mucoids of urine. This "substance A" was found on the matrix of all calcigerous stones, in the kidneys of patients who had stone disease, and in the urine of patients who formed calcium stones. It could also be found in the urine of patients who had renal inflammation due to infection, infarction, or cancer (Boyce, 1969; Keutel and King, 1964).

Moore and Gowland (1975) conducted extensive studies into immunologically distinct reactants of stone matrix and uromucoids of urine. They were not able to find a single distinct protein such as substance A but instead found three or four antigens unique to stones. They detected these "stone-specific antigens" in the urine of 85 per cent of patients who formed stones but in no urine of normal individuals. The exact relationship between these antigens, matrix A, and stone formation remains unclear.

In addition, Bichler and associates (1976) have challenged the observations that total uromucoid excretion is elevated in patients with active stone formation. These investigators found no significant difference in uromucoid excretion rates between 49 normal persons and 79 patients who formed stones. As noted previously, the uromucoid of patients who form stones does bind more calcium than that of normal persons (Foye et al., 1976). Matrix undoubtedly plays some role in stone formation. Whether it is active or passive, qualitative or quantitative, enhancing or inhibitory remains to be determined.

Inhibitors of Crystallization

Perhaps no aspect of urinary calculous disease has generated so much interest and confusion as the urinary inhibitors of crystallization. Elliot (1983) studied calcium oxalate solubility in urine. The solubility of calcium oxalate in urine is not greatly different in patients with stones and that in normal persons. For example, Elliot reports that the calcium oxalate solubility products in patients with active stone formation and in normal individuals were not significantly different.

In comparison, Robertson and Peacock (1972) have shown that those who form calcium stones tend to excrete considerably more oxalate and calcium than do normal persons, but the investigators also showed moderate overlap in the degree of saturation between normal groups and groups with stone formation. Many cystinuric patients do not form calculi. Therefore, in spite of the fact that these individuals have an excessive amount of cystine in the urine, for some reason they do not develop the processes of crystallization associated with urinary calculi. How can we explain the fact that some individuals with supersaturated urine seem to be capable of holding more crystallizable urinary substances in solution? The answer given by many investigators is a relative lack of crystallization inhibitors in the urine of those who form stones.

Inhibitors may be classified as predominantly organic or inorganic. Of the inhibitors within the organic group perhaps the most famous is the peptide inhibitor first described by Howard and colleagues (1967) and studied extensively by Robertson and colleagues (1969) and Smith (1989). This low-molecular-weight peptide enables the urine to hold in solution considerably greater amounts of calcium than is possible when it is absent.

These aforementioned investigators have indicated that patients who form stones have a significant lack of this inhibitor in the urine. The major criticism of this particular inhibitor is the fact that the test substrate is rachitic rat cartilage. Although the inhibitor studied may be effective in prohibiting calcification of rat cartilage, rat cartilage is as yet unreported as a component of human urinary calculi.

Later, Barker and associates (1974), working in the laboratory of Howard, published findings indicating that most inhibition that they found in urine could be accounted for by the polyelectrolyte interactivity of the multiple ions of urine. Some additional high-molecular-weight glycoproteins have been shown to inhibit calcium oxalate crystallization (Drach et al., 1983; White et al., 1983). Nakagawa and associates (1987) described an agent, nephrocalcin, which inhibits growth of calcium oxalate crystals and may be deficient in those who form stones.

Other types of organic inhibitors may be present. Foye and colleagues (1976) described a significant difference between the composition of uromucoids (matrix) in normal people and that in those who form stones. The uromucoid of the last group contains more sulfhydryl groups (–SH) than does that of the normal group. This increase in –SH is believed to explain the fact that the uromucoid of those who form stones binds more calcium than does that of normal individuals. Hence, normal uromucoid may not be inhibitory, but, in contrast to uromucoid from patients who form stones, it does not promote stones by excessive calcium binding. It is conceivable that particular types of mucoids may be very active in coating the surface of crystals that form in urine, particularly when crystals reach a certain size.

Crystal coating may inhibit stone formation by producing surface (zeta potential) charges that prevent further deposition of crystal or that inhibit aggregation (Scurr and Robertson, 1986). The individual coated crystals may then repel rather than aggregate (Riddick, 1968; Rollins and Finlayson, 1973; Sallis, 1987). As a related example, Schmidt Nielsen (1964) has published fascinating observations on the excretion of "gelatinous" urine by desert mammals. In this very concentrated urine, the crystals of oxalate that are excreted are uniformly coated by mucous substances that are similar to human matrix substances. Large crystals and stones do not occur.

Other organic substances undoubtedly have some importance in the inhibitory processes of urine (Angell and Resnick, 1989). Amino acids, specifically alanine, may be important in improving the solubility of calcium substances in some types of urinary lithiasis (Chow et al., 1973; Elliot and Eusebio, 1967). Alternatively, in humans, the contribution of these substances to the solubilization of stones seems minimal (Finlayson, 1974).

Urinary citrate, as mentioned previously, has a part in the solubilization of calcium, oxalate, and phosphate in urine (see Fig. 58–5). Certainly, citrate is found to be decreased in some patients who form urinary calculi that contain calcium or uric acid (Elliot, 1973a; Finlayson, 1974; King, 1967, 1971; Miller et al., 1958; Pak, 1987; Thomas, 1988; Welshman and McGeown, 1976; Williams, 1974 a and b). Urea increases the solubility of some components of urine, especially uric acid (Porter, 1966). However, urea does not seem to influence calcium precipitation (Finlayson et al., 1972).

Inorganic Inhibitors of Crystallization

Most inhibitors of crystallization that have been reported are related to inorganic elements that affect the calcium phosphate or calcium oxalate systems. Foremost among these are phosphates, especially pyrophosphate (Fleisch and Bisaz, 1964). Investigations leading to the elucidation of the effects of the –P–O–P–(pyrophosphate) structure were summarized by Fleisch (1965). Most subsequent reviews of inorganic inhibitors include pyrophosphate as one major component (Baumann and Wacker, 1979; Drach et al., 1983). In fact, Thomas (1975) believes that one of the major effects of oral administration of large doses of orthophosphate is the increased urinary excretion of pyrophosphate. Conversely, oral administration of pyrophosphate does not result in an increase in renal excretion of pyrophosphate. Therefore, no medications containing pyrophosphate have been devised for treatment of urinary lithiasis.

The action of phosphate as a crystal poison of calcification has been known for many years. Simkiss (1964) reviewed the multiple effects that phosphates may have on calcifying biologic systems and found that orthophosphates themselves do not appear to have a direct effect on urinary stone formation of the calcigerous type.

When it is excreted into urine in significant amounts,

magnesium, a divalent cation, tends to increase the solubility of calcium, phosphate, and perhaps oxalate (Moore and Gowland, 1975). A high calcium/magnesium ratio has been implicated as one of the causes of calcigerous renal calculi (King, 1967; Oreopoulos et al., 1975). Prien and Gershoff (1974) and Melnick and associates (1971) have used this finding to justify the administration of magnesium to many patients who chronically form calcigerous urinary calculi. These workers have reported a satisfactory decrease in the tendency toward calcium stone formation after therapy. This approach is discussed further in a later section.

As mentioned previously, some investigators have implicated trace metals in the inhibition of urinary stone formation, especially the calcigerous type of stone. Zinc seems to be the most frequently mentioned of these substances (Elliot and Eusebio, 1967; Elliot and Ribeiro; 1973).

In Figure 58–5, the cumulative effects of some organic or inorganic inhibitors on the solubilization of urinary calcium are shown. These effects are roughly additive, and therefore each contributes partly to the solubilization of calcium. For this reason, it is likely that calcium stone formers have deficiencies in not one but several of the inhibitors that should be present in urine (Drach, 1976b; Pak et al, 1985).

MODERN THEORIES OF ETIOLOGY

Now that epidemiology and the processes of crystallization, matrix and inhibitors have been reviewed, we can discuss the theories of the etiology of urinary stone formation (see Table 58–1).

Supersaturation/Crystallization

Uric acid or cystine calculi form whenever urine with a tendency to remain at an acid pH becomes oversaturated with uric acid or cystine. Stone growth or dissolution is directly and linearly related to this factor, as described further. Magnesium ammonium phosphate (struvite) calculi form when the product of the concentration of these ions exceeds the saturation product and when the urine remains alkaline for long periods. Therefore, three of the five major types of urinary calculi can be explained mostly by the first theory of stone formation—supersaturation of urine with a substance that can crystallize in urine at a given pH.

Inhibitor Deficiency

Supersaturation alone does not completely explain even these three types of calculi (uric acid, cystine, and struvite), and certainly not calcium phosphate or calcium oxalate stone formation. Many normal persons have urinary supersaturation with the substances mentioned previously. Crystals form, but the crystals remain small and are passed easily. We must then consider the effects of some types of inhibitors that prevent or at least limit crystal growth and aggregation in normal urine. Neither the supersaturation theory nor the inhibitor theory can stand alone. It seems necessary to combine both to have one cogent theory of stone formation. Robertson and colleagues (1976) approached such a theory for calcium oxalate urinary lithiasis. Their studies show that for calcium oxalate calculi, an index of supersaturation versus inhibition can be determined for an individual. In addition, patients who form stones have higher indices—that is, they show greater supersaturation and less inhibition of crystallization and stone formation.

Matrix Initiation

Where does the matrix fit in? Matrix, as mentioned previously, may inhibit crystal growth, interfere with crystal aggregation, and even enhance stone growth. At the present time, the uromucoid of normal persons is thought to be a beneficial inhibitor of crystallization and stone formation. In comparison, the matrix of those who form stones represents uromucoid with some qualitative defect that alters its ability to inhibit crystallization or even causes it to promote stone formation (Finlayson, 1974).

Intranephronic and Fixed Nucleation

We have discussed multiple theories of causation of urinary stones, whether formed of cystine, calcium, uric acid, or some other crystallizable substance. The proponents of the intranephronic theory of urinary stone disease believe that the disease begins within renal tubular cells. Excretion of multiple calcified nuclei from these cells into the urine allows the growth of crystals in the previously supersaturated urine. In such a theory, there is no need for a free nucleation phase. The ability to study these submicroscopic nuclei has been limited, however, and their importance in the genesis of stone disease is not yet understood. Intranephronic calculosis is probably most important in calcium stone disease.

Extranephronic and Free Particle Nucleation

Proponents of the extranephronic theory of urinary stone formation believe that all calculous disease begins in urine, outside the renal tubular cell. They believe that urinary supersaturation with a given element results in spontaneous crystallization of that element. Because crystal growth in urinary solutions does not proceed rapidly enough to postulate the formation of a single large mass that obstructs the ureter or bladder (Finlayson and Dubois, 1973; Miller et al., 1977), concepts of aggregation or agglomeration of spontaneously nucleated crystals must be advanced to explain formation of a larger mass. We know also that inhibitors of multiple organic or inorganic types exist in urine. It is theorized that these crystal inhibitors affect the surfaces of crystals and prevent them from aggregating or from

growing larger. Some investigators believe that one of these inhibitors may be uromucoid itself, or the agent, nephrocalcin (Nakagawa et al., 1987). Patients with stone disease lack nephrocalcin or some other significant component of inhibitors, or they produce additional components that decrease their inhibiting actions.

One of the major problems in the study of urinary lithiasis has been the difficulty of measuring the kinetics of crystallization: nucleation, growth, and aggregation of crystals of urinary calculi. At what point and how rapidly does nucleation occur? How fast does the crystal grow? Does aggregation occur or not? The approaches of Robertson and associates (1973, 1976), Gill and associates (1974), Lanzalaco and associates (1988), Miller and associates (1977), and Ryall and associates (1985) offer possibilities for thorough study of these aspects of urinary crystallization.

Summary of Crystallization Concepts

Whether nucleation, growth, or aggregation is the most important component in formation of urinary calculi is not yet known. One can surmise, however, from the massive amount of investigation that has been conducted, that basic crystallization processes are critical to the formation of urinary calculi. For this reason, we must now define those aspects of renal function that allow supersaturation of urine and thereby formation of urinary calculi. This theory of urolithiasis is an attempt to combine all the elements discussed previously.

First, renal function must be adequate for the excretion of excess amounts of crystallizable substances. In some instances, excess excretion is the result of some particular defect of renal tubular function (e.g., cystinuria).

Second, the urine must alter its pH to conform to that required to crystallize the substance. The net result of these first two requirements is the ability of the kidney to excrete an excessive amount of a given substance at a urinary pH that enhances precipitation of that substance.

Third, the urine must have a complete or a relative absence of a number of inhibitors of crystallization of the crystallizable components (see Fig. 58–5). It seems unlikely at the present time that a single inhibitor is responsible for solubilizing all urinary substances.

Fourth, the crystal mass must reside in the urinary system for a duration sufficient to allow growth or aggregation of the crystal mass to a size large enough to obstruct the urinary passage through which it is proceeding. Trapping of nuclei in the kidney or elsewhere provides the time for growth. Hence, stasis may have an important part in the genesis of urinary calculi if the crystal mass is retained in a particular position long enough to allow significant growth. This relationship with time is probably the reason that, as mentioned previously, the urinary system is built like an inverted cone.

These epidemiologic and physical chemistry observations form the bases of our understanding and treatment of almost all human urinary stone diseases. In the next sections, we assume that a patient has a certain defect, has formed a symptomatic calculus, and requires initial diagnosis and treatment of acute urinary lithiasis. Aspects of continued evaluation and treatment for specific types of stone disease are discussed.

ACUTE STONE EPISODE

General Observations

A urinary calculus usually "announces" its presence with an acute episode of renal or ureteral colic. Bladder colic differs from ureteral colic and is discussed separately in the section on bladder calculus. Uroliths create symptoms only when they become trapped in some segment of the upper urinary tract. First, stones may become impacted in a calyx of the upper urinary tract. Individual calyces may therefore become distended and painful and create hematuria. An alternative form of this process is the occurrence of stone in a calyceal diverticulum, which is usually a congenital abnormality (Middleton and Pfister, 1974), (Fig. 58–11).

The second area in which a calculus may become impacted is the ureteropelvic junction. It is here that the relatively large diameter of the renal pelvis (1 cm) abruptly decreases to that of the ureter (2 to 3 mm).

A third area of impaction is at or near the pelvic brim, where the ureter begins to arch over the iliac vessels posteriorly into the true pelvis.

The fourth area, especially in females, is the posterior pelvis, where the ureter is crossed anteriorly by the pelvic blood vessels and by the broad ligament.

Finally, the most constricted area through which the urinary calculus must pass is the ureterovesical junction (Fig. 58–12). These normal anatomic variations probably explain the frequency with which calculi become impacted in certain portions of the ureter more often than in others. The majority of impacted ureteral stones will be found in the pelvic portion of the ureter (Fig. 58–13) (Drach, 1978, 1983).

Numerous investigators have tried to relate the possibility of spontaneous passage of ureteral calculi to their size. To become impacted, calculi usually must have one diameter in excess of 2 mm. If the smaller diameter is less than 4 mm, spontaneous stone passage is likely (Fig. 58–14) (Drach, 1983; Prince and Scardino, 1960; Sandergard, 1956).

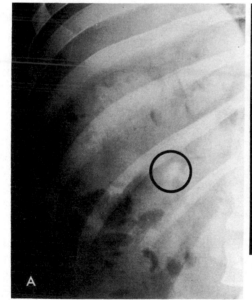
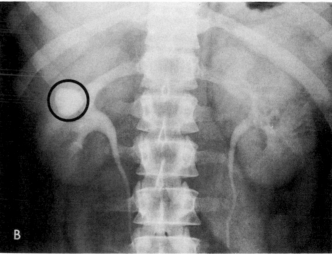
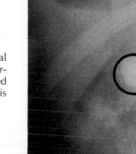

Figure 58–11. *A,* Pale milk-of-calcium stones *(circle)* within renal calyceal diverticulum. *B,* Iodinated contrast agent fills the diverticulum *(circle). C,* Plain film 24 hours after *B* reveals retained contrast and poor drainage. Segmental nephrectomy relieved this patient's intermittent right renal colic.

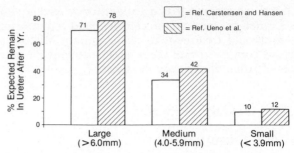

Figure 58–14. Combined data from two studies provide an estimate of percentages of stones first seen in the pelvic ureter and their likelihood of retention *for 1 year.* (From Drach, G. W.: Urol. Clin. North Am., 10:709, 1983.)

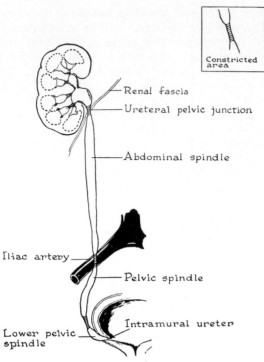

Figure 58–12. Points of constriction in a normal ureter.

Renal Colic

Renal colic is a symptom complex that is characteristic for the presence of upper urinary tract calculi. A typical episode occurs during the night or early morning hours, is abrupt in onset, and usually affects the patient while sedentary or at rest.

It is the partially obstructing, continuously moving calculus that appears to create the greatest amount of colic. The extreme crescendo of pain begins in the area of the flank, courses laterally around the abdomen, and generally radiates to the area of the groin and testicle in the male or to the labia majora and round ligament in the female. This radiation of pain may be related to the blood supply of the cord and testicular or ovarian vessels by the testicular or ovarian artery, which has its origin from the aorta very near the renal artery.

Autonomic nerve fibers that serve both kidney and testicle or ovary become involved in the transmission of pain sensations to the spinal cord and brain.

Research suggests that prostaglandins are involved in the genesis of pain of renal and ureteral colic (Wahlberg, 1983). More importantly, they seem also to be involved in renal repair after a stone episode (McDougal, personal communication, 1990).

As the stone moves to the mid-ureter, pain generally tends to radiate to the lateral flank and abdominal area. With impaction of the stone in a particular area of the ureter for a period of time, local inflammatory changes occur. The most painful area may be located around the impaction of the calculus. If the stone eventually moves toward the bladder, severe renal colic may once again occur. When ureteral stones are near the bladder, patients often develop the symptoms of urinary frequency and urgency.

Because the autonomic nervous system transmits visceral pain, confusion about the source of the pain is not uncommon and is related to the diffuse spreading of strong stimuli to other areas of similar anatomic innervation. The celiac ganglion serves both kidneys and stomach; therefore, nausea and vomiting are commonly associated with renal colic. In addition, ileus or other intestinal stasis associated with local irritation is not infrequent. Similarity of these symptoms to those of the gastrointestinal tract causes urinary lithiasis and colic to be confused with a number of abdominal diseases. Among these are gastroenteritis, acute appendicitis, colitis, and salpingitis.

Physical Signs

Physical signs of urinary calculous disease are characteristic. The first of these is the fact that the patient almost always has "moving irritation." That is, individuals with urinary lithiasis rarely can find comfort in any given position. They sit, stand, pace, recline, and move continuously in an attempt to "shake off" whatever it is that is creating discomfort.

Fever is rarely present unless urinary infection occurs along with the calculus. Pulse rate may be elevated by virtue of pain and agitation. Blood pressure is sometimes above normal in a patient in whom it has previously been normal.

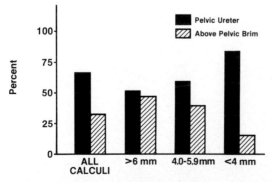

Figure 58–13. Distribution of ureteral calculi by size at time of presentation (253 patients). (From Drach, G. W.: Urol. Clin. North Am., 10:709, 1983. Data adapted from Carstensen, H. E. and Hansen, T. S.: Acta Chir. Scand. (Suppl.), 433:66, 1973.)

Grunting respirations occur, especially at the peak of colic, and may be similar to those of an individual who has respiratory distress.

Examination of the chest is necessary, and findings should be normal. Examination of the abdomen in general reveals moderate deep tenderness on palpation over the location of the calculus. In addition, the kidney may show moderate-to-marked tenderness, especially on palpation or fist percussion over the posterior flank.

Urinalysis

Urinalysis in most patients with urinary lithiasis reveals the presence of microscopic or gross hematuria. Some 10 per cent of patients do not demonstrate hematuria, especially if the calculus has created complete obstruction. In some instances of urinary calculus without pain, gross hematuria may be the only presenting complaint, or it may be discovered incidentally on routine physical examination. Although such painless hematuria may be due to other causes, silent urinary calculus remains one of the diseases that must be ruled out. Moderate pyuria may occur even in patients with uninfected urinary lithiasis. When significant numbers of pus cells are present in the urine, however, a thorough search for infection should be made. This is particularly true of females, in whom urinary infection is likely to be a common cause of urinary lithiasis.

Urinalysis sometimes reveals an additional finding that may be helpful in diagnosing the type of calculus present. On occasion, a patient who is in an active phase of urinary lithiasis will have in the urine crystals of the same type that are creating the calculus. Therefore, the observation of cystine, uric acid, or calcium oxalate crystals in the urine may be an indication of the type of calculus ultimately found.

Radiographic examination of the urinary tract is the next step in the evaluation of the patient with suspected urinary lithiasis. In fact, these findings form the cornerstone of the initial evaluation of the patient and establish, in general, the presence and severity of calculous disease.

Radiographic Examination

Plain Abdominal Films

In the initial evaluation, the first routine radiographs ordered are plain kidney-ureter-bladder (KUB) radiographs. A representative film is illustrated in Figure 58–15. Plain films of the abdomen often show densities that are not clearly stones but may represent other calcified densities, such as pelvic phleboliths. It is then helpful to obtain additional plain films in the right posterior oblique, left posterior oblique, or lateral position. Renal tomography without contrast material can also be very helpful.

In most patients, the position and outline of the kidneys can be seen on the plain films. The position of the ureter is characteristically parallel to the lateral processes of the lumbar spine. The ureter then crosses over the pelvic brim and turns somewhat laterally into

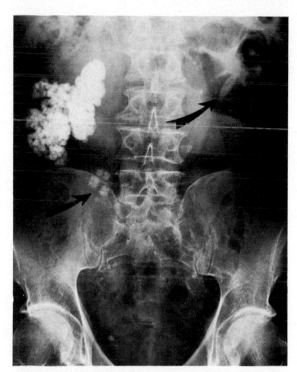

Figure 58–15. Multiple right renal, right ureteral *(arrow)*, and left renal *(arrow)* calculi appear on this plain abdominal film. Patient also had an obstructing left lower ureteral matrix calculus that is not visible.

the true pelvis (see Figs. 58–12 and 58–15). Therefore, the observation of a radiodense calculus in the areas of the kidney or along the course of the ureter, along with typical signs of colic and hematuria, may be sufficient for diagnosis of upper urinary stone.

Radiodensity of Calculi

Calculi that contain calcium, such as calcium oxalate and calcium phosphate calculi, are radiodense (Boyce et al., 1956; Emmett and Witten, 1971; Lalli, 1974). Roth and Finlayson (1973), through some unique radiographic techniques, have shown that calcium phosphate (apatite) stones are the most radiopaque and have a density like that of bone. Calcium oxalate calculi are almost as opaque. Magnesium ammonium phosphate (struvite) calculi are somewhat less radiopaque than calcium calculi. Cystine calculi must be considered partly radiodense. Roth and Finlayson estimate that cystine stones are approximately 0.45 times as radiopaque as calcium oxalate calculi. In addition, they note that cystine calculi are at least 40 times more opaque than uric acid stones.

Figure 58–16 compares calcium, magnesium, cystine, and uric acid calculi in a single radiograph. Figures 58–11 and 58–15 through 58–18 show the relative radiodensities of various stones on plain abdominal films of patients with bladder or upper tract calculi.

The degree of radiodensity is one factor in visualization of the calculus on the plain film, but the structure and configuration of the calculus also contribute. For example, calcium oxalate calculi must be at least 2-mm thick to appear on most radiographs. If the calculus

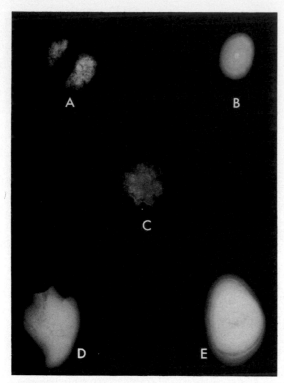

Figure 58–16. Radiodensities in air (to improve contrast) of five human calculi. *A,* Calcium oxalate. *B,* Calcium phosphate. *C,* Uric acid. *D,* Cystine. *E,* Magnesium ammonium phosphate. Note that only the uric acid calculus is truly radiolucent.

measures 1 × 2 mm in size, it can be seen only when the x-rays course through it parallel to the greatest diameter. For this reason, stones sometimes disappear in one plane of the radiograph and reappear in another. For cystine calculi, a degree of thickness approximating 3 to 4 mm is necessary for the stone to be visualized at all. Calculi of ammonium acid urate have slight radiodensity, but even large calculi of uric acid have no radiodensity at all, in comparison to surrounding soft tissues (Fig. 58–19).

Therefore, only calculi of relatively pure uric acid or of matrix (see Figs. 58–15 and 58–18) can be considered truly radiolucent. It is these calculi that create the greatest diagnostic problems based on plain abdominal films. For differentiation of these calculi, radiographic studies employing some type of contrast agent are necessary. The most common type of study performed in a patient with suspected renal or ureteral stones, who is not allergic to renal contrast material, is the intravenous urogram. Basic techniques for this study are discussed elsewhere in this text. Only those aspects of intravenous urography of special importance to urinary lithiasis are discussed.

Intravenous Urogram

Aside from the observation of a radiodense calculus somewhere in the path of the urinary tract, the first indication of the presence of urolithiasis is delay in the appearance of the contrast medium in the nephrogram following its injection. This finding implies obstruction by calculus. As Lalli (1974) and Van Arsdalen and colleagues (1990) point out, observation of such a delay indicates that the usual 5-, 10-, and 20-minute pyelographic films are not likely to be useful in defining the location and presence of the calculus. Therefore, it is better to extend the period of observation and obtain films at perhaps 20, 30, and 60 minutes. In this way, the patient does not experience the unnecessary inconvenience of reclining on the radiographic table for an excessive period of time and benefits from the decreased amount of radiation exposure. Delayed films may be obtained several hours or even 1 day following the injection of contrast material (see Fig. 58–18). Should there be difficulty in visualization after one dose of contrast agent, reinjection of the agent may be useful. If there is still no visualization, retrograde pyelography may be indicated (see Fig. 58–19).

Some physicians prefer infusion pyelography for detection of all types of urologic disorders. Occasional reports of spontaneous rupture of the renal pelvis or

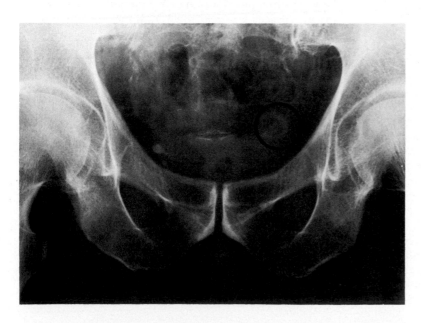

Figure 58–17. Matrix calculus of left lower ureter outlined faintly by iodinated contrast *(circle).* This type of calculus must also be considered radiolucent.

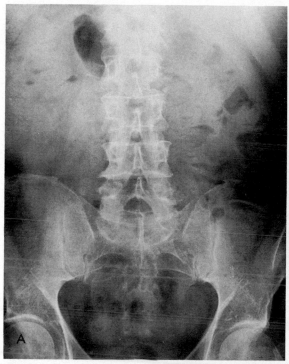

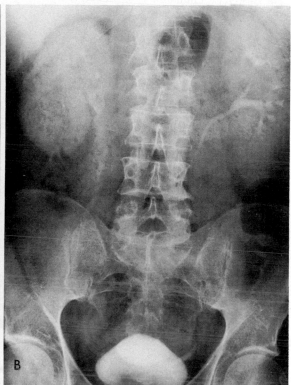

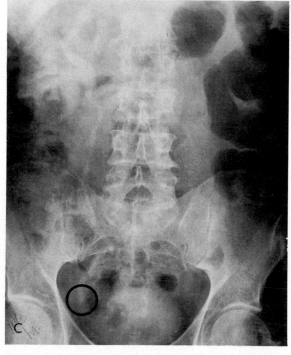

Figure 58–18. Value of delayed radiographs. *A,* KUB radiograph of a patient with acute right renal colic and hematuria. No obvious calculus. *B,* Radiograph 20 minutes after infusion of iodinated contrast material. Prolonged right nephrogram and poor right ureteral filling. *C,* Radiograph 11 1/2-hours after infusion. Mild right hydroureteronephrosis down to a small lucent filling defect *(circle).* Patient subsequently passed a 3-mm uric acid calculus.

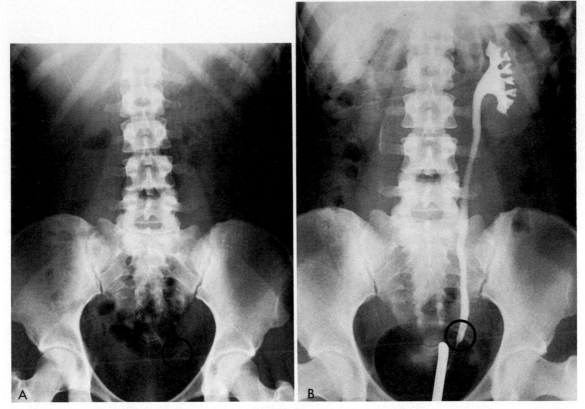

Figure 58–19. Retrograde pyelography (A and B) confirmed the presence of two ureteral cystine calculi (circles) obstructing the left ureter. Sepsis was present, and stones were removed by manipulation.

ureter due to obstructing calculus have appeared in the literature. However, I am impressed by the increased number of reports of spontaneous urinary extravasation following infusion pyelography (Amin and Howerton, 1974; Aubert, 1973; Borkowski and Czapliczki, 1974; Munster and Hunter, 1968; Quencer and Foster, 1972; Reece and Hackler, 1974; Silver et al., 1973; Van Regemorter and Hardy, 1973; Wart et al., 1973). To avoid this problem, it seems more useful and less challenging to perform repeated bolus injections of iodinated contrast material as necessary. In comparison, Claypool and colleagues (1975) have indicated that the infusion technique is likely to provide a definitive diagnosis more rapidly than bolus injection methods. Until extensive comparative information is available, it seems better at this time to rely on re-injection or other methods of visualization, such as computed tomography (CT) and ultrasound imaging. Combination of contrast radiography studies and CT studies can be very specific in defining stone location and type.

Computerized Tomography

This technique is especially useful in defining classically "radiolucent" uric acid calculi (Resnick et al., 1984). Studies without contrast precede those with contrast. Some investigators have attempted to use CT scanning to define the composition of stones, but this technique has been questioned (Van Arsdalen et al., 1990). Additional information on this technique is found in Chapter 10.

Ultrasound Scanning

Ultrasound scanning of the kidney, ureter, and bladder is useful. I have found it helpful in defining some relatively large urinary calculi. Figure 58–20 illustrates the ultrasound appearance of a relatively large calculus filling the pelvis of the kidney. The ultrasound scan also showed a significant renal substance and indicated an obstructed and a hydronephrotic kidney. This information led to the decision to treat the calculus by extracorporeal lithotripsy to preserve renal function. Newer methods of lithotripsy involve ultrasound imaging to view and control treatment. Increased use of this imaging modality within urology is likely.

Radioisotope Methods

Radioisotope renography and scanning have contributed to the diagnosis of obstruction and location of calculus in a number of patients, particularly those who are otherwise sensitive to contrast material. These techniques are demonstrated in Figure 58–21. In this patient, who was markedly sensitive to intravenous contrast agent, not only the location of the calculus but also the degree of urinary obstruction was clearly defined. The patient ultimately passed spontaneously a small calculus.

Retrograde Pyelography

In other instances, when radiographic, ultrasonic, or radioisotope methods are not successful, retrograde pye-

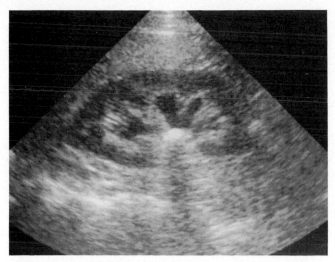

Figure 58–20. Longitudinal ultrasound scan of stone in renal pelvis of right kidney *(white object in center)*. Note acoustic shadowing beyond stone.

lography is necessary. This may be especially true in cases of relatively radiolucent calculi that are difficult to locate by other techniques. Such a case is illustrated in Figure 58–19. In this instance, the calculi were two small cystine calculi, which could be seen only with difficulty on plain films and were not clearly defined by intravenous urography or ultrasound.

Diagnostic and Treatment Decision Process

The progressive evaluation of symptomatology, physical examination, urinalysis, and imaging generally constitutes the preliminary examination of a patient with urinary calculous disease. After a urolith is diagnosed, the first decision requires assessment of the degree of seriousness of the disease process. Should one apply procedural therapy, such as endoscopy or lithotripsy, or wait for the stone to pass? I have reviewed some of these decision processes and indications (Fig. 58–22) (Drach, 1974b, 1983; Drach et al., 1989). Procedural insertion of a stent or removal of a stone is necessary when there is evidence of significant obstruction, progressive renal deterioration, refractory pyelonephritis, or unremitting pain. Stone obstruction of an infected kidney requires emergency procedural treatment, after stabilization of the patient.

Once this first decision is made, the majority of patients with urinary lithiasis require prompt therapy for pain relief. Most patients gain relief from the intramuscular injection of 50 to 100 mg of meperidine or 10 to 15 mg of morphine, depending on body size and severity of pain. Liberal use of narcotics to treat the pain of urolithiasis has resulted in some patients who feign symptoms. Most are addicts who are attempting to obtain drugs. Drug addicts most frequently relate a story that sounds too much like one from a textbook case. In addition, they are almost always "allergic" to intravenous contrast material and relay information that may indicate that previous stones are known to be radiolucent uric acid or matrix and therefore cannot be seen on plain radiographs. The absence of uric acid crystals or infection in the urine helps confirm one's suspicion of drug dependency.

The presence of hematuria in a patient who claims stone disease should not be taken as an absolute indication of the presence of this disease. In my experience, drug addicts have successfully added blood to their urine by incising the lateral edges of their fingers or biting the

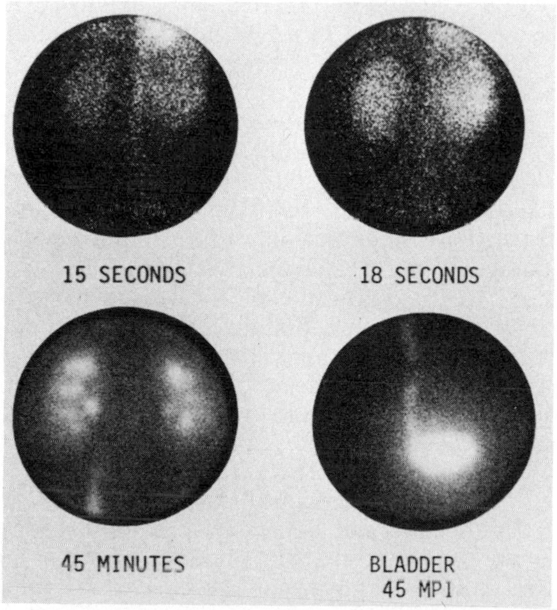

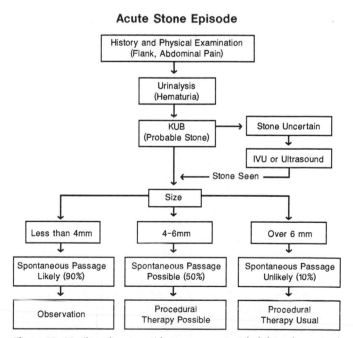

Figure 58–21. Radioisotopic renal scans may be helpful in detecting an obstructing calculus. Ureteral fullness near the bladder at 45 minutes in this very ill patient who was allergic to intravenous iodinated contrast material led to consideration of a right ureteral calculus.

Acute Stone Episode

History and Physical Examination (Flank, Abdominal Pain) → Urinalysis (Hematuria) → KUB (Probable Stone) → Stone Uncertain → IVU or Ultrasound → Stone Seen → Size

Size → Less than 4mm → Spontaneous Passage Likely (90%) → Observation

Size → 4–6mm → Spontaneous Passage Possible (50%) → Procedural Therapy Possible

Size → Over 6 mm → Spontaneous Passage Unlikely (10%) → Procedural Therapy Usual

Figure 58–22. Flow diagram with management probabilities for ureteral stones of various sizes.

inner edges of their cheeks and spitting into the urinary specimen, or even going so far as to insert a pin into the urethral meatus inside the glans penis.

However, once certain evidence of urinary calculus has been established, patients with stone disease are extremely thankful for whatever pain relief can be obtained.

Hospitalization may be necessary for those individuals who have so much gastrointestinal upset that they cannot retain food or fluids. In addition, they may become exhausted by the loss of sleep and other discomforts created by stone disease. Other patients may not be able to take or retain oral pain medication and may require narcotic injections at intervals frequent enough to require hospitalization.

It is an almost universal adage in urology that fluids must be forced on patients with stones, whether given intravenously or orally. Studies on urodynamics indicate that an increase in diuresis generally reduces the rate of ureteral peristalsis. If so, one questions whether forced water drinking serves to propel the stone through the urinary system or to decrease peristalsis, thereby inhibiting urinary colic. Experience with patients who have undergone percutaneous nephrostomy *and* shock wave lithotripsy reveals that they pass the stone fragments, even though no hydrostatic pressure or pain exists.

Some workers have advised antispasmodic or anti-inflammatory agents in the treatment of urinary calculous disease (Peters and Eckstein, 1975). In particular, aminophylline or indomethacin (Buck et al., 1983; Flannigan et al., 1983) therapy has been advised. I have attempted to provide these drugs on several occasions, with variable results. A long-term, carefully controlled study of these medications is necessary before they are accepted for this purpose. As noted previously, McDougal (personal communication, 1990) has expressed concern that nonsteroidal anti-inflammatory drugs may interfere with renal healing and function after a stone episode.

Most patients with urinary calculous disease do not require procedural treatment, surgery, or hospitalization and can be followed as outpatients. Because urinary calculi are often less than 4 to 5 mm in size and because the majority of these pass spontaneously (see Fig. 58–14), patients need only pain relief and instructions about recovery of the calculi.

The patient must understand that it is critical to recover any calculus or gravel that is passed. One of several commercially available funnel-like straining devices can be provided. In my experience, however, the simplest way for the patient to observe passage of a calculus is to urinate into a clear glass jar. The density of the calculus causes it to fall to the bottom. Because most calculi are larger than 1 mm, the patient can recognize and recover it. Stone analysis is performed on any calculus that is recovered, whether by the patient, at surgery, or by any other method. Stone analysis provides information about composition and allows planning of future therapy for the majority of patients with urinary calculous disease.

Other aspects of stone disease must be mentioned at this point: How long does the physician wait for passage of a calculus in a patient with partial or complete obstruction of the urinary tract before becoming concerned about significant damage to renal function? Does urinary obstruction due to calculus have any significant effect on the kidney?

Pathophysiology of Urinary Obstruction Associated with Lithiasis

One may divide the pathophysiologic effects of stone on the kidney and ureter into two categories as follows: (1) functional results of partial or complete obstruction and (2) results of local irritation. To these two categories must be added the associated effects of any infection, which will alter the effects of obstruction and local irritation.

Renal Function Changes

Renal or ureteral obstruction, partial or complete, produces a progressive decrease in excretory functions of the kidneys, according to studies performed in dogs. Little similar information in humans is available. After obstruction, a rapid redistribution of renal blood flow from medullary to cortical nephrons occurs. This redistribution results in a decrease in glomerular filtration rate (GFR) and renal plasma flow (RPF), reflecting a decrease in both glomerular and tubular function (Jones et al., 1989; Lackner and Barton, 1970). Finkle and Smith (1970) and Vaughan and associates (1971 a and b) observed similar decreases in function and agreed that these decreases resulted from reduced renal blood flow. Stecker and Gillenwater (1971) observed a significant concentration defect and reduced urinary acid excretion following partial ureteral obstruction, lasting up to 16 weeks in dogs.

Moody and co-workers (1975) divided renal response to ureteral occlusion into three phases: at 0 to 1½ hours, ipsilateral renal blood flow and ureteral pressures both rose; at 1½ to 5 hours, renal blood flow fell, while ureteral pressures continued to rise; and at 5 to 18 hours, renal blood flow and ureteral pressures both fell. Vaughan and associates (1970) showed further that contralateral renal blood flow increased as function and renal blood flow of the obstructed kidney decreased.

Obstruction results not only in decreased renal function but also in fairly rapid changes in ureteral peristaltic function. Gee and Kiviat (1975) observed hypertrophy of rabbit ureteral musculature after only 3 days of obstruction. If obstruction continued for 2 weeks, connective tissue deposits (scar) occurred between muscle bundles. Such changes were considered as marked at 8 weeks. Rose and colleagues (1975) observed the effects of chronic ureteral obstruction in 24 dogs. They concluded that chronic ureteral obstruction resulted in decreased peristalsis and decreased pressure generation. These workers noted that the presence of urinary infection in addition "totally impaired" ureteral function. Perhaps this is why fewer stones in patients with infection pass spontaneously (Westbury, 1974). Such infection must, of course, involve the obstructed kidney.

Pyonephrosis and pyelonephritis with stone create destructive renal changes, as described in other chapters. Obstruction by stone worsens these changes. Stone obstruction also inhibits the cure of pyelonephritis because decreased renal function results in decreased excretion of antibiotics and inhibits drainage of infected urine.

Relief of obstruction after 8 weeks results in a rapid increase in ipsilateral renal blood flow and partial reversal of functional defects (Vaughan et al., 1970, 1971 a and b). Finkle and co-workers (1970) proposed that measurement of tubular clearance of water (Tc H_2O), following mannitol diuresis, may be useful in assessing the amount of renal tubular function remaining after relief of chronic obstruction. Finkle and Smith (1970) believe that the major effects of obstruction are on the tubules. Stecker and Gillenwater (1971) and Jones and associates (1989) state, however, that the glomerular-tubular balance is maintained in the obstructed kidney and that relief of obstruction results in improvement of both glomerular filtration rate and renal plasma flow.

Of practical interest to the urologic surgeon is the answer to the question of how long to wait before treating the stone. If infection exists behind the obstruction, the answer is clear: relieve the obstruction as quickly as possible. If no infection exists and pain or discomfort is minimal, one must judge each case. With complete obstruction, it appears that renal deterioration (at least in dogs) begins within 18 to 24 hours. Within 5 days and certainly by 2 weeks, some irreversible renal functional loss has occurred. After 16 weeks of obstruction, only "slight recovery" can be expected (Stecker and Gillenwater, 1971). Partial obstruction modifies the aforementioned time periods but may still result in some irreversible functional damage. Schweitzer (1973) studied chronic partial obstruction in animals and concluded that renal damage occurs early. He suggested that intervention of some kind may well be necessary earlier than is usually practiced, if renal damage is to be avoided completely.

Analysis of Uroliths

Following treatment of the acute phase, stone recovery is of paramount importance. In their review of the incidence of urinary calculi, Burkland and Rosenberg (1955) asked urologists their opinion about the importance of stone analysis. The replies indicated that many urologists did not believe that analysis of calculi was important in planning treatment. It is hoped that this attitude has changed. Most medical therapy for stone disease is now based on analysis of calculi, and decisions about proper procedures for treatment require knowledge of stone composition (Dretler, 1990).

Based on information presented previously in this chapter, individuals who form calculi usually produce more than one during the course of their lives. To prevent the formation of future calculi, we must know the type usually found in that patient. Smith (1974a) has indicated that stone analysis is extremely important in planning therapy. Of the group of patients that he

placed in the "indeterminate activity" category, fully one third (37 per cent) developed a new calculus within the year following evaluation. One would suspect, therefore, that the incidence of repeat urinary calculus is significantly high. Estimates vary from 8 to 80 per cent.

Westbury (1974) indicated that the degree to which a patient is able to reproduce the pattern of chemical composition of the initial calculus depends to a large extent on the sterility of the urine. He states that "Excluding the presence of urinary infection for each patient liable to urolithiasis, there is an inherent set of factors which seem to determine the composition of all of the stones formed by that patient." As Westbury points out, it is only the advent of urinary infection that results in a change of composition of calculi in many patients. It is also important to determine whether the patient's infection was present prior to (and therefore causes) stone formation, or whether it was the result of catheterization, cystoscopy, or other manipulations necessary for treatment of the original stone. In the instance involving treatment, the patient develops a superimposed urinary infection that alters the type of stone, even though the original stone disease was of the non-infected type.

Methods

Many types of analysis of urinary calculi have been proposed (Table 58–2). The most common and most practical type for the clinical laboratory is chemical analysis, but this requires a trained and dedicated laboratory staff. Numerous investigators have pointed out that there are limitations to the use of qualitative chemical methodology for testing urinary calculi (Hazarika et al., 1974b; Hodgkinson et al., 1969; Laskowski, 1965; Murphy and Pyrah, 1962).

Schneider and co-workers (1973) compared chemical, x-ray defraction, infrared spectroscopy, and thermoanalytic procedures in analysis of urinary calculi. They found all of these methods accurate in detecting the components of urinary calculi. However, they thought that the chemical methods were best for practical use in the hospital laboratory—there was only a 2 per cent error in detection of components of calculi by this method.

Domanski (1937) has questioned the usefulness of

Table 58–2. METHODS OF STONE ANALYSIS

Chemical
   Qualitative "spot" tests*
   Quantitative analysis
   Chromatographic and autoanalyzer methods
Optical
   Binocular dissection microscopy with petrographic (polarization) microscopy
Instrumental
   Radiographic crystallography*
   Infrared spectroscopy*
   Thermoanalytic
   Scanning electron microscopy
   Transmission electron microscopy

*Commonly used methods

chemical analysis. He pointed out, for example, that although it was possible by chemical reaction to liberate ammonium from pure uric acid stones, ammonium was not really a significant component of most uric acid calculi. Carbonates also were often released from calculi in which they were not actually present, because the chemical test for carbonates was not accurate in the presence of oxalate.

Prien and Frondel (1947) pointed out clearly the difficulty of accurate identification and analysis of the components of urinary calculi by chemical techniques alone. They emphasized the greater accuracy of optical crystallography and x-ray crystallography. Therefore, the majority of precise analyses of urinary calculi have been performed with petrographic or more technical crystallographic methods. Prien and Frondel (1947), Prien and Prien (1968), and Prien (1963, 1974) have continuously updated their observations on petrographic analysis of urinary calculi. Sutor and colleagues (Sutor, 1968; Sutor and Scheidt, 1968) subsequently evaluated methods of crystallographic stone analysis that utilized x-ray and optical crystallography. They point out, for

example, that the x-ray defraction technique allows some minor components of mixed urinary calculi to go undetected. As much as 20 to 30 per cent of the lesser component may remain undetected, unless certain corrective factors are applied.

Many chemical and instrumental techniques of analysis, such as x-ray crystallography, are criticized because in preparation for such analysis the calculus is usually ground in a mortar and pestle. The nucleus and various layers of growth are thereby mixed.

In comparison, proponents of chemical analysis criticize optical crystallography because the observer selects only small portions of the stone for analysis. If the stone is not fractured or cut, only surface analysis is performed.

Elliot (1973a) therefore recommended optical crystallographic examination combined with initial careful dissection of the stone, under a binocular stereoscopic microscope. In this way separate layers and segments of the stone may be analyzed (Fig. 58–23). In calcium oxalate calculi, Elliot found that calcium oxalate monohydrate (whewellite) composed the nucleus or initiating

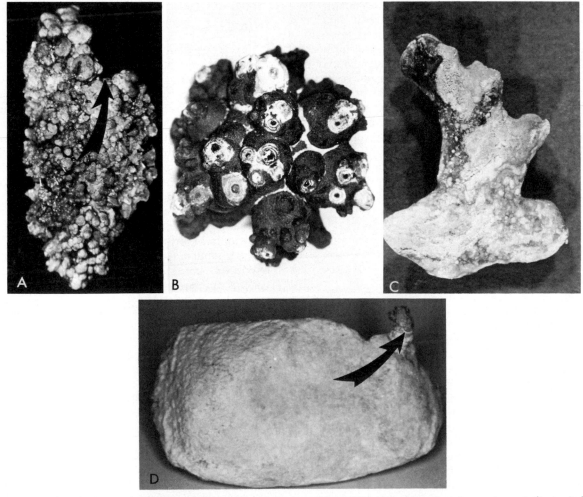

Figure 58–23. Examples of urinary calculi. *A,* Calcium oxalate monohydrate (whewellite). Actual size 5 × 8 mm. Arrow indicates indentation of point of attachment of stone to papilla. This is sometimes called a "mulberry stone." *B,* Uric acid calculus. Actual size 2.3 cm. Sometimes called a "jack stone." *C,* Staghorn calculus of magnesium ammonium phosphate (struvite). Actual size 4.5 × 7 cm. *D,* Bladder calculus of magnesium ammonium phosphate (struvite), which has formed on a piece of nonabsorbable suture *(arrow).* Patients who produced stones in *C* and *D* both had chronic urinary infections caused by *Proteus mirabilis.*

crystal of two thirds of all stones. The majority of surface deposits were composed of calcium oxalate dihydrate (weddellite).

These observations were confirmed by Bastian and Gebhardt (1974), who reported that whewellite was five times more frequent in the nucleus than weddellite. They also described nuclei of pure apatite overgrown with various forms of calcium oxalate or even uric acid (epitaxy). In addition, occasional nuclei of struvite, tricalcium phosphate (whitlockite), or cystine were found. Microanalysis revealed that the nuclei were composed of many small clumps of crystallites. They concluded that the initiation of stone disease was a process of aggregation, as discussed previously. None of these observations would have been possible if the stones had been pulverized for chemical analysis.

Laskowski (1965) has attempted to combine the most beneficial methods of optical crystallography with chemical analysis to give a definitive description of the calculus. He utilized the technique described by Elliot (1973a) for initial microdissection of the calculus, with subsequent petrographic examination under the polarizing microscope. He performed spot microchemical tests to confirm the presence or absence of particular ions. Using Elliot's methods, one can determine very precisely the composition of almost all urinary calculi without expensive instruments. Additional comments on the importance of analysis have been made by Berman (1975), Catalina and Cifuentes (1970), Finlayson (1974), Herring (1962), Lagergren (1955), Lonsdale (1968 b), Lonsdale and Sutor (1972), and Schmucki and Asper (1986). Sutor and Wooley (1969) have gone so far as to analyze calculi dating back to medieval times in London. Sutor and Wooley (1974 b) also performed an extensive geographic survey of urinary calculi (see previous section on geography), as did Mandel and Mandel (1989 a and b).

Infrared spectroscopic analysis of urinary calculi has been reported by Hazarika and Rao (1974 a), Kister and associates (1974), and Takasaki (1971, 1975, 1989). Thin-section transmission electron microscopic analysis of calculi has been reported by Meyer and co-workers (1971). Their analyses of uric acid, oxalate, and phosphate stones reveal that stone material is very finely divided and highly aggregated.

For the practicing urologist without access to large analytic laboratories, the most useful methods are chemical analysis and petrographic methods through the polarizing microscope. Because it is relatively simple to instruct laboratory personnel in these techniques, almost any small hospital laboratory or large clinic can have the ability to analyze urinary calculi. In comparison, for physicians with analytic facilities nearby or available by mail and certified by national agencies, it is more reliable to have these laboratories analyze stones.

Incidence of Types

Table 58–3 summarizes the observations of a number of investigators on reported incidence of urinary calculi as analyzed by various methods. Several points emerge. As noted in the section on geography, bladder calculi of uric acid may predominate in some specific areas with relative malnutrition and primitive development. But in most of the world today, the commonest types of calculus are calcium oxalate, calcium phosphate, or mixtures of the two. The relative proportion of uric acid calculi stays approximately the same the world over, except for India. Also, we see approximately the same proportions of cystine calculi. It seems that throughout the world, approximately the same percentage of population is afflicted with a given type of urinary lithiasis.

Also, although we have discussed several methods of analysis of urinary calculus components, they all tend to lead us to the same result—namely, the five basic types of urinary calculus. Only minor differences occur. For example, Herring (1962) reported calcium oxalate calculi collectively in his review and did not further separate them into those that were pure and those that were mixed calcium oxalate and calcium phosphate calculi. Similar results are reported by Schmucki and Asper (1986). Herring employed only crystallographic methods. As Sutor has discussed (Sutor, 1968; Sutor and Scheidt, 1968), there are limitations in x-ray crystallography for complete analysis of calculus components. As previously noted, there is a possibility of missing one

Table 58–3. SOME COMPARATIVE INCIDENCES OF FORMS OF URINARY LITHIASIS

Form of Lithiasis	Per Cent of Stones Analyzed					
	USA[1]	USA[2]	India[3]	Israel[4]	Japan[5]	Great Britain[6]
Pure calcium oxalate	33		86.1	14	17.4	39.4
Mixed calcium oxalate and phosphate	34	73	4.9	64	50.8	20.2
Pure calcium phosphate	6	8	1.9		3.2	13.2
Magnesium ammonium phosphate (struvite)	15	9	2.7	12	17.4	15.4
Uric acid	8	7.63	1.2	9	4.4	8
Cystine	3	0.88	0.4	2	1.0	2.8
Artifacts and other	1	1.5	2.6		5.8	1.0

[1]Prien, E.L., Sr., and Gershoff, S.F.: J. Urol., 112:509, 1974.
[2]Herring, L.C.: J. Urol., 88:545, 1962.
[3]Sharma, R.N., Shah, I., Gupta, S., Sharma, P., and Beigh, A.A.: Br. J. Urol., 64:564, 1989.
[4]Herbstein, F.H., Kleeberg, J., Shalitin, Y., et al.: Isr. J. Med. Sci., 10:1493, 1974.
[5]Takasaki, E.,: Calc. Tiss. Res., 7:232, 1971.
[6]Westbury, E.J.: Br. J. Urol., 46:215, 1974.

component if it represents 30 per cent or less of the total proportion of the calculus. Hence, Herring's approach to analysis may have resulted in some error in the quantitative analysis of urinary calculi.

Mixed urinary calculi, as can be seen from Table 58–3, are very common. Hodgkinson and Marshall (1975) performed extensive quantitative chemical analyses of pure and mixed urinary calculi. They showed clearly that calculi of mixed composition, which includes calcium oxalate, magnesium ammonium phosphate, and calcium phosphate, were prevalent in the Leeds population. The major component in the largest number of calculi was calcium oxalate. These investigators noted a decrease in the proportion of calcium phosphate and magnesium ammonium phosphate in the calculi studied between 1965 and 1974.

Urinary infection tends to increase the percentage of phosphate in a urinary calculus. So too does the presence of metabolic diseases, such as hyperparathyroidism, renal tubular acidosis, and medullary sponge kidney. All of these disease states result in a more alkaline urine. It is this alkalinity that is believed to contribute to the deposition of phosphate in calculi. Hodgkinson and Marshall presume that improved diagnosis and treatment of these metabolic conditions have contributed to the decreased proportions of phosphates in urinary calculi.

Knowledge of the percentage composition of a urinary calculus contributes to the ability to predict the most probable cause of that calculus. Therefore, it is critical that the laboratory be capable of providing accurate quantitative analysis of the calculus by suitable methods. Only then can the urologist and his colleagues formulate a therapeutic plan that will be useful in preventing future stone disease in that patient.

Pathologic Changes

Local changes created by stone include histopathologic evidence of inflammation and anatomic evidence of distortion. Locally, desquamation of epithelium, ulceration of the tissue contiguous to the calculi, and fibrosis may be observed. When a large stone occupies a thickened pelvis, interstitial fibrosis and leukocytic and round-cell infiltration are evident microscopically. Additional changes are influenced by the extent of obstruction of the outflow of urine from the renal pelvis.

Generally, the obstruction produced by the calculus at the outlet of the kidney is incomplete, but it still promotes the formation of intrarenal hydronephrosis. As the calculus enlarges, it assumes the configuration of the renal pelvis, and the urine usually courses about it into the ureter. This adaptability, along with the fibrosis and hypertrophy of the walls of the pelvis, explains the relative infrequency of pelvic dilatation (Hinman, 1979). Hydronephrosis is evidenced by blunting of the calyces and later by various degrees of dilatation of the individual calyces. Atrophy and destruction of renal parenchyma follow, and, as this process progresses, the dilated calyces stretch almost to the renal capsule. Progressive loss of the renal parenchyma occurs.

Infection is sometimes superimposed, and various

lesions such as calculous pyelonephritis, calculous pyohydronephrosis, and perinephritis may develop. With the introduction of infection, additional stones may form. Renal function is rapidly impaired, and renal parenchyma is destroyed more rapidly.

Calculous Pyelonephritis

Calculous pyelonephritis may become the most prominent lesion. With severe infection the renal pelvis is thickened, and miliary abscesses may develop in the swollen vascularized cortex of the kidney. With further ravages of infection, the cortex becomes thin, the infundibula of the calyces become obstructed, and localized areas of pyonephrosis are discernible, as the calyces become dilated. The kidney becomes adherent to adjacent tissue surfaces. When infection is chronic, the kidney is small and pale because of the fibrous tissue reaction.

Microscopically, the wall of the renal pelvis is thickened, the mucous membrane is edematous, and the desquamation of the epithelium and ulceration may occur. The tubules are filled with inflammatory debris and blood cells. Many of the tubules may be destroyed, as the renal cortex is thinned out. Interstitial fibrosis, round-cell infiltration, and localized areas of polymorphonuclear leukocytes occur.

Calculous pyohydronephrosis may develop when infection is superimposed on a kidney that is the site of calculous hydronephrosis.

Nephrocalcinosis

Nephrocalcinosis is the term applied to small diffuse calcifications distributed throughout the renal parenchyma. These calcifications usually occur in the renal papillae (Fig. 58–24). They are the result of congenital abnormalities of the kidney or of metabolic diseases, such as hyperparathyroidism.

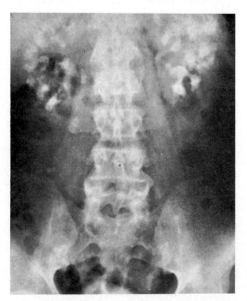

Figure 58–24. Nephrocalcinosis.

Replacement Lipomatosis (Xanthogranulomatous Pyelonephritis)

A kidney damaged by calculi may be the site of replacement lipomatosis. Roth and Davidson (1938) reviewed a series of 70 previously reported cases and added 37 new cases. They concluded that neither calculi nor inflammation was specific or necessary for the development of replacement lipomatosis. Of 33 cases reviewed by Kutzmann (1931), the coexistence of calculi and pyelonephritis was reported in 26. *Proteus mirabilis* is most often the causative agent (Goodman et al., 1979; Malek and Elder, 1978). Destruction of renal parenchyma appears to be a prerequisite for replacement lipomatosis. The fatty masses replace the destroyed tissue. CT scanning and ultrasonography have greatly improved the non-invasive diagnosis of this condition (Tolia et al., 1981; Subramanyam et al., 1982).

Squamous Cell Carcinoma

A striking relationship between urinary calculi and squamous cell carcinoma of the urinary system has been observed. Gilbert and McMillan (1934) presented a collective review of 55 cases of squamous cell carcinoma of the renal pelvis. In 1939, Higgins reviewed 59 cases and added five others, three of which were complicated by renal calculi. In a later collective review, Gahagan and Reed (1949) reported that calculi occurred in 48 of 106 cases of squamous cell carcinoma of the renal pelvis. This tumor is not limited to the upper tract—a large squamous cell carcinoma of the bladder can form adjacent to a large struvite calculus.

EVALUATION AND TREATMENT OF MEDICALLY ACTIVE TYPES OF URINARY LITHIASIS

Renal calculous disease that creates stones of pure calcium phosphate, magnesium ammonium phosphate, uric acid, and cystine accounts for about 30 per cent of all patients with urinary lithiasis. These stones result from conditions that are relatively simple to diagnose. Good therapeutic measures, such as special diets, fluids, drugs, manipulation, or surgery, are available. Similar but somewhat less effective therapy exists for the remaining 70 per cent of patients (those with calcium stones). In this section, we discuss aspects of treatment, except for procedural treatment and surgery. These last approaches are discussed under specific areas of the urinary tract in other sections of this textbook.

General Aspects of Diagnosis and Treatment

A single stone episode may be one of a series of recurrent stones in a given patient, or it may be the initial incident. Nevertheless, therapeutic steps are essentially the same (Fig. 58–25). The first step is to

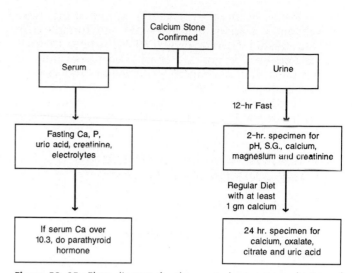

Figure 58–25. Flow diagram for the most elementary evaluation of patients with calcium stones, which can be done in the physician's office.

provide emergent, acute therapy, which is discussed earlier.

Categorization of stone-formation activity is made (Wilson, 1989). The main reason for this categorization is to decide whether immediate procedural intervention is necessary. The sizes of calculi that are likely to pass spontaneously have been discussed in the sections on incidence and on ureteral stones (see Fig. 58–14). Even very small calculi may become totally impacted in the ureter, causing pain, obstruction, and resultant kidney damage. Once the stone has passed or has been removed, one should consider a metabolic evaluation to discover and treat any prevalent causative factor. I prefer to evaluate patients after the first stone episode if they have a second stone seen on KUB, a family history of kidney stone disease, or other factors that increase risk of stone disease. Otherwise, I usually give general recommendations to increase fluid intake. I defer an evaluation until after a second stone episode.

Results of obstruction associated with urinary calculi have been discussed in the section on pathophysiology. If urinary infection is present, a more rapid deterioration of kidney function will occur. If a stone is associated with a urinary tract infection, the physician must decide whether the infection is the primary cause of the stone (as it is in most patients with struvite calculi) or if the infection is secondary to urinary manipulation or instrumentation for treatment of stone disease in the past (Holmgren et al., 1989). If infection is the primary cause, therapy is directed toward eradication of the infection and removal of the stone. Prevention of future calculi is dependent on the continued elimination of urinary infection and the maintenance of acidity of the urine. In the case in which infection is secondary, both infection and stone must usually be eliminated by surgery. However, the prophylactic plan must allow for control of both the infection and the primary urinary stone-forming process. The term "infection stones" refers only to those calculi that are caused primarily by the splitting of urea by bacteria in the urine, with subsequent elevation of urinary pH and formation of struvite crystals (Lerner et al., 1989). Stones that are not caused by infection are considered to be different from stones that are caused by infection and are not treated in the same way.

The evaluation and treatment of the patient who forms stones, based on stone analysis, are now reviewed.

STONES FORMING IN ACID URINE: CYSTINE AND URIC ACID

Uric Acid Lithiasis

Special Aspects of Epidemiology and Etiology

Early in development, humans suffered one significant genetic mutation as they branched off from the anthropoids. This mutation resulted in the disappearance of the enzyme uricase from human organs, especially the liver. As Gutman and Yu (1968) and Yu (1981) point out, this mutation left humans without the ability to convert the uric acid by-products of purine metabolism into the substance allantoin, which is freely water soluble when excreted by the kidneys.

Most animals filter uric acid through the glomerulus and rapidly reabsorb it through renal tubular cells. Uric acid recirculates through blood to the liver, where the enzyme uricase transforms it to allantoin. Allantoin then returns to the circulation and is excreted by the kidneys. Only the Dalmatian coach dog, of all mammals, has a risk of uric acid urinary lithiasis equal to that of humans, but it has a different enzymatic defect. The end result is that humans have levels of uric acid in their systems that are ten times greater than those of other mammals (Fanelli, 1977; Watts, 1976; Yu 1981).

Humans not only produce excessive, relatively water-insoluble uric acid but also excrete urine that is predominantly acid because of the acid end products of metabolism (Table 58–4). When uric acid enters human urine it exists in two forms: free uric acid and the urate salt, which forms a complex mostly with sodium. Sodium

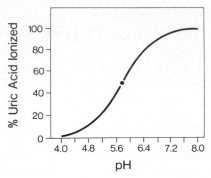

Figure 58–26. Dissociation of uric acid. At pK_a of 5.75, one half of uric acid is ionized as urate salts and is therefore soluble. As pH increases, more becomes ionized and soluble. (From Gutman, A. B., and Yu, T. F.: Am. J. Med., 45:756, 1968.)

urate is approximately 20 times more soluble in water than free uric acid. As Seegmiller (1973) notes: "The limited solubility of uric acid in acidic aqueous solution is obviously the most fundamental property responsible for its formation of renal calculi."

As noted in Figure 58–26, the pKa of uric acid is near 5.75. At that point, half of the uric ions exist as free uric acid and the other half are associated with other ions as the urate salt. Persistent excretion of urine below pH 5.75 contributes to increased concentration of the relatively insoluble uric acid. Peters and Van Slyke (1968) have calculated that urinary saturation with uric acid is achieved with 60 mg/L at pH 5.0 and 37°C, but urine at pH 6.0 can contain 220 mg/L (Fig. 58–27). The average male excretes approximately 400 mg of uric acid per day in a volume of slightly over a liter; therefore, urine is often supersaturated with uric acid. Fortunately, this uric acid is usually kept in solution through diurnal variations in urinary pH and through interaction with other molecules in the urine, probably mucoid molecules (Porter, 1966; Seegmiller, 1973; Sperling et al., 1965; Yu and Gutman, 1973) and urea.

Patients who persistently form uric acid stones often have prolonged periods of acidity in the urine. Normal individuals have variations in pH of urine that results, especially in daytime hours, in postprandial alkaline

Table 58–4. MAJOR URINARY ABNORMALITIES ASSOCIATED WITH SUPERSATURATION AND STONE

Type of Stone Former	pH*	Component
Cystine	Acid	Cystine excess
Uric acid	Acid	Relative uric acid excess
Calcium phosphate	Alkaline	Relative calcium excess
Calcium oxalate		
Idiopathic	†	Calcium and oxalate excess
Hyperoxaluric	†	Oxalate excess
Renal tubular acidosis	Alkaline	Perhaps calcium and phosphate excess
Magnesium ammonium phosphate (infected)	Very alkaline	Relative magnesium, ammonium, and phosphate excess

*Urinary pH that persists and promotes precipitation.
†Calcium oxalate precipitation occurs throughout pH range of normal urine.

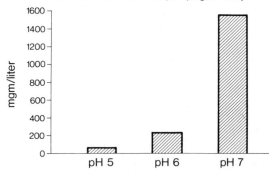

Amount of Uric Acid or Urate Suspended in Urine at Different pH (mgm/liter)

Figure 58–27. Amounts of uric acid or urate suspended by and soluble in 1 L of urine at three different pH levels. By comparison with Figure 58–26, note that the maximum solubility of uric acid is achieved near pH 7.

tides that take the pH well above 6.5. Urine in normal individuals also varies remarkably throughout the day in its content of acid or ammonium. Both represent acid excretion. Excretion of acid by the kidney may be summarized by the two equations explained in Figure 58–28.

At any given time, depending on the amount of acid presented to the kidney, the relative amounts of hydrogen ion or ammonium that are excreted may increase or decrease. In general, the processes of oxidation in the body result in the production of excess acidity, and therefore most urine excreted by the average human contains more free acid. For this reason, the mean urinary pH of the average individual is approximately one full pH unit lower than blood, or pH 6.4.

Marked changes in urine pH can also result from ingestion of acid or alkaline foods; environmental factors; and the presence of absence of diseases, such as respiratory illness, cardiac disease, and so forth. Diseases may result in a combination of reduced daily urinary volume and acid urine.

Patients with uric acid lithiasis have a tendency to maintain a urine pH of below 6.0, and often the pH is fixed at 5.0 (Cifuentes et al., 1973; Gutman and Yu, 1968; Rapaport et al., 1967; Thomas, 1975; Williams, 1974a; Yu and Gutman, 1973; Yu, 1981). Yu and Gutman postulate that the most likely explanation for persistent low urinary pH in these patients is a disturbance in the renal regulation of ammonium. Most such patients show a partial deficiency in renal production of ammonium. Less ammonium then becomes available for urine buffering.

In Figure 58–28, note that ammonium is produced from glutamine by enzymatic reactions in the renal tubular cell. It is excreted by diffusion through cell walls as NH_3. When it enters the renal tubular lumen, it quickly combines with a free ion of hydrogen, forming the nondiffusible NH_4 ion. The net result is buffering of urine to a more alkaline pH. Therefore, the acid load originally presented to the urine is converted to an alkaline load. In this way, the titratable acidity (free H ion) actually decreases, and the urine becomes less acid. If ammonium is not excreted, urine remains more acid.

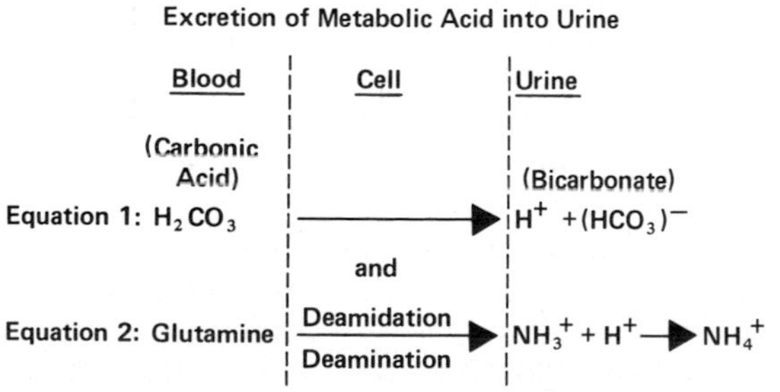

In summary, three factors must be involved in the creation of uric acid urolithiasis. First, there must be a relative hyperuricuria or chronic oversaturation of urine with uric acid. Second, such patients usually have a tendency toward excretion of excessively acid urine. Third, patients with uric acid urolithiasis often excrete a reduced volume of urine. Such patients may be chronically dehydrated by medication, by working in a hot environment, or by living in a hot climate (Atsmon et al., 1963; Toor et al., 1964, Sakhaee et al., 1987).

Awareness of these three factors immediately suggests three forms of therapy. First, an increase in daily fluid intake will increase urine output and dilute urinary uric acid. Second, an attempt should be made to alkalize the urine. Third, excessive uric acid excretion should be decreased.

Methods for performing this last alteration vary. As with many other elements in the urine, urinary uric acid arises from two sources, endogenous production within the tissues of the body and the exogenous diet. The relative contribution of these two sources to urinary uric acid varies in each individual. Zoller and Griebsch (1973) observed no difference in intestinal purine absorption in normal and hyperuricemic persons. Hyperuricemic persons, however, did demonstrate below-normal renal clearances of uric acid at any given level of plasma uric acid. These investigators also noted that, in spite of their observations on intestinal absorption, dietary limitation of purine intake (the precursor of most uric acid) did decrease serum and urinary uric acid levels. Similar results were obtained after administration of allopurinol.

Seegmiller (1973) reports that only one fourth of patients with hyperuricemic gout excrete excess uric acid when on a purine-free diet. Therefore, only one fourth of patients with this type of hyperuricemia can be producing excessive purine endogenously. In contrast, three fourths of these individuals probably acquire excess urinary uric acid from their diet. Controversy about this point exists, however. Cifuentes and colleagues (1973) do not believe that diet is important in control of uric acid lithiasis. May and Schindler (1973) and Breslau and associates (1988), reporting multiple observations in their patients, indicated that dietary control is important. Both diet and endogenous production are important in the control of uric acid lithiasis.

Classification of Uric Acid Lithiasis

By definition, if patients form uric acid calculi, the urine must be supersaturated with uric acid. They therefore have hyperuricuria. Because of the great variation in solubility of uric acid with variation in urinary pH, it is not possible to establish a precise definition of exactly how much uric acid per day can be considered excessive, without taking into consideration total urinary volume and urinary pH (see Figs. 58–26 and 58–27).

The upper limit of normal concentration for serum uric acid is reported by most laboratories to be between

Figure 58–28. Simplified presentation of excretion of metabolic acid end-products by urine. Free acid *(equation 1)* arrives at the kidney via blood as carbonic acid, traverses the renal cell, and enters the urine in ionized form. In urine, free acid is measured as pH by meters or paper strips. Some acid is bound in the form of glutamine *(equation 2)*, which is enzymatically cleaved within the renal cell to produce ammonia (NH_3^+), which diffuses rapidly into the urine. Here, the ammonia quickly combines with another H^+ to become ammonium (NH_4^+). Ammonium remains in the urine. Amounts contributed to acid excretion by ammonium are measured by determining the titratable acidity of urine. If little H^+ is excreted as ammonium (an alkaline ion), the urine maintains an acid pH.

6.5 and 7.0 mg/dl for men and about 5.5 mg/dl for women (Gutman and Yu, 1968). Based on serum levels, most workers tend to classify patients with uric acid lithiasis into two broad groups, those with hyperuricemia and those with normal serum uric acid concentration. Gutman and Yu (1968) and Seftel and Resnick (1990) further subdivide uric acid nephrolithiasis into four major categories.

Their first category is termed idiopathic uric acid lithiasis. The patients do not have hyperuricemia, and the amount of urinary excretion of uric acid per day is within normal rates. The major physiologic abnormality is a consistently low urine pH. Patients with chronic diarrheal states, those with ileostomies, and those who take medications to acidify urine may be included in this category (Williams, 1974a).

The second category includes uric acid nephrolithiasis associated with hyperuricemia, such as the Lesch-Nyhan syndrome. This disease is of interest because the patients have a definable deficiency in an enzyme, hypoxanthine-guanine phosphoribosyltransferase. DeVries and Sperling (1973) have also reported a mutation of a similar enzyme system in a family with a tendency toward gout. Therefore, there is an increasing belief that hyperuricemia associated with uric acid urolithiasis, such as gout, represents an inborn error of metabolism. In an additional group of patients in this category, there is myeloproliferative or other neoplastic disease with increased endogenous production of uric acid.

A third category consists of patients who develop uric acid lithiasis because of excessive loss of water to the environment. This may be due to excessive perspiration or to gastrointestinal losses such as that associated with ileitis, colitis, and similar conditions.

The fourth category includes patients who develop uric acid lithiasis because of ingestion of uricosuric drugs (salicylates, thiazides, and others) or overindulgence in foods high in purine and proteins (organ meats, sardines).

Of the foregoing categories, only one involves hyperuricemia. The other three involve only excessive urinary excretion of uric acid (hyperuricosuria) enhanced by consistent low volume and pH.

Evaluation of Patients

Evaluation of patients with uric acid lithiasis requires observation of daily urinary pH, conducted by measuring and recording the pH of every voiding with Nitrazine or other pH paper, determining the serum and urinary uric acid levels, assessing the degree of ingestion of dietary purines, and analyzing the work and play conditions for dehydration. If the patient has evidence of hyperuricemia, evaluation should include a brief survey to rule out myeloproliferative or neoplastic disease (Seftel and Resnick, 1990).

Special diagnostic aspects of uric acid lithiasis include recognition that this is the only solid urinary calculus that is radiolucent. In addition, uric acid lithiasis may be associated with urinary obstruction through showers of small crystals rather than a single large stone. For this reason, microscopic examination of the urine can be helpful both in diagnosing uric acid urolithiasis and in determining therapy success. Patients under medical control should not have evidence of uric acid crystals in the urine at any time.

Therapy

Most investigators agree on the regimen that should be used to treat such patients, with the possible exception of diet. Initial and immediate therapy involves instructing and testing of the patient to guarantee that he or she takes in enough fluids to ensure urinary output in excess of 1500 or even 2000 ml per day. In hot climates, this may require intake of enormous quantities of fluid. Higher urinary output also results in some increase in urinary pH because of the diuretic effects of water. Because the endogenous uric acid production continues at a basal rate in all individuals, it is best to advise the patient to consume a diet that limits protein intake to less than 90 g daily (see Appendix A). This amount is enough to maintain body protein balance.

If patients have the renal defect that produces consistently acid urine, they should be given medications to alkalize the urine to a level between pH 6.5 and 7.0. It is not necessary to alkalize the urine above pH 7.0. In fact, excessive alkalization may be detrimental. Patients may begin to form stones that precipitate in alkaline solution, such as apatite. Patients should be instructed to test the urine with Nitrazine or other suitable pH paper in order to maintain pH in the proper range. Uric acid calculi can be dissolved by nonsurgical therapy if the urine pH and uric acid are kept within the undersaturated range and if the patient has no other problem that makes surgery necessary (Sakhaee et al., 1983).

Medications for alkalization therapy include sodium bicarbonate, 650 mg or more every 6 to 8 hours, or comparable amounts of liquid preparations of balanced citrate in dosages of about 15 ml three times or four times daily (Drach, 1976a; Thomas, 1975). Sakhaee and co-workers (1983) recommend that potassium citrate solutions be given, because they may prevent formation of calcium stones in patients who form uric acid stones and are receiving alkali therapy. Freed (1975) suggested alkalization of urine with a regimen that combines sodium bicarbonate, 1 g three times a day, with administration of acetazolamide, 250 mg once a day. Hypertension and cardiovascular and renal problems due to sodium or potassium overload are thereby avoided.

Patients rarely cooperate with long-term administration of alkali; therefore, careful monitoring is essential. Long-term alkalization may not be necessary for control of most patients with uric acid stones. Dietary protein limitation and increased urinary output may suffice. Urinary alkalization seems advisable during periods when attempts at stone dissolution are under way.

If the patient has hyperuricemia, it is advisable that he or she be given allopurinol, 300 to 600 mg per day. This medication may be given as a single dose (tablet) or in divided doses. Allopurinol was originally developed for the treatment of gout and of hyperuricemia associated with malignant disease (Rundles et al., 1966). Occasional side effects may occur, including rash and activation of acute arthritis associated with primary gout. According to Gutman and Yu (1968), this activation of arthritis often occurs in spite of colchicine prophylaxis in doses of up to 1 mg per day or more. Other patients develop diarrhea or abdominal cramps. The incidence of these side effects ranges from 5 to 6 per cent (Gutman and Yu, 1968; Rundles et al., 1966; Thomas, 1975). To review, therapy of uric acid lithiasis requires increasing urinary volume, limiting dietary purines and protein, possibly alkalizing urine, and perhaps administering allopurinol.

Cystine Urinary Lithiasis

Special Aspects of Etiology

Cystinuria is an inherited defect in renal tubular reabsorption of four amino acids: cystine, ornithine, lysine, and arginine (see Table 58–4). Smith (1974b) has suggested use of the mnemonic COLA, as mentioned, to help remember these four amino acids. Cystinuria is inherited as an autosomal recessive trait. However, some individuals who are heterozygous for the disease do show evidence of excretion of excessive cystine and the other three dibasic amino acids in the urine. Some workers further divide this heterozygous form of cystinuria into separate forms. When it is completely recessive (type I), there is no amino aciduria. Incompletely recessive forms (types II and III) show increased urinary excretion of cystine in the range of 150 to 300 mg in 24 hours. These patients usually do not form calculi. Of the three alleles (I, II, and III), pure homozygotes and compound heterozygotes (e.g., I/III) usually form stones (Giugliani et al., 1985).

The amino acid transport defects exist both in the renal tubular cells and in the intestinal mucosa. Although patients with this disease sometimes have small stature, presumably due to excessive urinary loss of lysine, the only clinical symptom of importance is the occurrence of urinary calculi. The incidence of clinically evident cystinuria is believed to be approximately one per 20,000 (Smith, 1974b).

Methionine is probably the dietary precursor of cystine (Crawhall and Watts, 1968). Normal individuals in general excrete less than 100 mg of cystine in the urine per day. Because approximately 300 to 400 mg of cystine per L of urine is soluble within the pH range of 4.5 to 7.0 (Fig. 58–29), a normal individual rarely if ever exceeds the saturation concentration for cystine. In contrast, patients with homozygous cystinuria usually excrete amounts of cystine in excess of 600 mg per day. The upper limit of solubility of cystine per gram of creatinine appears to be 180 mg. Cystine, like uric acid, is much less soluble in acidic than in alkaline urine. It differs from uric acid in that its improved solubility becomes apparent only at pH levels above 7.2. Elevation of the pH to 7.8 almost doubles the solubility of cystine (see Fig. 58–29) (Dent and Senior, 1955).

Evaluation

Urinary stones of cystine should be suspected in the initial evaluation of individuals with family histories of

Amount of Cystine Suspended in Urine at Different pH (mgm/liter)

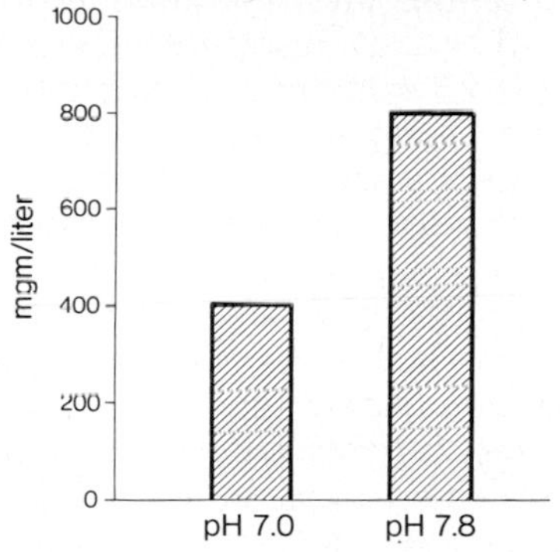

Figure 58–29. Elevation of urinary pH also improves the solubility of cystine. In contrast to uric acid (see Fig. 58–27), urine pH increasing from 7.0 to over 7.8 doubles the solubility of cystine. Therapy is therefore directed at attempting to keep the urinary pH near 8.

stone disease; in recurrent disease in those under 30 years of age (Pavanello et al., 1981); and in individuals who have radiographic evidence of slightly dense, laminated, ground-glass calculi (see Figs. 58–16 and 58–19). Cystine stones should always be considered whenever the characteristic hexagonal crystals are seen in urine. One screening test for cystinuria utilizing cyanide nitroprusside can detect concentrations of cystine in excess of approximately 75 mg/g creatinine (Smith, 1974b). False-positive reactions due to medications and positive test findings in non–stone-forming heterozygous cystinuric cases may produce confusing results. A confirmatory quantitative determination of total urinary cystine must be performed by chromatographic methods if the screening test result is positive. Knowledge of the total urinary cystine concentration also determines the amount of therapy necessary to prevent stone formation.

Therapy

One of the most helpful ways to devise therapy for cystinuria is to measure the total daily cystine excretion in urine. Most cystinuric patients who excrete 300 to 800 mg per day can be controlled by urinary dilution and alkalization similar to that given for uric acid lithiasis. Cystine solubility in urine increases two to three times at pH above 7.8 (see Fig. 58–29). Every attempt should be made to keep urinary pH above this level. Sodium bicarbonate, 12.6 g or more per 24 hours, in equally divided doses or 60 to 80 ml of balanced citrate solution per day in divided doses should provide adequate alkalization.

Fluid intake should continue around the clock and should ensure urinary output of 3 to 4 liters per day. Patients should drink two large glasses of water every 2 hours while awake and during sleep should awaken to drink once to force this amount of urine. If an increased urinary output doesn't awaken the patient to urinate, an alarm clock is set for this purpose.

Restriction of methionine is theoretically sound but results in a very unpalatable diet that most patients cannot tolerate. The resulting reduction in cystine excretion is small. Patients should not, however, overload the diet with methionine-containing proteins. Dietary methionine restriction, after consultation with a dietician, may be used as a last resort in patients who cannot obtain control by other methods of treatment.

It is seldom necessary to add D-penicillamine to the preventive treatment plan for these patients. However, D-penicillamine therapy may speed the attempts to dissolve cystine calculi. Up to 1.5 g per day of D-penicillamine in divided doses usually reduces pure urinary cystine excretion to below 400 mg per day. After administration of D-penicillamine, most urinary cystine combines with the D-penicillamine to form cystine-S-penicillamine, which is soluble in urine. Effectiveness of D-penicillamine can be assessed by testing a 24-hour urine specimen for free cystine with nitroprusside and for penicillamine disulfide with 3 per cent FeCl (Lotz et al., 1965). Unfortunately, many patients develop allergic or idiosyncratic reactions to penicillamine, including arthralgia, rash, nephrotic syndrome, or other manifestations. These complications plus high cost limit the use of D-penicillamine.

Several investigators have reported the utilization of alpha-mercaptopropionylglycine (MPG) to treat patients with cystinuria and stones (Johansson et al., 1980; Koide et al., 1982; Pak, 1987). Urinary cystine solubility and excretion are enhanced by formation of thiol disulfide compounds in a manner similar to that of D-penicillamine. In one report on the treatment of 35 patients (Koide et al., 1982), the dosages ranged from 600 to 1800 mg per day for stone dissolution and 300 to 1500 mg per day for prophylaxis. Complete or significant dissolution occurred in seven of 21 patients treated for this purpose. Side effects occurred in 16 patients, but most were able to adapt to the drug, when reintroduced to it gradually. This compound may be better tolerated than D-penicillamine. In summary, therapy for cystine stones includes greatly increased urinary volume, vigorous alkalization of urine, occasionally D-penicillamine or MPG, and rarely dietary restriction of methionine.

Stones of Urinary Infection

Special Aspects of Etiology

Calculi composed of magnesium ammonium calcium phosphate or struvite stones and those few due to carbonate-apatite are the subject of this portion of our discussion. Uric acid and cystine calculi are produced by simple physicochemical processes that occur with acidic urinary pH and associated hyperexcretion. The urine is therefore supersaturated with one or the other insoluble molecule. Magnesium ammonium phosphate stones are caused by a similar but opposite situation, owing to alkaline urinary pH. Clark and Nordin (1969) indicate in their introduction to a renal stone research symposium that "this type of stone (struvite) is also probably due to simple precipitation from supersaturated solution." Barnhouse (1968); Griffith and Musher (1973); and Lerner, Gleeson, and Griffith (1989) have greatly increased our knowledge about the physical chemistry in the production of struvite calculi. Our understanding of this disease has been a progressive deepening of an awareness that stones of infection are always associated with urea-splitting bacteria and subsequent elevation of urinary pH due to increased bacterial ammonium production (Fig. 58–30). In addition, these bacteria may participate actively in forming the structure of the stone by providing an initial "glycocalyx" (McLean et al., 1985).

Griffith (1979) and Lerner and co-workers (1989) reviewed and confirmed observations of previous investigators that the basic abnormality in the formation of struvite calculi is maintenance of a urinary pH of greater than 7.2 (Barnhouse, 1968; Elliot et al., 1959; Nemoy and Stamey, 1971; Priestley and Osterberg, 1936). The situation, as noted earlier, is opposite to that characteristic of uric acid and cystine calculi (see Table 58–4). In the case of magnesium ammonium phosphate (Mg-NH$_4$PO$_4$ • 6H$_2$O), urine is undersaturated at the normal mean physiologic pH of approximately 5.85 (Elliot et al., 1959). The presence of bacteria in the urine of the type that can split urea provides the conditions necessary for precipitation of magnesium ammonium phosphate (see Fig. 58–30) (Hugosson et al., 1990). Many of these calculi have small quantities of calcium phosphate mixed in the lattice (Hodgkinson and Marshall, 1975).

Struvite calculi account for the majority of staghorn calculi observed in urologic practice in most countries. These calculi can grow to immense size and indeed achieve the appearance of a true staghorn, as shown in Figures 58–23C and 58–31. Nemoy and Stamey (1971), Thompson and Stamey (1973), Jennis and co-workers (1970), and McLean and co-workers (1985) have reviewed previous studies and confirmed the fact that struvite and other urinary calculi not only are caused by action of bacteria on urine but also contain numerous infective bacteria within their structures. These investigators have also shown that the penetration of antibiotics into these stones is inadequate for cure; therefore, the presence of an infected urinary calculus acts as a source for continued urinary infection. As long as infected

**MAGNESIUM AMMONIUM PHOSPHATE (STRUVITE)
CALCULI: MECHANISMS OF FORMATION AND DISSOLUTION**

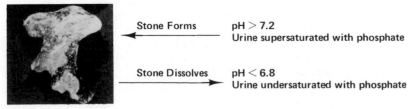

Stone Forms ⟵   pH > 7.2
Urine supersaturated with phosphate

Stone Dissolves ⟶   pH < 6.8
Urine undersaturated with phosphate

Figure 58–30. Factors in formation of magnesium ammonium phosphate (struvite) calculi related to persistent alkaline urine.

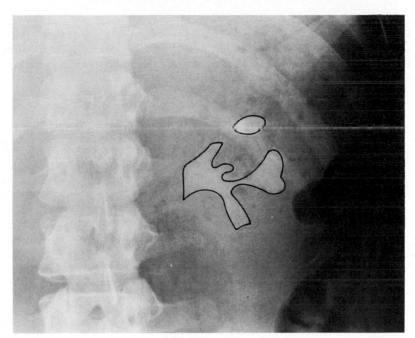

Figure 58–31. Struvite calculi *(outline)* may be relatively radiolucent and may be confused with cystine calculi. This calculus proved to be composed of pure struvite.

urinary stones exist anywhere in the urinary tract, it is unlikely that the urinary system can be sterilized by antibiotics or other methods.

Recurrence of struvite urinary calculi following surgical removal is usually due to retention of small fragments of stone within the kidney or to failure to eradicate urinary infection completely. Boyce and Elkins (1974) reviewed 100 consecutive surgical procedures to remove staghorn calculi. They report stone recurrence in 17.7 per cent of their patients. These investigators strongly emphasize that complete removal of every visible fragment of calculus is necessary during any procedure. Thereafter, patients must be observed carefully to keep the urinary tract totally free of infection forever. Hence, maintenance of a sterile urine is a very large part of any postsurgical plan for prevention of recurrence of infected staghorn urinary calculi (Drach, 1974b).

Two other urologic conditions appear to contribute to infection and to the tendency to form magnesium ammonium phosphate calculi. The first is the presence of a foreign body in the urinary tract (see Fig. 58–23D), and the second is neurogenic bladder associated with trauma, stroke, and similar conditions. Such patients often carry residual urine and frequently require urinary catheter drainage; subsequently, they acquire urinary infection. Infection plus catheter creates a situation that often results in magnesium ammonium phosphate calculi.

As an example of the interaction of infection and foreign body, Griffith and Musher (1973) in their series of struvite stone experiments used the foreign body method of Vermeulen and colleagues (1964, 1968) to create magnesium ammonium phosphate calculi on zinc discs placed in the bladders of rats that were infected with *Proteus* species. Hence, one cannot separate the effects of infection from those of foreign body. Dalton

and colleagues (1975) reviewed the literature regarding formation of struvite calculi on foreign body nuclei. Formation of foreign body calculi not associated with infection could be prevented by massive diuresis, which for humans would require approximately 15 liters of output per day. However, when infection is present even massive diuresis is of no help. These investigators listed over 30 separate agents that have acted as foreign body nuclei for urinary calculi. Among the most common are sutures (see Fig. 57–23D), and their investigation was concerned particularly with suture material. Nearly all types of suture material currently in use, including chromic catgut, have been demonstrated to support stone formation. Thus, the "prevention of suture exposure to the urinary stream seems prudent."

In patients with neurogenic bladder, recumbency and abnormalities of calcium and magnesium balance in urine supposedly contribute to stone disease. But investigations indicate that stone formation in such patients is not likely to be caused by excessive excretion of calcium, secondary hyperparathyroidism, or other metabolic effects (Burr, 1972; Burr and Walsh, 1974; Claus-Walker et al., 1973; Jennis et al., 1970). The most likely cause is urinary infection. This leads to persistent alkaline urine pH that results in urine supersaturation with magnesium ammonium phosphate (Holmgren et al., 1989). The formation product for struvite may be exceeded. Spontaneous nuclei of stones can thereby form.

If a catheter is also present, it represents the nucleus, and only the solubility product need be exceeded for struvite stone growth to occur. As shown in the simple chemical equation in Figure 58–30, an environment of constant elevation of urinary pH of over 7.2 is thereby achieved, at the concentrations of magnesium, ammonium, and phosphate in the urine of infected individuals at a body temperature of 37°C. No more is needed for growth of struvite crystals.

URINARY LITHIASIS: ETIOLOGY, DIAGNOSIS, AND MEDICAL MANAGEMENT

Classification of Infected Urinary Calculi

Infection as the cause of magnesium ammonium phosphate urinary calculi must be differentiated from infection as the result of treatment of previous calculi of different compositions (Hugosson et al., 1990). Cox (1974) has made this differentiation in his analysis of a series of patients who had urinary tract infection associated with renal lithiasis (Table 58–5). The table clearly distinguishes those patients with infections that caused stones from those with stones who acquire infections. A decision about whether infection occurred following treatment of a particular type of urinary calculus other than struvite is important in planning the therapy of the patient.

Westbury (1974) has pointed out that individuals who have had urinary calculi of a particular type are highly likely to have similar calculi caused by the same pathologic deficits. After infection, the composition of future calculi is not as clearly predictable. Therefore, admixtures of larger amounts of calcium phosphate and magnesium ammonium phosphate (struvite) become more common in the analyses of subsequent stones in infected patients (Hodgkinson and Marshall, 1975; Westbury, 1974).

Evaluation of Patients

Individuals with chronic urinary infections should always be considered to have a higher risk of formation of urinary calculi than individuals without such infections. For this reason, occasional radiographic evaluation of the urinary tract is advisable in patients with chronic infections. The majority of patients with clinical stone disease due to infection present with a clinical syndrome that is a combination of pain related to urinary obstruction from calculus and pain and fever related to acute urinary tract infection. The patients often have or have had indwelling urinary catheters. Foreign bodies must be suspected if there has been penetrating injury or abdominal surgery. Urinary infections must be documented by culture and identification of causative organisms. For proper treatment, drug sensitivities of these organisms should be determined by accepted techniques.

Therapy

In all patients with infected stones, the basis of therapy is either eradication or complete suppression of urinary tract infection. The majority of urea-splitting organisms are of the *Proteus* and *Providentia* species. However, organisms such as *Pseudomonas, Klebsiella, Staphylococcus* (especially *S. epidermidis*), and even *Mycoplasma* are capable of producing bacterial urease (Friedlander and Braude, 1974; Griffith et al., 1976b). *Escherichia coli* apparently does not produce urease (Griffith, 1979, Lerner et al., 1989).

Therapy should be directed toward long-term antibiotics, specific for the infecting organism. Treatment of chronically infected patients continues for months or years, not weeks. Stimulation of copious urinary output by ingestion of large amounts of fluids decreases urinary concentrations of magnesium, ammonium, and phosphate. The supersaturation of urine with these ions is also relieved. Restriction of dietary phosphate and a decrease in intestinal absorption of phosphate by administration of aluminum hydroxide gels (which bind intestinal phosphate) may be necessary to decrease urinary phosphate supersaturation (Appendix C) (Marshall and Green, 1952). Certainly, patients who have urinary infections and who are prone to struvite stone formation should not be given medications that contain magnesium or phosphate.

Whenever possible, foreign bodies should be removed. Newer techniques of management of neurogenic bladder by bladder training, intermittent catheterization, urinary diversion, or prosthetic valves (see Chapters 13 and 14) allow many patients who would have

Table 58–5. BACTERIOLOGIC DATA ON PATIENTS WITH RENAL LITHIASIS,
NORTH CAROLINA BAPTIST HOSPITAL, 1968–1970*

	Group 1†	Group 2	Group 3	Group 4
Number of patients in group	200	70	100	35
Per cent of patients infected	37	8	35	83
Infecting bacteria (no. of patients)				
E. coli	40 (54%)	4	13 (37%)	4 (13%)
Klebsiella	5	0	1	0
Enterobacteriaceae	3	0	2	2
P. mirabilis	7	0	10	10
Indole-positive Proteus‡	3	0	3	3
Pseudomonas	5	0	3	7
Staphylococcus	2	1	1	1
Enterococcus	4	1	1	1
Other or mixed	5	0	1	2

*From Cox, C. E.: Urol. Clin. North Am., 1:279, 1974.
†Patient groups:
   Group 1. Two hundred urologic patients without urolithiasis.
   Group 2. Seventy urologic patients with urolithiasis without prior instrumentation.
   Group 3. One hundred patients with urolithiasis with prior instrumentation.
   Group 4. Thirty-five patients with staghorn calculi. All but three had had previous instrumentation.
‡*Morganella morganii, Providencia rettgeri,* and *P. vulgaris.*

required catheters to be free of them. If catheters must be used, I have found that twice-daily irrigations with only 20 to 50 ml of solutions of 0.25 or 0.5 per cent acetic acid greatly reduce struvite encrustation and calculi. Teflon coating of latex catheters or pure silicone catheters or tubes also slows struvite encrustation. No material that is compatible with the body will "never" allow stone encrustation.

As noted by Nemoy and Stamey (1971), one cannot expect to clear the urinary tract as long as infected stones are present. For this reason, many patients with infected urinary calculi require surgical or procedural removal of such calculi. Aspects of these approaches to the treatment of stone disease are reviewed elsewhere in this text.

One aspect of medical treatment that has again achieved great importance is the dissolution of calculi by irrigation techniques. Acidic solutions proposed by Suby and associates (1942) and Suby and Albright (1943) have been used for many years. Mulvaney (1960) and later Mulvaney and Henning (1962) reported on hemiacidrin for dissolution of urinary calculi of struvite.

Nemoy and Stamey (1971), Blaivas and co-workers (1975), Jacobs and Gittes (1976) and Dretler and Pfister (1984a) reviewed the development of hemiacidrin irrigation and the problems associated with it. For many years, reports in the literature indicated that this agent was extremely toxic and may have caused death. However, these investigators state that in reviewing the literature, they believed that the majority of patients who had toxicity with this irrigation technique were actually afflicted with severe urinary infection and sepsis. All groups therefore now strongly recommend that the irrigation-dissolution technique be used only in a patient in whom the urinary tract infection is completely under control. Hypermagnesemia must also be avoided (Cato and Tulloch, 1974).

Albright and co-workers (1948) observed that citric acid solutions would disintegrate predominantly calcium (apatite) stones not only because of the acid pH of the solutions but also because of the formation of a calcium and citrate ion complex. Subsequent to the introduction of the "buffered" citrate solution by Albright, solutions G and M were developed by Suby.

Solution G contains citric acid monohydrate, 32.5 g; anhydrous magnesium oxide, 3.84 mg; anhydrous sodium carbonate, 4.37 g; and distilled water, 1000 ml. The pH of this solution is 3.95. Solution M is less acid (pH 4.6) than solution G and is made by adding 32.5 g of citric acid monohydrate, 3.84 g of anhydrous magnesium oxide, and 8.84 g of anhydrous sodium carbonate to 1000 ml of distilled water. These solutions have not always been effective in dissolving phosphate calculi. Mulvaney (1960), as noted, reported his experience with a new solvent designed especially for struvite and apatite calculi. This solution was called hemiacidrin (Renacidin). He stated that calcium phosphate, magnesium ammonium phosphate, and magnesium phosphate stones were soluble. The solvent appeared to have little effect on calcium oxalate and uric acid calculi.

The technique for management of irrigation in suitable patients is thoroughly outlined in the article by Nemoy and Stamey (1971) and in Stamey's text (1972). The package insert for hemiacidrin (10-per cent Renacidin) contains this warning: "It is contraindicated for therapy or preventive therapy above the ureteral-vesical junction; therefore, it is contraindicated for ureteral catheters or pyelostomy tubes or renal lavage for dissolving calculi." For these reasons, the composition of Suby's G and M solutions has also been given. Those individuals who do not wish to use Renacidin in the kidney may prefer to irrigate with one of Suby's solutions.

Whichever solution is chosen, the technique remains essentially the same as that described by Nemoy and Stamey. These workers state first that it is absolutely necessary that no irrigation be attempted until the urine is completely sterile. If surgery has been performed, a nephrostomy tube is left in place postoperatively. However, if the patient is in poor clinical condition and surgery is contraindicated, a percutaneous nephrostomy catheter may be inserted.

With either method, the renal pelvis is first irrigated with a sterile saline solution at a rate of 120 ml/hour for 24 to 48 hours, beginning on the 4th or 5th postoperative day. The height of irrigation is adjusted to the lowest level necessary to maintain the flow rate at 120 ml/hour. If there is leakage around a surgical drain or through the incision, irrigation is stopped until additional healing occurs. The patient is observed carefully for development of fever or any flank discomfort and for elevation of serum creatinine, magnesium, or phosphate levels (Dretler and Pfister, 1984a; Dretler et al., 1984b). Occurrence of any of these conditions requires immediate cessation of irrigation.

If after 48 hours the patient's condition remains satisfactory and if there is no infection, no leakage, and no fever or flank discomfort, irrigation with an appropriate solution is begun. Flow rate is continued at 120 ml/hour through the irrigation tube or catheter.

Nemoy and Stamey (1971) and Jacobs and Gittes (1976) and Palmer (1987) instruct their patients to stop the irrigation themselves if there is evidence of flank pain at any time.

The progress of irrigation is followed by obtaining radiographic tomographs of the calculi at intervals. Irrigation is continued for 24 to 48 hours after the last radiographically visible fragments have disappeared. In some instances, the rate of irrigation may be reduced to prevent irritation of the kidney or bladder, or sterile saline solutions may be alternated with irrigating solutions. Palmer and colleagues (1987) applied these concepts of treatment to outpatients.

These workers emphasize that the presence of infected urine, fever, or persistent flank pain is an absolute contraindication to continued irrigation. Treatment of urinary tract infection, maintenance of high fluid intake and output, and possible irrigation of calculi to dissolve them provide only partial answers to the questions about the medical treatment of infection stones. Some oral dissolution approaches have been reported but are still in the experimental phase.

Griffith and colleagues (1973, 1975, 1976a, 1979) have reported on the use of acetohydroxamic acid to inhibit the action of bacterial urease. This drug treatment results in decreased urinary pH, and about 60 per cent of patients show subsequent inhibition of the formation of struvite calculi and occasional dissolution of calculi that may be present. According to these workers, this medication is well tolerated. However, Rodman, Williams, and Jones (1987) have advised observation of such patients for thrombosis, tremors, other neurologic symptoms, and headaches. The usual dosage is 750 mg per day in divided doses. Andersen (1975) has reported on a similar urease inhibitor, benurestat.

The presence of obstruction by calculus in association with urinary infection requires immediate procedural relief of obstruction. Whether this relief is accomplished by insertion of ureteral catheter or stent, nephrostomy, or open surgery depends on the urologist's assessment of the patient's condition. Excretion of antibiotics by the obstructed kidney is severely limited, and therefore one cannot expect antibiotics to be effective in controlling the renal damage and sepsis associated with urinary infection complicated by obstruction due to stone.

Calcium Urinary Lithiasis

Special Aspects of Etiology

Table 58–3 indicates that calcium urinary calculi are the most common calculi worldwide. As noted, the incidence of bladder calculi decreased following improvement in nutrition and industrial advancement of many of the primitive societies of the world. The result has been a continuously increasing incidence of upper urinary tract calculi composed predominantly of calcium oxalate or of calcium oxalate and calcium phosphate. Hodgkinson and co-workers (1975) commented also on the relative decrease over the past centuries in the amount of phosphate found in mixed calculi. The proportion of the calcium oxalate in calculi is indeed increasing continuously and is most probably related to decreasing numbers of infection stones.

The three stones (uric acid, cystine, and struvite) discussed previously all form in accordance with simple chemical laws of pH-controlled precipitation in urine. In some cases, the presence of certain urine components increases the solubility of these substances above their solubility product. Nevertheless, if the concentration of their molecules rises above the respective formation product at a given pH and temperature of 37°C, precipitation of crystals occurs. When a large number of these molecules precipitate to form crystals, an object large enough to obstruct urinary passages, i.e., a stone, results, through aggregation or other processes mentioned previously.

For calcium oxalate and calcium phosphate calculi, it is the product of the two ions that predicts the propensity to crystallize. Marshall and Robertson (1976) have produced a nomogram that predicts crystallization when only the calcium and oxalate concentrations of urine are known. Hence, if the formation product for calcium phosphate is 35, the ratio of calcium to phosphate of either 1 to 35 or 35 to 1 may allow crystallization. In reality, such broad ratios allow inefficient crystallization and rarely occur in humans. Crystallization occurs with

ratios in the mid-range, such as 7 to 5 (Oreopoulos et al., 1975), which are found in human urine.

In an attempt to sort out the interrelationship of various theories and to place them in perspective with regard to diseases that are associated with calcium calculi (see Table 58–4), those observations associated only with idiopathic hypercalciuria are reviewed first. This includes a discussion of three types of absorptive hypercalciuria and renal leak hypercalciuria.

Second, a discussion is presented of those diseases that result in both hypercalcemia and hypercalciuria, such as hyperparathyroidism and others that may be confused with hyperparathyroidism.

Subsequently, we discuss those states associated with excessive excretion of urinary oxalate or hyperoxaluria. Two forms are illustrated. First, primary hyperoxaluria, the congenital disease in which individuals excrete enormous amounts of oxalate in the urine because of enzymatic defects in the kidneys and other body tissues. Second, acquired hyperoxaluria, the dietary or gastroenteric hyperoxaluria sometimes noted in patients who form recurrent oxalate urinary calculi.

Pure apatite urinary calculi (calcium phosphate) are discussed in the context of hypercalciuria. Once the etiologies of the various types of calcium urinary lithiasis are reviewed, patients are evaluated and classified in order to design appropriate therapy.

Calcium and the Kidney

Normal serum calcium concentration in humans averages 9.6 mg/dl. Of this, approximately 45 per cent is free ionic calcium, and 55 per cent is protein-bound, mostly to albumin. It is for this reason that measurement of total serum calcium concentration requires a knowledge of serum protein concentration. Direct measurement of serum ionized calcium is now more simple to perform, but it does not greatly improve the prediction of the amount of ionized calcium over that derived from the original nomogram of total serum calcium and serum protein (Fig. 58–32).

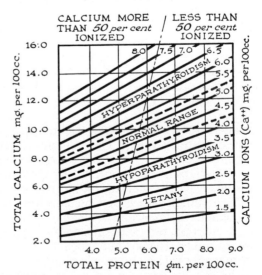

Figure 58–32. Chart for calculation of Ca^{++} ion concentration from total protein and total calcium of serum or plasma. (From McLean, F. C., and Hastings, A. B.: Am. J. Med. Sci., 189:602, 1935.)

Only free ionic serum calcium is filtered by the glomerulus. If effective renal blood flow is estimated at 600 ml/minute, about 47 g of calcium are filtered daily or about 32.4 mg/minute. Because normal individuals rarely excrete more than 200 mg/day, it is obvious that normal renal reabsorption of 98 or 99 per cent of calcium is excellent (Coe and Parks, 1988). In addition to conserving body calcium, this process also serves to produce a urine that is usually undersaturated with calcium. There is, however, a tubular maximum for reabsorption of calcium. When this is exceeded by an increased serum calcium load presented to the kidney, as in intestinal hyperabsorption or hyperparathyroidism, excessive renal calcium loss results (Copp, 1969; Kleeman et al., 1958). Hypercalciuria results (Henneman et al., 1958; Pak et al., 1974; Preminger et al., 1985).

Hypercalciuria and Calcium Urinary Lithiasis

Investigations of urinary lithiasis determined that substantial numbers of patients with idiopathic calcium stone disease excreted excessive amounts of calcium into the urine during any 24-hour period—they have hypercalciuria. Flocks (1939) described this first. For many years, most observations of hypercalciuria were based on the analyses of 24-hour urine collections. Perhaps the most difficult factor to reconcile with these daily observations is that the critical factor necessary for precipitation of calcium phosphate or calcium oxalate in urine is the instantaneous concentrations of the two elements in urine, not the 24-hour concentration (Marshall and Robertson, 1976).

The patient may exceed the formation product for these ions in urine in an interval of only 15 to 30 minutes. Nevertheless, rapid crystallization can occur, and, if it is associated with aggregation, trapping in the urinary system, or growth on previously formed nuclei, stone formation begins. Growth can continue even when supersaturation decreases to a relatively low level (at least greater than the solubility product). Hence, many classic studies that report hypercalciuria of 24-hour urinary specimens are now questioned. Is it possible to ascertain instantaneous hypercalciuria in patients who form stones unless one analyzes every urinary specimen? Chambers and Dormandy (1969) proposed just such an analysis, but most laboratories find it impractical. How can we resolve this dilemma?

Detection of Hypercalciuria

The variability of supersaturation of urine with calcium oxalate or calcium phosphate throughout the day has led to the development of numerous tests that attempt to detect hypercalciuria and thereby to estimate quickly the tendency of an individual to form stones. Some modifications, for example, test specimens from 2 or 4 hours of urine collection only (Drach, 1976b; Pak et al., 1975; Seftel and Resnick, 1990).

Previously, excretion rates per 24-hour day were routine, but some investigators (Finlayson, 1974; Robertson et al., 1976; Pak et al., 1974; and King, 1967 and 1971) have pointed out that excretion of urinary calcium throughout the day by patients who form stones varies so greatly that 24-hour specimens produce less information because of averaging. Various methods have been suggested to overcome these objections. Pak and co-workers (1975) initiated a brief test for absorptive hypercalciuria. The test utilizes only a 2-hour fasting and 4-hour postprandial urinary specimen. This test has since been modified to include 24-hour collections on a low (400 mg) and an unrestricted (over 1 g) calcium intake (Pak, 1987).

Chambers and Dormandy (1969), cited previously, have proposed a 20-hour "urinary series" in which every urinary specimen passed is analyzed for calcium, phosphorus, oxalate, and other ionic constituents. Broadus and colleagues (1978) proposed that a 24-hour urinary collection, while the patient is ingesting 1000 mg/day calcium, will reveal absorptive hypercalciuria if calcium excretion is more than 4 mg/kg/day.

Several laboratories have described collection of 24-hour urines, which are analyzed for many elements and factors. A "stone risk" based on that urine is generated for the patient (Pak et al., 1985). It describes the degree of saturation with calcium oxalate, uric acid, and so forth. This type of test is not as specific in defining hypercalciuria as are the aforementioned diet-controlled urinary tests.

Repeat studies that show decreased supersaturation can imply successful therapy; however, each method has its limitations and is not foolproof. Investigators continue to look for the test that will predict that significant hypercalciuria exists in the patient who has a tendency toward calcium lithiasis (Table 58–6).

Most clinicians must continue to rely on the analysis of 24-hour urine specimens to predict whether hypercalciuria exists. Table 58–6 lists some levels above which patients are said to be hypercalciuric. Note the considerable disagreement about the level of urinary calcium that must be exceeded for hypercalciuria to exist. Our problem is one of definition: We are really attempting to detect urinary supersaturation with calcium rather than only hypercalciuria. If one patient excretes 300 mg of calcium per day but the urine is not supersaturated at this level, perhaps this is not hypercalciuria for that patient. Perhaps "hypercalciuria" exists only when elevated urinary calcium levels result in urinary supersaturation and renal calcium deposition or stone formation. Hence, in the future, it is more likely that we will test for calcium supersaturation, as Pak and colleagues (1985) have done.

Once hypercalciuria is detected, it is useful to place the case in the proper category of causation of hypercalciuria. Six major causes exist (Table 58–7).

The first is absorptive hypercalciuria, which is the result of excessive intestinal absorption of calcium presented to the gut (Pak et al., 1974). Pak (1987) now subdivides this group into type I (hypercalciuric on a low-calcium diet) and type II (hypercalciuric on a normal calcium diet). He also defines a type III patient—hypercalciuria associated with hypophosphatemia and low tubular reabsorption of phosphorus. Hence, there are three subdivisions within absorptive hypercalciuria.

Table 58–6. WHEN IS THE PATIENT HYPERCALCIURIC?

Authors	Patient's Diet	Definition Males	Females
Coe, 1974	Not listed	>300 mg/day	>250 mg/day
Pak, 1974	400 mg calcium	>200 mg/day	>200 mg/day
Smith, 1974	1 g calcium	>275 mg/day	>250 mg/day
Williams, 1974b	Not listed	>300 mg/day	>250 mg/day
Nordin and colleagues, 1979	"When urinary excretion is excessive for dietary intake"		
Chambers and Dormandy, 1969	"If urine osmolality is over 530 milliosmols, any value >22 mg/dl"		
Finlayson, 1974	Whenever urine is "supersaturated with calcium" and another ion with which it may precipitate		
Thomas, 1975	Analysis of 24-hr calcium excretion is "not clinically useful"		
Broadus, 1978	1000 mg calcium >4 mg/kg/day, either sex		

The fourth cause is renal leak hypercalciuria, which results when renal tubules fail to reabsorb calcium normally, thereby losing or leaking calcium into urine (Coe and Davalach, 1974).

Fifth is the hypercalciuria of hyperparathyroidism, which occurs because excessive parathyroid hormone produces excessive resorption of bone. Intestinal calcium absorption may also be increased. The calcium load presented to the kidneys via the serum becomes too great to be efficiently reabsorbed, and excessive urinary calcium results.

Sixth, a particular subset of patients seems to have hypercalciuria in response to carbohydrate or glucose ingestion (Gluszek, 1988). An additional dietary test may be necessary to detect these individuals who excrete excessive urinary calcium after excessive carbohydrate intake. These patients develop a brief hypercalciuria after a high-carbohydrate meal, such as six donuts (Lemann et al., 1969; Thom et al., 1978). The mechanism is unclear, but some data suggest that the carbohydrate ingestion triggers a decreased renal reabsorption of calcium and hence a "renal leak" hypercalciuria in some patients who form oxalate stones and in their susceptible relatives (Gittes et al., 1967). Many other metabolic diseases result in hypercalciuria. Those associated with calcium stone disease are discussed later in this chapter.

The differentiation of any type of hypercalciuria depends first on the exclusion of known metabolic diseases or hyperparathyroidism. Then, distinction of absorptive hypercalciuria and renal leak hypercalciuria can be performed using the methods described by Pak (1987), Coe and Davalach (1974), Broadus and co-workers (1978), and Seftel and Resnick (1990). A composite summary

derived from their observations is presented in Tables 58–8 and 58–9.

Coe and associates (1982) and Lien and Keane (1983) question whether one can distinguish between different forms of hypercalciuria, such as "absorptive" or "renal leak." Both groups have concluded from studies of 27 and 52 patients, respectively, that the two defects may in reality be extremes of a continuum (Fig. 58–33). As Coe hypothesizes: "A uniform elevation of intestinal calcium absorption and a variable defect of renal calcium reabsorption could explain our results far better than the hypothesis of distinct absorptive and renal forms of hypercalciuria."

Finlayson (1974) and Pak (1987, 1989) have discussed hypercalciurias more extensively in their reviews.

Hyperparathyroidism

Hyperparathyroidism produces a combination of all previously described absorptive renal and bony calcium defects—hyperabsorption of calcium through the gut, increased reabsorption of bone, and increased renal loss of filtered calcium in spite of increased reabsorption (Kleeman et al., 1958). Other than elevated serum calcium level, the most significant diagnostic difference that distinguishes patients with hyperparathyroidism from those with absorptive hypercalciuria or renal leak

Table 58–7. HYPERCALCIURIAS OF UROLITHIASIS

Term	Presumed Cause
Intestinal hyperabsorption	Excessive intestinal absorption of calcium
Type I	When dietary calcium normal
Type II	When dietary calcium low
Type III	Phosphate leak
Renal leak	Failure of kidney to reabsorb tubular calcium
Bone resorption	Excessive calcium mobilized from bone
Carbohydrate load	Form of renal leak

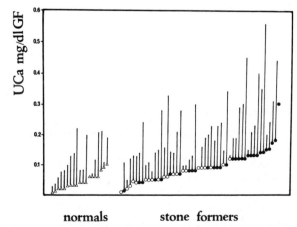

Figure 58–33. Fasting urinary calcium excretions (*baseline values*) and post–oral calcium load values (*vertical bars*) of normal persons and patients who form stones, ranked in ascending order. (0, normocalciuric; •, hypercalciuric patients). (From Lien, J., and Keane, P.: J. Urol., 129:401, 1983. By Williams & Wilkins, 1992.)

Table 58–8. GENERAL ASPECTS OF SEPARATION OF HYPERCALCIURIAS

Type of Hypercalciuria	Serum Calcium	Serum PTH	Fasting Urine Calcium	Bone Density	Intestinal Absorption
Primary hyperparathyroidism (bone-resorptive)	High	High	High	Low	High
Renal stones, absorptive	N1*	N1 or low	N1	N1	High
Renal stones, "renal leak"	N1	?	High	Low	N1
Renal stone, normocalciuric	N1	N1	N1	N1	N1

*N1 = Normal

hypercalciuria is a significant increase in serum parathyroid hormone levels.

Hyperparathyroidism can cause significant numbers of urinary calculi. Removal of the parathyroid glands eliminates the tendency toward urinary calculi in the majority of patients with this affliction (Harrison and Rose, 1973). However, older concepts of hyperparathyroidism now must include consideration of new factors that relate to calcium homeostasis and stone formation. These include the precise control of serum calcium concentrations by parathyroid hormone, thyrocalcitonin, vitamin D, and the renal hormone, 1,25-dihydroxycholecalciferol (1,25-DHCC) (Fig. 58–34). In addition, the importance of cyclic 3', 5'-adenosine monophosphate (AMP) as the intrarenal messenger for parathyroid hormone has been established (Chase and Aurbach, 1967). Urinary cyclic AMP (cAMP) determinations may aid the diagnosis of hyperparathyroidism (Murad and Pak, 1972; Stewart and Broadus, 1981).

Serum calcium concentration is regulated by a labile reservoir of calcium at the surface of the bone, which responds to increased or decreased parathyroid hormone (PTH) concentration. Parathyroid hormone is a relatively small polypeptide with a molecular weight of 9000, produced by the parathyroid gland. Purified PTH has both bone calcium mobilizing and renal phosphaturic actions. The effects of the hormone on bone and on kidneys probably are mediated through the formation of cAMP at the cell membrane. Through a combination of mobilization of calcium from the bone, increased renal tubular resorption of calcium, and increased intestinal absorption of calcium, increased serum PTH raises the serum calcium concentration. The hormone may have minor direct effects on the GI tract. Its major effect results from greater intestinal calcium absorption, by causing renal synthesis and release of 1,25-DHCC (see Fig. 58–34).

Physiologic studies indicate that the secretion of PTH by the parathyroid glands is controlled directly by the free serum calcium level. Hormone concentration increases when serum calcium level decreases and vice versa. Studies of the role of the phosphate ion in controlling PTH secretion show that the effect of phosphate is secondary to any effect produced on the serum calcium concentration. Hence, hyperphosphatemia stimulates the parathyroid glands only indirectly by inducing hypocalcemia, a mechanism that is probably involved in stimulating the parathyroid gland in chronic renal failure. The parathyroid glands store only small amounts of hormone; hence, they show a high rate of protein synthesis when stimulated by hypocalcemia.

Copp and colleagues (1962) demonstrated a hormone that they thought originated in the parathyroid gland. This hormone, which they called calcitonin, decreased blood calcium content. It was later shown that the calcium-lowering hormone came from the thyroid gland, and the name was changed to thyrocalcitonin (TCT). Parafollicular cells adjacent to the thyroid follicles produce TCT. This hormone appears to act directly on bone to inhibit calcium mobilization, an action that is antagonistic to but not dependent on the presence of PTH. Thyrocalcitonin appears to play only a minor role in calcium homeostasis in humans and may be secreted only at times of severe hypercalcemia. It functions independently of PTH (Gittes et al., 1967). Thyrocalcitonin may, however, be helpful as an agent for treating Paget's disease.

Knowledge concerning parathyroid hormone, TCT, and cAMP revolutionized the concepts of calcium metabolism and hyperparathyroidism. The role of the kidney in the function of these hormones and messengers was believed to be secondary, until it was discovered that the kidney was the major source of the active form of vitamin D_3, a substance called 1,25-DHCC. The final

Table 58–9. ORAL CALCIUM LOAD METHOD FOR DEFINING HYPERCALCIURIAS EXCLUDING CARBOHYDRATE-INDUCED HYPERCALCIURIAS*

Classification	Serum Calcium	Fasting Urine Calcium (mg/mg Cr)	Post Load Urine (mg/mg Cr)
Absorptive hypercalciuria	Normal	<0.11	>0.2
Renal leak hypercalciuria	Normal	>0.11	<0.2
Hyperparathyroidism	High (>10.3)	>0.11	>0.2
Normocalciuric nephrolithiasis	Normal	<0.11	<0.2
Normal control	Normal	<0.11	<0.2

*Modified from Pak, C.Y., Ohata, M., Lawrence, E.C., et al.: J. Clin. Invest., 54:387, 1974. By copyright permission of the American Society for Clinical Investigation. (Cr, creatinine.)

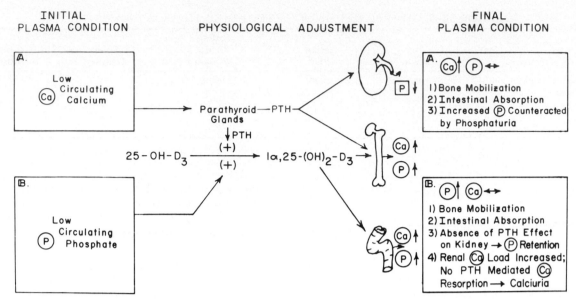

Figure 58–34. One model for homeostatic control of calcium and phosphate through the integrated functions of parathyroid hormone (PTH) and 1,25-dihydroxyvitamin D_3 (1,25-D_3, referred to in text as 1,25-DHCC). When either plasma calcium (A) or phosphate (B) is depleted, the kidneys are stimulated to convert circulating 25-hydroxyvitamin D_3 to 1,25-D_3. For calcium, this reaction is mediated by PTH, but for phosphate, no intermediary has been found. Combined results of PTH and 1,25-D_3 activities are shown for kidney, bone, and gut. The resulting adjustments in plasma for low calcium are shown in A, and those for low phosphate are shown in B. (From Haussler, M. R., et al.: Clin. Endocrinol., 5:151A, 1976. Blackwell Scientific Publications Limited.)

renal activation of its immediate precursor in blood, 25-hydroxycholecalciferol, results in "active" vitamin D_3, or 1,25-DHCC, by attachment of a hydroxyl at position 25. This vitamin acts primarily on the intestinal mucosa to promote calcium and phosphorus absorption by the gut. Vitamin D_3 does not require PTH to be active on intestinal mucosal cells, but it does require PTH to promote production by renal cells (DeLuca, 1976; Sherwood, 1988). Figure 58–34 represents the interrelationship of all these concepts.

In a given individual, the concentration of calcium is the most precisely controlled biologic component of the serum that has been studied to date (Copp, 1969; Drach and King, 1970; Harris, 1970; Sherwood, 1988). To maintain this serum calcium level, the body has three mechanisms—gut absorption of calcium, bone deposition and resorption of calcium, and renal and fecal excretion of calcium. Laboratory determination of serum calcium was imprecise. Precision has improved over the years, and therefore normal limits in serum have been defined (Harris, 1970).

At the present time, most hospital laboratories define the range as 9.0 mg/dl to 10.5 mg/dl. In one Mayo Clinic series (Keating, 1961), male patients in an older age group were found to have hyperparathyroidism even with serum calcium levels as low as 10.1 to 10.2 mg/dl. They noted a small regression of serum calcium level with age in males; therefore, the normal serum calcium level at age 20 can be at an upper limit of 10.2 mg/dl, whereas at age 80, an upper limit of normal is 10.0 mg/dl. In females, there is a slight increase in normal serum calcium levels with age. The upper limit of serum calcium at age 20 is 10.0 mg/dl, but the upper limit climbed slowly to 10.1 mg/dl at age 80. The upper limit of normal scrum calcium levels for most humans is

therefore at or below 10.2 mg/dl. This upper limit is much lower than that published by many laboratories. However, with improvements in analysis of serum calcium, it is likely that this level will continue to be shown to be an absolute upper limit for most humans.

Another concept that must be considered with regard to hyperparathyroidism is the degree of control that the parathyroid gland manifests over serum calcium. We are aware of the inverse control relationship between parathyroid hormone and serum calcium. This relationship is modified somewhat by thyrocalcitonin (although not much in humans) and by vitamin D_3. In general, elevation of serum calcium in normal humans results in suppression and decreased excretion of parathyroid hormone; this, in turn, results in adjustment of serum calcium to a lower level. Abnormally low levels of serum calcium lead to excretion of more parathyroid hormone, with the resultant tendency to increase serum calcium concentration to normal. The half-life of serum parathyroid hormone is believed to be about 20 minutes, which provides a quick reaction to changes in serum calcium levels.

Patients with hyperparathyroidism usually manifest abnormal control of serum calcium (Drach and King, 1970). Both the absolute level of serum calcium and the day-to-day control of serum calcium can be abnormal. Therefore, a patient who forms stones with hyperparathyroidism may have brief episodes of hypercalcemia interspersed with normocalcemic periods. As noted previously, the rise of serum calcium concentration above the normal limit increases the calcium load to the kidneys and may result in hypercalciuria and stone formation. For this reason, it has been proposed that urinary calculous disease due to "idiopathic" hypercalciuria may actually be an intermittent and intermediate form of hyperparathyroidism that is midway between normal and overt hyperparathyroidism. This hypothesis has not been proven.

One of the solutions to the problem of diagnosis of hyperparathyroidism was thought to be the measurement of serum immunoreactive parathyroid hormone. Unfortunately, this test has not been completely accurate. Great variations in measurement of parathyroid hormone by different laboratories have led to confusion. No suitable standard method or standard value exists; therefore, no comparisons can be made among laboratories. However, careful control of dietary calcium intake along with observation of the fasting serum calcium level with simultaneous measurement of serum parathyroid hormone has resulted in the designation of some normal zones for both. The elevation of serum calcium or parathyroid hormone level, or both, strongly suggests hyperparathyroidism. The work of Arnaud (1973) and Arnaud and Strewler (1981) has been critical in defining these relationships (Sherwood, 1988).

Based on the foregoing observations of the effects of PTH on serum or urinary components, a number of confirmatory tests have been devised for the diagnosis of hyperparathyroidism. The first and most important of these is multiple observations of serum calcium levels, sometimes over a prolonged period of time. On occasion, patients with urinary calculous disease have serum calcium concentrations that are clearly elevated and abnormal only intermittently. The concomitant presence of urinary calculous disease of calcium type (or on rare occasions, magnesium ammonium phosphate type) and any elevated serum calcium level are compelling reasons to suspect hyperparathyroidism.

A total of 53 serum calcium determinations were made over a period of 5 years in a patient who formed stones. It was only at the end of this period that overt hyperparathyroidism with hypercalcemia became evident. The patient underwent exploratory surgery, and a large parathyroid adenoma was removed. Stone formation ceased immediately. The patient has not had another urinary calculus in 21 years, whereas an average of one calculus was passed every 2 months prior to surgery. This case is presented to emphasize the fact that prolonged observations of serum calcium levels may be necessary to discover this disease (Johansson et al., 1975).

If elevated or even upper normal levels (over 10.1 mg/dl) of serum calcium are found, simultaneous determination of serum parathyroid hormone should be performed (Yendt and Cohanim, 1989). If both serum calcium and serum parathyroid hormone concentrations are elevated in the absence of other diseases that may cause these abnormalities, the diagnosis of hyperparathyroidism may be made (Arnaud and Strewler, 1981; Waterhouse and Heinig, 1976). In my opinion, the first consideration for treatment of this disease remains surgical, and a surgical consultant should be contacted. That consultant may advise medical management whether the patient is a poor candidate for surgery.

Other adjunctive tests have been proposed for diagnosis of hyperparathyroidism. Among these are the phosphate reabsorption test (Reynolds et al., 1960;

Schrott et al., 1972), the steroid suppression test (Strott and Nugent, 1968), the measurement of urinary cAMP (Murad and Pak, 1972), and many others (Sherwood, 1988). I agree with other reviewers that the false-positive and false-negative percentage of error (25 per cent) in all of these tests makes them of limited use as diagnostic indicators of parathyroid disease (Lafferty, 1981; Yendt and Cohanim, 1989).

Fewer patients with hyperparathyroidism now present with renal stones. Most are diagnosed after routine screening of multichannel blood profiles. If elevated serum calcium concentration exists, serum parathyroid hormone is measured. If both calcium and hormone levels are elevated, the patient has hyperparathyroidism. One must be very careful to exclude other diseases that may cause hypercalcemia in the absence of hyperparathyroidism, however (Table 58–10) (Smith, 1989). The final diagnosis of hyperparathyroidism is confirmed only by surgical exploration and demonstration of parathyroid adenoma or hyperplasia.

Renal histopathology resulting from hyperparathyroidism and nephrocalcinosis includes marked deposition of calcium, excreted calcium bodies, and other debris in the renal tubules. Two aspects to the renal disease process are evidenced. The first is a direct interference with the physiologic function of the kidney cells. If hypercalcemia caused by excess parathyroid hormone is relieved, this functional aspect of hyperparathyroidism can be reversed (Drach and Boyce, 1972). However, secondary mechanical and anatomic aspects of cell death and deposition of calcium in the kidney persist for long periods of time following relief of the hyperparathyroidism. Therefore, nephrocalcinosis of this disease may persist after treatment. In spite of this, the formation of new urinary calculi ceases in most patients following removal of the parathyroid adenoma or hyperplasia (Harrison and Rose, 1973; Stubbs and Myers, 1973).

Hypercalcemic Crisis

Acute parathyroid intoxication (parathyroid crisis) may necessitate emergency therapy for hypercalcemia if the patient is to be saved. Parathyroid crisis usually occurs when the serum calcium content approaches a level of 17 mg/dl or higher. It is characterized by a rapid pulse, progressive lethargy, nausea, vomiting, abdominal discomfort, and azotemia. When the serum calcium level reaches 20 mg/dl, respiratory distress, renal failure, and coma develop. The patient may die of cardiac arrest. Definitive treatment of parathyroid crisis requires para-

Table 58–10. SOME DISEASES THAT MAY BE ASSOCIATED WITH HYPERCALCEMIA AND HYPERCALCIURIA

Hyperparathyroidism	Metastatic malignant
Vitamin D intoxication	neoplasms
Idiopathic infantile	Leukemia
hypercalcemia	Lymphoma
Sarcoidosis	Milk-alkali sydrome
Multiple myeloma	Myxedema
Hyperthyroidism	Adrenal insufficiency

thyroidectomy. Serum calcium content may also be temporarily decreased by the intravenous administration of inorganic phosphates or sulfates. The mechanism by which inorganic phosphates lower the serum calcium level is not known, but it is not related to increased excretion of calcium in the urine. Inorganic phosphate may also be given orally, depending on how rapid an effect is needed. The usual daily dose of inorganic phosphate ranges from 1 to 3 g. In patients with renal failure, small doses should be provided to prevent hypotension and secondary acute tubular necrosis.

Intravenous administration of isotonic sodium sulfate solution (containing 38.9 g sodium sulfate decahydrate in water) will produce an increase in the urinary excretion of calcium. This increased calcium excretion may be due to an increased glomerular filtration rate produced by rehydration and the effect of sodium ion on calcium resorption in the proximal renal tubules or a complex effect of the nonresorbable sulfate anion on the renal tubule. Sodium sulfate produces a more rapid decrease in serum calcium content than does the administration of inorganic phosphates; sodium chloride produces a similar effect but to a lesser degree.

Other drugs that resolve hypercalcemia are furosemide (20-40 mg intravenously), ethacrynic acid, corticosteroids, mithramycin, calcitonin, and estrogens (Sherwood, 1988). One of the most rapid ways to effect reversal is hemodialysis. Paterson (1974) has reviewed all the foregoing methods and still recommends intravenous phosphates as the treatment of choice.

Other Diseases That May Cause Hypercalcemia and Hypercalciuria

A number of diseases increase serum concentration and urinary excretion of calcium and may be confused with hyperparathyroidism or idiopathic hypercalciuria (see Table 58–10). Although investigation of these diseases is beyond the practice of most urologists, one should be aware of their existence (Seftel and Resnick, 1990; Sherwood, 1988). Included in this disease group are idiopathic infantile hypercalcemia (Williams, 1974a), sarcoidosis (Ellman and Parfitt, 1960), multiple myeloma (Sherwood et al., 1967), hyperthyroidism (Williams, 1974a), leukemia (Sherwood et al., 1967), lymphoma (Sherwood et al., 1967), and milk-alkali syndrome (Smith, 1974a).

The diseases that are most important to and most likely to be seen by the urologist are vitamin D intoxication, immobilization syndrome, and renal tubular acidosis. Williams (1974a) confirms that, aside from idiopathic hypercalciuria and hyperparathyroidism, the diseases most commonly associated with calcium urolithiasis are renal tubular acidosis and vitamin D intoxication, but he also includes hyperthyroidism. A few of these more common diseases are briefly discussed.

VITAMIN D INTOXICATION. Excessive amounts of vitamin D or D_3 (more than 100,000 units per day for many months) ingested or injected will cause hypercalcemia and hypercalciuria. When administration of vitamin D is stopped, serum and urinary calcium levels return to normal slowly because large amounts of the vitamin are stored in fat. Stone formation also ceases.

IMMOBILIZATION SYNDROME. Abrupt total immobilization due to casts, traction, or quadriplegia may lead to marked loss of calcium from bone with resultant hypercalciuria. Space travel also causes immobilization syndrome. Treatment involves exercises when possible, avoidance of excessive calcium in the diet, forcing of fluids to provide urine output in excess of 2000 ml per day, and perhaps administration of oral orthophosphate if no urinary infection exists (Thomas, 1974). Stones associated with urinary infections should be treated as infection stones.

RENAL TUBULAR ACIDOSIS. In 1936, Butler, Wilson, and Farber described a clinical syndrome characterized by persistent dehydration, hyperchloremia, hypokalemia, metabolic acidosis, and nephrocalcinosis. This was the first clinical report of the syndrome now called distal renal tubular acidosis. It has a variety of other names, such as hyperchloremic acidosis, Butler-Albright syndrome, idiopathic acidosis, Lightwood's syndrome, and tubular insufficiency without glomerular insufficiency.

Renal tubular acidosis (RTA) results in an inability to excrete acid urine; the fasting urinary pH always exceeds 5.3 (see Table 58–4). Two forms of the disease exist, types I and II. Distal (type I) RTA probably results from decreased hydrogen ion secretion in the distal renal tubule with impairment of the conservation of fixed base. An acid load test reveals that the affected patients do not excrete metabolic acids normally (Caruana and Buckalew, 1988; Dretler et al., 1969). Distal tubular secretion of potassium increases in an attempt to offset the deficiency of hydrogen ion secretion, but this secretion does not compensate completely. Hydrogen ions nevertheless are retained, and excessive amounts of sodium, potassium, and calcium are lost into urine. One consequence is hypercalciuria.

With the continued loss of sodium in the urine, the serum sodium concentration is depressed, stimulating the osmoregulatory system to suppress the release of antidiuretic hormone. This produces water diuresis in an attempt to maintain iso-osmolarity of the body fluids.

Consequent to the increased loss of fluids, a contraction of extracellular fluid and intravascular volume occurs. As this contraction reaches a critical level, the volume control system is brought into action to maintain extracellular fluid volume. Contraction of plasma volume is a potent stimulus of aldosterone. Increased aldosterone elevates sodium and chloride resorption by the kidney in almost equal amounts, resulting in relative hyperchloremia, along with hypokalemia from potassium loss by the kidney. Serum CO_2 level is depressed. This group of defects, coupled with hydrogen ion retention, results in metabolic acidosis. Only type I patients form renal stones.

In review, the characteristic serum biochemical abnormalities resulting from type I RTA are a reduced serum CO_2 combining power, reduced P_{CO_2} and serum pH, hyperchloremia, and hypokalemia. The serum calcium and phosphorus levels are normal, but the urine is alkaline in the presence of hypercalciuria. These factors predispose the patient to formation of calculi, usually of calcium phosphate (Caruana and Buckalew, 1988; Dretler et al., 1969).

A subset of type I is now called type IV RTA. The patient shows an impaired ability to acidify the urine during basal testing but acidifies the urine in response to an acid load. Some patients with stone disease have this incomplete form of RTA in which metabolic acidosis is not present, and some acid in an acid load test can be excreted. Yet, these patients do not acidify the urine below pH 5.3 if tested in their everyday environments. Most also have hypercalciuria (Marquardt, 1973; Sommerkamp and Schwerk, 1973; Young and Martin, 1972), and some have hyperuricemia (Fellstrom et al., 1983).

Proximal (type II) renal tubular acidosis results from a defect in carbonic anhydrase of the proximal tubule. Severe renal bicarbonate wasting exists, but the patient does not form renal calculi.

Bone lesions of RTA are osteomalacic—there is a failure to calcify already formed osteoid matrix. Pseudofracture lines (described by Milkman, 1934) are not true fractures but localized linear areas of decreased bone formation bound on either side by areas of hyperostosis that suggest linear fractures.

Correction of metabolic acidosis and restoration of fixed base occur following administration of a balanced sodium citrate solution that may also contain potassium. Stone formation ceases with such therapy, although nephrocalcinosis may persist. The objectives of medical treatment are to relieve acidosis, to reduce hyperchloremia and hypercalciuria, and to improve renal reabsorption of calcium.

For maintenance therapy, an inexpensive mixture of Shohl's solution may be provided in divided doses. This liquid medication consists of 98 g of sodium citrate, 140 g of citric acid, and 1000 ml of water. When edema is present and sodium is to be avoided, or when potassium replacement is necessary, potassium citrate may be given in this prescription instead of sodium citrate. Albright's solution can be used as a substitute. It consists of 75 mg of sodium citrate, 25 g of potassium citrate, 140 g of citric acid, and 1000 ml of water. This solution is particularly effective when hypokalemia is present. Average dosages are 15 ml three or four times daily. When renal insufficiency is present, the patient must be closely observed for potassium intoxication and development of metabolic alkalosis. Because of the inherent inability of the kidneys to excrete acids, including chloride radicals, dietary salt should be restricted.

Claus-Walker and colleagues (1973) have shown that one of the significant differences between patients with calcium urinary lithiasis and normal individuals is a deficiency of potassium excretion in the urine. Patients with renal tubular acidosis, however, have excessive excretion of potassium in the urine, in exchange for the hydrogen that is retained in the system owing to the defect of the disease. Hence, urinary potassium does not seem to have any direct relationship to formation of calcium urinary calculi.

Calcium Urolithiasis Associated with Hyperoxaluria

We have seen in many conditions that the amount of urinary calcium may be elevated and may be associated with urinary calculi. The most common type of stone disease, however, is calcium oxalate urolithiasis. Many investigators emphasize the effect of increased urinary oxalate rather than calcium on the precipitation of calcium oxalate (Elliot, 1983; Hautmann et al., 1980; Menon and Mahle, 1983; Valyasevi and Dhanamitta, 1974; Yanagawa et al., 1983).

Robertson and co-workers (1969, 1972 a and b, 1973, 1974, 1976, 1978) have produced strong evidence that the amount of urinary oxalate at any given time is roughly ten times more important in determining the precipitation of calcium oxalate than the quantity of either calcium or phosphate in urine. Their reports indicate that one can actually distinguish those who form stones from those who do not by utilizing a biaxial comparison of the saturation of urine with calcium oxalate versus the presence of "inhibitor." These observations combine the supersaturation/crystallization and inhibitor theories.

Gill and colleagues (1974) utilized radioisotopic methods to measure the saturation of urine with calcium oxalate and to predict the propensity for growth of preformed calcium oxalate nuclei. Miller and associates (1977) have devised a system that measures directly the nucleation rate, growth rate, and total crystal mass of calcium oxalate crystals produced by urine specimens. Sarig and associates (1982) report a "diagnostic index" (DI) of calcium oxalate precipitation to estimate stone risk and to evaluate therapy in patients. Pak and colleagues (1985) trace the saturation of calcium oxalate in urine. Each of these methods provides some information that is useful in predicting calcium oxalate stone disease.

In most tests, the amounts of calcium, oxalate, phosphate, magnesium, sodium, and chloride in urine are determined in order to predict, by calculation, the saturation of urine with calcium oxalate or phosphate. Finlayson and colleagues (1973) measured only these components of urine and published a system of computer calculations that permit a fairly accurate estimation of the degree of calcium oxalate saturation of urine. This system, with modifications, continues to be used for practical investigations today (Hering et al., 1987).

One major factor that has been detrimental to the study of the effects of oxalate on urolithiasis has been the difficulty in analysis of oxalate, whether in serum or in urine. Methods for determination of oxalate in biologic systems may be roughly divided into four types. The first method is quantitation of oxalate by enzymatic reduction with oxalase and measurement of the carbon dioxide liberated by the reaction (Elliot et al., 1970). The margin of error in this method is about 5 per cent. The second method is an analysis performed by chromatographic titration (Hodgkinson, 1970). This analysis is somewhat more accurate but still does not give completely reproducible results, especially for determination of serum oxalate. Thirdly, radioisotopic dilution methods have also been devised. The fourth method, ion chromatography, has also been used.

However, analysis of duplicate samples of serum oxalate from the same specimen employing two different types of oxalate analysis does not give similar values. The amounts of oxalate in urine, however, are so much higher than those in serum that the present enzymatic and chromatographic or radioisotopic dilution techniques give values that are practical for clinical practice (Gregory, 1981).

Urinary oxalate has two major sources of origin in the human. The first is endogenous production by means of enzymatic cleavage of glyoxalate to form oxalic acid and glycine. The second source is absorption of excess oxalate via the gut from foods and liquids (Table 58–11) (Gregory, 1981). In serum, oxalate is found in very low amounts. Once excreted, urinary oxalic acid rapidly forms a complex with the multiple cationic salts and ions available and becomes oxalate salt. Oxalate is soluble when combined with most components of urine such as magnesium. Only when it forms a complex with calcium in high concentrations does it become insoluble. Then, crystalline precipitation of calcium oxalate occurs. As noted previously, this spontaneous precipitation occurs whenever the product of concentrations of calcium and oxalate exceeds the formation product (Marshall and Robertson, 1976; Pak, 1987). Calcium oxalate crystals may also grow on preformed nuclei whenever its solubility product is exceeded.

The importance of oxalate in the process cannot be denied. The upper limit of normal urinary excretion of oxalate for humans is approximately 35 mg/day. The upper limit of urinary excretion of calcium ranges between 200 and 300 mg/day, according to most investigators (see Table 58–6). An increase of one tenth in oxalate (to a level of 38.5 mg/day) equals an increase of ten times one tenth in urinary calcium (from 200 to 400 mg/day). The presence of 400 mg of calcium and 38.5 mg of oxalate in a 24-hour urine specimen with a volume of approximately 1.5 L would almost guarantee precipitation of calcium oxalate.

A peculiar difference is noted between those who form stones and those who do not form stones. A normal human, on occasion, can excrete 45 mg of oxalate and 300 mg of calcium per day. Indeed, these individuals produce multiple, small crystals of oxalate. However, the size of these crystals is limited to approximately 7 to 12 μ. Once the larger size is approached, additional small crystals are formed, but larger crystals do not grow or form by aggregation. It is only when this "small-crystal" system goes awry that urinary calculi form. As noted previously, calculus formation is presumably related to the formation of larger crystals, aggregates of crystals, and crystal masses that obstruct or occlude some portion of the urinary tract. Whether or not we accept the theory that excessive amounts of oxalate trigger calculi (see Fig. 58–7), we know that some conditions of hyperoxaluria result in calculi. We will review those processes of excessive oxalate excretion and calculi formation by examining first the disease condition known as primary hyperoxaluria.

HYPEROXALURIA. Primary hyperoxaluria is a congenital illness characterized by the endogenous formation of excessive amounts of oxalate in tissues without any associated pyridoxine deficiency. This rare congenital defect can be further separated into two types. Type I hyperoxaluria is labeled glycolic aciduria and is due to a deficiency of soluble 2-oxoglutarate: glyoxylate carboligase. Type II is called L-glyceric aciduria but results in similar findings of excessive urinary oxalate excretion. The enzymatic deficiency is D-glyceric dehydrogenase. Patients with primary hyperoxaluria and urinary stone disease often develop evidence of the disease in childhood. Extensive nephrocalcinosis and renal failure are present. Oral phosphates to treat this abnormality are discussed later, but no drug currently known alters the enzymatic defect. Treatment is not often successful (Hall et al., 1960; Hockaday et al., 1967; Watts, 1973). Most patients die prior to the age of 30.

Acquired hyperoxaluria is associated with enteric diseases. Patients with regional ileitis, colitis, and postoperative intestinal bypass have been demonstrated to excrete excessive amounts of oxalate in the urine (Dickstein and Frame, 1973; Fikri and Casella, 1975; Seftel and Resnick, 1990; Smith and Hofman, 1974). Rapid intestinal transit, shortness of bowel, and lack of bacterial activity in the bowel appear to contribute to excessive absorption of oxalate products. The turnover of oxalate in the serum is extremely rapid, and increased amounts of oxalate are excreted by the kidneys.

Because the effects of urinary oxalate on crystallization are ten times greater than the effects of calcium, according to the theory presented previously, and because a calcium-to-oxalate ratio of even 1 to 35 could result in stones, patients are extremely prone to develop urinary calculi even though calcium excretion levels may not be excessive.

If we add the fact that they are chronically dehydrated by diarrhea and tend to have relatively acid urine, it is not surprising that they form calculi easily. Reports have also been made that postoperative patients who have undergone a Bricker (ileal loop) procedure develop this type of calculous disease (Dretler, 1973; Koff, 1975; Rattiazzi et al., 1975; Singer et al., 1973).

IDIOPATHIC HYPEROXALURIA. Calculi associated with hyperoxaluria, for which a cause may be

Table 58–11. SOME LIQUIDS AND FOODS THAT CONTAIN LARGER AMOUNTS OF OXALATE*

Liquids

MODERATE AMOUNTS
Apple juice
Beer
Coffee
Cola
Cranberry juice
Grapefruit juice
Instant tea
HIGH AMOUNTS
Cocoa
Fresh tea

Foods

Almonds	Currants
Asparagus	Greens
Beets	Plums
Cactus fruits	Raspberries
Cashew nuts	Rhubarb
Concord grapes	Spinach
Cranberries	

*Modified from Thomas, W.C., Jr.: Urol. Clin. North Am., 1:261, 1974 and Gregory, J.G.: Urol. Clin. North Am., 8:331, 1981. (See also Appendix C.)

demonstrated, have been discussed so far. We now must consider those individuals who have "idiopathic" hyperoxaluria. As mentioned previously, the presence of oxalate in urine depends on endogenous production and oral intake. For each individual, there seems to be a characteristic basal level of production of oxalate.

On a regular diet without excessive ingested oxalate, most individuals do not have increased urinary oxalate concentrations (Drach, 1976b; Robertson and Peacock, 1972). However, if they eat or drink foods containing high amounts of oxalate, some patients experience rapid increases in urinary oxalate excretion. Examples of such high oxalate foods are given in Table 58–11. Ingestion of soluble oxalates in particular increases urinary excretion of oxalates in many patients.

Based on these facts, it is obvious that the best possible modification of oxalate excretion by a "normal" individual or an individual who forms stones with idiopathic disease is achieved mostly by limitation of oral oxalate intake. Unfortunately, this is not often successful (Gregory, 1981). At the present time, there is no known way to interfere with endogenous production of oxalate. Succinimide has been proposed, but Hodgkinson and associates (1975) surveyed the effects of this drug in animals and found relatively little response. Most continue to recommend limitation of dietary intake for control of oxalate excretion.

Ascorbic acid (vitamin C) ingestion leads to increased urinary oxalate excretion, and "megadose" vitamin C therapy has been implicated as a risk factor for urinary calculi (Conyers et al., 1985). Yet, high ascorbate excretion may falsely elevate urinary oxalate levels in certain assays, and it leads to no increased oxalate crystal deposition in animals (Singh et al., 1988). However, it seems prudent to advise patients who form calcium oxalate stones not to ingest more than 2 g of vitamin C per day.

Attempts to Estimate Activity of Calcium Stone Disease

An additional complexity in the study of calcium stone disease revolves around the fact that stones may be initiated and formed entirely of either calcium oxalate or calcium phosphate or, more commonly, of mixtures of the two components (see Table 58–3). Which component is critical in initiating the formation of stones? Several investigators have attempted to answer this question. Pak (1973, 1987) and his colleagues proposed that supersaturation of urine with calcium and phosphate followed by precipitation of brushite was the nucleus for formation of calcium stones. They not only substantiated this theory by in vitro testing in their own laboratories but also indicated that stone analyses often showed that the nidus of a calculus was indeed calcium phosphate, even though the surface growth was calcium oxalate (Elliot, 1973a; Prien, 1974). The form of phosphate that is present is apatite, however, not brushite, and not all stones have phosphate nuclei.

Other investigators have approached the problem of stone activity differently. As mentioned previously, Robertson and colleagues (1976) have proposed a method of evaluation in which the ionic activity products of urinary calcium, phosphorus, and oxalate are compared with the total amount of crystal inhibition present. When the ion product of these substances increases enough or the inhibition factors decrease enough, crystallization and presumably urinary stone formation occur.

Gill and colleagues (1974) have proposed a method of estimation of stone-forming activity in which a radioisotopic dilution procedure measures the degree of supersaturation of calcium and oxalate in urine. When urinary supersaturation of these patients reaches a critical point, therapy could be initiated. Sarig and colleagues (1982) have, as noted previously, devised a diagnostic index (DI) derived from the rapidity of calcium oxalate precipitation in urines. Those who are stone formers could be distinguished from normal individuals with an error rate of 13.5 per cent. The inverse error rate is 19.2 per cent.

Marshall and Barry (1973) observed that saturation of urine with calcium oxalate exists in patients with pure oxalate stones, but saturation with calcium phosphate and calcium oxalate exists in patients with mixed calculi. Hence, it becomes necessary to measure urine saturation with both components to correctly predict calcium stone formation activity.

Breslau and Pak (1980), Pak and associates (1985), and Pak (1987) have described methods for such estimation using an activity product ratio (APR) to predict saturation of urine with calcium oxalate or phosphate. They also estimate a formation product ratio (FPR) that gives an upper border for the limit of metastability of urine (see Fig. 58–6), or the point at which spontaneous nucleation of crystals will occur. This limit is found to be lower in those who form stones than in normal persons. This finding implies that afflicted patients have less crystallization inhibitor in the urine, or alternately, the inhibitors are less effective than those of normal persons (Nakagawa et al., 1987; Worchester et al., 1987).

All of these investigations attempt both to approach the problem of nucleation, growth, and aggregation of urinary calculi and to define those individuals who are actively forming calcium stones (i.e., they have a high risk of stone formation) (Pak et al., 1985). A tendency toward calcium urolithiasis persists for such a long period (Sutherland et al., 1985) that it is necessary to know, if possible, when patients are at high risk of stone formation. At that time, they can be treated with medication, whereas taking medication for 10 years to avoid the production of one calculus is not satisfactory to most patients. Perhaps we will soon be able to predict when stone formation becomes "active." Therapy can then be initiated or increased. Until then, we must simply apply our clinical judgment and treat those patients who have recurrent symptomatic calcium stone disease.

Classification of Patients with Calcium Urolithiasis

Therapy of calcigerous urinary calculi is based primarily on the identification of any primary factors that may cause disease. Therefore, patients are first categorized according to the presence of any other metabolic disease that may be contributing to the problem. Patients with hyperparathyroidism are treated by exploration and parathyroidectomy (Sherwood, 1988). Therapy for RTA consists of correction of the acidosis and potassium imbalance, including administration of bicarbonate and/or citrate solutions of sufficient quantity to bring serum pH back to normal.

Patients who develop calculi in association with other metabolic disease (see Table 58–10) should be treated for those diseases first. Stone formation usually ceases. Any residual stones can be treated subsequently. If none of the foregoing diseases is present, we must search for the defect likely to be associated with "idiopathic" calcium urinary calculi (see Table 58–8).

Evaluation of Patients with Calcium Urolithiasis

The minimum basic evaluation of any patient with calcium urolithiasis is presented in Table 58–12. Some commercially available packages now allow the performance of these serum (SMAC-20) and urinary (Pak et al., 1985) tests from any physician's office at a modest cost. Performance of the studies indicated will rule out the overt presence of most of the diseases mentioned in Table 58–10 and in previous portions of this section.

Utilizing these study results, patients with hyperparathyroidism, RTA, hyperoxaluria, hyperthyroidism, vitamin D intoxication, sarcoidosis, and hypercalciuria related to a hypercorticoid state (which may be drug-induced) can often be identified.

In some instances, however, certain metabolic diseases may be barely perceptible, as in "normocalcemic hyperparathyroidism" or "incomplete renal tubular acidosis." Such patients have usually been initially classified as having "idiopathic hypercalciuria." If stone formation continues in spite of apparently correct therapy, a complete metabolic evaluation by a team specializing in the study of calcium stone formation is usually advisable.

Table 58–12. LABORATORY EVALUATION OF THE PATIENT WITH METABOLICALLY ACTIVE CALCIUM UROLITHIASIS*

Serum	24 hr Urine
Creatinine	Creatinine
Sodium	Sodium
Potassium	Chloride
Carbon dioxide	Calcium
Chloride	Phosphorus
Calcium (fasting)†	Magnesium
Phosphorus	Citrate
Uric acid	Uric acid
Magnesium	Oxalate
Total protein	Culture
Albumin	Fasting pH ($\times$ 3)
Thyroid function tests	
Serum pH	

*Metabolically active–defined by Smith (1974a) as formation of more than one stone per year. Except for pH tests and culture, a 24-hour collection is preferred.
†Serum parathyroid hormone is determined if any serum calcium exceeds 10 mg/dl.

When a preliminary survey results in no obvious diagnosis of severe metabolic disease, a case is usually placed in the classification of "idiopathic hypercalciuria" or "acquired hyperoxaluria." Treatment is similar, and precise evaluation and classification beyond this point is at present not productive. Some hints may be gained from evaluation, however.

Figure 58–5 illustrates the cumulative effects on calcium solubility in urine of certain organic and inorganic inhibitors. Drach (1976b) and others have studied urinary constituents in patients who form stones. Patients who have "idiopathic" stone formation tend to have one or more urinary excesses or deficiencies that may promote formation of calcium stones. These include absorptive or renal leak hypercalciuria (Pak et al., 1974, 1975; Pak, 1987), hyperoxaluria due to dietary excess or intestinal disease (Smith, 1974a; Thomas, 1974), lack of urinary magnesium (Drach 1976b; Lehmann and Gray, 1989; Oreopoulos et al., 1975), and excessive uric acid (Coe and Raisen, 1973; Coe and Davalach, 1974; Coe and Parks, 1988). In general, patients are placed on some type of therapy directed at alleviating the most obvious abnormality found in the urine. As noted previously, Robertson and co-workers (1979b) have combined six of these urinary risk factors in urine into one "risk factor index," which seems to correlate well with incidence of recurrent stone formation. Pak and associates (1985) analyze for fifteen risk factors.

Therapy for Idiopathic Calcium Urolithiasis

A large group of individuals form idiopathic calcium oxalate/phosphate stones. They have some small urinary abnormality. Therapeutic advice to these patients has been extensive and variable over the years, but several general treatment factors are valid. The maintenance of a large fluid intake and high urinary output with avoidance of dehydration are critical preventive measures. Whenever the urinary concentration of calcium oxalate and phosphate can be reduced by increased water drinking, the risk of stone formation is reduced (Finlayson, 1974). Some patients, however, because of their lifestyle or because of excessive absorption or excretion of calcium, oxalate, or phosphate, are unable to increase their water drinking.

These patients should be advised to avoid excessive amounts of calcium and oxalate in their diets. The amount of phosphate in the diet does not seem to be critical, and excess dietary phosphate may actually bind gut calcium. A typical low-calcium, low-oxalate diet is included in Appendix B. Carbohydrate-induced hypercalciuria can be decreased by avoiding excessive dietary carbohydrate and by drinking fluids when eating carbohydrates. Interestingly, low-calcium, low-oxalate diets tend also to be low-carbohydrate diets.

In addition to the treatment cornerstones of increased fluid intake and dietary restriction, some medications may be helpful in the treatment of calcigerous urinary calculi. These drugs and their uses are summarized in Table 58–13. Controversy continues about whether commonly administered oral neutral phosphates, sodium

Table 58–13. DRUG TREATMENT FOR CALCIUM STONE DISEASE

Drug	Postulated Effect	Average Adult Dosage	Contraindications	Side Effects
Neutral phosphate	Increases solubility of calcium	500 mg 3 times a day	Urinary infection or poor renal function	Diarrhea
Cellulose phosphate	Binds calcium in gut	10 to 15 gm q.d.	Same as above	Diarrhea
Magnesium oxide or gluconate	Increases urinary magnesium; decreases urinary calcium	150 mg 4 times a day	Urinary infection or poor renal function	Diarrhea
Hydrochlorthiazide	Same as above	25 to 50 mg 2 times a day	Hypokalemia, other diuretics	Hypokalemia
Citrate	Increases citrate, lowers calcium	15 mEq 3 times a day	Renal insufficiency	Sodium retention
Allopurinol	Lowers serum uric acid	300 mg/day	Previous sensitivity	Activates gout

cellulose phosphate, or oral thiazides (Thomas, 1975; Pak, 1987; Yendt and Cohanim, 1973) constitute the better therapy for calcium urolithiasis. Table 58–14 attempts to summarize the pros and cons regarding these medications.

When thiazides are given as therapy for calcium urinary calculi, the response is usually based on decreased urinary calcium excretion. Hence, these drugs are especially helpful in hypercalciuric patients. This effect requires reduced vascular volume. Increased dietary salt intake and increased vascular volume negate the hypocalciuric effects of thiazides and promote hypercalciuria (Breslau et al., 1982). It is therefore advisable for patients who receive thiazide treatment to restrict dietary salt intake to that necessary in cooking.

Physicians sometimes question which medication should be selected initially in treating patients with stones. Table 58–15 summarizes a method I use, which is based on defects in the urine or serum as detected by a simple office protocol (Drach, 1976b, 1987). This protocol combines many of the testing practices of Pak (1987), Broadus and co-workers (1978), and Coe and Parks (1988). As Coe and Parks have stated: "In stone disease, everything is measurement. What the laboratory cannot tell you, you will not know; what it tells you in error, you will not correct by using your instincts, your medical experience or your art; what you take from your measurements directs your treatment."

One usually prescribes a drug that is designed to correct the most obvious urinary defect and is not otherwise contraindicated for that patient. Several other drugs have been proposed, especially in Europe. Cellulose phosphate has been used clinically in Europe and

is now used in the United States (Pak et al., 1974, 1987). Its mode of action is similar to that of neutral phosphate tablets—gut calcium is bound by phosphate and not absorbed. However, cellulose phosphate avoids the sodium or potassium overload that is sometimes associated with neutral phosphate tablets (Pak, 1987). One potential problem associated with any oral phosphate is that urinary oxalate excretion is apparently increased (Elliot et al., 1970).

Diphosphonates have also been proposed to prevent calcium urinary stones. Reports about these substances and their efficacy have not yet been proven (Ohata and Pak, 1974). Several potentially serious complications, especially osteomalacia, have been reported. Hence, we have a limited number of drugs that appear to affect calcium urolithiasis beneficially.

In most patients, however, the drugs listed in Table 58–13 have been effective in reducing the long-term incidence of urinary stone disease. Approximately 90 per cent of patients so treated may expect cessation of new stone formation (Coe, 1977; Coe and Parks 1988; Pak, 1987).

Investigators are still looking for the perfect treatment for stone disease. Perhaps the most frustrating aspect of stone disease is its intermittent activity (Table 58–16). Patients who are in treatment may decide that they are cured after several years and stop treatment, only to discover that the disease returns after medication and dietary treatment stop (Sutherland et al., 1985). Also, many experts believe that the overall incidence of calcium stone disease is increasing. More attention to specific etiologic factors; prediction of "activity of stone disease," such as "stone-risk profiles"; and development

Table 58–14. ORAL PHOSPHATES VERSUS THIAZIDES

Phosphates		Thiazides	
Benefits	*Problems*	*Benefits*	*Problems*
Urine calcium decreases	Diarrhea	Dosage once or twice daily	Hypokalemia
Urinary crystals decrease	Risk of infection	No diarrhea	Hyperuricemia
	Urine oxalate increased	No apparent risk if infection occurs	
	Large tablets	Urine calcium decreases	"Weakness"
	Gastritis		

Table 58–15. HINTS AT SELECTION OF PATIENTS FOR CALCIUM STONE THERAPY

Serum or Urinary Defect Found	Therapy Likely to Succeed
Hypercalcemia and hypercalciuria with elevated parathyroid hormone	Surgical removal of abnormal parathyroid glands
Hypercalcemia, hypervitaminosis D	Stop excessive vitamin D
Hypercalciuria, immobilization	Exercises, large fluid output, low-calcium diet
Hypercalciuria, hyperthyroidism	Treat hyperthyroidism
Hypercalciuria, hyperabsorption	Neutral or cellulose phosphates
Hypercalciuria, renal leak	Thiazides
Normocalciuria, low citrate	Oral citrates
Relative hypercalciuria, magnesium deficit	Magnesium oxide or gluconate
Hyperuricemia and hyperuricosuria with calcium urolithiasis	Allopurinol
Intestinal hyperabsorption, hyperoxaluria	Low oxalate diet plus citrate, magnesium gluconate

of specific therapeutic measures are necessary before calcium urolithiasis disease can be brought under control.

Rare Forms

Matrix Calculi

Matrix calculi are found predominantly in individuals with infections due to urease-producing organisms. *Proteus* species are especially likely to be associated with matrix calculi. Boyce (1968) has defined matrix calculi as those stones composed of coagulated mucoids with very little crystalline component. Several clinical reports of these stones have appeared (Allen and Spence, 1966; Mall et al., 1975). They are radiolucent and may be confused with uric acid calculi. However, their association with alkaline urinary tract infection usually assists in making a presumptive diagnosis, because uric acid calculi are usually formed in acid, sterile urine. In most instances, surgical manipulation is required for their removal, because they are not dissolved by any means yet known.

Ammonium Acid Urate Calculi

Two conditions predispose the patient to this rare type of stone, which accounts for about 0.2 per cent of all stones. The first is urealytic infection in the presence of excessive uric acid excretion, and the second is urinary phosphate deficiency plus the low fluid intake found in children of developing countries (Hsu, 1966; Klohn et al., 1986). Treatment involves eradication of infection and clearance of infected stone or restoration of normal phosphate metabolism (Klohn et al., 1986).

Hereditary Xanthinuria

Hereditary xanthinuria results in the production of xanthine calculus. This rare calculus is also radiolucent and may be confused with uric acid calculus. Radiographic crystallographic analysis of the stone is usually necessary to confirm this type of calculus. Quantitative urinary chromatography for xanthine reveals the presence of excessive excretion of this substance. No effective therapy exists (Dent and Philpot, 1954; Frayha et al., 1973; Pearlman, 1950). Occasionally, patients who are given allopurinol for treatment of uric acid urolithiasis or gout will begin to form xanthine calculi (Seegmiller, 1968) because allopurinol blocks conversion of xanthine to uric acid. The most specific therapy for xanthine stone appears to be increased urinary volume.

Silicate Calculi

Silicate urinary calculi occur in domestic animals with some degree of frequency (Joekes et al., 1973), but they are extremely rare in humans. Patients who have chronically taken large doses of silicate-containing antacids have developed small silicate calculi (Joekes et al., 1973; Haddad and Kouyoumdjian, 1986). Stone analysis is necessary to ascertain this type of calculus, although low

Table 58–16. ESTIMATION OF STONE DISEASE ACTIVITY AND NEED FOR TREATMENT*

Condition	Symptoms and Signs	Recommend
Surgically active	Renal colic Obstruction Infection Intractable pain	Urologic consultation for possible procedural treatment
Metabolically active	Formation of new stone within the past year Growth of known stone within the past year Documented passage of stone or gravel within the past year	Preventive measures†plus; specific drugs (Table 58–13)
Metabolically and surgically active	None of the above for 1 year	Preventive measures only†; observation
Indeterminate	Uncertain activity or period of observation less than 1 year	Preventive measures only†; observation

*After Smith, L.H.: Urol. Clin. North Am., 1:241, 1974a.
†Refers to increased daily urinary volume and appropriate diet. See text.

radiographic density may provide a hint about their composition. Treatment is directed toward the alteration of antacid therapy.

Triamterene Calculi

Triamterene is often given singly or in combination with hydrochlorothiazide in the treatment of hypertension. This combination tends to avoid potassium depletion, which may result from oral hydrochlorothiazide alone. Unfortunately, however, a few patients may incorporate triamterene into stones or have stones composed almost entirely of triamterene (0.4 per cent of 50,000 calculi) (Sorgel et al., 1985). Finlayson states that "From a kinetic viewpoint, it is fair to say that the percentage of triamterene in a stone is an index of the degree to which it accelerated stone growth." It seems, therefore, that triamterene should be used with great caution in those patients who form stones (Ettinger et al., 1980; Werness et al., 1982).

2,8-Hydroxyadenine Calculi

These very rare, radiolucent calculi occur in the presence of deficient adenine phosphoribosyl transferase, an inherited metabolic defect. Both homozygous and heterozygous genotypes have produced this condition. Treatment should be low-purine diet and oral allopurinol administration (Witten et al., 1983).

Spurious Calculi

Spurious or "fake" urinary calculi are not at all unusual. Most laboratories report that approximately 1 to 2 per cent of all calculi submitted are produced outside the human body. Sutor and O'Flynn (1973) reported one patient who inserted boiler scale into her bladder in order to mimic the production of urinary calculi. In this case it was observed that although matrix was not present when boiler scale was formed on the boiler, it did infiltrate the entire substance of the calculus after it had been placed in the bladder.

I was acquainted with a patient whose wife stated that she had extracted urinary calculi from his urethra, and the patient was thus convinced that he had calculi. It was only after confrontation with the fact that the calculi were composed of standard creekbed stones that the wife admitted that she had palmed the calculi, placed them in the urethra, and subsequently expelled them under the eyes of her husband.

The emergency rooms of North America's hospitals are occasionally visited by individuals who fake urinary calculous disease (usually due to "uric acid stones") for secondary gain to obtain drugs (Sharon and Diamond, 1974). As mentioned previously, the standard story of these individuals is that they know they have stone disease, uric acid stone disease, and that they are allergic to intravenous urogram dye.

A high degree of suspicion is in order when an individual from out of town arrives in the emergency room with this story, has a severe degree of pain, and dramatizes this pain to an excessive degree. Several

patients have developed a true Münchausen's syndrome and have traveled the United States with supposed stone disease (Atkinson and Earll, 1974). However, it is better for the physician to give an addict meperidine than to mistakenly withhold it from a true sufferer of ureteral colic.

URINARY LITHIASIS IN CHILDREN

Prior to this century, the major incidence of urinary lithiasis was bladder stones in children. As nations increased productivity and moved into the industrial age, average income and therefore food quality have improved. These events have resulted in the gradual disappearance of endemic bladder stone disease from previously afflicted populations. Such stones are now found mostly in North Africa, the Middle and Near East, Burma, Thailand, and Indonesia (Van Reen, 1981).

Most pediatric bladder calculi in endemic areas are composed of ammonium acid urate (Brockis et al., 1981), calcium oxalate, or mixtures thereof. Urine pH in such children is nearly always acidic in the absence of infection (Aurora et al., 1970). In the presence of infection, struvite stone becomes more common. Infection seems to be an unusual complication of an uninstrumented child with bladder stone. Perhaps the occurrence of such stones can be traced to the common practice in endemic areas of feeding infants human breast milk and cereal foods, such as polished rice or millet. Human breast milk, in contrast to cow's milk, is very low in phosphorus, as is polished rice (Andersen, 1962; Thalut et al., 1976). Such low-phosphate diets result in high peaks of urinary ammonia excretion (Brockis et al., 1981). Perhaps also important, Valyasevi and Dhanamitta (1974) showed that ingestion of vegetable oxalate contributed to the high degree of crystalluria often seen in these children. They fed the children oral neutral orthophosphate and stated that such supplementation ". . . practically eliminated (calcium oxalate) crystalluria and crystal clumping."

Anatomic urologic disease, such as obstruction and reflux, may coexist with bladder stone of nutritional etiology. Taneja and colleagues (1970) have recommended that such children undergo complete urologic study: voiding cystourethrogram, intravenous urography, and endoscopic examination. They base this recommendation on the occurrence of obstructive lesions in 38.5 per cent and reflux in 41 per cent of 52 afflicted children who were studied completely.

If we exclude endemic bladder calculi of children in developing countries, we observe that the majority of urinary stones of children affect the upper tracts, just as in adults. The subject of childhood urolithiasis in industrialized countries has been ably reviewed by a number of workers (see Borgmann and Nagel, 1982; Choi et al., 1987; Malek and Kelalis, 1975; Mitchell, 1981; Noe et al., 1983; O'Regan et al., 1982; Paulson, 1972, 1974; Steele et al., 1983).

It appears from the aforementioned reviews that the incidence of stones in patients under 15 or 16 years of age is about 7 per cent of all patients seen for stones (Borgmann and Nagel, 1982). The male:female ratio is 1:1, which differs from the 3:1 or 4:1 ratio of adults. Two major types of stones occur: (1) lower or upper tract stones associated with infection and neurogenic bladder or urologic anomaly and (2) "idiopathic" stones. Some 20 to 30 per cent of children with stones present with painless hematuria. Exclusion of stone disease becomes one of the most important aspects of the differential diagnosis of painless hematuria of children. Stapleton and colleagues (1984) propose that unexplained hematuria of children is related to hypercalciuria and may exist long before clinical stone disease becomes apparent.

In a preliminary study, Stapleton and colleagues (1982) studied 21 children who had uncomplicated calcium urolithiasis. These workers demonstrated that significant hypercalciuria occurred in children who form stones. It is necessary to set different limits and standards of calcium excretion for children, e.g., renal hypercalciuria if fasting UCa/UCr exceeded 0.21 and absorptive hypercalciuria if post-calcium load UCa/UCr exceeded 0.31. Perhaps this is the reason that many previous investigators did not report hypercalciuria in the studies of pediatric urolithiasis. Noe, who was a participant in the aforementioned study, subsequently reported that 91 per cent of 47 pediatric urinary stone patients had "factors causing or predisposing to stone disease (Noe et al., 1983)." Of these, 53 per cent had metabolic causes; 19 per cent, urologic anomalies; 15 per cent, infectious causes; and 4 per cent, immobilization syndrome. The remaining 9 per cent remain unexplained.

Children with urolithiasis also may have classic metabolic diseases, such as hyperparathyroidism, renal tubular acidosis, cystinuria (Pavanello et al., 1981), and primary hyperoxaluria, or diseases that produce an excessive excretion of uric acid, such as Lesch-Nyhan syndrome and leukemia. Any metabolic evaluation should include screening for these defects.

Adolescents are not spared urinary lithiasis. Rambar and MacKenzie (1978) studied 31 adolescents who had stones. In 13 per cent, the stones were related to inborn errors of metabolism, such as cystinuria or primary oxalosis. Three of these patients developed stones in transplanted kidneys. Some type of procedure was required in 22 (71 per cent) to relieve stone obstruction or a related problem.

Other investigators (Borgmann and Nagel, 1982; Noe et al., 1983) report the need for procedural intervention in 70 to 94 per cent of pediatric urolithiasis patients. Interestingly, once the surgical correction has been performed, the recurrence rate for stones in the pediatric age group seems to be lower than that for adults, or at least "no greater" than for adults (Diamond et al., 1989; Steele et al., 1983).

Diagnosis of urinary calculous disease in children is similar to that in adults. Findings include pain (although 20 to 30 per cent present with painless hematuria as noted earlier), hematuria, and radiologic evidence of calculi. One significant radiologic difference has been reported by Breatnach and Smith (1983). In a group of 50 children who had intravenous urography for calculi, "Increased nephrographic density was never seen" and "The adult intravenous urogram pattern of acute ureteric obstruction was not seen." Because 80 per cent of these children had associated urinary infections, generalized ureteral dilation and caliectasis were quite common and may have masked the typical radiologic signs of stone obstruction. The occurrence of lucent calculi (uric acid and, to some degree, cystine) requires urography. Radiolucency has been reported to approach 10 per cent of childhood calculi (Rambar and MacKenzie, 1978; Steele et al., 1983), but the more common incidence for radiolucent calculi in children approximates 3 to 4 per cent (Borgmann and Nagel, 1982).

Some physicians tend to avoid intravenous urography in younger children because of excessive radiation exposure. Certainly, genitalia and gonads should be shielded whenever possible. Higher degrees of radiation can be avoided by the performance of a tailored urogram. Only those radiographs necessary to make a proper diagnosis are taken. This technique requires the attention of the urologist or radiologist. Imaging by ultrasound methods can illustrate stones effectively, also.

Treatment of children is similar to that of adults and, as noted earlier, often includes initial procedural treatment or removal of stones and correction of any urinary defects. Most agree that thorough metabolic evaluation of children is warranted in order to discover the cause of the urolithiasis. Thereafter, appropriate therapy can be assigned. The usual admonitions to increase fluid intake and output seem universally accepted. Cystinuria, primary hyperoxaluria, hyperuricosuria, and rarer forms of stone disease respond to the specific therapies noted previously. Hypercalciuria has been treated by dietary limitation of calcium and oxalate with or without neutral orthophosphates (Noe et al., 1983). These investigators have also treated renal leak hypercalciuria with thiazides (2 mg/kg/day), but thiazide therapy in children has been questioned (Steele et al., 1983). Recurrence rates of stones in children vary according to the type (Diamond et al., 1989); an overall rate of 16 per cent was described, with a duration of recurrence that spanned 3 to 6 years. Long-term observation of children for recurrence becomes as important as that of adults.

SPECIFIC LOCATIONS OF CALCULI

Renal Calculi

Calculi too large to pass spontaneously range in size from 1 cm to the staghorn stones that occupy the renal pelvis and calyces. Minimally invasive therapy is usually necessary. Occasionally, in a patient in poor general health, an asymptomatic staghorn calculus may be discovered during the course of a general health examination. In such a patient, if the function of the second kidney is adequate, a conservative policy of observation may be advisable but only if it is clearly understood that if sepsis, pain, or evidence of decreased function should appear, intervention may be required (Dretler, 1990; Libertino et al., 1971).

Individual consideration of each patient's problem is necessary. The urologist's clinical judgment may be taxed to the utmost in some instances to determine whether to pursue a policy of watchful waiting or immediate intervention.

Bilateral renal calculi cause additional problems. In many instances, infection is present. Surgical or procedural intervention is not always advisable in a patient with bilateral stones. Aged persons with bilateral renal calculi may live fairly comfortably and eventually succumb to other disease. In such a patient, operation or intervention can be a hazardous procedure. In a younger patient with the same type of bilateral lithiasis, some type of intervention may be advisable in the hope of preserving renal function and of eliminating infection in the urinary tract.

Individualization of each patient's problem is essential in planning treatment for renal lithiasis. As a general rule, it is better to lean toward conservatism and preservation of renal function in regard to procedural treatment.

Ureteral Calculi—Some Specific Considerations

Site of Origin

Ureteral calculi originate in the kidney and then pass into the ureter. Their causes are thus the same as those of renal lithiasis. Calculi that develop primarily in the ureter are rare, perhaps because the smooth mucosal lining of the ureter is constantly bathed with urine. Accumulations of crystals are thereby promptly washed into the bladder. Reports indicate that in those rare instances in which ureteral stones are primary, they have been formed in association with ureteroceles, neoplasms, ureters with blind endings, ectopic ureters, sacculations, or dilated segments of the ureter proximal to a stricture.

Sites of Impaction

Certain anatomic characteristics determine where a stone may become impacted, as it moves down the ureter. The points of relative constriction discussed earlier in this section occur at or just below the ureteropelvic junction (see Figs. 58–12 and 58–13); where the ureter crosses the iliac vessels; at the base of the broad ligament in women and at the area of the vas deferens in men; where the ureter enters the external muscular coat of the bladder; and at the vesical orifice. Two points of angulation also are present: (1) at the place where the ureter crosses the iliac vessels and enters the true pelvis and (2) at the point where it enters the bladder.

Size, Weight, and Shape

The size of the ureteral calculus is of considerable importance clinically, but of equal importance is the caliber of the ureter below the stone. Calculi range in size from a few millimeters to 10 cm in length and width.

Stones that weigh more than 0.1 g, have a diameter of more than 1 cm, or are associated with urinary infection are not as likely to pass spontaneously (Sutor and Wooley, 1975). Some ureteral calculi become very large. Heath (1922) removed a calculus 2.5 by 15 cm that weighed 65.8 g. Tennant (1924) removed a ureteral stone that weighed 66 g. Joly (1931) cites one case reported by Federoff in which the calculus weighed 52 g. Despite occasional reports of giant stones, ureteral calculi are rarely more than 2 g in weight.

Their shape often varies according to the length of time the stone has been in the ureter. A calculus recently expelled from the kidney is usually round or ovoid. After stones have resided in the ureter for some time, the longitudinal diameter becomes much greater than the transverse. The stone also becomes more cylindrical in shape.

If the calculus resides inside a very dilated ureter, the stone may remain round, move freely in the ureter, and act as a ball valve. Multiple calculi may also remain round or ovoid in a dilated ureter. Alternately, they may become faceted as they rub beside one another in undilated ureters, in which free movement is not possible. Greatly elongated calculi in the pelvic portion of the ureter may even assume the curvature of this segment.

In the majority of patients, a single stone develops. In a series of 350 cases of ureteral calculi seen at the Cleveland Clinic, Higgins (1939) noted the presence of multiple ureteral stones in only seven and bilateral ureteral calculi in six patients. Braasch and Moore (1915) observed multiple stones in 17 patients in a series of 278 cases of ureteral stones.

Laterality

Ureteral calculi are almost equally frequent on the left and right sides, although in certain patients stone formation seems to be limited to one side. Kretschmer (1942), in a review of 500 cases, stated that 45.8 per cent of calculi were on the right side and 51.8 per cent, on the left. Two national studies on extracorporeal or percutaneous lithotripsy also reported a slight preponderance of left-sided stones (about 45 per cent right and 55 per cent left) (Drach et al., 1986; Segura et al., 1985). Bumpus and Thompson (1925) and Scholl (1936) reported that ureteral calculi were observed with equal frequency on the two sides. In Higgins's series, 47 per cent were present in the right ureter and 53 per cent in the left.

Composition

Because ureteral calculi originate in the kidney, they have the same chemical composition as renal stones. Small calculi of calcium oxalate occur most frequently. Uric acid, cystine, and struvite stones occur less commonly but can be more difficult to define because of their decreased radiodensity. If infection supervenes, layers of struvite may be formed over previously deposited substances such as uric acid. The unusual radiographic appearance of stones with "hollow" centers results.

Pathologic Changes Caused by Ureteral Calculi

Impaction of calculi in the ureter produces various pathologic changes influenced by the extent and duration of obstruction and the presence or absence of infection (see previous section on pathophysiology of obstruction).

Periureteritis and ureteritis may be pronounced in the area around the calculus. Calculi may rarely ulcerate through the ureter. At the site of impaction the ureter is usually fixed to the adjacent fat and contiguous structures by inflammatory changes. In early stages, the extent of linear dilatation of the ureter proximal to the calculus may be pronounced. In later stages, tortuosity develops and the ureter is thickened. Microscopically, round cell infiltration and fibrosis are observed. The degree of ureteral inflammation is also increased by infection, which also reduces ureteral peristalsis and may therefore contribute to greater dilatation of the ureter proximal to the calculus (Rose et al., 1975).

Symptoms

A calculus passing down the ureter often causes symptoms of colic, as previously described (see section Acute Stone Episode). Patients may experience a single attack of colic followed by the expulsion of the stone, or they may experience several episodes, as the calculus traverses the course of the ureter more slowly. The first pain is usually severe and occurs in the flank in the region of the costovertebral angle. Later, pain is sometimes felt in the region of the umbilicus and may follow the course of the ureter through the posterior abdomen, or it may be referred to the genitalia. As the stone nears the bladder, the patient may experience frequency, urgency, and strangury. Dysuria and tenesmus may be pronounced. The pain of renal colic may sometimes be referred to the perineum, bladder, penis, or testicles.

Stone impaction in the ureter may also cause atypical symptoms. Unusual referral of ureteral colic pain to the thigh, hip, or knee has been reported. In Higgins's series (1939), only 56 per cent of patients gave a fairly typical history of an attack of colic with subsequent intermittent pain or discomfort. On other occasions, the pain of colic may become relatively steady and fixed, although it is often aggravated by exertion. On the right side, pain caused by a ureteral stone may falsely suggest cholecystitis or appendicitis.

Roentgenographic Observations

In the review of 100 cases, Peterson and Holmes (1937) found that 96 per cent of the calculi were diagnosed through roentgenographic study and only 4 per cent were "invisible." Today, ultrasound imaging can reveal most of these radiographically invisible stones (Juul et al., 1987; Middleton et al., 1988). As noted, the shadow cast by a stone that has been in the ureter for some time is elongated and fusiform, with the long axis parallel to the course of the ureter.

If the stone cannot be seen and the procedure is not contraindicated by some other condition, excretory uro-

gram, ultrasound imaging, or radionuclide study should be obtained. The status of both kidneys is determined, and the degree of hydronephrosis and the intensity of obstruction of the kidney are implied from one of these studies. The degree of dilatation of the ureter above the calculus is noted.

Failure to visualize contrast medium or radioisotope when obstruction is complete does not signify that the kidney is destroyed and functionless. Significant renal function may return after obstruction is relieved, especially when the obstruction is recent. In many instances, enough information results from these studies to allow decisions to be made about immediate management of the patient. Dourmashkin (1945) stated that routine retrograde pyelography should be avoided in cases of calculous ureteral obstruction that cause no diagnostic problem and that may be evaluated by other means. Of a series of 1550 cases of ureteral calculi, retrograde pyelography was resorted to in only 118 cases, chiefly in patients with uric acid calculi or in those in whom the stone was not recognized immediately for various reasons. These observations remain typical nearly 50 years later.

It may be difficult to differentiate shadows cast by ureteral stones from those made by intestinal contents, mesenteric glands, phleboliths, atheromatous plaques, or lesions on the skin. Intestinal contents rarely cause confusion in the diagnosis if the patient is properly prepared before roentgenographic study. Mesenteric glands move with changes in position and usually do not have a uniform density. Phleboliths in pelvic veins may be confused with ureteral stones. Phleboliths usually are round and cast dense shadows lateral to the course of the normal ureter. Their centers are often radiolucent.

Factors That Influence Choice of Treatment

Few urologic problems require the weighing of so many factors as does treatment of an obstructing calculus in the ureter (Andersen, 1974; Drach, 1978, 1983; Dretler, 1990; Furlow and Bucchiere, 1976). The decision that must be made in each case includes whether some procedure should be performed for immediate relief of the obstruction; whether shock wave lithotripsy or stone manipulation should be done; or whether a period of watchful waiting should be undertaken. The most significant factors to be considered in making decisions about proper management of each case are detailed in the following discussion.

The economic status and occupation of the patient influence the type of treatment to be carried out. A sudden attack of recurrent ureteral colic in persons who work with machinery, engineers, or pilots may endanger their lives and the lives of those around them or dependent on them. A laborer who has a stone passing slowly down the upper ureter (with arrest of its progress from time to time occasioning severe attacks of colic) may frequently be restored more rapidly to gainful occupation with no greater financial burden when the calculus is removed by means of a simple manipulation or lithotripsy.

Duration of symptoms is another important factor. The patient who has had repeated episodes of severe colic deserves relief. When the symptoms and obstruction are of long duration, further delay in treatment may lead to irreparable renal damage. Should one wait 2 days or 2 weeks for spontaneous passage of a stone? In one older series of 350 cases of ureteral calculi, 54.1 per cent of the stones that passed spontaneously did so within 16 days after the patient was first examined (Higgins, 1939). Yet we know that the size of the calculus also influences the clinical course and the choice of treatment. As noted previously (see Fig. 58–14), the larger the calculus (over 4 mm), the less likely it is that it will pass spontaneously (Cartstensen and Hansen, 1973). These investigators also report that over 90 per cent of these small calculi will pass within 3 months.

Status of renal function is a prime consideration in making decisions about treatment for ureteral stones. When the excretory urogram or sonogram reveals slight hydronephrosis or dilatation of the ureter above the calculus, it signifies that the urine is flowing around the stone and that the stone is causing little obstruction. If repeat studies reveal little or no progress in the descent of the calculus but no worsening of obstruction, one may wait for spontaneous passage. Any progressive obstruction must be relieved. Cessation of pain does not always mean that obstruction has been relieved but may signify onset of complete obstruction. If there is any doubt about the degree of obstruction of an impacted stone, repeat intravenous urogram or radioisotope studies are indicated.

The preferred method of treatment for ureteral calculi should have as its prime objective the preservation of function of the kidney on the affected side. Clinical evidence of renal damage, which is confirmed by intravenous urograms indicating complete ureteral obstruction, or a progressively enlarging hydronephrosis sonographically, signifies that conservative treatment is unwarranted. Procedural intervention should be instituted promptly.

The degree of impaction also contributes to deciding on the course of treatment. A stone that remains in the same position week after week probably will not pass spontaneously. If the stone has not moved downward within a period of 2 weeks, watchful waiting should be abandoned and other methods of treatment should be instituted. The status of the opposite kidney must always be kept in mind. In patients with a solitary kidney, any continuing obstruction is grave and demands relief.

The age and general condition of the patient may influence the procedure to be advocated. Elderly, debilitated patients may not tolerate instrumentation or anesthesia well. Hence, anesthesia-free, noninvasive measures represent a possible best choice. In a child, because of the technical difficulty in passing a cystoscope of adequate size, the lack of complete cooperation, and the necessity for repeated administration of anesthetic, procedural surgery with minimal anesthetic is frequently the best approach.

In the presence of an obstructing calculus, infection is usually indicated by hyperpyrexia and leukocytosis. Prompt intervention with establishment of free drainage (percutaneous nephrostomy or insertion of a ureteral stent) is a lifesaving measure and may prevent the development of gram-negative bacteremia. In elderly men, associated disease such as prostatic hypertrophy may make cystoscopic manipulative procedures technically difficult. In such cases, lithotripsy "in situ" or after percutaneous nephrostomy drainage may be the preferred procedure.

In general, a small (< 6 mm) ureteral stone, accompanied by infrequent attacks of colic but not by infection or progressive hydronephrosis, may be observed in the hope that the stone will pass spontaneously. Progression of the calculus is noted by appropriate imaging studies, and the status of the kidney is periodically assured by means of roentgenographic or isotopic studies. If impaction or hydronephrosis occurs, active measures must be taken. Various drugs such as neostigmine and antispasmodics (e.g., atropine) have been used to facilitate the passage of the calculus. Aminophylline, oxyphenbutazone (Tandearil), and other agents have also been suggested (Holmlund, 1974; Lehtonen, 1973), but there are no clear reports of drug effectiveness in promoting stone passage (Peters and Eckstein, 1975; Rutishauser, 1971). Reports of the beneficial effects of glucagon are also inconclusive (Kahnoski et al., 1987). Hence, the results of drug treatment are inconsistent and vary considerably among different studies and urologists.

Manipulation

Braasch and Moore (1915) listed eight contraindications for manipulative treatment of ureteral calculi: (1) when the caliber of the stone exceeds 2 cm; (2) when there is considerable periureteritis; (3) when the kidney is either hydronephrotic or pyohydronephrotic; (4) when the stone is known to have been present for a long time; (5) when several unsuccessful attempts have already been made to remove it; (6) when cystoscopy is poorly tolerated; (7) when congenital anomalies of the genital organs are present; and (8) when a severe febrile reaction or acute pyelonephritis follows the first manipulative procedure. Today, each of these contraindications should caution the urologist. Yet, newer approaches to endoscopic manipulation of calculi allow nearly all ureteral stones to be approached by some form of manipulation (see Chapter 61).

Various mechanical devices have been recommended for stone manipulation. Procedures are discussed in detail in the following three chapters. The large number of instruments available today for the removal of ureteral stones indicates that no one instrument or method is suitable in all instances. Likewise, serious complications may result from the use of such instruments. Perforation of the ureter, ureteral avulsion, stricture, and stone basket incarceration may occur (Drach, 1978; Dretler, 1990).

Currently, the best management approach to small stones in the upper and middle thirds of the ureter in the absence of infection or significant obstruction is one of watchful waiting. If the calculus is 6 mm or less in diameter and moving spontaneously down the ureter, intervention should be delayed. If manipulation becomes advisable, endoscopic catheters, basket extractors, or contact lithotripters are employed. If the stone is in the upper or middle portion of the ureter and is producing complete obstruction, as shown by intravenous urography or another method, some type of procedural intervention is advocated.

The best opportunity to procedurally treat the ureteral stone exists when it reaches the true pelvis. If the stone progresses to the intramural ureter and does not pass spontaneously, a ureteral meatotomy is still an acceptable means of therapy. However, meatotomy may result in reflux or stricture. When manipulative procedures are not feasible for the reasons previously mentioned, and spontaneous expulsion cannot occur, extracorporeal shock wave lithotripsy may still be successful.

Recurrence

The results of procedural treatment for ureteral stone are usually satisfactory. True recurrence of stones in the ureter remains rare. An instance has been reported of a recurrence of primary stone in the ureter, perhaps associated with deposition of phosphates on a suture that had been passed into the lumen of the ureter during its closure after ureterolithotomy (Dalton et al., 1975). Most recurrent ureteral calculi originate in the kidney, however, and lodge again in various portions of the ureter.

The important features in the management of patients with ureteral calculi are prompt diagnosis; early removal of the calculus, whether spontaneously, by manipulative procedures, or by lithotripsy; adequate postoperative evaluation; and possibly prophylactic or specific therapy. These measures usually produce good results.

Surgical Treatment

See Chapter 65.

Vesical Calculi

As mentioned, in certain parts of the world the incidence of vesical calculi is high. In other areas, a steady and pronounced decrease in incidence of stones in the bladder has occurred since the 19th century, when vesical calculi were unusually prevalent. This decrease has been attributed to dietary and nutritional progress.

AGE. As an etiologic factor in calculi of the bladder, age incidence varies in different parts of the world. According to Joly (1931), in England and France during the 19th century, calculous disease was largely limited to children. Now, it is a disease of adults (Hodgkinson and Marshall, 1975). The decrease in vesical calculi in childhood is probably due to improvement in diet and nutrition (see Urinary Lithiasis in Children). In some areas of the world, such as Thailand and Indonesia, bladder calculi continue to occur in children.

SEX. Vesical calculus is predominantly a disease of males of all ages in all races and nationalities. In an older review of calculous disease of the bladder, Thompson (1921) stated that only 2 per cent of cases occurred in women. In the United States, the frequency of vesical calculi in men increases in those over 50. Vesical calculi appear to be definitely associated with obstruction of the bladder neck due to bladder neck contracture, prostatic enlargement, stricture of the urethra, or diverticulum of the bladder.

Hence, in men, factors that give rise to retention of urine, such as stricture of the urethra, prostatic hypertrophy, diverticulum of the bladder, cystoceles, and neurogenic bladder, are associated with the formation of vesical calculi. Urinary infection promotes formation of struvite stones in these patients. Other bladder stones are formed on foreign bodies, such as sutures or catheters, or on objects introduced into the bladder via the urethra by the patient (Fig. 58–35) (Dalton et al., 1975).

COMPOSITION. The composition of the calculus in the bladder is influenced by the pH and degree of saturation of the urine. In the United States, calcium oxalate is the most common constituent of calculi. In Europe, uric acid and urate stones are most prevalent. The bladder is more often infected than the kidney. Therefore, the proportion of struvite calculi due to bladder infection is higher than that of struvite calculi in the kidney.

Usually a single stone is observed in the bladder, but in the presence of retained urine, multiple stones—two or three to 100 or more—may be present in 25 to 30 per cent of cases (Fig. 58–36). Multiple stones are

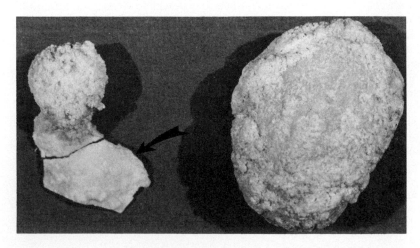

Figure 58–35. Bladder calculi of struvite removed from a patient who had had an indwelling Foley balloon retention catheter for 5 months. Catheter had been removed 3 months previously. Arrow points to thin portion of calculus, which fits the curvature of a catheter balloon.

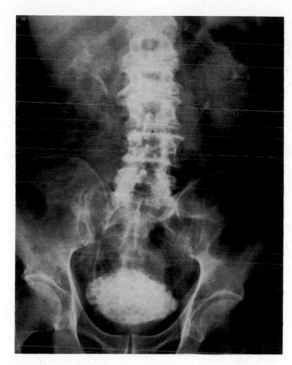

Figure 58–36. This patient with frequency, urgency, and microhematuria had a "normal" plain abdominal radiograph. Intravenous pyelogram revealed hundreds of small uric acid bladder calculi.

formed more frequently when there is a diverticulum of the bladder. Multiple stones may become faceted, and the size of the stones varies tremendously. Randall (1937) described a calculus weighing 1816 g. The longitudinal circumference was 48 cm and the transverse circumference was 40 cm. The bulk of the calculus was composed of calcium phosphate.

PATHOLOGIC CHANGES. In the presence of infection, a smooth stone may be present in the bladder for some time without causing inflammatory changes in the bladder wall. Generally, the calculus produces sufficient mechanical irritation to cause chronic inflammatory changes. With the introduction of infection, bullous edema, pronounced congestion, and ulceration appear.

When the calculus obstructs the urethral orifice, signs of back pressure are evident in the form of coarse trabeculation, with cellule and diverticulum formation. Pus may be noted on the floor of the bladder and on the stone. The bladder wall is thickened, and fibrous tissue reaction occurs in the muscular layer. In cases of long duration, pericystitis may occur, with adherence of the bladder to the adjacent fat in the pelvis. Rarely, perforation of the bladder may occur.

SYMPTOMS. In some patients, especially those with prostatic enlargement and residual urine, there may be no symptoms referable to the bladder calculus or calculi. In such patients, the complaints are predominantly those of prostatic obstruction, and the calculi are found during the course of urologic examination.

Typical symptoms of vesical stone are intermittent and painful voiding with terminal hematuria. Nonvoiding discomfort may be dull, aching, or sharp lower abdominal pain, which is aggravated by exercise and sudden movement. Severe pain usually occurs near the end of micturition, as the stone impacts on the bladder neck. Pain is also produced by the movement of the calculus as it strikes the base of the bladder. Relief may be afforded by assuming a recumbent position.

The pain may be referred to the tip of the penis, along the course of the second and third sacral nerves, or to the scrotum. In boys or girls, the pain may be referred to the perineum via the third and fourth sacral nerves. On occasion, referred pain may lodge in the back, the hip, or even the heel or sole of the foot.

Besides pain, there may be an interruption of the urinary stream from impaction of the stone in the internal urethral orifice. Frequency and dysuria are then usually present. Frequency of urination is enhanced by activity. Urgency is present in 40 to 50 per cent of patients, and interruption of the stream, in about 30 to 40 per cent of patients. In the presence of infection, the usual symptoms of cystitis are superimposed: nocturia occurs, urgency is increased, and terminal pain is pronounced. Priapism and nocturnal enuresis may occur in children.

Diagnosis of Vesical Calculus

HISTORY. Although a presumptive diagnosis may be tentatively made from a history of pain aggravated by exercise, interruption of the urinary stream, and terminal hematuria, these symptoms are not pathognomonic of this disease, for they may be produced by other lesions in the bladder.

PHYSICAL EXAMINATION. Physical examination is rarely of value in establishing a diagnosis, but instances have been cited in which a large stone was palpable on rectal, vaginal, or abdominal examination. Sensing the bladder stone by feeling it "clink" on a urethral sound is an age-old technique of detecting bladder stone.

LABORATORY FINDINGS. Albumin, erythrocytes, and leukocytes are usually found in the urine, but these are also commonly found with other lesions of the urinary tract. If infection has occurred, bacteria are often seen in the stained sediment or detected in the urinary culture.

ROENTGENOGRAPHIC STUDY. Often no evidence of vesical calculi is seen in plain roentgenograms because of the presence of uric acid in many of the calculi and because of overlying prostatic tissue (see Fig. 58–36). More than 50 per cent of bladder stones are not discernible on roentgenograms. Nichols and Lower (1933) reported that cystoscopic examination was the surest method for detecting vesical calculi, whereas roentgenography was better for detecting bladder diverticulum calculi.

The most accurate and certain means of diagnosis remains the cystoscopic examination. The absence of a shadow on the roentgenogram does not prove the absence of a vesical calculus.

Treatment

Because obstructive lesions and infections seem to play a role in the formation and enlargement of vesical calculi, their eradication will minimize the reoccurrence of stone. Obstruction must be relieved, bladder stasis corrected, and foreign bodies removed whenever possible.

Although satisfactory results for stone dissolution have been reported with the use of Suby's G or M solution, treatment is protracted and is now rarely employed. Renacidin may be employed to dissolve struvite or phosphate calculi and may prove beneficial in irrigating indwelling suprapubic or urethral catheters to prevent formation of calculus. It has produced little bladder irritability as a 10 per cent solution. Twice or thrice daily irrigations with 0.25 per cent or 0.5 per cent acetic acid solution also serve as beneficial prophylaxis against recurrent struvite calculi when indwelling catheters must be left. Uric acid calculi may be dissolved by irrigation with alkaline solutions.

Multiple procedural methods of treatment are available as discussed elsewhere. The choice of procedure is influenced by the age and physical condition of the patient, the size and hardness of the calculus, and the presence or absence of coexisting pathologic lesions involving the urethra, the bladder neck, or the bladder itself.

Calculi of the Prostate and Seminal Vesicles

Classification

True prostatic calculi are those that develop in the tissues or acini of the gland and are not to be confused with so-called false calculi that may be urinary calculi lodged in a dilated prostatic urethra or in a pouch of the urethra. Similarly, a calculus present in an abscess cavity or diverticulum that communicates with the urethra should not be considered a true prostatic calculus. It represents a urinary calculus that has formed within the anatomic area of the prostate.

Etiology

True prostatic calculi are formed by the deposition of calcareous material on corpora amylacea. Corpora amylacea are small round or ovoid bodies present in the alveoli of the prostate gland. They are rare in boys but frequent in men. Corpora amylacea have a laminated structure composed of lecithin and a nitrogenous substance of an albuminous nature, which is apparently formed around desquamated epithelial cells. Inorganic salts (calcium phosphate and calcium carbonate) impregnate the corpora amylacea, converting them into calculi. Sutor and Wooley (1974b) observed that "false" prostatic calculi probably arise from precipitation of salts found in normal prostatic fluid, that is, calcium and magnesium phosphates. Other workers have held that the corpora amylacea may serve only as nuclei. Infection also contributes to formation of some prostatic calculi.

Incidence

The frequency of prostatic calculi is not known because, in many instances, they are noted incidentally during a routine roentgenographic or ultrasonic survey. Joly (1931) observed 34 cases of prostatic calculi in a series of 636 cases of urinary calculi, an incidence of 5.3 per cent. Stones in the seminal vesicles are an extremely rare condition. White (1928) reported one case (not confirmed by vesiculotomy); the patient was 48 years old. White found only one other case reported in the literature. Prostatic calculi are rarely observed in boys and are infrequent in men less than 40 years of age. The majority occur in men aged 50 or more years.

Physical Characteristics

Prostatic calculi vary in number from one to several hundred. Generally, they are multiple and range in size from 1 to 4 mm in diameter. They are brownish gray and round or ovoid. Small stones are usually smooth, but large and multiple calculi occupying a single cavity may be definitely faceted. They are usually firm in consistency but can be readily crushed.

Calculi in the seminal vesicles may be single or multiple and are brown. The nucleus is composed of epithelial cells and a mucoid substance that is covered with lime salts. The stones are smooth and hard and range in size from 1 mm to 1 cm in diameter.

Composition

Generally, stones in the prostate are composed of calcium phosphate. Huggins and Bear (1944) observed that the organic components, which compose about 20 per cent of the calculus, include proteins (8 per cent), cholesterol (from 3.7 to 10.6 per cent), and citrate (from 0.17 to 2.9 per cent). True prostatic calculi are composed solely of calcium phosphate trihydrate (whitlockite) and carbonate (Sutor and Wooley, 1974b). Whenever such nuclei or nuclei of urinary stones become trapped in prostatic ducts, they are exposed to the urine and may therefore develop the same composition as urinary calculi. The amount of carbonate is somewhat less than that in bone. Otherwise, chemical and roentgenographic analyses show a close similarity between the inorganic constituents of prostatic calculi and bone salts. Huggins and Bear also stated that although corpora amylacea may occur in the anterior segment of the prostate, they occur mostly in the posterior segment.

Pathologic Changes

In the presence of minute calculi, the only pathologic change in the prostate may be chronic inflammation with areas of round cell infiltration. The acini may be filled with debris and desquamated epithelial cells, and the acini themselves may or may not be dilated.

When large calculi are present, the ducts and acini may be dilated, and the surrounding cavities may vary in size and shape. Their epithelial lining is absent, and round cell infiltration and fibrosis are observed between the acini. Occasionally, in the presence of a large calculus, little normal prostatic tissue is identifiable. Calculi are found either in the mouths of the ducts or deep in the gland. They are not usually observed in the adenomatous element of the gland but are adherent to the surface of a surgically removed adenoma. This explains the finding of calculi adjacent to the plane of enucleation of the adenoma at the time of suprapubic prostatectomy. Periprostatitis may occur along with possible abscess formation and eventual rupture into the urethra, when infection or suppuration is long standing. When a calculus is in the seminal vesicle, chronic inflammatory changes with fibrosis are usually present, and the duct may be completely blocked.

Symptoms

No symptoms are pathognomonic of calculous disease of the prostate gland. In many cases, there may be no suspicion of its presence. Symptoms, when present, may be due to prostatic hypertrophy, stricture of the urethra, or chronic prostatitis. Prostatic calculi contain and harbor bacteria, just as infected renal calculi do (Eykyn et al., 1974). In some instances, small prostatic calculi may be brought in by the patient after he has passed them spontaneously with the urine. The patient may complain of dull aching pain in the lower back, perineum, or penis. Difficulty in voiding, lack of force of the stream, and dribbling will occur if there is concomitant urethral stricture or prostatic hypertrophy. Sometimes, urethral discharge exists because of chronic prostatitis.

Hematuria is not usually observed, but terminal urinary bleeding may be present. Abscess formation due to calculi is uncommon. However, a patient with prostatic abscess has severe deep pain in the perineum and rectum that is aggravated by defecation. Temperature is elevated, and general constitutional symptoms may be pronounced. The prostate gland is exquisitely tender to palpation. If cystitis is present, dysuria, nocturia, and frequency of micturition occur. A stone in the seminal vesicle may be silent and produce no symptoms. In the cases reported, hematospermia, painful erections, and perineal discomfort at the time of ejaculation have occurred (Drach, 1975).

Physical Diagnosis of Prostatic Calculi

The diagnosis is usually established by rectal palpation of the prostate gland, urethroscopic examination, and

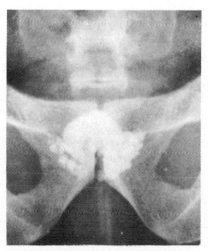

Figure 58–37. Prostatic calculi.

roentgenographic or ultrasonic study (Fig. 58–37). On rectal examination, the prostate gland may be enlarged in accordance with the patient's age. A discrete area of hardness or a digital sense of stone crepitation may be noted. More commonly, there may be no findings that suggest calculi.

Prostatic enlargement occurs in about 70 per cent of cases. The prostate is firm and movable, and the borders are well defined. Crepitation may be elicited in 18 to 20 per cent of cases and is usually most evident near the base of the gland. The consistency of the gland and its contour will vary. It may be smooth or nodular, firm or hard. In the presence of large calculi, localized areas of stony hardness are noted. In 18 to 22 per cent of cases, nodules are palpable, and the remaining tissue is of normal consistency. The nodules may be confused with prostatic carcinoma.

When a calculus is present in a seminal vesicle, the prostate is usually of normal consistency, and the involved vesicle is stony hard and fixed. Crepitation is elicited if multiple calculi are present.

Prostatic calculi, as noted, may be incorrectly interpreted as carcinoma on physical examination. The prostate gland with carcinomatous involvement is usually fixed, but in the presence of calculi is usually movable. In carcinoma of the prostate, the gland is stony hard, and extension toward the seminal vesicle is often demonstrable. Crepitation is absent in cases of carcinoma, and usually the tissue between any multiple nodules is not of normal consistency. Determination of serum acid phosphatase and prostate-specific antigen concentration, needle biopsy of the prostate, and ultrasonic scanning may help distinguish prostatic carcinoma from prostatic calculi.

Calculi in the prostate gland and seminal vesicles must also be differentiated from tuberculosis, which is more frequently observed in young than in old patients. One or both vesicles may be involved, and tuberculosis of the epididymis may be present.

Panendoscopic examination usually reveals only prostatic enlargement. Stones are seldom seen endoscopically in patients with prostatic calculi. Occasionally, a grating is felt upon passing the urethroscope. Rectal palpation of the prostate with the instrument in the urethra can confirm crepitation. A calculus sometimes protrudes into and obstructs the urethra.

Roentgenographic or ultrasonic study usually confirms diagnosis of prostatic calculi (see Fig. 58–37). Three characteristic types of shadows may be observed. Diffuse shadows may be generally distributed throughout the gland. Because such calculi are extremely small and occupy much of the gland, they are more likely to be related to chronic inflammatory processes such as tuberculosis. In other, more frequently observed types, there are so-called horseshoe or ring arrangements. In the ring type, the shadows surround a clear central portion formed by the central prostate (the adenoma of the urethra). In the horseshoe type, the stones are present laterally on both sides of the gland but are absent anterior to the urethra, as evidenced by the clear space that is the opening of the horseshoe. In still other instances, a large solitary calculus is observed, or the prostate gland appears to be completely replaced by calculus formation.

A diagnosis of stone in the seminal vesicle is made by rectal palpation, which demonstrates a hard, tender, smooth nodule in the vesicle. Large calculi may be revealed by roentgenographic study, which shows mottled shadows in the region of the vesicle, or by sonographic study.

Treatment

In patients with silent asymptomatic prostatic calculi, no treatment is indicated. Three methods of treatment are available when surgical relief is necessary.

Enthusiasm has been expressed of late for the precise transurethral removal of prostatic stones. This procedure may produce temporary relief, but it does not guarantee removal of all calculi, and recurrent stone formation may ensue. Combining ultrasonic observation of stone removal by transurethral surgery improves the urologist's ability to excise all visible calculi. It may be utilized in young patients to relieve pain and to avoid impairment of sexual activity or in the older patient who is a poor surgical risk. Suprapubic removal may be advocated in the presence of a large stone or stones or of significant prostatic hypertrophy. Perineal prostatotomy may be required for the removal of some deep stones. In the presence of multiple symptomatic calculi, total perineal prostatectomy and bilateral seminal vesiculectomy usually afford a cure.

Recurrence

Recurrence of prostatic calculi may follow prostatotomy if related diverticula are not obliterated or excised. New stones can form also in the remaining cavities of the gland. False recurrences—that is, stones overlooked at the time of the original operation—may be observed. Therefore, after operation, roentgenograms or sonograms should be obtained before the patient is dismissed from the hospital. True or new calculus formation may also occur after transurethral resection.

Urethral Calculi

In the Male

The majority of urethral calculi in the male consist of stones expelled from the bladder into the urethra. Rarely, a calculus may form primarily in the urethra when stricture is present, or it may form in a pouch or diverticulum that opens into the urethra.

INCIDENCE. Among the natives of developing countries, urethral calculi are common in children because stones of the bladder are also frequent. Otherwise, urethral calculi represent less than 1 per cent or all urinary stone disease.

POSITION AND COMPOSITION. A stone's progress through the normal urethra may be arrested in the prostatic urethra, the bulb, the anterior portion of the perineal urethra, the fossa navicularis, or the external meatus. The stone may also become impacted at the site of a urethral stricture. Englisch (1904), in a review of 361 cases, observed that in 41.2 per cent the stones were in the posterior urethra; in 18.8 per cent they were in the bulb; in 28.4 per cent they were in the scrotal and penile portions; and in 11.3 per cent they were in the fossa navicularis.

Calculi that migrate to the urethra obviously have the same constituents as bladder or upper urinary tract calculi, because they originate in either the bladder or the kidney. If there is associated infection, a primary urethral calculus is composed of struvite. Usually only a single stone is encountered.

SYMPTOMS. While urinating, the patient with a urethral calculus may experience a sudden stoppage and be therefore unable to empty the bladder. Dribbling also occurs. A patient may be able to palpate the stone within the scrotal or penile urethra. Pain occasioned by the stone may be rather severe and may radiate to the head of the penis. When the calculus is lodged in the posterior urethra, the pain is referred to the perineum or the rectum. When the calculus is lodged in the anterior urethra, the pain should be localized at the site of impaction. With increased effort and straining to void, the calculus may be expelled. Complete obstruction requires manipulation and temporary catheterization or, if that is not possible, immediate surgical or procedural removal of the stone.

A stone may be present in a diverticulum of the urethra for an extended period without producing symptoms. A urethral discharge may be observed–the result of the infection in the diverticulum. The patient may be aware of a lump that has gradually increased in size and hardness on the undersurface of the penis. This lump may at times become exquisitely tender. Usually, no change occurs in the caliber of the stream or urine, and no dribbling occurs.

DIAGNOSIS. Diagnosis may be established by palpation of the penis or the perineum. Rectal palpation may disclose the presence of a calculus in the posterior urethra. The tentative diagnosis may be confirmed by panendoscopic examination or roentgenography (Fig. 58–38). Likewise, a grating may be felt upon attempts to pass a sound.

TREATMENT. Treatment is influenced by the size, shape, and position of the calculus and by the status of the urethra. At times, a stone in the anterior urethra may be grasped and removed with forceps. Pressure is exerted simultaneously on the urethra proximal to the stone so that it is not forced into the bladder. A small stone may sometimes be gently massaged or milked outward, so that it can be expelled. Lithotripsy destruction and removal of a stone via the urethroscope may be advisable. When a stricture obstructs passage of the stone, a preliminary internal urethrotomy may be performed. However, when a large stone has been impacted for some time in the urethra, an external urethrotomy may be required. A calculus lodged in the fossa navicularis often can be removed by meatotomy.

A calculus recently impacted in the posterior urethra

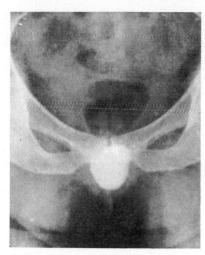

Figure 58–38. Calculus in a diverticulum of the urethra (female).

frequently can be pushed back into the bladder and then crushed. If the stone is large and definitely fixed, it may be removed by the perineal or suprapubic route, depending on the preference of the surgeon. A urethrovesical calculus is often best removed by the suprapubic route.

When the calculus occupies a urethral diverticulum, diverticulectomy and repair should be performed. In past years, recurrence within the diverticulum was frequently reported. At present, correction of urethral strictures, diverticulectomy, and adequate therapy to eradicate the infection are followed by extremely satisfactory results.

In the Female

The occurrence of urethral calculi in women is infrequent in comparison with that in men. This may be attributed to two factors—the short urethra in women that permits passage of any calculus and the infrequency of vesical calculi in women. Calculi in the female urethra are usually associated with a urethral diverticulum or a urethrocele (see Fig. 58–38). If the mouth of the diverticulum is wide, it is doubtful that calculus formation can occur. Stone formation in a diverticulum is usually due to urinary stasis and stagnation with infection, which allows the precipitation of urinary salts. Theoretically, therefore, the presence of a calculus in a diverticulum would presuppose a narrow opening between the urethra and the diverticulum.

SYMPTOMS AND DIAGNOSIS. The symptoms of urethral diverticulum, with or without calculus, are those of infection of the lower urinary tract, including frequency, dysuria, nocturia, pyuria, and in rare instances hematuria. Pain during coitus is a prominent symptom. Occasional discharge of pus may occur, giving the patient only temporary relief. Examination discloses a hard mass in the anterior vaginal wall in the area of the urethra.

TREATMENT. The treatment of a urethrocele or diverticulum containing a calculus is surgical, with ex-cision of the sac containing the calculus. The technique varies according to the preference of the operating surgeon.

Preputial Calculi

Three types of preputial calculi are noted. First are calculi arising from inspissated smegma that becomes impregnated with lime salts. These are soft in consistency, brown, and single or multiple. The second type includes calculi that form in stagnant urine retained in the sac because of phimosis. These may be multiple or single, round or faceted. They are composed of magnesium ammonium phosphate or calcium phosphate. Third are calculi that have been expelled from the bladder into the urethra and have gained entrance into the preputial sac by way of the urethral meatus or by ulceration through the fossa navicularis. Most of these calculi are grayish and composed of phosphates.

Preputial calculi usually form when phimosis is present. In this country, these calculi are rare, however, Thompson (1921) reported 116 cases. The condition is rarely observed in childhood. It is primarily a disease of adults. Although the patient may be aware of the presence of a lump for a considerable period, there may be no symptoms referable to the calculus. The usual symptoms are those of balanoposthitis. A discharge from the small opening in the foreskin; edema; and, in the late stages, ulceration may be present. Carcinoma may also coexist when the calculus has been present for a long time. The diagnosis is established by palpation of the stone.

When an acute infection is present, a dorsal slit should be performed to establish drainage. The ultimate treatment consists of circumcision.

ROLE OF PROCEDURES IN THE TREATMENT OF URINARY CALCULI

Approximately 50 per cent or more of patients with urinary calculous disease will, at some time or other, require treatment by procedural means. For this reason, development of an overall treatment plan is critical. It must include all aspects of the medical treatment of urinary calculi, including possible preoperative antibiotic therapy; adjustment of fluid intake; correction of dietary and metabolic abnormalities; and complete elimination of all obstructing calculi from the kidneys, ureters, and bladder so that postoperative preventive medical therapy may be effective.

If even small stone nuclei are left within the kidney, it is possible for new crystals to grow upon the surface of the retained nucleus and to re-create stone disease. Only by total eradication and prevention of stone formation in the patient can one achieve the goals of combined surgical and medical therapy and prevent further complications (Preminger et al., 1985).

FUTURE OUTLOOK

Major advances have taken place in the understanding of the etiology, diagnosis, and treatment of urinary calculous disease of all types. The cause of stone disease due to cystinuria, hyperuricosuria, or infection has been defined as simple physicochemical excesses of particular elements in the urine at a given pH and body temperature. Calcium oxalate and calcium phosphate urinary lithiasis may also be based on relatively simple physicochemical processes of supersaturation of urine with these substances. But whether calcium oxalate or calcium phosphate supersaturation is the sole initiating event is at present difficult to determine. Because these crystals often form in the urine of normal individuals, it is not likely that the simple precipitation of either element is the one causative factor in calcium stone disease. It seems much more likely that patients with calcium stone disease lack some limiting factor or inhibitor that prohibits the growth and aggregation of "normal" crystals before they are too large to be passed from the urinary tract (Nakagawa et al., 1987). Matrix may be important in this process as either a normal inhibitor or an abnormal initiator of stone growth.

Much still needs to be done in the discovery of new treatments for stone disease. Only two additional treatments have become popular in the United States since the mid 1980s, oral citrate for calcium stones and alpha-mercaptoglycine for cystine calculi. Many of our present drug treatments continue to be used empirically. Their mechanisms of action in improving urinary lithiasis are not known. Many drugs succeed despite paradoxical effects on urine components. For example, oral phosphate treatment of calcium oxalate urinary lithiasis reduces the concentration of urinary calcium, but it simultaneously increases the concentration of urinary oxalate and phosphate, which should enhance calcium oxalate or phosphate precipitation. May we presume that there is a greater degree of decrease in calcium than of increase in oxalate or phosphate? If so, how can we measure these differences? Robertson and colleagues (1976, 1983) may have given us a means to do this. The work of Pak and colleagues (1974, 1987) in defining precipitation of brushite as a possible factor in the initiation of urolithiasis may provide the answers to some of these questions.

Whatever the mode of medical treatment ultimately instituted, the major problem of urinary stone disease is the fact that the patients already have stone disease when they arrive at the physician's office. In many instances, they are already beyond the point of medical therapy, and procedural intervention is required. The real advances in treatment of stone disease will come when we can survey prospectively at reasonable cost all high-risk individuals and ascertain early in life the defects that may predispose them to urinary calculous disease. Perhaps approaches such as the diagnostic index of Sarig and co-workers (1982) and of Pak and co-workers (1985) will help us in the prospective detection of risk of urinary lithiasis. Based on this information, a plan of lifetime prophylaxis can be designed so that the significant morbidity and mortality of urinary lithiasis will not become problems for them (Scott, 1975).

Appendix A. LOW PURINE DIET*

Breakfast	
Fruit	1 serving
Cereal (no oatmeal)	1 serving
Eggs	2
Toast	1 slice
Butter or margarine	As desired
Beverage	Sanka, Kaffee Hag, or Postum
Milk	As desired
Cream	As desired
Sugar	As desired
Lunch	
Soup	1 serving (see list)
Cheese	2 ounces
Vegetable (cooked)	1 serving
Vegetable (raw)	1 serving
Bread	1 slice
Butter or margarine	As desired
Dessert	1 serving (see list)
Milk	1 glassful
Dinner	
Allowed soup	If desired
Meat, fish, fowl	2 ounces (twice weekly)
Potato	1 serving
Vegetable (cooked or raw)	1 serving
Bread	1 slice
Butter or margarine	As desired
Dessert	1 serving (see list)
Milk	1 glassful

Special Instructions
1. Avoid liver, sweetbreads, brains, and kidney. A 2-ounce portion of any other meat, fish, or fowl may be served twice weekly.
2. Serve cheese and eggs as meat substitutes. Fish roe and caviar may be used as desired.
3. Use 1–2 pints of milk daily.
4. Omit all meat extracts, broth soups, and gravies.
5. Omit the following vegetables entirely from the diet: Dried beans, lentils, dried peas, spinach.
6. Avoid coffee, tea, chocolate, and cocoa.
7. Omit alcoholic beverages of all kinds.
8. Use fruits of all kinds—fresh, canned, and dried.
9. Allow cereals of all kinds except oatmeal.
10. Soups allowed are milk soups made with any vegetables except those forbidden.
11. Desserts allowed are fruit, puddings, cake, ice cream, gelatin desserts or pie.
12. Beverages allowed are milk or buttermilk, and any decaffeinated coffee or cereal coffee.

*Carbohydrate—223, Protein—89, Fat—115: Cal. 2283.

Appendix B. LOW CALCIUM, LOW OXALATE DIET (300 mg calcium)

Food Groups	Foods Allowed	Foods to Avoid
Beverage	Carbonated beverages, cereal beverages; limit tea and coffee to 3 cups daily of either	Malted beverages, milk, milk drinks, chocolate beverages
Breads and cereals	White and wheat bread, refined cereals, crackers, rye or variety breads, donuts, pastries, sweet rolls	Any cereal enriched with calcium, such as instant-type hot cereals; cereals containing bran, such as All-Bran or Granola; pancakes, waffles, and other "quick breads"; breads containing bran; 100% whole wheat bread
Desserts	Gelatin desserts made of allowed foods, fruit ices, sherbets. Cakes, cookies, or other products not made from milk	Desserts made with milk, such as custard, pudding, ice cream, ice milk; cream pies and cream-filled baked products
Fats	Butter or margarine, cream (up to 1/3 cup daily), salad oils, cooking fat, nondairy creamer, cream cheese (up to 2 oz per day)	Half-and-half, sour cream (can be included in 1/3 cup allowance)
Fruit	Canned, cooked, or fresh fruit except those excluded, dried fruit (up to 1/2 cup daily)	Rhubarb,* cranberries,* plums,* gooseberries,* and raspberries*
Meat and meat substitutes	Meat, fish, and fowl except those excluded. Not more than 2 eggs daily, including those used in cooking†	Sardines, shrimp, and oysters; cheese—yellow, natural, and processed; white cheese, including cottage cheese and Parmesan cheese; yogurt
Potato or substitute	Potato, macaroni, noodles, spaghetti, refined rice	Whole grain rices
Soups	Broth, vegetable, or meat soup made from allowed foods	Bean or pea soup; cream or milk-based soups
Sweets and nuts	Candy without chocolate, almonds, or peanuts; honey, jam, jelly, syrups, and sugar; other nuts	Chocolate,* molasses, cocoa,* almonds, peanuts
Vegetables	Canned, cooked, or fresh vegetables or vegetable juice except those excluded	Asparagus,* dried beans and peas, broccoli, beet greens, swiss chard, collards, mustard greens, turnip greens, kale, spinach*
Miscellaneous	Salt, spices, and pepper (in moderation), vinegar	Cream sauce, milk gravy, peanut butter, ripe olives

*Foods high in oxalate.
†Robertson et al. (1979C) believe that limited animal protein intake also benefits calcium stone formers.

Appendix C. LOW PHOSPHATE DIET REGIMEN
(SHORR REGIMEN)*

1. Daily dietary intake of phosphorus restricted to less than 300 mg/day; calcium restricted to less than 700 mg/day.

2. Patient takes 40 ml of basic aluminum carbonate gel four times daily.

3. Fluid intake of at least 3000 ml/day and more as needed to keep urinary output at 2000 ml/day.

4. Analysis of urinary phosphorus excretion, which should be less than 250 mg/day, is done at intervals.

*Modified from Marshall, V. F., Lavengood, R. W., Jr., and Kelly, D.: Ann. Surg., 162:366, 1965.

REFERENCES

Albright, R., and Reifenstein, E. C., Jr. (Eds.): Parathyroid Glands and Metabolic Bone Disease. Baltimore, Williams & Wilkins, 1948.

Albright, F., Suby, H., and Sulkowitch, H. W.: In Albright, F., and Reifenstein, E. C., Jr. (Eds.): Parathyroid Glands and Metabolic Bone Disease. Baltimore, Williams & Wilkins, 1948.

Al-Dabbagh, T. G., and Fahadi, K.: Seasonal variations in the incidence of ureteric colic. Br. J. Urol., 49:269, 1977.

Allen, T. D., and Spence, H. M.: Matrix stone. J. Urol., 95:284, 1966.

Amin, M., and Howerton, L. W.: Spontaneous rupture of the ureter. South. Med. J., 67:1498, 1974.

Andersen, D. A.: The nutritional significance of primary bladder stone. Br. J. Urol., 34:160, 1962.

Andersen, D. A.: Environmental factors in the etiology of urolithiasis in urinary calculi. In Cifuentes, L., Rapado, A., and Hodgkinson, A. (Eds.): Urinary Calculi. International Symposium on Renal Stone Research. New York, S. Karger, 1973, p. 130.

Andersen, D. A.: Benurestat, a urease inhibitor for the therapy of infected urolithiasis. Invest. Urol., 12:381, 1975.

Andersen, E. E.: The management of ureteral calculi. Urol. Clin. North Am., 1:357, 1974.

Angell, A. H., and Resnick, M. I.: Surfact interaction between glycoseaminoglycans and calcium oxalate. J. Urol., 141:1255, 1989.

Arnaud, C. D.: Parathyroid hormone: Coming of age in clinical medicine. Am. J. Med., 55:577, 1973.

Arnaud, C. D., and Strewler, G. J.: Primary hyperparathyroidism. Semin. Nephrol., 1:376, 1981.

Atkinson, R. L., Jr., and Earll, J. M.: Munchausen syndrome with renal stones. JAMA, 230:89, 1974.

Atsmon, A., De Vries, A., and Frank, M.: Uric Acid Lithiasis. Amsterdam, Elsevier Publishing Co., 1963.

Aubert, J.: Calculous anuria and spontaneous rupture of the kidney pelvis. Importance of intravenous urography in the anuric patient. Acta Urol. Belg., 41:396, 1973.

Aurora, A. L., Teneia, O. P., and Gupta, D. N.: Bladder stone disease of childhood. II. A clinico-pathological study. Acta Paediatr. Scand., 59:385, 1970.

Bailey, R. R., Dann, E., Greenslade, N. F., Little, P. J., McRae, C. U., and Utley, W. L. F.: Urinary stones: A prospective study of 350 patients. N. Z. Med. J., 79:961, 1974.

Barker, L. M., Pallante, S. L., Eisenberg, H., Joule, J. A., Becker, G. L., and Howard, J. E.: Simple synthetic and natural urines have equivalent anticalcifying properties. Invest. Urol., 12:79, 1974.

Barnhouse, D. H.: In vitro formation of precipitates in sterile and infected urines. Invest. Urol., 5:342, 1968.

Bastian, H. P., and Gebhardt, M.: The varying composition of the nucleus and peripheral layers of urinary calculi. Urol. Res., 2:91, 1974.

Bateson, E. M.: Renal tract calculi and climate. Med. J. Aust., 2:111, 1973.

Baumann, J. M., and Wacker, M.: Experiences with the measurement of inhibitory activity of urine and crystallisation inhibitors by different techniques. Urol. Res., 7:183, 1979.

Becher, R. M., Bhupendra, M. T., and Newman, H. R.: Giant vesical calculus. JAMA, 239:2272, 1978.

Beck, C. W., and Mulvaney, W. P.: Apatitic urinary calculi from early American Indians. JAMA, 195:168, 1966.

Berman, L. B.: Renal geology. JAMA, 231:865, 1975.

Bichler, K. H., Kirchner, Ch., and Ideler, V.: Uromucoid excretion of normal individuals and stone formers. Br. J. Urol., 47:733, 1976.

Blacklock, N. J.: The pattern of urolithiasis in the Royal Navy. In Hodgkinson, A., and Nordin, B. E. C. (Eds.): Renal Stone Research Symposium. London, J. & A. Churchill, Ltd., 1969, p. 33.

Blaivas, J. G., Pais, V. M., and Spellman, R. M.: Chemolysis of residual stone fragments after extensive surgery for staghorn calculi. Urology, 6:680, 1975.

Borgmann, V., and Nagel, R.: Urolithiasis in childhood—a study of 181 cases. Urol. Int., 37:198, 1982.

Borkowski, A., and Czapliczki, M.: Nontraumatic extravasation from the ureter. Int. Urol. Nephrol., 5:271, 1974.

Boyce, W. H.: Organic matrix of human urinary concretions. Am. J. Med., 45:673, 1968.

Boyce, W. H.: Organic matrix of native human urinary concretions.

In Hodgkinson, A., and Nordin, B. E. C. (Eds.): Renal Stone Research Symposium. London, J. & A. Churchill, Ltd., 1969, p. 93.

Boyce, W. H., and Elkins, I. B.: Reconstructive renal surgery following anatrophic nephrolithotomy: Follow-up of 100 consecutive cases. J. Urol., 111:307, 1974.

Boyce, W. H., and King, J. S., Jr.: Crystal-matrix interrelations in calculi. J. Urol., 81:351, 1959.

Boyce, W. H., Garvey, F. K., and Strawcutter, H. E.: Incidence of urinary calculi among patients in general hospitals, 1948–1952. JAMA, 161:1437, 1956.

Boyce, W. H., King, J. S., and Fielden, M. L.: Total nondialysable solids (TNDS) of human urine. XIII. Immunological detection of a component peculiar to renal calculous matrix and to urine of calculous patients. J. Clin. Invest., 41:1180, 1962.

Braasch, W. F., and Moore, A. B.: Stones in the ureter. JAMA, 65:123, 1915.

Breatnach, E., and Smith, S. E. W.: The radiology of renal stones in children. Clin. Radiol., 34:59, 1983.

Breslau, N. A., and Pak, C. Y. C.: Urinary saturation, heterogeneous nucleation, and crystallization inhibitors in nephrolithiasis. In Coe, F. L., Brenner, B. M., and Stein, J. H. (Eds.): Nephrolithiasis. New York, Churchill-Livingstone, 1980.

Breslau, N. A., Brinkley, L., Hill, K. D., and Pak, C. Y. C.: Relation of animal protein–rich diet to kidney stone formation and calcium metabolism. J. Clin. Endocrinol. Metab., 66:140, 1988.

Breslau, N. A., McGuire, J. L., Zerwekh, J. E., and Pak, C. Y. C.: The role of dietary sodium on renal excretion and intestinal absorption of calcium and on vitamin D metabolism. J. Clin. Endocrinol., 55:369, 1982.

Broadus, A. E., Dominguez, M., and Barrter, F. C.: Pathophysiologic studies in idiopathic hypercalciuria: Use of an oral calcium tolerance test to characterize distinctive hypercalciuric subgroups. J. Clin. Endocrinol. Metab., 47:751, 1978.

Brockis, J. G., Bowyer, R. C., McCulloch, R. K., Taylor, T. A., Wisniewski, Z. S., et al.: Pathophysiology of endemic bladder stones. In Brockis, J. G., and Finlayson, B. (Eds.): Urinary Calculus. Littleton, M. A., PGS Publishing Co., 1981.

Buck, A. C., Lote, C. J., and Sampson, W. F.: The influence of renal prostaglandins on urinary calcium excretion on idiopathic urolithiasis. J. Urol., 129:421, 1983.

Bumpus, H. C., Jr., and Thompson, G. J.: Ureteral stones. Surg. Clin. North Am., 5:812, 1925.

Burkland, C. E., and Rosenberg, M.: Survey of urolithiasis in the United States. J. Urol., 73:198, 1955.

Burr, R. C.: Urinary calcium, magnesium, crystals and stones in paraplegia. Paraplegia, 10:56, 1972.

Burr, R. C., and Walsh, J. J.: Urinary calcium and kidney stones in paraplegia. Report of an attempted prospective study. Paraplegia, 12:38, 1974.

Butler, A. M., Wilson, J. L., and Farber, S. J.: Dehydration and acidosis with calcification at renal tubules. J. Pediatr., 8:489, 1936.

Cadoff, R. E., Drach, G. W., and LeBouton, J.: Specific gravity test strips used in monitoring urine concentrations of urolithiasis patients. J. Urol., 139:323, 1988.

Carr, R. J.: Aetiology of renal calculi: Micro-radiographic studies. In Hodgkinson, A., and Nordin, B. E. C. (Eds.): Renal Stone Research Symposium. London, J. & A. Churchill, Ltd., 1969, p. 123.

Cartstensen, H. E., and Hansen, T. S.: Stones in the ureter. Acta Chir. Scand. (Suppl.), 433:66, 1973.

Caruana, R. J., and Buckalew, V. M. Jr.: The syndrome of distal (Type 1) renal tubular acidosis. Clinical and laboratory findings in 58 cases. Medicine 67:84, 1988.

Catalina, R., and Cifuentes, L.: Calcium oxalate: Crystallographic analysis in solid aggregate in urinary sediment. Science, 169:183, 1970.

Cato, A. R., and Tulloch, A. G. S.: Hypermagnesemia in a uremic patient during renal pelvic irrigation with Renacidin. J. Urol., 111:313, 1974.

Chambers, R. M., and Dormandy, T. L.: Hypercalciuria—relative and absolute. In Hodgkinson, A., and Nordin, B. E. C. (Eds.): Renal Stone Research Symposium. London, J. & A. Churchill, Ltd., 1969, p. 233.

Chang-Ti, S., Lu-cheng, C., and Ke-han, H.: Assessment of urine saturation and inhibitory index in patients with calcium oxalate kidney stone and normals. Chinese Med. J., 100:935, 1987.

Chase, L. R., and Aurbach, G. D.: Parathyroid function and renal excretion of 3', 5'-adenylic acid. Proc. Natl. Acad. Sci. U. S. A., 58:518, 1967.

Choi, H., Snyder, H. M., III, and Duckett, J. W.: Urolithiasis in childhood: Current management. J. Pediatr. Surg., 22(2):158, 1987.

Chow, F. H., Hamar, D. W., Udall, R. H., et al.: Urinary calculi matrices and urine polyelectrolytes. Proc. Soc. Exp. Biol. Med., 144:912, 1973.

Churchill, D. N., Maloney, C. M., Bear, J., Bryant, D. G., Fodor, G., and Gault, M. H.: Urolithiasis—a study of drinking water hardness and genetic factors. J. Chron. Dis., 33.727, 1980.

Cifuentes, L., Rapado, A., Abehsera, A., et al.: Uric acid lithiasis and gout. In Cifuentes, L., Rapado, A., and Hodgkinson, A. (Eds.): Urinary Calculi. International Symposium on Renal Stone Research. Basel, S. Karger, 1973, p. 115.

Clark, P. B. and Nordin, B. E. C.: The problem of the calcium stone. In Hodgkinson, A., and Nordin, B. E. C. (Eds.): Renal Stone Research Symposium. London, J. & A. Churchill, Ltd., 1969, p. 1.

Claus-Walker, J., Campos, R. J., Carter, R. E., et al.: Electrolytes in urinary calculi and urine of patients with spinal cord injuries. Arch. Phys. Med. Rehabil., 54:109, 1973.

Claypool, H. R., Lind, T. A., Haber, K., and Freundlich, I.: Comparison of the drip infusion and bolus techniques in excretory urography as a routine examination. Ariz. Med., 32(7):552, 1975.

Clendening, L.: Sourcebook of Medical History. New York, Dover Publications, Inc., 1942, p. 14.

Coe, F. L.: Treated and untreated recurrent calcium nephrolithiasis in patients with idiopathic hypercalciuria, hyperuricosuria, or no metabolic disorder. Ann. Intern. Med., 87:404, 1977.

Coe, F. L., and Davalach, A. G.: Hypercalciuria and hyperuricosuria in patients with calcium nephrolithiasis. N. Engl. J. Med., 291:1344, 1974.

Coe, F. L., and Parks, J. A.: Pathophysiology of kidney stones and strategies for treatment. Hospital Practice, 185, Mar. 15, 1988.

Coe, F. L., and Raisen, L.: Allopurinol treatment of uric acid disorders in calcium stone formers. Lancet, 1:129, 1973.

Coe, F. L., Favus, M. J., Crockett, T., Strauss, A. L., Parks, J. H., Porat, A., Gantt, C. L., and Sherwood, L. M.: Effects of low-calcium diet on urine calcium excretion, parathyroid function and serum 1,24(OH)$_2$D$_3$ levels in patients with idiopathic hypercalciuria and in normal subjects. Am. J. Med. 72:25, 1982.

Coe, F. L., Margolis, H. C., Deutsch, L. H., and Strauss, A. L.: Urinary macromolecular crystal growth inhibitors in calcium nephrolithiasis. Min. Electrolyte Metab., 3:268, 1980.

Conyers, R. A., Bais, R., Rofe, A. M., Potezny, N., and Thomas, D. W.: Ascorbic acid intake, renal function, and urinary oxalate excretion. N. Z. J. Med. 15:353, 1985.

Copp, D. H.: Endocrine control of calcium homeostasis. J. Endocrinol., 43:137, 1969.

Copp, D. H., Cameron, E. C., Cheney, B. A., Davidson, A. G., and Henze, K. G.: Evidence for calcitonin—a new hormone from the parathyroid that lowers blood calcium. Endocrinology, 70:638, 1962.

Cox, C. E.: Symposium on renal lithiasis. Urinary tract infection and renal lithiasis. Urol. Clin. North Am., 1:279, 1974.

Crawhall, J. C., and Watts, R. W. E.: Cystinuria. Am. J. Med., 45:736, 1968.

Dalton, D. L., Hughes, J., and Glenn, J. F.: Foreign bodies and urinary stone. Urology, 6:1, 1975.

DeLuca, H. F.: Vitamin D endocrinology. Ann. Intern. Med., 85:367, 1976.

Dent, C. E., and Philpot, G. R.: Xanthinuria: Inborn error (or deviation) of metabolism. Lancet, 1:182, 1954.

Dent, C. E., and Senior, B.: Studies on the treatment of cystinuria. Br. J. Urol., 27:317, 1955.

DeVries, A., and Sperling, O.: Familial gouty malignant uric acid lithiasis due to mutant phosphoribosylpyrophosphate synthetase. Urologe[A], 12:153, 1973.

Diamond, D. A., Menon, M., Lee, P. H., Rickwood, A. M. K., and Johnston, J. H.: Etiological factors in pediatric stone recurrence. J. Urol., 142:606, 1989.

Dickstein, S. S., and Frame, B.: Urinary tract calculi after intestinal shunt operations for the treatment of obesity. Surg. Gynecol. Obstet., 136:257, 1973.

Domanski, T. J.: Renal calculi: A new method of qualitative analysis. J. Urol., 37.399, 1937.

Dourmashkin, R. L.: Cystoscopic treatment of stones in the ureter with special reference to large calculi based on a study of 1550 cases. J. Urol., 54:245, 1945.

Drach, G. W.: Baron Dupuytren, lithotomist (1777–1835). Invest. Urol., 11:424, 1974a.

Drach, G. W.: Symposium on renal lithiasis. Perioperative aspects of renal stone surgery. Urol. Clin. North Am., 1:299, 1974b.

Drach, G. W.: Prostatitis: Man's hidden infection. Urol. Clin. North Am., 2:499, 1975.

Drach, G. W.: Urolithiasis. In Conn, H. G. (Ed.): Current Therapy. Philadelphia, W. B. Saunders Co., 1976a, p. 552.

Drach, G. W.: Contribution to therapeutic decisions of ratios, absolute values and other measures of calcium, magnesium, urate or oxalate balance in stone formers. J. Urol., 116:339, 1976b.

Drach, G. W.: Stone manipulation: Modern usage and occasional mishaps. Urology, 12:286, 1978.

Drach, G. W.: Transurethral ureteral stone manipulation. Urol. Clin. North Am., 10:709, 1983.

Drach, G. W.: Epitome—integrated management of urinary stone disease. West. J. Med., 147:188, 1987.

Drach, G. W., and Boyce, W. H.: Nephrocalcinosis as a source for renal stone nuclei. Observations on humans and squirrel monkeys and on hyperparathyroidism in the squirrel monkey. J. Urol., 197:897, 1972.

Drach, G. W., and King, J. S.: Estimating aberrant homeostasis: Variance in serum calcium as an aid in diagnosis of hyperparathyroidism. Clin. Chem., 16:792, 1970.

Drach, G. W., Dretler, S., Fair, W., Finlayson, B., Gillenwater, J., Griffith, D., Lingeman, J., Newman, D.: Report of the United States Cooperative Study of Extracorporeal Shock Wave Lithotripsy. J. Urol., 135:1127, 1986.

Drach, G. W., Robertson, W. G., Scurr, D. S., and Randolph, A. D.: Pyrophosphate inhibition of calcium oxalate dihydrate crystallization in simulated urine: Continuous flow studies. World J. Urol., 1:146, 1983.

Dretler, S. P.: The pathogenesis of urinary tract calculi occurring after ileal conduit diversion. I. Clinical study. II. Conduit study. III. Prevention. J. Urol., 109:204, 1973.

Dretler, S. P.: Ureteral stone disease: Options for management. Urol. Clin. North Am., 17:217, 1990.

Dretler, S. P., Coggins, C. H., McIver, M. A., and Their, S. O.: The physiologic approach to renal tubular acidosis. J. Urol., 102:665, 1969.

Dretler, S. P., and Pfister, R. C.: Primary dissolution therapy of struvite calculi. J. Urol., 131:861, 1984a.

Dretler, S. P., Pfister, R. C., Newhouse, J. H., and Prien, E. L., Jr.: Percutaneous catheter dissolution of cystine calculi. J. Urol., 131:216, 1984b.

Duce, A. M., Jerez, E., Rapado, A., and Cajigal, R.: Intestinal absorption of oxalic acid in ileostomized patients. Acta Chir. Scand., 154:297, 1988.

Dyer, R., and Nordin, B. E. C.: Urinary crystals and their relation to stone formation. Nature, 215:751, 1967.

Elliot, J. S.: Structure and composition of urinary calculi. J. Urol., 109:82, 1973a.

Elliot, J. S.: In Cifuentes, L., Rapado, A., and Hodgkinson, A. (Eds.): Urinary Calculi. International Symposium on Renal Stone Research. Basel, S. Karger, 1973b, p. 24.

Elliot, J. S.: Calcium oxalate urinary calculi: Clinical and chemical aspects. Medicine, 62:36, 1983.

Elliot, J. S. and Eusebio, E.: Calcium oxalate solubility: The effects of trace metals. J. Invest. Urol., 9:428, 1967.

Elliot, J. S., and Ribeiro, M. E.: The urinary excretion of trace metals in patients with calcium oxalate urinary stone. Invest. Urol., 10:253, 1973.

Elliot, J. S., Ribeiro, M. E., and Eusebio, E.: The effect of oral phosphate upon the urinary excretion of oxalic acid. Invest. Urol., 7:528, 1970.

Elliot, J. S., Sharp, R. D., and Lewis, L.: The solubility of struvite in urine. J. Urol., 81:366, 1959.

Elliott, J. P., Jr.: A stone season. A ten-year retrospective study of 768 surgical stone cases with respect to seasonal variation. J. Urol., 114:574, 1975.

Ellis, H.: A History of Bladder Stone. Oxford, Blackwell, 1969.

Ellman, P., and Parfitt, A. M.: The resemblance between sarcoidosis with hypercalcemia and hyperparathyroidism. Br. Med. J., 2:108, 1960.

Emmett, J. L. and Witten, D. M.: Calculous disease of the genitourinary tract. *In* Clinical Urography. Philadelphia, W. B. Saunders Co., 1971, p. 607.

Englisch, J.: Über eigelagerte und eingesachte Stein der Harnröhre. Arch. Klin. Chir., 72:487, 1904.

Ettinger, A., Oldroyd, N. O., and Sorgel, F.: Triamterene urolithiasis. JAMA, 244:2443, 1980.

Eykyn, S., Bultitude, M. I., Mayo, M. E., and Lloyd-Davies, R. W.: Prostatic calculi as a source of recurrent bacteriuria in the male. Br. J. Urol., 46:527, 1974.

Fanelli, G. M.: Urate excretion. Annu. Rev. Med., 28:349, 1977.

Fellstrom, B., Backman, U., Danielson, B. G., Johansson, G., Ljunghall, S., and Wilkstrom, B.: Uricemia and urinary acidification in renal calcium stone disease. J. Urol., 129:256, 1983.

Fetter, T. L., and Zimskind, P. D.: Statistical analysis of patients with ureteral calculi. JAMA, 186:21, 1961.

Fikri, E., and Casella, R. R.: Hyperoxaluria and urinary tract calculi after jejunoileal bypass. Am. J. Surg., 129:334, 1975.

Finkle, A. L., and Smith, D. R.: Parameters of renal functional capacity in reversible hydroureteronephrosis in dogs. V. Effects of 7 to 10 days of ureteral construction on RBF-Kr, C-In, Tc-H_2O, C-PAH, osmolality, and sodium reabsorption. Invest. Urol., 8:299, 1970.

Finkle, A. L., Karg, S. J., and Smith, D. R.: Parameters of renal functional capacity in reversible hydroureteronephrosis in dogs. VI. Response to mannitol challenge by the chronically obstructed canine kidney and its clinical implication. J. Urol., 104:368, 1970.

Finlayson, B.: Symposium on renal lithiasis. Renal lithiasis in review. Urol. Clin. North Am., 1:181, 1974.

Finlayson, B.: Physicochemical aspects of urolithiasis. Kidney Int., 13:344, 1978.

Finlayson, B., and Dubois, L.: Kinetics of calcium oxalate deposition in vitro. Invest. Urol., 10:429, 1973.

Finlayson, B., and Reid, F.: The expectation of free and fixed particles in urinary stone disease. Invest. Urol., 15:442, 1978.

Finlayson, B., and Roth, R. A.: Appraisal of calcium oxalate solubility in sodium chloride and sodium–calcium chloride solutions. Urology, 1:142, 1973.

Finlayson, B., Roth, R., and Dubois, L.: Perturbation of calcium ion activity by urea. Invest. Urol., 10:138, 1972.

Finlayson, B., Roth, R. A., and Dubois, L.: Calcium oxalate solubility. *In* Cifuentes, L., Rapado, A., and Hodgkinson, A. (Eds.): Urinary Calculi. International Symposium on Renal Stone Research. Basel, S. Karger, 1973, p. 1.

Finlayson, B., Vermeulen, W., and Stewart, R. J.: Stone matrix and mucoprotein from urine. J. Urol., 86:355, 1961.

Flannigan, G. M., Clifford, R. P. C., Carver, R. A., Yule, A. G., Madden, N. P., and Towler, J. M.: Indomethacin—an alternative to pethidine in ureteric colic. Br. J. Urol., 55:6, 1983.

Fleisch, H.: Some new concepts on the pathogenesis and the treatment of urolithiasis. Urol. Int., 19:372, 1965.

Fleisch, H., and Bisaz, S.: The inhibitory effect of pyrophosphate on calcium oxalate precipitation and its relation to urolithiasis. Experientia, 20:276, 1964.

Flocks, R. H.: Calcium and phosphorus excretion in the urine of patients with renal or ureteral calculi. JAMA, 113:1466, 1939.

Flocks, R. H.: Prophylaxis and medical management of calcium urolithiasis: The role of the quantity and precipitability of the urinary calcium. J. Urol., 44:183, 1940.

Foye, W. O., Hong, H. S., Kim, C. M., and Prien, E. L., Sr.: Degree of sulfation in mucopolysaccharide sulfates in normal and stone forming urines. Invest. Urol., 14:33, 1976.

Frank, M., and DeVries, A.: Prevention of urolithiasis. Arch. Environ. Health, 13:625, 1966.

Frank, M., DeVries, A., Atsmon, A., et al.: Epidemiological investigation of urolithiasis in Israel. J. Urol., 81:497, 1959.

Frayha, R. A., Salti, L. S., Abuhaidar, G. I., et al.: Hereditary xanthinuria and xanthine urolithiasis: An additional three cases. J. Urol., 109:871, 1973.

Freed, S. Z.: The alternating use of an alkalizing salt and acetazolamide in the management of cystine and uric acid stones. J. Urol., 113:96, 1975.

Friedlander, A. M., and Braude, A. I.: Production of bladder stones by human T mycoplasmas. Nature, 247:67, 1974.

Furlow, W. L., and Bucchiere, J. J.: The surgical fate of ureteral calculi: Review of Mayo Clinic experience. J. Urol., 116:559, 1976.

Gahagan, H. O., and Reed, W. K.: Squamous cell carcinoma of the renal pelvis: Review of the literature. J. Urol., 62:139, 1949.

Gardner, B.: Studies of the zeta potential of cells and a silica particle in varying concentrations of albumin, calcium, sodium, plasma and bile. J. Lab. Clin. Med., 73:202, 1969.

Gee, W. F., and Kiviat, M. D.: Ureteral response to partial obstruction. Smooth muscle hyperplasia and connective tissue proliferation. Invest. Urol., 12:309, 1975.

Gilbert, J. B., and McMillan, S. F.: Cancer of the kidney: Squamous cell carcinoma of renal pelvis with special reference to etiology. Ann. Surg., 100:429, 1934.

Gill, W. B., Silvert, M. A., and Roma, M. J.: Supersaturation levels and crystallization rates of calcium oxalate from urines of normal humans and stone formers determined by a 14C-oxalate technique. Invest. Urol., 12:203, 1974.

Gittes, R. F., Wells, S. A., and Irvin, G. L., III: New role for the parathyroid glands in calcium homeostasis. J. Urol., 97:1082, 1967.

Giugliani, R., Ferrari, I., and Greene, L. J.: Heterozygous cystinuria and urinary lithiasis. Am. J. Med. Genet., 22:703, 1985.

Gluszek, J.: The effect of glucose intake on urine saturation with calcium oxalate, calcium phosphate, uric acid and sodium urate. Intl. Urol. Nephrol., 20:657, 1988.

Goldstein, A. E.: Familial urological diseases. Am. Surg., 17:221, 1951.

Goodman, M., Curry, T., and Russell, T.: Xanthogranulomatous pyelonephritis: A local disease with systemic manifestations. Medicine, 58:171, 1979.

Gram, H. C.: Heredity of oxalic urinary calculi. Acta Med. Scand., 78:268, 1932.

Gregory, J. G.: Hyperoxaluria and stone disease in the gastrointestinal bypass patient. Urol. Clin. North Am., 8:331, 1981.

Griffith, D. P.: Urease stones. Urol. Res., 7:215, 1979.

Griffith, D. P., and Musher, D. M.: Acetohydroxamic acid: Potential use in urinary infection caused by urea-splitting bacteria. Urology, 5:299, 1975.

Griffith, D. P., Bragin, S., and Musher, D. M.: Dissolution of struvite urinary stones. Experimental studies in vitro. Invest. Urol., 13:351, 1976a.

Griffith, D. P., Musher, D. M., and Campbell, J. W.: Inhibition of bacterial urease. Invest. Urol., 11:234, 1973.

Griffith, D. P., Musher, D. M., and Iten, C.: Urease: The primary cause of infection-induced urinary stones. Invest. Urol., 13:346, 1976b.

Gutman, A. B., and Yu, T. F.: Uric acid nephrolithiasis. Am. J. Med., 45:756, 1968.

Haddad, F. S., and Kouyoumdjian, A.: Silica stones in humans. Urol. Int., 41:70, 1986.

Hall, E. G., Scowen, E. F., and Watts, R. W.: Clinical manifestations of primary hyperoxaluria. Arch. Dis. Child., 35:108, 1960.

Hallson, P. C., and Rose, G. A.: Seasonal variations in urinary crystals. Br. J. Urol., 49:227, 1977.

Harris, E. K.: Distinguishing physiologic variation from analytic variation. J. Chron. Dis., 23:469, 1970.

Harrison, A. R., and Rose, G. A.: The late results of parathyroidectomy in patients with calculus or nephrocalcinosis. *In* Cifuentes, L., Rapado, A., and Hodgkinson, A. (Eds.): Urinary Calculi. International Symposium on Renal Stone Research. Basel, S. Karger, 1973, p. 354.

Hautmann, R., Lehmann, A., and Komor, S.: Calcium and oxalate concentrations in human renal tissue: The key to the pathogenesis of stone formation. J. Urol., 123:317, 1980.

Hazarika, E. Z., and Rao, B. N.: Spectrochemical analysis of urinary tract calculi. Indian J. Med. Res., 62:776, 1974a.

Hazarika, E. Z., Rao, B. N., Kapur, B. M., et al.: Lower urinary tract calculi analysed by x-ray diffraction and chemical methods. Indian J. Med. Res., 62:893, 1974b.

Heath, P. M.: Large ureteral calculus. Br. J. Surg., 10:153, 1922.

Hench, L. L.: Factors in protein-mineral epitaxis. *In* Finlayson, B., et al. (Eds.): Urolithiasis: Physical Aspects. Washington, National Academy of Sciences, 1972, p. 203.

Henneman, P. H., Benedict, P. H., Forbes, A. P., et al.: Idiopathic hypercalciuria. N. Engl. J. Med., 259:802, 1958.

Herbstein, F. H., Kleeberg, J., Shalitin, Y., et al.: Chemical and x-ray diffraction analysis of urinary stones in Israel. Isr. J. Med. Sci., 10:1493, 1974.

Hering, F., Briellmann, T., Luond, G., Guggenheim, H., Seiler, H., and Rutishauser, G.: Stone formation in human kidney. Urol. Res., 15:67, 1987.

Herring, L. C.: Observations of 10,000 urinary calculi. J. Urol., 88:545, 1962.

Herrman, G.: Nachweis der Beldung von Harnmucoid mit Hilfe der Immuno-Fluoreszenz. Verh. Dtsch. Ges. Inn. Med., 69:178, 1963.

Higgins, C. C.: Factors in recurrence of renal calculi. JAMA, 113:1460, 1939.

Hinman, F.: Directional growth of renal calculi. J. Urol., 121:700, 1979.

Hockaday, T. D. R., Clayton, J. E., Frederick, E. W., et al.: Primary hyperoxaluria. Medicine, 43:315, 1967.

Hodgkinson, A.: Determination of oxalic acid in biological material. Clin. Chem., 16:547, 1970.

Hodgkinson, A.: Uric acid disorders in patients with calcium stones. Br. J. Urol., 48:1, 1976.

Hodgkinson, A., and Marshall, R. W.: Changes in the composition of urinary tract stones. Invest. Urol., 13:131, 1975.

Hodgkinson, A., and Nordin. B. E. C.: Physical chemistry of calcium stone formation. Biochem. J., 122:5P, 1971.

Hodgkinson, A., Bissett, P., and Tye, J.: Effect of succinimide and other drugs on oxalate excretion by rats. Urol. Int., 30:465, 1975.

Hodgkinson, A., Peacock, M., and Nochalson, M.: Quantitative analysis of calcium containing urinary calculi. Invest. Urol., 6:549, 1969.

Holmes, G.: Worcestershire sauce and the kidneys. Br. Med. J., 3:252, 1971.

Holmgren, K., Danielson, B. G., Fellstrom, B., Ljunghall, S., Niklasson, F., and Wikstrom, B.: The relation between urinary tract infection and stone composition in renal stone formers. Scand. J. Urol. Nephrol. 23:131, 1989.

Holmlund, D.: Tanderil in the treatment of ureteral stone disease. Helv. Chir. Acta, 41:333, 1974.

Howard, J. E., Thomas, W. C., Barker, L. M., et al.: The recognition and isolation from urine and serum of a peptide inhibitor to calcification. Johns Hopkins Med. J., 120:119, 1967.

Hsu, T. G.: Ammonium acid urate lithiasis, experimental observations. J. Urol., 96:88, 1966.

Huggins, C., and Bear, R. S.: Course of prostatic ducts and anatomy: Chemical and x-ray diffraction analysis of prostatic calculi. J. Urol., 51:37, 1944.

Hugosson, J., Grenabo, L., Hedelin, H., Pettersson, S., and Seeberg, S.: Bacteriology of upper urinary tract stones. J. Urol., 143:965, 1990.

Inada, T., Miyazaki, S., Omori, T., et al.: Statistical study on urolithiasis in Japan. Urol. Int., 1:150, 1958.

Isaacson, L. C.: Urinary ionic strength, osmolality and specific conductivity. Invest. Urol., 5:406, 1968.

Jacobs, S. C., and Gittes, R. F.: Dissolution of residual renal calculi with hemiacidrin. J. Urol., 115:2, 1976.

Jennis, F., Larson, J. N., Neale, F. C., et al.: Staghorn calculi of the kidney: Clinical, bacteriological and biochemical features. Br. J. Urol., 42:511, 1970.

Joekes, A. M., Rose, G. A., and Sutor, J.: Multiple renal silica calculi. Br. Med. J., 1:146, 1973.

Johansson, G., Backman, U., Danielson, B. G., Fellstrom, B., Ljunghall, S., and Wikstrom, B.: Biochemical and clinical effects of the prophylactic treatment of renal calcium stones with magnesium hydroxide. J. Urol., 124:770, 1980.

Johansson, H., Thoren, L., Werner, I., et al.: Normocalcemic hyperparathyroidism, kidney stones, and idiopathic hypercalciuria. Surgery, 77:691, 1975.

Joly, J. S.: Stone and Calculous Disease of the Urinary Organs. St. Louis, C. V. Mosby Co., 1931.

Jones, D. A., Atherton, J. C., O'Reilly, P. H. Jr., Barnard, R. J., and George N. J. R.: Assessment of the nephron segments involved in post-obstructive diuresis in man, using lithium clearance. Br. J. Urol., 64:559, 1989.

Jordan, W. R., Finlayson, B., and Luxenberg, M.: Kinetics of early time calcium oxalate nephrolithiasis. Invest. Urol., 15:465, 1978.

Juul, N., Holm-Bentzen, M., Rygaard, H., and Holm, H. H.: Ultrasonic diagnosis of renal stones. Scand. J. Urol. Nephrol., 21:135, 1987.

Juuti, M., and Heinonen, O. P.: Incidence of urolithiasis and composition of household water in Southern Finland. Scand. J. Urol. Nephrol., 14:181, 1980.

Kahnoski, R. J., Lingeman, J. E., Woods, J. R., Eckley, R., Brooks-Bruun, J., and Coury, T. A.: Effectiveness of glucagon in the relief of ureteral colic following treatment by extracorporeal shock wave lithotripsy: A randomized double-blind trial. J. Urol., 137:1124, 1987.

Keating, F. R., Jr.: Diagnosis of primary hyperparathyroidism. Clinical and laboratory aspects. JAMA, 178:547, 1961.

Keutel, H. J.: Localization of uromucoid in human kidney and in sections of human kidney stones with the fluorescent antibody technique. J. Histochem. Cytochem., 13:155, 1965.

Keutel, H. J., and King, J. S., Jr.: Further studies of matrix substance A. Invest. Urol., 2:115, 1964.

King, J. S.: Etiologic factors involved in urolithiasis: A review of recent research. J. Urol., 97:583, 1967.

King, J. S.: Currents in renal stone research. Clin. Chem., 17:971, 1971.

Kister, R., Terhorst, B., and Greiling, H.: Analysis of renal calculi by means of IR-spectroscopy. Z. Klin. Chem. Klin. Biochem., 12:255, 1974.

Kleeman, C. R., Rockney, R. E., and Maxwell, M. H.: The effect of parathyroid extract (PTE) on the renal clearance of diffusible calculi. J. Clin. Invest., 37:907, 1958.

Klohn, M., Bolle, J. F., Reverdin, N. P., Susini, A., Baud, C.-A., and Graber, P.: Ammonium urate urinary stones. Urol. Res., 14:315, 1986.

Koff, S. A.: Mechanism of electrolyte imbalance following urointestinal anastomosis. Urology, 5:109, 1975.

Koide, T., Kinoshita, K., Takemoto, M., Yachiku, S., and Sonoda, T.: Conservative treatment of cystine calculi: Effect of oral alpha-mercaptopropionylglycine on cystine stone dissolution and on prevention of stone recurrence. J. Urol., 128:513, 1982.

Kretschmer, H. L.: Stone in the ureter: Clinical data based on 500 cases. Surg. Gynecol. Obstet., 74:1065, 1942.

Kutzmann, A. A.: Replacement lipomatosis of the kidney. Surg. Gynecol. Obstet., 52:690, 1931.

Lackner, H., and Barton, L. J.: Cortical blood flow in ureteral obstruction. Invest. Urol., 8:319, 1970.

Lafferty, F. W.: Primary hyperparathyroidism—changing clinical spectrum, prevalence of hypertension and discriminant analysis of laboratory tests. Arch. Intern. Med., 141:1761, 1981.

Lagergren, C.: Biophysical investigations of urinary calculi. Acta Radiol. (Suppl), 129:1, 1955.

Lalli, A. F.: Symposium on renal lithiasis. Roentgen aspects of renal calculous disease. Urol. Clin. North Am., 1:213, 1974.

Lanzalaco, A. C., Singh, R. P., Smesko, S. A., Nancollas, G. H., Sutrin, G., Binette, M., and Binette, J. P.: The influence of urinary macromolecules on calcium oxalate monohydrate crystal growth. J. Urol., 139:190, 1988.

Laskowski, D. E.: Chemical microscopy of urinary calculi. Anal. Chem., 37:1399, 1965.

Lehmann, J., Jr., and Gray, R. W.: Idiopathic hypercalciuria. J. Urol., 141:715, 1989.

Lehtonen, T.: Effect of aminophylline on passage of ureteral concretions. Ann. Chir. Gynaecol. Fenn., 62:90, 1973.

Lemann, J., Piering, W. F., and Lennon, E. J.: Possible role of carbohydrate-induced calciuria in calcium oxalate kidney stone formation. N. Engl. J. Med., 280:232, 1969.

Lerner, S. P., Gleeson, M. J., and Griffith, D. P.: Infection stones. J. Urol., 141:753, 1989.

Liao, L. L., and Richardson, K. E.: The metabolism of oxalate precursors in isolated perfused rat livers. Arch. Biochem. Biophys., 153:438, 1972.

Libertino, J. A., Newman, H. R., Lytton, B., et al.: Staghorn calculi in solitary kidneys. J. Urol., 105:753, 1971.

Lien, J., and Keane, P.: Urinary cAMP and calcium excretion in the fasting state and their response to oral calcium loading in patients with calcium urolithiasis. J. Urol., 129:401, 1983.

Lonsdale, K.: Epitaxy as a growth factor in urinary calculi and gallstones. Nature, 217:56, 1968a.

Lonsdale, K.: Human stones. Science, 159:1199, 1968b.

Lonsdale, K., and Sutor, D. J.: Crystallographic studies of urinary and biliary calculi. Sov. Phys. Crystallogr., 16:1060, 1972.

Lotz, M., Potts, J. T., and Bartter, F. C.: Rapid, simple method for determining effectiveness of D-penicillamine therapy in cystinuria. Br. Med. J., 2:521, 1965.

Malek, R. S., and Boyce, W. H.: Intranephronic calculosis: Its significance and relationships to matrix in nephrolithiasis. J. Urol., 109:551, 1973.

Malek, R. S., and Elder, J. S.: Xanthogranulomatous pyelonephritis: A critical analysis of 26 cases and of the literature. J. Urol., 119:589, 1978.

Malek, R. S., and Kelalis, P. P.: Pediatric nephrolithiasis. J. Urol., 113:545, 1975.

Mall, J. C., Collins, P. A., and Lyon, E. S.: Matrix calculi. Br. J. Radiol., 48:807, 1975.

Mandel, N. S., and Mandel, G. S.: Urinary tract stone disease in the United States veteran population. I. Geographical frequency of occurrence. J. Urol., 142:1513, 1989a.

Mandel, N. S., and Mandel, G. S.: Urinary tract stone disease in the United States veteran population. II. Geographical analysis of variations in composition. J. Urol., 142:1516, 1989b.

Marquardt, H.: Incomplete renal tubular acidosis with recurrent nephrolithiasis and nephrocalcinosis. Urologe [A], 12:162, 1973.

Marshall, R. W., and Barry, H.: Urine saturation and the formation of calcium-containing renal calculi: The effects of various forms of therapy. In Cifuentes, L., Rapado, A., and Hodgkinson, A. (Eds.): Urinary Calculi. International Symposium on Renal Stone Research. Basel, S. Karger, 1973, p. 164.

Marshall, R. W., and Robertson, W. G.: Nomograms for the estimation of the saturation of urine with calcium oxalate, calcium phosphate, magnesium ammonium phosphate, uric acid, sodium acid urate, ammonium acid urate and cystine. Clin. Chim. Acta, 72:253, 1976.

Marshall, V. F., and Green, J. L.: Aluminum gels with constant phosphorus intake for the control of renal phosphatic calculi. J. Urol., 67:611, 1952.

Mates, J.: External factors in the genesis of urolithiasis. In Hodgkinson, A., and Nordin, B. E. C. (Eds.): Renal Stone Research Symposium. London, J & A. Churchill, Ltd., 1969, p. 59.

May, P., and Schindler, E.: Methods and results of conservative treatment of uric acid stones. In Cifuentes, I., Rapado, A., and Hodgkinson, A. (Eds.): Urinary Calculi. International Symposium on Renal Stone Research. Basel, S. Karger, 1973, p. 111.

Mbonu, O., Attah, C., and Ikeakor, I.: Urolithiasis in an African population. Intl. Urol. Nephrol., 16:291, 1984.

McGeown, M. G.: Heredity in renal stone disease. Clin. Sci., 19:465, 1960.

McLean, R. J. C., Nickel, J. C., Noakes, V. C., and Costerton, J. W.: An in vitro ultrastructural study of infectious kidney stone genesis. Infect. Immun. 49:805, 1985.

Melnick, I., Landes, R. R., Hoffmann, A. A., et al.: Magnesium therapy for recurring calcium oxalate urinary calculi. J. Urol., 105:119, 1971.

Menon, M., and Mahle, C. J.: Urinary citrate excretion in patients with renal calculi. J. Urol., 129:1158, 1983.

Meyer, A. S., Finlayson, B., and Dubois, L.: Direct observation of urinary stone ultrastructure. Br. J. Urol., 43:154, 1971.

Middleton, A. W., Jr., and Pfister, R. C.: Stone-containing pyelocaliceal diverticulum: Embryogenic, anatomic, radiologic and clinical characteristics. J. Urol., 111:2, 1974.

Middleton, W. D., Dodds, W. J., Lawson, T. L., and Foley, W. D.: Renal calculi: Sensitivity for detection with US (ultrasound). Radiology, 167:239, 1988.

Milkman, L. A.: Multiple spontaneous idiopathic symmetrical fractures. Am. J. Roentgenol., 32:622, 1934.

Miller, G. H., Vermeulen, C. W., and Moore, J. D.: Calcium oxalate solubility in urine: Experimental urolithiasis, XIV. J. Urol., 79:607, 1958.

Miller, J. D., Randolph, A. D., and Drach, G. W.: Observations upon calcium oxalate crystallization kinetics in simulated urine. J. Urol., 117:342, 1977.

Mitchell, J. P.: Lithiasis in children. Editorial. Eur. Urol., 7:121, 1981.

Modlin, M.: The aetiology of renal stone: A new concept arising from studies on a stone-free population. Ann. R. Coll. Surg. Engl., 40:155, 1967.

Moody, T. E., Vaugh, E. D., Jr., and Gillenwater, J. Y.: Relationship between renal blood flow and ureteral pressure during 18 hours of total unilateral ureteral occlusion. Invest. Urol., 13:246, 1975.

Moore, S., and Gowland, G.: The immunological integrity of matrix substance A and its possible detection and quantitation in urine. Br. J. Urol., 47:489, 1975.

Mullin, J. W.: Crystallization, 2nd ed. Cleveland, CRC Press, 1972, p. 150.

Mulvaney, W. P.: The clinical use of Renacidin in urinary calcifications. J. Urol., 84:206, 1960.

Mulvaney, W. P., and Henning, D. C.: Solvent treatment of urinary calculi: Refinements in technique. J. Urol., 88:145, 1962.

Munster, A. M., and Hunter, J.: Urinary extravasation due to perforation of ureter by calculus. Arch. Surg., 97:632, 1968.

Murad, F., and Pak, C. Y. C.: Urinary excretion of adenosine 3',5'-monophosphate and guanosine 3',5'-monophosphate. N. Engl. J. Med., 286:1382, 1972.

Murphy, B. T., and Pyrah, L. N.: The composition, structure and mechanisms of the formation of urinary calculi. Br. J. Urol., 34:129, 1962.

Nakagawa, Y., Ahmed, M. A., Hall, S. L., Deganello, S., and Coe, F. L.: Isolation from human calcium oxalate renal stones of nephrocalcin, a glycoprotein inhibitor of calcium oxalate crystal growth. J. Clin. Invest., 79:1782, 1987.

Nemoy, N. J., and Stamey, T. A.: Surgical bacteriological and biochemical management of "infection stones." JAMA, 215:1470, 1971.

Nicar, M. J., Skurla, C., Sakhaee, K., and Pak, C. Y. C.: Low urinary citrate excretion in nephrolithiasis. Urology, 21:8, 1983.

Nichols, B. H., and Lower, W. E.: Roentgenographic Studies of the Urinary System. St. Louis, C. V. Mosby Co., 1933.

Noe, H. N., Stapleton, F. B., Jerkins, G., and Roy, S.: Clinical experience with pediatric urolithiasis. J. Urol., 129:1166, 1983.

Nordin, B. A., Hodgkinson, A., Peacock, M., and Robertson, W. G.: Urinary tract calculi. In Hamburger, J., Crosnier, J., and Grunfeld, J. P. (Eds.): Nephrology. New York, John Wiley & Sons, 1979.

Ohata, M., and Pak, C. Y. C.: Preliminary study of the treatment of nephrolithiasis (calcium stones) with diphosphonate. Metabolism, 23:1176, 1974.

O'Regan, S., Homsy, Y., and Mongeau, J. G.: Urolithiasis in children. Can. J. Surg., 25:566, 1982.

Oreopoulos, D. G., Walker, D., Akriotis, D. J., et al.: Excretion of inhibitors of calcification in urine. Part I. Findings in control subjects and patients with renal stones. Can. Med. Assoc. J., 112:827, 1975.

Ostergaard, A. H.: Analysis of a bladder stone in 1786. Acta Chir. Scand. (Suppl.), 433:25, 1973.

Pak, C. Y. C.: Hydrochlorothiazide therapy in nephrolithiasis. Effect on the urinary activity product and formation product of brushite. Clin. Pharmacol. Ther., 14:209, 1973.

Pak, C. Y. C.: Renal Stone Disease. Boston, Martinus Nijhoff Publishing, 1987.

Pak, C. Y. C., Delea, C. S., and Bartter, F. C.: Successful treatment of recurrent nephrolithiasis (calcium stones) with cellulose phosphate. N. Engl. J. Med., 290:175, 1974.

Pak, C. Y. C., Hill, K., Cintron, N. M., and Huntoon, C.: Assessing applicants to the NASA Flight Program for their renal stone-forming potential. Clin. Med., Feb. 1989, p. 157.

Pak, C. Y. C., Kaplan, R., Bone, H., et al.: A simple test for the diagnosis of absorptive, resorptive and renal hypercalciurias. N. Engl. J. Med., 292:497, 1975.

Pak, C. Y. C., Ohata, M., Lawrence, E. C., and Snyder, W.: The hypercalciurias: Causes, parathyroid functions and diagnostic criteria. J. Clin. Invest., 54:387, 1974.

Pak, C. Y. C., Skurla, C., and Harvey, J.: Graphic display of urinary risk factors. J. Urol., 134:867, 1985.

Palmer, J. M., Bishai, M. B., and Mallon, D. S.: Outpatient irrigation of the renal collecting system with 10 per cent hemiacidrin: Cumulative experience of 365 days in thirteen patients. J. Urol., 138:262, 1987.

Pantanowitz, D., Pollen, J. J., Politzer, W. M., and Van Blerk, P. J. P.: Urinary calculi. S. Afr. Med. J., 47:128, 1973.

Parry, E. S., and Lister, I. S.: Sunlight and hypercalciuria. Lancet, 1:1063, 1975.

Paterson, C. R.: Drugs for the treatment of hypercalcemia. Postgrad. Med. J., 50:158, 1974.

Paulson, D. F.: Symposium on renal lithiasis. The challenge of calculi in children. Urol. Clin. North Am., 1:365, 1974.

Paulson, D. F., Glen, J. F., Hughes, J., Roberts, L. C., and Coppridge, A. J.: Pediatric urolithiasis. J. Urol., 108:811, 1972.

Pavanello, L., Rizzoni, G., Dussini, N., Zacchello, G., and Passerini, G.: Cystinuria in children. Eur. Urol., 7:139, 1981.

Pearlman, C. K.: Xanthine urinary calculus. J. Urol., 64:799, 1950.

Peters, H. J., and Eckstein, W.: Possible pharmacological means of treating renal colic. Urol. Res., 3:55, 1975.

Peters, J. P., and Van Slyke, D. D.: Cited in Gutman, A. B., and Yu, T. F.: Uric acid nephrolithiasis. Am. J. Med., 45:756, 1968.

Peterson, H. O., and Holmes, G. W.: Roentgen analysis of 100 cases of ureteral calculi. Am. J. Roentgenol., 37:479, 1937.

Porter, P.: Colloidal properties of urates in relation to calculus formation. Res. Vet. Sci., 7:128, 1966.

Preminger, G. M., Peterson, R., Peters, P. C., and Pak, C. Y. C.: The current role of medical treatment of nephrolithiasis: The impact of improved techniques of stone removal. J. Urol., 134:6, 1985.

Prien, E. L., Sr.: Crystallographic analysis of urinary calculi: 23-year survey study. J. Urol., 89:917, 1963.

Prien, E. L., Sr.: The riddle of urinary stone disease. JAMA 216:503, 1971.

Prien, E. L., Sr.: Symposium on renal lithiasis. The analysis of urinary calculi. Urol. Clin. North Am., 1:229, 1974.

Prien, E. L., and Frondel, C.: Studies in urolithiasis: The composition of urinary calculi. J. Urol., 57:949, 1947.

Prien, E. L., Sr., and Gershoff, S. F.: Magnesium oxide–pyridoxine therapy for recurrent calcium oxalate calculi. J. Urol., 112:509, 1974.

Prien, E. L., and Prien, E. L.: Composition and structure of urinary stone. Am. J. Med., 45:654, 1968.

Priestley, J. T., and Osterberg, A. E.: The relationship between the chemical composition of renal calculi and associated bacteria. J. Urol., 36:447, 1936.

Prince, C. L., and Scardino, P. L.: A statistical analysis of ureteral calculi. J. Urol., 83:561, 1960.

Prince, C. L., Scardino, P. L., and Wolan, T. C.: The effect of temperature, humidity, and dehydration on the formation of renal calculi. J. Urol., 75:209, 1956.

Quencer, R. M., and Foster, S. C.: Perforated ureter secondary to a ureteral calculus: Report of a case. Radiology, 102:561, 1972.

Rahman, M. A., Rahman, B., and Perveen, S.: Studies on serum mucoproteins in patients with urinary calculi. Biomed. Pharmacother., 40:311, 1986.

Rambar, A. C., and MacKenzie, R. G.: Urolithiasis in adolescents. Am. J. Dis. Child., 132:1117, 1978.

Randall, A.: The origin and growth of renal calculi. Ann. Surg., 105:1009, 1937.

Rapaport, A., Crasswell, P. O., Husdan, H., From, G. L. A., Zweig, M., and Johnson, M. D.: The renal excretion of hydrogen ion in uric acid stone formers. Metabolism, 16:176, 1967.

Rattiazzi, L. C., Simmons, R. L., Markland, C., Casali, R., Kjellstrand, C. M., and Najarian, J. S.: Calculi complicating renal transplantation into ileal conduits. Urology, 5:29, 1975.

Reece, R. W., and Hackler, R. H.: Spontaneous rupture of the ureter. South. Med. J., 67:739, 1974.

Resnick, M. I., and Boyce, W. H.: Spherical calcium bodies in stone-forming urine. Invest. Urol., 15:449, 1978.

Resnick, M. I., Kursh, E. D., and Cohen, A. M.: Use of computerized tomography in the delineation of uric acid calculi. J. Urol., 131:9, 1984.

Resnick, M. I., Pridgen, D. B., and Goodman, H. O.: Genetic predisposition to formation of calcium oxalate renal calculi. N. Engl. J. Med., 278:1313, 1968.

Reynolds, T. B., Lamman, G., and Tupikova, N.: Re-evaluation of phosphate excretion tests in the diagnosis of hyperparathyroidism. Arch. Intern. Med., 106:48, 1960.

Riches, E.: The history of lithotomy and lithotrity. Ann. R. Coll. Surg. Engl., 43:185, 1968.

Riddick, T. M.: Control of Colloid Stability Through Zeta Potential. Wynnewood, PA., Livingston Publishing Co., 1968.

Rivera, J. V.: Urinary calculi in Puerto Rico. II. Seasonal incidence. Bull. Assoc. Med. Puerto Rico, 65:28, 1973.

Robertson, W. G., and Peacock, M.: Calcium oxalate crystalluria and inhibitors of crystallization in recurrent renal stone-formers. Clin. Sci., 43:499, 1972.

Robertson, W. G., and Peacock, M.: Review of risk factors in calcium oxalate urolithiasis. World J. Urol., 1:114, 1983.

Robertson, W. G., Hambleton, J., and Hodgkinson, A.: Peptide inhibitors of calcium phosphate precipitation in the urine of normal and stone-forming men. Clin. Chim. Acta, 25:247, 1969.

Robertson, W. G., Heyburn, P. J., Peacock, M., Hanes, F. A., and Swaminathan, R.: The effect of high animal protein intake on the risk of calcium stone-formation in the urinary tract. Clin. Sci., 57:285, 1979a.

Robertson, W. G., Peacock, M., and Heyburn, P. J.: Epidemiological risk-factors in calcium stone formation. Fortschr. Urol. Nephrol., 14:105, 1979b.

Robertson, W. G., Peacock, M., Heyburn, P. J., Hanes, F. A., Rutherford, A., et al.: Should recurrent calcium oxalate stone-formers become vegetarians? Br. J. Urol., 51:427, 1979c.

Robertson, W. G., Peacock, M., Heyburn, P. J., Marshall, D. H., and Clark, P. B.: Risk factors in calcium stone disease of the urinary tract. Br. J. Urol., 50:449, 1978.

Robertson, W. G., Peacock, M., Marshall, R. W., and Knowles, F.: The effect of ethane-1-hydroxy-1, 1-diphosphonate (EHDP) on calcium oxalate crystalluria in recurrent renal stone formers. Clin. Sci. Mol. Med., 47:13, 1974.

Robertson, W. G., Peacock, M., Marshall, R. W., Marshall, D. H., and Nordin, B. E. C.: Saturation-inhibition index as a measure of the risk of calcium oxalate stone formation in the urinary tract. N. Engl. J. Med., 294:249, 1976.

Robertson, W. G., Peacock, M., and Nordin, B. E. C.: Activity products in stone-forming and non–stone-forming urine. Clin. Sci., 34:579, 1968.

Robertson, W. G., Peacock, M., and Nordin, B. E. C.: Measurement of activity products in urine from stone-formers and normal subjects. In Finlayson, B., et al. (Eds.): Urolithiasis: Physical Aspects. Washington, National Academy of Sciences, 1972a, p. 79.

Robertson, W. G., Peacock, M., and Nordin, B. E. C.: Crystalluria. In Finlayson, B., et al. (Eds.): Urolithiasis: Physical Aspects. Washington, National Academy of Sciences, 1972b, p. 243.

Robertson, W. G., Peacock, M., and Nordin, B. E. C.: Inhibitors of the growth and aggregation of calcium oxalate crystals in vitro. Clin. Chim. Acta, 43:31, 1973.

Rodman, J. S., Williams, J. J., and Jones, R. L.: Hypercoagulability produced by treatment with acetohydroxamic acid. Clin. Pharmacol. Ther., 42:346, 1987.

Rollins, R., and Finlayson, B.: Mechanism of prevention of calcium oxalate encrustation by methylene blue and demonstration of the concentration dependence of its action. J. Urol., 110:459, 1973.

Rose, G. A., and Westbury, E. J.: The influence of calcium content of water, intake of vegetables and fruit and of other food factors upon the incidence of renal calculi. Urol. Res., 3:61, 1975.

Rose, G. A., Gillenwater, J. Y., and Wyker, A. T. L.: The recovery of function of chronically obstructed and infected ureters. Invest. Urol., 13:125, 1975.

Roth, L. J., and Davidson, H. B.: Fibrous and fatty replacement of renal parenchyma. JAMA, 111:233, 1938.

Roth, R., and Finlayson, B.: Observations on the radiopacity of stone substances with special reference to cystine. Invest. Urol., 11:186, 1973.

Rundles, R. W., Metz, E. N., and Silberman, H. R.: Allopurinol in the treatment of gout. Ann. Intern. Med., 64:229, 1966.

Rutishauser, G.: Etiology of ureteral colic. Ther. Umsch., 28:790, 1971.

Ryall, R. L., Hibberd, C. M., and Marshall, V. R.: A method for studying inhibitory activity in whole urine. Urol. Res., 13:285, 1985.

Sakhaee, K., Nicar, M., Hill, K., and Pak, C. Y. C.: Contrasting effects of potassium citrate and sodium citrate therapies on urinary chemistries and crystallization of stone-forming salts. Kidney Int., 24:348, 1983.

Sakhaee, K., Nigam, S., Snell, P., Hsu, M. C., and Pak, C. Y. C.: Assessment of the pathogenetic role of physical exercise in renal stone formation. J. Clin. Endocrinol. Metab., 65:974, 1987.

Sallis, J. D.: Glycosaminoglycans as inhibitors of stone formation. Miner. Electrolyte Metab., 13:273, 1987.

Sandergard, E.: Prognosis of stone in the ureter. Acta Chir. Scand. (Suppl.), 219:30, 1956.

Sarig, S., Garti, M., Azoury, R., Wax, Y., and Perlberg, S.: A method for discrimination between calcium oxalate kidney stone formers and normals. J. Urol., 128:645, 1982.

Schmidt-Nielsen, K. S.: Desert Animals: Physiological Problems of Heat and Water. Oxford, Oxford University Press, 1964.

Schmucki, O., and Asper, R.: Clinical significance of stone analysis. Urol. Int., 41:343, 1986.

Schneider, H. J., Berenyi, M., Hesse, A., et al.: Comparative urinary stone analyses. Quantitative chemical, x-ray diffraction, infrared spectroscopy and thermoanalytical procedures. Int. Urol. Nephrol., 5:9, 1973.

Scholl, A. J.: Stones in the kidney and ureter. In Cabot, B. (Ed.): Modern Urology. Philadelphia, Lea & Febiger, 1936, p. 598.

Schrott, H. G., Jubiz, W., Frailey, J., and Tyler, F. H.: Calcium infusion and phosphate deprivation tests in patients with primary hyperparathyroidism and with normocalcemia and nephrolithiasis. Metabolism, 21:205, 1972.

Schweitzer, F. A. W.: Intra-pelvic pressure and renal function studies in experimental chronic partial ureteric obstruction. Br. J. Urol., 45:2, 1973.

Schwille, P. O., Scholz, D., Schwille, K., Leutschaft, R., Goldberg, I., and Sigel, A.: Citrate in urine and serum and associated variables in subgroups of urolithiasis. Nephron, 31:194, 1982.

Scott, R.: Urinary tract stone disease. Classic studies. Urology, 6:667, 1975.

Scurr, D. S., and Robertson, W. G.: Modifiers of calcium oxalate crystallization found in urine. III. Studies on the role of Tamm-Horsfall mucoprotein and of ionic strength. J. Urol., 136:505, 1986.

Seegmiller, J. E.: Metabolic basis of renal lithiasis from over-production of uric acid. In Cifuentes, L., Rapado, A., and Hodgkinson, A. (Eds.): Urinary Calculi. International Symposium on Renal Stone Research. Basel, S. Karger, 1973, p. 89.

Seftel, A., and Resnick, M. I.: Metabolic evaluation of urolithiasis. Urol. Clin. North Am., 17:159, 1990.

Segura, J. W., Patterson, D. E., LeRoy, A. J., Williams, H. J., Jr., Barrett, D. M., Benson, R. C., Jr., May, G. R., and Bender, C. E.: Percutaneous removal of kidney stones: Review of 1,000 cases. J. Urol., 134:1077, 1985.

Seifert, H.: Epitaxy of macromolecules on quartz surfaces. In Peiser, H. S. (Ed.): Crystal Growth. Proceedings of an International Conference on Crystal Growth. New York, Pergamon Press, 1967, p. 543.

Sharma, R. N., Shah, I., Gupta, S., Sharma, P., and Beigh, A. A.: Thermogravimetric analysis of urinary stones. Br. J. Urol., 64:564, 1989.

Sharon, E., and Diamond, H. S.: Factitious uric acid urolithiasis as a feature of the Munchausen syndrome. Mt. Sinai J. Med., N.Y., 41:698, 1974.

Sherwood, L. M.: Diagnosis and management of hyperparathyroidism. Hosp. Pract., Mar., 30:9–10, 15, 1988.

Sherwood, L. M., O'Riordan, J. L. H., Aurbach, G. D., and Potts, J. T., Jr.: Production of parathyroid hormone by nonparathyroid tumors. J. Clin. Endocrinol., 27:140, 1967.

Shuster, J., Finlayson, B., Schaeffer, R., Sierakowski, R., Zoltek, J., and Dzegede, S.: Water hardness and urinary stone disease. J. Urol., 128:422, 1982.

Sierakowski, R., Finlayson, B., and Landes, R.: Stone incidence as related to water hardness in different geographical regions of the United States. Urol. Res., 7:157, 1978.

Sierakowski, R., Hemp, B., and Finlayson, B.: Water hardness and the incidence of urinary calculi. In Finlayson, B., and Thomas, W. C. (Eds.): Colloquium on Renal Lithiasis. Gainesville, University Presses of Florida, 1976.

Silver, T. M., Koff, S. A., and Thornbury, J.: An unusual pathway of urine extravasation associated with renal colic. Radiology, 109:537, 1973.

Simkiss, J.: Phosphates as crystal poisons of calcification. Biol. Rev., 39:487, 1964.

Singh, P. P., Sharma, D. C., Rathore, V., and Surana, S. S.: An investigation into the role of ascorbic acid in renal calculogenesis in albino rats. J. Urol., 139:156, 1988.

Singer, A. M., Bennett, R. C., Carter, N. G., and Hughes, E. S. R.: Blood and urinary changes in patients with ileostomies and ileorectal anastomoses. Br. Med. J., 3:141, 1973.

Smith, L. H.: Medical evaluation of urolithiasis. Etiologic aspects and diagnostic evaluation. Urol. Clin. North Am., 1:241, 1974a.

Smith, L. H.: Errors in membrane transport: Cystinuria, renal glycosuria and renal tubular acidosis. In Wintrobe, M. M., Thorn, G. W., Adams, R. D., Braunwald, E., Isselbacher, K. J., Petersdorf, R. G. (Eds.): Principles of Internal Medicine. 7th ed. New York, McGraw-Hill Book Co., 1974b, p. 600.

Smith, L. H.: Medical aspects of urolithiasis: An overview. J. Urol., 141:707, 1989.

Smith, L. H., and Hofman, A. F.: Acquired hyperoxaluria, urolithi-

asis, and intestinal disease: A new digestive disorder? Gastroenterology, 66:1257, 1974.

Smith, M. J. V., and Boyce, W. H.: Allopurinol and urolithiasis. J. Urol., 102:750, 1969.

Smith, M. J. V., Hunt, L. D., King, J. S., and Boyce, W. H.: Uricemia and urolithiasis. J. Urol., 101:637, 1969.

Sommerkamp, H., and Schwerk, W. B.: Incomplete tubular acidosis in recurrent urinary phosphate calculi. Urologe [A], 12:167, 1973.

Sorgel, F., Ettinger, B., and Benet, L. Z.: The true composition of kidney stones passed during triamterene therapy. J. Urol., 134:871, 1985.

Sperling, O., DeVries, A., and Kadem, O.: Studies on the etiology of uric acid lithiasis. IV. Urinary nondialyzable substances in idiopathic uric acid lithiasis. J. Urol., 94:286, 1965.

Stamey, T. A.: Urinary Infections. Baltimore, Williams & Wilkins Co., 1972.

Stapleton, F. B., Noe, H. N., Roy, A., and Jerkins, G.: Hypercalciuria in children with urolithiasis. Am. J. Dis. Child., 136:675, 1982.

Stapleton, F. B., Roy, S., III, Noe, H. N., and Jerkins, G.: Hypercalciuria in children with hematuria. N. Engl. J. Med., 310:1345, 1984.

Stecker, J. F., Jr., and Gillenwater, J. Y.: Experimental partial ureteral obstruction. I. Alteration in renal function. Invest. Urol., 8:377, 1971.

Steele, B. T., Lowe, P., Rance, C. P., Hardy, B. E., and Churchill, B. M.: Urinary tract calculi in children. Int. J. Pediatr. Nephrol., 4:47, 1983.

Stewart, A. F., and Broadus, A. E.: The regulation of renal calcium excretion: An approach to hypercalciuria. Annu. Rev. Med., 32:457, 1981.

Strott, C. A., and Nugent, C. A.: Laboratory tests in the diagnosis of hyperparathyroidism in hypercalcemic patients. Ann. Intern. Med., 68:188, 1968.

Stubbs, A. J., and Myers, R. T.: Experience with hyperparathyroidism. Surg. Gynecol. Obstet., 136:65, 1973.

Subramanyam, B. R., Megibow, A. J., Raghavendra, B. N., and Bosniak, M. A.: Diffuse xanthogranulomatous pyelonephritis: Analysis by computed tomography and sonography. Urol. Radiol., 4:5, 1982.

Suby, H. I., and Albright, F.: Dissolution of phosphatic urinary calculi by the retrograde introduction of a citrate solution containing magnesium. N. Engl. J. Med., 228:81, 1943.

Suby, H. I., Suby, R. M., and Albright, F.: Properties of organic acid solutions which determine their irritability to the bladder mucosa and the effect of magnesium ions in overcoming this irritability. J. Urol., 48:549, 1942.

Sugimoto, T., Funae, Y., Rübben, H., Nishio, S., Hautmann, R., and Lutzeyer, W.: Resolution of proteins in the kidney stone matrix using high-performance liquid chromatography. Eur. Urol., 11:334, 1985.

Sutherland, J. W., Parks, J. H., and Coe, F. L.: Recurrence after a single renal stone in a community practice. Miner. Electrolyte Metab., 11:267, 1985.

Sutor, D. J.: Difficulties in the identification of components of mixed urinary calculi using the ray method. Br. J. Urol., 40:29, 1968.

Sutor, D. J.: The nature of urinary stones. In Finlayson, B., et al. (Eds.): Urolithiasis: Physical Aspects. Washington, National Academy of Sciences, 1972, p. 43.

Sutor, D. J., and O'Flynn, J. D.: Matrix formation in crystalline material in vivo. In Cifuentes, L., Rapado, A., and Hodgkinson, A. (Eds.): Urinary Calculi. International Symposium on Renal Stone Research. Basel, S. Karger, 1973, p. 280.

Sutor, D. J., and Scheidt, S.: Identification standards for human urinary calculus components using crystallographic methods. Br. J. Urol., 40:22, 1968.

Sutor, D. J., and Wooley, S. E.: Composition of urinary calculi by x-ray diffraction. Collected data from various localities. VII. The Sir Henry Thompson collection of bladder stones from the Royal College of Surgeons, London. Br. J. Urol., 41:397, 1969.

Sutor, D. J., and Wooley, S. E.: Composition of urinary calculi by x-ray diffraction. Collected data from various localities. VIII. Leeds, England. Br. J. Urol., 42:302, 1970.

Sutor, D. J., and Wooley, S. E.: Composition of urinary calculi by x-ray diffraction. Collected data from various localities. IX–XI. Glasgow, Scotland; United States of America; and Sudan. Br. J. Urol., 43:268, 1971.

Sutor, D. J., and Wooley, S. E.: Composition of urinary calculi by x-ray diffraction. Collected data from various localities. XV–XVIII. Royal Navy; Bristol, England; and Dundee, Scotland. Br. J. Urol., 46:229, 1974a.

Sutor, D. J., and Wooley, S. E.: The crystalline composition of prostatic calculi. Br. J. Urol., 46:533, 1974b.

Sutor, D. J., Wooley, S. E., and Illingworth, J. J.: Some aspects of the adult urinary stone problem in Great Britain and Northern Ireland. Br. J. Urol., 46:275, 1974a.

Sutor, D. J., Wooley, S. E., and Illingworth, J. J.: A geographical and historical survey of the composition of urinary stones. Br. J. Urol., 46:393, 1974b.

Sutor, D. J., and Wooley, S. E.: Some data on urinary stones which were passed. Br. J. Urol., 47:131, 1975.

Suvachittanont, O., et al.: The oxalic acid content of some vegetables in Thailand, its possible relationships with the bladder stone disease. J. Med. Assoc. Thailand, 56:645, 1973.

Takasaki, E.: An observation on the analysis of urinary calculi by infrared spectroscopy. Calcif. Tissue Res., 7:232, 1971.

Takasaki, E.: An observation on the composition and recurrence of urinary calculi. Urol. Int., 30:228, 1975.

Takasaki, E.: Comparison of chemical compositions of multiple or recurrent urinary stones. Urol. Int., 44:160, 1989.

Taneja, O. P., Mall, M. P., and Mittal, K. P.: Urologic aspects of endemic bladder stones in children. Aust. N.Z. J. Surg., 40:130, 1970.

Tennant, C. E.: Ureteral stone of unusual size. JAMA, 82:1122, 1924.

Thalut, K., Rizal, A., Brockis, J. G., Bowyer, R. C., Taylor, T. A., and Wisniewski, Z. S.: The endemic bladder stones of Indonesia—epidemiology and clinical features. Br. J. Urol., 48:617, 1976.

Thom, J. A., Morris, J. E., Bishop, A., and Blacklock, N. J.: The influence of refined carbohydrate on urinary calcium excretion. Br. J. Urol., 50:459, 1978.

Thomas, W. C., Jr.: Kidney stones, urine, and cement. Md. Med. J., 37(11):861, 1988.

Thomas, W. C., Jr.: Symposium on renal lithiasis. Medical aspects of renal calculous disease. Treatment and prophylaxis. Urol. Clin. North Am., 1:261, 1974.

Thomas, W. C., Jr.: Clinical concepts of renal calculous disease. J. Urol., 113:423, 1975.

Thompson, J. C.: Urinary calculi at the Canton Hospital. Surg. Gynecol. Obstet., 32:44, 1921.

Thompson, R. B., and Stamey, T. A.: Bacteriology of infected stones. Urology, 2:267, 1973.

Thorwald, J.: The Century of the Surgeon. New York, Pantheon, 1956, p. 24.

Tolia, B. M., Iloreta, A., Freed, S. Z., Fruchtman, B., Bennett, B., and Newman, H. R.: Xanthogranulomatous pyelonephritis: Detailed analysis of 29 cases and a brief discussion of atypical presentations. J. Urol., 125:437, 1981.

Toor, M., Massry, S., Katz, A. I., and Agmon, J.: The effect of fluid intake on the acidification of urine. Clin. Sci., 27:259, 1964.

Transbol, I., and Frydendal, N.: Endocrine and metabolic aspects of urology. Aetiology of stone formation in 145 renal stone patients. Acta Chir. Scand. (Suppl.), 433:137, 1973.

Uhlmann, D. R., and Chalmers, B.: The energetics of nucleation. Indust. Eng. Chem., 57:19, 1965.

Valyasevi, A., and Dhanamitta, S.: Studies of bladder stone disease in Thailand, XVII. Effect of exogenous source of oxalate on crystalluria. Am. J. Clin. Nutr., 27:877, 1974.

Van Arsdalen, K. N., Banner, M. P., and Pollack, H. M.: Radiographic imaging and urologic decision making in the management of renal and ureteral calculi. Urol. Clin. North Am., 17:171, 1990.

Van Aswegen, C. H., Hurter, P., van der Merwe, C. A., and du Plessis, D. J. P.: The relationship between total urinary testosterone and renal calculi. Urol. Res., 17:181, 1989.

Van Reen, R.: Geographical and nutritional aspects of endemic stones. In Brockis, J. G., and Finlayson, B. (Eds.): Urinary Calculus. Littleton, MA, PSG Publishing Co., 1981.

Van Regemorter, G., and Hardy, J. C.: Extravasations at the level of the upper urinary tract. Acta Urol. Belg., 41:858, 1973.

Varghese, M., Rodman, J. S., Williams, J. J., Brown, A., Carter, D. M., Zerwekh, J. E., and Pak, C. Y. C.: Effect of ultraviolet B radiation treatments on calcium excretion and vitamin D metabolites in kidney stone formers. Clin. Nephrol., 31:225, 1989.

Vaughan, E. D., Jr., Sorenson, E. J., and Gillenwater, J. Y.: The renal hemodynamic response to chronic unilateral complete ureteral occlusion. Invest. Urol., 8:78, 1970.

Vaughan, E. D., Jr., Shenasky, J. H., II, and Gillenwater, J. Y.: Mechanism of acute hemodynamic response to ureteral occlusion. Invest. Urol., 9:109, 1971a.

Vaughan, E. D., Jr., Sorenson, E. J., and Gillenwater, J. Y.: Alterations in renal function immediately after release of acute total unilateral ureteral occlusion. Invest. Urol., 8:450, 1971b.

Vermeulen, C. W., and Lyon, E. S.: Mechanism of genesis and growth of calculi. Am. J. Med., 45:684, 1968.

Vermeulen, C. W., Lyon, E. S., and Gill, W. B.: Artificial urinary concretions. Invest. Urol., 1:370, 1964.

Vogel, V. J.: American Indian Medicine. Norman, University of Oklahoma Press, 1970.

Wahlberg, J.: The renal response to ureteral obstruction. Scand. J. Urol. Nephrol. (Suppl.), 73:1, 1983.

Walton, A. G.: Nucleation of crystals from solution. Science, 148:601, 1965.

Walton, A. G.: The Formation and Properties of Precipitates. New York, Interscience Publishing, 1967.

Wangensteen, O. H., Wangensteen, D. S., and Wiita, J.: Lithotomy and lithotomists: Progress in wound management from Franco to Lister. Surgery, 66:929, 1969.

Wart, F., Auvray, P., and Piront, A.: Extrarenal diffusion of contrast media during intravenous urography. Acta Urol. Belg., 41:564, 1973.

Watanabe, T.: Histochemical studies on mucosubstances in urinary stones. Tohoku J. Exp. Med., 107:345, 1972.

Waterhouse, C., and Heinig, R. E.: Parathormone function. N. Engl. J. Med., 294:545, 1976.

Watts, R. W.: Oxaluria. J. R. Coll. Physicians Lond., 7:161, 1973.

Watts, R. W.: Uric acid biosynthesis and its disorders. J. R. Coll. Physicians Lond., 11:91, 1976.

Welshman, S. G., and McGeown, M. G.: The relationship of the urinary cations calcium, magnesium, sodium and potassium, in patients with renal calculi. Br. J. Urol., 47:237, 1975.

Welshman, S. G., and McGeown, M. G.: Urinary citrate excretion in stone formers and normal controls. Br. J. Urol., 48:7, 1976.

Werness, P. G., Bergert, J. H., and Smith, L. H.: Triamterene urolithiasis: Solubility, pK, effect on crystal formation, and matrix binding of triamterene and its metabolites. J. Lab. Clin. Med., 99:254, 1982.

Wesson, M. B.: Renal calculi: Etiology and prophylaxis. J. Urol., 34:289, 1935.

Westbury, E. J.: Some observations on the quantitative analysis of over 1000 urinary calculi. Br. J. Urol., 46:215, 1974.

White, D. J., Jr., Christoffersen, J., Herman, T. S., Lanzalaco, A. C., and Nancollas, G. H.: Effects of urine pretreatment on calcium oxalate crystallization inhibition potentials. J. Urol., 129:175, 1983.

White, J. L.: Stones in the prostate and seminal vesicles. Texas J. Med., 23:581, 1928.

White, R. W., et al.: Minerals in the urine of stoneformers and their spouses. In Hodgkinson, A., and Nordin, B. E. C. (Eds.): Proceedings of the Renal Stone Research Symposium. London, J. & A. Churchill, Ltd., 1969.

Williams, H. E.: Nephrolithiasis. N. Engl. J. Med., 290:33, 1974a.

Williams, H. E.: Calcium nephrolithiasis and cellulose phosphate. N. Engl. J. Med., 290:224, 1974b.

Wilson, D. M.: Clinical and laboratory approaches for evaluation of nephrolithiasis. J. Urol., 141:770, 1989.

Witten, F. R., Morgan, J. W., Foster, J. G., and Glenn, J. F.: 2,8-Hydroxyadenine urolithiasis: Review of the literature and report of case in the United States. J. Urol., 130:938, 1983.

Worchester, E. M., Nakagawa, Y., and Coe, F. L.: Glycoprotein calcium oxalate crystal growth inhibitor in urine. Miner. Electrolyte Metab., 13:267, 1987.

Yanagawa, M., Ohkawa, H., and Tada, S.: The determination of urinary oxalate by gas chromatography. J. Urol., 129:1163, 1983.

Yendt, E. R., and Cohanim, M.: Clinical and laboratory approaches for evaluation of nephrolithiasis. J. Urol., 141:764, 1989.

Yendt, E. R., and Cohanim, M.: Ten years' experience with the use of thiazides in the prevention of kidney stones. Trans. Am. Clin. Climatol. Assoc., 85:65, 1973.

Young, J. D., Jr., and Martin, L. G.: Urinary calculi associated with incomplete renal tubular acidosis. J. Urol., 107:170, 1972.

Yu, T. F.: Urolithiasis in hyperuricemia and gout. J. Urol., 126:424, 1981.

Yu, T. F., and Gutman, A. B.: Relationship of renal production of ammonia to uric acid stone formation in primary gout. *In* Cifuentes, L., Rapado, A., and Hodgkinson, A. (Eds.): Urinary Calculi. International Symposium on Renal Stone Research. Basel, S. Karger, 1973, p. 101.

Zoller, N., and Griebsch, A.: Influence of various dietary purines on uric acid production. *In* Cifuentes, L., Rapado, A., and Hodgkinson, A. (Eds.): Urinary Calculi. International Symposium on Renal Stone Research. Basel, S. Karger, 1973, p. 84.

Research Seminars and Conferences, Proceedings

Cifuentes, L., Rapado, A., and Hodgkinson, A.: Urinary Calculi (Madrid, 1972). Basel, S. Karger, 1973.

Finlayson, B., and Thomas, W. C., Jr.: International Colloquium on Renal Lithiasis. Gainesville, University of Florida Press, 1976.

Finlayson, B., Hench, L. L., and Smith, L. H.: Urolithiasis, Physical Aspects. Washington, National Academy of Sciences, 1972.

Hodgkinson, A., and Nordin, B. E. C.: Renal Stone Research Symposium (Leeds, 1968). London, J. & A. Churchill, Ltd., 1969.

Schwille, P. O., Smith, L. H., Robertson, W. G., and Vahlensieck, W.: Urolithiasis and Related Clinical Research. New York, Plenum Press, 1985.

Smith, L. J., Robertson, W. G., and Finlayson, B.: Urolithiasis, Clinical and Basic Research. New York, Plenum Press, 1981.

Walker, V. R., Sutton, R. A. L., Cameron, E. C. B., Pak, C. Y. C., and Robertson, W. G.: Urolithiasis. New York, Plenum Press, 1989.

59
EXTRACORPOREAL SHOCK WAVE LITHOTRIPSY

David L. McCullough, M.D.

One of the great medical advances of all times is extracorporeal shock wave lithotripsy, ESWL. ESWL is a term registered by the Dornier Company, Marietta, Georgia. In this chapter, SWL is used to denote extracorporeal shock wave lithotripsy. Another term that is used is percutaneous lithotripsy or nephrolithotomy, symbolized by PCL.

SWL has greatly reduced the need for open stone surgery and PCL. It is estimated that SWL and endoscopic lithotripsy have reduced the need for open stone surgery to between 1 and 2 per cent of cases (Assimos, 1989B; Boyle et al., 1989). Combinations of SWL and PCL are often utilized in the treatment of staghorn calculi and other large stones. Precise indications for SWL, PCL, and open stone surgery are still being defined. The Guidelines Committee for Urinary Calculus Disease, appointed by the American Urological Association, should help determine the proper utilization of various treatment modalities and should complete its work by 1993.

HISTORY AND THEORY

Early Experiments

Forssmann and associates (1977) reported that mechanical breakdown on the surface of a solid occurs when the tensile force exceeds the comprehensive strength of the solid. When raindrops or small meteorites collide with the outer surfaces of aircraft, the pitting seen is thought to be due to shock wave generation by the collision. When brittle solids are immersed in fluids,

at the interface, shock waves traversing through the fluids exert a destructive effect on the solid by creating a strong tensile force on the solid (Chaussy et al., 1987). Chaussy, Eisenberger, Wanner, Hepp, Schmeidt, Forssmann, and others in the 1970s played a major role in the basic research of harnessing shock waves and their force into a clinically applicable delivery system to treat urinary calculi (Chaussy et al., 1987). This application took the form of an underwater shock wave. The underwater shock wave was generated by a spark gap electrical discharge contained within a Faraday cage to prevent electrical shock to the organism receiving the focused shock waves. Focusing was performed by fixing the spark plug within a semi-ellipsoid metal dish at F_1, shock wave first focal point. The semi-ellipsoid reflector focused the shock waves to the second focal point, F_2, where the energy converged on a small point (i.e., a calculus) designed to fracture the stone into small particles (Fig. 59–1).

Shock waves generated by such an electrohydraulic force are characterized by a very rapid onset and a gradual decline. They are not similar to ultrasound

I wish to thank Christian Chaussy, M.D., for training me in lithotripsy in Munich in 1984, and for his generosity in sharing his knowledge so willingly. I also thank the American Urological Association for the opportunity to serve as Chairman of the Lithotripsy Committee since 1984. Both of these opportunities have greatly enriched and stimulated my professional career in the area of urinary calculous disease.

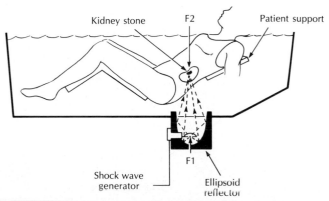

Figure 59–1. Lateral view of patient in gantry of Dornier HM-3 lithotriptor demonstrating focusing of shock wave (SW) from electrohydraulic power source (see text for explanation of F_1 and F_2).

waves, which are sinusoidal and have an alternating negative and positive deflection. The shock waves suffer very little alteration in water or body tissues in contrast to ultrasound waves.

The Dornier Company is a pioneer aerospace company whose early "flying boat" achieved wide notoriety in the earlier part of this century. The company was keenly interested in shock wave physics and employed a number of researchers in this area. Their early research involved the phenomenon of the collision of micrometeorites and raindrops against metal aircraft bodies, which caused pitting of the metal. This was found to be due to shock waves generated by such collisions. In 1984, I toured the German Dornier plant on Lake Constance, where the lithotriptor, HM-3, was manufactured.

Collaboration of the Dornier Company and the Institute of Surgical Research of the University of Munich was encouraged by the German government. Professors E. Schmeidt, F. Eisenberger, and C. Chaussy as well as others at the University of Munich worked on the project between 1974 and 1980. This collaboration culminated in a clinically testable lithotriptor, the HM-1 (Human Model number one).

On February 20, 1980, the first human SWL procedure was performed in Munich using the HM-1. By May 1982, 221 SWL treatments had been rendered to 206 patients (Chaussy et al., 1982). By that time, the HM-2 had evolved.

In October 1983, the HM-3 was installed in Stuttgart at a second center. By 1984, the HM-3 became commercially available after more than 1000 patients had been treated in Munich and Stuttgart. The unmodified HM-3 still is the most widely used lithotriptor in the world, a testimony to its excellent design, safety, and efficacy.

Types of Shock Wave Generators

Spark Gap

The spark gap generator is a spark plug which sits in a liquid medium and is powered by a high-kilovoltage generator (Fig. 59–2). The Dornier HM-3 machine uses between 12 and 24 kV in most clinical applications. It

was the first clinically proven lithotriptor. A number of competitive machines also use the spark gap shock wave generation concept. Shock waves generated in this fashion must be coordinated with the electrocardiographic monitor to prevent arrhythmias. Lithotriptors with spark gap electrodes employ a gating system so that they will discharge only during the refractory period of the heart cycle following the R wave (Carlson et al., 1986).

Piezoelectric

Lithotriptors using this type of shock wave generation have a high-frequency, high-voltage pulse, which excites a piezoelectric (ceramic) element. The elements are placed in a concave reflector (dish), and all the elements can be fired at once. Various machines have differing numbers of elements. The Wolf machine has about 3000 elements, whereas the EDAP has approximately 325. The shock waves converge at F_1 because the piezoelectric elements are positioned on a spherical dish (see Fig. 59–2). The focal region of the Wolf machine is approximately 4×8 mm. This small focal region plus lower peak pressures emanating from a wide aperture dish allow for a wide skin entry zone and truly "anesthesia-free" treatment (Fig. 59–3). The Diasonics machine utilizes a flat monoelement (piezoelectric mosaic) with shock waves that are focused by an elliptic aluminum lens. No cardiac arrhythmias are induced by this technology, which simplifies therapy and alleviates the need for electrocardiographic (ECG) triggering as with spark gap machines.

Electromagnetic

The Siemens Lithostar was the first lithotriptor to use this technology. It has been approved by the Food and Drug Administration (FDA). Shock waves are generated by electric currents which move a metallic membrane within a shock tube (see Fig. 59–2). Shock waves so generated are then focused by an acoustic lens to F_1 at the stone site. A water cushion transmits the shock waves into the body at the point where the cushion is coupled to the skin (Fig. 59–4). A respiratory gated system coordinating the patient's respiratory movements with delivery of the shock wave apparently enhances

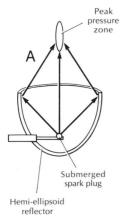

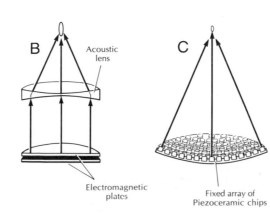

Figure 59–2. Diagrams of various power sources for shock wave (SW) generation. *A*, Spark-gap (electrohydraulic) generation of SW. Relatively large peak pressure zone. *B*, Electromagnetic generator with generation by rapid magnetic repulsion of a metal plate. SW is focused by a plastic acoustic lens. Smaller peak pressure zone at F_1 than at F_2 shown in *A*. *C*, Piezoelectric generation of SW. High voltage is applied to an array of ceramic chips placed on a curved dish. Simultaneous expansion generates a SW to small focal zone at F_1. (Reproduced with permission from Hospital Practice, p. 23, October 30, 1990.)

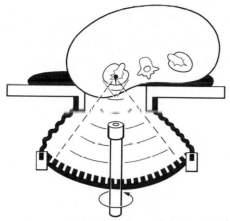

Figure 59–3. Diagram of Wolf Piezoelectric lithotriptor with ultrasonic imager in middle of piezoelectric array of ceramic chips. (Modified from figure supplied by Wolf Co.)

the efficacy of treatment. The Storz Modulith uses electromagnetic shock wave generation, but it uses a parabolic reflector.

Microexplosive

The Yachiyoda Company has developed the SZ-1 microexplosive lithotriptor. The shock waves are generated by lead azide pellet charges and are focused by an ellipsoid.

Lasers

Lasers have been employed in some machines to generate shock waves but, to my knowledge, they are not currently employed in any commercially available machine.

Coupling

The original Dornier HM-3 and the modified HM-3 spark gap lithotriptor use a water bath in which the

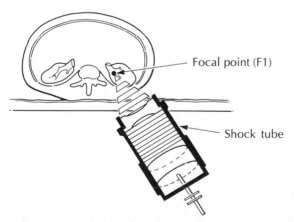

Focal point (F1)

Shock tube

Figure 59–4. Diagram of Siemens Lithostar electromagnetic lithotriptor. Machine has two shock tubes; only one is shown. Tube is coupled to skin with water cushion. Acoustic lens focuses SW on stone at F_1. (Modified from figure supplied by Siemens Co.)

patient is immersed in a chair-like device at a 30-degree angle to the plane of the floor with degassed water covering the patient up to breast level (see Fig. 59–1).

Subsequent Dornier models and those of other manufacturers have evolved into much more compact coupling devices that transmit shock waves through a relatively shallow fluid-filled cushion or tube, which abuts the skin adjacent to the kidney. Lithotriptors that have either a partial water bath or a full water bath include the following: Technomed Sonolith, Wolf Piezolith, and Yashiyoda SZ-1.

The trend is to eliminate the voluminous water bath and to have either a water cushion or a very abbreviated water bath. The original premise that the shock wave must be transmitted through a fluid medium coupled with the body (which, in turn, is mostly water) should be remembered.

Mechanisms of Stone Fracture by Shock Waves

As postulated by Forssmann and co-workers (1977), when the tensile force on the stone's surface exceeds the comprehensive force holding it together, disintegration of the brittle stone begins. Subsequent shock waves continue the process.

Once the shock wave hits the stone, its pressure front is split into compressive and tensile components (Fig. 59–5). The compressive component continues into the stone, while a reflected tensile component moves back toward the shock wave source (Chaussy et al., 1987). A high-pressure gradient occurs owing to these two forces and eventually causes the stone to begin disintegrating on the surface closest to the shock wave source. Some of the shock wave continues through the stone, and at the distant surface, the shock wave is reflected, creating another high-pressure gradient between tensile and compressive waves. Thus, the distant stone surface also begins to crumble. Finally, the remainder of the stone disintegrates. However, about 1 per cent of calcium-containing stones do not disintegrate. Many of these are monohydrate stones. Obviously, the greater the shock wave pressure, the greater is the compressive force.

Early Clinical Experience

Early clinical experience reported by the Munich team (Chaussy et al., 1982) was as follows. In a 27-month period from 1980 through 1982, 206 patients underwent 221 treatments. A minority, 39 per cent, had been previously operated on once or twice, and 15 patients required two treatments. The stone positions were as follows: 75 per cent, renal pelvis; 23 per cent, renal calyces; and 2 per cent, ureter. The stone compositions were as follows: 90 per cent, calcium oxalate; 5 per cent, struvite; and 5 per cent, various clinical compositions.

The follow-up results were as follows: 99 per cent, free of symptoms; 88.5 per cent, free of stones; 10.5 per cent, residual fragments, 3-month follow-up (usually in dilated lower pole calyces); and 1 per cent, open surgery.

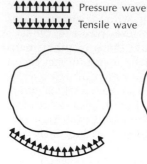 Pressure wave

Tensile wave

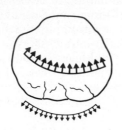 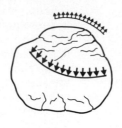

Figure 59–5. Mechanism of stone fragmentation. Arrows pointing up represent compressive forces; arrows pointing down represent tensile forces. Compressive forces fragment stone on side closest to power generation source, whereas on distant side compressive and reflected tensile forces effect fragmentation.

The last cases were ureteral stones. The stones were surrounded by an organic matrix, which prevented the disintegrated fragments from passing. The other two ureteral cases had good fragmentation and prompt passage. Later, two patients in the overall series required operative intervention because of obstruction by fragments, presumably steinstrasse. *Steinstrasse* is a term meaning "stone street," describing fragments stacked up or in a "log jam," wherein the fragments obstruct and line up in the ureter. Some pass spontaneously, others require intervention.

The aforementioned results electrified the urologic community worldwide, and many refused to believe them. The high-technological age had its impact on urology, and the "shock waves" from Munich literally shook the entire urologic community. This new technology was not a dream. It rapidly assumed a dominant position in the therapy of renal calculi. The lay press was suitably impressed by the Dornier Lithotriptor HM-1, and the "Munich Stonebuster" captured the imagination of suffering patients with renal stones worldwide.

Interest in the machine was keen in the United States, and the FDA appointed six centers to serve as clinical test sites in 1984: Methodist Hospital in Indianapolis, Baylor University in Houston, University of Florida in Gainesville, New York Hospital (Cornell) in New York, Massachusetts General Hospital in Boston, and the University of Virginia in Charlottesville. The first treatment in the United States was at Methodist Hospital in Indianapolis on February 23, 1984. The FDA approved the HM-3 for use in December 1984, after more than 2000 SWL treatments had been performed (Drach et al., 1986) (Fig. 59–6). By 1985, the HM-3 was approved in Japan.

Mobile HM-3 units hauled by tractor-trailer trucks were rapidly developed, thus moving the technology closer to the patients, especially in the more rural and sparsely populated areas of the United States. Skeptics who thought the transit of the machine over roads would make it inoperative much of the time were soon converted to believers, again a testimonial to the durability of the machine and the good design of the transporting truck.

There was great competition for HM-3 units by all types of entities. University medical centers, community hospitals, physician-owned outpatient units, physician-owned inpatient units, and combinations of all of the above developed variable ownership and utilization arrangements.

The demand for SWL training was immense and urgent. Originally, the Dornier Company proposed that it would help establish training centers at several institutions. A number of members of the American Urological Association (AUA) petitioned the AUA to take over the training and to establish sites and training criteria. This goal was accomplished, and sites were approved. Waiting lists were long; some training sites charged for training; and charges varied considerably. Some sites charged nothing. In my opinion, the training was generally good and the complication rate of SWL in the early days was reasonable and still is.

The HM-3 forever changed urology and was a prototype of how to implement new technology. This period of history is colorful and the subject of many tales. Urologists were eager to learn SWL and rightfully thought that they knew more about stone evaluation and overall therapy than any other group. A familiarity with fluoroscopy was a great asset in rapidly assimilating the technology. Many patients also required stents and ancillary urologic procedures, and generally, except for some percutaneous nephrostomies, urologists provided and continue to provide most of the SWL care in the United States for renal calculi.

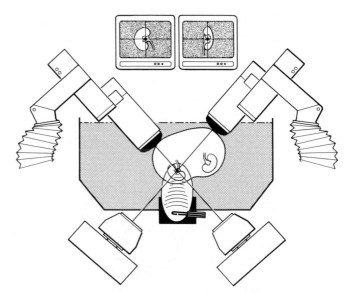

Figure 59–6. Drawing of Dornier HM-3 lithotriptor. Ellipsoid with spark plug at F_1. Stone in kidney at F_2. X-ray tubes beneath water-filled tub. Image intensifiers at top of tub abutting patient's skin. Twin monitors above showing localization of stone in cross-hairs at F_2 in two planes 90 degrees apart. (Modified from figure supplied by Dornier Co.)

EXPERIMENTAL BIOEFFECTS

Effect on Cells

Preliminary Work

The early work reported by the Munich team (Chaussy et al., 1982) produced the following data. After shocking 10 ml of whole blood at F_2 with a 1.5 cm³ focal zone, the free plasma hemoglobin level increased in a linear fashion relative to the number of exposures, and up to 400 mg hemoglobin/100 ml was measured after four shocks. However, after 20 exposures of the canine kidney, no increase in free hemoglobin level was discovered presumably due to the relatively small amount of blood going through the focal zone relative to the total blood volume of the dog. Later studies using 500 shock waves delivered to the kidney in six test dogs showed a slight increase in free plasma hemoglobin levels.

The same group reported no change in the ability of human lymphocytes to be stimulated either in the general mitogenic phytohemagglutinin or in the mixed lymphocyte culture. These lymphocytes, however, had only been subjected to two to five shock wave exposures prior to being cultured.

Later Studies

McCullough and colleagues (1989) used Chaussy's model to compare the bioeffects of an experimental Dornier lithotriptor (XL-1) with the HM-3 at a given voltage in shocking centrifuged red blood cells at F_2. Significantly more free hemoglobin was released when the XL-1 was used versus the HM-3, indicating greater cell damage. This is a rather simple way to compare cellular damage caused by various machines using different power levels.

Shock wave–induced cavitation effects appear to be a possible cause of tissue injury as reported by Fischer and co-workers (1988). Delius (1988) reported further evidence of cavitation-caused tissue injury and thought that a rapid fire rate of 100 shock waves per second caused greater damage than the same total number of shock waves given at 1 per second.

Randazzo and colleagues (1988) reported that, when 2000 shock waves were given to in vitro models of renal cell carcinoma, a significant decrease in viability, cell growth, and cell attachment was seen in comparison with normal human embryonic kidney cells subjected to the same treatment.

Elbers and associates (1988) found that SWL has no significant effect on bacterial viability. This result was determined by treating infected stones (previously removed by percutaneous extraction) with 2400 shock waves at 22 kV and by treating bacteria isolated in polypropylene tubes with 2000 shock waves at 22 kV.

Tissue culture and other in vitro systems have been used by a number of investigators to study the effects of SWL on cellular structure and function in addition to the original preclinical work by Randazzo and co-workers (1988), Drach (1989), and Landone and associates

(1989). Proximal and distal tubular cells in tissue culture were treated with the HM-3, and the viability of dissociated cells was not influenced by the voltage but rather by the number of shock waves (McAteer et al., 1989). Clayman and co-workers (1989b) compared the effects of shock waves generated by piezoelectric, electrohydraulic, and electromagnetic sources and found the effect on cell suspensions was an immediate decrease in cell viability. After the electrohydraulic lithotriptor was employed, the viable cells did not recover nearly as well as did the cells following electromagnetic and piezoelectric lithotripsy. After these energy sources were applied, nearly normal growth curves were achieved by recovery of the viable cells. Further comments are made in the discussion of the effects of SWL on neoplasms.

Evidence of tubular cellular effects of SWL on the kidney have been reported in studies of chemical changes discovered after SWL, namely, increased tubular enzymatic levels in both blood and urine (Assimos et al., 1989a; Jaegar and Constantinides, 1989; Karlin et al., 1989, 1990; Kishimoto et al., 1986). The effects have been seen in the immediate postlithotripsy period and generally are transient. Among the elevated enzymes are creatine phosphokinase, N-acetyl-beta-glucoaminidase, beta-galactosidase, gamma-glutamyl transpeptidase, and lactic dehydrogenase. Proteinuria of a transient nature in the nephrotic range has also been reported (Gilbert et al., 1988). Jaegar and Constantinides (1989) think that the damage from SWL generally occurs in the region of the proximal tubules.

Effect on Organs

Preclinical Experience

Chaussy and associates (1982) found that, in rats, even one thoracic shock wave caused massive hemoptysis. Microscopically, the tissue showed massive vascular and alveolar rupture. This effect could be blocked by a 0.3-cm thick Styrofoam sheet. This observation has been put to good use clinically in infants and children who have required SWL. However, even in some cases in which the lungs have been impacted by SWL, the temporary hemoptysis has cleared by 1 week without obvious sequelae (Kroovand et al., 1987).

Chaussy and co-workers (1982) reported that, in rats, ten shock waves delivered to the general abdominal cavity resulted in survival without clinical damage, as well as no microscopic or macroscopic changes at 24 hours through 14 days.

The Munich group found isolated petechial bleeding on the edge of the mesentery of eventrated intestines after two shock waves. No massive bleeding and no intestinal wall or serous lesions were observed. At 14 days, no ill effects were observed. Similar petechial findings in the liver after two shock waves were found. No animal deaths by 14 days were observed.

The aforementioned studies were basic prior to the preclinical animal trials. These investigators also determined serum chemistry values to ascertain if functional aberrations would occur in the organs adjacent to the kidney following shock wave exposure of the kidney. No difference in liver function tests, amylase, sodium, potassium, serum creatinine, or blood urea nitrogen levels was observed. Dogs received 500 shock waves to one kidney. The kilovoltage was not stated.

In a small series of six dogs, pre– and post–[99m] Tc-DMSA scans were performed. No significant differences between before and after scans 4 days and 14 days following shock wave exposure were noted. Interestingly, no macroscopic or microscopic organ changes were noted after 500 shock waves; this included kidneys. Later studies by others, usually using higher numbers of shock waves and variable kilovoltage have shown both microscopic and macroscopic changes in the kidney.

On the basis of these organ and cell studies, clinical trials were launched in Munich. Only the liberation of a small amount of free hemoglobin during in vivo experiments and lung trauma, which was preventable, were found to be adverse occurrences and were not thought to be significant enough to prevent clinical trials from beginning.

When these earlier experiments were performed in dogs, both ultrasound and fluoroscopy imaging systems were tried. At that time, fluoroscopy was determined to be the better system. Most renal calculi are radiopaque and visible on fluoroscopy. A two-axis fluoroscopy system was chosen with the two systems fixed at a 90-degree angle to each other on the HM-3 lithotriptor (see Fig. 59–6).

Later Experience

KIDNEY

Gross hematuria is nearly universally observed following SWL. Most workers think that hematuria is due to focal parenchymal injury and not to impacting fragments on the urothelium (Jaegar et al., 1988). Such bleeding is generally transient and self-limited.

The majority of kidneys exhibit swelling immediately after SWL with the Dornier HM-3 in the form of perinephric and intranephric fluid collections and perinephric tissue abnormalities. This finding can be documented by magnetic resonance imaging (MRI), computed tomography (CT), or ultrasound studies. When two MRI series are combined (Baumgartner et al., 1987; Kaude et al., 1985), 69 per cent of kidneys exhibited such acute changes. Corticomedullary junction changes were noted in 43 per cent, whereas subcapsular and/or perinephric fluid collections were noted in 40 per cent. Dyer and colleagues (1990) reported an increase in renal volume on MRI in 84 per cent of kidneys immediately after SWL treatment (P = .0001). Subcapsular bleeding or perinephric fluid collections were found in 32 per cent, and 32 per cent demonstrated fascial or perinephric prominence. However, at 3 months after treatment, the abnormal findings had returned to normal.

Rubin and associates (1987) reported on CT findings following SWL: 15 per cent had subcapsular hematomas, 4 per cent had intrarenal hematomas, and 64 per cent had a greater than 3 mm enlargement in anteroposterior diameter. Perinephric changes were seen in 70 per cent.

Abnormalities are not as commonly seen in ultrasound studies as in MRI or CT studies. Ultrasound abnormalities were noted in 6 per cent of cases (Kaude et al., 1987), and radionuclide abnormalities were noted in 46 per cent (Kaude et al., 1985).

When other lithotriptors with a smaller focal zone were used, such as the Wolf piezoelectric lithotriptor, only 5 per cent of patients had acute changes on MRI (Wilson et al., 1989).

The effect of shock waves on the kidneys appears to correlate with the number of shock waves, i.e., more damage with greater numbers of shock waves (Newman et al., 1987). The kilovoltage also appears to affect the kidney, with higher kilovoltage causing more changes.

Many studies have been performed on kidneys in a variety of experimental animals receiving SWL, including mice, rats, dogs, pigs, and New Zealand rabbits. Most of the studies demonstrate capillary and small vein damage, intraparenchymal hemorrhage, and tubular injury. Most studies of chronic changes demonstrate variable amounts of fibrosis occupying up to 1 per cent of renal volume along the path of the shock wave. Other changes that have been noted include focal calcifications, loss of nephrons, dilated veins, and acellular and hyalinized scars leading from the cortex to the medulla. The minipig is an especially good experimental model for this type of experiment because of its similarity to humans in body and kidney size and renal anatomy.

A large body of literature exists on this subject, some of which has been summarized by Lingeman and co-workers (1988). An incomplete list also includes other references previously cited as well as Neisius and co-workers (1989), Morris and co-workers (1989), Evan and co-workers (1989), Jaegar and co-workers (1988), Donovan and co-workers (1988), and Recker and co-workers (1988).

ORGANS OTHER THAN THE KIDNEY

McCullough and associates (1989) studied the effects of SWL on the solitary rat ovary to ascertain if there were gross effects on fetal morphology, numbers, or weight. They used the XL-1 Dornier experimental lithotriptor. No adverse effects were found. The results of this study cannot be necessarily transferred across species lines to humans. The study was done because of concern about potential effects on the ovary when treating ureteral stones in women of childbearing age.

In the same laboratory, Yeaman and colleagues (1989) studied the effects on immature rat epiphyseal growth plates with the broad experimental question as to whether SWL damages bone in pediatric patients. Years ago, radiation therapy to the kidney for Wilms' tumor was found to cause scoliosis in some patients. The question was "Does similar damage occur from SWL?" Again, acknowledging no definite pertinence across species, it was found that 44 per cent of rats exhibited growth plate abnormalities following SWL, whereas 17 per cent exhibited shortened limbs. This study used the fairly high powered XL-1 lithotriptor. No bone growth abnormalities have been reported in humans to my knowledge.

Haupt and associates (1990) reported that SWL delivered to chronic fractured limbs in experimental animals enhanced bone healing.

Moran and co-workers (1990) reported devastating effects of shock waves on chick embryos, which makes the point that has already become dogma—namely, SWL is absolutely contraindicated during pregnancy.

As pointed out in the early research by Chaussy and others, SWL will damage lungs unless the lungs are shielded by Styrofoam or are out of the shock wave field.

Sporadic reports of pancreatitis following SWL have been reported (Drach et al., 1986; Lingeman et al., 1988; Lingeman et al., 1986). No long-term adverse effects have been shown to exist in adjacent organs. No deleterious effects on the spinal cord were found in experimental animals (R. Newman in McCullough, 1987) or on the myocardium as a direct effect of shock waves (Assimos et al., 1989).

Other effects on organs are reviewed in the discussion of complications of SWL and their management.

Effect On Neoplasms

Many investigators have reported disruption and death of mammalian epithelial tumors by shock waves (Berens et al., 1989; Chaussy et al., 1986; Loening et al., 1988; Randazzo et al., 1988; Russo et al., 1986, 1987). Berens and associates (1989) reported additive effects of shock waves and chemotherapeutic drugs, such as doxorubicin, cisplatin, and cyclophosphamide, during in vitro experiments. Holmes and colleagues (1989) reported similar effects on an in vivo rat prostate cancer model. Shock waves alone were ineffective, but when combined with cisplatin, the results were additive. Also, in this experiment, the lungs of rats in which tumors were treated with shock waves were compared with those of control rats to ascertain if shock waves caused an increased rate of metastasis—they did not.

Holmes and co-workers (1988) also found that neutrophils treated with shock waves had transient cell membrane damage, which permitted entry of a chemotherapeutic agent briefly before the cells healed the membrane damage.

Whether shock waves will result in clinically applicable therapy for human neoplasms is open to question. A great deal has been learned about effects of shock waves on cells through this type of research.

IMAGING SYSTEMS IN CONJUNCTION WITH SWL

Fluoroscopy

The original Dornier machines—HM-1, HM-2, and HM-3—used two fluoroscopes mounted in a transverse plane to the long axis of the body at a 45-degree angle to the floor and at a 90-degree angle to each other, that is, a biplanar arrangement (see Fig. 59–6). This configuration results in precise localization of the stone at the F_2 location. Most urinary calculi are radiopaque, an advantage for fluoroscopy. Urologists are familiar with this technique. Special mounting devices are available to put over the image intensifiers to permit in-bath hard-copy films if desired. These fluoroscopic units are expensive and occasionally break down, which puts the machine out of commission until parts and service are available.

Radiation exposure to patients is a concern; usually, staff radiation danger is minimal. Newer machines have C-arm technology. Some machines still use biplanar fluoroscopy, sometimes lined up in the longitudinal plane rather than the transverse plane of the HM-3. This arrangement makes it simpler to localize stones along the course of the ureter.

Obviously radiolucent stones or poorly opacified stones are not seen well or at all with fluoroscopy. Placement of stents or instillation of radiopaque contrast medium intravenously or through ureteral catheters or nephrostomy tubes is often required for localization of such stones.

Plain Films

The Medstone machine uses hard-copy x-rays to image the stones plus a computer to converge F_2 on the stone.

Ultrasound Imaging

Many of the newer lithotriptors employ ultrasound as an imaging modality. Some machines have both fluoroscopy and ultrasound.

Radiopacity of the stone is not a factor with ultrasound. Most stones can be visualized with ultrasound if they are of sufficient size (greater than 2 to 3 mm) and are away from structures that can cause confusion. The best utilization of ultrasound is for stones greater than 3 mm, located at the ureteropelvic junction (UPJ) or within the kidney. Abernathy and colleagues (1989) reported that both urologists and radiologists were more accurate in detecting stone fragments less than 5 mm in size with ultrasound (68 per cent) than with a kidneys, ureters, bladder (KUB) (61 per cent) study. Others disagree with this finding. Upper and mid-ureteral stones are out of range for most ultrasound imaging systems, whereas lower ureteral stones in the juxta- and intravesical areas are often imaged and thus may be treated.

Difficulty may occur in determining when the stone has fragmented sufficiently with ultrasound. The main advantages of ultrasound are its lack of radiation, less cost, and less maintenance than fluoroscopy. Machines with ultrasound imaging are suitable for gallstone lithotripsy. About 85 per cent of gallstones are radiolucent, and the gallbladder is well visualized on ultrasound.

A fairly steep learning curve exists for most urologists using renal ultrasound. Renal ultrasound is more familiar to European urologists than to those in the United States. Ultrasound in prostate imaging is increasing the familiarity and expertise of many urologists in the United States with this technology.

Several machines have ultrasound plus fluoroscopy or hard-copy film capability to image all types of stones.

INDICATIONS AND CONTRAINDICATIONS FOR LITHOTRIPSY

Historical Considerations

During the FDA clinical trials in 1984, a number of contraindications were listed for the HM-3 machine (Spirnak et al., 1990). These contraindications included the following:

1. Children
2. Pregnant women
3. Urinary tract infection
4. Obstruction distal to the stone
5. Cardiac pacemaker
6. Renal artery calcification
7. Serum creatinine level greater than or equal to 3 mg/dl
8. Bleeding diathesis
9. Severe orthopedic deformities

Additional contraindications imposed by the Dornier Company because of the machine specifications included patient weight greater than 300 lb and height of less than 48 inches or more than 78 inches. Operators soon found that, in individuals whose anatomy was such that stones were greater than 13 cm from the ellipsoid (the distance of F_2 from the ellipsoid), such stones could not be placed in the cross hairs of the fluoroscopic monitors. Newman and associates (1988) studied this problem and reported that, if one could place the stone in the upper medial quadrant or lower outer quadrant of the monitors along a line drawn at a 25-degree angle to the cross hairs, then successful fragmentation could occur up to 10 cm away from F_2. This line was termed the "blast path." This work has enabled many overweight patients and some patients with horseshoe kidneys to experience successful lithotripsy under adverse circumstances (Locke et al., 1990).

Generally, if stones are not positioned at F_2, the efficacy of fragmentation is rapidly lost the farther away the stone is from F_2. On the HM-3, the F_2 focal point diameter is 1.5 cm. Stones located outside the cross hairs (with the exception of the "blast path" concept) are often insufficiently fragmented. At 2 cm away from F_2, the pressures are about 20 per cent of the pressures at F_2 (Hunter et al., 1986). Fragmentation of stones can be enhanced by increasing the kilovoltage and/or the number of shock waves (Hunter et al., 1986). If one employs higher kilovoltage and, therefore, greater pressure, the resultant fragments will be of larger size than if lower pressure is employed. Many operators start with lower kilovoltage to try to keep fragment size small and trauma less and reserve higher kilovoltage for the stones that are more difficult to fragment.

As experience was gained with the HM-3 after the

FDA trials were over, the number of contraindications declined rapidly.

Children less than 4 feet in height and children 20 lb or less in weight were successfully treated through gantry modification (Carson and Little, 1987; Kroovand et al., 1987; Newman et al., 1986). Those with severe orthopedic problems, such as myelodysplasia, were also successfully treated.

Patients with cardiac pacemakers were treated (Abber et al., 1988; Cooper et al., 1988; Langberg et al., 1987; Theiss et al., 1990). Most workers believe that a cardiologist or physician knowledgeable in pacemakers should be involved with such treatment and be ready to implant a transvenous pacemaker or to reprogram the pacemaker if it malfunctions (Drach et al., 1990).

Obstruction distal to the stone may be circumvented with double-J stents or ureteral catheters.

Patients who have stones associated with infection (struvite and some others) should have urine cultures performed and should receive pretreatment and appropriate antibiotics before, during, and after SWL. Active infections associated with fever should be controlled prior to SWL. Nephrostomy tubes and patent ureteral stents will prevent many potential septic problems in patients with stones associated with bacteria. Many lithotriptor operators leave double-J ureteral stents in for several weeks after a large volume of particles is created by SWL when treating stones (greater than 1 cm) to enhance passage of the fragments.

Care should be taken to avoid having renal artery calcifications and aortic aneurysms in the blast path or F_2. Vascular clips are apparently of no consequence. Abber and co-workers (1988) found no adverse effects of SWL on such clips applied to arteries distended to high pressures. Iliac vein thrombosis has been reported following SWL (Desmet et al., 1989). Keeler (1988) reported an iliac artery thrombosis following SWL of a lower ureteral stone; however, this finding is obviously very rare.

Pregnancy and uncontrolled coagulation parameters remain as absolute contraindications to SWL.

In machines other than the HM-3, weight per se of greater than 300 lb is not a contraindication; but, often, the stones cannot be imaged and treated at F_2 owing to the increased distance of the stone from the shock wave source and its ellipsoid or dish from F_2.

The issue of treating ureteral stones in the area of the ovary in women of childbearing age is unresolved. McCullough and associates (1989) reported no adverse effects on solitary rat ovary in terms of decreased fetal numbers, fetal weight, or gross fetal appearance of rats bred following SWL to the ovary. As mentioned previously, transfer of such data across species lines to humans is tenuous at best.

Children treated with SWL should have the lungs shielded by Styrofoam padding. Kilovoltage and number of shock waves should be as low as possible. Placement of wet towels or plastic intravenous fluid bags at the shock wave exit site on the abdomen may prevent severe ecchymosis from occurring (AUA, 1986; Kramolowsky et al., 1987).

Complications of SWL are discussed later in this chapter.

Types of Stones

Newman and colleagues (1988) reported their results in treating a variety of stones with different composition. Uric acid stones appeared to break up and be eliminated most readily with a stone-free rate of 85 per cent; struvite stones were also found to break up quite readily with a stone-free rate of 68 per cent. Calcium oxalate dihydrate stones fragmented well, with an 80 per cent stone-free rate, whereas the stone-free rate for monohydrate stones was 74 per cent. Calcium phosphate dihydrate (brushite) stones do not fragment readily, and success with these stones is often disappointing. They tend to fragment into large pieces. The stone-free rate for brushite stones was 53 per cent. Some smaller cystine stones fragment readily, whereas most large ones do not (Katz et al., 1990). Most urologists attempt PCL for cystine stones 2 cm or larger as initial treatment. Dretler (1988) has reported on variables in stone fragility that bear on the success of SWL. About 1 per cent of stones (other than cystine) do not fragment in the usual SWL patient mix. Many of these stones are composed of calcium monohydrate.

Some patients have benefited from post-SWL chemolysis delivered through percutaneous nephrostomy tubes (Schmeller et al., 1984; Van Arsdalen, 1987). Most of the stones have been composed of cystine or struvite. They are often remnants of calculi greater than 3 cm or of staghorn stones. Residual fragments are associated with a higher stone recurrence rate (Newman et al., 1988). Extraordinary efforts should be made to try to render the patient stone-free.

Great confusion exists in the literature over what constitutes successful treatment with SWL. Some investigators claim that stone fragments 4 mm or less in size are "clinically insignificant." I have seen a number of patients develop symptoms and ureteral obstruction from fragments this size.

Several years ago, the AUA Lithotripsy Committee proposed that a stone-free state is the only yardstick that is important as an end point. However, as mentioned earlier, one can then ask, "How was the diagnosis of a stone-free condition made?" One can use ultrasound, CT, or KUB (for radiopaque stones) to ascertain a stone-free condition (Coughlin et al., 1989). If one of these imaging studies is employed, it is probably sufficient for radiopaque stones. Obviously, ultrasound or CT will be needed to ascertain if nonradiopaque fragments have disappeared. An appropriate length of time should be allowed to elapse before declaring that a patient is or is not stone-free. Three months is most often the time permitted. Many fragments will pass within days or by 2 or 3 weeks after SWL. In my opinion, if fragments are still present at 3 months, it is unlikely that they will subsequently pass.

In nearly all series following SWL, the most common site of fragment retention is the lower calyceal site. Obviously, gravity plays an important role in this situation. A variety of schemes have been proposed to attack this problem, including irrigation through ureteral stents or nephrostomies; dangling of the shoulders from a bent waist position with the head down toward the floor from a bed (McCullough 1989); or hanging like a bat using boots with the whole body upside down, so-called inversion therapy (Brownlee et al., 1990). Stone fragments primarily located in the lower calyx are also difficult to pass. McDougall and associates (1989) reported a 57 per cent stone-free rate of lower calyceal stones of all sizes treated with SWL versus an 85 per cent stone-free rate treated with PCL. When 1-cm stones were compared, 66 per cent were cleared with SWL and 100 per cent were cleared with PCL. In spite of these statistics, most patients prefer an initial attempt with SWL.

In studying a number of reports, I have noted that most lithotriptor manufacturers report a greater than 95 per cent fragmentation rate at the initial SWL treatment. Most report a 65 to 75 per cent stone-free rate at 3 months. Generally, the smaller the stone, the greater the stone-free rate and fragmentation. Many workers have abandoned SWL as monotherapy for cystine stones greater than 2 cm in size, often preferring PCL which is occasionally combined with percutaneous chemolysis in combination therapy.

Size of Stones

Many investigators have categorized stones as less than or equal to 1 cm, 1 to 2 cm, 2 to 3 cm, and partial or complete staghorn calculi. Variations in stone size groups have confused the literature and made direct comparison between series difficult. Griffith and Valiquette (1987) proposed a classification system, but it has not achieved wide acceptance. Some schemes involve adding up the total linear distances of the stone's various components and its extension into calyces or infundibula. No universal system of size categorization has become dominant.

Stone-free success appears to be highly related to stone size. Stones less than or equal to 1 cm are ideal for SWL. A 90 per cent stone-free rate can often be achieved with such stones when they are located in the renal pelvis (Chaussy et al., 1982). As the size increases, the stone-free percentages start to decline. For stones averaging 1.2 cm, the stone-free rate obtained with treatment of solitary renal stones was 87 per cent (Riehle et al., 1987).

There appears to be a breakpoint of 3 cm and sometimes 2 cm for calcium-containing stones treated with SWL by many lithotritists in the United States. Stones above these dimensions are often treated with PCL monotherapy or preliminary PCL followed by SWL and a "second-look" PCL or irrigation after SWL. European urologists seem more willing to treat stones greater than or equal to 3 cm with SWL monotherapy one or more times (Constantinides et al., 1989). This finding may be related to reimbursement patterns or ability to keep patients in the hospital for longer periods in Europe.

The proper treatment of 3 cm or larger stones is a subject of considerable debate in lithotripsy at the present time. When patients are treated with SWL monotherapy, many urologists place an indwelling double-J stent to keep the kidney unobstructed and to enhance stone particle passage (Constantinides et al.,

1989). This procedure also seems to reduce the sepsis rate considerably. Gleeson and Griffith (1989) reported a stone-free rate of 43 per cent for stones 3 cm or larger using SWL monotherapy and did not recommend it for most patients with such stones.

Patients who had complete staghorn calculi treated with SWL monotherapy without any stents had only a 44 per cent stone-free rate at 6 months, and 63 per cent required rehospitalization (Constantinides et al., 1989). Approximately 48 per cent with incomplete staghorn calculi were stone-free at 6 months without double-J stents, and 85 per cent with double-J stents were stone-free. Lingeman and colleagues (1989) reported only a 31 per cent stone-free rate in staghorn stones treated with SWL monotherapy. The stone-free rate in many series appears to average about 50 per cent.

The success rate of open anatrophic nephrolithotomy for staghorn stones was 94 per cent (Boyce et al., 1974). With PCL monotherapy, between 80 per cent (Miller et al., 1988b) and 86 per cent (Winfield et al., 1988) were rendered stone-free. Combinations of PCL and SWL have achieved results of between 77 and 88 per cent in the treatment of complete staghorn stones (Eisenberger et al., 1985; Fuchs et al., 1988; Kahnoski et al., 1986; Schulze et al., 1989; Thomas et al., 1988a).

At the present time, I perceive that, in the United States, preliminary PCL followed by SWL and possible second-look PCL or irrigation is the most common way of treating 3 cm or larger stones. However, with more and more "anesthesia-free" machines appearing on the market, some patients prefer to avoid the more invasive, but probably more effective PCL. As mentioned previously, this area of lithotripsy is controversial.

Most United States and European urologists would probably treat stones of size 1.5 cm or less with SWL lithotripsy as monotherapy. Using this approach, some investigators have obtained quite good results on the order of 85 per cent stone-free at 3 months (Graff et al., 1988; Lingeman et al., 1986). These results were obtained with the Dornier HM-3, and about 1200 shocks were given. The retreatment rate was about 15 per cent. As attempts are made to reduce the pain experienced with SWL, various manufacturers have widened the aperture of the ellipsoids and reduced the power. This design reduces the pain, increases the retreatment rate, and results in a greater number of shock waves being utilized. When the modified HM-3 or HM-4 is used, the number of shock waves is increased to about 2100 and the stone-free percentages range from 55 to 95 per cent. The retreatment rate rises to approximately 15 to 30 per cent (range, 14 to 37 per cent) (Jocham et al., 1988; Kraft, 1989; Newman et al., 1989; Rassweiler et al., 1987; Siebold et al., 1988; Vogeli et al., 1989; Wilbert et al., 1988).

A higher number of shock waves are produced with the Siemens Lithostar (electromagnetic shock waves) than with the HM-3, with approximately 3600 shock waves used to achieve a stone-free rate of 70 per cent at 3 months, a retreatment rate of approximately 7 per cent, and a post-SWL auxillary procedure rate of 16 per cent (Clayman et al., 1989).

Piezoelectric lithotriptors have the advantage of being truly anesthesia-free with no general, spinal, epidural, or local anesthesia, or sedoanalgesia needed. The Wolf Piezoelectric 2300 and the EDAP LTO1 are being used worldwide. A stone-free rate of approximately 85 per cent has been reported at 3 months with a retreatment rate of greater than 30 per cent in most series. The number of shock waves necessary to achieve these results is about 3500 (Kiely et al., 1989; Marberger et al., 1988; McNicholas et al., 1989; Philip et al., 1988; Preminger and Erving, 1988; Segura et al., 1989; Vallacien et al., 1988; Zwergel et al., 1989).

A number of electrohydraulic lithotriptors are now being equipped with variable power (e.g., Technomed Sonolith, Dornier MPL 5000). These machines can be adjusted to deliver more or less power coupled with more or less anesthesia, as the need and clinical circumstances demand. As mentioned elsewhere, Newman and co-workers (1989) reduced the kilovoltage to the 12 to 14 range on an unmodified HM-3 and, with intravenous medication, were able to treat a number of patients successfully.

The Storz Modulith features variable power and a movable focal zone up to a depth of 15 cm on its electromagnetic power generation lithotriptor. The power can also be varied on the Siemens Lithostar electromagnetic lithotriptor.

Location of Stones

Stones in the kidney are readily treated with all types of lithotriptors with various types of imaging systems. Ultrasound-imaged machines readily detect all types of stones in the kidney. Fluoroscopic or hard-copy x-ray machines readily image radiopaque stones but require infusion of intravenous contrast medium or infusion of contrast medium through ureteral catheters or percutaneous nephrostomy tubes to localize other types of stones, such as uric acid stones, many cystine stones, and lightly opacified calcium-containing stones. Stones in horseshoe kidneys can be successfully treated with SWL plus adjunctive procedures in about 80 per cent of cases (Smith et al., 1989).

Radiopaque upper ureteral stones are treated in situ or by pushing them back into the kidney with retrograde maneuvers, such as forceful injection of saline, lidocaine jelly instillation and flushing, or "bumping up" the stone, with a variety of catheters as well as other techniques. Earlier series of upper ureteral stone therapy in situ with the HM-3 yielded successful results ranging from 60 to 85 per cent (Dretler et al., 1986; Fuchs et al., 1987; Miller et al., 1985; Mueller et al., 1986; Riehle et al., 1986). Tung and colleagues (1990) reported 75 per cent success rate with the EDAP machine. Most operators find it less difficult to image stones in the kidney and find that the success rate of fragmentation and stone-free rates are higher, approaching 100 per cent, when upper ureteral stones are managed by the "push up and smash" technique, wherein the stone is pushed up into the kidney and treated with SWL (Fuchs et al., 1988; Graff et al., 1988; Lingeman et al., 1987).

Stones that reside in the ureter between the ureteral

pelvic junction and where the ureter crosses over the pelvic bones are usually visualized on fluoroscopic machines. They are usually not visible on ultrasound. On the Dornier HM-3, it is often necessary to put a catheter up to or by the stone because, on one of the monitors, the opaque stones are often lost in the bony detail of the vertebrae. Rotation of the patient toward the treated side enhances visualization of the stone when using the HM-3 (Fuchs et al., 1987).

Most operators who treat ureteral stones in situ use a higher kilovoltage and more shock waves than those for kidney stones. To break up the stones, operators often use 22 to 24 kV and more than 2000 shock waves with the HM-3 model (Barr et al., 1990; Fuchs et al., 1987; Zehntner et al., 1989). However, some investigators have reported good results treating such stones in situ with no catheters up, catheters up to the stone, or catheters by the stone (Barr et al., 1990; Holden et al., 1989). Holden and associates (1989) have had an 88 per cent success rate with in situ treatment of ureteral stones with the Siemens Lithostar.

After the ureter passes over the pelvic bones, it is impossible to break up stones by having the shock waves enter from the backside of the patient and traverse through bone. It becomes necessary to treat the patient in the prone position. Several investigators (Jenkins and Gillenwater, 1988; Miller et al., 1988a) have had good success using such tactics in patients who often experienced failure during ureteroscopic attempts. A modified Stryker frame with an opening over the entry site for shock waves can be used (Jenkins and Gillenwater, 1988). The prone position is also chosen to treat some patients with horseshoe kidneys who cannot have the stones placed at F_2 in the conventional position (Locke et al., 1990). Some pelvic kidneys can also be treated in this fashion.

As the stones move into the lower ureter, several techniques have been successful with the HM-3. Miller and associates (1986) used the modified sitting position, which allows the shock waves to enter through the bony pelvic outlet with the patient sitting with the hips at a 90-degree angle to the vertebrae. Others have employed a supine approach (Becht et al., 1988; Chaussy et al., 1987; El-Faqih et al., 1988) and some, the "horse-riding" position (Ackaert et al., 1989). All of these approaches have about a 90 per cent success rate. Grace and colleagues (1989) and Netto and co-workers (1990) reported about the same success with in situ therapy with the Siemens Lithostar. Interestingly, the bowel rarely seems to be injured by any of these approaches, although a few isolated complications of this technique have been reported. Ackaert and colleagues (1989) noted transient anal blood loss in 7 per cent of patients. None required transfusion.

Often, it is necessary to have patients come in for a "positioning" trial prior to the definitive SWL treatment to determine the correct approach and the best imaging position. Lower ureteral, juxtavesical, and intramural stones are often imaged and treated with ultrasonic lithotriptors. Currently, considerable debate exists concerning the best way to treat lower ureteral stones. Ureteroscopic techniques are more than 95 per cent successful (Blute et al., 1988) and are generally less expensive, but they are more invasive and have a higher complication rate. The techniques are also extremely operator dependent. SWL is more expensive, probably less difficult to perform, and not as successful overall. Effects of shock waves on the ovary of a woman of childbearing age are unknown. Stones in the mid and upper ureter have, of course, been treated successfully by ureteroscopy. The higher the stone in the ureter, the less successful are the results with ureteroscopy. Kostakopoulos and co-workers (1989) reported ureteroscopic success rates of 38 per cent in the upper ureter, 50 per cent in the mid-ureter, and 96 per cent in the lower ureter. The converse appears to be true for SWL.

SWL has been utilized in novel ways, such as treatment of stones developed on metal staples in Kock pouches (Boyd et al., 1988), treatment of stones within entrapped stone baskets (Durano et al., 1988), and treatment of stones that have developed on double-J catheters thereby preventing their removal (Flam et al., 1990; Lupu et al., 1986).

Considerable debate exists as to whether ureteral stones can be treated as successfully without stents bypassing the stone as compared with stents bypassing the stones and creating a "water expansion chamber" alongside the stone. Reports from the United States (Barr et al., 1990) and from Europe (Becht et al., 1988) suggested that satisfactory results can be obtained without stent bypass. These findings create skepticism as to whether an expansion chamber of fluid being present alongside the stone is important. Many ureteral stones treated in situ take several weeks to pass. Success of SWL is difficult to predict from the immediate post-SWL radiograph taken following ureteral SWL because the fragments are intimately packed together.

Several series of in situ treatment of ureteral stones with the HM-3 are pertinent (Barr et al., 1990; Zehntner et al., 1989). According to the report by Barr and associates, an overall success rate of 97 per cent was achieved; 77 per cent had only one treatment. Approximately 78 per cent of ureteral stones treated were in the upper ureter, and 11 per cent were present in both the presacral and juxtavesical ureter. Eighty-two per cent had ureteral catheters present during the treatment. The catheter position or even the presence of the catheters at all was thought to be unimportant. Overall, 21 per cent had post-treatment interventions and 5 per cent had percutaneous nephrostomies placed. The average number of shock waves was 2248 versus 1382 in other series. Zehntner and co-workers (1989) reported a success rate of 96 per cent stone-free at 3 months following SWL of lower ureteral stones. Patients averaged 2340 shock waves per treatment and 7 per cent required retreatment; the overall auxillary procedure rate was 42 per cent.

Bladder stones have been successfully treated with one treatment (90 per cent success with one treatment) or two treatments (100 per cent success) using the Siemens Lithostar (Vandeursen and Baert, 1990).

Significance of Residual Fragments

As mentioned previously, uric acid, struvite, and calcium oxalate dihydrate stones usually fragment readily with SWL. Cystine stones, as well as calcium oxalate monohydrate and calcium phosphate dihydrate stones, are much more difficult to fragment. Cystine stones are composed of organic material.

Riehle and associates (1987) analyzed passed stone particle sizes following SWL. Most fragments passed were in the 0.9- to 1.4-mm range, whereas the largest particles in the samples were 1.4 and 2 mm. In only 15 per cent of cases were stone fragments that passed between 2.8 and 5.6 mm in size, and the larger fragments were usually composed of uric acid or struvite.

A question that is commonly asked is "Do small retained fragments following SWL make any difference?" Many contemporary urologists were trained to attempt removal of all fragments at open stone surgery and to believe that anything short of a stone-free condition was a failure.

As mentioned, most lithotriptor manufacturers quote a 65 to 70 per cent stone-free rate at 3 months after SWL. The initial FDA study quoted an overall stone-free rate of 66 per cent (Drach et al., 1986). The optimum size for a stone-free state is 1 cm or less. In the FDA study, 82 per cent with stones less than 1 cm were stone-free. As the stone size increased, the stone-free rate following treatment decreased with stones larger than 2 to 3 cm having a stone-free rate of about 53 per cent. If one has multiple stones, the stone-free rate decreases. In the FDA study, when 4 stones or more were present, the resulting stone-free rate was only about 30 per cent.

Newman and co-workers (1988) have analyzed the significance of residual fragments relative to subsequent stone growth. At 1 year, the recurrence rate was 8 per cent in those rendered stone free originally, and an additional 11 per cent developed stones between 1 and 2 years. If the patients were not originally stone-free following SWL, the recurrence rate was 22 per cent between 3 and 12 months post-SWL as well as between 1 and 2 years. Residual fragments appear to grow at a rate greater than the usual stone recurrence rate, which is about 10 to 15 per cent per year in untreated patients forming calcium stones (Coe, 1978; Ettinger, 1976; Marshall et al., 1975).

Newman and colleagues (1988) studied 1910 treated kidneys in the aforementioned study. The stone-free rate after SWL dropped from 80 per cent in up to 10 mm stones to about 60 per cent in stones greater than 30 mm. The stone-free rate of solitary stones dropped from about 85 per cent in the renal pelvis to about 70 per cent in the calyces. The stone-free rate for these stones in the lower calyx ranged from 80 per cent for stones up to 10 mm in size to 32 per cent for those 21 to 30 mm in size. Only 33 per cent of patients with calculi present in dilated calyces were rendered stone-free. The same percentage of patients with stones in medullary sponge kidneys were rendered stone-free. Only 50 per cent of cystine stone cases were stone-free when the stones were only 2 cm or less in size.

Newman and associates (1988) concluded that there is a significant difference ($p < .001$) between new stone growth in the stone-free group and in the group with residual fragments after SWL at the end of 1 year. This finding suggests that, if a stone-free status is not achieved

following SWL, accelerated new growth may occur. This result could be explained by the fragments serving as a nidus for new stone growth.

Patients with struvite stones subsequently rendered stone-free following SWL therapy had a recurrence at a rate of 9 per cent, whereas those with fragments remaining had a fragment growth of 29 per cent; however, the sample was small. Fragment growth rates were accelerated in the presence of infected urine.

In summary, some of the factors involved in reducing the likelihood of a stone-free status following SWL include the following (Newman et al., 1988):

1. Stone burden—multiple stones, stones greater than 2 cm in size, or staghorn stones.
2. Reduced clearance of fragments—lower calyceal location, marked hydronephrosis or scarring, calyceal diverticulum, horseshoe kidney.
3. Stone composition—cystine or hydroxyapatite/brushite.

Several investigators have presented evidence that, in patients with infectious stones who are treated perioperatively with appropriate antibiotics and in whom the fragments are small (< 2 mm), stone recurrence can be held to a minimum (Michaels et al., 1988; Sonda et al., 1988).

COMPLICATIONS

Renal Effects

No one really knows how many shock waves the human kidney can safely tolerate at a given kilovoltage. As mentioned, a number of investigators have reported swelling of the kidney and perinephric subcapsular and intranephric fluid collections in the majority of cases studied with MRI (Baumgartner et al., 1987; Dyer et al., 1990). The changes appear to revert to normal by 3 months. Several studies have demonstrated changes on renograms and scans, which appear to be of greater concern, with some immediate decrease in effective renal plasma flow measured by iodohippurate (Hippuran) renal scan in 30 per cent of kidneys treated with SWL (Kaude et al., 1985). Williams and co-workers (1988) found, at 17 to 21 months following SWL, a significant decrease in effective renal plasma flow. Chaussy, however, found a significant improvement in renal function 1 year following SWL. Also, at 4 years, no ill effects were noted following SWL in patients studied with ^{131}I hippurate scans (Chaussy et al., 1987) Thomas and associates (1988b) reported decreased renal plasma flow when more than 1600 shock waves were administered and warned against "casual overtreatment."

Nearly 100 per cent of renal stone treatment by SWL results in hematuria, which is thought to be due to blunt parenchymal trauma rather than to stone fragments traumatizing the urothelium like shrapnel. Such hematuria usually dissipates by 24 hours.

About 1 per cent of patients develop septic complications as a result of SWL (AUA, 1985; Roth and

Beckman, 1988). The incidence of these complications can be reduced by aggressively treating urinary tract infections prior to SWL. It is desirable to treat patients who have struvite stones with antibiotics before, during, and after SWL because they are likely to harbor bacteria, which often are liberated during SWL. Patients who have infectious stones and have had a large volume of fragments created by SWL are best treated with double-J stents or percutaneous nephrostomy drainage, which prevents urinary obstruction after SWL.

Steinstrasse is not very common, occurring in less than 5 per cent of cases in most series and in as low as 1 per cent in many series. Intervention following SWL for this condition is necessary in 6 to 35 per cent depending on stone size treated (AUA, 1986; Chaussy et al., 1986; Fedullo et al., 1988; Van Arsdalen, 1987). This condition, which means "stone street," exists when a series of fragments line up in the ureter like a logjam. Often, a larger "lead" fragment is responsible for the logjam. Many of these pass spontaneously. They must be watched carefully. Fedullo and colleagues (1988) reported that 75 per cent of steinstrasse cases occurred in the distal ureter; 18 per cent, in the proximal ureter; and 6 per cent, in the mid-ureter. They also reported that 75 per cent of interventions were endoscopic, and 35 per cent required intervention.

Indications for steinstrasse intervention are basically the same as those used for calculous obstruction of the ureter: pain, total obstruction, significant obstruction of a solitary kidney with rising creatinine levels, urosepsis, and failure to pass fragments within a reasonable time (Spirnak et al., 1990).

If the kidney is significantly obstructed, only short observation is prudent. If intervention is required, ureteroscopic treatment is often helpful with ureteral meatotomy; ureteroscopic lithotripsy with laser, ultrasound, or electrohydraulic probes; followed by stenting. Another quite acceptable strategy is to place a percutaneous nephrostomy tube and wait for the fragments to pass; they often do. Sometimes, combined percutaneous nephrostomy and ureteroscopic management of large steinstrasse (greater than one third of ureteral length) are required (Weinerth et al., 1989). Upper ureteral steinstrasse can occasionally be cleared by repeat SWL to the area of the "lead" fragment. Many urologists treating stones greater than 2 cm in size in the kidney place double-J stents prior to SWL and leave them in place until the majority of fragments pass. This prevents obstruction and sepsis and facilitates passage of fragments.

Many urologists obtain a plain film of the abdomen (KUB) about 2 weeks after SWL. Later, it is advisable to document that renal function is present. Many urologists do this about 1 month after SWL using a renogram, intravenous urogram, or ultrasound. Clinically significant perinephric or subcapsular hematomas occur in a small percentage of patients, for example, 0.66 per cent in the Indianapolis series of 3620 patients (Knapp et al., 1988). Interestingly, there was no correlation with kilovoltage or number of shock waves. Uncontrolled diabetes or hypertension, and use of nonsteroidal analgesics or aspirin are risk factors (Rius and Saltzman, 1990). Hematomas are rarely life-threatening, but occasionally, a nephrectomy is required (Donohue et al., 1989).

Renal failure of a temporary nature has been reported following SWL (Littleton et al., 1989). This complication appeared to be due to edema of the kidneys and not due to ureteral obstruction. Bilateral SWL at the same sitting obviously would be more likely to be associated with this problem, although a number of solitary kidneys have been successfully treated with SWL (Kulb et al., 1986). If bilateral treatment is planned at one sitting, one or both renal units should have stents or nephrostomy tubes placed prior to the procedure (Newman et al., 1988). Texter (1988) reported few adverse effects on previously poorly functioning kidneys. Permanent dysfunction is most often due to silent obstruction that went unnoticed during the post-SWL period.

Hypertension following SWL has been a lively topic among workers, evoking much debate. The incidence of new-onset hypertension in the general population each year is about 2 to 3.5 per cent in white men aged 25 to 54 years (Lingeman et al., 1990). In several series, patients treated with SWL were reported to have an approximately 8 per cent incidence of post-SWL hypertension (Lingeman et al., 1987; Williams et al., 1988). Other series reported no such increased incidence: Chaussy (1988), 1 per cent; Liedel and co-workers (1988), 3 per cent. The expected incidence in an age-related population followed for 40 months is approximately 3 per cent (Spirnak and Resnick, 1990). Lingeman and associates (1990) reported a very small (less than 1 mm) increase in diastolic blood pressure following SWL, which was thought to be significant. Of interest was that patients with ureteral stones treated with SWL had a higher incidence than did those with renal calculi. This finding is difficult to reconcile with the hypothesis that SWL may cause hypertension by causing small vessel changes in the kidney. Series that report hypertension in SWL-treated patients without control groups of the general population as well as patients with stones that pass without intervention, and patients with stones treated by percutaneous nephrolithotomy, pyelolithotomy, anatrophic nephrolithotomy, ureterolithotomy, or ureteroscopy are interesting, but they do not prove anything. It is difficult to assemble such control groups when SWL is so noninvasive.

It will be difficult to ever arrive at a definite answer to the question about SWL-associated hypertension. Sandlow and co-workers (1989) reported on patients undergoing multiple SWL treatments (two to five) and evaluated the incidence of hypertension. Of 112, 17 had an increase in mean blood pressure of at least 10 mm Hg, whereas 19 had a similar decrease. Germinale and associates (1989) concluded that no causal evidence for SWL-related hypertension exists, as did Zwergel and colleagues (1989). It is obvious, at least at this point in time, that the majority of patients treated with SWL have rapid and uneventful recovery with little morbidity in terms of hypertension.

Adjacent Organ Damage

The lungs are occasionally damaged by SWL. This damage usually occurs in patients with unusual anatomy, such as myelodysplastic infants and children. As previously mentioned, shielding the lungs with a thin piece of Styrofoam usually prevents such trauma. Patients who have had some damage and hemoptysis following SWL have recovered uneventfully within a week (Kroovand, 1987).

Several cases of pancreatitis have been reported (Drach et al., 1986; Lingeman et al., 1986). Some impacted pancreatic stones have been successfully treated with SWL (Meyer et al., 1989). One patient with gallstones demonstrated fragmentation following treatment of an upper pole renal calculus without sequelae (Michaels and Fowler, 1986).

Table 59–1 presents complications reported in more than 10,000 patients from 37 centers in the 1986 AUA Lithotripsy Committee Report.

Miscellaneous complications and sequelae are noted in the following discussion. Transient gastrointestinal erosions and mucosal bleeding have been reported (Ackaert et al., 1989; Cass and Anstad, 1988; Karawi et al., 1987). No adverse effects of SWL on the spinal cord in canines when using 2000 to 6000 shock waves were noted by Newman and associates (1987). No adverse effects on hearing were noted by Stoller and co-workers (1988). No damage to metal clips placed on aortic vessel branches or leakage from them after subjecting the aorta to SWL was observed by Abber and colleagues (1988).

Several patients with hemophilia have successfully undergone SWL (Christensen et al., 1989; Portney et al., 1987).

I am unaware of any reports concerning rupture of aortic or renal artery aneurysms following renal SWL. Most lithotritists do not knowingly treat such cases with SWL. However, there have been cases of iliac vein thrombosis (Desmet et al., 1989) and iliac artery thrombosis following SWL of lower ureteral calculi (Keeler et al., 1990).

The mortality of SWL was 0.02 per cent in a compilation of mortality and morbidity statistics by the AUA Lithotripsy Committee (1987) in more than 62,000 patients. Deaths were due to the following conditions: two pulmonary emboli, three myocardial infarctions, and one of each of the following, retroperitoneal hemorrhage, cerebrovascular accident (3 weeks), suicide (3 weeks), mesenteric thrombosis, respiratory arrest after a fall, complication of solvent irrigation after SWL, and unrecognized cancer of the gallbladder. Most of these deaths could not be blamed on SWL per se. This is a remarkably low mortality.

Care should be taken in positioning of the arms when treating a patient with the HM-3. Most operators allow the arms to dangle in the waterbath or use small inflatable "floaties" to allow the arms to float in the water. This precaution seems to prevent nerve palsies.

Patients with tracheostomies should be monitored closely when immersed in the HM-3 waterbath to prevent water entry into the trachea.

Proper strapping beneath patients lifted into and out of the waterbath of the HM-3 is also imperative.

Radiation Exposure

Obviously, ultrasound-imaged machines pose no radiation exposure risk to patients. Fluoroscopic or hardcopy x-ray–imaged machines do pose a risk.

Van Swearingen and co-workers (1987), Pollock (1987), Bush and co-workers (1987), and Griffith and co-workers (1989) reported on radiation exposure during SWL. Such exposure was not excessive as compared with conventional radiologic procedures, such as abdominal CT scans, coronary arteriography, and barium enemas as well as percutaneous nephrolithotomy. Radiation exposure appears to be operator-dependent and related to the learning curve. It can be lowered by making operators aware of their own personal utilization of x-rays, especially of excessive "quick-pick" images on the HM-3. In general, 1 minute of fluoroscopy time at 90 kV and 3.0 mA delivers approximately 3 rads. One quick-pick exposure lasting 500 milliseconds at 60 kV, 160 mA, delivers approximately 0.5 rad.

Relatively radiolucent stones and obesity contribute to higher levels of radiation exposure. Ureteral catheters passed up to the stone may help in localization. Keeping the fluoroscope turned off much of the time while moving the patient in the tub for long excursions is helpful. Keeping the balloons inflated against the patient and the image intensifiers close to the patient give better clarity. Radiation exposure in children should be reduced to the absolute minimum. It appears that radiation exposure to SWL technicians and anesthesiologists is minimal as long as they are several feet away from the HM-3 tub (Van Swearingen et al., 1987). Radiation exposure from SWL is less than that from PCL.

BILIARY LITHOTRIPSY

No lithotriptor in the United States has received FDA approval for treating gallstones in either the gallbladder or the common bile duct. Common duct stones have been successfully treated in about 80 per cent of cases both in the United States (Bland et al., 1989) and in Europe (Sauerbruch et al., 1986; Sauerbruch and Stern, 1989). This procedure is often performed in combination

Table 59–1. COMPLICATIONS OF TREATMENT WITH LITHOTRIPSY

	No. of Patients*
Pancreatitis (elevated amylase level)	2
Pancreatitis (clinical)	3
Hyperthermia (tub too hot)	1
Pneumonitis	6
Pulmonary embolus	4
Hemoptysis (children with myelodysplasia)	2
Cerebrovascular accident	3
Brachial palsy	4
Long thoracic nerve palsy	4
Falling off gantry	2
Retroperitoneal abscess	1
Strapped too tightly (could not be ventilated)	1

*Represents a patient population of more than 10,000.
Adapted from American Urological Association Ad Hoc Lithotripsy Committee Report, McCullough, D. L., Chairman, Baltimore, AVA, 1986.

with endoscopic sphincterotomy and fragment manipulation. This technique appears to be safer than open surgical removal of such common bile duct stones. Fluoroscopic imaging of such stones is performed with either a percutaneously placed biliary tube or a nasobiliary tube through which contrast medium is instilled.

Stones in the gallbladder can be imaged most simply with ultrasound. About 85 per cent of gallstones are radiolucent, thereby severely limiting the role of fluoroscopy in imaging such stones.

In the European experience, gallstones that are single and less than 3 cm in diameter are the most successfully treated with an 85 per cent stone-free rate at 8 to 12 months in combination with ursochenodeoxycholic acid oral adjuvant chemotherapy and a 97 per cent stone-free rate at 12 to 18 months (Sackman et al., 1988). Multiple stones had only a 40 per cent stone-free rate at 1 year. Overall, the stone-free rate at 12 to 18 months was 91 per cent. Complications included biliary colic in 33 per cent, cutaneous petechiae in 14 per cent, and transient gross hematuria in 3 per cent. One of the major problems is that, although the stones are frequently fragmented, the fragments have a difficult egress through the cystic ducts, through the tortuous valves of Heister.

Schoenfield and associates (1990) reported on the United States Dornier National Biliary Lithotripsy Study. A total of 600 symptomatic patients with three or fewer gallstones ranging in total size between 5 and 30 mm were treated with the Dornier MPL 9000, 95 per cent with intravenous sedoanalgesia and 5 per cent with no analgesia. The stones were fragmented in 97 per cent of all patients; in 47 per cent, the fragments were less than 5 mm in diameter. Only 21 per cent of patients treated with SWL plus Ursodiol (ursodeoxycholic acid bile acid adjuvant chemotherapy) and 9 per cent of those treated with SWL were stone-free at 6 months. Biliary pain, usually mild, occurred in 1.5 per cent, acute cholecystitis in 1 per cent, and acute pancreatitis in 1.5 per cent. Endoscopic sphincterotomy was performed in 0.5 per cent, and cholecystectomy was performed in 2.5 per cent. These results are obviously not very satisfactory.

At this time, the laparoscopic cholecystectomy appears to have moved to the forefront of new therapies for gallbladder stone management. Cholecystectomy has the advantage of removing the often diseased gallbladder. When stones are removed from the gallbladder that is left in situ, the recurrence rate is about 50 per cent.

Urologists have participated in a cooperative common bile duct SWL study in the United States (Bland et al., 1989). The techniques utilized in SWL of renal stones are quite transferable and applicable to common duct stones (McCullough, 1987b).

A number of lithotriptors that have both fluoroscopy and ultrasound imaging capability are capable of treating both urinary and biliary calculi. Stones in the gallbladder are usually treated with the patient in the prone position. Stones in the common duct can often be treated with the patient in the same position as that for renal lithotripsy.

ANESTHESIA

The original Dornier HM-3 lithotriptor required either regional or general anesthesia for the patient when operating in the 18 to 24 kV range with 1000 or more shock waves.

Epidural anesthesia has proved satisfactory for most SWL cases on the HM-3. It has been associated with few major complications. One disadvantage is the rather marked respiratory excursions of the kidneys, which often move the stone in and out of the shock wave energy path at F_2.

General anesthesia has been used as well with few complications. The variant of general anesthesia called high-frequency jet ventilation involves rapid bursts of anesthetic gases 1 to 200 times per second, which results in little, if any, respiratory excursion. This technique tends to keep the stone more in focus at F_2 (Warner et al., 1988). Its proponents claim that fewer shock waves are necessary because the stone is in focus nearly all of the time and that fragmentation is more complete. The argument appears to have merit.

Malhoutra (1986) reported an intercostal nerve block plus a regional block for SWL. Loening and colleagues (1987) reported local infiltration of lidocaine at the entry site region of shock waves in HM-3–treated patients and cited success in stoic individuals thus treated. Intravenous sedation in quadriplegic patients has been successfully performed (Spirnak et al., 1988). In Sweden, a patch of local anesthetic placed on the skin prior to SWL plus intravenous sedoanalgesia has proved helpful in HM-3–treated patients, especially when reduced power at 14 to 16 kV was applied (Petterson et al., 1989; Tiselius and Pettersson, 1989). Newman and associates (1989) reported on intravenous sedoanalgesia in combination with voltage in the 12 to 16 kV range on an unmodified HM-3 machine with good results. Clayman and co-workers (1989a) reported success in using the transcutaneous electrical nerve stimulator (TENS) unit for anesthesia with the Siemens Lithostar. They also employed oral sedation, intravenous sedoanalgesia, and general and epidural anesthesia.

Dornier has modified the HM-3 model in several ways in an attempt to make it less dependent on anesthesia. The ellipsoid aperture has been increased from 15.6 to 17.2 cm. The generator power has been reduced from 80 nF to 40 nF. A longer treatment time and more shock waves are usually necessary with this model (Graff et al., 1987; 1988b).

Many manufacturers now claim that the majority of patients treated with their machines require little intravenous sedoanalgesia or no anesthesia. The prospective buyer of such equipment should watch a given machine in use and form his or her own opinion about anesthesia requirements.

The piezoelectric machine by Wolf appears to be truly anesthesia-free (Marberger et al., 1988). The EDAP machine can be used to treat 90 per cent of patients without anesthesia. The majority, 72 per cent, of patients treated on the Diasonics machine required intravenous or intramuscular anesthesia with 6 per cent, epidural; 11 per cent, local; and 11 per cent, general

Table 59–2. ALTERNATIVE ENERGY SOURCES—MECHANICAL ASPECTS

Company/ Location	Machine	Energy Source	Focusing Shock Wave	Weight	Focal Distance (cm)	Pressure At Focal Point (bar)	Focal Zone (cm)	Generator Life Span (SW)	Shock Wave/ Patient Coupling
Siemens Medical	Lithostar	Electromagnetic	Acoustic lens	1000 lb (treatment table)	11.3	380	1.1 × 9.0	200,000	Water cushion
Systems/ F.R.G.	Lithostar Plus	Electromagnetic	Acoustic lens	—	—	650	—	200,000	Water cushion
Karl Storz Medical, Inc./ F.R.G.	Modulith SL-10 SL-20	Electromagnetic	Focusing lens (parabolic reflector)	1100 lb 2090 lb	15	200–2000	0.6 × 2.8	>1,000,000	Water cushion
Diasonics, Inc./ U.S.A.	Therasonic	Piezoelectric	Concave dish	1000 lb	12	650–800	0.25 × 3.0	>2,000,000	Water cushion
EDAP/France	LT-01	Piezoelectric	Concave dish	4343 lb (entire outfit)		900	0.3 × 2.0	>1,000,000	Water cushion
Richard Wolf, Inc./F.R.G.	Piezolith 2300	Piezoelectric	Concave dish	1166 lb	10–12 (from base of transducer)	600–1200	0.25 × 3.0	>2,000,000	Water/direct contact
Yachiyoda/Japan	SZ-1	Microexplosive	Ellipsoid	1540 lb	13.5	800	1.0 × 3.0	Unlimited (electrode has 300-shot life span)	Water/direct contact

Courtesy of R. V. Clayman, Washington University, Division of Urology, St. Louis, Missouri, August, 1990. (SW, shock waves.)

anesthesia. The factors that appear to make a machine anesthesia-free are a widened dish or ellipsoid aperture, which creates a wide shock wave skin entry radius, a reduced power generation by the shock wave generator, and a smaller focal zone.

Anesthesia-free appears to be a fairly casual term tossed around by vendors of machines. Certainly, a truly anesthesia-free machine is desirable from the patient's standpoint. However, the re-treatment rate appears to be at least 30 per cent for such machines; therefore, some of the anesthesia-free advantage is negated by a higher re-treatment rate. How such re-treatments should be reimbursed is also under discussion. Some think a global fee for SWL, which covers one or multiple treatments for a given stone, should be the standard. Another often overlooked issue is whether multiple treatments with a less powerful machine cause as much total trauma to the kidney as one treatment with a more powerful machine. Such issues are complex.

OVERVIEW OF NEW MACHINES

R. Clayman, at Washington University, St. Louis, Missouri, has compiled a masterful collection of data concerning all aspects of currently available lithotriptors. The tables containing this information are reproduced here with his permission.

Table 59–2 outlines the mechanical aspects of alternative energy source machines (those other than electrohydraulic).

Table 59–3 provides practical aspects of the alternative energy machines, such as room requirements, other needs, ease of setup, and portability.

Table 59–4 outlines the financial aspects of alternative energy source machines, including purchase price, service contracts, and disposable costs.

Table 59–5 provides information on the clinical aspects of such machines.

Results of stone treatment using alternative energy machines relative to stone size, stone position, stone-free rates, re-treatment rates, auxiliary treatments, and effectiveness quotient are presented in Table 59–6.

Clayman and co-workers (1989a) have introduced the "effectiveness quotient." Effectiveness quotient (EQ) is a term that they conceived in an attempt to compare one form of stone treatment with another or to compare one machine with another. It relates the stone-free rate to the incidence of additional therapy (e.g., repeat lithotripsy and auxiliary procedures) needed after the

Table 59–3. ALTERNATIVE ENERGY SOURCES—PRACTICAL ASPECTS

Company/Location	Machine	Room Requirements	Other Needs	Ease of Setup	Portability
Siemens Medical Systems/ F.R.G.	Lithostar Lithostar Plus	Dedicated room		Major room renovation	No
Karl Storz Medical, Inc./ F.R.G.	Modulith	Dedicated room (325 sq ft)	None		SL-10: Yes SL-20: No
Diasonics Inc./U.S.A.	Therasonic	Dedicated room (250 sq ft)	None	—	Yes
EDAP/France	LT-01	Dedicated room (225 sq ft)	208 Single-phase line; A/C 20,000 BTU; 30-amp line; sink with hot and cold running water	—	No
Richard Wolf, Inc./F.R.G., France	Piezolith 2300	Minimal (200 sq ft)	240 volts/20-amp line; water connections	Portable (8 hours to set up)	Yes
Yachiyoda/Japan	SZ-1	Minimal (250 sq ft)	Storage facility for microexplosive		No

Courtesy of R. V. Clayman, Washington University, Division of Urology, St. Louis, Missouri, August, 1990.

Table 59–4. ALTERNATIVE ENERGY SOURCES—FINANCIAL ASPECTS

Company/Location	Machine	Purchase Price ($)	Service Contract ($)*	Disposables
Siemens Medical Systems/F.R.G.	Lithostar	1.4×10^6	None	
	Lithostar Plus	1.3×10^6		
Karl Storz Medical, Inc./F.R.G	Modulith	1.0×10^6	98,500	None
Diasonics, Inc./U.S.A.	Therasonic	1.0×10^6	75,000	None
EDAP/France	LT-01	1.0×10^6	90,000 (quarterly visit)	None
Richard Wolf, Inc./F.R.G.	Piezolith 2300	0.995×10^6	90,000 (biannual visit)	None
Yachiyoda/Japan	SZ-1	$1.0–1.4 \times 10^6$	40,000 (monthly visit)	Detonating electrodes (300-shock life-span) microexplosive pellets

*Based on 700 patients treated per year.
Courtesy of R. V. Clayman, Washington University, Division of Urology, St. Louis, Missouri, August, 1990.

initial lithotripsy treatment. This value is calculated by the following formula:

$$EQ = \frac{\% \text{ stone-free}}{100\% + \% \text{ retreatment} + \% \text{ auxiliary procedures}} \times 100$$

Overall, the HM-3 machine was superior to all others in treating less than 1 cm and 1 to 2 cm stones with an overall EQ of 63 per cent. This quotient is probably the best way to compare various machines and therapies at this time.

Table 59–7 presents the mechanical aspects of electrohydraulic lithotriptors, such as the HM-3 and subsequent Dornier models, and the products of other manufacturers using the spark-gap technology.

Practical aspects of electrohydraulic lithotriptors are presented in Table 59–8.

Table 59–9 presents the financial aspects of such lithotriptors. Refurbished electrodes are now being marketed for the Dornier HM-3 by vendors other than the Dornier Company. A rather spirited debate is taking place as to whether such refurbished electrodes are equivalent to the original Dornier electrodes. The refurbished electrodes are less costly than the original electrodes. Both the newly produced Dornier electrodes and the refurbished electrodes are able to provide

greater numbers of shock waves than the original Dornier electrodes provided for the HM-3 model.

Clinical aspects of electrohydraulic lithotriptors are provided in Table 59–10, including date of FDA approval or lack thereof.

Results of treatment with electrohydraulic machines are presented in Table 59–11, which includes both renal and ureteral stone locations.

A tremendous amount of data is available for the treating physician, facility owner, referring physician, consumer, and third-party payer to digest. These tables should provide helpful information.

A prospective user, buyer, or patient should study the results of various machines and visit one or more lithotriptor centers to view a given machine in action.

No reliable method has been developed to compare the amount of renal trauma a given machine may generate on a given human patient. Because the machines are constantly changing with varying apertures and generator power, the whole field is constantly changing.

FINAL REFLECTIONS

SWL has provided a great number of patients suffering with stones a marvelous alternative to the more

Text continued on page 2178

Table 59–5. ALTERNATIVE ENERGY SOURCES—CLINICAL ASPECTS

Company/Location	Machine	FDA Approval	IDE Trials	Anesthesia	Procedural Time (min)	Other Capabilities	Stone Localization	Patient Positioning
Siemens Medical Systems/F.R.G.	Lithostar	9/88	Completed	IV sedation, TENS	60–83	Can be upgraded for biliary	Fluoroscopy	Movable table top
	Lithostar Plus		In progress	IV sedation	—	Biliary	Ultrasound	Move shock wave generator
Karl Storz Medical, Inc./F.R.G.	Modulith	No	Active (5/90)	IV sedation		Cystoscopy, PCN	SL-10: Ultrasound	Movable table top
						Ureteroscopy	SL-20: Ultrasound, fixed x-ray	
Diasonics, Inc./U.S.A.	Therasonic	No	Active (7/88)	IV sedation	60–90	Cystoscopy TUR	Fluoroscopy Ultrasound	Move shock wave generator
EDAP/France	LT-01	No	Completed	None (90%); IV sedation (10%)	67	Biliary	Ultrasound	Move shock wave generator
Richard Wolf, Inc./F.R.G.	Piezolith 2300	1/90	Completed (3/89)	None	45–55	Biliary Cystoscopy	Ultrasound	Move shock wave generator
Yachiyoda/Japan	SZ-1	No	No	None (90%)	90	Possibly biliary	Fluoroscopy (C-arm)	Movable chair

Abbreviations: FDA, Food and Drug Administration; IDE, investigational device exemption; IV, intravenous; TENS, transcutaneous electrical nerve stimulator; PCN, percutaneous nephrostomy; TUR, transurethral resection.
Courtesy of R. V. Clayman, Washington University, Division of Urology, St. Louis, Missouri, August, 1990.

Table 59–6. ALTERNATIVE ENERGY SOURCES—RESULTS

Company/ Location	Machine	Data Source	Stone Size (cm)	Upper Calyx SF (%)	Retx (%)	Aux (%)	EQ (%)	Middle Calyx SF (%)	Retx (%)	Aux (%)	EQ (%)	Lower Calyx SF (%)	Retx (%)	Aux (%)	EQ (%)	Pelvis SF (%)	Retx (%)	Aux (%)	EQ (%)
Siemens Medical Systems/ F.R.G.	Lithostar	Clayman, U.S.A. (123 cases)	<1					63	13	25	46	75	0	10	68	77	5	5	70
			1–1.9									68	4	24	53	50	21	21	35
	Lithostar Plus	Simon, Belgium (400 cases)	1.5					84	10	8	71					93	10	20	72
			1.5–2.5					66	(All		—					89	—	—	
			2.5					66	calyces)							46			
Karl Storz Medical, Inc./F.R.G.	Modulith																		
Diasonics, Inc./ U.S.A.	Therasonic	FDA trials		40				46				57				66			
EDAP/ France	LT-01	Kiely, Ireland (500 cases)	<1	59	37	0	43	80	26	0	64					78	36	0	57
			1–2	63	68	0	38	60	53	0	39					67	77	9	36
			>2–3 3													20	91	2	NA
Richard Wolf, Inc./F.R.G.	Piezolith 2300	Lacey, U.S.A. (47 cases)	1–2									23	13	4	20	50	33	17	33
Yachiyoda/ Japan	SZ-1	Kuwahara, Japan (229 cases)	<1					95	0	0	95					85	0	8	78
			1–2					62	35	19	40					84	26	16	59
			2.1–3					71	100	14	33					68	42	26	41
			>3					—	—	—	—					54	63	63	24

(Middle Calyx for Yachiyoda: All calyces)

Company/ Location	Machine	Data Source	Stone Size (cm)	Upper Ureter SF (%)	Retx (%)	Aux (%)	EQ (%)	Lower Ureter SF (%)	Retx (%)	Aux (%)	EQ (%)	Stone Size (cm)	Overall SF (%)	Retx (%)	Aux (%)	EQ (%)
		Mobley, U.S.A. (1850 cases)											77	17	19	56
Siemens Medical Systems/F.R.G.	Lithostar	Clayman, U.S.A. (123 cases)	<1	79	0	16	68					1	74	7	16	60
			1–1.9	89	38	11 12	60 52					1–1.9	65	12		
	Lithostar Plus	Simon, Belgium (400 cases)	1.5	96	20	12	73	84	20	26	58		80	17	14.5	61
Karl Storz Medical, Inc./F.R.G.	Modulith	Rassweiler, Germany (169 cases)											69	21	14	51
Diasonics, Inc./ U.S.A.	Therasonic	FDA trials		62									59			
EDAP/France	LT-01	Kiely, Ireland (500 cases)	1	68	38	6	47					1	72	29	2	55
			1–2	67	75	16	35					1–2	64	68	6	37
			2–3									2–3	9	87	17	4
Richard Wolf, Inc./ F.R.G.	Piezolith 2300	McNicholas, England (274 cases)	1–2									1–2	61	268	21	16
		Marberger, Austria (438 cases)										1.5	92	39	32	54
												1.5–2.5		74	47	50
												2.5	50	—	80	28
		Segura, U.S.A. (139 cases)										—	53	15	22	39
Yachiyoda/Japan	SZ-1	Kuwahara, Japan (229 cases)	<1	95	10	10	79	Unable to treat due to patient position				<1	92	4	6	84
			1–2	79	43	29	46					1–2	80	38	24	49
			2.1–3									2.1–3	69	77	35	33
			3													

Abbreviations: SF, stone-free rate; Retx, retreatment rate; Aux, auxiliary treatment rate; EQ, effectiveness quotient; FDA, Food and Drug Administration.
Courtesy of R. V. Clayman, Washington University, Division of Urology, St. Louis, Missouri, August, 1990.

Table 59–7. ELECTROHYDRAULIC LITHOTRIPSY—MECHANICAL ASPECTS

Company/Location	Machine	Method of Focusing Shock Wave	Weight (lb)	Focal Distance (cm)	Pressure at Focal Point (bar)	Focal Area (cm)	Electrode Life Span (SW)	Generator Life Span (SW)	Shock Wave/ Patient Coupling
Dornier Medical Systems, Inc./ F.R.G.	HM-3	Ellipsoidal reflector (15.6/17.2 cm aperture)		13.0	700–1300/600–1000	$1.5 \times 9.0/1 \times 4$	1500	600,000	Waterbath
	HM-4	Ellipsoidal reflector (15.6/17.1 cm)	3094	13	700–1300/600–1000	$1.5 \times 9/1 \times 4$	1500	1×10^6	Water membrane
	MFP 9000	Ellipsoidal reflector (21 cm)	4555	14	700–1300	0.3×2	1500	600,000	Water membrane
	MFL 5000	Ellipsoidal reflector (17.3 cm)		13	600–1000	1×4	1500	1×10^6	Water membrane
Technomed International, Inc./U.S.A.	Sonolith 3000	Ellipsoidal reflector (20.5 or 26 cm)	1650	13.5	700–1000	1.5×5.5	200,000	1×10^6	Water pool (30 gallons; patient stays dry)
Northgate Research, Inc./ U.S.A.	SD-3	Ellipsoidal reflector	1380	12.5	700–1000	1.5×3.0	2500	1×10^6	Water membrane
Medstone International/ U.S.A.	STS	Ellipsoidal reflector (15 cm)	1200 (console, 440)	15 (24.1, F_1–F_2)	350	1.5×12.0	2000	1×10^6	Water membrane
Direx Co./Israel	Triptor X1	Ellipsoidal reflector	209	12.5	1000	1.5×1.5	2400	500,000	Water membrane
Medas/Italy	Lithoring	Ellipsoidal reflector							Water membrane

Courtesy of R. V. Clayman, Washington University, Division of Urology, St. Louis, Missouri, August, 1990. (SW, shock waves.)

Table 59–8. ELECTROHYDRAULIC LITHOTRIPSY—PRACTICAL ASPECTS

Company/Location	Machine	Room Requirements	Other Needs	Ease of Setup	Portability
Dornier Medical Systems, Inc./F.R.G.	HM-3	Dedicated treatment and degassification facility (>30 m²)	Room for degassification equipment	Major room renovation; structural supports, floor/ceiling	No
	HM-4	Dedication room (>30 m²)			No
	MPL 9000	Dedicated room (>30 m²)			No
	MFL 5000	Dedicated room			No
Technomed International, Inc./ France	Sonolith 3000	Dedicated room (300 sq ft)	None	Minimal: 3.5 drains; H_2O source (hot and cold); 4kVA electrical connection	Yes
Northgate Research, Inc./U.S.A.	SD-3	Nondedicated room; portable (200 sq ft)		Simple–plug into electrical outlet (two 110-volt, 15-amp outlets)	Yes
Medstone International/ U.S.A.	STS	Dedicated room (300–400 sq ft)		Major room renovation: overhead x-ray system; 2 TV cameras in ceiling	No
Direx Co./Israel	Triptor X1	Nondedicated room *very* portable	Prepared water	Simple–plug into electrical outlet	Yes
Medas/Italy	Lithoring				

Courtesy of R. V. Clayman, Washington University, Division of Urology, St. Louis, Missouri, August, 1990.

Table 59–9. ELECTROHYDRAULIC LITHOTRIPSY—FINANCIAL ASPECTS

Company/Location	Machine	Purchase Price ($)	Service Contract ($)*	Disposables
Dornier Medical Systems, Inc./F.R.G.	HM-3	1.7×10^6		Nitrogen gas Electrodes Degassification supplies
	HM-4	1.5×10^6		Electrodes, nitrogen gas
	MPL 9000			Electrodes, nitrogen gas
	MFL 5000	1.35×10^6		Electrodes, nitrogen gas
Technomed International, Inc./France	Sonolith 3000	1.09×10^6	110,000 (quarterly visit)	None (long-lasting electrode, 200,000 shocks, is changed at time of routine service visit)
Northgate Research, Inc./ U.S.A.	SD-3	500,000 (kidney)	25–65,000 650,000 (dual purpose)	Electrodes
Medstone International/ U.S.A.	STS	1.375×10^6	1st year included (115–125,000/yr)	Electrodes, nitrogen gas
Direx Co./Israel	Triptor X1	200,000		Electrode
Medas/Italy	Lithoring			Electrode

Courtesy of R. V. Clayman, Washington University, Division of Urology, St. Louis, Missouri, August, 1990.

Table 59–10. ELECTROHYDRAULIC LITHOTRIPSY—CLINICAL ASPECTS

Company/ Location	Machine	FDA Approval	IDE Trials	Anesthesia	Procedural Time (min)	Other Capabilities	Stone Localization	Patient Positioning
Dornier Medical Systems, Inc./ F.R.G.	HM-3	12/84	Done	General spinal	17–37		Fluoroscopy	Movable patient stretcher
	HM-4	5/87	Done	IV sedation	60		Fluoroscopy	Movable patient stretcher
	MPL 9000	No	Pending	IV sedation	45	Biliary	Ultrasound/ optional fluoroscopy	
	MFL 5000	No	Pending	Oral, IV sedation	30–70	Percutaneous nephrostomy, cystoscopy, ureteroscopy	Fluoroscopy (ultrasound for biliary)	
Technomed International Inc./France	Sonolith 3000	6/89	Done	Epidural, spinal (Diatron II: 84% IV sedation)	62		Biliary lithotripsy to focus on stone	Move shock wave generator
Northgate Research Inc./ U.S.A.	SD-3	No	10/87	IV sedation, TENS (52%); epidural, spinal, general (48%)	60	Biliary stones (if dual purpose machine)	Ultrasound	Move shock wave generator
Medstone International/ U.S.A.	STS	4/88	Done	General, spinal IV sedation	44–118	Cystoscopy, IVP	Static radiographs stent placement	Movable top (or ultrasound)
Direx Co./Israel	Triptor X1	No	4/89	Epidural	30–45	Biliary	Fluoroscopy	Electrical table top movement
Medas/Italy	Lithoring	No	No	None, IV sedation	46	Biliary	Fluoroscopy/ ultrasound	Movable table top

Abbreviations: FDA, Food and Drug Administration; IDE, investigational device exemption; IV, intravenous; IVP, intravenous pyelogram; TENS, transcutaneous electrical nerve stimulator.

Courtesy of R. V. Clayman, Washington University, Division of Urology, St. Louis, Missouri, August, 1990.

Table 59–11. ELECTROHYDRAULIC LITHOTRIPSY—RESULTS

Company/ Location	Machine	Data Source	Stone Size (cm)	Upper Calyx SF (%)	Retx (%)	Aux (%)	EQ (%)	Middle Calyx SF (%)	Retx (%)	Aux (%)	EQ (%)	Lower Calyx SF (%)	Retx (%)	Aux (%)	EQ (%)	Pelvis SF (%)	Retx (%)	Aux (%)	EQ (%)
Dornier Medical Systems, Inc./F.R.G.	HM-3	Lingeman, U.S.A. (1024 cases)	≤2					75	6	7	66					87	10	7	74
	HM-4																		
	MPL 9000							(All calyces)											
	MFL 5000	Benkert, F.R.G. (415 cases)	1.45	88	17	—	<75	79	14	1.7	68	52	13	—	46	70	14	3.2	60
Technomed International, Inc./France	Sonolith 3000	U.S. Cooperative Study		50				30				41				43			
Northgate Research, Inc./U.S.A.	SD-3																		
Medstone International/ U.S.A.	STS	Cass, U.S.A. (1249 cases)	≤1	64	—	—	—	87	—	—	—	65	—	—	—	74	—	—	
			1.1–2	—				—				74	—	—	—	66	—	—	
			2.1–3	—				—				—	—	—	—	64	—	—	
		Hammond, U.S.A. (1374 cases)		91	4	—	<88	83	3	—	81	86	6	—	<81	99	1	4	94
Direx Co./Israel	Triptor X1	Livne, Israel (541 cases)		83	6	0	78					64	24	5	50				

Company/ Location	Machine	Data Source	Stone Size (cm)	Upper Ureter SF (%)	Retx (%)	Aux (%)	EQ (%)	Lower Ureter SF (%)	Retx (%)	Aux (%)	EQ (%)	Overall SF (%)	Retx (%)	Aux (%)	EQ (%)
Dornier Medical Systems, Inc./F.R.G.	HM-3	Kraft, U.S.A. (268 cases)	<2	80	14	28	56					79	3	3	75
		Lingeman, U.S.A. (1024 cases)	<1									77	5	12	66
			1–2									75	10	11	62
			2–3									43	33	27	27
			>3									29	31	46	16
	HM-4	Tailly, Belgium (483 cases)										85	38	4	60
		Kraft, U.S.A. (184 cases)										62	8	7	54
	MPL 9000														
	MFL 5000	Benkert, F.R.G. (415 cases)	1.45	96	20	11	73					70	15	—	61
		(Includes upper and lower ureteral stones)													
Technomed International, Inc./ France	Sonolith 3000	Smith, U.S.A. (160 cases)										46	4	6	42
		Worldwide										81	13	7	68
		Benson, U.S.A. (142 cases)										59	10	13	48
Northgate Research, Inc./U.S.A.	SD-3														
Medstone International/ U.S.A.	STS	Cass, U.S.A. (1249 cases)	≤1	84	—	—	—					70	—	—	—
			1.1–2.0	86	—	—	—								
		Hammond, U.S.A. (1374 cases)	<2	99	1	4	94	97	3	11	85	78	3	1	75
Direx Co./Israel	Triptor X1	Andrianne, Belgium (226 cases)		80	28	6	60					81	13	53	49
		Livne, Israel (541 cases)										75	24	7	57
Medas/Italy	Lithoring	Puppo, Italy (50 cases)										83	1.3	0	82

Abbreviations: SF, stone-free rate; Retx, retreatment rate; Aux, auxiliary treatment rate; EQ, effectiveness quotient.
Courtesy of R. V. Clayman, Washington University, Division of Urology, St. Louis, Missouri, August, 1990.

invasive forms of therapy. Dornier lithotriptors have been used to treat more than 2 million patients worldwide. However, there are definite limitations. One must generally rely on stone fragments to pass down the ureter, except when SWL is combined with a percutaneous approach. Many fragments lodge in lower calyces and do not pass. Patients who have large stones in kidneys with abnormal collecting systems have a low stone-free rate when treated with SWL monotherapy, which is about 40 per cent in several series (Gleeson and Griffith, 1989; Lingeman et al., 1989; Newman et al., 1988). Percutaneous removal, or combination therapy with SWL and either PCL or anatrophic nephrolithotomy seems preferable. Large cystine stones are not effectively treated with SWL. Stones existing in kidneys with ureteropelvic junction obstruction are better treated with open surgery or with PCL and endopyelotomy. Stones in calyceal diverticula are not successfully passed in 80 per cent of cases. In spite of these exceptions, most renal calculi and many ureteral calculi can be successfully treated with SWL with or without auxiliary procedures. Open stone surgery is required in only 1 to 3 per cent of cases at this point (Assimos et al., 1989b; Boyle et al., 1989).

Both short- and long-term complications of SWL need to be vigorously studied and eliminated as much as possible. Risk factors contributing to complications need to be further defined. Continued research into the positive and negative effects of shock waves on cell physiology is imperative.

Attempts should be made to reduce the cost of lithotripsy so that it may be more widely applied, especially to less affluent patients and countries.

The ease of and accessibility of SWL should not cloud the objective of discovering and treating the etiologic factors causing stones to form and recur. An ounce of prevention is still worth a pound of cure and is much less expensive.

In my opinion, the workers who developed principles involved in the Dornier lithotriptors, models HM-1 through HM-3, should someday receive the Nobel Prize in medicine for this monumental high-technology application of shock wave physics to urinary calculus therapy.

REFERENCES

Abber, J. D., Langberg, J., Mueller, S. C., et al.: Cardiovascular pathology and extracorporeal shock wave lithotripsy. J. Urol., 140:408, 1988.

Abernathy, B. B., Moins, J. S., Wilson, W. T., et al.: Evaluation of residual stone fragments following lithotripsy: Sonography v. radiography. In Lingeman, J. E., and Newman, D. M. (Eds.): Shock Wave Lithotripsy 2. New York, Plenum Press, 1989, p. 247.

Ackaert, K. S. J. W., Dik, P., Lock, M. T. W. T., et al.: Treatment of distal ureteral stones in the horse riding position. J. Urol., 142:955, 1989.

Al Karawi, M. A., Mohammed, A. E., El-Etaibi, K. E., et al.: Extrarenal shock wave lithotripsy (ESWL) induced erosions in upper gastrointestinal tract. Urology, 30:224, 1987.

American Urological Association Ad Hoc Lithotripsy Committee Report, McCullough, D. L., Chairman. Baltimore, Maryland, AUA, 1985.

American Urological Association Ad Hoc Lithotripsy Committee Report, McCullough, D. L., Chairman. Baltimore, Maryland, AUA, 1986.

American Urological Association Ad Hoc Lithotripsy Committee Report, McCullough, D. L., Chairman. Baltimore, Maryland, AUA, 1987.

Assimos, D. G., Boyce, W. H., Furr, E., et al.: Selective elevation of urinary enzyme levels after extracorporeal shock wave lithotripsy. J. Urol., 142:687, 1989a.

Assimos, D. G., Boyce, W. H., Harrison, L. H., et al.: Role of open stone surgery since extracorporeal lithotripsy. J. Urol., 142:2631, 1989b.

Barr, J. D., Tegtmeyer, C. J., and Jenkins, A. D.: In situ lithotripsy of ureteral calculi: Review of 261 cases. Radiology, 174:103, 1990.

Baumgartner, B. R., Dickey, K. W., Ambrose, S. S., et al.: Kidney changes after extracorporeal shock wave lithotripsy: Appearance on MR imaging. Radiology, 163:531, 1987.

Becht, E., Mohl, V., Neisius, D., et al.: Treatment of prevesical ureteral calculi by extracorporeal shock wave lithotripsy. J. Urol., 139:916, 1988.

Berens, M. E., Welander, C. E., Griffin, A. S., et al.: Effect of acoustic shock waves on clonogenic growth and drug sensitivity of human tumor cells in vitro. J. Urol., 142:1090, 1989.

Bland, K. I., Jones, R. S., Maher, J. W., et al.: Extracorporeal shock wave lithotripsy of bile duct calculi: An interim report of the Dornier BLS: Bile duct lithotripsy prospective study. Ann. Surg., 209:743, 1989.

Blute, M. L., Segura, J. W., and Patterson, D. E.: Ureteroscopy. J. Urol., 139:510, 1988.

Boyce, W. H., and Elkins, I. B.: Reconstructive renal surgery following anatrophic nephrolithotomy: Followup of 100 consecutive cases. J. Urol., 111:307, 1974.

Boyd, S. D., Everett, R. W., Schiff, W. M., and Fugelso, P. D.: Treatment of unusual Kock pouch urinary calculi with extracorporeal shock wave lithotripsy. J. Urol., 139:805, 1988.

Boyle, E. T., Segura, J. W., Patterson, D. E., et al.: The role of open stone surgery in stone disease. J. Urol., 141(4):293A, 1989.

Brownlee, N., Foster, M., Griffith, D. P., et al.: Controlled inversion therapy: An adjunct to the elimination of gravity-dependent fragments following extracorporeal shock wave lithotripsy. J. Urol., 143:1096, 1990.

Bush, W. H., Jones, D., and Gibbons, R. P.: Radiation dose to patient and personnel during extracorporeal shock wave lithotripsy. J. Urol., 138:716, 1987.

Carlson, C., Gravenstein, J., and Gravenstein, A.: Ventricular tachycardia during ESWL: Etiology, treatment, prevention. In Gravenstein, J., and Peter, K. (Eds.): Extracorporeal Shock Wave Lithotripsy for Stone Disease: Technical and Clinical Aspects. Stoneham, Butterworth, 1986, p. 101.

Carson, C. C., and Little, N.: The absolute and relative contraindications to extracorporeal shock wave lithotripsy. Probl. Urol., 1(4):604, 1987.

Cass, A. S., and Anstad, G. R.: Colonic injury with ESWL for an upper ureteral calculus. J. Urol., 139:851, 1988.

Chaussy, C. G.: ESWL: past, present, and future. J. Endourol, 2:97, 1988.

Chaussy, C. G., and Fuchs, G. J.: World experience with extracorporeal shock wave lithotripsy (ESWL) for the treatment of urinary stones: An assessment of its role after 5 years of clinical use. Endourology, 1:7, 1986.

Chaussy, C. G., and Fuchs, G. J.: Extracorporeal shock wave lithotripsy. Monogr. Urol., 4:80, 1987a.

Chaussy, C. G., and Fuchs, G. J.: Extracorporeal shock wave lithotripsy of distal ureteral calculi: Is it worthwhile? J. Endourol., 1:1, 1987b.

Chaussy, C. G., and Fuchs, G. J.: Extracorporeal shock wave lithotripsy (ESWL) for the treatment of upper urinary tract stones. In Gillenwater, J. Y., et al. (Eds.): Adult and Pediatric Urology, chap. 20. Chicago, Year Book Medical Publishers, Inc., 1987c, p. 605.

Chaussy, C. G., Randazzo, R. F., and Fuchs, G. J.: The effects of extracorporeal shock waves on human renal carcinoma cells and normal human embryonic kidney cells. J. Urol., 135:320A, 1986.

Chaussy, C., Schmeidt, E., Jochman, D., et al.: First clinical experiment with extracorporeally induced destruction of kidney stones by shock waves. J. Urol., 131:417, 1982a.

Chaussy, C. G., Schmeidt, E., Jochman, D., et al.: In Chaussy, C. (Ed.): Extracorporeal Shock Wave Lithotripsy. Munich, Karger Verlag, 1982b.

Chaussy, C. G., Schmeidt, E., Jocham, D., et al.: Extracorporeal shock wave lithotripsy (ESWL) for treatment of urolithiasis. Urology, 23:59, 1984.

Christensen, J. G., McCullough, D. L., and Cline, W. A., Sr.: Extracorporeal shock wave lithotripsy in hemophiliac patient. Urology, 33:424, 1989.

Clayman, R. V., McClennan, B. L., Garvier, T. J., et al.: Lithostar: An electromagnetic acoustic shock wave unit for extracorporeal lithotripsy. In Lingeman, J. E., and Newman, D. M.: Extracorporeal Shock Wave Lithotripsy 2. New York, Plenum Press, 1989a, p. 403.

Clayman, R. V., Preminger, G. M., Long, S., et al.: A comparison of in vitro cellular effects of shock waves generated by electrohydraulic, electromagnetic, and piesoelectric sources. J. Urol., 141:228A, 1989b.

Coe, F. L.: Nephrolithiasis: Pathogenesis and Treatment. Chicago, Year Book Medical Publishers, 1978.

Constantinides, C., Recker, F., Jaegar, P., et al.: Extracorporeal shock wave lithotripsy as monotherapy of staghorn renal calculi: 3 Years' experience. J. Urol., 142:1415, 1989.

Cooper, D., Wilkoff, B., Masterson, M., et al.: Effects of extracorporeal shock wave lithotripsy on cardiac pacemakers and its safety in patients with implanted cardiac pacemakers. PACE, 11:1607, 1988.

Coughlin, B. F., Risius, B., Streem, S. B., et al.: Abdominal radiograph and renal ultrasound versus excretory urography in the evaluation of asymptomatic patients after extracorporeal shock wave lithotripsy. J. Urol., 142:1419, 1989.

Delius, M.: This month in investigative urology: Effect of extracorporeal shock waves on the kidney. J. Urol., 140:390, 1988.

Desmet, W., Baert, L., Vandeursen, H., et al.: Iliac vein thrombosis after extracorporeal shock wave lithotripsy [letter to editor]. N. Engl. J. Med., 321:907, 1989.

Donohue, A. L., Linke, C. A., and Rowe, J. M.: Renal loss following extracorporeal shock wave lithotripsy. J. Urol., 142:809, 1989.

Donovan, J. M., Gunasekaran, G., and Drach, G. W.: Changes in rabbit renal physiology following extracorporeal shock wave treatment. In Lingeman, J. E., and Newman D. M. (Eds.): Shock Wave Lithotripsy. New York, Plenum Press, 1988, p. 347.

Drach, G. W.: Effects of shock waves on cells and tissues: Critical factors in the conduct of research. J. Urol., 141:964, 1989.

Drach, G. W., Dretler, S., Fair, W., et al.: Report of the United States Cooperative Study of Extracorporeal Shock Wave Lithotripsy. J. Urol., 135:1127, 1986.

Drach, G. W., Weber, C., and Donovan, J. M.: Treatment of pacemaker patients with extracorporeal shock wave lithotripsy: Experience from 2 continents. J. Urol., 143:895, 1990.

Dretler, S. P.: Stone fragility—a new therapeutic distinction. J. Urol., 139:1124, 1988.

Dretler, S. P., Keating, M. A., and Riley, J.: An algorithm for the management of ureteral calculi. J. Urol., 136:1190, 1986.

Durano, A. C., and Hanosh, J. J.: A new alternative for entrapped stone basket in the distal ureter. J. Urol., 139:116, 1988.

Dyer, R. B., Karstaedt, N., McCullough, D. L., et al.: Magnetic resonance imaging evaluation of immediate and intermediate changes in kidneys treated with extracorporeal shock wave lithotripsy. J. Lithotripsy Stone Dis., 2:302, 1990.

Eisenberger, F., Fuchs, G., Miller, K., et al.: Extracorporeal shock wave lithotripsy (ESWL) and endourology—an ideal combination for the treatment of kidney stones. World J. Urol., 3:41, 1985.

Elbers, J., Seline, P., and Clayman, R. V.: The effects of shock wave lithotripsy on urease-positive calculogenic bacteria. In Lingeman, J. E., and Newman, D. M. (Eds.): Shock Wave Lithotripsy. New York, Plenun Press, 1988, p. 391.

El-Faqih, S. R., Husain, I., Ekman, P. E., et al.: Primary choice of intervention for distal ureteric stones: Ureteroscopy or ESWL. Br. J. Urol., 62:525, 1988.

Ell, C., Kerzel, W., Heyden, N., et al.: Piezoelectric lithotripsy of gallstones. Lancet, 2:1149, 1987.

Ettinger, B.: Recurrent nephrolithiasis: Natural history and effect of phosphate therapy. Am. J. Med., 61:200, 1976.

Evan, A. P., McAteer, J. A., Steidle, C. P., et al.: Acute renal changes induced by ESW in the mini-pig. J. Urol., 141:233A, 1989.

Fedullo, L. M., Pollack, H. M., Banner, M. P., et al.: The development of steinstrasse after ESWL: Frequency, natural history, and radiologic management. AJR, 151:1145, 1988.

Fischer, N., Muller, H. M., Gulham, A., et al.: Cavitation effects: Possible cause of tissue injury during extracorporeal shock wave lithotripsy. J. Endourol., 2:215, 1988.

Flam, T. A., Brochard, M., Zerbib, M., et al.: Extracorporeal shock wave lithotripsy to remove calcified ureteral stents. Urology, 36:164, 1990.

Forssmann, B., Hepp., W., Chaussy, C. G., et al.: Eine Methode Zeer Beruhrungfreien Zertrummerung von Nieren-Steinen durch Stosswellen. Biomed. Tech. (Berlin), 22:164, 1977.

Fuchs, G. J.: Staghorn stone treatment with ESWL: The fate of residual stones. In Lingeman, J. E., and Newman, D. M. (Eds.): Shock Wave Lithotripsy. New York, Plenum Press, 1988, p. 101.

Fuchs, G. J., Chaussy, C. G., and Riehle, R. A.: Treatment of ureteral stones. In Riehle, R. A., and Newman, D. M. (Eds.): Principles of ESWL. New York, Churchill Livingstone, 1987, p. 159.

Fuchs, G. J., Chaussy, C. G., and Stenzl, A.: Current management concepts in the treatment of ureteral stones. J. Endourol., 2:107, 1988.

Germinale, F., Puppo, P., Battino, P., et al.: ESWL and hypertension: No evidence for causal relationship. J. Urol., 141:241A, 1989.

Gilbert, B. R., Riehle, R. A., and Vaughan, E. D.: Extracorporeal shock wave lithotripsy and its effects on renal function. J. Urol., 139:482, 1988.

Gleeson, M. J., and Griffith, D. P.: Extracorporeal shock wave monotherapy for large renal calculi. Br. J. Urol., 64:329, 1989.

Grace, P. A., Gillen, P., Smith, J. M., et al.: Extracorporeal shock wave lithotripsy with the Lithostar lithotripter. Br. J. Urol., 64:117, 1989.

Graff, J., Pastor, J., Funke, P. J., et al.: Extracorporeal shock wave lithotripsy for ureteral stones: A retrospective analysis of 417 cases. J. Urol., 139:513, 1988a.

Graff, J., Pastor, J., Herberhold, D., et al.: Technical modifications of the Dornier HM-3 Lithotripter with an improved anesthesia technique. World J. Urol., 5:202, 1987.

Graff, J., Schmidt, A., Pastor, J., et al.: New generator for low pressure lithotripsy with the Dornier HM-3: Preliminary experience of 2 centers. J. Urol., 139:904, 1988b.

Griffith, D. P., Gleeson, M. J., Politis, G., et al.: Effectiveness of radiation control for Dornier HM-3 lithotripter. Urology, 33:20, 1989.

Griffith, D. P., and Valiquette, L.: PICA/BURDEN: A staging system for upper tract urinary stones. J. Urol., 138:253, 1987.

Haupt, G., Haupt, A., Chvapil, M., et al.: Wound and fracture healing: New indication for extracorporeal shock waves [abstract A4]. J. Endourol., 4(Suppl 1):554, 1990.

Holden, D., and Rao, P. N.: Ureteral stones: The results of primary in situ extracorporeal shock wave lithotripsy. J. Urol., 142:37, 1989.

Holmes, R. P., Yeaman, L. I., Li, W. J., et al.: The combined effects of shock waves and cisplatin therapy on rat prostate tumor. In Lingeman, J. E., and Newman, D. M. (Eds.): Shock Wave Lithotripsy 2. New York, Plenum Press, 1989, p. 111.

Holmes, R. P., Yeaman, L. I., Taylor, R. G., Lewis, J. C., and McCullough, D. L.: Enhanced adriamycin uptake by neutrophils exposed to shock waves. J. Urol., 139:304A, 1988.

Hood, K., Kneightly, A., Dowling, R., et al.: Piezo ceramic lithotripsy of gallbladder stones: Initial experience in 38 patients. Lancet, 1:1322, 1988.

Hunter, P. T., Finlayson, B., and Hirkso, R. I.: Measurement of shock wave pressures used for lithotripsy. J. Urol., 136:733, 1986.

Jaegar, P., and Constantinides, C.: Canine kidneys: Changes in blood and urine chemistry after exposure to extracorporeal shock waves. In Lingeman, J. E., and Newman, D. M. (Eds.): Shock Wave Lithotripsy 2. New York, Plenum Press, 1989, p. 7.

Jaegar, P., Redha, F., Uhlschmid, G., et al.: Morphologic changes in canine kidneys following extracorporeal shock wave treatment. J. Endourol., 2:205, 1988.

Jenkins, A. D., and Gillenwater, J. Y.: Extracorporeal shock wave lithotripsy in the prone position: Treatment of stones in the distal ureter or anomalous kidney. J. Urol., 139:911, 1988.

Jocham, D., Liedl, B., Schuster, C., et al.: New techniques and developments in ESWL: Dornier HM-4 and MPL 9000. Urol. Res., 16:255A, 1988.

Kahnoski, R. J., Lingeman, J. E., Coury, T. A., et al.: Combined percutaneous and extracorporeal shock wave lithotripsy for staghorn calculi: An alternative to anatrophic nephrolithotomy. J. Urol., 135:679, 1986.

Karawi, M. A. A., Mohamed, A. R. E., El-Etaibi, K. E., et al.: Extracorporeal shock wave lithotripsy (ESWL)–induced erosions in upper gastrointestinal tract—Prospective study in 40 patients. Urology, 30:224, 1987.

Karlin, G. S., Schulsinger, D., Urivetsky, M., et al.: Absence of persisting parenchymal damage after extracorporeal shock wave lithotripsy as judged by excretion of renal tubular enzymes. J. Urol., 144:13, 1990.

Karlin, G. S., Urivetsky, M., and Smith, A. S.: Side effects of extracorporeal shock wave lithotripsy: Assessment of urinary excretion of renal enzymes as evidence of tubular injury. In Lingeman, J. E., and Newman, D. M. (Eds.): Shock Wave Lithotripsy 2. New York, Plenum Press, 1989, p. 3.

Katz, G., Lencorsky, A., Pide, D., et al.: Place of extracorporeal shock wave lithotripsy (ESWL) in management of cystine calculi. Urology, 36:124, 1990.

Kaude, J. V., Williams, C. M., Millner, M. R., et al.: Renal morphology and function immediately after extracorporeal shock wave lithotripsy. AJR, 145:305, 1985.

Kaude, J. V., Williams, J. E., Wright, P. G., et al.: Sonographic evaluation of the kidney following extracorporeal shock wave lithotripsy. J. Ultrasound Med., 6:299, 1987.

Keeler, L.: Presentation at American Lithotripsy Society Meeting. New Orleans, 1988.

Keeler, L., McNamara, T. C., Dorey, F. O., et al.: Extracorporeal shock wave lithotripsy for lower ureteral calculi: Treatment of choice. J. Endourol., 4:71, 1990.

Kiely, E. A., Ryan, P. C., McDermott, T. E., et al.: EDAP piezoelectric shock wave lithotripsy: Experience with 511 patients. In Lingeman, J. E., and Newman D. M. (Eds.): Shock Wave Lithotripsy 2. New York, Plenum Press, 1989, p. 371.

Kishimoto, T., Yamamato, K., Suginoto, T., et al.: Selective elevation of urinary enzyme levels after extracorporeal shock wave lithotripsy for upper urinary tract stones. Eur. Urol., 12:308, 1986.

Knapp, P. M., Kulb, T. B., Lingeman, J. E., et al.: Extracorporeal shock wave lithotripsy–induced perirenal hematomas. J. Urol., 139:700, 1988.

Kostakopoulos, A., Sofras, F., Karayiannis, A., et al.: Ureterolithotripsy: Report of 1000 cases. Br. J. Urol., 63:243, 1989.

Kraft, J. K.: Treatment results comparing the Dornier HM-3 and the Dornier HM-4. In Programs and Abstracts of the 5th Symposium on Shock Wave Lithotripsy, Indianapolis, 1989.

Kramolowsky, E. V., Willoughby, B. L., and Loening, S. A.: Extracorporeal shock wave lithotripsy in children. J. Urol., 137:939, 1987.

Kroovand, R. L.: Extracorporeal shock wave lithotripsy in the pediatric stone patient: Problems and results. Probl. Urol., 1(4):682, 1987.

Kroovand, R. L., Harrison, L. H., and McCullough, D. L.: Extracorporeal shock wave lithotripsy in childhood. J. Urol., 138:1106, 1987.

Kulb, T. B., Lingeman, J. E., Coury, T. A., et al.: Extracorporeal shock wave lithotripsy in patients with a solitary kidney. J. Urol., 136:786, 1986.

Landone, V. P., Morgan, T. R., Huryk, R. F., et al.: Cytotoxicity of high energy shock waves: Methodologic considerations. J. Urol., 141:965, 1989.

Langberg, J., Abber, J., Therroff, J. E., et al.: The effects of extracorporeal shock wave lithotripsy on pacemaker function. PACE, 10:1142, 1987.

Liedl, B., Jocham, D., Lunz, C., et al.: Five year follow-up of urinary stone patients treated with extracorporeal shock wave lithotripsy. J. Endourol., 2:157, 1988.

Lingeman, J. E., and Kalb, T. B.: Hypertension following extracorporeal shock wave lithotripsy. J. Urol., 137:154A, 1987.

Lingeman, J. E., McAteer, J. A., Kempson, S. A., et al.: Bioeffects of extracorporeal shock wave lithotripsy: Strategy for research and treatment. Urol. Clin. North Am., 15:507, 1988.

Lingeman, J. E., Newman, D. M., Mertz, J. H. O., et al.: Extracorporeal shock wave lithotripsy: The Methodist Hospital of Indiana experience. J. Urol., 135:1134, 1986.

Lingeman, J. E., Shirrell, W. L., Newman, D. M., Mosbaugh, P. G., Steele, R. E., and Woods, J. R.: Management of upper ureteral calculi with extracorporeal shock wave lithotripsy. J. Urol., 138:720, 1987.

Lingeman, J. E., Woods, J., Toth, P. D., et al.: The role of lithotripsy and its side effects. J. Urol., 141:793, 1989.

Lingeman, J. E., Woods, J., and Toth, P. D.: Blood pressure changes following extracorporeal shock wave lithotripsy and other forms of treatment for nephrolithiasis. JAMA, 263:1789, 1990.

Littleton, R. H., Melser, M., and Kupin, W.: Acute renal failure following bilateral extracorporeal shock wave lithotripsy in the absence of obstruction. In Lingeman, J. E., and Newman D. M. (Eds.): Shock Wave Lithotripsy 2. New York, Plenum Press, 1989, p. 197.

Locke, D. R., Newman, R. C., Sternbock, G. S., et al.: Extracorporeal shock-wave lithotripsy in horseshoe kidneys. Urology, 35:407, 1990.

Loening, S., Kramalowsky, E. V., and Willoughby, B.: Use of local anesthesia for extracorporeal shock wave lithotripsy. J. Urol., 137:626, 1987.

Loening, S. A., Mordon, A. H., Holmes, J., et al.: In vivo and in vitro effects of shock waves on Dunning prostate tumor. J. Urol., 139:563A, 1988.

Lupu, A. N., Fuchs, G. J., and Chaussy, C. G.: Calcification of ureteral stent treated by extracorporeal shock wave lithotripsy. J. Urol., 136:1297, 1986.

Malhoutra, V.: The use of regional block technique for extracorporeal shock wave lithotripsy. Endourology, 1:7, 1986.

Marberger, M., Turk, C., and Steinkogler, I.: Painless piezoelectric extracorporeal lithotripsy. J. Urol., 139:695, 1988.

Marshall, V. F., White R. H., Chaput de Saintonage, M., et al.: The natural history of renal and ureteral calculi. Br. J. Urol., 47:117, 1975.

McAteer, J. A., Evans, A. P., Hoak, R., et al.: Cell culture and in vitro systems to assess the bioeffects of ESWL. J. Urol., 141:228A, 1989.

McCullough, D. L.: Complications of ESWL. Probl. Urol., 1:604, 1987a.

McCullough, D. L.: The urologist's role in nonurologic use of ESWL—biliary stones. Probl. Urol., 1:694, 1987b.

McCullough, D. L.: Extracorporeal shock wave lithotripsy and residual stone fragments in lower calices. J. Urol., 141:140, 1989.

McCullough, D. L., Yeaman, L. D., Bo, W., et al.: Effects of shock waves on the rat ovary. J. Urol., 141:666, 1989.

McDougall, E. M., Denstedt, J. D., Brown, R. D., et al.: Comparison of extracorporeal shock wave lithotripsy and percutaneous nephrostolithotomy for the treatment of renal calculi in lower pole calices. In Lingeman, J. E., and Newman, D. M. (Eds.): Shock Wave Lithotripsy 2. New York, Plenum Press, 1989, p. 263.

McNicholas, T. A., Jones, D. J., and Russell, A.: Piezolithotripsy experience with Wolf Piezolith 2300. In Lingeman, J. E., and Newman D. M. (Eds.): Shock Wave Lithotripsy 2. New York, Plenum Press, 1989, p. 381.

Meyer, W. H., Soehendra, N., and Kosterhalfen, H.: Successful shockwave treatment of impacted pancreatic duct stones. J. Urol., 141:295A, 1989.

Michaels, E. K., and Fowler, J. E., Jr.: Inadvertent fracture of gallstones during extracorporeal shock wave lithotripsy. J. Urol., 136:1285, 1986.

Michaels, E. K., Fowler, J. E., Jr., and Mariano, M.: Bacteriuria following extracorporeal shock wave lithotripsy of infectious stones. J. Urol., 140:254, 1988.

Miller, K., Bachor, R., and Hautman, R.: Extracorporeal shock wave lithotripsy in the prone position: Techniques, indications, results. J. Endourol., 2:113, 1988a.

Miller, K., Bachor, R., and Hautman, R.: Percutaneous nephrolithotomy/ESWL versus ureteral stent/ESWL for the treatment of large renal calculi and staghorn stones: A prospective randomized study. In Lingeman, J. E., Newman, D. M. (Eds.): Shock Wave Lithotripsy. New York, Plenum Press, 1988b, p. 89.

Miller, K., Bubeck, J. R., and Hautman, R.: Extracorporeal shock wave lithotripsy of distal ureteral calculi. Eur. Urol., 12:305, 1986.

Miller, K., Fuchs, G., and Rossweiler, J.: Treatment of ureteral stone disease: The role of ESWL and endourology. World J. Urol., 3:53, 1985.

Moran, M. E., Sandock, D., and Drach, G. W.: Effects of high energy shock waves on chick embryo development. J. Urol., 143:167A, 1990.

Morris, J. S., Husmann, D. A., Wilson, W. T., et al.: Piezoelectric vs electrohydraulic lithotripsy: A comparison of morphologic alterations J. Urol., 141:228A, 1989.

Mueller, S. C., Wilbert, D., Thueroff, J. W., et al.: Extracorporeal shock wave lithotripsy of ureteral stones: Clinical experience and experimental findings. J. Urol., 135:831, 1986.

Neisius, D., Seitz, G., Gebhardt, T., et al.: Influence of shock wave number on canine renal morphology following treatment with piezoelectric lithotripsy using the Wolf Piezolith 2200. *In* Lingeman, J. E., and Newman, D. M. (Eds.): Shock Wave Lithotripsy 2. New York, Plenum Press, 1989, p. 23.

Netto, N. R., Jr., Lemos, G. C., and Claro, J. F. A.: In situ extracorporeal shock wave lithotripsy for ureteral calculi. J. Urol., 144:253, 1990.

Newman, D. M., Coury, T., Lingeman, J. E., et al.: Extracorporeal shock wave lithotripsy in children. J. Urol., 136:238, 1986.

Newman, D. M., Lingeman, J. E., Mosbaugh, P. G., et al.: Extracorporeal shock wave lithotripsy using only intravenous analgesia with an unmodified Dornier HM-3 Lithotripter. *In* Lingeman, J. E., and Newman, D. M. (Eds.): Shock Wave Lithotripsy 2. New York, Plenum Press, 1989, p. 411.

Newman, D. M., Scott, J. W., and Lingeman, J. E.: Two year followup of patients treated with extracorporeal shock wave lithotripsy. *In* Lingeman, J. E., and Newman, D. M. (Eds.): Shock Wave Lithotripsy. New York, Plenum Press, 1988, p. 159.

Newman, R. C., and Finlayson, B.: New developments in ESWL. AUA Update Series, 7:50, 1988.

Newman, R. C., Hackett, R., Senior, D., et al.: Pathologic effects of ESWL on canine renal tissue. Urology, 29:194, 1987.

Petterson, B., Tiselius, H. G., Anderson, A., et al.: Evaluation of extracorporeal shock wave lithotripsy without anesthesia using a Dornier HM-3 lithotripter without technical modification. J. Urol., 142:1189, 1989.

Philip, T., Kellett, M. J., Whitfield, H. N., et al.: Painless lithotripsy: Experience with 100 patients. Lancet, 2:41, 1988.

Pollock, H. M.: Radiation exposure and extracorporeal shock wave lithotripsy. J. Urol., 138:850, 1987.

Portney, K. L., Hollingsworth, R. L., Jordan, W. R., et al.: Hemophilia and extracorporeal shock wave lithotripsy: A case report. J. Urol., 138:393, 1987.

Preminger, G. M., and Erving J. H.: Piezoelectric lithotripsy: Initial experience with the Wolf 2200. *In* Lingeman, J. E., and Newman, D. M. (Eds.): Shock Wave Lithotripsy. New York, Plenum Press, 1988, p. 281.

Randazzo, R. F., Chaussy, C. G., Fuchs, G. J., et al.: The in vitro and in vivo effects of extracorporeal shock waves on malignant cells. Urol. Res., 16(6):419, 1988.

Rassweiler, J., Gumpinger, R., Moyer, R., et al.: Extracorporeal piezoelectric lithotripsy using the Wolf lithotripter versus low energy lithotripsy with the modified Dornier HM-3: A cooperative study. World J. Urol., 5:218, 1987.

Recker, F., Hofstadter, F., Davis, H. J., et al.: Morphological pathomechanism following extracorporeal shock wave lithotripsy in rat kidneys. *In* Lingeman, J. E., and Newman, D. M. (Eds.): Shock Wave Lithotripsy. New York, Plenum Press, 1988, p. 357.

Riehle, R. A., Carter, H., and Vaughan, E. D.: Quantitative and crystallographic analysis of stone fragments voided after extracorporeal shock wave lithotripsy. J. Endourol., 1:37, 1987.

Riehle, R. A., and Naslund, E. B.: Patient management and results after ESWL. *In* Riehle, R. A., and Newman, D. M. (Eds.): Principles of Extracorporeal Shock Wave Lithotripsy. New York, Churchill Livingstone, 1987, p. 121.

Riehle, R. A., Naslund, E. B., Fair, E., et al.: Impact of shock wave lithotripsy on upper ureteral calculi. Urology, 28:261, 1986.

Rius, H., and Saltzman, B.: Aspirin induced bilateral renal hemorrhage after extracorporeal shock wave lithotripsy: Implications and conclusions. J. Urol., 143:791, 1990.

Roth, R. A., and Beckman, C. F.: Complications of extracorporeal shock wave lithotripsy and percutaneous nephrolithotomy. Urol. Clin. North Am., 15:155, 1988.

Rubin, J. I., Arger, P. H., Pollock, H. M., et al.: Kidney changes after extracorporeal shock wave lithotripsy: CT evaluation. Radiology, 162:21, 1987.

Russo, P., Mies, C., Huryk, K., et al.: Histopathologic and ultrastructural correlates of tumor growth suppression by high energy shock waves. J. Urol., 137:338, 1987.

Russo, P., Stephenson, A. A., Mies, C., et al.: High energy shock waves suppress tumor growth in vitro and in vivo. J. Urol., 135:626, 1986.

Sackman, M., Delius, M., Sauerbruch, T., et al.: Shock wave lithotripsy of gallbladder stones: The first 175 patients. N. Engl. J. Med., 318:393, 1988.

Sandlow, J. I., Winfield, H. N., and Loening, S. A.: Blood pressure changes related to extracorporeal shock wave lithotripsy (ESWL). J. Urol., 141:242A, 1989.

Sauerbruch, T., Delius, M., Baumgartner, G., et al.: Fragmentation of gallstones by extracorporeal shock waves. N. Engl. J. Med., 314:818, 1986.

Sauerbruch, T., and Stern, M.: Fragmentation of bile duct stones by extracorporeal shock waves: A new approach to biliary calculi after failure of routine endoscopic measure. Gastroenterology, 96:146, 1989.

Schmeller, N. T., Kerating, H., Schuller, J., et al.: Combination of chemolysis and shock wave lithotripsy in the treatment of cystine renal calculi. J. Urol., 131:434, 1984.

Schoenfield, L. J., Berci, G., Carnovale, R. L., et al.: The effect of ursodiol on the efficacy and safety of extracorporeal shock wave lithotripsy of gallstones: The Dornier National Biliary Lithotripsy Study. N. Engl. J. Med., 323:1239, 1990.

Schulze, H., Hertle, L., Kutta, A., et al.: Critical evaluation of treatment of staghorn calculi by percutaneous nephrolithotomy and extracorporeal shock wave lithotripsy. J. Urol., 141:822, 1989.

Segura, J. W., Paterson, D. E., and LeRoy, A. J.: Continued experience with the Piezolith 2300: Extracorporeal piezoelectric lithotripsy. *In* Programs and Abstracts of the 5th Symposium on Shock Wave Lithotripsy, Indianapolis, 1989.

Siebold, J., Rossweiler, J., Schmidt, A., et al.: Advanced technology in extracorporeal shock wave lithotripsy—the Dornier MPL 9000 versus the upgraded Dornier HM-3. *In* Lingeman, J. E., and Newman, D. M. (Eds.): Shock Wave Lithotripsy. New York, Plenum Press, 1988, p. 231.

Smith, J. E., Van Arsdalen, K. N., and Hanno, P. M.: Extracorporeal shock wave lithotripsy treatment of calculi in horseshoe kidneys. J. Urol., 142:683, 1989.

Sonda, L. P., Wang, S., Ellis, J., et al.: Resolution of bacteriuria with infectious stones: Comparison of results employing newer treatment modalities. J. Endourol., 2.151, 1988.

Spirnak, J. P., Bodner, D., Udagashankar, S., et al.: Extracorporeal shock wave lithotripsy in traumatic quadriplegic patients: Can it be safely performed without anesthesia? J. Urol., 139:18, 1988.

Spirnak, J. P., and Resnick, M.: Extracorporeal shock wave lithotripsy. *In* Resnick, M. I., and Pak, C. Y. C. (Eds.): Urolithiasis: A Medical and Surgical Reference. Philadelphia, W. B. Saunders Co., 1990, p. 321.

Stoller, M. L., Thuroff, J. W., Grant, J. E., et al.: Audiometric evaluation of individuals exposed to sound waves from the Dornier HM-3 extracorporeal shock wave lithotripter. J. Urol., 139:871, 1988.

Texter, J. H.: The safety of extracorporeal shock wave lithotripsy in the high-risk patient and in the patient with compromised renal function. *In* Lingeman, J. E., and Newman, D. M. (Eds.): Shock Wave Lithotripsy. New York, Plenum Press, 1988, p. 127.

Theiss, M., Wirth, M. P., and Frohmuller, H. G. W.: Extracorporeal shock wave lithotripsy in patients with cardiac pacemakers. J. Urol., 143:479, 1990.

Thomas, R., Figuera, T. W., and Macaluso, J.: Advances in management of staghorn renal calculi. *In* Lingeman, J. E., and Newman, D. M. (Eds.): Shock Wave Lithotripsy. New York, Plenum Press, 1988a, p. 71.

Thomas, R., Sloane, B., and Roberts, J.: Effects of extracorporeal shock wave lithotripsy on renal function. J. Urol., 139:641A, 1988b.

Tiselius, H. G., and Petterson, B.: Experience with anesthesia-free shock wave lithotripsy using the unmodified Dornier HM-3 lithotripter. *In* Lingeman, J. E., and Newman, D. M. (Eds.): Shock Wave Lithotripsy 2. New York, Plenum Press, 1989, p. 417.

Tung, K. H., Tan, E. C., and Foo, K. T.: In situ extracorporeal shock wave lithotripsy for upper ureteral stones using the EDAP LT-01 lithotripter. J. Urol., 143:481, 1990.

Vallacien, G., Aviles, J., Munoz, R., Veillon, B., Charton, M., and Brisset, J. M.: Piezoelectric extracorporeal lithotripsy by ultrashort waves with the EDAP LT 01 device. J. Urol., 139:689, 1988.

Van Arsdalen, K. N.: Secondary procedures after ESWL. *In* Riehle, R. A., and Newman, D. M., (Eds.): Principles of Extracorporeal Shock Wave Lithotripsy. New York, Churchill Livingstone, 1987, p. 145.

Vandeursen, H., and Baert, L.: Extracorporeal shock wave lithotripsy monotherapy for bladder stones with second generation lithotripters. J. Urol., 143:18, 1990.

Van Swearingen, F. L., McCullough, D. L., Dyer, R., et al.: Radiation exposure to patients during extracorporeal shock wave lithotripsy. J. Urol., 138:18, 1987.

Vogeli, T., Mellin, H. E., and Ackerman, R.: High dosage extracorporeal shock wave lithotripsy with a modified Dornier HM-3 lithotripter. In Lingeman, J. E., and Newman, D. M. (Eds.): Shock Wave Lithotripsy 2. New York, Plenum Press, 1989, p. 247.

Warner, M. A., Warner, M. E., Buck, C. F., et al.: Clinical efficacy of high frequency jet ventilation during extracorporeal shock wave lithotripsy of renal and ureteral calculi: A comparison with conventional mechanical ventilation. J. Urol., 139:486, 1988.

Weinerth, J. L., Flatt, J. A., and Carson, C. C., III: Lessons learned in patients with large steinstrasse. J. Urol., 142:1425, 1989.

Whelan, J. P., Finlayson, B., Welch, J., et al.: The blast path: Theoretical basis, experimental data, and clinical application. J. Urol., 140:401, 1988.

Wilbert, D. M., Bichler, K. H., Strohmaier, W. L., et al.: Initial experience with the second generation lithotripter Dornier HM-4. Urol. Res., 16:262A, 1988.

Williams, C. M., Kaude, J. V., Newman, R. L., et al.: ESWL: Long-term complications. AJR, 150:311, 1988.

Wilson, W. T., Miller, G. L., Morris, J. S., et al.: Morphologic renal changes following piezoelectric lithotripsy or spark-gap lithotripsy. In Lingeman, J. E., and Newman, D. M. (Eds.): Shock Wave Lithotripsy 2. New York, Plenum Press, 1989, p. 19.

Winfield, H. N., Clayman, R. V., Chaussy, C. G., et al.: Monotherapy of staghorn renal calculi: A comparative study between percutaneous nephrolithotomy and extracorporeal shock wave lithotripsy. J. Urol., 139:895, 1988.

Yeaman, L. D., Jerone, C. P., and McCullough, D. L.: Effect of shock waves on structure and growth of the immature rat epiphysis. J. Urol., 141:670, 1989.

Zehntner, C., Casanova, G. A., Marth, D., et al.: Treatment of distal ureteral calculi with extracorporeal shock wave lithotripsy: Experience with 264 cases. Eur. Urol., 16:250, 1989.

Zwergel, T., Neisius, D., Zwergel, U., et al.: Hypertension in patients with extracorporeal lithotripsy of urinary stones: Incidence in first and second generation lithotripter treatment. J. Urol., 141:242A, 1989.

60
PERCUTANEOUS MANAGEMENT

Joseph W. Segura, M.D.

The first percutaneous nephrostomy done for the specific purpose of removing a kidney stone was performed by Fernström and Johannson in 1976. A few years later, Smith and colleagues (1979), at the University of Minnesota, began to remove selected stones in the renal pelvis and ureter through percutaneous nephrostomy tracts. By 1981, Alken and colleagues, in West Germany, and, in 1983, Wickham and colleagues, in the United Kingdom, were removing stones through matured percutaneous tracts. By the early 1980s, it was apparent that it was possible to remove renal stones safely and reliably through acutely dilated percutaneous tracts (Segura et al., 1983). Hospitalizations could now be shortened, and percutaneous stone removal (PL) could become another technique for the removal of surgical stones.

Over the next few years, PL became a standard and preferred procedure for management of a wide variety of surgical stones (Segura et al., 1985; White and Smith, 1984). The nearly concurrent development of shock wave lithotripsy and its acceptance throughout the world after 1984 have considerably reduced the role of PL. Still, PL has maintained its position as an important method for treatment of stones. In this chapter, we review the indications for a percutaneous approach to renal and ureteral calculi and discuss the surgical techniques.

INDICATIONS FOR PERCUTANEOUS STONE REMOVAL

In a wide variety of patients with stones, PL is strikingly successful. Despite its efficacy, the ubiquity of shock wave lithotripsy and its less invasive nature are such that the usual question is whether shock wave treatment should be selected. When the answer to this question is no, some other method should be employed and this is often PL. To address this issue, LeRoy and co-workers (1987) looked at the stones managed by percutaneous lithotripsy at the Mayo Clinic during the first year that shock wave lithotripsy was available (Table 60–1). This review generated insight into the kinds of cases that seem best managed by percutaneous ultrasonic lithotripsy (PL). We were also able to determine the percentage of patients treated by which technique. The data formed part of the input to the National Institutes of Health (NIH) Consensus Conference of 1988, which reflected an emerging agreement as to which patients should receive which method of stone management. Many situations occur in which the patient should

Table 60–1. INDICATIONS FOR PERCUTANEOUS TECHNIQUES IN 143 PATIENTS

	No. (%)
Obstruction	23 (16)
Ureteral, 4	
Ureteropelvic junction, 14	
Infundibular, 5	
Stone volume	66 (46)
Large pelvic stone volume, 17	
Staghorn, 18	
Combined ESWL and percutaneous, 31	
Body habitus	10 (7)
Patient too large, 7	
Patient too small, 1	
Scoliosis, 2	
Other modality failures	21 (15)
Ureteroscopic failures, ureteral stones, 4	
ESWL failures	
Stone did not break, 3	
Retained significant fragments, 12	
Hemorrhage after ESWL, 1	
Hypotension in bath, 1	
Miscellaneous	23 (16)
Cystine, 11	
Cardiac pacemaker, 4	
Calcified renal artery aneurysm, 1	
Indwelling nephrostomy tube, 3	
Patient requested percutaneous removal, 4	

From LeRoy, A. J., Segura, J. W., Williams, H. J., and Patterson, D. E.. Percutaneous renal calculus removal in an extracorporeal shock wave lithotripsy practice. J. Urol., 138:704, 1987. © by Williams & Wilkins, 1992.

be treated by PL. A number of factors bear on this decision. No single "best" method of management of all stones exists. The urologist should recognize which patients are likely to be benefited by which available technique.

Obstructive Uropathy

If an anatomic abnormality is present that will prevent stone fragments from passing spontaneously, shock wave lithotripsy is usually contraindicated. These situations are ideal for PL, inasmuch as the obstructive uropathy can often be corrected after stone removal employing endosurgical procedures (Fig. 60–1). Ureteropelvic junction (UPJ) obstruction may coexist with calculi in the collecting system. Such stones are best removed by percutaneous means because the obstruction can be treated by endopyelotomy, usually at the same time. Occasionally, it may not be obvious that the obstruction is secondary to edema from the stone rather than a primary UPJ obstruction. Sometimes, a jackstone calculus may suggest that the UPJ obstruction is primary rather than secondary.

Caliceal diverticula often contain stones, and their connections to the collecting system are usually such that broken fragments after shock wave lithotripsy will not only remain in the diverticula but the obstructive uropathy will remain untreated. Psihramis and Dretler (1987) reviewed a group of patients whose stone-containing diverticula were treated with shock wave lithotripsy. Although the stone-free rate was only 20 per cent, most of these patients became asymptomatic.

Lingeman and colleagues (1989) treated a similar patient group, but noted that with longer follow-up, symptoms recurred. Management of diverticular stones by PL with enlargement of the connection to the collecting system or obliteration of the diverticulum by electrocoagulation is the usual treatment today.

Previous surgery on the urinary tract generates scar tissue. One should consider whether this scar tissue will compromise stone passage. For example, the scarring from a ureteroneocystostomy or ureteroileal anastomosis may dictate that a PL be performed.

Stone Size

Although it is possible to treat large stones with shock wave lithotripsy, the high retreatment rates and the high residual stone rates make such treatment unattractive (Lingeman et al., 1989). PL is particularly effective with such stones because of its ability to remove large volumes of stoney material over a relatively short period of time. For this reason, if the stone is 3.0 cm or more, PL is preferred. We often use PL for stones in the 2.0 to 3.0 cm range, especially if other factors may compromise the utilization of shock wave lithotripsy.

Staghorn calculi constitute a special problem that has always tested surgical abilities. Most staghorn stones are composed of struvite, although stones composed of uric acid, calcium oxalate monohydrate, and especially cys-

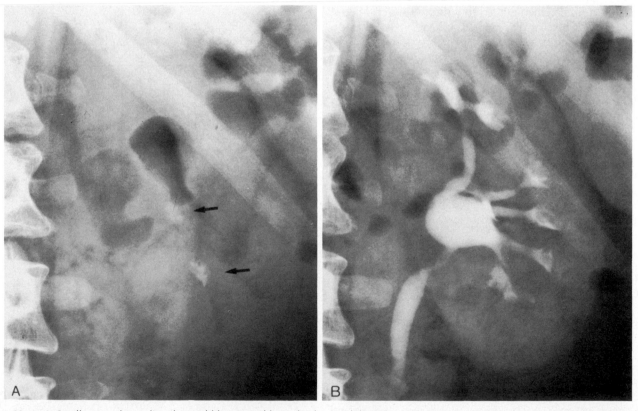

Figure 60–1. *A,* Small stones that ordinarily would be amenable to shock wave lithotripsy. *B,* Notice the ureteropelvic junction (UPJ). The patient clearly has a UPJ obstruction, which may prevent passage of the stones. This patient can be treated at the time of percutaneous stone removal.

tine occasionally fill enough of the collecting system to give it a staghorn appearance. Because most staghorn calculi are composed of struvite, they are infected, and as such no substitute exists for complete removal. This was true when all such stones were treated by open surgical removal, and it is true now. Failure to achieve complete stone removal allows the persistence of infection and the eventual regrowth of the stone.

Although excellent results can be achieved by percutaneous means alone, with stone-free rates of 85 to 90 per cent in experienced hands (Patterson et al., 1987), struvite staghorn stones are usually managed by a so-called combined technique of PL and shock wave lithotripsy (Fig. 60–2). This procedure takes advantage of the virtues of PL—rapid removal of large volumes of accessible stones and the ability of shock wave lithotripsy to treat small residual stones—in cases in which percutaneous access could be difficult or dangerous. Because experience has shown that passage of these now fragmented stones is inconsistent, they must be removed through a second percutaneous maneuver, usually through the same tract. Stone-free rates after combined treatment are no better than those after PL alone, but there is little question that this use of shock wave lithotripsy greatly simplifies the second endoscopic procedure.

It is a matter of clinical judgment as to whether a given staghorn calculus should be managed as discussed here or with nephrolithotomy. The need for multiple access tracts or the large size of the stone may mean that open surgery is the only practical way to remove the stone.

Anatomic Abnormalities

Some patients are so large or so constructed that shock wave lithotripsy is impossible because the stone

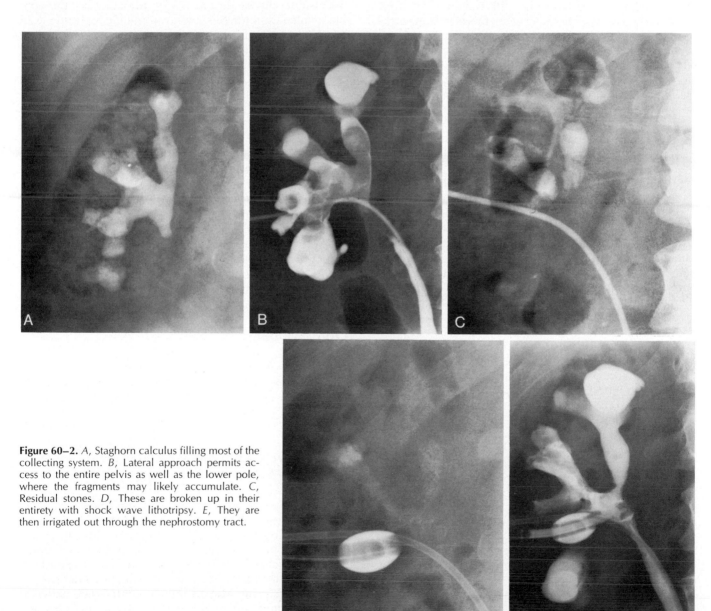

Figure 60–2. *A,* Staghorn calculus filling most of the collecting system. *B,* Lateral approach permits access to the entire pelvis as well as the lower pole, where the fragments may likely accumulate. *C,* Residual stones. *D,* These are broken up in their entirety with shock wave lithotripsy. *E,* They are then irrigated out through the nephrostomy tract.

cannot be placed in the focal point of the machine. Percutaneous removal will be possible if the distance from the skin to the stone is less than the length of the nephroscope or the sheath. Even then, it may be possible to remove the stone if the tract is matured and a flexible nephroscope employed. Sometimes, stones in these patients can be removed ureteroscopically. The flexible instrument with electrohydraulic lithotripsy is used to break up the stone, if it is not too large.

Stone Location

Stones located in the lower pole calyces are less likely to pass after shock wave breakup, particularly if the collecting system is grossly dilated or otherwise abnormal. If it is important that all fragments be removed, PL is probably preferable.

The accepted treatment for upper and mid-ureteral stones is shock wave lithotripsy. PL is chosen for stones in these locations generally when there is some other reason for PL. If necessary, a stone anywhere in the ureter can be removed after percutaneous access (Fig. 60–3). This point should be remembered when ureteral stones fragment after shock wave lithotripsy but do not pass and when occasional lower ureteral stones cannot be managed with ureteroscopy.

Stone Composition

Struvite stones should be treated with PL in order to be sure that all the fragments are removed. Stone composition is otherwise an important consideration due to the fact that hard stones will frequently not fragment into pieces small enough for spontaneous passage with minimal discomfort. This same hard stone may be equally difficult to remove with power lithotripsy after percutaneous access, but it will be possible to remove the pieces via PL, irrespective of how difficult it was to break up the stone.

The commonest hard renal stones are composed of calcium oxalate monohydrate. As these stones become larger, the more likely it is that multiple shock wave lithotripsy treatments or other instrumentation may be necessary. One should consider that it may be more cost-effective and actually less morbid to remove these stones with PL.

Brushite stones fragment poorly after shock wave lithotripsy. If these stones can be recognized prior to treatment, they should be managed by PL. These will appear rather dense on plain films, but the best indication of a brushite stone may be a history of passage or surgical removal of such a stone.

No group of patients benefits more from the nonsurgical removal of stones than those with cystine nephrolithiasis. These patients have often had multiple surgical procedures and despite medical treatment are likely to have surgical stones later in life.

These stones are not suited for shock wave lithotripsy, as they break up poorly. Many of them are so large that multiple shock wave lithotripsy treatments would be necessary even if they did respond. Ultrasonic lithotripsy is ideally suited to the management of patients with these stones, as large volumes of broken-up cystine stone can be readily removed. Some cystine stones respond to ultrasonic lithotripsy better than others. Although the reason is not clear, it may lie in the type of cystine stone. Bhatta and co-workers (1989) have identified two types of cystine crystal—rough and smooth. The rough variety seems to fragment easier than the smooth, which may be the explanation.

Knoll and associates (1988) reviewed a series of patients we had treated with PL for cystine nephrolithiasis. These 12 patients (13 kidneys) had a mean follow-up of nearly 2 years. Almost half had residual stones when they were discharged from the hospital. Attempts to clean out the kidney were not complete after the bulk of the material and the obstructive portion of the stone were removed, on the theory that medical treatment would now be practical. Few of these cases had dissolved the residual stones, despite appropriate medical therapy. The explanation for this finding is not clear. It may well be simply lack of compliance, but it may also be that these patients represent a particular metabolic subset, selected by their lack of response to the usual treatment. The corollary is that one cannot depend on medical treatment to clear the kidney. If the patient is to be free of stone, he or she will have to be made so at the time of PL.

Certainty of the Final Result

Residual stones are not acceptable for many patients. The most common example is the commercial airline pilot. However, many people find themselves considerably inconvenienced, for whatever reason, by the uncertainty as to whether a small fragment might pass. The very high stone-free rate after PL makes this method an ideal choice for such people.

Other Modality Failure

As mentioned, shock wave lithotripsy may fail or ureteroscopy may fail. Equally, stones may remain after an open surgical procedure. PL may retrieve these otherwise lost procedures.

TECHNIQUE OF PERCUTANEOUS STONE REMOVAL

The procedure may be divided into two parts: (1) access into the collecting system and (2) removal of the stone. Exactly how these two different procedures are done, their timing in relation to each other, and which surgical specialist performs which are not particularly germane to the outcome. The following procedures have worked well at the Mayo Clinic in nearly 2000 patients. Other common alternative methods are described when appropriate.

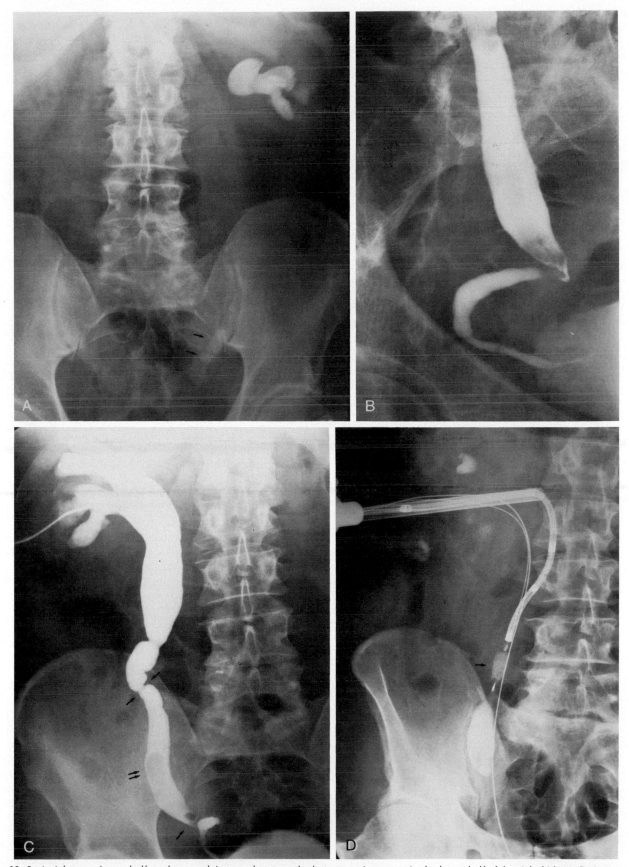

Figure 60–3. *A,* A large volume, half staghorn, calcium oxalate monohydrate stone is present in the lower half of the right kidney (Patient supine.). Stones are also in the ureter overlying the vessels. *B,* Marked angulation of the ureters is secondary to previous surgery. (Patient prone.) *C,* The renal stone is removed by percutaneous ultrasonic lithotripsy. (Patient prone.) *D,* The stone in the ureter engaged in the basket, and the large volume stone is destroyed with the electrohydraulic probe. (Patient prone.)

Access

The excretory urogram or retrograde pyelogram should be reviewed to determine the relationship of the stone to the collecting system and to determine the optimum access tract. If the goal is a caliceal stone or a diverticular stone, access should be through that particular calyx or diverticulum (Fig. 60–4). Otherwise, optimum access is generally through a lateral calyx, as this maneuver will enable a large amount of pelvic stone material to be removed and still permit access to the UPJ. An approach through the upper pole often assures access to the pelvis and UPJ, but the risk of pleural injury is significantly increased. If an optimum approach necessitates access above the 12th rib, one should proceed without hesitation. We have utilized a surpacostal approach in some 8 per cent of our patients without significant difficulty (see subsequent discussion).

The urogram should also be reviewed for gross renal abnormalities, as well as abnormalities of other organs that may compromise the procedure. Although PL is theoretically possible in any patient, in practice some anatomic abnormalities make PL impossible or unsafe. The retroperitoneal location of the kidney permits access through a posterolateral "window" (Fig. 60–5). Gross enlargement of the spleen, liver, or colon may be such that this window is closed so that safe access is not possible. Access should be performed under fluoroscopic or ultrasonic control. Fluoroscopic control is usual in the United States, and ultrasonic, more common in

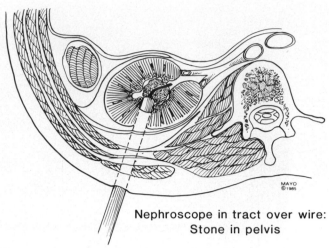

Nephroscope in tract over wire:
Stone in pelvis

Figure 60–5. Access is through a "window" in the posterior lateral flank. The nephroscope appears through a posterior calyx.

Europe. In our institution, this procedure is done using intravenous sedation and local anesthesia in the department of radiology.

The details of percutaneous access have been described elsewhere (LeRoy et al., 1984). Briefly, a Cope introducer system is most commonly employed. A 22-gauge needle is placed through the flank into the kidney at the point where access is desired. A small guide wire is passed through the needle, the tract enlarged, and the wire exchanged for larger wires until a .035 or .038 Linderquist-Ring (LR) torque wire is in the collecting system. It is very desirable that this wire be placed down the ureter as far as the pelvic ureter in order to minimize the possibility of inadvertent loss of the tract.

The patient is moved to the operating room, where the tract is dilated using general anesthesia. Dilatation proceeds under fluoroscopic control to 24 Fr., the size of the nephroscope we most commonly employ (Fig. 60–6). If an Amplatz sheath is used, dilatation should continue to 30 Fr. in order that the lumen of the sheath can accommodate the nephroscope.

Stone Removal

Small stones can be removed intact with forceps or basket. More commonly, some form of power lithotripsy is required to break the stone into manageable fragments. In general, we prefer ultrasonic lithotripsy for this purpose, because the pieces are removed as they are broken up. The action of the probe is that of a "jackhammer," battering the stone into progressively smaller pieces. The harder the stone, the more difficult this will be to do. Indeed, stones that are hard, as well as large, may require so much time to fragment that some other method of power lithotripsy is necessary. The electrohydraulic probe is the best choice. The 9 Fr. or the 5 Fr. probe will break pieces off the large stone, which can then be effectively attacked with the ultrasonic probe. Stone removal continues until the patient is free of stone or until it is necessary to stop the

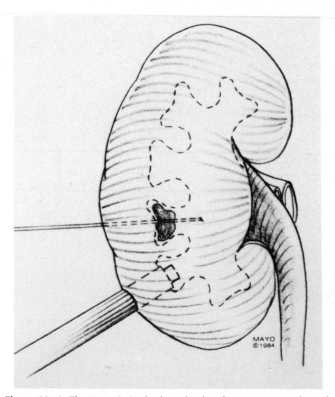

Figure 60–4. The stone is in the lateral calyx, but access was through the lower pole. This access will generate considerable difficulties, which could have been avoided by access through the calyx that contains the stone.

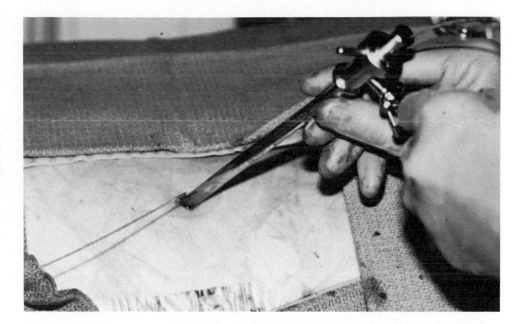

Figure 60–6. The 24 Fr. nephroscope is passed over a working wire. Note the second reserve or safety wire. This always remains in place to ensure safe access should the original tract be lost.

procedure. Common reasons for this include progressive bleeding which obscures the surgeon's vision so that the rate of stone removal is considerably slowed, and extravasation of irrigating fluid (see following discussion).

If the patient is not free of stone at the termination of the procedure, the nephroscope can safely be reinserted through the same tract after 48 hours. At this point, the tract is matured and bleeding has almost always stopped, so that removal of residual fragments is usually straightforward. As the size of the stones and complexity of these situations increase, the odds rise considerably that a second and occasionally a third treatment will be required.

At the end of the procedure, a straight catheter is left down the ureter and a nephrostomy tube is placed through the tract into the collecting system. My preference is a 22 Fr. Foley catheter with 2 to 3 ml of fluid in the balloon. Some have preferred smaller tubes, but this is large enough to maintain an adequate tract and permits blood and clots to drain readily. After 48 hours, a nephrostogram is obtained. If there are no leaks, the stent is removed and the nephrostomy tube clamped. If the patient tolerates this procedure, the tube is removed and the patient is discharged from the hospital. The drainage site will usually close within 24 hours. Time of disability varies; most patients return to average activity levels within a week or so. A return to vigorous activity should probably take place in another week.

RESULTS

The advent of shock wave lithotripsy has changed the definition of what constitutes a successful result. Considerable discussion has occurred about "clinically insignificant residual fragments" ("CIRF"), referring to broken up fragments of various sizes and their propensity for spontaneous passage. Because of a lack of unanimity as to the precise definition of CIRF, a consensus has emerged that the only true definition of success is a stone-free state. This point is an important consideration in measuring the effectiveness of PL against other methods of stone management.

If results are restricted to the best selected patients, i.e., those with the least difficult stones to access, stone-free rates of 98 to 99 per cent can be achieved (Brannen et al., 1985; Lingeman et al., 1989; Segura et al., 1985; White and Smith, 1984). As the size of the stone increases, and as the complexity of the situation increases, the stone-free rate drops to 75 to 80 per cent. Better results are achievable with greater effort, and it becomes a matter of judgment as to whether a given residual stone is worth the effort required to remove it.

COMPLICATIONS OF PERCUTANEOUS STONE REMOVAL

As with any other surgical procedure, problems may complicate any aspect of the percutaneous stone removal. One may conveniently divide events into three groups: (1) complications related to access, (2) complications related to tract dilatation, and (3) complications related to stone removal.

Complications Related to Access

The ultimate success of the procedure is a function of adequate access. Poor tract placement may make safe, expeditious stone removal an impossibility. Prudence dictates that a suboptimal access point should be changed prior to dilatation and lithotripsy.

The retroperitoneal position of the kidney permits access through a percutaneous window that enables entry into the kidney without trauma to adjacent peritoneal structures. Pathologic states and variations in normal anatomy may result in situations in which damage to adjacent organs can occur.

Spleen

Inadvertent perforation or damage to the spleen is unlikely in the average situation, but if splenomegaly is present to any degree, damage is possible. An enlarged spleen is often apparent on an abdominal plain film. Doubtful situations may be clarified by computed tomography (CT) scan.

Pleura

Whether injury to the pleura will ensue depends on a variety of factors. The kidney may be positioned more cephalad than usual. The pleural cavity may extend more inferiorly and posteriorly than average. The risk of injury is also a function of the frequency of upper pole approaches to the collecting system and whether or not the approach was above the 12th rib.

Most of the time, if access is below the 12th rib and if the kidney is in normal position, it is unlikely that the pleura will be injured. We have had only one proven case, but it seems likely that other, asymptomatic cases have occurred. In this case, there was a 15 per cent pneumothorax and a chest tube was not required. A patient managed elsewhere had a hematothorax, which necessitated a chest tube. Certainly a chest tube should be placed in any doubtful situation (Lange, personal communication, 1984).

Colon

In our experience, two patients have had an inadvertent injury to the colon (LeRoy et al., 1985). The close proximity of the colon to the kidney, the normal anatomic variations, and the occasional patient with pathologic enlargement of the colon make this a rare, but inevitable, event (Fig. 60–7).

Inspection of the abdominal plain film may identify the enlarged colon of the patient who may be at additional risk. Those who have undergone intestinal bypass procedures for morbid obesity appear to be prone to colonomegaly, apparently because of the larger volumes of stool and fluid passing through the colon.

In both of our cases, the colon was nicked. Contrast material clearly entered the colon, but no significant extraperitoneal or intraperitoneal extravasation of colonic contents occurred. The patients were managed by inserting a double-J stent into the collecting system to provide internal drainage of the kidney and by positioning the nephrostomy tube such that the colon was drained. This situation was continued for a week until contrast material placed through the "colostomy" tube no longer entered the renal collecting system. The colostomy tract had epithelialized and quickly closed over after the tube was removed. Vallancien and colleagues (1985) reported a case of more significant injury, which required open surgical repair.

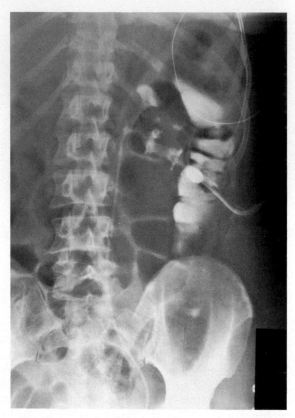

Figure 60–7. The colon was nicked at the time of percutaneous access, but virtually all of the stone was removed. The nephrostomy tube has been moved back into the colon to form a "colostomy" tube. Internal drainage of the urinary collecting system is affected by a double-J stent. After several days of drainage, the two areas seal off and the colocutaneous tract closes with removal of the stent.

Such cases are rare, and the risk seemingly difficult to predict. Situations in which this risk may be higher should be clarified with CT scanning.

Kidney

Optimum access traverses the bulk of the "meat" of the kidney to enter the collecting system through one of the calyces. Placement of the tract in a line too medial or too lateral may tear the parenchyma (Fig. 60–8). The pedicle or other large branch vessels may be injured if the access tract enters the collecting system medial to the calyces or if the tract exits the collecting system inadvertently. Proper placement of the tract through the calyx and infundibulum and into the renal pelvis minimizes the risk of such injury.

Despite these efforts, significant bleeding may occur during access and dilatation of the tract. This blood is most often venous and usually stops with tamponade from the dilators and from the nephrostomy tube itself. Arterial injury has occurred in some 0.5 per cent of our patients (Patterson et al., 1985). Why this happens is not clear but is probably a product of access too near a susceptible vessel coupled with the effects of dilatation and efforts to remove stone. Variations in the anatomy of the kidney together with limitations inherent in access

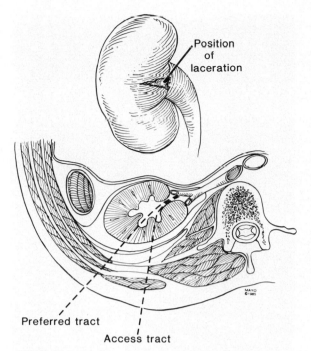

Figure 60–8. Tract placement was too lateral in this situation, which resulted in tearing of the thin renal parenchyma. Otherwise, the access was satisfactory. Although this patient was treated surgically, maturation of the tract and subsequent lithotripsy might have provided similar management results.

methods ensure that arterial injury will always be a real, if still rare, complication.

Sepsis

Many patients experience a rise in temperature after stone removal, although true sepsis is rare. Preoperative urine culture results will identify the patient who should be treated prior to the procedure. Special attention should be paid to those patients with infected stones. It also has been our practice to provide prophylactic antibiotics, usually a cephalosporin for these patients.

Complications Related to Tract Dilatation

The shorter the tract, the less difficult it is to dilate. As the tract lengthens, the guide wire is more likely to buckle, increasing the risk of being unable to complete dilatation. In obese patients, the kidney may be mobile enough that the dilators simply push the kidney away.

The dilators should usually be placed no further than the stone itself. The reason for this is that more aggressive dilatation could generate a perforation of the collecting system. Where the stone fills the entire pelvis, there may not be enough room for the stone and the dilator.

Rarely, some event may suggest that the procedure should be stopped at this point. After 48 to 72 hours of nephrostomy tube drainage, bleeding will have stopped

and the tract will be well epithelialized, permitting uncomplicated stone removal.

Complications Related to Stone Removal

Problems at the time of stone removal may be summarized as those related to bleeding, extravasation, inadvertent perforation of the collecting system, and incomplete stone removal.

Bleeding

Although a certain amount of bleeding occurs all throughout the procedure, significant blood loss may complicate the situation at any time. The most common type of bleeding is venous, which may be compared with the sinus bleeding that occurs with transurethral resection of the prostate. That this is the source of the bleeding is suggested by clearing of the field with irrigation fluid, but marked quantities of venous blood when the irrigation fluid is turned off. This finding usually also means intravascular extravasation is occurring and may be a reason to terminate the procedure (see subsequent discussion). This venous blood will flow through the nephrostomy tube in quantities that seem alarming. We have managed these problems by clamping the nephrostomy tube for 30 to 45 minutes (Fig. 60–9). This step allows a clot to form in the collecting system, tamponading the bleeding. Mannitol is given, and the tube is then opened. We have done this many times successfully without short-term or long-term complications.

Arterial bleeding is a more serious problem. This

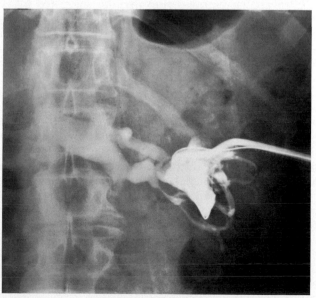

Figure 60–9. Contrast medium injected through the nephrostomy tube enters the venous system. This is managed by clamping the nephrostomy tube for 30 to 45 minutes, giving a diuretic, and then unclamping the tube.

bleeding may occur as an acute event at the time of lithotripsy but also may occur in the postoperative period up to a week or 10 days. The rapidity of blood loss, its red arterial character, and its lack of response to tamponade suggest injury to a significant vessel.

Arteriography should be performed immediately. This will confirm the diagnosis, usually revealing a pseudoaneurysm, but arteriography will also permit treatment of the problem by embolization of the offending artery. Surgery should be avoided if possible. Nephrectomy or partial nephrectomy may be the only alternative because of the emergent character of the situation. The incidence of this problem in our practice has been about 0.5 per cent. Most large series report an incidence of less than 1 per cent.

Our cases have been reviewed in detail by Patterson and associates (1985). Trauma was obviously a factor in some, but in others no untoward precipitating factor was apparent. The exact risk is unknown, because subclinical cases may have resolved spontaneously.

Extravasation

Normal saline should be used as the irrigation fluid to minimize adverse effects when extravasation occurs. Because we use the nephroscope sheath to tamponade the tract into the kidney, the irrigation fluid must pass out the suction lines attached to the nephroscope or flow down the ureter into the bladder and out the Foley catheter. When an Amplatz sheath is employed, most of the irrigation fluid travels out the sheath, rendering extravasation less likely. Despite the technical details, the operating personnel should monitor the quantity of irrigation fluid used and compare this amount with the quantity in various collecting bags. Discrepancies that cannot be accounted for should suggest the possibility of extravasation.

Intravascular extravasation may be suggested by venous bleeding (see previous discussion) and confirmed by injection of contrast medium (see Fig. 60–9). This finding usually means the procedure must be terminated for the day, otherwise large quantities of irrigation fluid will be rapidly absorbed.

Retroperitoneal extravasation is inevitable if the collecting system has been perforated (Fig. 60–10). If the perforation was identified when it was made, it may be possible to complete the procedure by rigorously controlling the amount of irrigation (Fig. 60–11). Sometimes, retroperitoneal extravasation may not be obvious unless it is noted that the kidney seems to be moving "away" from the flank and that the nephroscope must be placed farther in to access the stone. What constitutes significant extravasation will depend on the patient's general medical situation. Most adults in otherwise good health can absorb 1000 ml of normal saline without difficulty. For adults with borderline cardiac status or for small children, this might be a dangerous amount.

Intraperitoneal extravasation is rare. Two such patients were managed with diuretics and observation of electrolytes; Carson and Nesbitt (1985) managed two such patients with peritoneal taps.

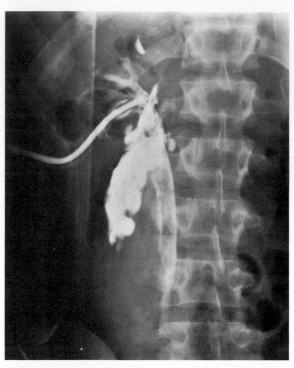

Figure 60–10. At least 2 L of fluid have been extravasated in the retroperitoneum. The defect in the pelvis and the retroperitoneal extravasation eventually resolved after several days of nephrostomy tube drainage, with no sequelae.

Retained Fragments

As in any method of stone management, the presence of residual fragments on a post-procedure plain film can be an unwanted finding. Reinsertion of the nephroscope through the tract, kept open by the nephrostomy tube, will permit removal of the stone fragments. One may decide that the effort necessary to remove these stones is not justified by the clinical situation. If a fragment large enough to obstruct the ureter should pass in the immediate post-procedure period, the tract may not close after the nephrostomy tube is removed.

Sometimes stones are extruded through the collecting system or are noted in the perinephric tissues outside the kidney. It has been our practice not to remove these stones, as experience has shown them to be clinically unimportant. Their main import has been to generate confusion on subsequent plain abdominal radiographs.

Long-Term Complications

The exact incidence of long-term complication is not known. We have not studied this factor in a systematic manner, but we have noted very few problems that seemingly could be related to the percutaneous procedure. Two patients developed mild UPJ obstructions not present previously that did not require treatment. In some patients who have required multiple procedures, there is difficulty dilating the tract, suggestive of the scar tissue present after an open operation. Marberger and associates (1984) studied 82 patients, followed

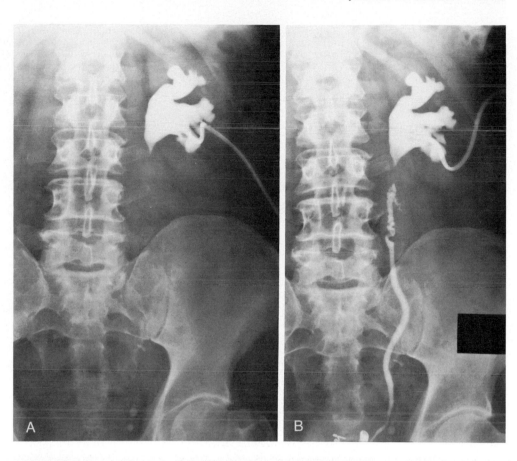

Figure 60–11. *A,* Nephrostogram after a percutaneous stone was removed shows no extravasation or contrast material below the ureteropelvic junction (UPJ). The patient experienced pain with clamping. *B,* Retrograde pyelogram revealed the ureter to be separated from the UPJ. This was repaired successfully 3 months later.

for up to 4 years after PL, and noted no abnormality or untoward result.

SUMMARY

Percutaneous surgery is an effective and safe method for the management of a wide variety of renal and ureteral stones. Today, it is selected mainly in certain specific situations in which the result justifies its invasive nature. Recognition of which patient can benefit from the procedure minimizes the number of other less successful attempts at stone removal and optimizes the chance that the problem will be managed safely, expeditiously, and economically.

REFERENCES

Alken, P., Hutschrenreiter, G., Günther, R., and Marberger, M.: Percutaneous stone manipulation. J. Urol., 125:463, 1981.

Bhatta, K. M., Prien, E. L., Jr., and Dretler, S. P.: Cystine calculi rough and smooth: a new clinical distinction. J. Urol., 142:937, 1989.

Brannen, G. E., Bush, W. H., Correa, R. J., Gibbons, R. P., and Elder, J. S.: Kidney stone removal: percutaneous versus surgical lithotomy. J. Urol., 133:6, 1985.

Carson, C. C., and Nesbitt, J. A.: Peritoneal extravasation during percutaneous lithotripsy. J. Urol., 134:725, 1985.

Fernström, I., and Johannson, B.: Percutaneous pyelolithotomy. A new extraction technique. Scand. J. Urol. Nephrol., 10:257, 1976.

Knoll, L. D., Segura, J. W., Patterson, D. E., LeRoy, A. J., and Smith, L. H.: Long-term follow-up in patients with cystine urinary calculi treated by percutaneous ultrasonic lithotripsy. J. Urol., 140.246, 1988.

Lange, P.: University of Minnesota, personal communication, 1984.

LeRoy, A. J., May, G. R., Bender, C. E., Williams, H. J., Jr., McGough, P. F., and Patterson, D. E.: Percutaneous nephrostomy for stone removal. Radiology, 151:607, 1984.

LeRoy, A. J., Segura, J. W., Williams, H. J., and Patterson, D. E.: Percutaneous renal calculus removal in an extracorporeal shock wave lithotripsy practice. J. Urol., 138:703, 1987.

LeRoy, A. J., Williams, H. J., Jr., Segura, J. W., Patterson, D. E., and Benson, R. C.: Colon perforation following percutaneous nephrostomy and renal calculus removal. Radiology, 155:83–85, 1985.

Lingeman, J. E., Jones, J. A., and Steidel, C. P.: ESWL vs. percutaneous management of calyceal diverticula. Presented at the 64th Annual Meeting of North Central Section AUA, Colorado Springs, October 27, 1990.

Lingeman, J. E., Smith, L. H., Woods, J. R., and Newman, D. M.: Urinary Calculi-ESWL, Endourology, and Medical Therapy. Philadelphia, Lea and Febiger, 1989.

Marberger, M., Stackl, W., Hruby, W., et al.: Late sequelae of ultrasonic lithotripsy of renal calculi. J. Urol., 133:170, 1984.

National Institutes of Health Consensus Conference. J. Urol., March, 1989.

Patterson, D. E., Segura, J. W., and LeRoy, A. J.: Long-term follow-up of patients treated by percutaneous ultrasonic lithotripsy for struvite staghorn calculi. J. Endourol., 1:777, 1987.

Patterson, D. E., Segura, J. W., LeRoy, A. J., et al.: The etiology and treatment of delayed bleeding following percutaneous lithotripsy. J. Urol., 133:447, 1985.

Psihramis, K. E., and Dretler, S. P.: Extracorporeal shock wave lithotripsy of calyceal diverticular calculi. J. Urol., 138:707–711, 1987.

Reddy, P. K., Hulbert, J. C., Lange, P. H., Clayman, R. V., Marcuzzi, A., Lapointe, S., Miller, R. P., Hunter, D. W., Castaneda-Zuniga, W. R., and Amplatz, K.: Percutaneous removal of renal and ureteral calculi: experience with 400 cases. J. Urol., 134:662, 1985.

Segura, J. W., Patterson, D. E., LeRoy, A. J., May, G. R., and Smith, L. H.: Percutaneous lithotripsy. J. Urol., 130:1051, 1983.

Segura, J. W., Patterson, D. E., LeRoy, A. J., Williams, H. J., Jr., Barrett, D. M., Benson, R. C., Jr., May, G. R., and Bender, C. E.: Percutaneous removal of kidney stones: review of 1000 cases. J. Urol., 134:1077, 1985.

Smith, A. D., Reinke, D. B., Miller, R. P., and Lange, P. H.: Percutaneous nephrostomy in the management of ureteral and renal calculi. Radiology, 133:49, 1979.

Vallancien, G., Capdeville, R., Veillon, B., Charton, M., and Brisset, J. M.: Colonic perforation during percutaneous nephrolithotomy: case report. J. Urol., 134:1185, 1985.

White, E. C., and Smith, A. D.: Percutaneous stone extraction from 200 patients. J. Urol., 132:437, 1984.

Wickham, J. E. A., Kellet, M. J., and Miller, R. A.: Elective percutaneous nephrolithotomy in 50 patients in an analysis of the technique results in complications. J. Urol., 129:904, 1983.

61
URETEROSCOPY

Jeffry L. Huffman, M.D.

The trend in medicine has been toward nonoperative or "minimally invasive" surgical procedures. This trend has been very apparent in orthopedics, otolaryngology, and urology. Often, minimally invasive endoscopic procedures replace surgical procedures. As part of this trend toward nonoperative therapy, there has been a steady increase in the number of endoscopic procedures performed within the upper urinary tract, including transurethral ureteroscopy, percutaneous nephroscopy, and antegrade ureteroscopy. This chapter discusses transurethral ureteroscopy and nephroscopy—employing both rigid and flexible instrumentation.

Ureteroscopy is an extension of cystoscopic techniques and involves similar indications. The main differences are related to the anatomy of the ureter and kidney compared with the lower tract, the smaller size of instrumentation, and the narrower safety margin for the prevention of complications.

The following major components of transurethral ureteroscopy that have contributed most to the success and safety of this procedure are discussed thoroughly in this chapter.

- An understanding of upper urinary tract anatomy as it is related to endoscopy of the ureter and kidney.
- A clarification of the indications for rigid and flexible ureteroscopy is presented. This subject is changing constantly relative to stone disease treatment, as more noninvasive shock wave lithotripsy devices are introduced.
- Rigid and flexible instruments continue to be improved and refined. Miniaturization of instruments and accessory devices has been a major step toward making the procedure more successful and safer.
- Less traumatic methods of ureteral dilation are available. Initial methods employed only nonguided bougies—modern methods employ pre-placed guide wires and balloon dilating catheters passed in a coaxial fashion over the wires.
- Methods of intraureteral lithotripsy have improved. Initially only ultrasonic lithotripsy probes were utilized routinely. Now, electrohydraulic probes and laser fibers are available.

- Recognition and management of complications have improved. Based on the experience of early investigators, most major complications can be prevented or at least recognized so that conservative treatment is still possible.

ANATOMY FOR TRANSURETHRAL URETEROSCOPY AND NEPHROSCOPY

A thorough knowledge of the anatomy of the kidney, intrarenal collecting system, and ureter enhances both the safety and success of ureteroscopic procedures. Although anatomic configuration and location of the ureter and renal pelvis vary from one patient to the next, certain endoscopic landmarks remain constant. Similar to the recognition of the bulbus urethra, verumontanum, bladder neck, and trigone in the lower urinary tract, the endoscopist must recognize the ureteral vesical junction, the pelvic brim, the ureteral pelvic junction, and the individual infundibula within the renal pelvis.

This section reviews the gross and microscopic anatomy of the kidney and ureter. A description of the endoscopic anatomy is also presented with an emphasis on the clinical correlation between anatomy of the collecting system and potential hazards encountered during endoscopic procedures performed in the ureter and kidney.

ANATOMIC RELATIONSHIPS OF THE KIDNEY

The right and left kidneys are retroperitoneal organs situated on either side of the vertebral column between the 12th thoracic vertebrae and the third lumbar vertebra (Bulger, 1983; Gray, 1973; Markee, 1966). The right kidney is slightly more caudal than the left, with its renal hilus being directly posterior to the descending portion of the duodenum. The right lobe of the liver covers the bulk of its anterior surface, and the hepatic flexure of the colon lies directly anterior to the lower pole. The upper pole of the right kidney is in direct contact with the adrenal gland.

Immediately anterior to the renal pelvis is the renal vein, which drains into the inferior vena cava medially, and the renal artery. Posteriorly, the kidney is in contact with the psoas quadratus lumborum and transversus abdominis muscles, from medial to lateral. The diaphragm and the 12th rib overlie the upper pole of the kidney posteriorly. The left kidney has somewhat different relationships. Posteriorly, the same muscles are encountered as for the right kidney. The diaphragm and the 12th rib overlie the upper pole. Anteriorly, the tail of the pancreas extends across the renal hilus and the inferior tip of the spleen covers its anterior border. The proximal jejunum and the splenic flexure of the colon extend across the lower pole of the left kidney anteriorly. The greater curvature of the stomach overlies the left upper pole and adrenal gland.

ANATOMIC RELATIONSHIPS OF THE URETER (Figure 61–1)

The ureter is an entirely retroperitoneal structure extending from the renal pelvis to the bladder. The ureter varies in length from 28 to 34 cm, with the right being about 1 cm shorter than the left (Davis, 1981). The abdominal portion of the ureter begins superiorly at the ureteral pelvic junction, where it is covered by the descending duodenum on the right and the beginning portion of the jejunum on the left. As the ureter courses inferiorly from the renal pelvis, it lies lateral to the inferior vena cava and anterior to the psoas major muscle and the genitofemoral nerve. The ureter then courses slightly, medially to cross the ventral surface of the transverse processes of the third to fifth lumbar vertebral bodies. It then crosses the bifurcation of the common iliac artery at the hypogastric artery. Near this

level it lies directly posterior to the right colic and ileocolic blood vessels and the terminal ileum on the right and the left colic vessels and the line of attachment of the sigmoid mesocolon on the left.

The pelvic portion of the ureter begins as it crosses the bifurcation of the common iliac vessels and enters the true pelvis. As it courses inferiorly, it lies ventral to the hypogastric artery and medial to the obturator nerve and artery. This portion of the ureter then runs slightly, laterally and posteriorly, along the lateral pelvic wall to the region of ischial spine. At this level the ureter bends medially and anteriorly to reach the bladder at the ureterovesical junction.

The ureterovesical junction is the narrowest portion of the ureter and corresponds to the entrance of the ureter through the detrusor hiatus in the bladder wall musculature. At this level, the ureters are approximately 5 cm apart. As the intramural ureter exits this muscular hiatus, it courses submucosally to approximately 2 cm within the bladder and ends at the ureteral orifice. This anatomic configuration of the submucosal ureter is thought to allow it to preserve its antireflux mechanism.

HISTOLOGIC STRUCTURE OF THE RENAL PELVIS AND URETER

The renal pelvis and ureter are thin-walled structures (1 to 2 mm when distended) composed of three layers: fibrous, muscular, and mucosal (Figs. 61–2 and 61–3) (Verlando, 1981). The outermost layer is the fibrous layer or tunica adventitia. This is a continuous fiber structure that runs from the renal sinus along the ureter and inserts into the fibrous coat of the bladder. The most distal aspect of this layer, as it inserts into the bladder, contains a specialized group of muscle fibers and fibrous tissue known as Waldeyer's sheath. Nerve fibers, lymphatics, and blood vessels are also contained in the tunica adventitia, which is joined externally by adipose tissue that surrounds the ureter.

The middle portion is the muscular layer or tunica

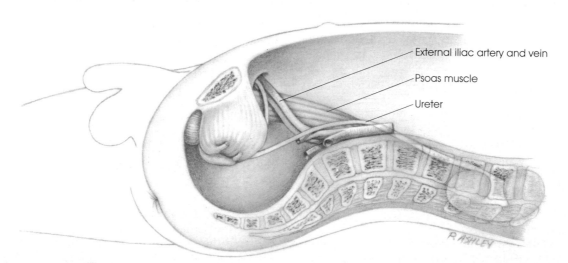

Figure 61–1. Lateral view of the bladder, ureter, and kidney. (From Huffman, J., Bagley, D., and Lyon, E. (Eds.): Ureteroscopy. Philadelphia, W. B. Saunders Co., 1988.)

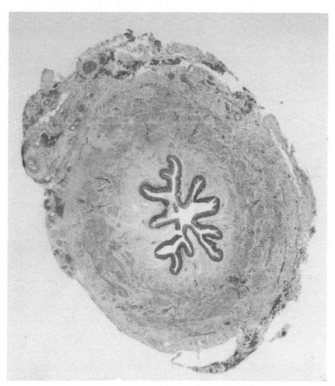

Figure 61–2. Histologic cross-section of normal mid-ureter (× 10).

muscularis. It consists of two poorly defined, thin layers in the renal pelvis and proximal ureter—the inner circular and outer longitudinal. Most often, these layers are indistinct and are found in small bundles, running in oblique directions separated by large amounts of connective tissue. Three distinct muscle layers are in the middle and distal ureter: inner longitudinal, middle circular, and outer longitudinal fibers. The inner longitudinal fibers are more developed near the bladder, and the circular fibers decrease in size at this level. Within the intramural ureter, the longitudinal muscle fibers also decrease in number and size as the ureteral orifice is approached.

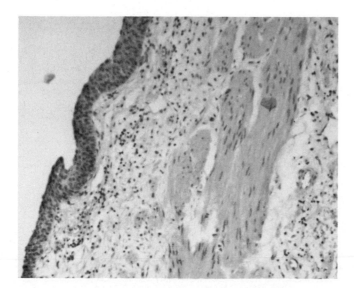

Figure 61–3. Histologic cross-section of normal renal pelvis (× 100).

In the submucosal ureter, there is only a semicircle of longitudinal fibers around the lateral aspect of the ureter with the medial portion having few muscle fibers at this level. This configuration helps to illustrate why great care must be taken in passing any instrument through this area when dilating the intramural tunnel. Perforation or submucosal false passages occur more easily at this level partly because of the sparse muscular coating.

The innermost lining of the ureter and renal pelvis is the mucosal layer. The anatomic features of this layer give rise to one of the unique properties of the ureter and pelvis: the ability to stretch and distend without rupturing. This layer consists of epithelium formed by transitional cells and subepithelium (lamina propria) formed by connective tissue. The epithelium becomes thicker in the distal ureter compared with that found in the minor calyces. The epithelium is approximately two cell layers thick in the calyces and becomes about five or six cell layers thick in the distal ureter near the bladder. The lamina propria contains dense collagenous tissue with many elastic fibers and is continuous with the renal interstitial tissue. The mucosal layer also contains many longitudinal folds or rugae. These give the nondistended or contracted ureter its characteristic star-shaped appearance when viewed endoscopically.

ENDOSCOPIC ANATOMY OF THE INTRARENAL COLLECTING SYSTEM

As urine is drained through the collecting ducts within the renal pyramids, it exits into the minor calyces via the renal papillae. The papillae form the apex of the renal pyramids and vary in number from four to 12 depending on the individual. Endoscopically, a papilla appears as a rounded cone with a pink, easily friable epithelium (Huffman et al., 1985a). The cupped minor calyx, surrounding each papilla, is called the calyceal fornix. Occasionally, more than one papilla may project into a minor calyx. These compound calyces occur more commonly in the upper pole. In a nondistended calyx, the papillae are very distinct and polypoid in nature. When the calyx is distended or appears "clubbed" radiographically, the papillae are less distinct and may be totally flattened.

The four to 13 minor calyces coalesce at their apices and empty into two or three major calyces, which drain directly into the renal pelvis. Endoscopically, upon entering the renal pelvis from the transureteral route, the bases of the major calyces leading to the upper, middle, and lower pole of the kidney are the first structures visible. They appear as cylindric openings branching from the pelvis. Often minor calyces are visible in the background. The tubular portion or infundibulum connects the apex to the base of each major calyx.

Separating the major calyces as they branch from the renal pelvis are carinae. Anatomically, these are similar in appearance to the branching of the trachea into the right and left main stem bronchi. However, there are usually two carinae separating the three major calyceal infundibula.

The endoscopic anatomy of the renal pelvis is extremely variable with many sizes, shapes, and locations. The renal pelvis is generally considered conical in shape. The apex of the cone represents the ureteral pelvic junction. Intrarenal pelves, lying entirely within the renal sinus, are small with short infundibula. Extrarenal pelves are usually capacious, lying entirely outside the renal sinus and often having long, narrow infundibula. The renal pelvis empties urine into the proximal ureter through the ureteral pelvic junction. This is one of the naturally narrower portions of the ureter. Endoscopically, it is identified as a junction between the relatively narrow ureter and the markedly more capacious renal pelvis. The movement of the pelvis and the proximal ureter with each respiratory excursion of the kidney is also apparent endoscopically. Usually, a lip of ureteral mucosa is visible within the lateral ureteral lumen near the ureteral pelvic junction. This anatomic landmark signifies the close proximity of the renal pelvis.

ENDOSCOPIC ANATOMY OF THE URETER

A normal ureter is relatively uniform in caliber and easily distensible; however, there are three naturally occurring relatively narrow sites within the lumen that are recognizable endoscopically—the ureteral pelvic junction, the pelvic brim region, and the ureterovesical junction. The degree of narrowing that is encountered endoscopically varies from one individual to another. Often the narrowing is not noticeable, however. Occasionally, the amount of narrowing is sufficient to prohibit passage of instruments without mechanical dilation.

Besides these anatomic regions, there are other landmarks to be observed. The portion of the ureter as it crosses the termination of the common iliac artery may often be seen pulsating, thus signifying the close approximation of the ureteral and arterial lumens.

As discussed previously, the approach to the proximal ureter is signified by movements with respiration. Each inspiration causes the diaphragm to push downward on the kidney, leading to simultaneous caudal movement of the renal pelvis and proximal ureter.

The junction between the fixed and mobile portions of the ureter has a characteristic appearance and signifies the close proximity of the renal pelvis. A bend or lip of mucosa corresponds to this junction. It is located in the posterolateral lumen and is accentuated during inspiration, becoming barely perceptible during expiration (Huffman et al., 1985a).

ENDOSCOPIC CORRELATION WITH ANATOMY

The clinical availability of small caliber flexible and rigid ureteroscopes has allowed the indications for ureteroscopy to expand greatly. Conversely, the number of unsuccessful procedures has diminished. Previously, the tortuous nature of the ureter did not lend itself well to many of the rigid instruments. However, smaller caliber instruments, especially the flexible variety, could be passed more reliably. Thus, anatomic size and configuration have become less restrictive with the newer and smaller flexible instruments.

Young muscular male patients often have a very hypertrophied psoas major muscle. This causes the abdominal ureter to be "pushed" more ventrally within the retroperitoneum. This ureter was very difficult to evaluate with the rigid ureteroscopes; however, with the flexible deflectable instruments, it is much simpler to transverse this deviation of the ureter and proceed into the kidney.

One must respect the delicate nature of the ureter when performing intraureteral procedures. Initial passage of a guide wire or cone-tipped ureteral catheter may perforate the mucosa and raise a mucosal flap, exposing the underlying submucosal tissue (Fig. 61–4). It is not difficult to pass a guide wire through the same area and dissect proximally within the ureter in the submucosa. A ureteroscope passed in the submucosal ureter would also dissect the ureteral mucosa away from the underlying submucosa and muscle with irrigation fluid. The mucosa derives its blood supply from underlying tissues, and thus when the mucosa is dissected away it would lose its blood supply.

The walls of the proximal ureter and renal pelvis are thinner than those of the distal ureter. The mucosal layers contain one to two cell layers versus four to five in the lower ureter. In addition, there are fewer muscle fibers proximally. Any ureteral dilation, biopsy, or instrument passage in this portion of the ureter is more likely to cause perforation. This problem is especially difficult when one attempts to perform balloon dilation in the proximal ureter or ureteral pelvic junction. It is much simpler to perforate these areas with balloon dilation than those in the lower ureters.

INDICATIONS FOR URETEROSCOPY
(Table 61–1)

Calculi

The most common indication for ureteroscopy is the endoscopic removal of ureteral and renal calculi (Bagley, 1988a). Initially, only small distal ureteral stones

---

Table 61–1. INDICATIONS FOR URETEROSCOPY

  I. Calculi removal
    A. Lower ureteral calculi
    B. Upper ureteral calculi
    C. Renal calculi
    D. Post ESWL steinstrasse
 II. Diagnosis
    A. Evaluation of radiographic filling defects or obstruction
    B. Evaluation of unilateral gross hematuria
    C. Evaluation of unilateral malignant cytology
    D. Surveillance following conservative treatment of an upper urinary tract tumor
III. Therapeutic procedures other than calculi
    A. Passage of a ureteral catheter for obstruction or fistula
    B. Removal of a foreign body
    C. Resection/fulguration of selected tumors
    D. Dilation/incision of strictures.

ESWL, extracorporeal shock wave lithotripsy.

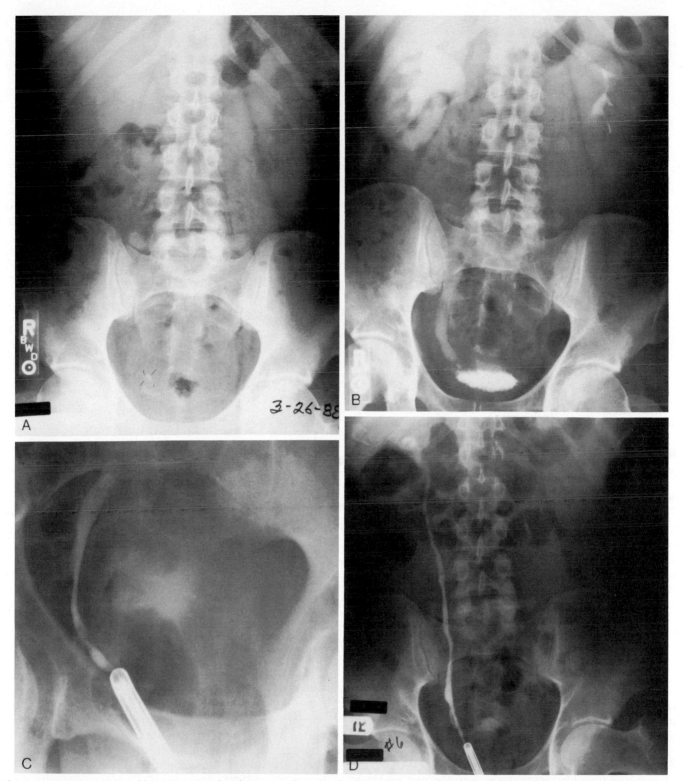

Figure 61–4. *A,* A 36-year-old man presented with severe right ureteral colic and was found to have an obstructing calculus. This preliminary radiograph demonstrates a 7 mm × 4 mm calculus in the region of the right lower ureter.

B, An excretory urogram was performed confirming the diagnosis. The radiograph was taken 2 hours and 10 minutes following the administration of contrast material and shows the stone to be lodged at the right ureteral vesical junction, with evidence of partial ureteral obstruction.

C, The patient was followed medically, with the hope that the stone would pass spontaneously. However, there was no progression of the stone. The patient continued to have intermittent episodes of severe right ureteral colic. Ureteroscopic stone removal was considered. Prior to the procedure, an occlusion tip, retrograde pyelogram was performed. The stone can be seen as a negative defect with contrast material proximal and distal. An area of concentric narrowing is observed just distal to where the stone is lodged.

D, A sequential radiograph is shown. The cone tip catheter advanced proximally a short distance, but now there appears to be a false lumen medial to the stone. Layering of contrast material is seen lateral and above the calculus, which most likely represents the true lumen, whereas the contrast medium represents dissection of the mucosa away from the remainder of the ureteral wall.

Illustration continued on following page

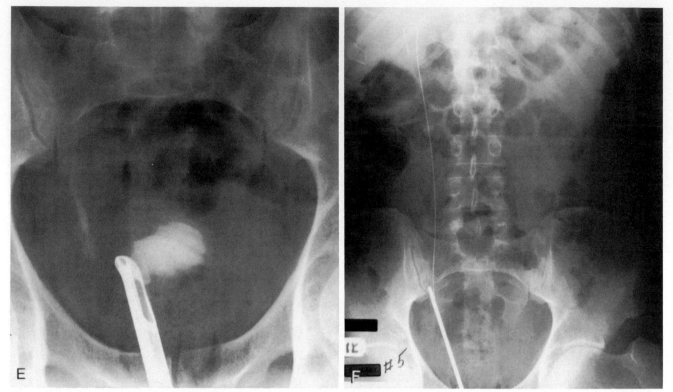

Figure 61–4 *Continued E,* A drainage film from the retrograde study confirms the presence of contrast material outside the lumen of the ureter. Residual contrast material is seen within the submucosa of the distal ureter adjacent to the stone.

F, A guide wire was inserted over which the ureteroscope was passed. The stone could not be identified with the rigid ureteroscope. Explanation for this phenomenon was that the guide wire was passed submucosally along with the rigid ureteroscope. This occurrence would explain why the stone could not be seen despite being confirmed to be in the vicinity of the stone by radiography. (From Huffman, J. L.: Ureteroscopic injuries to the upper urinary tract. Urol. Clin. North Am., 16:249–254, 1989.)

were amenable to ureteroscopic removal. However, the availability of rigid and flexible ureteroscopes combined with the feasibility of intraureteral lithotripsy (ultrasonic, electrohydraulic, and pulsed-dye laser) allows oversized calculi, located anywhere within the ureter or renal pelvis, to be considered for endoscopic retrieval.

Extracorporeal shock wave lithotripsy (ESWL) and percutaneous nephrostolithotomy are very effective methods for treatment of intrarenal and proximal ureteral calculi. Occasionally, these methods are also chosen to treat lower ureteral calculi. However, lower ureteral stones remain a definite indication for ureteroscopy. Upper ureteral calculi, especially those that are impacted in the ureter or those that have failed treatment by ESWL, may be amenable to "salvage" treatment by ureteroscopy (Fig. 61–5).

The success rates for ureteroscopic stone removal depend on the stone's size and location, the availability of ureteroscopic instrumentation, and the experience of the ureteroscopist. Early reported success rates for ureteroscopic stone retrieval in all locations of the ureter ranged from 57 to 95 per cent (Epple and Reuter, 1985; Ghoneim and El-Kappany, 1985; Green, 1985; Kahn, 1986; Keating et al., 1987; Khuri et al., 1985; Lyon et al., 1984; Seeger et al., 1988; Sosa et al., 1985). Success rates according to stone location vary from 22 to 60 per cent in the upper ureter, 36 to 83 per cent in the mid-ureter, and 84 to 99 per cent in the lower ureter (Huffman, 1988a).

In a large series of 346 ureteroscopic procedures performed at the Mayo Clinic, the success rate was 95 per cent for removing lower ureteral stones and 72 per cent for upper stones including mid and proximal third ureteral locations (Blute et al., 1988). Only eight patients (3 per cent) required ureterolithotomy.

Bagley (1990) reported successful removal of 62 calculi in 77 attempts (80.5 per cent), employing a variety of actively and passively deflectable flexible ureteroscopes. In nine of these patients, stones were repositioned to the lower ureter where they were removed with a rigid instrument. The successes included extraction of 22 of 23 intrarenal calculi.

Fragments of calculi resulting from ESWL may fill a portion of the ureter causing partial or complete obstruction. Usually, these fragments pass spontaneously with minimal discomfort; however, intervention may become necessary should the patient develop fever, persistent high-grade obstruction, or intractable pain. In these instances, ureteroscopy is a reliable method of removing the debris. The operating instrument with the ultrasonic probe is particularly helpful for fragmenting and removing the calculus debris (Fig. 61–6).

Suspicion of a Urothelial Tumor

Primary epithelial tumors of the upper urinary tract often pose a formidable diagnostic challenge. Unlike the

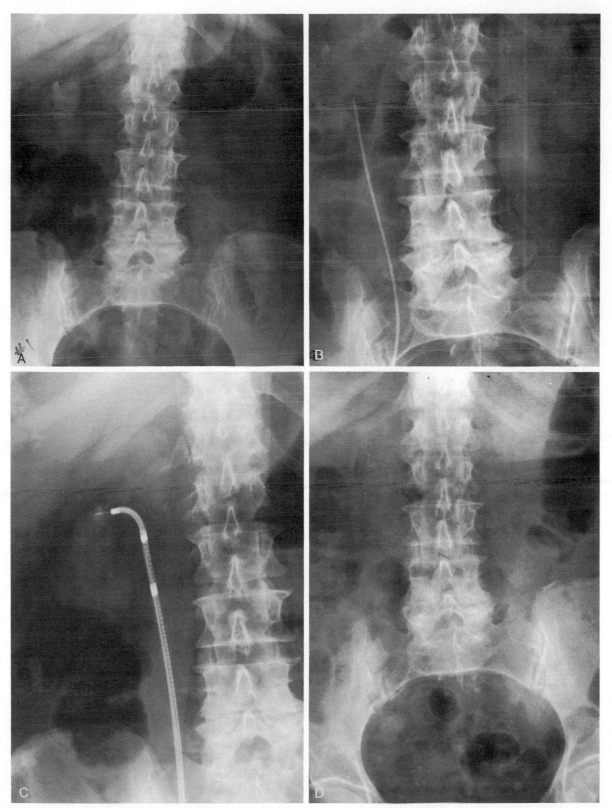

Figure 61–5. This kidney, ureter, bladder (KUB) radiograph reveals a 10 mm × 8 mm stone in the upper pole of the right kidney in a patient with recurrent flank pain and hematuria *(A)*. The patient underwent shock wave lithotripsy, which had little effect in fracturing the calculus *(B)*. A catheter had been inserted prior to this procedure to help localize the stone. Because of the failure to fragment the stone, flexible ureteroscopy was performed using an actively deflectable instrument. A 3 Fr. electrohydraulic lithotripsy probe was utilized to fragment the stone *(C)*, and the individual pieces were removed. Final abdominal radiograph shows that the patient has been rendered stone-free *(D)*. (From Huffman, J. L.: Flexible ureteroscopy. Probl. Urol., 3.420–434, 1989.)

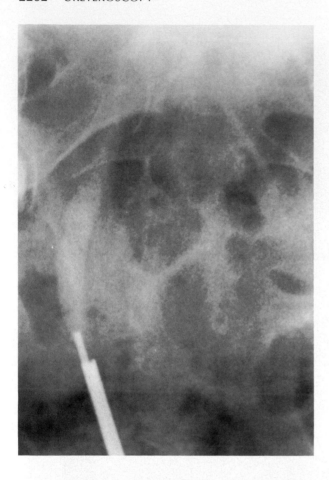

Figure 61–6. Following shock wave lithotripsy, stone fragments occasionally become lodged in the ureter causing obstruction. Ultrasonic lithotripsy performed through a rigid ureteroscope is an excellent means of removing these fragments. This radiograph shows a collection of stone particles in the right lower ureter. A rigid ureteroscope and an ultrasonic lithotripsy probe are inserted into the ureter to fragment the particles further and to remove them with suction through the probe.

cystoscopic approach to the diagnosis of bladder tumors, there previously has not been a satisfactory endoscopic method for the diagnosis of upper tract tumors. The ureteroscope has uses very similar to those of the cystoscope. These include diagnosis of upper tract tumors; surveillance of urothelium, following prior therapy; and, occasionally, primary treatment of selected tumors. The indications for diagnostic ureteroscopy are as follows: radiographic filling defect or obstruction (Fig. 61–7); tumor found cystoscopically near or at the ureteral orifice; unilateral upper tract hematuria; and upper tract urinary cytology findings suggestive of malignant cells (Gittes and Varaday, 1981; Huffman, 1985b).

The treatment approach for a patient with unilateral essential hematuria may be difficult. Gittes and Varaday (1981) showed the potential for diagnosis and localization of hematuria by operative nephroscopy. Bagley (1987) confirmed that this lesion, often a renal hemangioma, may be localized and treated by coagulation through the flexible ureteroscope or by total or partial nephrectomy.

Streem and colleagues (1986) analyzed the effects of adding rigid ureteroscopy to the standard methods for diagnosis of upper tract tumors. Using intravenous pyelography (IVP), retrograde pyelogram, computed tomography (CT), urinary cytology, and cystoscopy, the diagnosis of an upper tract tumor was realized in seven of 12 patients. Adding rigid ureteroscopy to the diagnostic regimen increased the accuracy to ten of 12 patients. The prime indication for flexible ureteroscopy

has been in the diagnosis within the kidney. The success rate of visualizing the entire intrarenal collecting system was 79 per cent in a prior published report; however, this rate continues to improve with experience (Bagley et al., 1987). Most lesions in the kidney require biopsy for confirmation of the pathology.

Besides the diagnosis and mapping of urothelial tumors, ureteroscopy has been utilized in following patients after segmental ureterectomies and in treating selected patients, especially those with isolated, low-grade, lower ureteral tumors and those with solitary kidneys in whom dialysis is not indicated, anesthesia is a risk, or renal insufficiency is of the extent that nephroureterectomy is not possible (Fig. 61–8) (Huffman, 1988b).

Passage of a Ureteral Catheter

In most instances, ureteral catheters are placed by standard cystoscopic methods. However, in some patients, ureteral tortuosity, obstruction, or iatrogenic false passage prohibits passage of a catheter. With a ureteroscopic direct vision approach, a catheter may pass. Ureteroscopy has also been found to be effective in managing ureterocutaneous fistula, enabling passage of a catheter or stent beyond the fistula site. In these instances, employing the 9.5 Fr. instrument with a 5 Fr. accessory channel or the smaller 8.5 Fr. instrument with a 3.5 Fr. channel has been most satisfactory (Huffman,

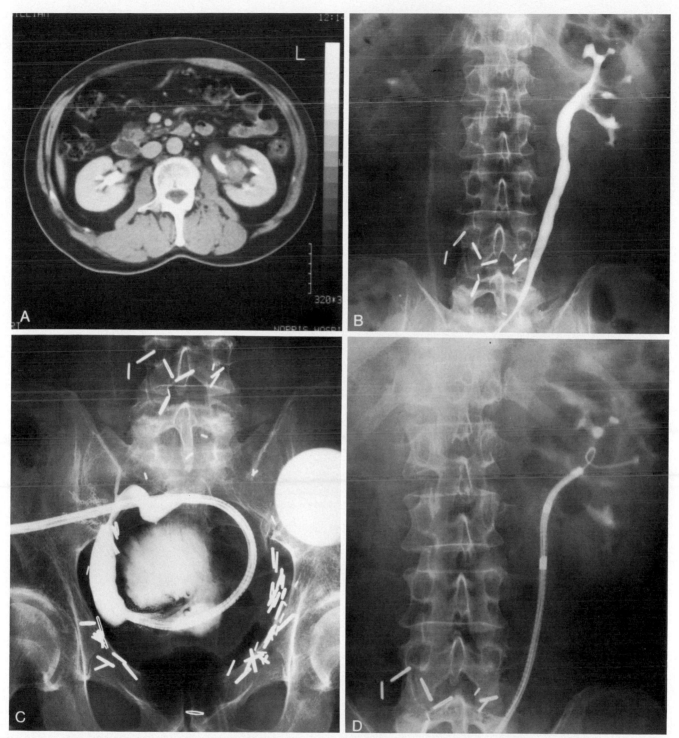

Figure 61–7. A 68-year-old man had previously undergone radical cystectomy, pelvic lymph node dissection, and creation of a continent urinary diversion for P2NO bladder carcinoma. He presented 4 years later with gross hematuria and was found to have bleeding from the upper urinary tract after endoscopy of the Kock pouch was performed. Urinary cytology findings were negative for malignant cells.

   A, Computed tomography (CT) scan was done. This selected view of the CT scan shows a probable mass in the renal pelvis of the left kidney.

   B, A retrograde study was then done through the afferent system of the continent diversion. A selected film from this retrograde study shows the same filling defect in the lateral portion of the renal pelvis.

   C, The flexible cystoscope in the afferent limb of the continent diversion is shown. This instrument was used to pass a guide wire directly into the left collecting system.

   D, The flexible ureteroscope was passed over a stiff guide wire that had been positioned in the kidney. After the guide wire was removed, the 3 Fr. biopsy forceps was inserted and tissue obtained. Biopsy findings confirmed a grade 2 to grade 3 transitional cell carcinoma of the left renal pelvis. The patient underwent a left nephroureterectomy. (From Huffman, J. L.: Flexible ureteroscopy. Probl. Urol., 3:420–434, 1989.)

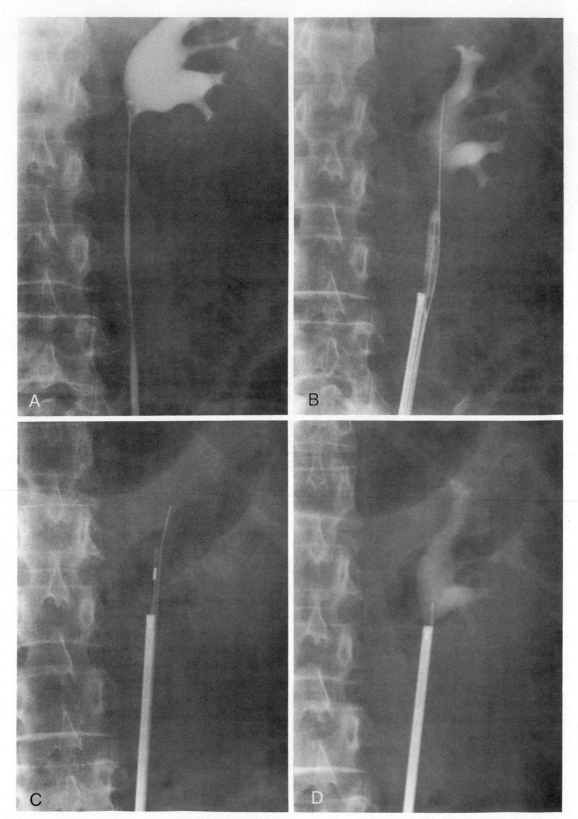

Figure 61–8. A 58-year-old woman presented with intermittent left flank pain. Excretory urograph showed a possible filling defect in the renal pelvis, but urinary cytology findings were negative for malignant cells.

  A, Retrograde pyelogram revealed a 1.5-cm irregular filling defect at the ureteropelvic junction with an otherwise normal collecting system.

  B, Passage of the diagnostic ureteroscope was prevented by proximal ureteral narrowing; therefore, a 4-mm dilating balloon was used.

  C, Rigid biopsy forceps extends from the operating ureteroscope.

  D, After biopsy and fulguration, a contrast study obtained via the ureteroscope shows no evidence of extravasation, obstruction, or residual filling defect. (From Huffman, J. L.: Ureteroscopic management of transitional cell carcinoma of the upper urinary tract. Urol. Clin. North Am., 15:419–424, 1988.)

1989a). These instruments are especially valuable in cases in which dilation of the orifice and tunnel is made impossible by prior trauma. These instruments often may be inserted directly into the orifice without prior dilation.

Retrieval of Foreign Bodies

Another indication for ureteroscopy is the retrieval of ureteral stents that have migrated or broken instrument parts, such as portions of stone baskets, that are retained in the ureter (Bagley, 1988a; Killeen and Bihrle, 1990). This is not a common indication and often this method of retrieval will be difficult because of associated ureteral edema and inflammation. The three-prong grasping forceps, alligator forceps, or stone basket should be selected for these retrievals.

Incision and Dilation of a Ureteral Stricture

Ureteroscopic methods may be employed to treat postoperative ureteral strictures. The process involves incising the region of narrowing under direct vision utilizing a rigid or flexible ureteroscope (Bagley et al., 1985; Inglis and Tolley, 1986; Clayman et al., 1990). The incision is made with either a cold knife ureterotome or a cutting electrode. The area may then be dilated with a 5-mm or 6-mm balloon catheter to complete the treatment. Incising the stricture allows controlled splitting of the ureter during the dilation process. An internal ureteral stent and/or a nephrostomy tube are left in place for 4 to 6 weeks, following the procedure. The long-term success of this technique remains to be determined, but preliminary results are encouraging. It offers definite advantages over repeated open surgery.

Ureteroscopy in Pregnancy

Ureteroscopy has very limited applications during pregnancy. The procedure may occasionally be required to help diagnose or treat a ureteral calculus. In general, the risks of medication, radiation exposure, and anesthesia limit endourology and open surgery procedures. SWL is contraindicated during pregnancy because of the potential harmful effects on the fetus.

Fortunately, most ureteral calculi diagnosed during pregnancy pass spontaneously. In a review by Cass and co-workers (1986), 18 of 24 pregnant patients with stones passed them spontaneously either during pregnancy (14) or after (four). Six patients required intervention for persistent pain (two), sepsis (three), and anuria (one). Intervention consisted of stone basket manipulation (two), open surgery (three), or placement of ureteral catheters (one).

The diagnosis of a stone during pregnancy is made difficult because of the desire to limit radiographic exposure, especially in the first trimester, and the inaccuracy of ultrasonography. Diagnostic ultrasonography is safe during pregnancy. However, the presence of renal pelvic dilation may not be due to an obstructing calculus, because upper tract dilation is often associated with pregnancy.

Rittenberg and Bagley (1988) have reported on flexible ureteroscopy in two pregnant patients. In one patient at 19 weeks' gestation, the procedure was utilized and excluded ureteral obstruction. In another patient at 35 weeks' gestation, a 6-mm obstructing calculus was removed successfully. Both procedures were performed without fluoroscopy. No detrimental effects were noted in the patient or the fetus.

Bakke and Ulvik (1988) have reported successful rigid ureteroscopy in eight patients with the duration of pregnancy ranging from 4 to 35 weeks. All patients were treated with the 11 Fr. rigid operating ureteroscope. The instrument was passed to the renal pelvis in all patients. Two were found to have excoriations and edema consistent with prior stone passage, one patient had only blood clots in the kidney, and one had no detected abnormalities. Four patients were found to have distal ureteral calculi, and these were removed successfully—two required ultrasonic lithotripsy before extraction. One pregnancy ended in an induced abortion at 8 weeks not associated with the procedure. The remaining seven women had normal babies.

Ureteroscopy in the Pediatric Patient

Ureteroscopy may occasionally be indicated in the pediatric patient for treatment of persistent ureteral calculi. Extreme caution is recommended when performing these procedures because of the smaller size of the child's upper urinary tract and the narrower safety margin. Certainly, small caliber instruments should be employed (6 to 8.5 Fr.) and fluoroscopy is limited.

Hill and associates (1990) reported on an 8.5 Fr. rigid ureteroscope in four children, 10 years of age or younger. In two patients, ureteral calculi were extracted successfully. One required fragmentation with laser lithotripsy. The other two patients underwent diagnostic ureteroscopy. In one, an area of stenosis was found and stented. In the other, ureteral polyps were found. The polyps were treated surgically after endoscopic diagnosis. In each patient, follow-up kidney function studies were normal. However, reflux was found by voiding cystogram in two patients. In this report, the importance of adhering to strict ureteroscopic technique, employing an isotonic irrigating solution, and maintaining a stent postoperatively for a minimum of 48 hours was stressed.

PREOPERATIVE PATIENT MANAGEMENT

The management of a patient before a ureteroscopic procedure includes a thorough history and physical examination, informed consent from the patient, and perioperative antibiotics (Huffman, 1988c). The preoperative patient history is especially important regarding prior pelvic surgery or radiation. Certainly, a previous radical prostatectomy or radical hysterectomy may leave the lower ureter fixed in the retroperitoneum and relatively immobile. A history of ureteral reimplantation or ureteral lithotomy also may make the ureter more difficult to manipulate.

The physical examination may provide clues that help predict potential problems in the procedure. A bimanual examination allows assessment of the mobility of the urethra, bladder, and lower ureter. Those structures that are immobile or "frozen" may not allow the straightening needed for passage of the rigid instrument and may be angulated, making flexible ureteroscopy more difficult.

The consent should inform the patient that ureteroscopy is a relatively new procedure without an extremely long follow-up period. Although the goal of ureteroscopy is to prevent an open operation, surgery may still be necessary if the procedure is unsuccessful or if complications arise. The majority of calculi can be removed in one procedure; however, the patient should be made aware that in order to attain a stone-free condition a second procedure, a percutaneous nephrostolithotomy or an open lithotomy, may be necessary.

It is incumbent upon the urologist to review all radiographic studies prior to ureteroscopy. It is also necessary to ensure that the radiographic studies are complete. For example, if the ureter distal to the calculus is not visualized well, it is essential to have a cone tip, retrograde pyelogram. This allows an appraisal of the ureteral tortuosity and caliber distal to the stone and helps identify the regions within the ureter that may be difficult to negotiate.

Perioperative antibiotics are required. Sterile urine is mandatory prior to the procedure, because intravasation of urine and irrigant is possible and sepsis has been a complication. Generally, patients are given a broadspectrum antibiotic (e.g., ampicillin and gentamycin) immediately prior to the procedure. Therapy is continued for several dosages following the procedure.

A general or regional anesthesia is normally required because of the pain when passing the instrument or dilating the lower ureter. Occasionally, if the ureter is capacious and a small caliber instrument employed, it may be possible to do the procedure using local anesthesia with intravenous sedation. This alternative is especially desirable in a patient undergoing endoscopic surveillance after undergoing an endoscopic removal of an upper tract tumor or in a patient after undergoing a segmental removal of the urinary tract. In these instances, flexible ureteroscopy is generally employed and little pain inflicted.

RIGID INSTRUMENTATION

Although first achieved by Young in 1912, rigid ureteroscopy was not performed routinely until Goodman (1977) and Lyon and co-workers (1978) independently demonstrated the feasibility of deliberate excursions into the ureter. The contributions and principles of Hopkins (1960) made this possible. His invention of the rod lens system enabled extremely effective light transmission through rigid endoscopes. It was then possible to construct instruments that were small enough to use in the ureter and that were still able to provide enough light for effective endoscopy.

The traditional rigid endoscopes prior to this time were constructed of a field lens system that consisted of a tube of air with thin lenses of glass. Objective lenses were at the distal tip of the endoscope. A succession of thin relay lenses refracted the rays of light through the instrument to the eyepiece, where they were magnified for the observer.

In 1960, Hopkins invented the rod lens system for rigid endoscopes that is employed currently. This system relays the image by a succession of rod lenses separated by air. The thin spaces of air serve as lenses, and the glass serves as spaces. The effect of this is twofold: (1) the total light transmitted is increased because of the higher refractive index of glass and (2) the rod lenses are simpler to mount than thin lenses.

A greater diameter lens may also be installed for a given endoscope sheath, thus again increasing light transmission. Another factor improving light transmission through the rod lens system for rigid endoscopes was an efficient multilayer antireflection coating on the surfaces of the lens. All these factors added together provide the modern rod lens endoscope with markedly increased light transmission.

Lyon and Goodman's procedures were performed initially with pediatric cystoscopes that were 9.5 Fr. in size. Although length was a limiting factor, these instruments could be used to examine the distal ureter and intramural tunnel in female patients and some male patients.

In conjunction with Lyon, Richard Wolf Medical Instruments designed an instrument modeled after a juvenile cystoscope, which was specified for ureteroscopy. This instrument had a working length of 23 cm and readily reached the distal ureter in male and female patients (Lyon et al., 1979). Several different rigid sheaths were available: 13.0, 14.5, and 16.0 Fr. with a 14.5 Fr. resectoscope sheath. The 13.0 Fr. instrument could be used only for observation. A total of 57 procedures were performed with these instruments between 1978 and 1981 with a success rate of 90 per cent. For the first time calculi were visualized directly in the ureter, engaged in a basket, and removed (Huffman et al., 1983).

This instrument was occasionally very difficult to pass into the ureteral orifice. Its beak was constructed without much bevel. In order to negotiate the orifice, the trigone had to be depressed while at the same time advancing the instrument. This requirement often resulted in a blind spot during insertion that prohibited visualization of the ureteral lumen. Not only was insertion difficult and time consuming but often it was impossible. False passages occasionally resulted because of the blind spot and subsequent improper alignment of the instrument.

Karl Storz Instruments in conjunction with Perez-Castro and Martinez-Pineiro (1980) made the next significant contribution to the field of rigid ureteroscopy. They introduced an instrument with a working length of

39 cm that could reach the renal pelvis in male and female patients after transurethral passage. Often called the ureterorenoscope or, more appropriately, the ureteropyeloscope, this instrument could examine the ureter and renal pelvis. The instrument had sheath sizes of 9 Fr. and 11 Fr. and each had a 5 Fr. working channel. The 9 Fr. sheath had an integral 0-degree telescope. In conjunction with the 11 Fr. sheath, interchangeable 0- and 70-degree telescopes with their bridges were available for visualization within the ureter and renal pelvis, respectively. An 11 Fr. resectoscope sheath that had a partially insulated beak with an inverted bevel allowed ureteroscopic resection.

Richard Wolf developed a similar instrument with a 41-cm working length in sheath sizes of 11.5 Fr. and 10.0 Fr. (Huffman et al., 1983). The larger operating sheath had a 5 Fr. channel for accessories, but the smaller sheath was for observation only. A resectoscope sheath was also designed that was 11.5 Fr. and had a completely insulated beak. Since that time, many new instruments have been introduced by several different manufacturers. The trend has been to reduce sheath size and still maintain an accessory channel for forceps, baskets, and intraureteral lithotripsy devices (Huffman, 1989). The introduction of fiberoptic imaging bundles within a rigid sheath has made this miniaturization possible (see Appendix A) (Dretler and Cho, 1989).

FLEXIBLE URETEROSCOPY

Flexible ureteroscopy has become a valuable addition to the diagnosis and treatment of many lesions in the upper urinary tract. The technique has extended the indications of rigid ureteroscopy and allows virtually any filling defect to be evaluated or any stone to be considered for removal from the ureter or kidney. The rapid advancement of this technology has been made possible by the development of effective ureteral dilation techniques and the manufacture of flexible ureteroscopes that are of small enough caliber to extend into the upper urinary tract.

FLEXIBLE URETEROSCOPIC INSTRUMENTATION

Marshall, in 1964, reported on a 3-mm fiberscope or ureteroscope that was passed transurethrally through a 26 Fr. cystoscope and then into the distal ureter where a ureteral stone was visualized at 9 cm. Although there was excellent transmission of light and images with this instrument, no methods were available for changing the direction of the tip of the instrument and for irrigation to provide a clear field of view and adequate distention of the ureter. The small size of this instrument, a necessity for passage through the ureter, prevented the incorporation of a deflecting mechanism and a channel for working instruments along with the imaging bundle. This size problem remains somewhat of a limiting factor today.

Takagi and associates began working in 1966 with a narrow flexible fiberoptic endoscope, which was 2.7 mm in diameter and 70 cm in length. In 1968, they reported on a patient undergoing an open operation in which the instrument was passed through the ureterotomy incision to visualize and photograph the renal pelvis and papillae. The difficulties of not having an irrigation system, or a deflecting mechanism were encountered. However, it became evident that it was possible to view portions of the urinary tract that could not be viewed through rigid cystoscopes.

Bush and colleagues also had been working with flexible instrumentation in the late 1960s. The instrument was inserted cystoscopically, like a ureteral catheter, and enabled visualization of the upper urinary tract. Irrigation was provided by means of a forced diuresis. Any manipulation was performed with accessories passed alongside the ureteroscope.

Successful treatment with a pyeloureteroscope passed transurethrally in 23 patients was reported by Takagi and co-workers in 1971. This instrument, an Olympus model KF, was 2 mm in diameter and 75 cm in length. The addition of a 2.5 cm angulating section at the distal end of the instrument enabled its passage into the ureteral orifice and through the intramural ureter in the same fashion as that of a ureteral catheter. The angulating section also allowed passage up the ureter and into the intrarenal collecting system with the aid of fluoroscopy. Despite having the advantage of a flexible tip, this instrument still did not have an irrigation system. As reported by Takagi, there were occasional problems with passage of the instrument through the intramural ureter that resulted in breakage of the glass fibers.

To circumvent this problem of insertion, these workers introduced a Teflon guide tube that was passed initially through a special cystoscope with an ocular lens system, which protruded at a 45-degree angle from the shaft. The angulation of the lens system helped prevent fracture of the glass fibers, as it was pushed through the cystoscope. A special deflecting bridge limited sharp angulation of the instrument, as it passed from the end of the cystoscope. The guide tube was passed into the bladder and engaged by the deflecting bridge. A ureteral catheter was then passed through the guide tube and into the ureteral orifice. Once the catheter was approximately 10 cm within the ureter, the guide tube was pushed over it in a coaxial fashion. The ureteral catheter was removed and replaced with the flexible pyeloureteroscope.

Takayasu and Aso (1974) reported a 100 per cent success rate in 19 patients, utilizing this guide tube method compared with an 80 per cent success rate in 50 patients prior to this method. However, the only irrigation system was provided either through the guide tube or by inducing diuresis. Therefore, observation was often difficult or impossible in the presence of hematuria.

Modern flexible ureteroscopes have been markedly improved by reducing sheath size, increasing channel size, and providing a deflecting mechanism in many designs. The two generic types of instruments are the passively deflectable and the actively deflectable (see Appendix B).

The passively deflectable design does not allow for purposeful movement of the tip, thus depending on a pre-placed guide wire for positioning within the urinary tract. The passively deflectable instruments are less expensive. They vary in size from 6 Fr. to 10 Fr. with an irrigation/accessory channel size directly proportional to the overall size. The actively deflectable instruments have the ability to be purposely turned within the urinary tract. They also have an irrigation/accessory channel for passage of stone baskets, grasping forceps, biopsy forceps, or guide wires. These actively deflectable instruments have been extremely helpful within the kidney, allowing the entire intrarenal collecting system to be visualized in a high percentage of patients.

URETERAL DILATION

It is advisable in most instances to dilate the ureteral orifice and intramural ureter prior to passage of the ureteroscope. Some of the smaller flexible or rigid instruments may be passed without prior dilation, depending on the size of the ureter. Although most orifices are approximately 3 mm in size, some are smaller because of anatomic variations. As the size is not predictable, most clinicians routinely dilate the orifice prior to a ureteroscopic procedure. Dilation expands the safety margin as the ureteroscopes are passed and allows larger fragments of calculi to be removed. Dilation to 14 Fr. or 15 Fr. is sufficient to allow passage of the operating instruments, and thus far all available experimental and clinical evidence suggests that dilation to this size has no detrimental effect on the structure or function of the orifice (Greene, 1944; Ford et al., 1984a; Huffman and Bagley, 1988). Hydraulic dilation, involving a pressurized pumping device, has been advocated. If not associated with intravasation of fluid, this method is also acceptable (Perez-Castro, 1988).

Dilation of the ureter is not new to urology. Lewis in 1906 described dilating the ureterovesical junction to facilitate passage of a ureteral stone. Many descriptions were provided in the literature of specific instruments and techniques for enlarging the distal ureteral lumen. Ureteral catheters of varying sizes and designs were probably the simplest. Dourmashkin (1945) described metal cone-tipped catheters passed into the orifice under direct vision to dilate the orifice to 20 Fr. to 24 Fr. The metal tips were interchangeable and attached to a flexible carrier. He also described dilating the orifice with rubber bags attached to catheters (Dourmashkin, 1926). The purpose of the dilation was to facilitate passage of ureteral calculi, thus dilation was to a size large enough to allow the calculi to pass.

Several techniques are currently in use that are acceptable methods of ureteral dilation (Bagley, 1988b). A ureteral catheter or an internal ureteral stent may be placed at least 1 day prior to the planned ureteroscopic procedure. This "subacute" method of ureteral dilation makes the ureteroscopy a two-stage procedure. The first stage of the procedure is the cystoscopic placement of

the catheter or stent. The ureter is passively dilated for 1 or more days. The ureteroscopy is performed in a second stage.

A more common method involves dilating the orifice immediately prior to the ureteroscopic procedure. This "acute" method of dilation allows the ureteroscopic procedure to be done in one stage. Methods of acute dilation include passage of progressively larger ureteral catheters (whistle tip, cone tip, or Braasch bulb) or successively larger metal cone-shaped bougies.

Both of these methods are performed without initial guide wire passage. Other methods are designed to be utilized in conjunction with a pre-placed floppy tip guide wire. These include graduated fascial dilators, olive-tipped metal dilators, and balloon dilating catheters.

Methods of Subacute or Passive Dilation of the Ureter

In 1980, Perez-Castro and Martinez-Pineiro described placing a catheter in the lumen of the ureter 24 hours prior to a planned ureteroscopic procedure. This was one of the early reports of successful ureteroscopy. In this case, the ureter was sufficiently dilated to accept the rigid ureteroscope. If the procedure is being done for stone removal the catheter is passed to a level above the obstructing calculus to relieve the ureteral colic and drain the upper urinary tract. The catheter is secured to a Foley catheter passed into the bladder and left in place for 1 to 3 days, depending on the patient's condition and the timing of the ureteroscopic procedure.

An internal ureteral stent may also be employed for passive dilation of the ureter prior to ureteroscopy. A double pigtail or double-J stent offers the advantage of being internalized with decreased risk of bacterial contamination when compared with a standard ureteral catheter.

Several disadvantages of this technique are noted. The major disadvantage is that it makes the ureteroscopic procedure a two-stage one, with added cost and time involved for the patient. In addition, the presence of the foreign body in the ureter and bladder does lead to a mucosal inflammation and an added risk of urinary tract infection. Passive dilation should not be done when diagnostic ureteroscopy is being performed. The catheter or stent may cause urothelial damage or inflammation and may thereby hinder the success of the ureteroscopic procedure.

Methods of Acute Dilation of the Ureter for Ureteroscopy

Many acceptable methods of acute cystoscopic dilation for ureteroscopy exist that have been proved in large series of patients. These methods include dilation with (1) successively larger ureteral catheters, (2) passage of metal bougies, and (3) balloon dilating catheters. Passage of progressively larger ureteral catheters or cone-shaped metal bougies is done without prior placement of a floppy tip guide wire. In comparison, dilation with fascial dilators, olive-shaped bougies, or balloon dilating catheters is performed after positioning a guide wire in the ureter. A dilating method over a pre-positioned guide wire has been the safest and most satisfactory. Although somewhat more cumbersome than passing a dilator directly, there are fewer false passages and intramural ureteral perforations with this method.

Acute Dilation with Ureteral Catheters

The cystoscope is passed into the bladder, and the orifice identified. Depending on the size of the orifice, a ureteral catheter is selected that can be passed without difficulty into the orifice. Generally, a 5 Fr. or 6 Fr. catheter is passed several centimeters above the orifice. The catheter is removed, and a larger catheter is passed in a similar fashion (1 Fr. to 2 Fr. larger). Dilation is carried out in this fashion until the orifice is dilated 12 Fr. to 15 Fr. Cone-tipped or Braasch bulb catheters may be needed for the larger sizes. It may be necessary to backload these into the catheterizing bridge of the cystoscope because of the large size of the tip. Alternatively, two catheters may be placed side by side in order to dilate to a larger size. Care must be taken with this technique not to perforate the ureter as the second catheter is passed.

Acute Dilation with Cone-Shaped Metal Bougies

Dilation with cone-shaped metal dilators has been done successfully for many years (Dourmashkin, 1945; Lyon et al., 1978). Initially, the tips were interchangeable and attached to a flexible carrier passed cystoscopically. The modern design has tips that are permanently attached to the carrier and are sized from 8 Fr. to 15 Fr. The larger sizes must be backloaded through the catheterizing bridge of the cystoscope.

These dilators are not guided and must be passed very carefully through the ureteral orifice (Fig. 61–9A to C). It is important to align the cystoscope and the dilator with the anticipated three-dimensional plane of the orifice and intramural ureter. The dilator is then slowly advanced through the orifice with gentle pressure. Usually, a slight "give" is perceived, as the dilator passes above the level of the detrusor hiatus of the bladder. Once it reaches this point in the ureter, it is removed and the next larger dilator inserted.

Acute Dilation over a Pre-Placed Guide Wire

Guided methods of ureteral dilation are preferable to nonguided. Initially, a 0.035- or 0.038-inch floppy tip

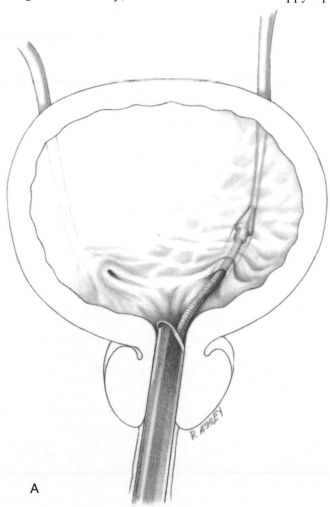

Figure 61–9. *A,* The cone-shaped dilator is advanced into the ureteral tunnel and must be carefully directed along the anticipated position of the ureteral lumen.
Illustration continued on following page

A

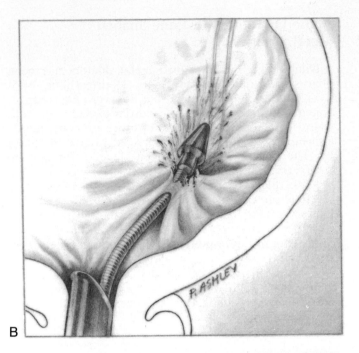

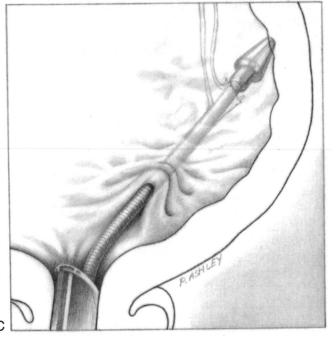

Figure 61–9 *Continued B* and *C,* Misdirection of the cone-shaped dilators results in perforation of the ureteral wall. *B,* Medial perforation in the intravesical segment may re-enter the bladder or may course submucosally. *C,* Lateral perforation passes into the perivesical tissue. (From Huffman, J., Bagley, D., and Lyon, E. (Eds.): Ureteroscopy. Philadelphia, W. B. Saunders Co., 1988.)

guide wire is passed cystoscopically into the ureter (Huffman et al., 1985b). This maneuver reduces the possibility of ureteral perforation because dilating instruments are passed over the wire in a coaxial fashion. In addition, the wire usually remains in position throughout the ureteroscopic procedure and later used to place an internal stent or open-end catheter at the completion of the procedure. Many types of guide wires are available for ureteroscopic procedures. It is helpful to have a variety of wires on hand, depending on the type of clinical situation that may be encountered. The hydrophylic-coated wires that become extremely "slippery" once brought into contact with saline solution are especially useful.

Flexible Fascial Dilators

Flexible dilating catheters similar to those employed to dilate nephrostomy tracts may be employed to dilate the ureteral orifice for ureteroscopy (Fig. 61–10). These are sized from 8 Fr. to 16 Fr. and are passed over a 0.038-inch guide wire. The smaller sizes may be passed under vision cystoscopically, but the larger ones must be passed under fluoroscopic guidance alone. Often, it is helpful to leave the sheath of the cystoscope in place when the larger sizes are selected. This step helps to keep the catheter straight without allowing it to buckle in the bladder or urethra.

A dilator sheathing system has been described that

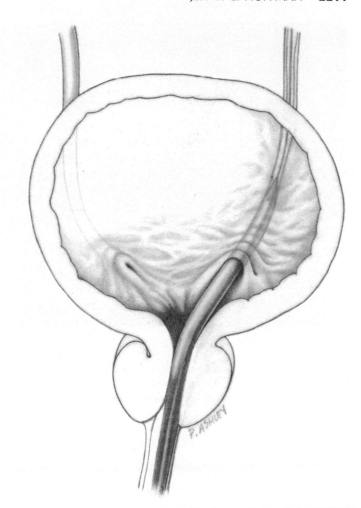

Figure 61–10. The graduated dilator is generally used in the intramural and distal ureter but can be placed more proximally with fluoroscopic control when necessary. (From Huffman, J., Bagley, D., and Lyon, E. (Eds.): Ureteroscopy. Philadelphia, W. B. Saunders Co., 1988.)

enables direct access into the ureter (Newman et al., 1985). This system consists of flexible fascial dilators from 6 Fr. to 17 Fr. The largest sized catheter is a sheath that is passed over the graduated dilators and then left in place while removing the inner catheters. The ureteroscope is passed through the sheath directly into the ureter.

The access sheath can also be inserted after dilation by other methods, such as those with balloons. With this technique, the orifice is dilated to 15 Fr. with a 5-mm balloon dilating catheter. The 15 Fr. sheath is then inserted into the ureter, utilizing the appropriately sized fascial dilator as a carrier. The inner catheter is removed, leaving the access sheath in place.

Although the access sheath system has the advantage of providing direct access into the ureter for ureteroscopy, it has several disadvantages. The distal ureter is obscured by the sheath and cannot be inspected with the ureteroscope. The size of the sheath (outer diameter) is larger than the size of the sheath of the ureteroscope, and this may lead to more damage to the ureter if left in place throughout the procedure. In addition, the proximal end of the sheath is not beveled and may cause significant trauma to the ureteral mucosa at this point.

When dilating with a guide wire method prior to stone removal, special precautions must be taken to help prevent stone migration. The guide wire may dislodge a stone positioned in the ureter and cause migration into the kidney. This occurs less commonly with stones lodged in the lower ureter, because this portion is posterior and therefore dependent relative to the upper ureter.

If the stone is lodged below the pelvic brim, one attempts cystoscopically to pass the guide wire proximal to the calculus; but if the stone is lodged above the pelvic brim, one passes the guide wire to a point immediately distal to the stone. Obviously, fluoroscopic control is essential if not mandatory to help guide these manipulations and assure proper guide wire position.

Stones that are impacted at the ureterovesical junction or within the intramural ureter pose a difficult problem for ureteral dilation. If it is possible to negotiate a guide wire, dilation up to the stone generally proceeds satisfactorily. Often with impacted stones, it is impossible to manipulate a guide wire cystoscopically above the stone. In these situations, the nonguided conical dilator is an excellent alternative. Dilation is performed up to the stone only. Although this may leave a segment of ureter inadequately dilated immediately distal to the stone, the amount is usually sufficient to allow insertion of the operating ureteroscope. The calculus is visualized and possibly removed without further manipulation. If a long segment of nondilated ureter remains between the

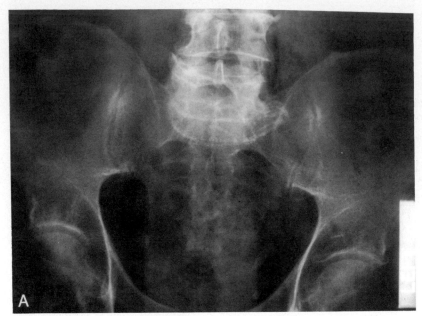

Figure 61–11. The ureteroscopic removal of impacted calculi is often very difficult. The stones become imbedded in the ureteral mucosa and often only a small portion of the stone is visible endoscopically.

A, This plain pelvic radiograph shows bilateral, large, distal ureteral stones. It was impossible to pass a guide wire cystoscopically. Therefore, the orifice was gently dilated with an 8 Fr. and a 10 Fr. metal cone-shaped dilator, which allowed passage of the 8.5 Fr. rigid ureteroscope.

instrument tip and the stone, a guide wire is passed alongside the stone under vision, the ureteroscope removed, and the cystoscope reinserted for further dilation.

Alternatively, in these instances of a distally impacted stone, a small caliber rigid instrument may be inserted directly into the orifice without dilating. Under vision, a guide wire is negotiated beyond the stone and the instrument removed. Dilation proceeds over the guide wire (Fig. 61–11).

BALLOON DILATION FOR URETEROSCOPY

The success of polyethylene balloons for transluminal dilation of arterial narrowings stimulated an interest in them in other areas of medicine. These balloons have been utilized to dilate the ureteral orifice and intramural ureter to facilitate ureteroscopy (Huffman et al., 1983; Huffman and Bagley, 1988). The advantage of the angioplasty-type balloon is that it provides controlled dilation by radially distributed pressure to a defined length of ureter. The expansion of this balloon is controlled by hand inflation to a predetermined maximum diameter.

Instrumentation for Balloon Dilation

Standard cystoscopes are needed for balloon dilation of the ureteral orifice and intramural tunnel. The only requirement is a catheterizing bridge that accepts at least 7 Fr. accessories. In addition to the balloon catheters discussed next, a syringe and radiographic contrast material (50 per cent solution) are needed for balloon inflation, along with a pressure gauge and fluoroscopy. The pressure gauge allows documentation of exact pressure for dilation and ensures against inflation above the maximum pressure rating of the balloon. Fluoroscopy adds to the safety of the technique by assuring guide wire positioning, balloon placement, and adequate inflation and deflation.

Selection of a Balloon Catheter

Many manufacturers offer balloon dilating catheters for ureteroscopy. Each is a product of high quality, but it is recommended to try several types and make an individual assessment. A properly sized guide wire accompanies most balloon dilating sets (0.038- or 0.035-inch). The most useful balloons for dilating the ureteral orifice and intramural tunnel have a 7 Fr. shaft size, 70 to 80 cm shaft length, 5- or 6-mm balloon inflated diameter, and 4 cm balloon length. These allow satisfactory dilation of the majority of orifices for ureteroscopy. A balloon with maximum inflation pressure of 15 atmospheres is usually sufficient for dilation of normal ureters. Generally, less than 10 atmospheres is needed. Occasionally, reimplanted ureters, scarred ureters, or strictured ureters may require high pressure balloons for dilation (Table 61–2).

Table 61–2. RESULTS OF BALLOON DILATION OF THE URETER IN 122 PATIENTS

	Number of Patients	(%)
Successful dilation for the ureteroscopic procedure	120	(98)
Pressure required—8 atmospheres or less	93	(78)
Pressure required—10–14 atmospheres	18	(15)
Pressure required—more than 15 atmospheres	9	(7)

From Huffman, J. L., and Bagley, D. H.: Balloon dilation of the ureter for ureteroscopy. J. Urol., 140:954–956, 1988.

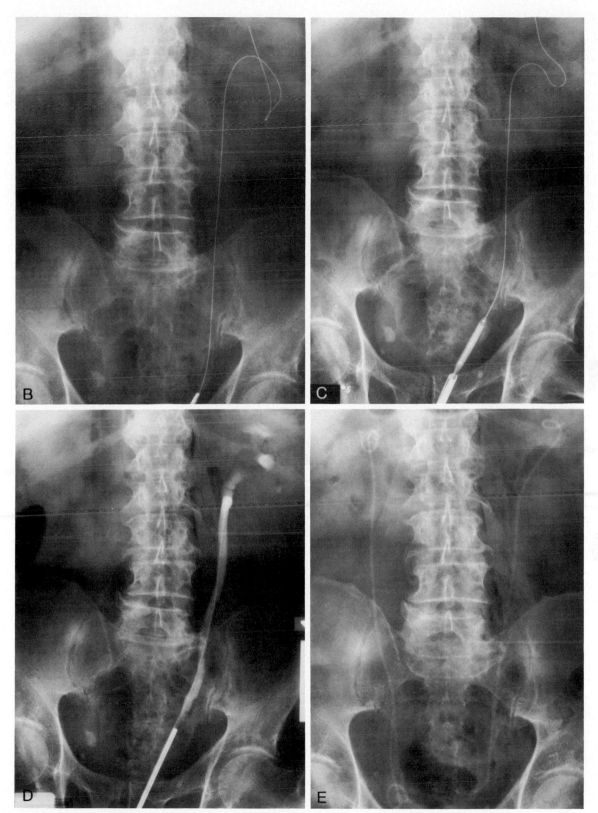

Figure 61–11 *Continued B*, Under direct vision, it was possible to pass a flexible tipped guide wire above the stone and into the renal pelvis. The ureteroscope was then removed and the cystoscope reinserted.

C, Balloon dilation was performed by passing the catheter over the guide wire. The end point of dilation is complete inflation of the balloon without any waisting or hourglass deformity. The operating ureteroscope was inserted, and the stone extracted completely with ultrasonic lithotripsy. Following removal of all stone particles, contrast material was injected through the ureteroscope.

D, Free flow of contrast material into the left ureter and kidney without evidence of extravasation or obstruction is shown. An internal stent was placed over the guide wire. This exact procedure was repeated to remove the right-sided stone.

E, A final radiograph shows internal stents in place bilaterally without any residual stone particles.

Table 61–3. METHOD OF BALLOON DILATION
OF THE URETER

1. A flexible tip guide wire is positioned cystoscopically and fluoroscopically in renal pelvis.
2. A balloon dilation catheter is placed over the wire and positioned across the orifice and intramural ureteral tunnel.
3. The balloon is inflated at a rate of 2 atmospheres per minute until all "waisting" is eliminated.
4. Once the balloon attains its complete cylindric shape, it is deflated completely and removed.

Technique of Balloon Dilation for Ureteroscopy (Table 61–3)

The technique of balloon dilation involves passing a standard cystoscope into the bladder. The orifice is identified, and the floppy end of the guide wire (sized according to the requirements of the balloon catheter) is inserted through the orifice and positioned in the renal pelvis.

The position of the guide wire is monitored fluoroscopically throughout the dilation process. Once the guide wire is positioned, the balloon catheter is passed over the wire and its radiopaque markers are positioned across the intramural ureteral tunnel and orifice. The proximal end of the balloon is visualized cystoscopically as it exits the ureteral orifice (Fig. 61–12). However, the distal end of the balloon cannot be seen and its position is judged fluoroscopically (see Fig. 61–11).

Once the dilating balloon is in the proper position, the balloon is inflated. Generally, a 50 per cent solution of radiographic contrast material is used to inflate the balloon in order for it to be visible fluoroscopically. A screw-type inflation syringe works very well. Inflation is carried out slowly at a rate of 2 atmospheres per minute, until all waisting of the balloon is removed. It is deflated completely before being removed over the guide wire. If the entire intramural ureter has not been dilated, the balloon is repositioned and dilation repeated. After the balloon is removed, the guide wire is left in place for the ureteroscopic procedure.

Dilation in the Supravesical Ureter

In some patients, dilation is required in a narrow portion of the upper ureter in order to pass the ureteroscope. A guide wire is passed through the ureteroscope and under vision. A small balloon catheter is then passed over the wire and positioned through the area of narrowing. The distal end of the balloon is judged to be in proper position by fluoroscopic guidance. The balloon is inflated in a similar fashion, as previously described, while watching endoscopically. Ureteroscope passage is attempted and if it is impossible, further dilation is needed. The smaller balloons are fragile, and it is suggested that they not be inflated prior to passage through the instrument. If redilation is needed after the balloon has been removed, the balloon should be checked for its integrity and re-molded, employing one of the plastic molds that accompanies the balloon in its package.

Precautions

Caution is advised during several parts of this procedure. The initial placement of the guide wire is crucial to success of the procedure. This must be done transluminally and not submucosally. The guide wire must pass smoothly into the renal pelvis and should not be forced. Its position in the pelvis is maintained as the balloon catheter is advanced in a coaxial fashion over the guide wire. If buckling occurs or the guide wire slips distally from its correct position, the end of the balloon catheter may perforate the ureter.

The balloon must be deflated completely before trying to advance or withdraw it. Moving a partially inflated balloon may avulse a portion of the ureteral mucosa. It is not unusual, however, to see a small amount of bleeding from the orifice after dilation.

If a balloon is utilized to dilate an area in the supravesical ureter, it is important to dilate the ureteral orifice first, prior to passing the balloon to more proxi-

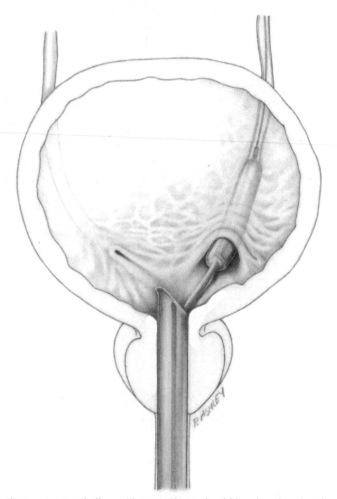

Figure 61–12. A balloon dilating catheter should be placed so that the entire intramural ureter and ureteral orifice are dilated. The proximal cylindric portion of the balloon should appear in the ureteral orifice. (From Huffman, J., Bagley, D., and Lyon, E. (Eds.): Ureteroscopy. Philadelphia, W. B. Saunders Co., 1988.)

mal areas of the ureter. Not dilating the orifice may preclude balloon withdrawal after it has been inflated in the upper ureter. The balloon may not resume its preinflation diameter, and it may not be possible to pull it out through a nondilated orifice.

INTRODUCING THE RIGID URETEROSCOPE

The rigid ureteroscope is inserted into the bladder with the techniques employed for rigid cystoscopy. Normal saline is selected for irrigation. Once in the bladder, the orifice is identified and the instrument aligned with the anticipated three-dimensional plane of the distal and intramural ureter, if it were extended from the ureteral orifice. In most instances, a guide wire will have been positioned in the ureter after dilation. The ureteroscope is passed along the wire into the orifice and advanced through the ureteral lumen. It is often helpful to rotate the rigid ureteroscope 90 to 180 degrees, as it enters the ureter. This maneuver enables the beveled tip of the instrument to "lift" the upper lip of the orifice and permit smooth insertion.

The ureteroscope is advanced in the ureter slowly while watching endoscopically. Visualization must be clear; any debris or blood should be removed with irrigation using a syringe attached to the instrument. If there is any question regarding location of the ureteroscope in the urinary tract, a small amount of dilute constrast material is injected through the instrument while watching fluoroscopically.

INTRODUCING THE FLEXIBLE URETEROSCOPE

Several techniques have been satisfactory for introduction of the flexible ureteroscope into the ureter and kidney (Bagley, 1988c). In most instances, this maneuver is done after dilation has been accomplished.

Guide Wire Method

After the dilation of the intramural ureter, a floppy tip heavy duty guide wire is passed into the lumen of the ureter or left in place. The cystoscope is removed, and the flexible ureteroscope is passed over the guide wire, which is placed through its working channel. The instrument is advanced over the guide wire and into the ureter, employing fluoroscopic monitoring to assure proper positioning and to assure that the guide wire or instrument does not buckle in the bladder (Fig. 61–13).

Flexible Introducer Sheath Method

Similar to the technique described by Takayasu and Aso (1974), a flexible guide tube can be passed into the ureter after dilation for the introduction of the flexible

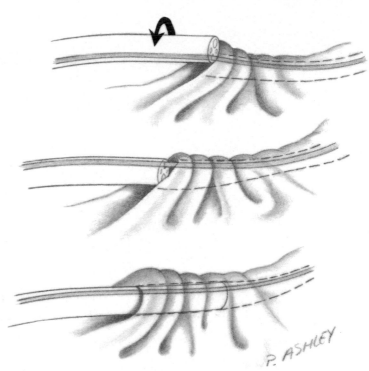

Figure 61–13. A guide wire can be used to guide flexible endoscopes into the ureteral orifice. Care should be taken as the tip approaches the orifice.

Because the channel is located eccentrically at the tip of the instrument, it may impinge on the lip of the orifice. The instrument should be turned to allow it to pass into the lumen. (From Huffman, J., Bagley, D., and Lyon, E. (Eds.): Ureteroscopy. Philadelphia, W. B. Saunders Co., 1988.)

instruments. After dilation of the ureter, a 12 Fr. or 14 Fr. flexible dilator with the guide tube as an outer sheath is passed into the ureter. The dilator is removed leaving the outer sheath in place. This acts as a conduit directly from outside the patient into the ureter for passage of the flexible instrument (Fig. 61–14).

Rigid Sheath Method

Smaller ureteroscopes may be passed directly through a rigid cystoscope and into the ureter. This technique is similar to that of passing a standard ureteral catheter cystoscopically. Although this method is quite fast and accurate, it may prove cumbersome to have the cystoscope sheath in place during the ureteroscopic procedure. In addition, the rigid sheath may damage the fragile flexible instrument as it exits the tip of the cystoscope.

Direct Insertion into the Ureter

A flexible ureteroscope may be directed into the ureteral orifice under vision. This method allows manual advancement of the instrument; however, the buckling of the flexible instrument in the bladder with coiling of its sheath is a possibility. The most common use for this insertion method is cutaneous ureterostomy.

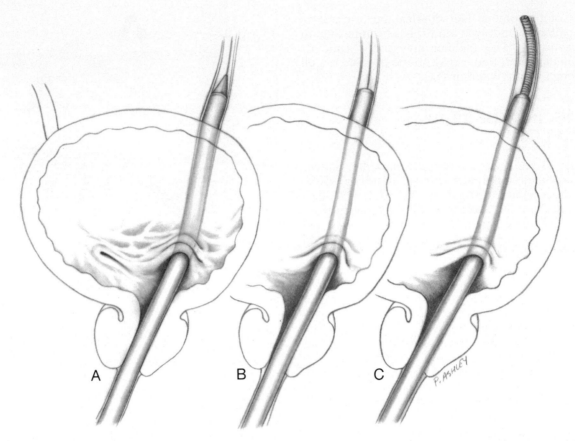

Figure 61–14. *A,* A flexible guide tube is passed over a graduated flexible ureteral dilator into the distal ureter. *B,* The guide wire may be left in place as the dilator is removed, or both the guide wire and dilator can be removed *(C),* leaving the sheath as a conduit from the urethra into the ureter for the flexible ureteroscope. (From Huffman, J., Bagley, D., and Lyon, E. (Eds.): Uteroscopy. Philadelphia, W. B. Saunders Co., 1988.)

PASSAGE OF THE FLEXIBLE URETEROSCOPE INTO THE UPPER URINARY TRACT

Once the ureteroscope is in the ureter, the irrigating fluid (0.9 per cent normal saline) is attached to the irrigation channel of the instrument and direct visual advancement performed. For the passively deflectable instrument, it is advisable to pass the instrument directly over the guide wire to the point where the stone or lesion to undergo biopsy is identified. Buckling and coiling of the flexible instruments may occur, and thus a stiff guide wire for passage or a guide tube may prove necessary. At this point, the guide wire is removed. Fluoroscopy is employed to ascertain the position of the tip of the instrument. Contrast material is added to the irrigating solution to identify the ureteral lumen and renal anatomy. The tip of the instrument may be adjusted slightly by torquing the sheath of the flexible scope with one hand.

Advancement of the actively deflectable instrument is slightly less difficult than that of the passively deflectable instrument. With one's right hand, the tip of the instrument is deflected with the lever toward the center of the lumen of the ureter or calyx. The left hand torques the sheath and positions the tip after it is deflected. Fluoroscopic positioning is mandatory. As one moves to higher levels in the urinary tract, contrast material is again injected to ascertain the position of the ureteral lumen relative to the tip of the instrument. For endoscopic diagnosis in the kidney, each individual calyx must be examined very carefully. Thus, fluoroscopy is utilized to make sure that the tip of the instrument is in the desired calyx.

PERFORMING PROCEDURES THROUGH THE FLEXIBLE URETEROSCOPES

Performing procedures through the flexible ureteroscopes requires a great deal of time and patience. The size of the irrigation/accessory channels is quite limited, thus the size of the accessory instrumentation is also quite small. As one inserts any accessory instrument through the flexible ureteroscope, the position of the tip will change slightly. The accessory instrument acts as a "stiffener" and tends to straighten the tip of the flexible ureteroscope.

Thus, fluoroscopy and constant visual monitoring are essential. The appropriate accessory devices must be available prior to the procedure. These must fit through the accessory channel, and they must be long enough for the flexible ureteroscope. A tight-fitting rubber nipple is helpful, because the amount of irrigating fluid that flows through the ureteroscope with an accessory instrument in place is quite small, and leakage makes visualization difficult. When an accessory instrument is in place, it is also helpful to have a mechanical irrigation device such as a hand syringe system or a blood pump to help ensure good adequate fluid flow and visualization within the collecting system. A variety of accessories are available for intrarenal surgery utilizing flexible instruments. These include stone baskets, grasping forceps, biopsy forceps, coagulating electrodes (both Bugbee and bipolar), electrohydraulic lithotripsy probes, and laser lithotripsy probes. Because accessory instruments change tip position when inserted, it is helpful to have them positioned in the field of view and ready for use before locating the stone.

REMOVAL OF LARGE URETERAL CALCULI

Following ureteral dilation, some calculi may be extracted intact without the need of intraureteral lithotripsy. The ureteroscope is advanced toward the stone usually alongside the guide wire placed to dilate the ureter. Upon visualizing the stone, a basket is advanced through the ureteroscope and the stone is engaged within its wires. A variety of baskets are available, depending on individual preference and instrument channel size. Baskets are made with spiral and double-snare design with either round or flat wires. They are sized from 1.7 to 4.5 Fr.

Once the stone is trapped within the wires of the basket, it is withdrawn as a unit with the ureteroscope. It is important to watch this process endoscopically to ensure that there is no binding between the stone and the ureteral wall. If binding does not occur, the stone is removed from the patient. The ureteroscope may then be reinserted to inspect the ureter for evidence of damage and to perform a retrograde ureterogram to inspect for extravasation or injury. An open-end catheter or internal stent is placed over the guide wire and left in place for a minimum of 24 hours. If binding occurs between the ureteral wall and stone, it is important not to pull on the basket any further because of the possibility of ureteral avulsion or injury. A method of intraureteral lithotripsy must be employed in order to fragment the stone and to allow safe extraction.

Ultrasonic Lithotripsy

Stones that are approximately 5 mm in size can often be extracted intact. However, stones that are too large to be pulled out intact must be fragmented. Ultrasonic lithotripsy techniques, successful in the bladder and in percutaneous approaches, may also be applied ureteroscopically (Huffman et al., 1983). High frequency vibrations of a rigid metal transducer provide the energy for stone fragmentation. The energy either fragments a stone completely or carves a path through the calculus, removing the smallest fragments by suction through its hollow central core.

The transducer depends on direct contact between its tip and the stone in order to cause fragmentation. For efficient disintegration, the stone must be secured within a basket and held in a fixed position to provide counter traction. The ultrasonic transducer produces heat while operating. The probe must therefore be cooled throughout the disintegration process to protect against thermal injury to the ureteral mucosa (Howards et al., 1974). Irrigation through the ureteroscope sheath provides an excellent means of cooling and dissipating heat. The irrigant flows in the sheath toward the tip of the probe and then flows out the probe suction port. It is also preferable to negotiate the stone, basket, and instrument into the more proximal ureter, which is usually dilated and more capacious, allowing better heat dissipation.

Technique of Ultrasonic Lithotripsy Using Standard Rigid Ureteroscope Sheaths

Standard rigid ureteroscopic sheaths can be employed effectively for ultrasonic lithotripsy. The disadvantage in using these sheaths rests in the necessity to remove the direct viewing telescope to allow room for passage of the ultrasonic transducer. The procedure is followed by tactile, audible, and fluoroscopic control.

The stone is pulled down against the tip of the instrument while watching endoscopically. The calculus should fill the entire visual field and occlude the end of the sheath. Thus, when the direct viewing telescope is removed and replaced with the ultrasound probe, it will touch the calculus at the end of the sheath. The basket is held in this position fixing the stone for ultrasonic fragmentation. At this point, the telescope is removed. The ultrasonic probe is inserted in place of the telescope and advanced slowly. When approaching the stone with the probe, the process is followed fluoroscopically. Tactile sensation and fluoroscopic visualization assure contact between the probe and stone. Irrigation is maintained through the sheath, and suction is applied to the probe.

The ultrasonic generator foot pedal is depressed, triggering the disintegration process. Only short bursts (10 to 15 seconds) are utilized after which the telescope is reinserted to assess progress. Steady pressure is applied to the probe until either the probe moves passed the stone (a "give" will be felt) or the 10- to 15-second time period is reached.

Often, the stone can be removed completely or partially after one application of the probe. If the stone is still too large to be extracted, further disintegration is required.

Technique of Ultrasonic Lithotripsy Using the Rigid Offset Viewing Telescope

The offset viewing telescope offers distinct advantages over the standard method; however, special precautions are necessary. The size of the ultrasonic probe is reduced

(1.5 mm) to enable simultaneous passage with the offset telescope. Thus, the size of the suction lumen within the probe is also reduced and the frequency with which its lumen becomes clogged by debris and stone fragments is increased. When the lumen is clogged, the continuous flow of irrigant stops and heat is allowed to build up along the probe. In this circumstance, the chance of thermal injury to the ureter becomes much higher. Therefore, patency of these probes must be maintained at all times during the disintegration process. The outflow of irrigant from the probe must be monitored constantly to assure patency.

It is helpful to have the calculus engaged in a stone basket to provide counter traction with the ultrasonic transducer. This facilitates the disintegration process and allows the fragments that are still trapped within the basket wires to be removed efficiently. In this instance, a basket 3 Fr. in size or less must be selected to allow simultaneous passage of the smallest ultrasonic probe.

The initial steps of engaging and positioning the calculus are similar to those for the standard sheath (Fig. 61–15). However, instead of replacing the telescope with the probe, the probe is applied directly to the stone while watching endoscopically. Again, irrigation is flowing through the sheath and suction is removing irrigant and fragments through the probe. The stone is either disintegrated completely or fragmented sufficiently to enable it to be pulled down the ureter (Fig. 61–16).

A solid wire probe for transurethral ultrasonic lithotripsy is also available from Karl Storz Medical Instruments (Chaussey et al., 1987). Although this probe is smaller and somewhat more powerful, it does not have a lumen. Thus, fragments are not removed through the probe and continuous irrigation for cooling is not possible.

Electrohydraulic Lithotripsy

A second method for fragmentation of oversized calculi is electrohydraulic shock wave lithotripsy (Raney and Handler, 1975; Goodfriend, 1984; Green, 1985; Huffman, 1988a; Willscher et al., 1988; Schoborg, 1989; Denstedt and Clayman, 1990). This method, using an

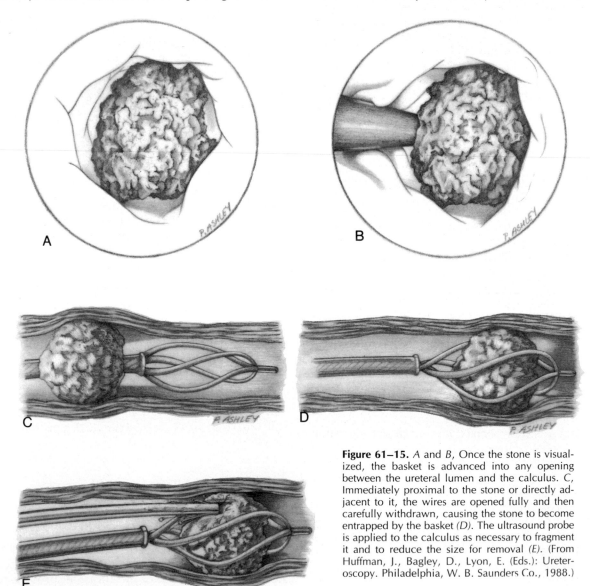

Figure 61–15. *A* and *B*, Once the stone is visualized, the basket is advanced into any opening between the ureteral lumen and the calculus. *C,* Immediately proximal to the stone or directly adjacent to it, the wires are opened fully and then carefully withdrawn, causing the stone to become entrapped by the basket *(D).* The ultrasound probe is applied to the calculus as necessary to fragment it and to reduce the size for removal *(E).* (From Huffman, J., Bagley, D., Lyon, E. (Eds.): Ureteroscopy. Philadelphia, W. B. Saunders Co., 1988.)

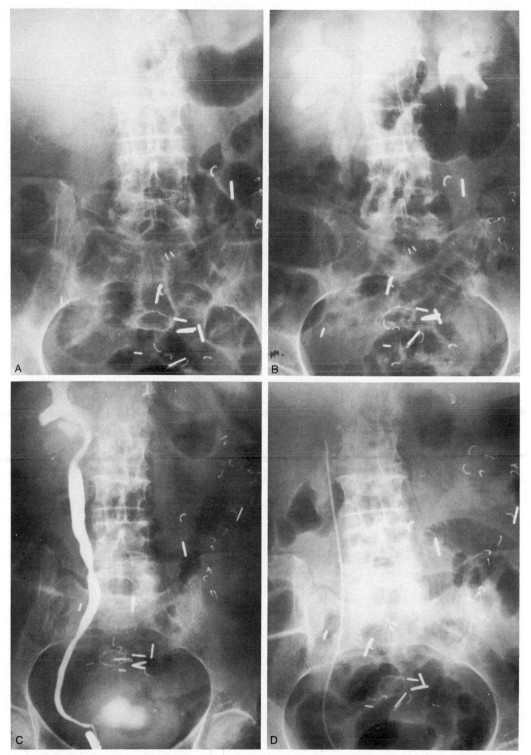

Figure 61–16. A 57-year-old woman who had previously undergone multiple intra-abdominal operations presented with severe right flank pain, a temperature of 103.5°F, and shaking chills. A plain abdominal film *(A)* followed by an excretory urogram *(B)* were done, which showed obstruction at the mid-portion of the right ureter by a 10 mm × 12 mm radiopaque calculus.

C, Initially, an occlusion tip retrograde ureteropyelogram was performed. This showed slight medial deviation of the mid-ureter and a narrowed region just distal to the site of stone impaction.

D, A 6 Fr. spiral tip catheter was passed beyond the calculus, and a brisk flow of cloudy urine was obtained.

Illustration continued on following page

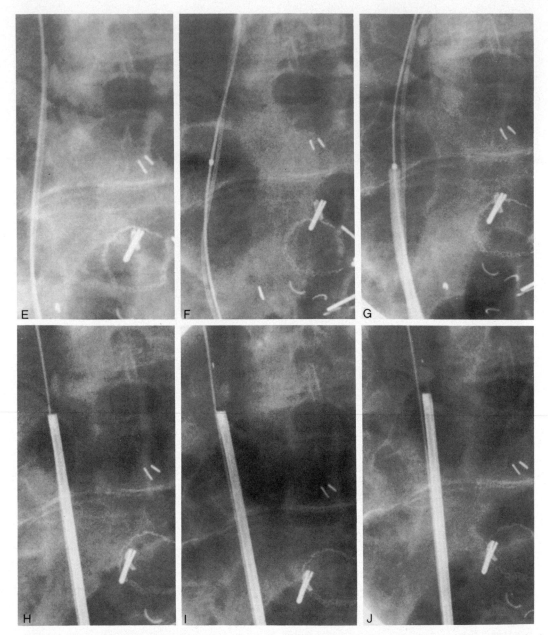

Figure 61–16 *Continued E,* Once the patient was stable clinically, endoscopic stone extraction was planned. This radiograph shows the poorly defined calculus near the vertebral body, with the tip of a spiral catheter alongside. A guide wire has also been passed cystoscopically beyond the calculus and is positioned in the renal pelvis.

F, A 10-cm by 5-mm ureteral balloon dilation catheter was then positioned across the intramural tunnel and lower ureter and was passed cystoscopically over the previously passed guide wire.

G, Inflation of the balloon was carried out, and the maneuver was watched both cystoscopically and fluoroscopically. A 3-ml syringe was used to inflate the balloon to approximately 100 psi.

H, The spiral tip catheter was removed and the operating offset ureteroscope inserted. This radiograph shows the tip of the ureteroscope 1 to 2 cm distal to the calculus.

I, A 3.5 Fr. stone basket is passed through the catheterizing port of the ureteroscope and positioned above the calculus.

J, The basket is opened and withdrawn to entrap the stone. This entire process is performed with visual control.

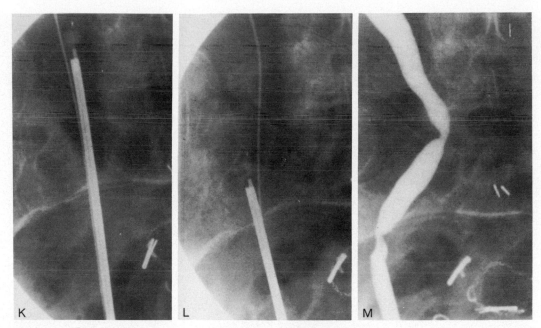

Figure 61–16 *Continued K,* This oversized stone could not be extracted intact; therefore, ultrasonic lithotripsy was necessary. Under direct vision, the ultrasonic probe was applied to partially fragment the calculus while it was held in position by the basket.

L, The calculus could then be pulled partially down the ureter; however, another area of narrowing prohibited passage into the bladder. Therefore, further disintegration was performed at this level.

M, The stone was removed and the instrument reinserted to check for any damage to the ureter or any residual stone fragments. A retrograde contrast study was performed. This film demonstrates the area of previous stone impaction in the mid-ureter. A ureteral catheter was left in place for 48 hours. (From Huffman, J., Bagley, D., and Lyon, E. (Eds.): Ureteroscopy. Philadelphia, W. B. Saunders Co., 1988.)

electrohydraulic shock wave generator and a coaxial probe, produces a shock wave that will cause cavitation and fragmentation when directed toward a calculus. In conjunction with miniaturization of rigid and flexible ureteroscopes, the sizes of electrohydraulic lithotripsy (EHL) probes are smaller and are currently available in sizes 1.6 to 5.0 Fr.

A potentially higher incidence of damage to the ureteral mucosa is a disadvantage. In addition, impacted calculi should not be fragmented by this method. The reported rate of perforation with EHL on nonimpacted ureteral calculi is 10 to 15 per cent. This rate would be higher if applied to impacted calculi that are often obscured by ureteral mucosa.

The advantages of this method are that the standard rigid and flexible ureteroscopes can be employed, the procedure is performed under direct visual control, and the stone size is effectively reduced to allow subsequent removal or passage of fragments. The cost of EHL instrumentation is substantially less than laser lithotripsy, thus making it preferred at many institutions (Denstedt and Clayman, 1990).

Technique of Electrohydraulic Ureteroscopic Lithotripsy

The rigid or flexible ureteroscope is manipulated into the ureter, and the calculus is approached utilizing the same technique and precautions described previously. Once the calculus is visualized, the coaxial probe is advanced to a point close to the stone but not quite in contact with it. The generator is set on single impulse (not continuous) and the foot pedal is depressed. Fol-

lowing stone fragmentation, the probe is removed and a stone basket inserted. All stone particles are sequentially removed, taking great care not to apply excessive irrigant that might cause migration of the fragments into less accessible intrarenal locations (Fig. 61–17). Initially it was thought that only 1/6 of normal saline irrigant would allow effective fragmentation with EHL. Subsequent studies have documented that normal saline is a satisfactory irrigant (Miller and Wickham, 1984).

Laser Lithotripsy

The most recently introduced method for intraureteral lithotripsy has been pulsed-dye laser lithotripsy (Watson and Wickham, 1986; Dretler et al., 1987 and 1989). This method employs a very small caliber electrode (250 to 320 μ) and a pulsed-dye laser (coumarin green). A laser light at 504 nanometers is emitted through a quartz fiber, 200 to 320 μ in size. The light is absorbed by the stone and a gaseous plasma formed on the stone surface. The plasma absorbs subsequent laser light, expands between the tip of the fiber and the stone surface, and generates an acoustic shock wave. This shock wave overcomes the tensile strength of the stone and fragmentation occurs. A very brief rise in temperature occurs on the stone surface but not nearly enough to cause any thermal injury to the surrounding mucosa.

Technique of Ureteroscopic Laser Lithotripsy

All operating room personnel, the patient, the anesthesiologist, and the urologist must wear protective eye

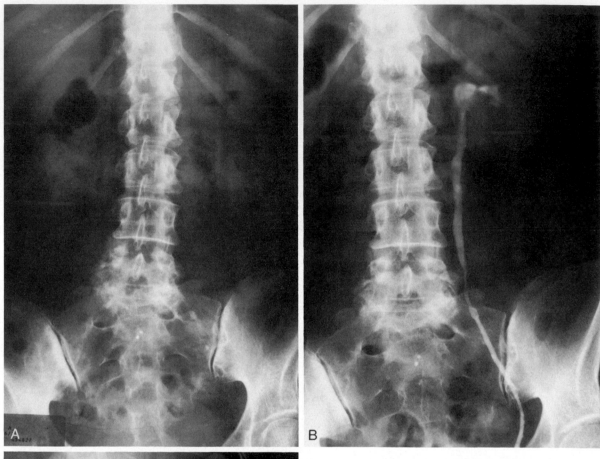

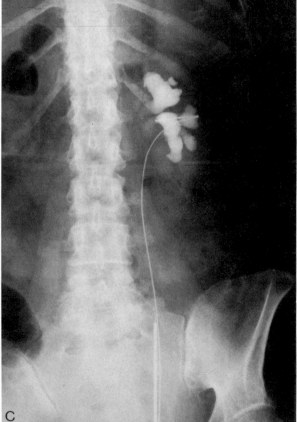

Figure 61–17. A 70-year-old female presented with a 9-month history of intermittent left flank pain. Excretory urography showed a high-grade obstruction of the left ureter near the L5-S1 vertebral body level due to a ureteral calculus. Ureteroscopic stone extraction was planned. Prior to the procedure a retrograde ureterogram was done.

A, A radiograph was taken initially, demonstrating a calcification in the region of the left ureter at the L5-S1 level.

B, The contrast study shows that the stone is located in the ureter at this level.

C, Following the retrograde study, a flexible tip guide wire was inserted, and a 6.9 Fr. rigid ureteroscope was passed along the wire to visualize the stone. The stone was fragmented with a 1.9 Fr. electrohydraulic lithotripsy probe passed through the rigid ureteroscope. Several small fragments of stone can be visualized near the tip of the probe extending from the instrument.

glasses when the laser is in use. An option for the urologist is to attach a protective eyepiece over the endoscope. However, eyeglasses are preferable in the rare event of breakage of the quartz fiber.

The stone is approached with any rigid or flexible ureteroscope that can accommodate the 200- or 320-μ fiber. Standard normal saline irrigation is employed. Once the stone is visualized, the laser fiber is passed through the endoscope until it makes contact with the stone. It is helpful to pass the fiber through a 3 Fr. or 4 Fr. open end catheter if the ureteroscope can accommodate this sized accessory. Alternatively, the stone may be engaged in a basket and held in position for subsequent laser fragmentation. This method is preferable, because it stabilizes the stone and avoids proximal stone migration.

The fiber must be in contact with the stone for effective fragmentation because of rapid dissipation of the laser energy. The laser is generally set at 60 to 80 millijoules of energy initially and raised, if necessary, for a hard stone. A repetition rate of 3 to 5 pulses per second is also selected. Laser lithotripsy is initiated by depressing the foot switch while watching endoscopically. A perceptibly louder, high-pitched ticking sound indicates stone fragmentation. The tip of the probe is maneuvered to make contact with different parts of the stone surface as fragmentation proceeds. The fragments may then be removed with a basket or forceps.

URETEROSCOPIC BIOPSY, RESECTION, AND FULGURATION

The biopsy of abnormalities within the ureter or pelvis is somewhat awkward for the endoscopist. This problem is due to the relationship of the instrument and forceps to the location of the tumors. In the bladder (a spherical structure), the forceps can be applied perpendicularly to the area of the biopsy. However, the ureter (a tubular structure) requires the forceps to be applied parallel to the ureteral mucosa.

Biopsy is performed during the initial pass of the ureteroscope. If an attempt is made to examine the entire upper tract and to then biopsy, the lesion may be traumatized or inadvertently avulsed during instrument passage. When the lesion is identified, the 3 Fr. or 5 Fr. cup forceps is carefully advanced with its jaws parallel to the ureter wall. The intraluminal portion of the lesion is then grasped with the jaws and pulled free from the ureter, applying gentle traction on the forceps (Fig. 61–18).

The size of the biopsy specimen obtained is minute, and the specimen should at once be placed into a fixative. Special notation is transmitted to the pathologists so that they are aware of the small size of the biopsy sample. A potential problem is losing the biopsy specimen as it is pulled through the instrument sheath. To avoid this problem, either remove the telescope first, thus providing more room within the sheath, or remove the entire scope including the forceps.

The technique of ureteroscopic resection is very similar to that of resection with a pediatric resectoscope. The instrument is also similar to that of a pediatric resectoscope, except for added length. The fine construction of the resectoscope loop provides excellent control over depth and location of resection (Fig. 61–19).

Basic transurethral electrosurgery principles are maintained. An irrigant, such as glycine or water, and the appropriate settings on the coagulation and cutting currents provide the most effective surgery with the least tissue injury.

The actual mechanics in resecting an upper tract tumor are different than those in the bladder or prostate. Only intraluminal tumor is resected, and no attempt is made to take deep arcing bites into the ureteral wall. For this reason, the tip of the resectoscope is positioned directly distal to the tumor. The loop is extended beyond the tumor. Prior to activating the power, the tissue is drawn back toward the tip insulation or directly outside.

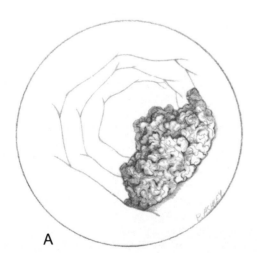
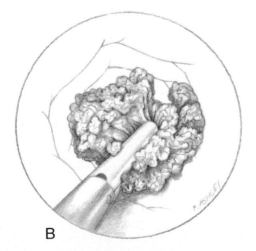

A   B

Figure 61–18. When a ureteral lesion is identified ureteroscopically, biopsy is performed during the initial pass of the instrument. The flexible cup forceps is extended from the sheath and opened parallel to the ureteral wall *(A)*. Once the tissue is within the jaws, the forceps is closed and gently pulled from the ureter *(B)*. (From Huffman, J., Bagley, D., Lyon, E. (Eds.): Ureteroscopy. Philadelphia, W. B. Saunders Co., 1988.)

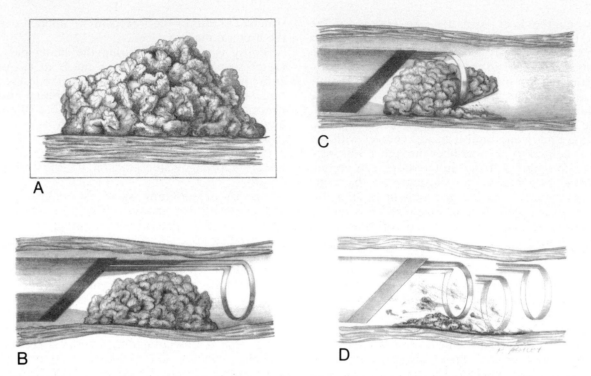

Figure 61–19. Ureteroscopic resection of a tumor *(A)*. The instrument is positioned immediately distal to the lesion, and the resectoscope loop is extended past the tumor *(B)*. Prior to activating the cutting power, the tissue is drawn into the sheath, thus minimizing the chance of ureteral injury *(C)*. The base of the tumor and any bleeding sites can be lightly fulgurated *(D)*. (From Huffman, J., Bagley, D., Lyon, E. (Eds.): Ureteroscopy. Philadelphia, W. B. Saunders Co., 1988.)

The power is started and the tissue resected. This method helps to ensure cutting only the desired tissue and prevents injury to the surrounding ureteral wall.

Following resection of all intraluminal tumor, the base of the lesion is lightly fulgurated with the resectoscope loop. Smooth to-and-fro movements are made to cauterize the region of the resected tumor.

Fulguration is also possible with a Bugbee or bipolar electrode. The probe is advanced through the sheath and gently positioned on the area to be fulgurated. With flowing irrigation, the coagulation current is activated. Irrigation is necessary to maintain clear visualization and to dissipate bubbles that are produced.

The operating instruments allow simultaneous passage of two working instruments, such as a stone basket and an ultrasonic lithotripsy probe. A grasping forceps may be passed in order to secure a polyp or other lesion, and a coagulating forceps may be inserted simultaneously to remove the lesion.

A neodymium-yttrium-aluminum-garnet (Nd:YAG) or KTP laser may also be utilized for tumor surveillance procedures. The advantages of laser technology include the small, flexible fibers that may be employed with flexible ureteroscopes and the hemostatic properties of laser energy.

The laser is also valuable in cases of lower ureteral tumors, in which standard electrocautery causes obturator nerve stimulation and resultant violent movement of the leg. Laser energy would avoid this complication. As with bladder tumors, it is important to obtain tissue for histologic examination if the laser is applied therapeutically.

PLACEMENT OF URETERAL CATHETER OR STENT AT THE END OF THE PROCEDURE

In most instances a temporary diversionary catheter or internal stent should be inserted after the ureteroscopic procedure. Many types of catheters may be utilized, including standard whistle tip catheters, single pigtail diversionary stents, open-end ureteral catheters, or double pigtail internal ureteral stents. The simplest method for insertion of the catheter or stent is directly over the guide wire, which is positioned in the ureter throughout the ureteroscopic procedure. If the guide wire has been removed, a wire should be reinserted through the ureteroscope prior to withdrawing the instrument from the ureter. Cystoscopic wire passage after ureteroscopy is often impossible. The tip of the wire may catch on a flap of mucosa raised during the ureteroscopic procedure. In these instances, it may become necessary to pass a small caliber ureteroscope in order to view the area directly and to pass the wire into the true lumen. This technique is the same as that employed for wire/stent/catheter placement for treatment of iatrogenic ureterocutaneous fistula. Fluoroscopy or a standard radiograph is employed to ensure proper position.

The catheter/stent is left in place for a short period of time if no ureteral injury has occurred. If there has been evidence of urinary extravasation, the stent is left for 2 to 3 weeks. If extravasation has been documented during the procedure a follow-up contrast study should be performed prior to removal of the stent.

COMPLICATIONS

The rapid development of endoscopic instruments for the upper urinary tract has expanded the urologist's ability to treat ureteral stones, tumors, and obstructions in this area. But similar to cystoscopy and transurethral resection of the prostate, ureteroscopy and percutaneous nephroscopy have been associated with iatrogenic injuries. Perforations of the prostatic capsule and formation of a urethral stricture certainly occur occasionally following transurethral resection of the prostate. Following endoscopic surgery within the bladder, there is an incidence of urethral stricture disease and bladder perforation. Thus, as one advances an endoscope proximally in the urinary tract into the ureter and kidney, similar types of complications and injuries may occur (Biester and Gillenwater, 1986; Carter et al., 1986; Kaufman, 1984; Kramolowsky, 1987; Lyon et al., 1984; Lytton et al., 1987; Schultz et al., 1987; Seeger et al., 1988; Sosa and Huffman, 1988).

A smaller margin of safety for endoscopic surgery in the ureter and kidney is noted, mainly because of the smaller anatomic size of the ureter compared with the urethra. As instrumentation is improved, with the addition of small caliber rigid endoscopes, dependable flexible ureteroscopes, and newer methods of intraureteral lithotripsy, this safety margin should widen. However, operator error, whether in judgment or technique, can still lead to complications. Therefore, it is incumbent upon the urologist to be familiar with the types of injuries that may occur, the appropriate means for diagnosing these injuries, and their treatment.

This section reviews the incidence of upper tract injuries and the possible etiologic factors in complications during endoscopy of the upper urinary tract. Treatment modalities for iatrogenic injuries are discussed, and various preventive measures emphasized.

Incidence of Complications

It is fortunate that complications of a ureteroscopic procedure do not occur frequently because, in part, of the caution taken by most endoscopists when performing ureteroscopy, with either rigid or flexible instrumentation. Injuries at the time of the procedure may be recognizable immediately, such as a perforation or an avulsion, but occasionally identification is delayed, as in the case of a ureteral stricture (Table 61–4). In a 1984 series involving original ureteroscopic investigators, the complication rate in 838 procedures was 4.5 per cent (Sosa and Huffman, 1988). These complications were due to mechanical injury to the ureter in 71 per cent (Table 61–5). The injuries included intraoperative perforation due to the guide wire or to the beak of an

Table 61–4. TYPES OF IATROGENIC URETERAL INJURIES

Immediate recognition	Delayed recognition
Perforation	Stricture
False passage	
Avulsion	

Table 61–5. COMPLICATIONS OF URETEROPYELOSCOPY*

Complications	Number of Cases	Percentage of All
Mucosal injury	13	34.2
Ureteral perforation	7	18.4
Ureteral bleeding	4	10.5
Extravasation	2	5.3
Stricture formation	1	2.6
Infection	11	29.0
Totals		
Number of Cases	838	
Complications (%)	38 (4.5)	
Mechanical injury (%)	27 (71.0)	
Infection (%)	11 (29.0)	

*Data compiled from the Third Congress of the International Society of Urologic Endoscopy. Karlsruhe, Federal Republic of Germany, August, 1984.

instrument or an accessory device, such as biopsy forceps. A false passage may occur in the ureter. This is a partial thickness injury to the ureteral wall, which does not extend through the adventitia of the ureter. An additional injury that is recognized immediately is avulsion of the ureter. This is without doubt the most severe complication.

Reviewing published reports throughout the urologic literature allows us to estimate the incidence of endoscopic injuries (Huffman, 1989b). These data, summarized in Table 61–6, compare the incidence of injury in 15 series, totaling 1696 ureteroscopic procedures. Injuries occurred in 9 per cent of all procedures, with 1.6 per cent requiring surgical interventions. These numbers are somewhat higher than those in the original reports and probably represent more accurate assessments.

Etiology

When one attempts to define the causes of iatrogenic injuries, it is important to consider the anatomy of the upper urinary tract (see Figs. 61–2 and 61–3). The intramural ureter and the supravesical ureter have much more muscular support than the proximal ureter or the renal pelvis. Also, the number of mucosal cell layers is substantially greater in the lower ureter (three to five) than it is in the renal pelvis (one to two). Thus, there is less likelihood of a complete perforation in the intramural tunnel or distal ureter than in the renal pelvis or proximal ureter. However, it is more common to have a false passage in these areas than in the upper ureter or renal pelvis.

The size and flexibility of the instruments are major determinants of the incidence of ureteral injury. A mucosal flap may become elevated with a cone-tipped catheter, guide wire, or beak of the instrument (see Fig. 61–4). This event was more common with the original instrumentation, which was larger and more difficult to insert. In addition, flexible instruments are less likely to cause a traumatic injury because they can accommodate to ureteral tortuosity, unlike their rigid counterparts.

The blood supply to the ureteral mucosa is also rather tenuous, which underscores the need to be aware of the possibility of dissecting the mucosa away from the mus-

Table 61–6. INCIDENCE OF URETERAL INJURIES WITH URETEROSCOPY

Author	Number of Procedures	Dilation	Perforations	Major Ureteral Injury	Stricture	Surgery
Aso	21	Yes	3	0	0	3
Schultz	100	Yes	4	0	1	4
Chaussey	118	89%	14 (12%)	0	1	1
Coptcoat	30	Yes	0	2 (7%)	0	2
Lytton	128	Yes	12 (9%)	1	1	4
Ford	48	Yes	0	0	0	0
Kramolowsky	142	Yes	24 (17%)	0	7	4
Keating	81	Yes	9	1	0	1
Lyon	242	Yes	0	1	0	1
El-Kappany	120	Yes	8	0	2	3
Hosking	58	Yes	16 (28%)	0	0	0
Carter	111	Yes	4	0	5	2
Tolley	46	Yes	1	0	2	
Blute	348	Yes	19	2	5	2
Seeger	105	Yes	Occasional	0	0	0
Total	1696		114 (7%)	7 (.4%)	24 (1.4%)	27 (1.6%)

From Huffman, J.L.: Injuries to the upper urinary tract. Urol. Clin. North Am., 16:249–254, 1989.

cularis, such as could result with submucosal dissection by the instrument (Lytton et al., 1987; Chang and Marshall, 1987). Coupled with factors such as prior radiation to the ureter, endoscopic manipulation may add to the incidence of devascularization and necrosis, with resulting stricture formation. Other possible causes for stricture formation following ureteroscopy include the initial balloon dilation, mucosal tears, extravasation, and thermal injury secondary to intraureteral lithotripsy. Certainly, stricture formation following ureteral dilation is a potential problem but has not been encountered very often. In several large series of patients followed for at least 6 months, no strictures have been identified because of the initial dilation (Lyon et al., 1984; Stackl and Marberger, 1986). Ureteral wall fibrosis could lead to stricture formation. Fibrosis may occur after a mucosal injury or urinary extravasation.

EHL, ultrasonic lithotripsy (Howards et al., 1974), and laser lithotripsy all have the potential of creating a thermal injury to the ureteral wall with secondary stricture formation. Each of these methods causes a local temperature elevation that, in the small confines of the ureteral lumen, may lead to thermal injury. It appears that EHL causes the greatest temperature increase. Certainly, this device has been associated with the greatest incidence of ureteral injury.

Other major determinants of ureteral injuries are poor patient selection and technique. These are more difficult to define but do play a role in many untoward events of ureteroscopy. Proper indications for intervention must be followed and safe methods employed. Inadequate dilation of the orifice and intramural ureter, or poor judgment, such as forcing an instrument or a catheter through a narrow area of the ureter, certainly may lead to injuries intraoperatively. Poor endoscopic visibility, if not corrected, may also lead to injuries. If the ureteral lumen is not visible, the chance of a misdirected instrument becomes greater. Improper or inadequate ureteral dilation prior to the procedure also increases the chance of an injury. With the advent of less traumatic balloon dilating catheters, there have been fewer perforations

of the intramural ureteral tunnel than with the metal bougie dilators (Huffman and Bagley, 1988).

Treatment of Ureteroscopic Complications

Fortunately, most ureteral injuries can be managed conservatively. The obvious exception is avulsion of the ureter, in which the treatment depends on the extent and location of the avulsion. If only the distal ureter is avulsed, a ureteral re-implant may be done with a psoas hitch or the Boari flap. With avulsion of the middle or proximal ureter, repair becomes more difficult and may require ureteral substitution with a bowel segment, autotransplantation, or nephrectomy.

Conservative or nonsurgical treatment generally suffices for other injuries (Benjamin, 1987). Once a perforation or false passage is recognized, stenting of the ureter with an internal ureteral stent or ureteral catheter will most likely allow complete resolution of the injury. If a stent or catheter cannot be inserted, it becomes necessary in most instances to insert a percutaneous nephrostomy tube, thus providing urinary diversion and drainage. Antibiotics are employed to assure sterilization of the urine. The time period of stenting or nephrostomy tube drainage is somewhat debatable; however, one acceptable approach is to divert for 6 weeks following documented perforation. Prior to removing the catheter, a contrast study is done to document complete healing.

Ureteral strictures may be managed conservatively, with endoscopic incision and balloon dilation. However, in some instances, open exploration and repair are required.

Prevention of Complications

The reports listed in Table 61–6 prove that ureteral injuries secondary to upper tract endoscopy do occur.

Table 61–7. PREVENTION OF URETEROSCOPIC INJURIES

1. Careful patient selection
2. Complete urologic work-up
3. Availability of essential instruments
4. Availability of fluoroscopy
5. Sound judgment in urologic procedures

However, several factors may lead to fewer injuries (Table 61–7). One important consideration is appropriate patient selection for ureteroscopy after a thorough evaluation. The selection should depend somewhat on individual endoscopic experience. For example, one should not treat a patient with an oversized upper ureteral calculus and attempt a difficult ureteroscopic extraction without having previously gained experience removing simpler, lower ureteral calculi.

In addition, a wide selection of instruments allows the urologist to perform the procedure more safely. An assortment of small and large caliber rigid and flexible instruments, along with a variety of baskets, forceps, and wires, provides more options if problems are encountered. The most common cause of ureteral avulsion is trying to extract a calculus that is too large for the ureter. In order to avoid this problem, a method of intraureteral lithotripsy (EHL, ultrasonic, laser) should be available.

Fluoroscopy is mandatory—a fixed, an overhead, or a C-arm unit is acceptable. Not only does fluoroscopy save time during all phases of the procedure, including balloon dilation, instrument passage, stone extraction, and stent passage, but it also adds to the margin of safety. For example, extravasation or guide wire malpositioning are detected immediately, allowing for quick intraoperative adjustments.

Sound judgment regarding endoscopic technique is imperative. One must be able to judge when to advance the instrument, when to pull on a stone in a basket, and when to terminate the procedure if necessary. Most instances of ureteral avulsion secondary to overzealous basket extractions can be avoided by good judgment based on available information and adequate experience.

SUMMARY

Kaufman reported a severe ureteral injury following ureteroscopy in 1984. His commentary summarizes the important messages in this section quite well as follows:

"The intent of this report is not to denigrate the splendid advances in nephroscopy and ureteroscopy, but rather to introduce a sobering message that the patient must be informed of the inherent risk of such procedures and that the urologist must be wary of the problems that might occur. Problems have been known ever since endoscopic instrumentation was first introduced, and every experienced urologist has had his share of problems associated with stone extraction and other endoscopic procedures. Traditional teaching in urology has been to eschew manipulation of stones in the upper two thirds of the ureter because the lumbar ureter is mobile

and more easily damaged by instrumentation than the pelvic segment. Endoscopic visualization of stones in the upper ureter allowing accurate grasping of calculi would appear at first to provide an element of security heretofore unachievable, but urologists nonetheless should be mindful of the hazards of any type of stone extraction from the upper ureter. Urologists must be ready and equipped to handle emergencies associated with new instruments and techniques, and the patients must be apprised of the exigencies. 'Caveat emptor' ([let the] buyer beware) could not be a more apt or timely maxim in our specialty."

Nonetheless, ureteroscopy has greatly aided many patients, and a large number of urologists have integrated this procedure into their daily practice. This procedure is no different than any other surgical procedure in that the urologist must be aware of the types of problems that may arise, the ways these problems can be prevented, and the type of treatments required should an injury occur.

REFERENCES

Aso, Y.: Use of flexible ureteroscopy to remove upper ureteral and renal calculi. J. Urol., 137:629–632, 1987.
Bagley, D. H.: Indications for ureteropyeloscopy. In Huffman, J., Bagley, D., and Lyon, E. (Eds.): Ureteroscopy. Philadelphia, W. B. Saunders Co., 1988a, pp. 17–30.
Bagley, D. H.: Dilation of the ureterovesical junction and ureter. In Huffman, J., Bagley, D., and Lyon, E. (Eds.): Ureteroscopy. Philadelphia, W. B. Saunders Co., 1988b, pp. 51–72.
Bagley, D. H.: Ureteropyeloscopy with flexible fiberoptic instruments. In Huffman, J., Bagley, D., and Lyon, E. (Eds.): Ureteroscopy. Philadelphia, W. B. Saunders Co., 1988c, pp. 131–155.
Bagley, D. H.: Removal of upper urinary tract calculi with flexible ureteropyeloscopy. Urology, 35:412–416, 1990.
Bagley, D. H., Huffman, J. L., and Lyon, E. S.: Flexible ureteropyeloscopy: Diagnosis and treatment in the upper urinary tract. J. Urol., 138:280–285, 1987.
Bagley, D. H., Huffman, J. L., Lyon, E. S., and McNamara, T.: Endoscopic ureteropyelostomy: opening the obliterated ureteropelvic junction with nephroscopy and flexible ureteropyeloscopy. J. Urol., 133:462, 1985.
Bakke, A., and Ulvik, N. M.: Ureterorenoscopy in pregnancy. Scand. J. Urol. Nephrol. (Suppl.), 110:243–244, 1988.
Benjamin, J. C., Donaldson, P. J., and Hill, J. T.: Ureteric perforation after ureteroscopy—conservative management. Urology, 29:623–624, 1987.
Biester, R., and Gillenwater, J. Y.: Complications following ureteroscopy. J. Urol., 136:380, 1986.
Blute, M. L., Segura, J. W., and Patterson, D. E.: Ureteroscopy. J. Urol., 139:510–512, 1988.
Bulger, R. E.: The urinary system. In Weiss, L. (Ed.): Histology—Cell and Tissue Biology. New York, Elsevier Biomedical, 1983, pp. 869–913.
Bush, I. M., Goldberg, E., Javadpour, N., Chakrobortty, H., and Morelli, F.: Ureteroscopy and renoscopy: a preliminary report. Chicago Med. School Q., 30:46, 1970.
Carter, S. St. C., Cox, R., and Wickham, J. E. A.: Complications associated with ureteroscopy. Br. J. Urol., 58:625–628, 1986.
Cass, A. S., Smith, C. S., and Gleich, P.: Management of urinary calculi in pregnancy. Urology, 28:370–372, 1986.
Chang, R., and Marshall, F. F.: Management of ureteroscopic injuries. J. Urol., 137:1132–1135, 1987.
Chaussy, C., Fuchs, G., Kahn, R., Hunter, P., and Goodfriend, R.: Transurethral ultrasonic ureterolithotripsy using a solid wire probe. Urology, 29:531–532, 1987.
Clayman, R. V., Basler, J. W., Kavoussi, L., and Picus, D. D.: Ureteronephroscopic endopyelotomy. J. Urol., 144:246–252, 1990.

Coptcoat, M. J., Webb, D. R., Kellett, M. J., Whitfield, H. N., and Wickham, J. E. A.: The treatment of 100 consecutive patients with ureteral calculi in a British stone center. J. Urol., 137:1122–1123, 1987.

Davis, J. E., Hagedoorn, J. P., and Bergmann, L. L.: Anatomy and ultrastructure of the ureter. *In* Bergmann, H. (Ed.): The Ureter. New York, Springer-Verlag, 1981, pp. 55–70.

Denstedt, J. D., and Clayman, R. V.: Electrohydraulic lithotripsy of renal and ureteral calculi. J. Urol., 143:13, 1990.

Dourmashkin, R. L.: Dilatation of the ureter with rubber bags in the treatment of ureteral calculi. Presentation of a modified operating cystoscope. A preliminary report. J. Urol., 15:449, 1926.

Dourmashkin, R. L.: Cystoscopic treatment of stones in the ureter with special reference to large calculi: based on the study of 1550 cases. J. Urol., 54:245–283, 1945.

Dretler, S. P.: An evaluation of ureteral laser lithotripsy: 225 consecutive patients. J. Urol., 143:267–273, 1990.

Dretler, S. P., and Cho, G.: Semirigid ureteroscopy: A new genre. J. Urol., 141:1314, 1989.

Dretler, S. P., Watson, G., Parrish, J. A., and Murray, S.: Pulsed-dye laser fragmentation of ureteral calculi: Initial clinical experience. J. Urol., 137:386, 1987.

El-Kappany, H., Gaballah, M. A., and Ghonheim, M. A.: Rigid ureteroscopy for the treatment of ureteric calculi: Experience in 120 cases. Br. J. Urol., 58:499–503, 1986.

Epple, W., and Reuter, H.: Ureterorenoscopy for diagnosis and therapy. Presented at XXth Congress Societe Internationale d'Urologie. Vienna, June, 1985.

Ford, T. F., Parkinson, M. C., and Wickham, J. E. A.: Clinical and experimental evaluation of ureteric dilatation. Br. J. Urol., 56:460–463, 1984a.

Ford, T. F., Payne, S. R., and Wickham, J. E. A.: The impact of transurethral ureteroscopy on the management of ureteric calculi. Br. J. Urol., 56:602–603, 1984b.

Ghoneim, M. A., and El-Kappany, H. A.: Ureteroscopy for the treatment of ureteral calculi. Presented at XXth Congress Societe Internationale d'Urologie. Vienna, June, 1985.

Gittes, R. F., and Varaday, S.: Nephroscopy in chronic unilateral hematuria. J. Urol., 126:2297, 1981.

Goodfriend, R.: Ultrasonic and electrohydraulic lithotripsy of ureteral calculi. Urology, 23:5–8, 1984.

Goodman, T. M.: Ureteroscopy with pediatric cystoscope in adults. Urology, 9:394, 1977.

Gray, H.: The urogenital system. *In* Goss, C. M. (Ed.): Anatomy of the Human Body. Philadelphia, Lea & Febiger, 1973, pp. 1265–1339.

Green, D. F., and Lytton, B.: Early experience with electrohydraulic lithotripsy of ureteral calculi using direct vision ureteroscopy. J. Urol., 133:767, 1985.

Greene, L. F.: The renal and ureteral changes induced by dilating the ureter. An experimental study. J. Urol., 52:505–521, 1944.

Hill, D. E., Segura, J. W., Patterson, D. E., and Kramer, S. A.: Ureteroscopy in children. J. Urol., 144:481–483, 1990.

Hopkins, H. H.: British patent 954,629, and U.S. patent 3,257,902; 1960.

Hosking, D. H., and Ramsey, E. W.: Rigid transurethral ureteroscopy. Br. J. Urol., 58:621–624, 1984.

Howards, S. S., Merrill, E., Harris, S., and Cohn, J.: Ultrasonic lithotripsy. Invest. Urol., 2:273–277, 1974.

Huffman, J. L.: Early experience with the 8.5 Fr. compact ureteroscope. Surg. Endosc., 3:164–166, 1989a.

Huffman, J. L.: Ureteroscopic injuries of the urinary tract. Urol. Clin. North Am., 16:45–65, 1989b.

Huffman, J. L.: Approach to upper tract calculi. *In* Huffman, J., Bagley, D., and Lyon, E. (Eds.): Ureteroscopy. Philadelphia, W. B. Saunders Co., 1988a, p. 85.

Huffman, J. L.: Ureteroscopic management of transitional call carcinoma of the upper urinary tract. Urol. Clin. North Am., 15:419–424, 1988b.

Huffman, J. L.: Preparation for a ureteroscopic procedure. *In* Huffman, J., Bagley, D., and Lyon, E. (Eds.): Ureteroscopy. Philadelphia, W. B. Saunders Co., 1988c, pp. 41–49.

Huffman, J. L., and Bagley, D. H.: Balloon dilation of the ureter for ureteroscopy. J. Urol., 140:954–956, 1988.

Huffman, J. L., Bagley, D. H., and Lyon, E. S.: Treatment of distal ureteral stones using a rigid ureteroscope. Urology, 20:574, 1982.

Huffman, J. L., Bagley, D. H., and Lyon, E. S.: Extending cystoscopic techniques into the ureter and renal pelvis—experience with ureteroscopy and pyeloscopy. JAMA, 250:2004, 1983.

Huffman, J. L., Bagley, D. H., and Lyon, E. S.: Normal anatomy of the ureter and kidney. *In* Bagley, D. H., Huffman, J. L., and Lyon, E. S. (Eds.): Urologic Endoscopy—A Manual and Atlas. Boston, MA, Little, Brown and Co., 1985a, pp. 13–18.

Huffman, J. L., Bagley, D. H., and Lyon, E. S.: Ureteral catheterization, retrograde ureteropyelography and self-retaining ureteral stents. *In* Bagley, D. H, Huffman, J. L., Lyon, E. S. (Eds.). Urologic Endoscopy—A Manual and Atlas. Boston, MA, Little, Brown and Co., 1985b, pp. 163–176.

Huffman, J. L., Bagley, D. H., Schoenberg, H. W., and Lyon, E. S.: Transurethral removal of large ureteral and renal pelvic calculi using ureteroscopic ultrasonic lithotripsy. J. Urol., 130:31–34, 1983.

Huffman, J. L., Morse, M. J., Bagley, D. H., Herr, H. W., Lyon, E. S., and Whitmore, W. F., Jr.: Endoscopic diagnosis and treatment of upper tract urothelial tumors—a preliminary report. Cancer, 55:1422–1428, 1985.

Inglis, J. A., and Tolley, D. A.: Ureteroscopic pyelolysis for pelviureteric junction obstruction. Br. J. Urol., 58:250, 1986.

Kahn, R. I.: Endourological treatment of ureteral calculi. J. Urol., 135:239, 1986.

Kaufman, J. J.: Ureteroscopic injury. Urology, 23:267–269, 1984.

Keating, M. A., Heney, N. M., Young, H. H., II, Kerr, W. S., Jr., O'Leary, M. P., and Dretler, S. P.: Ureteroscopy—the initial experience. J. Urol., 135:689–693, 1986.

Khuri, F. J., Peartree, R. J., Ruotolo, R. A., and Valvo, J. R.: Rigid ureteropyeloscopy. NY State J. Med., 85:205, 1985.

Killeen, K. P., and Bihrle, W.: Ureteroscopic removal of retained ureteral double-J stents. Urology, 35:354–359, 1990.

Kramolowsky, E. V.: Ureteral perforation during ureteroscopy. J. Urol., 138:36–38, 1987.

Lewis, B.: Trans. Am. Assoc. G.U. Surgeons, 1:124, 1906.

Lyon, E. S., Banno, J. J., and Schoenberg, H. W.: Transurethral ureteroscopy in men using juvenile cystoscopy equipment. J. Urol., 122:152, 1979.

Lyon, E. S., Huffman, J. L., and Bagley, D. H.: Ureteroscopy and pyeloscopy. Urology (Suppl.), 23:29, 1984.

Lyon, E. S., Kyker, J. S., and Schoenberg, H. W.: Transurethral ureteroscopy in women: a ready addition to urologic armamentarium. J. Urol., 119:35, 1978.

Lytton, B., Weiss, R. M., and Green, D. F.: Complication of ureteral endoscopy. J. Urol., 137:649–653, 1987.

Markee, J. E.: The urogenital system. *In* Anson, B. J. (Ed.): Morris' Human Anatomy. New York, McGraw-Hill, 1966, pp. 1457–1537.

Marshall, V. F.: Fiberoptics in urology. J. Urol., 91:110, 1964.

Miller, R. A., and Wickham, J. E. A.: Percutaneous nephrolithotomy: advances in equipment and endoscopic techniques. Urology (Suppl.), 23:2, 1984.

Newman, R. C., Hunter, P. T., Hawkins, I. F., and Finlayson, B.: A general ureteral dilator-sheathing system. Urology, 25:287, 1985.

Perez-Castro, E.: Ureteromat: method to facilitate ureterorenoscopy and avoid dilation. Urol. Clin. North Am., 15:315, 1988.

Perez-Castro, E., and Martinez-Pineiro, J. A.: Transurethral ureteroscopy—A current urological procedure. Arch. Esp. Urol., 33:445, 1980.

Raney, A. M., and Handler, J.: Electrohydraulic nephrolithotripsy. Urology, 6:439, 1975.

Rittenberg, M. H., and Bagley, D. H.: Ureteroscopic diagnosis and treatment of urinary calculi during pregnancy. Urology, 32:427–428, 1988.

Schoborg, T. W.: Efficacy of electrohydraulic and laser lithotripsy in the ureter. J. Endourol., 3:361, 1989.

Schultz, A., Kristenson, J. K., Bilde, T., and Eldrup, J.: Ureteroscopy: Results and complications. J. Urol., 137:865–866, 1987.

Seeger, A. R., Rittenberg, M. H., and Bagley, D. H.: Ureteropyeloscopic removal of ureteral calculi. J. Urol., 139:1180–1183, 1988.

Sosa, R. E., and Huffman, J. L.: Complications of ureteroscopy. *In* Huffman, J. L., Bagley, D. H., and Lyon, E. S. (Eds.): Ureteroscopy. Philadelphia, W. B. Saunders Co., 1988, p. 157.

Sosa, R. E., Huffman, J. L., Riehle, R. A., and Vaughan, E. D.:

Ureteropyeloscopy: Pitfalls and early complications of ureteral stone extraction. Presented at XXth Congress Societe Internationale d'Urologie. Vienna, June, 1985.

Stackl, W., and Marberger, M.: Late sequelae of the management of ureteral calculi with the ureterorenoscope. J. Urol., 136:386–389, 1986.

Streem, S. B., Pontes, J. E., Novick, A. C., and Montie, J.: Ureteropyeloscopy in the evaluation of upper tract filling defects. J. Urol., 136:383, 1986.

Takayasu, H., and Aso, Y.: Recent development for pyeloureteroscopy: Guide tube method for its introduction into the ureter. J. Urol., 112:176, 1974.

Takagi, T., Go, T., Takayasu, H., and Aso, Y.: Fiberoptic pyeloureteroscope. Surgery, 70:661, 1971.

Takagi, T., Go, T., Takayasu, H., and Hioki, R.: Small caliber fiberscope for visualization of the urinary tract, biliary tract, and spinal canal. Surgery, 64:1933, 1968.

Tolley, D. H., and Beynon, L. L.: Ureteroscopy. Br. J. Urol., 57:281–283, 1985.

Verlando, J. T.: Histology of the ureter. In Bergmann, H. (Ed.): The Ureter. New York, Springer-Verlag, 1981, pp. 13–54.

Watson, G. M., and Wickham, J. E. A.: Initial experience with a pulsed-dye laser for ureteric calculi. Lancet, 1:1357, 1986.

Willscher, M. K., Conway, J. F., Babayan, R. K., Morisseau, P., Sant, G. R., and Bertagnoll, A.: Safety and efficacy of electrohydraulic lithotripsy by ureteroscopy. J. Urol., 140:957–958, 1988.

Young, H. H., and McKay, R. W.: Congenital valvular obstruction of the prostatic urethra. Surg. Gynecol. Obstet., 48:509, 1929.

APPENDIX A

Rigid Ureteroscopy Instruments

Ultrasonic Lithotripsy Probes

Karl Storz Endoscopy: 2.5 mm (hollow); 1 mm (solid)
Richard Wolf Medical Instruments: 1.5 mm, 1.9 mm, 2.4 mm (hollow) (long and short lengths)
Circon ACMI: 1.8 mm (hollow)
Olympus: 1.5 mm (hollow) (long and short lengths)

Rigid Ureteroscopes—Long

Circon ACMI
Sheaths (interchangeable): 10 Fr. (0) and 12 Fr. (5)
Telescopes: 5-degree–straight
Integral sheath with Rigi-Flex, 5-degree telescope 12.7 Fr. (5.4/5 Fr.)
Integral sheath with straight, 5-degree telescope 6.9 Fr. (3.4/2.3 Fr.)

Rigid Ureteroscopes—Short

Sheaths (interchangeable): 10 Fr. (0), 12 Fr. (5)
Telescopes: 5-degree–straight
Integral sheath with Rigi-Flex, 5-degree telescope 12.7 Fr. (5.4/5 Fr.)
Resectoscope sheath (long and short): 12 Fr.
Electrodes: cutting and hook
Blades: cold knife

Candela
Miniscope: 7.2 to 11.9 Fr. (2.1/2.1 Fr.)

Rigid Ureteroscopes—Long

Olympus
Sheaths (interchangeable): 11 Fr. (3) and 13.5 Fr. (5/4)
Telescopes: 0- and 70-degree–straight and 0-degree Vari-flex

Rigid Ureteroscopes—Short

Sheaths (interchangeable): 10.5 Fr. (0), 11 Fr. (3), 13.5 Fr. (5/4 Fr.)
Telescopes: 0- and 70-degree–straight and 0-degree Vari-flex
Ureterotome sheath: 13.5 Fr. (3)
Blades: stricture/scalpel (long and short)

Rigid Ureteroscopes—Long

Karl Storz Endoscopy
Sheaths (interchangeable): 11.5 Fr. (4), 13.5 Fr. (5), 14 Fr. (6)
Telescopes: 6- and 70-degree–straight and 6-degree–angled
Integral sheaths with 6-degree telescope
   11.5 Fr. (4)–straight
   11.0 Fr. (3.7)–angled
   12.5 Fr. (6)–angled
   9.5 Fr. (4)–adjustable
Resectoscope sheath: 12 Fr.
Electrodes: cutting and coagulation
Blades: Cold knife

Rigid Ureteroscopes—Short

Sheaths (interchangeable) 11.5 Fr. (4) and 14 Fr. (6)
Telescopes: 6-degree–straight and 6-degree–angled

Rigid Ureteroscopes—Long

Richard Wolf Medical Instruments
Sheaths (interchangeable): 10.5 Fr. (3.5), 11.5 Fr.(5/3), 12.5 Fr. (5/3), 13.5 Fr. (6), 12.5 Fr. (5) (continuous flow)
Telescopes: 5-, 25-, 70-degree–straight and 5-degree–offset
Resectoscope sheath: 12 Fr.
Ureterotome sheath: 12 Fr.
Electrodes: hook, cutting, and coagulation
Blades: stricture scalpel, half-moon blade
Albarron bridge: 13.5 Fr. sheath only
Integral sheaths with 5-degree telescope:
   6.0 Fr. (3.3)–straight
   8.5 Fr. (3.5)–straight
   9.5 Fr. (5) –straight
   11.5 Fr. (5/3)–offset
Rigid Ureteroscopes—Short
Sheaths (interchangeable): 10.5 Fr. (3.5), 11.5 Fr. (5/3), 12.5 Fr. (5/3), 13.5 Fr. (6), 12.5 Fr. (5) continuous flow
Telescopes: 5-degree–straight and 5-degree–offset
Integral sheath with straight 5-degree telescope: 9.5 Fr. (5)

APPENDIX B

Flexible Ureteroscopes

A. Passively Deflectable

Manufacturer	Sheath size (Fr.)	Channel size (Fr.)	Deflection (Degrees)
Baxter	7	3.2	0
Microvasive	6	1.5 & 2.8	0
	8.5	1.5 & 3.2	0
	10	1.5 & 6.0	0
Storz	7	1.5	0
	9	3.5	0
Surgitek	7	1.5	0
	9	3.5	0
Wolf	7	1.5	0
	9	1.5	0

B. Actively Deflectable

Circon ACMI	9.8	3.6	160
	8.5	2.5	160
Olympus	10.8	3.6	100 & 160
	12.3	6.0	100 & 160
Storz	10.5	3.6	100 & 180
Surgitek	11.9	4.0	100 & 160
Wolf	12.0	4.2	90 & 180
	10.5	3.6	90 & 180

62

ENDOSURGICAL TECHNIQUES FOR THE DIAGNOSIS AND TREATMENT OF NONCALCULOUS DISEASE OF THE URETER AND KIDNEY

Ralph V. Clayman, M.D.
Louis R. Kavoussi, M.D.

MAGIC BULLETS AND THE CRAFT OF SURGERY

In 1910, Paul Ehrlich introduced the modern age of medicine with his concept of the "magic bullet": a drug (in this case salvarsan 606) capable of eradicating a disease process (syphilis) without harming the patient (Lyons and Petrucelli, 1978). Today, there is an extensive pharmacologic armamentarium that is capable of eliminating a variety of *systemic* diseases while incurring minimal or no damage to healthy tissues.

Traditionally, when surgical therapy is applied to disease affecting intra-abdominal organs, the price of this form of therapy is the creation of a large wound through normal tissue in order to access the site of disease. Oftentimes, the operation is indeed a "success" but the patient succumbs or is injured because of complications from establishing access to the site of illness: wound dehiscence, fasciitis, infection, and incisional hernia. Similarly, the pain, discomfort, and requisite lengthy convalescence of incisional surgery are again not disease related but rather related to the means of entry and exit from the area of disease.

Today, in urology and in many other surgical specialties, incisional surgery is being replaced by endoscopic

surgery (Wickham, 1987). Disease access is being achieved using rigid or flexible endoscopes passed along natural pathways (e.g., ureter, urethra, vein, artery, esophagus) or through keyhole incisions (Fig. 62–1). Surgical therapy is being rendered with diminutive instrumentation capable of incising and excising tissue or concretions, using electrocautery and ultrasonic, electrohydraulic, or laser energy. Indeed, fully 70 to 80 per cent of urologic practice has already become endoscopic in nature.

INSTRUMENTS OF CHANGE

The development of endosurgery in urology has been dependent on advances in three areas: *endoscopy* (rigid and flexible), *radiologic imaging,* and *miniaturization of endoscopic equipment* (e.g., electrocautery probes, lithotriptors, lasers). From these areas, the urologist has fashioned gun, sight, and bullet, thereby enabling one to target and treat a variety of surgical diseases affecting the upper urinary tract.

Advances in *radiologic imaging* of the urinary tract have been essential to the development of endosurgery. It is the newer imaging techniques in fluoroscopy, ultrasonography, and computed tomography that have given the urologist the ability to accurately locate and identify various conditions affecting the upper urinary tract and to access the kidney via either a percutaneous nephrostomy or ureteroscope.

This chapter is dedicated to Arthur D. Smith, whose energy, enthusiasm, and creativity provided the initial ongoing impetus to the field of endourology and whose advice remains a constant stimulus: "You're only as good as tomorrow."

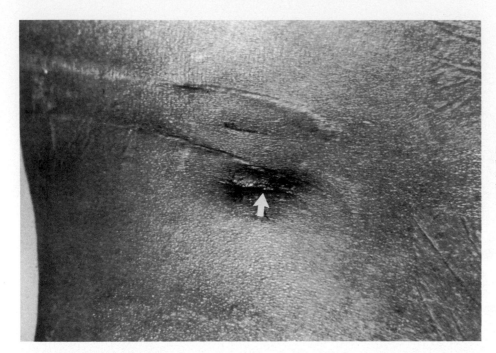

Figure 62–1. Flank incision in patient after two open nephrolithotomies compared with a minute incision *(arrow)* following percutaneous nephrolithotomy.

These advances in imaging were essential to the development and refinement of percutaneous renal access. In 1955, Goodwin, Casey, and Woolfe reported their initial experience with a percutaneous nephrostomy to drain an obstructed collecting system. Over the ensuing 20 years, marked advances in fluoroscopy and subsequently ultrasonography occurred such that by the early 1970s, percutaneous nephrostomy had largely replaced operative nephrostomy (Stables et al., 1971).

Subsequently, in 1976, Fernstrom and Johansson first utilized a fluoroscopically developed, percutaneous nephrostomy tract as a means of surgical access to the kidney for removal of a renal calculus. Currently, the nephrostomy tract has been adapted as a means of surgical access to a wide range of upper urinary tract diseases: strictures; renal cysts; calyceal diverticula; and, in rare cases, upper tract transitional cell cancer.

Fluoroscopy is also essential to the efficient and accurate use of the nephroscope and ureteroscope, particularly when examining the renal calyces. The intricacies of the intrarenal collecting system are such that a radiologic map is necessary both to plan a route to a particular calyx and to assess the completeness of an examination of the renal collecting system (Fig. 62–2). In this manner, the fluoroscope complements the nephroscope and ureteroscope, as it provides an ongoing dynamic localization of the endoscope within the renal landscape. The endoscope provides the visual detail of the surrounding urothelium of each infundibulum and calyx.

These advances in imaging capabilities were contemporary with developments in antegrade and retrograde endoscopy of the upper urinary tract. For viewing the kidney via the nephrostomy tract, specific side-viewing *rigid endoscopes* were developed along with lighter and smaller straight rigid endoscopes. However, even with the smallest rigid endoscopes, visualization of the collecting system was limited to the renal pelvis, ureteropelvic junction, and one or rarely two major calyces

(Wickham and Miller, 1983). This problem was subsequently overcome by the adaption for urologic use of *flexible fiberoptic* endoscopes. These were already developed for examination of the pulmonary tree and the biliary system. Thus, flexible bronchoscopes and choledochoscopes were passed into the nephrostomy tract in order to examine the entire renal collecting system. Within a few years, purpose-built flexible nephroscopes became available (Fig. 62–3) (Clayman, 1984).

Simultaneously with the endoscopic developments in antegrade nephroscopy, Lyon and associates, in 1978 and 1979, began their important studies in ureteroscopy employing pediatric cystoscopes to explore the distal ureter. Soon thereafter, in 1980, Perez-Castro and Martinez-Pineiro published their experience with a long rigid ureteroscope capable of examining the proximal ureter, renal pelvis, and upper pole calyces. However, as with rigid antegrade nephroscopy, retrograde ureteronephroscopy was limited by the rigid nature of the endoscope.

In order to overcome the physical limitations of rigid ureteroscopy, flexible fiberoptic endoscopes of 3.6 to 10.5 Fr. were produced (Bagley, 1987). At first, these endoscopes had a *passive* deflection system (Preminger and Kennedy, 1987). As such, the urologist could see the proximal ureter, renal pelvis, and upper pole calyces, but deflection of the endoscope into the middle or lower pole calyces could be done only by passing it over a preplaced guide wire. To overcome this problem, *active* deflection of the tip of the flexible endoscope was needed (Fig. 62–4). Initially, this feature necessitated the production of flexible ureteroscopes of impractically large size: 13 Fr. (Kavoussi and Clayman, 1989). However, with further refinements in the components of the fiberoptic bundle (development of 20-μ light-carrying fibers and 10-μ image-carrying fibers), 8.5 to 11.9 Fr. ureteronephroscopes with active tip deflection (arc of 160 to 180 degrees in one direction), secondary passive deflec-

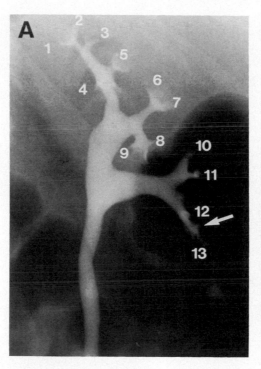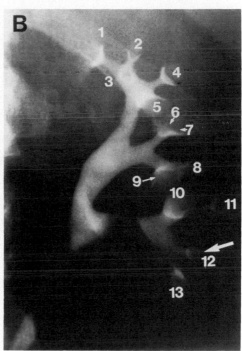

Figure 62–2. *A,* Anteroposterior view of renal collecting system. *B,* Oblique views of upper urinary tract are helpful when performing flexible nephroscopy or flexible ureteroscopy. Note how some of the calyces are better seen on the oblique view. Calyces 9 and 12 *(arrows)* are better seen in the oblique view.

tion, and working/irrigation channels of 2.6 to 4 Fr. became available (Kavoussi and Clayman, 1989). As a result, flexible ureteronephroscopy currently enables the urologist to visualize the entire calyceal collecting system in 65 to 85 per cent of patients (Bagley, 1987; Kavoussi et al., 1989).

In order to apply these new found access routes and endoscopes to the treatment of urologic disease processes, the urologist needed one further development: *diminutive (< 2 mm in diameter) auxiliary equipment.* These instruments fall into two broad categories: excisional and incisional. To completely or partially excise pathologic conditions, such as tumors or calculi in the kidney and ureter, the following instruments are available: resectoscope loops (only for the rigid 12.5 Fr. therapeutic ureteroscope), 2 Fr. stone baskets, 2.5 Fr., three-prong grasping forceps, 3 Fr. biopsy forceps, 3 Fr. retrieval forceps (rat tooth, alligator, mouse tooth), 2 Fr. two-prong grasping forceps, 2.4 Fr. ultrasonic lith-

otripsy probes (for rigid ureteroscopes only), 1.6 and 1.9 Fr. electrohydraulic lithotripsy probes, and 0.75 Fr. tunable dye laser lithotripsy probes. For the incision and fulguration of tissue, there are 4.5 Fr. cold knives (for rigid ureteroscopes only), 2 Fr. electrocautery probes with a 250-micron cutting tip, 1.2 Fr. neodymium-yttrium-aluminum-garnet (Nd:YAG) probes, and 1.2 Fr. potassium-titanyl-phosphate (KTP) laser probes (Clayman and Bagley, 1990).

METAMORPHOSIS OF UROLOGIC SURGERY

Bozzini's lichtleiter, developed in 1805, was the initial instrumentation in the realm of endoscopic urologic surgery. Impractical, cumbersome, and dangerous it took almost a century until Nitze in 1877 could create a more practical endoscope for exploring the lower urinary

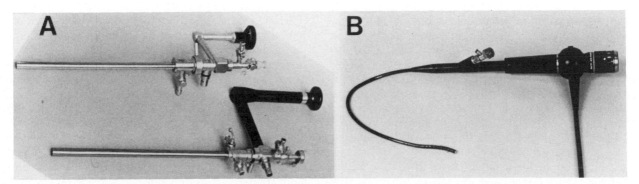

Figure 62–3. *A,* These rigid nephroscopes developed for nephroscopy are lighter than traditional cystoscopes. The tip of the endoscope is rounded to minimize the chance of perforating the intrarenal collecting system. The right angle viewing system keeps the central portion of the endoscope open for the direct introduction of the rigid ultrasound probe. *B,* Purpose-built flexible nephroscope with an outer diameter of 15 Fr. and a working port of 6 Fr. The tight turning radius allows for inspection of most or all of the upper urinary tract.

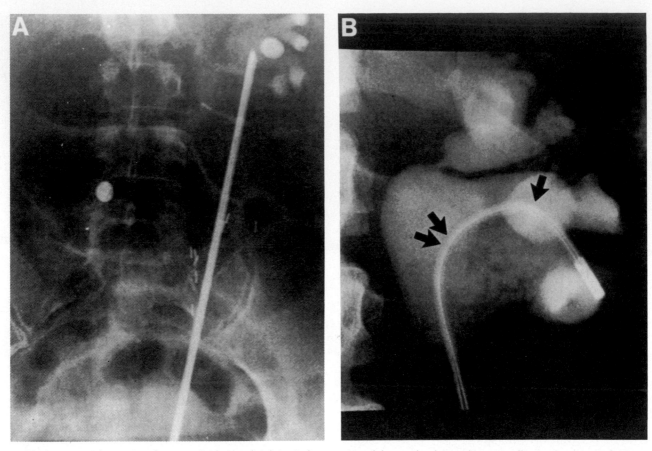

Figure 62–4. *A,* A rigid ureteronephroscope in the renal pelvis. Only a portion of the renal pelvis and upper collecting system can be inspected with this instrument. *B,* Flexible, deflectable ureteronephroscope allowing complete visualization of the pelvis and calyces (*one arrow,* primary active deflection; *two arrows,* secondary, passive deflection).

tract. The modern age of rigid cystoscopy began in the late 1940s and early 1950s, with the development of the electrocautery transurethral resectoscope and the discovery of the rod lens system and fiberoptic imaging/light-carrying technology of Harold Hopkins (Desnos, 1972; Wickham and Miller, 1983).

During the past 185 years, there has been a steady transition in the *lower* urinary tract from open to minimally invasive endoscopic procedures. Today, many lower tract, open surgical procedures have been supplanted by transurethral endoscopic counterparts: prostatectomy, cystolithotomy, suprapubic bladder drainage, urethroplasty, bladder neck contracture repair, and bladder tumor excision. This trend continues as urologists explore newer transurethral therapies for other urologic problems: transurethral fulguration and/or incision of bladder diverticula and injection of polytetrafluoroethylene (Polytef) or glutaraldehyde cross-linked bovine collagen to treat stress incontinence and ureteral reflux (Leonard et al., 1990; Orandi, 1977; Politano, 1978).

These "instruments of change" have also affected the treatment of the *upper* urinary tract; however, the transition has been more rapid. Indeed, in the past decade, minimally invasive endoscopic/fluoroscopic technology has replaced many formerly open surgical procedures: renal exploration for indeterminate masses,

renal and ureteral lithotomy, nephrostomy, renal cyst treatment, drainage of retroperitoneal collections (abscess and urinoma), and treatment of renal artery stenosis. Currently, other upper tract endoscopic therapies are being evaluated for the following conditions: ureteropelvic junction obstruction (both primary and secondary), infundibular stenosis, calyceal diverticula, ureteral strictures, and ureteroenteric strictures. The diagnosis and treatment of essential hematuria and the treatment of low grade, low stage transitional cell tumors of the upper urinary tract are also being considered.

In the future, endoscopic methods may be developed to deliver free tissue grafts or biologically compatible materials into the upper urinary tract for the treatment of ureteral strictures. In addition, the application of the laparoscope to urologic diseases will likely be expanded. Already, the laparoscope has been used successfully in urology to locate cryptorchid testicles, to treat symptomatic varicoceles, to perform pelvic node dissections in carcinoma of the prostate, and to remove the kidney in malignant and benign disease. Other applications of the laparoscope to ureteral and bladder pathology will likely soon follow.

Our generation of urologists is the beneficiary of the sum total of the aforementioned advances. From these tools, urologists have fashioned the gun (endoscope), sight (radiologic imaging), and bullet (auxiliary equipment) necessary to create an entirely new, minimally invasive subspecialty within urologic surgery—endourology. For urology, a "magic bullet" has come of age.

OVERVIEW

The remainder of this chapter is divided into four broad categories: percutaneous nephrostomy, diagnostic endourology, therapeutic endourology, and laparoscopy. This new technology is introduced in a developmental manner, ranging from simple to more complex procedures.

PERCUTANEOUS NEPHROSTOMY

Establishment of the percutaneous nephrostomy is essential in the treatment of acute upper urinary tract obstruction and is the first step in obtaining antegrade access to the kidney for a variety of procedures. In the treatment of upper urinary tract obstruction, the nephrostomy can be placed through any posterior calyx within the kidney. A lower pole approach is often selected, because it is usually infracostal, thereby precluding a pneumothorax/hydrothorax, and traverses the one surface (posterior-inferior) of the kidney that is not usually crossed by a major segmental renal artery. In

contrast, in performing a percutaneous therapeutic procedure (lithotomy, endopyelotomy), the precise placement of the nephrostomy site is essential to the success of the procedure. A *supracostal* puncture of the middle or upper portion of the kidney may be needed (Fig. 62–5) (Castaneda-Zuniga, 1984; Picus et al., 1986).

Patient Preparation

Prior to placement of a percutaneous nephrostomy, the urine should be sterile. In some cases, *due to the acute nature of the situation*, such as pyocalyx or pyonephrosis, a sterile urine cannot be achieved prior to emergency nephrostomy tube placement. Regardless, all patients should receive broad-spectrum parenteral antibiotics (most commonly, a cephalosporin or a combination of penicillin and aminoglycoside) prior to the nephrostomy procedure.

Also, if time permits, any bleeding diathesis or uncontrolled hypertension should be corrected before the percutaneous procedure. Anticoagulants, especially aspirin, must be stopped. The bleeding time, prothrombin time, platelet count, and partial thromboplastin time should be normal prior to proceeding. The patient should be normotensive, as this will decrease the chance of developing a perirenal hematoma or an extensive renal hemorrhage.

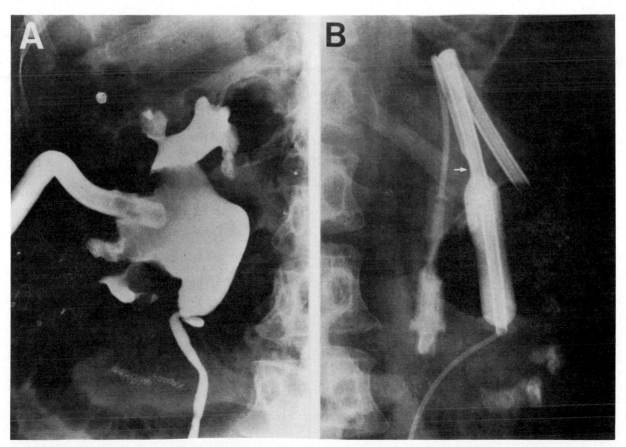

Figure 62–5. *A,* A nephrostomy tube placed percutaneously into a middle posterior calyx. *B,* At times, the nephrostomy tube may have to be placed supracostally, thus possibly traversing the pleural cavity. Note the bend in the tube *(arrow),* as it traverses over the rib. The tube shown here is a Kaye tamponade catheter.

All patients undergoing a percutaneous approach must understand the seriousness of the procedure. Accordingly, the patient should be made aware of the following potential complications: acute bleeding requiring transfusion (< 5 per cent), emergency embolization (< 0.5 per cent), possible nephrectomy (0.19 per cent), delayed hemorrhage (< 0.5 per cent), septicemia (< 1 per cent), failed access (< 5 per cent), periorgan injury (bowel perforation, splenic injury) (< 1 per cent), significant loss of functioning renal tissue (< 1 per cent), and in the case of an intercostal approach possible pleural effusion with the need for chest tube placement (12 per cent) (Picus et al., 1986).

Technique

The technique for performing a percutaneous nephrostomy is dependent on the surgeon's preference and the situation (drainage versus a percutaneous diagnostic/therapeutic procedure). With regard to the surgeon's preference, a *one-step procedure* refers to a nephrostomy and therapeutic procedure done in the operating room using the same anesthetic at the same time. A *two-step* procedure entails placement of a smaller nephrostomy tube in the radiology department followed by a nephrostomy tract dilation and a percutaneous therapeutic procedure in the operating room.

For the patient who requires a tube to drain a hydronephrotic or infected system, associated with distal obstruction, the nephrostomy procedure is quite straightforward. After giving appropriate parenteral antibiotics, the patient is moved to the fluoroscopy suite. The procedure is usually done utilizing intravenous sedation and local anesthesia.

In order to localize the hydronephrotic system, intravenous contrast material can be given. Alternatively, if the use of contrast material is contraindicated, a 22-gauge Chiba needle can be passed under ultrasonic or fluoroscopic control, approximately one or two fingerbreadths lateral to the first or second lumbar transverse process (Young, 1986a). The needle is initially passed deeply into the flank, attempting to puncture the renal pelvis. Intravenous connecting tubing is placed onto the hub of the needle; an empty 10-cc syringe is placed on the other end of the connecting tubing. As the Chiba needle is withdrawn, gentle suction is applied. When urine appears, direct instillation of contrast material will opacify the system for nephrostomy placement. Once the collecting system is visualized, a nephrostomy needle is passed via the lower pole into the collecting system (vide infra). The needle is positioned approximately four to six fingerbreadths from the spine.

In a case in which pyonephrosis is suspected, the path should be infracostal. In this situation, the only goal is to establish drainage. As such, an 0.038-inch Bentson guide wire is coiled in the system. Next, the nephrostomy tract is dilated minimally (10 Fr.). A nephrostomy tube is passed over the guide wire. Usually, a 10 Fr. or 12 Fr. pigtail catheter is secured at the skin level with two 2-0 silk sutures.

Alternatively, to facilitate the procedure, a back-loaded single stick nephrostomy system can be employed. A long, 22-gauge needle is passed through a shorter 19-gauge needle, which carries a 6 Fr. catheter (Young, 1986b). Once the collecting system is entered with the 22-gauge needle, the 19-gauge needle and then the 6 Fr. sheath can be serially slid off the nephrostomy needle, thereby establishing immediate access and drainage. If desired, the 6 Fr. catheter can be left in place; however, in most cases, the 6 Fr. catheter is used to pass a 0.035-inch guide wire into the collecting system. A *locking* Cook-Cope loop-type nephrostomy tube (8.2, 10, 12, or 14 Fr.) is positioned as the nephrostomy tube (Fig. 62–6) (Young, 1986b).

A variety of smaller nephrostomy tubes are available to drain a perirenal abscess. To drain an acutely obstructed collecting system, an 8.2 Fr. to 12 Fr. pigtail nephrostomy tube can be used (Young, 1986b). The tube comes in two basic forms: nonlocking and locking. The nonlocking tube relies upon the strength of the pigtail itself for retention (biliary urinary drainage catheter or BUD). In contrast, the locking tube has a suture running the length of the catheter. The suture exits the tip of the catheter and then re-enters the shaft of the catheter, just distal to the point where the tip is deformed as it coils to create a pigtail (see Fig. 62–6). After passage of the catheter into the collecting system, the tip is allowed to assume a pigtail configuration. The locking suture is pulled taut, thereby fixing the pigtail to the distal shaft of the nephrostomy tube.

A knob on the hub of the tube is turned 180 degrees. This action locks the suture and hence the pigtail in place. This type of tube offers excellent security; however, when removing a locking nephrostomy tube, the suture must be released by either returning the know to its neutral position or cutting the catheter and suture just below the hub. If the cutting is done, it is essential that the entire suture be retrieved along with the nephrostomy tube. If resistance is met in attempting to remove a locking nephrostomy tube, the metal obturator should be *gently* reintroduced in order to straighten the pigtail directly or as the tube is pulled backward onto the metal obturator. The metal obturator should not be forcibly introduced.

For a patient requiring a diagnostic/therapeutic nephrostomy tract, it is extremely helpful to intially place a *retrograde ureteral catheter*. The retrograde catheter may be placed with a rigid or a flexible cystoscope, with the patient in a dorsal lithotomy, supine, or prone position. In the prone position, a flexible cystoscope is used. This approach, which is more simply done in females, decreases the procedural time by 15 minutes as the patient does not need to be turned to access the flank (Clayman et al., 1987a). In addition, the prone position provides the urologist with two sterile fields: one for the ureteral catheter and one for the percutaneous nephrostomy (Fig. 62–7) (Clayman et al., 1987a). The retrograde ureteral catheter allows for opacification of the collecting system and provides for drainage of the collecting system should the procedure need to be stopped, owing to a false passage of the collecting system or an inability to place the nephrostomy tube. In addition, the retrograde ureteral catheter facilitates subse-

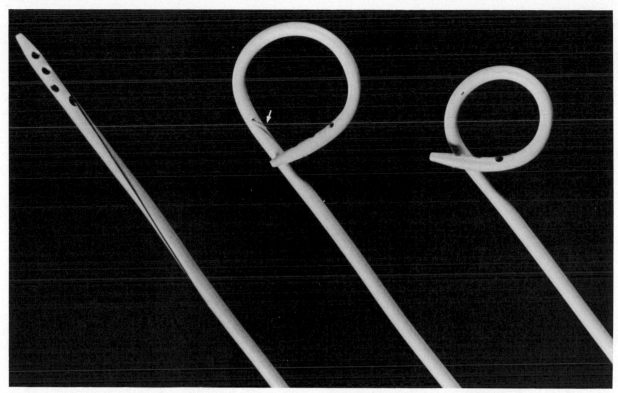

Figure 62–6. Locking pigtail nephrostomy catheter. Note the suture running the length of the locking catheter. When the catheter is in position, the obturator and guide wire, which keep the catheter straight, are removed. The pigtail that subsequently forms is locked in position by pulling on the suture (arrow) and turning a locking knob on the shaft of the catheter. The pigtail is then drawn against the shaft of the catheter and will not straighten unless the suture is released or cut.

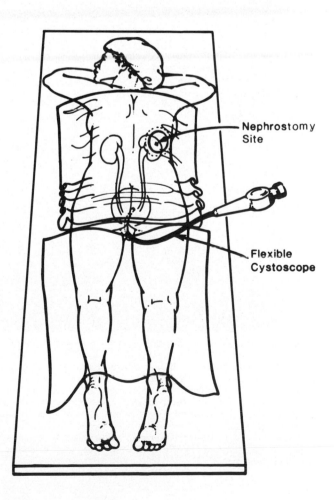

Figure 62–7. Diagram demonstrating prone flexible cystoscopy using the flexible cystoscope to pass a guide wire for percutaneous stone removal. Also note the sterile field over the planned nephrostomy site. This decreases procedural time and decreases the risk of dislodging any anesthesia monitoring equipment during the procedure. Also, the sterility of the perineal and flank field is preserved. (From Clayman, R. V., Bub, P., Haaff, E., et al.: J. Urol., 137:65, 1987. © By Williams & Wilkins, 1992.)

quent endoscopic identification of the ureteropelvic junction and provides for placement of a retrograde "through-and-through" guide wire for subsequent nephrostomy tube insertion and establishment of an antegrade ureteral catheter (Castaneda-Zuniga, 1984).

After placement of the retrograde ureteral catheter, with the patient in a *prone* position, 10 cc of room air or CO_2 is slowly instilled through the retrograde catheter, thereby outlining the posterior calyces (Fig. 62–8). Alternatively, ionic (Conray 400, i.e., 66.8 per cent sodium iothalamate) or non-ionic (Optiray 320, i.e., 68 per cent ioversal) may be used. However, because the contrast material is denser than air or urine, it will usually outline only the anterior calyces and renal pelvis in the prone patient.

The percutaneous nephrostomy is most simply and safely achieved utilizing a C-arm fluoroscopy unit (Fig. 62–9). As such, the following description applies to a *C-arm monitored procedure.* A small skin incision is

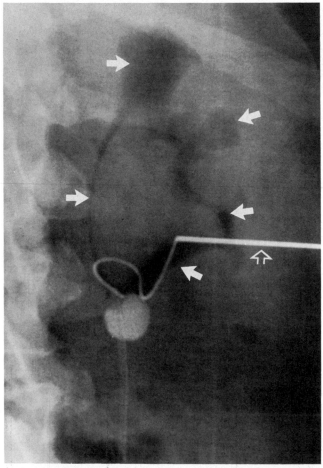

Figure 62–8. Air pyelogram. Air (5 to 10 cc) has been used to outline the collecting system *(white arrows)* in a patient with a complete staghorn calculus. Note how the air fills out the upper pole calyces, which lie superiorly and posteriorly when the patient is in the prone position. A 7 Fr. retrograde occlusion balloon catheter is in the ureter; the 11.5-mm balloon has been inflated with contrast material and pulled caudal to occlude the ureteropelvic junction. An 18-gauge nephrostomy needle *(open arrow)* has been passed into a lower pole posterior calyx. A 0.035-inch floppy tip guide wire has been passed through the nephrostomy needle. The guide wire is just beginning to coil in the renal pelvis.

made directly over the desired calyx of entry. An 18-gauge nephrostomy needle is positioned in the incision until it lies tip over hub, i.e., on the radiograph, the entire needle appears only as a radiodense dot overlying the air or contrast filled calyx. The needle is advanced in a straight path, under fluoroscopic control, for approximately 5 cm into the flank, thereby fixing its trajectory. At this point, the C-arm is rotated to a near lateral position. The lateral view of the needle makes its entire shaft and tip clearly visible. The tip of the needle can then be monitored fluoroscopically, as it is advanced toward the calyx (Fig. 62–10) (Castaneda-Zuniga, 1984).

Some resistance to passage of the needle occurs, as the renal capsule is encountered and punctured. Once the renal capsule is pierced, the needle should move with respiration because its tip resides within the renal parenchyma. As the calyx is punctured, there is again a sensation of resistance to passage of the needle followed by a "give" or loss of resistance, as the needle tip pops across the urothelium and enters the calyceal space. The needle is advanced another 1 to 2 cm, under fluoroscopic control (C-arm in lateral view position), until its tip lies in the center of the calyx (Castaneda-Zuniga, 1984).

Two other types of fluoroscopy units can be utilized for percutaneous nephrostomy: cephalocaudal movement and fixed (i.e., x-ray tube does not move) (see Fig. 62–9). These are both stationary units and less satisfactory than the C-arm, which provides the physician with multiple views of the collecting system in a variety of planes. With either stationary unit, the procedure for nephrostomy includes placement of a retrograde ureteral catheter and opacification of the collecting system as previously described. However, with the cephalocaudal or fixed fluoroscopy unit, it is necessary to roll the patient into a prone oblique position until the selected posterior calyx lies directly perpendicular to the x-ray tube. The calyx is then imaged en face. The nephrostomy needle is positioned, tip over hub (it should appear as a radiodense dot), directly over the calyx. The needle is advanced 5 cm into the flank to fix its trajectory. If a cephalocaudal unit is being employed, the x-ray tube can now be moved until the tip of the needle appears to be farthest from the calyx. The needle can be advanced under fluoroscopic control until the tip is seen to enter the calyx.

Alternatively, if a fixed fluoroscopy unit is being used, the physician must rely on the aforementioned "feel" of the needle, as it passes through the resistance of the renal capsule and urothelium to enter the "free space" of the calyx. This maneuver is significantly more difficult and requires a higher level of skill (Castaneda-Zuniga, 1984).

Ultrasonography can also be helpful in puncturing the collecting system. This technique provides for continuous real-time monitoring of the procedure in multiple planes without involving any radiation. With the ultrasound transducer, the selected calyx can be located and under continuous ultrasound monitoring, the tip of the needle can be advanced directly into the calyx (Fig. 62–11) (Thuroff and Alken, 1987). However, once the nephrostomy needle is passed into the collecting system,

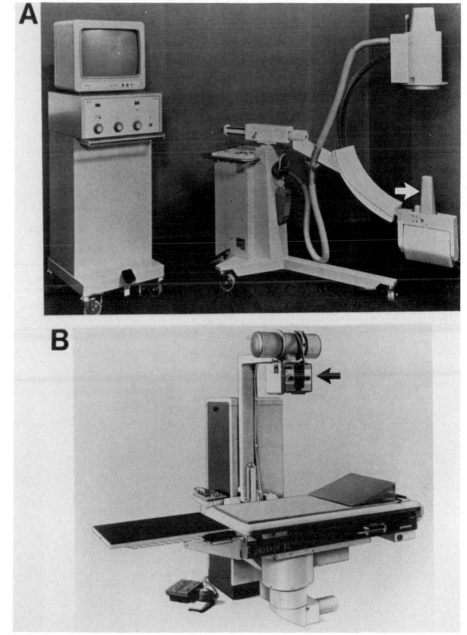

Figure 62–9. *A,* C-arm fluoroscope unit. The x-ray tube *(arrow)* is placed beneath the patient. The equipment is arranged with a last image hold and an electronic reduction. These features can decrease radiation exposure to the patient and operator by 40- and 150-fold, respectively, compared with an overhead system. *B,* In this stationary fluoroscope unit, the x-ray tube lies above the patient *(arrow),* thereby exposing the operator to significantly more radiation. The tube can only be moved in a cephalocaudal plane, thereby limiting the operator's ability to visualize the nephrostomy tract.

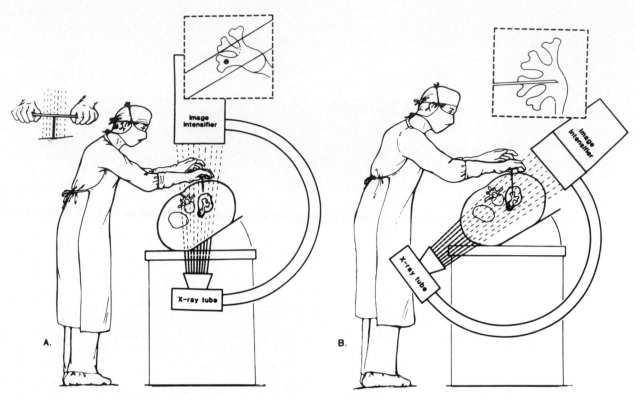

Figure 62–10. *A,* The nephrostomy needle is positioned over the desired calyx. The needle should appear as a dot on the fluoroscopy screen *(inset). B,* The calyx is lined up in the lateral view with a C-arm fluoroscope. As the needle is advanced, its path can be monitored as it enters the calyx *(inset).* (From Clayman, R. V., and Castaneda-Zuniga, W. R.: Techniques in Endourology: A Guide to Percutaneous Removal of Renal and Ureteral Calculi. Chicago, Year Book Medical Publishers, 1986.)

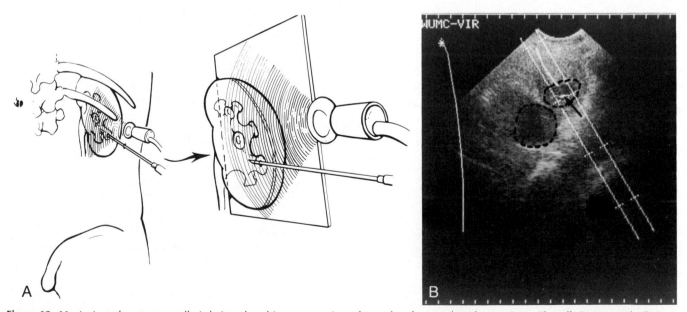

Figure 62–11. *A,* A nephrostomy needle is being placed into a posterior calyx under ultrasound guidance. (From Thuroff, D. W., and Alken, P.: Endourology, 2:1, 1987.) *B,* Ultrasound study shows the needle *(arrow)* entering a calyx *(outlined)* of a hydronephrotic kidney.

the remainder of the procedure is completed under fluoroscopic control.

After entering the collecting system, the next task is to secure a guide wire in the calyx or renal pelvis. The obturator of the needle is withdrawn, and a floppy tip guide wire (0.035-inch Bentson) or plastic guide wire (0.035-inch Terumo or glide wire) can be advanced into the collecting system and, if possible, maneuvered down the ureter. Alternatively, the guide wire can be coiled in the renal pelvis or secured in the calyx farthest from the site of entry (i.e., for a lower pole entry, the guide wire is coiled in the upper pole). The needle is removed, and a shovel-shaped 13.5 Fr. fascial incising needle is passed into the flank to cut the lumbodorsal fascia. This needle is passed twice. The second time it is rotated so that the blades are 90 degrees to the plane of the first pass. Next, semirigid plastic fascial dilators are passed (6, 8, and 10 Fr.). An 8 Fr./10 Fr. dilator/sheath assembly is introduced. The dilator is removed and through the 10 Fr. sheath, a second guide wire is passed into the collecting system (Fig. 62–12). A 5 Fr. angiographic catheter can be passed over the second guide wire. The 10 Fr. sheath is removed. The 5 Fr. angiographic catheter and the second guide wire are fixed to the skin with a 2-0 silk suture, thereby becoming the "safety guide wire and safety catheter." The remaining guide wire is now labeled the "working guide wire," as it is used for subsequent dilation of the nephrostomy tract (Castaneda-Zuniga, 1984).

Percutaneous access to the kidney may also be obtained in a *retrograde fashion* with the system developed by Hawkins and associates (1984) or by Lawson and associates (1983). In this approach, a 7 Fr. or 9 Fr. guiding ureteral catheter is passed retrograde and positioned into the calyx of interest. A 3 Fr. needle-containing catheter is then passed through the retrograde ureteral catheter. The 0.017-inch puncture wire needle is pushed through the kidney and through the retroperi-

toneal tissue, until it exits the skin of the flank. Once through-and-through access is achieved (i.e., urethral meatus to flank), dilation of the tract is similar to that for antegrade access (vide infra) (Hawkins et al., 1984; Lawson et al., 1983).

Dilation of the nephrostomy tract can be accomplished with a variety of instruments (Fig. 62–13). The semirigid Amplatz dilators or metal telescoping dilators are quite effective (Coleman, 1986; Marberger et al., 1982). Ireton (1990) has written about a modified Otis urethrotome to enlarge the nephrostomy tract. However, balloon dilation of the nephrostomy tract to 30 to 36 Fr. seems to be the quickest and safest modality (see Fig. 62–13) (Clayman et al., 1983a). The balloon dilator, often backloaded with a 30 Fr. Amplatz sheath, is passed over the working guide wire until the tip of the balloon catheter enters the calyx. The radiopaque marker on the balloon is positioned within the calyx. If this opaque marker is passed deeper into the renal pelvis, the calyceal infundibulum is unnecessarily traumatized when the balloon is inflated. The balloon is inflated with a syringe capable of developing pressures in the 10 to 12 atmospheres range (LeVeen or power injector), following which the 30 Fr. Amplatz sheath is advanced over the inflated balloon and into the collecting system (Fig. 62–14). The balloon is deflated and removed.

Alternatively, the sheath can be positioned utilizing a coaxial system. The balloon is deflated and removed, and an 8 Fr. Amplatz catheter is advanced over the working guide wire. A 28 Fr. Amplatz dilator is passed over the 8 Fr. catheter. A 28 Fr. Amplatz sheath is pushed over its 28 Fr. dilator, until the sheath enters the collecting system. The 28 Fr. dilator is removed. In passing the large 28 Fr. sheath, the tip of the sheath should just enter the collecting system. Attempts to put the sheath directly on the calculus may result in an anterior false passage of the collecting system.

After percutaneous intrarenal surgery, a nephrostomy

Figure 62–12. Introducer catheter. *A,* Safety guide wire introducer (Amplatz type) is passed over the initial guide wire. *B,* The 8 Fr. obturator is removed from the 10 Fr. sheath. *C,* The second (i.e., "working") wire is introduced through the 10 Fr. sheath of the introducer catheter. *D,* The 10 Fr. sheath of the introducer catheter. *E,* 8 Fr. obturator of the introducer catheter. (From Clayman, R. V., and Castaneda-Zuniga, W. R.: Techniques in Endourology: A Guide to Percutaneous Removal of Renal and Ureteral Calculi. Chicago, Year Book Medical Publishers, 1986.)

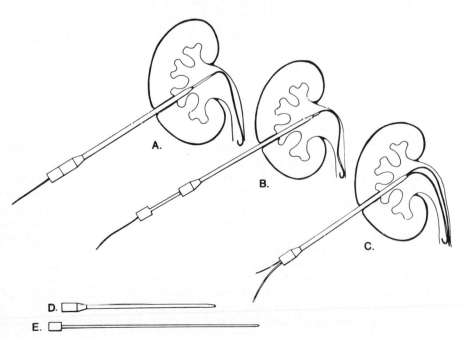

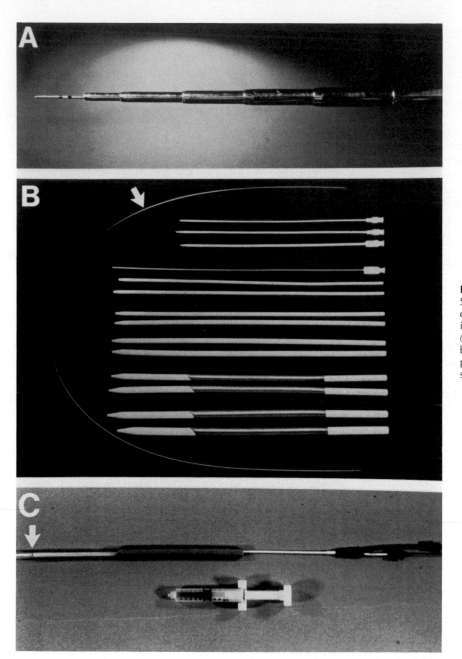

Figure 62–13. *A,* Metal telescoping dilators. *B,* Semi-rigid fascial dilators: coaxial system. After dilating to 10 Fr., each of the remaining dilators is passed over the 8 Fr., long Amplatz catheter *(arrow). C,* A 10-mm nephrostomy tract dilating balloon *(arrow)* (backloaded) with a 10-mm Amplatz sheath. A LeVeen high pressure inflation syringe is in the foreground.

tube that offers excellent drainage, retention, and tamponade is requisite. This can be achieved with a variety of catheters usually of a 22 Fr. size: Foley urethral, Malecot, or Councill. The modified Malecot catheter has an introducer that collapses the wings of the catheter to facilitate its passage; it also has an end hole, so that the catheter can be passed over a pre-existing guide wire. Likewise, the Councill catheter, with its precut end hole, can be passed directly over a guide wire.

To further secure the Councill catheter in the collecting system, it can be passed over a 5 Fr. or 7.1 Fr. straight or pigtail catheter that has in turn been passed over a pre-existing guide wire that reaches the bladder. The 5 Fr. or 7.1 Fr. catheter serves as an antegrade ureteral catheter. The Councill catheter is secured to the antegrade ureteral catheter with a side arm adapter, the end of which fits tightly into the end of the Councill catheter. The upper portion of the side arm adapter can be turned until it locks tightly onto the pigtail catheter. This ability provides two means of holding the Councill nephrostomy tube in the system: the balloon of the nephrostomy tube itself and the side arm adapter, which fixes the nephrostomy tube to the antegrade pigtail ureteral catheter. A tongue blade is taped at the juncture of the ureteral connectors, side arm adapter (where the 7.1 Fr. pigtail exits), and proximal end of the Councill catheter. This maneuver precludes any pulling on the connectors, which could dislodge the ureteral catheter. Alternatively, a one piece nephrostent can be placed. In this adaptation of a Cummings tube, the antegrade ureteral catheter is an extension of the nephrostomy portion of the catheter. When these tubes are used, the tip of the ureteral portion of the tube must enter the bladder or else the tip of the catheter will traumatize

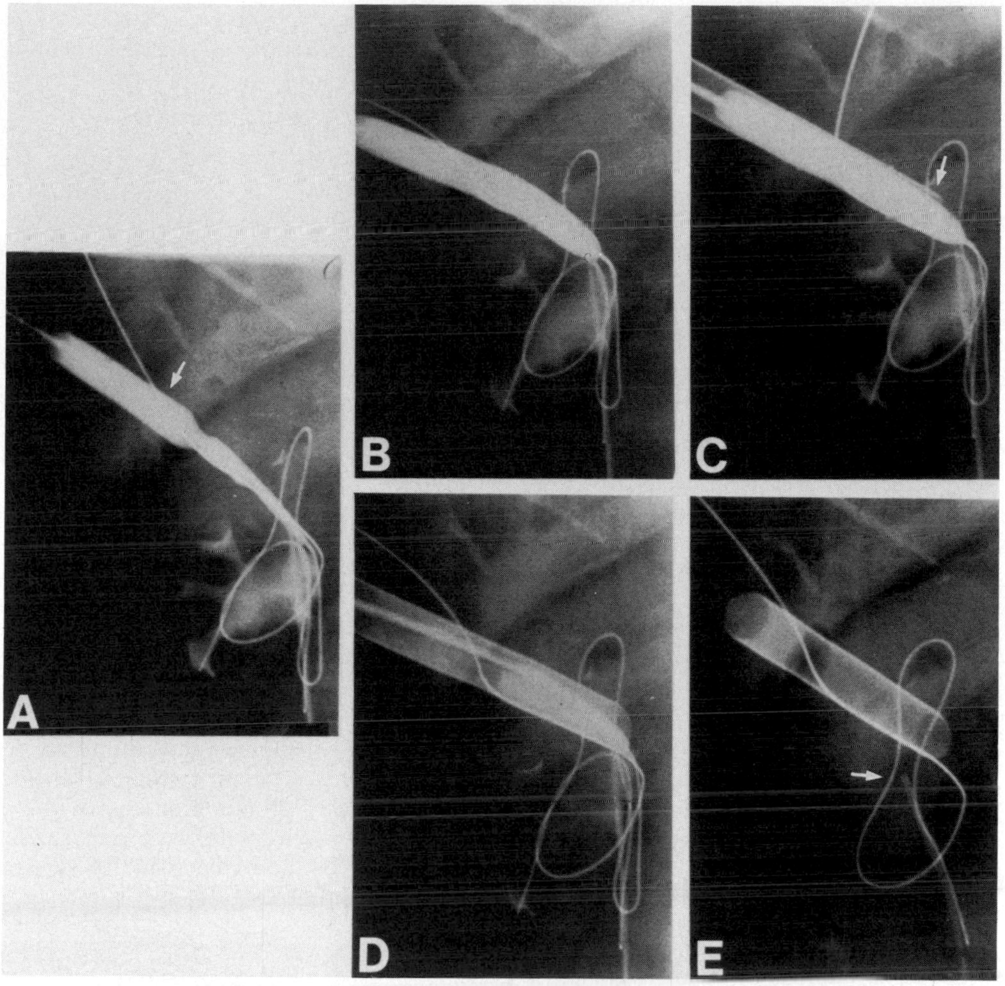

Figure 62–14. *A,* A 10-mm dilating balloon *(arrow)* is being inflated in the nephrostomy tract. *B,* The balloon has been fully inflated. *C,* Over the balloon a 30 Fr. Amplatz nephrostomy sheath *(arrow)* is advanced. *D,* After advancing the 30 Fr. sheath into the collecting system, the nephrostomy balloon is deflated and removed. *E,* The 30 Fr. sheath lies in the collecting system and provides a direct conduit to the kidney for passage of the nephroscope. The *safety* guide wire *(arrow)* lies *outside* of the Amplatz sheath. It is covered by a 5 Fr. angiographic catheter and sewn to the skin with a 2-0 silk suture.

the ureteral urothelium. Transient obstruction may then occur when the nephrostent is removed.

All nephrostomy tubes are secured to the flank. This step can be done by placing a plastic disc and tape or by sewing the tube to the flank with one or preferably two, 2-0 silk sutures. The suture method is recommended. A dressing of gauze sponges covered by laparotomy pads is placed. The dressing can be secured most simply with one large piece of adhesive cut to cover the entire dressing and flank (Cover-Roll), or it can be secured with Montgomery straps. Dense layers of adhesive tape are discouraged. They can cause marked skin irritation or blisters on removal.

With regard to nephrostomy tubes, *the one type of catheter that must always be immediately available to the urologist performing a percutaneous procedure is a 14 Fr. Kaye tamponade balloon catheter* (Fig. 62–15) (Kaye and Clayman, 1986). This particular tube is essential when brisk hemorrhage is encountered. Once placed and inflated to its full 42 Fr. size, it provides immediate and effective tamponade of the tract and satisfactory drainage of the collecting system. As with the previously described nephrostomy tube, it is recommended to pass this catheter over a pre-existing *multiholed* 5 Fr. or 7 Fr. antegrade ureteral catheter and to use a side arm adapter to secure the hub of the Kaye catheter to the ureteral catheter. To preclude kinking, the tube as it exits the skin should be smoothly draped over a roll of Kerlix. Usually, 2 days later, the Kaye tube can be deflated under fluoroscopic control. If there is no nephrostomy tract bleeding, it can be fluoroscopically exchanged for a more comfortable and smaller standard nephrostomy tube (Kaye and Clayman, 1986).

Results and Complications

Using the aforementioned antegrade or retrograde approaches, percutaneous drainage or access to the kidney can be achieved in over 90 per cent of patients (Stables et al., 1971). The complications associated with percutaneous nephrostomy, especially if performed only for drainage purposes (i.e., ≤ 10 Fr. nephrostomy tract), are minimal and usually minor in nature. The problems increase when therapeutic endosurgical procedures necessitate a larger (28 to 30 Fr.) nephrostomy tract, an extensive intrarenal manipulation, or a supracostal approach. Complications directly attributable to the establishment of a larger nephrostomy tract include the following: hemorrhage, perforation (i.e., false passage) of the renal parenchyma or collecting system, pneumothorax/hydrothorax, infection, injury to neighboring organs, allergic reaction to contrast medium, acute loss of the nephrostomy tract, and dislodgement of the nephros-

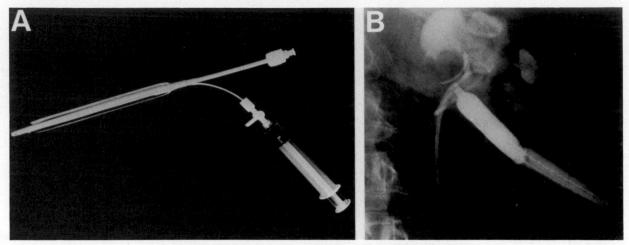

Figure 62–15. *A*, A 14 Fr. Kaye tamponade balloon is critical when performing percutaneous work. When bleeding is encountered it can be inflated to 42 Fr. to provide immediate hemostasis with satisfactory drainage of the collecting system. This tube should be dressed over a gauze roll to avoid kinking. *B*, Kaye tamponade balloon entering the lower pole of the kidney.

tomy tube (Clayman et al., 1984; Coleman et al., 1984b; Winfield and Clayman, 1985). Hemorrhage is best managed by immediate tamponade. In this regard, placement of a large nephrostomy tube or of a Kaye catheter is invariably effective. Only in rare cases will angiography with arterial embolization or open surgical therapy be necessary (<0.1 per cent) (Fig. 62–16) (Clayman et al., 1984). Similarly, delayed bleeding (i.e., after nephrostomy tube removal) is rare (0.5 per cent); however,

this problem usually requires angiographic embolization (Clayman et al., 1984c).

Perforation of the collecting system occurs commonly (20 to 30 per cent); it is managed by the simple placement of the nephrostomy tube. The tear in the collecting system typically resolves within 48 hours, provided proper drainage of the collecting system (via nephrostomy tube or ureteral catheter) is established (Winfield and Clayman, 1985).

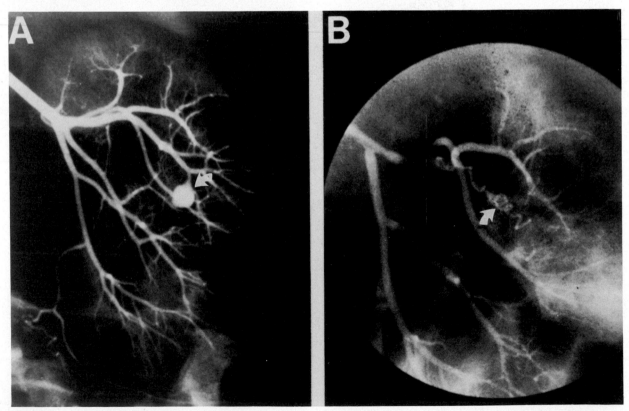

Figure 62–16. *A*, Arteriogram of a patient who developed macroscopic hematuria several weeks following percutaneous stone removal. A pseudoaneurysm of a segmental renal artery is present *(arrow)*. *B*, Embolization with a Gianturco coil *(arrow)* was immediately effective.

In a supracostal approach (i.e., 11th intercostal space), a pleurotomy may occur in upward of 12 per cent of cases (Picus et al., 1986; Young et al., 1985). This complication is more commonly associated with a hydrothorax than a pneumothorax following percutaneous nephrostolithotomy. Chest tube placement and drainage allow the pleura to seal along the nephrostomy tract such that the chest tube can usually be removed within 48 hours. Reports of an ensuing chronic nephropleural fistula are rare (A. D. Smith, personal communication).

Infection is rare provided antibiotic prophylaxis is administered (a penicillin derivative and an aminoglycoside). In all elective circumstances, the urine should be sterile prior to percutaneous nephrostomy. Oral antibiotics are routinely continued for 1 week after the nephrostomy tube is removed.

Injury to the spleen, duodenum, and colon have all been reported as a result of percutaneous nephrostomy. Colonic injury occurs most frequently because of the retrorenal colon overlying the lower pole of the kidney (Hopper et al., 1987; LeRoy et al., 1985). This circumstance is potentially more likely among patients with a megacolon or malpositioned kidney (i.e., jejunal-ileal bypass, ulcerative colitis, horseshoe kidney). In these patients, a preoperative computed tomograph (CT) scan is recommended in order to properly plan the nephrostomy tract. Overall, whereas only 2 per cent of patients have a retrorenal colon when supine, this increases to 10 per cent when patients are prone, the position routinely used for percutaneous nephrostomy. In most cases, the problem is simply managed by pulling the nephrostomy tube posteriorly until it is in the colon (colostomy tube) and placing an external retrograde ureteral catheter to drain the renal pelvis and divert the urine. Only if the patient has signs of peritonitis is a colostomy indicated.

Severe reactions to contrast material are rare (<0.2 per cent), especially since the contrast material is usually instilled directly into the collecting system and not intravenously. If a problem is anticipated based on the patient's history, the preprocedural administration of prednisone and antihistamine is recommended. For a minor allergic reaction, an antihistamine (diphenhydramine hydrochloride, 50 mg, IM) is given; for a severe allergic reaction, epinephrine (0.3 to 0.5 ml of 1:1000, subcutaneously) is recommended (Winfield and Clayman, 1985; Siegle and Lieberman, 1978).

Acute loss of the nephrostomy tract during the procedure is best prevented by use of a "safety" guide wire. If the tract is lost during the procedure, it can be probed with a Terumo guide wire; however, a repeat puncture is usually necessary. In this circumstance, the value of preprocedural placement of a retrograde ureteral catheter is immediately apparent. This catheter can be used either to aid in opacification of the collecting system for a second puncture or to drain the system should the second attempt at percutaneous nephrostomy fail.

Delayed displacement of the nephrostomy tube (i.e., postoperatively) is most likely in obese patients or in those with supracostal nephrostomy tubes. In these patients, a locking pigtail catheter or, preferably, a nephroureteral stent system that extends to the bladder is recommended. Tube dislodgement is approached similarly to a lost nephrostomy tract: initial gentle probing with a Terumo guide wire, which if unsuccessful leads to a repeat puncture and creation of a new nephrostomy tract.

Another concern with regard to percutaneous access to the kidney is the amount of damage to functional renal parenchyma. Employing detailed histologic studies and planimetry, in pigs, the degree of cortical loss from a percutaneous nephrostomy of 36 Fr. has consistently been estimated to be < 0.15 per cent of the total renal cortical surface (Clayman et al., 1987b). Indeed, in a meticulous canine study, Webb and Fitzpatrick (1977) estimated that with a standard 24 Fr. nephrostomy tract, less than 140 nephrons were injured. This is in agreement with the 1-mm postnephrostomy scar noted at nephrectomy in two patients who had undergone placement of a 30 Fr. nephrostomy tract 4 and 2 months prior to kidney removal (Tailly, 1988).

DIAGNOSTIC ENDOUROLOGY

Two areas in which endosurgical techniques can be utilized for diagnostic purposes are essential hematuria and lesions within the collecting system (i.e., nonopaque filling defect noted on intravenous urography). In both situations, when noninvasive radiologic evaluation is inconclusive, the ureteroscope becomes the primary means of diagnosis.

Essential Hematuria

A case of essential hematuria (i.e., macroscopic hematuria localized to the left or right supravesical collecting system) is a true diagnostic challenge (Table 62–1). Before any invasive studies are initiated, a thorough history and physical examination are necessary to alert the urologist to the possibility of a medical renal disease or a systemic condition (i.e., sickle cell anemia, glomerulopathy, diabetes with associated papillary necrosis) that may result in hematuria (McMurtry et al., 1987). Next, it is important to complete a laboratory evaluation of coagulation parameters, hemoglobin electrophoresis or sickle cell preparation, serum creatinine level, urine culture, urine cytology, and fresh urinalysis. The value of the urinalysis can be enhanced by examining the urinary sediment with a phase-contrast microscope. The shape of the red blood cells can help differentiate the bleeding into glomerular, nonglomerular, or urothelial origin. Smooth surfaced and round red blood cells are indicative of active bleeding, usually from a site along the urothelium (i.e., nonglomerular due to tumor, stone, or inflammation), whereas red blood cells with blebs or intracellular phase dense aggregates are more indicative of glomerular/tubular pathology (Fairley and Birch, 1982). A Coulter counter analysis has been shown to be quite helpful in distinguishing the origin of red blood

Table 62–1. LATERALIZING ESSENTIAL HEMATURIA: EVALUATION

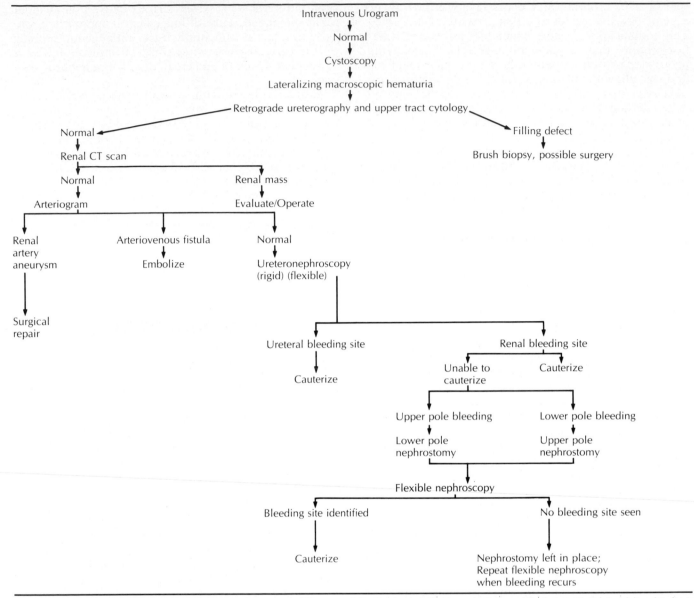

From Clayman, R. V., and Bagley, D. H.: Ureteronephroscopy. *In* Gillenwater, J. Y., Grayhack, J. T., Howards, S. S., and Duckett, J. W. (Eds.): Adult and Pediatric Urology. Chicago, Year Book Medical Publishers, 1990.)

cells in the urinary tract. Those cells of glomerular origin were dysmorphic, whereas red blood cells of urothelial origin were isomorphic (Sayer et al., 1990). This analysis accurately discriminated between glomerular/tubular and nonglomerular/urothelial bleeding in 97 per cent of patients with microhematuria and may be of value in those with macroscopic hematuria (Sayer et al., 1990).

Radiologic studies in patients with essential hematuria include a plain film of the abdomen along with an intravenous urogram to identify a calculus or a filling defect within the collecting system. To rule out a parenchymal renal mass, an ultrasound or CT study is recommended. Following these noninvasive steps, a retrograde ureterogram is performed on the affected side. In some cases, this study may have been done at the time of the initial cystoscopy when the bleeding was localized to the upper tract. During the cystoscopic examination, it is important to look for any bladder pathology (i.e., a small bladder tumor or vesical calculus), which might

alert the examiner to the possibility of a similar upper tract process.

The role of arteriography is controversial. The possibility of a "leaking" renal artery aneurysm or a large arteriovenous malformation continues to cause urologists to order arteriograms. However, these lesions are extremely rare (<1 per cent), and this type of problem usually is accompanied by blood loss sufficient to result in passage of clots and in acute anemia (Mariani, 1989).

Endoscopically, the rigid and flexible ureteroscopes have become the primary means for examining the upper urinary tract in a patient with essential hematuria (Bagley and Allen, 1990). An antegrade percutaneous approach is indicated if ureteroscopy cannot be performed or if ureteroscopy fails to establish a diagnosis (Bagley and Allen, 1990). In reports on patients with essential hematuria, antegrade percutaneous nephroscopy was not necessary (Bagley and Allen, 1990; Kumon et al., 1990).

Technique

The patient should be bleeding at the time of the examination. However, if the bleeding is brisk, it becomes more difficult to identify a lesion given the slow flow of irrigant through the ureteroscope. If no lesion is found at the initial examination, the patient is asked to return during an episode of bleeding so that ureteroscopy can be immediately repeated.

The ureteroscopic evaluation of the patient with essential hematuria is a systematic procedure (Fig. 62–17). First, the distal ureter is examined directly with a short, rigid ureteroscope (7.2 Fr. size) to rule out any ureteral pathology. Following this, a 0.035-inch floppy tip guide wire is advanced to the point where inspection of the distal ureter with the short rigid ureteroscope ended. A *flexible actively deflectable* ureteroscope is advanced over the guide wire, to the point where inspection with the rigid endoscope ended and the guide wire is removed. However, if the flexible endoscope will not pass into the distal ureter, a 4-mm or 5-mm high pressure (i.e., rated to 15 atmospheres) ureteral dilating balloon must be utilized to dilate the already inspected portion of the distal ureter.

The flexible endoscope is advanced along the middle and proximal ureter always under direct vision. Next, the ureteropelvic junction is examined, followed by the renal pelvis, upper pole calyces, middle calyces, and lower pole calyces, in that order (Fig. 62–18). In this regard, it is helpful to inject approximately 10 to 15 ml of Optiray 320 (1:1 dilution with normal saline) or another non-ionic contrast material through the irrigation port of the endoscope in order to outline the collecting system. The non-ionic contrast material will not adversely affect the cellular morphology seen in urine collected for cytology (Andriole et al., 1989). On the fluoroscopic screen, the collecting system can be traced out with a water soluble marking pen and each calyx can be numbered. The urologist can then mark off each calyx as it is entered and record in which calyx any pathologic lesion is noted. Only *after* completely inspecting the entire collecting system should any therapeutic maneuvers be undertaken.

Among patients with essential hematuria, it is important to avoid causing any iatrogenic injury to the collecting system; hence, the aforementioned carefully ordered and described technique for ureteroscopy. In this respect, the fluoroscopic passage of a guide wire into the collecting system *in advance of the ureteroscope*, invariably causes small petechial lesions within the renal pelvis (Fig. 62–19). Likewise, prior placement of an indwelling ureteral stent will result in pelvic edema and pyelitis, which may obscure the site of essential hematuria. Similarly, during ureteroscopy, it is important to maintain a low inflow pressure of irrigant (≤ 40 cm H_2O) in order to preclude bleeding from a torn fornix. If the lower pole calyces are inadvertently examined first, the deflected shaft of the endoscope may traumatize the ostium of the upper pole infundibulum, creating iatrogenic lesions (see Fig. 62–19) (Clayman and Bagley, 1990).

In the rare event that an antegrade approach is selected, the nephrostomy tube is placed in a lower pole, infracostal calyx. Nephroscopy at the time of nephrostomy tube placement is usually fruitless because of the iatrogenic bleeding from the nephrostomy tract. In this case, it is best to place a 20 Fr. nephrostomy tube, discharge the patient and wait until the patient is again bleeding. Nephroscopy is then performed through a mature (i.e., ≥ 7-day-old) nephrostomy tract on an outpatient basis under minimal intravenous sedation (McMurtry et al., 1987).

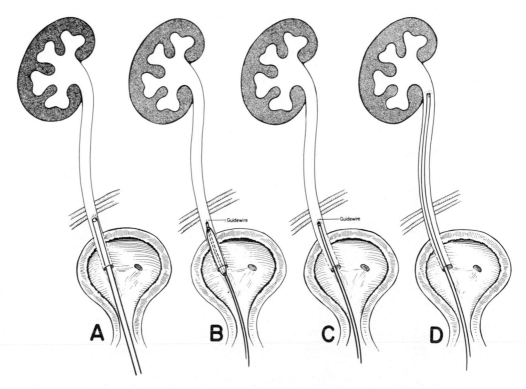

Figure 62–17. Recommended sequence for upper tract examination in order to preclude iatrogenic lesions during endoscopy for essential hematuria.

A, The lower ureter is cleared of any lesions by passing a small diagnostic rigid ureteroscope (i.e., 6.9 Fr. to 7.2 Fr.) without dilating the distal ureter.

B, A 0.035-inch guide wire is passed to the most cephalad point in the ureter that was directly visualized by the rigid ureteroscope. The distal ureter is balloon dilated to 12 to 15 Fr.

C, The 9.4 Fr. to 10.8 Fr. flexible actively deflectable ureteroscope is passed over the guide wire. The guide wire has not been passed above the distal ureter.

D, The guide wire is withdrawn, and the flexible ureteronephroscope is advanced up the ureter under direct endoscopic control. At no time has a guide wire preceded the direct visual inspection of any area of the ureter or renal collecting system.

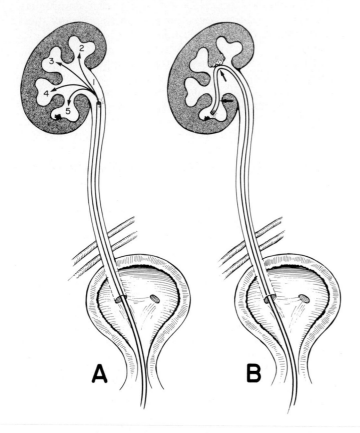

Figure 62–18. *A*, The entire upper urinary tract is examined in an orderly sequence (1 to 5). *B*, A tumor is noted in a lower pole calyx. Note the area of bruising where the passive deflection section of the endoscope abutted the upper pole infundibulum. If the lower pole were examined first, this area of iatrogenic injury could be misinterpreted as a pathologic lesion. Lower and upper arrows point to active and passive deflection portions of the endoscope, respectively.

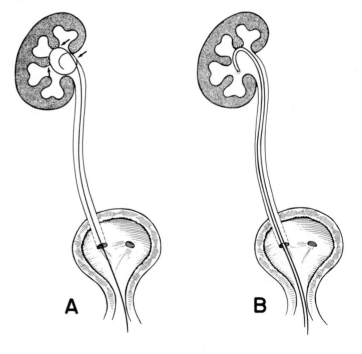

Figure 62–19. *A*, If the guide wire is coiled in the renal pelvis prior to endoscopic inspection, multiple diminutive petechial lesions *(arrows)* are created, which can be mistaken as the cause of essential hematuria. *B*, As the flexible endoscope is deflected off the upper pole infundibulum, bruising of the urothelium will occur. As such, if the lower pole were examined prior to (instead of after) the upper pole calyces, the resulting iatrogenic injury could again be erroneously identified as the site of bleeding.

Results

In patients with macroscopic or microscopic hematuria the site of bleeding is attributable to the upper urinary tract in only 10 per cent (Mariani et al., 1989). Among these individuals, the most common problem is a renal/ureteral calculus (42 per cent). Medical renal disease (medullary sponge kidney, glomerulonephritis, papillary necrosis, and pyelonephritis), renal cell cancer, and transitional cell cancer account for 19 per cent, 10 per cent, and 7 per cent, respectively. Other more rare diagnoses (<1 per cent) include renal cyst, renal arteriovenous fistula, and uteropelvic junction obstruction (Mariani et al., 1989).

However, by the time a patient with essential hematuria presents for *ureteroscopy*, the basic radiographic studies have been completed and the diagnosis of urolithiasis or tumor has been eliminated. As such, in this highly select patient group, the most common lesion found during *ureteroscopic examination* is a discrete or diffuse (albeit in 1 or 2 calyces) small vascular abnormality (hemangioma, usually at the tip of a renal papilla, and arteriovenous malformations) (Fig. 62–20) (Table 62–2). This abnormality was the problem in 85 per cent of patients studied from several urologists' experience (Bagley and Allen, 1990; Gittes and Varady, 1981; Kavoussi et al., 1989; Kumon et al., 1990; Patterson et al., 1984). The vascular lesions were located all along the collecting system (Bagley and Allen, 1990). These lesions are usually located directly on a papilla and can

be seen either as a prominent vessel traversing the top of the papilla or as a mulberry-type collection of diminutive vessels (hemangioma). Interestingly, of 76 patients with essential hematuria requiring ureteroscopy, only one patient had a transitional cell cancer and only two patients had calculi missed by the usual radiographic studies. In no patient in any of these series was the site of bleeding localized to the ureter or was the bleeding secondary to a renal artery aneurysm or other life-threatening vascular abnormality.

Intrarenal/Intraureteral Mass

The differential diagnosis of a *nonopaque* mass within the collecting system is vast (Tables 62–3 and 62–4) (Clayman and Bagley, 1990; Clayman et al., 1983b; Eklund and Gothlin, 1976; Malek et al., 1975). The major differential diagnosis is between transitional cell cancer and uric acid urolithiasis. In this respect, a thorough medical history is helpful (Davidson, 1990; Segal et al., 1978). Certainly a history of gout (uric acid stones), transitional cell cancer of the bladder, analgesic abuse (papillary necrosis), or prolonged use of tobacco products (transitional cell cancer) each may be suggestive of the diagnosis. In addition, the following conditions or symptoms may be associated with a radiographic filling defect within the upper collecting system: insulin-dependent diabetes mellitus (emphysematous pyelone-

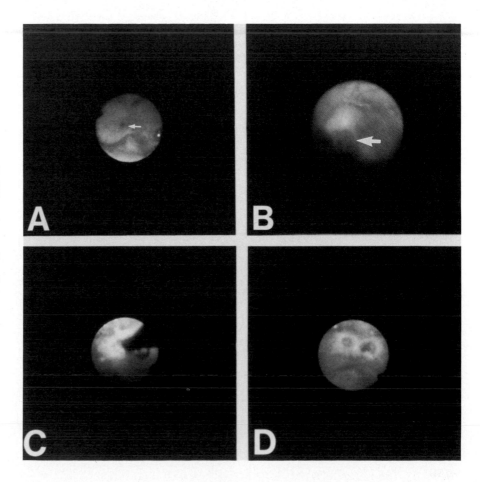

Figure 62–20. Endoscopic view of a small hemangioma found in a patient with benign essential hematuria. (From Bagley, D. H., and Allen, J.: J. Urol., 143:549, 1990.)

A, Overview of compound papilla with lesion noted *(arrow).*

B, Close-up view of hemangioma *(arrow).*

C, Electrofulguration of hemangioma with a 3 Fr. electrode.

D, Immediate result after fulguration reveals that the hemangioma has been completely cauterized.

Table 62–2. ESSENTIAL HEMATURIA: DIAGNOSIS AND TREATMENT

Authors	Number of Patients	Method of Nephroscopy	Ureteroscopy	Diagnosis Unilateral Discrete Vascular Abnormality	Diffuse Vascular Abnormality	Stone	Tumor	No Diag-nosis	Treatment	Re-bleed	Average Mean Follow-up Range (months)
Gittes and Varady, 1981	12	Operative (12)	None	5	7	0	0	0	Nephrectomy (1) Partial nephrectomy (11)	None	—
Patterson et al., 1984	4	Percutaneous (3)	Rigid (4)	1	3	0	0	0	Fulguration (4) Nephroscope (3) Ureteroscope (1)	None	5 2–10
McMurtry et al., 1987	8	Percutaneous (7)	Rigid (2) Flexible (1)	4	3	1	0	0	Fulguration (8) Nephroscope (7) Ureteroscope (1)	25% (4–6 mo.)	6 2–41
Kavoussi et al., 1989	8	None	Flexible (6)	Not specified		0	0	0	Fulguration (6) Ureteroscope (6)	12% (7 mo.)	11 7–18
Bagley et al., 1990	32	None	Flexible (30)	14	9	1	1	5	Fulguration (16) Nephroureterectomy (1) Stone removal (1)	8% (1/12) discrete abnormality 100% (4/4) diffuse abnormality	—
Kumon et al., 1990	12	None	Flexible (12)	9	1	0	0	2	Fulguration Ureteroscope (9)	None	10.3 6–21
Summary	**76**			49%	36%	3%	1%	9%		13%	

Table 62–3. RADIOLUCENT FILLING DEFECTS IN THE UPPER URINARY TRACT: DIFFERENTIAL DIAGNOSIS

Common Entities

	Renal Pelvis and Ureter
Tumor	Transitional cell cancer
Urolithiasis	Uric acid calculi
Blood clot	Trauma/tumor
Air	Iatrogenic (retrograde ureterogram)
Infection/inflammation	Papillary necrosis
	Fungal ball

Uncommon Causes

	Renal Pelvis	*Ureter*	*Both Pelvis and Ureter*
Tumors	Leukemic infiltrate Angiomyolipoma Multiple myeloma Lymphoma Wilms' tumor Renal cell cancer Cyst		Fibroepithelial polyp Squamous cell cancer Adenocarcinoma Leukoplakia Amyloid Sarcoma Connective tissue tumors Metastatic tumors
Urolithiasis			Matrix Xanthine
Blood clot			Coagulopathy Nephritis Anticoagulants
Air			Enteric fistula Gas-forming organism
Congenital			Vessel crossing Ectopic papilla End-of-calyx
Vascular	Renal artery aneurysm Vascular impression (vessel crossing renal pelvis/upper pole infundibulum)	Vascular (lower pole vessel, ovarian vein)	Arteriovenous fistula
Infection/inflammation	Pyelitis cystica	Ureteritis cystica	Tuberculosis Malacoplakia Helminths Fistula
Foreign body			Iatrogenic

From Clayman, R. V., Lange, P. H., and Fraley, E. E.: Cancer of the upper urinary tract. *In* Javadpour, N. (Ed.): Principles and Management of Urologic Cancer, 2nd ed. Baltimore, Williams & Wilkins, 1983.

phritis or papillary necrosis), immunosuppression (fungal mass), analgesic abuse (papillary necrosis), recurrent urinary tract infections with bacterial suppression (fungal mass), pneumaturia (ureteropelvic enteric fistula or fungal infection), or recent genitourinary tract manipulation (iatrogenic air or foreign body).

An extremely important part of the evaluation is a *fresh* urinalysis. It is recommended that the physician perform the urinalysis. If the urine pH is above 6.5, the likelihood of a uric acid stone becomes extremely remote (pKa of uric acid = 5.75) (Holmes, 1980). Likewise, the properly performed urinalysis can be helpful in assessing the likelihood of other, less common entities, such as hyphae (e.g., fungal ball); pyuria and bacteriuria (e.g., urinary tract infection with a gas-producing organism, emphysematous pyelonephritis, and ureteropelvic enteric fistula), or hematuria (e.g., blood clot and urothelial tumor). The urine specimen is also sent for bacterial and fungal cultures as well as for cytology and flow cytometry. Although cytology can help determine the presence of an upper tract transitional cell cancer, a negative finding is *not* diagnostic of a benign process. Indeed, 60 per cent of patients with a low-grade transitional cell cancers and even 10 per cent of patients with high-grade tumors will demonstrate urine cytology and/or flow cytometry study findings that are "normal" (Denovic et al., 1982; Melamed, 1984; Sarnacki, et al., 1971).

Radiographic studies may be helpful in determining the nature of the lesion. The urologist is usually first alerted to the problem by examining an intravenous urogram that reveals a *negative filling defect* within the supravesical urinary tract. Clubbing of the calyces and the classic "ring sign" of an absent papilla are instrumental in making a diagnosis of papillary necrosis (Malek et al., 1975). Air, stone, sloughed renal papilla, or blood clot should readily move as the patient changes position during the radiographic examination. In contrast, a tumor, unless it is on a stalk, should remain fixed in its position. Similarly, contrast material will usually surround a stone or blood clot but not *completely* surround a tumor. The outline of an air bubble or a uric

Table 62–4. RADIOLUCENT FILLING DEFECT IN THE UPPER URINARY TRACT EVALUATION

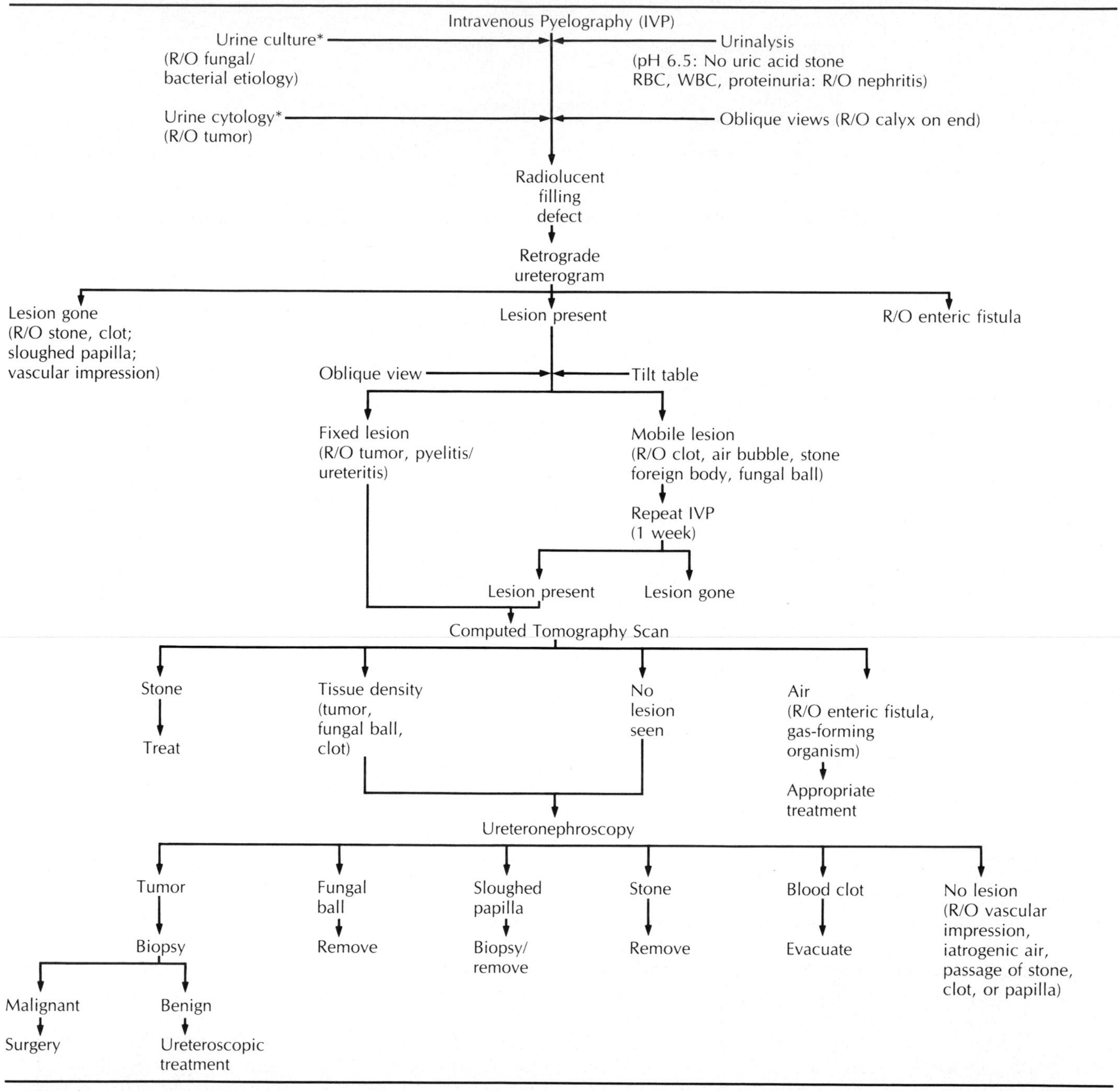

Intravenous Pyelography (IVP)

Urine culture* — (R/O fungal/ bacterial etiology)

Urinalysis (pH 6.5: No uric acid stone RBC, WBC, proteinuria: R/O nephritis)

Urine cytology* — (R/O tumor)

Oblique views (R/O calyx on end)

Radiolucent filling defect

Retrograde ureterogram

Lesion gone (R/O stone, clot; sloughed papilla; vascular impression)

Lesion present

R/O enteric fistula

Oblique view — Tilt table

Fixed lesion (R/O tumor, pyelitis/ ureteritis)

Mobile lesion (R/O clot, air bubble, stone foreign body, fungal ball)

Repeat IVP (1 week)

Lesion present   Lesion gone

Computed Tomography Scan

| Stone | Tissue density (tumor, fungal ball, clot) | No lesion seen | Air (R/O enteric fistula, gas-forming organism) |

Treat

Appropriate treatment

Ureteronephroscopy

| Tumor | Fungal ball | Sloughed papilla | Stone | Blood clot | No lesion (R/O vascular impression, iatrogenic air, passage of stone, clot, or papilla) |

| Biopsy | Remove | Biopsy/ remove | Remove | Evacuate | |

Malignant   Benign

Surgery   Ureteroscopic treatment

(R/O, rule out.)
*With a positive urine cytology, sterile urine, and a soft tissue filling defect, a surgical procedure for suspected transitional cell cancer is indicated.
From Resnick, M. I.: Radiolucent filling defects. *In* Resnick, M. I., Caldarmone, A. A., and Sprinak, J. P. (Eds.): Decision Making in Urology. St. Louis, C. V. Mosby Co., 1985.

acid stone is smooth and sharp, whereas the outline of a tumor is often irregular. If the intravenous urogram is repeated 1 to 2 weeks later, air (especially iatrogenic), sloughed papilla, or blood clot will usually have passed, whereas a tumor or stone will still be present.

A major boon to resolving the diagnostic dilemma of lesions in the upper urinary tract was the development of ultrasonography and CT. When ultrasonography is used, the characteristic acoustic shadowing associated with a stone is diagnostic (Fig. 62–21). With CT, the density of a uric acid stone (> 300 Hounsfield (HU) units; calcium stones are usually > 500 HU on a scale of ± 1000) distinguishes it from the lower density of a transitional cell tumor (30 to 40 HU), a blood clot (30 to 55 HU), and a papilla or fungal ball (20 to 40 HU) (Fig. 62–22) (Federle et al., 1981; Healy et al., 1984; Pollack et al., 1981). Of the two studies, CT is more helpful; however, CT is of diagnostic value in only 50 per cent of these cases (Pollack et al., 1981).

Additional differential radiographic signs may be appreciated on a retrograde ureterogram. With a stalk-bound transitional cell tumor of the ureter, there may be a "goblet sign" produced as the tumor is propelled upward by the retrograde flow of injected contrast material (Fig. 62–23) (Clayman et al., 1983b; Goldman and Gatewood, 1990). At the same time as a retrograde ureterography, under fluoroscopic control, a ureteral catheter can be passed and washings of the lesion can be obtained for cytology and/or flow cytometry. In addition, a tissue brush or a stone basket may be passed retrograde up to the lesion, under fluoroscopic control, and a sample of any tissue lesion can be obtained for cytology or, rarely, histologic evaluation (Gill et al., 1979).

When the CT or ultrasound study fails to reveal a calculus and the urine cytology findings are benign or merely suspicious, the next step is ureteronephroscopy. However, if the urine cytology findings are positive, the decision to proceed with ureteroscopy or nephroureterectomy is controversial. Although the nephroureterectomy is usually recommended, Bagley reported a 17 per cent incidence of *false-positive* urine cytology findings among patients with noncalculous lesions of the upper urinary tract. Total reliance on urine cytology, there-

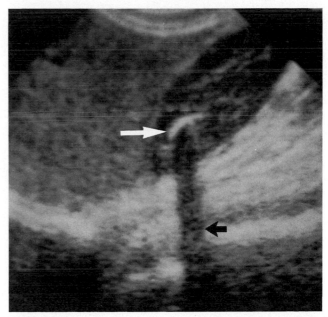

Figure 62–21. Ultrasound demonstrating stone. Note the increased echogenicity and decreased, through transmission of the soundwave (i.e., "acoustic shadowing"). (*White arrow,* stone; *black arrow,* acoustic shadowing.)

fore, may result in an unnecessary nephroureterectomy (Bagley and Rivas, 1990).

Technique

Unlike essential hematuria, the exact location of the lesion is already known. As such, the ureteroscopic procedure can begin with obtaining a retrograde ureterogram using *non-ionic* contrast material. Distortion of the morphology of subsequent cytologic samples is much less if isotonic contrast material is used (Andriole et al., 1989). Ureteroscopy involves dilation of the ureter to a size that is 2 to 3 Fr. larger than the ureteroscope. Usually, a 4-mm or 5-mm ureteral dilating balloon suffices (Bagley et al., 1987). If the lesion is in the distal ureter, a rigid ureteroscope is needed; whereas, if the lesion is in the middle or lower calyces, a flexible

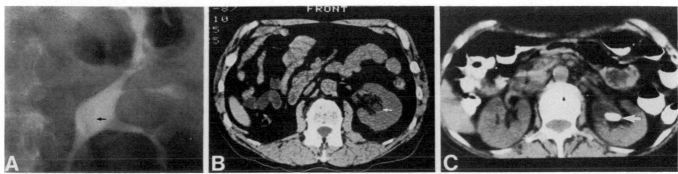

Figure 62–22. *A,* This radiograph depicts a smooth-surfaced filling defect *(arrow)* in the renal pelvis, presumed to represent a uric acid calculus.
B, The noncontrast computed tomography (CT) scan reveals that the lesion in the renal pelvis has a density compatible with tissue *(arrow)* rather than calculus. Subsequent ureteroscopy and biopsy established the diagnosis of a low-grade transitional cell cancer.
C, In a similar case in which a noncalcified filling defect was present on an intravenous urogram, the CT scan clearly shows a dense lesion *(arrow)* compatible with a uric acid calculus.

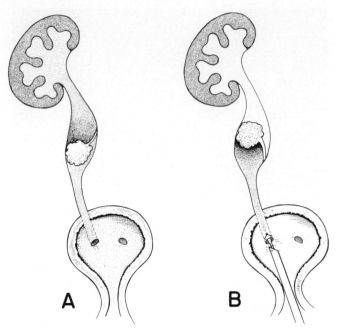

Figure 62–23. *A,* A transitional cell tumor on a stalk is seen on an intravenous urogram. The tumor lies below its attachment to the ureter. *B,* A retrograde ureterogram displaces the tumor cephalad. As such, the tumor is pushed cephalad until it now lies above its urothelial attachment. The contrast material fills out the widened area where the tumor initially resided and spreads out on either side of the tumor thereby creating the "goblet" sign.

ureteroscope is needed (Bagley et al., 1987). In general, for ureteral lesions above the iliac vessels or any renal lesion, the flexible, deflectable ureteronephroscope is preferred.

While passing the ureteroscope, one should endeavor to produce the fewest abrasions to the collecting system in order to avoid the hypothetic problem of creating areas "potentially" favorable to tumor seeding. Likewise, a ureteral perforation is to be avoided at all costs, as it might result in the extravasation of tumor cells into the periureteral area and the potential retroperitoneal seeding of tumor cells. Accordingly, if the ureteroscope does not pass easily, it is advisable to terminate the procedure and place an indwelling ureteral stent. Ureteroscopy can be repeated in a week, at which time the ureteroscope can usually be more easily passed because of the passive ureteral dilation associated with the indwelling stent.

Normal saline is employed as the irrigant under gravity flow (40 cm above the table). Pressurized flow is avoided. The low pressure on the irrigant should preclude any forniceal tears through which tumor cells could again hypothetically enter the systemic circulation.

With ureteroscopy, as at times with cystoscopy, the endoscopist must rely more on the appearance of the lesion than on the final histologic report in order to make a correct diagnosis. The classic appearance of a papillary tumor is known to urologists, whereas a smooth-walled pedunculated lesion may represent a fibroepithelial polyp. A freely floating lesion may be a papilla, a blood clot, or a fungal ball. A sloughed papilla has a dull gray appearance as opposed to the white gelatinous appearance of a fungal mass or the bright

(fresh) or dark (old) red appearance of a blood clot. However, the endoscopist should be aware of the possibility that the CT or ultrasound study may have missed a calculus.

If despite having the ureteroscope at the radiographic site of the lesion, no lesion is present, the filling defect within the renal pelvis may be secondary to a crossing vessel. In this case, contrast material can be gently injected through the endoscope. The lesion will be seen fluoroscopically; however, when the collecting system is distended with contrast material, the filling defect, if it is a crossing vessel, will disappear. Likewise, if the ureteroscope is positioned at the area of the filling defect, when the contrast material is slowly aspirated, arterial pulsations can often be noted at the site of the filling defect. This sequence of a "disappearing" and "reappearing" lesion is diagnostic of a crossing renal vessel impressing upon the renal pelvis (Bagley et al., 1987). If no lesion is seen despite careful ureteroscopy, it is possible that the lesion was a stone, sloughed papilla, or blood clot that subsequently passed.

To biopsy an upper tract lesion, a 3 Fr. biopsy forceps is passed, opened under endoscopic control, and advanced into the lesion until the surface of the lesion is visibly deformed by the biopsy forceps (Fig. 62–24). At this point, the jaws are closed upon the lesion and the closed forceps and ureteroscope are withdrawn for 1 to

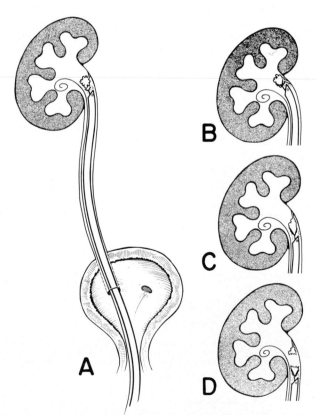

Figure 62–24. *A,* The biopsy forceps is opened.

B, The biopsy forceps is pushed deeply into the tumor, thereby visibly deforming the surface of the tumor. The tumor is pinned against the wall of the pelvis and the forceps is closed.

C and *D,* By withdrawing the closed forceps and the ureteroscope 2 to 3 cm as a unit, a larger piece of the tumor is obtained than if the closed forceps were to be immediately pulled into the 3.6 Fr. port of the ureteroscope.

2 cm as a unit. This maneuver enables the endoscopist to obtain a larger sample of the lesion than if the forceps were immediately withdrawn into the endoscope. If a ureteral access sheath has been placed, the entire endoscope with the biopsy forceps extended can be withdrawn. Otherwise, the forceps must be pulled through the working/irrigation channel and portions of the specimen lying outside the immediate jaws of the biopsy forceps may be lost along the biopsy channel. This biopsy technique can improve the per cent of specimens suitable for pathologic diagnosis from 30 to 80 per cent (Kavoussi et al., 1989).

From a practical standpoint, to biopsy a lesion in the upper urinary tract can be difficult. The specimens obtained with a 3 Fr. biopsy forceps are small. Also, the stiffness of the biopsy forceps decreases the deflection of the tip of the flexible ureteroscope making access to the lesion more difficult. Furthermore, *with the 3 Fr. instrument in place*, it may be necessary to momentarily pressurize the flow of irrigant ($\leq$ 150 mm Hg) in order to be able to still visualize the lesion. After the first biopsy, bleeding from the lesion may further obscure the examiner's field of view.

Ideally, 5 to 6 biopsy samples are obtained. Several of the samples are placed in saline or Bouin's solution. Bouin's solution provides for improved nuclear detail (J. Huffman, personal communication). A detailed description of the site of origin of the biopsy specimens should be sent to the pathologist. In some cases, it is helpful to invite the pathologist to the operating room to personally view the macroscopic findings. The remaining samples are sent to the cytologist. In addition, following the biopsy procedures, washings are performed with saline through the irrigation channel of the endoscope. The low pressure jet of saline is aimed directly at the lesion. These directed washings are also examined by the cytologist.

Other maneuvers that can be performed through the ureteroscope to help diagnose the type of tumor include brushing the lesion and basketing a sample of the lesion. For the former, small brushes are available and the lesion can be brushed under endoscopic control. Likewise, for the latter, basketing the lesion is feasible provided one is certain of the tissue-like nature of the lesion. The stone basket can be opened alongside the lesion and twirled within the lesion to obtain a tissue sample. If the lesion is on a stalk, the entire tumor can be at times entrapped and extracted, provided it is not too large (<10 mm).

Results

Noninvasive diagnostic studies are rarely definitive in the patient with an upper urinary tract lesion. Confirmatory ureteroscopy is necessary to obtain an accurate diagnosis. In this regard, in one series, CT failed to image 43 per cent of the calculi and 64 per cent of the transitional cell tumors. Similarly, ultrasound failed to provide diagnostic information in all of the patients studied who had calculi and in 83 per cent of patients who had tumors detected by ureteroscopy (Bagley and Rivas, 1990). Furthermore, cytology alone is not reliable. Indeed, among the transitional cell tumors noted in

Bagley's series, cytology resulted in a 65 per cent false-negative diagnosis. Even more worrisome was a false-positive cytology in 17 per cent of individuals with upper tract lesions (Bagley and Rivas, 1990). While providing more accurate information, brush biopsy/cytology under fluoroscopic control is also not wholly definitive. In one study, although a $\geq$ class III cytology (i.e., $\geq$ dysplasia) was associated with transitional cell cancer in each case, 12 per cent of cases with a "normal" brush cytology were shown to have transitional cell cancer (Sheline et al., 1989). Among patients with filling defects, ureteroscopy is often essential for establishing a definitive diagnosis.

In reports of upper urinary tract lesions examined ureteroscopically, the most common diagnoses are calculus (18 to 44 per cent) and low-grade transitional cell carcinoma (16 to 40 per cent) (Bagley et al., 1987; Kavoussi et al., 1989). However, the presence of a "filling defect" in association with macroscopic hematuria is more indicative of the diagnosis of a transitional cell tumor. Approximately 25 per cent of lesions are due to benign anatomic abnormalities: vascular impression, edema, and pyelitis.

Of note is the absence of any lesion, at the time of ureteroscopy, in upward of 16 per cent of patients (Bagley et al., 1987; Bagley and Rivas, 1990; Kavoussi et al., 1989). In these cases, a benign free-floating lesion has been passed in the urine or the filling defect was a "pseudotumor" due to an eccentric papilla. Other less common findings include fungal ball, papillary necrosis, pyelitis cystica, peripelvic/intrarenal cyst, renal adenocarcinoma, fibroepithelial polyps, and inverted papilloma.

THERAPEUTIC ENDOUROLOGY

Four broad categories exist in which endosurgical techniques have a therapeutic role: drainage of retroperitoneal collections (urinoma, abscess, lymphocele, and hematoma), treatment of intrarenal collections (cyst, abscess, calyceal diverticulum, and fungal concretion), essential hematuria, and upper urinary tract strictures (infundibular, ureteropelvic junction, and ureteral). In addition, an endosurgical approach can be of benefit in two relatively rare, albeit difficult, situations: ureteroenteric strictures and inoperable vesicocutaneous fistulas. Also, this technology can be helpful for the renal transplant patient with a ureteral stricture or a ureteral fistula. The most controversial application of the newer minimally invasive technology is in the patient with low-grade, upper tract transitional cell cancer. The role of endosurgery in this patient is still in the process of being determined.

Retroperitoneal Collections

Endosurgical Management of a Urinoma (Uriniferous Pseudocyst)

A retroperitoneal urinoma occurs most commonly following renal trauma (Morano and Burkhalter, 1985;

Portela et al., 1979). Other causes of urinoma are secondary to ureteral obstruction with attendant calyceal forniceal rupture and complication of an endosurgical procedure. There is one caveat: a left-sided urinoma must be distinguished from a pancreatic pseudocyst, as the therapy is quite different.

The retroperitoneal urine collection, by virtue of its size, may cause considerable discomfort. Because of the lipolytic effect of urine, over the next 2 to 5 days, perinephric fat disappears and an inflammatory reaction follows. The urine collection becomes encapsulated in a fibrous sac within 3 to 6 weeks (Healy et al., 1984; Lang and Glorioso, 1986; Morano and Burkhalter, 1985; Thompson et al., 1976).

Initial studies should include an intravenous pyelography (IVP) or an antegrade nephrostogram, a retrograde ureterogram and/or a CT scan with contrast agent to identify the three factors necessary for a urinoma to form: (1) a ureteral obstruction, (2) an extravasation from the collecting system, and (3) a functioning kidney. The initial CT attenuation values of approximately 10 to 20 HU may increase after administration of intravenous contrast material (Healy et al., 1984). Also, unlike a hematoma or an abscess cavity, the CT attenuation values throughout the urinoma are homogeneous (Lang and Glorioso, 1986). In addition, the CT scan yields important data about the exact location and extent of the urinoma, with regard to the retroperitoneal and peritoneal cavities and the kidney, ureter, and fascial planes.

TECHNIQUE. Percutaneous drainage of a urinoma is performed under ultrasound or CT guidance. The creatinine concentration in the fluid should be identical with the urine creatinine concentration. A 10 Fr. catheter–bearing needle (biliary urinary drainage catheter with a locking pigtail) can be directed into the urinoma. The cavity is drained, and the catheter is left indwelling. The fluid obtained can be analyzed for creatinine and amylase and cultured.

In some instances, no communication between the collecting system and urinoma is identifiable and no evidence of ureteral obstruction is found. In these cases, drainage from the urinoma usually ceases within 48 to 72 hours and the cavity rapidly decreases in size. A contrast-medium injection via the urinoma catheter is helpful to determine if the cavity has collapsed. Once the cavity is no larger than the drainage catheter itself, and is shown radiographically not to communicate with the collecting system, the catheter can be removed.

If ureteral obstruction is present or if over a several day period, the cavity continues to drain without a decrease in the amount of fluid, it becomes necessary to drain the affected collecting system. In this case, a retrograde ureterogram and placement of an indwelling ureteral stent or a percutaneous nephrostomy are needed to help divert the urine from the fistulous tract. In most cases, the communication will spontaneously close.

In the rare circumstance in which the fistula persists despite adequate drainage of the urinoma and renal collecting system, ureteroscopy or antegrade nephroscopy is indicated. The tract can be biopsied to rule out a malignancy and fulgurated. Fulguration may be successful in stimulating scarring of the fistula; however, experience with this approach is scant. In these cases, surgical exploration and formal closure of the fistulous tract may be necessary.

RESULTS. The largest report on treatment of urinomas is by Thompson and associates (1976) in which 16 patients were treated surgically. Half of them required nephrectomy. The other half underwent surgical drainage of the urinoma with at times resection of the urinoma wall and placement of a nephrostomy tube.

To date, there are only anecdotal reports of percutaneous drainage of urinomas (Morano and Burkhalter, 1985). According to Lang and Glorioso (1986), obstructive urinomas can be successfully treated in more than 90 per cent of patients by percutaneous drainage and relief of the obstruction. Likewise for nonobstructive (i.e., traumatic) urinomas, drainage of the cavity and establishment of upper tract continuity (stent) are usually successful. This appears to be a reasonable first step provided that the urinoma can be completely drained, (i.e., not multiloculated) and that ureteral or percutaneous drainage of the obstructed collecting system is simultaneously established. To date, there are no reports regarding the need for sclerotherapy in these patients.

Perinephric Abscess

Perinephric abscess is most commonly associated with disruption of a corticomedullary intranephric renal abscess. This finding is usually seen in conjunction with prior urologic surgery, urolithiasis, or diabetes mellitus (60 to 90 per cent of cases) (Edelstein and McCabe, 1988; Thorley et al., 1974). The most common symptoms of a retroperitoneal abscess are fever (90 per cent) and flank pain (40 to 50 per cent) (Saiki et al., 1982). A palpable flank mass occurs in 9 to 47 per cent (Edelstein and McCabe, 1988; Gerzof and Gale, 1982; Goldman et al., 1977; Salvatierra et al., 1967; Sheinfeld et al., 1987). In the 1960s, the predominant organism associated with hematogenous infection was *Staphylococcus aureus*; however, the offending organism is today most commonly a gram-negative bacterium (*Escherichia coli* or *Proteus mirabilis*) (Thorley et al., 1974; White et al., 1985). The diagnosis of this entity is best done with CT or ultrasonography (Haaga et al., 1977; Jaques et al., 1986; Weigert et al., 1985). However, CT is preferred, as it is more accurate in diagnosing an intra-abdominal abscess (90 per cent) than ultrasonography, and CT is more effective in defining the extent of the abscess in its relationship to other retroperitoneal structures. On CT scan, the typical appearance of a perinephric abscess is that of a soft tissue mass ($\leq$ 20 HU), with a thick wall that may be enhanced with intravenous contrast material ("rind sign") (Gerzof and Gale, 1982; Haaga et al., 1977; Sheinfeld et al., 1987). The gallium scan and indium-labeled white blood cells may also be of benefit.

TECHNIQUE. Prior to ultrasound or CT examination, the patient should receive broad-spectrum parenteral antibiotics (e.g., ampicillin and aminoglycoside). Next, a 21-gauge needle can be passed percutaneously under ultrasound or CT guidance into the abscess cavity. This puncture provides the physician with important information: determination of the presence of infection and consistency of purulent contents (if it's too thick, it cannot be drained) (Gerzof et al., 1985). It is essential that the abscess be punctured below the 12th rib in order to preclude an inadvertent pleurotomy. If the pleural cavity is traversed, significant pleural effusion and possible empyema may ensue (Albala et al., 1990). Likewise, the peritoneal cavity should be avoided.

Next, an 18-gauge needle is passed. Fluid is drained from the abscess and sent to the laboratory for aerobic, anaerobic, and fungal cultures. If the fluid is thick and drains poorly, or if the cavity is multiloculated, an open operation is necessary to properly drain and debride the abscess cavity. However, if the fluid is relatively thin and drains well, then at the same time as the diagnostic ultrasound or CT study, a catheter (e.g., 8 Fr. or 10 Fr. biliary urinary drainage catheter with a locking pigtail on a 12 Fr. or 14 Fr. double lumen sump drain: Van-Sonnenberg or Ring-McClean catheter) can be left in the abscess cavity or collecting system (i.e., nephrostomy tube) to permit drainage (Fig. 62–25) (Elyaderani and Moncman, 1985; Gerzof and Gale, 1982; Haaga, 1990). Although the catheters (7 Fr. to 14 Fr.) that come with a needle can be placed in a single step, positioning of the double lumen catheters requires some dilation of the tract. The double lumen catheter helps decrease clogging and can be used for infusion and drainage of saline or antibiotic solution. With directed antibiotic coverage, this therapy often will resolve the abscess.

Usually within 5 to 7 days, drainage from the abscess ceases (Caldamone and Frank, 1980; Cronan et al., 1980). However, if drainage initially decreases, then begins to increase and becomes clear, a urinary fistula must be suspected (Caldamone and Frank, 1980; Cronan et al., 1980). Prior to removing the drainage tube, a radiographic study of the cavity can be done by gently injecting contrast material into the drainage catheter. If

the cavity has decreased to the size of the catheter, the catheter can be removed. When a large cavity persists, a sclerosant may be instilled, provided there is no communication with the collecting system. Most commonly, tetracycline or 95 per cent ethanol has been chosen for this purpose. The sclerosant effect of tetracycline (50 mg/ml) is attributed to its acid pH of 2 to 3.5. The tetracycline is instilled under gravity drainage into the cavity following which the tube is clamped for 15 minutes. The process is repeated on a weekly basis until the only cavity remaining is that which immediately surrounds the pigtail of the drainage tube. At this point, the tube is withdrawn (White et al., 1985). Alternatively, 95 per cent ethanol may be used as described under sclerosant therapy for renal cysts. However, the combined sclerosant and antibacterial characteristics of tetracycline make it an ideal choice for treating a persistent retroperitoneal abscess cavity.

Oral antibiotics, appropriate for the responsible bacterium, are given throughout this period and for 1 to 3 weeks after removal of the drainage tube. Repeat urine cultures and repeat CT scans are necessary at 1- and 3-month intervals to rule out recurrent infection or reappearance of a retroperitoneal fluid collection.

Absolute contraindications to a percutaneous approach are few. An uncorrectable or uncorrected bleeding diathesis precludes percutaneous drainage. Likewise, suspicion of a hydatid cyst or a renal artery aneurysm is a direct contraindication to this approach (Gerzof and Gale, 1982).

RESULTS. Perinephric abscess is a life-threatening entity. Left undrained, despite antibiotic administration, the mortality rate approaches 80 per cent (Altemeyer and Alexander, 1961). Even with traditional surgical therapy (nephrectomy or drainage), the mortality is 11 to 22 per cent and significant morbidity is 35 per cent (Thorley et al., 1974). The need for initial or subsequent nephrectomy following surgical drainage is 25 to 50 per cent (Edelstein and McCabe, 1988; Salvatierra et al., 1967). Recurrence rates after surgery are 20 per cent

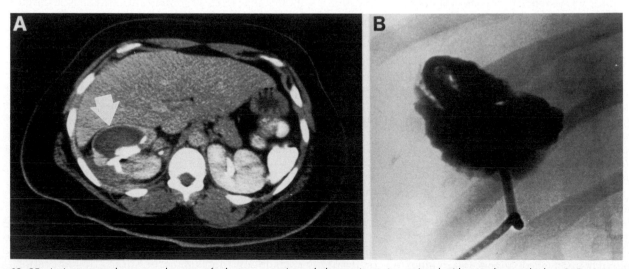

Figure 62–25. A, A computed tomography scan of a large retroperitoneal abscess (arrow) associated with a staghorn calculus. B, Drainage tube in the abscess cavity. The tube has been passed such that it is subcostal. In this case, a supracostal puncture is contraindicated for fear of bacterial contamination of the pleural space.

(Edelstein and McCabe, 1988; Elyaderani and Moncman, 1985; Haaga, 1977; Haaga, 1990; Jacques et al., 1986; Salvatierra, et al., 1967). For a perinephric abscess, the complication of sepsis, pleural fistula, bleeding, or need for surgical intervention is seen in 3 to 22 per cent (Edelstein and McCabe, 1988; Gerzof et al., 1985). The subsequent nephrectomy rate is still high—40 per cent—and reflects the poor function of these diseased kidneys (Edelstein and McCabe, 1988). However, recurrences are relatively rare, i.e., 1 to 4 per cent for all abdominal/retroperitoneal abscesses drained percutaneously (Gerzof et al., 1985).

The results of percutaneous drainage of retroperitoneal abscesses are particularly good. Haaga (1977, 1990) has reported successful drainage in 39 collected cases of perinephric abscess. This mirrors the 86 per cent success rate for percutaneous drainage of all types of intra-abdominal abscesses (Gerzof et al., 1985; Jaques et al., 1986). Overall, the success rate is higher for single than for loculated abscesses, 82 per cent versus 45 per cent (Gerzof et al., 1985). Despite this less invasive procedure, the perinephric abscess is still a life-threatening process, and a mortality rate of 8 per cent is reported for patients undergoing percutaneous therapy (Haaga, 1990).

Unfavorable factors for a percutaneous approach include fungal infection; calcification of the mass; thick purulent material; multiloculated abscess; markedly diseased nonfunctioning kidney, which is an indication for a nephrectomy; and infected hematoma. If an enteric fistula is the source of the retroperitoneal abscess, an open surgical repair is necessary (Elyaderani and Moncman, 1985). An air-fluid level within the abscess is identified on CT scan in half of these cases (Jaques et al., 1986).

Lymphocele

Although lymphocele is a complication noted after a variety of procedures, it is the urologic surgeon who most often must manage this problem. Lymphoceles are noted after any extensive retroperitoneal node dissection (testis, kidney, prostate, or bladder cancer) and after renal transplantations (1.2 to 14 per cent) (Braun et al., 1974; Brockis et al., 1978; Morin and Baker, 1977; Mueller et al., 1984; Schweizer et al., 1972; Skinner et al., 1982; White et al., 1985). The following symptoms usually are the result of compression of adjacent structures (ureter, colon, and iliac vessels) by the lymphocele: hydronephrosis, ipsilateral lower extremity edema, constipation, decreased bladder volume, and abdominal mass. In transplant patients, a lymphocele may cause a rise in creatinine concentration due to ureteral obstruction (Brockis et al., 1978).

Initial evaluation of these masses includes CT scans or ultrasonography, either of which is suitable for outlining the lesion (Spring et al., 1981). A definitive diagnosis can be made by needle aspiration of the collection. In the drained, pale yellow or clear fluid, lymphocytes can be detected. The values of creatinine and other electrolytes reflect those of serum values, as opposed to the high creatinine, high potassium, and low sodium values in urinoma. The levels of cholesterol and protein are often lower than those in serum (Braun et al., 1974). If the disruption of the lymphatic chain is farther cephalad in the retroperitoneum (celiac axis area), a chylous fluid collects. This material is cloudy and has a high content of triglycerides and proteins.

TECHNIQUE. Under CT or ultrasound guidance, a 20- or 22-gauge needle is guided into the cystic collection (Mueller et al., 1984). The fluid obtained is sent to the laboratory for serum electrolytes, creatinine, protein, triglyceride, cholesterol, culture, and cytologic evaluations. Blood and urine samples are obtained for similar chemical evaluations. If more than 150 ml is aspirated, an 8 to 14 Fr. locking-type, pigtail catheter (Cope loop, VanSonnenberg sump, or other tube) is guided into the cavity (White et al., 1985). At 1 to 10 days, contrast material is instilled via the catheter to assess the size of the cavity. When the cavity has collapsed around the catheter and drainage is < 10 ml/day, the catheter can be removed. However, if higher outputs continue, sclerotherapy with tetracycline can be tried (≤50 ml of 50 mg tetracycline/ml left in place for 15 minutes) (White et al., 1985).

RESULTS. Simple aspiration of a lymphocele appears sufficient for smaller collections (<150 ml). However, for the larger lymphocele, it is usually not effective (<20 per cent success) (Braun et al., 1974). In this case, a drainage tube is necessary. Drainage should cease, anytime from days to months. Otherwise, sclerotherapy with tetracycline can be attempted. The method is successful in 82 per cent; however, drainage may not cease for up to 4 months after catheter placement (White et al., 1985). In addition, if the collection has multiple loculations, the success of aspiration is markedly diminished.

Open surgical drainage and intraperitoneal marsupialization are generally more effective than aspiration (94 per cent success) (Brockis et al., 1978). The locules of the lymphocele are each opened, and the collection is made to communicate with the peritoneal cavity by excising the peritoneal wall of the lymphocele and mobilizing a tag of omentum, which is secured within the lymphocele itself. Of note is a recurrence rate of 25 per cent and a 10 per cent incidence of lymphocele infection (Braun et al., 1974; Morin and Baker, 1977; Schweizer et al., 1972; Spring et al., 1981).

Of interest is a case report by McCullough of laparoscopic drainage and marsupialization of a post-transplant lymphocele. This approach resolved the problem, and the patient was discharged from the hospital on the first postoperative morning (McCullough, 1990). The impact of laparoscopic surgery on lymphocele therapy awaits further reports.

Hematoma

A retroperitoneal hematoma is most commonly the consequence of blunt renal trauma. Other causes include penetrating renal trauma, anticoagulant therapy, vascular lesion, and tumor or surgical complications (percutaneous surgery, renal biopsy). The symptoms include flank mass and discomfort, at times ureteral obstruction may also occur. The diagnosis is best made by a CT scan, which can both demonstrate the extent of the hematoma and differentiate between a retroperitoneal and subcapsular collection. The last is of greater concern, as it may result in decreased renal function. The attenuation values for a hematoma may vary from +18 to +40 HU (±1000 HU scale) (Pollack et al., 1981). Fortunately, these lesions rarely require therapy

The natural history of a retroperitoneal hematoma is slow spontaneous resolution of the mass. However, if the hematoma is overly large (i.e., compromising respiratory function), expanding, impairing renal function, or associated with hypotension, embolization or surgical exploration and drainage are indicated. In some cases, angiographic localization and embolization of the offending vessel may be helpful to end the acute hemorrhage. However, if the amount of retroperitoneal hematoma is sufficiently large (i.e., impaired renal function or compromised respiratory function), surgical evacuation of the clot is necessary. Percutaneous procedures in these cases are more meddlesome than therapeutic, because the blood clot is too thick and loculated to drain (Schaner et al., 1977). Likewise, in patients with spontaneous renal hemorrhage in whom there is no history of anticoagulation, vasculitis, or trauma, surgical radical nephrectomy is recommended because 50 to 70 per cent will be found to have diminutive renal cell cancers (Kendall et al., 1988).

Intrarenal Collections

Renal Cysts

Upward of 25 per cent of adults over the age of 40 years have radiographically detectable renal cysts (≥ 1 cm) (Laucks and McLachlan, 1981). These cysts increase slowly in size and number as an individual ages; by the age of 60 years, 33 per cent have cysts with an average size ≥ 2 cm (Dalton et al., 1986; Laucks and McLachlan, 1981). Symptoms attributable to renal cysts include flank pain, usually secondary to hemorrhage into a cyst; microscopic hematuria; obstruction; or renin-mediated hypertension. However, only 8 per cent of cysts result in significant symptoms.

Among patients with polycystic kidney disease, the following problems are more frequent: flank pain (30 per cent), pyelonephritis (30 per cent), urolithiasis (34 per cent), hypertension (21 per cent), perinephric abscess (8 per cent), mass (15 per cent), macroscopic hematuria (19 per cent), and renal failure (17 per cent) (Delaney et al., 1985).

TECHNIQUE. In the symptomatic patient, therapy is best achieved by percutaneous drainage during monitoring with ultrasound, fluoroscopy, or CT. Utilizing one of these imaging modalities, the cyst is identified and a nephrostomy-type needle is placed into the center of the cyst. The cyst contents are drained and sent to the laboratory for cytologic studies, cultures, and chemical evaluation (protein, lactate dehydrogenase, creatinine) (Fig. 62–26). A thin, clear, yellow fluid is indicative of a benign cyst, whereas a sanguineous fluid may

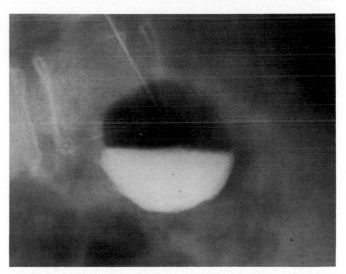

Figure 62–26. A large symptomatic cyst filled with air and contrast material to assure no communication with the collecting system. Note the smooth walls of the cyst indicative of its benign nature.

be associated with a traumatic puncture or a neoplasm. Contrast material is injected into the cyst (i.e., cystogram) to be certain it does not communicate with the collecting system. Also, on the cyst injection, the walls should appear smooth, indicating the absence of a tumor within the lining of the cyst.

Provided the cyst appears to be benign and isolated from the collecting system, percutaneous drainage and sclerosis of the cyst can be undertaken. The cyst is drained following which ethanol (equal to 25 per cent of cyst volume) is instilled into the cyst and left for 10 to 20 minutes. The ethanol is then withdrawn (Bean, 1981; Ozgun et al., 1988). Alternative sclerotherapy can be achieved by injection of 5 to 10 ml of bismuth phosphate (Table 62–5) (Holmberg and Hietala, 1989; Zachrisson, 1982). In these circumstances, the agent is left in the cyst.

An absolute contraindication to percutaneous sclerosis is a parapelvic (sic: peripelvic) or communicating pyelovenous cyst (i.e., communicates with renal pelvis or infundibulum of a major calyx) (Abeshouse and Abeshouse, 1963). Among these patients, a formal percutaneous approach should be undertaken. First, the cyst is punctured with a nephrostomy needle such that the puncture site is either along the peripheral (i.e., thin) or parenchymal wall of the cyst. Then, either a *direct* or *indirect* endoscopic approach may be taken to the collecting system.

In the *direct* approach, a retrograde ureteral catheter is passed and the collecting system is opacified via the ureteral catheter by injecting contrast material mixed with indigo carmine and sorbitol (50 ml sorbitol, 25 ml contrast material, and 1 to 2 ml indigo carmine). Next, the radiologist can try to direct the needle that is in the cyst (clear or straw-colored fluid) through the anterior cyst wall and into the opacified renal pelvis (blue-stained urine). Next, the transcystic nephrostomy tract is dilated, and a 30 Fr. Amplatz working sheath is placed.

Alternatively, after a needle/catheter has been passed

Table 62–5. RENAL CYSTS: DRAINAGE AND SCLEROTHERAPY

Authors	Agent	Number of Cysts	Cyst with ≥ 50% Reduction in Size	Cyst Disappearance (%)	Follow-up Data
Holmberg and Hietala, 1989	No intervention	62	0%	0	27 ≥ 24 mos.
Dalton et al., 1986			(7% >50% increase in size)		
Raskin et al., 1975	Drainage	15	13%	—	5-48 mos.
Wahlqvist et al., 1966		26	15%	19	≥ 19 mos.
Holmberg and Hietala, 1989		57	20%	4	25 pts. ≥ 24 mos.
Vestby, 1967	Pantopaque (3-6	18	28%	56	10 ≥ 1 yr.
Raskin et al., 1975	ml)	56	68%	—	28 pts. ≥ 2 yr.
Zachrisson, 1982	Bismuth	73	100%	—	33 pts ≥ 2 yr.
Holmberg and Hietala, 1989	phosphate (5-10 ml)	59	24%	51	37 pts. ≥ 2 yr.
Bean, 1981	Ethanol 95%	34	—	97	16 pts. > 1 yr.
Holmberg and Hietala, 1989	(25% of cyst volume × 20 minutes)	22	—	100	4 pts. > 6 mos.

Pts, patients.

into the cyst, an *indirect* approach can be taken. In this case, a separate nephrostomy tract is placed into the collecting system pointed as much as possible at the cyst. The interior of the cyst is opacified via the previously placed nephrostomy needle. A mixture of contrast material and indigo carmine mixed in *sorbitol* is used. This step will facilitate identification of the cyst and will aid any subsequent electrocautery incision into the cyst.

The next step is to operate on the cyst wall. The thin renal pelvic wall of the cyst can be *incised* (i.e., direct approach) or sharply entered and *excised* (i.e., indirect approach) with a cutting electrode (Collings knife) or resectoscope loop. The opening between the cyst and the collecting system is thus widened, thereby marsupializing the cyst into the renal pelvis (Hulbert et al., 1988c). Next, a roller electrode is utilized via a 24 Fr.

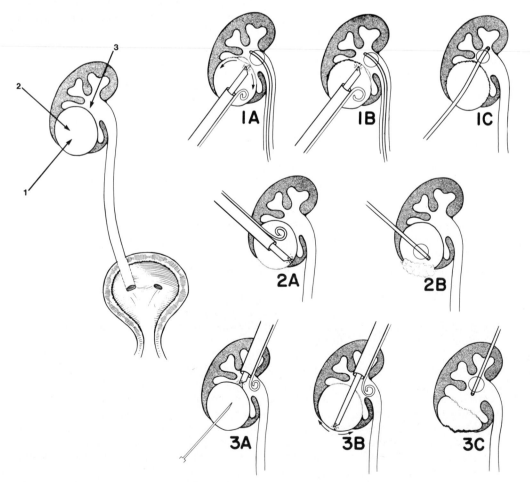

Figure 62–27. Three approaches for endoscopic therapy of a renal cyst.

1. Direct approach: transcystic. A, Cyst is directly punctured and a 30 Fr. Amplatz sheath is placed. The cyst wall abutting the renal pelvis is resected. B, The remaining cyst wall is fulgurated. C, The nephrostomy tube traverses the cyst.

2. Direct approach: transparenchymal. A, Cyst is punctured through the renal parenchyma. A 30 Fr. Amplatz sheath is placed. The cyst wall abutting the retroperitoneum is resected. B, A tube is placed in the cyst, and no communication is evident with the renal pelvis.

3. Indirect approach. A, The collecting system is entered away from the cyst. A 30 Fr. Amplatz sheath is placed. An 18-gauge needle is passed into the cyst to help distend its renal pelvic wall. The cyst is sharply entered and marsupialized into the renal pelvis. B, The far wall of the cyst is fulgurated. C, A nephrostomy tube is placed.

or 26 Fr. resectoscope, to fulgurate the walls of the cyst to encourage subsequent obliteration of the cystic cavity (Fig. 62–27). Alternatively, one may elect to not puncture the renal pelvis and instead of marsupializing the cyst, the thin peripheral wall of the cyst is resected, thereby effectively decorticating the cyst (see Fig. 62–27) (Hubner et al., 1990).

Following a direct approach to the cyst, a nephrostomy tube is placed through the cyst cavity and into the renal pelvis. With the indirect approach, the nephrostomy tube resides within the renal pelvis but does not cross or enter the cyst. The nephrostomy tube can be removed when a nephrostogram reveals no extravasation and satisfactory obliteration of the cystic cavity, which may require days to weeks.

Another, albeit more tedious endoscopic approach to the peripelvic cyst, is with the ureteroscope (Fig. 62–28) (Kavoussi et al., 1991a). In this case, a small percutaneous nephrostomy tube (8 Fr.) is first placed into the cyst. Next, a flexible or rigid ureteroscope is advanced into the renal pelvis. By filling the cyst with a mixture of sorbitol, radiographic contrast material, and indigo carmine and by alternately injecting and aspirating fluid into the cyst, the undulating wall of the cyst can be identified as it is filled and drained. If a flexible ureteroscope is being employed, a small electrode (2 Fr. or 3 Fr.) or Nd:YAG laser probe (400 μ) can be used to sharply enter the cyst, following which the cyst wall can be further incised. Alternatively, with the rigid ureteroscope, a cold knife can be utilized to enter the cyst. Next, the inner surface of the cyst wall is fulgurated with an electrocautery probe or a Nd:YAG laser (20 watts). However, fulguration of the cyst lining via the ureteroscope is tedious because of the necessarily small size of the instruments.

RESULTS. Simple cyst drainage is effective in curing only 4 to 19 per cent of lesions (see Table 62–5) (Holmberg and Hietala, 1989; Wahlquist and Grumstedt, 1966). For the symptomatic patient, sclerotherapy is indicated. Initial experience with iophendylate (Pantopaque) was successful (Vestby, 1967). However, sclerosis therapy with ethanol is even more effective (Ozgun et al., 1988). In a series of 22 cysts, all cysts treated with ethanol completely resolved and had not recurred at follow-up 3 months later. Also, cysts as large as 600 cc have been effectively sclerosed, with this approach.

Reports of an endoscopic approach have appeared sporadically in the literature (Chehval et al., 1990; Eickenberg, 1985; Hulbert et al., 1988c). Hubner and colleagues (1990) reported one of the largest experiences and noted a 93 per cent success rate. However, this approach is far more invasive and no more successful than ethanol injection. The endoscopic approach is therefore largely limited to peripelvic or communicating renal cysts.

Kavoussi and associates (1991a) reported treating small cysts ureteroscopically in three patients. The less invasive nature of the procedure is appealing; however, it is currently limited to relatively small cysts. In general, for cysts not amenable or not responsive to percutaneous sclerotherapy, the next step is a percutaneous approach.

Renal Abscesses

Intrarenal abscesses are either intraparenchymal (i.e., lobar nephronia or infected renal cyst) or confined to the collecting system as a result of calyceal obstruction with associated urosepsis (pyocalyx with an obstructing infection stone). The responsible organism is most commonly a gram-negative bacterium, such as *E. coli* or *Proteus* (Kaneti and Hertzanu, 1987; Sadi et al., 1988). The major risk of intraparenchymal lesions is life-threatening urosepsis and septicemia. However, some patients with infected renal cysts may present with minimal symptoms: mild flank discomfort and low-grade fever.

A patient with an intracollecting system abscess (i.e., a pyocalyx or pyonephrosis secondary to distal obstruction), usually from a struvite calculus, presents with an *acute* septicemia or a *chronic* condition, with minimal symptoms. In the *acute* case, *emergency* drainage of the obstructed collecting system is indicated. Any delay in establishing drainage can be fatal. However, in the *chronic* situation, the patient's symptoms may be so

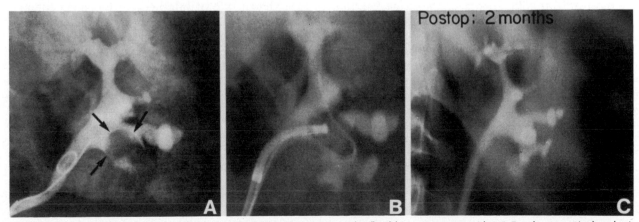

Figure 62–28. *A,* Intrapelvic cyst *(arrow)* noted on retrograde ureterogram. *B,* The flexible ureteroscope with a 3 Fr. electrosurgical probe is used to incise the cyst and fulgurate its interior. *C,* Postoperative intravenous urogram 2 months later reveals complete resolution of the cyst. (From Clayman, R. V., and Bagley, D. H.: Ureteronephroscopy. *In* Gillenwater, J. Y., Grayhack, J. T., Howards, S. S., and Duckett, J. W. (Eds.): Adult and Pediatric Urology, Chicago, Year Book Medical Publishers, 1990.)

minimal that the diagnosis is not initially entertained. Indeed, the individual may be afebrile and complain of only a slight amount of flank discomfort. These patients may have mild leucocytosis. The urine culture is often sterile. The clue to the underlying pathology is obtained from an intravenous urogram revealing a calculus but *nonvisualization* of the affected calyx (i.e., "missing" or "phantom" calyx) (Brennan and Pollack, 1979; Meretyk et al., 1991a).

Other signs of an intrarenal abscess on the intravenous urogram include perirenal gas, calculi, and nonfunction of the affected kidney. The abscess itself can best be outlined by CT or ultrasonography. Overall, CT is more accurate (in particular, more sensitive) than ultrasound in localizing the lesion and defining the surrounding anatomy (Haaga, 1990). As opposed to the ill-defined wedge-shaped lesions of lobar nephronia, the renal abscess has a well-defined thick-walled margin. The CT density (i.e., 2 to 25 HU on a $\pm$ 1000 HU scale) is often greater than that of a simple cyst. On ultrasound, these infected collections are hypoechoic with poor development of the posterior wall of the lesion. Intralesional debris may produce ultrasonically detectable intralesional echoes (Weigert et al., 1985).

TECHNIQUE. The most important therapeutic measure with regard to a renal abscess is drainage (see Percutaneous Nephrostomy, discussion of retroperitoneal abscess). Currently, treatment can be most rapidly done with percutaneous drainage. The added benefit of this approach is the minimal morbidity incurred, because the entire procedure can be performed using local anesthesia with minimal intravenous sedation.

Initially, a 22-gauge needle is passed into the renal abscess under CT or ultrasound guidance. Upon confirmation of the abscess (i.e., return of purulent material), a 7 Fr. or 8 Fr. catheter is placed utilizing a trocar or guide wire technique (Meretyk et al., 1991a).

The recommended approach is an *infracostal* puncture and drainage of the affected calyx, especially if the affected calyx is in the upper pole. The rationale behind this approach is to avoid an incidental pleurotomy. In order to perform an infracostal puncture, the needle may need to be steeply angled cephalad, thereby making the tract inadequate for subsequent stone removal. After 5 to 7 days of antibiotic coverage, the urine cultured from the bladder and the abscess drainage catheter is usually sterile. At this point, shock wave lithotripsy or percutaneous stone removal can be safely pursued (Meretyk et al., 1991a). Attempts at retrograde drainage via ureteral catheter are not recommended. This approach requires significant anesthesia, is more invasive, and provides less effective drainage (i.e., smaller catheter) than a percutaneous antegrade approach. Also, placement of the catheter into the affected calyx may be difficult if there is a site of distal obstruction (e.g., stone, stricture).

RESULTS. Results of percutaneous drainage of infected renal cysts have been satisfactory. The overall success rate is 82 per cent (22 collected cases), with a complication rate (sepsis, bleeding, secondary nephrectomy or recurrent abscess) of 18 per cent. Among these 22 cases, there have been two deaths (Cronan et al.,

1984; Gerzof et al., 1985; Haaga, 1990; Jaques et al., 1986).

The key factor affecting the outcome of the percutaneous approach is whether the abscess is simple or loculated. In the simple abscess case, percutaneous drainage yields success rates over 80 per cent. In the loculated abscess, a successful percutaneous outcome is noted in only 45 per cent. The presence of air within the mass indicates that the purulent contents may be thick and less amenable to percutaneous drainage (Haaga et al., 1977; Jaques et al., 1986). In addition, fungal infections or infected hematomas respond poorly to percutaneous drainage. In the case of a fungal renal abscess, drainage plus irrigation of the abscess cavity with amphotericin B (50 mg/L/day) may be necessary to achieve a satisfactory result (Haaga, 1990).

Among patients with urolithiasis and complicating pyocalyx/pyohydronephrosis, adherence to the aforementioned principles can effect an excellent result: drainage of the abscess and successful treatment of the calculus. However, in one series in which two patients were managed with supracostal (11th intercostal space) puncture, pulmonary complications resulted. In one individual, a massive pleural effusion developed, requiring prolonged chest tube drainage. A second individual developed empyema and needed open drainage. Also, in one individual in whom the diagnosis of a "phantom" calyx was missed, outpatient extracorporeal shock wave lithotripsy was performed. Immediate urosepsis and septicemia ensued, necessitating an emergency hospital admission with subsequent percutaneous drainage of the calyx and delayed percutaneous stone removal (Fig. 62–29) (Albala et al., 1990; Meretyk et al., 1991a).

Calyceal Diverticula

The calyceal diverticulum is a relatively rare entity, diagnosed in 4.5 per 1000 intravenous urograms. The diverticulum arises from the fornix of a minor calyx and hence is lined with transitional cell epithelium. Approximately a third to a half of these lesions cause symptoms such as pain, infection, hematuria, and those of calculi (Timmons et al., 1975). In general, surgical intervention is indicated in one third of patients, although a 1.4 per cent annual rate of intervention has been cited (Abeshouse and Abeshouse, 1963; Timmons et al., 1975). In contradistinction to a hydrocalyx, the calyceal diverticulum is believed to be a congenital rather than an acquired lesion. The surgical approach to these lesions involves either excision or marsupialization of the diverticulum with occlusion of the neck of the diverticulum by suture or electrocautery. However, the walls of the diverticulum may be scarified using electrocautery. If the diverticulum is large, a partial nephrectomy may be necessary (Abeshouse and Abeshouse, 1963). Over the past decade, the treatment for calyceal diverticula has become less invasive. Currently, a percutaneous approach appears to be favored (Fig. 62–30) (Clayman and Castaneda-Zuniga, 1984; Hulbert et al., 1988).

TECHNIQUE. The first step in the percutaneous approach to a calyceal diverticulum is the cystoscopic placement of a retrograde ureteral catheter. A 0.035-

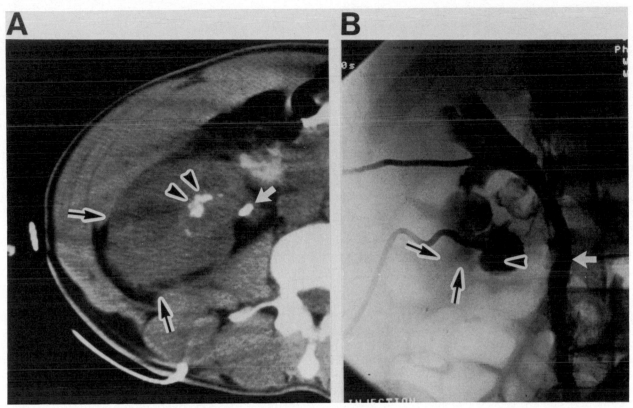

Figure 62–29. *A,* At 24 hours after extracorporeal shock wave lithotripsy, the patient presented with urosepsis. A computed tomography (CT) scan reveals stone debris *(arrowheads),* a nephrostent in the ureter *(white arrow),* and a large dilated lower pole calyx *(black arrows).*
   B, A percutaneous tube was placed into the lower pole calyx; purulent material was drained. Via the two tracts, the stone material was percutaneously removed and continuity between the lower pole infundibulum and the renal pelvis was re-established. (*White arrow,* nephrostent; *black arrow,* outline of pyohydrocalyx; *black arrowhead,* location of stone debris.) The arrows correspond to the level of the CT film shown in *A.*

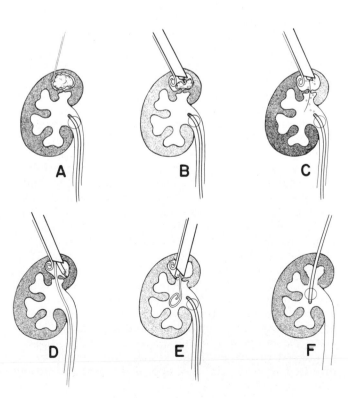

Figure 62–30. *A,* Large upper pole calyceal diverticulum with a stone. *B,* The diverticulum has been punctured directly. Ultrasonic lithotripsy is used to remove the calculus. *C,* Air injected retrograde is used to identify the diverticular neck. A guide wire is passed across the diverticular neck. *D,* An electrocautery probe is used to fulgurate the walls of the diverticulum. *E,* The electrocautery probe is now used to incise the neck of the diverticulum. *F,* A transdiverticular nephrostomy tube is placed.

inch floppy tip guide wire is passed retrograde. Over this guide wire, a 7 Fr., 11.5-mm occlusion balloon is passed into the renal pelvis. Next, a fluoroscopically guided puncture is made directly into the calyceal diverticulum itself, utilizing an 18-gauge nephrostomy needle. The guide wire is coiled in the diverticulum as the neck of the diverticulum is usually too small to cannulate. If the diverticulum is particularly large, a second guide wire can be placed (see Percutaneous Nephrostomy), thereby providing the surgeon with both a "safety" and a "working" guide wire. The tract into the diverticulum is dilated with a 10-mm balloon dilator. Dilating the tract with shear dilators (i.e., Amplatz coaxial system, separate Teflon dilators, or metal telescoping dilators) is more difficult and may result in an anterior false passage of the diverticulum. A 10-mm Amplatz sheath is placed into the diverticulum, following which the rigid nephroscope is introduced. Any calculus present is treated by either intact removal or ultrasonic nephrolithotripsy (Clayman and Castaneda-Zuniga, 1984).

Next, the occlusion balloon on the retrograde ureteral catheter is inflated and the catheter is pulled caudad until it gently occludes the ureteropelvic junction. Saline stained with indigo carmine, CO_2, or room air is gently instilled through the retrograde ureteral catheter while the surgeon examines the interior of the calyceal diverticulum with the rigid or flexible nephroscope. Blue fluid or air bubbles can be seen traversing the neck of the diverticulum. If these are not seen, the Amplatz sheath may be too deep into the diverticulum. The sheath should be carefully withdrawn 1 to 2 cm under endoscopic control, while the assistant continues to gently instill fluid or air into the retrograde ureteral catheter. Once the neck of the diverticulum is visualized, a 0.035-inch floppy tip guide wire or a plastic (i.e., Terumo) guide wire can be passed across the neck of the diverticulum and coiled in the renal pelvis (see Fig. 62–30) (Clayman and Castaneda-Zuniga, 1984).

The neck of the diverticulum can now be treated. This can be done most simply by balloon dilation of the neck of the diverticulum with an 8-mm, 4-cm long ureteral dilating balloon. However, some urologists prefer to cut the neck of the diverticulum under direct vision with either a cold knife (i.e., direct vision urethrotome) or an electrocautery probe (2 Fr. or 3 Fr. Greenwald electrode). In electrocautery, the metal guide wire should be covered with a 5 Fr. angiographic catheter so that no electrical current will be transmitted by the guide wire. Several shallow incisions (2 to 4 mm) are made in the neck of the diverticulum in a radial fashion (12, 3, 6, and 9 o'clock). A solitary deep cut into the diverticular neck should be avoided, as this may result in significant hemorrhage (Clayman and Castaneda-Zuniga, 1984).

After opening the neck of the diverticulum, a large bore (22 Fr.) nephrostomy tube is placed such that its shaft traverses the diverticulum and the tip of the catheter lies in the renal pelvis (see Fig. 62–30). The nephrostomy tube can be removed as early as 3 days after the procedure (Hulbert et al., 1986). Indeed, prolonged drainage of the kidney and stinting of the diverticular neck do not appear to improve results (Hulbert et al., 1988a).

An alternative and perhaps simpler method is to percutaneously approach the diverticulum directly and remove the calculus. At this point, the neck of the diverticulum is identified and thoroughly cauterized with a 3 Fr. or 5 Fr. electrocautery probe (J. Segura, personal communication). Next the walls of the diverticulum are cauterized, utilizing a roller electrode. A 22 Fr. nephrostomy tip is placed only to tamponade the nephrostomy tract. The tip of the catheter enters the calyceal diverticulum. Nothing traverses the neck of the diverticulum. The renal parenchyma is barely traversed, and the renal collecting system is never entered. The "calycostomy" tube is removed on the following morning provided there is no drainage. This approach most closely resembles previously described conservative surgical therapy for calyceal diverticula.

In addition to the previously described methods, in patients with large diverticula, additional therapy may be necessary. Specifically, just prior to opening the neck of the diverticulum, the walls of the diverticulum can be fulgurated using a straight or roller electrode (see Fig. 62–30). This scarification of the wall may further hasten the collapse of the diverticulum. It is best to do this *prior to incising the neck of the diverticulum,* so that the electrocoagulation can be accomplished in a clear endoscopic field (Hulbert et al., 1987).

Three other endosurgical alternatives are possible for treating a calyceal diverticulum: indirect percutaneous approach, ureteroscopic approach, and extracorporeal shock wave lithotripsy. An *indirect percutaneous approach* can be problematic. A usually nonhydronephrotic collecting system must be punctured. Next, the surgeon must locate the diminutive communication between the calyceal diverticulum and the collecting system. Following this step, the neck must be opened and the diverticulum entered. However, incising the neck of the diverticulum often results in bleeding, which obscures the surgeon's vision. Any calculus must be removed. This maneuver can be extremely difficult because of the indirect approach. As such, the indirect approach is mentioned solely to discourage its use.

Problems, similar to those of an indirect percutaneous approach, are also encountered with *ureteroscopic attempt* to treat a calyceal diverticulum. A flexible ureteroscope is usually necessary. Even if the diverticulum is in the upper pole of the kidney in a female patient there still may not be enough room to maneuver the rigid endoscope to enable the surgeon to successfully identify the neck of the diverticulum. Next, the neck of the diverticulum must be cannulated and then dilated or incised. This maneuver also requires considerable manipulation. For *balloon dilation,* usually a guide wire must be passed across the neck of the diverticulum, the ureteroscope removed, and a balloon catheter passed over the guide wire into the diverticulum. Occasionally, under fluoroscopic guidance, a 4-mm balloon can be passed through the rigid ureteroscope after the lens is withdrawn.

Alternatively, *incising* the neck of the diverticulum requires a 2 Fr. electrocautery probe or a Nd:YAG laser probe. If a rigid ureteroscope is being used, a cold knife is needed (Fig. 62–31). Entering the diverticulum by direct incision may result in bleeding, which rapidly

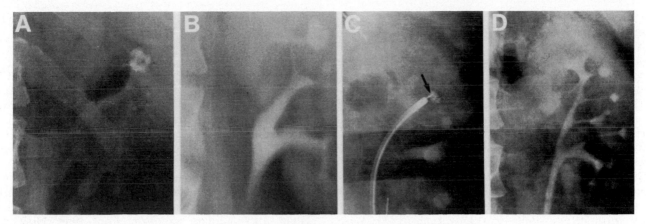

Figure 62–31. *A,* A stone is present in the upper pole of the left kidney on this plain film of the abdomen.
B, The stone is located in a calyceal diverticulum as seen on this intravenous urogram.
C, A flexible ureteroscope with a 3 Fr. electrode is being used to incise the neck of the diverticulum *(arrow).* Subsequently, the ureteroscope could be passed into the diverticulum. The calculus was fragmented using a 250-μ pulsed dye laser probe.
D, At 2 months postoperatively, the neck of the diverticulum is widely patent providing excellent drainage of the diverticulum. The stone fragments have passed. (From Clayman, R. V., and Bagley, D. H.: Ureteronephroscopy. *In* Gillenwater, J. Y., Grayhack, J. T., Howards, S. S., and Duckett, J. W. (Eds.): Adult and Pediatric Urology, Chicago, Year Book Medical Publishers, 1990.)

obscures the surgeon's vision. When a calculus is identified, it must be grasped directly (if it is <7 mm) or fragmented with a pulsed dye laser or an electrohydraulic lithotripsy probe. If the diverticulum is capacious, electrocoagulation of its wall should be done, which can be difficult and tedious. Given all of these technical difficulties, it is not surprising that to date reports of ureteroscopic treatment of calyceal diverticula have been largely anecdotal (Hulbert et al., 1987; Mikkelsen et al., 1989).

One other modality has been examined for treating a stone-containing calyceal diverticulum: extracorporeal shock wave lithotripsy (SWL). Although the stone can be disintegrated with shock waves, the treatment does not eliminate the diverticulum. Also, because of the small caliber of the diverticular neck, the stone fragments may not clear unless the neck has been ureteroscopically cannulated and balloon dilated prior to SWL (Fuchs and David, 1989).

RESULTS. In comparing all of the endosurgical methods for treating a calyceal diverticulum, it becomes quite clear that an antegrade (i.e., direct puncture) percutaneous approach is safe and most effective. In reports on a direct approach, the calculus has been removed in upward of 100 per cent and the diverticulum has been successfully obliterated in 85 per cent of patients (Eshghi et al., 1987; Hulbert et al., 1988a). The indirect methods have all provided poorer results. Indeed, Hulbert and colleagues (1986) noted that in three patients approached with indirect punctures, the diverticula were still present in all three on follow-up radiographic studies, 4 to 14 months later.

The nonpercutaneous alternatives have produced similarly disappointing results. Using an ureteroscopic approach, Mikkelsen and co-workers (1989) could only successfully treat two of six calyceal diverticula. In one of the successful cases, two ureteroscopic procedures were required because of postoperative bleeding from the diverticulum. Similarly, with SWL as front line therapy, Psihramis and Dretler (1987) noted that 70 per cent of patients became asymptomatic after treatment.

However, 80 per cent still had stone fragments within the diverticula at the time of follow-up. In all patients studied, the diverticula remained intact.

Fuchs and David (1989) have combined SWL with ureteroscopy for dilation of the calyceal neck and stone extraction in 15 patients with stone-containing calyceal diverticula. Their overall stone-free rate of 73 per cent is an improvement over SWL monotherapy; however, it is not as effective as an antegrade approach. Likewise, there was no direct treatment of the underlying stone-forming diathesis other than dilation of the neck of the diverticulum.

Fungal Bezoar

Candida pyelonephritis (associated with cortical abscesses and/or diffuse involvement of the medullary rays) and asymptomatic *Candida* infestation of the urine can both be associated with the development of intrarenal fungal concretions (Beland and Piette, 1973). The pseudomycelia that are characteristic of *Candida albicans* may aggregate to form a significant mass within the renal pelvis. Similarly, *Torulopsis glabrata* can form a fungal conglomeration albeit without pseudohyphae. In these patients, the masses consist of fungus, necrotic tissue, inflammatory cells, and on occasion stone matrix (Abramowitz et al., 1986; Beland and Piette, 1973).

Patients who are especially predisposed to developing fungal bezoars are those who have diabetes mellitus, who use antibiotics chronically, who have urinary tract catheters, and who are immunosuppressed (Schonebeck and Ansehn, 1972). About half the reported cases of fungal concretions are in diabetic patients (Dembner and Pfister, 1977). Upward of 20 per cent of renal transplant patients may develop funguria (Schonebeck and Ansehn, 1972). These individuals may be septic, may develop problems directly attributable to the obstructive properties of the fungal bezoar itself, or may remain asymptomatic (Beland and Piette, 1973; Schonebeck and Ansehn, 1972).

The diagnosis of a fungal concretion is suspected when

an intravenous urogram or a retrograde ureterogram reveals a noncalcified "filling defect" within the renal pelvis. The pseudomycelia or yeast forms characteristic of a *Candida* infection can be noted on a freshly prepared urinalysis. A urine culture will likewise reveal the presence of *C. albicans* or *T. glabrata*.

Therapy for the fungal concretion involves two simultaneous approaches. In the preoperative or seriously ill patient, a course of amphotericin B or 5-fluorocytosine is initiated. Once adequate serum levels are obtained, topical irrigation of the affected collecting system with amphotericin B (50 mg/L at 25 to 50 ml/hour) can be given via either two retrograde ureteral catheters (one for inflow; one for outflow) or an antegrade nephrostomy tube (Blum, 1966; Harrach et al., 1970; Wise, 1990). Alternatively, once antibiotic coverage has resulted in sterile urine cultures, the bezoar can be removed percutaneously or by open surgery (Karlin et al., 1987).

TECHNIQUE. The percutaneous removal of a fungal bezoar requires meticulous attention to detail (Table 62–6). Initially, two retrograde ureteral catheters are placed. The renal pelvis is irrigated with amphotericin B (50 mg/L) to decrease the hypothetic possibility of retroperitoneal seeding of the fungus. The percutaneous nephrostomy technique follows the same principles for placement of a nephrostomy tract as previously described. An infracostal lower pole approach to the renal pelvis is secured; a "working" and "safety" guide wire are secured. A supracostal approach is never used, as traversal of the pleural cavity could result in a fungal empyema. Because the goal is to minimize both the manipulation of the renal parenchyma and the potential of retroperitoneal extravasation, dilation of the tract is most simply done with a 10-mm nephrostomy tract dilating balloon. In an effort to limit retroperitoneal extravasation, of urine and fragments of the fungal concretion, a 30 Fr. Amplatz sheath is positioned in the collecting system.

The fungal bezoar has a gray-white or yellow-gray appearance. The consistency is similar to a blood clot. If it is < 1.5 cm, it can be extracted intact from the collecting system; however, for the larger concretions, the suction on the ultrasonic lithotriptor probe is most useful for bezoar evacuation. The flexible nephroscope is helpful to ensure complete removal of all fungal concretions from the collecting system.

At the end of the procedure, a 22 Fr. Councill catheter is secured as a nephrostomy tube. Approximately 50 ml of a solution of 50 mg of amphotericin per liter is immediately flushed (by gravity pressure) through the nephrostomy tube. One of the two ureteral catheters is removed. On postoperative day one, a nephrostogram is obtained. If there are no extravasations and no remaining concretions, irrigation with amphotericin B (50 mg/L at 50 ml/hour) is performed via the ureteral catheter for 48 to 72 hours (Wise, 1990). Provided the urine culture is free of *Candida*, the ureteral catheter and nephrostomy tube can be removed on postoperative day 3 or 4. However, if the nephrostogram reveals any remaining "filling defects," repeat of flexible and rigid

nephroscopy may be necessary to render the kidney bezoar-free.

RESULTS. In general, reports of fungal bezoars are rare (Schonebeck and Ansehn, 1972). Indeed, in a review of the literature, Schonebeck and Ansehn (1972) noted only 24 cases of upper tract fungal concretions; to this list, they added five more cases from their own experience. Presence of an upper tract fungal bezoar in association with an unrelieved ureteral obstruction has a mortality rate in the 80 per cent range. However, placement of ureteral catheters with and without irrigation with amphotericin B as well as *surgical* removal of the fungal concretion is curative, albeit in a small number of reviewed cases (Beland and Piette, 1973; Blum, 1966; Gillam and Wadelton, 1958; Harrach et al., 1970).

Given the infrequent occurrence of this problem, it is not surprising that there is a paucity of experience with regard to the percutaneous management and removal of fungal concretions (Abramowitz et al., 1986; Dembner and Pfister, 1977; Karline et al., 1987). Over the last 10 years, approximately ten cases of percutaneous therapy for renal fungal bezoars have been reported. In some cases (i.e., few and small fungal aggregates) this has involved only the establishment of a percutaneous nephrostomy for drainage. In others, with larger fungal masses, the bezoar has been either fragmented (with a guide wire) or extracted directly (Bartone et al., 1988; Blum, 1966; Harrach et al., 1970; Irby et al., 1990). In this limited group of patients, successful treatment has occurred in almost all (> 80 per cent) with minimal attendant morbidity and mortality. Of particular interest is the report by Bartone and associates (1988) of successful application of these techniques in neonates with urinary candidiasis.

Essential Hematuria

As previously noted, during an *endoscopic evaluation* the most common cause of benign essential hematuria is an *anatomic site-specific* vascular abnormality or malformation. The vascular lesions are scattered throughout the kidney without a single area of predominance (Bagley and Allen, 1990).

TECHNIQUE. The procedure for identifying the site of bleeding was previously described under Diagnostic Endourology. After endoscopic site-specific localization, treatment is effectively and efficiently rendered by direct fulguration of the lesion. This procedure is accomplished with a monopolar electrocautery probe (2 Fr. or 3 Fr. with a 250- or 600-μ tip, 50 watts, pure coagulation), a bipolar electrocautery unit, or a Nd:YAG laser probe (400 μ fiber, 20 watts). After fulguration, irrigant flow (sorbitol or saline) through the ureteroscope is stopped. If there is no further bleeding, the endoscope is removed. An indwelling ureteral stent is placed for 2 to 3 days to preclude obstructive ureteral edema due to the dilation of the distal ureter.

RESULTS. The result of endoscopic fulguration is excellent provided the lesion is solitary (i.e., anatomically localized). Minimal renal damage and usually im-

Table 62–6. PERCUTANEOUS EXTRACTION OF FUNGAL BEZOAR

| Authors | Sex | Age | Symptoms | | DM* | Renal Transplant | Immuno-suppression | History of Lithiasis or Renal Surgery | Method | Urine Culture | Long-term Follow-up |
			Fever	Flank Pain							
Karlin et al., 1987	F	49	Yes	Yes	Yes	No	No	Yes	Percutaneous extraction/ systemic and percutaneous irrigation with amphotericin B	*Candida albicans* *Pseudomonas aeruginosa*	—
Abramowitz et al., 1986	F	72	Yes	No	Yes	No	No	No	Percutaneous extraction	*Torulopsis glabrata*	Sterile urine culture at 4 mos.
Doemeny et al., 1988	F	65	Yes	Yes	Yes	No	No	No	Percutaneous extraction	*Torulopsis glabrata*	—
Ireton et al., 1985	F	49	Yes	No	No	Yes	Yes	Yes	Percutaneous extraction	*Candida albicans*	6 mos.
Irby et al., 1990	M	28	—	—	Yes	No	No	No	Percutaneous extraction	*Candida albicans*	—
	M	50	—	—	Yes	No	No	No	Percutaneous extraction	*Aspergillus*	Required nephrectomy

*DM, diabetes mellitus.

mediate cessation of the bleeding are noted. The durability of this approach is also excellent. Follow-up information has revealed a low incidence of recurrent hemorrhage among patients in whom a single site of hemorrhage due to a vascular abnormality was treated (Bagley and Allen, 1990; McMurtry et al., 1987; Patterson et al., 1984). However, re-bleeding is quite common, if the source of hematuria appears to be diffuse (Bagley and Allen, 1990).

Other therapeutic options for site-specific hemorrhage are seldom necessary. Embolization is reserved for only those patients with well-defined vascular lesions identified on arteriograms. These are most commonly seen in patients with acute or delayed bleeding, following percutaneous procedures: an injured segmental renal artery or renal vein unresponsive to tamponade (acute injury) and an arterial pseudoaneurysm or arteriovenous malformation (delayed hemorrhage) (see Fig. 62–16). Surgical exploration for essential hematuria is indicated only as a salvage procedure when all of the aforementioned attempts at endoscopic/radiologic therapy fail. In these cases, a partial or total nephrectomy is often necessary to stop the hemorrhage (Lanno et al., 1979).

The results of an endosurgical approach are less certain when a definite lesion is not located (e.g., medical renal diseases: acute tubular necrosis, diabetic nephropathy, glomerulonephritis, IgA nephropathy, vasculitis, systemic lupus erythematosus). Fulguration of multiple areas of "inflammation" may be effective but usually only for a brief period of time. Some patients (i.e., those with sickle cell hemoglobinopathy) may be better treated with irrigation of the collecting system with 1 per cent silver nitrate, which produces a caustic protein precipitant (Bahnson, 1987). In this situation, 10 ml of the 1 per cent silver nitrate solution can be slowly instilled into the system via a single retrograde catheter once or twice until the effluent becomes clear. With this regimen, Bahnson (1987) noted successful termination of hematuria in three patients with sickle cell trait, who remained free of recurrent bleeding for an average of 13 months. Alternatively, a trial with intravenous and then oral epsilon amino caproic acid (4 to 24 gm/day; recommended oral dosage, 150 mg/kg for 3 weeks), an inhibitor of plasminogen activation, can be given (Immergut and Stevenson, 1965; Nash and Henry, 1984; Stefanini et al., 1990).

Strictures of the Upper Urinary Tract

AN OVERVIEW OF ENDOINCISION FOR UPPER URINARY TRACT STRICTURE

"In evaluating one's clinical results, I think the relief of symptoms is a very poor guidepost. I think, unless we can demonstrate better renal drainage, we have not accomplished the success which we hope to."

R. B. HENLINE
JULY 1, 1947
AMERICAN UROLOGICAL ASSOCIATION ANNUAL MEETING

In the field of endourology, there is no more difficult area in which to establish a preoperative diagnosis and to judge a postoperative result than that of upper urinary tract strictures. The *diagnosis* of a stricture itself may often be in doubt. *Anatomic* obstruction as noted on an intravenous urogram may not represent *functional* obstruction as delineated by a diuretic washout renogram or a Whitaker bladder/renal pelvis pressure study. Indeed, it is only the documented functional obstruction that mandates corrective surgery.

Also, the urologist must be careful to examine the characterization of each stricture in the reported patient population. Coexisting conditions may result in a transient stricture. For example, a renal pelvic calculus or a urinary tract infection may result in inflammation sufficient to obstruct the ureteropelvic junction. However, this problem will usually resolve spontaneously upon removal of the calculus or appropriate antibiotic therapy. In this setting, the "success" of an endoincision becomes inflated. A preponderance of postirradiation ureteral strictures in a series may also negatively prejudice the results. Both the length and location of a stricture influence the success of an endoincision. Short (< 1 cm) strictures at the proximal or distal ureter fare better than longer strictures at the middle ureter.

It is also difficult to ascertain the *success* of an endoincision. Subjective and objective follow-up should be carefully differentiated. Although a telephone call to the patient or to the primary physician can provide some data as to how the patient has fared, these data, unaccompanied by objective studies, are seriously flawed. For example, complaints of minor musculoskeletal back discomfort may negatively prejudice results, whereas many patients (upward of 25 per cent) with significant recurrent stricture disease may actually be asymptomatic, thereby falsely improving the results. As such, objective *functional* tests of patency, such as the diuretic washout renogram or the Whitaker test, although not ideal, still may provide more accurate information on the ultimate outcome of the procedure. Alone, the IVP can be misleading, because the hydronephrosis associated with chronic uteropelvic junction obstruction in the adult usually does not resolve. Certainly, among these patients, when a postoperative IVP is suggestive of recurrent obstruction, a functional test should follow.

Another problem in evaluating the outcome of an endoincision is to discern the *permanence* of the "successful" endoincision. Unlike stone disease in which the result is immediately evident, with obstructive uropathy, it may take 6 months to a year before one can be confident that the problem has resolved. Short follow-up (< 6 months) usually provides overly optimistic results. In a series of endoureterotomy patients, late failure (> 6 months) occurred in 15 per cent, thereby lowering the overall success rate from 79 per cent to 64 per cent (Meretyk et al., 1990).

Also, incomplete patient follow-up data may likewise result in inaccurate conclusions. To have a series of 100 patients undergoing endoincisions and report follow-up information on only 50 patients in all of whom the procedure "succeeded" provides one with the uneasy task of attempting to decide whether the success rate is actually 100 per cent or perhaps only 50 per cent. Do the failures seek self-exile in the care of another physician or do the successes merely declare independence from the "healing" profession? It should not be left to the individual to ferret out this information.

Diagnosis of Obstruction of the Upper Urinary Tract

The classic symptom of obstruction of the upper urinary tract is flank discomfort exacerbated by intake of fluids or of natural (e.g., alcohol) or pharmacologic diuretics. Interestingly, many patients (upward of 25 per cent) may be pain-free, the diagnosis being made during the evaluation for serendipitously discovered urolithiasis or urosepsis. The incidental discovery of ureteropelvic junction obstruction may lead to repair, if compromise of renal function is documented during conservative follow-up management (Gillenwater, 1987).

The objective diagnosis of obstruction of the upper urinary tract can, at times, be quite difficult. The IVP, with delayed films, will usually show the point of obstruction. However, this is only an anatomic abnormality and not necessarily a functional obstruction. Indeed, the collecting system may appear to be narrowed at a particular point, yet the patient is asymptomatic. In order to differentiate between anatomic and functional obstruction, the two tests available are, as mentioned, the diuretic washout renogram and the Whitaker renal pelvic/bladder differential pressure study.

With the diuresis renogram (furosemide [Lasix] washout), [131]I Hippuran (o-iodohippurate), [123]I Hippuran, or technetium-99m diethylenetriamine pentaacetic acid (DTPA) is given, and renal images are taken at 2, 5, 10, 15, 20, 25, and 30 minutes (Talner, 1990). If the curve appears to demonstrate obstruction, furosemide (0.5 mg/kg to 1.0 mg/kg) is given intravenously at 30 minutes. After furosemide administration, in a normal nonobstructed situation, with two kidneys, 50 per cent of the radionuclide tracer should drain from the kidney within 10 minutes. If it takes longer than 20 minutes, obstruction is likely (Fig. 62–32). Drainage times between 10 and 20 minutes are considered equivocal for obstruction (Talner, 1990). Problems in interpretation of the diuretic washout renogram usually result in a false-positive conclusion. This interpretation is due to medical renal disease, renal artery disease, or massive hydronephrosis, because these conditions may blunt the response to furosemide or affect the dilution of the excreted radionuclide (Maizels et al., 1986; O'Reilly et al., 1979; Talner, 1990).

In cases in which the diuretic washout renogram is equivocal, a renal perfusion pressure flow study (i.e., Whitaker test) can be performed (Fig. 62–33) (Newhouse et al., 1981; Whitaker, 1979). This invasive study involves placement of a needle (20- or 22-gauge) or a small nephrostomy tube (8 Fr.) into the renal collecting system. A urethral catheter is also placed to drain the bladder. The collecting system is perfused via the percutaneously placed needle or catheter at a rate of 10 ml/minute with dilute contrast material. After the collecting system is fully distended, separate pressure readings of the renal pelvis and the bladder are recorded every 5 minutes until a steady pressure is reached in both areas. If the difference in the pressure between the renal pelvis and bladder is less than 13 to 15 cm H_2O, the system is unobstructed. In contrast, a renal pelvis/bladder pressure differential greater than 22 cm H_2O indicates obstruction. A pressure difference of 15 to 22 cm H_2O is considered equivocal. To further test the patency of the system, the inflow can be increased to 15 ml/minute; in this case, the normal differential pressure should be ≤ 18 cm H_2O (Newhouse et al., 1981).

Two sources for error in the Whitaker test are the presence of extravasation during the test and failure to completely fill the renal pelvis *system* before obtaining pressure readings. If the obstruction is positional in nature, it may not be evident during the Whitaker test, as the patient is in the prone position. Each of these problems can result in a false-negative result (O'Reilly, 1986).

Overall, the diuretic washout renal scan and the

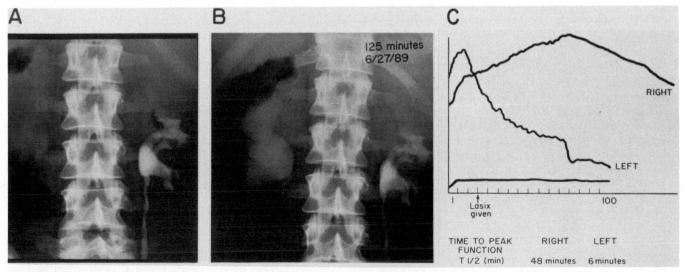

Figure 62–32. *A* and *B*, Intravenous urogram in a 37-year-old female with intermittent right flank pain. A marked delay occurs in visualization of the right collecting system.

C, Furosemide (Lasix) washout renogram demonstrating normal clearance from the left kidney but a prolonged clearance of radionuclide from the right kidney with a half-life of 48 minutes.

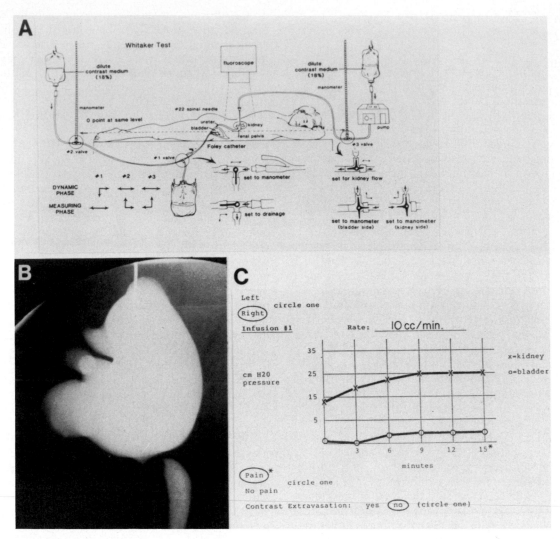

Figure 62–33. *A*, The set up for a Whitaker test. Through the needle in the renal pelvis, fluid is perfused at a constant rate. Once the collecting system is fully distended, the pressure is simultaneously measured in the bladder and renal pelvis. (From Clayman, R. V., and Castaneda-Zuniga, W. R.: Techniques in Endourology: A Guide to Percutaneous Removal of Renal and Ureteral Calculi. Chicago, Year Book Medical Publishers, 1986.)

B, In this Whitaker test, the collecting system is fully distended. The uteropelvic junction is markedly narrowed. At 10 ml/min, the pressure differential is 22 cm H₂O, indicating significant obstruction.

C, Graph of the Whitaker test showing that after a steady state was reached at 9 minutes, the pressure differential remained elevated (22 cm).

Whitaker test are complementary. Although a normal diuretic washout renal scan is a reliable indicator of a nonobstructed system, an abnormal result must be viewed with caution. In this case, a Whitaker test is indicated, as it will help discern the positive renal scan from a false-positive one (O'Reilly, 1986). Indeed, in 9 to 30 per cent of patients, a positive diuretic washout renal scan is discredited by a concomitantly normal perfusion pressure flow study. The patient usually has marked hydronephrosis or a poorly functioning kidney. Conversely, the Whitaker test may be clinically unreliable in 15 per cent of patients. The ideal situation, especially in the patient with marked hydronephrosis or decreased renal function (< 20 per cent of total), is to perform both studies, because agreement between the two examinations, which occurs in 40 to 60 per cent, is the most clinically reliable situation (Krueger et al., 1980).

Infundibular Stenosis: Endoinfundibulotomy

Infundibular stenosis and hydrocalyx are usually an acquired condition associated with inflammation, obstructive calculus, spasm of a major calyceal sphincter, or prior renal surgery (Abeshouse and Abeshouse, 1963). Rarely, infundibular stenosis may be caused by an upper pole crossing segmental renal artery (Fraley's syndrome) (Eshghi et al., 1987; Fraley, 1969). If one suspects the presence of an obstructing crossing segmental renal artery, an arteriogram should be obtained prior to any endourologic therapeutic maneuvers, because this condition mandates an open surgical repair (Eshghi, et al., 1987). Also, the hydrocalyx should not be confused with a calyceal diverticulum because the treatments are very different. At times this distinction can be made only by nephroscopy, because the presence (hydrocalyx) or absence (calyceal diverticulum) of a renal papilla is diagnostic. Although an endoscopic approach may be attempted in the patient with a stenotic infundibulum and hydrocalyx, an open surgical approach (usually partial nephrectomy) has the highest success rate (Abeshouse and Abeshouse, 1963). However, in patients with a calyceal diverticulum, a percutaneous approach with attendant fulguration of the cavity is recommended.

TECHNIQUE. The percutaneous antegrade technique for infundibular stenosis is initially similar to the approach for calyceal diverticulum (Fig. 62–34). Initially, a retrograde ureteral occlusion balloon catheter is placed. The balloon is inflated in the renal pelvis and pulled caudally to place it snugly against the ureteropelvic junction. Via the flank, the hydrocalyx is punctured directly and a 0.035-inch floppy tip guide wire is coiled in the affected calyx. The nephrostomy tract into the hydrocalyx is dilated with a 10-mm nephrostomy balloon, and an Amplatz 10-mm sheath is placed into the calyx. Careful inspection with the rigid or flexible

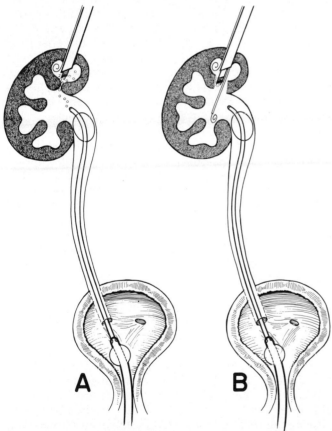

Figure 62–34. A, Arrangement for endoscopic treatment of an upper pole stenotic infundibulum. Note the retrograde occlusion balloon catheter in the ureter, the safety wire coiled in the hydrocalyx, and the CO_2 from the ureteral catheter bubbling across the stenotic infundibulum. Via the 30 Fr. Amplatz sheath, a 12 Fr. therapeutic short ureteroscope with an insulated tip has been introduced. A 0.035-inch guide wire is poised at the identified infundibular neck.

B, A guide wire and 5 Fr. angiographic catheter have been passed across the stenotic infundibulum. A 2 Fr. electrode is passed via the 12 Fr. short therapeutic ureteroscope. The electrode is being used to make multiple 1- to 2-mm radial incisions (3, 6, 9, 12 o'clock) (pure cut, 50 to 100 watts) into the stenotic infundibulum.

nephroscope enables the endoscopist to visualize the stenotic infundibulum and cannulate it with a 0.035-inch floppy tip or Terumo guide wire. This second (i.e., working) guide wire is coiled in the renal pelvis or, if possible, passed down the ureter. If difficulty is encountered in locating the mouth of the infundibulum, CO_2, air, or saline mixed with a small amount of indigo carmine can be infused via the retrograde occlusion balloon catheter (see Fig. 62–34). Usually, bubbles or blue fluid can be seen entering the calyx via the stenotic infundibulum.

The infundibular narrowing can be resolved in any number of ways. The least difficult approach is to dilate the infundibulum to 8 mm with ureteral balloon passed over the working guide wire. Alternatively, the infundibulum can be cut under endoscopic control with a cold knife via a direct vision urethrotome or using a Nd:YAG laser. In the last case, only the bare wire should be in place because the laser energy will melt any interposed catheters. Alternatively, a 2 Fr. or 3 Fr. electrocautery probe can be used. In that case, a 5 Fr. angiographic catheter is passed over the working guide wire to insulate it. The incision should be made in several places along the infundibulum: specifically, three or four, 2-mm incisions are made in a radial (12, 3, 6, and 9 o'clock) fashion along the mouth of the infundibulum. A single deep cut is to be avoided—this may result in marked bleeding. Before making an incision, the area to be incised should be carefully inspected for the presence of any arterial pulsations.

After the incision is completed, the patency of the infundibulum can be further gauged by passing an 8-mm dilating balloon catheter across the incised infundibulum. The balloon should inflate to 24 Fr. at low pressure (< 1 atm). Next, a 22 Fr. or 24 Fr. Councill catheter is passed into the system to serve as a nephrostomy tube. A side hole is cut just proximal to the retention balloon in order to help drain the affected calyx. The Councill catheter is passed over the working guide wire, such that the tip of the catheter lies in the renal pelvis and the shaft of the catheter traverses the incised calyx. This catheter is left in place for 4 to 6 weeks.

Alternatively, a 7 Fr./14 Fr. variable-sized indwelling stent can be placed, such that one end of the pigtail is in the affected calyx and the 14 Fr. portion of the stent traverses the incised infundibulum. In this case, only a 10 Fr. BUD catheter serves as the nephrostomy tube. The coil of the nephrostomy tube is placed in the calyx or in the renal pelvis. A nephrostogram is obtained 2 to 3 days later. If there is no extravasation, the nephrostomy tube is removed under fluoroscopic control. The indwelling 7 Fr./14 Fr. stent is removed via the bladder 4 to 6 weeks later.

Another therapeutic approach to infundibular stenosis is retrograde via the ureteroscope. In this case, a Terumo or floppy tip guide wire is passed retrograde via the ureteroscope, across the narrowed infundibulum and coiled in the affected calyx. The ureteroscope is removed. Next, under fluoroscopic monitoring, an 8-mm balloon catheter with no tip is passed. The balloon is passed until it straddles the stenotic infundibulum. The balloon is inflated and deflated two or three times. Each inflation cycle lasts for five to ten minutes. A 10 Fr. or 7 Fr./14 Fr. indwelling ureteral stent is placed with one coil residing in the affected calyx and the 10 Fr. or 14 Fr. shaft traversing the infundibulum. Alternatively, if it is deemed necessary to incise the infundibulum (i.e., waist does not resolve with the dilating balloon), then accomplishing this via the ureteroscope can be quite difficult. In this case, a cold knife can be used if a rigid endoscope is in place. For the flexible ureteroscope, a Nd:YAG laser probe, a KTP laser probe, or a 2 Fr. or 3 Fr. electrocautery probe can be utilized. As discussed, a 5 Fr. catheter must cover the safety guide wire. As with an antegrade approach, multiple shallow radial incisions are recommended. However, in this situation, any bleeding that is encountered will immediately obscure the field and usually cause termination of the procedure, as the irrigant flow via the ureteroscope is much less than the flow through the nephroscope. At the end of the procedure, a 10 Fr. or 7 Fr./12 Fr. double pigtail indwelling ureteral stent is placed.

Problems similar to those of the retrograde approach are encountered, if an *indirect* percutaneous approach is attempted. Puncturing the collecting system through an unaffected calyx and trying to approach the stenotic infundibulum in a retrograde fashion with a nephroscope is tedious and less rewarding than a direct antegrade approach. As with the calyceal diverticulum, this approach should be avoided.

RESULTS. Reported series of endoinfundibulotomy are few (Eshghi et al., 1987). Commonly, calyceal diverticula are mixed with the problems of infundibular stenosis and hydrocalyx, such that the "true" success rate may appear overly sanguine (Table 62–7) (Eshghi et al., 1987; Janetschek, 1988). Schneider and co-workers (1989) reported a 66 per cent success rate in four patients with infundibular stenosis; however, the length of follow-up in these patients was not stated. My experience with two patients with acquired infundibular stenosis has been unsuccessful. More experience and a clearer reporting of data (e.g., calyceal diverticulum versus true hydrocalyx and differentiation of acquired versus congenital hydrocalyx) are needed in order to accurately determine the outcome of an endosurgical procedure in the patient with this relatively rare condition.

Ureteropelvic Junction (UPJ) Obstruction: Endopyelotomy

The surgical correction of UPJ obstruction spans a century of operations both creative and effective. In 1886, Friedrich Trendelenburg performed the first reconstructive procedure for UPJ obstruction. The patient succumbed in the postoperative period (Murphy, 1972). The first successful pyeloplasty was reported by Ernest Kuster in 1891. He repaired the pelvis using a dismembered plastic UPJ procedure (Murphy, 1972). Subsequently, myriad operations were devised to repair the obstruction: renal pelvic plication, Y-V advancement, the Anderson-Hynes dismembered pyeloplasty, the Culp flap, and the Scardino flap. Of all these, perhaps

the renal pelvic plication is the most intriguing. Not a single suture was placed across the UPJ area; rather, gathering sutures were positioned near the UPJ area in order to transpose the renal pelvis more cephalad until the UPJ assumed a dependent position. With almost all of the aforementioned approaches, success rates in the 80 to 90 per cent range were reported, albeit, rarely with attendant long-term functional follow-up studies (Scardino and Scardino, 1984).

Endopyelotomy is truly a contemporary of pyeloplasty. Indeed, the basis for the technique was developed well before the classic operations of Foley, Anderson, Hynes, and others. In 1909, Joachim Albarran in France described a procedure he entitled "ureterotome externe," in which a scarred or narrowed ureter was incised through its entire thickness following which a catheter was placed in the ureter and a large drain was placed in the retroperitoneum (Murphy, 1972). The incised ureter was left to heal in situ or sutures could be used to close the periureteric tissues over the stent.

Keyes brought this technique to the United States in 1915 (Murphy, 1972). However, it wasn't until the 1940s that Davis (1943) popularized this approach and renamed it: the intubated ureterotomy. In his technique, after opening the ureter, a stent was placed and a few "loose" sutures were employed to guide the growth of the incised ureter around the indwelling tube. The cut ureteral edges were not coapted. The stent was removed in 4 to 5 weeks. Success with this approach in 47 patients was achieved in 89 per cent and 60 per cent based on subjective and objective follow-up, respectively, with a mean follow-up of 1 to 2 years (Davis, 1943; Davis et al., 1948). It appears that while contracture plays a role, urothelium and hyperplastic ureteral smooth muscle regenerate, with or without a stent. Without a stent, a retroperitoneal drain is placed. Drainage usually ceases within 5 days, indicating a watertight urothelial covering (Hamm and Weinberg, 1955; Webb et al., 1957). Indeed, peristalsis returns to the incised area in approximately 6 weeks (Hamm and Weinberg, 1955; Hamm and Weinberg, 1956; Mahoney et al., 1962; Oppenheimer and Hinman, 1955; Webb et al., 1957). Despite the initial enthusiastic interest in this method, use of the intubated ureterotomy began to wane when more aesthetically pleasing and more effective methods of surgical pyeloplasty were described.

In 1983, Wickham and Miller, at the Institute of Urology in London, brought Albarran's procedure into the modern era. The nephrostomy tract and a Sachs urethrotome were used to percutaneously incise an obstructed UPJ from the inside outward, thereby accomplishing the same effect as that in Albarran's procedure, only via a 1-cm flank incision. Wickham named the procedure *pyelolysis.* An indwelling stent was left in place for 4 weeks. Success with this approach was achieved in 65 per cent (Ramsey et al., 1984). Interestingly, at about this same time (1982), Kadir, White, and Engel reported successful balloon dilation of a secondary UPJ.

Subsequently, Smith popularized an endourologic incisional approach in the United States. He renamed the procedure an *endopyelotomy* (Greek tome—to cut), as

Table 62-7. ENDOSURGICAL THERAPY FOR CALYCEAL ABNORMALITIES

Authors	Patients with a Calyceal Abnormality	Calyceal Diverticula	Hydrocalyx Infundibular Stenosis	Associated Stones (%)	Method of Treatment	Stent Size	Catheter Duration	Outcome		
								Stone Free (%)	Calyceal Problem Corrected (%)	Follow-up
Percutaneous Approach										
Schneider et al., 1989	6	0	6	?	Antegrade PCN: cold knife		3–6 wk	?	66	?
Eshghi et al., 1987	14	Not stated	Not stated	86	Antegrade Cold knife (8) Dilation (4) Dissection (2)		3 days–2 wk	100	86	?
Hulbert et al., 1988a	17	17	0	100	Antegrade PCN (14) Retrograde PCN (3) Dilation (17) Fulguration of diverticular wall (1)		2 wk	100	80 (all failures had a retrograde (indirect) approach	9 mos. (avg.) (3–15 mos.)
Janetschek, 1988	14	3	11	43	Antegrade PCN: Hot knife				—	—
Overall	51									
SWL Approach										
Psihramis and Dretler, 1987	10	10	0	100	ESWL monotherapy	—	—	20	0	5.9 mos. (all ≥ 3 mos.)
Fuchs and David, 1989	15	12	3	100	Retrograde URS: Balloon dilation to 15 F of calyceal neck × 10 min. Double-J stent (one end in affected calyx)		3 wk	73	7 (27% with decrease in diverticular size)	7.4 mos.
Surgical Approach										
Abeshouse et al., 1963	126	126	—	36	Open surgery Excision 25% Incision 17% Partial nephrectomy: 25% Nephrectomy 28% Other: 5%	—	—	100	100	Operative mortality 1

indeed one is incising the renal pelvis under endoscopic control (Badlani et al., 1986; Karlin et al., 1988; Motola et al., 1990). Smith's success rate of 87.5 per cent was remarkably similar to that of Davis.

With all of these various operations, the question arises as to the etiology of adult primary UPJ obstruction. The most accepted hypothesis is that of an *intrinsically* "diseased" UPJ area. Indeed, Hanna and others have shown that the pathology of the obstructed UPJ is, at least in part, due to the presence of dysfunctional muscle cells, secondary to excessive intercellular deposits of collagen, incapable of properly propelling urine (Hanna et al., 1976a, 1976b; Murnaghan, 1958; Whitaker, 1976).

However, an *extrinsic* cause for UPJ obstruction is noted in one third of cases. Usually, this is due to a branching lower pole renal artery. However, simple division of the compressing vessel or of any associated fibrous band is rarely sufficient to resolve the obstruction (Whitaker, 1976). This problem is in large part due to the fibrous replacement noted in the area of the UPJ above the level of the obstruction. Given the foregoing data, it would appear that any procedure short of an open operative repair in which the UPJ area is excised or surgically displaced should fail. As such, the endopyelotomy is an ongoing conundrum: an endoscopic procedure that succeeds but cannot be explained by the available literature on the accepted pathophysiology of UPJ obstruction. Obviously, further research in this area is needed.

TECHNIQUE. If a balloon dilation is to be performed, a retrograde guide wire is passed beyond the UPJ. Next, an 8- to 10-mm, dilating balloon catheter (rated to 10 to 15 atm) is passed retrograde, until the balloon straddles the UPJ. The balloon is inflated until the waist at the UPJ disappears, usually within 10 to 20 seconds. The balloon is left inflated for 1 minute (Beckman and Roth, 1987). If no waist is seen, the balloon can be deflated and re-inflated for up to three cycles. A 7 to 8 Fr. double pigtail stent is placed and left for a 6- to 8-week period. A urethral catheter is placed but removed the following morning (O'Flynn et al., 1989).

For endopyelotomy, the initial step in performing an antegrade procedure is the *retrograde* passage of a 0.035-inch floppy tip or Terumo guide wire. Next, a percutaneous nephrostomy is performed into an upper or middle *posterior* calyx in order to provide a straight line, direct access to the UPJ. With the cold knife endopyelotomy technique, the nephrostomy tract is dilated and a 30 Fr. Amplatz sheath is placed. A second (i.e., working) guide wire is now advanced, albeit *antegrade*, through the UPJ. The knife of the direct vision urethrotome or a pyelotome (hooked blade) may be used to cut in between the "rails" of the guide wires (Fig. 62–35) (Karlin and Smith, 1988; Van Cangh et al., 1989).

If electrocautery is selected to make the endopyelotomy, a smaller nephrostomy tract can be created (18 Fr. biliary sheath). The electrocautery probe can be utilized through a 12 Fr. short, rigid ureteroscope with an insulated sheath. In this case, a second guide wire is not passed antegrade into the ureter. Next, a 6-mm ureteral dilating balloon is passed over the initial retrograde guide wire until the balloon straddles the UPJ area. The balloon is inflated (with a mixture of contrast material and a few drops of indigo carmine) to less than 1 atmosphere. The incision in the UPJ is made alongside

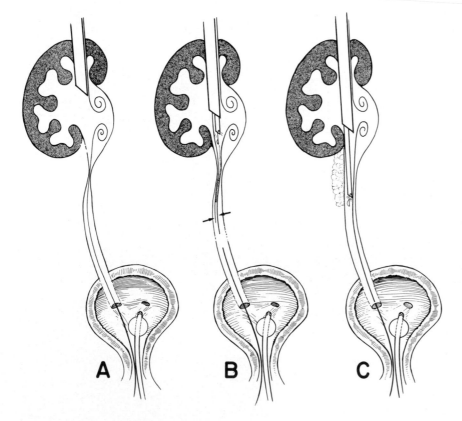

Figure 62–35. *A*, For an endopyelotomy, the nephrostomy tract is placed through an upper pole or middle posterior calyx. A retrograde guide wire has been passed across the stenotic uteropelvic junction (UPJ).

B, A second guide wire has been passed, albeit antegrade, across the stenotic UPJ, thereby providing a clear guide for incising the UPJ (*arrows* point to the two guide wires). Endoscope with cold knife is in place.

C, A straight cold knife has been used to incise the UPJ until normal ureter can be seen distally. The incision is made through the full thickness of the ureter until retroperitoneal fat is clearly visible. Hatch marks outline the planned site of incision along the posterolateral border of the ureter.

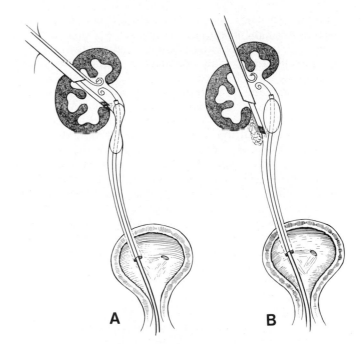

Figure 62–36. A, Endopyelotomy using a short therapeutic ureteroscope and electrocautery. Note how the balloon, inflated to ≤ 1 atm, clearly outlines the area of obstruction. B, The incision is made posterolaterally and carried down along the balloon to 1 cm distal to the UPJ obstruction. The depth of the incision is through the full thickness of the ureter, such that retroperitoneal fat is clearly seen.

the balloon with the electrocautery unit (2 Fr. or 3 Fr. electrode; 50 to 100 watts; pure cut). The inflated balloon facilitates incising the UPJ area because it places the UPJ tissue under tension, providing for a more controlled incision (Fig. 62–36).

In all cases, the incision in the UPJ is made through the full thickness of the ureter, until retroperitoneal fat is clearly seen (Karlin and Smith, 1988). The incision is made along the posterolateral border of the UPJ and is carried caudally for approximately 1 cm beyond the point of UPJ obstruction. To confirm the adequacy of the incision, dilute contrast material is instilled via the endoscope—there should be rapid extravasation of con-

trast material through the incised UPJ (Fig. 62–37). To further confirm the adequacy of the incision, an 8-mm ureteral dilating balloon can be passed over one of the guide wires until the balloon straddles the UPJ area. If the UPJ has been properly incised, the 8-mm balloon should inflate to full size at low pressure (< 1 atm).

When the UPJ obstruction is of a secondary rather than a primary nature, dense scar tissue may be encountered. A deeper incision than normal may be necessary to access retroperitoneal fat. If, despite a generous incision, no fat is seen, it may be worthwhile to inject 3 to 5 ml of triamcinolone (40 mg/ml) into the scar tissue bordering the incision in the UPJ area (R. V. Clayman,

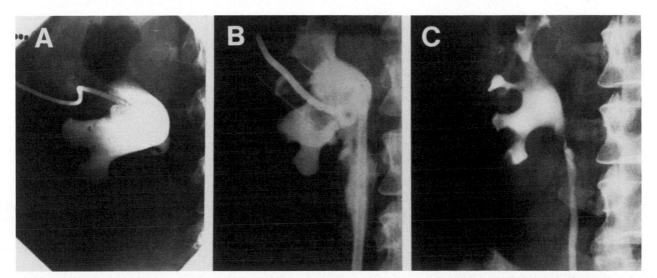

Figure 62–37. A, Positive Whitaker test finding in a patient with uteropelvic junction (UPJ) obstruction. Note the hooking of the UPJ and lack of filling of the ureter.

B, At the completion of an antegrade endopyelotomy using electrocautery, there is marked extravasation of contrast material from the area of the incision. A nephrostomy tube and a 14 Fr./7 Fr. indwelling stent are in place.

C, An intravenous urogram 6 months later shows that the UPJ area, albeit irregular, is patent. No remaining hydronephrosis is noted. The patient is asymptomatic.

unpublished data). A 3 Fr. Greenwald needle or standard cystoscopic needle can be chosen for this purpose. However, it is as yet undetermined whether the injection of triamcinolone is truly beneficial in reducing recurrent scarring of the UPJ area.

Following the procedure, the incised UPJ may be stented in one of two manners (Fig. 62–38). A nephrostent may be placed. This catheter is 14 Fr. along the nephrostomy portion and along the portion that traverses the UPJ area. The distal portion of the stent is 7 Fr. and forms a pigtail in the bladder (Badlani and Smith, 1988). Alternatively, an indwelling ureteral stent may be placed along with a separate nephrostomy tube (6 to 8 Fr. indwelling stent alongside a 4 Fr. angiographic catheter) (Van Cangh et al., 1989). A variable size indwelling ureteral stent has become available. This indwelling stent has a 7 Fr. pigtail on either end; however, half of the stent's shaft is 14 Fr. and the rest of the shaft is 7 Fr. After an endopyelotomy, the stent is placed such that the 14 Fr. portion traverses the incised UPJ (Clayman and Picus, 1988).

On the 2nd postoperative day, a nephrostogram is obtained. If this study shows no evidence of extravasation, the nephrostent can be capped. If an indwelling stent was placed, the nephrostomy tube can be removed. This should be done under fluoroscopic monitoring in order to avoid dislodgement of the indwelling ureteral stent. The nephrostent or indwelling ureteral stent is removed 4 to 6 weeks later. Follow-up studies usually consist of a furosemide washout renogram or an intravenous urogram 3 to 4 weeks after the stent has been removed.

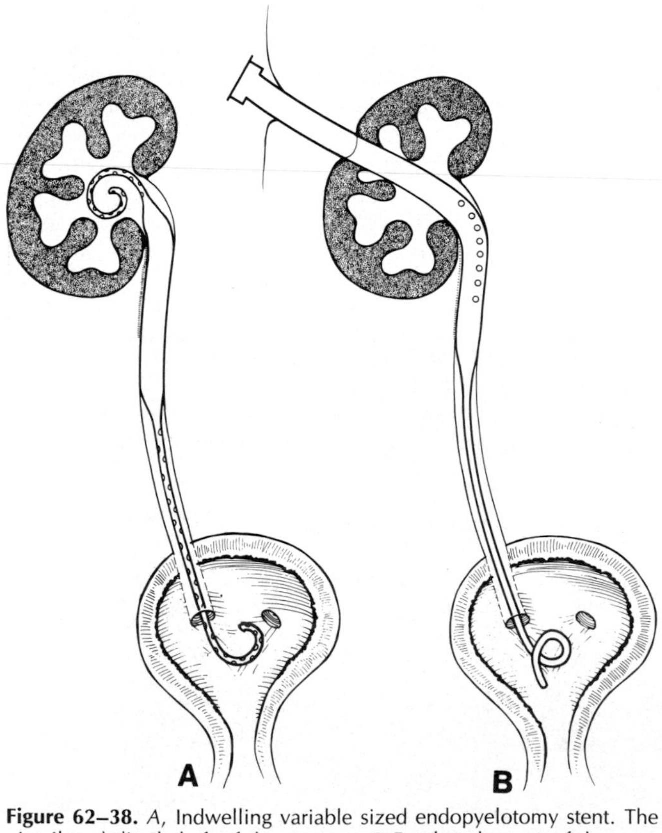

A *retrograde* approach to endopyelotomy is possible employing the rigid or flexible ureteroscope (see Fig. 62–39) (Clayman et al., 1990b; Inglis and Tolley, 1986; Korth and Kuenkel, 1988). Although a cold knife is available for use with the rigid ureteroscope, it can be extremely difficult, especially in males, to maneuver the rigid endoscope up to the UPJ area in order to make the necessary incision. In contrast, accessing the UPJ area is simpler with the flexible ureteroscope. The available cutting modalities for the flexible ureteroscope are electrocautery, Nd:YAG laser, and KTP laser. To date, experience with endopyelotomy via a flexible ureteroscope has largely been limited to electrocautery (Clayman et al., 1990b).

The technique for performing a retrograde endopyelotomy is similar to that for antegrade approach (Fig. 62–39). Often, a small (8 to 10 Fr.) nephrostomy tube has been placed as part of a Whitaker test. The nephrostomy tube provides for excellent drainage from the renal pelvis during ureteroscopy. It also allows for the passage of a through-and-through 260-cm exchange guide wire at the end of the case. The guide wire is retrieved from the renal pelvis with the ureteroscope and pulled antegrade along the ureter and out the urethra. With a through-and-through guide wire, it is simpler to position an indwelling stent, especially if a 7 Fr./14 Fr. stent is being placed. Also, the nephrostomy tube provides for postoperative drainage of the renal pelvis, thereby decreasing the chances of urine extravasation and urinoma formation.

To accomplish a retrograde endopyelotomy, the first step is to position a retrograde 0.035-inch floppy tip guide wire beyond the UPJ and coil it in the renal pelvis. If electrocautery is to be utilized, a 5 Fr. angiographic catheter is passed over the guide wire. The distal ureter is dilated as necessary (usually to 15 Fr.) in order to pass the ureteroscope. Ureteral dilation may not be needed, if an indwelling stent is placed for 1 week before the procedure (Thomas and Cherry, 1990). The endopyelotomy incision is begun at the lower end of the UPJ and continued cephalad until the capacious renal pelvis is entered. The incision is carried through the full thickness of the ureter until retroperitoneal fat is seen. At the end of the procedure, the 260-cm exchange guide wire is retrieved from the nephrostomy tube and the ureteroscope is withdrawn. Then, an 8-mm ureteral dilating balloon may be passed to check the adequacy of the incision. The balloon should fully inflate in the area of the incision at low pressure (< 1 atm). Next, an indwelling ureteral stent is passed retrograde. This stent may be an 8 Fr. or the previously described 7 Fr./14 Fr. A urethral catheter is placed to drain the bladder.

The care of the patient following retrograde endopyelotomy is similar to that following antegrade endopyelotomy. On postoperative day 2, a nephrostogram is obtained. If there is no extravasation, the nephrostomy

Figure 62–38. *A,* Indwelling variable sized endopyelotomy stent. The pigtail and distal shaft of the stent are 7 Fr., but the part of the stent that traverses the ureteropelvic junction (UPJ) area is 14 Fr. The stent is removed via the bladder at the end of 6 weeks. *B,* Smith nephrostent for use after endopyelotomy. The UPJ area is stented by the 14 Fr. portion of the stent, while the 8.2 Fr. portion of the stent traverses the normal ureter. The 14 Fr. nephrostomy portion of the stent is left capped for the ensuing 6 weeks.

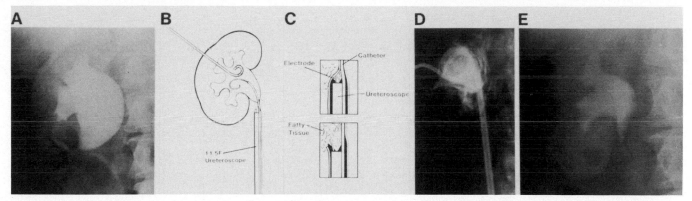

Figure 62–39. *A,* Preoperative intravenous pyelography (IVP) revealing right uteropelvic junction (UPJ) obstruction. *B,* Rigid therapeutic ureteroscope (insulated tip) in place with a 2 Fr. electrosurgical probe extended. Note the 8 Fr. nephrostomy tube left in place after the positive Whitaker test findings. *C,* Incision is made through the full thickness of the ureter until retroperitoneal fat is seen. *D,* Extravasation of contrast material from the endopyelotomy site. *E,* IVP completed 5 months after the retrograde endopyelotomy reveals a patent UPJ. The patient is asymptomatic. (From Clayman, R. V., and Picus, D.D.: Urol. Clin. North Am., 15:433, 1988.)

tube can be removed under fluoroscopic monitoring. If extravasation is present, the nephrostomy tube is left open to drainage and the nephrostogram can be repeated, on an outpatient basis, in 1 week. The urethral catheter is also removed on the 2nd postoperative day. The patient can usually be discharged from the hospital on the 3rd postoperative morning. Alternatively, if the retrograde endopyelotomy has been done without preplacement of a nephrostomy tube, the patient can be discharged on the same day as the procedure or on the following morning. In these patients, the urethral catheter is left in place. An outpatient cystogram is performed 2 to 3 days later. If there is no ureteral reflux or extravasation, the urethral catheter is removed.

In complete obstruction of the UPJ, the area of stenosis can still be overcome with endourologic techniques. A combined retrograde ureteroscopic and antegrade percutaneous nephroscopic approach is necessary. The technique is similar to that described for the endosurgical treatment of complete obstruction of the proximal ureter (see subsequent discussion) (Bagley et al., 1985; Hulbert, 1990; Korth and Kuenkel, 1988). In some patients, a permanent indwelling ureteral stent is placed to preclude recurrent occlusion. However Korth (5 cases) and Hulbert (4 cases) have both reported successful durable recanalization despite stent removal (Bagley et al., 1985; Hulbert, 1990; Korth and Kuenkel, 1988).

Some controversy has arisen as to the best type of cutting modality for incising the UPJ. Concern has been expressed with regard to possible tissue damage from employing electrocautery to make incisions in the UPJ area. Of interest is that data from Korth, Smith, and Van Cangh, in which only a cold knife was utilized to make the endopyelotomy, are similar to independent reports from Meretyk and Hulbert, in which monopolar electrocautery was utilized (2 Fr. and 3 Fr. electrocautery probes) (Hulbert et al., 1988b; Karlin et al., 1988; Kuenkel and Korth, 1990; Meretyk et al., 1990; Van Cangh et al., 1989). Current clinical data regarding a bipolar electrocautery system, Nd:YAG laser, or KTP laser to make an incision in the UPJ are lacking.

Laboratory data in pigs reveal that larger electrocautery probes (5 Fr., pure cut at 100 watts) and, to some extent, 3 Fr. probes cause considerably more periincisional injury than a cold knife, Nd:YAG laser, or KTP laser. However, the monopolar 2 Fr. electrocautery probe with a 250-μ cutting surface produces an incision similar in appearance to a cold knife or laser incision (Dierks et al., 1990). Obviously, considerably more work in this area is needed, given the various electrocautery probe sizes and power settings.

RESULTS. The results of endourologic therapy for UPJ obstruction have been excellent. Of note, although smaller in number (< 100 reported cases), the results with a balloon dilation of the UPJ have been quite acceptable. Success with primary and secondary UPJ obstruction is in the 68 to 73 per cent range. With this technique, the operative time is less, morbidity is minimal, and if performed in a retrograde manner, hospitalization time can be reduced to 1 day or even less as an outpatient (Table 62–8) (Kadir et al., 1982; O'Flynn et al., 1989).

By far the largest endourologic experience (> 400 cases) has been with *antegrade* endopyelotomy. Smith, Korth, van Cangh, Brannen, and Clayman have all reported success rates in the 72 to 87 per cent range (Brannen et al., 1988; Karlin et al., 1988; Kuenkel and Korth, 1990; Meretyk et al., 1990; Motola et al., 1990; Van Cangh et al., 1989). The success rate appears to be durable. The average duration of follow-up in the reported series is from 1 to 3 years (see Table 62–8). The majority of failures occur within 3 months of the procedure (Brannen et al., 1988; Karlin et al., 1988; Kuenkel and Korth, 1990; Meretyk et al., 1990; Motola et al., 1990; Van Cangh et al., 1989). There does not appear to be a significant difference in success rates for primary versus secondary UPJ obstruction (Karlin et al., 1988; Meretyk et al., 1990; Motola et al., 1990).

Although the success with a *retrograde* approach is similar to that with the antegrade, technical difficulties are discouraging and delayed complications occur that detract from the initial attractiveness of a retrograde approach. The average procedural time for a retrograde

Table 62–8. ENDOPYELOTOMY: URETEROPELVIC JUNCTION (UPJ) OBSTRUCTION

Authors	Patients	Approach	Method of Incision	Stent Size	Stent Duration (weeks)	Overall (%)	1° UPJ (%)	2° UPJ (%)	Hospital Stay (days)	2° Pyeloplasty (%)	2° Nephrectomy (%)	Average Follow-up
Endopyelotomy												
Badlani, Karlin, and Smith, 1988	156	Endopyelotomy antegrade	Cold knife (pyelotome)	12–14	6	87	87	86	6.2	13	0	3 years (all > 6 mos.)
Brannen et al., 1988	10	Endopyelotomy antegrade	Cold knife (pyelotome)	8–10	6–8	80	80	—	4.1	0	0	> 3 mos.
Kuenkel and Korth, 1990	175	Endopyelotomy antegrade	Cold knife (Sachs urethrotome)	10–14	3–6	78	83	75	—	—	0	12 mos.
Meretyk, Clayman, et al., 1990	23	Endopyelotomy antegrade	Hot knife (1 mm and 0.6 mm tips)	14	6	78	—	—	4	9	0	22 mos. (2–39 mos.)
	20	Endopyelotomy retrograde				80	—	—	3.4	5	5	17 mos. (4–36 mos.)
Ramsay, Wickham et al., 1984	28	Endopyelotomy antegrade	Cold knife (Sachse urethrotome)	8–10	4–10	65	61	80	—	32	—	18 mos. (9–48 mos.)
Van Cangh et al., 1989	47	Endopyelotomy antegrade	Cold knife (urethrotome)	10–12	6	72	—	—	6.7	2	0	16 mos. (4–56 mos.)
Overall	459					82			4–6	13	0.3	> 12 mos.
Balloon Dilation												
Beckman, Roth, and Bihrie, 1989	11	Balloon dilation	—	8–10	4–8	73	86	50	—	—	—	10 mos. (2–22 mos.)
O'Flynn et al. 1989	31	Balloon dilation		7–8	6–8	68	—	—	4.3	10	20	10 mos. (3–30 mos.)
Surgery												
Scardino and Scardino, 1984	2481	Open pyeloplasty		—	—	88	—	—	8–10	2	3	

*Brannen et al., 1988; Karlin and Smith, 1988.

endopyelotomy is 188 minutes (Clayman et al., 1990b). In addition, a small nephrostomy tube did not, in our experience, decrease the analgesic requirements of the patient in the postoperative period. More worrisome was the development of distal ureteral strictures in 20 per cent of our patients (Clayman et al., 1990b).

Thomas and Cherry (1990) reported a *retrograde* approach to endopyelotomy. In this series, all patients had indwelling ureteral stents placed for 1 week prior to the procedure to allow the normal ureter to passively dilate. No nephrostomy tube was placed. After 1 week, the stent was removed and an ureteroscopic endopyelotomy was performed. One immediate advantage of this method is that the procedure can be completely done on an outpatient basis. Long-term follow-up data are as yet unavailable.

Patient selection for endopyelotomy has been controversial. The fear of incising a posterior crossing vessel (i.e., segmental lower pole renal artery) is to date unfounded. No doubt, these vessels have likely been incised, but to date reports of large retroperitoneal hematomas are lacking. However, in our experience, retroperitoneal hematomas have occurred. In this regard, electrocautery permits one to both perform an endopyelotomy and coagulate any retroperitoneal vessels that are encountered or inadvertently incised.

Concern over the effectiveness of this procedure in a patient with a "high insertion" of the ureter into the renal pelvis has been addressed by van Cangh and associates (1989). The procedure appears to be effective in these individuals. However, in selecting an adult patient for an endopyelotomy, there are two circumstances in which results are less favorable. First, the presence of chronic massive hydronephrosis is an undesirable situation (Badlani et al., 1988). The patient needs tailoring of the renal pelvis in order to ensure proper drainage. Currently, this can only be done surgically. This problem accounted for 30 per cent of the failures in the series reported by Badlani, Karlin, and Smith (1988). Secondly, in a patient with poor renal function, the incised UPJ has a tendency to scar. As such, prior to endopyelotomy, a renal scan is recommended. If the contribution to total renal function of the affected kidney is less than 20 per cent, it is advisable to place an indwelling stent or an 8 Fr. nephrostomy tube. If after 2 to 4 weeks of unobstructed status, the function of the affected kidney remains at less than 20 per cent, the kidney likely should be removed. In our experience, functionally compromised, obstructed kidneys had a greater tendency to fail endopyelotomy. The reason for this poorer result is as yet undetermined (Meretyk et al., 1990).

Several intraoperative/postoperative problems cause a negative impact on the outcome of an endopyelotomy. In Smith's series, 3 per cent of patients had intraoperative problems (hemorrhage, ureteral avulsion) that necessitated an immediate open procedure (Badlani et al., 1988). Other problems include urinoma, hematoma, and urinary tract infection. The postoperative formation of a urinoma is problematic. As such, it is important to properly drain the collecting system after endopyelotomy. To this end, a nephrostomy tube, ureteral stent, and urethral catheter are recommended at least for the initial 48 hours following endopyelotomy. In most cases, the collecting system rapidly seals. In over 80 per cent of patients, the nephrostogram on the 2nd postoperative morning reveals an intact collecting system. Another problem is the development of a postoperative perirenal hematoma, which can at times be massive. The patient may require blood transfusions (Fig. 62–40). In the series of Meretyk and Clayman, two patients developed retroperitoneal hematomas sufficient to warrant blood transfusions in both. The procedure failed in both individuals (Meretyk et al., 1990). A sterile urine must be maintained throughout the postoperative period. An oral antibiotic can be given nightly throughout the 4- to 6-week period of stenting and for 2 weeks after the stent is removed. A urine culture is obtained 3 weeks and 6 weeks after the procedure. The urine should be sterile prior to removal of the ureteral stent. In order to

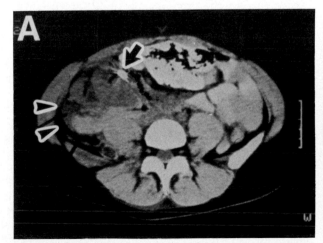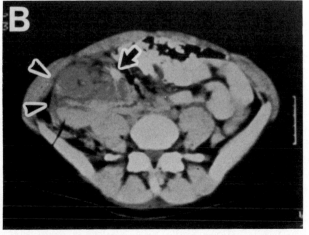

Figure 62–40. *A* and *B,* Massive retroperitoneal hematoma following retrograde endopyelotomy is shown in these two noncontrast computed tomography (CT) scans. The kidney was located low in the retroperitoneum. Note the stent in the ureter *(arrow).* The hematoma is outlined by the arrowheads. A total of 4 units of blood were transfused. Ultimately, an open pyeloplasty was successful.

maintain a sterile urine immediately following stent removal, continuance of an oral antibiotic for 1 to 2 weeks is reasonable.

Questions have been asked about the role of endopyelotomy in the pediatric population. Experience in this age group is scant. Towbin and colleagues (1987) reported on endopyelotomy in three patients with primary UPJ obstructions, ages 11 to 18 years. After utilizing electrocautery to make the incision, a 16 Fr. indwelling stent was left in place for 6 to 10 weeks. The procedure was successful in two patients in a subjective follow-up at 10 and 27 months. In the third patient, the stent migrated distally and the procedure failed. This patient was later salvaged with a standard dismembered pyeloplasty (Towbin et al., 1987). Kavoussi reported on four children, ages 6 1/2 weeks to 5 years with *secondary* UPJ obstruction in all of whom an endopyelotomy was successful; objective follow-up ranged from 1.5 to 3 years. However, two patients required two procedures, and the endopyelotomy itself was lengthy (average, 210 minutes) (Kavoussi et al., 1991b).

Ureteral Strictures: Endoureterotomy

In dealing with ureteral strictures, it is helpful to divide the ureter into three unequal areas: the proximal ureter ($\leq$3 cm below the UPJ), the distal ureter ($\leq$5 cm above the ureteral orifice), and the middle ureter. By this classification, the majority of the ureter falls under the designation of middle ureter. However, most strictures seem to occur in the proximal or, more commonly, in the distal lengths of the ureter. This finding is largely due to the fact that the predominant cause of a ureteral stricture is iatrogenic ureteroscopy, gynecologic surgery, or ureteral surgery.

TECHNIQUE. Three general endosurgical techniques exist for treating ureteral strictures: catheter dilation, balloon dilation, and endoincision (Banner and Pollack, 1984; Beckman et al., 1989; Eshghi et al., 1989b; Gothlin et al., 1988; Lang, 1984; Smith, 1988). In each situation, the first step is to pass a guide wire beyond the stricture until its tip is coiled in the renal pelvis (Coleman et al., 1984). The simplest guide wire to pass under these circumstances is often a 0.035-inch Terumo. Its plastic construction and lubricatory coating greatly facilitate its passage through even a very tight ureteral stricture. The surface of this guide wire must always be kept *wet*. Once this guide wire has been passed, a 5 Fr. angiographic catheter can be passed over it. The Terumo guide wire is then exchanged for a stiffer guide wire, such as a 0.035-inch Bentson guide wire or the most rigid guide wire available, a 0.035-inch Amplatz super stiff guide wire.

Catheter dilation of the ureter has been practiced for many years (Hunner, 1924). Today, catheter dilation is performed with multiple tapered, tipped ureteral dilators that are sequentially passed over the guide wire. In this case, it is often helpful to exchange the floppy tip guide wire for a stiffer guide wire, such as a 0.038 inch heavy duty guide wire or an Amplatz super stiff guide wire. The ureteral stricture can be dilated up to 14 Fr. Following the dilation, an 8 Fr. indwelling ureteral stent

is placed for up to 6 weeks (Witherington and Shelor, 1980). However, Witherington and Shelor noted several cases in which serial, rather than solitary, ureteral dilations to 7 to 8 Fr. (i.e., 4 to 5 times over 1 month) without long-term stenting succeeded in resolving a posthysterectomy ureteral stricture.

Balloon dilation of ureteral strictures followed closely upon Gruntzig and associates' original description in 1979 of balloon dilation (9 to 11.1 Fr. balloon, 4 to 5 atm, 3 to 4 seconds of inflation) of the coronary vessels. In 1980, Pingoud and associates reported on a 12 Fr. Gruntzig balloon to dilate a malignant ureteral stricture, following which an indwelling ureteral stent was placed.

For balloon dilation, an 8-mm ureteral dilating balloon rated to at least 10 atmospheres is passed over the guide wire until it traverses the stricture. Employing a high pressure inflation syringe (LeVeen or similar device) and an inline pressure gauge, the balloon is inflated until the waist of the stricture disappears. The balloon pressure should never exceed the manufacturer's listed maximum pressure or else the balloon might rupture and harm the ureter. At this point, a variety of suggestions are offered. One reasonable course of action is to leave the balloon inflated for 1 minute, deflate the balloon, and repeat the entire cycle one or two additional times. An indwelling ureteral stent (standard 7 Fr. or 8 Fr. or a 7 Fr./14 Fr.) is then placed. The stent is usually left in place for 4 to 6 weeks (Table 62–9) (Banner and Pollack, 1984; Beckman et al., 1989; Johnson et al., 1987).

For performing an endoincision, the same cutting modalities can be utilized that were discussed for performing an endopyelotomy: cold knife, electrocautery probe, Nd:YAG laser, and KTP laser. However, the majority of cases have been done with a cold knife (see Table 62–9). Korth and Kuenkel (1988) have developed a cold knife, flexible ureterotome for incising strictures in the middle portion of the ureter. Similarly, Selikowitz (1990) developed a diminutive 4.5 Fr. coaxial cold knife. Netto and colleagues (1990) reported on ureteroscopic back-cutting endoscopic scissors, in which the outer edges of the blades of the scissors have been sharpened. Upon passing the scissors beyond the stricture, the blades are opened and the open scissors is drawn antegrade through the stricture, thereby incising the stricture in two places. Electrocautery probes (2 Fr. or 3 Fr.) have been selected by only a few urologists (Kavoussi et al., 1990). To date, reports on lasers are anecdotal (Nd:YAG) or unavailable (KTP).

For a *proximal* ureteral stricture, the method of incision is similar to an endopyelotomy in all respects (Fig. 62–41) (Hulbert et al., 1988b). The goal is to marsupialize the stricture into the renal pelvis. The stricture is approached *antegrade* via a percutaneous nephrostomy tract. Rigid instrumentation is used: direct vision urethrotome, pyelotome, or short 12 Fr. rigid ureteroscope with an operating sheath for use with a cold knife, back-cutting scissors or with an insulated sheath for use with a 2 Fr. or 3 Fr. electrocautery probe. The incision is made along the posterolateral surface of the ureter through the full thickness of the stricture until retroperitoneal fat is seen. The incision is carried caudad

Table 62–9. ENDOSURGERY FOR URETERAL STRICTURES: BALLOON DILATION RESULTS

Authors	Patients	Approach	Stent Size (Fr.)	Stent Duration	Patent (%)	Follow-up (mos.)
Balloon Dilation						
Banner and Pollack, 1984	44	4 mm balloon	7-10	4 days-3 mos.	48	—
Beckman et al., 1989	17	4-8 mm balloon	7-10	4-8 wks.	82	1-40 mos.
Johnson et al., 1987	30	4-10 mm balloon	6-10	2 days-mos.	58	≥ 6 mos.
Lang et al., 1988	127	4-6 mm balloon	7-10	3-6 wks.	50	≥ 15 mos.
Netto et al., 1990	19	4-6 mm balloon	8.5	2-8 wks.	53	≥ 18 mos.
Chang and Marshall, 1987	11	5-8 mm balloon	8-16	4-8 wks.	88	10 mos. (avg.)
O'Brien et al., 1988	24	4-6 mm balloon	—	—	45	2-36 mos.
Kramolowsky et al., 1989	20	5-10 mm balloon	6-12	6 wks.	64	22 mos.
Overall	294	4-10 mm	6-10	2 days-mos.	55	> 6 mos.
Endoureterotomy						
Meretyk et al., 1990b	16	Incision: electrocautery	14	3-6 wks.	63	3-22 mos. (avg., 12 mos.)
Schneider et al., 1989	12	Incision: cold knife	—	3-6 wks.	75	7-23 mos. (mean, 13 mos.)
Eshghi et al., 1989	40	Incision: cold knife	6-10	4-6 wks.	88	—
Overall	68	—	6-14	3-6 wks.	79	≥ 12 mos.
Surgical Repair						
Kramolowsky et al., 1989	11	Surgical repair	5-7	2.5 wks.	91	21 mos. (avg.)
Smith, 1988	36	Surgical	—	—	97	—
Overall	47				96	

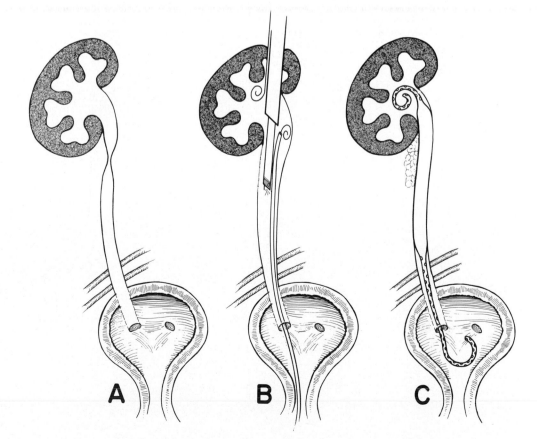

Figure 62–41. Endoureterotomy of a proximal ureteral stricture.

A, Proximal ureteral stricture: the stricture and the uteropelvic junction (UPJ) are in close proximity.

B, A hot knife incision is being made on the posterolateral surface of the ureteral stricture using a 2 Fr. electrode passed through a 12 Fr. insulated therapeutic ureteroscope.

C, Two days following the endoincision, a nephrostogram is performed. If there is no extravasation, the nephrostomy tube is removed. The ureteral stent (7 Fr./14 Fr.) is left in place for 6 weeks.

for 1 cm beyond the stricture. The cephalic portion of the incision extends into the renal pelvis. Following the incision, a 14 Fr. nephrostent or an indwelling ureteral stent (7 Fr. or 8 Fr. double pigtail or a 7 Fr./14 Fr. variable size stent) and a small 10 Fr. nephrostomy tube is placed. A urethral catheter drains the bladder for 24 to 36 hours. Two days later, a nephrostogram is performed. If the nephrostogram reveals an intact collecting system, the nephrostent can be capped; if an indwelling ureteral stent is present, the nephrostomy tube can be removed. The nephrostent or ureteral stent is maintained for a total of 4 to 6 weeks.

For the *distal* ureteral stricture, the goal is to marsupialize the stricture into the bladder (Fig. 62–42) (Cubelli and Smith, 1987). The site of the stricture according to the aforementioned classification is at the ureteral orifice, intramural tunnel, or just at or slightly beyond the ureterovesical junction. A 0.035-inch guide wire (Bentson or Terumo) is first passed, and the tip of the guide wire is coiled in the renal pelvis. The stricture is approached retrograde. This approach can be done with a cold knife urethrotome. The ureter is opened from the inside outward into the bladder or retroperitoneum by cutting along the previously placed guide wire at the 12-o'clock position. Alternatively, a 6-mm or 8-mm ureteral dilating balloon catheter can be passed over the guide wire until the balloon straddles the stricture. Next, the balloon is inflated to less than 1 atmosphere, using a solution of radiographic contrast material stained with indigo carmine, thereby delineating the area of the stricture.

The incision is made with a standard Iglesias resectoscope equipped with a Collings or Orandi electrocautery knife. In this case, the incision is made from outside the ureter inward onto the inflated blue balloon. The incision is continued cephalad for approximately 1 cm above the area of narrowing. The end point is the presence of fat, indicating that the incision has been extended through the ureterovesical junction. At this point, an 8-mm balloon should be fully inflatable at less than 1 atmosphere of pressure, indicating that the stricture has been deeply incised. A 7 Fr. or 8 Fr. standard indwelling ureteral stent or a 7 Fr./14 Fr. indwelling ureteral stent is placed. If the last stent is chosen, the 14 Fr. portion is placed so that it traverses the incised stricture. A urethral catheter is placed; *the patient is discharged from the hospital with the urethral catheter in place*. One week later, an outpatient cystogram is obtained, if there is no extravasation, the urethral catheter is removed. The ureteral stent is maintained for 4 to 6 weeks.

The *middle* ureteral stricture is the most difficult obstruction to treat endosurgically (Fig. 62–43). In this case, the extent of the endoincision is normal ureter on either end. The endoscope is the rigid ureteroscope, if the stricture is between the lower border of the distal ureter and the level of the iliac vessel crossing. The rigid or flexible ureteroscope is selected when the stricture lies between the iliac vessel crossing and the upper border of the proximal ureter. Any of the aforementioned cutting modalities can be employed through the rigid ureteroscope; however, the flexible ureteroscope

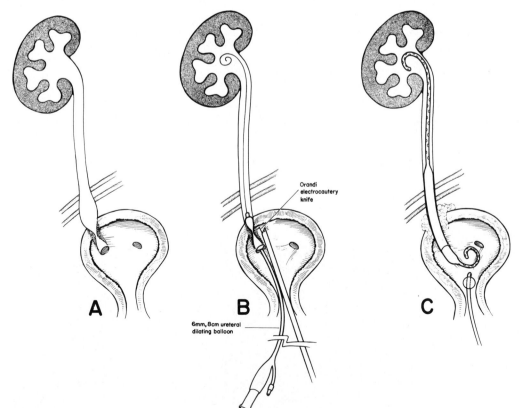

Figure 62–42. Distal ureteral stricture.

A, Distal ureteral stricture in the intramural tunnel.

B, A 0.035-inch Bentson guide wire is advanced to the renal pelvis, followed by placement of a 6-mm dilating balloon. The balloon is filled to ≤ 1 atm with a mixture of contrast material and indigo carmine, thereby outlining the stricture. An Orandi electrocautery knife is used through a standard resectoscope sheath to incise the ureteral tunnel anteriorly from the ureteral orifice up to and through the detrusor muscle.

C, A 7 Fr./14 Fr. indwelling stent is placed such that the 14 Fr. portion traverses the distal ureter. It is left in place for 6 weeks. A urethral catheter is left in place usually for 1 week.

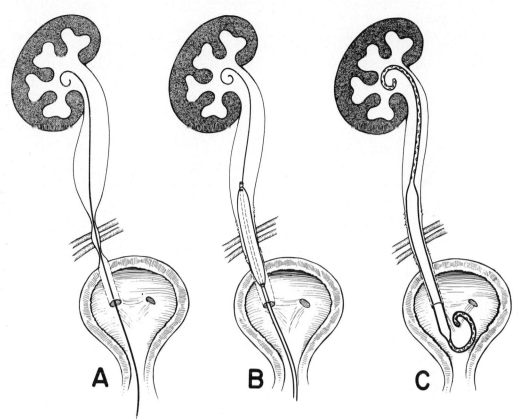

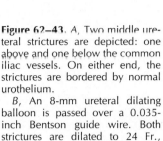

Figure 62–43. *A,* Two middle ureteral strictures are depicted: one above and one below the common iliac vessels. On either end, the strictures are bordered by normal urothelium.

B, An 8-mm ureteral dilating balloon is passed over a 0.035-inch Bentson guide wire. Both strictures are dilated to 24 Fr., thereby tearing the urothelium and spreading (tearing) the scar tissue. Alternatively, the more cephalad stricture could be incised via the flexible nephroscope (antegrade) or flexible ureteroscope (retrograde), and the more caudal stricture could be incised using the short rigid ureteroscope passed retrograde.

C, A 7 Fr./14 Fr. indwelling stent is left in place for 6 weeks.

can only allow passage of the electrocautery or laser probe.

The site of the incision depends on the exact location of the stricture in the middle ureter. Above the iliac vessel crossing, the incision is made posterolateral. Directly overlying the iliac vessels, the incision is made anteriorly. Below the iliac vessels, the incision is made directly medial to avoid the branches of the internal iliac artery and vein traveling along the lateral surface of the ureter (Figs. 62–44 and 62–45). As described previously, the incision should be deep enough to expose retroperitoneal or periureteral fat. The incision is extended proximally and distally for 1 cm beyond the stricture. An indwelling stent is placed: a 7 Fr. or 8 Fr. double pigtail stent or a 7 Fr./14 Fr. stent. A urethral catheter is left in place for 2 days. No nephrostomy tube is placed. The stent is left in place for 4 to 6 weeks.

A more difficult situation occurs when the ureteral obstruction is *complete* (Bagley, 1990). In this case, neither a contrast agent nor a guide wire can be made to traverse the stricture. A nephrostomy tract must therefore be established. The exact limits of the total occlusion are defined by a combined nephrostogram and retrograde ureterogram. If the occlusion is short (< 1 cm), an endosurgical approach can be tried; however, if the occlusion is long (> 1 cm), an open surgical procedure is recommended (Bagley, 1990). However, Bagley (1990) has reported successful recannulation of complete ureteral obstructions as long as 5 cm.

When *complete obstruction* occurs in the *proximal or middle ureter,* a new opening can be made by passing a flexible nephroscope or a short rigid 12 Fr. ureteroscope

via the nephrostomy tract and a flexible ureteroscope via the ureter. The light from the antegrade endoscope is disconnected, and the light from the retrograde ureteroscope is sought. When the glow through the obstructing tissue is light pink to white and the C-arm fluoroscope shows the tips of the two endoscopes to be aligned in at least two planes, a direct incision (rigid endoscope, cold knife/flexible endoscope, electrocautery) of the ureter can be made via the nephroscope at the brightest point of light. The light on the nephroscope is then reconnected to look for the guide wire passed through the retrograde ureteroscope. This procedure can also be done in reverse, with the light disconnected from the ureteroscope, and the light from the nephroscope sought. In this case, the incision is made via the ureteroscope. However, it appears to be simpler to make an incision with the larger or rigid endoscope passed antegrade through the nephrostomy tract whenever possible.

After contact is established, a 260-cm, 0.035-inch exchange guide wire is passed via the ureteroscope and retrieved by the nephroscope, thereby providing a through-and-through guide wire (Kavoussi et al., 1990b). A 5 Fr. angiographic catheter is passed over the guide wire in preparation for an electrocautery incision. If need be, the incision is deepened alongside the 5 Fr. catheter until retroperitoneal fat is seen. An 8-mm balloon catheter is passed and inflated (<1 atm) to gauge the adequacy of the incision (Fig. 62–46).

Alternatively, a 5 Fr. or an 8 Fr. staight tip angiographic catheter is passed retrograde. A stiff guide wire (Lunderquist) or stylet (rocket wire with a sharp tip

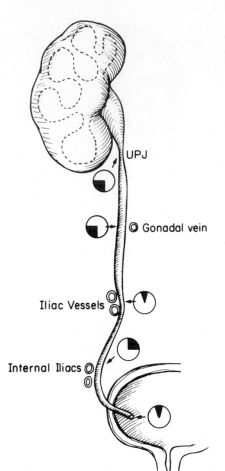

Figure 62–44. Endoureterotomy. The site of the incision *(black quadrant)* is dependent on the location of the stricture. (From Eshghi, M.: AUA Update Series, Volume 8, Lesson 38, 1989.)

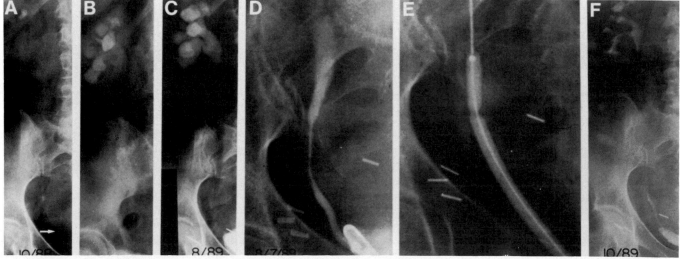

Figure 62–45. Distal ureteral stricture: endoureterotomy.

A and *B*, October, 1988: Distal ureteral calculus *(arrow)* with associated ureteral obstruction and hydronephrosis on an intravenous urogram. The calculus was surgically removed.

C, August, 1989: The patient returned complaining of flank discomfort. An intravenous urogram reveals marked hydronephrosis.

D, A retrograde ureterogram reveals narrowing of the distal ureter.

E, A 6-mm ureteral dilating balloon inflated to 1 atm more clearly delineates the stricture. The stricture was subsequently incised using a rigid insulated, therapeutic ureteroscope and an electrocautery probe.

F, October, 1989: Two months following the endoureterotomy, an intravenous urogram reveals a satisfactory *early* result with no hydronephrosis and flow of contrast material through the distal ureter.

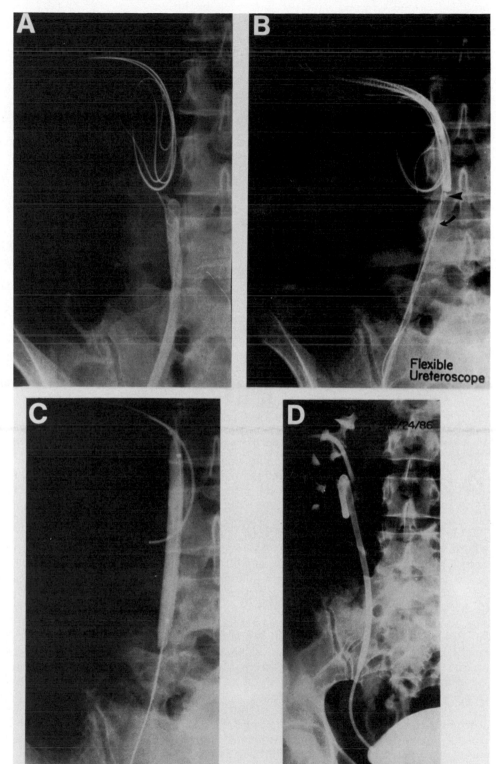

Figure 62–46. Complete ureteral obstruction: Endosurgical therapy.

A, Complete proximal ureteral obstruction following an endopyelotomy. The retrograde ureterogram reveals no communication with the renal pelvis. A percutaneous nephrostomy was placed, and a guide wire is seen coiled in the capacious renal pelvis. A retrograde guide wire is coiled in the ureter.

B, A flexible nephroscope with a 3 Fr. electrosurgery probe *(arrowhead)* has been passed antegrade; a flexible ureteroscope *(arrow)* has been passed retrograde. In this case, the tip of the flexible nephroscope was fluoroscopically aligned with the tip of the flexible ureteroscope. Then, the light to the flexible nephroscope was turned off. The illumination from the flexible ureteroscope could be seen through the intervening tissue as a bright pink light. The intervening tissue was incised using a 3 Fr. electrocautery probe, thereby uncovering the tip of the ureteroscope (i.e., "cut-to-the-light" procedure). A 260-cm, 0.035-inch exchange guide wire was passed through the ureteroscope and retrieved by the nephroscope.

C, The incised stricture was balloon dilated with an 8-mm, 8-cm long dilating balloon.

D, A percutaneous nephrostomy tube was left in place for 2 days. An indwelling 7 Fr./14 Fr. stent was left in place for 6 weeks. In this case, the stricture recurred following removal of the stent. An open pyeloplasty was subsequently successful.

from the Lawson retrograde nephrostomy kit) can be passed through the retrograde catheter and its indentation upon the ureteral tissue noted with the antegrade nephroscope. The wire can then be forced across the occluded ureter, grasped with the antegrade nephroscope, and pulled out through the nephrostomy tract, thereby establishing a through-and-through guide wire. At this point, the stricture can be balloon dilated or incised, as previously described. An indwelling standard 7 Fr. or 8 Fr. pigtail stent or a 7 Fr./14 Fr. stent is placed. A nephrostomy tube and urethral catheter are positioned. Two days after the procedure, a nephrostogram is obtained. If there is no extravasation, the nephrostomy tube and the urethral catheter can be removed. The nephrostomy tube is removed under fluoroscopic monitoring. If there is extravasation, these catheters are left in place for 1 week and the studies repeated on an outpatient basis. The indwelling ureteral stent is left in place for 12 weeks (Bagley, 1990).

If the site of *total occlusion* is in the *distal ureter*, a nephrostomy tube is placed. The approach to this problem can be solely fluoroscopic or a combination of fluoroscopy and endoscopic incision. In the fluoroscopic approach, via a percutaneous nephrostomy, a stiff guide wire (Lunderquist) or a sharpened wire, such as the rocket wire from a retrograde percutaneous access kit, is passed antegrade to the site of obstruction (Chao et al., 1987; Lang, 1984). The bladder is filled with contrast material. Using the C-arm, the tip of the antegrade guide wire is maneuvered until it is pointed directly at the bladder in both the anterior-posterior and lateral planes. The guide wire is then forcibly advanced into the bladder. Next a 4- to 8-mm, 4-cm long, polyethylene balloon can be passed antegrade and used to dilate the obstructed site. It is left inflated for 10 minutes and exchanged for a 10 Fr. or larger antegrade biliary urinary drainage or Cope loop catheter. Additional drainage holes are created along the shaft of the catheter where it traverses the renal pelvis. This nephrostent is removed 6 weeks later.

If an endoscopic approach is selected, the flexible endoscope is passed antegrade down to the site of obstruction, or a guide wire is manipulated down the ureter and a 6-mm or 8-mm ureteral dilating catheter with a short tip or no tip is passed over the guide wire to the level of obstruction. The balloon can be inflated with contrast material mixed with indigo carmine. Next, an Iglesias resectoscope with a Collings knife, an Orandi knife, or a direct vision urethrotome is passed via the urethra. Using the fluoroscope, the retrograde endoscope is positioned until it directly overlies the endoscope or the contrast medium–containing balloon. If the first method is chosen, the light in the retrograde endoscope (i.e., cystoscope) is turned off and the incision is made to the bright light coming from the antegrade endoscope. Alternatively, if the contrast agent–filled balloon is selected as a target, the fluoroscope is used to align the cystoscope over the 5 Fr. catheter or balloon. An incision is directed toward the balloon filled with material and contrast indigo carmine (Fig. 62–47). Once the nephroscope or antegrade balloon catheter is uncovered in the proximal ureter, a 260-cm, 0.035-inch ex-

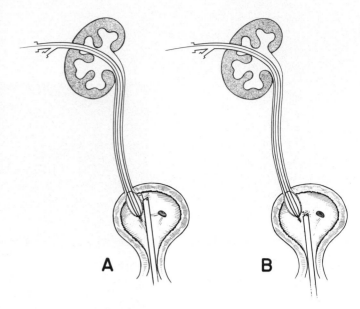

Figure 62–47. Distal ureteral obstruction complete.

A, A 0.035-inch guide wire has been advanced via a percutaneous nephrostomy until its tip lies at the cephalad border of a distal ureteral occlusion. A 6-mm ureteral dilating balloon (no tip) has been advanced over the guide wire and inflated. An Orandi electrosurgical knife has been aligned under fluoroscopic guidance, such that the tip of the knife directly overlies the inflated balloon.

B, The overlying tissue has been incised, thereby uncovering the balloon. At this point, a 260-cm exchange guide wire is passed antegrade through the balloon catheter and pulled via the cystoscope through the urethra. An indwelling stent and nephrostomy tube or a nephrostent is positioned across the incised stricture. The stent is removed after 6 weeks.

change guide wire is passed and retrieved via the urethra, thereby providing a through-and-through guide wire. As previously described, an indwelling stent, nephrostomy tube, and ureteral catheter are placed. In this circumstance, however, while the nephrostomy tube is removed on postoperative day 2 (provided a nephrostogram reveals no extravasation), the urethral catheter is left indwelling for a full week. At 1 week, on an outpatient basis, a cystogram is obtained. If there is no extravasation, the urethral catheter is removed. The indwelling ureteral stent remains in place for 4 to 6 weeks (Cubelli and Smith, 1987).

The injection of triamcinolone (40 mg/ml) into the stricture bed may be helpful if the scar tissue is particularly dense or if, despite a deep incision, no retroperitoneal fat is seen. A 3 Fr. Greenwald ureteroscopic or a larger cystoscopic needle is selected. Approximately 5 ml of triamcinolone (40 mg/ml) is injected. It is helpful to have a LeVeen pressure syringe connected to the needle so that the triamcinolone can forcibly be injected into the scarred tissues (Fig. 62–48). The triamcinolone is slowly absorbed over 3 months; its peak effect is at 3 weeks. In theory, the triamcinolone serves as a catalyst for endogenous collagenase, thereby limiting collagen formation. Although triamcinolone administration has received favorable comments in association with treating contractures at the bladder neck, no data prove its efficacy in treating ureteral strictures (Damico et al., 1973; Farah et al., 1979).

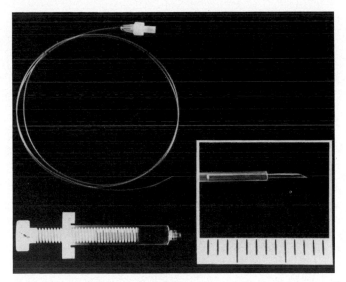

Figure 62–48. A 3 Fr. Greenwald injection needle (*inset*, closeup of the < 1 mm needle) used for triamcinolone injection. A LeVeen pressure syringe is helpful to forcibly inject the medication into the scarred area.

RESULTS. The results with endosurgery for ureteral strictures are quite variable (Hulbert et al., 1988). Catheter dilation can be quite successful. In 1924, Hunner reported on 100 patients with ureteral strictures, treated by catheter dilation between 1910 and 1918. Overall, 29 per cent "were cured" and 65 per cent were improved. Recommendations at that time were to dilate the ureter up to 19 to 23 Fr. No indwelling stents were placed (Hunner, 1924). Witherington and Shelor (1980) reported on four patients with strictures occurring following hysterectomy. Catheter dilation to 7 to 8 Fr. was uniformly successful in this highly select patient population (follow-up, 4 months to 3 years).

Overall durable "success" rates (follow-up >1 year) for balloon dilation and endoincision are similar: 50 to 60 per cent (Gothlin et al., 1988; Johnson et al., 1987; Lang and Glorioso, 1988; O'Brien et al., 1988). Two major reasons exist for this vast range of success rates: the nature of the stricture and the design of the study itself. The differences among the strictures treated are also vast: the length of the stricture, the etiology of the stricture, and the location of the stricture all may vary. These factors significantly influence the final result. Currently, the most important determinant of the outcome of an endoureterotomy appears to be the length of the stricture. Strictures longer then 1 cm rarely respond well to an endosurgical approach (11 to 18 per cent), whereas the success rate for balloon dilation of ≤1 cm strictures is 90 to 100 per cent in three series comprising 41 patients (Chang et al., 1987; Netto et al., 1990).

Another, albeit lesser, factor that causes an impact on the outcome of endoureterotomy is the etiology of the strictured area. Intrinsic ureteral strictures are currently most commonly (upward of 75 per cent) caused by postoperative fibrosis following open pelvic surgery or a ureteroscopic procedure (Netto et al., 1990). Other causes of intrinsic ureteral strictures include inflammatory processes associated with schistosomiasis, retroperitoneal fibrosis, or tuberculosis; malignancy; and radiation (ischemic injury) (Johnson et al., 1987; Kramolowsky et al., 1989; Netto et al., 1990). A stricture due to an ischemic problem appears to respond less well than a benign nonischemic stricture—40 per cent versus 58 per cent (Lang, 1984; O'Brien et al., 1988). Those strictures that are of a proximal or distal nature and can be marsupialized at either their upper or lower border into the renal pelvis or bladder have a better success rate than strictures that are mid-ureteral and bounded by normal caliber ureter on either end: 80 per cent versus 25 per cent (Meretyk et al., 1991b). Indeed, in Smith's series, all four patients with a mid-ureteral stricture failed balloon dilation.

The duration of a stricture prior to therapy appears to have little impact on subsequent outcome. Initially, it was believed that the age of a stricture would directly impair the success of an endoureterotomy (Beckman et al., 1989; Lang and Glorioso, 1988). In this regard, Beckman and colleagues (1989) noted that treatment of strictures of ≤ 3 months' duration, resulted in an 88 per cent success rate versus 67 per cent, if the stricture was present more than 3 months. However, when the aforementioned factors of stricture length and vascular supply and location are taken into consideration, the duration of the stricture appears to have little or no effect on the subsequent outcome of an endoureterotomy (Finnerty et al., 1984; Netto et al., 1990). Indeed, success has been recorded with strictures as old as 18 months, and failures have been recorded with strictures diagnosed within 8 weeks of the initiating event (Netto et al., 1990).

Another major reason for the vast range in the reported "success" with endosurgery for ureteral strictures is the nature of the studies themselves. The aforementioned response modifiers are usually not all taken into account in any one series. Ischemic or nonischemic; short or long; distal, proximal, or middle ureteral strictures of varying duration are mixed together in a nondescript potpourri of ureteral pathology. Next, variables occur in both the method of balloon dilation or endoincision and the postoperative management. In the method, the size of the balloon (4 to 8 mm), duration of inflation (15 seconds to 60 minutes), number of inflation cycles (1 to 3), and duration of stent placement (2 days to 2 months) are different in each reported series (Banner and Pollack, 1984; Chang et al., 1987; Coleman et al., 1984a; Finnerty et al., 1984; Johnson et al., 1987; Kramolowsky et al., 1989; Lang and Glorioso, 1988; Netto et al., 1990; O'Brien et al., 1988). With regard to the endoincision, the method may vary among cold knife, electrocautery, and laser.

Furthermore, the use of triamcinolone as a modifier of scar formation may influence the outcome. In one report, injection of triamcinolone was associated with a 86 per cent incidence of ureteral patency at 11 months versus only 33 per cent at 22 months in patients who did not receive triamcinolone (Kavoussi et al., 1991b; Meretyk et al., 1991b). With respect to postoperative management, the size (7 Fr./14 Fr.), composition (Silastic, polyurethane), and duration (0 days to 3 months) of the indwelling ureteral stent may vary greatly and may cause an independent impact upon the outcome (Banner and Pollack, 1984; Chang et al., 1987; Finnerty et al., 1984; Glanz et al., 1983; Johnson et al., 1987). Indeed, some workers have not placed an indwelling stent at all after endoureterotomy (Reimer et al., 1981).

In the various studies on endosurgical therapy for ureteral strictures, the means for evaluating a successful outcome vary greatly. Subjective follow-up, while not difficult to secure, is hardly reliable. In contrast, *objective* follow-up is often difficult to obtain. Regarding subjective follow-up, in one series of ureteral strictures, 25 per cent of patients were asymptomatic *at the time of presentation* (Kavoussi et al., 1990; Meretyk et al., 1991b). A lack of symptoms referable to obstruction postoperatively does not necessarily imply a patent ureter. In contrast, objective data are usually scant and too close to the time of the surgical procedure to be reliable. In this regard, follow-up of only a few months is not sufficient to judge the outcome of the procedure. In Meretyk and Clayman's series, 15 per cent of patients undergoing an endoincision experienced a failed procedure between 6 and 12 months postoperatively. The difference in results is impressive. In this series, the procedure would have been considered successful in 79 per cent if the study were ended after 3 postoperative months. However, only a 64 per cent success was recorded when objective follow-up information was extended to 1 year (Kavoussi et al., 1991b; Meretyk et al., 1991b).

Unlike endopyelotomy, endourologic therapy for ureteral strictures is still in a process of evolution. Although the endopyelotomy data are quite reproducible among various institutions, the balloon dilation and endoureterotomy data remain highly variable. More detailed studies with meticulous long-term follow-up data and proper separation of strictures according to length, etiology, location, and duration are necessary to better define the indications for an endourologic approach. At present, this procedure is most applicable for those ureteral strictures that are short in length (<1 cm), not associated with radiation or other ischemic injury, and preferably located in the proximal or distal ureter. If these circumstances do not apply, then, at present, the better method of repair is an open surgical approach.

Extension of endosurgical therapy to "unfavorable" strictures is currently being pursued. Clayman and Denstedt (1989) have reported on four patients with long distal strictures (5 to 7 cm) in whom a patch of urothelium was cystoscopically harvested from the bladder (up to 2 cm × 4 cm in size). This patch of urothelium was defatted and sewn onto a 7 Fr. ureteral stent (urothelium facing the stent). The graft-bearing stent was positioned in the bed of the stricture, such that the graft free of urothelium would overlie the incised area. The stent was removed 6 weeks later. In two patients, a larger stent (7 Fr./14 Fr.) was placed for an additional 6 weeks. Follow-up beyond 1 year is available in two patients; in both, the ureter is patent. However, while of interest, these investigators to date have been unable to provide any data showing that the grafted tissue actually was incorporated into the ureter in any fashion. Future developments in the area of biologically compatible

prosthetics in combination with cell and tissue culture may eventually render an acceptable ureteral substitute.

Other Applications

Ureteroenteric Strictures: Endoureterotomy

An ureteroenteric stricture occurs in 4 to 8 per cent of patients who are undergoing urinary conduit procedures (Engel, 1969; Schmidt et al., 1973). Insidious in onset, a potential harbinger of recurrent and unresectable cancer, and requiring an often difficult open surgical repair, the ureteroenteric stricture is a difficult entity to treat. However, in properly selected patients, the endosurgical therapy of these strictures can offer a successful alternative to open surgical therapy (Meretyk et al., 1990c).

In dealing with a ureteroenteric stricture, the initial evaluation is designed to answer the question: Is the stricture the result of benign scar tissue formation or secondary to recurrent malignant disease? As such, the following diagnostic studies are obtained: an intravenous urogram, a radiographic contrast study of the conduit (i.e., loopogram), and in patients with a history of malignant disease a CT of the abdomen and pelvis, along with a chest radiograph and a bone scan. For further evaluation of the degree of obstruction and the remaining renal function in the affected kidney, a Whitaker pelvic/bladder pressure study and a furosemide washout renogram are indicated, respectively. The bladder pressure study, in combination with the loopogram, will also help delineate the degree and length of the stricture. In addition, endoscopy is helpful to rule out recurrent malignant disease in the conduit, at the site of the ureteroenteric anastomosis.

If the stricture is *complete or of malignant origin*, the goal of endourologic therapy is to place a retrograde *external* ureteral catheter. The ureteral drainage catheter is changed on an outpatient basis every 3 to 4 months (Horgan et al., 1988). However, if the stricture is *benign* and *partial,* the goal of endosurgical therapy is to reestablish continuity in such a manner that a permanent indwelling stent is not necessary.

TECHNIQUE. Prior to endosurgical therapy for a ureteroenteric stricture, the patient is advised of the following potential problems: the less than 60 per cent success rate, the possibility of hemorrhage necessitating transfusion and emergency open surgery, the possible loss of the kidney, and the possible creation of an ureteroenteric fistula (Meretyk et al., 1990). Preoperative preparation includes a sterile urine culture and the administration of parenteral antibiotics, usually ampicillin and aminoglycoside.

The position of the patient must allow access both to the flank on the affected side and to the stoma of the conduit. The patient is thus usually placed in a flank position, with the affected side superior (Fig. 62–49). Both the flank and the stoma are prepared and draped. An effective procedure is to use two nephrostomy drapes; one is placed over the planned nephrostomy

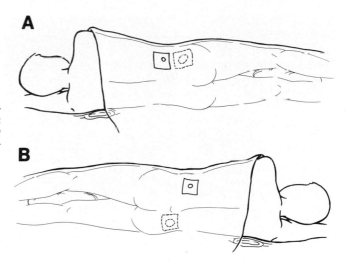

Figure 62–49. *A,* Patient positioned for endoureterotomy of right ureteroenteric stricture (*dotted circle,* ileal stoma on anterior abdominal wall; *solid circle,* nephrostomy site). *B,* Patient positioned for endoureterotomy of left ureteroenteric stricture (*dotted circle,* ileal stoma on anterior abdominal wall; *solid circle,* nephrostomy site).

site, and a second is placed directly over the abdominal stoma.

As with other upper urinary tract strictures, there are two methods and two approaches for management of an ureteroenteric stricture: balloon dilation and endoincision with an antegrade or a retrograde approach (Figs. 62–50 and 62–51). *Balloon dilation* is by far the older and simpler of the two techniques (Banner and Pollack, 1984; Lang, 1984). A guide wire is passed either antegrade via a small nephrostomy tract or retrograde at the time of looposcopy. The preferred guide wire for this purpose is a 0.035-inch Terumo glide wire, usually with

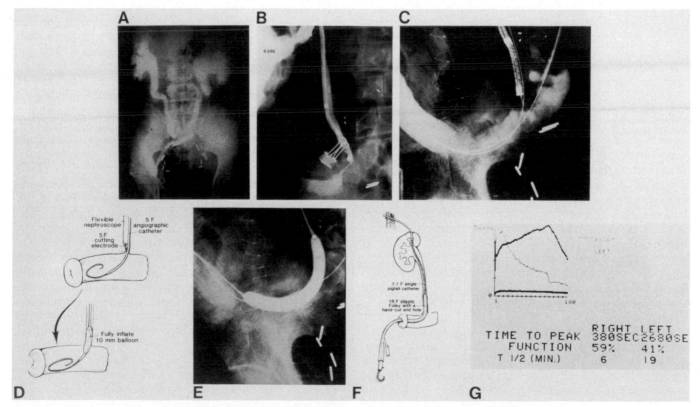

Figure 62–50. Steps in performing an endoincision of ureteroenteric stricture via an *antegrade* approach.

A, Bilateral ureteroenteric anastomotic strictures occurring 10 years after a total exenteration for rectal cancer (June 1985).

B, Antegrade approach is performed with a flexible nephroscope. An antegrade ureterogram outlines the stricture.

C, A 3 Fr. electrosurgery probe is used to incise the stricture under direct endoscopic control. The incision is continued until the ileal conduit is entered.

D, A diagram depicting the incision of the stricture and subsequent balloon dilation of the area.

E, The incised stricture is balloon dilated to ensure the adequacy of the incision.

F, The endoincision is stented with an 18 Fr. catheter for 6 weeks.

G, A renal scan, 14 months later, reveals acceptable clearance on the right and slightly prolonged clearance on the left. The patient is asymptomatic and the creatinine serum is normal. (From Kramolowsky, E. V., Clayman, R. V., and Weyman, P. J.: J. Urol., 137:390, 1987. © By Williams & Wilkins, 1992.)

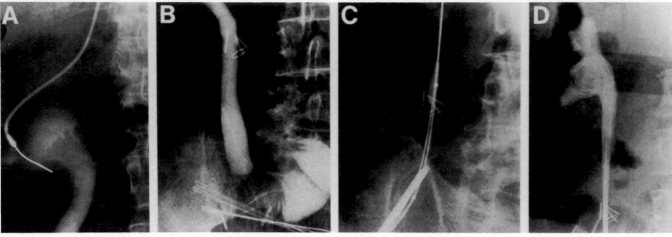

Figure 62–51. A retrograde approach to a ureteroenteric stricture.

A and *B*, Antegrade nephrostogram demonstrates ureteroenteric stricture. *A*, Nephrostomy needle in kidney; *B*, distal ureter at ureteroenteric juncture.

C, The stricture was incised via a retrograde approach. In this figure, a 3 Fr. Greenwald needle is being used to inject the area of the incision with triamcinolone (40 mg/ml).

D, Two retrograde pigtail catheters (each 8 Fr.) have been positioned with their distal coils in the renal pelvis. No nephrostomy tube is placed. The shaft of each pigtail exits the stoma to preclude obstruction from mucus. Holes are only in the coiled pelvic portions of the pigtail catheters.

an angled tip. A torque control device enables the urologist to rotate the Terumo guide wire without difficulty. This extremely lubricatory wire has a tendency to bypass even the tightest strictures. When passed retrograde, the guide wire is coiled in the renal pelvis; however, if an antegrade approach is taken, the tip of the guide wire is passed into the loop, where it can be retrieved with an endoscope, thereby creating a through-and-through Terumo guide wire. The last situation provides more control over the collecting system.

Next, a 5 Fr. angiographic catheter is passed over the Terumo guide wire, and the Terumo guide wire is exchanged for a 0.035-inch Amplatz super stiff guide wire (retrograde approach) or a 0.035-inch, 260-cm exchange guide wire (antegrade approach). The 5 Fr. angiographic catheter is removed. A 6-mm or an 8-mm balloon dilating catheter is passed over the guide wire, until it straddles the stricture. The dilating balloon, which should be rated to at least 15 atmospheres, is slowly inflated with a pressure syringe (LeVeen type). Once the waist (i.e., stricture) disappears, the balloon is left inflated for 1 minute; the balloon is deflated, and the inflation/deflation cycle may be repeated once or twice.

Following this, when a *retrograde* approach is used, a 10 Fr. to 16 Fr. single pigtail catheter is passed retrograde over the Amplatz super stiff guide wire and positioned in the renal pelvis. The flush end of the pigtail catheter, as it exits the stoma, can be sewn with a 2-0 Prolene to the peristomal skin to prevent its premature dislodgement. When an *antegrade* approach is used, the 10 Fr. to 16 Fr. pigtail catheter is placed, as described, and a nephrostomy tube (8 Fr.) is also positioned. At 2 to 3 days, a stentogram is obtained. If the collecting system is intact, the nephrostomy tube is removed. The 16 Fr. pigtail catheter is either removed after 6 weeks or exchanged under fluoroscopic control

after 3 to 4 months, dependent on whether the stricture was benign and partial or malignant and complete (Meretyk et al., 1991c).

Prior to performing an *endoincision* of an ureteroenteric stricture, the patient should also undergo a complete mechanical and antibiotic bowel preparation. The possibility of an inadvertent enterotomy exists, and if the bowel has been properly prepared, this problem may be handled conservatively by simply stenting the ureter with a 10 Fr. to 16 Fr. pigtail drainage catheter. In the case of significant bleeding, an open procedure may be necessary. The ureteroenteric problem could then be repaired at the same time and, if need be, a new conduit created.

For performing an endoincision of an ureteroenteric stricture, a *retrograde* approach is simpler (see Fig. 62–51) (Meretyk et al., 1991c). Paradoxically, the initial step in a retrograde approach is to secure control of the kidney via an 8 Fr. nephrostomy catheter. A guide wire (usually an 0.035-inch Terumo glide wire) can then be passed antegrade, across the area of stricture and into the conduit. If this is not possible, a nephrostomy tube should still be placed in order to allow for repeated injection of indigo carmine–stained saline to enable the endoscopist to localize the narrowed ureteroenteric anastomosis.

Endoscopy of the conduit is performed with a rigid endoscope (i.e., direct vision Sachs urethrotome or a 12 Fr. short rigid therapeutic ureteroscope). If a guide wire has not been passed antegrade, attempts are made to pass a guide wire retrograde and coil its tip in the renal pelvis. The endoscope is removed and then reinserted alongside the guide wire. A 6-mm ureteral dilating balloon catheter is passed either antegrade or retrograde, until the balloon straddles the stricture. The balloon is inflated with 50:50 contrast agent:saline stained with indigo carmine, to 1 atmosphere, to outline the stricture on the fluoroscope. Next, the balloon is deflated and the area of the stricture is deeply incised with a cold knife via the rigid endoscope.

Alternatively, the balloon can be left inflated and an incision made along the balloon, using a 2 Fr. or 3 Fr. Greenwald electrode. The incision should extend through the entire thickness of the ureter. Occasionally, retroperitoneal fat can be seen. The incision is continued cephalad until the dilated normal ureter is identified. Usually, the ureteroenteric stricture is quite short (< 1 cm), and it is not difficult to discern "normal ureter" because of its marked proximal dilation. At the completion of the incision, the 6-mm or 8-mm balloon is reinflated to be certain that at low pressure (i.e., 1 atm), the previously strictured area completely expands. A 10 Fr. (or if available, a 16 Fr.) single pigtail catheter is passed over the guide wire and its pigtail end is positioned in the renal pelvis. The pigtail catheter, as it exits the stoma, is secured to the peristomal skin with a 2-0 Prolene suture.

Under no circumstances should any of the currently available *internal* ureteral stents be placed. These catheters have drainage holes all along the shaft; as such, they may become occluded with mucus. The resulting obstruction may lead to fatal urosepsis (Walther et al., 1985). The external ureteral catheter only has drainage holes in the portion that resides within the renal pelvis.

At the end of the procedure, the urinary drainage appliance is placed over the cut end of the pigtail catheter and affixed in its usual manner to the skin. An 8 Fr. nephrostomy catheter is also placed. Two days postoperatively, with the patient still receiving parenteral antibiotics, a nephrostogram is performed. If there is no extravasation, the nephrostomy tube can be removed, *under fluoroscopic guidance.* The retrograde pigtail catheter can be removed or exchanged 6 weeks postoperatively, depending on the goal of therapy. During the 6-week period and for 2 weeks after stent removal, the patient takes a nightly antibiotic tablet, usually nitrofurantoin or a trimethoprim-sulfamethoxazole combination.

When a retrograde approach cannot be performed because of the tortuosity of the conduit or failure to identify and cannulate the stenotic ureteroenteric anastomosis, an *antegrade* approach is necessary (Fig. 62–50) (Meretyk et al., 1991c). The nephrostomy tract is placed in an upper or a middle posterior calyx in order to provide a direct line of access to the ureteropelvic junction. The nephrostomy tract is dilated and an 18 Fr. or 24 Fr. Amplatz sheath is placed, dependent on whether a flexible nephroscope (15 Fr.) or a flexible ureteroscope (9.4 Fr.) is to be used to traverse the collecting system and the dilated proximal ureter. The flexible endoscope is passed. Under direct inspection, the lumen of the strictured ureter is identified and a 0.035-inch Terumo guide wire is passed into the stricture and coiled in the conduit. A rigid endoscope is passed via the abdominal stoma into the conduit, and the guide wire is grasped and pulled until its tip exits the stoma (i.e., a through-and-through guide wire). The flexible nephroscope or ureteroscope is withdrawn and passed again via the sheath, albeit alongside the through-and-through guide wire. Over the through-and-through guide wire, a 5 Fr. angiographic catheter is passed and the Terumo guide wire is traded for a 0.035-inch, 260-cm exchange guide wire. The 5 Fr. catheter is exchanged for a 6-mm or an 8-mm balloon dilating catheter, which is positioned so that the balloon straddles the stricture. The balloon is inflated with dilute radiographic contrast material stained with indigo carmine to ≤1 atmosphere using a LeVeen syringe connected to an inline pressure gauge. Next, with the balloon inflated, a 2 Fr. or 3 Fr. electrocautery probe is passed via the flexible endoscope and an incision is made along the ureter until the conduit is entered. To date, a laser has not been used to make this type of incision.

The incision is made through the full thickness of the ureter. Often, retroperitoneal fat can be seen. An 8-mm ureteral dilating balloon or a 10-mm nephrostomy dilating balloon is passed retrograde over the through-and-through guide wire, until the new balloon straddles the incised stricture. The balloon should *fully* inflate at only 1 to 2 atmospheres. This indicates that the depth of the incision into the stricture is sufficient. As previously described, a nephrostomy tube, in this case a 10 Fr. pigtail or 22 Fr. Councill catheter, is placed, along with a separate retrograde 10 Fr. to 16 Fr. pigtail catheter. The postoperative regimen is identical to that described for the retrograde approach.

If the scar tissue is particularly dense, 3 to 5 ml of triamcinolone (40 mg/ml) may be injected into the bed of the incised stricture. This step is done with a 3 Fr. Greenwald needle, which is mounted on a flexible shaft (see Fig. 62–48). It is helpful to inject the scar tissue utilizing a LeVeen pressure syringe, as otherwise the scar tissue may be too dense to allow the triamcinolone to penetrate. Although conceptually appealing, the benefit of this maneuver remains unproven (Meretyk et al., 1991c).

If the obstruction is *complete,* a combined antegrade/retrograde approach is required. In this case, a rigid endoscope is passed via the bowel conduit and a flexible ureteroscope or flexible nephroscope is passed via the nephrostomy tract. The light from the antegrade endoscope is turned off. The examiner then seeks the light coming from the rigid retrograde endoscope within the conduit. When the tips of the two endoscopes are fluoroscopically close (<1 cm), the initial pink hue transilluminating the intervening tissue should appear almost white. In this regard, a C-arm fluoroscope is essential because the position of the tips of the endoscopes must be viewed in *two* projections to ensure that they are indeed aligned and proximate in the same plane.

At this point, several methods can be selected to reestablish a communication between the ureter and the conduit. The stiff end of a 0.035-inch, 260-cm exchange guide wire can be passed via the antegrade flexible endoscope, guided fluoroscopically and endoscopically to perforate the brightest (i.e., "white") area of light, and thereby enter the conduit (Muench et al., 1987). Alternatively, a 2 Fr. or 3 Fr. electrocautery probe can be employed via the flexible antegrade endoscope to "cut to the light" and uncover the rigid retrograde endoscope. A third approach is to turn off the light of the rigid retrograde endoscope while maintaining the light of the flexible endoscope (see Fig. 62–46). If the conduit is not tortuous, a cold knife urethrotome can be utilized via the retrograde endoscope to cut to the white light cast by the antegrade flexible endoscope.

If a recommunication is established between the ureter and enteric conduit, a 0.035-inch, 260-cm exchange guide wire is passed via the flexible antegrade endoscope, grasped via the retrograde rigid endoscope, and pulled through the stoma of the conduit, thereby providing a through-and-through guide wire. However, if the recommunication is established from the conduit to the ureter, the flexible antegrade ureteroscope can be maneuvered across the newly developed ureteroenteric juncture until the ureteroscope resides in the distal portion of the conduit. Now a 0.035-inch, 260-cm exchange guide wire is passed via the flexible endoscope and out the stoma. Subsequent dilation or incision of the stricture is accomplished, as previously described for an incomplete stricture of an ureteroenteric anastomosis.

The ureteroenteric stricture is the most difficult to approach endourologically. No landmarks, as with an endopyelotomy or typical endoureterotomy, are noted to guide the urologist as to where to make the incision. Accordingly, it is important for the surgeon to review the original operative notes in order to determine if the conduit is intraperitoneal or retroperitoneal. The incision in the ureter should be deepened very slowly *under constant endoscopic monitoring* in order to avoid inadvertent injury to an underlying artery or the bowel. If during the incision, it appears as though one is again seeing urothelium, this is more than likely the serosal surface of the adjoining bowel.

If the bowel is entered, placement of the ureteral pigtail drainage catheter across the incised stricture and into the renal pelvis should be done immediately. The fistula will usually close spontaneously over several weeks (Meretyk et al., 1991c). If excessive bleeding is encountered, an 8-mm ureteral dilating balloon can be placed over the through-and-through guide wire until it straddles the incised stricture, and the balloon is inflated.

Tamponade will usually stop the bleeding. With excessive bleeding, it is helpful to leave the through-and-through guide wire in place. A separate nephrostomy tube is positioned alongside the through-and-through guide wire. With a suture, the through-and-through guide wire can be sewn to the skin of the flank and with a side-arm adapter, it can be secured to the hub of the balloon tamponade catheter, thereby maintaining the proper position of the inflated balloon tamponade catheter. The balloon can usually be deflated, 2 days later, removed, and a 10 Fr. to 16 Fr. pigtail catheter placed retrograde. The through-and-through guide wire can also be removed. However, postoperatively, if despite the aforementioned measures, signs of peritonitis develop or hemodynamics become unstable, immediate open exploration and repair of any enterotomy or vascular injury are necessary.

All of these strictures are at the ureteroenteric anastomosis. As such, as with a proximal or distal ureteral stricture, the surgeon is marsupializing the stricture into a larger structure: in this case, the enteric conduit. Also, in this regard, among patients with a conduit, strictures occurring in the left ureter, as it passes beneath the sigmoid mesentery, are best managed with balloon dilation or open surgery. Endoincision in this area is fraught with potential complications: enterotomy into the sigmoid colon lying anteriorly or arteriotomy or venotomy into the aorta or vena cava lying posteriorly.

RESULTS. Reports on the surgical results of treating ureteroenteric strictures are scant. In one report of a total of seven patients (with 33 months' objective follow-up), the patency rate was 89 per cent. However, the complication rate in this series was high. Indeed, in these seven patients, two (29 per cent) required reoperation in the immediate postoperative period for urine leakage from the conduit or ureteroenteric anastomosis (Kramolowsky et al., 1988).

In 1982, Martin and co-workers (1982), as well as Dixon and colleagues (1982), published reports of successful *balloon dilation* of ureteroenteric strictures in four patients (Table 62–10). However, since then, only a few series of balloon dilation of ureteroenteric strictures have been reported (Banner and Pollack, 1984; Chang et al., 1987; Lang, 1984). In these studies, the size of the balloon for dilation varied from 5 to 12 mm,

Table 62–10. URETEROENTERIC STRICTURES: ENDOSURGICAL THERAPY

Authors	Patients	Size Balloon (Fr.)	Stent Size (Fr.)	Stent Duration	Patency (%)	Follow-up
Balloon Dilation						
Shapiro et al., 1988	37	12-30	8-10	1-6	16	≥ 12 mos.
Chang et al., 1987	6	15-24	8-16	5-12	33	≥ 11 mos. (avg. 14 mos.)
O'Brien et al., 1988	6	12-18	—	—	17	≥ 12 mos.
Beckman et al., 1989	5	12-24	7-10	4-8	60	≥ 20 mos. (mean, 22 mos.)
Overall	54				22	all ≥ 11 mos.
Endoincision						
Meretyk et al., 1990c	15	30-36 (calibration)	12-22	4-28	57	≥9 mos. (avg. 29 mos.)
Surgical Repair						
Kramolowsky et al., 1988	9	—	7-8	—	89	≥ 24 mos. (avg. 33 mos.)

the number of cycles of dilation varied from one to three (during one session or over several days) (Martin et al., 1982), and the balloon was left inflated for anytime from 30 seconds to 15 minutes (Banner and Pollack, 1984; Chang et al., 1987; Kramolowsky et al., 1987). The stent size varied from 5 Fr. to 24 Fr. (on average 8 Fr. to 14 Fr.) and the duration of stent placement was from 4 days to 3 months (average, 6 weeks).

Follow-up at approximately 6 months showed a patency rate of 58 per cent; however, longer follow-up revealed an ongoing deterioration of patency with time: 33 per cent patent at 11 months and only 0 to 10 per cent at 1 year (Chang et al., 1987; Kramolowsky et al., 1987; Lang, 1984; Shapiro et al., 1988). Of note, in none of the reports was any significant morbidity incurred with balloon dilation.

With regard to *endoincision* of ureteroenteric strictures, Kramolowsky and co-workers (1988) and subsequently Meretyk and co-workers (1991c) at Washington University reported the largest series. Among 19 ureteroenteric strictures in 15 patients, 25 per cent of the strictures were managed only by placement of a permanent external ureteral stent because of the presence of metastatic disease or the complete obliteration of the ureteroenteric anastomosis. Of the remaining 14 strictures, all were treated by endoincision usually via an antegrade approach employing a 2 Fr. or 3 Fr. monopolar electrocautery probe. The average procedural time was 175 minutes. Blood loss was minimal in all patients, estimated at (50 to 200 ml). Among these patients, long-term objective follow-up (average, 2.5 years; all patients, > 9 months postoperative) revealed a patency rate of 57 per cent.

Of those patients who experienced a failed procedure, a third (i.e., two patients) developed metastatic disease within a year, a third (i.e., two patients) were too debilitated to undergo an open repair and were managed with a long-term external retrograde ureteral stent, and a third (i.e., two patients) would have been candidates for an open surgical correction. Of these two patients, one patient experienced restricture of the anastomosis soon after endosurgery and was advised to have an open procedure; however, he refused. He continues with a long-term external ureteral catheter. The other patient developed restricturing of the left ureteroileal anastomosis *4.5 years* after endoincision. This restricturing was managed with a balloon dilation, and the ureter has remained patent 12 months following the second endourologic procedure. Complications with an endoincision occurred in 7 per cent (ureteroenteric fistula managed conservatively and closing without intervention). No blood transfusions were necessary in any of the patients.

In sum, with the aforementioned techniques and guidelines, only 7 to 13 per cent of all patients presenting with ureteroenteric strictures would have required open surgical procedures.

Vesicocutaneous Fistulas

Few problems are as vexing to surgeon and patient alike as inoperable vesicovaginal or vesicocutaneous fistulas resulting from pelvic malignancy. This situation most often occurs in women with recurrent or inoperable cervical or uterine cancer (34 per cent of cases) or in males with bladder cancer (18 per cent of cases) or prostate cancer (8 per cent of cases) in whom the tumor has eroded into the floor of the bladder (Darcy et al., 1987; Gunther et al., 1982; Gunther et al., 1979; Kinn et al., 1986; Papanicolaou et al., 1985; Reddy et al., 1987; Smith et al., 1987). The constant leakage of urine results in the maceration and eventual destruction of the perineal skin with ensuing infection, discomfort, and malodor.

TECHNIQUE. Although bilateral nephrostomy tubes can divert the urine, enough urine traverses the ureter to result in continued leakage. Nephrostomy tube drainage can become a solution only when it is coupled with concomitant occlusion or diversion of the ureters. A variety of endosurgical solutions are available to accomplish this goal by either an *indirect intraluminal* (i.e., transrenal percutaneous nephrostomy) or a *direct extraluminal* (i.e., retroperitoneal), approach to the ureter (Moldwin and Smith, 1988).

The earliest attempt to obstruct the ureters in such patients was via an *intraluminal* approach. This maneuver can be accomplished by (1) the fluoroscopic placement of an obstructing foreign body, (2) the instillation of a sclerosing agent, and (3) the application of electrocautery to the ureteral wall. A multitude of foreign bodies have been developed to achieve ureteral occlusion. Initially, a nondetachable 13-mm balloon was placed fluoroscopically in the ureter along with a nephrostomy tube. However, this provided only temporary relief as problems of ureteral necrosis, pain, and urine extravasation developed (Papanicolaou et al., 1985). Accordingly, Gunther in 1982 developed a 20-mm detachable latex balloon that could be inflated in the mid-ureter and then disengaged from its introducing catheter.

A silicone elastomer, silicone fluid, 1 gm/ml of tantalum powder (for opacification), and a couple of drops of catalyst M (to activate the silicone) were instilled into the balloon to a volume of 1 ml (Gunther et al., 1982). The mixture eventually solidified within the balloon. A similar approach, using a detachable silicone "olive" has been described by Brandl (1987). Gaylord and Johnsrude (1989) have reported on the success of multiple 8 mm × 5 cm and 5 mm × 3 cm Gianturco coils plus a gelatin sponge (3/8-inch thick × 3/4-inch long × 1/4-inch wide) material to successfully occlude the ureter. Of all the types of occlusive foreign bodies, the last appears to be the simplest yet effective method.

Other indirect methods to achieve ureteral occlusion involve the injection of sclerosing fluids. In one approach, isobutyl-2-cyanoacrylate plus iodized oil [Lipiodol (contrast agent)] was instilled into the distal ureter after first inflating a balloon catheter in the mid-ureter in order to isolate the proximal ureter and renal pelvis from the sclerosing agent. After a 1-minute "set time," the balloon was deflated and removed, leaving the newly formed ureteral plug of glue in place (Gunther et al., 1979).

By far the simplest and perhaps safest intraluminal approach to achieving ureteral occlusion is by electrocautery applied directly to the inner wall of the ureter under direct endoscopic (i.e., antegrade nephroscopy) monitoring. In this technique, developed by Reddy and associates (1987), a 20-Fr. nephrostomy tract is created. Next, a 15 Fr. flexible nephroscope is passed via this tract into the proximal ureter. Through the nephroscope, a 5 Fr. electrode is passed and the ureteral lumen is circumferentially cauterized (Valley Laboratory setting of 4—pure coagulation current), for a distance of 2 cm along the most proximal portion of the ureter. As the mucosa is cauterized, it should turn white. The operative time for the coagulation process is in the range of 15 minutes (Fig. 62–52) (Reddy et al., 1987).

A bipolar electrode, bearing a 4-mm balloon, has been developed to induce electrocautery cicatrization of the ureter. The 2-cm long balloon is mounted on a 7 Fr. shaft and placed in the ureter over a 0.035-inch guide wire. The 4-mm balloon is inflated to 2 atmospheres, and the two gold bipolar electrodes are activated (40 watts) for 5 to 10 seconds. To date, this unit has only undergone animal testing; however, the occlusion of swine ureters was uniformly complete and long lasting. Clinical trials are anticipated in the near future. This approach might allow for the entire procedure to be performed with local anesthesia via a diminutive (≤ 10 Fr.) nephrostomy tract (Kopecky et al., 1989).

Two *direct extraluminal* approaches are possible to occlude the ureter in patients with incurable vesicovaginal fistulas: creation of a cutaneous ureterostomy and direct extraluminal occlusion of the ureter. Smith and co-workers (1987) have used a 34 Fr. retroperitoneal tract to approach the ureter. A percutaneous nephrostomy is created, and contrast material is instilled into the proximal ureter. Under C-arm fluoroscopy, a nephrostomy type needle is guided into the dilated, opacified ureter and a guide wire is passed into the kidney and retrieved via the nephrostomy tract. A 34 Fr. tract is developed in the retroperitoneum, and a finger digitally mobilizes the ureter for about a 10- to 15-cm length. The ureter is grasped with a Babcock clamp and brought to the skin surface. The ureter is divided, and the distal segment is sutured closed. The proximal end of the ureter is sewn to the skin as a conventional ureterostomy. A cutaneous U-loop nephroureterostomy tube is now placed. All patients in whom this method has been performed have been thin and the ureters have been tortuous.

With a similar approach to that of Smith, Amplatz and colleagues have also chosen a 30 Fr. retroperitoneal tract to directly approach the middle ureter (Darcy et al., 1987). Via a previously established nephrostomy tract, a guide wire is passed into the ureter. Long forceps are passed through the retroperitoneal 30 Fr. Amplatz sheath in order to free the ureter from the surrounding retroperitoneal fat. A self-closing, spring-activated clip is then applied to the ureter (Darcy et al., 1987).

RESULTS. The occurrence of a vesicovaginal or vesicocutaneous fistula in the patient with a pelvic malignancy is often the final degrading event in a life that has already become nigh intolerable. The resulting malodor and perineal ulceration force these individuals into a state of self-exile precisely at the time when they are in greatest need of both professional care and familial compassion. The aforementioned minimally invasive techniques can substantially add to the quality of the brief life that remains.

As can be seen from Table 62–11, many of these individuals succumb to underlying disease within a short period of the development of their urinary tract fistula. Accordingly, any therapy rendered must be simple, preferably on an outpatient basis, involve minimal anesthesia, and yet be highly and immediately effective. In this regard, only two of the aforementioned methods can be strongly recommended: occlusion with Gianturco coils and gelatin sponge or endoscopic application of electrocautery to the ureter. Both therapies are less

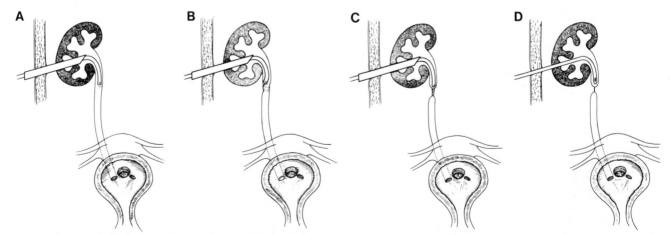

Figure 62–52. *A*, A fungating cervical carcinoma has eroded into the posterior wall of the bladder resulting in a large vesicovaginal fistula. A percutaneous nephrostomy has been used to place a 24 Fr. Amplatz sheath. A 15 Fr. flexible nephroscope has been passed into the proximal ureter.

B, A 5 Fr. electrosurgical probe (75 watts, coagulating current) is used to circumferentially fulgurate the right ureteral wall for a distance of 2 cm.

C, Immediately after fulguration, the proximal right ureter is just barely patent.

D, The right proximal ureter has completely closed; the kidney is drained via a 20 Fr. nephrostomy tube. A similar procedure would be simultaneously performed on the right kidney, thereby resolving any urine leakage from the fistula.

Table 62–11. ENDOUROLOGY: URETERIC OCCLUSION

Authors	Approach	Method	Nephrostomy Tube (Fr.)	Patients	Ureter Successfully Occluded (%)	Procedures Per Patient	Complications	Follow-up
Gunther et al., 1979	Intraluminal	Butyl-2 cyanoacrylate instillation	Yes (10-12)	3	100	2-3	Delayed plug expulsion and leakage	—
Kinn et al., 1986	Intraluminal	Polidocanol intramural injection nylon plugs	Yes (24-26)	15	67	1-2	Nausea, pain at injection site; 46% with plug migration	8 mos. (mean) (58% died at mean of 7 mos. of primary disease)
Papanicolaou et al., 1985	Intraluminal	Nondetachable balloon	Yes (7-8)	3	33	1	Bleeding necessitating nephrectomy	≤4 wks.
Gunther et al., 1982	Intraluminal	Detachable silicone-filled balloon	Yes	7	100	1	(1) Balloon ruptured	2.9 mos. (avg., 2-6 mos.)
Gaylord et al., 1989	Intraluminal	Gianturco coils with gelatin sponges	Yes (8-12)	5	100	1	2 UTI (responded to oral antibiotics)	9 mos. (1-22 mos.)
Reddy and Sidi, 1990	Intraluminal	5 F. probe via 15 F. flexible nephroscope to fulgurate proximal ureter	Yes (20)	4	100	1	0	2-21 mos. (three died at 2, 3, and 21 mos.)
Smith et al., 1987	Extraluminal	Percutaneous ureterostomy	Yes (34)	2	100	1	None	72 mos.
Darcy et al., 1987	Extraluminal	Percutaneous applied ureteral clip	Yes (30)	1	100	1	None	6 mos.

UTI, upper tract infection.

expensive, less time-consuming, and require a lesser degree of anesthesia than any of the described alternatives. Indeed, endoscopic ureteral fulguration can now be achieved utilizing one of the 9.4 Fr. flexible ureteroscopes with a 3 Fr. electrode, thereby precluding the need to even dilate the nephrostomy tract beyond 10 Fr. In our opinion, endoscopic electrofulguration is perhaps the better initial therapy as the ureter is occluded proximally rather than distally, thereby avoiding a stagnant standing column of urine and the potential development of a urinary tract infection.

Endourologic Management of Complications of Renal Transplantation

Patients undergoing renal transplantations are at risk for developing a variety of urinary tract problems: urolithiasis, ureteral strictures (3 per cent), ureteral fistulas, and funguria with associated fungal concretions (Oosterhof et al., 1989). Each of these problems can be approached endourologically. Urolithiasis in the transplant patient can be managed by standard percutaneous techniques as discussed in Chapter 60. For ureteral strictures, antegrade catheter or balloon dilation from 4 mm to 10 mm using the *aforementioned* techniques and placement of a 6 to 12 Fr. internal stent for 6 to 8 weeks can be helpful in treating ureteral strictures, especially if they are in the distal ureter. Success rates for this approach range from 50 to 79 per cent (Oosterhof et al., 1989; Streem et al., 1986; Voegeli et al., 1988).

The placement of a percutaneous nephroureterostomy tube can be beneficial in resolving a postoperative ureteral fistula. Streem and colleagues (1986) noted a satisfactory response in two of three patients managed in this way. In markedly immunocompromised patients, the percutaneous approach has been helpful in managing fungal complications. Fungal growths within the collecting system can be extracted and topical antifungal agents (e.g., amphotericin B) can be administered via the nephrostomy tube (see previous discussion dealing with fungal bezoars) (Wise et al., 1982).

Relief of Noncalculous Renal Obstruction: Indwelling Ureteral Stents

Patients with noncalculous renal obstructions who require internal diversion with a ureteral stent generally fall into two categories: nonoperable benign stricture disease due to patient debility or previously failed attempts at repair and malignant obstruction (most commonly due to gynecologic cancer or prostate cancer. Temporary relief can be achieved with an indwelling ureteral stent. The stent can be changed on an outpatient basis every 3 to 4 months for an indefinite period of time.

The preferred stent is one made of silicone or of a C-flex construction (Marx et al., 1988). Inflammation and epithelial ulceration in a canine model are minimal with these types of stents. Likewise, the fractures seen with the older polyurethane stents are less likely with silicone stents (Marx et al., 1988). The pigtail or figure 4–tip configuration appears to provide the best retention (Fig. 62–53) (McDougall et al., 1990). Usually, a 6 Fr. or 7 Fr. size is suitable. To date, no studies have been done

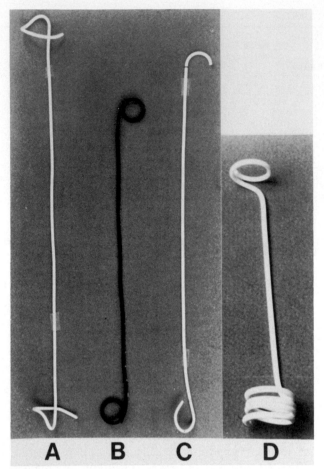

Figure 62–53. A variety of configurations of the end of the indwelling stent including (A) figure 4; (B) pigtail; (C) "J"; and (D) coil configuration.

regarding the drainage characteristics of the myriad stents available. The urologist must choose among stents with no side holes in the body of the stent, stents with side holes all along the stent, and stents with a series of grooves cut along the outer surface.

TECHNIQUE. The length of the stent needed can be most accurately determined by measuring the length of the ureter during fluoroscopy. This measurement can be done by passing a floppy tip guide wire to the level of the renal pelvis and then kinking the guide wire at the urethral meatus. The guide wire is withdrawn, until the tip reaches the level of the symphysis pubis (fluoroscopic monitoring) or the ureteral orifice (combined fluoroscopic and endoscopic monitoring). The guide wire is kinked again at the level of the urethral meatus and then withdrawn. The distance between the two kinks in the guide wire is the actual length of the ureter (Elyanderani, 1986). All stents are measured and labeled by the *length of the straight portion of the stent*. A stent that is 1 to 2 cm longer than the measured ureter is placed to allow for the stent to reach the bladder without difficulty (Elyanderani, 1986).

Alternatively, the length of the ureter on a radiograph from an intravenous urogram series can be measured. In this case, 10 per cent should be subtracted from the

ureteral length in order to allow for magnification artifacts from the radiograph.

Another method to estimate the necessary stent length for a given patient is based on the patient's height; however, this is routinely an overestimate of the length of the stent needed. For patients 5 feet 2 inches and taller: subtract 2 from their height in inches and place a stent that is 20 cm plus the results of the subtraction. If the stent suggested is an odd length, the stent size is rounded off to the next higher even number. For example, for patients: ≤5 feet 2 inches = 20 cm stent; 5 feet 2 inches to ≤5 feet 4 inches = 22 cm stent; >5 feet 4 inches to ≤5 feet 6 inches = 24 cm stent; >5 feet 6 inches to ≤5 feet 8 inches = 26 cm stent; >5 feet 8 inches to ≤6 feet = 28 cm stent; and >6 feet = 30 cm stent.

Placement can be most simply accomplished by passing a *closed-ended* stent with its prepackaged guide wire through the cystoscope. This is guided up to the renal pelvis under combined endoscopic and fluoroscopic control. Alternatively, with an *open-ended* stent, a guide wire is first passed to the renal pelvis via the cystoscope and the stent is advanced over the guide wire and through the cystoscope. A pusher moves the stent over the guide wire until the stent enters the renal pelvis. If this maneuver is done under cystoscopic guidance, the end of the stent can be clearly seen during its passage. Withdrawal of the guide wire permits either end of the stent to assume its retentive configuration (i.e., J, pigtail, or figure 4).

In certain patients, especially in those with malignant obstructions, the stent may buckle as it crosses the iliac vessels or the stent may not pass through the area of obstruction. In this situation, the following technique is helpful (Fig. 62–54) (McDougall et al., 1990). Under cystoscopic and fluoroscopic control a guide wire is passed to the renal pelvis. If the floppy tip Bentson guide wire will not pass, a lubricatory glide wire (Terumo) may be used (Suzuki et al., 1989). This plastic wire, when wet, is extremely slick. Also, because of its plastic construction, it will not kink. Once the Terumo guide wire is passed, a 5 Fr. angiographic catheter *preflushed with saline* should be passed so that this guide wire can be exchanged for a stiffer guide wire, such as a 0.035-inch Bentson heavy duty or 0.035-inch Amplatz super stiff guide wire. Next, the cystoscope is removed and over the guide wire an 8 Fr. dilator and a 10 Fr. sheath are passed (Amplatz 8 Fr./10 Fr. set). The 8 Fr. dilator is withdrawn. The stent is advanced over the guide wire and through the sheath. A metal-tipped pusher further advances the stent through the 10 Fr. sheath. The wire is withdrawn so that a coil of the stent forms in the renal pelvis. Next, the metal-tipped pusher is positioned at the superior border of the symphysis pubis in males and at the inferior border of the symphysis pubis in females (lower if a cystocele is present). The 10 Fr. sheath is withdrawn under constant fluoroscopic monitoring. The metal tip of the pusher is never advanced beyond the symphysis or else the end of the stent may be pushed into the ureteral tunnel necessitating ureteroscopic retrieval. The guide wire is retracted until the curl in the lower end of the stent begins to

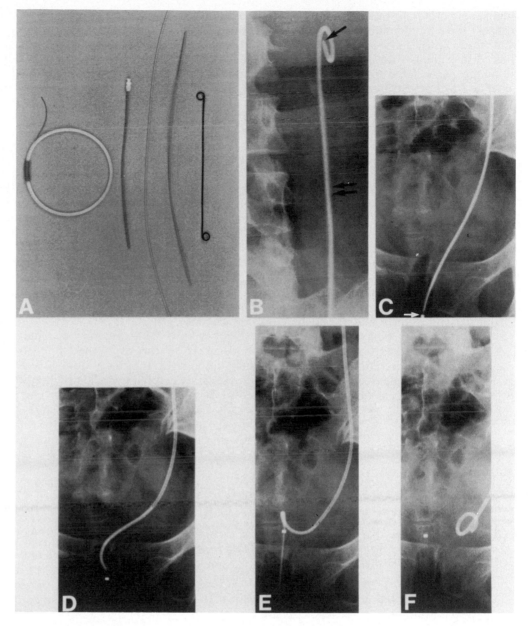

Figure 62–54. Ureteral stent placement under fluoroscopic guidance.

A, Set up: 0.035-inch floppy tip, 145-cm guide wire; 10 Fr. Amplatz sheath; 8 Fr. Amplatz catheter; metal tip pusher; and stent.

B, After placement of the 10 Fr. Amplatz sheath *(double arrow),* the stent has been advanced over the guide wire and the distal end of the guide wire has been withdrawn 5 cm to allow the coil in the stent to form *(single arrow).*

C, The metal tip pusher *(arrow),* in the female patient, is positioned at the inferior margin of the symphysis pubis. (In the male, the pusher is positioned at the upper border of the symphysis pubis.) The 10 Fr. Amplatz sheath has been removed under fluoroscopic control to prevent inadvertently moving the pusher too far up the ureter.

D and *E,* As the guide wire is withdrawn, the lower coil of the stent deforms the floppy tip of the guide wire. At this point, the pusher can be safely advanced because the floppy tip end of the guide wire is so malleable that the advancement of the pusher will no longer move the stent up the ureter.

F, The guide wire has been withdrawn. The lower pigtail of the stent has formed in the bladder. The tip of the metal tip pusher is still visible in the bladder. The pusher can now be removed.

form. This means that the floppy portion of the guide wire is now in the lower pigtail. The metal-tipped pusher can now be advanced slightly into the bladder, as the stent will now buckle into the bladder rather than advance up the ureter, because the floppy portion of the guide wire is all that is left in the pusher and the distal end of the stent. The guide wire is now completely withdrawn, thereby allowing the curl in the end of the stent to form in the bladder (see Fig. 62–54).

At times, in patients with cancer or dense periureteral scar tissue, during attempted passage of the 8 Fr. dilator and 10 Fr. sheath, either or both may actually buckle into the bladder. To overcome this, the Luer fitting on the back end of the 10 Fr. sheath can be cut off. A rigid 17 Fr. or 20 Fr. panendoscope sheath (without the rod lens) can be passed over the 8 Fr. dilator and 10 Fr. sheath, to the level of the ureteral orifice. The metal panendoscope sheath will now prevent the 8 Fr. dilator

and 10 Fr. sheath from buckling into the bladder. The 8 Fr. dilator is advanced beyond the area of narrowing, followed by passage of the 10 Fr. sheath. The 8 Fr. dilator is withdrawn, and the stent is passed as previously described.

Stent drainage in the patient with obstruction from *benign* disease is usually excellent. The stent needs to be exchanged every 3 to 4 months. Stent patency can be affirmed with *voiding* cystography; however, the absence of reflux is not necessarily an indication of stent obstruction (false-negative rate of 50 per cent) (Weinstein and Saltzman, 1990).

In contrast, among patients with hydronephrosis due to *malignant* obstruction, the first decision must be whether to relieve the obstruction at all. This is a judgment that should be reached by the patient in consultation with the physician. The placement of indwelling stents in this case is difficult. Also stents with malignant ureteral obstructions (i.e., retroperitoneal cancer) have a tendency to obstruct much sooner. Docimo and Dewolf (1989) noted that 43 per cent of stents placed in patients with malignant obstructions failed to drain properly. This problem is more apparent with smaller (6 Fr.) than larger (7 Fr.) stents (68 per cent versus 33 per cent).

In the patient with a malignant ureteral obstruction, if the stent repeatedly blocks, it is necessary to place a percutaneous nephrostomy. If both kidneys are obstructed by a malignancy, the better functioning of the two kidneys should be percutaneously drained. Placement of bilateral nephrostomy tubes should be reserved only for the patient who must undergo potentially nephrotoxic chemotherapy.

From the patient's standpoint, all stents result in significant morbidity: irritative voiding symptoms, hematuria (without passage of blood clots), and occasional flank pain during micturition. Indeed, even with the newer silicone stents, flank discomfort may occur in upward of 50 per cent and lower tract symptoms of frequency and dysuria may occur in 25 to 60 per cent (Bregg and Riehle, 1988; McDougall et al., 1990; Pollard and Mac Farland, 1988). Attempts to decrease these symptoms with anticholinergics are usually unsuccessful. In the extreme case, the short-term (i.e., several days) administration of belladonna and opiate suppositories is effective.

Upper Tract Transitional Cell Carcinoma

"For many decades, it has been demonstrated that the local excision of a bladder tumor of low-grade and low-stage is a very adequate way to eliminate the problem without endangering the patient. We can also say that local excision of a tumor of the upper urinary tract that is known to be of low-grade is the optimal treatment for it."

R. F. GITTES, 1980

No area of endosurgery is more controversial than the application of newer endoscopic techniques to transitional cell carcinoma affecting the ureter (TCCU) or renal pelvis (TCCP). The rationale behind this therapy is based on the conservative approach to low-grade, low-stage bladder cancer. Certainly for superficial transitional cell carcinoma of the bladder (TCCB), a transurethral approach is acceptable; whereas, cystectomy and urinary diversion are reserved only for those individuals with high-grade or muscle-invasive disease (Catalona, 1987). When bladder tumors that initially developed as superficial or low-stage disease recur, they do so as low-grade and superficial tumors in upward of 85 to 90 per cent of patients (Kaye and Lange, 1982). The question then arises: why can't a similar minimally invasive therapeutic approach be applied to transitional cell carcinoma affecting the upper urinary tract?

Objections to an endoscopic approach to upper tract cancer center on five issues: (1) importance of renal preservation, (2) accuracy of diagnosis (i.e., grade/stage), (3) tumor implantation, (4) subsequent surveillance, and (5) incidence of recurrent disease. In the patient with two kidneys, why spare the tumor-bearing renal unit? Transitional cell cancer occurs bilaterally and metachronously in the renal pelvis in only 1 to 2 per cent of patients (Clayman et al., 1983b). The removal of a kidney in the adult patient population is well tolerated. Although proteinuria may slowly develop, no associated increase occurs in the frequency of renal failure or hypertension among individuals with an iatrogenic solitary kidney. This observation is well documented in patients who survive radical nephrectomy for renal cell cancer and in those who are renal donors (Fotino, 1989; Wishnow et al., 1990). Renal preservation appears to be a laudable goal; however, the reality of the situation is not supportive of this goal.

The *accuracy of the diagnosis* of a superficial, noninvasive lesion is of paramount importance. In this regard, it is of note, that whereas 85 per cent of bladder cancers appear as low-grade superficial disease, only 40 per cent of renal pelvic and 50 to 60 per cent of ureteral tumors initially appear as low-grade, noninvasive disease (Batata et al., 1975; Johansson and Wahlquist, 1979; Wagle et al., 1974).

The accuracy of a diagnosis of superficial/noninvasive disease in the upper tract is wanting. Neither urine cytology nor flow cytometry are reliable. Although helpful in revealing high-grade tumors, negative urine cytology findings may occur in 60 per cent of patients with low-grade disease and in 10 per cent of patients with high-grade lesions (Sarnacki et al., 1971). Flow cytometry, which measures cellular DNA and RNA content, is also not infallible. A false-negative histogram commonly occurs with predominantly diploid tumors. This problem is noted in 66 per cent of superficial "papillomas" and in 8 per cent of invasive lesions (Denovic et al., 1982; Melamed, 1984).

Furthermore, transitional cell cancer affecting the renal pelvis, unlike ureteral TCC, is often not a solitary lesion. Overall, 30 per cent of these tumors may be multicentric at the time of presentation (Huffman, 1988; Mazeman, 1976). Likewise, in a patient with a low-grade (1, 2), low-stage (O, A) renal pelvic tumor, the tumor may be associated with urothelial dysplasia in the renal pelvis in 90 per cent and with actual carcinoma in situ in 3 to 9 per cent (Nocks et al., 1982). Likewise, a low-grade/low-stage ureteral tumor may be associated with urothelial dysplasia and carcinoma in situ in other areas of the ureter in 50 per cent and 9 to 13 per cent, respectively (Heney et al., 1981). These pathologic changes may be missed during an endoscopic approach. In those series in which an endoscopic diagnosis was followed by surgical extirpation, the error in undergrading/understaging renal pelvic tumors was 60 per cent. In the ureter, tumor grade and stage were correctly diagnosed ureteroscopically (Huffman et al., 1985a; Huffman, 1990). Because of the extremely thin muscle layer of the ureteral and pelvic walls, it is oftentimes impractical to endosurgically stage the tumor for fear of perforating the renal pelvis or ureter.

Another significant concern is the possibility of *tumor implantation* after endosurgical procedures. Implantation may take two forms: (1) confined within the upper tract collecting system and (2) retroperitoneal. Any urothelial abrasion may provide a fertile site for tumor implantation. This finding has been demonstrated in an animal model by Soloway and Masters (1980). In their study, cauterization of part of the mouse bladder increased implantation of transitional cell tumors by fourfold. The same problem may apply during ureteroscopy or nephroscopy of an upper tract tumor. With ureteroscopy, the dilation of the distal ureter and passage of the rigid or flexible ureteroscope may result in multiple abrasions along the ureter. Similar problems may occur with antegrade nephroscopy. However, reports of this problem are as yet unpublished. Superficial studding of the ureter with transitional cell tumors has been noted in one individual at 9 months following a percutaneous procedure for a low-grade renal pelvic tumor (Meretyk et al., 1991d). Prior to the procedure, the patient underwent diagnostic ureteroscopy. Whether this effect is coincidence (i.e., the natural history of the tumor) or consequence is difficult to discern.

Retroperitoneal perforation and subsequent tumor implantation may occur with either a ureteroscopic or percutaneous approach. From a ureteroscopic standpoint, this effect may be more likely when the tumor is treated by resection with an electrocautery loop than by a Nd:YAG laser. Concerns over retroperitoneal implantation become even greater if a percutaneous approach is selected to treat the tumor. Surgical pyelotomy to resect a transitional cell tumor has been shown to result in retroperitoneal seeding and recurrent extrarenal disease in upward of 11 per cent of patients (retroperitoneal recurrence noted at 6 months and 3 years) (Tomera et al., 1982).

Despite the small size of the nephrostomy tract, it is not unreasonable to believe that a similar problem of retroperitoneal or nephrostomy tract implantation may eventuate after a percutaneous approach. The chances of this problem occurring would obviously be increased if during the procedure there was an anterior false passage of the renal pelvis. Indeed, Orihuela and Smith (1988) have noted one case of a retroperitoneal recurrence of transitional cell cancer following a percutaneous approach. However, Guz and co-workers (1990), in a series of 14 patients who were undergoing percutaneous nephrostomy to drain a malignant obstruction (13 cases) or resect an upper tract transitional cell cancer (one case), grossly noted no seeding of the nephrostomy tract at 1 to 121 months' follow-up (average 27.8 months). Likewise, other investigators have independently noted among their patients who were undergoing percutaneous endosurgery for upper tract TCC, no patient experienced a retroperitoneal or nephrostomy tract recurrence (Blute et al., 1989; Huffman, 1990; Nurse et al., 1989). However, most patients in these series have been followed for a relatively brief period of time, usually less than 2 years. A 5-year follow-up period will be necessary to fully evaluate whether concerns over tract seeding or retroperitoneal recurrence can be laid to rest. In this regard, it is important for these patients to undergo periodic surveillance CT of the retroperitoneum.

The next issue among patients treated with an endoscopic approach is surveillance. Simply stated, if one is to treat upper tract cancer similar to the way bladder cancer is treated, the surveillance for both types of TCC should be similar. Upward of 85 per cent of recurrences after resection of an initial bladder tumor occur within the 1st year of follow-up (Loening et al., 1980; Varkarakis et al., 1974). As such, a routine in which cystoscopy is performed every 3 months for at least the first 1 to 2 years, and then every 6 months for 1 to 2 years, and then annually thereafter appears to be reasonable (Droller, 1986; Varkarakis et al., 1974). This regimen is reinstituted if a recurrent tumor occurs during the follow-up period. In further support of surveillance ureteroscopy are data on the inadequacy of upper tract radiographic studies for detecting small transitional cell recurrences (Huffman et al., 1985a). In his experience, recurrent tumors have been detected endoscopically that were not deleted radiographically. Intravenous urography or retrograde ureterography alone is no more an acceptable replacement for surveillance ureteroscopy than cystography is an acceptable replacement for follow-up cystoscopy among patients with TCC of the bladder.

However, if surveillance ureteronephroscopy is the price of endoscopic therapy, the price may be too high. For the 50-year-old patient with an average life expectancy, surveillance ureteroscopy, under the best of circumstances (i.e., assuming no recurrences), might result in over 30 separate outpatient or short hospital stay ureteroscopic procedures, complete with ureteral dilation and the need to place an indwelling ureteral stent for 2 to 3 days. The longest reported follow-up of a patient undergoing endoscopic resection of upper tract TCC is 6.5 years. During that time period, there were 14 general anesthetics given for 14 surveillance ureteroscopies and fulguration of six low-grade upper tract TCC recurrences (Huffman et al., 1985b). As such, the overall expense and convalescence (i.e., total time off from work and overall discomfort) of an endourologic approach might well exceed that of nephroureterectomy. Furthermore, after a percutaneous approach for TCCP it might be prudent to include an annual CT study of the retroperitoneum to rule out a retroperitoneal recurrence. Only in this manner can retroperitoneal disease secondary to tumor cell extravasation at the time of the procedure be detected early. However, this would again add to the overall cost of this "less invasive" approach and increase the time lost from gainful employment.

Based on the earlier series of simple nephrectomy for TCCP, it is reasonable to anticipate rapid and likely multiple *recurrences* among patients undergoing endoscopic therapy. Indeed, recurrent transitional cell tumors develop in a retained ureteral stump in 30 per cent of patients (48 per cent after simple nephrectomy and 24 per cent after nephrectomy, with subtotal ureterectomy) (Mazeman, 1976; Strong et al., 1976). These recurrent tumors are of a higher grade in approximately 25 per cent of patients (Mazeman, 1976; Strong et al., 1976). Obviously, the more urothelium that remains intact, the higher the incidence of recurrence. In a series of endoscopic therapy, 46 per cent of 11 patients developed a recurrent tumor in the renal pelvis and/or ureter within 9 months of the procedure (Orihuela and Smith, 1988). In another series, 38 per cent of patients experienced an upper tract recurrence within a 21-month follow-up period (Huffman et al., 1985a).

For all of these reasons, the urologist interested in endoscopic therapy for upper tract TCC is cautioned. Much additional data and longer term follow-up data are needed before such therapy can be recommended. For the time being, endosurgery for upper tract TCC should be limited to individuals with a *solitary* kidney and a low-grade, apparently low-stage disease confined to a single, small (i.e., < 1 cm) focus or to those too ill to undergo standard surgical therapy. For the majority of patients with TCC of the upper urinary tract, distal ureterectomy or nephroureterectomy, dependent upon the location of the tumor, remains the treatment of choice.

Technique for Endourologic Therapy of Upper Tract Transitional Cell Cancer

The choice of an endosurgical approach to an upper tract TCC is dependent on the location and size of the tumor. Presumably, the tumor should be a solitary, low-grade lesion. High-grade or multiple lesions are better handled by an ablative surgical approach, even if this results in an anephric state. If the lesion is < 1 cm in the ureter or kidney, a *retrograde ureteroscopic* (rigid in the ureter or flexible in the kidney) is reasonable. However, for a large tumor in the renal pelvis or ureteropelvic junction, an *antegrade percutaneous* approach is recommended. Both approaches have unique advantages and disadvantages. The ureteroscope provides for a completely "closed" approach. The collecting system, unless inadvertently perforated during the procedure, remains intact. However, the ureteroscopic instrumentation is diminutive. Although Nd:YAG fulguration of a small lesion is straightforward, fulguration of a larger tumor can be difficult.

Furthermore, there are concerns, albeit largely unrealized, regarding implantation of tumor cells with seeding of the distal ureter due to the "beaking" effect resulting from passage of the endoscope and the process of ureteral dilation prior to ureteroscopy. In contrast, a percutaneous approach necessitates perforation of the collecting system with the attendant concerns over "seeding" of the retroperitoneum with tumor cells. However, the instrumentation used in the percutaneous approach is the standard resectoscope and biopsy equipment used in the bladder, thereby greatly facilitating biopsy and lesion removal. This factor helps to more accurately grade and stage the tumor.

For the ureteroscopic approach to upper-tract, low-grade TCC, the type of endoscope and, hence, the method of resection are, to a large degree, dependent on the location of the tumor. As previously stated, these tumors should be < 1 cm. For tumors in the distal ureter in males (i.e., below the iliac vessel crossing) or anywhere along the ureter, medial wall of the pelvis, or upper calyx in females, the rigid ureteroscope can be used. However, if the tumor is anywhere above the iliac vessels in the male or in the lower or middle calyces in the female, a flexible ureteroscope is needed.

An initial (i.e., safety) guide wire is passed retrograde until it *just* reaches the renal pelvis. Excessive coiling of the wire in the renal pelvis is to be avoided because this can result in undesirable urothelial abrasions. Using an 8 Fr./10 Fr. Amplatz introducer system, a second 0.035-inch, floppy tip (i.e., working) guide wire is placed. If electrocautery is applied, the safety guide wire is covered with a 5 Fr. angiographic catheter, when the laser is to be used, the guide wire is left uncovered. The distal ureter is dilated over the working guide wire, with a ureteral dilating balloon that is only 2 to 3 Fr. larger than the ureteroscope. The goal is to cause as little trauma to the normal ureter as possible. The irrigant pressure is maintained at ≤ 40 cm H_2O to prevent renal backflow and hypothesized vascular entry of tumor cells.

If a *rigid* endoscope is chosen, the tumor can be resected with a small electrocautery loop until it is flush with the muscular layer. The base of the tumor can be biopsied for staging purposes and fulgurated with the Nd:YAG laser. Alternatively, if the tumor is small enough, a biopsy specimen can be taken and through the rigid ureteroscope, a 400-μ Nd:YAG laser probe can fulgurate the tumor, at 25 to 30 watts.

If a *flexible* ureteroscope is being utilized, a cold cup biopsy of the tumor is taken for diagnostic purposes. The tumor cannot be resected because there are no resection loops for the flexible endoscope. Hence, either an electrocautery probe or a Nd:YAG laser is utilized to fulgurate the tumor. The laser is preferred; however, if with the 400-μ laser probe the tip of the flexible endoscope cannot be deflected sufficiently to treat the tumor, a 2 Fr. or 3 Fr. Greenwald electrode may be needed. The electrocautery probes are more malleable than the laser probes.

At the end of the ureteroscopic procedure, cold cup biopsy samples can be taken of the tumor base (if not too thin) and of the peritumor area. Next, a withdrawal retrograde ureterogram is obtained to rule out extravasation. An indwelling ureteral stent is placed along with a urethral catheter. The urethral catheter is removed the next morning; the ureteral catheter is usually removed 3 to 5 days later, on an outpatient basis.

The *antegrade percutaneous* method for resecting a low-grade, presumably low-stage tumor of the renal pelvis or proximal ureter must be carefully planned. Initially, a 7 Fr. retrograde ureteral occlusion balloon (11.5 mm) catheter is passed to the renal pelvis. The balloon is inflated in the renal pelvis and gently pulled caudal to occlude the ureteropelvic junction. Air or contrast material can be instilled via the retrograde catheter to opacify the collecting system. The nephrostomy tract is made such that it is in a direct line with the tumor, yet enters the collecting system as remote from the tumor as possible. The nephrostomy tract is established under C-arm fluoroscopic control in an effort to avoid an anterior false passage and extravasation. The nephrostomy tract is dilated with a 10-mm nephrostomy tract balloon dilator, and an Amplatz working sheath is placed. This maneuver should result in the least amount of trauma to normal urothelium and should protect the tract from subsequent extravasation during the procedure.

The resection of the tumor may be done in several

ways. A standard resectoscope can be used and the tumor resected and evacuated piece by piece. The base of the tumor can be separately biopsied and fulgurated. Alternatively, a no touch technique can be employed with the Nd:YAG laser set at 25 to 30 watts. The entire tumor is treated with the laser, and the tumor fronds are removed with cold cup biopsy forceps and sent for histologic analysis. The base of the tumor is biopsied and treated with the Nd:YAG laser. Following resection of the tumor, random biopsy samples of the surrounding urothelium in four separate peritumor quadrants and biopsy samples of any other suspicious areas of urothelium are recommended. An indwelling nephrostomy tube is placed. This is usually removed 2 to 5 days later, provided a nephrostogram reveals no evidence of extravasation. The retrograde ureteral occlusion balloon catheter is removed at the end of the procedure (Fig. 62–55).

Based on independent reports by Gittes and Meretyk and their co-workers, thiotepa can be instilled into the retrograde ureteral catheter just prior to creation of the nephrostomy tract in the patient who is undergoing endourologic therapy for upper tract TCC. At the end of the procedure and for 2 to 3 days during the early postoperative period, thiotepa has been instilled via the indwelling nephrostomy tube. Unfortunately, tumor re-currence was not prevented; however, retroperitoneal implantation has not been noted albeit during brief follow-up (Gittes, 1980; Meretyk et al., 1991d). Orihuela and Smith (1988) have reported using bacille Calmette-Guérin (BCG) instillations via the nephrostomy tract after the nephrostogram has shown no evidence for extravasation.

RESULTS. The results of endosurgical management of upper tract TCC are remarkably similar to open conservative therapy for upper tract transitional cell disease (Table 62–12) (Blute et al., 1989; Huffman et al., 1985a, 1990; Nurse et al., 1989; Orihuela and Smith, 1988). Overall, ureteral tumors appear to respond somewhat better than pelvic tumors to endosurgical management. Ureteral tumors are usually treated ureteroscopically. The recurrence rate in TCCU cases at approximately 2 years (15 per cent) and the progression to open ablative surgery (13 per cent) are both low. In contrast, the renal pelvic tumor is more commonly approached percutaneously, especially if it is larger than 1 cm. In the TCCP patients the incidence of multicentricity, the associated urothelial dysplasia, and the more vast and at times poorly accessible urothelium of the renal pelvis "conspire" against definitive endosurgic treatment. Recurrence and open surgery rates at 2 years in TCCP patients (30 per cent) are twice those in patients

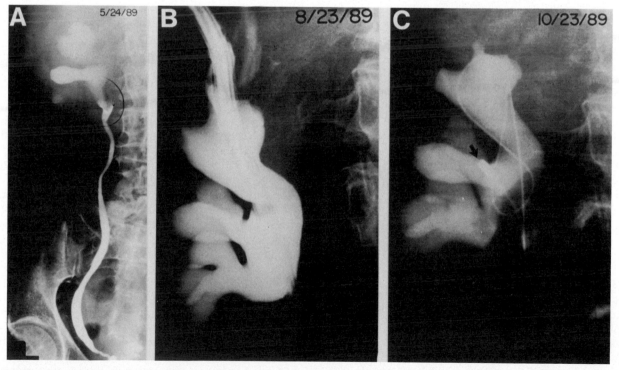

Figure 62–55. *A,* Retrograde ureterogram reveals a filling defect at the ureteropelvic junction *(circle).* A ureteroscopic biopsy sample showed that the tumor was a grade 2 papillary transitional cell carcinoma.

B, A percutaneous approach was used to resect the tumor. Note that access has been achieved via an upper pole calyx, distant from the lesion itself. The nephrostogram reveals no anterior extravasation, and the lesion is now absent. The external antegrade ureteral stent was exchanged for an indwelling stent, following which the nephrostomy tube was removed.

C, Two months later, a retrograde ureterogram showed no recurrent lesions. However, surveillance ureteroscopy performed at the same time revealed a radiographically undetectable 2- to 3-mm papillary tumor *(arrow),* treated with the Nd:YAG laser. In this case, a follow-up intravenous urogram, 1 year later, revealed a recurrent tumor in the renal pelvis. Before any further therapy could be rendered, the patient died from a cardiac event. The autopsy report on the right kidney revealed *recurrent superficial grade 3 transitional cell cancer at the ureteropelvic junction.* In addition, new tumors were noted in the calyceal system, mid-ureter, and bladder (dome and left kidney wall). No evidence of metastatic disease was noted.

Table 62–12. ENDOSURGICAL THERAPY/OPEN CONSERVATIVE SURGERY FOR
UPPER TRACT TRANSITIONAL CELL CARCINOMA

Authors	Patients	Approach	Adjunctive Local Therapy	Local Recurrence (%)	Open Surgical Ablation (%)	Metastases (%)	Follow-up (mos.)
Endosurgical Therapy							
Orihuela and Smith, 1988	4 (pelvis)	Percutaneous	No	75	25	0	19
	7 (pelvis)	Percutaneous	Yes (BCG (6); mitomycin C(1))	29	29	14*	22
Nurse, Woodhouse et al., 1989	15	Percutaneous	Iridium wire (4000-4500 cGy) (14); mitomycin C(1)	39	33	0	24
Blute, Segura et al., 1989	8 (pelvis)	Percutaneous (3)	—	0	0	0	18
	13 (ureter)	Ureteroscopy (5)	—	20	0	0	28
		Ureteroscopy (13)	—	15	0	0	21
Huffman, 1990	5	Percutaneous and ureteroscopy	—	40	40	0	>12
Huffman, Bagley, et al., 1985a	8	Ureteroscopy	Mitomycin C(1)	38	13	0	21
Surgical Therapy							
Wallace, 1981	7 (pelvis)	Local excision	—	35	NA	29	9.6 yrs.
	7 (ureter)	Segmental ureterectomy	—	14	NA	0	5.9 yrs.
Mazeman, 1976	23 (pelvis)	Local excision	—	35	NA	—	>12
	50 (ureter)	Segmental/distal ureterectomy	—	6	NA	—	>12

*Retroperitoneal recurrence. (NA, not applicable.)

with ureteral tumor (15 per cent) (see Table 62–12). Interestingly, reports of distant metastatic disease or seeding of the nephrostomy tract are nil. To date, there has been only one reported retroperitoneal recurrence (Orihuela and Smith, 1988). However, the follow-up periods in both TCCU and TCCB are still relatively brief (1 1/2 to 2 1/2 years).

With regard to topical chemotherapy, it would appear that BCG administration in the upper urinary tract is relatively safe and effective. In Orihuela and Smith's series of 14 patients (1988), seven patients received BCG (two to eight doses). At 22 months' follow-up (range, 8 to 29 months), two of their patients (29 per cent) who received BCG had topical recurrences. Both of these individuals underwent successful nephroureterectomy, and there were no deaths in this group. In the non-BCG group (four patients) the results were less favorable: the recurrence rate was 75 per cent within the first 9 months of follow-up. Two of these patients died within 19 months of the initial percutaneous procedure.

Additional favorable reports with topical BCG in patients with upper tract TCC have been supplied independently in single case reports (pyeloileostomy, pyelovesicostomy) (Herr, 1985; Ramsey and Soloway, 1990). Both patients were given five or six weekly doses of BCG and followed beyond 1 year. The lesions in both of these cases responded to BCG despite the fact that they were both of a high-grade nature (carcinoma in situ and grade 3). At present, the necessary length of contact time of the BCG with the upper tract urothelium is unknown. Presumably, the contact time is quite limited because there are no reports of taking measures to cause retention of BCG in the upper tract collecting system. Recommendations for retention of the BCG range from as brief as 10 minutes to as long as 2 hours (Herr, 1985; Ramsey and Soloway, 1990).

At present, it would appear that the ideal candidate for endoscopic therapy of upper tract TCC would be a patient with a low-grade, solitary, papillary *ureteral* tumor (< 1 cm) or a low-grade solitary *renal pelvic* or calyceal solitary lesion (< 1 cm) in a solitary kidney or a patient with pre-existing renal compromise in whom cytology findings are negative and with no prior or present TCC of the bladder. Furthermore, the endosurgical therapy of pelvic tumors appears to be improved if the patient is given a course of postoperative topical BCG to the affected upper tract.

The extension of endosurgical therapy for TCC of the ureter and especially of the renal pelvis/calyces to patients with two kidneys without pre-existing renal compromise remains controversial. Initial experience in the ureter with this approach appears to be favorable. Indeed, for low-grade ureteral tumors, the recurrence rate is low and the progression to open surgical ablation is in the 13 per cent range. Also, the endoscopic staging of ureteral tumors appears to be accurate. However, these sanguine results do not extend to renal pelvic tumors. Indeed, the recurrence rate and the need for open surgical ablation for TCCP is twice that for TCCU. Also, the endoscopic understaging with TCCP is high: 60 per cent. Follow-up periods in both TCCU and TCCP patient groups are still quite brief. Until more lengthy follow-up data are available, the *standard surgical treatment* for upper tract TCC continues to be the accepted first line approach to the majority of cases of TCC of the renal pelvis or ureter. Currently, this therapy is more effective and in the long term less expensive and less time consuming than the endosurgical alternatives of minimally invasive therapy and ongoing surveillance.

EVALUATING THE NEW TECHNOLOGY

Each of the aforementioned techniques requires proof of efficacy before its surgical counterpart is superseded. Professional acceptance of any of the described procedures must be based on carefully performed, long-term studies from which the success, morbidity, and cost of each endosurgical procedure can be calculated. Such data are now available for endopyelotomy, percutaneous treatment of calyceal diverticula, evaluation of essential hematuria, and endoscopic determination of soft tissue lesions of the upper urinary tract. In each of these instances, the endosurgical approach offers equivalent efficacy and less morbidity than its surgical alternative. However, such is not the case for endoureterotomy, endoinfundibulotomy, or endoincision of ureteroenteric strictures. Although less morbid, each of these procedures is less efficacious than its standard surgical counterpart. The patient must be counseled accordingly.

The role of endourology in treating upper tract TCC is quite unsettled. In this situation, the data are extremely scant. Furthermore, the substitution of an endosurgical procedure for a standard surgical excision may prove fatal. All too often, there is only one chance to cure the patient with TCCP/TCCU. Until more data are available, an open surgical procedure is strongly recommended in all but the most unusual situations (i.e., low-grade tumor in the ureter or pelvis/calyces of a solitary kidney).

ON THE HORIZON

Urologic laparoscopy is on the horizon. All of urologic surgery can be divided into two broad categories: endosurgery or intraluminal (done from within a structure: cystoscopy, ureteroscopy, and nephroscopy) and exosurgery or extraluminal (performed on the outer surface of an organ or structure: nephrectomy, ureterectomy, prostatectomy, and lymph node dissection). This chapter concentrates only on advances in endosurgery. The next step is to use the laparoscope to also transform exosurgery into a minimally invasive technique. Just as percutaneous nephrostomy was described for almost 25 years before it was adapted to the treatment of urolithiasis, so diagnostic and operative laparoscopy have been available for over 80 and 50 years, respectively (Gunning, 1977; Semm, 1987). Indeed, laparoscopy was initially performed in 1901 with a Nitze cystoscope. However, urologists have only recently become involved with this technology (Gunning, 1977).

Technique

For simple diagnostic procedures, intravenous sedation is sufficient anesthesia. For longer therapeutic procedures, a general anesthetic is needed. All patients so treated receive preoperative antibiotics. In the operating room, the patient is placed in a supine position and the abdomen is prepared and draped. A nasogastric tube is needed only if a lengthy, therapeutic procedure is being performed. For diagnostic laparoscopy, a blood type and screen suffices; whereas, if an extensive procedure (i.e., pelvic lymph node dissection) is planned, a blood type and cross for two units should be done.

To perform laparoscopy, it is first necessary to obtain a pneumoperitoneum (Semm, 1987). A specially designed Veress needle is passed into the abdominal cavity via an infraumbilical midline approach. The abdomen is insufflated with carbon dioxide (4.5 to 6 L). The pressure within the abdomen is maintained between 10 and 15 mm Hg. Next, 5.5-mm and 11-mm or 12-mm airtight laparoscopic trocars and their associated sheaths are passed across the abdominal wall. Through one 11-mm sheath, a large endoscope is inserted and connected to a television camera so that the image can be clearly seen by all operating room personnel (Fig. 62-56). Through the other sheaths, a variety of grasping, cutting, laser, morcellation, and electrocautery instruments can be passed. The number and position of sheaths are dependent on the task. For diagnostic laparoscopy, a single sheath is often all that is needed. For therapeutic laparoscopy, two to five additional sheaths may be placed in order to dissect or resect a variety of tissues: cryptorchid testicle, ureter, and pelvic lymph nodes. At the end of the procedure, the sheaths are removed. The 11-mm skin sites are closed with a simple fascial suture and a skin Steri-Strip. The 5 mm incisions are closed using just a Steri-Strip. Most patients are able to return home on the day of surgery or the following morning.

LAPAROSCOPY

Reports of urologic laparoscopy first appeared in the literature in 1976 (Cortesi et al., 1976). At that time and until recently, the predominant application of the laparoscope in urology was to aid the pediatric urologist in the evaluation of patients with nonpalpable testes (Lowe et al., 1984; Manson et al., 1985). Via the diagnostic laparoscope (i.e., 0° telescope), the spermatic cord if present and internal inguinal ring can be identified. The diagnosis of anorchia can be confirmed by the presence of blind-ending spermatic vessels. When a testicle was found, this information was beneficial in planning the subsequent orchiopexy. In three series, a laparoscopic approach was successful in identifying the location of a cryptorchid testicle in 94 per cent of 66 boys (Das, 1988; Lowe et al., 1984; Manson et al., 1985). Children as young as 15 months have been successfully examined laparoscopically.

It wasn't until the general surgeon popularized the laparoscope for performing cholecystectomy that the urologist took notice of the potential operating capabil-

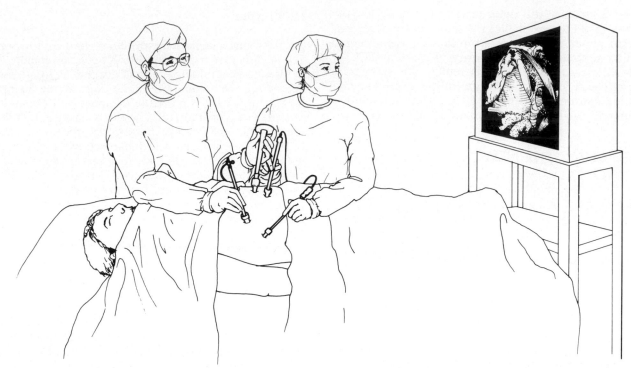

Figure 62–56. Laparoscopy procedure. The laparoscopic image (right renal artery and its segmental branches) is displayed on the television screen via a camera that couples directly to the laparoscope. Two individuals are present: the surgeon and the camera operator. There are four trocars in the CO_2-distended abdomen.

ities of this technology (Reddick, 1988). Early results were largely anecdotal. Specifically, in 1979, Wickham used the laparoscope to retroperitoneally approach and remove a ureteral calculus. Later, in 1985, Eshghi and colleagues utilized a laparoscope to successfully guide a transabdominal percutaneous approach to a pelvic kidney laden with a staghorn calculus. However, the first adult urologic procedure to be done in a large scale was pelvic lymph node dissection prior to extripative surgery or radiation therapy for prostate cancer. The pioneering efforts in this area were by Schuessler, Vancaillie, and Griffith in 1990 (Griffith et al., 1990; Schuessler et al., 1991). In their reports, 12 bilateral lymph node dissections were successfully accomplished without significant morbidity. An average of 7 nodes were removed on each side. The average operating time was 148 minutes; however, with experience, the surgical time can be decreased to 90 minutes. Patients were usually discharged after a 24-hour hospital stay.

Winfield and associates have adapted the laparoscope for performing other urologic procedures (Winfield, 1990; Winfield and Ryan, 1990). From a clinical standpoint, they have been successful in performing laparoscopic varicocelectomy. In their studies (personal communication), the spermatic vessels can be clearly delineated and the spermatic veins cleanly dissected and ligated (Liga clips). The spermatic veins are divided just as they join the vas immediately superior to the internal inguinal ring. The patient is usually discharged on the same day as the procedure.

Also, McCullough and associates (1990) reported the successful incision and drainage of a post-transplant lymphocele employing a laparoscopic approach. A window of overlying peritoneum was excised from the lymphocele, and a tag of omentum was dissected and transposed into the lymphocele cavity where it was fixed in place with Liga clips. The patient recovered rapidly and was discharged from the hospital the next morning. A follow-up CT scan, 7 weeks postoperatively, revealed no reaccumulation of the lymphocele.

Clayman and associates have reported on laparoscopic nephrectomy (Clayman et al., 1990a and 1991). In ten clinical cases, the entire intact kidney was removed (in one case, an overlying cap of perirenal fat and Gerota's fascia was included with the specimen) (Fig. 62–57). The kidney, once freed from its vascular and retroperitoneal attachments, was entrapped in a surgical sack that was passed into the abdomen and then drawn up to the undersurface of the abdominal wall via the drawstring on the sack. An electrical instrument for tissue morcellation was introduced into the sack, and the entire kidney was fragmented and aspirated within 10 minutes. The sack and morcellation instrument were designed such that contact of the probe with the wall of the nylon sack caused no damage to the integrity of the sack itself. Although the procedure times were excessive (4 to 7 hours), the patients were discharged from the hospital on the 6th and 7th postoperative days, respectively. They were back to their normal routine by postoperative day 10 and 14, respectively. One of the patients required only a single dose of analgesics throughout the postoperative period.

These few reports on laparoscopy are but the first steps in what may eventually become a standard part of

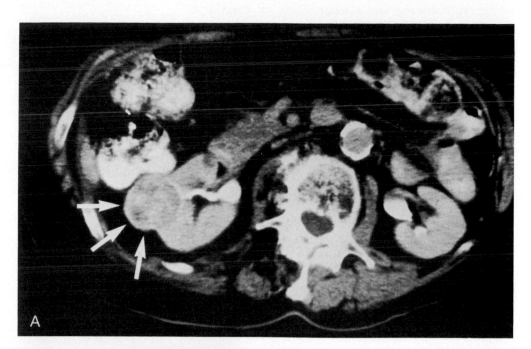

Figure 62–57. *A*, Computed tomography scan revealing a 3-cm right lower pole renal tumor.

B, Laparoscopic nephrectomy. In this laparoscopic view, the kidney (with a 3-cm renal tumor) has been entirely freed from its ureteral, retroperitoneal, and vascular attachments. Gerota's fascia and the perirenal fat overlying the tumor remain intact. A surgical sack was passed into the abdominal cavity, and the kidney was maneuvered into the sack. The neck of the sack was pulled up to the skin surface, thereby trapping the kidney on the underside of the anterior abdominal wall. A tissue morcellation instrument was then used to evacuate the tissue. The final pathology revealed a grade 1 granular cell cancer of the kidney.

C, Abdomen of patient 2 months following laparoscopic nephrectomy. There are two 5-mm port sites *(small arrows)* and three 11-mm port sites evident *(larger arrows)*. (From Clayman, R. V., Kavoussi, L. R., Soper, N. J., et al.: J. Urol., In Press.)

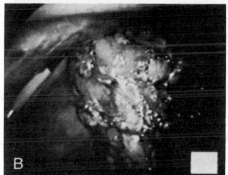

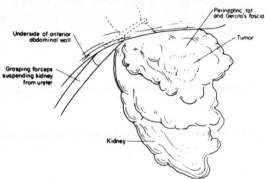

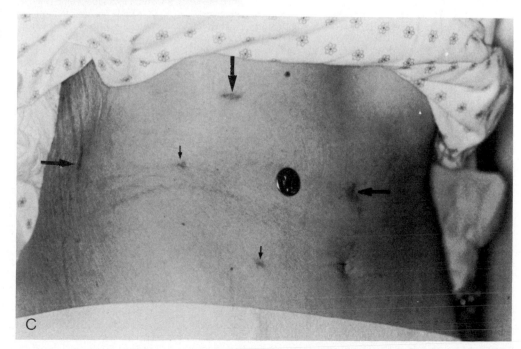

urologic surgery. The performance of currently open surgical procedures via a laparoscope or endoscope continues to be very appealing. To achieve the same beneficial effects as incisional surgery without incurring the discomfort and disfigurement of a major incision and to reduce the hospitalization and morbidity of a given procedure are attainable goals. The next decade will be an exciting time for urologists, as our specialty and our patients enjoy the benefits of numerous technologic advances both in endosurgery and exosurgery. To this end, our future beams brightly.

REFERENCES

Abeshouse, B. S., and Abeshouse, G. A.: Calyceal diverticulum: A report of sixteen cases and review of the literature. Urol. Int., 15:329, 1963.

Abramowitz, J., Fowler, J. E., Jr., Falhuni, K., et al.: Percutaneous identification and removal of fungus ball from renal pelvis. J. Urol., 135:1232, 1986.

Albala, D., Meretyk, S., Clayman, R. V., et al.: Percutaneous procedures for purulent perirenal/renal processes: Pleural precautions. J. Urol., 145:235A, 1991.

Altemeyer, W. A., and Alexander, J.: Retroperitoneal abscess. Arch. Surg., 83:512, 1961.

Andriole, G. L., McClennan, B. L., Picus, D., et al.: The effect of low osmolar contrast material on the interpretation of urinary cytology specimens. J. Urol., 139:177A, 1989.

Badlani, G., Eshghi, M., and Smith, A. D.: Percutaneous surgery for ureteropelvic junction obstruction (endopyelotomy): Technique and early results. J. Urol., 135:26, 1986.

Badlani, G., Karlin, G., and Smith, A. D.: Complications of endopyelotomy: Analysis in series of 64. J. Urol., 140:473, 1988.

Badlani, G. H., and Smith, A. D.: Stent for endopyelotomy. Urol. Clin. North Am., 15:445, 1988.

Bagley, D. H.: Active versus passive deflection in flexible ureteroscopy. J. Endourol., 1:15, 1987.

Bagley, D. H.: Endoscopic ureteroureterostomy. J. Urol., 143:235A, 1990.

Bagley, D. H., and Allen, J.: Flexible ureteropyeloscopy in the diagnosis of benign essential hematuria. J. Urol., 143:549, 1990.

Bagley, D. H., Huffman, J. L., and Lyon, E. S.: Flexible ureteropyeloscopy: Diagnosis and treatment in the upper urinary tract. J. Urol., 138:280, 1987.

Bagley, D. H., Huffman, J., Lyon, E., et al.: Endoscopic ureteropyelotomy. Opening the obliterated ureteropelvic junction with nephroscopy and flexible ureteropyeloscopy. J. Urol., 133:462, 1985.

Bagley, D. H., and Rivas, D.: Upper urinary tract filling defects: Flexible ureteroscopic diagnosis. J. Urol., 143:1196, 1990.

Bahnson, R. B.: Silver nitrate irrigation for hematuria from sickle cell hemoglobinopathy. J. Urol., 137:1194, 1987.

Banner, M. P., and Pollack, H. M.: Dilation of ureteral stenoses: Techniques and experience in 44 patients. Am. J. Roentgenol., 143:789, 1984.

Banner, M. P., Pollack, H. M., Amendola, M. A., et al.: [Letter to the editor.] Percutaneous extraction of renal fungus ball. Am. J. Radiol., 152:1342, 1988.

Bartone, F. F., Hurwitz, R. S., Rojas, E. L., et al.: The role of percutaneous nephrostomy in the management of obstructing candidiasis of the urinary tract in infants. J. Urol., 140:338, 1988.

Batata, M. A., Whitmore, W. F., Jr., Hilaris, B. S., Tokita, N., and Grabstald, H.: Primary carcinoma of the ureter: A prognostic study. Cancer, 35:1626, 1975.

Bean, W. J.: Renal cysts: Treatment with alcohol. Radiology, 138:329, 1981.

Beckman, C. F., and Roth, R. A.: Secondary ureteropelvic junction stricture: Percutaneous dilation. Radiology, 164:365, 1987.

Beckman, C. F., Roth, R. A., and Bihrie, W., III: Dilation of benign ureteral strictures. Radiology, 172:437, 1989.

Beland, G., and Piette, Y.: Urinary tract candidiasis: Report of a case with bilateral ureteral obstruction. Can. Med. Assoc. J., 108:472, 1973.

Blum, J. A.: Acute monilial pyelohydronephrosis: report of a case successfully treated with amphotericin B continuous renal pelvis irrigation. J. Urol., 96:614, 1966.

Blute, M. L., Segura, J. W., Patterson, D. E., et al.: Impact of endourology on diagnosis and management of upper urinary tract urothelial cancer. J. Urol., 141:1298, 1989.

Brandl, H.: Percutaneous ureteral occlusion with silicone olive. Fifth World Congress on Endourology and ESWL, Cairo, Egypt, 1987, p. 90.

Brannen, G. E., Bush, W. H., and Lewis, G. P.: Endopyelotomy for primary repair of ureteropelvic junction obstruction. J. Urol., 139:29, 1988.

Braun, W. E., Banowsky, L. H., Straffon, R. A., et al.: Lymphoceles associated with renal transplantation: Report of 15 cases and review of the literature. Am. J. Med., 57:714, 1974.

Bregg, K., and Riehle, R. A.: Morbidity associated with indwelling internal stents inserted prior to shock wave lithotripsy. J. Urol., 139:265A, 1988.

Brennan, R. E., and Pollack, H. M.: Nonvisualized ("phantom") renal calyx: causes and radiological approach to diagnosis. Urol. Radiol., 1:17, 1979.

Brockis, J. G., Hulbert, J. C., Patel, A. S., et al.: The diagnosis and treatment of lymphoceles associated with renal transplantation. Br. J. Urol., 50:307, 1978.

Caldamone, A. A., and Frank, I. N.: Percutaneous aspiration in the treatment of renal access. J. Urol., 123:92, 1980.

Castaneda-Zuniga, W. R.: Establishing access: The percutaneous nephrostomy. In Cayman, R. V., and Castaneda-Suniga, W. R. (Eds.): Techniques in Endourology: A Guide to the Percutaneous Removal of Renal and Ureteral Calculi. Chicago, Year Book Medical Publishers, 1984, p. 73.

Catalona, W. M.: Bladder cancer. In Gillenwater, J. Y., Grayhack, J. T., Howards, S. S., and Duckett, J. W. (Eds.): Adult and Pediatric Urology. Chicago, Year Book Medical Publishers, 1987, pp. 1000.

Chang, R., Marshall, F. F., and Mitchell, S.: Percutaneous management of benign ureteral strictures and fistulas. J. Urol., 137:1126, 1987.

Chao, P. W., Glanz, S., Gordon, D. H., et al.: Percutaneous ureteroneocystotomy for treatment of postoperative distal-ureteral stricture. J. Endourol., 1:55, 1987.

Chehval, M. J., Nepute, J. Q., and Purcell, M. H.: Nephroscopic obliteration of an obstructing peripelvic renal cyst in conjunction with stone removal. J. Endourol., 4:259, 1990.

Clayman, R. V.: Rigid and flexible nephroscopy. In Clayman R. V., and Castaneda-Zuniga, W. R. (Eds.): Techniques in Endourology: A Guide to the Percutaneous Removal of Renal and Ureteral Calculi. Chicago, Year Book Medical Publishers, 1984a, p. 153.

Clayman, R. V., and Bagley, D. H.: Ureteronephroscopy. In Gillenwater, J. Y., Grayhack, J. T., Howards, S. S., and Duckett, J. W. (Eds.): Adult and Pediatric Urology. Chicago, Year Book Medical Publishers, 1990c.

Clayman, R. V., Basler, J. W., Kavoussi, L., et al.: Ureteronephroscopic endopyelotomy. J. Urol., 144:246, 1990b.

Clayman, R. V., Bub, P., Haaff, E., et al.: Prone flexible cystoscopy: An adjunct to percutaneous stone removal. J. Urol., 137:65, 1987a.

Clayman, R. V., and Castaneda-Zuniga, W. R.: Calyceal diverticulum. In Techniques in Endourology: A Guide to the Percutaneous Removal of Renal and Ureteral Calculi. Dallas, Heritage Press, 1984b, p. 45.

Clayman, R. V., Castaneda-Zuniga, W. R., Hunter, D. W., et al.: Rapid balloon dilatation of the nephrostomy tract for nephrostolithotomy. Radiology, 147:884, 1983a.

Clayman, R. V., and Denstedt, J. D.: New technique: Ureteronephroscopic urothelial endoureteroplasty: Case report. J. Endourol., 3:425, 1989.

Clayman, R. V., Elbers, J., Miller, R. P., et al.: Percutaneous nephrostomy: Assessment of renal damage associated with semirigid (24F) and balloon (36F) dilation Invest. Urol., 138:203, 1987b.

Clayman, R. V., Kavoussi, L. R., Long, S. R., et al.: Laparoscopic nephrectomy: Initial report of pelviscopic organ ablation in the pig. J. Endourol., 4:247, 1990a.

Clayman, R. V., Kavoussi, L. R., Letter, R. E., Soper, N. J., et al.: Laparoscopic nephrectomy. Initial case report. N. Engl. J. Med., 19:1370, 1991.

Clayman, R. V., Kavoussi, L. R., Soper, N. J., et al.: Laparoscopic nephrectomy: Initial case report. J. Urol., 146:1, 1991.

Clayman, R. V., Lange, P. H., and Fraley, E. E.: Cancer of the upper urinary tract. In Javadpour, N. (Ed.): Principles and Management of Urologic Cancer, 2nd ed. Baltimore, Williams & Wilkins, 1983b, p 544.

Clayman, R. V., and Picus, D. D.: Ureterorenoscopic endopyelotomy: Preliminary report. Urol. Clin. North Am., 15:433, 1988.

Clayman, R. V., Surya, V., Hunter, D., et al.: Renal vascular complications associated with percutaneous removal of renal calculi. J. Urol., 132:228, 1984c.

Coleman, C. C.: Percutaneous nephrolithotomy: Dilation techniques. In Amplatz, K. and Lange, P. H. (Eds.): Atlas of Endourology. Chicago, Year Book Medical Publishers, 1986, p. 131.

Coleman, C. C., Kimura, Y., Castaneda-Zuniga, W. R., et al.: Interventional techniques in the ureter. Sem. Intervent. Radiol., 1:24, 1984a.

Coleman, C. C., Kimura, Y., Reddy, P., et al.: Complications of nephrostolithotomy. Semin. Intervent. Radiol., 1:70, 1984b.

Cortesi, N., Ferrari, P., Zambarda, E., et al.: Diagnosis of bilateral abdominal cryptorchidism by laparoscopy. Endoscopy, 8:33, 1976.

Cronan, J. J., Amic, E. S., and Dorfman, G. S.: Percutaneous drainage of renal abscess. J. Urol., 123:92, 1980.

Cronan, J. J., Armiag, E. S., Jr., and Dorfman, G. S.: Percutaneous drainage of renal abscesses. Am. J. Radiol., 142:351, 1984.

Cubelli, V., and Smith, A. D.: Transurethral ureteral surgery guided by fluoroscopy. Endourology, 2:8, 1987.

Dalton, D., Neiman, H., and Grayhack, J. T.: The natural history of simple renal cysts: A preliminary study. J. Urol., 135:905, 1986.

Damico, C. F., Mebust, W. K., Valk, W. L., et al.: Triamcinolone: Adjuvant therapy for vesical neck contracture. J. Urol., 110:203, 1973.

Darcy, M. D., Jung, G. B., Smith, T. P., et al.: Percutaneously applied ureteral clips: Treatment of vesicovaginal fistula. Radiology, 163:819, 1987.

Das, S., and Amar, A. D.: The impact of laparoscopy on modern urologic practice. Urol. Clin. North Am., 15:537, 1988.

Davidson, A. J.: Chronic parenchymal disease. In Pollack, H. (Ed.): Clinical Urography. Philadelphia, W. B. Saunders Co., 1990, p. 2278.

Davis, D. M.: Intubated ureterotomy: A new operation for ureteral and ureteropelvic stricture. Surg. Gynecol. Obstet., 76:513, 1943.

Davis, D. M.: Intubated ureterotomy. J. Urol., 66:77, 1951.

Davis, D. M., Strong, G. H., and Drake, W. M.: Intubated ureterotomy: Experimental work and clinical results. J. Urol., 59:851, 1948.

Delaney, V. B., Adler, S., Bruns, F. J., et al.: Autosomal dominant polycystic kidney disease: Presentation, complications, and prognosis. Am. J. Kidney Dis., 5:104, 1985.

Dembner, A. G., and Pfister, R. C.: Fungal infection of the urinary tract: demonstration by antegrade pyelography and drainage by percutaneous nephrostomy. Am. J. Roentgenol. 129:415, 1977.

Denovic, M., Darzynkiewicz, A., Kostryrka-Claps, M. L., et al.: Flow cytometry of low stage bladder tumors. Cancer, 48:109, 1982.

Desnos, E.: The nineteenth century. In Murphy, L. J. T. (Ed.): The History of Urology. Springfield, IL, Charles C Thomas, 1972, p. 180.

Dierks, S. M., Clayman, R. V., Kavoussi, L. R., et al.: Intraureteral surgery: Appropriate cutting modality. J. Endourol., 4:S114, 1990.

Dixon, G. D., Moore, J. D., and Stockton, R.: Successful dilatation of ureteroileal anastomotic stenosis using Gruntzig catheter. Urology, 19:555, 1982.

Docimo, S. G., and Dewolf, W. C.: High failure rate of indwelling ureteral stents in patients with extrinsic obstruction. Experience at two institutions. J. Urol., 142:277, 1989.

Doemeny, J. M., Banner, M. P., Shapiro, M. J., et al.: Percutaneous extraction of renal fungus ball. Am. J. Radiol., 150:1331, 1988.

Droller, M. J.: Transitional cell cancer: Upper tracts and bladder. In Walsh, P. C., Gittes, R. F., Perlmutter, A. D., and Stamey, T. A. (Eds.): Campbell's Urology, 5th ed. Philadelphia, W. B. Saunders Co., 1986, p. 1382.

Edelstein, H., and McCabe, R. E.: Perinephric abscess: Modern diagnosis and treatment in 47 cases. Medicine, 67:118, 1988.

Eickenberg, H. U.: Percutaneous surgery of renal cysts. J. Urol., 133:200A, 1985.

Eklund, L., and Gothlin, J.: Angiography in carcinoma of the renal pelvis and the ureter. Acta Radiol. Diagn., 17:676, 1976.

Elyaderani, M. K.: Antegrade percutaneous ureteral stent insertion. In Smith, A. D., Castaneda-Zuniga, W. R., and Bronson, J. G.

(Eds.): Endourology: Principles and Practice. New York, Thieme Inc., 1986, p. 274.

Elyaderani, M. K., and Moncman, J.: Value of ultrasonography, fine needle aspiration and percutaneous drainage of perinephric abscesses. South. Med. J., 78:685, 1985.

Engel, R. M.: Complications of bilateral uretero-ileo cutaneous urinary diversion: A review of 208 cases. J. Urol., 101:508, 1969.

Eshghi, M., Franco, I., Schwalb, D., et al.: Cold knife endoureterotomy of 40 strictures. Seventh World Congress on Endourology and ESWL, Kyoto, Japan. [Abstract P6-4.] November 27–30, 1989b.

Eshghi, M.: Endoscopic incisions of the urinary tract. AUA Update Series, Volume 8, Lesson 37 to 39, 1989a.

Eshghi, M., Roth, J. S., and Smith, A. D.: Percutaneous transperitoneal approach to a pelvic kidney for endourological removal of staghorn calculus. J. Urol., 134:525, 1985.

Eshghi, M., Tuong, W., Fernandez, R., et al.: Percutaneous (endo) infundibulotomy. J. Endourol., 1:107, 1987.

Fairley, K. F., and Birch, D. F.: Hematuria: A simple method for identifying glomerular bleeding. Kidney Int., 21:105, 1982.

Farah, R. N., DiLoreto, R. R., and Cerny, J. C.: Transurethral resection combined with steroid injection in treatment of recurrent vesical neck contracture. Urology, 13:395, 1979.

Federle, J. P., McAninch, J. W., Kaiser, J. A., et al.: Computed tomography of urinary calculi. Am. J. Radiol., 136:255, 1981.

Fernstrom, I., and Johansson, B.: Percutaneous pyelolithotomy. Scand. J. Urol. Nephrol., 10:257, 1976.

Finnerty, D. P., Trulock, T. S., Berkman, W., et al.: Transluminal balloon dilation of ureteral stricture. J. Urol., 131:1056, 1984.

Fotino, S.: The solitary kidney: a model of chronic hyperfiltration in humans. Am. J. Kidney Dis., 13:88, 1989.

Fraley, E. E.: Dismembered infundibulopyelostomy: Improved technique for correcting vascular obstruction of the superior infundibulum. J. Urol., 101:144, 1969.

Fuchs, G.J., and David, R.D.: Flexible ureterorenoscopy, dilation of narrow caliceal neck, and ESWL: A new, minimally invasive approach to stones in caliceal diverticula. J. Endourol., 3:255, 1989.

Gaylord, G. M., and Johnsrude, I. S.: Transrenal ureteral occlusion with Gianturco coils and gelatin sponge. Radiology, 172:1047, 1989.

Gerzof, S. C., Johnson, W. C., Robbins, A. H., et al.: Expanded criteria for percutaneous abscess drainage. Arch. Surg., 120:227, 1985.

Gerzof, S. G., and Gale, M. E.: Computed tomography and ultrasonography for the diagnosis and treatment of renal and retroperitoneal abscesses. Urol. Clin. North Am., 9:185, 1982.

Gill, W. B., Chen-tai, L., and Bibbo, M.: Retrograde brush biopsy of the ureter and renal pelvis. Urol. Clin. North Am., 6:573, 1979.

Gillam, J. F. E., and Wadelton, D. H.: A case of renal moniliasis. Br. Med. J., 1:985, 1958.

Gillenwater, J. Y.: In Gillenwater, J. Y., Grayhack, J. T., Howards, S. S., and Duckett, J. W. (Eds.): Hydronephrosis in Adult and Pediatric Urology. Chicago, Year Book Medical Publishers, 1987, p. 691.

Gittes, R. F.: Management of transitional cell carcinoma of the upper tract: Case for conservative local excision. Urol. Clin. North Am., 7:559, 1980.

Gittes, R. F., and Varady, S.: Nephroscopy in chronic unilateral hematuria. J. Urol., 126:297, 1981.

Glanz, S., Gordon, P. H., Butt, K., et al.: Percutaneous transrenal balloon dilatation of the ureter. Radiology, 149:101, 1983.

Goldman, S. M., and Gatewood, O. M.: Neoplasms of the renal collecting system, pelvis and ureters. In Pollack, H. M. (Ed.): Clinical Urography. Philadelphia, W. B. Saunders Co., 1990, p. 1327.

Goldman, S. M., Minkin, S. D., Naraval, D. C., et al.: Renal carbuncle: the use of ultrasound in its diagnosis and management. J. Urol., 118:525, 1977.

Goodwin, W. E., Casey, W.,C., and Woolfe, W.: Percutaneous trocar (needle) nephrostomy in hydronephrosis. JAMA, 157:891, 1955.

Gothlin, J. H., Gadcholt, G., Farsund, T., et al.: Percutaneous antegrade dilatation of distal ureteral strictures and obstruction. Eur. J. Radiol., 8:217, 1988.

Griffith, D. P., Schuessler, W. W., and Vancaille, T. H.: Laparoscopic lymphadenectomy—A low morbidity alternative for staging pelvic malignancies. J. Endourol., 4(Suppl. 1):S-84, 1990.

Gruntzig, A. R., Senning, A., and Siegenthaler, W. E.: Nonoperative dilation of coronary-artery stenosis: percutaneous transluminal coronary angioplasty. N. Engl. J. Med., 301:61, 1979.

Gunning, J. E.: History of laparoscopy. *In* Phillips, J. M., and Carson, S. L. (Eds.): Laparoscopy. Baltimore, Williams & Wilkins, 1977, p. 6.

Gunther, R., Klose, R., and Alken, P.: Transrenal ureteral occlusion with a detachable balloon. Radiology, 142:521, 1982.

Gunther, R., Marberger, M., and Klose, R.: Transrenal ureteral embolization. Radiology, 132:317, 1979.

Guz, B., Streem, S. B., Novick, A. C., et al.: Role of percutaneous nephrostomy in patients with upper tract transitional cell carcinoma. J. Urol., (In press).

Haaga, J. R.: Imaging intra-abdominal abscesses and nonoperative drainage procedures. World J. Surg., 14:204, 1990.

Haaga, J. R., Alfidi, R. J., and Harvilla, T. R.: CT detection and aspiration of abdominal abscess. Am. J. Roentgenol., 128:465, 1977.

Hamm, F. C., and Weinberg, S. R.: Renal and ureteral surgery without intubation. J. Urol., 73:475, 1955.

Hamm, F. C., and Weinberg, S. R.: Experimental studies of regeneration of the ureter without intubation. J. Urol., 75:43, 1956.

Hanna, M. K., Jeffs, R. D., Sturgess, J. M., et al.: Ureteral structure and ultrastructure. I. The normal human ureter. J. Urol., 116:718, 1976a.

Hanna, M. J., Jeffs, R. D., Sturgess, J. M., et al.: Ureteral structure and ultrastructure. II. Congenital ureteropelvic junction obstruction and primary obstructive megaureter. J. Urol., 116:725, 1976b.

Harrach, L. B., Burkholder, G. V., and Goodwin, W. E.: Renal candidiasis—A cause of anuria. Br. J. Urol., 42:258, 1970.

Hawkins, I. F., Jr., Hunter, P., Leal, J., et al.: Retrograde nephrostomy for stone removal: Combined cystoscopic/percutaneous technique. Am. J. Radiol., 143:299, 1984.

Healy, M. E., Teng, S. S., and Moss, A. A.: Uriniferous pseudocyst? Computed tomographic findings. Radiology, 153:757, 1984.

Heney, N. M., Nocks, B. N., Daly, J. J., et al.: Prognostic factors in carcinoma of the ureter. J. Urol., 125:632, 1981.

Herr, H. W.: Durable response of a carcinoma in situ of the renal pelvis to topical bacillus Calmette-Guerin. J. Urol., 134:531, 1985.

Holmberg, G., and Hietala, S. O.: Treatment of simple renal cysts by percutaneous puncture and instillation of bismuth phosphate. Scand. J. Urol. Nephrol., 23:207, 1989.

Holmes, E. W., Jr.: Uric acid nephrolithiasis. *In* Coe, F. L. (Ed.): Nephrolithiasis. Contemporary Issues in Nephrology, #5. New York, Churchill Livingstone, 1980, pp. 188–208.

Hopper, K. D., Sherman, J. L., Luethke, J. M., et al.: The retrorenal colon in the supine and prone patient. Radiology, 162:443, 1987.

Horgan, J., Cubelli, V., Lee, W. J., et al.: Endourologic stenting of ureteroileal anastomotic stricture: Cope modification. J. Endourol., 1:275, 1988.

Hubner, W., Pfab, R., et al.: Renal cysts: Percutaneous resection with standard urologic instruments. J. Endourol., 4:61, 1990.

Huffman, J. L.: Ureteroscopic management of transitional cell carcinoma of the upper urinary tract. Urol. Clin. North Am., 15:419, 1988.

Huffman, J. L.: Endoscopic management of upper urinary tract urothelial cancer. J. Endourol., 4:S-141, 1990.

Huffman, J. L., Bagley, D. H., Lyon, E. S., et al.: Endoscopic diagnosis and treatment of upper tract urothelial tumors. A preliminary report. Cancer, 55:1422, 1985a.

Huffman, J. L., Morse, M. J., Herr, H. W., et al.: Ureteropyeloscopy: the diagnostic and therapeutic approach to upper tract urothelial tumors. World J. Urol., 3:58, 1985b.

Hulbert, J. C.: Percutaneous endoscopic management of the completely obliterated ureteropelvic junction. J. Endourol., 4:S142, 1990.

Hulbert, J. C., Hernandez, J., Hunter, D. W., et al.: Current concepts in the management of pyelocaliceal diverticula. J. Endourol., 2:11, 1988a.

Hulbert, J. C., Hunter, D., and Castaneda-Zuniga, W. R.: Classification of and techniques for the reconstitution of acquired strictures in the region of the ureteropelvic junction. J. Urol., 140:468, 1988b.

Hulbert, J. C., Hunter, D., Young, A. T., et al.: Percutaneous intrarenal marsupialization of a perirenal cystic collection—endocystolysis. J. Urol., 139:1039, 1988c.

Hulbert, J. C., Lapointe, S., Reddy, P. K., et al.: Percutaneous endoscopic fulguration of a large volume caliceal diverticulum. J. Urol., 138:116, 1987.

Hulbert, J. C., Reddy, P. K., Hunter, D. W., et al.: Percutaneous

techniques for the management of caliceal diverticula containing calculi. J. Urol., 135:225, 1986.

Hunner, G. L.: End results in one hundred cases of ureteral stricture. J. Urol., 12:295, 1924.

Immeregut, M. A., and Stevenson, T.: The use of epsilon amino caproic acid in the control of hematuria associated with hemoglobinopathies. J. Urol., 93:110, 1965.

Inglis, J. A., and Tolley, D. A.: Ureteroscopic pyelolysis for pelviureteric junction obstruction. Br. J. Urol., 58:250, 1986.

Irby, P. B., Stoller, M. L., and McAninch, J. W.: Fungal bezoars of the upper urinary tract. J. Urol., 143:447, 1990.

Ireton, R. C.: Percutaneous nephrostomy tract incision using modified Otis urethrotome. Urol. Clin. North Am., 17:95, 1990.

Ireton, R. C., Krieger, J. N., Rudd, T. G., et al.: Percutaneous endoscopic treatment of fungus ball obstruction in a renal allograft. Transplantation, 39:453, 1985.

Janetschek, G.: Percutaneous intrarenal surgery for calyceal stones, infundibular stenosis, calyceal diverticula, and obstruction of the ureteropelvic junction. J. Urol., 139:187A, 1988.

Jaques, P., Mauro, M., Safrit, H., et al.: CT features of intraabdominal abscesses. Am. J. Roentgenol., 146:1041, 1986.

Johansson, S., and Wahlquist, L.: A prognostic study of urothelial renal pelvic tumors. Cancer, 43:2525, 1979.

Johnson, D. C., Oke, E. J., Dunnick, R. N., et al.: Percutaneous balloon dilation of ureteral strictures. Am. J. Roentgenol., 148:181, 1987.

Kadir, S., White, R. I., Jr., and Engel, R.: Balloon dilatation of a ureteropelvic junction obstruction. Radiology, 143:263, 1982.

Kaneti, J., and Hertzanu, Y.: Renal abscess owing to *Salmonella* septicemia: Percutaneous drainage. J. Urol., 138:395, 1987.

Karlin, G. S., Badlani, G. H., and Smith, A. D.: Endopyelotomy versus open pyeloplasty: Comparison in 88 patients. J. Urol., 140:476, 1988.

Karlin, G. S., Rich, M., Lee, W., et al.: Endourological management of upper-tract fungal infection. J. Endourol., 1:49, 1987.

Karlin, G. S., and Smith, A. D.: Endopyelotomy. Urol. Clin. North Am., 15:433, 1988.

Kavoussi, L. R., and Clayman, R. V.: Flexible endoscopy of the urinary tract. Part II. AUA Update Series, Lesson 6, Volume VIII. American Urological Association, Inc., Office of Education, 1989, p. 43.

Kavoussi, L. R., Clayman, R. V., and Basler, J.: Flexible actively deflectable fiberoptic ureteronephroscopy. J. Urol., 142:949, 1989.

Kavoussi, L. R., Clayman, R. V., Mikkelsen, D. J., et al.: Ureteronephroscopic marsupialization of obstructing peripelvic renal cyst. J. Urol., (In press), 1991a.

Kavoussi, L. R., Dierks, S., Clayman, R., et al.: Endoureterotomy: Ureteronephroscopic treatment of ureteral strictures. J. Endourol., 4:S113, 1990.

Kavoussi, L. R., Meretyk, S., Dierks, S. M., et al.: Endopyelotomy for secondary ureteropelvic junction obstruction in the pediatric population. J. Urol., 145:345, 1991b.

Kaye, K. W., and Clayman, R. V.: Tamponade nephrostomy catheter for percutaneous nephrostolithotomy. Urology, 27:441, 1986.

Kaye, K. W., and Lange, P. H.: Mode of presentation of invasive bladder cancer: Reassessment of the problem. J. Urol., 128:31, 1982.

Kendall, A. R., Senay, B. A., and Coll, M. E.: Spontaneous subcapsular renal hematoma: Diagnosis and management. J. Urol., 139:246, 1988.

Kinn, A., Ohlsen, H., Brehmer-Andersson, E., et al.: Therapeutic ureteral occlusion in advanced pelvic malignant tumors. J. Urol., 135:29, 1986.

Kopecky, K. K., Steidle, C. P., Eble, J. N., et al.: Endoluminal radio-frequency electrocautery for permanent ureteral occlusion in swine. Radiology, 170:1043, 1989.

Korth, K., and Kuenkel, J.: Unusual applications of ureteroscopy. Urol. Clin. North Am., 15:459, 1988.

Kramolowsky, E. V., Clayman, R. V., and Weyman, P. J.: Endourologic management of ureteroileal anastomotic strictures. Is it effective? J. Urol., 137:390, 1987.

Kramolowsky, E. V., Clayman, R. V., and Weyman, P. J.: Management of ureterointestinal anastomotic strictures: Comparison of open surgical and endourological repair. J. Urol., 139:1195, 1988.

Kramolowsky, E. V., Tucker, R. D., and Nelson, C. M. K.: Management of benign ureteral strictures: Open surgical repair on endoscopic dilation? J. Urol., 141:285, 1989.

Krueger, R. P., Ash, J. M., Silver, M. M., et al.: Primary hydrone-phrosis: Assessment of diuretic renography, pelvis perfusion pressure, operative findings, and renal and ureteral histology. Urol. Clin. North Am., 7:231, 1980.

Kuenkel, M., and Korth, K.: Endopyelotomy: Results after long-term follow-up of 135 patients. J. Endourol., (In press).

Kumon, H., Tsugawa, M., Matsumura, Y., et al.: Endoscopic diagnosis and treatment of chronic unilateral hematuria of uncertain etiology. J. Urol., 143:554, 1990.

Lang, E. K.: Antegrade ureteral stenting for dehiscence, strictures, and fistulae. Am. J. Roentgenol., 143:795, 1984.

Lang, E. K., and Glorioso, L. W., III: Management of urinomas by percutaneous drainage procedures. Radiol. Clin. North Am., 24:551, 1986.

Lang, E. K., and Glorioso, L. W., III: Antegrade transluminal dilation of benign ureteral strictures: Long term results. Am. J. Roentgen., 150:131, 1988.

Lano, M. D., Wagoner, R. D., and Leary, F. J.: Unilateral essential hematuria. Mayo Clin. Proc., 54:88, 1979.

Laucks, S. P., Jr., and McLachlan, M. S. F.: Aging and simple cysts of the kidney. Br. J. Radiol., 54:12, 1981.

Lawson, R. K., Murphy, J. B., Taylor, A. J., et al.: Retrograde method for percutaneous access to kidney. Urology, 22:580, 1983.

Leonard, M. P., Canning, D. A., Epstein, J. I., et al.: Local tissue reaction to the subureteral injection of glutaraldehyde cross-linked bovine collagen in humans. J. Urol., 143:1209, 1990.

LeRoy, A. J., Williams, H. J., Jr., Bender, C. E., et al.: Colon perforation following percutaneous nephrostomy and renal calculus removal. Radiology, 155:83, 1985.

Loening, S., Narayana, A., Yoder, L., et al.: Factors influencing the recurrence rate of bladder cancer. J. Urol., 123:29, 1980.

Lowe, D. H., Brock, W. A., and Kamplan, G. W.: Laparoscopy for localization of nonpalpable testes. J. Urol., 131:728, 1984.

Lyon, E. S., Banno, J. J., and Schoenberg, H. W.: Transurethral ureteroscopy in men using juvenile cystoscopy equipment. J. Urol., 122:152, 1979.

Lyon, E. S., Kyker, J. S., and Schoenberg, H. W.: Transurethral ureteroscopy in women: A ready addition to the urologic armamentarium. J. Urol., 119:35, 1978.

Lyons, A. S., and Petrucelli, R. J., II: Infection. *In* Medicine: An Illustrated History. New York, Harry N. Abrams, 1978, p. 561.

Mahoney, S. A., Koletsky, S., and Persky, L.: Approximation and dilatation: The mode of healing of an intubated ureterostomy. J. Urol., 88:197, 1962.

Maizels, M., Firlit, C. F., Conway, J. J., et al.: Troubleshooting the diuretic renogram. Urology, 28:355, 1986.

Malek, R. S., Aguilo, J. T., and Hattery, R. R.: Radiolucent filling defects of the renal pelvis: Classification and report of unusual cases. J. Urol., 114:508, 1975.

Manson, A. L., Terhune, G., Jordan, J. R., et al.: Preoperative laparoscopic localization of the nonpalpable testis. J. Urol., 134:919, 1985.

Marberger, M., Stackl, W., and Hruby, W.: Percutaneous litholapaxy of renal calculi with ultrasound. Eur. Urol., 8:236, 1982.

Mariani, A. J., Mariani, M. C., Macchioni, C., et al.: The significance of adult hematuria: 1000 hematuria evaluations including a risk-benefit and cost-effectiveness analysis. J. Urol., 141:350, 1989.

Martin, E. C., Fankuchen, E. I., and Casarella, W. J.: Percutaneous dilatation of ureteroenteric strictures or occlusions in ileal conduits. Urol. Radiol., 4:19, 1982.

Marx, M., Bettmann, M. A., Bridges, S., et al.: Effects of various indwelling ureteral catheter materials on normal canine ureter. J. Urol., 139:180, 1988.

Mazeman, E.: Tumors of the upper urinary tract calyces, renal pelvis and ureter. Eur. Urol., 2:120, 1976.

McCullough, C. S., Soper, N. J., Clayman, R. V., et al.: Laparoscopic drainage of a post-transplant lymphocele. Transplantation, 51:725, 1991.

McDougall, E. M., Denstedt, J. D., and Clayman, R. V.: Comparison of patient acceptance of polyurethrane vs. silicone indwelling ureteral stents. J. Endourol., 4:79, 1990.

McMurtry, J. M., Clayman, R. V., and Preminger, G. M.: Endourologic diagnosis and treatment of essential hematuria. J. Endourol., 1:145, 1987.

Melamed, M. R.: Flow cytometry of the urinary bladder. Urol. Clin. North Am., 11:599, 1984.

Meretyk, S., Clayman, R. V., Kavoussi, L. R., et al.: Caveat emptor: Calyceal stones and the missing calyx. J. Urol., (In preparation), 1991a.

Meretyk, S., Clayman, R. V., Kavoussi, L. R., et al.: Endoureterotomy for treatment of ureteral strictures. J. Urol. (In preparation), 1991b.

Meretyk, S., Clayman, R. V., Kavoussi, L. R., et al.: Endourological treatment of ureteroenteric anastomotic strictures: Long-term follow-up. J. Urol., 145:723, 1991c.

Meretyk, S., Kavoussi, L. R., and Clayman, R. V.: Changing concepts in the approach to upper tract urothelial tumors. (In preparation), 1991d.

Meretyk, S., Meretyk, I., Kavoussi, L. R., et al.: Ureteronephroscopic vs. antegrade endopyelotomy for treatment of ureteropelvic junction obstruction. J. Endourol., 4:S141, 1990.

Mikkelsen, D. J., Kavoussi, L. R., Clayman, R. V., et al.: Advances in flexible deflectable ureteronephroscopy (FDU): Intrarenal surgery. J. Urol., 141:192A, 1989.

Moldwin, R. M., and Smith, A. D.: Percutaneous management of ureteral fistulas. Urol. Clin. North Am., 15:453, 1988.

Morano, J. U., and Burkhalter, J. L.: Percutaneous catheter drainage of post-traumatic urinoma. J. Urol., 134:319, 1985.

Morin, M. E., and Baker, D. A.: Lymphocele: a complication of surgical staging of carcinoma of the prostate. Am. J. Radiol., 129:333, 1977.

Motola, J. A., Badlani, G. H., and Smith, A. D.: Endopyelotomy: Long-term follow-up of 156 cases. J. Endourol., 4:S139, 1990.

Mueller, P. R., van Sonnenberg, E., and Ferrucci, J. T., Jr.: Percutaneous drainage of 250 abdominal abscesses and fluid collections. II. Current procedural concepts. Radiology, 151:343, 1984.

Muench, P. J., Haynes, C. B., Raney, A. M., et al.: Endoscopic management of the obliterated ureteroileal anastomosis: J. Urol., 137:277, 1987.

Murnaghan, G. F.: The mechanism of congenital hydronephrosis with reference to the factors influencing surgical treatment. Ann. R. Coll. Surg. Eng., 23:25, 1958.

Murphy, L. J. T.: The Kidney. *In* The History of Urology. Springfield, IL, Charles C Thomas, 1972, p. 201.

Nash, D. A., and Henry, A. R.: Unilateral essential hematuria: Therapy with epsilon aminocaproic acid. Urology, 23:297, 1984.

Netto, N. R., Jr., Ferreira, U., Lemos, G. C., et al.: Endourological management of ureteral strictures. J. Urol., 144:631, 1990.

Newhouse, J. H., Pfister, R. C., Hendren, W. H., et al.: Whitaker test after pyeloplasty: Establishment of normal ureteral perfusion pressures. Am. J. Radiol., 137:223, 1981.

Nocks, B. N., Heney, N. M., Daly, J. J., et al.: Transitional cell carcinoma of the renal pelvis. Urology, 19:472, 1982.

Nurse, D. E., Woodhouse, C. R. J., Kellett, M. J., et al.: Percutaneous removal of upper tract tumors. World J. Urol., 7:131, 1989.

O'Brien, W. M., Maxted, W. C., and Pahira, J. J.: Ureteral stricture: Experience with 31 cases. J. Urol., 140:737, 1988.

O'Flynn, K., Hehin, M., McKelvie, G., et al.: Endoballoon rupture and stenting for pelviureteric junction obstruction: Technique and early results. Br. J. Urol., 64:572, 1989.

Oosterhof, G. O. N., Hoitsma, A. J., and Debruyne, F. R. J.: Antegrade percutaneous dilation of ureteral strictures after kidney transplantation. Transplant Int., 2:36, 1989.

Oppenheimer, R., and Hinman, F., Jr.: Ureteral regeneration: Contracture vs. hyperplasia of smooth muscle. J. Urol., 74:476, 1955.

Orandi, A.: Transurethral fulguration of bladder diverticulum: New procedure. Urology, 10:30, 1977.

O'Reilly, P. H.: Diuresis renography 8 years later: An update. J. Urol., 136:993, 1986.

O'Reilly, P. H., Lawson, R. S., and Testa, H. J.: Idiopathic hydronephrosis: The diuresis renogram: A new non-invasive method of assessing equivocal pelviureteral junction obstruction. J. Urol., 121:1531, 1979.

Orihuela, E., and Smith, A. D.: Percutaneous treatment of transitional cell carcinoma of the upper urinary tract. Urol. Clin. North Am., 15:425, 1988.

Ozgun, S., Cetin, S., and Ilken, Y.: Percutaneous renal cyst aspiration and treatment with alcohol. Int. Urol. Nephrol., 20:481, 1988.

Papanicolaou N., Pfister, R. C., and Yoder, I. C.: Percutaneous occlusion of ureteral leaks and fistulae using nondetachable balloons. Urol. Radiol., 7:28, 1985.

Patterson, D. E., Segura, J. W., Benson, R. C., Jr., et al.: Endoscopic evaluation and treatment of patients with idiopathic gross hematuria. J. Urol., 132:1199, 1984.

Perez-Castro Ellendt, E., and Martinez-Pineiro, J. A.: Transurethral ureteroscopy: A current urological procedure. Arch. Esp. Urol., 33:445, 1980.

Picus, D. D., Weyman, P. J., Clayman, R. V., et al.: Intercostal-space nephrostomy for percutaneous stone removal. Am. J. Rad., 147:393, 1986.

Pingoud, E. G., Bagley, D. H., Zeman, R. K., et al.: Percutaneous antegrade bilateral ureteral dilatation and stent placement for internal drainage. Radiology 134:780, 1980.

Politano, V. A.: Periurethral teflon injection for urinary incontinence. Urol. Clin. North Am., 5(2):415, 1978.

Pollack, H. M., Arger, P. H., Banner, M. P., et al.: Computed tomography of renal pelvic filling defects. Radiology, 138:645, 1981.

Pollard, S. G., and MacFarland, R.: Symptoms arising from double-J ureteral stents. J. Urol., 139:37, 1988.

Portela, L. A., Patel, S. K., and Callahan, D. H.: Pararenal pseudocyst (urinoma) as complication of percutaneous nephrostomy. Urology, 13:570, 1979.

Preminger, G. M., and Kennedy, T. J.: Ureteral stone extraction utilizing nondeflectable flexible fiberoptic ureteroscopes. J. Endourology, 1:31, 1987.

Psihramis, K. E., and Dretler, S. P.: Extracorporeal shock wave lithotripsy of caliceal diverticula calculi. J. Urol., 138:707, 1987.

Ramsey, J. C., and Soloway, M. S.: Instillation of bacillus Calmette-Guerin into the renal pelvis of a solitary kidney for the treatment of transitional cell carcinoma. J. Urol., 143:1220, 1990.

Ramsey, J. W. A., Miller, R. A., Kellet, M. J., et al.: Percutaneous pyelolysis: Indications, complications, and results. Br. J. Urol., 56:586, 1984.

Raskin, M. M., Poole, D. O., Roen, S. A., et al.: Percutaneous management of renal cysts: results of a four year study. Radiology, 1150:551, 1975.

Reddick, E. J.: Laparoscopic laser cholecystectomy: Short hospital stay, minimal scarring. Laser Practice Report, 1S–3S, 1988.

Reddy, P. K., Moore, L., Hunter, D., et al.: Percutaneous ureteral fulguration: A nonsurgical technique for ureteral occlusion. J. Urol., 138:724, 1987.

Reddy, P. K., and Sidi, A. A.: Endoscopic ureteral occlusion for urinary diversion in patients with lower urinary tract fistulas. Urol. Clin. North Am., 17:103, 1990.

Reimer, D. E., and Oswalt, G. C., Jr.: Iatrogenic ureteral obstruction treated with balloon dilation. J. Urol., 126:689, 1981.

Resnick, M. I.: Radiolucent filling defects. In Resnick, M. I., Caldarmone, A. A., and Sprinak, J. P. (Eds.): Decision Making in Urology. New York, C. V. Mosby Co., 1985, p. 18.

Sadi, M. V., Nardozza, A., Jr., and Gianotti, I.: Percutaneous drainage of retroperitoneal abscesses. J. Endourol., 2:293, 1988.

Saiki, J., Vaziri, N. D., and Barton, C.: Perinephric and intranephric abscesses: A review of the literature. West. J. Med., 136:96, 1982.

Salvatierra, O., Jr., Bucklew, W. B., and Morrow, J. W.: Perinephric abscess: A report of 71 cases. J. Urol., 98:296, 1967.

Sarnacki, C. T., McCormack, L. J., Kiser, W. S., et al.: Urinary cytology and the clinical diagnosis of urinary tract malignancy: A clinicopathological study of 1400 patients. J. Urol., 106:761, 1971.

Sayer, J., McCarthy, M. P., and Schmidt, J. D.: Identification and significance of dysmorphic versus isomorphic hematuria. J. Urol., 143:545, 1990.

Scardino, P. T., and Scardino, P. L.: Obstruction of the ureteropelvic junction. In Bergman, H. (Ed.): The Ureter. New York, Springer-Verlag, 1984, p. 697.

Schaeffer, A. J., and Grayhack, J. T.: Surgical management of ureteropelvic junction obstruction. In Walsh, P. C., Gittes, R. F., Perlmutter, A. D., and Stamey, T. A. (Eds.): Campbell's Urology, 5th ed. Philadelphia, W. B. Saunders Co., 1986, p. 2505.

Schaner, E. G., Balow, J. E., and Doppman, J. L.: Computed tomography in the diagnosis of subcapsular and perirenal hematoma. Am. J. Radiol., 128:83, 1977.

Schmidt, J. D., Hawtrey, C. E., Flocks, R. H., et al.: Complications, results, and problems of ileal conduit diversions. J. Urol., 109:210, 1973.

Schneider, A. W., Busch, R., Otto, V., et al.: Endourological management of 41 stenosis in the upper urinary tract using the cold knife technique. J. Urol., 141:208A, 1989.

Schonebeck, J., and Ansehn, S.: The occurrence of yeast-like fungi in the urine under normal conditions and in various types of urinary tract pathology. Scand. J. Urol. Nephrol., 6:123, 1972.

Schuessler, W. W., Vancaillie, T. G., Reich, H., et al.: Transperitoneal endosurgical lymphadenectomy in patients with localized prostate cancer. J. Urol., 145:988, 1991.

Schweizer, R. T., Cho, S., Korentz, S. L., et al.: Lymphoceles following renal transplantation. Arch. Surg., 104:42, 1972.

Segal, A. J., Spataro, R. F., Linke, C. A., et al.: Diagnosis of monopaque calculi by computed tomography. Radiology, 129:447, 1978.

Selikowitz, S. M.: New coaxial ureteral stricture knife. Urol. Clin. North Am., 17:83, 1990.

Semm, K.: Endoscopic Abdominal Surgery. Chicago, Year Book Medical Publishers, 1987, p. 499.

Shapiro, M. J., Banner, M. P., Amendola, M. A., et al.: Balloon catheter dilation of ureteroenteric strictures: Long-term results. Radiology, 168:385, 1988.

Sheinfeld, J., Erturk, E. R. F., and Cockett, A. T. K.: Perinephric abscess: Current concepts. J. Urol., 137:191, 1987.

Sheline, M., Amendola, M. A., Pollack, H. M., et al.: Fluoroscopically guided retrograde brush biopsy in the diagnosis of transitional cell carcinoma of the upper urinary tract: Results in 45 patients. Am. J. Radiol., 153:313, 1989.

Siegle, R. L., and Lieberman, P.: A review of untoward reactions to iodinated contrast material. J. Urol., 119:581, 1978.

Skinner, D. G., Melamud, A., and Lieskovsky, G.: Complications of thoracoabdominal retroperitoneal lymph node dissection. J. Urol., 127:1107, 1982.

Smith, A. D.: Management of iatrogenic ureteral strictures after urological procedures. J. Urol., 140:1372, 1988.

Smith, A. D., Moldwin, R. M., and Karlin, G. S.: Percutaneous ureterostomy. J. Urol., 138:286, 1987.

Soloway, M. S., and Masters, S.: Urothelial susceptibility to tumor cell implantation—Influence of cauterization. Cancer, 46:1158, 1980.

Spring, D. B., Schroeder, D., Babu, S., et al.: Ultrasonic evaluation of lymphocele formation after staging lymphadenectomy for prostatic carcinoma. Radiology, 141:479, 1981.

Stables, D. P., Ginsberg, N. I., and Johnson, M. L.: Percutaneous nephrostomy: A series and review of the literature. Am. J. Roentgenol., 130:75, 1971.

Stefanini, M., English, H. A., and Taylor, A. E.: Safe and effective, prolonged administration of epsilon aminocaproic acid in bleeding from the urinary tract. J. Urol., 143:559, 1990.

Streem, S. B., Novick, A. C., Steinmuller, D. R., et al.: Percutaneous techniques for the management of urological renal transplant complications. J. Urol., 135:456, 1986.

Strong, D. W., Pearse, H. D., Tank, E. S., Jr., et al.: The ureteral stump after nephroureterectomy. J. Urol., 115:654, 1976.

Suzuki, K., Tanaka, T., Ikeda, R., et al.: Terumo guidewire in endourologic treatment. J. Endourol., 3:69, 1989.

Tailly, G.: Tract healing after percutaneous nephrolithotomy. J. Endourol., 2:71, 1988.

Talner, L. B.: Obstructive uropathy. In Pollack, H. M. (Ed.): Nuclear Medicine Techniques in Clinical Urography. Philadelphia, W. B. Saunders Co., 1990, p. 1570.

Thomas, R., and Cherry, R.: Ureteroscopic endopyelotomy for management of ureteropelvic junction obstruction. J. Endourol., 4:S141, 1990.

Thompson, I. M., Ross, G., Jr., Habib, E. H., et al.: Experiences with 16 cases of pararenal pseudocyst. J. Urol., 116:289, 1976.

Thorley, J. D., Jones, S. R., and Sanford, J. P.: Perinephric abscess. Medicine, 53:441, 1974.

Thuroff, J. W., and Alken, P.: Ultrasound for renal puncture and fluoroscopy for tract dilation and catheter placement: A combined approach. Endourology, 2:1, 1987.

Timmons, J. W., Jr., Malek, R. S., Hattery, R. R., et al.: Caliceal diverticulum. J. Urol., 114:6, 1975.

Tomera, K. M., Leary, F. J., and Zincke, H.: Pyeloscopy in urothelial tumors. J. Urol., 127:1088, 1982.

Towbin, R. B., Wacksman, J., and Ball, W. S.: Percutaneous pyeloplasty in children: Experience in three patients. Radiology, 163:381, 1987.

Van Cangh, P. J., Jorion, J. L., Wese, F. X., et al.: Endoureteropyelotomy: Percutaneous treatment of ureteropelvic junction obstruction. J. Urol., 141:1317, 1989.

Varkarakis, M. J., Gaeta, J., Moore, R. H., et al.: Superficial bladder tumor: Aspects of clinical progression. Urology, 4:414, 1974.

Vestby, G. W.: Percutaneous needle-puncture of renal cysts: New method in therapeutic management. Invest. Radiol., 2:449, 1967.

Voegeli, D. R., Crummy, A. B., McDermott, J. C., et al.: Percutaneous dilation of ureteral strictures in renal transplant patients. Radiology, 169:185, 1988.

Wagle, D. G., Moore, R. H., and Murphy, G. P.: Primary carcinoma of the renal pelvis. Cancer, 33:1642, 1974.

Wahlqvist, L., and Grumstedt, B.: Therapeutic effect of percutaneous puncture of simple renal cyst. Acta Chir. Scand., 132:340, 1966.

Wallace, D. M. A., Wallace, D. M., Whitfield, H. N., et al.: The late results of conservative surgery for upper tract urothelial carcinomas. Br. J. Urol., 53:537, 1981.

Walther, P. J., Robertson, C. N., and Paulson, D. F.: Lethal complications of standard self-retaining ureteral stents in patients with ileal conduit urinary diversion. J. Urol., 133:851, 1985.

Webb, D. R., and Fitzpatrick, J. M.: Percutaneous nephrolithotripsy: A functional and morphological study. J. Urol., 134:587, 1985.

Webb, E. A., Smith, B. A., Jr., and Price, W. E.: Plastic operations on the ureter without intubation. J. Urol., 77:821, 1957.

Weigert, F., Schulz, V., and Kromer, H. D.: Renal abscess: Report of a case with sonographic urographic, and CT evaluation. Eur. J. Radiol., 5:224, 1985.

Weinstein, D., and Saltzman, B.: Predicting patency of double pigtail ureteral stents using cystography. J. Endourol., 1990.

Whitaker, R. H.: An evaluation of 170 diagnostic pressure flow studies of the upper urinary tract. J. Urol., 121:602, 1979.

Whitaker, R. H.: Pathophysiology of ureteric obstruction. In Williams, D. I. (Ed.): Scientific Foundations of Urology. London, Blackwell Scientific, 1976, p. 18.

White, M., Mueller, P. R., Ferucci, J. T., et al.: Percutaneous drainage of postoperative abdominal and pelvic lymphoceles. Am. J. Radiol., 145:1065, 1985.

Wickham, J. E. A.: The surgical treatment of renal lithiasis. In Urinary Calculous Disease. New York, Churchill Livingstone, 1979, p. 145.

Wickham, J. E. A.: Percutaneous pyelolysis. In Wickham, J. E. A., and Miller, R. A.: Percutaneous Renal Surgery. New York, Churchill Livingstone, 1983, p. 148.

Wickham, J. E. A.: Minimally invasive surgery. J. Endourology, 1:71, 1987.

Wickham, J. E. A., and Miller, R. A.: Nephroscopy: Endoscopic instruments and their accessories. In Wickham, J. E. A., and Miller, R. A. (Eds.): Percutaneous Renal Surgery. New York, Churchill Livingstone, 1983, p. 45.

Winfield, H.: Laparoscopy for the urologist. Eighth World Congress on Endourology and ESWL, August, 1990.

Winfield, H. W., and Clayman, R. V.: Complications of percutaneous removal of renal and ureteral calculi. Part I. World Urology Update Series, Volume 2, Lesson 37, 1985.

Winfield, H. N., and Ryan, K. G.: Experimental laparoscopic surgery: Potential clinical applications in urology. J. Endourol., 4:37, 1990.

Wise, G. J.: Amphotericin B in urological practice. J. Urol., 144:215, 1990.

Wise, G. J., Kozinn, P. J., and Goldberg, P.: Amphotericin B as a urologic irrigant in the management of noninvasive candiduria. J. Urol., 128:82, 1982.

Wishnow, K. I., Johnson, D. E., Preston, D., et al.: Long-term serum creatinine values after radical nephrectomy. Urology, 35:114, 1990.

Witherington, R., and Shelor, W. C.: Treatment of postoperative ureteral stricture by catheter dilation. A forgotten procedure. Urology, 16:592, 1980.

Young, A. T.: Percutaneous nephrostomy: Opacification of collecting system. In Amplatz, K., and Lange, P. H. (Eds.): Atlas of Endourology. Chicago, Year Book Medical Publishers, 1986a, p. 39.

Young, A. T.: Percutaneous nephrostomy: Puncture techniques. In Amplatz, K., and Lange, P. H. (Eds.): Atlas of Endourology. Chicago, Year Book Medical Publishers, 1986b, p. 55.

Young, A. T., Hunter, D. W., Castaneda-Zuniga, W. R., et al.: Percutaneous extraction of urinary calculi: Use of the intercostal approach. Radiology, 154:633, 1985.

Zachrisson, L.: Simple renal cysts treated with bismuth phosphate at the diagnostic puncture. Acta Radiol. Diagn., 23:209, 1982.

XIV
UROLOGIC
SURGERY

63
PERIOPERATIVE CARE

Charles B. Brendler, M.D.

Since this chapter was first written in 1984, there have been major changes in perioperative care that have had an impact on patients with urologic disorders. Because nearly all patients are now admitted either on the day of the surgical procedure or at most 1 day before, the responsibility for preoperative evaluation and preparation of patients for surgery lies increasingly with the urologist. Because it is no longer possible to obtain preoperative inpatient consultations, the urologist must recognize potential risk factors that may affect perioperative morbidity and must supervise preoperative planning and treatment in an outpatient setting. In addition, the urologist must keep abreast of continued improvements in perioperative care to achieve the best results.

PERIOPERATIVE CARDIAC CARE

Preoperative Assessment

Multifactorial Risk Assessment

The first multifactorial index of cardiac risk in noncardiac surgery was published in 1977 (Goldman et al., 1977). The nine clinical factors in the index were found to have independent predictive value for risk of cardiac complications and were weighted with "risk points" to allow a preoperative estimate of the risk of perioperative cardiac mortality and morbidity (Table 63–1). Factors that were found not to be independent risk predictors included hypertension, diabetes, stable angina, smoking, peripheral vascular disease, and hypercholesterolemia.

The index assigns patients to one of four classes according to level of risk. Thirty-eight of the 53 risk points are derived directly from cardiac conditions, and 28 of the 53 points are reversible. Since this index was derived, it has been prospectively evaluated at other institutions (Detsky et al., 1986) and has been shown to separate patients into risk groups reliably (Table 63–2). Congestive heart failure and recent myocardial infarc-

Table 63–1. MULTIFACTORIAL INDEX OF CARDIAC RISK IN NONCARDIAC SURGERY

Parameter	Points
History	
Myocardial infarction within 6 months	10
Age over 70 years	5
Physical Examination	
S_3 or jugular venous distention	11
Important aortic stenosis	3
Electrocardiogram	
Rhythm other than sinus or sinus plus atrial premature beats on last preoperative electrocardiogram	7
More than five premature ventricular beats per minute at any time preoperatively	7
Other	
Poor general medical status*	3
Intraperitoneal, intrathoracic, or aortic surgery	3
Emergency operation	4
Total	53

*Electrolyte abnormalities (potassium < 3.0 mEq/L or HCO_3 < 20 mEq/L); renal insufficiency (blood urea nitrogen > 50 mg/dl or creatinine > 3.0 mg/dl); abnormal blood gases (PO_2 < 60 mm Hg or PCO_2 > 50 mm Hg); abnormal liver status (elevated serum aspartate transaminase or signs on physical examination of chronic liver disease); or any condition that has caused the patient to be chronically bedridden.

From Goldman, L., Caldera, D. L., Nussbaum, S. R., et al.: Reprinted by permission from the New England Journal of Medicine 297:845–850, 1977.

tion (<6 months) remain the two strongest predictors of perioperative cardiac morbidity.

Diagnostic Testing

12-LEAD ELECTROCARDIOGRAM. The value of the preoperative electrocardiogram (ECG) for predicting perioperative cardiac morbidity is controversial. Goldman and colleagues found that ECG abnormalities had no significant predictive value (Goldman et al., 1978). A later study found that an abnormal preoperative ECG was the best diagnostic predictor of adverse cardiac outcome, even more predictive than preoperative exercise stress test changes. Specifically, ST-T wave ischemic or nonspecific changes and intraventricular conduction delays were the abnormalities that occurred most frequently in the patients with adverse outcomes

Table 63-2. MAJOR COMPLICATION RATES IN STUDIES IN WHICH THE MULTIFACTORIAL RISK INDEX WAS ANALYZED

Class	Definition (Points)	Goldman Unselected Noncardiac Surgery Patients > 40 Years Old		Zeldin Unselected Noncardiac Surgery Patients > 40 Years Old		Detsky Referrals for Preoperative Medical Consultation		Jeffrey Abdominal Aortic Aneurysm Surgery	
I	0-5	5/537	(1%)	4/590	(1%)	8/134	(6%)	4/56	(7%)
II	6-12	21/316	(7%)	13/453	(3%)	6/85	(7%)	4/35	(11%)
III	13-25	18/130	(14%)	11/74	(15%)	9/45	(20%)	3/8	(38%)
IV	≥ 26	14/18	(78%)	7/23	(30%)	4/4	(100%)	0	
All patients:		58/1001	(6%)	35/1140	(3%)	27/268	(10%)	11/99	(11%)

Adapted from Goldman, L.: J. Cardiothorac. Anesth., 1:237-244, 1987.

(Carliner et al., 1985). Further study is necessary, but at present all patients older than age 40 undergoing major urologic procedures should have a preoperative ECG.

CHEST RADIOGRAPHY. The presence of cardiomegaly on the chest x-ray film indicates a low ejection fraction (<0.40) in more than 70 per cent of patients with coronary artery disease (Mangano, 1987). Because a low preoperative ejection fraction predicts perioperative cardiac morbidity, radiographic cardiomegaly may also predict such morbidity (Foster et al., 1986). A tortuous or calcified aorta on a preoperative chest x-ray film has also been reported to be a predictor (Goldman et al., 1977). In general, however, routine chest radiography is not indicated in noncardiac surgery except for patients with pre-existing cardiopulmonary disease.

EXERCISE STRESS TESTING. Exercise stress testing is relatively inexpensive, is noninvasive, and is highly predictive of subsequent cardiac events when ST changes are (1) characteristic; (2) large (>2.5 mm); (3) immediate (first 1 to 3 minutes); (4) sustained into the recovery period; or (5) associated with subnormal increases in blood pressure (Mangano, 1990). One study reported that 27 per cent of patients with a negative history and normal preoperative ECG had a positive exercise stress test, and 26 per cent of these patients developed a perioperative myocardial infarction (Cutler et al., 1981). Such asymptomatic patients will escape identification by risk factor analysis and thus may benefit from preoperative exercise stress testing. A later study, however, found that preoperative stress testing did not independently predict cardiac risk in noncardiac surgical patients over age 40 (Carliner et al., 1985). At present, exercise stress testing has limited value for generalized screening of healthy asymptomatic patients.

AMBULATORY ECG MONITORING. Ambulatory ECG monitoring has proved to be successful in detecting ST-T changes in patients with coronary artery disease. In one study, 200 patients undergoing peripheral vascular surgery were monitored perioperatively by means of a real-time ambulatory ECG device. Nine patients suffered acute perioperative myocardial infarctions within the first 48 hours after surgery. All nine patients displayed evidence of silent myocardial ischemia during the perioperative period, and there were no perioperative myocardial infarctions among patients who did not experience silent ischemia. Multivariate analysis of perioperative risk factors revealed that preoperative silent myocardial ischemia and angina at rest were the only significant predictors of perioperative myocardial infarction. Thus, preoperative ambulatory ECG monitoring in high-risk patients is a practical and effective method of predicting patients at risk for myocardial infarction. Such patients may benefit from pretreatment with beta-blocking agents, nitrates, and calcium channel–blocking agents to limit myocardial ischemia (Pasternack et al., 1989).

OTHER DIAGNOSTIC TESTS. Evaluation of cardiac risk in asymptomatic patients without a previous history of cardiac disease should include only a multivariate risk factor analysis and a 12-lead ECG. In patients with a history of cardiac disease, chest radiography, exercise stress testing, and ambulatory ECG monitoring should be considered. Additional diagnostic tests that may be of value for high-risk patients include precordial echocardiography, radionuclide imaging, magnetic resonance imaging, and cardiac catheterization. Radionuclide cardiography is a noninvasive test that measures left ventricular function accurately. In high-risk patients with heart failure or severe ischemic heart disease, there is a significantly higher risk of cardiovascular complications when the left ventricular ejection fraction is abnormal (Pedersen et al., 1990). Radionuclide imaging with dipyridamole and thallium-201 has been found to be superior to both risk factor analysis and echocardiographic measurement of left ventricular function in detecting coronary artery disease in patients undergoing operation for aortic aneurysm. Scintigraphy not only is highly predictive of perioperative cardiac morbidity, but also identifies a significant number of patients with occult coronary artery disease otherwise undetected who benefit from preoperative coronary revascularization (McEnroe et al., 1990). Although these diagnostic tests are seldom indicated for asymptomatic patients, they should be considered for high-risk patients.

Perioperative Management

Congestive Heart Failure

Patients with no prior history of congestive heart failure are at low risk for the development of postoperative pulmonary edema or congestive heart failure. On the other hand, patients with clinical heart failure (New York Heart Classification III/IV) have little or no cardiac reserve and have a greater risk for cardiac morbidity and mortality. Patients with an S_3 gallop or jugular venous distention who are undergoing noncardiac surgical procedures have a 20 per cent incidence of perioperative cardiac mortality (Goldman et al., 1977). In a study of patients undergoing elective surgery who had suffered myocardial infarctions in the previous year, congestive heart failure was the most significant risk factor for cardiac mortality in the patients who died after appendectomy and the only significant risk factor for cardiac mortality in patients undergoing hip surgery (Dirksen and Kjøller, 1988). Conversely, patients with compensated congestive heart failure do not have an increased risk for surgically related cardiac complications. It is recommended, therefore, that patients with severe congestive heart failure undergo corrective treatment with digitalis, diuretics, and vasodilators before undergoing surgery.

The indications for preoperative administration of digitalis include (1) a prior history of congestive heart failure, (2) cardiac dysfunction with evidence of impaired ventricular performance, (3) nocturnal angina, (4) atrial fibrillation or flutter with a rapid ventricular response, and (5) frequent episodes of paroxysmal atrial or junctional tachycardia (Mason, 1974). Digitalis is not recommended on the basis of either advanced age or the presence of coronary artery disease alone. Digitalis should be started several days before surgery so that an adequate therapeutic level can be achieved.

Additional therapeutic measures that may be used in patients with congestive heart failure include the administration of diuretics to decrease the ventricular fluid load and the use of cardiotonic and vasodilating agents, such as isoproterenol, dopamine, and nitroprusside, to improve myocardial function. Patients receiving beta-blockers should continue to use them perioperatively. Withdrawal may precipitate serious myocardial ischemia, and perioperative administration of these agents has beneficial antiarrhythmic effects and protects against myocardial ischemia. Beta-blockers should be continued throughout the perioperative period and should be administered parenterally if necessary (Frishman, 1987).

Myocardial Infarction

The incidence of myocardial infarction after noncardiac surgery in the general population is about 0.5 per cent (Roberts and Tinker, 1988). A perioperative infarction rate of 1.1 per cent has been reported in patients with coronary artery disease, and a nonfatal infarction rate of 1.8 per cent in patients over age 40 with or without a history of coronary artery disease (Foster et al., 1986). Reinfarction rates in patients who have sustained a previous myocardial infarction greater than 6 months previously have been reported between 5 and 8 per cent. However, patients who undergo surgery within 3 months after a myocardial infarction have up to a 37 per cent incidence of reinfarction (von Knorring, 1981). In one study, the overall reinfarction rate was reduced to 1.9 per cent, increasing to only 5.7 per cent when the previous infarction was recent (<3 months), with aggressive intraoperative monitoring and extended stay in an intensive care unit (Rao et al., 1983).

Perioperative myocardial infarction usually occurs in the first postoperative week and is silent in about 50 per cent of patients. The mortality from an initial myocardial infarction is about 20 to 30 per cent, whereas the mortality from a recurrent myocardial infarction is between 50 and 80 per cent. Careful preoperative surveillance is therefore mandatory in patients with a previous history of myocardial infarction. A strategy that combines daily clinical evaluation with a routine ECG on the day of operation and on the first and second postoperative days has a 96 per cent sensitivity rate in detecting infarctions. Strategies that combine clinical evaluation, ECG, and cardiac isoenzymes have similar sensitivity rates, but higher false-positive rates (Charlson et al., 1988).

Because of the high mortality associated with a recurrent myocardial infarction, elective surgery should be postponed for at least 3 months, and preferably 6 months, after an infarction. Because about 50 per cent of recurrent myocardial infarctions are clinically silent, patients who have had a recent myocardial infarction and must undergo surgical procedures should be monitored closely in an intensive care unit for several days postoperatively. A continuous ECG, blood pressure monitoring with an arterial catheter, and evaluation of left ventricular function with a pulmonary arterial (Swan-Ganz) catheter may be required. Hypoxia should be avoided, and electrolyte and acid-base disorders should be corrected promptly to decrease the incidence of arrhythmias. Arrhythmias should be treated by use of appropriate drugs, by the insertion of a cardiac pacemaker, or by the application of direct current countershock when necessary (Baesl and Buckley, 1983).

Local anesthesia can be administered during the first 6 months after a myocardial infarction (Backer et al., 1980), and cystoscopy can be performed safely with local anesthesia without cardiac complications. The risk of perioperative infarction after transurethral resection of the prostate is less than 0.5 per cent, and this procedure has been performed safely within the first 6 months after a myocardial infarction (Ashton et al., 1989). Nevertheless, it would seem reasonable to postpone any elective surgery requiring general or regional anesthesia for 6 months.

Patients with stable angina and without a prior history of myocardial infarction do not have an increased perioperative cardiac risk (Goldman et al., 1978). Patients with unstable or post-infarction angina have a markedly increased risk and should undergo coronary angiography before undergoing urologic surgery. Such patients may require cardiac revascularization, either with angioplasty or coronary bypass surgery, before elective procedures.

Arrhythmias

PREOPERATIVE ARRHYTHMIAS. Sinus bradycardia is often not a pathologic rhythm but is commonly encountered because of a drug effect, that is, beta-blockers or digoxin. If the cause cannot be determined, patients should undergo further evaluation, including exercise stress testing and possible administration of atropine, to determine if the heart rate can be elevated above 100 beats per minute. Patients with sick sinus syndrome should be considered for placement of a permanent pacemaker depending on associated symptoms (Rose et al., 1979).

Premature atrial contractions are usually benign, but they may reflect a decreased cardiac reserve, which may increase cardiac risk. Patients with ventricular arrhythmias are at increased risk when undergoing surgery, and the presence of complex ventricular ectopy on preoperative evaluation necessitates cardiologic consultation for possible underlying cardiac disease. Although occasional premature ventricular contractions may not require treatment, frequent premature ventricular contractions or potentially dangerous ventricular extrasystoles (multifocal, salvos, or occurring on the preceding T wave) do require treatment. If treatment is required, the initial treatment is intravenous lidocaine given as a bolus of 50 to 100 mg, followed by a continuous infusion of 1 to 4 mg/minute (Sakima, 1990).

INTRAOPERATIVE ARRHYTHMIAS. Premature ventricular contractions occur commonly during operation and usually are of little clinical significance. They often are precipitated by inadequate ventilation and increased adrenergic stimulation and can be treated by decreasing the concentration of anesthetic agent, hyperventilation, decreased administration of catecholamines, and decreased manipulation of vital organs. Ventricular tachyarrhythmias should be treated with antiarrhythmic agents, because they may cause circulatory depression or ventricular fibrillation (Sakima, 1990).

POSTOPERATIVE ARRHYTHMIAS. Supraventricular tachycardia occurs in about 4 per cent of surgical patients postoperatively (Goldman et al., 1978). Atrial fibrillation is the most common supraventricular tachyrhythmia and accounts for about half of the cases. Preoperative factors that are associated with the development of postoperative arrhythmias include age greater than 70 years; major thoracic, abdominal, or vascular operations; and the presence of pulmonary rales. Patients who develop postoperative arrhythmias frequently have one or more of the following associated problems: congestive heart failure, a history of a previous myocardial infarction, cardiac tamponade, a hematocrit of less than 30 per cent, hypotension, hypokalemia, metabolic acidosis, hypernatremia, hypoxia, or fever. Although the mortality associated with the arrhythmia alone is minimal, the overall mortality associated with these underlying conditions approaches 50 per cent (Goldman, 1978). A summary of antiarrhythmic therapy is provided in Table 63–3.

Valvular Heart Disease

Aortic stenosis is the cardiac valvular lesion associated with the greatest risk of cardiac morbidity in patients undergoing noncardiac surgery; severe aortic stenosis is associated with a 13 per cent risk of perioperative mortality (Goldman, 1978). The narrowing of the aortic valve restricts the ability of the cardiac output to increase in response to vasodilation or blood loss. Furthermore, left ventricular hypertrophy results in impaired ventricular compliance and impaired diastolic filling. Such

patients tolerate hypovolemia, tachycardia, and atrial fibrillation poorly. In patients with aortic and mitral valve insufficiency, the left ventricle is subjected to high fluid loads that can lead to impairment of contractility; in patients with mitral stenosis, tachycardia associated with the stress of surgery can lead to decreased cardiac output because of delayed emptying of the left atrium. Although the risks are not as great as those in patients with aortic stenosis, all patients with severe valvular disease should be considered for invasive hemodynamic monitoring, and careful attention should be given to fluid management. Patients with serious valvular dysfunction, particularly aortic stenosis, should undergo corrective heart surgery before undergoing elective noncardiac surgery (Lee and Goldman, 1990). All patients with valvular heart disease should receive antibacterial prophylaxis before undergoing any surgical procedure (see section on perioperative infections).

Patients with prosthetic heart valves have an increased risk for thromboembolic disease associated with cessation of anticoagulation therapy. This risk is greatest in patients with older caged-disc prosthetic mitral valves because of associated left atrial enlargement and atrial fibrillation. Patients with prosthetic aortic valves should discontinue using oral anticoagulants 2 to 3 days preoperatively; surgery can proceed when the prothrombin time is between 1 and 2 seconds above the control value. Intravenous heparin is started 12 to 24 hours postoperatively and is continued until anticoagulation with oral warfarin (Coumadin) has been achieved. Patients with prosthetic mitral valves should discontinue oral anticoagulation 2 days before operation but should be admitted to the hospital and receive continuous intravenous heparin until 6 hours preoperatively and should resume

Table 63–3. THERAPY OF ARRHYTHMIAS

Arrhythmias	Therapy (In Order of Preference)
Supraventricular arrhythmias	
Paroxysmal supraventricular tachycardia	Carotid sinus massage, digoxin, verapamil, quinidine, procainamide
Atrial flutter	Cardioversion, digoxin, quinidine, procainamide
Atrial fibrillation	Cardioversion, quinidine, procainamide, disopyramide (to maintain sinus rhythm); digoxin, propranolol, verapamil (to control ventricular response)
Ventricular arrhythmias	
PVCs*, emergency	Lidocaine, procainamide, bretylium
PVCs, chronic	Quinidine, procainamide, disopyramide, combinations (see later)
Tachycardia	Lidocaine, procainamide, bretylium, cardioversion
Combination therapy for suppression of ventricular ectopy	Quinidine or procainamide (type I agents) with mexiletine or tocainide (type Ib agents) Quinidine or procainamide with propranolol in patients without congestive heart failure
Digitalis-induced arrhythmias	Lidocaine, diphenylhydantoin

*PVCs, premature ventricular contractions.

heparin 12 hours postoperatively. Any residual elevation in the prothrombin time should be normalized with fresh frozen plasma or vitamin K. The use of intravenous heparin in the perioperative period has the advantages of a rapid onset of action and the potential for rapid reversibility in case of hemorrhage (Katholi et al., 1978).

Hypertension

Although it is desirable for patients to be normotensive before the surgery, patients with diastolic blood pressures less than 120 mm Hg do not have an increased risk of cardiac complications (Goldman and Caldera, 1979). Patients with diastolic blood pressures greater than 120 mm Hg do have an increased risk at surgery, mainly because they may have wider and more frequent changes of blood pressure while they are under anesthesia. Patients whose normal systolic blood pressure falls by more than one third for as little as 10 minutes during surgery have an increased incidence of cardiovascular complications (Goldman and Caldera, 1979). As with beta-adrenergic blockers, other antihypertensive agents should be continued until the time of surgery and should not be withdrawn preoperatively. Clonidine, a central-acting antiadrenergic agent, deserves special mention, because abrupt cessation of this drug may precipitate severe hypertension. Patients receiving clonidine who will not be able to resume oral medications for several days postoperatively should discontinue taking clonidine 2 weeks preoperatively and should start alternative therapy (Blaschke and Melmon, 1980). Patients receiving diuretics should be evaluated preoperatively for possible hypokalemia and hypovolemia.

Intraoperatively, both tracheal intubation and emergence from anesthesia are associated with increased catecholamine secretion and transient increases in heart rate and blood pressure. This stress response is frequently exaggerated in hypertensive patients and produces an increase in myocardial oxygen demand and possible myocardial ischemia. In hypertensive patients, a single small oral dose of a beta-adrenergic–blocking agent such as labetalol, atenolol, or oxprenolol given with the premedication can reduce the risk of intraoperative myocardial ischemia (Stone et al., 1988).

Postoperatively, blood pressure should be regulated with parenteral agents until oral medications can be resumed. Alpha-adrenergic–blocking drugs, such as phentolamine, and direct-acting vasodilators, such as nitroglycerine and nitroprusside, are commonly used to treat postoperative hypertension. Nifedipine, a calcium channel blocker, may also be used, but because no intravenous preparation is available, its effects are not titratable. Nicardipine is a new, short-acting calcium channel blocker and a potent vasodilator that can be given intravenously. Studies have shown that nicardipine is extremely effective in the treatment of postoperative hypertension (Goldberg et al., 1990; Kaplan, 1990).

Pacemakers

Permanent pacemakers should be checked preoperatively to be sure they are capturing consistently and firing at the stated rate. Direct electromagnetic interference of a permanent demand pacemaker by the use of electrocautery during surgery may cause pacemaker inhibition. This is of particular concern in patients undergoing transurethral resection, and certain precautions are necessary to protect patients in this situation. First, in patients who are pacemaker dependent (i.e., complete heart block), the pacemaker should be changed preoperatively from a demand to a fixed mode. Second, the diathermy plate should be positioned as far away from the pacemaker as possible, usually on the thigh or the buttocks. Third, the active tip of the electrocautery should remain at least 15 cm away from the pacemaker, because ventricular fibrillation can be induced if the electrocautery current is conducted down the lead to the heart. Fourth, the duration of each cautery burst should be limited as much as possible. Fifth, a temporary pacemaker as well as antiarrhythmic agents should be available in the operating room in case a problem develops (Simon, 1977).

Cardiovascular Effects of Anesthesia

All anesthetic agents produce some degree of myocardial depression, which may result in perioperative heart failure or cardiogenic shock (Kaplan and Dunbar, 1979). This depression may occur at levels of anesthetic that produce only light anesthesia. Halothane produces the greatest myocardial depression, and nitrous oxide the least. Narcotics have a variable effect on myocardial function. Morphine and fentanyl have minimal depressant activity, but meperidine has a marked depressant effect (Lee et al., 1976). Barbiturates produce vasodilatation and have little myocardial depressant action except in large doses. Benzodiazepines such as valium and midazolam are generally free of cardiovascular effects except when administered by rapid infusion (Stanley et al., 1976).

Anesthetic agents may also precipitate cardiac arrhythmias. Arrhythmias frequently occur during induction of anesthesia, intubation, and extubation because of associated blood pressure changes, hypoxia, hypercapnea, and endogenous catecholamine release. The incidence of arrhythmias is greater in patients with a history of heart disease.

Regional anesthesia is not necessarily safer than general anesthesia in terms of cardiac risk. Regional anesthesia has two potential disadvantages. First, it may produce hypotension by sympathetic blockade, and second, it is not as reversible as general anesthesia if cardiac problems develop intraoperatively. Local anesthesia is usually safe, although local anesthetic agents may produce myocardial depression when administered in large doses (Beattie, 1990).

Hemodynamic Monitoring

Arterial Pressure Monitoring

INDICATIONS. Direct blood pressure monitoring is indicated (1) when there may be rapid changes in blood pressure as a result of underlying cardiac disease; (2) when patients are expected to lose large volumes of blood or can be expected to have sudden changes in blood pressure because of the nature of the surgical procedure (e.g., that for pheochromocytoma); and (3) after an operation, when unstable patients receive intravenous infusions of vasopressor or vasodilating agents (Merritt, 1990).

TECHNIQUES. Continuous blood pressure monitoring can be done by either noninvasive or invasive techniques. Noninvasive techniques include oscillotonometry, Doppler ultrasonography, and plethysmography. A relatively new method of noninvasive blood pressure measurement is based on photoelectric measurement of pressure and volume in the finger. A small pneumatic finger cup is inflated to a pressure equal to the arterial transmural pressure. An infrared transmission plethysmograph signal on one side of the finger and a photoelectric detector on the opposite side track the relative arterial volume instantaneously. Computerized algorithms allow the small cup to maintain transmural pressure at 0 so that cup pressure then equals arterial blood pressure. The plethysmogram produced by these measurements is displayed on a monitor screen and closely resembles an arterial wave form. Hypothermia, hypovolemia, low cardiac output, proximal arterial constriction, and the use of vasoconstrictors may make these devices unreliable. However, if these limitations can be overcome, this form of monitoring could become of major intraoperative significance (Boehmer, 1987).

Direct arterial monitoring is preferable whenever hemodynamic instability is anticipated and when repeated arterial blood sampling is required. Arterial puncture causes significant discomfort to patients, and percutaneous arterial samples may be inaccurate because of admixture of small amounts of venous blood (Sheldon and Leonard, 1983).

The usual technique for the placement of an arterial catheter involves percutaneous insertion of a Teflon catheter over a thin needle into the nondominant radial artery. Alternative sites of arterial cannulation should be considered if there is insufficiency of the ulnar artery or palmar arch. In adults and children, alternative sites include the axillary, femoral, and dorsalis pedis arteries, and in infants the umbilical and temporal arteries may be used.

COMPLICATIONS. Complications of arterial cannulation include (1) hand ischemia; (2) radial artery thrombosis; (3) arterial embolization; and (4) heparin-induced thrombocytopenia. The patency of the palmar arch should be tested before radial artery cannulation to determine the patency of the ulnar artery and palmar arch. Arterial catheters should be removed as soon as possible and whenever thrombosis or ischemia is noted. The risk of arterial embolization can be reduced by using a continuous infusion rather than bolus administration of heparin to maintain catheter patency and by never irrigating the arterial cannula forcefully (Sheldon and Leonard, 1983).

Central Venous Pressure Monitoring

INDICATIONS. The main indication for measurement of central venous pressure is to provide a dynamic assessment of volume status. The most direct method of assessing circulatory volume and left ventricular function is by measurement of left atrial pressure via a left atrial catheter, which must be inserted at the time of open heart surgery. Alternatively, left ventricular end-diastolic pressure can be measured with a pulmonary arterial catheter inserted into the pulmonary arterial capillary bed (Swan and Ganz, 1975).

Central venous pressure measurements are unreliable for assessing intravascular volume and left ventricular function in patients with cardiorespiratory disease, in whom left ventricular and right ventricular function may differ significantly. In the absence of cardiorespiratory disease, however, there is a close correlation between the two measurements. Despite its limitations, the measurement of central venous pressure usually provides a useful first approximation of the adequacy of blood volume and ventricular function.

TECHNIQUES. Central venous pressure catheters are inserted via a percutaneous approach into the basilic, external jugular, internal jugular, or subclavian vein. Techniques of catheter insertion have been described in detail elsewhere, with excellent diagrams (Sheldon and Leonard, 1983).

COMPLICATIONS. Complications of central venous catheter placement include (1) catheter misplacement, (2) pneumothorax, (3) hydrothorax, and (4) cardiac erosion with resultant tamponade. A chest radiograph must be obtained after insertion of a central venous pressure catheter to determine that the catheter is in the correct position and that a pneumothorax does not exist. Misplacement of the catheter can be corrected either by repositioning the catheter over a guide wire or by passing a Fogarty catheter within the central venous pressure cannula; the balloon of the catheter is inflated and the cannula is flow directed into the correct position (Schaefer and Geelhoed, 1980).

Pulmonary Arterial Pressure Monitoring

INDICATIONS. Pulmonary arterial pressure monitoring is indicated for clinical situations in which there is a disparity between left ventricular and right ventricular function. In these conditions, central venous pressure measurements are unreliable, and measurements of pulmonary arterial and pulmonary wedge pressures must be relied on to provide information about intravascular volume and left ventricular function. Changes in pulmonary arterial pressure accurately reflect changes in left atrial pressure, and there is a close correlation between an elevation in pulmonary wedge pressure above 18 to 20 mm Hg and radiologic evidence of pulmonary congestion (Del Guercio and Cohn, 1980).

TECHNIQUE. A pulmonary arterial, or Swan-Ganz, catheter usually is inserted percutaneously via an internal jugular or a subclavian approach. After the catheter has been introduced, it is advanced under fluoroscopic guidance or by monitoring the pressure at the tip of the catheter to determine its position. After the catheter enters the heart, the balloon at its end is inflated with air to facilitate flow guidance through the right ventricle and pulmonary artery. As the catheter is advanced further, the balloon becomes wedged in the pulmonary capillary bed. The catheter is withdrawn slightly and is positioned so that wedging is achieved only on full inflation of the balloon. Pulmonary wedge pressure normally varies between 5 and 12 mm Hg. After insertion of a Swan-Ganz catheter, a chest roentgenogram should be obtained to check the position of the catheter tip, and daily chest films should be obtained to monitor for possible catheter migration. Patency of the catheter is achieved by a continuous slow infusion of heparinized saline (Sheldon and Leonard, 1983).

COMPLICATIONS. The complications associated with the use of pulmonary arterial catheters include technical problems such as catheter misplacement and pneumothorax. In addition, 80 per cent of patients undergoing insertion of a pulmonary arterial catheter experience cardiac arrhythmias as the catheter is advanced through the right ventricle. These arrhythmias usually are self-limiting and resolve when the catheter passes into the pulmonary artery. It is important to monitor the ECG and to treat any serious arrhythmias promptly (Elliott et al., 1979).

Pulmonary infarction, arterial thrombosis, and arterial embolization have resulted from insertion of pulmonary arterial catheters. Perforation of the pulmonary artery has also been reported; it is a rare but devastating complication with a 50 per cent mortality (Barash et al., 1981). To minimize the risk of arterial perforation, the catheter balloon should never be inflated with fluid, the balloon should not be inflated too distally in the pulmonary capillary bed, and inflation of the balloon for measurement of pulmonary wedge pressure should be kept to a minimum (Kelley et al., 1981).

Damage to both tricuspid and pulmonary valves has been reported from withdrawal of the catheter through the right-hand chambers of the heart with the catheter balloon inflated (O'Toole et al., 1979). This report reemphasizes the importance of never inflating the catheter balloon with anything other than air.

Cardiac Output and Mixed Venous Oxygen Saturation

Placement of a pulmonary arterial catheter allows for direct measurement of cardiac output by a thermodilution technique. Measured cardiac output values are normalized by dividing the cardiac output by the body surface area and expressing the results in liters per minute per square meter. A normal cardiac index varies between 2.7 and 4.3 L/minute/m². Values between 2.2 and 2.7 L/minute/m² indicate subclinical myocardial depression; values between 1.8 and 2.2 L/minute/m² are associated with clinical myocardial depression; and values less than 1.8 L/minute/m² reflect cardiac insufficiency (Forrester et al., 1976).

Placement of a pulmonary arterial catheter also makes possible the measurement of mixed venous oxygen saturation, which is an additional parameter to assess the adequacy of peripheral perfusion. The mixed venous oxygen saturation is usually measured by blood sampling directly from the pulmonary arterial catheter. Alterna-

tively, an indwelling fiberoptic oxymeter can be placed on the pulmonary arterial catheter, which allows for a continuous digital readout. The mixed venous oxygen saturation correlates closely with cardiac output (De la Rocha et al., 1978). Values between 60 and 70 per cent are associated with adequate peripheral perfusion; values between 50 and 60 per cent suggest myocardial depression; and values between 40 and 50 per cent reflect circulatory failure (Kazarian and Del Guercia, 1980).

Pulse Oximetry

Adequate oxygenation is essential during all surgical procedures; hypoxia accounts for the majority of surgical deaths. A number of monitoring devices are currently used to assess the adequacy of oxygenation throughout the perioperative period. Pulse oximetry measures the oxygen saturation of hemoglobin and has greatly decreased the need for direct measurement of arterial blood gases. The pulse oximeter utilizes a finger probe, which combines the principles of photoelectric plethysmography and oximetry (New, 1985). The ratio of absorbance of oxygenated to reduced hemoglobin at 2 monochromatic wavelengths (660 and 940 nm) allows calculation of the per cent saturation of hemoglobin. The usefulness of pulse oximetry may be limited by motion, low hemoglobin values, intravenous dyes, fiberoptic and infrared light sources, electrocautery, and settings in which venous flow has a pulsatile quality, as with tricuspid regurgitation. Nevertheless, pulse oximetry has proved to be the best oxygenation monitor to date (Merritt, 1990).

Capnography

Infrared sensitive filters and photocells can be used to measure carbon dioxide levels in expired gas to provide an accurate measure of the adequacy of ventilation. The measurement of end-tidal concentration of carbon dioxide is recommended for ensurance of adequate ventilatory support, intraoperatively as well as postoperatively. End-tidal samples of respiratory gases can be analyzed at the bedside by mass spectroscopy. The cost of this equipment, however, has limited its use, and end-tidal carbon dioxide monitoring is most commonly done by using an infrared detection system. The accuracy of this system can be validated intermittently by direct measurement of carbon dioxide in arterial blood (Merritt, 1990).

PERIOPERATIVE PULMONARY CARE

Preoperative Assessment and Management

Initial Evaluation

The initial evaluation of respiratory status in patients without a previous history or symptoms of pulmonary disease should include only a history and physical examination. Important historical considerations include smoking, the presence of a productive cough or wheezing, exercise tolerance, previous exposure to general anesthesia, and the possibility of a recent upper respiratory tract infection. Significant physical findings include orthopnea or dyspnea at rest, pauses during speech caused by dyspnea, and wheezes with augmented breathing (Jackson, 1988).

A preoperative chest radiograph should be obtained for patients with a previous history or symptoms of cardiopulmonary disease and for patients over 50 years old with a history of smoking. Preoperative chest radiographs seldom show significant pathologic changes and infrequently result in a change in perioperative management. In a recent prospective study, the preoperative chest x-ray film led to a modification in perioperative management in only 5 per cent of patients having radiography; conversely, in only 0.07 per cent of patients not having preoperative radiography was it thought in retrospect that such a study would have been potentially useful (Charpak, 1988).

The ECG is an insensitive measure for detecting pulmonary disease, but the ECG findings of right ventricular hypertrophy are specific, and an ECG should be obtained in patients with a history of chronic obstructive pulmonary disease (COPD). The ECG may also reveal arrhythmias, which occur frequently in the perioperative period in patients with COPD (Brashear, 1984).

Although pulmonary function testing has measurable benefit in predicting outcome in candidates for lung resection, its value for patients undergoing abdominal surgical procedures has not been established. In patients undergoing upper-abdominal surgery, spirometry is recommended only for cigarette smokers or for patients who have respiratory symptoms that have not been previously evaluated. In patients undergoing lower-abdominal and pelvic surgery, the risk of pulmonary complications is much lower, and routine pulmonary function testing appears unlikely to result in treatment that will alter outcome. In urologic surgery, pulmonary function testing appears indicated only for patients undergoing major abdominal or flank procedures who have a history of cigarette smoking, marked obesity, or previously unevaluated pulmonary symptoms (Zibrak et al., 1990).

Arterial blood gas measurements are usually indicated only for patients with abnormal pulmonary function test results. In patients with COPD, an elevated arterial partial pressure of carbon dioxide, rather than the forced expiratory volume in 1 second, appears to be the most important factor predicting postoperative pulmonary complications (Hotchkiss, 1988).

Pulmonary Risk Factors

CIGARETTE SMOKING. Cigarette smokers and patients with chronic pulmonary disease have a 3- to 4-fold increased risk for postoperative pulmonary morbidity, and a 7- to 10-fold higher mortality rate (Fowkes et al., 1982). Patients with a history of 20 pack-years of smoking and patients currently smoking more than 10 cigarettes a day have an increased risk of developing pulmonary complications (Pearce and Jones, 1984). Patients with restrictive lung disease generally do better than patients with obstructive disease, because patients with restrictive disease maintain an adequate maximal expiratory flow rate, which allows a more effective cough with less retention of sputum.

SITE OF INCISION. The site of the surgical incision also affects pulmonary risk. Except for thoracotomy incisions, upper-abdominal incisions are associated with the highest incidence of atelectasis because of reduced diaphragmatic excursion and suppressed coughing and deep breathing related to incisional pain. In one study, 25 per cent of patients who had upper-abdominal incisions developed pulmonary complications, whereas all patients who had pulmonary complications after lower-abdominal incisions either had pre-existing lung disease or were cigarette smokers (Forthman and Shepard, 1969). Subcostal incisions are associated with fewer pulmonary complications and better pulmonary mechanical ventilation than are midline incisions (Garcia-Valdecasas et al., 1988).

LENGTH OF PROCEDURE. Anesthesia time in excess of 3 hours is associated with increased pulmonary complications, but the reason for this association remains unexplained (Roukema et al., 1988).

POOR PREOPERATIVE NUTRITION. Protein-depleted patients demonstrate a significant reduction in respiratory muscle strength, vital capacity, and peak expiratory flow rate. The risk of developing pneumonia is significantly higher in protein-depleted patients, and efforts should be made to correct this risk factor before elective surgery (Windsor and Hill, 1988).

OBESITY. Severe obesity (>250 per cent of predicted body weight) is associated with a greatly increased risk of pulmonary complications (Ray et al., 1983). Obesity results in decreased expiratory reserve volume, decreased functional reserve capacity, ventilation-perfusion inequality, intrapulmonary shunting, impaired oxygenation, and increased breathing work. Increased gastric volume and decreased gastric pH in obese patients may result in extensive lung injury if aspiration occurs perioperatively (Pasulka et al., 1986).

AGE. Age alone is not a risk factor for pulmonary complications, and older patients whose pulmonary function is comparable to that of younger patients do not experience increased pulmonary morbidity. Overall, there is a higher incidence of pulmonary complications in older patients because of the prevalence of pulmonary disease and associated abnormalities in pulmonary function (Grodsinsky et al., 1974).

Preoperative Measures to Decrease Pulmonary Risk

In patients with pre-existing lung disease, cessation of smoking and the preoperative use of antibiotics and bronchodilators result in a significant reduction in postoperative pulmonary complications. Cigarette smoking should be discontinued at least 8 weeks before surgery. Patients who discontinue smoking less than 8 weeks before surgery actually have a higher risk of developing pulmonary complications than patients who continue to smoke up to the time of surgery. This result may be due to the acute absence of the irritating effect of cigarette smoke, which may further decrease postoperative coughing and result in a greater risk of pulmonary complications. However, patients who discontinue smoking more than 8 weeks preoperatively have a significantly lower complication rate, and patients who have ceased smoking for more than 6 months have a pulmonary morbidity similar to that of patients without a smoking history (Warner et al., 1989).

Patients with acute respiratory infections should be treated with antibiotics, and elective surgery should be delayed until the infections are resolved. Similarly, preoperative preparation of COPD patients can dramatically reduce postoperative pulmonary complications and should include aggressive use of bronchodilators, antibiotics, and chest physiotherapy. Newer broncodilating agents such as ipratropium bromide (Atrovent), a derivative of atropine, are administered by inhalation and have little systemic absorption (Easton et al., 1986). Beta-adrenergic agonists are more effective than aminophylline in the treatment of acute bronchospasm and can be administered safely in large doses (Hotchkiss, 1988). Preoperative treatment with corticosteroids is beneficial in patients with asthma (Pien et al., 1988). Chest physiotherapy begun preoperatively significantly lowers pulmonary morbidity (Castillo and Hass, 1985).

Patients who require intensive care postoperatively benefit from preoperative psychologic preparation and orientation to an intensive care environment. This preparation results in decreased pain and narcotic usage postoperatively and may reduce the length of hospitalization. Preoperative instruction in pulmonary therapy and deep breathing exercises is also beneficial.

Pulmonary Effects of Anesthesia and Surgery

General anesthesia reduces functional residual capacity (FRC) from 15 to 25 per cent below awake, supine values (Dueck et al., 1988). This result is thought to be due to compression of lung tissue caused by anesthesia-induced changes in the shape and motion of the chest wall (Brismar et al., 1985). There is a progressive decrease in FRC during anesthesia, probably because of spontaneous atelectasis secondary to ventilation with decreased tidal volumes (Harman and Lillington, 1979). Decreased FRC is associated with impaired oxygenation and shunting. The magnitude of shunting depends on the amount of atelectasis that develops, and atelectasis is greater in smokers and obese patients (Miller and Martin, 1990).

A number of physiologic changes occur postoperatively after general anesthesia, which also contribute to the development of atelectasis and pulmonary morbidity. Tidal volume, forced expiratory volume in 1 second, and FRC are all decreased in the postoperative period, more after abdominal or thoracic incisions than after lower-abdominal procedures (Meyers et al., 1975). These changes result from breathing in the supine

position, postoperative pain, the administration of narcotics, and other factors that reduce diaphragmatic excursion, including abdominal distention, pneumoperitoneum, and constrictive bandages (Harman and Lillington, 1979). The normal pattern of ventilation is altered postoperatively, resulting in a decreased number of sigh breaths and an increased risk of atelectasis. Narcotics, atropine, and the use of increased inspired oxygen concentrations impair mucociliary function, which results in retention of pulmonary secretions (Tisi, 1979).

Regional anesthesia commonly is assumed to be associated with a lower risk of pulmonary complications than is general anesthesia, but this assumption has not been proved. General anesthesia has the advantage that it allows continuous control of the airway and pulmonary secretions. Although the incidence of wheezing is lower in patients having regional anesthesia than in those having general anesthesia with intubation, it is not less than in patients having general anesthesia without intubation. Postoperative deterioration of pulmonary function is virtually universal but appears to be related to the surgical site rather than to the type of anesthesia (Beattie, 1990).

Postoperative Pulmonary Care

The primary goal of postoperative respiratory therapy is to prevent atelectasis and subsequent pneumonia by maintaining or restoring lung volume. To achieve this goal, a number of approaches have been developed: (1) aggressive postoperative analgesia; (2) incentive spirometry; (3) intermittent positive-pressure breathing devices; (4) continuous positive airway pressure (CPAP) by mask; and (5) chest physiotherapy (Hotchkiss, 1988).

Aggressive Postoperative Analgesia

Aggressive pain control in the postoperative period can reduce postoperative pulmonary complications. New approaches to postoperative analgesia include (1) epidural administration of narcotics or local anesthetics; (2) intrathecal administration of narcotics; (3) patient-controlled administration of narcotics or use of continuous-infusion devices; and (4) infusion of local anesthetics into intercostal nerves. There have now been several studies demonstrating that epidural analgesia and intrathecal morphine increase patient compliance and performance in both incentive spirometry and chest physiotherapy, thus reducing pulmonary morbidity (Yeager et al., 1987). Improved pain control is also achieved with patient-controlled administration of narcotics and the use of continuous-infusion devices (Hull, 1988). The use of intercostal nerve blocks after biliary surgery through a subcostal incision reduces postoperative pulmonary complications by 50 per cent and should be strongly considered for urologic patients having flank or intercostal incisions (Engberg and Wiklund, 1988).

Incentive Spirometry

The incentive spirometer is the most effective mechanical aid for promoting maximal inspiration and preventing atelectasis. Patients, however, must be instructed in their use. For the device to be effective, the patient must take a maximal inspiration and hold it for 2 to 3 seconds, and this procedure should be done 10 times an hour while the patient is awake. After patients have been properly instructed, the device can be left at the bedside for hourly use (Hotchkiss, 1988).

Intermittent Positive-Pressure Breathing Devices

Positive-pressure breathing was initially reported to be effective in decreasing atelectasis, but subsequent studies have failed to demonstrate its efficacy, and it has generally been replaced by incentive spirometry (Graham and Bradley, 1978). However, these devices may still be of value for patients who are unable to generate increased inspiratory volumes because of abnormal chest wall mechanics or inspiratory weakness. Patients with kyphoscoliosis or neuromuscular disease are examples of patients who may benefit from use of these devices as opposed to incentive spirometry, in combination with chest physiotherapy (Hotchkiss, 1988).

Continuous Positive Airway Pressure

Although CPAP is often used in the treatment of patients who are intubated, it is now possible to deliver CPAP by using a tight-fitting, flexible face mask. CPAP has been well documented to be highly effective in increasing FRC, and studies have shown that mask CPAP is much more effective in the treatment of atelectasis than conventional therapy alone. Mask CPAP is generally well tolerated by patients. The major complication is forcing air into the stomach, with subsequent vomiting and aspiration. Therefore, only transparent face masks should be used and only patients who are alert and able to protect the airway should be treated with this technique (Andersen et al., 1980).

Chest Physiotherapy

Chest physiotherapy is indicated for patients with COPD undergoing upper-abdominal surgery. When chest physiotherapy is performed by well-trained physical therapists, there is strong evidence that it is highly effective in reducing postoperative atelectasis (Castillo and Hass, 1985).

Ancillary Measures

Other measures may help to prevent atelectasis. Early mobilization is desirable because the supine position is associated with decreased lung volume. Appropriate fluid management to avoid overhydration with subsequent pulmonary congestion or dehydration with drying of mucous secretions is important. Bronchodilators may be effective in reducing atelectasis, even in patients without airway disease. Antibiotics are indicated for patients with acute bronchitis or pneumonia. Narcotics should be used cautiously to avoid respiratory depres-

sion. Also, patients with COPD and a hypoxic respiratory drive should receive oxygen in low concentrations to avoid respiratory depression (Gilmour, 1983).

Mechanical Ventilation

Indications

The usual indication for positive-pressure ventilation is acute respiratory failure manifested by a partial pressure of carbon dioxide (P_{CO_2}) greater than 50 mm Hg and a blood pH less than 7.30, or by profound hypoxia with a partial pressure of oxygen (P_{O_2}) less than 60 mm Hg and a fraction of inspired oxygen (F_{IO_2}) greater than 60 per cent. The primary goal of mechanical ventilation is to achieve satisfactory blood oxygenation at the lowest possible F_{IO_2}. Ancillary goals include providing adequate airway humidification and removing pulmonary secretions (Gilmour, 1983).

Physiology

A spontaneously breathing person normally takes 10 to 15 sighs per hour to ventilate dependent lung tissue. Patients receiving fixed-volume positive-pressure ventilation from a mechanical ventilator thus require larger tidal volumes to prevent atelectasis. The tidal volume in adults is set between 10 and 15 ml/kg and is delivered at a rate of 8 to 10 breaths per minute to achieve a minute volume between 8 and 15 L. Children older than 10 years are managed similarly to adults, but infants and younger children need a higher minute volume and are ventilated at a rate between 20 and 25 breaths per minute (Shapiro, 1981).

The F_{IO_2} is normally set to achieve a P_{O_2} between 60 and 90 mm Hg. An important exception is the level for patients with a hypoxic respiratory drive, in whom a lower P_{O_2} may be desirable to avoid respiratory depression. Oxygen toxicity becomes a concern when an F_{IO_2} of greater than 50 per cent is required to achieve an acceptable P_{O_2}, and some form of continuous distending pressure is required to facilitate oxygen delivery without further increasing the F_{IO_2} (Gilmour, 1983).

A mechanical ventilator should usually be used in the assist-control mode, and the sensitivity should be set so that the respirator is triggered easily by the patient's own inspiratory efforts. Patients should be able to take additional breaths with minimal effort to avoid psychologic disturbance and because increased breathing efforts may result in atelectasis (Gilmour, 1983).

Complications

DECREASED CARDIAC OUTPUT. Positive airway pressure increases intrathoracic pressure, thereby decreasing venous return and cardiac output. Any maneuver that increases intrathoracic pressure, such as increasing tidal volume or applying continuous airway-distending pressure, may result in a further decrease in cardiac output. Fortunately, the relationship between airway and intrathoracic pressures is modified by pulmonary compliance, so that a stiff, noncompliant lung does not transmit pressure to the same degree as does a healthy lung. Therefore, impairment of cardiac output is less severe in patients with respiratory disease, who may require increased intrathoracic pressure to achieve satisfactory oxygen delivery, than in patients with normal pulmonary function (Colgan et al., 1979).

DISTURBANCE OF VENTILATION-PERFUSION BALANCE. Ventilation and perfusion are normally distributed primarily to dependent lung tissue. Mechanical ventilation results in a disturbance of the ventilation-perfusion balance for a number of reasons. First, patients receiving positive-pressure ventilation frequently have pulmonary disease. The dependent sections of the lung are usually the most diseased and have greater resistance to airflow as well as decreased compliance. Second, the supine position decreases the functional residual capacity and increases airway resistance principally in dependent lung tissue. Third, diaphragmatic excursion is reduced in patients receiving mechanical ventilation, and the weight of the abdominal contents may further impair the normal ventilation of dependent lung segments. These factors affect perfusion less than ventilation, and ventilation-perfusion imbalance therefore results. This imbalance can be overcome somewhat by periodically placing patients who are using mechanical ventilators in a prone position to improve ventilation of dependent lung segments (Douglas et al., 1977).

BAROTRAUMA. A third major complication of mechanical ventilation is barotrauma, which results either from mechanical trauma to the tracheobronchial tree or from overdistention of the lung. The risk of overdistention and subsequent pneumothorax is increased by the use of continuous airway-distending pressure (Gilmour, 1983).

RESPIRATORY ALKALOSIS. A fourth major complication of mechanical ventilation is acute respiratory alkalosis related to inappropriate hyperventilation. Respiratory alkalosis can result in decreased cardiac output, decreased cerebral blood flow, increased cardiac irritability, and a shift in the oxyhemoglobin curve to the left (Shapiro, 1981). The etiology of respiratory alkalosis can be psychologic, iatrogenic, or reflex. Psychologic hyperventilation is managed by sedation, and iatrogenic hyperventilation can be corrected by adjusting the ventilatory rate. Reflex hyperventilation arises from either the lungs or the central nervous system and may be difficult to treat. Some patients may respond to increased tidal volume or positive end-expiratory pressure, but usually some measure to increase alveolar ventilation is required. These measures include changing to intermittent mandatory ventilation (IMV) or lowering the ventilatory support rate, adding dead space to the respirator, or using muscle relaxants (Gilmour, 1983).

Use of Continuous Distending Pressure

Continuous distending pressure refers to the continuous elevation of transpulmonary pressure above baseline levels, and it is achieved by the techniques of positive end-expiratory pressure and CPAP. The goal of continuous distending pressure is to minimize abnor-malities in the ventilation-perfusion balance and thus allow delivery of oxygen to the tissues at a lower FIO_2. The increase in transpulmonary pressure results in an increased FRC, which allows recruitment of noncompliant lung units and prevents their collapse between breaths. Continuous distending pressure also splints small airways and inhibits atelectasis during ventilation.

Continuous distending pressure is associated with several complications. The further increase in transpulmonary pressure above that of mechanical ventilation alone results in a further decrease in venous return and cardiac output. Again, this effect may be less marked in patients with chronic pulmonary disease than in those with normal lungs because of the decreased compliance in diseased pulmonary tissue. Furthermore, decreased venous return may be desirable in patients with pulmonary congestion (Colgan et al., 1979).

Two other complications of continuous distending pressure result from overdistention of alveoli. The first is alveolar rupture. Second, overdistention of lung segments may cause compression of adjacent capillaries, which, through a Starling resistor effect, stimulates a redistribution of pulmonary blood flow. This effect may result in increased pulmonary vascular resistance and right ventricular failure.

Continuous distending pressure is usually used with the goal of maintaining a PO_2 between 60 and 90 mm Hg with an FIO_2 of less than 50 per cent. Alternatively, continuous distending pressure can be used with the goal of maintaining a shunt fraction of less than 15 per cent. This value may require continuous distending pressures in excess of 50 cm H_2O. This method requires more careful cardiovascular monitoring and is not recommended for the routine postoperative patient (Gilmour, 1983).

Intermittent Mandatory Ventilation

IMV was introduced about 15 years ago as an alternative to spontaneous respiration with a T-piece as a means of weaning patients from the respirator. With the T-piece, patients ventilate on their own for increasing intervals of time, whereas with IMV patients continue to use the respirator but provide an increasing fraction of the minute ventilation by spontaneous breaths.

IMV has several advantages over continuous mechanical ventilation. First, spontaneous breaths are achieved with a decrease in intrathoracic pressure, and, therefore, they promote venous return and cardiac output and allow higher levels of continuous distending pressure to be used. IMV may also result in decreased barotrauma, improved distribution of ventilation, and, by allowing patients to breath on their own, better regulation of acid-base balance (Civetta, 1981).

The technique of IMV usually involves maintaining a pH between 7.35 and 7.45, with a minute ventilation of less than 10 L and a respiratory rate of less than 30 breaths per minute. PO_2 is maintained between 60 and 90 mm Hg by altering the FIO_2 and continuous distending pressure. The results of IMV are generally satisfactory, but it can result in increased respiratory work, which may delay weaning from the ventilator (Smith, 1981).

Weaning

Although it is desirable to wean patients from a ventilator as soon as possible, there are advantages to leaving patients with respiratory insufficiency intubated during the immediate postoperative period. These include (1) increased ability to suction airway secretions; (2) easier application of distending airway pressures; and (3) decreased risk of aspiration (Hotchkiss, 1988). Patients can be left intubated but allowed to continue spontaneous ventilations on a CPAP circuit. The major disadvantage of prolonged intubation is development of respiratory muscle atrophy, which begins within 24 to 48 hours after intubation.

Two tests correlate well with the ability of a patient to be weaned from the respirator: vital capacity and maximal inspiratory force (Pontoppidan et al., 1977). A vital capacity greater than 15 ml/kg and a maximal inspiratory force greater than -20 cm H_2O are acceptable values for weaning. It is inadvisable to wean patients with a vital capacity of less than 10 ml/kg, a respiratory rate greater than 30 breaths per minute, or a minute volume greater than 10 L. Patients with an alveolar-arterial oxygen gradient greater than 300 mm Hg on 100 per cent oxygen or with a dead space/tidal volume ratio of greater than 0.6 are also poor candidates for weaning. Adjunctive measures for successful weaning include adequate hydration, vigorous pulmonary therapy, and careful monitoring by periodic arterial blood gas determinations (Gilmour, 1983).

ANESTHESIA AND ANALGESIA

General Versus Regional Anesthesia

Mortality

Multiple controlled studies have demonstrated that in patients undergoing acute hip surgery regional anesthesia decreases early postoperative mortality (Valentin et al., 1986). Mortality data from other procedures are few and inconclusive, except for one study demonstrating significantly reduced mortality in high-risk patients undergoing thoracic, abdominal, or vascular procedures under an epidural anesthetic (Yeager et al., 1987). Further controlled trials of regional versus general anesthesia are needed.

Cardiac Complications

Regional anesthesia is associated with decreased cardiac morbidity in high-risk patients undergoing surgery within 3 months after myocardial infarction (Reiz et al., 1982). Despite concern about the development of serious hypotension and myocardial ischemia after a high regional anesthetic blockade, cardiac output is well maintained during induced hypotension under epidural anesthesia in the absence of cardiac depressants and increased vagal activity. Perioperative demands on the heart are also reduced by regional anesthesia, probably because of the diminished catecholamine response to surgery (Bowler et al., 1986).

Pulmonary Complications

Although it has not been proved, evidence suggests that regional anesthesia is better than general anesthesia in preserving FRC postoperatively (Catley et al., 1985). Use of regional anesthesia may also result in a decreased incidence of pulmonary infections (Cuschieri et al., 1985). Once again, further controlled studies are necessary.

Blood Loss

Regional anesthesia is associated with significantly reduced bleeding in patients undergoing hysterectomy, lower-limb vascular surgery, and hip replacement (David et al., 1987). Regional anesthesia results in a 35 per cent reduction in blood loss during retropubic prostatectomy (Hendolin et al., 1981) and an 18 per cent reduction in blood loss after transurethral prostatectomy, although this latter reduction did not achieve statistical significance (McGowan and Smith, 1980).

Thromboembolic Complications

Multiple studies have demonstrated a significant decrease in both deep venous thrombophlebitis and pulmonary embolism for operations below the umbilicus performed under regional anesthesia; no benefit has been observed for upper-abdominal surgery (McKenzie et al., 1985).

In summary, strong evidence indicates that regional anesthesia should be the anesthesia of choice in patients undergoing surgery below the umbilicus. Although further controlled studies are necessary, regional anesthesia appears to reduce perioperative morbidity and to have no serious disadvantages in comparison with general anesthesia (Scott and Kehlet, 1988).

Malignant Hyperthermia

Malignant hyperthermia is an inherited human skeletal muscle disorder and is one of the main causes of death related to anesthesia. The reported incidence varies from 1 in 12,000 in children to 1 in 40,000 in adults (Britt, 1985). Malignant hyperthermia is probably inherited as an autosomal dominant trait; data suggest that the disease is likely caused by mutations in the ryanodine receptor gene on chromosome 19 (MacLennan et al., 1990).

The disease is usually brought on by certain inhalational anesthetics and depolarizing muscle relaxants. Symptoms include high fever, muscle rigidity, acidosis, and hyperkalemia. The pathophysiology is uncertain; one theory is that a malfunctioning sarcoplasmic reticulum causes a derangement in skeletal muscle fibers, which is followed by an increase in the level of intracellular ionized calcium.

The diagnosis of malignant hyperthermia is made by the caffeine/halothane muscle contracture test. In patients with a previous history of malignant hyperthermia or a strong family history of this disease, inhalational agents such as halothane and depolarizing muscle relaxants such as succinylcholine should be avoided. The fatality rate for this condition was formerly as high as 70 per cent, but it has been reduced to about 10 per cent with prompt recognition and treatment with dantrolene sodium (Dantrium), a skeletal muscle relaxant (Dubrow et al., 1989).

Analgesia

Epidural Analgesia

Placement of an indwelling epidural catheter at surgery allows continued analgesia through the postoperative period that can be administered either intermittently or via continuous infusion. In one study of children and adolescents, patients receiving intermittent epidural morphine required significantly less narcotic than those receiving parenteral morphine. No complications were attributable to the epidural catheters (Amaranath et al., 1989). Similar success has been reported in patients with urologic disorders who receive continuous epidural morphine postoperatively. The most frequent complications were hypotension, which was easily corrected by administration of additional intravenous fluids, and pruritus secondary to morphine, which was relieved by use of antihistamines or low doses of naloxone. Other problems included disconnection of the epidural tubing resulting in infection and prolonged urinary retention, which can be reduced by leaving a urethral catheter in place until epidural anesthesia has been discontinued (Schwartz et al., 1989).

Patient-Controlled Analgesia

Patient-controlled analgesia (PCA) was described in 1968 (Sechzer, 1968). PCA is administered intermittently by a pump, and numerous studies have shown that it provides adequate analgesia with few reported side effects (Eisenbach et al., 1988). PCA can be administered either intravenously or through an epidural catheter. Complications with PCA are rare; the most common complication is respiratory depression, which may be severe (White, 1987). In a study that compared PCA with conventional parenteral analgesia with morphine in patients undergoing cholecystectomy, there were no significant differences in the amount of analgesic used, recovery of bowel function, or length of hospitalization. Urinary retention occurred less frequently in patients using PCA, perhaps because of lower peak serum concentrations of morphine (Rogers et al., 1990). Early experience with epidural PCA is quite favorable.

Intercostal Blockade

Intercostal blockade can effectively relieve upper-abdominal pain, and intercostal blocks placed at the end of surgery can prevent the need for additional analgesia for many hours (Engberg, 1975). Intercostal blockade with local anesthetic is recommended for all urologic patients having unilateral flank incisions. Bilateral blockade may result in respiratory limitation and should be

avoided in patients with poor pulmonary reserve (Jakobson and Ivarsson, 1977). Pneumothorax is also an occasional complication of intercostal nerve block (Moore, 1975).

Butorphanol

Butorphanol (Stadol) is a parenteral synthetic benzomorphan analgesic that has greater analgesic potency than either morphine or meperidine and is associated with decreased respiratory depression, urinary retention, gastrointestinal spasticity, and addiction. It has been successfully used to treat renal colic without adverse side effects, and it can be administered successfully via PCA (Henry, 1986).

Rectal Analgesics

Studies have demonstrated that both nonsteroidal anti-inflammatory drugs (Thind and Sigsgaard, 1988) and morphine (Hanning et al., 1988) when administered as rectal suppositories can provide effective analgesia. These suppositories can be prepared as sustained-release preparations designed to provide a constant concentration of analgesic, which may require the addition of smaller supplementary doses of analgesic to counter transient increases in pain. Although not indicated in patients who have undergone radical pelvic surgery because of possible rectal perforation, this technique of analgesia merits further evaluation.

THROMBOEMBOLIC DISEASE

Incidence

Nearly all clinically significant pulmonary emboli originate in the deep veins of the legs (Hovig, 1977). It is difficult to estimate the incidence of deep venous thrombosis (DVT) by physical examination, because at least 50 per cent of venous thrombi in the leg are clinically silent (Moser et al., 1977). The incidence can be more accurately determined with radioactive iodine–labeled fibrinogen scanning or venography. By using these techniques, the incidence of DVT in patients undergoing urologic surgery has been found to be between 30 and 60 per cent (Kutnowski et al., 1977). The incidence is highest in patients undergoing open prostatectomy, with estimates varying from 30 to 80 per cent (Coe et al., 1978). The incidence of DVT is considerably lower in patients undergoing transurethral prostatectomy but is still between 7 and 10 per cent (Arsdalen et al., 1983).

The incidence of nonfatal pulmonary embolism in urologic patients is also underestimated by physical examination. Although 3 per cent of patients develop clinical evidence of pulmonary embolism after open prostatectomy (Vandendris et al., 1980), this value increases to 22 per cent when perfusion lung scans are routinely obtained (Allgood et al., 1970). The incidence of fatal pulmonary embolism is obviously much lower than the incidence of nonfatal pulmonary embolism, but it has been reported to be as high as 1 to 2 per cent after open urologic procedures (Holbraad et al., 1976).

Risk Factors

The duration of anesthesia is a major risk factor contributing to thromboembolic disease, and the incidence of DVT increases markedly when anesthesia time is greater than 1 hour. This increase is due in part to venous stasis associated with the use of muscle relaxants (Kakkar, 1975). Other risk factors for thromboembolic disease include age greater than 60 years, the presence of malignant disease, the use of estrogens, and the period and degree of immobility after surgery (Moser, 1983).

Diagnosis

The principal tests used to diagnose DVT are radioactive iodine–labeled fibrinogen scanning, impedance plethysmography, duplex ultrasonography, and contrast venography. The diagnosis of pulmonary embolism is usually made with a perfusion-ventilation scan.

Fibrinogen I 125 Scanning

Fibrinogen I 125 scanning is based on the principle that fibrinogen is incorporated into an actively forming thrombus. Radiolabeled fibrinogen is injected intravenously, and the legs are scanned with a hand-held detector. Fibrinogen scanning is unreliable for detecting thrombi in the upper thigh because of the large pelvic blood pool (Moser, 1983). It is an extremely sensitive technique, however, for detecting thrombi in the calf and lower thigh (the locations at which the majority of thrombi form), and the results correlate well with venography (Kakkar, 1975). The technique is most reliable when the fibrinogen is injected while thrombi are actively forming, and false-negative results may be obtained with older thrombi that are no longer incorporating fibrinogen. Fibrinogen uptake may also be limited by previous treatment with heparin (Moser et al., 1977). Fibrinogen scanning has been replaced by duplex ultrasonography.

Impedance Plethysmography

Impedance plethysmography is useful for detecting venous thrombosis above the knee. It is much less sensitive than radiolabeled fibrinogen scanning for detecting calf thrombi. Furthermore, the sensitivity of fibrinogen scanning and impedance plethysmography in combination is only 50 per cent when compared with venography (Cruickshank et al., 1989). As with fibrinogen scanning, impedance plethysmography is infrequently done today, having been replaced by duplex ultrasonography.

Duplex Ultrasonography

Duplex scanning using real-time B-mode imaging with pulsed Doppler ultrasonography has been shown to accurately diagnose DVT with an overall sensitivity of 86 per cent and a specificity of 97 per cent, which are comparable to venography (Barnes et al., 1989). Duplex ultrasonography can be done at the bedside, is noninvasive, and can be repeated easily. Detection of calf vein thrombosis appears more difficult with this technique than more proximal thrombosis, but it has an overall accuracy of 95 per cent (Flinn et al., 1989).

Contrast Venography

Contrast venography has been the "gold standard" method to diagnose DVT. It is an invasive technique, however, which may be difficult to perform, particularly when repeated examinations are required. Venography should probably be reserved for times when radiolabeled fibrinogen scanning and duplex ultrasonography are unavailable or when the results of these studies are equivocal (Caprini and Natonson, 1989).

Perfusion-Ventilation Scans

The diagnosis of pulmonary embolism may also be difficult to establish on clinical grounds because many cases are clinically silent, and the signs and symptoms often vary. The lung perfusion scan is a useful screening technique, and normal results rule out pulmonary embolism. An abnormal scan, however, may not be diagnostic of pulmonary embolism, because many cardiopulmonary conditions can alter regional pulmonary blood flow and give rise to segmental perfusion defects (Moser et al., 1977).

The specificity of the perfusion scan can be enhanced by combining it with a ventilation scan. The patient inhales a radioactive labeled gas such as ^{133}Xe, and the pattern of distribution of the isotope on the ventilation scan is compared with the pattern of distribution on the perfusion scan. In pulmonary embolism this scan reveals areas that are ventilated but not perfused, the so-called ventilation-perfusion mismatch (Alderson et al., 1979).

Ventilation-perfusion scans may be unreliable for diagnosing pulmonary embolism if the scan is abnormal only in areas in which the chest radiograph is also abnormal. This may occur with a pulmonary infiltrate or pleural effusion. In these cases one must rely on pulmonary angiography to establish the diagnosis with certainty (Moser, 1983).

Prophylaxis

Physical Measures

AMBULATION. Most physical measures to decrease DVT fail to overcome the fact that 50 per cent of thrombi develop during the surgical procedure. Although early ambulation has been shown to decrease venous thrombosis after myocardial infarction (Miller et al., 1976), its efficacy for surgical patients has not been established. For ambulation to be effective, the patient must either stand at the bedside or walk. Sitting in a chair or on the edge of the bed with the legs dangling serves only to promote venous stasis and to increase the risk of venous thrombosis (Rose, 1979). Leg elevation and leg exercises have not been shown to provide effective prophylaxis.

COMPRESSION STOCKINGS. Elastic, graded compression stockings are probably of little benefit, and poorly fitting stockings may compress the popliteal area and thigh and promote venous stasis (Moser, 1983). Newer compression stockings that provide a pressure gradient to the leg, with the highest pressure at the ankle and the lowest pressure at the thigh, may be more effective for increasing venous flow (Ishak and Morley, 1981). Compression stockings should be applied before surgery to help counteract venodilation and associated venous stasis that occur with the onset of anesthesia (Caprini and Natonson, 1989).

PNEUMATIC COMPRESSION DEVICES. The most effective physical measure to decrease venous thrombosis is the pneumatic sequential compression device. This external plastic boot has six pneumatic chambers that circumscribe the leg throughout its length. A variable pressure ranging from 30 to 50 mm Hg develops in each chamber and progresses up the leg in a sequential fashion. The boot is inflated for 10 to 15 seconds every minute.

It is recommended that sequential compression devices be applied the night before surgery and kept on until the patient is fully ambulatory. Studies have shown that these devices markedly increase femoral vein blood flow velocity without producing excess compression or pockets of stasis within the leg (Borow and Goldson, 1981). In addition, the devices produce a significant increase in fibrinolytic activity, as reflected by measurement of euglobulin lysis time (Inada et al., 1988). Furthermore, the devices have been shown to increase venous capacitance and outflow when applied only unilaterally. Thus, in addition to its mechanical effect, pneumatic compression may alter systemic venous and hemodynamic function through a thus far unexplained humoral or neurogenic mechanism (Blackshear et al., 1987).

Regardless of the mechanism of action, these sequential compression devices are undoubtedly extremely effective in preventing DVT. In one study, the incidence of fibrinogen uptake–detected DVT was reduced from 20.8 per cent in control patients to 2.6 per cent in patients wearing these devices (Caprini et al., 1983). Several other prospective trials, including one of urologic patients, have all shown that these devices significantly reduce the incidence of DVT (P < .001) (Butson, 1981; Clarke-Pearson et al., 1984; Coe et al., 1978). They should be used routinely for all patients undergoing open abdominal or pelvic operations of greater than 1 hour duration (Caprini and Natonson, 1989).

Regional Anesthesia

Regional anesthesia also reduces the incidence of DVT. Although general anesthesia reduces blood flow in the legs by about 50 per cent, regional anesthesia increases blood flow (Modig et al., 1980). In a study of patients undergoing elective hip surgery, fibrinogen up-take–detected DVT developed in 31 per cent of patients receiving general anesthesia compared with only 9 per cent receiving epidural anesthesia (P = .026). In addition, although not statistically significant, there was a 9 per cent incidence of pulmonary embolism in the general anesthesia group compared with a 3 per cent incidence in the regional anesthesia group (Wille-Jorgensen et al., 1989). For this reason alone, regional anesthesia is preferable to general anesthesia when possible in patients undergoing major pelvic surgery.

Pharmacologic Measures

Pharmacologic measures to decrease DVT have included the use of volume expanders, antiplatelet drugs, and anticoagulants. Dextran, a volume expansion agent, has been used extensively worldwide, particularly in orthopedic surgery, but has not achieved general acceptance in the United States. The reasons for this include the possibility of fluid overload, interference in the typing and cross-matching of blood, a deleterious interaction with fibrin that can result in bleeding, and occasional anaphylactic reactions (Caprini and Natonson, 1989).

ANTIPLATELET THERAPY. Although antiplatelet therapy, specifically aspirin derivatives, is of value in the prophylaxis of certain arterial occlusive diseases such as transient ischemic attacks and myocardial infarction, it has not been shown to be effective in the prevention of venous thromboembolic disease (Caprini and Natonson, 1989).

PROTHROMBINOPENIC AGENTS. Prothrombinopenic agents such as warfarin and dicumarol effectively prevent DVT. However, they are associated with an increased incidence of postoperative bleeding that, on rare occasions, has been fatal (Salzman and Davies, 1980). Data suggest that therapeutic efficacy can be maintained and bleeding complications reduced if the prothrombin time is maintained at 1.4 times control (Kakkar and Adams, 1986). Nevertheless, because the effect of these agents can be reversed only by use of fresh frozen plasma in emergency situations, most surgeons have been reluctant to use them.

LOW-DOSE HEPARIN. There is now conclusive evidence that subcutaneous low-dose heparin effectively reduces both DVT and pulmonary embolism. Although the international multicenter trial concluded in 1975 that prophylactic heparin effectively reduced the incidence of fatal pulmonary embolism (Kakkar, 1975), low-dose heparin prophylaxis has been and continues to be underutilized. The reasons for this are that one must treat between 200 and 300 patients to prevent one fatal pulmonary embolism, and that there is concern about the risk of increased perioperative bleeding. Nevertheless, several published studies have analyzed data from multiple prospective trials demonstrating that subcutaneous low-dose heparin provides safe and effective prophylaxis against both DVT and pulmonary embolism. One study pooled data from 24 randomized trials and documented a 0.2 per cent incidence of fatal pulmonary embolism among treated patients versus 0.7 per cent in controls (P < .001) (Clagett and Reisch, 1988). Another study found a significant decrease in the incidence of DVT in patients receiving heparin (P < .0001) and a decreased incidence of both fatal and nonfatal pulmonary embolism (P < .02) (Collins et al., 1988). In patients undergoing elective hip surgery, heparin prophylaxis reduces the rate of fatal pumonary embolism from 2.0 to 0.07 per cent (Bergqvist et al., 1988).

Although the use of low-dose heparin does result in some increase in perioperative bleeding, it appears that this effect does not result in increased morbidity. In fact, many double-blind studies have demonstrated no difference in either blood loss or transfusion requirements in patients receiving heparin compared with controls (Kiil et al., 1978). When results from multiple prospective trials were pooled, the incidence of major hemorrhage was identical (0.33 per cent) among heparin-treated and control patients, although the incidence of wound hematomas was significantly (P < .001) more frequent with heparin-treated patients (6.3 per cent) compared with control patients (4.1 per cent) (Clagett and Reisch, 1988). In another study, heparin prophylaxis again resulted in a greater incidence of hemorrhagic complications, but none were fatal (Bergqvist et al., 1988). Although not usually used in patients undergoing transurethral resection of the prostate, low-dose heparin does not increase operative blood loss in this procedure (Wilson et al., 1988).

LOW-MOLECULAR-WEIGHT HEPARIN PREPARATIONS. The anticoagulant activity of heparin is highly dependent on its molecular weight. Thus, a heparin preparation with low molecular weight has a weak effect on thrombin inhibition and only slightly increases the activated partial thromboplastin time; at the same time, it effectively blocks thrombin activation by inhibition of factor X_a. Low-molecular-weight heparin preparations, therefore, are associated with less bleeding risk and have been demonstrated to be equally effective to standard calcium heparin preparations in the prevention of thrombosis. In addition, low-molecular-weight heparin preparations need to be administered only once daily, which makes them more convenient and comfortable to give than the traditional twice daily calcium heparin preparations (Speziale et al., 1988). A prospective multicenter trial of patients undergoing major general surgical procedures demonstrated that low-molecular-weight heparin (Fragmin) given once daily was as effective as standard calcium heparin given twice daily (Caen, 1988). Other studies have reported similar results and have demonstrated that use of this preparation is not associated with an increased risk of either hemorrhage or wound hematomas (Encke et al., 1988; Fricker et al., 1988). Low-molecular-weight heparin is administered as a single daily subcutaneous dose of 2500 units. Treatment should be started 2 hours before surgery and continued until the patient is fully ambulatory.

Although the use of subcutaneous heparin has been associated with prolonged lymphatic drainage in patients undergoing major pelvic surgery, this is usually of no clinical significance provided pelvic drains are left in place until heparin has been discontinued and pelvic drainage has ceased.

DIHYDROERGOTAMINE. There is evidence that another prophylactic agent, dihydroergotamine, may further reduce venous thrombosis. This agent increases venous tone and venous blood flow (Lange and Echt, 1972). A multicenter trial demonstrated that the combination of dihydroergotamine and low-dose heparin was more effective than low-dose heparin alone (Multicenter Trial Committee, 1984). Nevertheless, this combination has not been used extensively, perhaps because of concern about the use of an ergot derivative in the presence of hypertension, cardiac disease, or arterial occlusive disease. There have been no controlled trials of this combination in urologic patients.

Summary

In patients younger than 40 years of age undergoing minor surgical procedures, thromboembolic prophylaxis should include only the use of graded compression stockings and early ambulation. All patients older than 60 years of age and those older than 40 with an additional risk factor such as malignancy, obesity, trauma, or a history of prior thrombosis should be treated with sequential compression devices. In addition, the data strongly suggest that these patients should also be treated with subcutaneous heparin, although this practice is certainly not usual among most urologists. However, for patients older than 60 years of age with one of the additional previously mentioned risk factors, subcutaneous low-molecular-weight heparin in combination with sequential compression devices is recommended throughout the perioperative period (Caprini and Natonson, 1989).

Treatment of Thromboembolism

The initial treatment of both DVT and pulmonary embolism is intravenous heparin, which is usually administered as a continuous infusion of 1000 units per hour. Alternatively, heparin may be given in boluses of either 5000 units every 4 hours, 7500 units every 6 hours, or 10,000 units every 8 hours. Although continuous infusion is the most popular method, it has not been shown to have any advantage in terms of efficacy or safety over bolus administration (Salzman et al., 1975). Intravenous heparin is continued for at least 7 days and longer in patients who remain immobilized or who have other associated risk factors. In the past it has been recommended that patients with pulmonary embolism receive an initial bolus of 15,000 to 20,000 units of heparin and that heparin be infused at an increased rate during the first 24 hours of therapy, but it is uncertain whether these additional measures are necessary (Moser, 1980).

The therapeutic effect of heparin is monitored by measurement of either the partial thromboplastin time (PTT) or the activated partial thromboplastin time (aPTT), and these values are usually maintained in the twice-normal range. It has been argued that measurement of PTT or aPTT is unnecessary, because coagulation parameters may not reflect the efficacy of therapy and because the risk of bleeding with heparin is primarily related to other coexistent risk factors (Nelson et al., 1982).

In patients with DVT for whom anticoagulation is contraindicated, placement of a Greenfield filter into the vena cava should be considered (Greenfield, 1984). These filters are implanted via the right internal jugular vein or, alternatively, through the femoral vein. They can be positioned with the use of local anesthesia and fluoroscopic control and can be positioned in less than 1 hour. In one study there were no intraoperative complications related to filter implantation, no migration of the filters, and no cases of inferior vena caval occlusion. The devices effectively prevented fatal pulmonary embolism (Vaughn et al., 1989).

Surgery is rarely indicated for treatment of thromboembolic disease. Pulmonary embolectomy is performed only when there is massive pulmonary thromboembolism that has been documented by angiography and that is associated with profound hypotension. Results of such surgery have been dismal (Moser, 1983).

After the treatment of acute postoperative thromboembolism, patients who have persistent risk factors should continue anticoagulant therapy. Oral warfarin and low-dose subcutaneous heparin are the drugs commonly used. Warfarin is given in a dosage sufficient to maintain the prothrombin time at approximately 1.5 to 2 times control values (Hull et al., 1982). Heparin is administered at doses of 7500 to 10,000 units subcutaneously every 12 hours (Bynum and Wilson, 1979). The optimal duration of therapy has not been established. Some believe that therapy should continue until all risk factors have resolved, whereas others treat patients empirically for 3 months to 1 year postoperatively (Moser, 1983).

PERIOPERATIVE MANAGEMENT OF PATIENTS WITH RENAL INSUFFICIENCY

This section deals with the preoperative evaluation of renal function and the perioperative management of patients with renal insufficiency. The evaluation and management of acute and chronic renal failure are discussed in Chapter 55.

Preoperative Assessment

Evaluation of Renal Function

In patients with renal insufficiency the glomerular filtration rate (GFR) correlates with the surgical risk of postoperative renal failure and associated extrarenal morbidity. Because it is dependent on other factors, the blood urea nitrogen (BUN) value does not provide the best estimate of GFR. Patients with an increased dietary protein intake, hypercatabolism, or intestinal bleeding may have an elevated BUN concentration; conversely, patients with a decreased dietary protein intake, polyuria, or severe liver disease may have a decrease in

BUN that is unrelated to GFR (Burke and Gulyassy, 1979).

Because the serum creatinine concentration does not depend on either protein load or urinary flow rate, its measurement provides a more accurate estimate of GFR. Serum creatinine level is dependent, however, on muscle mass. A serum creatinine concentration of 1.5 mg/dl may reflect a normal GFR in a muscular young male but may be associated with as much as a 75 per cent reduction in the GFR in an older, malnourished patient with muscular wasting. In general, however, serum creatinine concentration accurately reflects perioperative changes in creatinine clearance (Charlson et al., 1989).

Creatinine clearance correlates most closely with the GFR, but it is sometimes unreliable because of inaccuracy in obtaining a complete 24-hour urine collection. A 4-hour collection of urine is more easily obtained and in a well-hydrated patient provides a reasonable estimation of creatinine clearance. In situations in which timed collections of urine are not feasible, a rough estimate of creatinine clearance can be obtained by dividing the serum creatinine value into 100. This simple calculation is more reliable in young patients, and a more accurate estimate for all patients is provided by the formula

$$\text{Creatine clearance} = \frac{(140 - \text{age [years]}) \times \text{body weight (kg)}}{72 \times \text{serum creatinine (mg/dl)}}$$

Adjustment for females equals 15 per cent less (Cockcroft and Gault, 1976).

Renal Insufficiency and Surgical Risk

In all patients, GFR decreases intraoperatively and in the immediate postoperative period (Kono et al., 1981). In one study, 23 per cent of patients undergoing elective general, vascular, or gynecologic surgery experienced an increase in serum creatinine concentration of greater than 20 per cent during the first 6 postoperative days. In one half of these patients, these increases were sustained for greater than 48 hours, and in many patients renal function had not returned to its initial level by time of discharge. Patients who sustained such a deterioration were at risk for nonoliguric renal failure if they had a subsequent insult (i.e., hypotension, reoperation, angiography, or use of aminoglycosides) (Charlson et al., 1989).

Patients with mild renal insufficiency and a GFR between 50 and 75 ml/minute have an increased risk of developing perioperative renal failure. Patients with a moderate reduction in GFR to between 25 and 50 ml/minute have an even greater risk and require close attention to perioperative fluid and electrolyte balance and may require adjustments in drug dosages. Patients with a GFR below 25 ml/minute have an increased risk of developing associated extrarenal complications such as hyperkalemia, pneumonia, wound complications, hypotension, hypertension, hemorrhage, hypoventilation, and sepsis (Pinson et al., 1986).

Preoperative Management

Fluid and Electrolytes

SODIUM AND WATER. Patients with renal insufficiency are usually able to maintain normal sodium and water balance until renal function is severely reduced. As GFR decreases, however, patients may lose the ability to respond to acute shifts in sodium and water. They may not be able to handle the large amounts of sodium and water often administered during surgery and may have an increased risk of developing fluid overload and congestive heart failure in the perioperative period. Careful observation is required throughout the first postoperative week because of reabsorption of "third space" fluid into the intravascular compartment (Miller, 1990). Conversely, patients with salt-wasting nephropathy have an increased risk of perioperative volume depletion and may require increased amounts of intravenous saline to avoid dehydration and subsequent renal deterioration (Tasker et al., 1974).

Hyponatremia occurs commonly in patients with renal insufficiency and generally reflects an excess of free water rather than a deficiency of sodium. Hyponatremia becomes clinically significant when the serum sodium level falls below 125 mEq/L because of the risk of cerebral edema. Prompt treatment is required with either diuretics and hypertonic saline or dialysis. Hypernatremia is uncommon in renal insufficiency and usually reflects volume depletion (Burke and Gulyassy, 1979).

POTASSIUM. Hyperkalemia is potentially a major problem in patients with renal insufficiency who are undergoing surgery. Although under normal conditions patients are able to maintain potassium balance until the GFR falls below 10 ml/minute, surgery increases the risk of hyperkalemia because of the increased endogenous and exogenous potassium load. Endogenous sources of potassium include rhabdomyolysis, surgical tissue trauma, and hemolysis. Exogenous sources include intravenously or orally administered potassium, total parenteral nutrition, and blood transfusions (Burke and Gulyassy, 1979). In addition, acidosis frequently occurs during the perioperative period, and it causes a rise in serum potassium level of 0.6 mEq/L for every 0.1 unit decrease in serum pH (Kunau and Stein, 1979).

The serum potassium level should be normalized before surgery. Acute hyperkalemia may be precipitated by hypercapnea and acidosis associated with induction of anesthesia, and patients with pre-existing hyperkalemia have an increased risk for ventricular arrhythmias and cardiac death (Kasiske and Kjellstrand, 1983). Elective operations should be postponed if the serum potassium level exceeds 5.5 mEq/L. Patients whose serum potassium value exceeds 6.5 mEq/L require prompt treatment to prevent cardiac arrhythmias.

The treatment of hyperkalemia is outlined in Table 63–4. Calcium chloride antagonizes the effect of potassium on the myocardium; insulin and glucose produce an intracellular shift of potassium. Administration of sodium bicarbonate and infusion of epinephrine are less effective and lower the serum potassium level in only 50 per cent of patients (Blumberg et al., 1988). Although ion-exchange resins are commonly used to treat hyperkalemia, they may cause extensive ischemic colitis and death in uremic patients (Lillemoe et al., 1987). Hemodyalysis is the most effective method to rapidly lower the serum potassium level (Blumberg et al., 1988).

Hypokalemia occurs commonly and most often results from diuretic therapy. Although renal failure is seldom the cause, hypokalemia should be corrected cautiously in patients with renal failure to avoid precipitating acute hyperkalemia and cardiac arrhythmias. Elective surgery should be postponed if the serum potassium value is less than 3 mEq/L. Potassium should be replaced orally if possible but can be administered intravenously when necessary. It should not be replaced at a rate greater than 10 to 15 mEq/hour without careful ECG monitoring. Hypokalemia in the postoperative period is usually due to the loss of potassium and hydrochloric acid from the gastrointestinal tract (Burke and Gulyassy, 1979).

OTHER ELECTROLYTES. Hypocalcemia and hypophosphatemia occur commonly in patients with renal insufficiency and are generally well tolerated. Hypercalcemia occurs less frequently and is associated with secondary hyperparathyroidism. Hypermagnesemia also occurs commonly, especially in patients receiving antacids or cathartics. Serum magnesium levels greater than 3 mEq/L are associated with an increased risk of cardiac arrhythmias, respiratory paralysis, and prolonged muscle relaxation after anesthesia (Burke and Gulyassy, 1979).

Acid-Base Balance

Patients with renal insufficiency frequently have metabolic acidosis because of an inability to excrete a normal acid load and to regenerate bicarbonate. Although metabolic alkalosis is seldom of renal origin, it occurs commonly in the postoperative period because of gastrointestinal losses. Metabolic alkalosis is usually corrected by the kidneys, and patients with renal insufficiency may be unable to compensate adequately (Burke and Gulyassy, 1979).

Both acidosis and alkalosis represent serious risks and should be corrected before elective surgery is undertaken. In addition, patients with metabolic acidosis related to renal insufficiency may compensate for this problem by chronic hyperventilation. If hyperventilation is not maintained during anesthesia, patients may develop a worsening metabolic acidosis, which, in turn, may precipitate acute hyperkalemia and fatal cardiac complications (Goggin and Joekes, 1971).

Hematologic Considerations

Anemia is common in patients with severe renal insufficiency primarily because of the decreased production and action of erythropoietin, but other factors include gastrointestinal bleeding, hemolysis, and deficiencies of iron and folate (Fisher, 1980). These patients usually are well adjusted to hematocrits between 18 and 24 per cent because of increased production of 2,3-diphosphoglycerate (2,3-DPG). 2,3-DPG causes a shift in the oxyhemoglobin dissociation curve to the right,

Table 63–4. TREATMENT OF HYPERKALEMIA

Agent	Mechanism	Route of Administration and Dose	Onset of Action	Comments
Calcium chloride	Antagonizes effect of potassium on myocardium	Intravenous bolus or drip	Immediate	Avoid in digitalized patients. Give under ECG control
Sodium bicarbonate	Intracellular potassium shift	Intravenous bolus or drip	Immediate	May cause volume overload if used in large quantities
Insulin and glucose	Intracellular potassium shift	Intravenous bolus or drip; 1 unit regular insulin for every 2 g of glucose	Within minutes	
Sodium polystyrene (Kayexalate)	Removal of potassium	Oral: 30 g Rectal: 60 g Give with sorbitol	1–2 hours	
Hemodialysis and peritoneal dialysis	Removal of potassium		Immediate	Hemodialysis much faster

From Kasiske, B., and Kjellstrand, C. M.: Perioperative management of patients with renal failure. Urol. Clin. North Am., 10:35, 1983.

which facilitates oxygen delivery to the tissues (Mac-Donald, 1977). Preoperative transfusions are not usually required in these patients and may precipitate volume overload and congestive heart failure. Patients with lesser degrees of renal insufficiency or those whose renal failure is of short duration are more susceptible to complications from anemia, and these patients may require preoperative transfusions to a hematocrit above 30 per cent (Czer and Shoemaker, 1978). Alternatively, administration of human recombinant erythropoietin to dialysis patients produces a dose-dependent increase in hematocrit to normal values (Eschbach et al., 1987). The main disadvantage of erythropoietin therapy is exacerbation of hypertension in some patients, but this effect is more than offset by their increased appetite and sense of well-being (Erslev, 1987).

Patients with moderate or severe renal insufficiency are also at risk for increased perioperative hemorrhage, primarily from abnormal platelet function. The best laboratory test to assess this risk is the bleeding time. The degree of abnormality of the bleeding time correlates closely with the degree of renal insufficiency, whereas the prothrombin time, partial thromboplastin time, and platelet count usually are normal. Patients with levels of BUN greater than 100 mg/dl should undergo dialysis before surgery to decrease the risk of perioperative hemorrhage (Kasiske and Kjellstrand, 1983). In some patients, dialysis is not effective in normalizing the bleeding time, and these patients may respond to the administration of cryoprecipitate (Janson et al., 1980) or desmopressin (Mannucci et al., 1983), both of which shorten bleeding time, increase circulating levels of factor VIII/von Willebrand antigen, and decrease blood loss in dialysis patients undergoing surgical procedures. Preoperative transfusion above 30 per cent also shortens bleeding time and reduces bleeding in dialysis patients (Livio et al., 1982).

Drug Therapy

The degree of renal insufficiency correlates closely with the development of adverse drug reactions, and the administration of drugs in the perioperative period to patients with renal failure deserves careful consider-

ation. Drug dosages must be decreased in accordance with the degree of renal impairment, particularly for drugs that are normally excreted unchanged by the kidneys, but drugs that are not excreted by the kidneys must also be administered cautiously if the effects of these agents are synergistic with the effects of uremia. Such agents include anticoagulants, sedatives, analgesics, and tranquilizers. Prolonged respiratory depression can occur in patients with renal failure who are receiving standard doses of morphine because of the accumulation of pharmacologically active metabolites of morphine produced by the liver and ineffectively cleared by the kidney (Chauvin et al., 1987).

Drug levels can be adjusted either by decreasing the drug dosage or by increasing the dose interval. Nomograms are available for many of the commonly used drugs, and serum levels should be followed when administering drugs with high potential toxicity. Associated hepatic disease and congestive heart failure increase the risk of potential drug toxicity. Drugs commonly used in the perioperative period, with recommended dosage modifications for patients with renal failure, are given in Table 63–5.

AMINOGLYCOSIDES. Aminoglycosides remain one of the major causes of acute renal insufficiency. Nephrotoxicity can be reduced by using nomograms to calculate proper loading and maintenance dosages and by following drug levels in the serum. The serum creatinine level should be measured at least every other day while aminoglycosides are being administered and for 4 to 6 days after therapy. Creatinine clearance should be measured periodically in patients receiving prolonged aminoglycoside therapy (Burke and Gulyassy, 1979).

RADIOCONTRAST AGENTS. Although the use of intravascular radiographic contrast agents has been associated with nephrotoxicity, the frequency with which this toxicity occurs is probably much less than previously believed. Diabetics with pre-existing renal insufficiency (serum creatinine level > 1.7 mg/dl) have about a 10 per cent risk of mild nephropathy (transient increase in serum creatinine value > 50 per cent) after receiving contrast material compared with about a 2 per cent risk for similar patients who do not receive contrast material. However, nondiabetic patients with either normal renal function or only mild renal insufficiency have little risk

Table 63–5. MODIFICATIONS OF MAINTENANCE THERAPY FOR PATIENTS WITH RENAL FAILURE FOR DRUGS OFTEN USED IN THE PERIOPERATIVE PERIOD*†

Drug	Dosage Modification for Glomerular Filtration Rate of‡		Remarks
	10–15 ml/min	*10 ml/min*	
Digoxin	Minor	Moderate	Use 70% of normal loading dose
Magnesium or calcium antacids	Moderate	—	If CrCl§ < 25, check [Mg^{2+}] or [Ca^{2+}]; do not use if CrCl < 10
Cimetidine	Minor	Moderate	If CrCl < 10 give no more than 300 mg q 12 h
Thiazides	—	—	Ineffective if CrCl < 30
Furosemide	None	None	Doses > 400 mg ineffective, potentially ototoxic
Triamterene, spironolactone	—	—	Avoid in patients with renal failure; may cause hyperkalemia
Barbiturates			In uremic patients use with caution; may cause excessive central nervous system depression
Narcotics	None	Minor	
Benzodiazepines			
Phenothiazines			
Succinylcholine	None	None	Increases [K$^+$]; use with caution if [K$^+$] is elevated
Gallamine	—	—	Avoid if CrCl < 50
Penicillin G	Minor	< 3 million U/d	Potassium salt contains 1.7 mEq potassium/million units
Ampicillin	Minor	Moderate	
Nafcillin	None	Minor	
Carbenicillin	Minor	Moderate	Contains 4.7 mEq sodium/g
Cephalothin	Minor	Moderate	
Cephalexin	Minor	Moderate	
Cephazolin	Moderate	Major	Consult available nomogram
Doxycycline	None	None	Avoid use of all other tetracyclines in patients with renal failure
Aminoglycosides	Moderate	Major	Consult available nomogram; measure blood levels

*Normal loading dose should be used, unless noted.
†Use of peritoneal or hemodialysis may require further adjustments.
‡Approximate adjustments are minor, 0.5–0.75; moderate, 0.25–0.5; major, 0.1–0.25 of normal maintenance dosages.
§CrCl in milliliters per minute.
From Burke, G. R., and Gulyassy, P. F.: Surgery in the patient with renal disease and related electrolyte disorders. Med. Clin. North Am., 63:1191, 1979.

of clinically significant contrast-induced nephropathy (Parfrey et al., 1989).

The risk of contrast-induced nephrotoxicity can be greatly reduced by preventing or correcting dehydration before the administration of radiocontrast agents (Eisenberg et al., 1981). Patients at risk, particularly diabetics with renal insufficiency, should not have fluid intake restricted before the administration of radiocontrast agents, and supplemental intravenous fluids should be given if necessary. Use of cathartics and enemas should be minimized. Multiple radiologic studies should not be scheduled consecutively to prevent a cumulative effect on renal function.

Conventional radiographic contrast agents contain iodine, are highly osmolar, and are highly charged—characteristics that are believed to contribute to both the nephrotoxicity and the allergic reactions associated with these agents. New contrast agents have been developed that have lower osmolarity and are nonionic yet retain sufficient iodine to provide satisfactory radiographic visualization. The principal disadvantage of these new agents is their cost, which is about 15 to 25 times that of comparable amounts of ionic contrast material. Although some experimental studies have demonstrated that these nonionic contrast agents are less nephrotoxic than ionic contrast agents, a recent randomized controlled trial demonstrated that nonionic contrast agents were not more effective than conventional ionic agents in preventing nephrotoxicity (Schwab

et al., 1989). Nevertheless, it appears prudent to use nonionic contrast material for diabetic patients with pre-existing renal insufficiency, as well as for patients who previously demonstrated an allergic reaction to iodinated contrast agents.

Intraoperative Management

Fluids and Diuretics

Patients with renal insufficiency are more likely to develop fluid and electrolyte problems associated with surgery. Many patients have a diminished capacity to excrete free water. Because surgery and anesthesia cause the release of antidiuretic hormone, which further decreases the excretion of free water, these patients have an increased risk of developing fluid overload and congestive heart failure. Conversely, patients with severe renal insufficiency may have a decreased ability to concentrate urine and thus have an increased risk of developing volume depletion. It is essential, therefore, to monitor fluid and electrolyte levels closely in patients with renal impairment (Kasiske and Kjellstrand, 1983).

In the past, some physicians have advocated routine preoperative salt loading in patients with renal insufficiency to prevent further perioperative deterioration of renal function. Salt loading is no longer routinely recommended, because it may result in fluid overload and congestive heart failure. Although all patients should be adequately hydrated at the time of surgery, the administration of supplemental intravenous saline is advisable only for patients with salt-wasting nephropathy (Tasker et al., 1974).

Diuretics should be administered prophylactically during surgery to patients with renal insufficiency to increase the GFR and thereby decrease the risk of further renal deterioration (Kasiske and Kjellstrand, 1983). Both mannitol and furosemide have a beneficial effect on renal function, and it has been recommended that patients with renal insufficiency receive a continuous intravenous infusion of these two diuretics during the perioperative period (Nuutinen et al., 1978). Five hundred milliliters of a 20 per cent mannitol solution is prepared, to which is added furosemide, the amount of which is calculated as 100 mg multiplied by the serum creatinine value (e.g., if the serum creatinine value is 4 mg/dl, $100 \times 4 = 400$ mg of furosemide). The solution is infused at a rate of 20 ml/hour during surgery, and the rate is then tapered over the first 6 to 12 hours postoperatively. The infusion is slowed if excessive diuresis results. Urine volume is replaced with 0.45 per cent saline containing 20 to 40 mEq of potassium chloride per liter. Serial serum and urine electrolyte levels are measured, and the sodium and potassium content of the replacement fluid is adjusted accordingly (Kasiske and Kjellstrand, 1983). The infusion is discontinued if the patient becomes anuric or oliguric because of potential mannitol toxicity (Borges et al., 1982).

Anesthetic Agents and Muscle Relaxants

The use of inhalational agents for patients with renal insufficiency is generally safe, because excretion of these agents is independent of renal function. These drugs may produce a mild decrease in urine volume, free water clearance, and GFR, but these effects are transitory and usually of no clinical significance. Methoxyflurane is an exception; it is nephrotoxic and should not be used for patients with renal insufficiency. Preanesthetic agents such as morphine and meperidine may depress renal function slightly, but moderate doses can be given safely. Anticholinergics such as atropine have little effect on renal function and also are safe to use (Kasiske and Kjellstrand, 1983).

Traditional nondepolarizing muscle relaxants such as *d*-tubocurarine and pancuronium are 50 to 100 per cent excreted by the kidneys; they can be administered safely in reduced doses to patients with renal insufficiency, but there is a significant risk of prolonged residual neuromuscular blockade. The newer short-acting nondepolarizing agents vecuronium and atracurium are not excreted by the kidneys, and their use should reduce the incidence of neuromuscular respiratory failure in uremic patients (Upton et al., 1982). The depolarizing agent succinylcholine can be given safely during induction but should not be administered as a continuous infusion. It has active metabolites that are dependent on renal excretion and that may thus accumulate in patients with renal failure. Furthermore, succinylcholine elevates serum po-

tassium levels by about 0.5 mEq/L in all patients and should be avoided in patients with elevated potassium levels (Kasiske and Kjellstrand, 1983). Gallamine is excreted totally by the kidneys and is contraindicated in patients with renal failure (Sirotzky and Lewis, 1978).

Postoperative Management

The fluid and electrolyte balance of patients with renal insufficiency should be monitored carefully during the postoperative period. Volume assessment may necessitate placement of a central venous or Swan-Ganz catheter, as well as daily measurement of the patient's weight and monitoring of fluid input and output. In patients with normal renal function, diuresis usually begins 24 to 48 hours postoperatively as patients regain the ability to excrete free water. In patients with renal insufficiency, this normal physiologic response must be distinguished from inappropriate fluid loss related to nephrogenic diabetes insipidus or renal salt wasting. These conditions can be differentiated by careful monitoring of intravascular volume and measurement of serum and urinary electrolyte levels (Vaughan and Gillenwater, 1973).

Patients with renal failure may have delayed wound healing, and skin sutures should be left in place a few extra days. Proper nutrition is important, not only to facilitate wound healing but also to reduce the frequency of infections that occur more commonly in uremic patients. Nutrition should preferably be provided orally or via nasogastric tube feedings. If oral nutrition is not feasible, however, patients should have parenteral nutrition promptly, even if this measure necessitates dialysis to prevent fluid overload (Kasiske and Kjellstrand, 1983).

Surgery in Patients Having Chronic Dialysis

Patients undergoing chronic dialysis have an increased surgical risk, but with careful management the mortality in this group of patients can be reduced to between 1 and 3 per cent (Wiehle et al., 1981). Fluid and electrolyte problems must be corrected preoperatively in these patients. Patients should have dialysis within 24 hours before surgery to optimize fluid status and to reduce the incidence of perioperative hemorrhage, hyperkalemia, hypotension, and acidosis. If blood transfusions are necessary, hyperkalemia resulting from transfusion must be corrected during dialysis before surgery. Because dialysis requires anticoagulation that may induce thrombocytopenia, minimal heparinization should be used during dialysis on the day preceding surgery and for all dialysis sessions required during the first week after surgery. Minimal heparinization is associated with fewer bleeding complications than the older technique of regional heparinization, which involved the simultaneous infusion of heparin and protamine (Swarts, 1981). Postoperatively, it is desirable to postpone dialysis for 48 hours because of the increased risk of bleeding and then to resume dialysis every 2 to 3 days as required (Kasiske and Kjellstrand, 1983).

Hyperkalemia is of particular concern in patients having chronic dialysis. The surgeon should attempt to minimize tissue trauma and to avoid blood transfusions. If transfusions are required, it is preferable to administer fresh blood to decrease the potassium load. It is important to monitor serum pH as well as potassium level, because acidosis causes an extracellular shift of potassium.

Patients undergoing dialysis often have associated hypertension. Antihypertensive medications should be continued until the time of surgery and resumed immediately thereafter. When it is not possible to administer oral medications, blood pressure may be regulated by using intravenous agents such as hydralazine and furosemide, which preserve renal blood flow. Hydralazine may cause tachycardia and should be administered cautiously in patients with coronary artery disease. Sodium nitroprusside may be given as a continuous infusion to control hypertension (Kasiske and Kjellstrand, 1983).

Patients having dialysis may develop pericarditis in the postoperative period, and preoperative dialysis may help to prevent this complication. Heart auscultation should be performed daily during the postoperative period to detect a pericardial rub. If pericarditis is discovered, it should be treated by daily dialysis with minimal heparinization.

Patients undergoing dialysis also have an increased risk of perioperative thrombosis of the hemodialysis access site, probably resulting from decreased blood flow and hypercoagulability associated with surgical stress. A blood pressure cuff should never be placed on the arm above the access site. Thrombosis of external shunts may be prevented by continuous infusion of heparin at a low rate into both limbs of the cannula (Kasiske and Kjellstrand, 1983).

HEMATOLOGIC CONSIDERATIONS IN UROLOGIC SURGERY

This section deals with areas of hematology that are of particular concern to the urologist: anemia, transfusions, coagulation mechanisms and disorders, and management of intraoperative bleeding. Hematologic disorders such as white blood cell diseases, which are not commonly encountered by the urologist, are not discussed.

Anemia

Evaluation

Mild to moderate degrees of anemia do not increase the risk of elective surgery but should be evaluated to determine the etiology. A careful history should be obtained, with particular attention to a possible family history of anemia or other blood disorders, bleeding associated with previous dental or surgical procedures, and factors that suggest chronic blood loss, such as heavy menstrual periods, gastrointestinal bleeding, and the use of drugs, most commonly aspirin and alcohol. Physical examination should include a fecal examination for occult blood and examination of the peripheral blood smear. Other physical findings may include brittle nails, stomatitis, and a red and raw tongue associated with iron deficiency anemia; peripheral neuritis and a pale, smooth tongue seen in patients with vitamin B_{12} deficiency; and hepatomegaly, ascites, and spider angiomas seen in patients with chronic hepatic disease (Watson-Williams, 1979).

Anemias are classified on the basis of red blood cell morphology by using the mean corpuscular volume and mean corpuscular hemoglobin content. The mean corpuscular volume normally varies between 82 and 100 fl per cell, and the mean corpuscular hemoglobin content varies between 30 and 35 g/dl of blood. The reticulocyte count is a measure of the percentage of new blood cells seen in the peripheral smear and should be corrected for the degree of anemia to more accurately reflect the response of the bone marrow to anemia. The corrected reticulocyte percentage index is calculated by multiplying the reticulocyte percentage by the hematocrit value (packed red blood cell volume) and dividing the product by 45. The reticulocyte percentage index is normally between 1 and 2 per cent but may be as high as 7 per cent in patients with severe hemolytic anemia (Watson-Williams, 1979).

Iron Deficiency Anemia

Iron deficiency anemia is the most common cause of anemia. In this condition both the mean corpuscular volume and the mean corpuscular hemoglobin content are decreased, resulting in a microcytic hypochromic peripheral smear. The reticulocyte percentage index is less than 1 per cent. Iron deficiency anemia may be distinguished from other microcytic hypochromic anemias by the findings of decreased serum iron level, increased total iron-binding capacity, and decreased serum ferritin level. Because iron deficiency anemia usually reflects chronic blood loss, one should never simply treat the anemia without searching for the underlying cause. If iron deficiency anemia is associated with a positive stool guaiac test, elective surgical procedures should be postponed until the possibility of a gastrointestinal malignancy has been investigated.

Treatment of iron deficiency anemia is often required in the postoperative period, most commonly by administration of 325 mg of ferrous sulfate orally twice daily. The serum hemoglobin concentration starts to rise about the seventh day of treatment and increases about 0.2 g/dl every day thereafter. If more rapid treatment is required, iron dextran can be given parenterally. Alternatively, administration of recombinant human erythropoietin quickly elevates the hematocrit and represents another alternative to homologous transfusion (Levine et al., 1989).

Megaloblastic Anemia

Megaloblastic anemia is most commonly seen in association with a deficiency of folic acid or vitamin B_{12}

(pernicious anemia) and is suggested by the presence of red blood cell macrocytes (increased mean corpuscular volume), macrovalocytes, nucleated red blood cells, megaloblasts with considerable poikilocytosis and anisocytosis, hypersegmented neutrophils, and a reduction in platelets in the peripheral blood smear. The diagnosis can be confirmed by measurement of red blood cell folate concentration, serum vitamin B_{12} level, and/or a positive Schilling test. Folic acid deficiency can be corrected by oral administration of 1 mg of folic acid per day in most patients unless there is a concomitant malabsorption syndrome. Vitamin B_{12} is most frequently given intramuscularly (it also can be given intravenously), initially at a dose of 1000 g for two or three doses and at 100 g/month for life when the diagnosis is pernicious anemia. If a malabsorption syndrome or dietary deficiency is present and can be corrected, total-body stores can be replaced with either folate or vitamin B_{12} in several weeks to a few months.

Hemolytic Anemia

Hemolytic anemia is suggested by the finding of an increased reticulocyte percentage index without associated blood loss. Hemolytic anemias are classified as either immune or nonimmune on the basis of the Coombs' test, which determines the presence of human globulin coating the red blood cells. A positive Coombs' test result indicates an immune hemolytic anemia that may be due to autoimmune antibodies, drug-induced antibodies, or a transfusion reaction. Coombs' test–negative anemias can be classified further by testing of red blood cell fragility. Increased fragility is associated with hereditary spherocytosis and elliptocytosis. Decreased fragility is observed in abnormal hemoglobin disorders, such as sickle cell disease and thalassemia. Normal red blood cell fragility is seen in lead poisoning and alcoholism (Watson-Williams, 1979).

Transfusions

Indications

The optimal hematocrit value for surgery is one that achieves a balance between increased oxygen transport and decreased blood viscosity and appears to be between 30 and 33 per cent (Czer and Shoemaker, 1978). Two other factors, cardiac output and the oxygen dissociation curve, affect oxygen delivery to the tissues and should be considered in assessing the need for perioperative blood transfusions. Patients with a hemoglobin value of 10 g/dl must develop a cardiac output twice that of patients with a hemoglobin value of 14 g/dl to deliver the same amount of oxygen to the tissues. Patients with coronary artery disease who are unable to increase cardiac output may require higher hemoglobin levels to withstand the stress of surgery. When transfusing such patients, it is advisable to administer packed red blood cells at a low rate to avoid fluid overload and congestive heart failure (Lunsgaard-Hansen, 1975).

In patients with chronic anemia, there is a shift of the oxygen dissociation curve to the right, which facilitates the release of oxygen to the tissues. This shift is mediated by an increased amount of 2,3-DPG in the red blood cells. Patients with chronic anemia, therefore, may not require perioperative transfusion provided that intravascular volume is normal and cardiac function is not impaired (Spence et al., 1990).

Transfusion of stored whole blood or packed red blood cells does not immediately increase oxygen availability to the tissues to the extent indicated by a rising hemoglobin level because 2,3-DPG must be regenerated in the red blood cells after transfusion. There is about a 50 per cent recovery of 2,3-DPG within 4 hours, but normal oxygen delivery may not be achieved for 24 hours. Furthermore, 24 hours is required to readjust total blood volume and validate a successful increase in hemoglobin levels. Therefore, preoperative transfusions should ideally be completed 24 hours before surgery (Watson-Williams, 1979).

Complications

EARLY COMPLICATIONS. The incidence of adverse reactions occurring within the first 4 days after blood transfusion is approximately 5 per cent (Baker and Nyhus, 1970). Hemolytic reactions are classified as either immediate or delayed. Immediate reactions result from the transfusion of incompatible blood and carry a mortality as high as 35 per cent. Immediate reactions usually result from physician error and are totally avoidable. Delayed hemolytic reactions occur several days to weeks after transfusion and are much milder, with an associated mortality of less than 2 per cent (Walter, 1971). Delayed reactions result from stimulation of a pre-existing antibody that was not detected at the time of compatibility testing; at present these reactions are not preventable (Solanki and McCurdy, 1978). The risk of delayed reactions is increased by previous blood transfusions and pregnancy.

Allergic reactions are most often caused by leukocyte antigens and occur in 2 to 3 per cent of patients receiving transfusions. Symptoms include a temperature of lower than 39°C, erythema, and itching. Pyrogenic reactions are associated with a temperature of higher than 39°C and have a bacterial or immunologic etiology. These reactions fortunately have become rare because of more careful storage and handling of blood (Collins, 1983).

Several complications are associated with transfusions of large volumes. Hypocalcemia may result from the increased citrate load, and supplemental intravenous calcium may be required in patients receiving multiple transfusions (Denlinger, 1978). Microembolization of blood particulate matter to the lungs may cause adult respiratory distress syndrome. The efficacy of transfusion microfilters in preventing this complication is controversial (Geelhoed, 1978). Multiple transfusions also result in depletion of platelets and coagulation factors, particularly factors V and VIII, which are labile in storage, and these patients may have an increased tendency to bleed (Sherman, 1978).

LATE COMPLICATIONS. In spite of enhanced detection of donors carrying hepatitis B virus, hepatitis secondary to blood transfusion results in 3000 deaths per year in the United States (Watson-Williams, 1979). Most of these cases are caused by a virus other than hepatitis A or B virus, and the incubation period is between 14 and 140 days. Patients may also develop chronic active hepatitis after transfusion (Gradey, 1978). Other diseases, such as mononucleosis and cytomegalovirus infection, can be transmitted by transfusion (Lerner and Sampliner, 1977).

With universal testing for the human immunodeficiency virus (HIV), the risk of a patient's contracting acquired immunodeficiency disease from a blood transfusion is presently extremely low, in the range of 0.001 per cent. Of greater concern is the risk to surgical personnel from accidental exposure to blood. In a study in a high-risk hospital, the theoretical risk of HIV infection in surgical personnel was calculated to be 0.125 per year, or one infection every 8 years. Although this rate may not seem high, it nevertheless represents a major life-threatening occupational hazard for surgical personnel practicing at hospitals with a high prevalence of HIV infection. Of the precautionary measures undertaken to reduce intraoperative blood exposure, wearing double sets of gloves seems to be most effective and should be adopted as routine practice. The use of face shields and waterproof garments also significantly reduces the risk of mucocutaneous exposure. On the other hand, perception of the risk of HIV infection was not associated with a decreased risk of occupational exposure, and there was no evidence on that basis to justify preoperative HIV testing (Gerberding et al., 1990).

There is increasing evidence that blood transfusions are associated with changes in immune system function leading to some degree of immunosuppression. In patients undergoing operation for cancer, a trend toward early recurrence in transfused patients has been noted for several tumors. In patients with colorectal cancer, a 5-year disease-free survival of 84 per cent was found for patients not having perioperative transfusions compared with 51 per cent for those having such transfusions (Burrows and Tartter, 1982). A similar trend of poorer survival has been found in transfused patients undergoing surgery for breast cancer, lung cancer, soft tissue sarcoma, cervical cancer, and head and neck cancer. In renal cell carcinoma, the only urologic malignancy evaluated, the results are controversial, with one study finding no effect of transfusion on survival and another finding a survival advantage in nontransfused patients that was not quite statistically significant ($P < .08$) (Schriemer et al., 1988). Patients undergoing operations for colorectal cancer who receive transfusions have a higher incidence of infectious complications than such patients who do not receive transfusions (Tartter, 1988). The mechanism by which blood transfusions alter the immune system remains unclear, but transfusions may decrease natural killer cell activity and thus reduce the capacity to eliminate blood-borne tumor cells.

Alternatives to Transfusion

AUTOLOGOUS BLOOD. Dramatic changes have occurred in blood collection and transfusion practices in recent years because of the infectious and immunosuppressive complications associated with transfusions. The supply of homologous blood peaked in 1986 and has not increased subsequently. Conversely, donations of autologous blood increased 13-fold between 1982 and 1987 (Surgenor et al., 1990). Guidelines documenting the appropriate number of autologous units that should be collected before a specific elective surgical procedure are presently being established (Axelrod et al., 1989).

ERYTHROPOIETIN. Administration of recombinant human erythropoietin significantly increases the amount of autologous blood that can be collected before surgery. In one study, only 1 of 23 patients treated with erythropoietin was unable to donate at least four units within 3 weeks, compared with 7 of 24 control patients. Patients treated with erythropoietin also had significantly higher hematocrits and reticulocyte levels. No serious complications resulted from erythropoietin administration; in particular, no erythropoietin antibodies were detected before or 1 month after the study (Goodnough et al., 1989).

AUTOTRANSFUSION. Although autotransfusion is usually performed for patients undergoing cardiac surgery, it may also be feasible for patients undergoing urologic procedures. In a study of patients undergoing radical cystectomy, an autotransfusion machine was used to aspirate blood from the operative field. The blood was then anticoagulated, filtered, and centrifuged. Packed erythrocytes were then immediately reinfused into the patient. Although there has been some concern that this technique may disseminate cancer cells, there has been no evidence to support this concern. At present autotransfusion is cost-effective only if two or more units of blood are retrieved (Hart et al., 1989).

Coagulation Mechanisms and Disorders

Early Events

The early hemostatic events after vascular injury include constriction of bleeding vessels and formation of a platelet plug. Platelets adhere to exposed subendothelial tissue and aggregate within 2 to 3 minutes after injury. The platelet plug must be solidified by subsequent fibrin deposition or it will distintegrate spontaneously and bleeding will resume (Owen and Walter Bowie, 1983).

Coagulation Pathways

Coagulation may be initiated by two mechanisms, the so-called intrinsic and extrinsic pathways. These pathways are initiated by different factors, but they ultimately merge into a final common pathway that results in the production of prothrombin, fibrinogen, and ultimately a fibrin clot. Figure 63–1 summarizes the coagulation pathways. The intrinsic pathway involves the interaction of platelet phospholipids with a number of plasma coagulation proteins and calcium. Four protein activation factors that are sequentially activated by the contact of plasma with a foreign surface are required to initiate the pathway. After activation and interaction with platelets and calcium, factors VIII and IX initiate

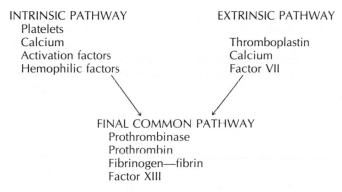

INTRINSIC PATHWAY
   Platelets
   Calcium
   Activation factors
   Hemophilic factors

EXTRINSIC PATHWAY

   Thromboplastin
   Calcium
   Factor VII

FINAL COMMON PATHWAY
   Prothrombinase
   Prothrombin
   Fibrinogen—fibrin
   Factor XIII

Figure 63–1. Overall coagulation pathways. (From Owen, C. A., Jr., and Walter Bowie, E. J.: Urol. Clin. North Am., 10:77, 1983.)

the final common pathway that ultimately results in the production of fibrin (Owen and Walter Bowie, 1983).

The extrinsic pathway is so called because it was believed originally that prothrombin could be converted into thrombin by the interaction of tissue juices (thromboplastin) and calcium alone. We now know that three other plasma proteins, factors V, VII, and X, are also required (Owen and Walter Bowie, 1983).

Evaluation of Hemostatic Competence

HISTORY AND PHYSICAL EXAMINATION. A careful history is critical to assess hemostatic competence. The history may reveal the presence of a coagulation disorder that otherwise may be missed by routine laboratory screening. It is insufficient simply to inquire about easy bruising or bleeding because the patient may not be aware of these phenomena. Specific questions regarding family history, previous dental extractions and surgical procedures, nosebleeds, menstrual bleeding, and drug history must be asked. The physical examination is also important and may reveal fundal hemorrhages, petechiae and ecchymoses, and hematomas and hemarthroses (Watson-Williams, 1979).

PLATELET FUNCTION. The adequacy of the number of platelets can be assessed from the peripheral blood smear (5 to 10 platelets per oil immersion field), and if the number is normal, a formal platelet count usually is unnecessary. Platelet function is assessed by the bleeding time, which is the time it takes for bleeding to stop after skin puncture and which correlates with the formation of a platelet plug. A normal bleeding time is less than 7 minutes but may vary depending on the technique used. The bleeding time is prolonged in patients with a deficient number of platelets, patients with an abnormality in platelet function (e.g., patients with von Willebrand's disease), and patients with an acquired abnormality of platelet function (e.g., patients with uremia or an abnormality caused by aspirin ingestion) (Owen and Walter Bowie, 1983).

Aspirin interferes with platelet function by irreversibly acetylating platelet cyclo-oxygenase for the life of the platelet, which is about 10 days. In patients undergoing coronary artery surgery, those receiving aspirin have significantly more postoperative bleeding, which results in increased transfusions and reoperations for control of

hemorrhage (Sethi et al., 1990). Although it has not been proved for other surgical procedures, it seems prudent for patients undergoing any elective surgery to discontinue taking aspirin at least 10 days before surgery. Other nonsteroidal anti-inflammatory drugs such as ibuprofen have less severe effects on platelet function but should be discontinued 7 to 10 days before surgery if possible. If any doubt exists about platelet function, a measure of bleeding time should be obtained before surgery.

INTRINSIC PATHWAY. The intrinsic pathway of coagulation is evaluated by the PTT or the aPTT. Both tests measure the coagulation time when partial thromboplastin and calcium are added to the patient's plasma. They differ only in that in the aPTT test activation is induced before the partial thromboplastin and calcium are added to the plasma, whereas in the PTT test the activation occurs after the partial thromboplastin is added. The PTT and aPTT are prolonged if there is a deficiency of any of the coagulation proteins with the exception of factor VII. The PTT and aPTT are most sensitive to reductions in factors VIII, IX, XI, and XII. The most common congenital abnormalities involving the intrinsic pathway are deficiencies of factor VIII:C (hemophilia A), factor VIII:AgvWB (von Willebrand's disease), and factor IX (hemophilia B or Christmas disease) (Owen and Walter Bowie, 1983).

EXTRINSIC PATHWAY. The extrinsic coagulation pathway is assessed by the prothrombin time, which is performed by adding a thromboplastic emulsion and calcium to plasma. The prothrombin time is prolonged by a deficiency in factors II, V, VII, and X (Owen and Walter Bowie, 1983).

The initial laboratory tests that should be obtained to screen for a coagulation disorder are a peripheral blood smear (to estimate platelet numbers), a PT, and an aPTT. If either the PT or the aPTT is prolonged, examination for the presence of a circulating anticoagulant is indicated. If there is no circulating anticoagulant present, a deficiency state most likely exists, and assay of individual factors is required to specify the deficiency state (Watson-Williams, 1979).

Specific Coagulopathies

INHERITED DISEASES. Any of the coagulation factors may be lacking on an inherited basis. Deficiency states of factors VIII and IX are transmitted by sex-linked inheritance; all the others have an autosomal mode of inheritance.

All the inherited coagulation disorders are rare except for classic hemophilia and von Willebrand's disease. Both are related to a deficiency of a part of the factor VIII complex. Classic hemophilia (sex-linked recessive) is caused by a lack of the clotting portion of the complex (VIII:C), whereas von Willebrand's disease (autosomal dominant) is caused by a deficiency of the high-molecular-weight carrier protein (VIII:AgvWB) (Owen, 1981). Von Willebrand's protein has two important functions. First, it is necessary for platelet adherence, and patients with von Willebrand's disease have a prolonged bleeding time. Second, the liver will not release

VIII:C unless VIII:AgvWB is present (Owen and Walter Bowie, 1983). Classic hemophilia is inherited as a sex-linked recessive disease and occurs almost exclusively in men. Von Willebrand's disease has an autosomal mode of inheritance. Both diseases are characterized by a normal prothrombin time and an abnormal PTT or aPTT, but they may be distinguished from each other by the pattern of inheritance and the increased bleeding time associated with von Willebrand's disease.

Surgical management of patients with classic hemophilia and von Willebrand's disease has changed dramatically since the introduction of factor VIII on a commercial basis in 1970. It is usually possible to administer a sufficient quantity of factor VIII so that patients with these diseases can undergo required surgical procedures. The risk of surgical bleeding and the need for factor VIII replacement are determined by the degree of factor VIII deficiency in the individual patient. Patients undergoing minor surgery usually require a level of factor VIII that is 30 to 35 per cent of normal, and patients undergoing major surgery require a level that is 50 per cent or greater of normal (Mazza et al., 1970).

Patients with hemophilia and von Willebrand's disease usually are treated with cryoprecipitate. Factor VIII and von Willebrand's factor replacement are initiated 1 hour before surgery and are administered at regular intervals during the next several days. Because the metabolism of these factors is increased during the postoperative period, patients may require administration of cryoprecipitate as frequently as every 6 to 8 hours. Subsequently, the administration of cryoprecipitate may be extended to every 8 to 12 hours, after the bleeding time and the clinical response are reviewed (Gilchrist et al., 1980). Both cryoprecipitate and fresh frozen plasma have the same risk of disease transmission. However, the advantage of cryoprecipitate over plasma is that equal amounts of the necessary clotting factors can be administered to patients in a much smaller volume of fluid (Cameron and Kobrinsky, 1990).

Desmopressin (1-desamino-8-D-arginine-vasopressin) also increases factor VIII and von Willebrand's factor levels (Mannucci et al., 1983) and is currently being investigated as an alternative to transfusion of blood products for the management of these diseases. Desmopressin has been demonstrated to reduce blood loss during spinal fusions (Kobrinsky et al., 1987) and after cardiac surgery (Saltzman et al., 1986) and is currently being evaluated for patients with bleeding diatheses (Cameron and Kobrinsky, 1990).

Unfortunately, about 5 to 10 per cent of patients with classic hemophilia have an associated antibody to factor VIII. This antibody is identified by measurement of factor VIII levels that are quite low and by the failure of fresh plasma added to the patient's plasma to correct the PTT. Patients with antibodies to factor VIII have a severe risk of developing hemorrhage and usually are not candidates for any elective surgical procedures (Pintado et al., 1975).

ACQUIRED DISEASES. In contrast to inherited disorders, acquired coagulopathies usually are multifactorial in origin. Two specific entities, vitamin K deficiency and disseminated intravascular coagulation (DIC), are discussed here. Vitamin K is necessary for hepatic synthesis of coagulation precursors to form factors II, VII, IX, and X and proteins C, S, and Z. The most common abnormality related to vitamin K is not deficiency of the vitamin but pharmacologic blockade of its hepatic function caused by warfarin and other prothrombinopenic agents. These drugs prevent the liver from synthesizing functional coagulation factors from their precursor forms (Owen and Walter Bowie, 1983).

Hemorrhagic disease of the newborn results from a deficiency of vitamin K. Because vitamin K can be obtained only from its production by intestinal bacteria or by the ingestion of green leafy plants, vitamin K deficiency can occur in surgical patients whose diets have been restricted or who have received antibiotic bowel preparations in anticipation of intestinal surgery. In addition, some second- and third-generation cephalosporin antibiotics antagonize normal vitamin K metabolism. Vitamin K deficiency also occurs in patients with biliary obstruction or fistulas (Owen and Walter Bowie, 1983).

Patients with vitamin K deficiency have prolongation of both the prothrombin time and the PTT or aPTT. Vitamin K deficiency can be corrected preoperatively by administration of 10 mg of vitamin K subcutaneously every 12 hours. Three doses are usually sufficient (Watson-Williams, 1979).

DIC is a consumption coagulopathy manifested by spontaneous simultaneous widespread thrombosis and hemorrhage. The massive coagulation is followed by generalized fibrinolysis and increased bleeding, and a more appropriate name for this condition might be "intravascular clotting with fibrinolysis" (Owen and Walter Bowie, 1983). Acute DIC may be precipitated by shock, septicemia, transfusions of mismatched blood, amniotic fluid embolism, snake bite, and other unrelated conditions. A chronic, less severe form of DIC is seen in patients with large metastatic cancers (Sun et al., 1974).

In urologic patients, DIC usually occurs as a result of sepsis. The diagnosis should be suspected clinically in a patient with widespread purpura oozing from venipuncture sites and bleeding from mucous membranes. Associated laboratory findings include a decreased platelet count, elevation of both the prothrombin time and the PTT or aPTT, and increased fibrinogen-fibrin split products resulting from fibrinolysis (Watson-Williams, 1979).

The treatment of DIC should be directed primarily at correcting the underlying cause of the condition. Administration of fresh plasma or cryoprecipitate may help to restore clotting factors after the underlying problem has been corrected. The administration of heparin may be effective because fibrinolytic activity may diminish spontaneously after fibrin formation is blocked (Owen and Walter Bowie, 1979). The administration of aminocaproic acid (Amicar) is useful only for treating isolated fibrinolysis. Its administration to patients with DIC may lead to further widespread thrombosis (Naeye, 1962).

Sickle Cell Disease

Although it is not a coagulation disorder, sickle cell disease is commonly encountered by urologists in dealing with patients with papillary necrosis and priapism. Patients with sickle cell disease have an increased risk of developing perioperative thrombosis. The risk can be decreased by maintenance of adequate oxygenation, hydration, and normal body temperature. In addition, exchange transfusions are recommended for surgical patients with sickle cell disease to lower the percentage of abnormal cells to below 50 per cent (Morrison and Wiser, 1976). Sickle cell trait is not associated with increased surgical risk, and no special precautions are necessary (Sears, 1978).

Jehovah's Witnesses

Occasionally urologists are faced with the dilemma of operating on Jehovah's Witness patients who cannot accept either homologous or autologous transfusions. Operations can probably be done safely, regardless of the initial hemoglobin value, as long as blood loss is kept below 500 ml. In a study of Jehovah's Witness patients who underwent major elective surgery, mortality was 3.2 per cent in patients with preoperative hemoglobin values greater than 10 g/dl compared with 5 per cent in patients with levels between 6 and 10 g/dl. There was no mortality if estimated blood loss was less than 500 ml, regardless of preoperative hemoglobin level (Spence et al., 1990).

Management of Intraoperative Bleeding

Venous bleeding after pelvic surgery can be excessive and difficult to control, and urologists should be aware of techniques to manage excessive bleeding. Although not new, pelvic packing remains a time-honored technique that is simple, effective, and safe, provided the packs are removed within 48 to 72 hours postoperatively. In one study, 28 per cent of patients developed either abdominal or perineal wound infections after pelvic packing for rectal surgery, but no patient developed a deep infection requiring surgical drainage (Zama et al., 1988).

Newer techniques to control pelvic bleeding include the use of fibrin glue and the argon beam coagulator. Fibrin glue is a biologic adhesive prepared from equal amounts of cryoprecipitate and bovine thrombin. Equal volumes are sprayed through separate plastic syringes into the pelvis either alone or in combination with an agent such as absorbable gelatin sponge (Gelfoam) or microfibrillar collagen hemostat (Avitene). A fibrin hemostatic plug is formed that effectively controls both low-pressure venous bleeding and small-arterial bleeding (Malviya and Deppe, 1989). The argon beam coagulator uses argon gas, which is inert and nonconducting, to blow away the surface blood from the bleeding vessels. This allows an electrical current to effectively coagulate diffuse pelvic bleeding. The argon beam coagulator may also be effective in controlling hemorrhage in other urologic procedures such as partial nephrectomy and in difficult situations such as hemorrhagic cystitis secondary to cyclophosphamide use (Quinlan et al., 1990).

ENDOCRINE CONSIDERATIONS

Diabetes Mellitus

Serum glucose levels should be well controlled before surgery; elective surgery in an uncontrolled diabetic patient is seldom justified. Blood glucose levels should be maintained between 125 and 250 mg/dl during the perioperative period to decrease the incidence of infections (Bagdade, 1976) and to facilitate wound healing (Goodsen and Hunt, 1977). To achieve this goal, a number of regimens for administering insulin during the perioperative period have been proposed (Meyers et al., 1986; Taitelman et al., 1977; Walts et al., 1981). Regardless of the technique used, therapy must reflect the fact that insulin requirements change frequently during the perioperative period. The stress of surgery may increase insulin requirements resulting from hyperglycemia caused by the release of epinephrine and cortisol (Baesl and Buckley, 1983). Regional anesthesia and high-dose narcotics can significantly reduce intraoperative increases in stress-related hormone levels (Pflug and Halter, 1981). Insulin requirements may decrease after surgical treatment of an established infection, such as a perinephric abscess (White and Kumagai, 1979). Although it is desirable to control blood glucose levels within reasonable limits to reduce perioperative complications, overzealous regulation may result in fatal hypoglycemia.

Preoperatively, the patient usually receives one half of the usual morning insulin dose as NPH insulin at 7 A.M. on the morning of surgery. An intravenous infusion of a 5 per cent glucose solution is begun 2 hours preoperatively at a rate of 100 ml/hour. Intraoperatively, blood glucose levels should be measured every hour. It is particularly important to follow blood glucose levels during prolonged surgery, because hypoglycemia is difficult to diagnose in the anesthetized patient.

There are several regimens to control glucose levels intraoperatively, including intravenous insulin boluses based on blood glucose levels (Walts et al., 1981), hourly intravenous insulin (Meyers et al., 1986), continuous insulin infusions (Goldberg et al., 1981), and simultaneous infusion of insulin and glucose (Thomas et al., 1984). Although there are few data comparing these regimens, it appears that continuous insulin infusions offer potentially superior glycemic control but require monitoring of blood glucose levels and alteration of the infusion rate as needed. Although simultaneous infusion of insulin and glucose has been reported to reduce the risk of hypoglycemia, the results are controversial (Bowen et al., 1982) and the regimen is quite cumbersome, because the entire infusate must be changed to alter the insulin-to-glucose ratio (King and Snyder, 1990).

Postoperatively, hyperglycemia is managed by the supplemental administration of subcutaneous insulin, as shown in Table 63–6. Supplemental insulin requirements should be measured by blood levels rather than urinary glucose levels, which may be inaccurate. Human or purified pork insulin preparations are recommended to minimize antibody production and the potential devel-

Table 63–6. MANAGEMENT OF POSTOPERATIVE HYPERGLYCEMIA IN THE DIABETIC PATIENT

Blood Glucose Level (mg/dl)	Percentage of Normal Morning Insulin Dose (Subcutaneous)*
<250	None
250–300	10
300–400	20
>400	25

*Regular insulin dosage administered at 4- to 6-hour intervals according to serum glucose level.

From Izenstein, B., Dhuhy, R., and Williams, G.: Endocrinology. *In* Vandan, L. (Ed.): To Make the Patient Ready for Anesthesia. Menlo Park, Ca., Addison-Wesley Co., 1980.

opment of insulin resistance or allergy (Molitch, 1982). The time of peak effect of previously administered intermediate-acting insulin should be kept in mind when administering supplemental regular insulin.

During the early postoperative period when patients are unable to eat, an intravenous infusion that provides 50 to 100 g of glucose per day should be continued. Blood glucose levels should be measured every 6 hours, and patients should receive regular insulin as required. After insulin requirements have stabilized, blood glucose determinations may be necessary only in the early morning and in the midafternoon.

After the patient has resumed a preoperative diet, intravenous fluids may be discontinued, and the patient may be managed with an intermediate-acting insulin such as NPH, which is administered as a single dose in the morning. Blood glucose levels should be checked at 3 P.M., and adjustment of the morning insulin dose may be required, as shown in Table 63–7.

Diabetic patients who are not insulin dependent are easier to manage because they are not as likely to develop ketoacidosis or hyperosmolar dehydration. Patients taking oral hypoglycemic agents should not be given the medication on the morning of surgery. An intravenous infusion containing 5 per cent glucose is begun 2 hours before surgery. Blood glucose levels should be measured in the recovery room and on the afternoon of surgery, and regular insulin should be administered as required to maintain blood glucose levels below 250 mg/dl. Patients who are able to eat after surgery usually do not require supplemental insulin, and they can resume oral medication either on the evening after surgery or the next morning. Patients who are unable to eat for several days will probably require supplemental regular insulin. Diabetic patients who are managed by dietary restrictions alone usually do not require supplemental insulin during the perioperative period (King and Snyder, 1990).

Diabetic patients have an increased risk for complications in the perioperative period. In one study, 7 per cent of diabetic patients undergoing surgery had cardiac complications. The significant predictors of cardiac mortality were (1) pre-existing congestive heart failure or valvular heart disease and (2) age older than 75 years. Eleven per cent of patients had noncardiac complications. Three significant clinical predictors were identified: (1) diabetic end-organ disease (retinopathy, neu-ropathy, or nephropathy), (2) congestive heart failure or valvular disease, and (3) peripheral vascular disease associated with infection. Four per cent of patients died postoperatively, and death was predicted only by the presence of major cardiac risk factors such as congestive heart failure or valvular heart disease. It is interesting that neither the severity of the diabetes nor the degree of glucose control correlated with perioperative morbidity or mortality (MacKenzie and Charlson, 1988).

Hyperthyroidism

Hyperthyroidism must be recognized preoperatively to prevent perioperative morbidity associated with this condition. In addition to the common findings of increased sweating, vasodilatation, and tachycardia, more subtle manifestations include weight loss, listlessness, apathy, and psychiatric abnormalities. Preoperative screening tests include a serum thyroxine interpreted with a triiodothyronine resin uptake to correct for changes in binding proteins and a serum triiodothyronine level for confirmation of hyperthyroidism (Goldmann, 1987).

In a patient with hyperthyroidism, preoperative examination should include careful evaluation of the airway for tracheal compression or deviation by a large goiter, a chest x-ray film, and possibly laryngoscopy to assess vocal cord movement (Mercer and Eltringham, 1985). The anesthesiologist should give special attention to eye care to prevent corneal ulceration, because 5 per cent of hyperthyroid patients have proptosis.

Hyperthyroidism results in increased cardiac output and heart rate and may cause arrhythmias. Propylthiouracil, iodine, hydrocortisone, and beta-adrenergic blockers decrease thyroid hormone levels or block peripheral effects (King and Snyder, 1990). Before these drugs were used routinely, thyroid storm (thyrotoxicosis) developed in as many as one third of hyperthyroid patients undergoing thyroidectomy, with a high mortality (McArthur et al., 1974). Symptoms of thyroid storm include fever, tachycardia, and severe hypotension. Treatment includes use of iodine, steroids, and propranolol, with additional supportive measures of intravenous fluids, oxygen, and mechanical cooling devices. Despite modern therapy, thyroid storm remains a dangerous complication with significant mortality (Eriksson et al., 1977).

Table 63–7. ADDITIONAL MORNING INSULIN DOSE AFTER STABILIZATION OF REQUIREMENTS

3 P.M. Blood Glucose Level (mg/dl)	Percentage of Morning Insulin Dose (Subcutaneous)
200–300	None
300–400	20 as intermediate insulin
>400	20 as intermediate insulin and 20 as regular insulin

From Izenstein, B., Dhuhy, R., and Williams, G.: Endocrinology. *In* Vandan, L. (Ed.): To Make the Patient Ready for Anesthesia. Menlo Park, Ca., Addison-Wesley Co., 1980.

Hypothyroidism

As with hyperthyroidism, the diagnosis of hypothyroidism requires a high index of suspicion. Symptoms include lethargy, cold intolerance, hoarseness, constipation, dry skin, impaired memory, and apathy. Physical findings include hoarseness, periorbital edema, thinning of the eyebrows, brittle hair, dry skin, goiter, hypothermia, bradycardia, and prolonged relaxation of the deep tendon reflexes (Murkin, 1982). The diagnosis is established by a low thyroxine level and an elevated thyroid-stimulating hormone level.

Hypothyroidism results in a decreased metabolic rate, myocardial depression, depressed respiratory drive, impaired renal function, and altered mental status. Although plasma levels of triiodothyronine, thyroxine, and thyroid-stimulating hormone can be corrected fairly quickly, reversal of organ-specific abnormalities may take weeks to months. Therefore, replacement of thyroid hormone is usually accomplished slowly, and only emergency surgical procedures should be performed before correction of thyroid hormone status (King and Snyder, 1990).

Adrenal Insufficiency

The normal response of the body to stress is to increase adrenal production of cortisol. Normally, 15 to 25 mg of cortisol is produced by the adrenal glands daily, but under severe stress cortisol production may increase to between 250 and 300 mg daily. Adrenocortical insufficiency may develop not only in patients with primary adrenal or pituitary failure but also in patients who have received exogenous steroid therapy in the previous year for the treatment of other diseases. Patients with steroid suppression are likely to develop acute adrenocortical insufficiency during the perioperative period unless they receive supplemental steroids.

The intravenous adrenocorticotropic hormone (ACTH) stimulation test is a safe and reliable means of evaluating the hypothalamic-pituitary-adrenal axis before surgery in patients who have received glucocorticoid therapy. Measurement of the cortisol response to 250 μg of adrenocorticotropic hormone is an excellent predictor of the maximal cortisol response. Markedly impaired cortisol secretion during surgery is unlikely if a normal adrenal response to this hormone is demonstrated preoperatively (Kehlet and Binder, 1973).

The indications for supplemental perioperative steroid therapy are as follows: (1) chronic adrenal insufficiency, (2) continuous treatment with topical steroids for greater than 1 month in the previous 6 months (Rabinowitz et al., 1977), and (3) treatment with systemic steroids for greater than 1 week in the past 6 months (Gran and Pahle, 1978), (4) current steroid therapy, (5) anticipated bilateral adrenalectomy, and (6) anticipated unilateral adrenalectomy for a cortisol-producing tumor (Baesl and Buckley, 1983).

Patients with suspected steroid suppression should receive 100 mg of hydrocortisone intravenously at midnight and at 6 A.M. on the day of operation and 100 mg

Table 63–8. RELATIVE ANTI-INFLAMMATORY AND SODIUM-RETAINING POTENCIES OF GLUCOCORTICOIDS

Drug	Potency	Sodium Retention
Cortisone acetate	0.8	0.8
Hydrocortisone	1	1
Prednisone	4	0.8
Prednisolone	4	0.8
Methylprednisolone	5	0.5
Dexamethasone	25	0

From Baesl, T. J., and Buckley, J. J.: Preoperative assessment, preparation for operation, and postoperative care. Urol. Clin. North Am., 10:3, 1983.

every 6 hours for the first 24 hours postoperatively. Supplemental hydrocortisone is decreased to 50 mg every 6 hours for the next 24 hours and is further decreased to 25 mg every 6 hours during the following 24 hours. Supplemental glucocorticoids are then tapered to a maintenance dosage over the next 3 to 5 days. Serum cortisol levels return to normal with 72 hours in control patients, and supplemental steroids in patients with steroid suppression usually are unnecessary after this time. Steroid supplementation should be continued, however, in patients with surgical complications, such as sepsis or ileus, which increase the cortisol demand (Baxter and Tyrell, 1981).

The relative anti-inflammatory and sodium-retaining potencies of various glucocorticoids are shown in Table 63–8. Cortisone acetate is a poor choice for steroid replacement because it is rapidly metabolized to inactive hormones and is absorbed erratically after intramuscular administration (Kehlet et al., 1974).

NUTRITIONAL SUPPORT OF THE UROLOGIC PATIENT

About 50 per cent of patients undergoing major surgery are malnourished (Bistrian et al., 1975), and nutritional depletion is associated with increased surgical morbidity and mortality (Mullen, 1981). Malnutrition results in delayed wound healing, increased frequency of wound infections, decreased vital organ function, decreased immunocompetence, increased occurrence of sepsis, prolonged ileus, and more frequent respiratory infections and pulmonary insufficiency (Mullen et al., 1979; Reinhardt, 1980; Seltzer et al., 1979). These problems are related to a loss of body protein. Depletion of one quarter of the body's nitrogen content, which corresponds to a decrease of one third of body weight, is fatal. Nutritional problems are common in geriatric patients and patients with renal failure or cancer—groups of patients with whom the urologist deals frequently. It is important, therefore, that the urologist be aware of nutritional requirements and be familiar with methods of nutritional evaluation and support.

Nutritional Requirements

Calories

An individual's daily caloric requirement is about 25 kcal/kg body weight. The demands of surgery result in an increased caloric requirement to about 30 to 35 kcal/kg body weight, and severely burned or septic patients may require as much as 50 kcal/kg body weight. Carbohydrates and protein both provide 4 kcal/g, and fats provide 9 kcal/g (Teasley et al., 1983).

Protein

Between 1.5 and 2 g of protein per kilogram body weight is required daily to preserve lean body mass. Protein consists of amino acids that are either nonessential or essential. The former can be manufactured by the body, whereas the latter cannot and must be supplied in the diet (Hensle, 1983).

Fats

Fatty acids can also be classified as nonessential and essential. The three essential fatty acids are linoleic acid, arachidonic acid, and linolenic acid. Only linoleic acid is absolutely essential, because a fatty acid deficiency will not develop if it alone is provided (McDougal, 1983).

Vitamins and Minerals

Vitamins must be provided daily, particularly water-soluble vitamins because they are depleted rapidly. Minerals such as sodium, potassium, calcium, magnesium, and phosphate must be provided daily, and trace metals such as zinc, copper, magnesium, and iodine must be provided periodically (McDougal, 1983).

Overall Nutritional Planning

The goals of nutritional therapy are to protect body protein stores and to provide adequate calories. Although it is important to preserve body protein, excessive administration of protein should be avoided because it may result in an elevation of the BUN and altered hepatic and renal transport in critically ill patients. For each gram of protein administered, 25 kcal of carbohydrate or fat should be provided, and it is important to supply a balance of both carbohydrate and fat to satisfy the body's energy demands. Carbohydrate is usually administered as glucose, and although glucose provides only 4 kcal/g, it has a protein-sparing effect. Supplying up to 700 kcal/day as glucose provides maximal protection of body protein. A further increase in glucose does not increase protein sparing, and it is impossible to maintain a positive nitrogen balance with glucose alone. Fats provide 9 kcal/g, but they do not have as great a protein-sparing effect as do carbohydrates (McDougal, 1983).

Nutritional Evaluation

Preoperative Evaluation

Preoperative evaluation of nutritional status is easy and inexpensive and should be done in all patients who are undergoing major surgery. The basic evaluation includes only a determination of weight loss and measurements of the lymphocyte count and the serum albumin. Additional tests are required only when uncertainty about nutritional status persists after these basic tests have been done.

WEIGHT LOSS. All patients should be asked about possible recent weight loss. Patients who have lost up to 10 lb in the preceding 3 months are assumed to be mildly malnourished. A weight loss of 10 to 20 lb reflects moderate malnutrition, and a weight loss of more than 20 lb indicates severe malnutrition. Absolute weight loss may underestimate the degree of malnutrition because there is an accumulation of extracellular fluid when body protein is metabolized that may offset total-body weight loss. The use of a height-weight index may be helpful in assessing weight loss, but the index is often inaccurate for obese patients (McDougal, 1983).

LYMPHOCYTE COUNT. The lymphocyte count reflects visceral protein status and is normally greater than 2000/mm^3. A value between 1200 and 2000/mm^3 reflects mild malnutrition, a value between 800 and 1200/mm^3 indicates moderate malnutrition, and a value less than 800/mm^3 is associated with severe malnutrition (Seltzer et al., 1979).

SERUM ALBUMIN LEVEL. Serum albumin level also reflects visceral protein status and normally is greater than 3.5 g/dl. A value between 3 and 3.5 g/dl indicates mild malnutrition, a value between 2.5 and 3 g/dl reflects moderate malnutrition, and a value less than 2.5 g/dl is associated with severe malnutrition (Reinhardt et al., 1980).

SERUM TRANSFERRIN LEVEL. Serum transferrin and other plasma proteins such as prealbumin and retinol-binding protein have a shorter half-life than albumin and have been investigated as potential indicators of malnutrition. Normal serum transferrin values are above 200 mg/dl, and values less than 170 mg/dl have been associated with an increased risk of sepsis and death (Blackburn et al., 1977). More recently, the value of transferrin in assessing nutritional status has been challenged, and its utility at present is controversial (Roza et al., 1984).

SKIN TEST ANTIGENS. The use of skin test antigens may be helpful when uncertainty about nutritional status exists after weight loss, serum albumin level, and total lymphocyte count have been assessed. Failure to respond to recall skin test antigens such as mumps, *Candida,* and streptokinase-streptodornase (SK-SD) indicates severe malnutrition (Meakins et al., 1977).

OTHER TESTS. Measurement of the circumference of the middle upper arm and determination of the creatinine excretion index are tests used to evaluate lean body mass or muscle protein stores. The triceps skin fold thickness is used to assess fat stores (McDougal, 1983).

PROGNOSTIC NUTRITIONAL INDEX. Several multivariate indices have been developed to better select patients who may benefit from preoperative parenteral nutrition. One index based on total lymphocyte count, albumin and transferrin levels, and delayed hypersensitivity was found to predict postoperative sepsis and surgical mortality (Harvey et al., 1981). Another index based on multimetabolic markers identified high-risk patients who had a nearly 60 per cent mortality as opposed to a 3 per cent mortality for low-risk patients (Mullen et al., 1979). One study used an index based on serum albumin level, delayed hypersensitivity, and triceps skin fold thickness to identify high-risk patients undergoing major abdominal surgery (Smith and Hartemink, 1988).

Assessing Response to Therapy

A response to therapy is indicated by weight gain and normalization of the lymphocyte count and plasma protein levels. Albumin, which is present in large quantities and has a low fractional synthesis rate, is a good indicator of chronic nutritional deficiency but a poor indicator of acute nutritional changes. Therefore, rapid-turnover plasma proteins such as prealbumin and retinol-binding protein are more useful as indicators of response to improved nutrition (Fleck, 1989). Recovery of skin test hypersensitivity is also a useful measure of nutritional response. About 50 per cent of cancer patients who have negative skin test results convert to a positive status after nutritional repletion, and those patients who convert to a positive status respond better to surgery and chemotherapy (Daly et al., 1980). It may take 2 to 3 weeks of therapy before an objective response is noted, and elective surgery should be postponed as long as necessary. It has been recommended that an objective end point such as testing of skeletal muscle function be used rather than an arbitrary number of days to determine the preoperative end point for parenteral nutrition (Meguid et al., 1989).

The response to nutritional therapy can be assessed daily by determination of body weight and nitrogen balance. Changes in body weight accurately reflect nutritional therapy provided that the patient is not overloaded with fluid. Nitrogen balance can be calculated readily. Eighty per cent of the nitrogen lost in the urine is excreted as urea, and about 1.25 g of nitrogen is excreted per day in the feces and through the skin. The daily nitrogen loss can be calculated, therefore, by multiplying the amount of urea excreted in the urine in 24 hours by a factor of 1.25 and adding 1.25 g to account for fecal and skin losses. The daily nitrogen intake can be calculated by the dietary service. Nitrogen balance is determined by subtracting the daily nitrogen loss from the daily nitrogen intake (McDougal, 1983).

Effects of Parenteral Nutrition on Postoperative Outcome

Parenteral nutrition has not been shown to be of value in normally nourished or mildly malnourished patients (Detsky et al., 1987). Indeed, parenteral nutrition may be harmful to some patients because it may be associated with a higher incidence of sepsis (Brister et al., 1984). In moderately to severely malnourished patients, however, parenteral nutrition significantly reduces perioperative morbidity and mortality. One study reported a 9 per cent mortality in patients receiving combined preoperative and postoperative parenteral nutrition compared with a 47 per cent mortality in patients receiving postoperative therapy alone (Mullen et al., 1980). In another study, malnourished patients receiving preoperative nutritional support had a 21 per cent incidence of septic complications compared with a 53 per cent incidence in control patients (Bellantone et al., 1988). In a prospective trial of patients undergoing gastrointestinal surgery for solid tumors, 7 to 10 days of preoperative parenteral nutrition resulted in a significant reduction of postoperative wound infections and a decrease in other major complications as well as in mortality (Meguid et al., 1989). Although there are few data for urologic patients, perioperative nutritional support seems advisable for malnourished patients undergoing radical cystectomy and urinary diversion who are deprived of oral nutrition for at least 7 to 10 days after surgery.

Methods of Nutritional Support

Enteral Nutrition

Enteral nutrition is associated with fewer complications and can provide a more balanced physiologic diet than intravenous nutrition. Enteral nutrition can be accomplished via a feeding tube, a gastrostomy, or a feeding jejunostomy. The newer small-caliber Silastic mercury-tipped feeding tubes are well tolerated by patients. A variety of commercially prepared solutions can provide about 1 kcal/ml and cause fewer gastrointestinal side effects than older preparations (Hensle, 1983).

Enteral diets are either nonelemental or elemental. Nonelemental diets consist of undigested and minimally digested protein hydrolysates, fat, and carbohydrates. Elemental diets consist of medium-chain triglycerides, glucose, and amino acids. Nonelemental preparations are less expensive, have a lower osmolality, and are preferable to elemental preparations if the intestinal tract is not diseased. Elemental diets are bulk-free and are better tolerated in patients with gastrointestinal problems (Fairfull-Smith et al., 1980). Severely malnourished patients may have altered gastrointestinal absorption related to a decrease in the height of the mucosal brush border and a decrease in the height of the columnar epithelium, and they may have decreased gastrointestinal motility caused by overgrowth of anaerobic bacteria. These patients should initially be given an elemental diet until these changes associated with starvation have been reversed (Viteri and Schneider, 1974).

Enteral feedings are administered by continuous infusion. They are begun at a concentration of one-half strength at a rate of 50 to 75 ml/hour. The volume is increased as tolerated to provide 2000 to 3000 ml/day. The concentration or rate should be reduced if the patient develops abdominal cramps, diarrhea, or diaphoresis. Diarrhea may also be controlled by the administration of paregoric in doses of 5 ml (McDougal, 1983).

Isosmotic Intravenous Nutrition

Isosmotic intravenous nutrition is an ideal means of preserving normal metabolic function in short-term situations after trauma or surgery in which the gastrointestinal tract cannot be used. The advantages of using isosmotic solutions instead of hypertonic solutions are that they can be administered by peripheral vein and that the rate of infusion may be adjusted rapidly without affecting serum osmolality. Isosmotic infusions may be termporarily discontinued so that colloids, medications, and blood may be administered as required. Unfortunately, a positive nitrogen balance cannot be achieved with isosmotic solutions alone, because the number of calories required would precipitate fluid overload. Therefore, long-term intravenous hyperalimentation requires the use of hypertonic solutions (McDougal, 1983).

A solution commonly used for isosmotic intravenous nutrition consists of a liter solution containing 500 ml of a 10 to 20 per cent dextrose solution and 500 ml of a 7 per cent amino acid solution. This balanced glucose and amino acid solution provides maximal protein sparing while maintaining optimal hepatic, renal, and cardiac function. Additional calories are supplied via administration of 500 ml of fat emulsions (Intralipid) once or twice per day.

Hyperosmotic Intravenous Nutrition

Hyperosmotic intravenous nutrition was developed by Dudrick and colleagues in 1968. Standard solutions contain 1000 cal and 6 g of nitrogen per liter and are a mixture of 50 per cent dextrose and 7 per cent amino acid solutions. Electrolytes, trace elements, and vitamins are added to the solution as required. Essential fatty acids in the form of Intralipid are administered two or three times weekly.

Hyperosmotic intravenous solutions are about 2 osmolar and must be administered through a central venous catheter. A percutaneous subclavian or internal jugular catheter is sufficient for short-term use, but a Broviac or a Hickman catheter is required for long-term hyperalimentation. These catheters are inserted into the superior vena cava and are tunneled across the anterior chest wall to exit midway between the sternum and the nipple. These catheters have been maintained for as long as 14 months in children and 21 months in adults (McDougal, 1983). Central venous catheters must be inserted under strict aseptic conditions and must be kept sterile at all times. Blood, additional fluid, and medications cannot be given through a hyperalimentation catheter, and the line should never be used to measure central venous pressure.

Intravenous hyperalimentation is begun at a rate of 50 ml/hour. The rate is increased gradually to avoid hyperglycemia, and insulin is added to the solution as required to maintain a blood glucose level of less than 200 mg/dl. Eventually, 3 to 4 L of solution may be infused per day, which provides 3000 to 4000 kcal. Patients receiving intravenous hyperalimentation must be followed carefully. Serum glucose and osmolality should be monitored closely, particularly when begin-

ning therapy, to prevent hyperosmolar dehydration. Serum electrolyte, BUN, creatinine, calcium, and phosphate levels should be assessed daily, and the serum magnesium level should be checked twice weekly (McDougal, 1983).

The complications of hyperosmotic intravenous nutrition can be divided into three categories: technical, infectious, and metabolic. Technical complications are related to catheter insertion and include pneumothorax, hydrothorax, brachial plexus injury, arterial laceration, venous thrombosis, air embolism, arrhythmias, and cardiac tamponade. The frequency of technical complications is inversely related to the experience of the person inserting the hyperalimentation catheter (Cerra, 1987).

Previously, infectious complications occurred in 10 to 30 per cent of patients receiving intravenous hyperalimentation. Infection usually arises in the dermal tunnel created at the time of catheter insertion. The incidence of infection increases with the length of time the catheter is in place and is more common when polyvinyl chloride catheters are used. With more careful preparation of solutions and sterile technique for inserting and maintaining catheters, the incidence of infectious complications has been reduced to between 1 and 3 per cent (Schlichtig and Ayres, 1988).

The most serious metabolic complication of intravenous hyperalimentation is hyperosmolar nonketotic dehydration and coma, which occurs when blood glucose levels exceed 500 mg/dl. This condition has a mortality approaching 50 per cent and must be treated aggressively by administering large doses of insulin and fluid and by decreasing the rate of infusion. Conversely, excess insulin may cause hypoglycemia when parenteral nutrition is slowed or discontinued (Fischer and Freund, 1983).

Hyperalimentation can also cause alterations in amino acid metabolism, which result in hyperchloremic metabolic acidosis, azotemia, and hyperammonemia. If glucose is provided in excess, insulin release is stimulated, which induces hepatic lipogenesis with subsequent fatty infiltration of the liver, cholestatic jaundice, and elevated serum levels of very-low-density lipoproteins. This complication can usually be avoided by using fat to replace one third of the glucose calories (Meguid et al., 1984). Other metabolic abnormalities result from improper amounts of nutrients in the intravenous solution, and these problems usually are minor and corrected easily. Vitamin, mineral, trace metal, and essential amino acid deficiencies all can occur and usually cause no clinical problems when corrected promptly (Deutschman, 1990).

Intravenous Nutrition and Renal Failure

Acute Renal Failure

The mortality associated with acute renal failure can be reduced by 50 per cent by providing adequate calories and essential amino acids. Protein restriction and supplementation with essential amino acids result in a less rapid increase in BUN, which is associated with de-

Table 63–9. DIETARY PROTEIN RESTRICTION IN RENAL FAILURE

GFR (ml/min)	Daily Protein Allowance (g)
< 10	40
10–15	50
16–20	70
21–25	90

From Hensle, T. W.: Nutritional support of the urologic patient. Curr. Trends Urol., 1:157, 1981.

creased catabolism, increased wound healing, and decreased duration of renal failure (Abel et al., 1973).

Chronic Renal Failure

Surgical patients with chronic renal failure benefit from protein restriction and supplementation with essential amino acids. This therapy results in improvement in anemia associated with renal insufficiency, decreased BUN, and a positive nitrogen balance. It is not necessary to restrict protein until the GFR is less than 25 ml/minute. Recommended protein allowances for lower GFR values are shown in Table 63–9. Patients having dialysis must be allowed extra protein in the diet, because they lose between 6 and 10 g of free amino acids during each hemodialysis session and between 6 and 10 g of protein during each peritoneal dialysis session. Intravenous hyperalimentation is not a substitute for dialysis, but the combination of hyperalimentation and dialysis results in maximal protein synthesis, which may produce a positive nitrogen balance (Hensle, 1983).

PERIOPERATIVE INFECTIONS

Urinary Tract Infections

Prophylaxis

The majority of perioperative urinary tract infections are caused by bladder catheterization. The frequency of bacteriuria in patients requiring short-term (24 to 48 hours) postoperative catheterization is about 6 per cent; however, symptomatic urinary tract infections develop in only 1 per cent of such patients. The risk of infection increases with the duration of catheterization, and even with careful management about 50 per cent of patients will have urinary tract infections after 10 days of catheterization (Nickel et al., 1989).

Preservation of a closed drainage system reduces the risk of urinary tract infections in catheterized patients. Although continuous bladder irrigation with antiseptic solutions does not reduce infections, continuous saline irrigation via a three-way catheter reduces the need for manual bladder irrigations and thus may lower the risk of urinary tract infections.

Other measures to reduce the risk of urinary tract infections associated with catheterization have not been effective. Application of antimicrobial agents at the urethral meatus has been ineffective, and cleansing the meatus with soap and water is associated with an increased risk of infection (Burke et al., 1981). Instillation of antiseptic solutions into the urinary drainage bag delays the onset of bacteriuria in the bag itself, but the bag is an infrequent source of urinary tract infection (Pien and Landers, 1983).

The diagnosis and treatment of established urinary tract infections are discussed in Chapter 17.

Antibiotic Prophylaxis in Transurethral Prostatectomy

The efficacy of perioperative antibiotic prophylaxis in patients undergoing transurethral prostatectomy has been controversial. Some studies have shown that antibiotic prophylaxis reduces the incidence of perioperative infections, whereas others have shown no benefit (Gibbons et al., 1978). Routine use of antibiotics may result in selection of resistant organisms, which may require parenteral antibiotic therapy after the catheter has been removed, thus prolonging hospitalization. Several studies, however, have shown that a single dose of antibiotic administered intravenously 1 hour before transurethral surgery lowers the incidence of perioperative urinary tract infections and is not associated with emergence of resistant organisms. Appropriate antibiotics include either a combination of ampicillin and gentamicin, or ciprofloxacin, or a third-generation cephalosporin (Bremner et al., 1988; Christensen et al., 1989; Cox, 1989).

Prophylactic antibiotics should be administered routinely to patients with either indwelling catheters or pre-existing urinary tract infections. Such patients have a high risk of developing bacteremia associated with transurethral surgery and should receive perioperative antibiotics (Cafferkey et al., 1982). Patients undergoing transurethral surgery should also receive a single dose of antibiotics before catheter removal, because catheter manipulation may precipitate bacteremia (Kiely et al., 1989).

Prophylaxis for Prostatic Needle Biopsy

Transrectal needle biopsy of the prostate has been associated with a high incidence of bacteremia, and patients undergoing this procedure frequently were hospitalized for prophylactic intravenous antibiotics. The development of smaller needles introduced with a spring-loaded gun has reduced the incidence of infection. Nevertheless, patients undergoing this procedure should receive oral broad-spectrum antibiotics that provide gram-negative and anaerobic coverage. Antibiotics are not required in patients undergoing either transrectal needle aspiration or transperineal needle biopsy of the prostate unless the urine is infected (Packer et al., 1984).

Prophylaxis for Subacute Bacterial Endocarditis

Patients who have a history of valvular heart disease or who have a prosthetic valve or joint should receive prophylactic antibiotics before urologic instrumentation. Because *Enterococcus* is the organism usually responsible for endocarditis, patients at risk should receive ampicillin, 1 g, and gentamicin, 1.5 mg/kg (not to exceed 80 mg), either intravenously or intramuscularly 30 to 60 minutes before any genitourinary procedure. Patients allergic to penicillin should receive vancomycin, 1 g intravenously, instead of ampicillin. Although it is recommended that such patients receive two additional doses of these antibiotics at 8-hour intervals after the procedure, this method is frequently impractical because many of these procedures are done on an outpatient basis. Patients should be given ampicillin, 500 mg orally at 6 and 12 hours after these procedures; with this regimen, the incidence of endocarditis is extremely low (American Heart Association Committee, 1977).

Prophylaxis for Intestinal Surgery

Patients undergoing urologic procedures that involve entry into the intestinal tract, particularly the distal ileum or colon, should undergo bowel preparation. The standard preparation involves a combination of dietary restriction, cathartics and enemas, and oral antibiotics to reduce bacterial flora (Nichols, 1982). This routine for bowel preparation is outlined in Table 63–10.

The development of isotonic whole-gut lavage solutions has reduced the time required for preoperative bowel preparation. GoLYTELY is the most commonly used solution and contains two primary components, polyethylene glycol and sodium sulfate base, both of which are poorly absorbed from the gastrointestinal tract. Polyethylene glycol is a functional osmotic agent that does not allow absorption or secretion of water. Sodium sulfate base and additional electrolytes are added to balance the solution to equal the body's natural concentrations. The ultimate result is negligible net water loss and electrolyte movement that reduces the risk of dehydration. GoLYTELY can be used safely and effectively not only in adults, but also in infants and children (Konings, 1989).

Table 63–10. BOWEL PREPARATION FOR ELECTIVE COLORECTAL OPERATIONS

Preoperative day 3	Clear liquid or minimum-residue diet; bisacodyl, 1 capsule orally at 6 P.M.
Preoperative day 2	Clear liquid or minimum-residue diet; magnesium sulfate, 30 ml of 50 per cent solution (15 g) orally at 10 A.M., 2 P.M., and 6 P.M.; saline enemas at bedtime until return is clear
Preoperative day 1	Clear liquid diet; magnesium sulfate (in dose above) at 10 A.M. and 2 P.M.; supplemental intravenous fluids as needed; no enemas; neomycin-erythromycin base, 1 g orally at 1 P.M., 2 P.M., and 11 P.M.
Operative day	Rectum evacuated at 6:30 A.M.; operation at 8 A.M.

From Nichols, R. L.: Prophylaxis for elective bowel surgery. *In* Wilson, S. E., Finegold, S. M., and Williams, R. A. (Eds.): Intra-abdominal Infection. New York, McGraw-Hill Book Co., 1982. Copyright © 1982 by McGraw Hill, Inc. Used by permission of McGraw-Hill Book Co.

Whole-gut lavage is usually done by administering 4 to 6 L of GoLYTELY on the day before surgery. Alternatively, it can be administered as 1 L every 12 hours on the 2 days before surgery, thus reducing cramping and diarrhea associated with conventional laxatives (Soballe and Greif, 1989). The use of lavage solutions also decreases the length of dietary restriction necessary to prepare the intestine. Patients are placed on a low-residue diet 2 days before surgery and a clear liquid diet on the day before surgery. Enemas are unnecessary (Wolff et al., 1988).

The usual antibiotic prophylaxis for intestinal surgery includes oral neomycin and erythromycin base, which have little systemic absorption. Several studies have shown that single preoperative doses of metronidazole in combination with a cephalosporin are equally effective (Klin and Dahlgren, 1989; Raahave et al., 1988). Alternatively, the new quinolone antibiotics can be used prophylactically and are effective against staphylococci and a wide spectrum of gram-negative bacteria. They are relatively ineffective, however, against streptococci and anaerobic bacteria (Nord, 1989).

The use of orthograde lavage solutions and single-dose preoperative intravenous antibiotics, along with the elimination of harsh cathartics, multiple enemas, and multiple-dose oral antibiotics, now allows bowel preparation to be done almost entirely on an outpatient basis. It is advisable, however, to admit patients on the day before surgery for administration of intravenous fluids that night.

Pulmonary Infections

Prophylaxis

Lower respiratory tract infections account for about 15 per cent of all nosocomial infections and are particularly common after prolonged anesthesia. The risk of developing pulmonary infections can be reduced by using aseptic technique during intubation and endotracheal suctioning and by maintaining sterile respiratory support equipment. Respiratory isolation procedures should be initiated in patients with pulmonary infections to prevent cross-infection to other patients (Alexander, 1983).

Diagnosis

Pneumonia is usually readily diagnosed because it produces consolidation of pulmonary tissue seen on a chest roentgenogram. A tracheal aspirate should be obtained daily in all intubated patients and a Gram stain performed. An early pneumonia may be detected when the Gram stain findings change from scattered inflammatory cells to dense neutrophils and bacteria. Sputum cultures from nonintubated patients are usually worthless because of pharyngeal contamination. When pneumonia is suspected, transtracheal aspiration can be performed to obtain a reliable culture. Renal transplant patients and other immunosuppressed patients are prone to develop nonbacterial pneumonias, and transbronchial or open pulmonary biopsies may be required to establish the diagnosis (Alexander, 1983).

Treatment

Pneumonias can usually be eradicated with pulmonary therapy and antibiotics. Empiric antibiotic therapy should include both gram-positive and gram-negative coverage. A more precise antibiotic regimen may be initiated when the results of the sputum cultures have been obtained (Alexander, 1983).

Wound Infections

Prophylaxis

Removal of hair from the incision site should be done immediately before surgery. Usually a razor is used, but, alternatively, electric clippers or a depilatory can be used. The skin should not be shaved on the night before surgery because small lacerations may become infected, which increases the risk of wound infections.

Although skin disinfection in the operating room reduces the risk of wound infections, there is no evidence that either preoperative total-body showering or incision site scrubs with disinfectant agents before surgery provides any additional benefit (Garibaldi et al., 1988). Immediately before surgery, a 10-minute scrub with an antiseptic agent has been traditional, but shorter periods may suffice with newer antiseptic agents, particularly when applied to smaller operative fields. Hexachlorophene, chlorhexidine, and povidone-iodine all have been used; of these, povidone-iodine is the most popular and hexachlorophene the least effective (Alexander, 1983).

The conventional scrub for the surgeon involves washing the hands and forearms with an antiseptic agent for 5 to 10 minutes. Unfortunately, this standard technique frequently leaves the hands dry and irritated, especially if a scrub brush is used. Ironically, such skin irritation fosters the very growth of bacteria that the scrub is intended to prevent. Evidence suggests that alternative preparation with an antiseptic foam combining hexachlorophene with ethyl alcohol for 2 minutes is associated with a 0.3 per cent incidence of wound infection compared with previously reported estimates of 3 to 5 per cent with standard surgical scrubs (Rubio, 1987).

Although intraincisional application of antibiotics in contaminated wounds reduces wound infection rates in both experimental and clinical investigations, it does not appear to provide any additional benefit to that achieved with systemic antibiotics (Moesgaard et al., 1989). Similarly, plastic skin drapes have not been effective in reducing wound infections, even when impregnated with iodophor. Plastic drapes may shelter and allow bacteria to proliferate, and, thus, a larger bacterial inoculum is available to enter the wound when the drape is removed. Plastic drapes are recommended, however, to exclude contaminated sites, such as a colostomy, from the operative field (Dewan et al., 1987).

Systemic antibiotic prophylaxis for clean surgical procedures is controversial and usually unnecessary, but it is indicated for either clean-contaminated or contaminated cases (Rotman et al., 1989). In operations involving the large intestine, broad-spectrum coverage against both gram-negative and anaerobic bacteria should be used; a combination of gentamicin and metronidazole is effective (Lau et al., 1988). Third-generation cephalosporins have not been as effective when used alone because of the emergence of anaerobic infections (Keighley, 1988). When a third-generation cephalosporin is used, cephalothin is preferable to cefazolin because of better activity against *Staphylococcus aureus*, but it should again be used in combination with metronidazole (Kernodle et al., 1990).

Wound closure is best done by using a continuous nonabsorbable monofilament suture; it is at least as effective as interrupted suture techniques in preventing wound dehiscence and is associated with an extremely low rate of wound infections (Gallup et al., 1989). Although surgical incisions are generally sealed after 48 hours, wound resistance to infection increases progressively until the fourth or fifth postoperative day. It is advisable, therefore, to maintain a sterile dressing over the wound site until that time. Wet dressings must be changed in a sterile manner, because they will promote bacterial proliferation. After the surgical dressing has been removed, the dry wound coagulum should be left undisturbed, because it provides resistance to exogenous infection. Painting the incision with an antiseptic solution and application of an antibiotic ointment are contraindicated because they may disrupt this defensive barrier (Alexander, 1983).

Contaminated wounds should be managed with delayed primary or secondary closure to reduce the risk of wound infection. A reactive vascular network develops along the wound edges, and this network provides increasing resistance to infection, which becomes maximal about the fifth postoperative day. Delayed primary closure can be accomplished at this time without risking later infection (Edlich et al., 1969).

Diagnosis

Wound infections usually occur between the 5th and 10th postoperative days. Infections that occur within 48 hours postoperatively are caused by either a hemolytic streptococcus or a clostridium. Wound infections may cause pain and erythema over the surgical incision, but often the presentation is less obvious and is manifested by constitutional symptoms such as fever and tachycardia. The diagnosis is made by probing the wound; any purulent material should be cultured for both aerobic and anaerobic bacteria, and a Gram stain should be obtained to guide immediate antibiotic therapy (Allo and Simmons, 1983).

Treatment

The treatment of superficial wound infections involves incision and drainage along with local wound care. The use of antibiotics for superficial wound infections remains controversial. Treatment of deeper wound infections involves administration of broad-spectrum antibiotics along with drainage of purulent material and débridement of devitalized tissue. Antibiotic therapy should be initiated before surgical manipulation of a wound because of the risk of bacteremia and septic shock. Initial antibiotic coverage usually should include an aminoglycoside for gram-negative organisms and metronidazole or a third-generation cephalosporin with broad anaerobic activity. Wound infections that occur within 48 hours postoperatively should be treated with penicillin for streptococci and clostridia. Antibiotic therapy can be modified depending on the results of the wound cultures (Allo and Simons, 1983).

Failure to eradicate an infection with drainage and antibiotic therapy suggests a deep-seated infection such as an abdominal or retroperitoneal abscess. Further tests including an ultrasound examination or a computed tomography scan should be obtained to establish the diagnosis, and it may be possible to drain a deep abscess through a percutaneous catheter inserted under radiographic control (Van Sonnenberg et al., 1982).

Gram-Negative Bacteremia and Septic Shock

Incidence

Gram-negative bacteremia occurs in more than 1 of every 100 hospital admissions in the United States (McCabe and Treadwell, 1983). It is a condition that urologists should recognize and treat promptly, because more than half of the cases result from urologic procedures. Gram-negative bacteremia is one of the most frequent causes of death resulting from hospital-acquired infection. The mortality rate associated with bacteremia alone varies up to 40 per cent; septic shock is associated with mortality rates of up to 80 per cent (Hanno and Wien, 1981).

Etiology

Gram-negative bacteremia accounts for about 70 per cent of septicemias. Mixed gram-positive and gram-negative infections account for another 10 to 20 per cent. Gram-positive bacteremia has become much less common because of earlier recognition and treatment of gram-positive infections (Schwartz and Cerra, 1983). *Escherichia coli* is the single most common causative organism. It causes about 30 per cent of cases and is associated with the best prognosis (Hanno and Wein, 1981). The *Klebsiella-Enterobacter-Serratia* family is the next most common group of organisms and accounts for about 20 per cent of cases (McCabe and Treadwell, 1983).

Pathophysiology

The pathophysiology of gram-negative bacteremia is complicated and not completely understood. A brief discussion is included here; for greater detail the reader is referred to the appropriate references (Hanno and Wien, 1981; McCabe and Treadwell, 1983; Schwartz

and Cerra, 1983). The cell wall of gram-negative bacilli is composed of a lipid-carbohydrate complex termed lipopolysaccharide. This complex acts as an endotoxin, and considerable emphasis has been placed on this substance and its role in the pathophysiology of gram-negative bacteremia. Studies have indicated that this endotoxin is only partially responsible for the pathophysiologic changes that occur in this condition. Intact bacilli or endotoxin stimulates the complement system, which results in the production of two vasoactive anaphylatoxins, C3a and C5a. These activated complement components stimulate the production of bradykinin, which produces the vasodilation and increased vascular permeability observed in gram-negative bacteremia. Bradykinin also results in increased production of prostaglandins E_2 and F_2. Prostaglandins and endorphins may contribute to the hypotension associated with this condition (Peters et al., 1981). Intact bacteria or endotoxin may also initiate the activation of Hageman factor, which, in turn, stimulates sequential activation of other components of the coagulation system, resulting in DIC and fibrinolysis.

The two major consequences of these complicated interactions are reduction in vascular tone and failure of oxygen extraction by the tissues. Gram-negative bacteremia is thus usually associated with increased cardiac output and decreased peripheral resistance (Schwartz and Cerra, 1983). In addition to cardiac failure, hypoxia and altered vascular permeability result in a loss of the functional integrity of alveolar-capillary membranes in the lung. This loss may result in pulmonary edema and the adult respiratory distress syndrome, or "shock lung," which is one of the major causes of death in patients with bacteremia (Hanno and Wien, 1981).

Diagnosis

The early symptoms of gram-negative bacteremia may be subtle and may include only those of fever, altered sensorium, or tachypnea. The astute clinician who is alerted by these early signs will act promptly and usually will be able to prevent the disastrous complications of septic shock. As bacteremia progresses, the patient develops tachycardia and hypotension associated with increased cardiac output and decreased peripheral vascular resistance. Central venous pressure is usually normal or increased (Hanno and Wien, 1981).

Laboratory findings include changes in the white blood cell count, which is initially depressed and then elevated. A coagulopathy is suggested by a decreased platelet count and is confirmed by a decrease in serum fibrinogen and an elevation in fibrin split products. Arterial blood gases indicate respiratory alkalosis initially and metabolic acidosis subsequently. Increasing levels of serum lactic acid are associated with a poor prognosis. Derangement of cellular function may give rise to hyperkalemia and hyponatremia (Hanno and Wien, 1981).

Treatment

Gram-negative bacteremia demands prompt, aggressive treatment to prevent septic shock. Blood, urine, and other appropriate cultures should be obtained, and broad-spectrum antibiotics should be administered immediately after obtaining these cultures. Antibiotics should include an aminoglycoside, a third-generation cephalosporin, and metronidazole to provide maximal gram-negative as well as gram-positive and anaerobic bacterial coverage (McCabe and Treadwell, 1983).

Treatment of hypotension associated with bacteremia may require large volumes of crystalloid because of the decreased peripheral vascular resistance. Intravenous fluids must be administered judiciously, particularly in the elderly, to avoid fluid overload and congestive heart failure. A Swan-Ganz pulmonary arterial catheter may be helpful in guiding fluid therapy (Hanno and Wien, 1981).

Patients with persistent hypotension after adequate volume replacement require administration of vasoactive agents. Dopamine is the drug of first choice, because in low doses it increases renal blood flow and cardiac output without increasing heart rate or peripheral vascular resistance (Hanno and Wien, 1981).

Patients with hypoxemia may require supplemental oxygen, and mechanical ventilatory support may be necessary. Patients with adult respiratory distress syndrome may require large doses of positive end-expiratory pressure to facilitate oxygen delivery (McCabe and Treadwell, 1983).

Other ancillary treatment measures include the administration of intravenous sodium bicarbonate to correct metabolic acidosis and the use of digitalis in patients with heart failure. Corticosteroids remain controversial in the treatment of septic shock. Their reported actions included vasodilation with improved renal blood flow, a positive inotropic effect, decreased platelet aggregation, and stabilization of lysosomal membranes in the injured cell. Steroids appear to be more effective when they are administered early in the course of the disease (Hanno and Wien, 1981).

After immediate therapeutic measures have been initiated, the cause of the bacteremia should be determined. If a focus of infection such as an abscess is identified, it should be drained as soon as possible after initial resuscitation of the patient (Schwartz and Cerra, 1983).

UROLOGIC SURGERY IN PREGNANCY

Urologic surgery in pregnancy should be restricted to emergency procedures and generally is limited to the management of urinary tract calculi. The incidence of calculous disease is no greater during pregnancy, but the symptoms are often attributed to another cause, and the diagnosis frequently is not made until after delivery (Coe et al., 1978). A brief discussion of the diagnosis and management of urinary tract calculi in pregnancy is presented here.

Diagnosis

Radiographic evaluation of the urinary tract during pregnancy should be limited to emergency situations.

When obstructive uropathy secondary to calculous disease is suspected, an intravenous pyelogram should be performed. The hazards of radiation exposure during pregnancy have been exaggerated, and the risk is far outweighed by the potential clinical benefits derived from a properly indicated examination.

The evidence suggests that harmful radiation effects to the fetus are associated with radiation exposure in excess of 50 rad. This dose is far in excess of that associated with the usual intravenous pyelogram, which has a radiation dosage of less than 1 rad. Although radiation is most hazardous to the fetus during the first trimester, a radiation dose of up to 5 rad that would result from an extensive radiologic procedure is still safely tolerated, and interruption of a pregnancy because of previous radiation exposure is seldom justified (Swartz and Reichling, 1978).

Although the risk of radiation is small, the radiation dose to the fetus incurred with an intravenous pyelogram can be reduced as much as 40-fold by careful radiographic technique (Bruwer, 1976). The number of films should be limited to a scout film, a 15-minute film, and a delayed film if necessary. This two- or three-film examination will demonstrate an obstructing calculus and will document the degree of obstruction. The x-ray beam should be collimated to the point of interest, and proper beam filtration should be used to limit radiation scatter. Placing the patient in the prone rather than the supine position further limits radiation exposure to the fetus because the roentgen rays are attenuated by the spine and the thick posterior abdominal wall. Application of compression bands around the maternal abdomen may further reduce fetal radiation exposure by decreasing the thickness of the maternal abdomen and also results in less radiation scatter and an improved radiographic image. The use of fast films with short exposure times and high-speed radiographic screens also decreases radiation exposure (Stern, 1982). Finally, the use of low kilovoltage of about 60 to 70 kV affords better contrast and more detailed information than those obtained with a higher kilovoltage of about 120 kV. Although the radiation dose to the skin is higher with lower kilovoltage, the radiation dose to deeper tissues and the fetus is no different (Fisher and Russell, 1975).

Alternative diagnostic modalities include ultrasonography and radionuclide renography. Both techniques are less reliable than intravenous urography but are associated with less radiation exposure. Ultrasonography is accurate in detecting renal calculi but is less reliable in detecting obstructing ureteral calculi. Furthermore, it may be difficult to distinguish physiologic hydronephrosis associated with pregnancy from pathologic hydronephrosis associated with an obstructing calculus (Freed, 1982). The radionuclide renogram is also somewhat less reliable than the intravenous pyelogram but can provide valuable information regarding renal function and the presence of obstruction. Renography is particularly accurate during the first and second trimesters of pregnancy. Physiologic obstruction may be confused with pathologic obstruction in about 10 to 20 per cent of cases during the third trimester (Wax, 1982).

Treatment

Although it is desirable to avoid surgery during pregnancy, obstructing urinary stones usually can be safely removed during any stage of pregnancy. The risk of spontaneous abortion associated with surgery is greatest during the third trimester, and pelvic surgery for distal ureteral calculi can be extremely difficult because of the enlarged uterus and engorged vasculature (Freed, 1982).

Several alternatives for management of obstructing urinary tract calculi may obviate or delay the need for surgery during pregnancy. Most stones are small and should be given time to pass spontaneously as long as the clinical situation permits. It is often possible to insert a double-J catheter into the obstructed ureter beyond the stone; the insertion is made easier if the patient lies on her side opposite the side of the stone to reduce compression of the ureter by the fetus. If it is successfully passed, the double-J catheter can be left in place until the completion of pregnancy. Endoscopic extraction of distal ureteral calculi is also possible during any phase of pregnancy. Alternatively, an obstructing distal ureteral stone may be milked into the bladder by transvaginal compression (Farkas and Firstater, 1979). Ureteral calculi that are too large to manipulate may be treated with percutaneous nephrostomy drainage until pregnancy has been completed, and these stones can be treated safely thereafter.

MISCELLANEOUS

Several perioperative problems have not been addressed previously and are discussed briefly in this section.

Acute Pseudo-Obstruction of the Colon (Ogilvie's Syndrome)

Pseudo-obstruction of the colon was first described by Ogilvie in 1948 and is characterized by massive colonic dilation without any anatomic obstruction. The condition most likely results from interruption of parasympathetic innervation from S2–S4 to the distal colon. Although the point of pseudo-obstruction is the distal colon, the condition most dramatically affects the cecum, because it is the most distensible segment of the large bowel.

In urologic patients, Ogilvie's syndrome occurs most often after pelvic surgery and may be caused by pressure on the sigmoid colon from a retractor placed at the time of pelvic lymphadenectomy. Thus, the sigmoid colon should be padded carefully when retracting it. In a patient with severe postoperative ileus, an abdominal film should be obtained immediately. If the cecum is more than 12 cm in diameter, immediate decompression is required to prevent perforation. Colonoscopy is usually successful in treating this condition, but a cecostomy is sometimes necessary to prevent cecal perforation. The mortality in nonperforated cases is 25 per cent but

increases to about 50 per cent with intestinal perforation (Bauer and Overgaard, 1988).

Compartment Syndrome

Patients in the lithotomy position are particularly prone to developing compartment syndrome. This syndrome occurs when the closing pressure in the arterioles of the legs that supply compartmental muscles is exceeded. Decreased blood flow, decreased ability to meet the tissue's metabolic demands, and edema result. The edema further increases the compartmental pressure, which then reduces blood flow, and a destructive cycle begins.

Prophylactic measures to prevent compartment syndrome include frequent repositioning of the legs, with stirrups that support both the thigh and the lower leg and avoiding ankle dorsiflexion, which increases compartmental pressure. Most important, a prolonged lithotomy position should be avoided whenever possible. Patients undergoing cystectomy with simultaneous urethrectomy should be kept in the supine position until the legs are raised for the urethrectomy. The legs are returned to the supine position after the urethrectomy has been completed (Adler et al., 1990).

Pelvic Lymphoceles

Pelvic lymphoceles usually occur after lymphadenectomy and renal transplantation. Surgery has been the usual treatment, with reported success rates of 50 to 70 per cent for external drainage and 90 per cent for peritoneal marsupialization. Needle aspiration has been demonstrated to be safe and effective, but most studies report a recurrence rate of 80 to 90 per cent. One study has demonstrated that percutaneous treatment with instillation of povidone-iodine through a catheter into the lymphocele cavity for 30 minutes twice daily is also effective. The major disadvantage of this technique is the time involved, with the average patient requiring treatment for 25 days. The technique is worth remembering, however, particularly for high-risk surgical patients with large postoperative lymphoceles (Gilliland et al., 1989).

Postoperative Confusion

As many as 35 per cent of preoperative cognitively intact elderly patients become mildly confused and 15 per cent become severely confused postoperatively. This confusion can be a major problem for urologists who deal with a large number of elderly patients. All such patients should be investigated for reversible medical disorders including alcohol or drug withdrawal, electrolyte imbalances, myocardial infarction, infection, hypoxia, hypotension, and acute thiamine deficiency. All medications should be continuously evaluated for possible side effects. Effective orientation techniques include repetitive statements regarding person, place, and time; maintenance of body image by tactile stimulus or physical movement; soothing sensory stimulation, such as music; and repeated explanations and explorations of foreign objects such as intravenous lines, catheters, and oxygen masks. If sedation is required, neuroleptics such as haloperidol or short-acting benzodiazepines should be used in small doses. Restraints should be used sparingly and only when necessary, because they often increase agitation and confusion and thus accomplish the opposite result for which they were intended. When confusion clears, the episode should be discussed thoroughly with the patient and the family to allay fears (Pousada and Leipzig, 1990).

Perioperative Peripheral Nerve Lesions

Urologists may sometimes encounter postoperative ulnar nerve palsy. Ulnar nerve lesions are among the most common focal peripheral neuropathies and can be a recurrent problem in patients undergoing abdominal and pelvic surgery. Ulnar nerve injuries occur most often when the patient's arm is abducted and pronated, which makes the ulnar nerve more vulnerable to external pressure. Available electrophysiologic data suggest that the lesion occurs at the cubital tunnel, the fibrous opening between the two heads of the flexor carpi ulnaris. The ulnar nerve is best protected by placing the patient's arms above the head, with the elbows partially flexed. This position may increase the risk of brachial plexus injury, but such injury can be prevented if marked extension at the shoulder is avoided. If the arms must be abducted, it is better to place them in a supinated rather than a pronated position (Dawson and Krarup, 1989).

REFERENCES

Abel, R. M., Beck, C. H., Jr., Abbott, W. M., et al.: Improved survival from acute renal failure after treatment with intravenous essential L-amino acids and glucose. N. Engl. J. Med., 288:695, 1973.

Adler, L. M., Loughlin, J. S., Morin, C. J., et al.: Bilateral compartment syndrome after a long gynecologic operation in the lithotomy position. Am. J. Obstet. Gynecol., 126:1271, 1990.

Alderson, P. O., Lee, H., Summer, W. R., et al.: Comparison of Xe-133 washout and single breath imaging for detection of ventilation abnormalities. J. Nucl. Med., 20:917, 1979.

Alexander, J. W.: Infection, host resistance, and antimicrobial agents. In Dudrick, S. J., et al. (Eds.): Manual of Preoperative and Postoperative Care. Philadelphia, W. B. Saunders Co., 1983, p. 106.

Allgood, R. J., Cook, J. H., Weedn, R. J., et al.: Prospective analysis of pulmonary embolism in the postoperative patient. Surgery, 68:116, 1970.

Allo, M., and Simmons, R. L.: Surgical infectious disease and the urologist. Urol. Clin. North Am., 10:131, 1983.

Amaranath, L., Andrish, J. T., Gurd, A. R., et al.: Efficacy of intermittent epidural morphine following posterior spinal fusion in children and adolescents. Clin. Orthop. Related Res., 249:223, 1989.

American Heart Association Committee: Prevention of bacterial endocarditis. Circulation, 56:139A, 1977.

Andersen, J. B., Olesen, K. P., Eikard, B., et al.: Periodic continuous positive airway pressure, CPAP, by mask in the treatment of atelectasis. Eur. J. Respir. Dis., 61:20, 1980.

Ashton, C. M., Lahart, C. J., and Wray, N. P.: The incidence of perioperative myocardial infarction with transurethral resection of the prostate. J. Am. Geriatr. Soc., 37:614, 1989.

Axelrod, F. B., Pepkowitz, S. H., and Goldfinger, D.: Establishment of a schedule of optimal preoperative collection of autologous blood. Transfusion, 29:677, 1989.

Backer, C. L., Tinker, J. H., Robertson, D. M., et al.: Myocardial infarction following local anesthesia for ophthalmic surgery. Anesth. Analg., 59:257, 1980.

Bacsl, T. J., and Buckley, J. J.: Preoperative assessment, preparation for operation, and routine postoperative care. Urol. Clin. North Am., 10:3, 1983.

Bagdade, J. D.: Phagocytic and microbial function in diabetes mellitus. J. Endocrinol., (Suppl.) 83:27, 1976.

Baker, R. J., and Nyhus, L. M.: Diagnosis and treatment of immediate transfusion reaction. Surg. Gynecol. Obstet., 130:665, 1970.

Barash, P. G., Nardi, D., Hammond, G., et al.: Catheter induced pulmonary artery perforation. J. Thorac. Cardiovasc. Surg., 82:5, 1981.

Barnes, R. W., Nix, M. L., Barnes, C. L., et al.: Perioperative asymptomatic venous thrombosis: Role of duplex scanning versus venography. J. Vasc. Surg., 9:251, 1989.

Bauer, T., and Overgaard, K.: Acute pseudo-obstruction of the colon in a kidney-transplanted patient (Ogilvie's syndrome). Int. Urol. Nephrol., 20:85, 1988.

Baxter, J. D., and Tyrell, J. B.: The adrenal cortex. In Felig, P., et al. (Eds.): Endocrinology and Metabolism. New York, McGraw-Hill Book Co., 1981, p. 462.

Beattie, C.: Regional versus general anesthesia. In Breslow, M. J., Miller, C. F., and Rogers, M. C. (Eds.): Perioperative Management. St. Louis, C. V. Mosby Co., 1990, p. 108.

Bellantone, R., Doglietto, G. B., Bossola, M., et al.: Preoperative parenteral nutrition in the high risk surgical patient. JPEN, 12:195, 1988.

Bergqvist, D., Jendteg, S., Lindgren, B., et al.: The economics of general thromboembolic prophylaxis. World J. Surg., 12:349, 1988.

Bistrian, B. R., Blackburn, G. L., Sherman, M., et al.: Therapeutic index of nutritional depletion in hospitalized patients. Surg. Gynecol. Obstet., 141:512, 1975.

Blackburn, G. L., et al.: Nutritional and metabolic assessment of the hospitalized patient. JPEN, 1:11, 1977.

Blackshear, W. M., Prescott, C., LePain, F., et al.: Influence of sequential pneumatic compression on postoperative venous function. J. Vasc. Surg., 5:432, 1987.

Blaschke, T. F., and Melmon, K. L.: Antihypertensive agents and the drug therapy of hypertension. In Goodman, A. G., Goodman, L. S., and Gilman, A. (Eds.): Goodman and Gilman's Pharmacological Basis of Therapeutics. 6th ed. New York, Macmillan Publishing Co., 1980.

Blumberg, A., et al.: Effect of various therapeutic approaches on plasma potassium and major regulating factors in terminal renal failure. Am. J. Med., 85:507, 1988.

Boehmer, R. D.: Continuous, real time, non-invasive monitor of blood pressure: Penaz methodology applied to the finger. J. Clin. Monit., 3:282, 1987.

Borges, H. F., Hocks, J., and Kjellstrand, C. M.: Mannitol intoxication in patients with renal failure. Arch. Intern. Med., 142:63, 1982.

Borow, M., and Goldson, H.: Postoperative venous thrombosis: evaluation of five methods of treatment. Am. J. Surg., 141:245, 1981.

Bowen, D. J., et al.: Perioperative management of insulin-dependent diabetic patients. Use of continuous intravenous infusion of insulin-glucose-potassium solution. Anesthesiology, 37:852, 1982.

Bowler, G. M. R., Wildsmith, J. A., and Scott, D. B.: Epidural administration of local anaesthetics. In Cousins, M. J., Phillips, G. D. (Eds.): Acute Pain Management. Clinics in Critical Care Medicine. Edinburgh, Churchill Livingstone, 1986, p. 187.

Brashear, R. E.: Arrhythmias in patients with chronic obstructive pulmonary disease. Med. Clin. North Am., 68:969, 1984.

Bremner, D., Brown, M., Girdwood, A., et al.: Antibiotic prophylaxis in transurethral resection of the prostate with reference to the influence of preoperative catheterization. J. Hosp. Infect., 12:75, 1988.

Brismar, B., Hedenstierna, G., Lundquist, H., Strandberg, A., Svensson, L., and Tokics, L.: Pulmonary densities during anesthesia with muscular relaxation—A proposal of atelectasis. Anesthesiology, 62:422, 1985.

Brister, S. J., Chin, R. C. J., Brown, R. A., et al.: Clinical impact of intravenous hyperalimentation on esophageal carcinoma: Is it worthwhile? Ann. Thorac. Surg., 38:618, 1984.

Britt, B. A.: Malignant hyperthermia. Can. Anaesth. Soc. J., 32:666, 1985.

Bruwer, A.: If you are pregnant, or if you think you might be . . . . Editorial. AJR, 127:696, 1976.

Burke, G. R., and Gulyassy, P. F.: Surgery in the patient with renal disease and related electrolyte disorders. Med. Clin. North Am., 63:1191, 1979.

Burke, J. P., Garibaldi, R. A., Britt, M., et al.: Prevention of catheter-associated urinary tract infections: Efficacy of daily meatal care regimens. Am. J. Med., 70:655, 1981.

Burrows, L., and Tartter, P. I.: Effect of blood transfusions on colonic malignancy recurrence rate. Letter. Lancet, 2:662, 1982.

Butson, A. R. C.: Intermittent pneumatic calf compression for prevention of deep venous thrombosis in general abdominal surgery. Am. J. Surg., 142:525, 1981.

Bynum, L. J., and Wilson, J. E., III: Low dose heparin therapy in the long-term management of venous thromboembolism. Am. J. Med., 67:553, 1979.

Caen, J. P.: A randomized double-blind study between a low molecular weight heparin Kabi 2165 and standard heparin in the prevention of deep vein thrombosis in general surgery. A French multicenter trial. Thromb. Haemost., 59:216, 1988.

Cafferkey, M. T., Falkiner, F. R., Gilespie, W. A., et al.: DM: antibiotics for the prevention of septicaemia in urology. J. Antimicrob. Chemother., 9:471, 1982.

Cameron, C. B., and Kobrinsky, N.: Perioperative management of patients with von Willebrand's disease. Can. J. Anaesth., 37:341, 1990.

Caprini, J. A., Chuker, J. L., Zuckerman, L., et al.: Thrombosis prophylaxis using external compression. Surg. Gynecol. Obstet., 156:599, 1983.

Caprini, J. A., and Natonson, R. A.: Postoperative deep vein thrombosis: Current clinical considerations. Semin. Thromb. Hemost., 15:244, 1989.

Carliner, N. H., Fisher, M. L., Plotnick, G. D., et al.: Routine preoperative exercise testing in patients undergoing major noncardiac surgery. Am. J. Cardiol., 56:51, 1985.

Castillo, R., and Hass, A.: Chest physical therapy: Comparative efficacy of preoperative and postoperative treatment in the elderly. Arch. Phys. Med. Rehabil., 66:376, 1985.

Catley, D. M., Thornton, C., Jordan, C., et al.: Pronounced episodic desaturation in the postoperative period. Its association with ventilatory pattern and analgesic regime. Anesthesiology, 65:20, 1985.

Cerra, F. B.: Hypermetabolism, organ failure, and metabolic support. Surgery, 101:1, 1987.

Charlson, M. E., MacKenzie, C. R., Ales, K., et al.: Surveillance for postoperative myocardial infarction after noncardiac operations. Surg. Gynecol. Obstet., 167:407, 1988.

Charlson, M. E., MacKenzie, C. R., Gold, J. P., et al.: Postoperative changes in serum creatinine. When do they occur and how much is important? Ann. Surg., 209:328, 1989.

Charpak, Y., Blery, C., Chastang, C., et al.: Prospective assessment of a protocol for selective ordering of preoperative chest x-rays. Can. J. Anaesth., 35:259, 1988.

Chauvin, M., Sandouk, P., Scherrmann, J. M., et al.: Morphine pharmacokinetics in renal failure. Anesthesiology, 66:327, 1987.

Christensen, M. M., Nelsen, K. T., Knes, J., et al.: Brief report: Single-dose preoperative prophylaxis in transurethral surgery. Am. J. Med., 87:258S, 1989.

Civetta, J. M.: Goal directed respiratory therapy. ASA Refresher Course 110, 1981.

Clagett, G. P., and Reisch, J. S.: Prevention of venous thromboembolism in general surgical patients. Ann. Surg., 208:227, 1988.

Clarke-Pearson, D. L., Creasman, W. T., Coleman, R. E., et al.: Perioperative external pneumatic calf compression as thromboembolism prophylaxis in gynecologic oncology: Report of a randomized controlled trial. Gynecol. Oncol., 18:226, 1984.

Cockcroft, D. W., and Gault, M. H.: Prediction of creatinine clearance from serum creatinine. Nephron, 16:31, 1976.

Coe, F. L., Parks, J. H., and Lindheimer, M. D.: Nephrolithiasis during pregnancy. N. Engl. J. Med., 298:324, 1978.

Colgan, F. J., Barrow, R. E., and Fanning, G. L.: Continuous positive pressure breathing and cardiorespiratory function. Anesthesiology, 34:145, 1979.

Collins, J. A.: Blood and blood products. In Dudrick, S. J., et al. (Eds.): Manual of Preoperative and Postoperative Care. Philadelphia, W. B. Saunders Co., 1983, p. 137.

Collins, R., Scrimgeour, A., Yusuf, S., et al.: Reduction in fatal pulmonary embolism and venous thrombosis by perioperative administration of subcutaneous heparin. N. Engl. J. Med., 318:1162, 1988.

Cox, C. E.: Comparison of intravenous ciprofloxacin and intravenous cefotaxime for antimicrobial prophylaxis in transurethral surgery. Am. J. Med., 87:252S, 1989.

Cruickshank, M. K., Levine, M. N., Hirsh, J., et al.: An evaluation of impedance plethysmography and ^{125}I-fibrinogen leg scanning in patients following hip surgery. Thromb. Haemost., 62:830, 1989.

Cuschieri, R. J., Morran, C. G., Howie, J. C., and McArdle, C. S.: Postoperative pain and pulmonary complications: Comparison of three analgesic regimes. Br. J. Surg., 72:495, 1985.

Cutler, B. S., Wheeler, H. B., Paraskos, J. A., et al.: Applicability and interpretation of electrocardiographic stress testing in patients with peripheral vascular disease. Am. J. Surg., 141:501, 1981.

Czer, L. S. C., and Shoemaker, W. C.: Optimal hematocrit value in critically ill postoperative patients. Surg. Gynecol. Obstet., 147:363, 1978.

Daly, J. M., Dudrich, S. J., and Copeland, E. M.: Intravenous hyperalimentation. Effect on delayed cutaneous hypersensitivity in cancer patients. Ann. Surg., 192:587, 1980.

David, F. M., McDermott, E., Hickton, C., et al.: Influence of spinal and general anaesthesia on haemostasis during total hip arthroplasty. Br. J. Anaesth., 59:561, 1987.

Dawson, D. M., and Krarup, C.: Perioperative nerve lesions. Arch. Neurol., 46:1355, 1989.

De la Rocha, A. G., Edmonds, J. F., Williams, W. G., et al.: Importance of mixed venous oxygen saturation in the care of critically ill patients. Can. J. Surg., 21:227, 1978.

Del Guercio, L. R. M., and Cohn, J. D.: Monitoring operative risk in the elderly. JAMA, 243:1350, 1980.

Denlinger, J. K.: Calcium metabolism during blood transfusion and citrate toxicity. In Brzica, S. M., Jr. (Ed.): Blood Transfusion Dilemmas. Washington, D.C., American Association of Blood Banks, 1978, p. 45.

Detsky, A. S., Baker, J. P., O'Rourke, K., et al.: Perioperative parenteral nutrition: A meta-analysis. Ann. Intern. Med., 107:195, 1987.

Detsky, A. S., Abrams, H. B., Forbath, N., et al.: Cardiac assessment for patients undergoing noncardiac surgery. A multifactorial clinical risk index. Arch. Intern. Med., 146:2131, 1986.

Deutschman, C.: Protein-energy malnutrition in the perioperative period. In Breslow, M. J., Miller, C. F., and Rogers, M. C. (Eds.): Perioperative Care. St. Louis, C. V. Mosby Co., 1990, p. 436.

Dewan, P. A., Van Ru, A. M., Robinson, R. G., et al.: The use of an iodophor-impregnated plastic incise drape in abdominal surgery—A controlled clinical trial. Aust. N.Z. J. Surg., 57:859, 1987.

Dirksen, A., and Kjoller, E.: Cardiac predictors of death after noncardiac surgery evaluated by intention to treat. BMJ, 297:1011, 1988.

Douglas, W. W., Rehder, K., Beynen, F. M., et al.: Improved oxygenation in patients with acute respiratory failure. The prone position. Am. Rev. Respir. Dis., 115:559, 1977.

Dubrow, T. J., Wackym, P. A., Abdul-Rasool, I. H., et al.: Malignant hyperthermia: Experience in the prospective management of eight children. J. Pediatr. Surg., 24:163, 1989.

Dudrick, S. J., Wilmore, D. W., Vars, H. M., et al.: Long-term parenteral nutrition with growth development and positive nitrogen balance. Surgery, 64:135, 1968.

Dueck, R., Prutow, R. J., Davies, N. J., Clausen, J. L., and Davidson, T. M.: The lung volume at which shunting occurs with inhalation anesthesia. Anesthesiology, 69:854, 1988.

Easton, P. A., Jadue, C., Dhingra, S., et al.: A comparison of the bronchodilating effects of a beta-2 adrenergic agent (albuterol) and an anticholinergic agent (ipratropium bromide) given by aerosol alone or in sequence. N. Engl. J. Med., 315:735, 1986.

Edlich, R. F., Rodgers, W., Kasper, G., et al.: Studies in the management of the contaminated wound. Am. J. Surg., 117:323, 1969.

Eisenbach, J., Grice, S., and Dewan, D.: Patient-controlled analgesia following cesarean section: A comparison with epidural and intramuscular narcotics. Anesthesiology, 68:444, 1988.

Eisenberg, R. L., Bank, W. O., and Hedgock, M. W.: Renal failure after major angiography can be avoided with hydration. AJR, 136:859, 1981.

Elliott, C. G., Zimmerman, G. A., and Clemmen, T. P.: Complications of pulmonary artery catheterization in the care of the critically ill patient. Chest, 76:647, 1979.

Encke, A., Breddin, K., Biegholdt, M., et al.: Comparison of a low molecular weight heparin and unfractionated heparin for the prevention of deep vein thrombosis in patients undergoing abdominal surgery. Br. J. Surg., 75:1058, 1988.

Engberg, G.: Single-dose intercostal nerve blocks with etidocaine after upper abdominal surgery. Acta Anaesthesiol. Scand. (Suppl.), 60:43, 1975.

Engberg, G., and Wiklund, L.: Pulmonary complications after upper abdominal surgery: Their prevention with intercostal blocks. Acta Anaesthesiol. Scand., 32:1, 1988.

Eriksson, M., Rubenfeld, S., Garber, A. J., et al.: Propranolol does not prevent thyroid storm. N. Engl. J. Med., 296:263, 1977.

Erslev, A.: Erythropoietin coming of age. N. Engl. J. Med., 316:101, 1987.

Eschbach, J. W., et al.: Correction of the anemia of end-stage renal disease with recombinant erythropoietin: Results of a combined phase I and II clinical trial. N. Engl. J. Med., 316:73, 1987.

Fairfull-Smith, R., Abunassar, R., Freeman, J. B., et al.: Rational use of elemental and nonelemental diets in hospitalized patients. Ann. Surg., 192:600, 1980.

Farkas, A., and Firstater, M.: Transvaginal milking of lower ureteric stones into the bladder. Br. J. Urol., 51:193, 1979.

Fischer, J. E., and Freund, H. R.: Central alimentation. In Fischer, J. E. (Ed.): Surgical Nutrition. Boston, Little, Brown & Co., 1983.

Fisher, A. S., and Russell, J. G. B.: Radiography in Obstetrics. London, Butterworth & Co., 1975.

Fisher, J. W.: Mechanisms of the anemia of chronic renal failure. Nephron, 25:106, 1980.

Fleck, A.: Plasma proteins as nutritional indicators in the perioperative period. Br. J. Clin. Pract. (Suppl.), 63:20, 1989.

Flinn, W. R., Sandager, G. P., Cerullo, L. J., et al.: Duplex venous scanning for the prospective surveillance of perioperative venous thrombosis. Arch. Surg., 124:901, 1989.

Forrester, J. S., Diamond, G., Chatterjee, K., et al.: Medical therapy of acute myocardial infarction by application of hemodynamic subsets. N. Engl. J. Med., 295:1356, 1976.

Forthman, H. J., and Shepard, A.: Postoperative pulmonary complications. South. Med. J., 62:1198, 1969.

Foster, E. D., Davis, K. B., Carpenter, J. A., et al.: Risk of noncardiac operation in patients with defined coronary disease: The Coronary Artery Surgery Study (CASS) registry experience. Ann. Thorac. Surg., 41:42, 1986.

Fowkes, F. G. R., et al.: Epidemiology in anaesthesia. III. Mortality risk in patients with coexisting physical disease. Br. J. Anaesth., 54:819, 1982.

Freed, S. Z.: Urinary tract calculi in pregnancy. In Freed, S. Z., and Herzig, N. (Eds.): Urology in Pregnancy. Baltimore, Williams & Wilkins Co., 1982, p. 135.

Fricker, J. P., Vergnes, Y., Schach, R., et al.: Low dose heparin versus low molecular weight heparin (Kabi 2165, Fragmin) in the prophylaxis of thromboembolic complications of abdominal oncological surgery. Eur. J. Clin. Invest., 18:561, 1988.

Frishman, W. H.: Beta-adrenergic blocker withdrawal. Am. J. Cardiol., 59:26F, 1987.

Gallup, D. G., Talledo, O. E., and King, L. A.: Primary mass closure of midline incisions with a continuous running monofilament suture in gynecologic patients. Obstet. Gynecol., 73:675, 1989.

Garcia-Valdecasas, J. C., et al.: Subcostal incision versus midline laparotomy in gallstone surgery: A prospective and randomized trial. Br. J. Surg., 75:473, 1988.

Garibaldi, R. A., Skolnick, D., Lerer, T., et al.: The impact of preoperative skin disinfection on preventing intraoperative wound contamination. Infect. Control Hosp. Epidemiol., 9:109, 1988.

Geelhoed, G. W.: Microembolization in blood transfusion. A non-disease for which we have a cure. In Brzica, S. M., Jr.: Blood Transfusion Dilemmas. Washington, D.C., American Association of Blood Banks, 1978, p. 35.

Gerberding, J. L., Littell, C., Tarkington, A., et al.: Risk of exposure of surgical personnel to patients' blood during surgery at San Francisco General Hospital. N. Engl. J. Med., 322:1788, 1990.

Gibbons, R. P., Stark, R. A., Correa, R. J., Jr., et al.: The prophylactic use—or misuse—of antibiotics in transurethral prostatectomy. J. Urol., 119:381, 1978.

Gilchrist, G. S., Hagedorn, A. B., Owen, C. A., Jr., et al.: Management of patients with von Willebrand's disease undergoing surgical procedures. In Mamen, E. F., Barnhart, M. I., Lusher, J. M., and Walshe, R. T. (Eds.): Review of Hematology. Vol. I. Treatment of Bleeding Disorders with Blood Components. Westbury, N.Y., P.J.D. Publications, 1980, p. 83.

Gilliland, J. D., Spies, J. B., Brown, S. B., et al.: Lymphoceles: Percutaneous treatment with povidone-iodine sclerosis. Radiology, 171:227, 1989.

Gilmour, I. J.: Perioperative respiratory care. Urol. Clin. North Am., 10:65, 1983.

Goggin, M. J., and Joekes, A. M.: Gas exchange in renal failure. I. Dangers of hyperkalemia during anaesthesia. Br. Med. J., 2:244, 1971.

Goldberg, M. E., Clark, S., Joseph, J., et al.: Nicardipine versus placebo for the treatment of postoperative hypertension. Am. Heart J., 119:446, 1990.

Goldberg, N. J., et al.: Insulin therapy in the diabetic surgical patient: Metabolic and hormone response to low dose insulin infusion. Diabetes Care, 4:279, 1981.

Goldman, L., and Caldera, D.: Risks of general anesthesia and elective operation in the hypertensive patient. Anesthesiology, 50:285, 1979.

Goldman, L., Caldera, D. L., Nussbaum, S. R., et al.: Multifactorial index of cardiac risk in noncardiac surgical procedures. N. Engl. J. Med., 297:845, 1977.

Goldman, L., Caldera, D. L., Southwick, F. S., et al.: Cardiac risk factors and complications in noncardiac surgery. Medicine, 57:357, 1978.

Goldmann, D. R.: Surgery in patients with endocrine dysfunction, preoperative consultation. Med. Clin. North Am., 71:499, 1987.

Goodnough, L. T., Rudnick, S., Price, T. H., et al.: Increased preoperative collection of autologous blood with recombinant human erythropoietin therapy. N. Engl. J. Med., 321:1163, 1989.

Goodsen, W. H., and Hunt, T. K.: Studies on wound healing in experimental diabetes mellitus. J. Surg. Res., 22:221, 1977.

Gradey, C. F.: Transfusion and hepatitis update in '78. Editorial. N. Engl. J. Med., 298:1413, 1978.

Graham, W., and Bradley, D.: Efficacy of chest physiotherapy and intermittent positive pressure breathing in the resolution of pneumonia. N. Engl. J. Med., 299:624, 1978.

Gran, L., and Pahle, J. A.: Rational substitution therapy for steroid-treated patients. Anaesthesia, 33:59, 1978.

Greenfield, L. J.: Current indications for and results of Greenfield filter placement. J. Vasc. Surg., 1:502, 1984.

Grodsinsky, C., Brush, B. E., and Ponka, J. L.: Postoperative pulmonary complications in the geriatric age group. J. Am. Geriatr. Soc., 22:407, 1974.

Hanning, C. D., Vickers, A. P., Smith, G., et al.: The morphine hydrogel suppository. A new sustained release rectal preparation. Br. J. Anaesth., 61:221, 1988.

Hanno, P. M., and Wien, A. J.: Management of septic shock. Am. Urol. Assoc. Update Ser., 1:3, 1981.

Harman, E., and Lillington, G.: Pulmonary risk factors in surgery. Med. Clin. North Am., 63:1289, 1979.

Hart, O. J., Klimberg, I. W., Wajsman, Z., et al.: Intraoperative autotransfusion in radical cystectomy for carcinoma of the bladder. Surg. Gynecol. Obstet., 168:302, 1989.

Harvey, K. B., et al.: Biological measures of the formulation of a hospital prognostic index. Am. J. Clin. Nutr., 34:2013, 1981.

Hendolin, H., Mattila, M. A. K., and Poikolainen, E.: The effect of lumbar epidural analgesia on the development of deep venous thrombosis of the legs after open prostatectomy. Acta Chir. Scand., 147:425, 1981.

Henry, H. H., II: Urological applications of butorphanol tartrate: Postoperative pain and renal colic. Acute Care, 12:22, 1986.

Hensle, T. W.: Nutritional support of the surgical patient. Urol. Clin. North Am., 10:109, 1983.

Holbraad, L., Thybo, E., and VeNits, H.: A controlled investigation of the value of anticoagulant therapy in cases of prostatectomy. Scand. J. Urol. Nephrol., 10:39, 1976.

Hotchkiss, R. S.: Perioperative management of patient with chronic obstructive pulmonary disease. Int. Anesthesiol. Clin., 26:134, 1988.

Hovig, O.: Source of pulmonary emboli. Acta Chir. Scand. Suppl., 478:42, 1977.

Hull, C. J.: Control of pain in the perioperative period. Br. Med. Bull., 4:341, 1988.

Hull, R., Delmore, T., Carter, C., et al.: Adjusted subcutaneous heparin versus warfarin sodium in the long-term treatment of venous thrombosis. N. Engl. J. Med., 306:189, 1982.

Inada, K., Koike, S., Shirai, N., et al.: Effects of intermittent pneumatic leg compression for prevention of postoperative deep venous thrombosis with special reference to fibrinolytic activity. Am. J. Surg., 155:602, 1988.

Ishak, M. A., and Morley, K. D.: Deep venous thrombosis after total hip arthroplasty: A prospective controlled study to determine the prophylactic effect of graded pressure stockings. Br. J. Surg., 68:429, 1981.

Jackson, C. J.: Preoperative pulmonary evaluation. Arch. Intern. Med., 148:2120, 1988.

Jakobson, S., and Ivarsson, I.: Effects of intercostal nerve blocks (etidocaine 0.5%) on chest wall mechanics in cholecystectomized patients. Acta Anaesthesiol. Scand., 21:497, 1977.

Janson, P. A., Jubelirer, S. J., Weinstein, M. J., et al.: Treatment of the bleeding tendency in uremia with cryoprecipitate. N. Engl. J. Med., 303:1318, 1980.

Kakkar, V. V.: Prophylaxis of venous thromboembolism. Proc. R. Soc. Med. 68:263, 1975.

Kakkar, V. V., and Adams, B. A.: Preventive and therapeutic approach to venous thromboembolic disease and pulmonary embolism—Can death from pulmonary embolism be prevented? J. Am. Coll. Cardiol., 8:146B, 1986.

Kaplan, J. A.: Clinical considerations for the use of intravenous nicardipine in the treatment of postoperative hypertension. Am. Heart J., 19:443, 1990.

Kaplan, J. A., and Dunbar, R. W.: Anesthesia for noncardiac surgery in patients with cardiac disease. In Kaplan, J. A. (Ed.): Cardiac Anesthesia. New York, Grune & Stratton, 1979, p. 377.

Kasiske, B. L., and Kjellstrand, C. M.: Perioperative management of patients with chronic renal failure and postoperative acute renal failure. Urol. Clin. North Am., 10:35, 1983.

Katholi, R. E., Nolan, S. P., and McGuire, L. B.: The management of anticoagulation during noncardiac operations in patients with prosthetic heart valves. Am. Heart J., 96:163, 1978.

Kazarian, K. K., and Del Guercia, L. R. M.: The use of mixed venous blood gas determinations in traumatic shock. Ann. Emerg. Med., 9:179, 1980.

Kehlet, H., and Binder, C.: Value of an ACTH test in assessing hypothalamic-pituitary-adrenocortical function in glucocorticoid-treated patients. Br. Med. J., 2:147, 1973.

Kehlet, H., Nistrup-Madsen, S., and Binder, C.: Cortisol and cortisone acetate in parenteral glucocorticoid therapy. Acta Med. Scand., 195:421, 1974.

Keighley, M. R. B.: Infection: Prophylaxis. Br. Med. Bull., 44:374, 1988.

Kelley, T. F., Morris, G. C., Crawford, E. S., et al.: Perforation of the pulmonary artery with Swan-Ganz catheters. Ann. Surg., 193:686, 1981.

Kernodle, D. S., Classen, D. C., Burke, J., and Kaiser, A. B.: Failure of cephalosporins to prevent Staphylococcus aureus surgical wound infections. JAMA, 263:961, 1990.

Kiely, E. A., McCormack, T., Cafferkey, M. T., et al.: Study of appropriate antibiotic therapy in transurethral prostatectomy. Br. J. Urol., 64:61, 1989.

Kiil, J., Axelsen, F., et al.: Prophylaxis against postoperative pulmonary embolism and deep-vein thrombosis by low-dose heparin. Lancet, 1:1115, 1978.

King, L. W., and Snyder, D. S.: Diabetes and other endocrine disorders. In Breslow, M. J., Miller, C. F., and Rogers, M. C. (Eds.): Perioperative Management. St. Louis, C. V. Mosby Co., 1990, p. 292.

Klin, P -A., and Dahlgren, S.: Oral prophylaxis with neomycin and erythromycin in colorectal surgery. Arch. Surg., 124:705, 1989.

Konings, K.: Preop use of golytely in pediatrics. Pediatr. Nurs., 15:473, 1989.

Kono, K., Philbin, D. M., Coggins, C. H., et al.: Renal function and stress response during halothane and fentanyl anesthesia. Anesth. Analg., 50:552, 1981.

Kunau, R. T., and Stein, J. H.: Disorders of potassium metabolism.

In Earley, L. E., and Gottschalk, C. W. (Eds.): Strauss and Welt's Diseases of the Kidney. 3rd ed. Boston, Little, Brown & Co., 1979.

Kutnowski, M., Vandendris, M., Steinberger, R., et al.: Prevention of postoperative deep-vein thrombosis by low-dose heparin in urological surgery. A double blind randomized study. Urol. Res., 5:123, 1977.

Lange, L., and Echt, M.: Comparative studies on drugs which increase venous tone using noradrenaline, ethyl-adrianol, dihydroergotamine and horse chestnut extract. Fortschr. Med., 90:1161, 1972.

Lau, W. Y., Chu, K. W., Poon, G. P., et al.: Prophylactic antibiotics in elective colorectal surgery. Br. J. Surg., 75:782, 1988.

Lee, G., DeMaria, N. A., Amsterdam, E. A., et al.: Comparative effects of morphine, meperidine and pentazocine on cardio-circulatory dynamics in patients with acute myocardial infarction. Am. J. Med., 60:949, 1976.

Lee, T. H., and Goldman, L.: Cardiac risk assessment for individual patients. In Breslow, M. J., Miller, C. F., and Rogers, M. C. (Eds.): Perioperative Management. St. Louis, C. V. Mosby, 1990, p. 26.

Lerner, P. I., and Sampliner, J. E.: Transfusion-associated cytomegalovirus mononucleosis. Ann. Surg., 185:406, 1977.

Levine, E. A., Rosen, A. L., Sehgal, L. R., et al.: Treatment of acute postoperative anemia with recombinant human erythropoietin. J. Trauma, 29:1134, 1989.

Lillemoe, K. D., et al.: Intestinal necrosis due to sodium polystyrene (Kayexalate) in sorbitol enemas: Clinical and experimental support for the hypothesis. Surgery, 101:267, 1987.

Livio, M., et al.: Uraemic bleeding: Role of anaemia and beneficial effect of red cell transfusions. Lancet, 2:1013, 1982.

Lunsgaard-Hansen, P.: Blood transfusion and a capillary function. In Ikkala, E., and Nykanen, A. (Eds.): Transfusion and Immunology. Helsinki, International Society of Blood Transfusions, 1975, p. 121.

MacDonald, R.: Red cell 2,3-diphosphoglycerate and oxygen affinity. Anaesthesia, 32:544, 1977.

MacKenzie, C. R., and Charlson, M. E.: Assessment of perioperative risk in the patient with diabetes mellitus. Surg. Gynecol. Obstet., 167:293, 1988.

MacLennan, D. H., Duff, C., Zorzato, F., et al.: Ryanodine receptor gene is a candidate for predisposition to malignant hyperthermia. Nature, 343:559, 1990.

Malviya, V. K., and Deppe, G.: Control of intraoperative hemorrhage in gynecology with the use of fibrin glue. Obstet. Gynecol., 73:284, 1989.

Mangano, D. T.: Preoperative assessment. In Kaplan, J. A. (Ed.): Cardiac Anesthesia. Vol. I, 2nd ed. New York, Grune & Stratton, 1987, p. 341.

Mangano, D. T.: Perioperative cardiac morbidity. Anesthesiology, 72:153, 1990.

Mannucci, P. M., et al.: Desamino-8-D-arginine vasopressin shortens the bleeding time in uremia. N. Engl. J. Med., 308:8, 1983.

Mason, D. T.: Cardiovascular management. In Mason, D. T. (Ed.): Essays in Medicine. New York, Medcom Publishers, 1974.

Mazza, J. J., Bowie, E. J. W., Hagedorn, A. B., et al.: Antihemophilic factor VIII in hemophilia: Use of concentrates to permit major surgery. JAMA, 211:1818, 1970.

McArthur, J. W., et al.: Thyrotoxic crisis: An analysis of the 36 cases seen at the Massachusetts General Hospital during the past twenty-five years. JAMA, 134:868, 1974.

McCabe, W. R., and Treadwell, T. L.: Gram-negative bacteremia. Monogr. Urol., 4:193, 1983.

McDougal, W. S.: Surgical nutrition. Am. Urol. Assoc. Update Ser., 2:16, 1983.

McEnroe, C. S., O'Donnell, T. F., Yeager, A., et al.: Comparison of ejection fraction and Goldman risk factor analysis to dipyridamole-thallium 201 studies in the evaluation of cardiac morbidity after aortic aneurysm surgery. J. Vasc. Surg., 11:497, 1990.

McGowan, S. W., and Smith, G. F. N.: Anaesthesia for transurethral prostatectomy. Anaesthesia, 35:847, 1980.

McKenzie, P. J., Wishart, H. Y., Gray, I., et al.: Effect of anaesthetic technique on deep vein thrombosis. Br. J. Anaesth., 57:853, 1985.

Meakins, J. L., Pietsch, J. B., Bubenick, O., et al.: Delayed hypersensitivity: Indicator of acquired failure of host defenses in sepsis and trauma. Ann. Surg., 186:241, 1977.

Meguid, M. M., Curtas, M. S., McGuid, V., et al.: Effects of preoperative TPN on surgical risk—Preliminary status report. Br. J. Clin. Pract. (Suppl.), 63:53, 1989.

Meguid, M. M., et al.: Reduced metabolic complications in total parenteral nutrition: Pilot study using fat to replace one third of glucose calories. JPEN, 6:304, 1984.

Mercer, D. M., and Eltringham, R. J.: Anesthesia for thyroid surgery. Ear Nose Throat J., 64:375, 1985.

Merritt, W. T.: Monitoring modalities. In Breslow, M. J., Miller, C. F., and Rogers, M. C. (Eds.): Perioperative Management. St. Louis, C. V. Mosby Co., 1990, p. 64.

Meyers, E. F., et al.: Perioperative control of blood glucose in diabetic patients: A two-step protocol. Diabetes Care, 9:40, 1986.

Meyers, J. R., Lembeck, L., O'Kane, H., et al.: Changes in functional residual capacity of the lung after operation. Arch. Surg., 110:576, 1975.

Miller, C. F.: Renal failure. In Breslow, M. J., Miller, C. F., and Rogers, M. C. (Eds.): Perioperative Management. St. Louis, C. V. Mosby Co., 1990, p. 327.

Miller, C. F., and Martin, J. L.: Changes in lung function following anesthesia and surgery. In Breslow, M. J., Miller, C. F., and Rogers, M. C. (Eds.): Perioperative Management. St. Louis, C. V. Mosby Co., 1990, p. 194.

Miller, R. R., Lies, J. E., and Carretta, R. F.: Prevention of lower extremity venous thrombosis by early mobilization. Ann. Intern. Med., 84:700, 1976.

Modig, J., Malmberg, P., and Karlstrom, G.: Effect of epidural versus general anaesthesia on calf blood flow. Acta Anaesthesiol. Scand., 24:305, 1980.

Moesgaard, F., Nielsen, M. L., Hjortrup, A., et al.: Intraincisional antibiotic in addition to systemic antibiotic treatment fails to reduce wound infection rates in contaminated abdominal surgery. Dis. Colon Rectum, 32:36, 1989.

Molitch, M. E.: Endocrinology. In Molitch, M. E. (Ed.): Management of Medical Problems in Surgical Patients. Philadelphia, F. A. Davis Co., 1982.

Moore, D. C.: Intercostal nerve block for postoperative somatic pain following surgery of thorax and upper abdomen. Br. J. Anaesth., 47:284, 1975.

Morrison, J. E., and Wiser, W. L.: The use of prophylactic partial exchange transfusion in pregnancies associated with sickle cell hemoglobinopathy. Obstet. Gynecol., 48:516, 1976.

Moser, K. M.: Pulmonary thromboembolism. In Isselbacher, K. J., et al. (Eds.): Harrison's Principles of Internal Medicine. 9th ed. New York, McGraw-Hill Book Co., 1980.

Moser, K. M.: Thromboembolic disease in the patient undergoing urologic surgery. Urol. Clin. North Am., 10:101, 1983.

Moser, K. M., Brach, B., and Dolan, G. F.: Clinically suspected deep venous thrombosis of the lower extremities. JAMA, 237:2195, 1977.

Mullen, J. L.: Consequences of malnutrition in the surgical patient. Surg. Clin. North Am., 61:465, 1981.

Mullen, J. L., et al.: Prediction of operative morbidity and mortality by preoperative nutritional assessment. Surg. Forum, 30:80, 1979.

Mullen, J. L., et al.: Reduction of operative morbidity and mortality by combined preoperative and postoperative nutritional support. Ann. Surg., 192:604, 1980.

Multicenter Trial Committee: Dihydroergotamine-heparin prophylaxis of postoperative deep vein thrombosis: A multicenter trial. JAMA, 251:2960, 1984.

Murkin, J. M.: Anesthesia and hypothyroidism: A review of thyroxine physiology, pharmacology, and anesthetic implications. Anesth. Analg., 61:371, 1982.

Naeye, R. L.: Thrombotic state after a hemorrhagic diathesis, a possible complication of therapy with epsilonaminocaproic acid. Blood, 19:694, 1962.

Nelson, P. H., Moser, K. M., Stoner, C., et al.: Risk of complications during intravenous heparin therapy. West. J. Med., 136:189, 1982.

New, W.: Pulse oximetry. J. Clin. Monit., 1:126, 1985.

Nichols, R. L.: Prophylaxis for elective bowel surgery. In Wilson, S. E., Finegold, S. M., and Williams, R. A. (Eds.): Intra-abdominal Infection. New York, McGraw-Hill Book Co., 1982.

Nickel, J. C., Feero, P., Costerton, J. W., et al.: Incidence and importance of bacteriuria in postoperative, short-term urinary catheterization. Can. J. Surg., 32:131, 1989.

Nord, C. E.: Surgical prophylaxis and treatment of surgical infections with quinolones. Rev. Infect. Dis., 11:S1287, 1989.

Nuutinen, L. S., Kairaluoma, M., Tuononen, S., et al.: The effect of furosemide on renal function in open heart surgery. J. Cardiovasc. Surg., 19:471, 1978.

O'Toole, J. D., Wurtzbacher, J. J., Wearner, N. E., et al.: Pulmonary-valve injury and insufficiency during pulmonary artery catheterization. N. Engl. J. Med., 301:1167, 1979.

Owen, C. A., Jr.: Factor VIII terminology. Letter. Lancet, 2:359, 1981.

Owen, C. A., Jr., and Walter Bowie, E. J.: Disorders of coagulation. Urol. Clin. North Am., 10:77, 1983.

Packer, M. G., Russo, P., and Fair, W. R.: Prophylactic antibiotics and Foley catheter use in transperineal needle biopsy of the prostate. J. Urol., 131:687, 1984.

Parfrey, P. S., Griffiths, S. M., Barrett, B. J., et al.: Contrast material-induced renal failure in patients with diabetes mellitus, renal insufficiency, or both. N. Engl. J. Med., 320:143, 1989.

Pasternack, P. F., Grossi, E. A., Baumann, F. G., et al.: The value of silent myocardial ischemia monitoring in the prediction of perioperative myocardial infarction in patients undergoing peripheral vascular surgery. J. Vasc. Surg., 10:617, 1989.

Pasulka, P. S., et al.: The risks of surgery in obese patients. Ann. Intern. Med., 104:540, 1986.

Pearce, A. C., and Jones, R. M.: Smoking and anesthesia: Preoperative abstinence and perioperative morbidity. Anesthesiology, 61:576, 1984.

Pedersen, T., Kelbaek, H., and Munck, O.: Cardiopulmonary complications in high-risk surgical patients: The value of preoperative radionuclide cardiography. Acta Anaesthesiol. Scand., 34:183, 1990.

Peters, W. P., Johnson, M. W., Friedman, P. A., et al.: Pressor effect of naloxone in septic shock. Lancet, 1:529, 1981.

Pflug, A. E., and Halter, J. B.: Effect of spinal anesthesia on adrenergic tone and the neuroendocrine responses to surgical stress in humans. Anesthesiology, 55:120, 1981.

Pien, F. D., and Landers, J. Q.: Indwelling urinary catheter infections in small community hospital. Role of urinary drainage bag. Urology, 22:255, 1983.

Pien, L. C., Grammer, L. C., and Patterson, R.: Minimal complications in a surgical population with severe asthma receiving prophylactic corticosteroids. J. Allergy Clin. Immunol., 82:696, 1988.

Pinson, C. W., et al.: Surgery in long-term dialysis patients: Experience with more than 300 cases. Am. J. Surg., 151:567, 1986.

Pintado, T., Taswell, H. F., and Bowie, E. J. W.: Treatment of life-threatening hemorrhage due to acquired factor VIII inhibitor. Blood, 46:535, 1975.

Pontoppidan, H., Wilson, R. S., Rite, M. A., et al.: Respiratory intensive care. Anesthesiology. 47:96, 1977.

Pousada, L., and Leipzig, R. M.: Rapid bedside assessment of postoperative confusion in older patients. Geriatrics, 45(5):59, 1990.

Quinlan, D. M., Brendler, C. B., and Naslund, M. J.: Urological applications of the argon beam coagulator. J. Urol., (in press).

Raahave, D., Hesselfeldt, P., and Pedersen, T. B.: Cefotaxime I.V. versus oral neomycin-erythromycin for prophylaxis of infections after colorectal operations. World J. Surg., 12:369, 1988.

Rabinowitz, I. N., Watson, W., and Farber, E. M.: Topical steroid depression of the hypothalamic-pituitary-adrenal axis in psoriasis vulgaris. Dermatologica, 154:321, 1977.

Rao, T. K., Jacobs, K. H., El-Etr, A. A.: Reinfarction following anesthesia in patients with myocardial infarction. Anesthesiology, 59:499, 1983.

Ray, S., et al.: Effects of obesity on respiratory function. Am. Rev. Respir. Dis., 128:501, 1983.

Reinhardt, G. F., et al.: Incidence and mortality of hypoalbuminemic patients in hospitalized veterans. JPEN, 4:357, 1980.

Reiz, S., Balfors, E., Sorensen, M. B., et al.: Coronary haemodynamic effects of general anaesthesia and surgery. Modification by epidural analgesia in patients with ischaemic heart disease. Reg. Anaesth., 7(S4):8, 1982.

Roberts, S. L., and Tinker, J. H.: Cardiovascular disease. In Brown, D. L. (Ed.): Risk and Outcome in Anesthesia. Philadelphia, J. B. Lippincott, 1988, p. 33.

Rogers, D. A., Dingus, D., Stanfield, J., et al.: A prospective study of patient-controlled analgesia. Am. Surg., 56:86, 1990.

Rose, S. D.: Prophylaxis of thromboembolic disease. Med. Clin. North Am., 63:1205, 1979.

Rose, S. D., Gorman, L. C., and Mason, D. T.: Cardiac risk factors in patients undergoing noncardiac surgery. Med. Clin. North Am., 63:1271, 1979.

Rotman, N., Hay, J. M., Lacaine, F., et al.: Prophylactic antibiotherapy in abdominal surgery. Arch. Surg., 124:323, 1989.

Roukema, J. A., Carol, E. J., and Prins, J. G.: The prevention of pulmonary complications after upper abdominal surgery in patients with noncompromised pulmonary status. Arch. Surg., 123:30, 1988.

Roza, A. M., Tuitt, D., and Shizgal, H. M.: Transferrin—a poor measure of nutritional status. JPEN, 8:523, 1984.

Rubio, P. A.: Septisol antiseptic foam: A sensible alternative to the conventional surgical scrub. Int. Surg., 72:243, 1987.

Sakima, N. T.: Arrythmias including SSS/heart block. In Breslow, M. J., Miller, C. F., and Rogers, M. C. (Eds.): Perioperative Management. St. Louis, C. V. Mosby, 1990, p. 249.

Salzman, E., Weinstein, M., Weintraut, R., et al.: Treatment with desmopressin acetate to reduce blood loss after cardiac surgery: a double blind randomized trial. N. Engl. J. Med., 314:1402, 1986.

Salzman, E. W., and Davies, G. C.: Prophylaxis of venous thromboembolism: Analysis of cost effectiveness. Ann. Surg., 191:207, 1980.

Salzman, E. W., Deykin, D., Shapiro, R. M., et al.: Management of heparin therapy: Controlled prospective trial. N. Engl. J. Med., 292:1046, 1975.

Schaefer, C. F., and Geelhoed, G. W.: Redirection of misplaced central venous catheters. Arch. Surg., 115:789, 1980.

Schlichtig, R., and Ayres, S. M.: Nutritional Support of the Critically Ill. Chicago, Year Book Medical Publishers, 1988.

Schriemer, P. A., Longnecker, D. E., and Mintz, P. D.: The possible immunosuppressive effects of perioperative blood transfusion in cancer patients. Anesthesiology, 68:422, 1988.

Schwab, S. J., Hlatky, M. A., Pieper, K. S., et al.: Contrast nephrotoxicity: A randomized controlled trial of a nonionic and an ionic radiographic contrast agent. N. Engl. J. Med., 320:149, 1989.

Schwartz, B. R., Gregg, R. V., Kessler, D. L., et al.: Continuous postoperative epidural analgesia in management of postoperative surgical pain. Urology, 34:349, 1989.

Schwartz, R. A., and Cerra, F. B.: Shock: A practical approach. Urol. Clin. North Am., 10:89, 1983.

Scott, N. B., and Kehlet, H.: Regional anaesthesia and surgical morbidity. Br. J. Surg., 75:299, 1988.

Sears, D. A.: The morbidity of sickle cell trait: A review of the literature. Am. J. Med., 64:1021, 1978.

Sechzer, D. H.: Objective measurement of pain. Anesthesiology, 29:209, 1968.

Seltzer, M. H., et al.: Instant nutritional assessment. JPEN, 3:157, 1979.

Sethi, G. K., Copeland, J. G., Goldman, S., et al.: Implications of preoperative administration of aspirin in patients undergoing coronary artery bypass grafting. J. Am. Coll. Cardiol., 15:15, 1990.

Shapiro, B. A.: Airway pressure therapy for acute restrictive pulmonary pathology. In Critical Care: State of the Art 1981. Fullerton, Ca., Society for Critical Care Medicine, 1981.

Sheldon, C. A., and Leonard, A. S.: Hemodynamic monitoring. Urol. Clin. North Am., 10:19, 1983.

Sherman, L. A.: Alterations in hemostasis during massive transfusion. In Nusbacher, J. (Ed.): Massive Transfusion. Washington, D.C., American Association of Blood Banks, 1978, p. 53.

Simon, A. B.: Perioperative management of the pacemaker patient. Anesthesiology, 46:127, 1977.

Sirotzky, L., and Lewis, E. J.: Anesthesia related muscle paralysis in renal failure. Clin. Nephrol., 10:38, 1978.

Smith, R. A.: Respiratory care. In Miller, R. D. (Ed.): Anesthesia. New York, Churchill Livingstone, 1981.

Smith, R. C., and Hartemink, R.: Improvement of nutritional measures during preoperative parenteral nutrition in patients selected by the prognostic nutritional index: A randomized controlled trial. JPEN, 12:587, 1988.

Soballe, P. W., and Greif, J. M.: Preoperative whole-gut lavage vs. traditional three-day bowel preparation in left colon surgery. Milit. Med., 154:198, 1989.

Solanki, D., and McCurdy, P. R.: Delayed hemolytic transfusion reactions: An often missed entity. JAMA, 239:729, 1978.

Spence, R. K., Carson, J. A., Poses, R., et al.: Elective surgery without transfusion: Influence of preoperative hemoglobin level and blood loss on mortality. Am. J. Surg., 159:320, 1990.

Speziale, F., Verardi, S., Taurino, M., et al.: Low molecular weight heparin prevention of post-operative deep vein thrombosis in vascular surgery. Pharmatherapeutica, 5:261, 1988.

Stanley, T. H., Bennett, G. M., Lorser, E. A., et al.: Cardiovascular effects of diazepam and droperidol during morphine anesthesia. Anesthesiology, 44:255, 1976.

Stern, W. Z.: Diagnostic imaging of the urinary tract in pregnancy. In Freed, S. Z., and Herzig, N. (Eds.): Urology in Pregnancy. Baltimore, Williams & Wilkins, 1982, p. 48.

Stone, J. G., Foex, P., Sear, J. W., et al.: Myocardial ischemia in untreated hypertensive patients: Effect of a single small oral dose of a beta-adrenergic blocking agent. Anesthesiology, 68:495, 1988.

Sun, N. C. J., Bowie, E. J. W., Kazmier, F. J., et al.: Blood coagulation studies in patients with cancer. Mayo Clin. Proc., 49:636, 1974.

Surgenor, D. M., Wallace, E. L., Hao, S. H. S., et al.: Collection and transfusion of blood in the United States, 1982–1988. N. Engl. J. Med., 322:1646, 1990.

Swan, H. J. C., and Ganz, W.: Use of a balloon flotation catheter in critically ill patients. Surg. Clin. North Am., 55:501, 1975.

Swarts, R. D.: Hemorrhage during high-risk hemodialysis using controlled heparinization. Nephron, 28:65, 1981.

Swartz, H. M., and Reichling, B. A.: Hazards of radiation exposure for pregnant women. JAMA, 239:1907, 1978.

Taitelman, U., Reece, E. A., and Bessman, A. N.: Insulin in the management of the diabetic surgical patient. JAMA, 237:658, 1977.

Tartter, P. I.: Blood transfusion and infectious complications following colorectal cancer surgery. Br. J. Surg., 75:789, 1988.

Tasker, P. R. W., MacGregor, G. A., and deWardener, H. E.: Prophylactic use of intravenous saline in patients with chronic renal failure undergoing major surgery. Lancet, 2:911, 1974.

Teasley, K. M., Lysne, J., Nuwer, N., et al.: Nutrition and metabolic support of the surgical patient. Urol. Clin. North Am., 10:119, 1983.

Thind, P., and Sigsgaard, T.: The analgesic effect of indomethacin in the early post-operative period following abdominal surgery. Acta Chir. Scand., 154:9, 1988.

Thomas, D. J. B., et al.: Insulin-dependent diabetes during the perioperative period. Anaesthesia, 39:629, 1984.

Tisi, G. M.: Preoperative evaluation of pulmonary function. Am. Rev. Respir. Dis., 119:293, 1979.

Upton, R. A., et al.: Renal and biliary elimination of vecuronium (ORG NC 45) and pancuronium in rats. Anesth. Analg., 61:313, 1982.

Valentin, N., Lomholt, B., Jensen, J. S., et al.: Spinal or general anaesthesia for surgery of the fractured hip. Br. J. Anaesth., 58:284, 1986.

Van Arsdalen, K., Smith, M. J., Barnes, R. W., et al.: Deep vein thrombosis and prostatectomy. Urology, 21:461, 1983.

Vandendris, M., Kutnowski, M., Futeral, B., et al.: Prevention of postoperative deep-vein thrombosis by low-dose heparin in open prostatectomy. Urol. Res., 8:219, 1980.

Van Sonnenberg, E. F., Ferrucci, J. T., Mueller, P. R., et al.: Percutaneous radiographically guided catheter drainage of abdominal abscesses. JAMA, 247:190, 1982.

Vaughan, E. D., and Gillenwater, J. Y.: Diagnosis, characterization and management of post-obstructive diuresis. J. Urol., 109:286, 1973.

Vaughn, B. K., Knezevich, S., Lombardi, A. V., et al.: Use of the Greenfield filter to prevent fatal pulmonary embolism associated with total hip and knee arthroplasty. J. Bone Joint Surg., 71A:1542, 1989.

Viteri, F. E., and Schneider, R. E.: Gastrointestinal alterations in protein-calorie malnutrition. Med. Clin. North Am., 58:1487, 1974.

von Knorring, J.: Postoperative myocardial infarction: A prospective study in a risk group of surgical patients. Surgery, 90:55, 1981.

Walter, C. W.: Blood donors, blood and transfusion. In Kinney, J. M., et al. (Eds.): Manual of Preoperative and Postoperative Care. Philadelphia, W. B. Saunders Co., 1971, p. 139.

Walts, L. F., et al.: Perioperative management of diabetes mellitus. Anesthesiology, 55:104, 1981.

Warner, M. A., Offord, K. P., Warner, M. E., et al.: Role of preoperative cessation of smoking and other factors in postoperative pulmonary complications: A blinded prospective study of coronary artery bypass patients. Mayo Clin. Proc., 64:609, 1989.

Watson-Williams, E. J.: Hematologic and hemostatic considerations before surgery. Med. Clin. North Am., 63:1165, 1979.

Wax, S. H.: The use of the radioisotope renogram in pregnancy. In Freed, S. Z., and Herzig, N. (Eds.): Urology in Pregnancy. Baltimore, Williams & Wilkins Co., 1982, p. 64.

White, P. F.: Mishaps with patient controlled analgesia. Anesthesiology, 66:81, 1987.

White, V. A., and Kumagai, L. F.: Preoperative endocrine and metabolic considerations. Med. Clin. North Am., 63:1321, 1979.

Wiehle, S. P., Banowsky, L. H., Nicastro-Lutton, J. J., et al.: Pretransplant bilateral nephrectomy and adjuvant operations. Urology, 18:349, 1981.

Wille-Jorgensen, P. W., Christensen, S. W., Bjerg-Nielsen, A., et al.: Prevention of thromboembolism following elective hip surgery. Clin. Orthop., 247:163, 1989.

Wilson, R. G., Smith, D., Paton, G., et al.: Prophylactic subcutaneous heparin does not increase operative blood loss in transurethral resection of the prostate. Br. J. Urol., 62:246, 1988.

Windsor, J. A., and Hill, G. L.: Risk factors for postoperative pneumonia. Ann. Surg., 208:209, 1988.

Wolff, B. G., Beart, R. W., Dozois, R. R., et al.: A new bowel preparation for elective colon and rectal surgery. Arch. Surg., 123:895, 1988.

Yeager, M. P., Glass, D. D., Neff, R. K., et al.: Epidural anesthesia and analgesia in high-risk surgical patients. Anesthesiology, 66:729, 1987.

Zama, N., Fazio, V. W., Jagelman, D. G., et al.: Efficacy of pelvic packing in maintaining hemostasis after rectal excision for cancer. Dis. Colon Rectum, 31:923, 1988.

Zibrak, J. D., O'Donnell, C. R., and Marton, K.: Indications for pulmonary function testing. Ann. Intern. Med., 112:763, 1990.

64
THE ADRENALS

E. Darracott Vaughan, Jr., M.D.
Jon David Blumenfeld, M.D.

HISTORICAL BACKGROUND

The understanding of the essential physiologic role of the adrenal glands has evolved from the initial description in *Opuscula Anatomica* in 1563 (Eustachius, 1563) to the elegant biochemical analysis of adrenal secretory products and precise radiologic imaging studies currently available (Vaughan and Carey, 1989a).

Despite earlier recognition of the presence of the adrenals and the division into cortex and medulla (Cuvier, 1800–1805), it was not until the precise observations of Addison in 1855 that the essential role of these glands was recognized in patients who died with adrenal destruction secondary to tuberculosis. Soon thereafter, Brown-Sequard (1856) performed bilateral adrenalectomies in animals and predicted that the adrenals were essential for life.

Hyperfunction of the adrenal cortex was not documented until 1912 with the definitive report on 11 patients describing the now classic characteristics of Cushing's syndrome being reported in 1932 in patients with basophilic adenomas of the pituitary (Cushing, 1912, 1932). However, it was not until the purification of adrenocortical extracts that adrenalectomized animals could be maintained; the adrenal cortex was then documented as the site of critical and essential steroid production (Hartman et al., 1927). Progressive and sequential advances in the understanding of adrenal steroid production (Scott, 1990) have led to the development of precise diagnostic tests (Dolan and Carey, 1989) to identify patients with Cushing's syndrome (Siragy et al., 1989), adrenocortical forms of hypertension (Biglieri et al., 1990), congenital adrenal hyperplasia (New and Speiser, 1989), adrenal carcinoma (Vaughan and Carey, 1989b), and other adrenal disorders.

Frankel first described a medullary adrenal tumor in 1886. London physiologists demonstrated a pressor substance from the adrenal medulla, which they named adrenalin (Oliver and Sharpey-Schafer, 1895). Subsequently, John Abel coined the term epinephrine (Abel, 1897), and Kohn described the chromaffin system (Kohn, 1902). In 1912, the pathologist Pick formulated the descriptive term pheochromocytoma from the Greek *phaios* (dark or dusty) and *chroma* (color) to describe adrenal medullary tumors with their chromaffin reaction (Pick, 1912).

The development of precise urinary and plasma tests led to the accurate identification of patients with adrenal medullary disorders (Reckler et al., 1989). Moreover, it is particularly in the identification and localization of pheochromocytomas that imaging techniques have become highly accurate and essential (Kazam et al., 1989; Markisz and Kazam, 1989).

The diagnosis of the major adrenal disorders is now actually simpler than in the past because of precise diagnostic assays and radiologic tests. The evaluation of a patient for a potential adrenal disorder can be performed efficiently, usually without hospitalization by a practicing urologist knowledgeable in adrenal disease. Moreover, the surgical approaches are well within the expertise of the urologist and are now precisely described (Libertino and Novick, 1989; Scott, 1990; Vaughan and Carey, 1989a; Vaughan, 1991).

This chapter reviews concisely the relevant adrenal anatomy, pathology, and physiology that serve as the bases for the clinical, biologic, and radiologic diagnoses of the major adrenal disorders. In addition, current medical and surgical strategies are reviewed. The adrenal disorders of neuroblastoma and congenital adrenal hyperplasia are reviewed in detail in the pertinent chapters and are mentioned only briefly in this chapter.

ANATOMY, HISTOLOGY, AND EMBRYOLOGY

The adrenal glands are paired retroperitoneal organs that lie within perinephric fat at the anterosuperior and medial aspects of the kidneys. They measure up to 5 cm

Acknowledgment is made to all the contributors to the text, *Adrenal Disorder*, edited by E. D. Vaughan, Jr. and R. M. Carey, which served as the basis for much of this present chapter.

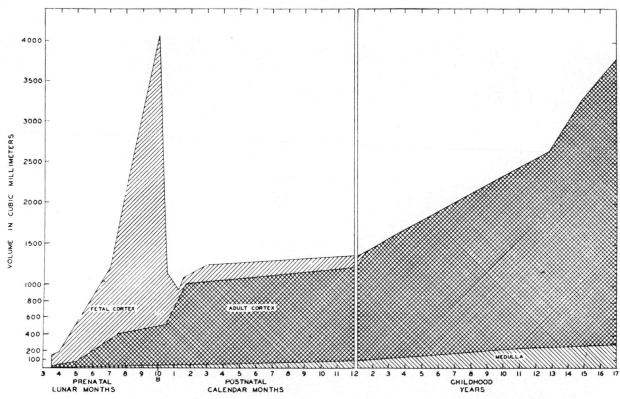

Figure 64–1. Growth of the adrenal cortex including the fetal cortex in utero and after birth. A striking decrease occurs in the size of the fetal cortex after birth and a gradual increase in the adult cortex with aging. (From Bethune, J. E.: The adrenal cortex. A Scope monograph. The Upjohn Co., Kalamazoo, Mich.)

in length by 3 cm in width, and are 1 cm thick. In the healthy nonstressed adult, the glands weigh about 5 g each. In contrast, the adrenal weight at birth is quite large (5 to 10 g) because of the fetal adrenal cortex, which may play a major role in fetal embryogenesis and homeostasis (Fig. 64–1) (Pepe and Albrecht, 1990). The

fetal adrenal regresses rapidly during the first 6 weeks of life (Scott et al., 1990) but is susceptible to adrenal hemorrhage at the time of birth, a condition now readily diagnosed by magnetic resonance imaging (MRI) (Fig. 64–2).

Sectional imaging has given us a better understanding

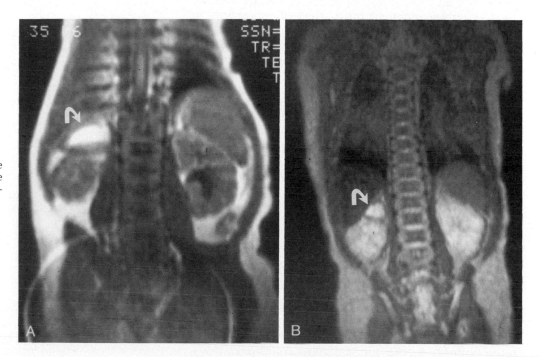

Figure 64–2. Adrenal hemorrhage (A) bright on magnetic resonance imaging (arrow) showing later resolution (B).

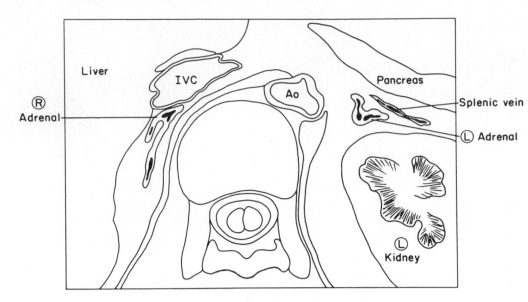

Figure 64–3. Line schematic of an anatomic specimen showing position of the adrenal glands in relation to the diaphragm, inferior vena cava, and kidneys. (From Vaughan, E. D., Jr., and Carey, R. M. (Eds.): Adrenal Disorders. New York, Thieme Medical Publishers Inc., 1989.)

of the precise appearance of the adrenals. Both glands are flattened anteriorly with a thick central ridge and thinner medial and lateral rami (Kazam et al., 1989). Cortical infoldings, especially seen on sagittal sections, may be confused for small adenomas especially in primary aldosteronism in which the lesions are small.

The right adrenal lies above the kidney posterolateral to the inferior vena cava (IVC). The anterior surface is in immediate contact with the inferior posterior surface of the liver. Thus, from an anterior approach, the anterior surface of the adrenal can be exposed by remaining extraperitoneal and by gently lifting the liver cephalad, the inferior vena cava being medial. The posterior surface of both adrenals is in contact with the posterior diaphragm (Fig. 64–3). Both adrenals lie more posteriorly as they follow the lumbar curve of the spine, thus falling away from the surgeon for the superior dissection.

The left adrenal is in more intimate contact with the kidney, and the main left renal artery often lies deep to the left adrenal vein as it enters the left renal vein. The gland overlies the upper pole of the kidney with its anterior surface and medial aspect behind the pancreas and splenic artery (see Fig. 64–3). The anterior surface of the left adrenal can be exposed by remaining retroperitoneal and by gently retracting the spleen within the peritoneum cephalad. Division of the splenorenal ligament facilitates this dissection.

The adrenals have a delicate and rich blood supply estimated to be 6 to 7 ml/g/min, without a dominant single artery. The inferior phrenic artery is the main blood supply with additional branches from the aorta and the renal artery (Fig. 64–4) (Pick and Anson, 1940; Anson et al., 1947). The small arteries penetrate the gland in a circumferential stellate fashion, leaving both anterior and posterior surfaces avascular. The venous drainage is usually a common vein on the right exiting the apex of the gland and entering the posterior surface of the IVC; this vein is short and fragile and the most common source of troublesome bleeding during right adrenalectomy (Fig. 64–5). The left vein empties directly into the left renal vein about 3 cm from the IVC and often opposite to the gonadal vein (Johnstone, 1957).

Not well recognized is the left inferior phrenic vein, which typically communicates with the adrenal vein but then courses medially and can be injured during dissection of the medial edge of the gland.

The adrenal cortex develops from mesoderm and the medulla from neuroectoderm. During the 5th week of development, mesothelial cells located between the root of the mesentery and the developing gonad proliferate and invade the mesenchyme. These cells form the fetal cortex, while a second migration of cells forms the definitive cortex; an additional cell type comes from mesonephric origin (Crowder, 1957). The intimate relationship with developing gonad, kidney, and adrenal generally explains the finding of ectopic or aberrant

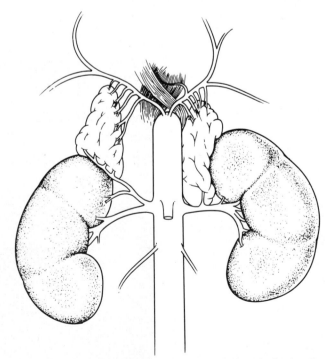

Figure 64–4. Arterial supply of left and right adrenal glands. (From Vaughan, E. D., Jr., and Carey, R. M.: Adrenal Disorders. New York, Thieme Medical Publishers Inc., 1989.)

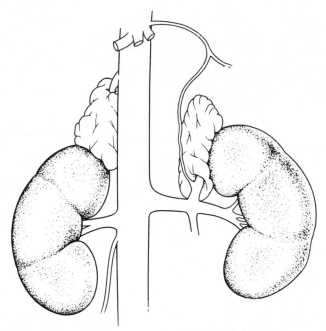

Figure 64–5. Venous drainage of left and right adrenal glands with particular attention to the intercommunicating vein on the left, which is medial and drains into the phrenic system. (From Vaughan, E. D., Jr., and Carey, R. M.; Adrenal Disorders. New York, Thieme Medical Publishers Inc., 1989.)

adrenal tissue. Heterotopic adrenal tissue is usually associated with the kidney but is also reported to be associated with the broad ligament, gonadal vessels, spermatic cord, canal of Zuck, uterus, testis, and sites of peritoneal attachment (Culp, 1959; Schechter, 1968).

Microscopically, the mature adrenal cortex constitutes 90 per cent of the gland and is divided into three zones: zona glomerulosa, zona fasciculata, and zona reticularis (Fig. 64–6). Zonation is complete by 18 months, although adult configuration is not reached until 10 to 12 years (Moore et al., 1989). The zona glomerulosa is less prominent in humans than in other species and is the site of aldosterone production. The zonae fasciculata and reticularis form a single functional zone that produces glucocorticoids, androgens, and estrogens.

The adrenal medulla is derived from cells of the neural crest that migrate at the 7th week to form collections, which enter the fetal cortex leaving nodules of neuroblasts scattered throughout the cortex. Neuroblastic cortical nodules regress as the medulla forms, but they can persist and should not be confused with an in situ neuroblastoma. By the 20th week, there is a primitive medulla but the distinct medulla is not present until atrophy of the fetal cortex.

The medulla is soft currant jelly–like and can be bluntly dissected free from cortex for adrenal medullary

Figure 64–6. Section of an adrenal (left) of a man and (right) of a 6-month-old infant. Mallory azan stain. About × 105. (From Maximow and Bloom. Textbook of Histology. By permission from Don W. Fawcett, M. D.)

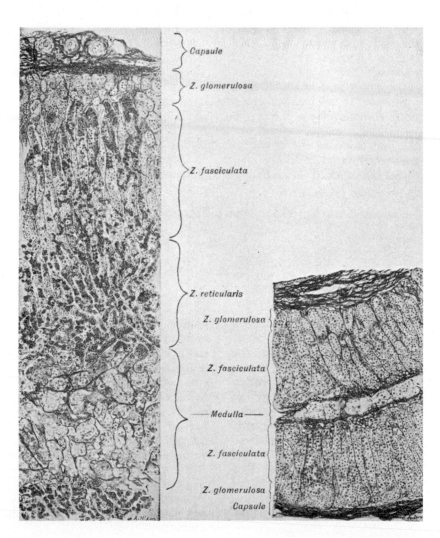

transplantation (Madrazo et al., 1987). The medulla produces both norepinephrine and epinephrine, with the reaction facilitated in the presence of glucocorticoids. The chromaffin cells are polyhedral, arranged in cords, and richly ennervated. Epinephrine- and norepinephrine-secreting cells are distinct (Tannenbaum, 1970).

ADRENAL PHYSIOLOGY

The adrenal can be thought of functionally as two distinct organs: cortex and medulla. Each has its own unique physiology and hormonally active secretory products.

Adrenal Cortex

From a common precursor the zones of the adrenal cortex produce a series of steroid hormones that have an array of actions, including salt retention, metabolic homeostasis, and adrenarche development. The basic steroid structure of pregnenolone as derived from cholesterol is shown (Fig. 64–7). The zona glomerulosa is the only source of the major mineralocorticoid aldosterone, which regulates sodium resorption in the kidney, and gut, and salivary and sweat glands (Carey, 1986). The other zones produce and secrete cortisol, the major glucocorticoid in humans and the principal androgens dehydroepiandrosterone (DHEA), dehydroepiandrosterone sulfate (DHEAS), and androstenedione. The pathways for production of these steroids are shown (Figs. 64–8 and 64–9). The rate-limiting step for the formation of all these hormones is the production of pregnenolone (see Fig. 64–7) (Nelson, 1980).

As is discussed in detail elsewhere in this text, it is the deficiency of one of the five enzymes necessary to convert cholesterol to cortisol that leads to the family of diseases termed congenital adrenal hyperplasia (New

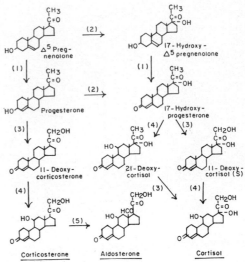

Figure 64–8. Corticosteroid synthesis in the adrenal cortex. Enzyme systems are numbered: (1) β-hydroxysteroid dehydrogenase: Δ5-oxosteroid isomerase complex, (2) C-17-hydroxylase, (3) C-21-hydroxylase, (4) C-11-hydroxylase, (5) C-18-hydroxylase. The Δ signifies a double bond, and the attached number shows its position in the nucleus. (From Dluhy, R. G., and Gittes, R. F.: The Adrenals. *In* Walsh, P. C., Gittes, R. F., Perlmutter, A. D., and Stamey, T. A. (Eds.): Campbell's Urology, 5th ed. Philadelphia, W. B. Saunders Co., 1986.)

and Speiser, 1989; Speiser et al., 1991). The presenting symptom complexes are dependent on the specific enzyme deficiency, the lack of necessary pituitary feedback, and the resultant adrenal hyperplasia and proximal precursor excess.

The excess of one or numerous steroid products gives the characteristic signs and symptoms of Cushing's syn-

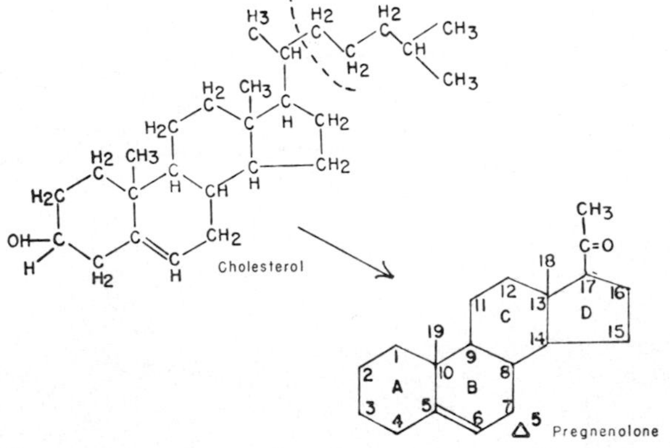

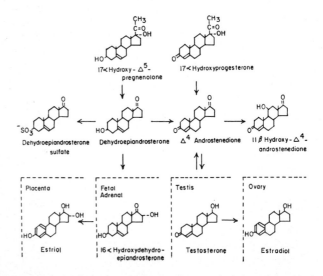

Figure 64–9. Sex hormone synthesis. The upper portion of the scheme shows the synthesis of adrenal androgens. The lower panel shows conversion of androstenedione to testosterone (testis, adrenal cortex, and, to a small degree, the liver); 16 α-hydroxylation of dehydroepiandrosterone by the fetal adrenal and conversion to estrogen in the placenta; and conversion of androgen to estrogen in the ovary. Note that the initial steps in sex hormone synthesis are the same in all these organs. (From Dluhy, R. G., and Gittes, R. F.: The Adrenals. *In* Walsh, P. C., Gittes, R. F., Perlmutter, A. D., and Stamey, T. A. (Eds.): Campbell's Urology, 5th ed. Philadelphia, W. B. Saunders Co., 1986.)

Figure 64–7. Conversion of cholesterol to pregnenolone. The cholesterol formula shows the complete steroid structure; the pregnenolone formula shows the conventional representation of the steroid molecule with the rings designated by letter and the carbon atoms numbered. (From Dluhy, R. G., and Gittes, R. F.: The Adrenals. *In* Walsh, P. C., Gittes, R. F., Perlmutter, A. D., and Stamey, T. A. (Eds.): Campbell's Urology, 5th ed. Philadelphia, W. B. Saunders Co., 1986.)

drome, primary hyperaldosteronism (Conn's syndrome), or adrenal carcinoma.

Now that these pathways have been established clearly it is possible to perturb purposely the system for diagnostic purposes. Thus, the system can be stimulated with adrenocorticotropic hormone (ACTH) to search for adrenal insufficiency; suppressed with dexamethasone, a synthetic glucocorticoid, to identify different types of Cushing's syndrome; or interrupted with a drug like metyrapone, which inhibits the enzyme 11β-hydroxylase, thus decreasing circulating cortisol and thereby stimulating the hypothalamic-pituitary axis to increase ACTH (Dolan and Carey, 1989).

Regulation of Hormone Release

The regulation of cortical steroid release involves a complex interaction of the hypothalamus, pituitary gland, and adrenal gland. ACTH is a 39 amino acid polypeptide that exerts a major influence on the adrenal cortex (Hoffman, 1974). ACTH is produced from a large protein (290 amino acids) termed proopiomelanocortin (POMC). Other POMC-derived peptides include β-lipotropin (β-LPH), α-melanocyte stimulating hormone (α-MSH), β-melanocyte stimulating hormone (β-MSH), β-endorphin, and methionine enkephalin (Fig. 64–10) (Mains and Eipper, 1980; Tepperman and Tepperman, 1987). ACTH secretion is characterized by an inherent diurnal rhythm leading to parallel changes in cortisol and ACTH (Fig. 64–11) (Krieger, 1975; Orth et al., 1967). The absence of the normal diurnal variation of plasma cortisol is a critical finding in a patient with Cushing's syndrome. ACTH secretion is stimulated by stress with studies leading to the concept of a releasing factor—corticotropin releasing factor (CRF) is a 41 amino acid, linear peptide (Speiss et al., 1981; Vale et al., 1981), which stimulates ACTH release as well as other POME products, probably working through a cAMP-dependent process requiring calcium (Vale, 1981). Other stimulators of ACTH include vasopressin, oxytocin, epinephrine, angiotensin II, vasoactive intestinal peptide (VIP), serotonin, gastrin-releasing peptide atrial natriuretic factor (ANF), and gamma-aminobutyric acid (GABA) (Antoni, 1986). Finally, ACTH secretion is reciprocally related to the circulating cortisol level.

Fortunately, the plasma level of ACTH can now be measured by radioimmunoassay and bioassay. Clinicians utilizing the radioimmunoassay must be aware that nu-

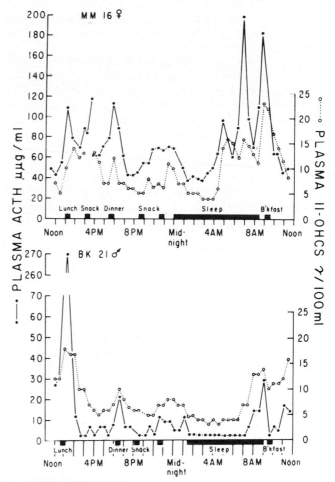

Figure 64–11. Circadian rhythm of plasma 11-OHCS and ACTH. Characterization of the normal temporal pattern of plasma corticosteroid levels. (Adapted from Kreiger et al.: J. Clin. Endocrinol. Metab., 32:269, 1971. © The Endocrine Society.)

merous antibodies to different portions of the ACTH molecule are available, thus the assay may not be measuring the biologically active portion of the peptide. Thus, the specific assay utilized must be clearly understood when interpreting an ACTH value.

Adrenal androgen production in the zonae reticularis and fasciculata is also under the influence of ACTH, but other mechanisms are involved. DHEA level rises following administration of ACTH; a later elevation of DHEAS level occurs, presumably because of the slow peripheral conversion (Vaitukaitis et al., 1969). However there clearly are situations whereby adrenal androgen stimulation is disassociated from ACTH. These include adrenarche, puberty, aging, fasting, and stress (Parker and Odell, 1980). Hence, there is evidence for a cortical androgen stimulating hormone (CASH), which may regulate adrenal androgen production (Parker et al., 1983).

In contrast to glucocorticoids and adrenal androgens, the primary physiologic control of aldosterone secretion is angiotensin II (Laragh et al., 1960; Laragh and Sealey, 1991). ACTH control is secondary. The physiology of the renin-angiotensin-aldosterone system is thoroughly reviewed in Chapters 3 and 55. A clear knowledge of

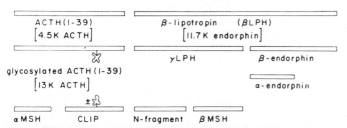

Figure 64–10. Structural relationships of peptides with a parental compound of proopiomelanocortin. (Adapted from Eipper, B. A., and Mains, R. E.: Endocr. Rev., 1:2, 1980. © The Endocrine Society.)

the system is mandatory in order to understand the pathophysiology and to evaluate the patients with primary hyperaldosteronism.

The critical sensor of the venin-angiotensin-aldosterone system (RAAS) resides in the juxtaglomerular apparatus within the kidney. Thus, in response to a variety of stimuli but primarily decreased renal perfusion (Fig. 64–12), there is renin release, angiotensin II formation, and subsequent aldosterone secretion resulting in sodium retention in an attempt to restore renal perfusion (Fig. 64–13). Conversely, if there is sodium retention then renin secretion is suppressed, aldosterone secretion falls, and urinary sodium rises. The inverse relationship found between plasma renin activity (PRA) or aldosterone and urinary sodium excretion in normal volunteers is shown in Figure 64–14.

A second less potent stimulus for aldosterone release is potassium, thus there is a second cybernetic system for the control of serum potassium involving the RAAS (Laragh and Sealey, 1991). Hypokalemia blunts the adrenal ability to synthesize aldosterone and can result in the lowering of the plasma aldosterone to a normal range in a patient with hypokalemia and hyperaldosteronism (Herf et al., 1979). A notion that a hypothalamic or pituitary aldosterone stimulating factor (ASF) similar

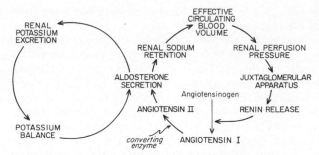

Figure 64–13. Control of aldosterone secretion by means of interrelationships between the potassium and renin-angiotensin feedback loops. (From Dluhy, R. G., and Gittes, R. F.: The Adrenals. *In* Walsh, P. C., Gittes, R. F., Perlmutter, A. D., and Stamey, T. A. (Eds.): Campbell's Urology, 5th ed. Philadelphia, W. B. Saunders Co., 1986.)

to CRF exists, although the factor has not yet been purified (Carey et al., 1984).

Hormonal Actions

All steroid hormones diffuse passively into cells and then bind to the amino terminal end of a high affinity protein receptor in the cystosol to form a steroid-receptor complex. The complex slowly converts to an active form and then migrates to the nucleus (Rousseau et al., 1972). In the nucleus, a second activation results in a stimulation of transcription, which is regulated by interaction with a specific group of steroid-regulated genes, resulting in new RNA and specific protein synthesis (Johnson and Baxter, 1987).

In addition, glucocorticoids have a non-nuclear pathway that is important in the control of ACTH. The numerous activities of this pathway include inhibition of prostaglandin synthesis, inhibition of calcium flux, inhibition of cAMP protein kinase, and others (Hubbard et al., 1990).

Glucocorticoids are essential for life, even following mineralocorticoid replacement. Glucocorticoids exert their effects on a wide spectrum of cellular metabolism,

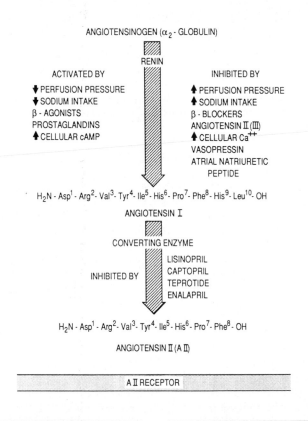

Figure 64–12. Factors activating and inhibiting the renin-angiotensin-aldosterone system.

Table 64–1. EFFECTS AND IMPLICATIONS OF GLUCOCORTICOIDS

Effects	Clinical Implications
Enhance skeletal and cardiac muscle contraction	Absence results in weakness
Cause protein catabolism	Excess results in wastage and weakness
Inhibit bone formation	Excess decreases bone mass
Inhibit collagen synthesis	Excess causes thin skin and fragile capillaries
Increase vascular contractility and decrease permeability	Absence makes it difficult to maintain blood pressure
Have anti-inflammatory activity	Exogenous steroid useful in treating inflammatory diseases
Have anti-immune system activity	Exogenous steroids useful in treating transplantation and various immune diseases
Maintain normal glomerular filtration	Absence reduces glomerular filtration

From Howards, S. S., and Carey, R. M.: The adrenals. *In* Gillenwater, J. Y., Grayhack, J. T., Howards, S. S., and Duckett, J. W. (Eds.): Adult and Pediatric Urology, 2nd ed. Chicago, Year Book Medical Publishers, 1991.

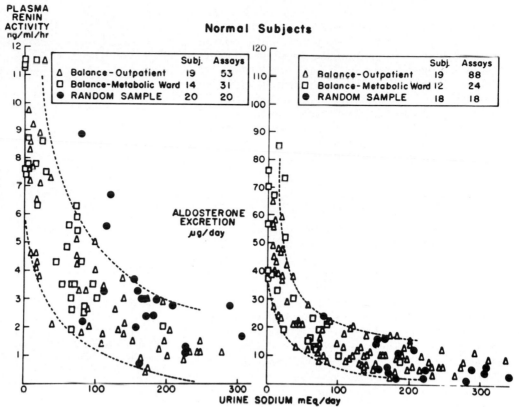

Figure 64–14. Relation of renin activity in plasma samples obtained at noon, and the corresponding 24-hour urinary excretion of aldosterone, to the concurrent daily rate of sodium excretion. For these normal subjects, the data describe a dynamic hyperbolic relationship between each hormone and sodium excretion.

The dynamic fluctuations in renin in response to changes in sodium intake help to maintain constant blood pressure in the presence of wide changes in sodium balance. The renin and aldosterone responses work together in the kidney to conserve or eliminate sodium in response to changes in dietary sodium intake.

Subjects who were studied while on random diets outside the hospital or on carefully controlled diets in the hospital exhibited similar relationships—a finding that validates the use of this nomogram in the study of outpatients or subjects who were not on controlled diets. (From Laragh, J. H., et al.: In Hypertension Manual. Stoneham, Butterworth, Yorke Medical Publishers, 1974, p. 313.)

including accumulation of glycogen in the liver and muscle, enhanced gluconeogenesis, impaired peripheral glucose utilization, muscle wasting and myopathy, osteopenia, and numerous interactions with other hormones (Table 64–1) (Howards and Carey, 1991).

Aldosterone accounts for 95 per cent of adrenal mineralocorticoid activity and serves to maintain sodium and potassium balance as previously stated. The active sites include the kidney, gut, salivary glands, and sweat glands. In all sites, there is the effect of stimulating sodium reabsorption and the increased secretion of potassium and hydrogen via activation of Na^+, K^+, ATPase activity, or activation of permease in the luminal membrane (Biglieri et al., 1990).

Adrenal androgens are only weakly active in contrast to testosterone and appear to be relevant only in pathologic states, such as congenital adrenal hyperplasia, in which there may be excess production.

Metabolism

The release of these steroids and their metabolism and route of excretion play a critical role in our understanding of the tests utilized to diagnose adrenal disorders.

In the circulation, 80 per cent of cortisol is bound to corticosterone-binding globulin (CBG, transcortin); 10 to 15 per cent is bound to albumin; and 7 to 10 per cent is free.

Thus, variations in binding proteins influence the total plasma cortisol value but not the free cortisol, which is metabolically active (Baxter and Tyrrell, 1981). Accu-

rate plasma cortisol assays are now available, utilizing the fluorometric assay (Nielson and Asfeldt, 1967) or the radioimmunoassay (Krieger, 1979). Thus, the diurnal variation of plasma cortisol (see Fig. 64–11) or its response to dexamethasone suppression has evolved as critical tests in the evaluation of patients for possible Cushing's syndrome (Siragy et al., 1989). Urinary-free cortisol can also be utilized as a screening test, although about 3.3 per cent of lean, obese, or chronically ill individuals will have elevated values and values are not well established in children (Crapo, 1979). Difficulties have also been found in establishing upper limits of 17-hydroxysteroid secretion. They are most valuable in evaluating normal adrenal function, particularly when looking for adrenal insufficiency or congenital adrenal hyperplasia in which 17-hydroxysteroid levels are low, except for 11-hydroxylase levels, which are high.

The precise control of adrenal androgens is not totally understood, although there is some ACTH control. Peripheral conversion of DHEA to DHEAS contributes to the DHEAS level (Nelson, 1980). DHEA does show some diurnal variation. DHEA is not produced in significant quantities by other tissues except occasionally in polycystic ovarian disease and gonadal androgen-producing tumors (GAPT) (Nelson, 1980; Osborn and Yannone, 1971). Patients with high DHEA levels also have high 17-ketosteroids, whereas those with virilization due to elevated testosterone do not. Elevated levels of DHEA, androstenedione, or 17-ketosteroids out of proportion to glucocorticoid production call to mind the diagnosis of adrenal carcinoma (Cohn et al., 1986). Of these tests of adrenal androgen function, the plasma

DHEAS value is more commonly used today and is more accurate than the androstenedione value.

Aldosterone, the major sodium-retaining hormone secreted by the zona glomerulosa, is poorly bound to albumin and plasma protein (Laragh and Sealey, 1991) and has a short half-life of 20 to 30 minutes. Plasma aldosterone can be measured by radioimmunoassay. The plasma value has to be related to the sodium status of the patient and should be measured in conjunction with the PRA. Equally accurate is the urinary aldosterone excretion analyzed in a similar fashion (see Fig. 64–14).

Adrenal Medulla

The adrenal medulla is composed of large chromaffin cells, which primarily secrete epinephrine but also secrete norepinephrine and dopamine. The fact that the cells stain brown when exposed to chromium salts as the result of oxidation of epinephrine and norepinephrine is the derivation of the term chromaffin cell (Fig. 64–15). The enzyme phenylethanolamine-*N*-methyltransferase (PNMT), which catalyzes the methylation of norepinephrine to form epinephrine is almost solely localized to the adrenal medulla (Axelrod, 1962). Thus, if there is excessive production of both norepinephrine and epinephrine the offending lesion is almost always within the adrenal and not other sites of chromaffin tissue. Data suggest that high levels of glucocorticoids are necessary to maintain high levels of PNMT and thus epinephrine secretion (Wurtman, 1965). These observations would explain the unique location of the adrenal medulla and the central venous drainage system within the adrenal bathing the medullary cells with high levels of glucocorticoids.

Catecholamine synthesis begins with dietary tyrosine and phenylalanine, which are the substrates (Fig. 64–16). Catecholamine synthesis occurs in the adrenal, the central nervous system, and the adrenergic nerve terminals. Activation and suppression of tyrosine hydroxylase activity are the major regulators of catecholamine biosynthesis (Levitt et al., 1965) and may be influenced by the adrenal cortex (Mueller et al., 1970). Norepi-

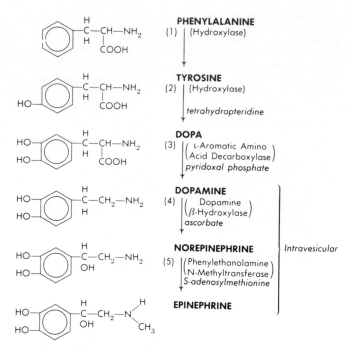

Figure 64–16. Enzymatic pathway for dopamine, norepinephrine, and epinephrine synthesis. Enzymes are in parentheses; cofactors are in italics. (Adapted from Goodman, A. G., Goodman, L. S., and Gillman, A. (Eds.): The Pharmacologic Basis of Therapeutics. 6th ed. New York, Macmillan, 1980, p. 72.)

nephrine is the major catecholamine secreted by sympathetic neurons. Studies of healthy humans indicate that plasma dopamine accounts for 13 per cent of the free catecholes; epinephrine, 14 per cent; and norepinephrine, 73 per cent (Manger and Gifford, 1990).

Catecholamines are stored in separate vesicles along with ATP, chromogranins, and the enzyme dopamine β-hydroxylase. Stimulation of the preganglionic sympathetic nerves during stress, pain, cold, heat, asphyxia, hypotension, hypoglycemia, and sodium depletion increases catecholamine release (Lewis, 1975). Following stimuli, the contents of the vesicles are released by exocytosis (Winkler and Smith, 1975). In addition, catechols may be released without sympathetic stimulation and possibly without exocytosis—a phenomenon postulated in patients with pheochromocytomas.

Catecholamine Metabolism

Catecholamines are rapidly removed from the circulation with a plasma half-life less than 20 seconds (Ferrerira and Vane, 1967). The metabolic pathways for catecholamines are shown in Figure 64–17. Neuronal re-uptake is of major importance in the removal of norepinephrine from the synaptic gap for re-release and has been termed uptake (Iverson, 1975). Catecholamines are degraded by the action of both catechol-*O*-methyltransferase (COMT) and by monoamine oxidase (MAO) (see Fig. 64–17), with either enzyme beginning the degradative process. The primary metabolite in the urine is vanillylmandelic acid (VMA) with metanephrine, normetanephrine, and their derivatives contributing to total metabolic products, which are often meas-

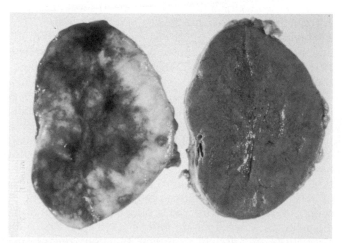

Figure 64–15. Pheochromocytoma showing chromaffin reaction *(right)*.

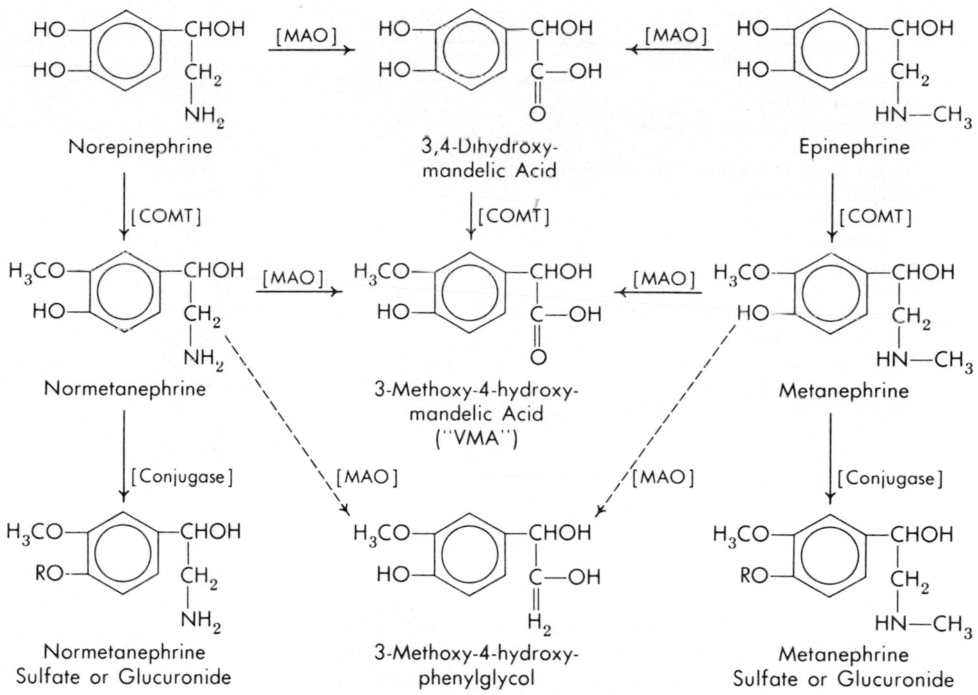

Figure 64–17. Metabolic fate of the catecholamines. Enzymes are in brackets; COMT is catechol-O-methyltransferase, and MAO is monoamine oxidase. VMA is also known as vanillylmandelic acid. (Adapted from Goodman, A. G., Goodman, L. S., and Gillman, A. (Eds.): The Pharmacologic Basis of Therapeutics, 6th ed. New York, Macmillan, 1980, p. 77.)

ured while evaluating patients with pheochromocytomas (Reckler et al., 1989).

Catecholamine Actions

Catecholamines exert varied effects by stimulating specific cellular receptors (adrenoreceptors), which are protein-binding sites (Table 64–2). The diversity of effects of circulating catecholamines on various organs acting at specific receptors accounts for the diversity of symptoms exhibited by patients with pheochromocytomas. Moreover, different tumors can produce different proportions of norepinephrine, epinephrine, or dopamine.

The actions of epinephrine and norepinephrine are not totally independent and are dose dependent. Hence, the classification of naturally occurring adrenergic hormones as alpha or beta or as a blocking agent, such as an "alpha-l-antagonist," is useful but does not fully characterize the activity of the hormone or antagonist in all clinical settings.

CUSHING'S SYNDROME

Cushing's syndrome is the term utilized to describe the symptom complex caused by excess circulating glucocorticoids (Cushing, 1912; 1932). The term is all encompassing and includes patients with pituitary hypersecretion of ACTH, Cushing's disease, which accounts for 75 to 85 per cent of patients with endogenous Cushing's; patients with adrenal adenomas or carcinomas; and patients with ectopic secretion of ACTH (Table 64–3) or CRF, about 20 per cent of ACTH-dependent disease (Table 64–3) (Carpenter, 1986; Hardy, 1982; Howlet et al., 1985; Meador et al., 1962; Scott, 1990).

The entity is rare, occurs most often in young adults, and is more common in females. An exogenous source of Cushing's syndrome should always first be excluded, because therapeutic steroids are the most common cause. Often, the patient does not even realize she is utilizing a steroid-containing preparation, especially

Table 64–2. CATECHOLAMINE RECEPTORS

Adrenoreceptors
Alpha Adrenergic

Alpha$_1$	Postsynaptic agonists Vascular smooth muscle—vasoconstriction Prostate—contraction Liver glycogenesis
Alpha$_2$	Presynaptic—inhibit norepinephrine release Postsynaptic—agonist Large veins—venoconstrictor Brain—decrease sympathetic outflow Pancreas—inhibit insulin secretion Gut—relaxation Adipocyte—inhibit lipolysis

Beta Adrenergic

Beta$_1$	Heart—inotrophic and chromotrophic effect Adipocyte—lipolysis Kidney—stimulate renin release
Beta$_2$	Lung—bronchodilatation Vascular smooth muscle—vasodilatation Liver—gluconeogenesis Uterus—relaxation Gut—relaxation

Dopaminergic

DA$_1$	Vascular—vasodilatation
DA$_2$	Presynaptic—inhibit norepinephrine release

Table 64–3. SOURCES OF ECTOPIC ACTH IN 100 CASES

Tumor	Number
Carcinoma of lung	52
Carcinoma of pancreas (including carcinoid)	11
Thymoma	11
Benign bronchial adenoma (including carcinoid)	5
Pheochromocytoma	3
Carcinoma of thyroid	2
Carcinoma of liver	2
Carcinoma of prostate	2
Carcinoma of ovary	2
Undifferentiated carcinoma of mediastinum	2
Carcinoma of breast	1
Carcinoma of parotid gland	1
Carcinoma of esophagus	1
Paraganglioma	1
Ganglioma	1
Primary site uncertain	3

From Scott, H. W., Jr.: *In* H. W. Scott, (Ed.). Surgery of the Adrenal Glands. Philadelphia, J. B. Lippincott Co., 1990.

Table 64–4. CLINICAL MANIFESTATIONS OF CUSHING'S SYNDROME

	All[1] %	Disease[2] %	Adenoma/Carcinoma[3] %
Obesity	90	91	93
Hypertension	80	63	93
Diabetes	80	32	79
Centripetal obesity	80	—	—
Weakness	80	25	82
Muscle atrophy	70	34	—
Hirsutism	70	59	79
Menstrual abnormal/sexual dysfunction	70	46	75
Purple striae	70	46	36
Moon facies	60	—	—
Osteoporosis	50	29	54
Early bruising	50	54	57
Acne/pigmentation	50	32	—
Mental changes	50	47	57
Edema	50	15	—
Headache	40	21	46
Poor healing	40	—	—

[1]Hunt and Tyrell, 1978.
[2]Wilson, 1984.
[3]Scott, 1973. From Scott, H. W., Jr.: *In* Scott, H. W. (Ed.): Surgery of the Adrenal Glands. Philadelphia, J. B. Lippincott Co., 1990.

creams or lotions (Champion, 1974; Flavin and Fredricksen, 1983). The manifestations of the disease are legion and are the result of the manifold actions of glucocorticoids (see Table 64–1). There are few diseases in which the clinical appearance of the patient can be as useful in suspecting the diagnosis (Figs. 64–18 and 64–19). Old photographs are helpful in documenting the recent changes in appearance that have occurred. The more common clinical manifestations of Cushing's syndrome found in several series of patients are shown in Table 64–4. The clinical findings do not distinguish patients with Cushing's disease from those with adrenal adenomas or carcinomas. Most patients with ectopic ACTH do not present with the typical features (Bagshaw, 1960) but exhibit cachexia due to underlying tumor as well as hypertension, hypokalemic alkalosis,

and skin pigmentation (Bagshaw, 1960; Schambelan et al., 1971). Virilization in the female or feminization in the male should raise the question of adrenal carcinoma, although more patients will present with traditional manifestations of glucocorticoid excess (Luton et al., 1990).

The goals of managing patients with Cushing's syndrome have been articulated by investigators who have a longstanding interest in this disease: (1) lowering daily cortisol secretion to normal, (2) eradication of any tumor threatening health, (3) producing no permanent endo-

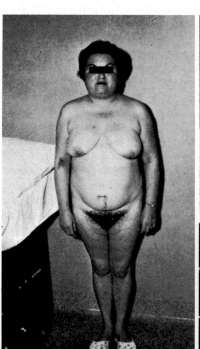
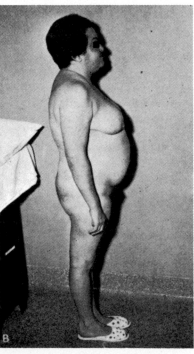

Figure 64–18. *A,* A 34-year-old female with Cushing's syndrome. The patient shows truncal obesity and mild hirsutism. *B,* Note that cutaneous striae and ecchymoses are absent, in contrast to most cases shown in textbooks. (From Dluhy, R. G., and Gittes, R. F.: The Adrenals. *In* Walsh, P. C., Gittes, R. F., Perlmutter, A. D., and Stamey, T. A. (Eds.): Campbell's Urology, 5th ed. Philadelphia, W. B. Saunders Co., 1986.)

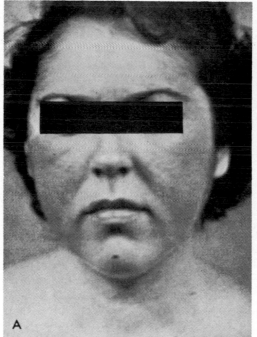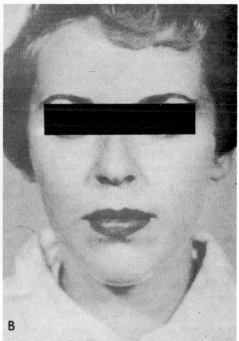

Figure 64–19. *A*, Woman, aged 23 years, 6 months after the development of moon face and other early signs of Cushing's syndrome due to an adrenocortical adenoma on the left side. *B*, Same patient 6 months after surgical removal of adenoma of the adrenal cortex. (From Harrison, J. H.: Surgery of the adrenals. In Davis, L. (Ed.): Christopher's Textbook of Surgery. Philadelphia, W. B. Saunders Co.)

crine deficiency and (4) avoiding permanent dependence on medications (Orth and Liddle, 1971). Obviously, all of these goals cannot be met in all patients; however, they serve as a thoughtful frame of reference. To initiate evaluation, the etiology of Cushing's syndrome in a given patient must be established.

Laboratory Diagnosis

A panoply of tests of glucocorticoid function have evolved that are utilized to establish the presence of Cushing's syndrome and to distinguish between pituitary and adrenal causes as well as ectopic ACTH secretion (Dolan and Carey, 1989). Moreover, medical institu-

tions have developed their own set of tests, which time has proved most helpful, particularly in the sometimes difficult task of distinguishing bilateral adrenal hyperplasia from adenoma. The diagnostic scheme that we have found useful is shown in Figure 64–20.

In the patient suspected of having Cushing's syndrome on clinical grounds, we advocate first determining the presence or absence of the normal circadian rhythm in plasma cortisol by obtaining ambulatory A.M. and P.M. plasma cortisol levels. Following ACTH release (see Fig. 64–10), healthy subjects show the characteristic rise in plasma cortisol in the morning with a fall to less than 5 ng/dl in the evening (Fig. 64–21). Patients with Cushing's syndrome lose the diurnal variation (Besser and Edwards, 1972) or show some variations but at higher

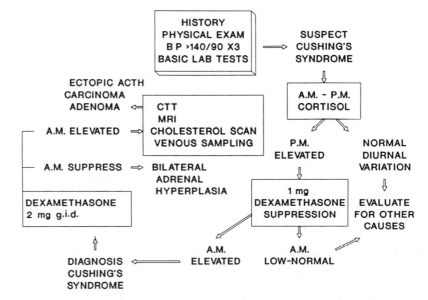

Figure 64–20. Identifying Cushing's syndrome. (From Vaughan, E. D., Jr.: Diagnosis of adrenal disorders in hypertension. World J Urol., 7:111–116, 1989.)

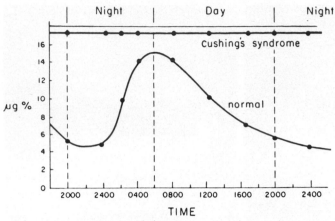

Figure 64–21. Circadian rhythm in cortisol secretion of plasma in normal subject contrasted with absence of rhythm in patient with Cushing's syndrome. (From Bergland, R. M. and Harrison, T. S.: Pituitary and adrenal. In Schwartz, S. I. (Ed.): Principles of Surgery, 3rd ed. New York, McGraw-Hill, 1979, p. 1493.)

basal levels (Glass et al., 1984). An alternative first line screening test is the measurement of 24-hour urinary-free cortisol with the normal value being somewhat dependent on the specific laboratory but generally being below 80 µg/24 hour (Eddy et al., 1973).

The next and most valuable test is the dexamethasone suppression test as developed by Liddle (1960). Pituitary ACTH secretion is regulated with a negative feedback inhibition by cortisol. Liddle utilized the synthetic steroid dexamethasone, 30 times as potent as cortisol to study the pituitary feedback mechanism in patients with suspected Cushing's syndrome. In normal subjects 0.5 mg orally every 6 hours for 2 days causes a dramatic fall in 17-hydroxycorticosteroid, urinary-free cortisol, or plasma cortisol (< 5 ng/dl). A simplification of the test is to administer a single 1 mg oral dose between 2300 and 2400 hours and to measure the plasma cortisol level between 0800 and 0900 hours (Fig. 64–22) (Paulotos et al., 1965; Sarvin et al., 1968). However, the test is less reliable than the formal "low-dose" 2-day test as described previously, especially in obese patients. Patients with Cushing's syndrome show resistance to suppression to low-dose dexamethasone. This failure of suppression has been found to be characteristic of all patients with Cushing's syndrome studied by Scott and Orth (1990).

Patients are now diagnosed as having Cushing's syndrome, and it is necessary to determine the etiology. Thus, they are given "high-dose dexamethasone" (2 mg every 6 hours for 2 days) and plasma cortisol or urinary-free cortisol levels are measured. In patients with pituitary disease (Cushing's disease), there should be a 50 per cent or greater suppression of cortisol. Patients with adrenal adenomas or carcinomas and most patients with ectopic ACTH fail to suppress (Carpenter, 1986). Errors in interpretation can occur (Siragy et al., 1989), and if the clinical suspicion is high further testing should be carried out.

Other variations in dexamethasone suppression include a high-dose (8 mg) overnight suppresion test (Tyrell et al., 1986) or continuous infusion (Biemond et al., 1990). However, the standard tests usually suffice.

The measurement of ACTH would intuitively appear to be a simpler method of differentiating pituitary (high ACTH) from adrenal (low ACTH) disease, and indeed this is the case. However, ACTH determinations are not widely available and there is different antibody specificity as discussed. ACTH measurements are useful in detecting ectopic ACTH secretion in a patient who does not fully suppress cortisol production with high-dose dexamethasone. In Cushing's disease, ACTH is suppressed with the high dose, whereas ectopic ACTH shows a persistent high level.

At this point, despite the availablity of numerous other stimulatory or inhibitory tests (Dolan and Carey, 1989), the dramatic advances in radiologic localizing tests usually make further biochemical studies unnecessary (Dunnick, 1990; Kazam et al., 1989; Korobkin, 1989; Newhouse, 1990; Mezrich et al., 1986; Reinig et al., 1986).

Radiographic Localization

The development of computer-aided sectional imaging and magnetic resonance imaging has revolutionized adrenal imaging. Accordingly, older tests such as intravenous urography with tomography, ultrasound, and adrenal arteriography and venography are only rarely utilized today. In general, computed tomography (CT) has become the initial imaging procedure.

In patients with Cushing's disease additional information can be obtained with CT or magnetic resonance imaging (MRI) of the sella turcica in search of a pituitary adenoma (Fig. 64–23) (Mitty and Yeh, 1982). CT may also be utilized to detect primary tumors in patients with ectopic ACTH production.

Patients with hyperplasia can show diffuse thickening

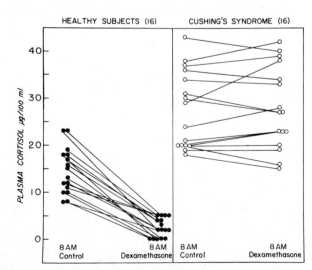

Figure 64–22. The rapid dexamethasone suppression test distinguishes patients with Cushing's syndrome from healthy subjects or other obese subjects. Note the overlap in cortisol levels between the two groups before suppression. The patients with very high basal cortisol levels were those with ectopic ACTH production by a nonendocrine tumor as the underlying cause. (From Melby, J.: N. Engl. J. Med., 285:735, 1971. Reprinted with material from the New England Journal of Medicine.)

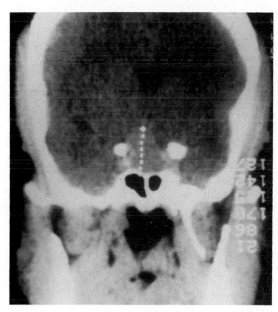

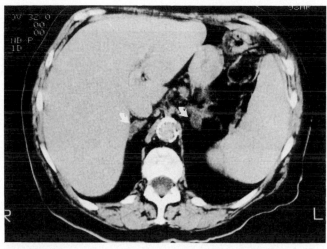

Figure 64–25. Computed tomography scan showing a patient with macronodular adrenal hyperplasia.

Figure 64–23. Computed tomography scan of a chromophobe adenoma in the sella turcica of a patient with Cushing's syndrome presenting with hyperpigmentation, headaches, and a visual field defect. (From Dluhy, R. G., and Gittes, R. F.: The Adrenals. *In* Walsh, P. C., Gittes, R. F., Perlmutter, A. D., and Stamey, T. A. (Eds.): Campbell's Urology, 5th ed. Philadelphia, W. B. Saunders Co., 1986.)

and elongation of the adrenal rami (Fig. 64–24) or, unfortunately, prominent glands bilaterally which fall within normal range (Kazam et al., 1989). A second variant, found in 10 to 20 per cent of cases, is nodular cortical hyperplasia characterized by multinodularity of both adrenals (Fig. 64–25). The CT appearance does not distinguish between patients with glucocorticoid excess or idiopathic hyperaldosteronism (pseudo-primary hyperaldosteronism), owing to bilateral adrenal hyperplasia. The small size (< 2 cm) and multiplicity of the nodules as well as the bilateral distribution are the

distinguishing features from Cushing's adenomas. Rarely, patients with macronodular hyperplasia develop autonomous glucocorticoid secretion and may require adrenalectomy.

Adrenal adenomas are usually larger than 2 cm, solitary, and associated with atrophy of the opposite gland. The density is low because of the high concentration of lipid. Sonography and study after contrast showing enhancement avoid misdiagnosis of an adrenal cyst (Fig. 64–26) (Huebener and Treugut, 1984).

Adrenal carcinomas are often indistinguishable from adenomas except for the larger size > 6 cm (Fig. 64–27) (Belldegrun, 1989). Necrosis and calcification are also more common in association with adrenal carcinoma but are not diagnostic. Clearly, large irregular adrenal lesions with invasion represent carcinoma; however, metastatic carcinoma to the adrenal has the same appearance.

MRI is not usually necessary in patients with Cushing's syndrome unless adrenal carcinoma is suspected. In that clinical setting, the signal intensity may be much

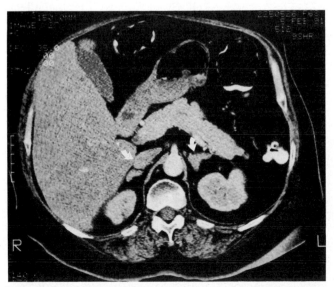

Figure 64–24. Computed tomography scan showing bilateral adrenal hyperplasia in a patient with Cushing's disease.

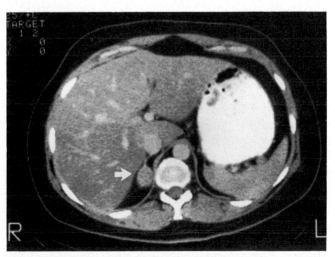

Figure 64–26. Computed tomography scan of a patient with right adrenal adenoma.

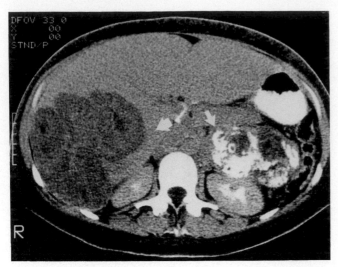

Figure 64–27. Computed tomography scan of a patient with a calcified left adrenal carcinoma and hepatic metastasis.

higher than that in liver (Reinig et al., 1986). MRI also may provide useful information concerning adjacent organ or vascular invasion.

Adrenal cortical scanning with iodinated cholesterol agents is no longer routinely utilized but can be helpful in differentiating functional adrenal tissue from other retroperitoneal lesions (Kazerooni et al., 1990; Sarkar et al., 1977) and in identifying residual cortical tissues.

Treatment

Cushing's Disease and Ectopic ACTH

When recalling the goals of management of Cushing's syndrome as outlined by Liddle, it is obvious that precise diagnosis is critical. Accordingly, in the patient with ectopic ACTH syndrome, treatment is directed to the primary tumor. Reduction of secretion of functional steroids by utilization of blocking agents can further ameliorate symptoms. Agents utilized include aminoglutethimide, which blocks the conversion of cholesterol to pregnenolone; and metyrapone, which blocks the conversion of 11-desoxycortisol to cortisone and ketoconazole, the antifungal agent that blocks cytochrome P450-mediated side chain cleavage and hydroxylation at both the early and late steps in steroid biosynthesis (Farwell et al., 1988; Loose et al., 1988). Patients given aminoglutethimide must be observed for adrenocortical insufficiency because aldosterone production is also impaired. Metyrapone does not usually result in salt wasting at the usual dose of (250 to 500 mg, three times daily) because of increased production of deoxycorticosterone—a potent mineralocorticoid (see Figs. 64–8, and 64–9) (Scott and Orth, 1990).

The synthesis of cortisol in 1950 (Wendler et al., 1950) led to the availability of replacement steroids not only for patients with Addison's disease but also following bilateral adrenalectomy for Cushing's disease. Thus, bilateral adrenalectomy through a bilateral posterior approach became utilized in patients with severe Cush-

ing's disease. Generally, patients did well with resolution of the disease (Scott et al., 1977, 1990). However, 10 to 20 per cent of patients subsequently developed pituitary tumors, usually chromophobe adenomas perhaps caused by the lack of hypothalamic/pituitary feedback and high ACTH and related compounds (Cohen et al., 1978; Nelson et al., 1958). This entity termed Nelson's syndrome may arise many years following bilateral adrenalectomy. Thus, patients must be followed with the determination of ACTH levels and the evaluation of the sella turcica (Fig. 64–28).

The development of pituitary irradiation subsequently limited the utilization of bilateral adrenalectomy for Cushing's disease beginning in the 1950s (Orth and Liddle, 1971). However, long-term follow-up revealed about a third of patients were cured, a third improved, and a third failed to respond. The results appear to be better in children (Jennings et al., 1977). Irradiation is useful to treat Nelson's syndrome. Heavy particle proton beam therapy may be more effective but also is more likely to induce panhypopituitarism (Burch, 1985).

In 1971, Hardy reported his experience with transphenoidal hypophysial microsurgery for removal of pituitary adenomas with preservation of pituitary function. Subsequently, this technique evolved as the single most effective and safest treatment of Cushing's disease. The cure rates are 85 to 95 per cent, the results immediate, the complications low, and the recurrences rare (Bigos et al., 1980; Styne et al., 1984; Wilson, 1984). Patients often have transient decreases in cortisol levels and may need replacement therapy and monitoring for some months (Fitzgerald et al., 1982). Transient diabetes mellitus may also occur.

Cushing's Syndrome During Pregnancy

Cushing's syndrome during pregnancy has been reported in only about 50 cases (Mulder et al., 1990) because of the menstrual irregularities characteristic of the disease. Of cases reported, 59 per cent have been ACTH independent and 33 per cent ACTH dependent. The others were not classified. During normal pregnancy plasma cortisol binding protein and plasma protein bound and unbound cortisone levels rise; however, the normal diurnal variation persists (Siragy et al., 1989). Urinary-free cortisol level also rises slightly. Moreover, there is some resistance to dexamethasone suppression that progresses with each trimester; however, there remains some suppression so that the total absence of suppression to low-dose dexamethasone is compatible with Cushing's syndrome.

Obviously, imaging studies are contraindicated during pregnancy especially in the 1st trimester. We have utilized MRI to identify an adenoma in a pregnant patient with Cushing's syndrome (Fig. 64–29).

Both fetal and maternal morbidity is reduced with treatment. Surgical removal of an adenoma can be successfully achieved during pregnancy, as was done in our patient, especially during the 2nd trimester. Alternatively, some patients have been treated with metyrapone or transpheroidal adenomectomy when indicated (Casson et al., 1987).

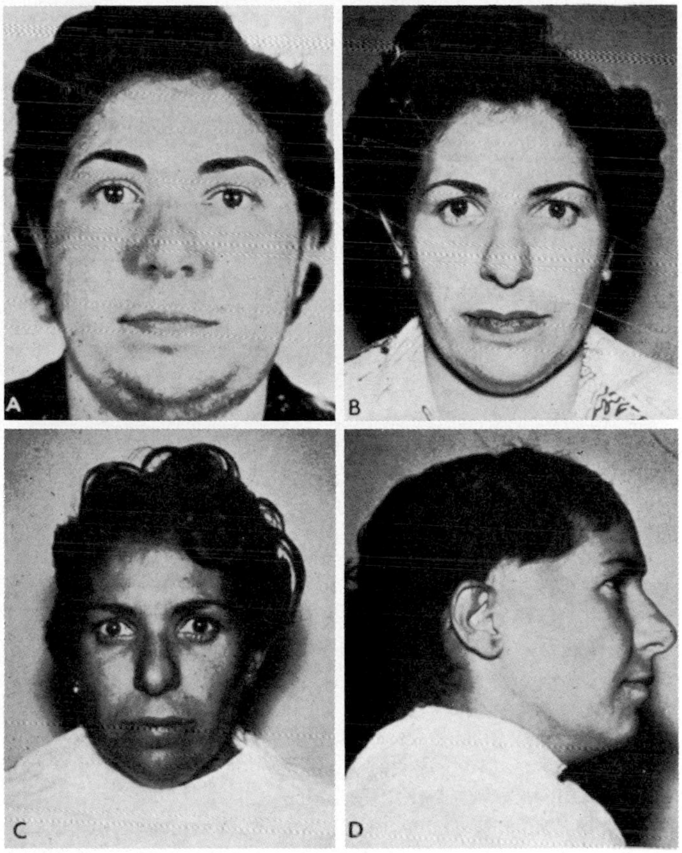

Figure 64–28. *A,* Full-face view of a patient with hyperadrenocorticism in 1954, treated by total adrenalectomy at that time. *B,* The same patient 6 months after total adrenalectomy showing striking improvement. All symptoms and signs of Cushing's syndrome had disappeared. *C,* Deep pigmentation, headache, and failing vision supervened in 1957; emergency craniotomy was necessary after radiation therapy. *D,* Disappearance of pigmentation is shown in the facial view after removal of chromophobe adenoma of pituitary by Dr. Donald Matson. (From Rothenberg, R. E. (Ed.): Reoperative Surgery, New York, McGraw-Hill, 1969.)

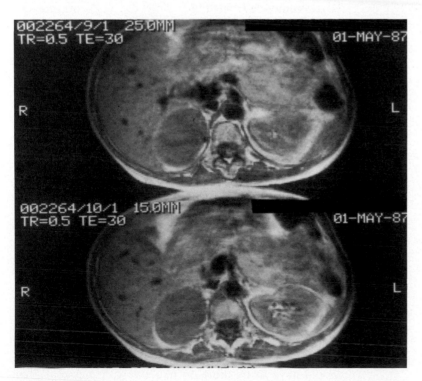

Figure 64–29. *A* and *B,* Magnetic resonance T1 and T2 weighted images of patient who developed Cushing's syndrome during pregnancy showing the large right adrenal adenoma. (From Vaughan, E. D., Jr., and Carey, R. M. (Eds.): Adrenal Disorders. New York, Thieme Medical Publishers Inc., 1989.)

Fortunately, because of the low transplacental transfer of adrenal corticosteroids the fetus is not affected in most cases and does not require steroid replacement following birth.

Adrenal Adenoma

Adrenal adenomas causing Cushing's syndrome are treated by surgical removal, which is discussed in the section concerning adrenal surgery.

ADRENAL CARCINOMA

Adrenal carcinoma is a rare disease and has a poor prognosis (Luton et al., 1990; Vaughan and Carey, 1989). The incidence is estimated as one case per 1.7 million, accounting for 0.02 per cent of cancers and 0.2 per cent of all cancer deaths (Brennan, 1987; Nader et al., 1983; Plager, 1984).

A practical subclassification for adrenal carcinomas is according to their ability to produce adrenal hormones. The varieties of functioning tumors are shown in Table 64–5. Most tumors secrete multiple compounds. In a series of Luton and co-workers (1990), 79 per cent of adrenal tumors were functional—a higher percentage than previously reported probably due to more sensitive assays. In addition, nonfunctional tumors may become functional or a tumor may subsequently produce multiple hormones (Arteaga et al., 1984; Grunberg et al., 1982). Moreover, tumors may produce metabolites that are nonfunctional or in such low amounts so as not to cause physiologic changes. Thus, while convenient, a classification of tumors by product is somewhat contrived, and debate exists as to whether or not "nonfunctioning" tumors carry a worse prognosis for the patient than functioning tumors (Heinbecker et al., 1957; Lewinsky et al., 1974).

Incidentally Discovered Adrenal Masses

The increased utilization of abdominal ultrasound and CT scanning is leading to the frequent finding of a unexpected adrenal mass or an "incidentaloma" (Belldegrun et al., 1986; Belldegrun and deKernion 1989).

Table 64–5. CLASSIFICATION OF ADRENAL CARCINOMA

Functional

    Cushing's syndrome
    Virilization in females
        Increased DHEA 17-ketosteroids
        Increased testosterone
    Feminizing syndrome in males
    Hyperaldosteronism
    Mixed combination of above

Nonfunctional

DHEA, dehydroepiandrosterone.

Adrenal malignancies are usually larger than 6 cm in size. Belldegrun and co-workers, reviewing six series, found that 105 of 114 adrenocortical carcinomas were more than 6 cm in size (Bertagna and Orth, 1981; Heinbecker et al., 1957; Knight et al., 1960; Lewinsky et al., 1974; Sullivan et al., 1978). Accordingly, solid adrenal lesions of more than 6 cm should be considered malignant until proved otherwise by exploration and adrenalectomy.

The problem arises in the management of incidentally found adrenal lesions smaller than 6 cm. Unsuspected adrenal masses have been detected on 0.6 to 1.3 per cent of upper abdominal computed axial tomographic (CAT) studies (Abecassis et al., 1985; Copeland, 1983; Ross and Aron, 1990). Moreover, the prevalence of benign, clinically silent, adrenal adenomas found on autopsy series ranges from 1.4 to 8.7 per cent (Hedeland et al., 1968; Russi et al., 1945). In contrast, occult nonfunctioning adrenocortical carcinoma is rarely found on autopsy. Accordingly, attention has turned to the appropriate management of the incidentaloma (Belldegrun 1989; Copeland, 1983; Prinz, 1982; Ross and Aron, 1990).

One approach is shown in Table 64–6. Several points do not engender controversy. First, there is agreement that all patients with solid adrenal masses should undergo biochemical assessment. If biochemical abnormalities are identified, the lesions should be treated appropriately as described elsewhere in this chapter— usually by removal of the offending lesion. However, the extent of the biochemical evaluation has been reviewed (Ross and Aron, 1990). A selective approach has been outlined, which markedly limits cost without sacrificing diagnostic accuracy. A very limited evaluation is recommended, including only the tests to rule out pheochromocytoma, potassium levels in hypertensive cases, and glucocorticoid evaluation only in the presence of clinical stigmata of Cushing's syndrome or virilization. Because of the likelihood of nonfunctioning solid lesions larger than 6 cm being malignant, these lesions should be removed. CT scanning may underestimate the size of an adrenal lesion, and we suggest that exploration be performed when the lesion is more than 5 cm on CT or MRI (Cerfolio and Vaughan, 1991). In addition, the smaller tumors were often nonspherical. Perhaps a volume index should be established to describe tumor size. Furthermore, lesions clearly proved to be cystic by CAT, MRI, or cyst puncture, which is often not necessary, can also be followed (Fig. 64–30).

The controversy arises in the management strategy for the solid adrenal lesion smaller than 5 cm in size. Glazer and co-workers have suggested that adrenalectomy be considered for solid lesions more than 3 to 4 cm in size (Glazer et al., 1982). Prinz and associates (1982) have also suggested a surgical approach, especially in younger patients. Copeland challenges the "3- to 4-cm" criterion and suggests observation for all patients with nonfunctioning lesions less than 6 cm in size. These workers estimate that over 4000 adrenalectomies would have to be done on patients with masses 1.5 cm in diameter or larger to remove one carcinoma. However, it is undeniable that most of the major reviews of

Table 64–6. INCIDENTALLY FOUND ADRENAL MASS

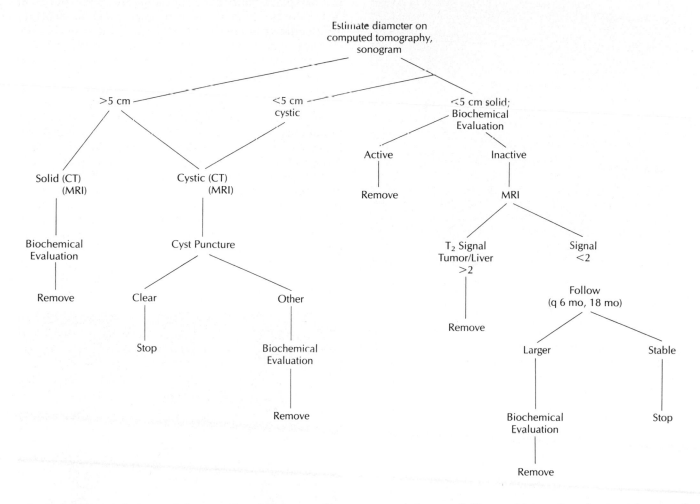

adrenal malignancies reveal the occasional lesion smaller than 6 cm.

The 3- to 6-cm solid, nonfunctioning adrenal mass incidentally found remains the major area of controversy. Certainly on statistical ground, the majority will be benign. However, the occasional one will be malignant and potentially curable, a situation not frequently encountered in patients with adrenal carcinomas. An additional test that may prove of utility is MRI, whereby a high (greater than two tumor/liver intensity) on T2 images suggest that the lesion is not a benign adenoma (Fig. 64–31) (Reinig et al., 1986).

Myelolipoma

In the past, these nonfunctioning benign lesions were incidentally found at autopsy. They are generally small (<5 cm), unilateral, asymptomatic, and benign, containing hematopoietic and fatty elements (DelGaudio and Solidoro, 1986, 1991).

The lesion has been recognized with increasing frequeny, because it has a characteristic appearance on CAT scanning that establishes the diagnosis and excludes the need for surgical exploration. The exception may be the case of the vary large lesion (Fig. 64–32), in which confusion with a necrotic adrenal carcinoma could exist (Wilhelmus et al., 1981).

The etiology of the lesion is unknown but may be a part of a group of entities characterized by deposition of myeloid and adipose tissue (Papavasiliou et al., 1990). Patients have been predominantly obese with a 1.75:1.0

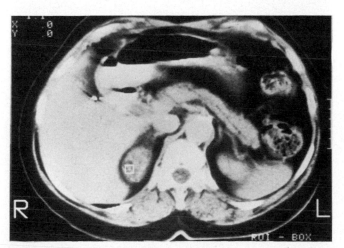

Figure 64–30. Computed tomography scan of patient with a 5-cm nonfunctioning adrenal mass found incidentally.

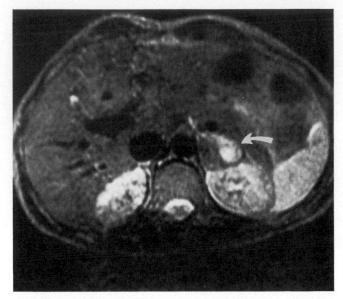

Figure 64–31. Ganglioneuroma. Nonfunctioning left adrenal tumor, bright on T2, found incidentally.

male:female ratio. Pain is the most common presenting symptom. The lesions are rarely calcified or hormonally active. However, hormonal levels should be obtained, because coexisting cortical adenoma and myelolipoma have been reported (Vyberg and Sestof, 1986).

Adrenal Metastasis

Actually, primary adrenocortical carcinoma is less common than metastatic tumors to the adrenal. In a series of 500 autopsy cases, Willis (1952) found adrenal metastasis in 9 per cent. Specifically, the adrenal has been found to be a site of metastasis in over 50 per cent of patients with melanomas and carcinomas of the breast and lung; 40 per cent with renal cell carcinomas; and in order of frequency carcinomas of the contralateral adrenal, bladder, colon, esophagus, gallbladder, liver, pancreas, prostate, stomach, and uterus (Bullock and Hirst, 1953).

Now that adrenal imaging with CAT and MRI is commonplace, more adrenal lesions are identified earlier in the course of patients with cancer (Thomas et al., 1982). Management is obviously predicated on the underlying malignancy. The major clinical point is not to confuse a metastatic adrenal lesion for a primary adrenal process. Generally, the adrenal lesion is part of the clinical picture of diffuse metastatic disease. However, long-term survival following adrenalectomy and aggressive treatment of the primary process has been reported in patients with pulmonary carcinoma and adrenal metastasis (Reyes et al., 1990; Twomley et al., 1982). Moreover, the finding of an unsuspected adrenal mass should heighten the clinical suspicion of a neoplasm elsewhere. The MRI pattern not characteristic of a benign adenoma raises the index of suspicion for metastatic disease (Fig. 64–33) (Reinig et al., 1986). Adrenal insufficiency has been reported secondary to both benign adenomas and bilateral adrenal metastases (Sheeler et al., 1983).

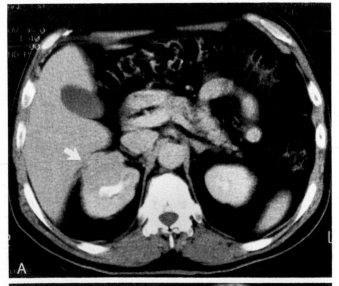

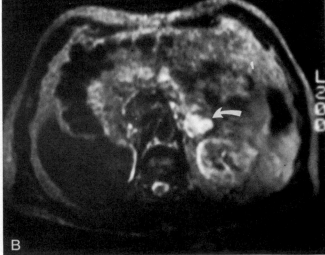

Figure 64–33. *A,* Computed tomography scan showing a left renal cell carcinoma. *B,* Subsequent right adrenal metastasis with high intensity. Pathology proved by excision.

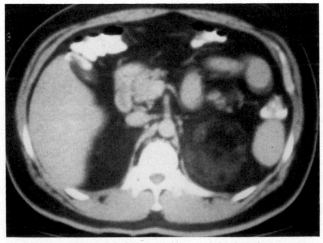

Figure 64–32. Myelolipoma, left adrenal.

Benign Adenoma

The difficulty in discriminating by pathologic examination adenoma from carcinoma is a major problem for pathologists (Amberson and Gray, 1989). All large adrenal lesions do not behave biologically as carcinomas. Some lesions that appear benign on histologic evaluation will eventually metastasize. Hence, as discussed previously, surgical removal is recommended for all lesions larger than 5 cm in size.

Weiss (1984) has compared the histology of 43 clinically benign and malignant adrenal tumors. Utilizing a multifactorial analysis of nine criteria, he was able to differentiate metastasizing from nonmetastasizing tumors.

Klein and co-workers (1985) have reported that flow cytometry accurately demonstrated aneuploid stem lines in four cases classified histologically as carcinoma. We have also found that all but one patient exhibiting subsequent metastatic disease have had aneuploid primary tumors. However, other patients who have as of yet not demonstrated metastatic disease have also shown aneuploid patterns (Amberson et al., 1987). In contrast, only one patient with a diploid pattern has developed metastatic disease (Fig. 64–34). Accordingly, flow cytometry may prove to be a valuable tool in the prediction of potential biologic activity of large adrenal cortical lesions.

Functional Tumors

Cushing's Syndrome

Cushing's syndrome has been discussed in detail—adrenal carcinoma being one of the causes of corticosteroid excess. This form of functional tumor is the commonest in its pure form or with associated virilization. In a study comparing the clinical and laboratory studies of patients with Cushing's syndrome due to adenoma and carcinoma, Bertagna and Orth (1981) found that virilization without evidence of cortisol excess was indicative of carcinoma except in children. Other clinical parameters were not helpful except for hirsutism, being more common in patients with carcinoma. Thin skin, purple striae, thin hair, and temporal hair loss were more common in patients with adenomas. From a metabolic standpoint, 17-ketosteroid (Forbes and Albright, 1951) as well as DHEAS levels (Yamaji et al., 1984) are often high in patients with carcinomas, usually in conjunction with elevated glucocorticoid production (Luton et al., 1990). Patient prognosis is poor.

Testosterone-Secreting Adrenal Cortical Tumors

Virilization is the hallmark of Cushing's syndrome secondary to adrenal carcinoma. However, virilization in the absence of elevated urinary 17-ketosteroids is very uncommon and should raise the possibility of testosterone-secreting ovarian or adrenal lesions (Im-

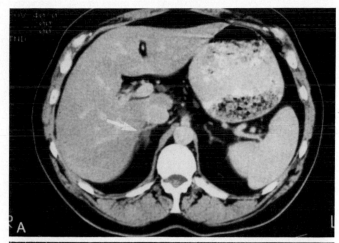

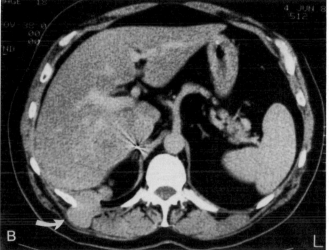

Figure 64–34. Patient with a small right aldosterone-producing adenoma *(A)*, which was malignant and recurred in the adrenal bed and at the site of the flank incision *(B)*. Disease caused death of patient.

perato-McGinley et al., 1981). Of the two sites of origin, adrenal cortical tumors that secrete testosterone are exceedingly rare. Most adrenal tumors have been adenomas, but several have been ganglioneuromas with Leydig cell nodules (Aguirre and Sculley, 1983) or a Leydig cell adenoma (Trost et al., 1981). The majority of tumors have been found in adult females, although cases in adult males and in children have been reported. The testosterone secretion can be autonomous, under gonadotropin control (Werk et al., 1973) or under ACTH control (Trost et al., 1981).

In contrast to the other tumors described in this chapter, these tumors are usually small, less than 6 cm, and they behave in a benign fashion. However, in a review of 47 documented cases of testosterone-producing neoplasms, eight were virilizing carcinomas (Gabrilove et al., 1981; Mattox and Phelan, 1987).

Estrogen-Secreting Adrenal Cortical Tumors

Most feminizing tumors occur in males 25 to 50 years old, and in contradistinction to testosterone-secreting tumors, they are usually larger, often palpable, and highly malignant (Gabrilove et al., 1965). Characteristically, the patients present with gynecomastia. In addition, they may exhibit testicular atrophy, impotence, or decreased libido. In one of our cases, the clinical presentation was infertility and oligospermia.

These tumors secrete androstenedione, which is converted peripherally to estrogens. Other steroids may also be secreted, and the clinical picture may be mixed with associated cushingoid features.

Of these tumors, 80 per cent have been malignant. Half the patients with this disease expire within 18 months of diagnosis. The 3-year survival is less than 20 per cent.

The prime therapy is surgical, usually utilizing a thoracoabdominal approach with wide excision of the tumor, adjacent organs, if necessary, and regional lymph nodes. Despite wide resection, the patient's prognosis remains poor, and no effective adjunctive therapy has been developed to date.

Aldosterone-Secreting Adrenal Cortical Carcinoma

Primary hyperaldosteronism is almost always due to a small benign solitary adenoma, Conn's syndrome, or bilateral adrenal hyperplasia. However, the syndrome in its pure form may rarely be caused by adrenal carcinoma (Vaughan et al., 1989b). In fact, in most cases with evidence of mineralocorticoid excess and hypokalemia due to adrenal carcinoma, there are also signs of abnormalities in glucocorticoid or androgen secretion.

On review of the cases, the striking difference between the tumors found in these patients and in those with Conn's syndrome due to benign adenomas is the size of the tumor. Benign adenomas are rarely larger than 3 cm in size. In contrast, all but two reported aldosterone-secreting carcinomas were larger than 3 cm (Vaughan et al., 1989c). Accordingly, the clinical and biochemical syndrome of hyperaldosteronism and the CT evidence of a large adrenal mass should strongly suggest carcinoma. Similar to most of the other patients with tumors as described, these patients do poorly despite initial resection of the tumor. Adjunctive therapy is ineffective.

Adrenal Cortical Carcinoma in Children

Adrenal cortical carcinoma composes only 0.002 per cent of all childhood malignancies (Young and Miller, 1975) and only 6 per cent of childhood malignant adrenal tumors—the majority being neuroblastomas (Stewart et al., 1984) (see Chapter 54). However, despite the somewhat tenuous feeling that survival is better in children, double that in adults, the entity is still highly lethal and refractory to adjunctive therapy, although adequate trials have not been carried out (Kay et al., 1983).

In contrast to adults, most of these tumors in children are hormonally active, and perhaps earlier detection is the reason for their better survival. The clinical syndromes include Cushing's syndrome, commonly due to carcinoma—not adenoma—in children, virilization in females, and isosexual precocious puberty in males. Evaluation follows the same lines as that described in adults with careful examination for steroid precursors and by-products. These may be of later use as tumor markers following initial tumor removal. In addition to recurrence, the late occurrence of other tumors has also been reported (Andler et al., 1978).

Management of Adrenocortical Carcinoma

Except for testosterone-secreting tumors, adrenocortical carcinomas are highly malignant with both local and hematogenous spread and a 5-year survival rate of less than 30 per cent (Brennan, 1987; Luton et al., 1990; Venkatesh et al., 1989). In the series by Richie and Gittes, 1980, the most common sites of metastasis were lung, liver, and lymph nodes. A large autopsy study of 132 cases showed metastases to lungs (60 per cent), liver (50 per cent), lymph nodes (48 per cent), bone (24 per cent), and pleura and heart (10 per cent) (Didolkar et al., 1981). In addition, these tumors often extend directly into adjacent structures, especially the kidney. The treatment is surgical removal of the primary tumor with attempt to remove the entire lesion even if resection of adjacent organs (e.g., kidney and spleen) are necessary as well as resection of local lymph nodes en bloc. Following surgical removal of functioning adrenal tumors, the patient can be followed with appropriate hormonal levels as markers for tumor recurrence.

Medical Therapy

Despite the current accuracy in anatomic and biochemical definition of adrenal carcinoma, many patients present with metastatic disease. Most patients with locally resectable disease eventually succumb to recurrent local or distant disease. The search for effective adjunctive therapy has been frustrating; radiation therapy has not been useful except for palliation (Percarpio and Knowlton, 1976). In addition, conventional chemotherapy, although not widely studied in a systematic fashion, has not been effective.

The most success reported has been with the adrenolytic drug (1,1-dichloro-2-[o-chlorophenyl]-2-[p-chlorophenyl]ethane) (o,p'-DDD) or mitotane (Bergerstal et al., 1960). This DDT derivative has been shown to induce tumor response in 34 per cent (Hutter et al., 1966) and 61 per cent (Lubitz et al., 1973) in two large series. The major use has been for patients with metastatic disease, and despite the response rates given, survival time has not been prolonged in all reported series (Hoffman and Mattox, 1972; Luton et al., 1990). Moreover, the usual treatment regimen is to increase the dosage to 8 to 10 g per day until toxicity occurs. Toxicity that is significant includes gastrointestinal, neurologic, and dermatologic disorders, most of which regress upon cessation of therapy. One patient has been reported who remained in remission for 5 years during mitotane therapy without intolerable side effects (Jarabak and Rice, 1981). Hence, rarely long-term remission can be induced by the drug.

During management, adrenal insufficiency can occur, and cortisol and aldosterone levels should be monitored. Because of the high fat solubility of the drug, traces of it can be found several months after the drug has been discontinued, warranting continued steroid monitoring during this period.

An unresolved issue is early adjunctive mitotane in patients without evidence of residual local or metastatic disease following surgical removal of the tumor. Schteingert and co-workers (1982) have demonstrated prolonged survival in a small group of patients treated in this fashion and early reoperation for recurrent disease. In summary, the overall response to o,p'DDD has been disappointing and other agents are being studied such as suramin, the antiparasitic agent. The antifungal drug ketoconazole, which has an adrenolytic effect, has also induced regression in metastatic adrenal carcinoma (Contreras et al., 1985), as have cisplatin and etoposide (Johnson and Greco, 1986).

Thus, drugs such as mitotane, ketoconazole, metyrapone, and aminoglutethimide may help relieve the devastating symptoms of glucocorticoid or mineralocorticoid excess. However, little evidence exists that survival is extended in most cases.

Whether the new antiglucocorticoid agent mifepristone (RU486) and the somatostatin analogues (Invitti, 1990) will be significant remains to be studied (Segal, 1990).

ADRENAL CYSTS

These are usually unilateral lesions discovered incidentally during imaging procedures or surgery and at autopsy. Calcifications may be found in approximately 15 per cent of cases and need not imply malignancy. Endothelial or lymphangiomatous cysts account for nearly 45 per cent of these lesions and are usually small, measuring 0.1 to 1.5 cm in diameter. Adrenal pseudocysts that lack an epithelial lining are the next most common variety (39 per cent) and most likely represent encapsulated residua of previous adrenal hemorrhages. Pseudocysts may become massive and may cause symptoms because of the compression of adjacent structures (Fig. 64–35). The acute hemorrhage in the case shown was readily distinguished by MRI (see Fig. 64–35). Parasitic cysts due to echinococcal disease (7 per cent) and true epithelial cysts (9 per cent) account for the remainder of adrenal cysts (Kazam et al., 1989).

ADRENAL INSUFFICIENCY

Adrenal insufficiency is rarely encountered in the practice of urology. Because it is potentially fatal if not

recognized, the salient features of the entity are worthy of review.

Addison's disease is rare, the death rate being approximately 0.3 per 100,000 with the most common cause being either tuberculosis or adrenal atrophy (Dunlop, 1963; Eason et al., 1982; Irvine and Barnes, 1972). Other causes include malignant infiltration (Cedermark et al., 1977), sarcoidosis (Irvine and Barnes, 1972; Rickards and Barrett, 1954), histoplasmosis (Crispel et al., 1956), North American blastomycosis (Fish et al., 1960), South American blastomycosis (Osa et al., 1981), and coccidioidomycosis (Moloney, 1952). The general term adrenal atrophy actually refers to a pathologic process of lymphocytic adenitis with fibrosis (Maisey and Stevens, 1969). However, from a clinical point of view, symptoms of adrenal insufficiency usually appear in hospitalized patients in whom the history of the long-term use of exogenous steroids has not been obtained and the acute withdrawal from steroids has occurred.

The symptoms and signs of chronic adrenal insufficiency are nonspecific and may be associated with numerous other diseases (Table 64–7). Similarly, abnormalities determined with routine laboratory tests are also nonspecific. The most common abnormalities are hyponatremia and hyperkalemia, with at least one electrolyte abnormality being found in 99 of 108 patients in one series (Nerup, 1974). However, the classic triad of hyponatremia, hyperkalemia, and azotemia was present in only 50 to 60 per cent of cases. Hypercalcemia may also be an initial abnormality. Other endocrine disorders, including hyperthyroidism or hypothyroidism (17 per cent), diabetes mellitus (12 per cent), gonadal dysfunction (12 per cent), and hypothyroidism (5 per cent) occur in about 10 to 30 per cent of patients with Addison's disease (May et al., 1989).

Table 64–7. SIGNS AND SYMPTOMS OF CHRONIC ADDISON'S DISEASE[a] AND ACUTE ADRENAL INSUFFICIENCY[b]

Number	Per Cent	Symptom
435/462[a]	94	Weakness, tiredness, fatigue
393/438	90	Weight loss
303/351	86	Anorexia
178/268	66	Nausea, vomiting
100/164	61	Unspecified gastrointestinal complaints
35/127	28	Abdominal pain
44/246	18	Diarrhea
15/94	16	Muscle pain
24/168	14	Salt craving
24/166	14	Orthostatic hypotension, dizziness, or syncope
4/33	12	Lethargy, disorientation
165/165[b]	100	Severe clinical deterioration
98/140	70	Fever
20/31	64	Nausea, vomiting
21/46	46	Abdominal or flank pain
59/165	36	Hypotension
9/28	32	Abdominal distention
25/96	26	Lethargy, obtundation
55/122	45	Hyponatremia
21/83	25	Hyperkalemia

From May, M. E., Vaughan, E. D., Jr., and Carey, R. M.: Adrenocortical insufficiency—clinical aspects. In Vaughan, E. D., Jr., Carey, R. M. (Eds.): Adrenal Disorders. New York, Thieme Medical Publishers, Inc., 1989.

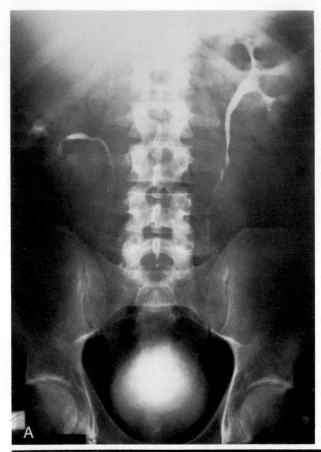

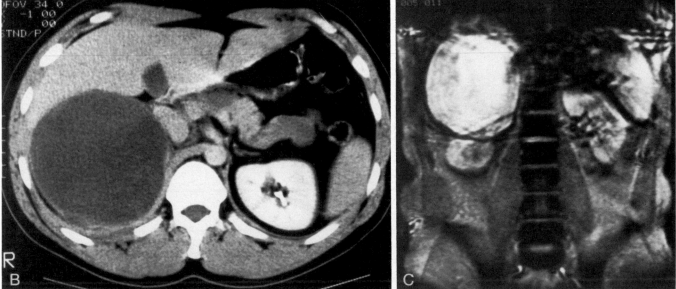

Figure 64–35. *A*, Massive right adrenal cyst. The patient presented with fever, pain, and anemia. *B*, Computed tomography scan of cyst. *C*, Bright hemorrhage into the lumen, cyst proved at exploration, shown on magnetic resonance image.

The symptoms of acute adrenal insufficiency "crisis," usually due to withdrawal of exogenous steroids, sepsis, bilateral adrenal hemorrhage, or postadrenalectomy, differ somewhat from those of Addison's disease, particularly fever that occurs in 70 per cent of patients (see Table 64–7) (Liu et al., 1982). Abdominal pain is also often present and may be due to unilateral or bilateral adrenal hemorrhage, which can be diagnosed by CT (Liu, 1982) or MRI (Falke et al., 1987).

The critical test to confirm the presence of Addison's disease is the demonstration of a failure to increase plasma (Perkoff et al., 1954) or urinary corticosteroid level into the normal range with ACTH infusions (Renold et al., 1952). A provocative test is particularly important because there are numerous reports of patients with primary adrenal insufficiency having normal-based plasma cortisol or urinary 17-hydroxycorticoid levels (May et al., 1989). Plasma ACTH levels may be

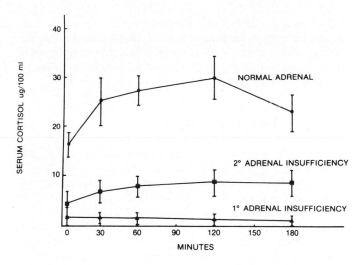

Figure 64–36. Serum cortisol response and response to ACTH infusion in normal persons and in patients with primary and secondary adrenal insufficiency and adrenal insufficiency. (From Vaughan, E. D., Jr., and Carey, R. M. (Eds.): Adrenal Disorders. New York, Thieme Medical Publishers Inc., 1989.)

markedly elevated, but such an assay is not always available. The simplest screening test is the rapid ACTH test, whereby plasma cortisol levels are measured before and 60 minutes after 0.25 mg of cosyntropin is given intravenously; cortisol levels should be > 18 μg/dl at 60 minutes (Fig. 64–36) (Speckard et al., 1971). A patient with a relative or an absolute lack of ACTH may respond normally to cosyntropin but not respond properly to surgical stress (Jasani et al., 1968; Kehlet and Binder, 1973). However, most of these patients tolerate surgical stress without steroid coverage. If treatment is mandated in a patient with suspected adrenal insufficiency, the ACTH stimulation test can be performed when treatment is with the synthetic steroid dexamethasone (Sheridan and Mattingly, 1975). Other more definitive but more complex and longer infusion tests also can be utilized (Dolan and Carey, 1989).

The treatment of acute or chronic adrenal insufficiency is obviously the acute administration of glucocorticoids. In acute adrenal crisis, stress level dexamethasone (8 to 12 mg per day) is given along with replacement saline (Smith and Byrne, 1981) and a simultaneous ACTH stimulation test to confirm the diagnosis (Sheridan and Mattingly, 1975).

The treatment of chronic Addison's disease is maintenance therapy—approximately 30 mg of hydrocorti-sone plus 0.05 to 0.1 μg fluorohydrocortisone per day orally, or a synthetic steroid (Table 64–8).

Replacement therapy following unilateral adrenalectomy is discussed elsewhere. However, the same guidelines pertain and it is helpful to maintain patients on dexamethasone so that the ACTH test can be utilized to follow the recovery of the contralateral gland.

Selective Adrenal Insufficiency

Selective hypoaldosteronism is rare and usually is due to hyporeninemia or functional "hypoaldosteronism" due to tubular insensitivity to normal aldosterone levels (Schambelan et al., 1972; Williams et al., 1983). The urologist will occasionally observe this phenomenon in an adult or a child who exhibits unexplained hyperkalemia following relief of chronic obstructive uropathy, especially in association with azotemia (Kozeny et al., 1986; Pelleya et al., 1983; Schambelan et al., 1980).

Other selective hypoaldosteronism may occur from primary disturbances of the zona glomerulosa. Congenital primary hypoaldosteronism may be sporadic or familial (May et al., 1989).

Selective familial glucocorticoid deficiency has been well described, almost totally in the pediatric literature

Table 64–8. COMPARISON OF HALF-LIFE AND BIOLOGIC ACTIVITY OF VARIOUS NATURAL AND SYNTHETIC STEROIDS

Compound	Biologic Half-Life (h)	Plasma Half-Life (h)	Equivalent Dose (mg)	Relative Sodium-Retaining Activity
Cortisone*	8–12	0.5	25	0.8
Cortisol (hydrocortisone)	8–12	1.5	20	1.0
Prednisone*	12–36	1	5	0.8
Prednisolone	12–36	2–4	5	0.8
6-Alpha-methylprednisolone	12–36	1–3	4	0.5
Dexamethasone	36–72	2–3	0.75	0–2
Betamethasone	36–72		0.60	0
Deoxycorticosterone†			0	20
9-Alpha-fluorohydrocortisone			2	125–400
Aldosterone		0.2	0.1	400

*Require hepatic metabolism for bioactivity.
†Inactivated upon oral administration. (From May, M. E., Vaughan, E. D., Jr., and Carey, R. M.: Adrenocortical insufficiency—Clinical aspects. In Vaughan, E. D. Jr., and Carey, R. M. (Eds.): Adrenal Disorders. New York, Thieme Medical Publishers, Inc., 1989.)

(May et al., 1989). The clinical presentation is dominated by recurrent hypoglycemia, both fasting and reactive with subsequent seizures. The children usually have normal findings of electrolytes, which often delays the proper diagnosis.

HYPERALDOSTERONISM

The term primary hyperaldosteronism was originally coined by Conn (1955a, b) to describe the clinical syndrome characterized by hypertension, hypokalemia, hypernatremia, alkalosis, and periodic paralysis due to an aldosterone-secreting adenoma. As precise methodology for quantifying the components of the renin-angiotensin-aldosterone system (RAAS) has become available, the syndrome of primary hyperaldosteronism is now identified by the combined findings of hypokalemia, suppressed plasma renin activity (PRA), and high urinary and plasma aldosterone levels in hypertensive patients. Moreover, the term primary aldosteronism should be extended to contain a family of adrenal forms of hyperaldosteronism, including but not exclusive to adrenal adenomas (Biglieri et al., 1990; Brownie, 1990).

Thomas Addison first associated the syndrome of weakness, prostration, dehydration, and coma to adrenal insufficiency. Subsequently, Loeb and co-workers (1933) demonstrated renal sodium wastage in patients with Addison's disease and in dogs with adrenal insufficiency, as well as the therapeutic effect of sodium replacement.

The first demonstration by Hench and associates, in 1949, that cortisol administration restored sodium balance and initiated kaliuresis as well as reversing characteristics of glucocorticoid deficiency led to the hypothesis that cortisol was the sole and omnipotent adrenal cortical hormone. However, the variances among glucocorticoid excess; Cushing's syndrome; and toxicity from excess administration of the mineralocorticoid, 11-deoxycorticosterone, led Luetscher and associates to search for the presence of another steroid. Such activity was demonstrated in large amounts in patients exhibiting renal sodium retention (Deming and Luetscher, 1950; Luetscher and Johnson, 1954). This substance also exhibited sodium-retaining activity in adrenalectomized rats. At about the same time Simpson, Tate, and their associates began a series of studies that were to culminate in the isolation and identification of 18-oxycorticosterone, electrocortin, or aldosterone (Simpson et al., 1954). The clinical impact of this information is best described in Conn's own words (Conn, 1977):

"In April, 1954, a 34-year-old female patient with a bizarre constellation of clinical and laboratory manifestations was presented to me on ward rounds. They included periodic paralysis, intermittent muscular weakness, episodic tetanic manifestations, polydipsia and nocturnal polyuria, headache, hypertension, positive Chvostek and Trousseau signs, hypokalemia, hypernatremia, alkalosis, alkaline urine with mild proteinuria, and a ward note suggesting a diagnosis of hyperventilation tetany.

Although that morning at the bedside I made the correct diagnosis, namely, excessive activity of the, then, newly described adrenal steroid, electrocortin, I was not unaware of the raised eyebrows and of the slow to-and-fro motion of the heads of my staff. It required 8 months of continuous metabolic study of that patient to put all the multiple manifestations satisfactorily into the syndrome that I then called 'primary aldosteronism.' It was only then that I mounted sufficient courage to request adrenal exploration for indications that had never before been employed. My head rang with the objections of my associates: 'What if it turns out to be simple potassium-losing nephritis?' But it did not turn out that way and, with time, the so-called potassium-losing nephritis has turned out, in most cases, to be primary aldosteronism."

Pathophysiology

The normal physiology of the RAAS including the stimuli for aldosterone release has been reviewed in Chapters 3 and 55. When aldosterone is secreted in amounts inappropriately high for the state of sodium balance, there is additional sodium reabsorption by the distal nephron (O'Neil, 1990; Verrey, 1990). Extracellular sodium is increased and is accompanied by water so that isotonicity is maintained. Mild increases in serum sodium may occur, and accompanying hypokalemia and mild alkalosis are characteristic. The sodium accumulation is usually gradual and is dependent on the availability of sodium and the degree of hyperaldosteronism. However, after a gain of about 1.5 kg of extracellular fluid, there is diminished proximal tubular reabsorption of sodium, and the phenomenon of "renal escape" occurs (Espiner et al., 1967). The mechanism of renal escape remains unclear but there appears to be decreased sodium reabsorption at sites not responsible for the initial sodium reabsorption. Escape is associated with increased renal arterial pressure and increased atrial natriuretic factor, which may play critical roles (Atlas, 1991; Haas and Knox, 1990; Rocco et al., 1990). This limitation of sodium retention explains the characteristic clinical findings in patients with primary aldosteronism of mild hypertension, the rarity of malignant hypertension, and the absence of edema.

In contrast to the escape from further aldosterone-induced sodium retention, there is no "escape" from potassium loss. In addition, aldosterone increases potassium secretion from all sites in which it enhances sodium absorption: renal tubule, sweat and salivary glands, and intestine. Hence, overactivity of aldosterone can be determined by analyzing salivary electrolyte content (Wotman et al., 1970) or transluminal potential differences across the intestine (Carey et al., 1974). Aldosterone also increases renal tubular secretion of hydrogen ion, which escapes mainly as ammonium ion. The alkalosis that ensues appears to correlate with the degree of potassium depletion. Taken together, these physiologic derangements explain the clinical and biochemical findings of patients with hyperaldosteronism. However, at the present time, the clinical syndrome as first described by Conn is rarely observed because we are more suspicious of this entity in hypertensive patients and now usually establish the diagnosis and treatment earlier in the evolution of the disease.

The response of PRA to the aldosterone-induced sodium retention and blood pressure elevation is the cornerstone of early diagnosis of the entity (Fig. 64–37). Accordingly, the normal renal juxtaglomerular responses to increased blood pressure (the baroreceptor mechanism) and the increased distal delivery of sodium chloride (the macula densa mechanism) result in suppression of PRA (Conn et al., 1964). Moreover, the PRA remains low even in the presence of sodium depletion or acute furosemide administration (Carey et al., 1972; Spark and Melby, 1968; Weinberger et al., 1979). This observation is in marked contrast to the elevated PRA seen in patients with secondary aldosteronism, usually due to renal arterial or parenchymal disease. In this last clinical setting, the oversecretion of aldosterone is secondary to the excess production of angiotensin II, stimulating the adrenal zona glomerulosa (see Chapter 55).

The ability to measure urinary and plasma aldosterone has given further insight to abnormalities of aldosterone secretion (Dolan and Carey, 1989). Hence, the oversecretion of aldosterone is not suppressed by sodium loading (Espiner et al., 1967; Weinberger, 1979) as in healthy subjects. Conversely, with ambulation, patients with an aldosterone-producing adenoma (APA) do not exhibit the characteristic rise in aldosterone secretion found in healthy subjects, and there may be a paradoxical fall in plasma aldosterone levels (Ganguly et al., 1981; Herf et al., 1979). This last observation helps to differentiate patients with APA from those with idiopathic hyperaldosteronism (IHA) (also termed pseudoprimary hyperaldosteronism) (Baer et al., 1970) due to bilateral adrenal hyperplasia, in which the rise in circulating aldosterone persists (Herf et al., 1979; Weinberger et al., 1979). These observations highlight the autonomous secretion that is present in patients with APA and begin to highlight the differences in the pathophysiology of APA and IHA (Biglieri et al., 1990).

Patients with bilateral adrenal hyperplasia (IHA) exhibiting hyperaldosteronism present with the same clinical and biochemical abnormalities as those with APA. However, differentiation between the two groups is important, because it is generally accepted that patients with IHA are not cured of hypertension by subtotal or even total bilateral adrenalectomy (Baer et al., 1970; Biglieri et al., 1990; Lim et al., 1986). Accordingly, the treatment of choice is medical rather than surgical in most cases of bilateral hyperplasia.

The pathogenesis of adrenal nodular hyperplasia remains uncertain, but the fact that the lesions are bilateral suggests the presence of some stimulus other than angiotensin II or ACTH inducing adrenal hyperplasia and hyperaldosteronism. In this regard, the observations of Carey and co-workers (1984) that aldosterone-stimulating factor is elevated in this entity is intriguing. Aldosterone-stimulating factor is a glycoprotein of anterior pituitary origin, which differs from derivatives of pro-opiomelanocortin, which may also stimulate aldosterone.

Less common types of bilateral adrenal hyperplasia have also been identified (Biglieri et al., 1990). A small subset of patients experience the suppression of aldosterone secretion with the administration of large doses of 11-deoxycorticosterone acetate (DOCA). This entity has been termed DOCA-suppressible idiopathic hyperaldosteronism, or indeterminate hyperaldosteronism (Ind HA). Correction of hypertension and hypokalemia with dexamethasone identifies the glucocorticoid-remediable form of hyperaldosteronism dexamethasone-suppressible hyperaldosteronism (DSH).

Banks and co-workers (1984) have identified a subset of patients with bilaterally increased aldosterone secretion who are cured by bilateral adrenalectomy. This entity has been termed primary adrenal hyperplasia, and patients show autonomy of aldosterone secretion as found in patients with adenomas (Irony et al., 1988). At times, in patients with bilateral hyperplasia, we have found that one gland is dominant. Unilateral adrenalectomy will ameliorate or eliminate the symptoms.

In summary, a family of entities fall under the general rubric of idiopathic hyperaldosteronism, characterized by bilateral adrenal hyperplasia. Fortunately, although there is incomplete understanding of the pathophysiology of these lesions, the anatomic entity can readily be identified by CAT and adrenal vein sampling for aldosterone.

Clinical Characteristics

The incidence of primary aldosteronism is low, less than 1 to 2 per cent of the hypertensive population, and

Figure 64–37. Hyperaldosteronism may be seen in association with elevated (secondary) or depressed (primary) levels of plasma renin activity. In primary aldosteronism an adrenal neoplasm or bilateral hyperplasia is the initiating event. Secondary aldosteronism is most commonly seen in edematous disorders (e.g., cirrhosis, renal failure), in which the elevated renin levels are a physiologic adjustment to a contracted blood volume; it is also present in renal artery stenosis, secondary to the stimulus of elevated levels of renin and angiotensin II. (From Dluhy, R. G., and Gittes, R. F.: The Adrenals. In Walsh, P. C., Gittes, R. F., Perlmutter, A. D., and Stamey, T. A. (Eds.): Campbell's Urology, 5th ed. Philadelphia, W. B. Saunders Co., 1986.)

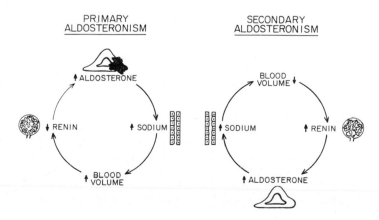

Table 64–9. AGE DISTRIBUTION OF 266 TUMORS OF THE ADRENAL CORTEX IN HYPERALDOSTERONISM WITH LOW PLASMA RENIN

Adrenal Changes (No. of Cases)	Sex	Age (Years)							Total
		15–20	*21–30*	*31–40*	*41–50*	*51–60*	*61–70*	*>70*	
Adenoma (241)	Female	6	16	59	67	17	5	1	171
	Male	2	7	20	28	9	3	1	70
Carcinomas (25)	Female	—	2	5	3	5	1	—	16
	Male	—	1	4	1	2	1	—	9

From Neville, A. M., and O'Hare, M. J.: The Human Adrenal Cortex. Pathology and Biology—An Integrated Approach. New York, Springer-Verlag, 1982.

aldosteronism occurs predominantly in females (70 per cent). The clinical findings in patients with hyperaldosteronism are primarily due to the hypokalemic state. They include, in approximate order of frequency, muscular weakness, nocturia, frontal headaches, polydipsia, parathesias, visual disturbances, temporary paralysis, cramps, and tetany. Traditionally, the determination of hypokalemia has been used as the screening test for the entity.

In the review of 51 cases reported by Weinberger and co-workers (1979), the serum potassium value was less than 4 mEq/L in every patient. However, 11 patients (22 per cent) had serum potassium concentrations of 3.6 mEq/L or greater. In a prospective study of 80 patients with primary aldosteronism (70 adenoma/10 hyperplasia), 22 patients (17 APA/5 IHA) had serum K^+ of more than 3.5 mEQ/L on a low-sodium diet (UnaV = 10 mEQ/L). Ten patients remained normokalemic (6 APA/5 IHA) despite sodium loading (Bravo et al., 1983). Indeed, the concept of normokalemic hyperaldosteronism had previously been recognized by Conn and co-workers (1966). If the patient is normokalemic, the characteristic symptoms of the disease are absent. It is rare for a patient today to exhibit all the features first described by Conn. Hypokalemia may be absent in a patient who has restricted dietary sodium intake. The observant patient may recognize that he or she is less weak when restricting salt intake. Accordingly, we do not believe that screening for the disease is adequate, unless the patient remains normokalemic while on a high-sodium diet (> 10 g/day).

Because the sodium retention is limited by the escape phenomenon, patients do not exhibit edema, and hypertension is often but not always mild. This form of volume hypertension is usually not malignant (Tarazi et al., 1973). The physical signs and symptoms of primary hyperaldosteronism are not always distinguished from essential hypertension without appropriate laboratory studies.

Adrenal adenomas causing primary hyperaldosteronism are usually small unless malignant (most less than 4 cm), and there is a left-side predominance (Table 64–9).

No specific familial associations have been identified in most cases, except in some subsets of patients with bilateral hyperplasia (Weinberger et al., 1979). Although the mean age of patients with APA in Weinberger's series was 42.3 ± 8.12 years, in the same series the overlap in patients with IHA is obvious. The age distribution of 266 tumors in patients with hyperaldosteronism as reported by Neville and O'Hare is shown in Table 64–10.

Diagnostic Studies

The diagnostic studies described are designed to accomplish two goals: to screen the large hypertensive population for primary hyperaldosteronism and to distinguish the patients with adrenal adenoma from those with bilateral hyperplasia. The absence of a reliable clinical picture of hyperaldosteronism has led to a battery of tests suggested to accomplish these goals. Our approach is shown in Figure 64–38.

Screening Tests

Certainly unprovoked hypokalemia is the hallmark of hyperaldosteronism, but as already discussed, serum K^+

Table 64–10. HYPERALDOSTERONISM

Weights of 151 Adrenal Adenomas			Weights of 25 Adrenal Carcinomas	
Weight (g)	*No.*	*Per Cent*	*Weight (g)*	*No.*
<2	51	(34)	<30	1
2–4	36	(24)	30–100	5
4–5	16	(11)	100–200	3
5–10	26	(17)	200–500	4
10–20	11	(7)	500–1000	6
20–30	3	(3.5)	1000–2000	5
>30	8	(3.5)	>2000	1
Total	151	(100)		

SITE DISTRIBUTION OF ADRENAL ADENOMAS IN 218 PATIENTS

	No. of Patients		
Site	*Male*	*Female*	**Total**
Single			
Right adrenal	22	37	59
Left adrenal	25	70	95
Bilateral	2	1	3
Unknown	14	40	54
Subtotal	63 (91%)	148 (93%)	201 (92%)
Multiple			
Right adrenal	4	2	6
Left adrenal	1	8	9
Bilateral	1	1	2
Unknown	—	—	—
Subtotal	6 (9%)	11 (7%)	17 (8%)
Total	69 (30%)	159 (70%)	218 (100%)

From Neville, A. M., and O'Hare, M. J.: The Human Adrenal Cortex. Pathology and Biology—An Integrated Approach. New York, Springer-Verlag, 1982.

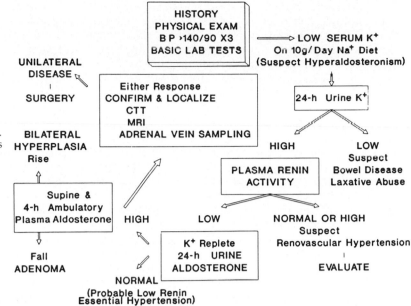

Figure 64–38. Identifying primary hyperaldosteronism. (From Vaughan, E. D., Jr.: Diagnosis of adrenal disorders in hypertension. World J. Urol., 7:111–116, 1989.)

levels between 3.5 and 4.0 mEq/L are commonly found in patients subsequently proved to have primary aldosteronism. Patients with essential hypertension may exhibit hypokalemia. Monitoring serum K^+ following salt loading lowers the false-negative normokalemic finding, but the entity of normokalemic primary aldosteronism is well recognized (Bravo et al., 1983; Weinberger et al., 1979). In addition, following sodium loading, patients with primary aldosteronism excrete more sodium and potassium in the urine. However, these metabolic balance studies are too complex to be utilized as screening tests. Adjunctive measurements of salivary sodium/potassium ratios are also too cumbersome and inaccurate to be utilized as screening tests (Christlieb et al., 1971; Espiner et al., 1967; Wotman et al., 1970).

A combination of studies is necessary to identify the entity accurately. The first breakthrough followed the ability to accurately determine PRA. In 1964, Conn demonstrated the suppression of PRA in patients with primary aldosteronism. At that time, a major diagnostic dilemma was distinction of patients with primary aldosteronism from patients with excessive secretion of aldosterone secondary to primary renal disease and oversecretion of renin (secondary hyperaldosteronism). This single measurement has survived the test of time as critical to the differentiation of patients with these two disorders (McDougal et al., 1990; Streeten et al., 1979; Vaughan et al., 1989c; Weinberger et al., 1979). The test has subsequently been refined by demonstrating that the PRA remains low in patients with primary hyperaldosteronism despite sodium depletion (Baer et al., 1970), ambulation (Ganguly et al., 1973), and the administration of furosemide (Carey et al., 1972). However, 25 per cent of patients with essential hypertension exhibit low PRA (Brunner et al., 1972). Although most of these patients are normokalemic, additional screening tests were necessary.

The development of an accurate methodology to measure plasma aldosterone has led to accurate screening. Elevated plasma or urinary aldosterone level indexed against urinary sodium excretion, measured following sodium loading in combination with previously demonstrated low PRA during sodium depletion, is the biochemical hallmark of the entity (see Fig. 64–14). This measurement does not distinguish patients with APA from those with IHA. It is also possible to screen with an acute sodium load. The measurement of plasma aldosterone concentration after the intravenous infusion of 2L of normal saline over 4 hours has proved to be highly accurate in the hands of several investigators. Weinberger and co-workers (1979) found that plasma aldosterone concentration was often within the normal range during ambulation without sodium loading (Weinberger et al., 1979). Markedly suppressed serum K^+ may impair aldosterone secretion. Thus, a low serum K^+ should be corrected prior to measurement of aldosterone (Herf et al., 1979).

The combination of hypokalemia, low PRA during sodium restriction or furosemide administration, an 18-OH corticosterone >50 ng/dl (Biglieri, 1990), and elevated plasma aldosterone concentration following sodium loading accurately identifies most patients with hyperaldosteronism (see Fig. 64–38).

Fortunately, the development of a number of tests to lateralize aldosterone production and excretion to one adrenal gland coupled with radiographic studies now provides a highly accurate means by which to differentiate patients with APA from those with IHA. In healthy subjects, a rise in PRA level occurs on standing accompanied by a rise in plasma aldosterone levels. This same response also occurs in patients with essential hypertension. This same response in PRA and aldosterone is also observed in patients with IHA, although the PRA is significantly lower than in healthy subjects. However, in APA a parallel decrease in aldosterone and cortisol reflects the predominant influence of ACTH in the absence of angiotensin II stimulation (Biglieri, 1990; Bravo et al., 1983; Ganguly et al., 1973; Herf et al.,

1979). Obviously, but not in most patients with APA, this physiologic test does not preclude further lateralization studies. However, a drop in plasma aldosterone concentration after 4 hours of ambulation strongly suggests APA. In contrast, the diurnal variation of plasma aldosterone concentration was not found to be of value (Herf, 1979).

Lateralizing Tests

APAs are usually small, and they often defied identification by studies such as intravenous pyelography, retroperitoneal air insufflation, and arteriography. The first major advance in this regard followed the demonstration that it was relatively simple to catheterize the adrenal veins for radiocontrast retrograde injection, outlining the venous circulation of the adrenal (Bucht et al., 1964). Obviously, larger tumors are most easily visualized, but clearly many APA can be visualized by this method. However, inaccuracies of venography and reports of inadvertent adrenal infarction led to a search for more accurate tests (Fisher et al., 1971).

The ability to measure plasma aldosterone concentration added a new and highly useful dimension to adrenal vein catheterization (Dunnick et al., 1982; Geisinger et al., 1983; Horton and Finck, 1972). The major problems encountered involve the difficulty in catheterizing the short right adrenal vein, the risk of trauma, the dilution of blood by blood from nonadrenal sources, and the episodic changes in aldosterone secretion coincident with changes in cortisol (Weinberger et al., 1979). Most of these problems can be controlled by careful catheter localization, simultaneous plasma cortisol measurements to document appropriate catheter placement, collecting blood by gravity flow, or collecting during ACTH administration. Weinberger and co-workers have found this last maneuver to increase sensitivity of aldosterone production to such an extent that their technique consistently identified patients with APA.

Adrenal vein sampling of aldosterone remains the cornerstone for localization of aldosterone production. In patients with APA there is a high aldosterone concentration from the involved gland with contralateral suppression of aldosterone from the normal gland. In contrast, in IHA, there is bilateral secretion, albeit it is asymmetric in some cases. The results of the various lateralizing studies, as reviewed by Weinberger and colleagues, are shown in Table 64–11.

Table 64–11. RESULTS OF LOCALIZATION STUDIES

	Unilateral Adenoma
Blood pressure response to adrenalectomy	
Normotensive	26/38
No change	0/38
Adrenal venography*	16/27
Adrenal scan*	13/28
Adrenal hormones*	35/35
Postural decline in plasma aldosterone*	23/32

*Positive/total. (From Weinberger, M. H., Grim, C. E., Hollifield, J. W., Kem, D. C., Ganguly, A., Kramer, N. J., June, H. Y., Wellman, H., and Donohue, J. P.: Primary aldosteronism: Diagnosis localization and treatment. Ann. Intern. Med., 93:86, 1979.)

The problems with adrenal vein sampling and the search for a noninvasive test led to the development of a radioiodinated analogue of cholesterol, which concentrated in the adrenal. In 1971, Beirwaltes reported visualization of human adrenal glands utilizing ^{131}I-6-iodomethyl-19-nor-cholesterol. However, despite refinements, the accuracy of adrenal scanning has been limited by both subjective interpretation and asymmetric uptake in both healthy subjects and patients with primary aldosteronism. The unreliability of the test in relation to other modalities as found by Weinberger and co-workers is shown in Table 64–11. In summary, scanning now holds an adjunctive role when other tests are inconclusive and clearly has been superseded by CAT (Dunnick et al., 1982; Geisinger et al., 1983; Kazam et al., 1989; White et al., 1980).

CT has evolved as the most accurate anatomic test for adrenal disease. Earlier, the small lesions of APA could not be defined by CT, but further refinements in technology allow a highly accurate identification of APA as small as 1 cm. CT coupled with adrenal venous sampling for plasma aldosterone has become our preferred technique for localization. In contrast, small adrenal lesions are often not well visualized with adrenal MRI (Newhouse, 1990).

Treatment—Medical Management

Patients with APA should be managed with excision of the adrenal gland containing the adenoma, whereas patients with IHA should be managed with medical therapy—usually spironolactone (Aldactone). The rationale is based on the observation that both the metabolic abnormalities and the hypertension are alleviated, following uniadrenalectomy in 70 to 80 per cent of patients with APA. Patients with IAH usually do not become normotensive following partial or total bilateral adrenalectomy. Moreover, patients with APA frequently require higher doses of spironolactone for correction of both hypertension and hypokalemia. Accordingly, the studies previously listed to differentiate APA from IAH are of more than academic interest. Rarely, we have seen patients with bilateral hyperplasia and asymmetric aldosterone secretion with the major aldosterone production issuing from a markedly larger hyperplastic adrenal gland. In this setting, unilateral adrenalectomy has resulted in cure of the metabolic derangement and hypertension. Whether this observation means that occasionally a hyperplastic gland can develop an "autonomous" dominant nodule is conjectural (Banks et al., 1984).

Hence, spironolactone, 100 to 400 mg per day, is the treatment of choice for most patients with bilateral hyperplasia or for those who refuse surgical exploration. The blood pressure response to spironolactone has been suggested as a screening test for primary hyperaldosteronism (Conn et al., 1964). However, patients with low renin essential hypertension also respond well to spironolactone (Vaughan et al., 1973).

Patients with APA are generally recommended to have uniadrenalectomy unless there are major medical complications. It is our practice to prepare the patients preoperatively with spironolactone, 100 to 400 mg/day for 3 to 4 weeks, to lower blood pressure and correct hypokalemia. Whether spironolactone enhances the recovery of renin secretion by the kidney or contralateral adrenal aldosterone secretion is unclear (Morimoto et al., 1970).

PHEOCHROMOCYTOMA

Pheochromocytoma is an uncommon entity but one that has fascinated both clinicians and investigators who have worked together to derive effective means for detection, localization, and management (Bravo and Gifford, 1984; Manger and Gifford, 1990). Although the causative factor of hypertension in less than 1 per cent of the hypertensive population, detection is mandatory not only for the potential of cure of the hypertension but also to avoid the potentially lethal effects of the unrecognized tumor.

Clinical manifestations of pheochromocytoma are all due to the physiologic effects of the amines produced by the lesion. Epinephrine and norepinephrine are similar as regards their metabolic action, though epinephrine is more potent. The symptom complex manifested by the patient will depend somewhat on the secretory products, both type and amount, including the more unusual products dopa and dopamine as well as a variety of peptides produced from amine precursor uptake and decarboxylation (APUD) type cells (Pearse, 1971; Bolande, 1974). The peptides are ACTH, somatostatin, serotonin, enkephalins, calciotonin, vasoactive intestinal polypeptide, neuropeptide, lipotropin, β-endorphin, and dynorphin (Robertson, 1990). Small tumors generally bind catecholamine poorly. Thus, the severity of symptoms, despite the small size of these tumors, results from direct release of most of catecholamines directly into the circulation. Large lesions have high catecholamine content but bind them well and metabolize substantial quantities directly within the tumors. Thus, only relatively small amounts of the vasoactive amines mixed with large amounts of inactive metabolites are secreted (see Fig. 64–17).

Signs and Symptoms

Signs and symptoms of patients with pheochromocytoma, all secondary to secretion of the neurohumoral agents, epinephrine and norepinephrine, may be extraordinarily variable. In all reported series, hypertension is by far the most consistent sign (Tables 64–12 and 64–13). Of 106 patients reported by Van Heerden and colleagues (1982) 84 per cent were hypertensive. As a sign itself, hypertension may have a variability of manifestations. The three common patterns are as follows:

1. *Sustained hypertension*—37 per cent of Van Heerden's patients manifest sustained hypertension with little fluctuation—much as in patients with essential hypertension. This form is most common in children and patients with multiple endocrine adenoma type II.

Table 64–12. SYMPTOMS REPORTED BY 76 PATIENTS (ALMOST ALL ADULTS) WITH PHEOCHROMOCYTOMA ASSOCIATED WITH PAROXYSMAL OR PERSISTENT HYPERTENSION

Symptoms	Per Cent Paroxysmal (37 Patients)	Per Cent Persistent (39 Patients)
Symptoms Presumably Due to Excessive Catecholamines or Hypertension		
Headache (severe)	92	72
Excessive sweating (generalized)	65	69
Palpitations ± tachycardia	73	51
Anxiety or nervousness (± fear of impending death, panic)	60	28
Tremulousness	51	26
Pain in chest, abdomen (usually epigastric), lumbar regions, lower abdomen, or groin	48	28
Nausea ± vomiting	43	26
Weakness, fatigue, prostration	38	15
Weight loss (severe)	14	15
Dyspnea	11	18
Warmth ± heat intolerance	13	15
Visual disturbances	3	21
Dizziness or faintness	11	3
Constipation	0	13
Paresthesia or pain in arms	11	0
Bradycardia (noted by patient)	8	3
Grand mal	5	3

Manifestations Due to Complications
Congestive heart failure ± cardiomyopathy
Myocardial infarction
Cerebrovascular accident
Ischemic enterocolitis ± megacolon
Azotemia
Dissecting aneurysm
Encephalopathy
Shock
Hemorrhagic necrosis in a pheochromocytoma

Manifestations Due to Coexisting Diseases or Syndromes
Cholelithiasis
Medullary thyroid carcinoma ± effects of secretions of serotonin, calcitonin, prostaglandin, or ACTH-like substance
Hyperparathyroidism
Mucocutaneous neuromas with characteristic facies
Thickened corneal nerves (seen only with slit lamp)
Marfanoid habitus
Alimentary tract ganglioneuromatosis
Neurofibromatosis and its complications
Cushing's syndrome (rare)
Von Hippel-Lindau disease (rare)
Virilism, Addison's disease, acromegaly (extremely rare)

Symptoms Caused by Encroachment on Adjacent Structures or by Invasion and Pressure Effects of Metastases

From Manger, W. M., and Gifford, R. W., Jr.: Pheochromocytoma. In Laragh, J. H., and Brenner, B. M. (Eds.). Hypertension Pathophysiology Diagnosis and Management. New York, Raven Press, 1990.

2. *Paroxysmal hypertension*—"dramatic attacks" of hypertension, usually associated with other signs and symptoms, punctuating the patient's usual asymptomatic, normotensive status. This pattern more readily provokes the suspicion of and work-up for the possibility of an underlying pheochromocytoma and was reported to affect 47 per cent of the patients. Females are more likely than males to manifest paroxysmal hypertension.

3. *Sustained hypertension with superimposed paroxysms*—the phenomenon is self-explanatory. Manger and

Table 64–13. SIGNS OBSERVED IN PATIENTS WITH PHEOCHROMOCYTOMA

Blood Pressure Changes

± Hypertension ± wide fluctuations (rarely, proxysmal hypotension or hypertension alternating with hypotension)

Hypertension induced by physical maneuver such as exercise, postural change, or palpation and massage of flank or mass elsewhere

Orthostatic hypotension ± postural tachycardia

Paradoxical blood pressure response to certain antihypertensive drugs; marked pressor response with induction of anesthesia

Other Signs of Catecholamine Excess

Hyperhidrosis

Tachycardia or reflex bradycardia, very forceful heartbeat, arrhythmia

Pallor of face and upper part of body (rarely flushing; mottled cyanosis)

Anxious, frightened, troubled appearance

Hypertensive retinopathy

Dilated pupils (very rarely exophthalmos, lacrimation, scleral pallor, or injection; pupils may not react to light)

Leanness or underweight

Tremor (± shaking)

Raynaud's phenomenon or livedo reticularis (occasionally puffy, red, cyanotic hands in children); skin of extremities wet, cold, clammy, or pale; gooseflesh; occasionally cyanotic nail beds

Fever

Mass Lesion (Rarely Palpable)

Tumor in abdomen or neck (pheochromocytoma, chemodectoma, thyroid carcinoma, or thyroid swelling that is very rare and only during hypertensive paroxysm)

Signs Caused by Encroachment on Adjacent Structures or by Invasion and Pressure Effects of Metastases

Manifestations Related to Complications or to Coexisting Diseases or Syndromes

From Manger, W. M., and Gifford, R. W., Jr.: Pheochromocytoma. *In* Laragh, J. H., Brenner, B. M. (Eds.): Hypertension Pathophysiology Diagnosis and Management. New York, Raven Press, 1990.

Gifford (1990) have reported a 50 per cent incidence of this manifestation. Scott reported 66 per cent (Scott et al., 1976; Scott et al., 1990).

The frequency of attacks among patients is quite variable, ranging from a few times per year to multiple daily episodes. Their duration may be minutes to hours, usually with rapid onset and slower subsidence. One or more episodes a week occur in 75 per cent of patients. Daily attacks, or more than one attack each day, occur in nearly all other patients. Among patients with pheochromocytoma, half experience symptoms for a duration of less than 15 minutes. In 80 per cent of patients, attacks last less than an hour. With passage of time after the initial appearance of symptoms, frequency of attacks tends to increase, although severity may or may not change.

Attacks may occur in the absence of recognizable stimuli. However, a multitude of associated factors have been reported: compression of the tumor elicited by massage, physical exercise, particularly a certain posture or lying in a certain position, and direct trauma. Similar precursors of attacks are the wearing of tight clothing, straining to defecate or to void, micturition itself, bladder distention, sexual intercourse, laughing, sneezing, coughing, retching, Valsalva maneuver, and hyperventilation, which cause increased intra-abdominal pressure. Foods that are rich in tyramine may elicit attacks: beer, wine, and aged cheese. Potentially provocative drugs are tyramine, histamine, epinephrine and norepinephrine, nicotine, glucagon, tetraethylammonium, methacholine, succinylcholine, phenothiazine, ACTH, saralasin, other angiotensin II analogues, and beta blockers such as propranolol.

Additional signs and symptoms are numerous but not specific. Among these are headaches, sweating, pallor or flushing, palpitations, tachycardia, abdominal and/or chest pain, and postural hypotension. Also common are weakness, nausea, emesis, and anorexia. Profound psychologic changes are frequently observed. The occasional patient, in whom the diagnosis has not been recognized, has sometimes been referred for psychiatric evaluation of what was thought to have been functional symptoms.

Some patients have been symptomatic for years before diagnosis. Others may present with convulsions, cerebrovascular accidents, and coma. Others have died of massive intracranial bleeding. The appearance of sudden, severe hypertension during the induction of anesthesia or during the course of a surgical procedure may herald underlying pheochromocytoma.

Patients may have pheochromocytomas without manifesting hypertension. About 10 per cent of pheochromocytomas are found in normotensive patients (Scott et al., 1976). On occasion, during a severe paroxysmal attack, blood pressure may be unobtainable. Herein, the patient is not hypotensive. Marked peripheral vasoconstriction occurs; therefore, one cannot measure the blood pressure with a sphygmomanometer. Hypertension may also be modest in nature, less serious than other signs and symptoms. Flushing, pallor, and signs of hypermetabolism closely mimic the classic appearance of thyrotoxicosis, leading to surgery of the thyroid gland before recognition of the underlying cause of the disease process.

Many reports exist of pheochromocytoma diagnosed during pregnancy (Fudge et al., 1980; Schenker et al., 1971). Symptoms commonly mimic those of eclampsia, preeclampsia, and toxemia. Headache, visual disturbances, palpitations, diaphoresis, and hypertension (paroxysmal or sustained) are common. According to Fudge and associates (1980), the diagnosis of pheochromocytoma in association with pregnancy has been made prior to delivery in only one third of patients. All too often it is only with stress of labor and delivery, although more commonly during the postpartum period, that resultant fulminant hypertension or shock leads to the diagnosis of an underlying pheochromocytoma (Hume, 1960). Maternal and infant mortality rates exceed 40 per cent. Despite a history of prior successful pregnancy, in the presence of hypertension, the diagnosis of pheochromocytoma should be considered in the pregnant patient with labile or postural hypertension, congestive heart failure, or arrhythmias. Appropriate diagnostic studies must be carried out.

Pheochromocytoma may be the underlying causative agent in patients afflicted by other various disease states with conditions that may result from excess catecholamine secretion. Common manifestations are cerebrovascular accident, encephalopathy, retinopathy, congestive heart failure, cardiomyopathy, dissecting aneurysm, shock, renal failure, azotemia, ischemic enterocolitis, and megacolon. Conversely, numerous entities mimic some of the symptoms and signs of pheochromocytoma (Table 64–14).

One specific entity that has gained more recognition is catecholamine-induced cardiomyopathy (Imperato-McGinley et al., 1987). Experimentally injected catecholamines can cause foci of myocardial necrosis, with inflammation and fibrosis (Rosenbaum et al., 1988; Van Vliet et al., 1966). These patients may have a reduction in blood pressure due to a global reduction in myocardial pump functions, considered to be due to both a down regulation of beta receptors and a decrease of viable myofibrils (Sardesai et al., 1990). Fortunately, the lesion is usually reversible with the combination of alpha-blockade and alpha-methylparatyrosine (Imperato-McGinley et al., 1987). All patients with pheochromocytoma should have a complete cardiac evaluation with echocardiograms and radionuclide scans prior to corrective surgery.

An appreciable number of pheochromocytomas have been found in association with several disease entities and hereditary syndromes (see Table 64–14). Tank and co-workers (1982) estimate that 95 per cent of pheochromocytomas are sporadic in occurrence but that the remaining 5 per cent have a familial pattern. However, 10 per cent is often reported. Calkins and Howard (1947) published the first report of familial pheochromocytoma. Familial transmission is believed to be through autosomal dominance, with a locus on chromosome 10 (Simpson et al., 1987) found in the subset designated multiple endocrine neoplasia (MEN), type 2.

Familial pheochromocytomas may be divided into different types of genetic abnormalities. In 1961, Sipple described the combination of pheochromocytoma and medullary carcinoma (MCT) of the thyroid that came to be known as Sipple's syndrome. In subsequent years, as more cases came to light, new terminology—MEA (multiple endocrine adenopathy) or MEN—has been popularized as has a subclassification system: MEA I, MEA II, and MEA III or MEA IIb (Raue et al., 1985). Pheochromocytomas occur in MEA II, a triad including pheochromocytoma, MCT, and parathyroid adenomas. The last may be a secondary phenomenon. The parafollicular cells of MCT elaborate thyrocalcitonin. The resulting decrease in serum calcium concentration leads to parathyroid stimulation with subsequent hyperplasia or development of adenomas. Pheochromocytoma may also be a part of MEN III, which also includes MCT, mucosal neuromas, thickened corneal nerves, alimentary tract, ganglioneuromatosis, and frequently a marfanoid habitus (Manger and Gifford, 1990).

Recognition of MEA II and aggressive evaluation of MEA II kindreds are mandatory. Carney and associates (1976) report 22 per cent mortality from complications of pheochromocytoma in a review of 149 patients with MEA II. MCT has an expected incidence of 50 per cent in MEA II kindred.

The neuroectodermal dysplasias are a group of related diseases: Von Recklinghausen's disease (neurofibromatosis), tuberous sclerosis, Sturge-Weber syndrome, and Von Hippel-Lindau disease. All are strongly familial

Table 64–14. DIFFERENTIAL DIAGNOSIS*

All hypertensives (sustained and paroxysmal)
Anxiety, tension states, psychoneurosis, psychosis
Hyperthyroidism
Paroxysmal tachycardia
Hyperdynamic beta-adrenergic circulatory state
Menopause
Vasodilating headache (migraine and cluster headaches)
Coronary insufficiency syndrome
Acute hypertensive encephalopathy
Diabetes mellitus
Renal parenchymal or renal arterial disease with hypertension
Focal arterial insufficiency of the brain
Intracranial lesions (with or without increased intracranial pressure)
Autonomic hyperreflexia
Diencephalic seizure and syndrome
Toxemia of pregnancy (or *eclampsia with convulsions*)
Hypertensive crises associated with monoamine oxidase inhibitors
Carcinoid
Hypoglycemia
Mastocytosis
Familial dysautonomia
Acrodynia
Neuroblastoma; ganglioneuroblastoma; ganglioneuroma
Neurofibromatosis (with or without renal arterial disease)
Adrenocortical carcinoma
Acute infectious disease

Rare causes of paroxysmal hypertension (*acute medullary hyperplasia, acute porphyria, lead poisoning,* tabetic crisis, encephalitis, *clonidine withdrawal,* hypovolemia with inappropriate vasoconstriction, pulmonary artery fibrosarcoma, port hypersensitivity, dysregulation of hypothalamus, *tetanus, Guillain-Barré syndrome, factitious*)

Fortuitous circumstances simulating pheochromocytoma
Conditions sometimes associated with pheochromocytoma
  Coexisting disease or syndromes
    Cholelithiasis
    Medullary thyroid carcinoma
    Hyperparathyroidism
    Mucosal neuromas
    Thickened corneal nerves
    Marfanoid habitus
    Alimentary tract ganglioneuromatosis
    Neurofibromatosis
    Cushing's syndrome
    Von Hippel-Lindau disease
    Polycythemia
    Virilism, Addison's disease, acromegaly
  Complications
    Cardiovascular disease†
    Cerebrovascular disease
    Renovascular disease
    Circulatory shock
    Renal insufficiency
    Hemorrhagic necrosis of pheochromocytoma†
    Dissecting aneurysm†
    Ischemic enterocolitis with or without intestinal obstruction†

*Conditions in italics may have increased excretion of catecholamines and/or metabolites.
†Patient may present as having abdominal or cardiovascular catastrophe.
From Manger, W. M., and Gifford, R. W., Jr.: Pheochromocytoma. *In* Laragh, J. H., and Brenner, B. M. (Eds.): Hypertension Pathophysiology Diagnosis and Management. New York, Raven Press, 1990.

and associated with each other and with pheochromocytoma.

The prevalence of pheochromocytoma in patients with neurofibromatosis is reported as 1 to 2 per cent. Of those patients with pheochromocytoma, 5 per cent have Von Recklinghausen's disease. Kalff and associates (1982), having seen ten patients with pheochromocytoma and neurofibromatosis, reviewed the sample population, selecting patients with both Von Recklinghausen's disease and hypertension. They found 17 such patients, 53 per cent of whom had pheochromocytomas.

Pheochromocytoma is distinctly less common than the other neuroectodermal dysplasias (Kalff et al., 1982). The rare association of a somatostatin-rich duodenal carcinoid tumor and pheochromocytoma has also been reported (Wheeler et al., 1986).

The increased incidence of pheochromocytomas in association with the neuroectodermal dysplasias and MCT may be explained by the APUD cell system of Pearse. The APUD cells derive from the neural crest of the embryo, sharing common ultrastructural and cytochemical features and elaborating amines by precursor uptake and decarboxylation (Bolande, 1974; Pearse, 1971). The products of these cells have been previously listed. Immunochemical techniques showing both neuron-specific enolase and chromogranin A in a variety of polypeptide hormone-producing tissues support the concept of the APUD system (Fig. 64–39) (Lloyd et al., 1984; O'Connor et al., 1983).

Children

Manifestations of pheochromocytoma in children vary somewhat from those in adults. Headache, nausea and/or vomiting, weight loss, and visual complaints occur more commonly in children than in adults. Manger reports polydypsia, polyuria, and convulsions—rarely observed in adults—occurring in 25 per cent of children. Puffy, red, and cyanotic appearance of the hands is reported in 11 per cent of children. Of children with pheochromocytomas, 90 per cent have sustained hypertension. Paroxysmal hypertension occurs in less than 10 per cent of children (Manger and Gifford, 1977).

In contrast to adults, children manifest a higher incidence of familial pheochromocytomas (10 per cent) and bilaterality (24 per cent). Multiple pheochromocytomas have been reported in children with an incidence of 15 to 32 per cent, and extra-adrenal location of pheochromocytomas has been reported in 15 to 31 per cent of the children (Glenn et al., 1968). Glenn and co-workers (1968) believed that on a histologic basis, there was a higher incidence of malignant pheochromocytomas in children. Stackpole's review found a random distribution of age at diagnosis among the males. In females the diagnosis was made in 62 per cent during menarche (Stackpole et al., 1963).

Laboratory Diagnosis of Pheochromocytoma

The clinical diagnosis of pheochromocytoma is based on the subjective evaluation of signs and symptoms. Laboratory confirmation of the clinical diagnosis is man-

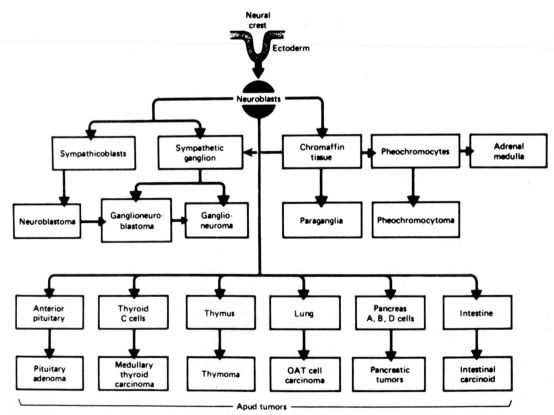

Figure 64–39. Ectodermal origin of APUD (i.e., amine precursor uptake and decarboxylation) tumors. (From Manger, W. M., and Gifford, R. W., Jr.: Pheochromocytoma. *In* Laragh, J. H., and Brenner, B. M. (Eds.): Hypertension Pathophysiology Diagnosis and Management. New York, Raven Press, 1990.)

datory and may be divided into two general categories: biochemical diagnosis and radiologic diagnosis (Fig. 64–40).

Confirmation of the diagnosis is by demonstrating elevated levels of catecholamines in the blood or urine, which occur in 95 to 99 per cent of patients with pheochromocytoma. Extremely accurate assays exist (Dolan and Carey, 1989; Manger and Gifford, 1990). However, there are a considerable number of foods and drugs that can affect urinary levels of catecholamines or breakdown products (Table 64–15). Plasma catecholamines are highly responsive to stress, activity, blood loss, and other stimuli.

Because of the severe consequences of the undiagnosed pheochromocytoma, it is recommended that all hypertensive patients be screened. Measurement of urinary catecholamines and vanillylmandelic acid (VMA) is less reliable (Manger and Gifford, 1990).

Rarely, the concentrations of plasma and urinary catecholamines and their metabolites are not elevated, especially if the patient is normotensive at the time of study. In this clinical setting, if there is a high index of suspicion, imaging studies with ^{131}I-metaiodobenzylguanidine (Shapiro, 1985), MRI (Newhouse, 1990), or repeating sampling when the patients are hypertensive is indicated. Provocative tests with histamine, glucagon, or phentolamine are rarely used (Dolan and Carey, 1989).

In contrast, some patients with essential hypertension and signs or symptoms of pheochromocytoma will have slightly elevated plasma catecholamine levels, probably representing a neurogenic component to the hypertension. The clonidine suppression test distinguishes these patients (Bravo et al., 1981; Karlberg and Hedman, 1986). Following a single 0.3-mg oral dose of clonidine, patients with neurogenic hypertension at rest show a 50 per cent fall in plasma norepinephrine level, whereas patients with pheochromocytoma do not.

Whether an elevation of catecholamines in platelets (Zweifler and Julius, 1982) or a decrease in beta-adrenoreceptors on leucocytes (Valet et al., 1987) in patients with pheochromocytoma will be sufficiently sensitive and specific remains to be determined.

Radiologic Tests

Similar to other adrenal tumors, the development of sectional imaging was a major advancement in the diagnosis and localization of pheochromocytoma (Kazam et al., 1989). For adrenal pheochromocytomas, the CT accuracy for detection is over 90 per cent (Abrams et al., 1982; Thomas et al., 1980) and rapidly replaced angiography, venography, and ultrasonography for extraadrenal pheochromocytoma, in which the detection is less (about 75 per cent). However, CT does not aid in differentiating pheochromocytomas from other adrenal lesions or in predicting malignancy. Accordingly, CT has been suggested as the initial imaging procedure.

We have been impressed with the multiple uses of the MRI scan in patients with pheochromocytoma. The test appears to be as accurate as CT in identifying lesions,

while also having a characteristic bright, "light bulb" image on T2 weighted study (Fig. 64–41) (Reinig, 1986). In addition, sagittal and coronal imaging can give excellent anatomic information concerning the relationship between the tumor and the surrounding vasculature as well as the draining venous channels (Figs. 64–42 and 64–43). As MRI technology improves, it is likely that it will become the initial imaging study.

An alternative approach that is also useful at times, particularly in the search for residual or multiple pheochromocytoma, is the metaiodobenzylguanidine (MIBG) scan that images medullary tissue (Shapiro et al., 1985). In the experience in 400 cases, the developers of the technique found a 78.4 per cent sensitivity in primary sporadic tumors, 92.4 per cent in malignant lesions, and 94.3 per cent in familial cases, giving an overall sensitivity of 87.4 per cent with 99 per cent specificity. Thus, the test may be more sensitive than

Table 64–15. EFFECTS OF DRUGS AND INTERFERING SUBSTANCES ON CONCENTRATIONS OF URINARY CATECHOLAMINES AND METABOLITES*

Upper Limit of Normal (Adult) (mg/24 h)		Effects	
		Increases Apparent Value	*Decreases Apparent Value*
Catecholamines		Catecholamines	Fenfluramine
Epinephrine	0.02	Drugs containing	(large doses)
Norepinephrine	0.08	catecholamines	
Total	0.10	Isoprenolol	
Dopamine	0.20	(isoproterenol)†	
		Levodopa	
		Methyldopa	
		Labetalol†	
		Tetracyclines†	
		Erythromycin†	
		Chlorpromazine†	
		Other fluorescent substances† (e.g., quinine, quinidine, bile in urine)	
		Rapid clonidine withdrawal	
		Ethanol	
Metanephrines		Catecholamines	Methylglucamine
Metanephrine	0.4	Drugs containing	(in Renovist,
Normetanephrine	0.9	catecholamines	Renografin,
Total	1.3	Monoamine oxidase inhibitors	etc.)
		Benzodiazepines	Fenfluramine
		Rapid clonidine withdrawal	(large doses)
		Ethanol	
Vanillymandelic acid	6.5	Catecholamines (minimal increase)	Clofibrate
		Drugs containing catecholamines (minimal increase)	Disulfiram
			Ethanol
		Levodopa	Monoamine oxidase inhibitors
		Nalidixic acid†	Fenfluramine
		Rapid clonidine withdrawal	(large doses)

*As determined by most reliable assays.
†Probably spurious interference with fluorescence assays.
(From Manger, W. M., and Gifford, R. W., Jr.: Pheochromocytoma. In Laragh, J. H., and Brenner, B. M. (Eds.): Hypertension Pathophysiology Diagnosis and Management. New York, Raven Press, 1990.)

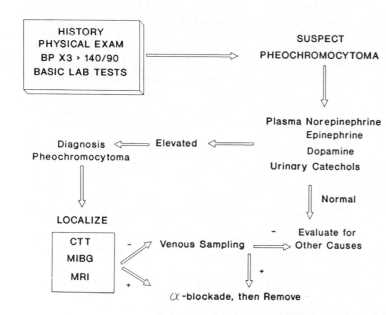

Figure 64–40. Identifying pheochromocytoma. (From Vaughan, E. D., Jr.: Diagnosis of adrenal disorders in hypertension. World J. Urol., 7:111–116, 1989.)

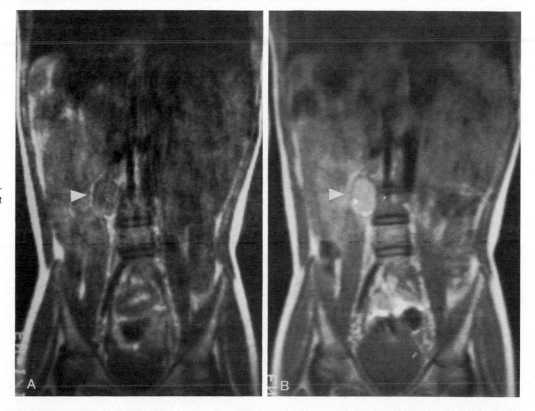

Figure 64–41. Extra-adrenal pheo-chromocytoma showing a bright T2 image *B*.

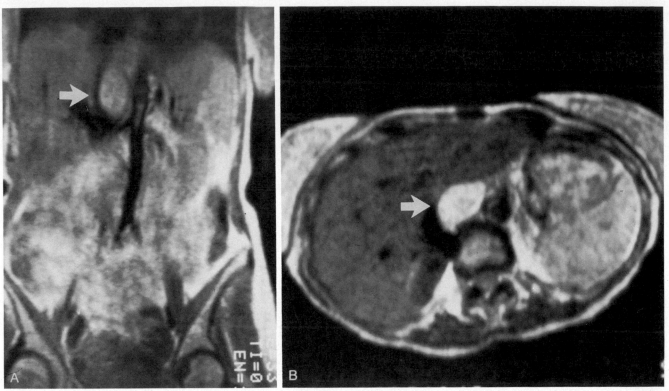

Figure 64–42. Magnetic resonance image of pheochromocytoma. Right adrenal arising from the medial limb, which grew medial to the inferior vena cava above the celiac axis under the caudate lobe of the liver and was missed at first abdominal exploration. Intra-aortico-caval location is clearly seen on these films.

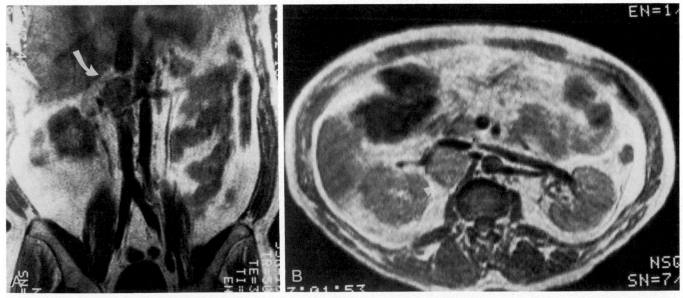

Figure 64–43. Magnetic resonance image of recurrent pheochromocytoma with an excellent demonstration of anterior crossing right renal vein, feeding lumbar vein, and involvement of right renal artery.

CT in patients with extra-adrenal lesions. The isotope may be picked up by other APUD cell–type tumors. In a smaller series involving children, the MIBG scan findings were positive in all cases (Deal et al., 1990). In summary, the MIBG scan is highly sensitive and is a useful tool, especially if CT and MRI findings are negative or confusing (Fig. 64–44).

Sequential venous sampling has been utilized successfully to identify small extra-adrenal lesions.

Preoperative Management

There is unanimity of opinion that surgical extirpation is the only effective treatment for pheochromocytoma. The one accepted exception to this principle is treatment late in pregnancy. The patient should be treated with alpha-adrenergic blockade via oral administration of phenoxybenzamine until the fetus has reached maturity. At this point, cesarean section with tumor excision in one operation should be carried out, without allowing the patient to undergo the stress of vaginal delivery.

In the past, one of the most controversial issues in the management of patients with pheochromocytoma was whether or not to employ pharmacologic blockade preoperatively (Boutros et al., 1990). We do not believe that there is an issue at the present time. The evolution of an accurate localization test weakens the argument that alpha-blockade limits the ability to identify the lesion at the time of exploration.

Moreover, the greater stability of the patient with adequate preoperative preparation greatly facilitates the procedure for both surgeon and anesthesiologist as well as increasing the safety to the patient.

At our institution, the preoperative medical preparation is of utmost importance to provide an ideal anesthetic and operative environment. The perioperative course will be smoother with adequate preoperative preparation. Phenoxybenzamine hydrochloride (Dibenzyline), a long-acting alpha-adrenergic blocker, controls the blood pressure in patients with pheochromocytoma. The initial divided dose of 20 to 30 mg is given orally and is increased by 10 to 20 mg per day, until the blood

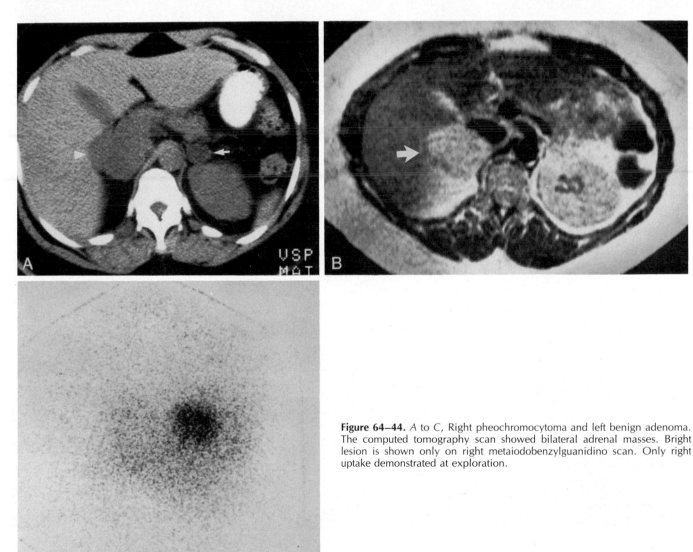

Figure 64–44. *A* to *C*, Right pheochromocytoma and left benign adenoma. The computed tomography scan showed bilateral adrenal masses. Bright lesion is shown only on right metaiodobenzylguanidino scan. Only right uptake demonstrated at exploration.

pressure has been stabilized and there is mild postural hypotension. Usually, a dose of 40 to 100 mg per day is required.

Beta-adrenergic blockers, such as propranolol, have been added to alpha blockers to prepare patients for anesthesia and surgery. Beta blockers protect against arrhythmias and permit reduction in the amount of alpha-adrenergic blockers necessary to control blood pressure (Ross et al., 1967). Beta blockers have also been given when tachyphylaxis to alpha blockers occurs. However, they must be used carefully (Salem and Ivankovic, 1969). Beta-adrenergic blocker should be administered only when alpha blockade is established. Beta blockade alone may cause a marked rise in the total peripheral vascular resistance secondary to unopposed alpha-adrenergic activity. Accordingly, we do not routinely prepare patients with propranolol. A beta-adrenergic blocker is provided only when cardiac arrhythmias are prominent. Propranolol is given orally in doses of 20 to 40 mg three or four times daily. Labetalol, an alpha- and beta-adrenergic blocking agent, has been utilized but may not control hypertension (Briggs et al., 1978; Rosen et al., 1976).

Alpha-methylparatyrosine (metyrosine, a tyrosine hydroxylase inhibitor) has been recommended in addition to phenoxybenzamine and/or propranolol during preparation of the patient for anesthesia and surgery (Engleman et al., 1968; Sjoerdsma et al., 1965). Metyrosine decreases the rate of catecholamine synthesis—the conversion of tyrosine to dihydroxyphenylalanine (DOPA). Adverse effects include crystalluria, sedation, diarrhea, anxiety, psychic disturbance, and extrapyramidal signs. Experience with alpha-methylparatyrosine is limited, although its combination with alpha-adrenergic blockade has been recommended (Perry et al., 1990). We therefore do not use it routinely. We reserve the drug for patients who have myocarditis, multiple catecholamine-secreting paragangliomas, or resistance to alpha-adrenergic blockers. Alpha-methylparatyrosine is given in doses of 0.5 to 1.0 g orally three or four times daily and is usually started prior to surgery (Reckler et al., 1989). The dose is determined by repeat catecholamine evaluations.

Prazosin, a specific postsynaptic alpha$_1$-adrenergic blocker, has gained rapid acceptance as an effective antihypertensive agent. The drug has been evaluated in the medical management of patients with pheochromocytoma either alone (Wallace and Gill, 1978) or in combination with a beta blocker. However, we have experience with four patients who were prepared with prazosin alone for surgical removal of adrenal pheochromocytoma. The control of blood pressure was effective preoperatively but was not adequate during surgical removal of the tumor. Marked blood pressure elevations were present in all four patients. In contrast to phenoxybenzamine that binds irreversibly to alpha-adrenergic receptors, prazosin blockade is reversible and may be overwhelmed by the surge in catecholamine secretion during intubation and surgical manipulation. We have since abandoned prazosin in preparing patients for anesthesia and surgery (Nicholson et al., 1983).

In addition to the alpha- and beta-blocking agents, it is important that the state of hydration and blood volume be evaluated, because many patients have decreased intravascular volume. Crystalloids or blood transfusion may be needed to raise the intravascular volume to accommodate the expanded vascular bed produced by alpha-blocking agents. To avoid this potential problem, patients are given two units of packed cells and receive a liter of 5 per cent glucose in Ringer's lactate preoperatively, although blood has been omitted lately in some cases for fear of acquired immune deficiency syndrome transmission. The alpha-blocking agent and beta-blocking agent (if used) should be used up to and including the day of surgery.

Anesthetic Management*

Anesthetic management of the patient undergoing surgical removal of a pheochromocytoma is directed toward control of the cardiovascular system (Robertson et al., 1990). Close monitoring is of utmost importance and includes attention to the electrocardiogram, blood pressure (arterial line for continuous arterial pressure reading), urinary output, and central venous pressure. A Swan-Ganz catheter may be employed to measure pulmonary capillary wedge pressure if the patient has left ventricular dysfunction.

Induction with sodium pentothal has been used in almost every case of pheochromocytoma reported. Virtually all inhalational agents have been administered for the maintenance of anesthesia. Uncontrolled hypertension, severe hypotension, and cardiac arrhythmias are the problems that must be anticipated. The anesthesiologist must be prepared to treat each condition that may occur. Severe hypertension may occur during intubation and manipulation of the tumor. Hypertension may also be precipitated by increased intra-abdominal pressure during transfer to the operating table, coughing, or surgical preparation. Therefore, adequate depth of anesthesia is necessary during all these maneuvers. Patients with pheochromocytomas have been successfully anesthetized with a variety of agents including diethylether, methoxyflurane, halothane, enflurane, isoflurane, and neuroleptanesthesia with droperidol and fentanyl (Innovar). Although diethylether is alleged to liberate catecholamines, tachycardia and cardiac arrhythmias were not major problems when it was administered.

Of the current agents, halothane is undesirable because it is associated with a high incidence of serious ventricular arrhythmias in the presence of an excess of circulating catecholamines. Many workers have reported favorably on neuroleptanesthesia with a combination of droperidol and fentanyl for removal of pheochromocytoma. Droperidol antagonizes the pressor effects of the catecholamines and prevents dysrhythmia by either alpha blockade or local anesthetic action. Bittar (1979), however, described hypertensive crisis following Innovar administration to patients with pheochromocytomas.

The safest anesthetics available appear to be enflurane and isoflurane. Both have provided good results. Enflu-

---

*From Reckler, J. M., Vaughan, E. D., Jr., Tjeuw, M., Carey, R. M.: Pheochromocytoma. *In* Vaughan, E. D., Jr., and Carey, R. M. (Eds.): Adrenal Disorders. Thieme Medical Publishers, Inc., New York, 1989.

rane decreases myocardial irritability. However, 2 per cent of enflurane is metabolized to inorganic fluoride, which has potential toxicity in patients with pre-existing kidney disease. The small amount of free fluoride levels do not damage normal kidneys, but Mazze and associates have suggested that these low levels could cause deterioration of renal function in a patient with pre-existing renal disease.

Isoflurane, an isomer of enflurane, also decreases myocardial irritability, but it is more resistant to metabolism. Only 0.2 per cent is metabolized. Systemic hypertension was controlled with isoflurane alone or in combination with phentolamine (Regitine) or nitroprusside. Accordingly, isoflurane appears to be the anesthetic of choice (Suzukawa et al., 1983).

Neuromuscular blocking agents selected for surgery for pheochromocytoma have included succinylcholine, d-tubocurarare, and pancuronium. Gallamine has been generally avoided because of its anticholinergic action and resulting tachycardia.

Succinylcholine can lower the cardiac excitability threshold and cause arrhythmia. Small amounts of d-tubocurarare block arrhythmias induced by succinylcholine. This is probably due to ganglion-blocking effects of d-tubocurarare. Tumor catecholamines may be released by d-tubocurarare through its histamine release. However, clinically, both succinylcholine and d-tubocurarare have been successful. Pancuronium does release histamine and has no ganglion-blocking effect in humans.

Both lidocaine and propranolol have been utilized for treatment of arrhythmias during surgery. Intravenous (IV) lidocaine, 1 mg per kg, is effective to treat ventricular arrhythmias, and propranolol, 1 to 2 mg IV bolus is effective to control sinus tachycardia. Arrhythmias often disappear spontaneously when hypertension is controlled.

Nitroprusside and phentolamine are the drugs most often administered for management of hypertensive episodes during the stress of anesthesia and exploration. We prefer phentolamine, because it is effective in controlling blood pressure, is short-acting, and is theoretically more physiologic, as it is an alpha-adrenergic blocker. Nitroprusside is given to phentolamine-resistant patients. If immediate lowering of the blood pressure is desired, nitroprusside is also used.

When the blood supply of the tumor has been curtailed, a fall in circulatory catecholamine levels may result in hypotension. Volume replacement is the treatment of choice, with careful cardiovascular monitoring. If vasopressors are needed, norepinephrine (Levophed) in low dosages may be administered. When the circulation is stabilized and the vascular volume approaches normal, the vasopressor can be discontinued.

ADRENAL SURGERY

Surgical Options

There are numerous approaches to the adrenal gland (Table 64–16). The proper approach depends on the

Table 64–16. SURGICAL OPTIONS

Disease	Approach
Primary hyperaldosteronism	Posterior (left or right)
	Modified posterior (right)
	11th Rib (left > right)
	Posterior Transthoracic
Cushing's adenoma	11th Rib (left or right)
	Thoraco-abdominal (large)
	Posterior (small)
Cushing's disease	Bilateral posterior
Bilateral hyperplasia	Bilateral 11th Rib (alternating)
Adrenal carcinoma	Thoracoabdominal
	11th rib
	Transabdominal
Bilateral adrenal ablation	Bilateral posterior
Pheochromocytoma	Transabdominal Chevron
	Thoracoabdominal
	(large—usually right)
	11th rib
Neuroblastoma	Transabdominal
	11th rib

From Vaughan, E. D., Jr.: Adrenal surgery. In Marshall, F. (Ed.): Operative Urology. Philadelphia, W. B. Saunders Co., 1991.

underlying cause of the adrenal pathology, the size of the adrenal, the side of the lesion, the habitus of the patient, and the experience and preference of the operating surgeon (Vaughan, 1991). In some cases, options and a careful review of all these variables are required before a choice is made. Thus, each case should be considered individually, although there are preferred approaches for given diseases. For example, the posterior or modified posterior approach is preferred for small well-localized lesions. An abdominal approach is utilized for a patient with multiple pheochromocytoma. In contrast, a large adrenal carcinoma may require a thoracoabdominal approach and a well-localized large pheochromocytoma may best be excised through a similar incision if there is no evidence for multiple lesions.

Operative Techniques

Before describing specific techniques, some unifying concepts warrant attention. Adequate visualization with the wearing of head lamps is critical. Hemostasis should be rigorously maintained. The operator should bring the adrenal down by initially exposing the cranial attachments and by dividing the rich blood supply between right angle clips, utilizing the forceps cautery for additional control. The blood supply bounds the gland in a stellate fashion. It is often simplest to begin dissection laterally, identifying the vascular supply and then working around the cranial edge of the gland. Interestingly, the posterior surface of the adrenal is usually devoid of vasculature. The gland then can be drawn caudally with gentle traction on the kidney. The gland is extremely friable and fractures easily, which causes troublesome bleeding. In essence, the patient should be dissected from the tumor, a concept particularly true for a pheochromocytoma in which the gland should not be manipulated and early venous control is preferred.

Posterior Approach

The posterior position can be utilized for either bilateral adrenal exploration or unilateral removal of small tumors (Fig. 64–45). In the past, all patients with primary aldosteronism were explored in this fashion because of the inability to localize the lesion. Today, localization is mandatory before exploration is recommended. The bilateral approach is primarily utilized for ablative total adrenalectomy. The options for incisions are shown, and generally rib resection is preferable to obtain high exposure. Following standard subperiosteal rib resection, care must be taken with the diaphragmatic release. The pleura should be avoided, and the diaphragm swept cranially.

The fibrofatty contents within Gerota's fascia are swept away from the paraspinal musculature exposing a subdiaphragmatic "open space," which is the apex of the resection. The liver, within the peritoneum, is dissected off the anterior surface of the adrenal, and the cranial blood supply divided. Medially, on the right, the IVC is visualized. The short, high adrenal vein, entering the cava in dorsolateral fashion, is identified and can be clipped or ligated. The adrenal can be drawn caudally by traction on the kidney. Care must be taken to avoid apical branches of the renal artery. On the left, the approach is similar with division of the splenorenal ligament giving initial lateral exposure.

The posterior approach can also be modified for a transthoracic adrenal exposure through the diaphragm (Novick et al., 1989). However, we rarely find this more extensive approach necessary for small adrenal tumors.

Modified Posterior Approach

Although the posterior position has the advantages of rapid adrenal exposure and low morbidity, there are definite disadvantages. The jackknife position may impair respiration, the abdominal contents are compressed posteriorly, and the visual field is limited. The advantage of the posterior approach is primarily for control of the short, right adrenal vein (Fig. 64–46); therefore, we have developed a modified approach for right adrenalectomy (Vaughan and Phillips, 1987).

The approach is based on the anatomic relationship of the right adrenal, which lies deeply posterior and high in the retroperitoneum behind the liver (see Fig. 64–46). In addition, the short, stubby right adrenal vein enters the IVC posteriorly at the apex of the adrenal. Hence, we utilize an approach that is posterior but with the patient in a modified position, similar to that for a Gil-Vernet dorsal lombotomy incision (see Fig. 64–46)

Figure 64–45. Posterior approach to the adrenals. (From Vaughan, E. D., Jr.: Adrenal surgery. In Marshall, F. F. (Ed.): Operative Urology. Philadelphia, W. B. Saunders Co., 1991.)

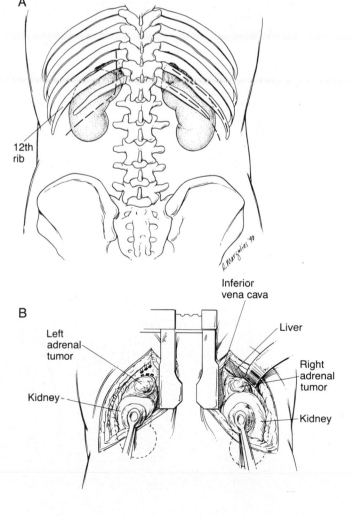

(Gil-Vernet, 1965). The patient is placed in this position, and the 11th or 12th rib are resected with care to avoid the pleura. The diaphragm is resected off the underlying peritoneum and liver and should be sharply dissected free in order to gain mobility. Similarly, the inferior surface of the peritoneum, closely associated with the liver, is sharply dissected from Gerota's fascia, which is gently retracted inferiorly.

The adrenal becomes visible in the depth of the incision, as the final hepatic attachments are divided. A lateral space can be found exposing the posterior abdominal musculature. The adrenal lies against the paraspinal muscles and multiple small adrenal arteries that actually course behind the IVC, emerge over these muscles, and are clipped and divided (see Fig. 64–46). At this point, the adrenal can usually be moved against

the paraspinal musculature exposing the IVC below the adrenal gland.

The major advantage of this approach is that the adrenal vein is also identified without difficulty, because it emerges from the segment of the IVC exposed and courses up to the adrenal, which now rises toward the operating surgeon. In other flank or anterior approaches, the adrenal vein resides in its posterior relationship, requiring caval rotation with the chance of adrenal vein avulsion. After adrenal vein exposure, it is doubly tied and divided or clipped with right angle clips and divided (see Fig. 64–46).

The adrenal can now be retracted inferiorly for division of the remaining arteries and total removal. The wound is not drained and is closed with interrupted 0 polydioxanone sutures.

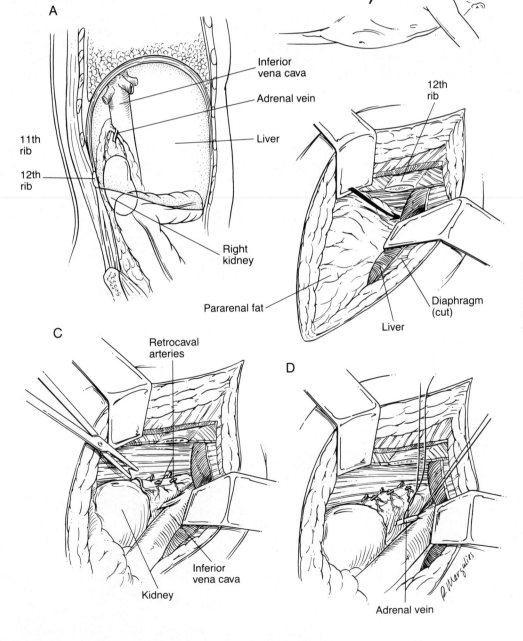

Figure 64–46. Modified posterior approach to the right adrenal. (From Vaughan, E. D., Jr.: Adrenal surgery. In Marshall, F. F. (Ed.): Operative Urology. Philadelphia, W. B. Saunders Co., 1991.)

We select this technique for all patients with right adrenal aldosterone-secreting tumors and for other patients with benign adenomas less than 6 cm. We do not recommend the approach in the patient with pheochromocytoma or malignant adrenal neoplasm.

Flank Approach

The standard extrapleural, extraperitoneal 11th rib resection is excellent for either left or right adrenalectomy (Fig. 64–47) (Riehle and Lavengood, 1985). This approach is described in detail elsewhere, and the adrenal dissection is described here (Chapter 65).

Following the completion of the incision, the lumbocostal arch is utilized as a landmark showing the point of attachment of the posterior diaphragm to the posterior abdominal musculature. Gerota's fascia containing the adrenal and kidney can be swept medially.

On the right side, the liver within the peritoneum is lifted off the anterior surface of the adrenal (see Fig. 64–47). Quite often, the adrenal gland cannot be identified precisely until these maneuvers are performed. One should not attempt to dissect into the body of the adrenal or to dissect the inferior surface of the adrenal off the kidney. The kidney is quite useful for retraction.

The dissection should continue from lateral to medial along the posterior abdominal and diaphragmatic musculature with precise ligation or clipping of the small but multiple adrenal arteries (Fig. 64–48). While the operator clips these arteries, with one hand, the opposite hand is utilized to retract both adrenal and kidney inferiorly. With release of the superior vasculature, the adrenal becomes visualized.

Following the release of the adrenal from the superior vasculature, it is helpful to expose the IVC and to divide the medial arterial supply, allowing mobilization of the cava for better exposure of the high posterior adrenal vein. This vein then is again doubly tied or clipped and divided. Patients with large adrenal carcinomas or pheochromocytomas may require en bloc resections of the adrenal and kidney, following the principles of radical nephrectomy.

A major deviation from this technique is utilized in patients with pheochromocytoma, in whom the initial dissection should be aimed toward early control and division of the main adrenal vein on either side. Obviously, in this clinical setting, the anesthesiologist should be notified when the adrenal vein is divided because there will often be a marked drop in blood pressure even if the patient is adequately hydrated and treated with alpha-adrenergic blockade.

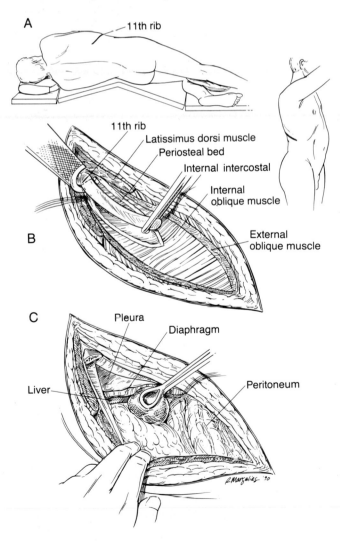

Figure 64–47. Eleventh rib resection for exposure of right adrenal. (From Vaughan, E. D., Jr.: Adrenal surgery. In Marshall, F. F. (Ed.): Operative Urology. Philadelphia, W. B. Saunders Co., 1991.)

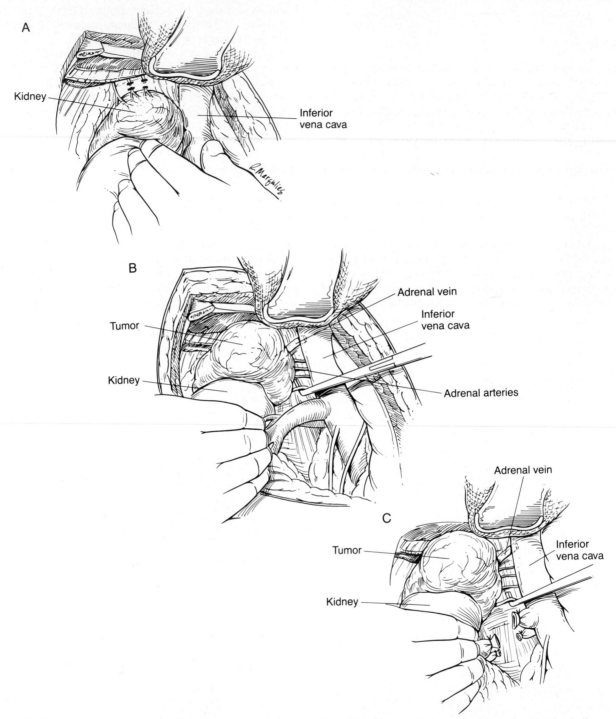

Figure 64–48. Exposure of right adrenal with and without nephrectomy. (From Vaughan, E. D., Jr.: Adrenal surgery. In Marshall, F. F. (Ed.): Operative Urology. Philadelphia, W. B. Saunders Co., 1991.)

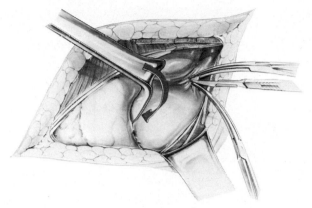

Figure 64–49. Release of splenorenal ligament early in exposure of left adrenal. (From Vaughan, E. D., Jr.: Adrenal surgery. In Marshall, F. F. (Ed.): Operative Urology. Philadelphia, W. B. Saunders Co., 1991.)

On the left side, the lumbocostal arch also is utilized as a landmark. Gerota's fascia can be swept medially and inferiorly, giving exposure to the splenorenal ligament, which should be divided to avoid splenic injury (Fig. 64–49). While the surgeon works anteriorly, the spleen and pancreas within the peritoneum can be lifted cranially, exposing the anterior surface of the adrenal gland. The superior dissection is performed first, drawing the adrenal and kidney down inferiorly. On the left medially, the phrenic branch of the venous drainage

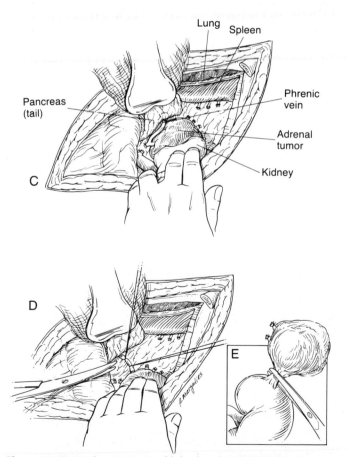

Figure 64–50. Further exposure of left adrenal including phrenic vein. (From Vaughan, E. D., Jr.: Adrenal surgery. In Marshall, F. F. (Ed.): Operative Urology. Philadelphia, W. B. Saunders Co., 1991.)

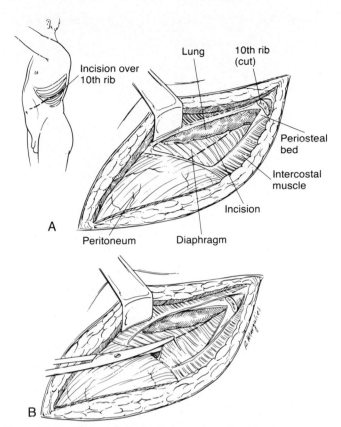

Figure 64–51. Thoracoabdominal approach to the left adrenal. (From Vaughan, E. D., Jr.: Adrenal surgery. In Marshall, F. F. (Ed.): Operative Urology. Philadelphia, W. B. Saunders Co., 1991.)

must be carefully clipped or ligated (Fig. 64–50). This vessel is not noted in most surgical atlases and can cause troublesome bleeding if divided. The medial dissection along the crus of the diaphragm and aorta will lead to the renal vein, and finally the adrenal vein is controlled, doubly tied, and divided. The adrenal is then removed from the kidney with care to avoid the apical branches of the renal artery (see Fig. 64–50).

Following removal of the adrenal, inspection should be made for any bleeding. Also, inspection of the diaphragm for pleural tear and inspection of the kidney should be done. The incision is closed without drains with interrupted 0 polydioxanone sutures.

Thoracoabdominal Approach

The thoracoabdominal 9th- or 10th-rib approach is utilized for large adenomas, some large adrenal carcinomas, and well-localized pheochromocytomas especially on the right side. The incision and exposure is standard (Fig. 64–51), with a radial incision through the diaphragm and a generous intraperitoneal extension. The techniques described for adrenalectomy with the 11th-rib approach are utilized.

Transabdominal Approach

The transabdominal approach is commonly chosen for patients with pheochromocytomas, for pediatric patients, and for some patients with adrenal carcinomas.

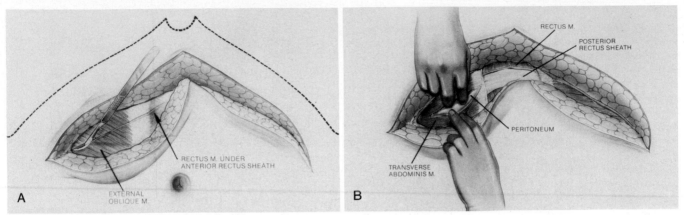

Figure 64–52. Chevron incision. (From Vaughan, E. D., Jr.: Adrenal surgery. In Marshall, F. F. (Ed.): Operative Urology. Philadelphia, W. B. Saunders Co., 1991.)

The obvious concept is to have the ability for complete abdominal exploration to identify either multiple pheochromocytomas or adrenal metastases.

We utilize the transverse or chevron incision, which we believe gives better exposure of both adrenal glands than does a midline incision (Fig. 64–52). The rectus muscles and lateral abdominal musculature are divided exposing the peritoneum. Upon entering the peritoneal cavity, the surgeon should gently palpate the para-aortic areas and the adrenal areas. Close attention is paid to blood pressure changes, in an attempt to identify any unsuspected lesions if the patient has a pheochromocytoma. This maneuver is less important today because we have excellent localization techniques, as previously discussed. In fact, with precise preoperative localization of the offending tumor, the chevron incision does not

need to be completely symmetric and can be limited on the contralateral side.

If the patient has a lesion on the right adrenal the hepatic flexure of the colon is reflected inferiorly. The incision is made in the posterior peritoneum lateral to the kidney and carried superiorly, allowing the liver to be reflected cranially (Fig. 64–53). Incision in the peritoneum is carried downward, exposing the anterior surface of the IVC to the entrance of the right renal vein. Once the cava is cleared, there are often one or two accessory hepatic veins that should be secured (Fig. 64–54). These veins are easily avulsed from the cava and can cause troublesome bleeding. Ligation of these veins gives 1 to 2 cm of additional caval exposure, which often is quite useful during the exposure of the short posterior right adrenal vein. Small accessory adrenal

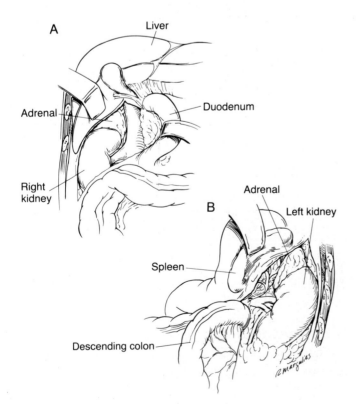

Figure 64–53. Exposure of right adrenal and left adrenal utilizing a transabdominal approach. (From Vaughan, E. D., Jr.: Adrenal surgery. In Marshall, F. F. (Ed.): Operative Urology. Philadelphia, W. B. Saunders Co., 1991.)

veins may also be encountered. The cava is rolled medially, exposing the adrenal vein, which should be doubly tied or clipped and divided (see Fig. 64–54).

As mentioned, the surgeon should inform the anesthesiologist when the vein is ligated in a patient with a pheochromocytoma because a precipitous fall in blood pressure can occur at this point, requiring volume expansion or even vasopressors. Following control of the adrenal vein, it is then simplest to proceed with the superior dissection lifting the liver off the adrenal and securing the multiple small adrenal arteries arising from the inferior phrenic artery, which is rarely seen. The adrenal can then be drawn inferiorly with retraction on the kidney. The adrenal arteries traversing to the adrenal from under the cava can be secured with right-angle clips. The final step is removing the adrenal from the kidney.

The left adrenal vein is simpler to approach, because it lies lower, partially anterior to the upper pole of the kidney. The adrenal vein empties into the left renal vein. Accordingly, on the left side the colon is reflected medially, exposing the anterior surface of Gerota's capsule. The initial dissection should be directed toward identification of the renal vein (see Fig. 64–53). In essence, the dissection is the same as that utilized for a radical nephrectomy for renal carcinoma. Once the renal vein is exposed, the adrenal vein is identified and doubly ligated and divided. Following this maneuver, the pancreas and splenic vasculature are lifted off the anterior surface of the adrenal gland. Because of additional drainage from the adrenal into the phrenic system, we generally would carry on farther with the medial dissection and control of the phrenic vein. We would then work cephalad and lateral to release the splenorenal ligament and the superior attachments of the adrenal. The remaining dissection is carried out as previously described (Fig. 64–55).

Following removal of the tumor, regardless of size, careful inspection is made to ensure hemostasis and the absence of injury to adjacent organs. Careful abdominal exploration is carried out after which the wound is closed with the suture material of choice. No drains are utilized.

Patients with multiple endocrine adenopathy, a familial history of pheochromocytoma, or pediatric patients should be considered at high risk for multiple lesions. It is hoped that the preoperative evaluation would identify these lesions. Regardless, a careful abdominal exploration should be carried out.

In patients with suspected malignant pheochromocytomas, en bloc dissections may be necessary in order to obtain adequate margins, a concept that is also true of patients with adrenal carcinomas (Fig. 64–56).

The results of adrenal surgery are extremely satisfying to both the treating physicians and patients. Rarely in medicine do we have a better understanding of the underlying pathophysiology than with adrenal disorders. Moreover, we have highly sophisticated analytic and radiographic diagnostic techniques that confirm our clinical impression. Elegant surgical approaches have been developed to the adrenal, which can be individualized for the specific clinical setting and can be successfully performed at minimum risk to the patient.

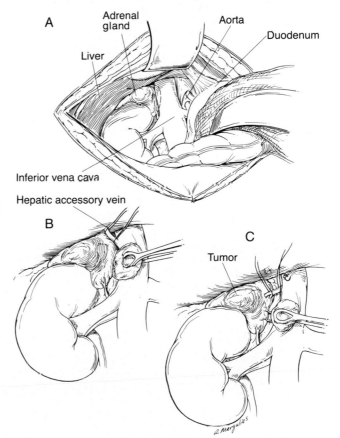

Figure 64–54. Further transabdominal exposure of the right adrenal with ligation of an accessory right hepatic vein. (From Vaughan, E. D., Jr.: Adrenal surgery. In Marshall, F. F. (Ed.): Operative Urology. Philadelphia, W. B. Saunders Co., 1991.)

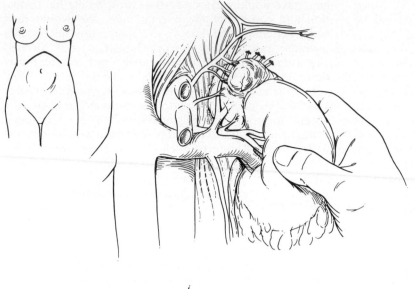

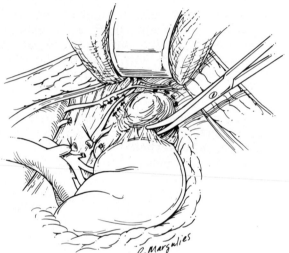

Figure 64–55. Further exposure, left adrenal. (From Vaughan, E. D., Jr.: Adrenal surgery. In Marshall, F. F. (Ed.): Operative Urology. Philadelphia, W. B. Saunders Co., 1991.)

Figure 64–56. Large pheochromocytoma. Magnetic resonance image provides excellent visualization of the left renal vein, leading to early ligation of the left adrenal vein. Nephrectomy required.

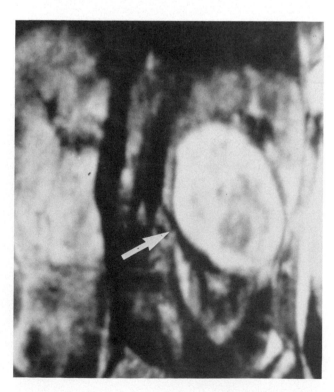

REFERENCES

Abecassis, M., McLoughlin, M. J., Langer, B., and Kudlow, J. E.: Serendipitous adrenal masses: Prevalence, significance, and management. Am. J. Surg., 149:783, 1985.

Abel, J. J., and Crawford, A. C.: On the blood-pressure raising constituent of the suprarenal capsule. Johns Hopkins Hosp. Bull., 8:151, 1897.

Abrams, H. L., Siegelman, S., Adams, D. F., Sanders, R., Fineberg, H. J., Hessel, S. J., and McNeil, B. J.: Computed tomography versus ultrasound of the adrenal gland: A prospective study. Radiology, 143:121, 1982.

Addison, T.: On the constitutional and local effects of disease of the suprarenal capsules. London Samuel Highley, 1855.

Aguirre, P., and Scully, R. E.: Testosterone-secreting adrenal ganglioneuroma containing Leydig cells. Am. J. Surg. Pathol., 7:699, 1983.

Amberson, J. B., and Gray, G. F.: Adrenal pathology in adrenal disorders. In Vaughan, E. D., Jr., and Carey, R. M. (Eds.): Adrenal Disorders. New York, Thieme Medical Publishers, Inc., 1989.

Amberson, J. B., Vaughan, E. D., Jr., Gray, G. F., and Naus, G. J.: Flow cytometric analysis of nuclear DNA from adrenocorticoid tumors: A retrospective study using paraffin-imbedded tissue. Cancer, 59:2091, 1987.

Andler, W., Havers, W., Stambolis, C., Medrano, J., and Stolman, N. B.: Renal cell carcinoma following irradition therapy for adrenal cortical carcinoma. J. Pediatr., 93:634, 1978.

Angermeier, K. W., and Montie, J. E.: Perioperative complications of adrenal surgery. Urol. Clin. North Am., 16:597–606, 1989.

Anson, B. J., Caldwell, E. W., Pick, J. W., and Beaton, L. E.: The blood supply of the kidney suprarenal gland and associated structures. Surg. Gynecol. Obstet., 84:313, 1947.

Antoni, F.: Hypothalamic control of adrenocorticotropin secretion: Advances since the discovery of 41-residue corticotropin-releasing factor. Endocr. Rev., 7:351, 1986.

Artega, E., Biglieri, E. G., Kater, C. E., Lopez, J. M., and Schambelan, M.: Aldosterone-producing adrenocortical carcinoma preoperative recognition and course in 3 cases. Ann. Intern. Med., 101:316, 1984.

Atlas, S. A., and Maack, T.: Atrial natriuretic factor. In Windhager, E. E. (Ed.): Handbook of Physiology. New York, Oxford University Press, 1991.

Axelrod, J.: Purification and properties of phenylethanolamine-N-methyl transferase. J. Biol. Chem., 237:1657, 1962.

Baer, L., Sommers, S. C., Krakoff, L. R., Newton, M. A., and Laragh, J. H.: Pseudoprimary aldosteronism: An entity distinct from true primary aldosteronism. Circ. Res. (Suppl.), 27:203, 1970.

Bagshaw, E. K. D.: Hypokalemia carcinoma and Cushing's syndrome. Lancet, 2:284, 1960.

Banks, W. A., Kastin, H. A., Biglieri, E. G., and Ruiz, E. A.: Primary adrenal hyperplasia: A new subset of primary hyperaldosteronism. J. Clin. Endocrinol. Metab., 58:783, 1984.

Baxter, J. D., and Tyrell, J. B.: The adrenal cortex. In Endocrinology and Metabolism. New York, McGraw-Hill, 1981, p. 408.

Beierwaltes, W. H., Lieberman, L. M., Ansari, A. N., and Nishiyama, H.: Visualization of human adrenal glands in vivo by scintillation scanning. JAMA 216:275–277, 1971.

Belldegrun, A., and deKernion, J. B.: What to do about the incidentally found adrenal mass. World J. Urol., 7:117–120, 1989.

Belldegrun, A., Hussain, S., Seltzer, S. E., Loughlin, K. R., Gittes, R. F., and Richie, J. P.: The incidentally discovered adrenal mass: a therapeutic dilemma—BWH experience 1976–1983. Surg. Gynecol. Obstet., 163:203, 1986.

Bergenstal, D. M., Hurtz, R., Lipsett, M. B., and Moy, R. H.: Chemotherapy of adrenal cortical cancer with o,p'DDD. Ann. Intern. Med., 53:672, 1960.

Bergland, R. M., and Harrison, P. S.: Pituitary and adrenal. In S. I. Schwartz (Ed.): Principles of Surgery. New York, McGraw-Hill, 1983.

Berkoff, G. T., Sandberg, A. A., Nelson, D. H., and Tyler, F. H.: Clinical usefulness of determination of circulating 17-hydroxycorticosteroid levels. Arch. Intern. Med., 93:1, 1954.

Bertagna, C., and Orth, D. N.: Clinical and laboratory findings and results of therapy in 58 patients with adrenocortical tumors admitted to a single medical center (1951 to 1978). Am. J. Med. 71:855–875, 1981.

Besser, G. M., and Edwards, C. R. W.: Cushing's syndrome. J. Clin. Endocrinol. Metab., 1:451, 1972.

Biemond, P., DeJong, F. H., and Lamberts, F. W. J.: Continuous dexamethasone infusion for 7 hours in patients with Cushing's syndrome—A superior differential diagnostic test. Ann. Intern. Med., 112:738, 1990.

Biglieri, E. G., Irony, I., and Kater, C. E.: Adrenocortical forms of human hypertension. In J. H. Laragh, and B. M. Brenner (Eds.): Hypertension: Pathophysiology Diagnosis and Management. New York, Raven Press, 1990.

Bigos, S. T., Somma, M., Rasio, E., Eastman, C. E., Lanthier, A., Johnston, H. H., and Hardy, J.: Cushing's disease: Management by transphenoidal pituitary microsurgery. J. Clin. Endocrinol. Metab., 50:348, 1980.

Bittar, D. A., and Innova, R.: Induced hypertensive crisis in patients with pheochromocytoma. Anesthesiology, 50:366, 1979.

Bolande, R. P.: The neurocrestopathias: A unifying concept of disease arising in neurocrest maldevelopment. Hum. Pathol., 5:409, 1974.

Boutros, A. R., Bravo, E. L., Zanettin, G., Straffon, R. A.: Perioperative management of 63 patients with pheochromocytoma. Cleve. Clin. J. Med., 57:613–617, 1990.

Bravo, E. L., and Gifford, R. W., Jr.: Pheochromocytoma: Diagnosis, localization and management. N. Engl. J. Med., 311:1298, 1984.

Bravo, E. L., Tarazi, R. C., Dustan, H. P., Fouad, F. M., Textor, S. C., Gifford, R. W., and Vidt, D. G.: The changing clinical spectrum of primary aldosteronism. Am. J. Med., 74:641, 1983.

Bravo, E. L., Tarazi, R. C., Fouad, F. M., Vidt, D. G., and Gifford, R. W., Jr.: Clonidine-suppression test: A useful aid in the diagnosis of pheochromocytoma. N. Engl. J. Med., 305:623, 1981.

Brennan, M. F.: Adrenocorticoid carcinoma. Cancer, 37:348, 1987.

Briggs, R. S. J., Birtwell, A. J., and Pohl, J. E. F.: Hypertensive response to labetalol in pheochromocytoma. Lancet, 1:1045, 1978.

Brown-Sequard, C. E.: Recherches experimentales sur la physiologie et la pathologie des capsules surrenales. Arch. Gen. Med., 2:385, 572, 1856.

Brownie, A. C.: The adrenal cortex and hypertension DOCA/salt hypertension and beyond. In Hypertension Pathophysiology Diagnosis and Management. J. H. Laragh, and B. M. Brenner (Eds.): New York, Raven Press, 1990.

Brunner, H. R., Laragh, J. H., Baer, L., Newton, M. A., Goodwin, F. T., Krakoff, L. R., Bard, R. H., and Buhler, F. R.: Essential hypertension: Renin and aldosterone, heart attack and stroke. N. Engl. J. Med., 286:441, 1972.

Bucht, H., Bergstrom, J., Lindholmar, G., Wijnbladh, H., and Hokfelt, B.: Catheterization of left adrenal vein for contrast injection and steroid analysis in a case of Conn's syndrome. Acta Med. Scand., 176:233, 1964.

Bullock, W. K., and Hirst, A. E.: Metastatic carcinoma of the adrenal. Am. J. Med. Sci., 226:521, 1953.

Burch, W. M.: Cushing's disease. A review. Intern. Med., 145:1106, 1985.

Calkins, E., and Howard, J. E.: Bilateral familiar pheochromocytoma with paroxysmal hypertension: Successful surgical removal of tumors in two cases, with discussion of certain diagnostic procedures and physiological considerations. J. Clin. Endocrinol. Metab., 7:475, 1947.

Carey, R. M., Douglas, J. G., and Schweikert, J. R.: The syndrome of essential hypertension with suppressed plasma renin activity: Normalization of blood pressure with spironolactone. Arch. Intern. Med., 130:849, 1972.

Carey, R. M., Estratopolous, A. D., Peart, W. S., and Wilson, G. A.: Effect of aldosterone on colonic potential difference in renal electrolyte excretion in normal man. Clin. Sci. 46:488, 1974.

Carey, R. M., and Sen, S.: Recent progress in the control of aldosterone secretion. Rec. Prog. Hormone. Res., 42:251, 1986.

Carey, R. M., Sen, S., Dolan, L. M., Malchoff, C. D., and Bumpus, S. M.: Idiopathic hyperaldosteronism: A powerful role for aldosterone-stimulating factor. N. Engl. J. Med., 311:94, 1984.

Carney, J. A., Sizemore, G. W., and Sheps, G. S.: Adrenal medullary disease in multiple endocrine neoplasia type 2. Am. J. Clin. Pathol., 66:279, 1976.

Carpenter, P. C.: Cushing syndrome: Update of diagnosis and management. Mayo Clin. Proc., 61:49, 1986.

Casson, I. F., Davis, J. C., Jeffreys, R. V., Silas, H., Williams, J., and Belchetz, P. E.: Successful management of Cushing's disease during pregnancy by transsphenoidal adenectomy. Clin Endocrinol., 27:423–428, 1987.

Cedermark, B. J., Blumenson, L. E., Pickering, J. W., Holyoke, D. E., and Elias, E. G.: The significance of metastasis to the adrenal glands in adenocarcinoma of the colon and rectum. Surg. Gynecol. Obstet., 144:537, 1977.

Cerfolio, R. J., and Vaughan, E. D., Jr.: The accuracy of computed tomography in predicting adrenal tumor size. In press.

Champion, P. K.: Cushing's syndrome secondary to abuse of dexamethasone nasal spray. Arch. Intern. Med., 134:750, 1974.

Christlieb, A. R., Espiner, E. A., Amsterdam, E. A., Yagger, P. I., Dobrzinsky, S. J., Lauler, D. P., and Hickler, R. B.: The pattern of electrolyte excretion in normal and hypertensive subjects before and after saline infusions. A simple electrolyte formula for the diagnosis of primary aldosteronism. Am. J. Cardiol., 27:595, 1971.

Cohen, K. L., Noth, R. H., and Pechinski, T.: Incidence of pituitary tumors following adrenalectomy. A long-term follow-up study of patients treated for Cushing's disease. Arch. Intern. Med., 138:575, 1978.

Cohn, K., Gottesman, L., and Brennan, M.: Adrenocortical carcinoma. Surgery, 100:1170, 1986.

Conn, J. W.: Primary hyperaldosteronism. A new clinical syndrome. J. Lab. Clin. Med., 45:3, 1955a.

Conn, J. W.: Primary aldosteronism. J. Lab. Clin. Med., 45:661, 1955b.

Conn, J. W.: Primary aldosteronism. In Hypertension: Physiopathology and Treatment. New York, McGraw-Hill, 1977.

Conn, J. W., Cohen, E. L., and Rovner, D. R.: Suppression of plasma renin activity in primary aldosteronism: Distinguishing primary from secondary aldosteronism in hypertensive disease. JAMA, 190:125, 1964.

Conn, J. W., Rovner, D. R., Cohen, E. L., and Nesbit, R. M.: Normokalemic primary aldosteronism: Its masquerade as "essential" hypertension. JAMA, 195:111, 1966.

Contreras, P., Rojas, H. A., Biagini, L., Gonzalez, P., and Massardo, T.: Regression of metastatic adrenal carcinoma during paliative ketoconazole. Lancet, 2:151, 1985.

Copeland, P. M.: The incidentally discovered adrenal mass. Ann. Intern. Med., 98:940, 1983.

Crapo, L.: Cushing's syndrome. A review of diagnostic tests. Metabolism, 28:955, 1979.

Crispel, K. R., Parson, W., Hamlin, J., and Hollifield, G.: Addison's disease associated with histoplasmosis. Am. J. Med., 20:23, 1956.

Crowder, R. E.: The development of the adrenal gland in man. Carnegie Contrib. Embryol., 36:193, 1957.

Culp, O. S.: Adrenal hetertopia: A survey of the literature and a report of a case. J. Urol., 41:303, 1959.

Cushing, H.: The Pituitary Body and its Disorders: Clinical States Produced by Disorders of the Hypophysis Cerebri. Philadelphia, J. B. Lippincott Co., 1912.

Cushing, H.: The basophil adenomas of the pituitary body and their clinical manifestations (pituitary basophilism): Johns Hopkins Hosp. Bull., 50:137, 1932.

Cuvier, G. L. C. F. D., Baron: Lecons d'Anatomie Comparee. Five volumes. Paris, Baudonin, 1800–1805.

Deal, J. E., Sever, P. S., Barratt, T. M., and Dillon, M. J.: Pheochromocytoma—investigation and management of 10 cases. Arch. Dis. Child., 65:269–274, 1990.

DelGaudio, A., and Solidoro, G.: Myelolipoma of the adrenal gland: Report of 2 cases with the review of the literature. Surgery, 99:293, 1986.

DelGaudio, A., and Solidoro, G.: Myelolipoma of the adrenal gland: Two further observations and update of literature. J. Urol., In press.

Deming, Q. B., and Leutcher, J. A., Jr.: Bioassay of desoxycorticosterone-like material in urine. Proc. Soc. Exp. Biol. Med., 73:171, 1950.

Didolkar, M. S., Bescher, A. R., Elias, E. G., and Moore, R. H.: Natural history of adrenal cortical carcinoma: A clinical pathologic study of 42 patients. Cancer, 47:2153, 1981.

Dolan, L. M., and Carey, R. M.: Adrenal cortical and medullary function: Diagnostic tests. In E. D. Vaughan Jr., and R. M. Carey (Eds.): Adrenal Disorders. New York, Thieme Medical Publishers Inc., 1989, p. 81.

Dunlop, D.: 86 cases of Addison's disease. Br. Med. J., 2:887, 1963.

Dunnick, N. R., Doppman, J. L., Gill, J. R., Jr., Strott, C. A., Keiser, H. R., and Brennan, M. F.: Localization of functional adrenal tumors by computed tomography and venous sampling. Radiology, 142:429, 1982.

Dunnick, N. R.: Adrenal imaging: Current status. Am. J. Radiol., 154:927, 1990.

Eason, R. J., Croxson, M. S., Perry, M. C., and Somerfield, S. D.: Addison's disease, adrenal autoantibodies and computerized adrenal tomography. NZ Med. J., 95:569, 1982.

Eddy, R. L., Jones, A. L., Gilliland, P. F., Ibarra, J. D., Jr., Thompson, J. O., and McMurray, J. F.: Cushing's syndrome: A perspective study of diagnostic methods. Am. J. Med., 55:621, 1973.

Engelman, K., Horowitz, D., Jequier, E., and Sjoerdsma, A.: Biochemical and pharmacologic effects of alpha-methyl-tyrosine in man. J. Clin. Invest., 47:577, 1968.

Espiner, E. A., Tucci, J. R., Yagger, P. I., and Lauler, D. P.: Effect of saline infusions on aldosterone secretion and electrolyte excretion in normal subjects and patients with primary aldosteronism. N. Engl. J. Med., 277:1, 1967.

Eustachius, B.: Opuscula anatomica Venice vicentius luchinus. 1563.

Falke, T. H. M., Strakel, T. E., Sandler, M. P.: Magnetic resonance imaging of the adrenal glands. Radio Graphses, 7:343, 1987.

Farwell, A. P., Devlin, J. T., and Stewart, J. A.: Total suppression of cortisol excretion by ketoconazole in the therapy of the ectopic adrenocorticotropic hormone syndrome. Am. J. Med., 84:1063, 1988.

Ferrerira, S. H., and Vane, J. R.: Half lives of peptides and amines in the circulation. Nature, 215:1237, 1967.

Fish, R. G., Takaro, T., and Lovell, M.: Coexistent Addison's disease and American blastomycosis. Am. J. Med., 28:152, 1960.

Fisher, C. E., Turner, F. A., and Horton, R.: Remission of primary hyperaldosteronism after adrenal venography. N. Engl. J. Med., 285:334, 1971.

Fitzgerald, P. A., Aron, D. C., Findling, J. W., Brooks, R. M., Wilson, C. D., Forsham, P. H., and Tyrell, J. B.: Cushing's disease transient adrenal insufficiency after selective removal of the pituitary microadenomas. Evidence for pituitary origin. J. Clin. Endocrinol. Metab., 54:413, 1982.

Flavin, D. K., Fredrickson, P. A., and Richardson, J. W.: An unusual manifestation of drug dependence. Mayo Clin. Proc., 58:764, 1983.

Forbes, A. P., and Albright, F.: A comparison of the 17-keto steroid excretion in Cushing's syndrome associated with adrenal tumor and with adrenal hyperplasia. J. Clin. Endocrinol. Metab., 11:926, 1951.

Fränkel, F.: Ein fall von doppelseitigen vollig latent verlaufenen Nebennierentumor und gleichseitigen Nephritis mit Veranderungen am circulations—Apparat und Retinitis. Arch. Pathol. Anat., 103, 1886.

Fudge, T. L., McKinnon, W. M. P., and Geary, W. L.: Current surgical management of pheochromocytoma during pregnancy. Arch. Surg., 15:1224, 1980.

Gabrilove, J. L., Seeman, A. T., and Saba, T.: Virilizing adrenal adenoma with studies on the steroid content of the adrenal venous effluent and review of the literature. Endocrinol. Rev., 2:462, 1981.

Gabrilove, J. L., Sharma, D. C., Waitz, H. H., and Dorfman, R.: Feminizing adrenal cortical tumors in the male: A review of 52 cases including a case report. Medicine, 44:37, 1965.

Ganguly, A., Dowdy, A. J., Luetscher, J. A., and Melada, G. A.: Anamolous postural response of plasma aldosterone concentration in patients with aldosterone-producing adrenal adenomas. J. Clin. Endocrinol. Metab., 36:401, 1973.

Ganguly, A., Grim, C. E., and Weinberger, M. H.: Anomalous postural aldosterone response in glucocorticoid-suppressible hyperaldosteronism. N. Engl. J. Med., 305:991, 1981.

Geisinger, M. A., Zelch, M. G., Bravo, E. L., Risius, B. F., O'Donovan, P. B., and Borkowski, G. P.: Primary hyperaldosteronism: comparison of CT, adrenal venography and venous sampling. AJR, 141:299, 1983.

Gil-Vernet, J.: New surgical concepts in removing renal calculi. Urol. Int., 20:255–262, 1965.

Glass, A. R., Zavadil, A. P., Halberg, F., Cornelissen, G., and Schaef, M.: Circadian rhythm of serum cortisol in Cushing's disease. J. Clin. Endocrinol. Metab., 59:161, 1984.

Glazer, H. S., Weyman, P. J., Sagal, S. S., Levitt, R. G., and McClennan, R. L.: Nonfunctioning adrenal masses: Incidental discovery on computed tomography. AJR, 139:81, 1982.

Glenn, F., Peterson, R. E., and Mannix, H., Jr. (Eds.): Surgery of the Adrenal Glands. New York, MacMillan, 1968.

Grunberg, S. M.: Development of Cushing's syndrome and virilization after presentation of a nonfunctioning adrenocortical carcinoma. Cancer, 50:815, 1982.

Haas, J. A., and Knox, F. G.: Mechanism for escape from salt-retaining effects of mineralocorticoids: Role of the nephrons. Semin. Nephrol., 10:380, 1990.

Hardy, J.: Transphenoidal hypophysectomy. J. Neurosurg., 34:582, 1971.

Hardy, J.: Cushing's disease—50 years later. Can. J. Neurol. Sci., 9:375, 1982.

Hartman, F. A., MacArthur, C. G., and Hartman, W. E.: A substance which prolongs the life of adrenalectomized cats. Proc. Soc. Exp. Biol. Med., 25:69, 1927.

Hedeland, H., Ostberg, G., and Hokfeld, B.: On the prevalence of adrenal cortical adenomas in an autopsy and autopsy material in relation to hypertension and diabetes. Acta Med. Scand., 184:211, 1968.

Heinbecker, P., O'Neal, L. W., and Ackerman, L. V.: Functioning and nonfunctioning adrenocortical tumors. Surg. Gynecol. Obstet., 105:21, 1957.

Hench, P. S., Kendall, E. C., Slocumb, C. H., and Polley, H. F.: The effect of a hormone of the adrenal cortex (17-hydroxy-11-dehydrocorticosterone: compound E) and of pituitary adrenocorticotropic hormone on rheumatoid arthritis. Proc. Staff Meetings Mayo Clin., 24:181–197, 1949.

Herf, S. M., Teates, D. C., Tegtmeyer, C. J., Vaughan, E. D., Jr., Ayers, C. R., and Carey, R. M.: Identification and differentiation of surgically correctable hypertension due to primary aldosteronism. Am. J. Med., 67:397, 1979.

Hoffman, D. L., and Mattox, V. L.: Treatment of adrenal cortical carcinoma with o,p'DDD. Med. Clin. North Am., 50:999, 1972.

Hoffman, K.: Relations between chemical structure and function of adrenocorticotropin and melanocyte stimulating hormones. Handbook of Physiology, Endocrinology, Vol. 4. The pituitary and its neuroendocrine control, section 7, part 2. American Physiologic Society, Washington, D.C., 1974.

Horton, R., and Finck, E.: Diagnosis and localization in primary aldosteronism. Ann. Intern. Med., 76:885, 1972.

Howards, S. S., and Carey, R. M.: The adrenals. In Gillenwater, J. Y., Grayhack, J. T., Howards, S. S., and Duckett, J. W. (Eds.): Adult and Pediatric Urology, 2nd ed. Year Book Medical Publishers, Chicago, 1991.

Howlet, T. A., Rees, L. H., and Besser, G. M.: Cushing's syndrome. J. Clin. Endocrinol. Metab., 14:911, 1985.

Hubbard, M. M., Kulaylat, M. M., and Amabumrad, N. N.: Adrenocorticoids—physiology regulation function and metabolism. In Scott, H. W. Jr. (Ed.): Surgery of the Adrenal Glands. Philadelphia, J. B. Lippincott Co., 1990.

Huebener, K. H., and Treugu, T. H.: Adrenocortex dysfunction CT findings. Radiology, 150:195, 1984.

Hume, T. M.: Pheochromocytoma in the adult and in the child. Am. J. Surg., 99:458, 1960.

Hunt, T. K., and Tyrell, J. B.: Cushing's syndrome: Hypercortisolism. In Friesen, S. R. (Ed.): Surgical Endocrinology: Clinical Syndromes. Philadelphia, J. B. Lippincott Co., 1978.

Hutter, A. M., and Kayhoe, D. E.: Adrenal cortical carcinoma. Results of treatment with o,p'DDD in 138 patients. Am. J. Med., 41:581, 1966.

Imperato-McGinley, J., Gautier, T., Ehlers, K., Zullo, M. A., Goldstein, D. S., and Vaughan, E. D., Jr.: Reversibility of catecholamine-induced dilated cardiomyopathy in a child with a pheochromocytoma. N. Engl. J. Med., 316:793–797, 1987.

Imperato-McGinley, J., Young, I. S., Huang, T., Dreyfus, J. C., III, Reckler, J. M., and Peterson, R. E.: Testosterone secreting adrenal cortical adenomas. Int. J. Gynaecol. Obstet., 19:421, 1981.

Invitti, E. C., DeMartin, M., Banin, A., Biolini, M., and Cavagnini, F.: Treatment of Cushing's syndrome with the long-acting somatostatin analogue SMS 201-995 (Sandostatin). Clin. Endocrinol., 32:275, 1990.

Irony, I., Kater, C. E., Arteaga, E., and Biglieri, E. G.: Characteristics of correctable subtypes of primary aldosteronism. Am. J. Hyperten., 1:50A, 1988.

Irvine, W. J., and Barnes, E. W.: Adrenocortical insufficiency. J. Clin. Endocrinol. Metab., 1:549, 1972.

Iverson, L. L.: Uptake of circulating catecholamines. In Blaschko, H., Sayers, G., and Smith, A. D. (Eds.): Handbook of Physiology. Washington, D.C., American Physiological Society, p. 713, 1975.

Jarabak, J., and Rice, K.: Metastatic adrenal cortical carcinoma. Prolonged regression with mitotane therapy. JAMA, 246:1706, 1981.

Jasani, M. K., Freeman, P. A., Boyle, J. A., Reid, A. M., Diver, M. J., and Buchanan, W. H.: Studies of the rise in plasma 11-hydroxycorticosteroids in corticosteroid-treated patients with rheumatoid arthritis during surgery: Correlations with the functional integrity of the hypothalamic-pituitary-adrenal axis. Q. J. Med., 37:407, 1968.

Jennings, A. S., Liddle, G. W., and Orth, D. N.: Results of treating childhood Cushing's disease with pituitary radiation. N. Engl. J. Med., 29:957, 1977.

Johnson, D. H., and Greco, F. A.: Treatment of metastatic adrenal cortical carcinoma with cisplatin and etoposide (vp16). Cancer, 58:2198, 1986.

Johnson, L. K., and Baxter, J. D.: Regulation of gene expression by glucocorticoid hormones: Early effects preserved in isulin chromatin. J. Biol. Chem., 254:1991, 1987.

Johnstone, F. R.: The suprarenal veins. Am. J. Surg., 94:615, 1957.

Junqueira, L. C., and Ncearneir, O. J.: Adrenal islets of Langerhans, parathyroids and pineal body. In Junqueira, L. C., and Carneiro, J. (Eds.). Basic Histology, 4th ed. Los Altos, California, Lange Medical Publications, 1983.

Kalff, V., Shapiro, B., Lloyd, R., Sisson, J. C., Holland, K., Makajo, M., and Beierwaltes, W. H.: The spectrum of pheochromocytoma in hypertensive patients with neurofibromatosis. Arch. Intern. Med., 142:209, 1982.

Kaplan, N. M., Kramer, N. J., Holland, O. B., Sheps, S. G., and Gomez-Sanchez, C.: Single-voided urine metanephrine assays in screening for pheochromocytoma. Arch. Intern. Med., 137:190, 1977.

Karlberg, B. E., and Headman, L.: Value of clonidine suppression test in the diagnosis of pheochromocytoma. Acta Med. Scand. (Suppl.), 714:15, 1986.

Kay, R., Schumacker, O. P., and Pank, E. S.: Adrenal cortical carcinoma in children. J. Urol., 130:1130, 1983.

Kazam, E., Engel, I. A., Zirinsky, K., Auh, J. H., Rubenstein, W. A., Reckler, J. M., and Markisz, J. A.: Sectional imaging of the adrenal glands, computed tomography and ultrasound. In Vaughan, E. D., Jr., and Carey, R. M. (Eds.): Adrenal Disorders. New York, Thieme Medical Publishers Inc., 1989.

Kazerooni, E. A., Sisson, J. C., Shapiro, B., Gross, M. D., Driedger, A., Hurwitz, G. A., Mattar, A. G., and Petry, N. A.: Diagnostic accuracy and pitfalls of (iodine-131) 6-beta-iodomethyl-119-norcholesterol (np59) imaging. J. Nucl. Med., 31:526, 1990.

Kehlet, H., and Binder, C.: Value of an ACTH test in assessing hypothalamic-pituitary-adrenal cortical function in glucocorticoid-treated patients. Br. Med. J., 2:147, 1973.

Klein, F. A., Kay, S., Ratliff, J. E., White, F. K. H., and Newsome, H. H.: Flow cytometric determinations of ploidy and proliferation patterns of adrenal neoplasms: An adjunct to histological classification. J. Urol., 9:33, 1985.

Knight, C. D., Trichel, B. E., and Mathews, W. R.: Nonfunctioning carcinoma of the adrenal cortex. Ann. Surg. 151:349–358, 1960.

Korobkin, M.: Overview of adrenal imaging/adrenal CT. Urol. Radiol., 11:221, 1989.

Kozeny, G. A., Hurley, R. M., Vertuno, L. L., Bansal, V. K., Zeller, W. P., and Hano, J. E.: Hypertension, mineralocorticoid-resistant hyperkalemia, and hyperchloremic acidosis in an infant with obstructive uropathy. Am. J. Nephrol., 6:476–481, 1986.

Kreiger, D. T.: Rhythms of ACTH and corticosteroid secretion in health and disease and their experimental modification. J. Steroid Biochem., 6:785, 1975.

Kreiger, D. T.: Plasma ACTH and corticosteroids. In deGroot, L. (Ed.): Endocrinology. New York, Grune & Stratton, 1979.

Kreiger, D. T., Allen, W., Rizzo, F., and Kreiger, H. P.: Characterization of the normal temporal pattern of plasma corticosteroid levels. J. Clin. Endocrinol. Metab., 32:266, 1971.

Laragh, J. H., Angers, M., Kelly, W. G., et al.: The effect of epinephrine, norepinephrine, angiotensin II, and others on the secretory rate of aldosterone in man. JAMA, 174:234, 1960.

Laragh, J. H., and Sealey, J. E.: The renin-angiotensin-aldosterone system and the renal regulation of sodium, potassium, and blood pressure homeostasis. In Windhager, E. E. (Ed.): Handbook of Physiology. New York, Oxford University Press, 1991.

Levitt, M., Spector, S., Sjoredsma, A., Udenfriend, S.: Elucidation of the rate-limiting step in norepinephrine biosynthesis in the profuse guinea pig heart. J. Pharmacol. Exp. Ther., 148:1, 1965.

Lewinsky, B. S., Grigor, K. M., Symington, T., and Nelville, A. M.: The clinical and pathologic features of "non-hormonal" adrenocortical tumors. Report of 20 new cases and review of the literature. Cancer, 33:778, 1974.

Lewis, G. P.: Physiological mechanisms controlling secretory activity of adrenal medulla. In Blaschko, H., Sayers, G., and Smith, A. D. (Eds.): Handbook of Physiology. Washington, D.C., American Physiological Society, 1975, p. 309.

Libertino, J. A., and Novick, J. E.: Adrenal surgery. Urol. Clin. North Am., 16, 1989.

Liddle, G. W.: Test of pituitary-adrenal suppressibility in the diagnosis of Cushing's syndrome. J. Clin. Endocrinol. Metab., 20:1539, 1960.

Lim, R. C., Nakayama, D. T., Biglieri, E. G., Schambelan, M., and Hunt, T. K.: Primary aldosteronism: Changing concepts and diagnosis and management. Am. J. Surg., 152:116, 1986.

Liu, L., Haskin, M. E., Rose, L. A., and Beemus, C. E.: Diagnosis of bilateral adrenal cortical hemorrhage by computerized tomography. Ann. Intern. Med., 97:720, 1982.

Lloyd, R. V., Shapiro, B., and Sisson, J. C.: An immunohistochemical survey of pheochromocytomas. Arch. Pathol. Lab. Med., 108:541, 1984.

Loeb, R. F.: Effect of sodium chloride in treatment of patients with Addison's disease. Proc. Soc. Exp. Biol. Med., 380:8, 1933.

Loose, D. S., Kan, P. B., Hirst, M. A., Marcus, R. A., and Feldman, D.: Ketoconazole blocks adrenal steroidogenesis by inhibiting cytochrome P450-dependent enzymes. J. Clin. Invest., 71:1495, 1983.

Lubitz, J. A., Freeman, L., and Okun, R.: Mitotane use in inoperable adrenal cortical carcinoma. JAMA, 223:1109, 1973.

Luetscher, J. A., Jr., and Johnson, B. B.: Observations on the sodium-retaining corticoid (aldosterone) in the urine of children and adults in relation to sodium balance and edema. J. Clin. Invest., 23:1441, 1954.

Luton, J. - P., Cerdas, S., Billaud, L., Thomas, G., Guilhaume, B., Bertagna, X., Laudat, M. - H., Louvel, A., Chapuis, Y., Blondeau, P., Bonnin, A., and Bricaire, H.: Clinical features of adrenocortical carcinoma, prognostic factors, and the effect of mitotane therapy. N. Engl. J. Med., 322:1195, 1990.

McDougal, W. S., Kirchner, F. K., Jr., Scott, H. W., Jr., and Nadeau, J. H.: Primary aldosteronism (Conn's syndrome). In Scott, H. W., Jr. (Ed.): Surgery of the Adrenal Glands. Philadelphia, J. B. Lippincott Co., 1990.

Mador, C. K., Liddle, G. W., Island, D. P., Nicholson, W. E., Lucas, C. P., Nuckton, J. G., and Leutscher, J. A.: Cause of Cushing's syndrome in patients with tumors arising from "non-endocrine" tissue. J. Clin. Endocrinol. Metab., 22:693, 1962.

Madrazo, I., Drucker-Colin, R. H., Diaz, V., Martinez-Mata, J., Torres, C., and Becerril, J. J.: Open microsurgical autograph of adrenal medulla to the right caudate nucleus into patients with intractable Parkinson's disease. N. Engl. J. Med., 316:3831, 1987.

Mains, R. E., and Eipper, B. A.: Structure and biosynthesis of proadrenocorticotropin/endorphin and related peptides. Endocr. Rev., 1:1, 1980.

Maisey, I., and Stevens, A.: Addison's disease at Guys Hospital: A pathologic study. Guys Hosp. Rep., 118:373, 1969.

Manger, W. M., and Gifford, R. W., Jr.: Pheochromocytoma. New York, Springer-Verlag, 1977.

Manger, W. M., and Gifford, R. W., Jr.: Pheochromocytoma. In Laragh, J. H., and Brenner, B. M. (Eds.): Hypertension Pathophysiology Diagnosis and Management. New York, Raven Press, 1990.

Markisz, J. A., and Kazam, E.: Magnetic resonance imaging of the adrenal glands. In Vaughan, E. D., Jr., and Carey, R. M. (Eds.): Adrenal Disorders. New York, Thieme Medical Publishers Inc., 1989.

Mattox, J. H., and Phelan, S.: The evaluation of adult females with testosterone-producing neoplasms of the adrenal cortex. Surg. Gynecol. Obstet., 164:98, 1987.

Mazze, R. I., Calverley, R. K., and Smith, N. T.: Inorganic fluoride and nephrotoxicity: Prolonged enflurane and halothane anesthesia in volunteers. Anesthesiology, 46:265–271, 1977.

Meador, C. K., Liddle, G. W., Island, D. P., et al.: Cause of Cushing's syndrome in patients with tumors arising from "nonendocrine tumors." J. Clin. Endocrinol. Metab., 22:693, 1962.

Melby, J.: Assessment of adrenocortical function. N. Engl. J. Med., 285:735–739, 1971.

Mezrich, R., Banner, M. P., and Pollack, H. M.: Magnetic resonance imaging of the adrenal glands. Urol. Radiol., 8:127, 1986.

Mitty, H. A., and Yeh, H. C.: Radiology of the Adrenals for Sonography and CT. Philadelphia, W. B. Saunders Co., 1982.

Moloney, B. J.: Addison's disease due to chronic disseminating coccidioidomycosis. Arch. Intern. Med., 90:869, 1952.

Moore, M., Amberson, J. B., Kazam, E., Vaughan, E. D., Jr.: Anatomy, histology, embryology. In Vaughan, E. D., Jr., and Carey, R. M. (Eds.): Adrenal Disorders. New York, Thieme Medical Publishers Inc., 1989.

Morimoto, S., Hakeda, R., and Murakami, M.: Does prolonged pretreatment with large dosage of spironolactone hasten a recovery from juxtaglomerular-adrenal suppression in primary aldosteronism? J. Clin. Endocrinol. Metab., 31:659, 1970.

Mueller, R. A., Thoenen, H., and Axelrod, J.: Effect of the pituitary and ACTH on the maintenance of basal tyrosine hydroxylase activity in the rat adrenal gland. Endocrinology, 86:751, 1970.

Mulder, W. J., Berghout, A., and Wiersinga, W. M.: Cushing's syndrome during pregnancy. Neth. J. Med., 36:234–241, 1990.

Nader, S., Hickey, R. C., Sellin, R. V., and Samaan, N. A.: Adrenal cortical carcinoma: the study of 77 cases. Cancer, 52:707, 1983.

Nelson, D. H., Meakin, J. W., Dealy, J. B., Jr., and Matson, D. D., Emerson, K., Jr., and Thorn, G. W.: ACTH-producing tumor of the pituitary gland. N. Engl. J. Med., 259:161, 1958.

Nelson, D. H.: The adrenal cortex: physiological function and disease. Major Probl. Intern. Med., 18:15, 1980.

Nerup, J.: Addison's disease—clinical studies. A report of 108 cases. Acta Endocrinol., 76:127, 1974.

Neville, A. M., and O'Hare, M. J.: The Human Adrenal Cortex. Pathology and Biology—An Integrated Approach. New York, Springer-Verlag, 1982.

New, M. I., and Speiser, P. W.: Disorders of adrenal steroidogenesis. In Vaughan, E. D., Jr., and Carey, R. M. (Eds.): Adrenal Disorders. New York, Thieme Medical Publishers Inc., 1989.

Newhouse, J. H.: MRI of the adrenal gland. Urol. Radiol., 12:1, 1990.

Nicholson, J. P., Vaughan, E. D., Jr., Pickering, T. G., Resnick, L. M., Artusio, J., Kleinert, H. D., Lopez-Ovejero, J. A., and Laragh, J. H.: Pheochromocytoma and prazosin. Ann. Intern. Med., 99:477–479, 1983.

Nielson, E., and Asfeldt, V. H.: Studies on the specificity of fluorimetric determination of plasma corticosteroids. Scand. J. Clin. Lab. Invest., 20:185, 1967.

Novick, A. C., Straffon, R. A., and Kaylor, W.: Posterior transthoracic approach for adrenal surgery. J. Urol., 141:254, 1989.

O'Connor, D. T., Burton, D., and Deftos, L. J.: Immunoreactive human chromogranin A in diverse polypeptide hormone producing human tumors and normal endocrine tissue. J. Clin. Endocrinol. Metab., 57:1084, 1983.

Oliver, G., and Sharpey-Schafer, E. A.: The physiological effects of extracts on the suprarenal capsules. J. Physiol. (London), 18:230, 1895.

O'Neil, R. G.: Aldosterone regulation of sodium and potassium transport in the cortical collecting duct. Sem. Nephrol., 10:365, 1990.

Orth, D. N., Island, D. P., and Liddle, G. W.: Experimental alteration of the circadian rhythm in plasma cortisol concentration in man. J. Clin. Endocrinol. Metab., 27:549, 1967.

Orth, D. N., and Liddle, G. W.: Results of treatment in 108 patients with Cushing's syndrome. N. Engl. J. Med., 285:243, 1971.

Osa, S. R., Peterson, R. E., and Roberts, S. B. R. B.: Recovery of adrenal reserve following treatment of disseminated South American blastomytosis. Am. J. Med., 71:298, 1981.

Osborn, R. H., and Yannone, M. E.: Plasma androgens in the normal and androgenic female. Obstet. Gynecol. Surg., 26:195, 1971.

Papavasiliou, C., Gouliamos, A., Deligiorgi, E., Vlahos, L., and Cambouris, T.: Masses of myeloadipose tissue: Radiological and clinical considerations. Int. J. Radiat. Oncol. Biol. Phys., 19:985–993, 1990.

Parker, L., and Odell, W.: Control of adrenal androgen secretion. Endocr. Rev., 1:392, 1980.

Parker, L. N., Lifrak, E. T., and Odell, D.: A 60,000 molecular weight human pituitary glucopeptide stimulates adrenal androgen secretion. Endocrinology, 113:2092, 1983.

Paulotos, F. C., Smilo, R. P., and Forchamp, H.: A rapid screening test for Cushing's syndrome. JAMA, 193:720, 1965.

Pearse, A. G., and Polak, J. M.: Cytochemical evidence for the neural crest origin of mammalian ultimobranchial C cells. Histochemie, 27:96, 1971.

Pelleya, R., Oster, J. R., and Perez, G. O.: Hyporeninemic hypoaldosteronism, sodium wasting and mineralocorticoid-resistant hyperkalemia in two patients with obstructive uropathy. Am. J. Nephrol., 3:223–227, 1983.

Pepe, G. J., and Albrecht, E. D.: Regulation of the primate fetal adrenal cortex. Endocr. Rev., 11:151, 1990.

Percarpio, B., and Knowlton, A. H.: Radiation therapy of adrenal cortical carcinoma. Acta Radiol. [Ther.] (Stockh.) 15:288, 1976.

Perkoff, G. T., Sandberg, A. A., Nelson, D. H., and Tyler, F. H.: Clinical usefulness of determination of circulation 17-hydroxycorticosteroid levels. Arch. Intern. Med., 93:1–8, 1954.

Perry, R. R., Keiser, H. R., Norton, J. A., Wall, R. T., Robertson, C. N., Travis, W., Pass, H. I., Walther, M. M., and Linehan, W. M.: Surgical management of pheochromocytoma with the use of metyrosine. Ann. Surg., 212:621–628, 1990.

Pick, J. W., and Anson, B. J.: The inferior phrenic artery: origin and suprarenal branches. Anat. Rec., 78:413, 1940.

Pick, L.: Das Ganglioma embryonale sympathicum. Klin. Wochenschr., 19:16, 1912.

Plager, J. E.: Carcinoma of the adrenal cortex: Clinical description, diagnosis and treatment. Int. Adv. Surg. Oncol., 7:329, 1984.

Prinz, R. A., Brooks, M. H., Churchill, R., Graner, J. L., Lawrence, A. M., Paloyan, E., and Sparagana, M.: Incidental asymptomatic adrenal masses detected by computed tomographic scanning—is operation required? JAMA, 248:701, 1982.

Raue, F., Frank, K., Meybeir, H., and Ziegler, R.: Pheochromocytoma in multiple endocrine neoplasia. Cardiology, 72 (Suppl.):147, 1985.

Reckler, J. M., Vaughan, E. D., Jr., Tjeuw, M., and Carey, R. M.: Pheochromocytoma. In Vaughan, E. D., Jr., and Carey, R. M. (Eds.): Adrenal Disorders. New York, Thieme Medical Publishers Inc., 1989.

Reinig, J. W., Doppelman, J. L., Dwyer, A. J., Johnson, A. R., and Knop, R. H.: Adrenal masses differentiated by MR. Radiology, 158:81, 1986.

Renold, A. E., Jenkins, D., Forsham, P. H., and Thorn, G. W.: The use of intravenous ACTH: A study in quantitative adrenocortical stimulation. J. Clin. Endocrinol. Metab., 12:763, 1952.

Reyes, J., Parvez, Z., Nemoto, P., Regal, A. - M., and Takita, H.: Adrenalectomy for adrenal metastases from lung carcinoma. J. Surg. Oncol., 44:32, 1990.

Richie, J. P., and Gittes, R. F.: Carcinoma of the adrenal cortex. Cancer, 45:1957, 1980.

Rickards, A. G., and Parrett, G. M.: Non-tuberculous Addison's disease and its relationship to giant cell granuloma and multiple glandular disease. Q. J. Med., 43:403, 1956.

Riehle, R. A., Jr., and Lavengood, R. W.: An extrapleural approach with rib removal for the 11th rib flank incision. Surg. Gynecol. Obstet., 161:276–279, 1985.

Robertson, D.: The adrenal medulla and adrenomedullary hormones. In Scott, H. W. (Ed.): Surgery of the Adrenal Glands. Philadelphia, J. B. Lippincott Co., 1990.

Robertson, D., Oates, J. A., Jr., and Berman, M. L.: Preoperative and anesthetic management of pheochromocytoma. In Scott, H. W. (Ed.): Surgery of the Adrenal Glands. Philadelphia, J. B. Lippincott Co., 1990.

Rocco, S., Opocher, G., Carpene, G., and Mantero, F.: Atrial natriuretic peptide infusion in primary hyperaldosteronism renal hemodynamic and hormonal effects. Am. J. Hyperten., 3:688, 1990.

Rosen, A. E., Brown, J. J., and Lever, A. F.: Treatment of pheochromocytoma and of clonidine withdrawal hypertension with labetalol. Br. J. Clin. Pharmacol., 3 (Suppl. 3):809, 1976.

Rosenbaum, J. S., Billingham, M. E., and Ginsberg, R.: Cardiomyopathy in a rat model of pheochromocytoma morphological and functional alterations. Am. J. Cardiovasc. Pathol., 1:389, 1988.

Ross, E. J., Prichard, B. N. C., Kaufman, L., Robertson, A. I. G., and Harries, B. J.: Preoperative and operative management of patients with pheochromocytoma. Br. Med. J., 1:191, 1967.

Ross, N. S., and Aron, D. C.: Hormonal evaluation of the patient with an incidentally discovered adrenal mass. N. Engl. J. Med., 323:1401, 1990.

Rousseau, G. G., Baxter, J. D., and Tomkins, G. M.: Glucocorticoid receptors. Relationship between steroid binding and biological effects. J. Mol. Biol., 67:99, 1972.

Russi, S., Blumenthal, H. T., and Gray, S. H.: Small adenomas of the adrenal cortex in hypertension and diabetes. Arch. Intern. Med., 76:284, 1945.

Salem, M. R., and Ivankovic, A. D.: Management of phentolamine-resistant pheochromocytoma with beta adrenergic blockade. Br. J. Anaesth., 41:1087–1090, 1969.

Sardesai, S. H., Mourant, A. J., Sivathandon, Y., Farrow, R., and Gibbons, D. O.: Pheochromocytoma and catecholamine-induced myocardopathy presenting as heart failure. Br. Heart J., 63:234, 1990.

Sarkar, S. D., Cohen, E. L., Beierwaltes, W. H., Ice, R. D., Cooper, R., and Gold, E. M.: A new and superior adrenal imaging agent 131I-6B-iodo-methyl-19-nor-cholesterol (np-59) evaluation in humans. J. Clin. Endocrinol. Metab., 45:353, 1977.

Sarvin, C. T., Bray, G. A., and Idelson, B. A.: Overnight suppression test with dexamethasone in Cushing's syndrome. J. Clin. Endocrinol. Metab., 28:422, 1968.

Scasheeler, L. R., Myers, J. H., Eversman, J. J., and Taylor, H. C.: Adrenal insufficiency secondary to carcinoma metastatic in the adrenal gland. Cancer, 52:1312, 1983.

Schambelan, M., Sebastin, A., Biglieri, E. G., Brust, N. L., Chang, B. C., Harai, J., and Slater, K. L.: Prevalence pathogenesis and functional significance of aldosterone deficiency in hyperkalemic patients with chronic renal insufficiency. Kidney Int., 17:89, 1980.

Schambelan, M., Slaton, P. E., Jr., and Biglieri, E. G.: Mineralocorticoid production in hyperadrenocortism. A role in pathogenesis of hypokalemic alkalosis. Am. J. Med., 51:299, 1971.

Schambelan, M., Stockigt, J. R., and Biglieri, E. G.: Isolated hypoaldosteronism in adults, a renin deficiency syndrome. N. Engl. J. Med., 287:573, 1972.

Schechter, D. C.: Aberrant adrenal tissue. Ann. Surg., 167:421, 1968.

Schenker, J. G., and Chowers, I.: Pheochromocytoma and pregnancy. Obstet. Gynecol. Surg., 26:739, 1971.

Schteingert, D. E., Motazedi, A., Noonan, R. A., and Thompson, N. W.: Treatment of adrenal carcinomas. Arch. Surg., 117:1142, 1982.

Scott, E. M., Thomas, A., McGarrigle, H. H. G., and Lachelin, G. C. L.: Serial adrenal ultrasonography in normal neonates. J. Ultrasound Med., 9:279, 1990.

Scott, H. W., Jr.: Tumors of the adrenal cortex and Cushing's syndrome. Seventh National Cancer Conference Proceedings. Philadelphia, J. B. Lippincott Co., 1973.

Scott, H. W., Jr.: Historical background of the adrenal glands. In Scott, H. W. (Ed.): Surgery of the Adrenal Glands. Philadelphia, J. B. Lippincott Co., 1990a.

Scott, H. W., Jr.: In Scott, H. W. (Ed.): Surgery of the Adrenal Glands. Philadelphia, J. B. Lippincott Co., 1990b.

Scott, H. W., Jr., Liddle, G. W., Mulherin, J. L., Jr., McKenna, T. J., Stroup, S. L., and Rahmy, R. K.: Surgical experience with Cushing's disease. Ann. Surg., 185:524, 1977.

Scott, H. W., Jr., Oates, J. A., Nies, A. S., Burko, H., Page, D. L., and Rhamy, R. K.: Pheochromocytoma: present diagnosis and management. Ann. Surg., 183:587, 1976.

Scott, H. W., Jr., and Orth, D. N.: Hypercortisolism (Cushing's syndrome). In Scott, H. W. (Ed.): Surgery of the Adrenal Glands. Philadelphia, J. B. Lippincott Co., 1990.

Scott, H. W., Jr., Van Way, C. W., III, Gray, G. F., and Sussman, C. R.: Pheochromocytoma. In Scott, H. W. (Ed.): Surgery of the Adrenal Glands. Philadelphia, J. B. Lippincott Co., 1990.

Sealey, J. E., and Laragh, J. H.: Measurement of urinary aldosterone excretion in man. In Laragh, J. H. (Ed.): Hypertension Manual. New York, Yorke Medical Books, 1974.

Segal, S. J.: Mifepristone (RU486). N. Engl. J. Med., 322:691, 1990.

Selem, M. R., and Ivankovic, A. D.: Management of phentolamine-resistant pheochromocytoma with beta-adrenergic blockade. Br. J. Anaesth., 41:1087, 1969.

Shapiro, B., Copp, J. E., Sisson, J. C., Ayer, T. L., Wallis, J., and Beierwaltes, W. H.: Iodine-131 metaiodobenzylguanidine for the locating of suspected pheochromocytoma: Experience in 400 cases. J. Nucl. Med., 26:576, 1985.

Sheeler, L. R., Myers, J. H., Eversman, J. J., and Taylor, H. C.: Adrenal insufficiency secondary to carcinoma metastatic to the adrenal gland. Cancer, 52:1312–1316, 1983.

Sheridan, P., and Mattingly, P.: Simultaneous investigative treatment of suspected acute adrenal insufficiency. Lancet, 2:676, 1975.

Simpson, N. E., Kidd, K. K., and Goodfellow, P. J.: Assignment of multiple endocrine neoplasia type 2a to chromosome 10 by linkage. Nature, 328:528, 1987.

Simpson, S. A., Tait, J. R., Wettstein, A., Neher, R., von Euw, J., Schindler, O., and Reichstein, T.: Konstitution des aldosterons des neuen. Mineralocorticoids Experientia, 10:132, 1954.

Sipple, J. H.: The association of pheochromocytoma with carcinoma of the thyroid gland. Am. J. Med., 31:163, 1961.

Siragy, H. M., Vaughan, E. D., Jr., and Carey, R. M.: Cushing syndrome. *In* Vaughan, E. D., Jr., and Carey, R. M. (Eds.): Adrenal Disorder. New York, Thieme Medical Publishers Inc., 1989.

Sjoerdsma, A., Engelman, K., Spector, S., and Undenfriend, S.: Inhibition of catecholamine synthesis in man with alpha-methyl-tyrosine, an inhibitor to tyrosine hydroxylase. Lancet, 1:1092, 1965.

Smith, M. G., and Byrne, A. J.: An Addisonian crisis complicating anesthesia. Anesthesia, 36:681, 1981.

Spark, R. F., and Melby, J. C.: Aldosteronism and hypertension: The spironolactone response test. Ann. Intern. Med., 69:685, 1968.

Speckard, P. F., Nicoloff, J. T., and Bethune, J. E.: Screening for adrenocortical insufficiency with corticosyntrophin. Arch. Intern. Med., 128:761, 1971.

Speiser, P. W., Agdere, L., Ueshiba, H., White, P. C., and New, M. I.: Aldosterone synthesis in salt-wasting congenital adrenal hyperplasia with complete absence of adrenal 21-hydroxylase. N. Engl. J. Med., 324:145–149, 1991.

Speiss, J., Rivier, J., Rivier, C., and Vale, W.: Primary structure of corticotropin-releasing factor from ovine hypothalamus. Proc. Natl. Acad. Sci. (USA), 78:6517, 1981.

Stackpole, R. H., Melicow, M. M., and Uson, A. C.: Pheochromocytomas in children. J. Pediatr., 63:315, 1963.

Stewart, D. R., Jones, P. H., and Jolley, S. A.: Carcinoma of the adrenal gland in children. J. Pediatr. Surg., 9:59, 1974.

Streeten, D. H. P., Tomycz, N., and Anderson, G. H., Jr.: Reliability of screening test for the diagnosis of primary aldosteronism. Am. J. Med., 67:403, 1979.

Styne, D. M., Grumbach, M. M., Kaplan, S. L., Wilson, C. B., and Cante, F. A.: Treatment of Cushing's disease in childhood and adolescence by transphenoidal microadenomectomy. N. Engl. J. Med., 310:889, 1984.

Sullivan, M., Boileau, M., Hodges, C. V.: Adrenal cortical carcinoma. J. Urol., 120:660–665, 1978.

Sutton, M. G., Sheps, S. G., and Lie, J. T.: Prevalence of clinically unsuspected pheochromocytoma: A review of a 50-year autopsy series. Mayo Clin. Proc., 56:354, 1981.

Suzukawa, M., Michaels, I. A. L., Ruzbarsky, J., Koprivac, J., and Kitahata, L. M.: Use of isoflurane during resection of pheochromocytoma. Anesth. Analg., 62:119, 1983.

Tank, E. S., Gelbard, M. K., and Blank, B.: Familial pheochromocytomas. J. Urol., 128:1013, 1982.

Tannenbaum, M.: Ultrastructural pathology of the adrenal medullary tumor. *In* Sommers, S. C. (Ed.): "Pathology Annual." Appleton-Century-Crofts, New York, Vol. 5, pp. 145–171, 1970.

Tarazi, R. C., Ibrahim, M. M., Bravo, E. L., and Dustan, H. P.: Hemodynamic characteristics of primary aldosteronism. N. Engl. J. Med., 289:1330, 1973.

Tepperman, J., and Tepperman, H.: *Metabolic and Endocrine Physiology,* 5th ed. Chicago, Year Book Medical Publishers, 1987.

Thomas, J. L., Barnes, P. A., Bernardino, M. E., and Lewis, E.: Diagnostic approaches to adrenal and renal metastases. Radiol. Clin. North Am., 20:531, 1982.

Thomas, J. L., Bernardino, M. E., Samaan, N. A., and Hickey, R. C.: CT of pheochromocytoma. A.J.R., 135:477, 1980.

Trost, B. N., Koenig, M. P., Zimmerman, A., Zachmann, M., and Muller, J.: Virilization of a post-menopausal woman by a testosterone-secreting Leydig cell type adrenal adenoma. Acta Endocrinol., 98:274–282, 1981.

Twomey, P., Montgomery, C., and Clark, O.: Successful treatment of adrenal metastasis from large-cell carcinoma of the lung. JAMA, 248:581, 1982.

Tyrrell, J. B., Findling, J. W., Aron, D. C., Fitzgerald, P. A., and Forshamp, H.: An overnight high dose dexamethasone suppression test for rapid differential diagnosis of Cushing's syndrome. Ann. Intern. Med., 104:180, 1986.

Vaitukaitis, J. L., Dale, S. L., and Malby, J. C.: Role of ACTH in the secretion of free dehydroepiandrosterone and its sulfate ester in man. J. Clin. Endocrinol. Metab., 29:1443, 1969.

Vale, W., Speiss, J., Rivier, C., and Rivier, J.: Characterization of a 41 residue ovine hypothalmic peptide that stimulates secretion of corticotropin and beta endorphin. Science, 213:1394, 1981.

Valet, P., Damas-Michael, C., Chamontin, B., Durand, D., Gaillard, G., Salvador, M., and Montastruc, J. L.: Adrenoreceptors in the diagnosis of pheochromocytoma. Lancet, 2:337, 1987.

Van Heerden, J. A., Sheps, S. G., Hamberger, B., Sheedy, P. F.,

Poston, J. G., ReMine, W. H.: Pheochromocytoma: current status and changing trends. Surgery, 91:367, 1982.

Van Vliet, P. D., Burchell, H. B., and Titus, J. L.: Focal myocarditis associated with pheochromocytoma. N. Engl. J. Med., 274:1102, 1966.

Vaughan, E. D., Jr.: Diagnosis of adrenal disorders in hypertension. World J. Urol., 7:111–116, 1989.

Vaughan, E. D., Jr.: Adrenal surgery. *In* Marshall, F. F. (Ed.): Atlas of Urologic Surgery. Philadelphia, W. B. Saunders Co., 1991.

Vaughan, E. D., Jr., and Carey, R. M.: Adrenal Disorders. New York, Thieme Medical Publishers Inc., 1989a.

Vaughan, ED., Jr., and Carey, R. M.: Adrenal carcinoma. *In* Vaughan, E. D., Jr., and Carey, R. M. (Eds.): Adrenal Disorders. New York, Thieme Medical Publishers Inc., 1989b.

Vaughan, E. D., Jr., Atlas, S., and Carey, R. M.: Hyderaldosteronism. *In* Vaughan, E. D., Jr., and Carey, R. M. (Eds.): Adrenal Disorders. New York, Thieme Medical Publishers Inc., 1989c.

Vaughan, E. D., Jr., and Phillips, H.: Modified posterior approach for right adrenalectomy. Surg. Gynecol. Obstet., 165:453–455, 1987.

Vaughan, E. D., Jr., Laragh, J. H., Gavras, I., Bueller, F. R., Gavras, H., Brunner, H. R., and Baer, L.: Volume factor in low and normal renin essential hypertension. Am. J. Cardiol., 32:523, 1973.

Venkatesh, S., Hickey, R. C., Sellin, R. V., Fernandez, J. F., and Samaan, N. A.: Adrenal cortical carcinoma. Cancer, 64:765, 1989.

Verrey, F.: Regulation of gene expression by aldosterone in tight epithelia. Sem. Nephrol., 10:410, 1990.

Vyberg, M., and Sestof, T. L.: Combined adrenal myelolipoma and adenoma associated with Cushing's syndrome. Am. J. Clin. Pathol., 86:541, 1986.

Wallace, J. M., and Gill, D. P.: Prazosin in the diagnosis and treatment of pheochromocytoma. JAMA, 240:2752, 1978.

Weinberger, M. H., Grim, C. E., Hollifield, J. W., Kem, D. C., Ganguly, A., Kramer, N. J., June, H. Y., Wellman, H., and Donohue, J. P.: Primary aldosteronism: Diagnosis, localization and treatment. Ann. Intern. Med., 93:86, 1979.

Weiss, J. M.: Comparative histologic study of 43 metastasizing and non-metastasizing adrenal cortical tumors. Am. J. Surg. Pathol., 8:163, 1984.

Wendler, N. L., Graber, R. P., Jones, R. E., and Tischler, M.: Synthesis of 11 hydroxylated steroids: 17 hydroxycorticosterone. J. Am. Chem. Soc., 72:5793, 1950.

Werk, E. E., Jr., Sholiton, L. J., and Kalejs, L.: Testosterone-secreting adrenal adenoma under gonadotropin control. N. Engl. J. Med., 289:767–770, 1973.

Wheeler, M. H., Curley, I. R., and Williams, E. D.: The association of neurofibromatosis, pheochromocytoma, and somatostatin-rich aduodenal carcinoid tumor. Surgery, 100:1163, 1986.

White, E. A., Schambelan, M., Rost, L. R., Biglieri, E. G., Moss, A. A., and Korobkin, M.: Use of computed tomography in diagnosing the cause of primary aldosteronism. N. Engl. J. Med., 303:1503–1507, 1980.

Wilhelmus, J. L., Schrodt, G. R., Alberhasky, M. T., and Alcorn, M. O.: Giant adrenal myelolipoma: Case report and review of the literature. Arch. Pathol. Lab. Med., 105:532, 1981.

Williams, F. A., Jr., Schambelan, M., Biglieri, E. G., and Carey, R. M.: Acquired primary hypoaldosteronism' due to an isolated zona glomerulosa defect. N. Engl. J. Med., 309:1623–1627, 1983.

Willis, R. A.: The Spread of Tumors in the Human Body, 2nd ed. St. Louis, C. V. Mosby Co., 1952.

Wilson, C. B.: A decade of pituitary microsurgery. J. Neurosurg., 61:814, 1984.

Winkler, H., and Smith, A. D.: The chromaffin granule and the storage of catecholamines. *In* Blaschko, H., Sayers, G., and Smith, A. D. (Eds.): Handbook of Physiology. Washington, D.C., American Physiological Society, p. 321, 1975.

Wotman, S., Baer, L., Mendel, I. D., and Laragh, J. H.: Submaxillary potassium concentration in true and pseudoprimary hyperaldosteronism. Arch. Intern. Med., 129:248, 1970.

Wurtman, R. J., and Axelrod, J.: Adrenalin synthesis: Control by the pituitary gland and adrenoglucosteroids. Science, 150:1464, 1965.

Yamaji, T., Ishibashi, M., Sekihara, H., Itabashi, A., and Yanaihara, P.: Serum dehydroepiandrosterone sulfate in Cushing's syndrome. J. Clin. Endocrinol. Metab., 59:1164, 1984.

Young, J. L., Jr., and Miller, R. W.: Incidence of malignant tumors in U.S. children. J. Pediatr., 86:254, 1975.

Zweifler, A. J., and Julius, S.: A diagnostic test in patients with elevated plasma catecholamines. N. Engl. J. Med., 306:8, 1982.

65
SURGERY OF THE KIDNEY

Andrew C. Novick, M.D.
Stevan B. Streem, M.D.

HISTORICAL ASPECTS

The first nephrectomies were probably performed serendipitously. Early reports of removal of large ovarian tumors indicate that surgeons were occasionally surprised to find kidneys included in the specimens. Definitive renal surgery was first performed in 1869 by Gustav Simon, who carried out a planned nephrectomy for treatment of a ureterovaginal fistula. The operation was preceded by an extensive experimental investigation of uninephrectomy in dogs to demonstrate that they could survive normally with only one kidney. This application of an experimental model to a clinical problem was the forerunner of the method by which many current surgical procedures were developed.

In 1881, Morris was the first to perform nephrolithotomy in an otherwise healthy kidney, and he later defined the terms nephrolithiasis, nephrolithotomy, nephrectomy, and nephrotomy. The first partial nephrectomy was performed in 1884 by Wells for removal of a perirenal fibrolipoma. In 1887, Czerny was the first to use partial nephrectomy for excision of a renal neoplasm. Kuster performed the first successful pyeloplasty (a dismembered procedure) in 1891 on the solitary kidney of a 13-year-old boy. In 1892, Fenger applied the Heincckc-Mukulicz principle for pyloric stenosis to ureteropelvic junction obstruction. In 1903, Zondek emphasized the importance of a thorough knowledge of the renal arterial circulation when performing partial nephrectomy.

There was great controversy among early surgeons regarding the relative merits of retroperitoneal versus transperitoneal exposure of the kidney. Kocher performed an anterior transperitoneal nephrectomy through a midline incision as early as 1878. A transverse abdominal incision was employed in 1913 by Berg, who also mobilized the colon laterally to expose the great vessels and thus secure the renal pedicle with greater safety. Berg was able to remove vena caval tumor thrombi through a cavotomy after control of the veins by vascular clamps. Rehn actually reimplanted the con-

tralateral renal vein after resecting the inferior vena cava in 1922. However, the high incidence of peritonitis and other abdominal complications led most urologists to adopt a retroperitoneal flank approach to the kidney during the first half of this century. During the late 1950's, the development of safe abdominal and vascular surgical techniques led to a revival of the anterior approach in patients undergoing renal surgery (Culp, 1961; Poutasse, 1961).

SURGICAL ANATOMY

The kidneys are paired vital organs located on either side of the vertebral column in the lumbar fossa of the retroperitoneal space. Each kidney is surrounded by a layer of perinephric fat which is in turn covered by a distinct fascial layer termed gerota's fascia. Posteriorly, both kidneys lie on the psoas major and quadratus lumborum muscles. They are also in relationship with the medial and lateral lumbocostal arches and the tendon of the transversus abdominis. Posteriorly and superiorly, the upper pole of each kidney is in contact with the diaphragm (Fig. 65-1).

A small segment of the anterior medial surface of the right kidney is in contact with the right adrenal gland. However, the major anterior relationships of the right kidney are the liver, which overlies the upper two thirds of the anterior surface, and the hepatic flexure of the colon, which overlies the lower one third. The second portion of the duodenum covers the right renal hilum.

A small segment of the anterior medial surface of the left kidney is also covered by the left adrenal gland. The major anterior relationships of the left kidney are the spleen, body of the pancreas, stomach, and splenic flexure of the colon.

The kidney has four constant vascular segments that are termed apical, anterior, posterior, and basilar (Boyce, 1967). The anterior segment is the largest and extends beyond the mid plane of the kidney onto the posterior surface. A true avascular line exists at the

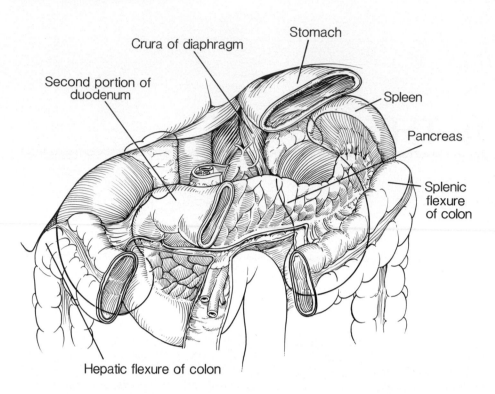

Crura of diaphragm

Stomach

Second portion of duodenum

Spleen

Pancreas

Splenic flexure of colon

Hepatic flexure of colon

Figure 65–1. The anatomic relationship of the kidneys to the surrounding structures. The liver is retracted superiorly in this illustration.

junction of the anterior and posterior segments, on the posterior surface of the kidney.

Each vascular segment of the kidney is supplied by one or more major arterial branches (Fig. 65–2). Although the origin of the branches supplying these segments may vary, the anatomic position of the segments is constant (Graves, 1954). All segmental arteries are end-arteries with no collateral circulation; therefore, when performing renal surgery, failure to preserve one of these branches will lead to devitalization of functioning renal tissue. Most individuals have a single main artery to each kidney originating from the lateral aspect of the aorta just below the superior mesenteric artery. Multiple renal arteries occur unilaterally and bilaterally in 23 per cent and 10 per cent of the population, respectively.

The normal renal venous anatomy is depicted in Fig. 65–3. The left and right renal veins both terminate in the lateral aspect of the inferior vena cava. The left renal vein is longer and has a thicker muscular layer than the right renal vein. Several important nonrenal branches empty into the left renal vein. These are the gonadal vein inferiorly, the left adrenal vein superiorly, and one or two large lumbar veins posteriorly. No significant branches drain into the right renal vein. Multiple renal veins are less common than multiple renal arteries.

The renal venous drainage system differs significantly from the arterial blood supply in that the intrarenal venous branches intercommunicate freely between the various renal segments. Ligation of a branch of the renal vein, therefore, will not result in segmental infarction of the kidney because collateral venous blood supply will provide adequate drainage. This factor is important clinically, because it enables one to obtain surgical access to structures in the renal hilus by ligating and dividing small adjacent or overlying venous branches. This ability allows major venous branches to be completely mobilized and freely retracted in either direction to safely expose the renal hilus, with no vascular compromise of renal parenchyma.

With regard to the intrarenal collecting system, there are eight to ten major calyces that open into the renal pelvis (Fig. 65–4). The apical segment has one major calyx that lies in the mid-frontal plane and receives two minor calyces, which are lateral and medial. The basilar segment has a single major calyx in the median plane and receives two minor calyces, which are anterior and posterior. Three major calyces in the anterior segment enter the renal pelvis at a 20-degree angle to the mid-frontal plane; three major calyces in the posterior segment enter the renal pelvis at a 75-degree angle to the mid-frontal plane.

PREOPERATIVE PREPARATION

A thorough preoperative evaluation is important in patients who are undergoing renal surgery because of the special positions in which the patients may have to be placed intraoperatively and because of the systemic disturbances that may occur secondary to renal infections and impairment of renal function.

Cardiorespiratory function is evaluated by eliciting any history of heart disease, chest pain, smoking, or respiratory distress on exertion. An electrocardiogram, chest radiograph, and complete blood count should be obtained on all patients. The flank position with lateral flexion of the spine is known to cause embarrassment of ventilatory capacity. The venous return may be significantly diminished in this position, resulting in hypotension. Therefore, alternatives to the flank approach

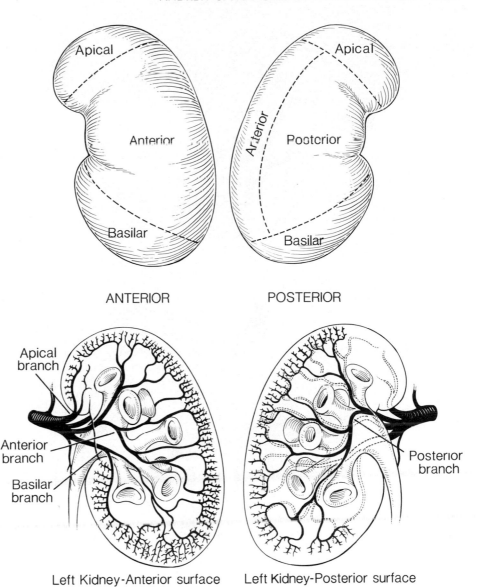

Figure 65–2. The vascular segments of the left kidney, as shown in the anterior and posterior projections, and the corresponding segmental arterial supply to each segment.

Left Kidney-Anterior surface   Left Kidney-Posterior surface

should be used whenever possible in the patient with a decreased pulmonary reserve. Preoperative pulmonary function studies and blood gas analyses are mandatory in patients suspected of having impaired respiratory function. In the event of the latter, an anterior surgical approach with the patient in the supine position is preferred.

Regardless of the surgical incision, respiration may be seriously impaired postoperatively because of the transection of the upper abdominal or flank muscles and, occasionally, the removal of a rib. Also, the upper poles of the kidneys encroach on the undersurface of the diaphragm, and the removal of a large upper pole renal mass may interfere temporarily with its function. Preoperative breathing exercises, alleviation of bronchospasm, cessation of smoking, and evaluation of cardiopulmonary function are helpful in improving respiratory function and in preventing postoperative cardiorespiratory problems.

Bleeding tendencies are assessed by examination of platelet function and coagulation factors. Patients should

be questioned about excess alcohol intake and ingestion of drugs, such as aspirin, that can influence blood clotting.

A thorough anatomic examination of the urinary tract should be made in all patients undergoing renal surgery. Available studies include intravenous pyelography, cystoscopy, retrograde pyelography, ureteroscopy, cystourethrography, computed tomography (CT), ultrasonography, magnetic resonance imaging (MRI), renal arteriography, and renal venography. These tests are reviewed in detail in Chapter 10. Their usefulness in evaluating patients for specific renal operations is described in subsequent sections of this chapter.

Overall renal function is evaluated by estimation of the serum creatinine level and either endogenous creatinine clearance or iothalamate glomerular filtration rate. Differential renal function can be assessed noninvasively with computerized isotope renography using Hippuran I 131 or technetium-99m. Hippuran I 131 is cleared by both glomeruli and tubules and is most useful for measuring unilateral renal dysfunction when overall

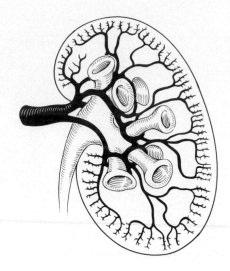

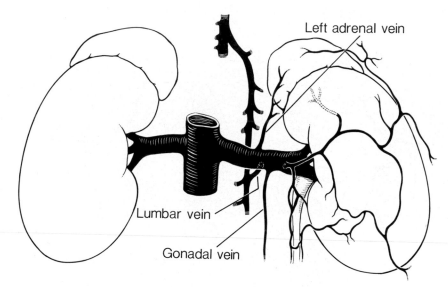

Left adrenal vein

Lumbar vein

Gonadal vein

Figure 65–3. The normal renal venous anatomy, including branches of the left renal vein, is shown below. The intrarenal venous drainage parallels the segmental arterial supply and is depicted above for the left kidney.

renal function is normal. Technetium chelated with diethylenetriaminepenta-acetic acid (DTPA) is filtered only by the glomeruli and is thus more helpful in assessing differential renal perfusion. Both of these isotopes are excreted in the urine. In the presence of obstruction, parenchymal concentration is obscured by the high concentration of isotope in the accumulated urine. Selective ureteral catheterization to determine differential renal function is an invasive study, which is currently rarely utilized.

Patients with either upper or lower urinary tract infection should receive organism-specific antibiotic therapy preoperatively. With suspected or proven upper tract infection, antibiotic therapy of at least 48 hours is indicated prior to renal surgery. Severe bacteremia can occur during an operation on an infected kidney, with significant resulting morbidity and potential mortality.

Percutaneous embolization of the kidney is occasionally helpful prior to performing radical nephrectomy for large renal malignancies. The major value of this adjunct is in a patient with an arterialized vena caval tumor thrombus or with a medial extension of tumor that interferes with early ligation of the renal artery. Currently, absolute ethanol injected directly into the renal artery appears to be the most satisfactory material for angioinfarction. Subsequent transient flank pain is common and often requires analgesic medication for control.

Patients are often concerned about how the removal of a kidney will affect remaining renal function. Following nephrectomy for unilateral renal disease, the opposite kidney undergoes compensatory hypertrophy. The glomerular filtration rate is ultimately maintained at 75 per cent of the normal value (Aperia, 1977; Robitaille, 1985). Following unilateral nephrectomy with a normal contralateral kidney, several long-term studies have shown no increase in hypertension or proteinuria, stable overall renal function, and normal life expectancy (Anderson, 1968; Goldstein, 1956; Kretschmer, 1943). This information should be shared with patients to alleviate their anxiety prior to surgery.

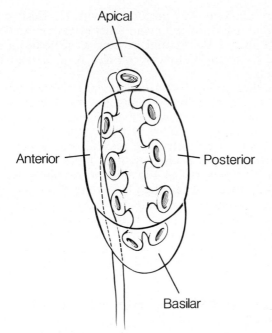

Apical

Anterior

Posterior

Basilar

Figure 65–4. The intrarenal collecting system in relation to major vascular segments of the kidney.

INTRAOPERATIVE RENAL ISCHEMIA

Temporary occlusion of the renal artery is necessary for a variety of operations, such as partial nephrectomy, renal vascular reconstruction, anatrophic nephrolithotomy, and traumatic renal injury repair. In such cases, temporary arterial occlusion not only diminishes intraoperative renal bleeding but also improves access to intrarenal structures by causing the kidney to contract, reducing renal tissue turgor. Performance of these operations requires an understanding of renal responses to warm ischemia and available methods of protecting the kidney, when the period of arterial occlusion exceeds that which may be safely tolerated.

Renal Tolerance to Warm Ischemia

Because renal metabolic activities are predominantly aerobic, the kidney is very susceptible to damage from warm ischemia. Almost immediately following renal arterial occlusion, energy-rich adenosine triphosphate (ATP) within the kidney cells begins to break down into monophosphate nucleotide in order to provide the energy required for maintenance of structural and functional cellular integrity (Collins, 1977; Collste, 1971). When energy sources have been depleted, cellular membrane transport mechanisms fail, causing an influx of salt and water, which ultimately results in severe cellular edema and cell death.

The extent of renal damage following normothermic arterial occlusion depends on the duration of the ischemic insult. Canine studies have shown that warm ischemic intervals of up to 30 minutes can be sustained with eventual full recovery of renal function (Ward, 1975).

For periods of warm ischemia beyond 30 minutes, there is generally significant immediate functional loss. Late recovery of renal function is either incomplete or absent. Histologically, renal ischemia is most damaging to the proximal tubular cells, which may show varying degrees of necrosis and regeneration. The glomeruli and blood vessels are generally spared.

Human tolerance to warm renal ischemia very closely parallels that of experimental canine observations. In general, 30 minutes is the maximum tolerable period of arterial occlusion before permanent damage is sustained. In some clinical situations, the latter admonition may not apply, and a longer period of ischemia may be safely tolerated. The solitary kidney is more resistant to ischemic damage than the paired kidney, although precise limits have not been defined (Askari, 1982). Another situation that may enhance renal tolerance to temporary arterial occlusion is the presence of an extensive collateral vascular supply. This is generally observed only in patients with renal arterial occlusive disease (Schefft, 1980).

Another determinant of renal ischemic damage is the method employed to achieve vascular control of the kidney. Animal studies have shown that functional impairment is least when the renal artery alone is continuously occluded. Continuous occlusion of both the renal artery and vein for an equivalent time interval is more damaging, because this prevents retrograde perfusion of the kidney through the renal vein and may produce venous congestion of the kidney (Leary, 1963; Neely, 1959; Schirmer, 1966). Intermittent clamping of the renal artery with short periods of recirculation is also more damaging than continuous arterial occlusion, possibly because of the release and trapping of damaging vasoconstrictor agents within the kidney (McLaughlin, 1978; Neely, 1959; Schirmer, 1966; Wilson, 1971). Animal studies have further demonstrated that manual renal compression to control intraoperative hemorrhage is more deleterious than simple arterial occlusion (Neely, 1959).

Prevention of Ischemic Renal Damage

Several general adjunctive measures should be employed in all patients who are undergoing operations that involve a period of temporary renal arterial occlusion. These include generous preoperative and intraoperative hydration, prevention of hypotension during the period of anesthesia, avoidance of unnecessary manipulation or traction on the renal artery, and intraoperative administration of mannitol. These measures help to limit postischemic renal injury by ensuring optimal perfusion with absence of cortical vasospasm at the time of arterial occlusion. This practice allows uniform restoration of blood flow throughout the kidney when the renal artery is unclamped. Mannitol is most effective when given 5 to 15 minutes prior to arterial occlusion (Collins, 1980) and is beneficial by increasing renal plasma flow, decreasing intrarenal vascular resistance, minimizing intracellular edema, and promoting osmotic diuresis when the renal circulation is restored

(Nosowsky, 1963). Systemic or regional heparinization prior to renal arterial occlusion is not necessary, unless there is existing small vessel or parenchymal renal disease.

When the anticipated period of intraoperative renal ischemia is longer than 30 minutes, additional specific protective measures are indicated to prevent permanent damage to the kidney. Local hypothermia is the most efficacious and commonly employed method for protecting the kidney from ischemic damage. Lowering renal temperature reduces energy-dependent metabolic activity of the cortical cells, with a resultant decrease in both the consumption of oxygen and the breakdown of ATP (Harvey, 1959; Levy, 1959). The optimum temperature for hypothermic in situ renal preservation is 15°C, based on canine experiments conducted by Ward (1975). In clinical renal surgery, it is difficult to achieve uniform cooling to this level because of the temperature of adjacent tissues and the need to have a portion of the kidney exposed to perform the operation. For practical reasons, a temperature of 20 to 25°C is simpler to maintain and represents a compromise that renders renal surgery technically feasible, still allowing a renal preservative effect. Both animal and human studies have shown that this level of hypothermia provides complete renal protection from up to 3 hours of arterial occlusion (Kyriakidis, 1979; Luttrop, 1976; Marberger, 1978; Petersen, 1977; Stubbs, 1978; Wagenknecht, 1977; Wickham, 1967).

In situ renal hypothermia can be achieved with external surface cooling or with perfusion of the kidney with a cold solution instilled into the renal artery. Either method is equally effective; however, perfusion is an invasive technique that requires direct entry into the renal artery (Abele, 1981; Farcon, 1974; Kyriakidis, 1979; Leary, 1963). Surface cooling of the kidney is a simpler and more widely used method, which has been accomplished by a variety of techniques such as surrounding the kidney with ice slush (Gibbons, 1976; Metzner, 1972; Stubbs, 1978), immersing the kidney in a cold solution (Mitchell, 1959), or applying an external cooling device to the kidney (Cockett, 1961). These methods all require complete renal mobilization to achieve effective surface cooling.

Most urologists currently prefer cooling with ice slush for surface renal hypothermia because of its relative ease and simplicity. The mobilized kidney is surrounded with a rubber sheet on which sterile ice slush is placed to completely immerse the kidney. An important caveat with this method is to keep the entire kidney covered with ice slush for 10 to 15 minutes, immediately after occluding the renal artery and before commencing the renal operation. This amount of time is needed to obtain core renal cooling to a temperature (approximately 20°C) that optimizes in situ renal preservation. During performance of the renal operation, invariably large portions of the kidney are no longer covered with ice slush and, in the absence of adequate prior core renal cooling, rapid rewarming and ischemic renal injury can occur. This technique is very effective for in situ renal preservation. Stubbs and associates (1978) reported 30 patients with a solitary kidney in whom anatrophic nephrolithotomy was performed with ice slush surface hypothermia; despite a mean renal artery clamp time of longer than 2 hours, and as long as 4 hours in some cases, renal function was completely preserved in all patients.

Another approach to in situ renal preservation that does not involve hypothermia has been pretreatment with one or more pharmacologic agents to prevent postischemic renal failure (Novick, 1983). Agents that have been tested include vasoactive drugs, membrane-stabilizing drugs, calcium channel blockers, and others that act to preserve or replenish intracellular levels of ATP. A review of this field is beyond the scope of this chapter, however. Experimental studies have shown that several of these agents can help to prevent postischemic renal failure. However, thus far, no pharmacologic regimen has proved to be as effective as local hypothermia for ischemic intervals of 2 hours or more.

SURGICAL APPROACHES TO THE KIDNEY

Exposure of the kidney during surgery must be adequate to perform the operation and to deal with any possible complications. This factor is particularly important in renal surgery, because the kidney is deeply placed in the upper retroperitoneum with access limited by the lower ribs, liver, and spleen. Injuries to large renal vessels may be difficult to control or repair through small incisions, particularly in the presence of a large tumor or inflamed perinephric tissues. Poor exposure renders the operation unnecessarily difficult and leads to excessive retraction, with bruising of the muscles and possible injury to the intercostal nerves, which can increase postoperative pain.

Factors to consider in selecting an appropriate incision for renal surgery include the (1) operation to be performed, (2) underlying renal pathology, (3) previous operations, (4) concurrent extrarenal pathology that requires another operation to be done simultaneously, (5) need for bilateral renal operations, and (6) body habitus. Physical abnormalities in the patient, such as kyphoscoliosis, or severe pulmonary disease may also dictate that certain approaches, such as the standard flank incision, not be selected. The kidney may be approached by one of four principal routes: (1) extraperitoneal flank, (2) dorsal lumbotomy, (3) abdominal incision, and (4) thoracoabdominal incision. The indications, the relative advantages, and the technical performance of each approach are reviewed next, separately.

Flank Approach

This approach provides good access to the renal parenchyma and collecting system (Woodruff, 1955). It is an extraperitoneal approach and involves minimal disturbance to other viscera. Contamination of the peritoneal cavity is avoided, and drainage of the perirenal space is readily established. This approach is particularly

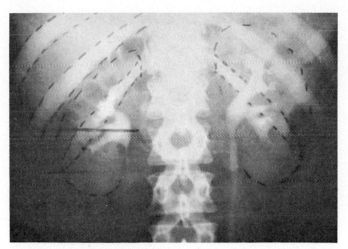

Figure 65–5. The right kidney is traversed at its midpoint by the 12th rib. The ideal incision is chosen by drawing a horizontal line from the hilum to the lateral rib cage.

useful in the obese patient. Most of the panniculus falls forward, making this incision relatively straightforward even in the very large person. The principal disadvantage of the flank incision is that exposure in the area of the renal pedicle is not as good as that in the anterior transperitoneal approach. In addition, the flank incision may prove unsuitable for the patient with scoliosis or cardiorespiratory problems.

The most commonly chosen flank approach to the kidney is through the bed of the 11th or 12th rib (Bodner, 1950; Hess, 1939; Hughes, 1949). The choice of rib depends on the position of the kidney and on whether the upper or lower pole is the site of disease. With a flank incision, the midportion of the wound and the site of maximum exposure are in the midaxillary line. Access in the posterior part, at the neck of the rib, is limited by the sacrospinalis muscle. The appropriate level of the incision is therefore best determined by drawing a horizontal line on the urogram from the hilum of the kidney to the most lateral rib that it intersects (Fig. 65–5). When access to the upper renal pole is required, the rib above is selected.

The patient is placed in the lateral position after anesthesia and endotracheal tube insertion. The back should be placed fairly close to the edge of the operating table to ensure unimpeded access by the surgeon. The patient should be positioned so that the tip of the 12th rib is over the kidney rest. The bottom leg is flexed to 90 degrees, with the top leg straight to maintain stability. A pillow is placed between the knees, and a sponge pad is placed under the axilla to prevent compression of the axillary vessels and nerves. The patient is secured in this position with a wide adhesive tape passed over the greater trochanter and attached to the movable portion of the table (Fig. 65–6). The extended upper arm can be supported on a padded Mayo stand, which is adjusted to the appropriate height to maintain the arm in a horizontal position with the shoulder rotated slightly forward.

Flexion of the table and elevation of the kidney rest should be performed slowly and may be delayed until the surgeon is ready to make the skin incision in order to minimize the time the patient spends in this position. The flexion increases the space between the costal margin and iliac crest and puts the flank muscles and skin on tension. Care must be taken with patients who have stiff spines to ensure that their extremities remain in contact with the table, because their range of lateral flexion is limited. This position may not be well tolerated in elderly patients or in those with impaired cardiopulmonary function, because it results in decreased venous return due to compression of the inferior vena cava and the dependent position of the legs. This position also limits aeration of the lung on the dependent side. It is important to determine the patient's blood pressure after he or she has been turned to the side and again after the table has been flexed and the kidney rest elevated. The rest may have to be lowered and the table straightened, if hypotension is observed.

The flank incision is made directly over the appropriate rib, beginning at the lateral border of the sacrospinalis muscle (Fig. 65–7). A left-sided 12th rib incision is demonstrated in Figures 65–7 to 65–12. After dividing the external oblique, latissimus dorsi, and slips of the underlying serratus posterior inferior muscles (see Fig. 65–8), the periosteum over the rib is incised with a scalpel or by diathermy. The flat periosteal elevator is used to reflect the periosteum off the rib (see Fig. 65–9). Mobilization of the periosteum is completed by separating it from the inner aspect of the rib, using a Doyen elevator (see Fig. 65–10). The proximal end of

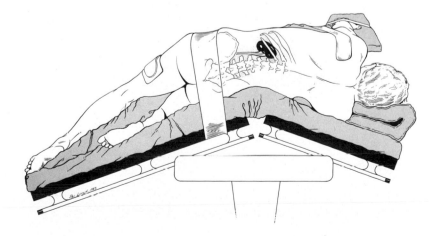

Figure 65–6. Position of the patient for the flank approach. Note the axillary pad. The kidney rest may be elevated if further lateral extension is needed.

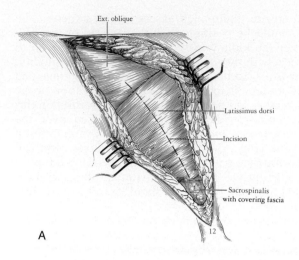

A

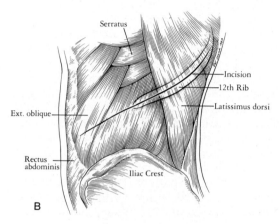

B

Figure 65–7. *A*, Left flank incision. Anterior edge of the latissimus dorsi muscle overlies the posterior edge of the external oblique muscle. *B*, The relationship of the 12th rib to the overlying muscles is depicted.

Figure 65–8. The muscles in the posterior part of the wound have been divided to expose the rib for incision of the periosteum.

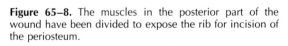

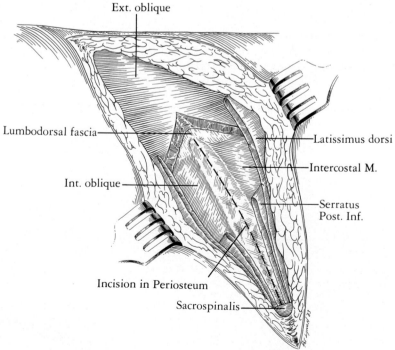

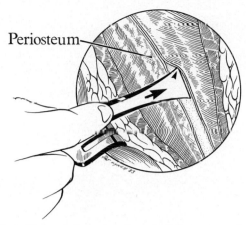

Figure 65–9. The periosteum is reflected off the upper surface of the rib. Note the periostial elevator is moved distally or downward on the upper edge of the rib against the direction of the intercostal muscle fibers.

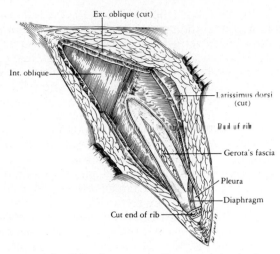

Figure 65–11. The rib has been resected, exposing the diaphragm and pleura in the posterior part of the wound. The slips of the diaphragm inserting into the rib have been divided allowing the pleura to be displaced upward. An incision is made through the periosteal bed of the wound to expose Gerota's fascia.

the rib is then transected as far back as possible with the guillotine rib resector. The retracted muscle mass is allowed to fall back over the sharp cut edge, protecting the operator from injury. The rib is grasped with a Kocher clamp and is separated from the muscles attached anteriorly by sharp dissection to complete its removal.

When the 11th rib is resected, attention must be directed toward the pleural reflection, which crosses its lower border at the junction of the anterior and middle thirds and occupies the posterior part of the wound, as it lies on the lower fibers of the diaphragm. The pleura may be reflected upward by sharply dividing the fascial attachments to the diaphragm. Alternatively, the lower fibers of the diaphragm can be detached from their insertions into the posterior inner aspect of the 12th rib. This maneuver allows the lower diaphragm and pleura to be retracted upward, out of the wound.

An incision is now made through the periosteal bed of the rib to expose Gerota's fascia (see Fig. 65–11). The incision is completed anteriorly by incising the lumbar fascia and inserting two fingers into the peri-

nephric space to push the underlying peritoneum forward. The lateral peritoneal reflection is peeled off the undersurface of the anterior abdominal wall and transversalis fascia, by sweeping it forward with the fingers. The external and internal oblique muscles are divided by incising them sharply or by electrocautery, while they are tented up over the two fingers inserted below the transversus muscle (see Fig. 65–12). A little upward pressure will control bleeding from the severed vessels, allowing them to be clamped or cauterized by the assistant. This procedure should expose the intercostal neurovascular bundle, as it courses forward and downward between the internal oblique and transversus muscles. The transverse fibers of the transversus muscle may

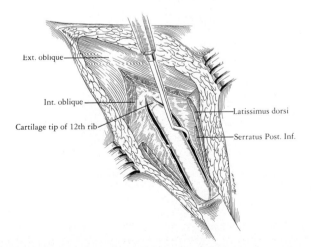

Figure 65–10. The periosteum is dissected off the rib, using a Doyen periosteal elevator, prior to resection of the rib.

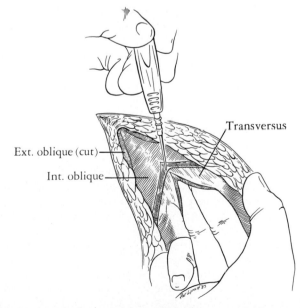

Figure 65–12. Two fingers are inserted into the incision in the posterior part of the transversus muscle to sweep the peritoneal reflection forward and divide the anterior abdominal muscles.

be split by blunt dissection below the nerve, allowing it to fall away with the upper margin of the incision.

A Finochietto retractor maintains the exposure. The blades of the retractor are placed over moistened gauze sponges to avoid breaking a rib. The perinephric space is entered by incising Gerota's fascia posteriorly to avoid injury to the peritoneum. Care should be taken to avoid injury to the iliohypogastric and ilioinguinal nerves, as they emerge from behind the lateral border of the psoas muscle and pass down over the anterior surface of the quadratus lumborum in the renal fossa.

The incision is closed by careful approximation of the corresponding muscle and fascial layers. To facilitate this procedure, the kidney rest is lowered and the table is returned to the horizontal position. Care must be taken to avoid inclusion of any intercostal nerves or branches during closure of the transversus muscle. Injection of 0.5 per cent bupivacaine (Marcaine) into the fascial sheath around the intercostal nerves as they emerge from the intervertebral foramina is helpful in diminishing postoperative pain and involuntary splinting of the lower chest. Drains are usually brought out posteriorly, through a separate stab incision below the wound.

Occasionally, a subcostal flank incision is indicated for surgery on the lower renal pole or upper ureter, for insertion of a nephrostomy tube, for drainage of a perinephric abscess. It has the disadvantage of being rather low in relation to the usual position of the kidney, which makes access to the pedicle and renal pelvis more difficult. Exposure may be hampered by the iliac crest and subcostal nerve. The subcostal incision does not have disadvantages in children, in whom it provides good access to the kidney, because the lower ribs are soft and simply displaced upward.

The subcostal incision is begun at the lateral border of the sacrospinalis muscle where it crosses the inferior edge of the 12th rib and is carried forward about a fingerbreadth below the lower border of the last rib onto the anterior abdominal wall. The medial end of the incision is curved slightly downward, as it passes the midaxillary line to avoid the subcostal nerve and may be extended as far as the lateral border of the rectus abdominis muscle. The extent of the incision is modified, depending on the location of the kidney and the nature of the disease.

With a subcostal incision, the latissimus dorsi muscle is divided in the posterior part of the wound to expose the posterior edge of the external oblique muscle (Fig. 65–13). The serratus posterior inferior muscles, arising from the lumbar fascia and inserting into the lower four ribs, are divided in the posterior portion of the wound. The external oblique muscle is divided anteriorly. The fused layers of the lumbodorsal fascia are now exposed, as they give origin to the internal oblique and transversus muscles. After the internal oblique muscle is divided, the transversus is separated bluntly either above or below the subcostal nerve, depending on the course of the nerve in relation to the incision (Fig. 65–14). Every effort should be made to avoid injury to the intercostal nerves, which may cause persistent postoperative pain or bulging in the flank due to paresis of the denervated

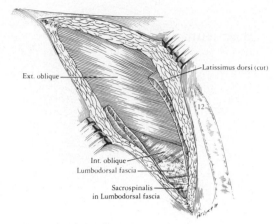

Figure 65–13. Left subcostal incision. The latissimus dorsi muscle has been divided to expose the lumbodorsal fascia and posterior aspects of the abdominal muscles.

muscle. The lumbar fascia and the lateral border of the sacrospinalis may need to be incised to improve exposure in the posterior part of the wound. Division of the costotransverse ligament, as it passes up to the neck of the 12th rib, will allow the rib to be retracted upward to further improve the exposure. The closure is as described previously for a flank incision.

Dorsal Lumbotomy

The dorsal lumbotomy incision is a useful approach for removal of a small kidney, bilateral nephrectomy in the patient with end-stage renal disease, open renal biopsy, pyeloplasty, pyelolithotomy, and upper ureterolithotomy when the stone is firmly impacted (Gil-Vernet, 1965; Novick, 1980). This approach offers several advantages when performing these operations (Gardiner, 1979). Unlike the standard flank incision, no muscles are transected and access to the kidney is obtained by

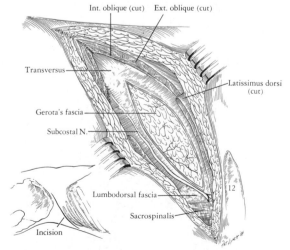

Figure 65–14. The lumbodorsal fascia and transversus muscles have been divided to expose Gerota's fascia. The subcostal nerve and vessels pierce the lumbodorsal fascia posteriorly and course forward on the transversus muscle.

incising the posterior fascial layers. This approach is more rapid, provides a strong wound closure with less postoperative pain, and obviates anterolateral bulging of the abdomen that commonly results from flank incisions. With detachment of the costovertebral ligament, the 12th rib can be retracted widely and laterally, rendering resection of the rib unnecessary. The dorsal lumbotomy approach is also advantageous in patients with prior abdominal or flank operations on the kidney, because it permits dissection of fresh tissue planes. The major disadvantage of the dorsal lumbotomy is the limited access to the kidney and renal vessels, which can pose a problem if there are intraoperative complications such as migration of a calculus or injury to major renal vessels with bleeding.

When bilateral nephrectomy is done, the patient is placed in the prone position with the table flexed to increase the distance between the 12th rib and the iliac crest. In this position, the patient is supported over the sternum and pubis so that there is free excursion of the anterior abdominal wall to prevent embarassment of respiration and venous return. For unilateral renal operations, the patient may be placed in the lateral position with the table flexed to extend the lumbar region. In this position, a sandbag is placed between the abdomen and the table for support and to help push the kidney posteriorly.

A vertical lumbar incision is made along the lateral margin of the sacrospinalis muscle. The incision begins at the upper margin of the 12th rib superiorly and follows a gentle lateral curve to the iliac crest inferiorly (Fig. 65–15A). The incision is carried through the lumbodorsal fascia just lateral to the sacrospinalis and quadratus lumborum muscles, which are then retracted medially to approach the renal fossa (Fig. 65–15B). The transversalis fascia is incised to expose the kidney contained within Gerota's fascia (see Fig. 65–15C). Exposure of the kidney is thus obtained without transection of any muscle fibers. If additional superior exposure is needed, the costovertebral ligamentous attachment of the 12th rib is divided to allow lateral and superior retraction of the rib (see Fig. 65–15D and E). The kidney can be mobilized and delivered down into the incision, provided the lower third of the kidney is located below the 12th rib on preoperative radiographs. However, for high-lying or enlarged kidneys, the dorsal lumbotomy approach is cumbersome and either a flank or an anterior incision will provide better exposure. To close the incision, the retracted muscles are allowed to return to their original position and the lumbodorsal fascia is reapproximated.

Abdominal Incision

The principal advantage of the abdominal approach is that exposure in the area of the renal pedicle is excellent. The principal disadvantage is the somewhat longer period of postoperative ileus and the possible long-term complication of intra-abdominal adhesions, leading to bowel obstruction. The choice between a vertical or transverse type of abdominal incision is determined by the patient's anatomy and the disease entity. A vertical incision is simpler and quicker to perform and repair, as it involves only division of the linea alba or the anterior and posterior layers of the rectus sheath rather than several muscle layers. The vertical incision may be utilized in a patient with a narrow subcostal angle and is preferred in a patient with a renal injury, because it allows better access for inspection of the remainder of the abdominal contents for associated injuries. A transverse incision is preferable for the patient with a wide subcostal angle and for the exploration or removal of renal mass lesions (Chute, 1967). This incision provides better access to the lateral and superior portion of the kidney. A unilateral subcostal incision can be extended across the midline as a chevron incision to provide excellent exposure of both kidneys along with the aorta and inferior vena cava.

When employing an anterior subcostal incision, the patient is in the supine position with a rolled sheet beneath the upper lumbar spine. The incision begins approximately one to two fingerbreadths below the costal margin in the anterior axillary line and then extends with a gentle curve across the midline, ending at the midportion of the opposite rectus muscle. The incision is carried through the subcutaneous tissues to the anterior fascia, which is divided in the direction of the incision. In the lateral aspect of the incision, a portion of the latissimus dorsi muscle is divided. The external oblique muscle is divided, exposing the fibers of the internal oblique muscle (Fig. 65–16A). The rectus, internal oblique, and transversus abdominis muscles are divided along with the posterior rectus sheath (Fig. 65–16B and C). The peritoneal cavity is entered in the midline, and the ligamentum teres is divided (Fig. 65–16D).

The bilateral subcostal incision is performed as previously described for the unilateral incision, except that both sides are involved (Fig. 65–17). It extends from one anterior axillary line to the opposite anterior axillary line, with a gentle upward curve as it crosses the midline. This incision provides better exposure of both kidneys than a midline incision, particularly in an obese patient with a wide subcostal angle. The disadvantage is that it involves extensive transection of the abdominal wall musculature.

An extraperitoneal anterior subcostal approach may be useful to perform open renal biopsy or nephrectomy, particularly when there has been a previous intra-abdominal procedure or when there is a possibility that the patient may require postoperative peritoneal dialysis (Lyon, 1958). The peritoneal cavity is not entered, thereby minimizing postoperative ileus and the chance of an intra-abdominal complication. Reflection of the peritoneum off the anterior abdominal wall may at times be difficult, and access to the renal pedicle may be less satisfactory than that with a transperitoneal incision. The patient is placed in a semioblique position with a rolled sheet beneath the side in which the incision is to be made. The muscle layers are divided as they are for a unilateral subcostal incision, except that the peritoneal cavity is not entered. The peritoneum is mobilized intact from the undersurface of the lateral musculature and

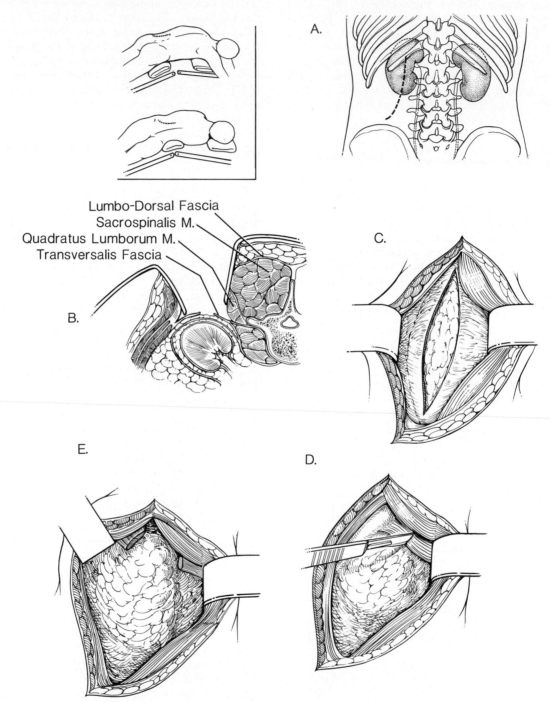

Lumbo-Dorsal Fascia
Sacrospinalis M.
Quadratus Lumborum M.
Transversalis Fascia

Figure 65–15. *A to E,* The dorsal lumbotomy incision (see text for description of procedure).

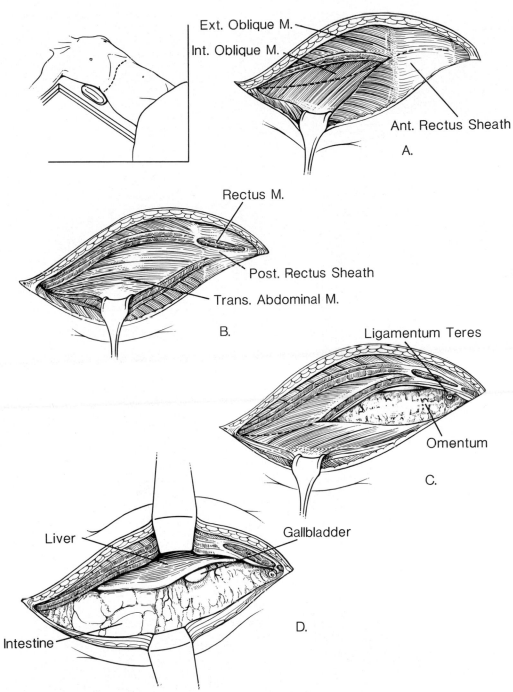

Figure 65–16. *A* to *D*, Unilateral anterior subcostal transperitoneal incision (see text).

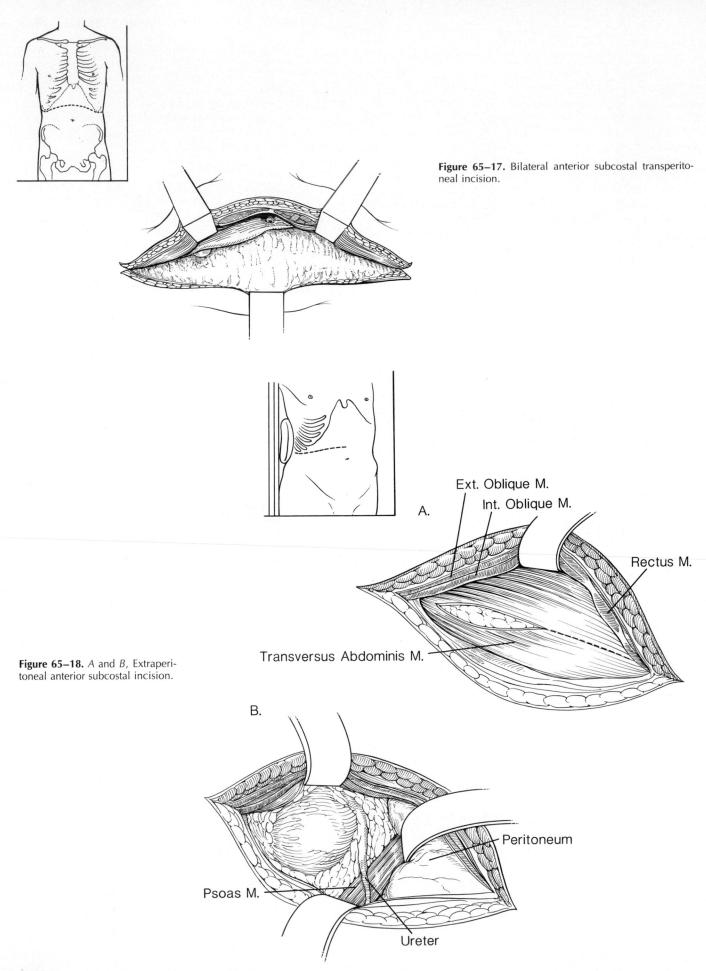

Figure 65–17. Bilateral anterior subcostal transperitoneal incision.

Ext. Oblique M.

Int. Oblique M.

A.

Rectus M.

Transversus Abdominis M.

Figure 65–18. *A* and *B*, Extraperitoneal anterior subcostal incision.

B.

Peritoneum

Psoas M.

Ureter

rectus sheath and is then retracted medially to expose the retroperitoneal space (Fig. 65–18).

When employing a midline upper abdominal incision, the patient is placed supine on the operating table with a rolled sheet beneath the upper lumbar spine. The incision extends from the xiphoid to the umbilicus and can be extended around the umbilicus on either side, if necessary. The incision is carried down through the subcutaneous tissues to the linea alba, which is the midline fusion of the tendinous fibers of the anterior rectus sheath. The linea alba is divided to expose the extraperitoneal fat and peritoneum which is then entered (Fig. 65–19).

A paramedian incision is another type of vertical abdominal incision, which may be preferred, because the separate closure of the two layers of the rectus sheath makes the wound more secure. The incision is made about 3 cm lateral to the midline to provide an adequate margin of rectus sheath medially (Fig. 65–20). The anterior sheath is divided and reflected medially off the underlying muscle by sharp division of the tendinous

intersections. The free medial edge of the muscle is retracted laterally to allow the posterior rectus sheath and peritoneum to be incised (Fig. 65–21). An extraperitoneal approach to the kidney can also be made through a paramedian incision by carefully reflecting the peritoneum off the posterior rectus sheath, after it has been divided (Tessler, 1975).

Thoracoabdominal Incision

The thoracoabdominal approach is desirable for performing radical nephrectomy in patients with large tumors involving the upper portion of the kidney (Chute, 1956; Clarke, 1958; Khoury, 1966; Middleton, 1973). It is particularly advantageous on the right side, where the liver and its venous drainage into the upper vena cava can limit exposure and impair vascular control as the tumor mass is being removed. Less need exists for a thoracoabdominal incision on the left side, because the spleen and pancreas can usually be readily elevated

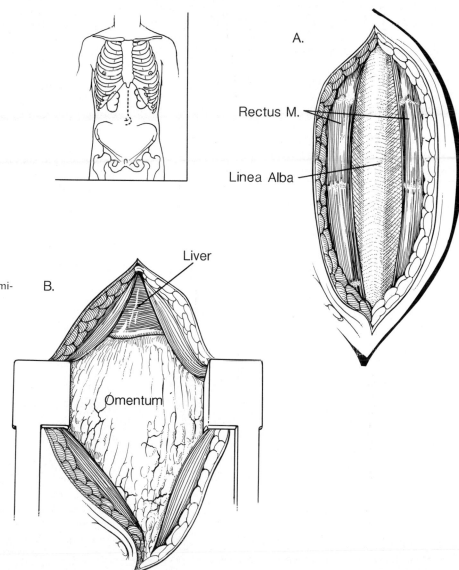

Figure 65–19. *A* and *B,* Midline upper abdominal incision.

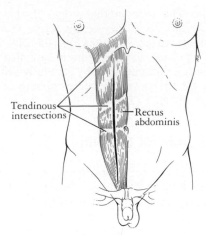

Figure 65–20. Right paramedian incision with division of the anterior rectus sheath.

away from the tumor mass. The thoracoabdominal incision optimizes exposure of the suprarenal area. Nevertheless, because it involves additional operative time and greater potential pulmonary morbidity, we reserve this approach for a patient in whom the additional exposure over that provided by an anterior subcostal incision is considered important to achieve complete and safe tumor removal.

The patient is placed in a semioblique position, with a rolled sheet placed longitudinally beneath the flank. The lower leg is flexed and the upper one is extended with a pillow beneath the legs. The pelvis assumes a more horizontal position, being tilted only about 10 to 15 degrees, which allows free access to the anterior abdominal wall. The incision is begun in the eighth or ninth intercostal space, near the angle of the rib, and is

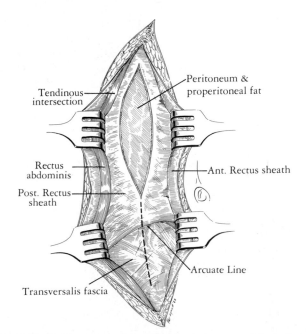

Figure 65–21. The rectus abdominis muscle is retracted laterally and the posterior rectus sheath and transversalis fascia are then incised to expose the properitoneal space.

carried across the costal margin to the midpoint of the opposite rectus muscle, just above the umbilicus. The incision is carried down to the fascia, which is divided in the direction of the incision (Fig. 65–22A). The latissimus dorsi, external oblique, rectus, and intercostal muscles also divided in the direction of the incision. The costal cartilage between the tips of the adjacent ribs is divided (Fig. 65–22B). The pleura in the posterior portion of the incision is opened to obtain complete exposure of the diaphragm (Fig. 65–22C).

The diaphragmatic incision is begun at the periphery about 2 cm inside its attachment to the chest wall, with the incision then being carried around circumferentially to the posterior aspect of the diaphragm (Fig. 65–22D). In doing this, at least 2 or 3 cm of diaphragm must be left attached to the rib cage to allow later reconstruction. By dividing the diaphragm in a circumferential manner from anterior to posterior, damage to the phrenic nerve is avoided. This procedure also creates a diaphragmatic flap, which can be pushed into the chest to provide complete exposure of the liver, which is then simply retracted upward (Fig. 65–22E). If further mobilization of the liver is needed, the right triangular ligament and coronary ligament can be incised to mobilize the entire right lobe of the liver upward. This maneuver provides excellent additional exposure of the suprarenal vena cava. Medial to the ribs, the internal oblique and transversus abdominis muscles are divided and the peritoneal cavity is entered. The colon and duodenum are mobilized medially, and the liver is retracted upward to expose the kidney and great vessels (Fig. 65–22F).

At the completion of the procedure, the abdominal viscera are replaced in their anatomic position. The diaphragm is repaired with interrupted 2-0 silk mattress sutures with the knots tied on the undersurface. The chest wall is reapproximated by passing 0 polyglycolic sutures around the ribs, above and below. These sutures should be passed on a tapered needle to avoid cutting any vessels, with care taken to avoid the neurovascular bundle. Prior to closing the pleura, a 20 Fr. chest tube is placed in the pleural cavity and brought out through a stab wound below the incision in the posterior axillary line. The transected muscle and fascial layers are reapproximated separately. The chest tube is connected to an underwater drain and is usually removed 24 to 48 hours postoperatively, provided no persistent leakage of air is evident and a chest radiograph shows satisfactory lung expansion.

SIMPLE NEPHRECTOMY

Indications

Simple nephrectomy is indicated in the patient with an irreversibly damaged kidney due to symptomatic chronic infection, obstruction, calculus disease, or severe traumatic injury. It is occasionally appropriate to remove a functioning kidney involved with one of these conditions when the patient's age or general condition is too poor to permit a reconstructive operation, provided that the opposite kidney is normal. Nephrectomy

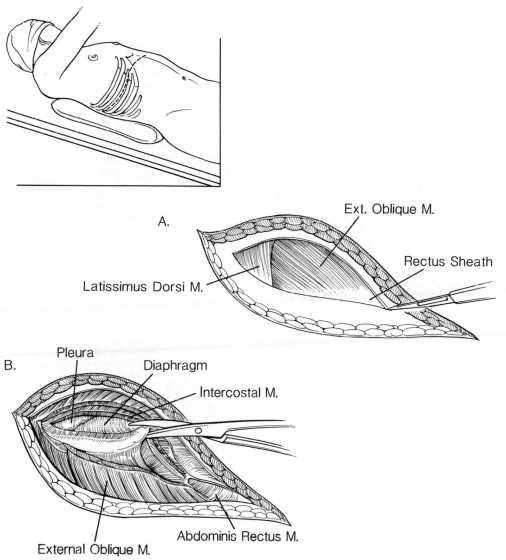

A.

Ext. Oblique M.

Rectus Sheath

Latissimus Dorsi M.

B.

Pleura

Diaphragm

Intercostal M.

External Oblique M.

Abdominis Rectus M.

Figure 65–22. *A–F,* Right thoracoabdominal incision (see text for description of procedure).

Illustration continued on following page

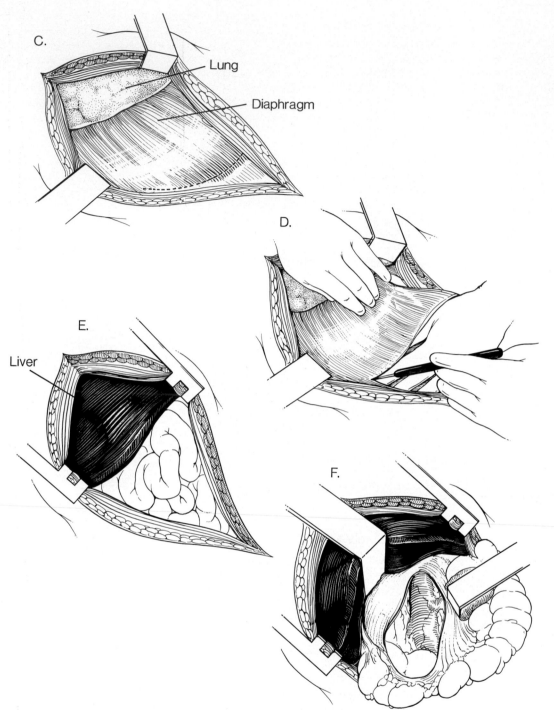

C.
Lung
Diaphragm

D.

E.
Liver

F.

Figure 65–22 *Continued*

may also be indicated to treat renovascular hypertension due to noncorrectable renal artery disease or to severe unilateral parenchymal damage due to nephrosclerosis, pyelonephritis, reflux, or congenital dysplasia.

Simple nephrectomy can be performed through a variety of incisions. An extraperitoneal flank approach is usually preferable when the kidney is chronically infected, when the patient is obese, or when multiple prior abdominal operations have been performed. A subcapsular approach is indicated when severe perirenal inflammation or adhesions obscure anatomic relationships between the kidney and the surrounding structures. A transperitoneal approach is preferable in a patient who cannot tolerate the flank position, in a patient who has end-stage renal disease and is undergoing bilateral nephrectomy, and in a patient who has a traumatic renal injury in which early access to the pedicle is necessary. The transperitoneal approach is also useful when multiple operations have been performed previously through the flank, with resulting dense adhesions around the kidney.

Flank Approach

Once the perinephric space is entered, access to the kidney is obtained by incising Gerota's fascia on the lateral aspect of the kidney to avoid injury to the overlying peritoneum (Fig. 65–23A). The plane of cleavage between the perinephric fat and the renal capsule is usually developed without difficulty. The kidney is mobilized by blunt dissection and, on the left side, the pancreas and duodenum are carefully reflected medially along with the peritoneum. The ureter is identified during mobilization of the lower renal pole. It is preferable to divide the ureter after ligation of the pedicle to avoid congestion of the kidney. The kidney is now pulled downward, and the upper pole is dissected free. Normally a separate compartment is in Gerota's fascia for the adrenal gland, which enables it to be readily separated from the upper pole.

The kidney is now pulled laterally to identify the renal artery and vein, which are separated from surrounding fatty and lymphatic tissues by blunt dissection (Fig. 65–23B). Whenever possible, it is preferable to secure the vessels individually away from the hilus, and the artery should always be ligated first. The renal vein is usually visualized without difficulty and is mobilized by ligating and dividing the gonadal, adrenal, and lumbar branches. The vein can be retracted to expose the artery, which lies posteriorly. Alternatively, the renal artery can be approached posteriorly by mobilizing the kidney and retracting it up into the wound. The renal artery and vein are individually secured with 2-0 silk ligatures and are then divided (Fig. 65–23C). The ureter is now

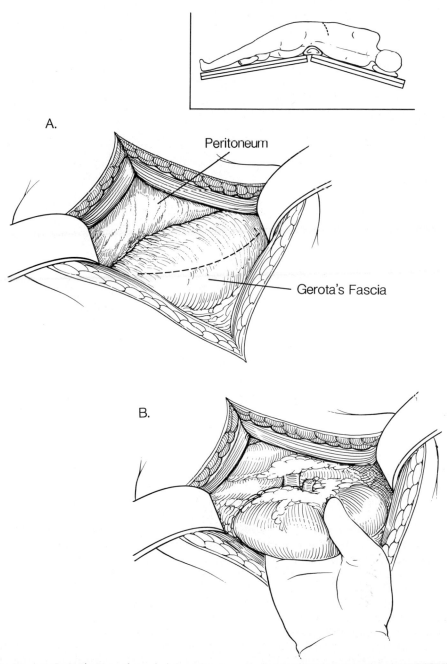

A.

Peritoneum

Gerota's Fascia

B.

Figure 65–23. *A* to *D*, Technique of simple left nephrectomy through an extraperitoneal flank incision (see text).
Illustration continued on following page

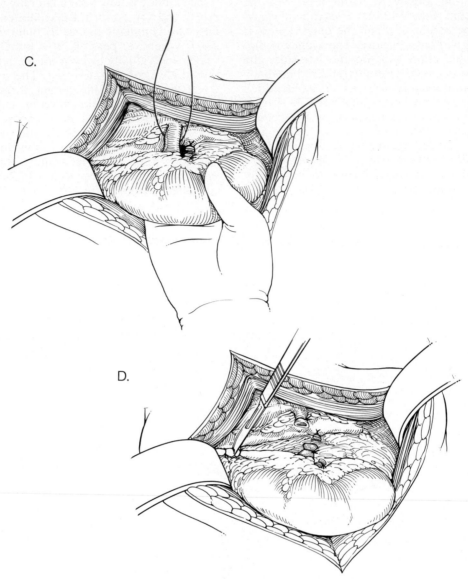

Figure 65–23 *Continued*

clamped and divided, and the distal end is ligated with 2-0 chromic catgut suture to complete the nephrectomy (Fig. 65–23*D*).

Subcapsular Technique

Subcapsular nephrectomy is indicated when severe perirenal inflammation precludes satisfactory dissection between the kidney and surrounding structures (Kimbrough, 1953; Kittredge, 1958). After the retroperitoneal space has been entered, the renal capsule is identified and a longitudinal incision is made over the lateral surface of the kidney (Fig. 65–24*A*). Once the capsule has been entered, a plane is developed between the renal parenchyma and capsule over the entire surface of the kidney down to the level of the hilus (Fig. 65–24*B* and *C*). The renal parenchyma is retracted laterally to expose the major renal vessels as they enter the hilus. Vascular branches are ligated and transected as far

laterally as possible to allow satisfactory proximal control of each branch (Fig. 65–24*D*). The upper ureter is ligated and divided to complete the nephrectomy.

Transperitoneal Approach

When performing transperitoneal simple nephrectomy, a subcostal incision is made and the peritoneal cavity is entered. On the left side, the colon, pancreas, and spleen are reflected upward and medially to expose the left renal vein. A self-retaining ring retractor is useful to maintain exposure of the surgical field (Fig. 65–25*A*).

The renal vein and artery are mobilized, ligated, and transected (Fig. 65–25*B*). The artery is occluded first to avoid excessive blood loss into the kidney. The kidney is then mobilized laterally, superiorly, and inferiorly by sharp and blunt dissection. It is best to initiate the dissection laterally to obtain maximum mobilization

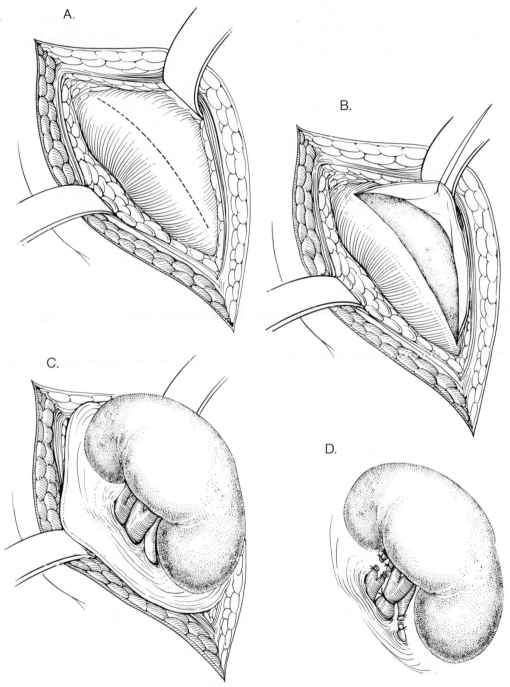

A.

B.

C.

D.

Figure 65–24. *A* to *D*, Technique of subcapsular nephrectomy (see text).

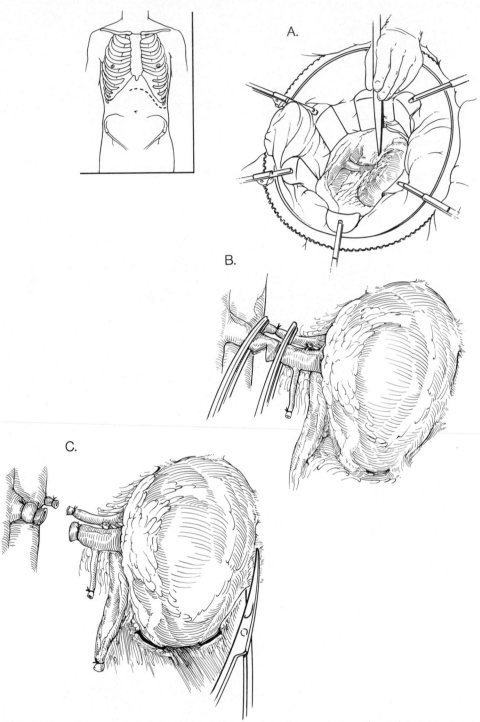

Figure 65–25. *A* to *C*, Technique of transperitoneal simple nephrectomy through an anterior subcostal incision (see text for description of procedure).

before approaching the posterior renal hilus where friable lumbar veins may be present (Fig. 65–25C). In cases of severe perirenal fibrosis, it may be necessary to remove some of the posterior psoas fascia together with the kidney. After complete renal mobilization, the ureter is ligated and divided to complete the nephrectomy.

RADICAL NEPHRECTOMY

Indications and Evaluation

Radical nephrectomy is the treatment of choice for patients with localized renal cell carcinoma (Robson, 1969; Skinner, 1971). The preoperative evaluation of patients with renal cell carcinoma has changed considerably in recent years because of the advent of new imaging modalities, such as ultrasonography, CT scanning, and MRI. In many patients, a complete preliminary evaluation can be performed employing these noninvasive modalities. Renal arteriography is no longer routinely necessary prior to performing radical nephrectomy. All patients should undergo metastatic evaluations, including chest radiographs, abdominal CT scans, and occasionally bone scans. The bone scans are necessary only in patients with bone pain or elevated serum alkaline phosphatase levels. Radical nephrectomy is occasionally done in patients with metastatic disease to palliate severe associated local symptoms or to allow entry into a biologic response modifier protocol, or it is done concomitant with resection of a solitary metastatic lesion.

Involvement of the inferior vena cava with renal cell carcinoma occurs in 3 to 7 per cent of cases and renders the task of complete surgical excision more complicated (Schefft, 1978). Yet, operative removal offers the only hope for cure and, when there are no metastases, an aggressive approach is justified. Five-year survival rates of 40 to 68 per cent have been reported after complete surgical excision (Libertino, 1987; Neves, 1987; Novick, 1990; Skinner, 1989). The best results have been achieved when the tumor does not involve the perinephric fat and regional lymph nodes (Cherrie, 1982). In planning the appropriate operative approach for tumor removal, it is essential for preoperative radiographic studies to define accurately the distal limits of a vena caval tumor thrombus.

Renal cell carcinoma involving the inferior vena cava should be suspected in patients who have lower extremity edema, varicocele, dilated superficial abdominal veins, proteinuria, pulmonary embolism, right atrial mass, or nonfunction of the involved kidney. Currently, MRI is the preferred diagnostic study for demonstrating both the presence and distal extent of inferior vena cava involvement (Goldfarb, 1990; Pritchett, 1987). Inferior vena cavography is reserved for the patient in whom an MRI study is either nondiagnostic or contraindicated. Renal arteriography is particularly helpful in patients with renal cell carcinoma involving the inferior vena cava because, in 35 to 40 per cent of cases, distinct arterialization of a tumor thrombus is observed. When this finding is present, preoperative embolization of the

kidney often causes shrinkage of the thrombus, which facilitates its intraoperative removal. When adjunctive cardiopulmonary bypass with deep hypothermic circulatory arrest is considered, coronary angiography is also performed preoperatively (Belis, 1989). If significant obstructing coronary lesions are found, these can be repaired simultaneously during cardiopulmonary bypass.

Standard Technique

Radical nephrectomy involves preliminary ligation of the renal artery and vein followed by en bloc removal of the kidney and adrenal gland outside of Gerota's fascia. A complete regional lymphadenectomy is performed from the diaphragmatic hiatus to the origin of the inferior mesenteric artery (Robson, 1969). Although lymphadenectomy allows for more accurate pathologic staging, the therapeutic value remains controversial. Perhaps the most important aspect of radical nephrectomy is removal of the kidney outside Gerota's fascia, because capsular invasion with perinephric fat involvement occurs in 25 per cent of patients.

The surgical approach for radical nephrectomy is determined by the size and location of the tumor as well as by the habitus of the patient. The operation is usually performed through a transperitoneal incision to allow abdominal exploration for metastatic disease and early access to the renal vessels with minimal manipulation of the tumor. We prefer an extended subcostal or a bilateral subcostal incision for most patients. A thoracoabdominal incision is chosen for patients with large upper pole tumors (Fig. 65–26). We occasionally employ an extraperitoneal flank incision to perform radical nephrectomy in elderly patients or in patients with small tumors who are also classified as poor risks.

When performing radical nephrectomy through a subcostal transperitoneal incision, a thorough exploration for metastatic disease is done after opening the abdominal cavity. On the left side, the colon is reflected

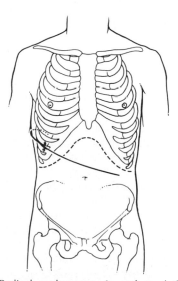

Figure 65–26. Radical nephrectomy is performed through either a bilateral subcostal or throracoabdominal incision.

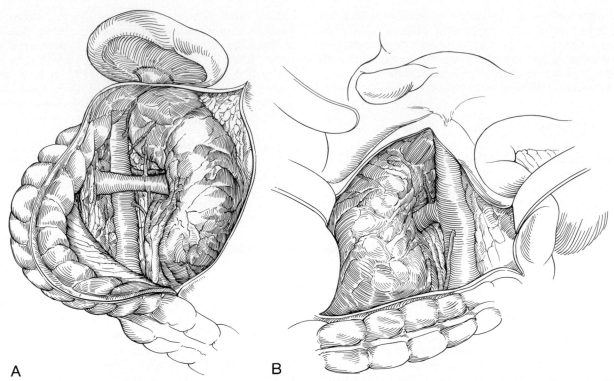

A   B

Figure 65–27. After entering the peritoneal cavity, the colon is reflected medially to expose the left *(A)* or right *(B)* kidney and great vessels. (From Novick, A. C., Streem, S. B., and Pontes, E. (Eds.): Stewart's Operative Urology, 2nd ed. Baltimore, Williams & Wilkins, 1989.)

medially to expose the great vessels. This procedure is facilitated by division of the splenocolic ligaments, which also helps to avoid excessive traction and injury to the spleen. On the right side, the colon and duodenum are reflected medially to expose the vena cava and aorta (Fig. 65–27).

The operation is initiated with dissection of the renal pedicle. On the right side, the renal vein is short and care must be taken not to injure the vena cava. The right renal artery may be mobilized lateral to the vena cava or, with a large medial tumor, between the vena cava and the aorta (Fig. 65–28).

On the left side, the renal vein is quite long as it passes over the aorta. The vein is mobilized completely by ligating and dividing gonadal, adrenal, and lumbar tributaries. The vein can be retracted to expose the artery posteriorly, which is then mobilized toward the aorta (Fig. 65–29). The renal artery is ligated with 2-0 silk ligatures and divided, and the renal vein is then similarly managed (Fig. 65–30).

The kidney is mobilized outside Gerota's fascia with blunt and sharp dissection as needed. Remaining vascular attachments are secured with nonabsorbable sutures or metal clips. The ureter is then ligated and divided to complete the removal of the kidney and adrenal gland (Fig. 65–31).

The classic description of radical nephrectomy includes the performance of a complete regional lymphadenectomy. The lymph nodes can be removed en bloc with the kidney and adrenal gland or separately, following the nephrectomy. The lymph node dissection is begun at the crura of the diaphragm just below the origin of the superior mesenteric artery. A readily

definable periadventitial plane is seen close to the aorta that can be entered. The dissection may then be carried along the aorta and onto the origin of the major vessels, to remove all the periaortic lymphatic tissue. Care must be taken to avoid injury to the origins of the celiac and

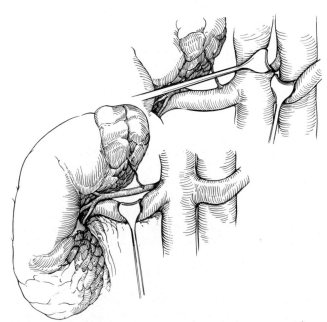

Figure 65–28. The right renal artery may be mobilized lateral to the vena cava or between the vena cava and the aorta. (From Novick, A. C., Streem, S. B., and Pontes, E. (Eds.): Stewart's Operative Urology, 2nd ed. Baltimore, Williams & Wilkins, 1989.)

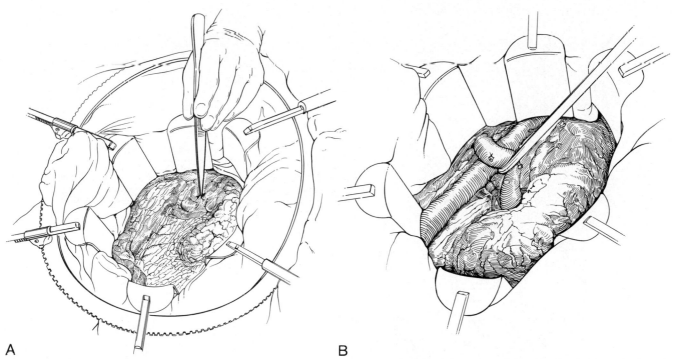

A   **B**

Figure 65–29. *A*, A self-retaining ring retractor is inserted to maintain exposure. *B*, The left renal vein is mobilized by ligating its major branches to expose the artery posteriorly. (From Novick, A. C., Streem, S. B., and Pontes, E. (Eds.): Stewart's Operative Urology, 2nd ed. Baltimore, Williams & Wilkins, 1989.)

superior mesenteric arteries superiorly, as they arise from the anterior surface of the aorta. The dissection of the periaortic and pericaval lymph nodes is then carried downward en bloc to the origin of the inferior mesenteric artery. The sympathetic ganglia and nerves are removed together with the lymphatic tissue. The cisterna chyli is identified medial to the right crus. Entering lymphatic vessels are secured to prevent the development of chylous ascites.

A thoracoabdominal incision is preferable when performing radical nephrectomy for a large upper pole tumor. This approach is demonstrated in Figures 65–32 to 65–34 for a right-sided tumor. Once the liver has been retracted upward into the chest, the hepatic flexure of the colon and the duodenum are reflected medially to expose the anterior surface of the kidney and great

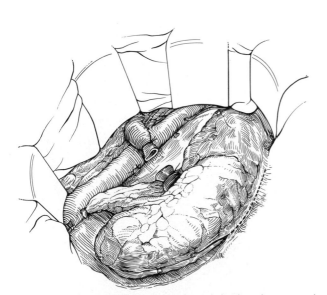

Figure 65–30. After securing the pedicle and dividing the ureter, the kidney is mobilized outside Gerota's fascia. (From Novick, A. C., Streem, S. B., and Pontes, E. (Eds.): Stewart's Operative Urology, 2nd ed. Baltimore, Williams & Wilkins, 1989.)

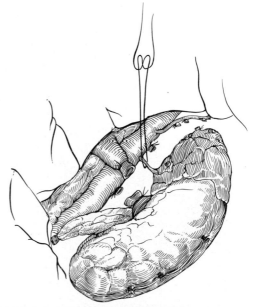

Figure 65–31. Remaining medial vascular attachments are secured and divided to complete the nephrectomy. (From Novick, A. C., Streem, S. B., and Pontes, E. (Eds.): Stewart's Operative Urology, 2nd ed. Baltimore, Williams & Wilkins, 1989.)

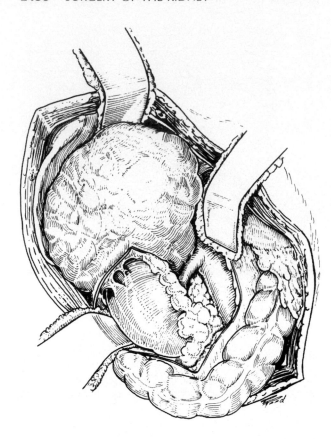

Figure 65–32. Exposure of a large right upper pole tumor through a thoracoabdominal incision. (From Novick, A. C., Streem, S. B., and Pontes, E. (Eds.): Stewart's Operative Urology, 2nd ed. Baltimore, Williams & Wilkins, 1989.)

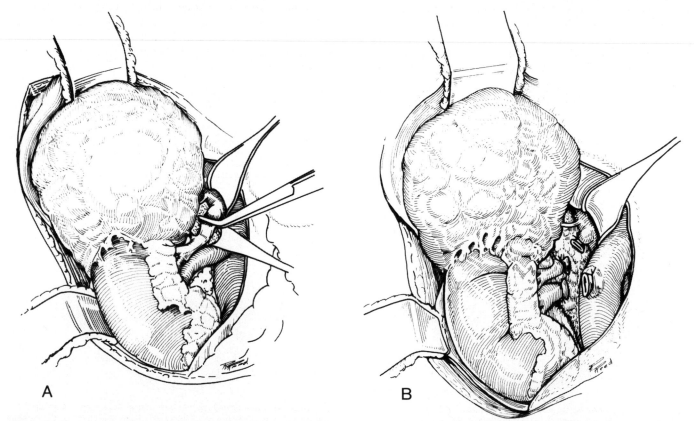

A

B

Figure 65–33. A and B, The renal artery and vein are secured and divided. (From Novick, A. C., Streem, S. B., and Pontes, E. (Eds.): Stewart's Operative Urology, 2nd ed. Baltimore, Williams & Wilkins, 1989.)

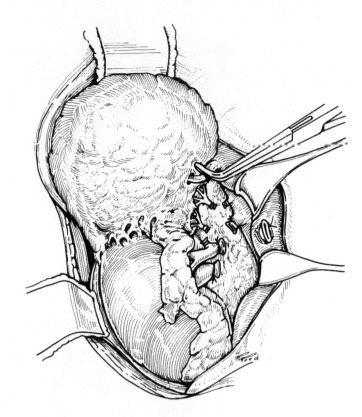

Figure 65–34. The vena cava is retracted medially to expose the remaining superior vascular attachments, which are secured and divided. (From Novick, A. C., Streem, S. B., and Pontes, E. (Eds.): Stewart's Operative Urology, 2nd ed. Baltimore, Williams & Wilkins, 1989.)

vessels (see Fig. 65–32). The renal artery is secured with 2-0 silk ligatures and divided, and the renal vein is then similarly managed (see Fig. 65–33). The ureter and right gonadal vein are ligated and divided, and the kidney is mobilized outside Gerota's fascia. Downward and lateral traction of the kidney exposes the superior vascular attachments of the tumor and adrenal gland. Exposure of these vessels is also facilitated by medial retraction of the inferior vena cava (see Fig. 65–34). Care is taken to preserve small hepatic venous branches entering the vena cava at the superior margin of the tumor mass. The tumor mass is then gently separated from the undersurface of the liver to complete the resection.

Management of Retroperitoneal Hemorrhage

During performance of radical nephrectomy, intraoperative hemorrhage can occur from the inferior vena cava or its tributaries. The urologist should be familiar with methods of preventing and controlling this problem. In most cases, vena caval hemorrhage is caused by the laceration or avulsion of large yet fragile veins entering the vena cava at predictable locations. Lumbar veins enter the posterolateral aspect of the vena cava at each vertebral level. Undue traction on the cava can result in their avulsion with troublesome bleeding. To prevent this, care should be taken to retract the vena cava very gently with curved vein retractors during its dissection. If additional mobilization is necessary, these veins should be dissected free from surrounding structures, ligated, and divided. In ligating venous tributaries

entering the vena cava, 3-0 to 4-0 suture material should be used. The ligatures should not be tied too tightly, as this can cause shearing through the fragile venous wall with further hemorrhage. After the ligature has been applied, it should not be pulled too tightly before the ends of the ligature are cut, to prevent avulsing the entrance of the vein into the vena cava.

A second predictable bleeding site is the entry of the right gonadal vein into the anterolateral surface of the vena cava. This is an extremely thin-walled vein, and excessive traction or mobilization of the cava at this level can lead to its avulsion, with resulting hemorrhage.

A third predictable site of bleeding lies at the level of the renal veins, where large lumbar veins often course posteriorly from the left renal vein just lateral to the aorta or from the posterior aspect of the vena cava, close to the entry of the right renal vein. Injudicious mobilization of the renal veins, without consideration of these fragile and often large caliber veins, can result in severe hemorrhage that may be difficult to control.

A fourth predictable site of bleeding is at the level of the right adrenal vein, which enters the inferior vena cava. This vein is large, friable, frequently lies higher than expected, and must be carefully dissected free from surrounding structures to avoid avulsion from the vena cava.

Excessive hemorrhage can also be prevented by careful dissection in proper tissue planes along the vena cava. This maneuver may be difficult when tumor involves the vena cava, but usually a plane can be established along the vena cava wall which, if followed, allows safe and relatively bloodless exposure. One should follow the general principle of isolating a relatively normal

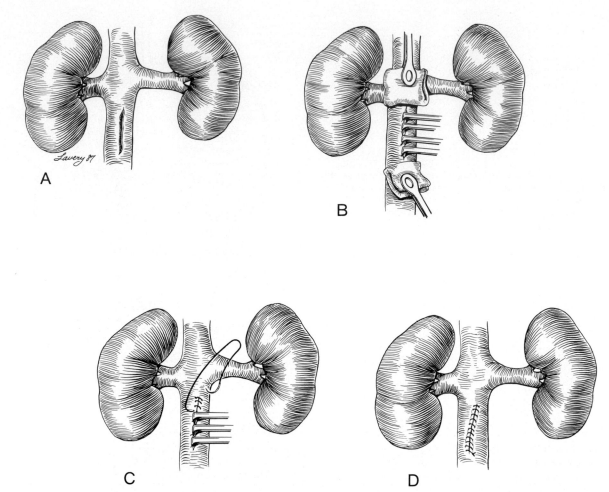

Figure 65–35. *A* to *D*, Technique for repairing extensive laceration of the inferior vena cava. (From Novick, A. C., Streem, S. B., and Pontes, E. (Eds.): Stewart's Operative Urology, 2nd ed. Baltimore, Williams & Wilkins, 1989.)

area of vena cava and working upward or downward from that area to expose the diseased portion.

If inadvertent lacerations of vena cava or avulsions of entering veins occur, control of hemorrhage can be accomplished by a variety of techniques. Direct pressure on the site of bleeding gives immediate control until additional exposure can be gained, the field properly illuminated, and additional suckers or retractors brought in if necessary. When the laceration involves the anterior or lateral caval wall and is of considerable length, it can be readily controlled by applying a series of Allis clamps over the edges of the laceration in serial fashion. The edges of the laceration are then oversewn with running 5-0 vascular suture material (Fig. 65–35).

If avulsion of an entering lumbar vein is the cause of bleeding, the vena cava should be rolled medially, with digital compression above and below the site of bleeding, until the posterolateral entry of the avulsed vein is exposed. This vein is then grasped with one or two Allis clamps, which can be applied as tractors to bring the avulsion into better view for oversewing with vascular suture material. Persistent bleeding can occur from the proximal end of an avulsed lumbar vein, which may retract into the psoas muscle and thereby be difficult to secure. This situation can be controlled in some cases by grasping the end of the vein with a hemostat and

twisting the hemostat to bring the end of the vein into better view for suture ligation (Fig. 65–36). If this maneuver is not possible, bleeding can be controlled by inserting a figure-of-eight 2-0 silk suture through the muscle overlying the vein.

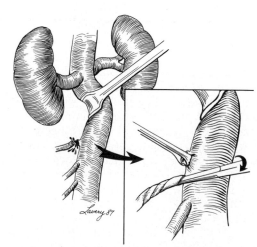

Figure 65–36. Technique for securing ends of lumbar vein avulsed from inferior vena cava. (From Novick, A. C., Streem, S. B., and Pontes, E. (Eds.): Stewart's Operative Urology, 2nd ed. Baltimore, Williams & Wilkins, 1989.)

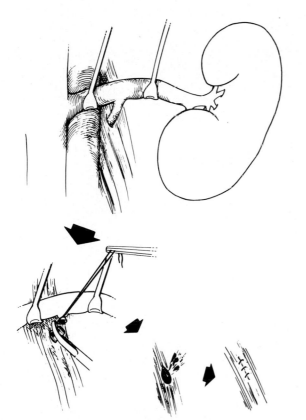

Figure 65–37. Technique for securing ends of lumbar vein avulsed from the left renal vein. (From Novick, A. C., Streem, S. B., and Pontes, E. (Eds.): Stewart's Operative Urology, 2nd ed. Baltimore, Williams & Wilkins, 1989.)

Bleeding from large lumbar veins entering the posterior aspect of the left renal vein or the posterior wall of the vena cava near the entry of the right renal vein can be particularly troublesome (Fig. 65–37). Further mobilization of the vena cava and renal veins is often needed while compression is maintained on the bleeding site. It may be necessary to apply a Satinsky side clamp across the entry of the renal vein, as well as a distal bulldog clamp beyond the bleeding point in the renal vein, in order to control the hemorrhage and to allow closure of the venous defect. Mobilization and gentle rotation of the vena cava and/or renal veins may also be necessary to gain optimal exposure. In this situation, the distal entry of the lumbar vein into the posterior musculature can cause troublesome bleeding and must be controlled as previously described.

Radical Nephrectomy with Infrahepatic Vena Caval Involvement

Four levels of vena caval involvement in renal cell carcinoma are characterized, according to the distal extent of the tumor thrombus (Fig. 65–38). A bilateral subcostal transperitoneal incision usually provides excellent exposure for performing radical nephrectomy and removal of a perirenal or infrahepatic inferior vena cava thrombus. For extremely large tumors involving

the upper pole of the kidney, a thoracoabdominal incision may alternatively be chosen. After the abdomen is entered, the colon is reflected medially and a self-retaining ring retractor is inserted to maintain exposure of the retroperitoneum (Fig. 65–39A). The renal artery and the ureter are ligated and divided, and the entire kidney is mobilized outside Gerota's fascia, leaving the kidney attached only by the renal vein (Fig. 65–39B and C). During the initial dissection, care is taken to avoid unnecessary manipulation of the renal vein and vena cava.

The vena cava is completely dissected from surrounding structures above and below the renal vein, and the opposite renal vein is also mobilized. It is essential to obtain exposure and control of the suprarenal vena cava above the level of the tumor thrombus. If necessary, perforating veins to the caudate lobe of the liver are secured and divided to allow separation of the caudate lobe from the vena cava. This maneuver can allow an additional 2 to 3 cm length of vena cava to be exposed superiorly. The infrarenal vena cava is then occluded below the thrombus with a Satinsky venous clamp. The opposite renal vein is gently secured with a small bulldog vascular clamp. In preparation for tumor thrombectomy, a curved Satinsky clamp is placed around the suprarenal vena cava above the level of the thrombus (Fig. 65–39D).

The anterior surface of the renal vein is incised over the tumor thrombus, and the incision is continued posteriorly with scissors, passing just beneath the thrombus (Fig. 65–39E). In most cases, there is no attachment of the thrombus to the wall of the vena cava. After the renal vein has been circumscribed, gentle downward traction is exerted on the kidney to extract the tumor thrombus from the vena cava (Fig. 65–39F). After removal of the gross specimen, the suprarenal vena caval clamp may be released temporarily, as the anesthetist applies positive pulmonary pressure. This maneuver can ensure that any small remaining fragments of thrombus are flushed free from the vena cava. When the tumor thrombectomy is completed, the cavotomy incision is repaired with a continuous 5-0 vascular suture (Fig. 65–39G).

In occasional cases, direct caval invasion of the tumor occurs at the level of the entrance of the renal vein at varying distances. This finding requires resection of a portion of the vena caval wall. Narrowing of the caval lumen by up to 50 per cent will not adversely affect maintenance of caval patency. If further narrowing appears likely, caval reconstruction can be performed with a free graft of pericardium.

In some patients, more extensive direct growth of tumor into the wall of the vena cava is found at surgery. The prognosis for these patients is generally poor, particularly when hepatic venous tributaries are also involved. The decision to proceed with radical surgical excision must be carefully considered. Several important principles must be kept in mind when undertaking en bloc vena caval resection. Resection of the infrarenal portion of the vena cava usually can be done safely, because an extensive collateral venous supply will have developed in most cases. With right-sided kidney tu-

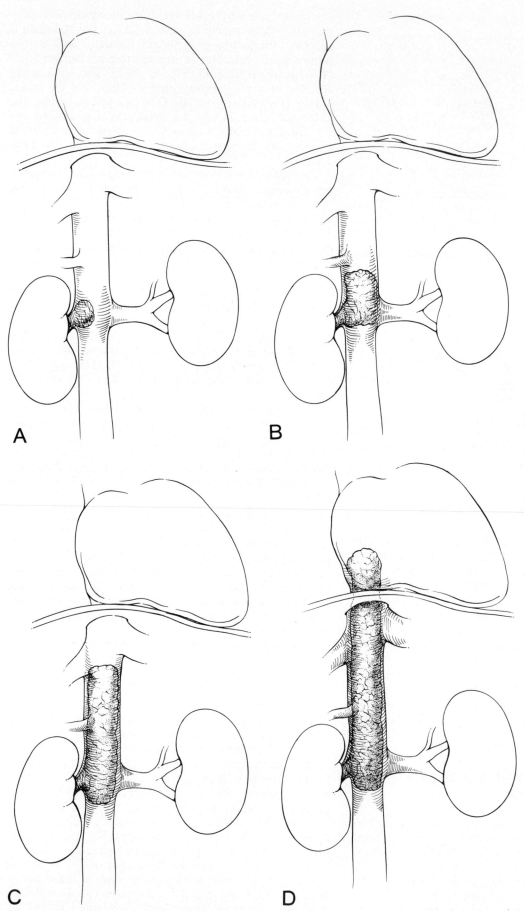

Figure 65–38. Classification of inferior vena caval tumor thrombus from renal cell carcinoma according to the distal extent of the thrombus, as *(A)* perirenal, *(B)* infrahepatic, *(C)* intrahepatic, and *(D)* suprahepatic. (From Novick, A. C., Streem, S. B., and Pontes, E. (Eds.): Stewart's Operative Urology, 2nd ed. Baltimore, Williams & Wilkins, 1989.)

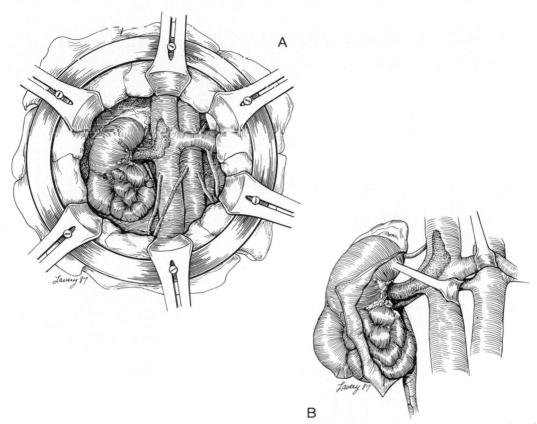

Figure 65–39. *A to G,* Technique of radical nephrectomy and vena caval tumor thrombectomy with infrahepatic tumor thrombus (see text for description). (From Novick, A. C., Streem, S. B., and Pontes, E. (Eds.): Stewart's Operative Urology, 2nd ed. Baltimore, Williams & Wilkins, 1989.)

Illustration continued on following page

mors, resection of the suprarenal vena cava is also possible, provided the left renal vein is ligated distal to the gonadal and adrenal tributaries, which then provide collateral venous drainage from the left kidney. With left-sided kidney tumors, the suprarenal vena cava cannot be resected safely because of the paucity of collateral venous drainage from the right kidney. In such cases, right renal venous drainage can be maintained by preserving a tumor-free strip of vena cava augmented (Fig. 65–40), if necessary, with a pericardial patch. Alternatively, the right kidney can be autotransplanted to the pelvis or an interpositional graft of saphenous vein can be placed from the right renal vein to the splenic, inferior mesenteric, or portal vein.

Radical Nephrectomy with Intrahepatic or Suprahepatic Vena Caval Involvement

In patients with renal cell carcinoma and an intrahepatic or a suprahepatic inferior vena cava thrombus, the difficulty of surgical excision is significantly increased. In such cases, the operative technique must be modified because it is not possible to obtain subdiaphragmatic control of the vena cava above the tumor thrombus. Several different surgical maneuvers have been employed to provide adequate exposure, prevent severe

bleeding, and achieve complete tumor removal in this setting (Cummings, 1979; Foster, 1988; Novick, 1980; Skinner, 1989).

One described technique for obtaining vascular control involves temporary occlusion of the suprahepatic intrapericardial portion of the inferior vena cava. To reduce hepatic venous congestion and troublesome back-bleeding, the porta hepatis and superior mesenteric artery are also temporarily occluded (Skinner, 1989). A disadvantage of this approach is that occlusion of the latter vessels can be safely tolerated for only 20 minutes. This approach is also not applicable in cases of tumor extension into the right atrium. At the Cleveland Clinic, we prefer to employ cardiopulmonary bypass with deep hypothermic circulatory arrest for patients with intrahepatic and suprahepatic tumor thrombi (Marshall, 1986). Our initial experience with this approach in 43 patients has been quite favorable (Novick, 1990). The relevant technical aspects are subsequently described.

A bilateral subcostal incision is used for the abdominal portion of the operation. After confirming resectability, a median sternotomy is made (Fig. 65–41). Intraoperative monitoring is accomplished with an arterial line, a multiple lumen central venous pressure catheter, and a pulmonary artery catheter. Nasopharyngeal and bladder temperatures are monitored. Anesthesia is induced with fentanyl, sufentanil, or thiopental and is maintained with a narcotic inhalation agent (Welch, 1989).

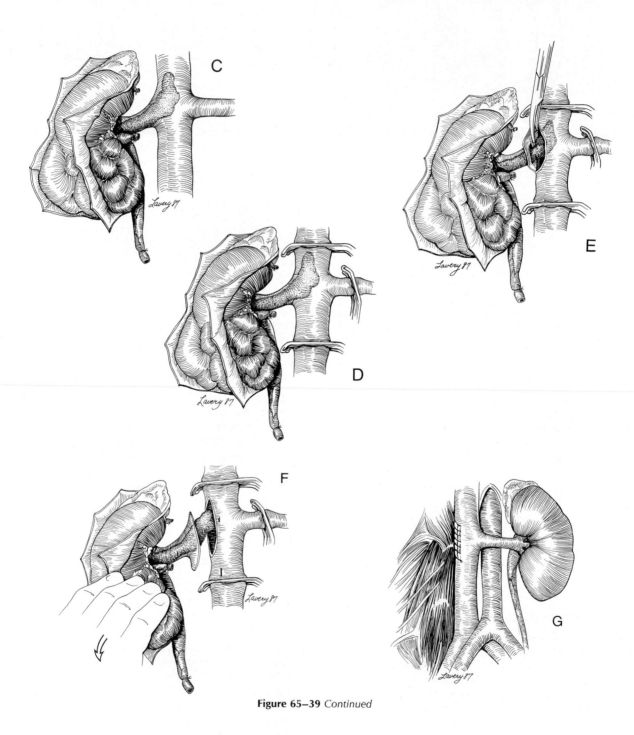

Figure 65-39 *Continued*

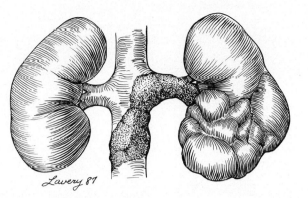
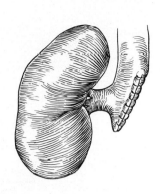
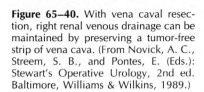

Figure 65–40. With vena caval resection, right renal venous drainage can be maintained by preserving a tumor-free strip of vena cava. (From Novick, A. C., Streem, S. B., and Pontes, E. (Eds.): Stewart's Operative Urology, 2nd ed. Baltimore, Williams & Wilkins, 1989.)

The kidney is completely mobilized outside Gerota's fascia with division of the renal artery and ureter, such that the kidney is left attached only by the renal vein. The infrarenal vena cava and contralateral renal vein are also exposed. Extensive dissection and mobilization of the suprarenal vena cava are not necessary with this approach. Adequate exposure is somewhat more difficult to achieve for a left renal tumor. Simultaneous exposure of the vena cava on the right and the tumor on the left is not readily accomplished simply by reflecting the left colon medially. We have dealt with this situation by transposing the mobilized left kidney anteriorly, through a window in the mesentery of the left colon, while leaving the renal vein attached. This maneuver yields excellent exposure of the abdominal vena cava with the attached left renal vein and kidney. Precise retroperitoneal hemostasis is essential before proceeding with cardiopulmonary bypass because of the risk of bleeding associated with systemic heparinization.

The heart and great vessels are now exposed through the median sternotomy. Heparinization is completed, ascending aortic and right atrial venous cannulae are

placed, and cardiopulmonary bypass is initiated (Fig. 65–42). When the heart fibrillates, the aorta is clamped and crystalloid cardioplegic solution is infused. Under circulatory arrest, deep hypothermia is initiated by reducing arterial inflow blood temperature to as low as 10°C. The head and abdomen are packed in ice during the cooling process. After approximately 15 to 30 minutes, a core temperature of 18 to 20°C is achieved. At this point, flow through the perfusion machine is stopped and 95 per cent of the blood volume is drained into the pump with no flow to any organ. The tumor thrombus can now be removed in an essentially bloodless operative field. An incision is made in the inferior vena cava at the entrance of the involved renal vein, and the ostium is circumscribed. When the tumor extends into the right atrium, the atrium is opened at the same time (Fig. 65–43A). If possible, the tumor thrombus is removed intact with the kidney. Frequently, this step is not possible because of the friability of the thrombus and its adherence to the vena caval wall. In such cases, piecemeal removal of the thrombus from above and below is necessary. Occasionally, a venous Fogarty catheter can be inserted into the vena cava to assist in extraction of the thrombus. Under deep hypothermic circulatory arrest, the entire interior lumen of the vena cava can be directly inspected to ensure that all fragments of thrombus are completely removed. The vena cava is closed with a continuous 5-0 vascular suture, and the right atrium is closed (Fig. 65–43B).

As soon as the vena cava and right atrium have been repaired, rewarming of the patient is initiated. If coronary artery bypass grafting is necessary, this procedure is done during the rewarming period. Rewarming takes 20 to 45 minutes and is continued until a core temperature of approximately 37°C is obtained. Cardiopulmonary bypass is then terminated. Decannulation takes place, and protamine sulfate is administered to reverse the effects of the heparin. Platelets, fresh-frozen plasma, desmopressin acetate, or their combination may be provided when coagulopathy is suspected (Harker, 1986). Mediastinal chest tubes are placed, but the abdomen is not routinely drained.

Complications

Following radical nephrectomy, postoperative complications occur in approximately 2 per cent of patients,

Figure 65–41. Surgical incision for performing radical nephrectomy with removal of suprahepatic vena caval tumor thrombus. (From Novick, A. C., Streem, S. B., and Pontes, E. (Eds.): Stewart's Operative Urology, 2nd ed. Baltimore, Williams & Wilkins, 1989.)

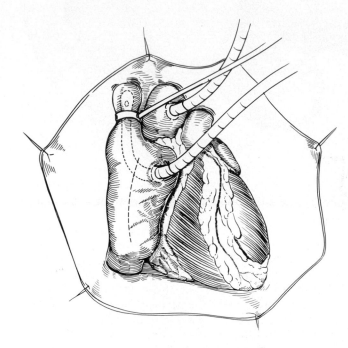

Figure 65–42. Cannulas are placed in the ascending aorta and right atrium in preparation for cardiopulmonary bypass. The planned incision into the right atrium is shown. (From Novick, A. C., Streem, S. B., and Pontes, E. (Eds.): Stewart's Operative Urology, 2nd ed. Baltimore, Williams & Wilkins, 1989.)

A.

B.

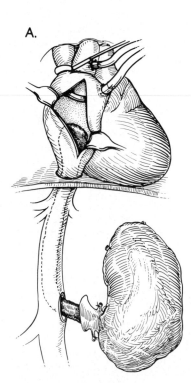

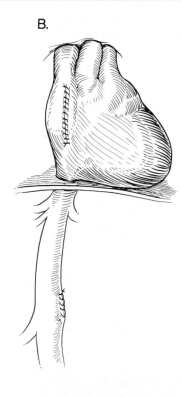

Figure 65–43. *A,* The ostium of the renal vein is circumferentially incised, and the right atrium is opened. *B,* Following removal of the tumor thrombus, the atriotomy and venacavotomy incisions are closed.

and the operative mortality rate is approximately 2 per cent (Swanson, 1983). Systemic complications may occur after any surgical procedure. These include myocardial infarction, cerebrovascular accident, congestive heart failure, pulmonary embolism, atelectasis, pneumonia, and thrombophlebitis. The incidence of these problems can be reduced by adequate preoperative preparation, avoidance of intraoperative hypotension, appropriate blood and fluid replacement, postoperative breathing exercises, early mobilization, and elastic support of the legs both during and after surgery.

An intraoperative gastrointestinal injury should always be checked for during the procedure, and lacerations should be repaired and drained. Tears of the liver may be repaired with mattress sutures. Splenic injuries usually require splenectomy, although small lacerations may be managed by application of avitene or oxycel. Injuries to the tail of the pancreas, which may occur with left radical nephrectomy, are best managed by partial amputation.

A particularly distressing postoperative complication is the development of a pancreatic fistula due to unrecognized intraoperative injury to the pancreas. This complication is usually manifested in the immediate postoperative period with signs and symptoms of acute pancreatitis and drainage of alkaline fluid from the incision. A CT scan of the abdomen will demonstrate a fluid collection in the retroperitoneum. Fluid draining from the incision should be analyzed for the presence of amylase pH. Treatment involves either percutaneous or surgical drainage of the fluid collection to avoid the development of a pancreatic pseudocyst or abscess (Spirnak, 1984; Zinner, 1974). The majority of fistulae close spontaneously, with the establishment of adequate drainage. Because the healing of a pancreatic fistula is usually a slow process, the patient is also supported with hyperalimentation. Surgical closure by excising the fistulous tract and creating an anastomosis between the pancreas and a Roux-en-Y limb of the jejunum is only occasionally necessary in patients with prolonged drainage.

Another gastrointestinal problem that may occur includes a generalized ileus or a functional obstruction caused by a localized ileus of the colon overlying the operated renal fossa. Oral feedings should not be given until adequate bowel sounds are present and the patient has flatus. Nasogastric suction is given in more severe cases. When a prolonged period of ileus is anticipated, or when the patient is in a poor nutritional state, parenteral hyperalimentation should be instituted.

Secondary hemorrhage may occur following radical nephrectomy and is manifested by pain, signs of shock, abdominal or flank swelling, and drainage of blood through the incision or drain site. Bleeding may be from the kidney or renal pedicle but is occasionally from an unrecognized injury to a neighboring structure, such as the spleen, liver, or mesenteric vessel. Patients should be given blood and fluid replacement as needed. In most cases, it is best to reopen the wound, evacuate the hematoma, and secure the bleeding point. In the event of diffuse bleeding from a clotting disorder, it may be necessary to temporarily pack the wound with gauze,

which can then be gradually removed after 24 to 48 hours.

Pneumothorax may occur during thoracoabdominal or flank incisions. Pleural injuries are usually recognized immediately and repaired with a running 3-0 or 4-0 chromic suture. Prior to complete closure of the incision, a red rubber catheter is inserted into the pleural cavity and a pursestring suture is tied around the catheter. The anesthesiologist is then asked to hyperinflate the patient's lungs. With hyperinflation and suction on the catheter, air and fluid in the hemithorax are forced out through the red rubber catheter, which is then removed. The pursestring suture is secured. An alternative method is to place the distal end of the catheter in a basin of water. As the anesthesiologist hyperinflates the lung, air and fluid are forced out of the pleural cavity through the red rubber catheter and into the basin of water. When the pleura is entered, a chest radiograph should be obtained in the recovery room to ensure adequate reexpansion of the lung. A pneumothorax greater than 10 per cent or tension pneumothorax or one causing respiratory distress requires insertion of a chest tube.

Postoperative atelectasis is common in radical nephrectomy and is probably secondary to the positioning of the patient during the procedure. This complication is a common cause of fever postoperatively and may be effectively treated with pulmonary physiotherapy, including deep breathing, coughing, and incentive spirometry.

Infection is another common complication encountered in the postoperative period. Superficial wound infections are best managed by removal of skin sutures or staples to allow for drainage. Deeper infections must be treated by the establishment of adequate drainage and the administration of appropriate antibiotics for systemic manifestations of the infection. If the drainage is persistent and profuse, the possibility of a retained foreign body or a fistulous communication with the intestine should be considered. Accumulations of lymph or serous fluid in the renal fossa or pleura are best managed expectantly, unless they are causing respiratory embarrassment. Such accumulations may become infected or may be complicated by bleeding if treated by needle aspiration.

Temporary renal insufficiency may develop postoperatively after ligation of the left renal vein in conjunction with right radical nephrectomy and extraction of a vena caval tumor thrombus (Clark, 1961; Pathak, 1971). Renal failure in this setting is probably secondary to venous obstruction and usually resolves as drainage improves with the development of venous collaterals, although temporary hemodialysis may occasionally be needed. It is always preferable, if possible, to preserve left renal venous drainage into the vena cava to diminish the risk of this complication. As previously mentioned, ligation of the right renal vein leads to permanent and complete renal failure.

When a flank incision is selected to perform nephrectomy, an incisional hernia or bulge may occur postoperatively. The intracostal nerve lies immediately below the corresponding rib between the internal oblique and the transverse abdominal muscle. At surgery, an effort should be made to spare this nerve by dissecting both proximally and distally, enabling careful padding and retraction of the nerve out of the operative field, because transection may lead to muscle denervation. Postoperatively, muscle denervation with flank bulging must be differentiated from a flank incisional hernia, which is rare. In the latter instance, a fascial defect is usually palpable.

PARTIAL NEPHRECTOMY FOR MALIGNANCY

Although radical nephrectomy remains the treatment of choice for the patient with localized renal cell carcinoma and a normal opposite kidney, partial nephrectomy is the treatment of choice when localized renal cell carcinoma is present bilaterally or in a solitary functioning kidney (Bazeed, 1986; Jacobs et al., 1979; Marberger, 1981; Novick, 1989; Smith, 1984; Topley, 1984; Zincke, 1985). In such patients, partial nephrectomy allows complete surgical excision of the primary tumor, preserving sufficient renal parenchyma to avoid the need for renal replacement therapy. The indications for partial nephrectomy have been expanded to include the patient with localized renal cell carcinoma and a functioning opposite kidney, when that kidney is involved with a disorder (e.g., calculi, diabetes, pyelonephritis, nephrosclerosis) that might cause progressive renal functional impairment in the future (Novick, 1989). Partial nephrectomy is also indicated in the management of occasional patients with renal pelvic transitional cell carcinoma or Wilms' tumor, when preservation of functioning renal parenchyma is a clinically relevant consideration (Ziegelbaum, 1987; Zincke, 1984).

A variety of surgical techniques are available for performing partial nephrectomy in patients with malignancy. These include simple enucleation, polar segmental nephrectomy with preliminary ligation of the appropriate renal arterial branch, wedge resection, major transverse resection, and extracorporeal partial nephrectomy with renal autotransplantation. All of these techniques require adherence to basic principles of early vascular control; avoidance of ischemic renal damage; complete tumor excision with free margins; precise closure of the collecting system; careful hemostasis; and closure or coverage of the renal defect with adjacent fat, fascia, oxycel, or with peritoneum.

Patients who are undergoing partial nephrectomy for malignancy should be studied preoperatively with standard catheter renal arteriography to delineate the main renal artery and its branches. Knowledge of the number and location of these vessels helps greatly in removing the tumor with minimal blood loss and injury to adjacent parenchyma (Novick, 1987). In most patients, intravenous digital subtraction angiography does not provide satisfactory visualization of the renal artery branches (Zabbo, 1984).

In the majority of cases, it is possible to perform partial nephrectomy for malignancy in situ by choosing an operative approach that optimizes exposure of the kidney and by combining meticulous surgical technique with an understanding of the renal vascular anatomy in relation to the tumor. We employ an extraperitoneal flank incision through the bed of the 11th or 12th rib for all of these operations. This incision allows the surgeon to operate on the mobilized kidney almost at skin level and provides excellent exposure of the peripheral renal vessels. With an anterior transperitoneal incision, the kidney is invariably located in the depth of the wound, and the surgical exposure is simply not as good.

When performing in situ partial nephrectomy for malignancy, the kidney is mobilized inside Gerota's fascia. However, the perirenal fat around the tumor is left undisturbed. For small polar or peripheral renal tumors, it may not be necessary to temporarily occlude the renal artery. In most cases, however, partial nephrectomy is most effectively performed after temporary renal arterial occlusion. The last measure not only limits intraoperative bleeding but, by reducing renal tissue turgor, improves access to intrarenal structures. Because the anticipated period of arterial occlusion patients undergoing partial nephrectomy for malignancy usually is longer than 30 minutes, additional protection from postischemic renal injury is necessary, as described earlier in this chapter.

In patients with renal cell carcinoma or transitional cell carcinoma, partial nephrectomy is contraindicated in the presence of lymph node metastasis, because the prognoses for these patients are poor. Enlarged or suspicious-looking lymph nodes should be biopsied before initiating renal resection. When partial nephrectomy is performed, after excision of all gross tumor, absence of malignancy in the remaining portion of the kidney should be verified intraoperatively by frozen-section examinations of biopsy specimens obtained at random from the renal margin of excision. If such biopsy specimens demonstrate residual tumor, additional tissue must be removed to ensure a complete excision.

Simple Enucleation

Some renal cell carcinomas are completely surrounded by a distinct pseudocapsule of fibrous tissue that can allow relatively avascular tumor removal by enucleation with maximal conservation of renal tissue (Vermooten, 1950). These are generally small and low-grade lesions. The technique of enucleation involves circumferentially incising the parenchyma around the tumor, identifying the plane between the pseudocapsule and adjacent uninvolved parenchyma, and bluntly shelling out the lesion with the blunt end of a scalpel (Fig. 65–44) (Graham, 1979). For in situ enucleation of peripheral tumors, it is generally unnecessary to occlude the renal artery, and the few transected blood vessels at the base of the enucleation can simply be ligated with 4-0 chromic sutures. While these ligatures are being inserted, the physician can control surface bleeding by gentle digital compression of the parenchyma. Fat or oxycel can be placed into the cavity, and the margins of the parenchyma can be sutured together to further assure complete hemostasis.

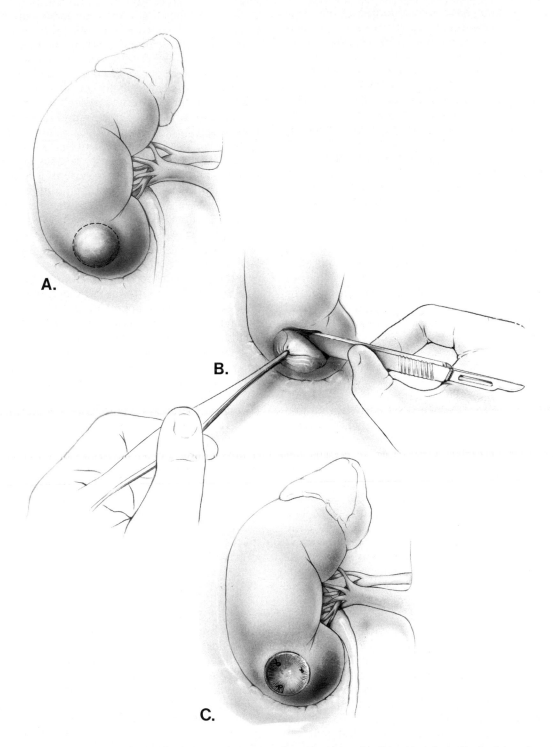

Figure 65—44. *A* to *C*, Technique of enucleation for tumors with a surrounding pseudocapsule. (From Novick, A. C.: Partial nephrectomy for renal cell carcinoma. Urol. Clin. North Am., 14:419, 1987.)

The technique of enucleation should be used only for renal cell carcinomas that are surrounded completely by distinct pseudocapsules. The presence of such tumor encapsulation is difficult to establish preoperatively, and histopathologic studies have shown defects in the pseudocapsule with microscopic tumor invasion in many cases (Marshall, 1986; Rosenthal, 1984). Therefore, the most judicious practice is to excise the tumor with a surrounding margin of normal parenchyma whenever possible. The technique of enucleation has limited indications and is currently reserved primarily for patients with von Hippel-Lindau disease who generally present with multiple low-stage encapsulated tumors involving both kidneys (Spencer, 1988). The advantages of enucleation in this clinical setting are that it is simple and rapid to perform, renal arterial occlusion is usually not necessary, and multiple tumors can be removed with maximal preservation of functioning renal parenchyma.

Segmental Polar Nephrectomy

In a patient with malignancy confined to the upper or lower pole of the kidney, partial nephrectomy can be performed by isolating and ligating the segmental apical or basilar arterial branch while allowing unimpaired perfusion to the remainder of the kidney from the main renal artery. This procedure is illustrated in Figure 65–45 for a tumor confined to the apical vascular segment. The apical artery is dissected away from the adjacent structures, ligated, and divided. Often, a corresponding venous branch is present, which is similarly ligated and divided. An ischemic line of demarcation will then generally appear on the surface of the kidney and will outline the segment to be excised. If this area is not obvious, a few milliliters of methylene blue can be directly injected distally into the ligated apical artery to better outline the limits of the involved renal segment. An incision is then made in the renal cortex at the line of demarcation, which should be at least 1 to 2 cm away from the visible edge of the cancer. The parenchyma is divided by sharp and blunt dissection, and the polar segment is removed. In cases of malignancy, it is not possible to preserve a strip of capsule beyond the parenchymal line of resection for use in closing the renal defect.

Often, a portion of the collecting system will have been removed with the cancer during a segmental polar nephrectomy. The collecting system is carefully closed with interrupted or continuous 4-0 chromic sutures to ensure a watertight repair. Small transected blood vessels on the renal surface are identified and ligated with shallow figure-of-eight 4-0 chromic sutures. The edges of the kidney are reapproximated as an additional hemostatic measure, using simple interrupted 2-0 or 3-0 chromic sutures inserted through the capsule and a small amount of parenchyma. Before these sutures are tied, perirenal fat or oxycel can be inserted into the defect for inclusion in the renal closure. If the collecting system has been entered, a Penrose drain is left in the perinephric space.

Wedge Resection

Wedge resection is an appropriate technique for removing peripheral tumors on the surface of the kidney, particularly ones that are larger or not confined to either renal pole. Because these lesions often encompass more than one renal segment, and because this technique is generally associated with heavier bleeding, it is best to perform wedge resection with temporary renal arterial occlusion and surface hypothermia.

In performing a wedge resection, the tumor is removed with a 1- to 2-cm surrounding margin of grossly normal renal parenchyma (Fig. 65–46). The parenchyma is divided by a combination of sharp and blunt dissection. Invariably, the tumor extends deeply into the kidney, and the collecting system is entered. Often, prominent intrarenal vessels are identified as the parenchyma is being incised. These may be directly suture-ligated at that time, while they are most visible. After excision of the tumor, the collecting system is closed with interrupted or continuous 4-0 chromic sutures. Remaining transected blood vessels on the renal surface are secured with figure-of-eight 4-0 chromic sutures. Bleeding at this point is usually minimal, and the operative field can be kept satisfactorily clear by gentle suction during placement of hemostatic sutures.

The renal defect can be closed in one of two ways (Fig. 65–46). The kidney may be closed upon itself by approximating the transected cortical margins with simple interrupted 2-0 or 3-0 chromic sutures, after placing a small piece of oxycel at the base of the defect. If this is done, there must be no tension on the suture line and no significant angulation or kinking of blood vessels supplying the kidney. Alternatively, a portion of perirenal fat may simply be inserted into the base of the renal defect as a hemostatic measure and sutured to the parenchymal margins with interrupted 4-0 chromic. After closure or coverage of the renal defect, the renal artery is unclamped and circulation to the kidney is restored. A Penrose drain is left in the perinephric space.

Major Transverse Resection

A transverse resection is done to remove large tumors that extensively involve the upper or lower portion of the kidney. This technique is performed using surface hypothermia after temporary occlusion of the renal artery. Major branches of the renal artery and vein supplying the tumor-bearing portion of the kidney are identified in the renal hilus, ligated, and divided (Fig. 65–47A). If possible, this should be done before temporarily occluding the renal artery to minimize the overall period of renal ischemia.

After occluding the renal artery, the parenchyma is divided by blunt and sharp dissection, leaving a 1- to 2-cm margin of grossly normal tissue around the tumor (Fig. 65–47B). Transected blood vessels on the renal surface are secured as previously described, and the hilus is inspected carefully for remaining unligated seg-

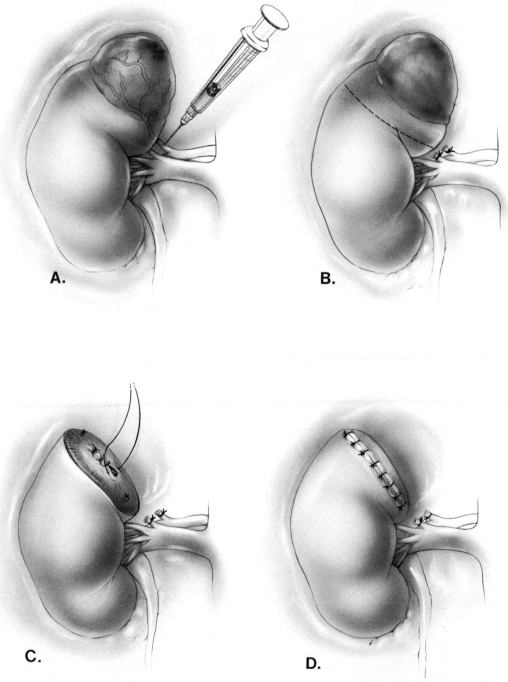

Figure 65–45. *A* to *D,* Technique of segmental (apical) polar nephrectomy with preliminary ligation of apical arterial and venous branches. (From Novick, A. C.: Partial nephrectomy for renal cell carcinoma. Urol. Clin. North Am., 14:419, 1987.)

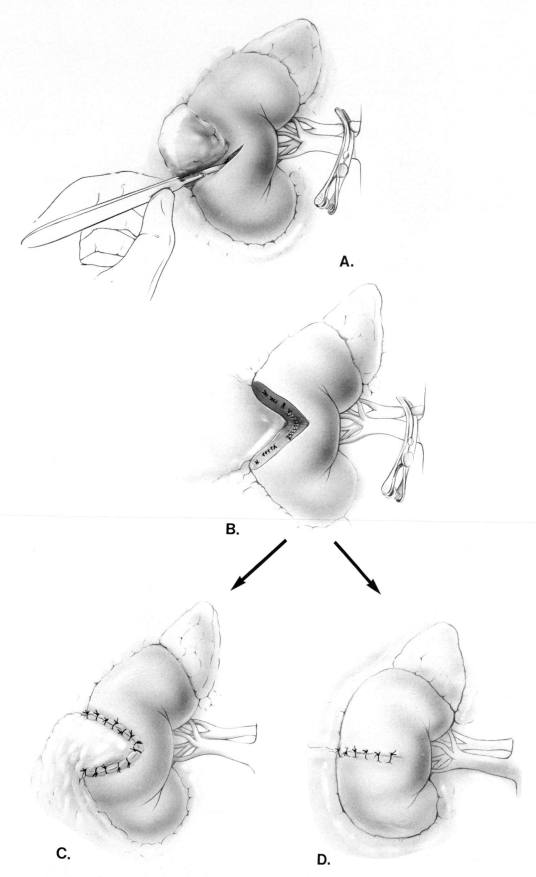

Figure 65–46. *A* to *D*, Technique of wedge resection for a peripheral tumor on the surface of the kidney. The renal defect may be closed upon itself *(D)* or covered with perirenal fat *(C)*. (From Novick, A. C.: Partial nephrectomy for renal cell carcinoma. Urol. Clin. North Am., 14:419, 1987.)

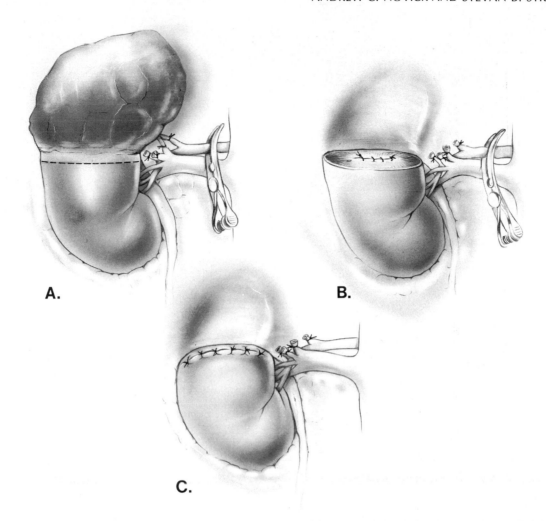

Figure 65–47. *A* to *C,* Technique of transverse resection for a tumor involving the upper half of the kidney (see text for description of procedure). (From Novick, A. C.: Partial nephrectomy for renal cell carcinoma. Urol. Clin. North Am., 14:419, 1987.)

mental vessels. An internal ureteral stent may be inserted if extensive reconstruction of the collecting system is necessary. If possible, the renal defect is sutured together with one of the techniques previously described (Fig. 65–47C). If this suture cannot be placed without tension or without distorting the renal vessels, a piece of peritoneum or perirenal fat is sutured in place to cover the defect. Circulation to the kidney is restored, and a Penrose drain is left in the perirenal space.

Extracorporeal Partial Nephrectomy and Autotransplantation

Extracorporeal partial nephrectomy can allow removal of complex renal tumors that would otherwise be considered inoperable. This technique involves increased operative time with greater potential morbidity and, therefore, should be reserved for the occasional patient with a large, hypervascular central tumor that is not amenable to in situ excision (Novick, 1989; Zincke, 1985). The advantages of an extracorporeal approach in such cases include an optimum exposure, a bloodless surgical field, an ability to perform a more precise operation with maximum conservation of renal parenchyma, and a greater protection of the kidney from prolonged ischemia. Some data also suggest that postoperative local tumor recurrence is less common with this approach than with partial nephrectomy in situ (Jacobs, 1979).

Extracorporeal partial nephrectomy and renal autotransplantation are generally performed through a single midline incision. In heavy or obese patients, an anterior subcostal transperitoneal incision is combined with a separate, lower quadrant, transverse semilunar incision. The kidney is mobilized and removed outside Gerota's fascia with ligation and division of the renal artery and vein as the last steps in the operation (Fig. 65–48 A). Immediately after dividing the renal vessels, the removed kidney is flushed with 500 ml of a chilled intracellular electrolyte solution and is submerged in a basin of ice slush saline solution to maintain hypothermia. Under these conditions, if warm renal ischemia has been minimal, the kidney can safely be preserved outside the body for as much time as needed to perform extracorporeal partial nephrectomy.

If possible, it is best to leave the ureter attached in such cases to preserve its distal collateral vascular sup-

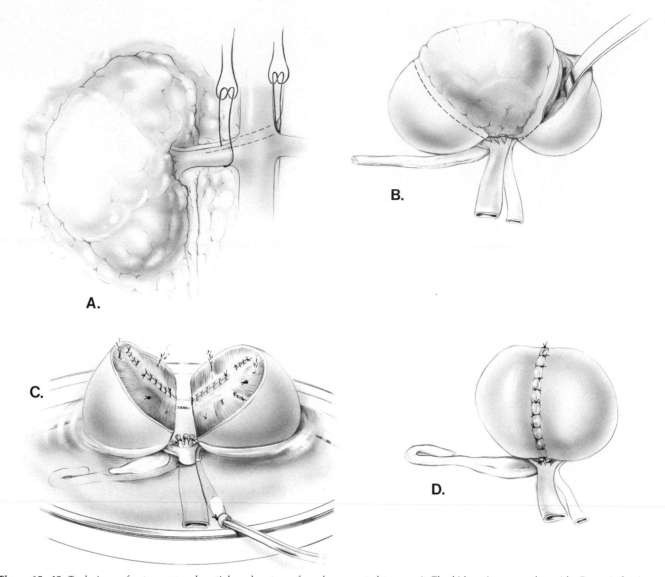

Figure 65–48. Technique of extracorporeal partial nephrectomy for a large central tumor. *A*, The kidney is removed outside Gerota's fascia. *B*, The tumor is excised extracorporeally while preserving the vascular branches to uninvolved parenchyma. *C*, Pulsatile perfusion or reflushing identify the transected blood vessels. *D*, The kidney is closed upon itself. (From Novick, A. C.: Partial nephrectomy for renal cell carcinoma. Urol. Clin. North Am., 14:419, 1987.)

ply, particularly with large hilar or lower renal tumors in which complex excision may unavoidably compromise the blood supply to the pelvis, ureter, or both. When this procedure is done, the extracorporeal operation is performed on the abdominal wall. If the ureter is left attached, it must be occluded temporarily to prevent retrograde blood flow to the kidney when it is outside the body. Often, unless the patient is thin, working on the abdominal wall with the ureter attached is cumbersome because of the tethering and restricted movement of the kidney. If these are observed, the ureter should be divided and the kidney placed on a separate workbench. This practice will provide better exposure for the extracorporeal operation and, as this is being done, a second surgical team can be simultaneously preparing the iliac fossa for autotransplantation. If concern exists about the adequacy of ureteral blood supply, the risk of postoperative urinary extravasation can be diminished

by restoring urinary continuity through direct anastomosis of the renal pelvis to the retained distal ureter.

Extracorporeal partial nephrectomy is done with the flushed kidney preserved under surface hypothermia. The kidney is first divested of all perinephric fat to appreciate the full extent of the neoplasm. Because such tumors are usually centrally located, dissection is generally begun in the renal hilus with identification of major segmental arterial and venous branches. Vessels clearly directed toward the neoplasm are secured and divided, and those supplying uninvolved renal parenchyma are preserved. The tumor is then removed by incising the capsule and parenchyma to preserve a 1- to 2-cm surrounding margin of normal renal tissue (Fig. 65–48*B*). Transected blood vessels visible on the renal surface are secured, and the collecting system is closed as described for in situ partial nephrectomy.

At this point, the renal remnant may be re-flushed or

placed on the pulsatile perfusion unit to facilitate identification and suture ligation of remaining potential bleeding points (Fig. 65–48C). The kidney can be alternately perfused through the renal artery and vein to ensure both arterial and venous hemostasis. Because the flushing solution and perfusate lack clotting ability, there may continue to be some parenchymal oozing, which can safely be ignored. If possible, the defect created by the partial nephrectomy is closed by suturing the kidney upon itself to further ensure a watertight repair (Fig. 65–48D).

Autotransplantation into the iliac fossa is done, employing the same vascular technique as that in renal allotransplantation. Urinary continuity may be restored with ureteroneocystostomy or pyeloureterostomy, leaving an internal ureteral stent in place. When removal of the neoplasm has necessitated extensive hilar dissection of vessels supplying the renal pelvis, an indwelling nephrostomy tube is also left for postoperative drainage. After autotransplantation, a Penrose drain is positioned extraperitoneally in the iliac fossa away from the vascular anastomotic sites.

Complications

Complications of partial nephrectomy include hemorrhage, urinary fistula formation, ureteral obstruction, renal insufficiency, and infection. Significant intraoperative bleeding can occur in patients who are undergoing partial nephrectomy. The need for early control and ready access to the renal artery is emphasized. Postoperative hemorrhage may be self-limiting, if confined to the retroperitoneum, or it may be associated with gross hematuria. The initial management of postoperative hemorrhage is expectant with bed rest, serial hemoglobin and hematocrit determinations, frequent monitoring of vital signs, and blood transfusions as needed. Angiography may be helpful in some patients to localize actively bleeding segmental renal arteries, which may be controlled via angioinfarction. Severe intractable hemorrhage may necessitate re-exploration with early control of the renal vessels and ligation of the active bleeding points.

Postoperative urinary flank drainage after a partial nephrectomy is common and usually resolves as the collecting system closes with healing. Persistent drainage suggests the development of a urinary cutaneous fistula. This diagnosis can be confirmed by determination of the creatinine level of the drainage fluid, and intravenous injection of indigo carmine with subsequent appearance of the dye in the drainage fluid. The majority of urinary fistulas resolve spontaneously if there is no obstruction of urinary drainage from the involved renal unit. If the perirenal space is not adequately drained, a urinoma or abscess may develop. An intravenous pyelogram or a retrograde pyelogram should be obtained to rule out obstruction of the involved urinary collecting system. In the event of hydronephrosis or persistent urinary leakage, an internal ureteral stent is placed. If this is not possible, a percutaneous nephrostomy may be inserted. The majority of urinary fistulas resolve spontaneously

with proper conservative management, although this may take several weeks in some cases. A second operation to close the urinary fistula is rarely necessary.

Ureteral obstruction can occur after partial nephrectomy because of postoperative bleeding into the collecting system with resulting clot obstruction of the ureter and pelvis. This obstruction can lead to temporary extravasation of urine from the renal suture line. In most cases, expectant management is appropriate and the obstruction resolves spontaneously with lysis of the clots. When urinary leakage is excessive, or in the presence of intercurrent urinary infection, placement of an internal ureteral stent can help to maintain antegrade ureteral drainage.

Varying degrees of renal insufficiency often occur postoperatively when partial nephrectomy is performed in a patient with a solitary kidney. This insufficiency is a consequence of both intraoperative renal ischemia and removal of some normal parenchyma along with the diseased portion of the kidney. Such renal insufficiency is usually mild and resolves spontaneously with proper fluid and electrolyte management. Also, in most cases, the remaining parenchyma undergoes compensatory hypertrophy that serves to further improve renal function. Severe renal insufficiency may require temporary or permanent hemodialysis, and the patient should be aware of this possibility preoperatively. In a review of 100 patients who underwent partial nephrectomy for renal cell carcinoma, temporary and permanent renal failure occurred postoperatively in seven patients (7 per cent) and three patients (3 per cent), respectively (Novick, 1989).

Postoperative infections are usually self-limiting if the operative site is well drained and in the absence of existing untreated urinary infection at the time of surgery. Unusual complications of partial nephrectomy include transient postoperative hypertension and aneurysm or arteriovenous fistula in the remaining portion of the parenchyma (Rezvani, 1973; Snodgrass, 1964).

PARTIAL NEPHRECTOMY FOR BENIGN DISEASE

Partial nephrectomy is also indicated in selected patients with localized benign pathology of the kidney (Leach, 1980). The indications include (1) hydronephrosis with parenchymal atrophy or atrophic pyelonephritis in a duplicated renal segment; (2) calyceal diverticulum complicated by infection, stones, or both; (3) calculus disease with obstruction of the lower pole calyx or segmental parenchymal disease with impaired drainage (Bates, 1981; Papathanassiadis, 1966); (4) renovascular hypertension due to segmental parenchymal damage or noncorrectable branch renal artery disease (Aoi, 1981; Parrott, 1984); (5) traumatic renal injury with irreversible damage to a portion of the kidney (Gibson, 1982); and (6) removal of a benign renal tumor, such as an angiomyolipoma or oncocytoma (Maatman, 1984).

The preoperative considerations are similar to those in a patient who is undergoing partial nephrectomy for malignancy. In most cases, renal arteriography should

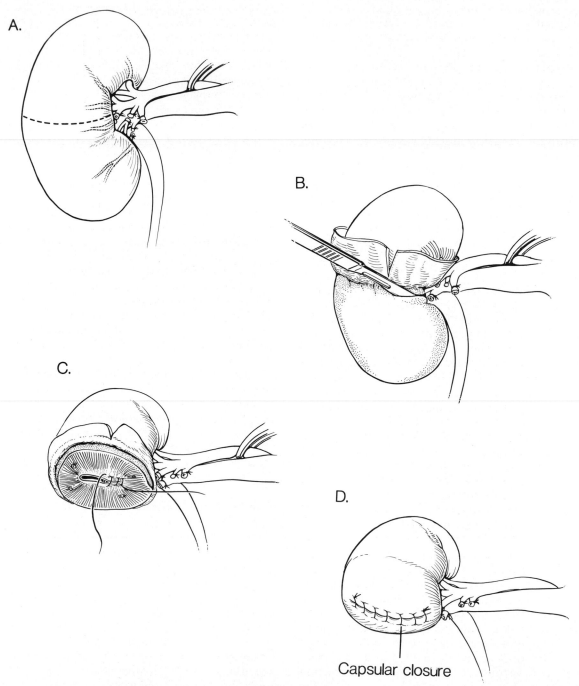

Figure 65–49. *A* to *D*, Technique of transverse renal resection for a benign disorder. The renal capsule from the diseased parenchyma is preserved and used to cover the transected renal surface.

be performed to delineate the main and segmental renal arterial supply. The same measures should be taken to minimize intraoperative renal damage from ischemia. The preferred surgical approach is usually through an extraperitoneal flank incision, except for cases of renal trauma, which are best approached anteriorly. The surgical techniques are also similar to those previously described for malignant renal disease.

When performing an apical or a basilar partial nephrectomy for benign disease, the segmental apical or basilar arterial branch is secured. The parenchyma is divided at the ischemic line of demarcation, without the need for temporary renal arterial occlusion. More complex transverse or wedge renal resections are best performed with temporary renal arterial occlusion and ice slush, surface hypothermia. When employing the technique of transverse renal resection for a benign disorder, the renal capsule is excised and reflected off the diseased parenchyma for subsequent use in covering the renal defect (Fig. 65–49). The technical aspects of partial nephrectomy for benign disease are otherwise the same as those described for malignancy with adherence to the same basic principles of appropriate vascular control, avoidance of ischemic renal damage, precise closure of the collecting system, careful hemostasis, and closure or coverage of the renal defect.

Heminephrectomy in Duplicated Collecting Systems

Because the indications for partial nephrectomy in this clinical setting are usually hydronephrosis and parenchymal atrophy of one of the two segments, the demarcation of the tissue to be removed is usually very evident. The atrophic parenchyma lining the dilated system can be further delineated by pyelotubular backflow with blue dye, if the ureter is ligated and the affected collecting system is distended by the blue dye under pressure. In such a case, there is also often a dual arterial supply with distinct segmental branches to the upper and lower halves of the kidney. Segmental arterial and venous branches to the diseased portion of the kidney are ligated and divided. After preserving a strip of renal capsule, the parenchyma is divided at the observed line of demarcation. Minimal bleeding is usual from the renal surface, and temporary occlusion of the arterial supply to the nondiseased segment is often unnecessary. No entry should occur into the collecting system over the transected renal surface, which is then closed or covered as previously described.

RENAL STONE DISEASE

The surgical management of renal stone (calculus) disease has changed dramatically since the introduction of percutaneous and extracorporeal shock wave technology. Clearly, well over 95 per cent of patients who previously required "open" operative intervention may now be managed with these less invasive modalities, either alone or in combination (Assimos et al., 1989).

Although technologic advances have changed the manner in which urologic surgeons approach renal calculi, the basic indications for intervention remain the same. These include obstruction, pain, infection, or significant hematuria associated with the stone, or stone growth despite appropriate medical therapy. Within these clinical settings, the indications for open operative intervention are much more confined and include the following:

- An associated anatomic abnormality requiring open operative intervention.
- A stone so large and extensive that in the judgment of an experienced urologic surgeon, a single open operative procedure would, with less risk, more likely render the patient stone-free than would the option of multiple percutaneous and extracorporeal shock wave procedures.
- Failure of, or contraindication to, both extracorporeal shock wave lithotripsy and percutaneous nephrostolithotomy.

Radiographic and Renal Function Evaluation

In most cases, intravenous urography is the initial radiographic study obtained. Ideally, adequate anatomic and functional information will be provided. Specifically, the number, size, and location of the stones will be evident from this study alone. Oblique views and nephrotomograms should be included both before and after injection of contrast material.

At times, renal function may be compromised from either intrinsic renal disease or obstruction, so that intravenous urography does not allow adequate visualization of the upper tracts. In those cases, retrograde or antegrade pyelography can delineate the renal anatomy. When obstruction is found, an internal stent or a percutaneous nephrostomy tube should remain indwelling to relieve symptoms, enhance treatment of any associated infection, and allow recovery of renal function. For selected patients, further assessment of renal function may be attained with a differential renal function scan (computerized renogram), utilizing technetium 99-DTPA.

Planning of surgical intervention for complex stone disease may also include a CT scan obtained both before and after intravenous contrast material injection, because this scan will provide valuable information regarding the three-dimensional location of the stone. CT scanning also allows evaluation of the renal cortical thickness, which is especially useful when consideration is being given to an ablative procedure such as partial or total nephrectomy. Currently, standard catheter angiography has only a limited role in the preoperative evaluation of patients with stones. When information regarding the number and location of the main renal arteries is desired, intra-arterial or intravenous digital subtraction angiography will generally be adequate (Zabbo et al., 1988).

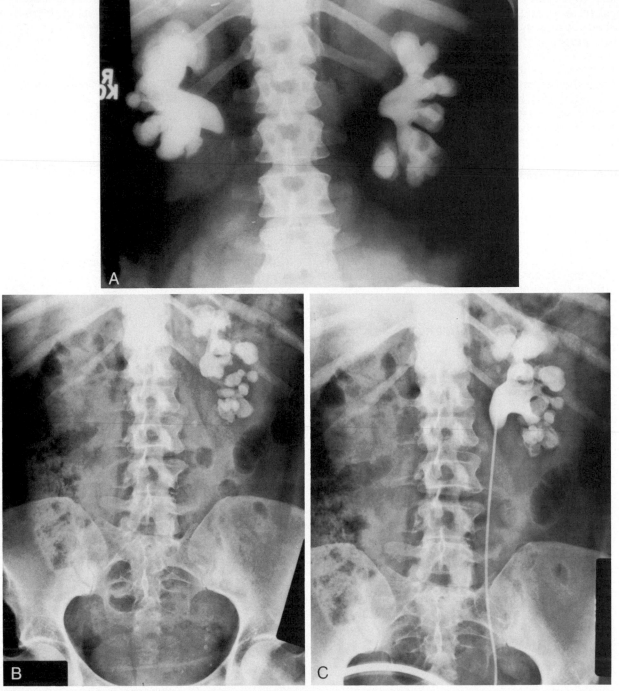

Figure 65–50. *A*, Scout film reveals bilateral staghorn calculi. However, there is no infundibular stenosis. Therefore, a combination of percutaneous nephrostolithotomy and extracorporeal shock wave lithotripsy is an excellent contemporary treatment option.

B and *C*, Scout film reveals staghorn calculus on the left side. In contrast to the patient in *A*, the retrograde study reveals multiple areas of relative infundibular narrowing. Therefore, significant debulking would be difficult without multiple percutaneous tracts. In addition, multiple sessions of extracorporeal shock wave lithotripsy may also be required. In such a case, anatrophic nephrolithotomy still provides a reasonable therapeutic option.

Anatrophic Nephrolithotomy

Although the approach to managing staghorn calculi has changed dramatically, the rationale for intervention remains the same. Most staghorn calculi are composed of magnesium-ammonium-calcium phosphate and are associated with chronic urinary tract infection that is virtually impossible to irradicate as long as the stone is present. Although a controlled, prospective study of conservative medical management versus operative intervention has yet to be done, strong clinical evidence exists that, in all but those who have the poorest risks for surgery, renal function and overall clinical status are improved by removing the stone (Blandy and Singh, 1976; Rous and Turner, 1977; Vargas et al., 1982).

The majority of staghorn calculi, even extensive ones, can and should be managed by combinations of percutaneous "debulking" and extracorporeal shock wave lithotripsy (Kahnoski et al., 1986; Schulze et al., 1986; Streem et al., 1987). Occasionally, however, specific circumstances may dictate open operative intervention, although in our experience such an approach to staghorn calculi is recommended only rarely. The most frequent relative indication for an open procedure is the finding of a massive, complete staghorn calculus with multiple dumbbell-shaped infundibulocalyceal extensions, associated with relatively narrow infundibula (Fig. 65–50). In such cases, the option of a single, open operative procedure, especially in a previously unoperated kidney, may be a reasonable one when weighed against the alternative of multiple percutaneous tracts just to attain significant debulking and the need for multiple additional sessions of extracorporeal shock wave lithotripsy and possible percutaneous chemolysis. In these cases, the open operative approach of choice is the anatrophic nephrolithotomy, initially described by Boyce and Smith in 1967.

Complete radiographic and renal function evaluation is accomplished as previously outlined. Because most of these stones are associated with chronic infection, it is important to search for underlying anatomic or functional urinary tract abnormalities predisposing the patient to infection. Metabolic evaluation should also be performed because a significant proportion of struvite stones form secondarily (Resnick, 1981). Vigorous treatment of associated urinary tract infection is an important part of the preoperative care. Intravenous antibiotics are generally begun 36 to 48 hours prior to surgery. Adequate intravenous hydration is also a standard part of the immediate preoperative regimen.

The technique of anatrophic nephrolithotomy follows the basic principles set forth by Boyce and Smith (1967). Essentially, all stone is to be removed through an incision that is least traumatic to overall renal function. Because temporary occlusion of the renal artery is required for a bloodless field, the kidney must be protected from an ischemic insult. Areas of true, functionally significant infundibular stenosis must be addressed to provide adequate drainage from all parts of the collecting system.

A flank approach is chosen, with resection of the 11th or 12th rib. Medially, the incision should extend to the lateral border of the rectus muscle. The peritoneum is reflected medially to gain access to the retroperitoneum. The proximal ureter is identified and surrounded with a vessel loop to prevent distal migration of any stone fragments during the subsequent nephrolithotomy. The kidney is completely mobilized, leaving only the renal pedicle and ureter intact. A surgical tape placed around the upper and lower poles at this time provides a useful sling to facilitate handling of the kidney. Medial retraction of the kidney then affords exposure to the hilar vessels posteriorly, where the renal artery is dissected free and surrounded with a vessel loop (Fig. 65–51). Mannitol, 12 to 15 g, is now given intravenously to help protect the kidney from the subsequent period of ischemia. The renal artery is further dissected until the anterior and posterior divisional branches are identified. Generally, the first major branch of the main renal artery represents the posterior division. This dissection is required to precisely identify the junction of the blood supply to the anterior and posterior segments of the kidney. As first described by Brodell in 1901 and then delineated further by Graves in 1954, this junction, at the surface of the kidney, generally lies on the posterior aspect, approximately two thirds of the distance from the hilum to the true lateral border of the kidney (Fig. 65–52).

A vascular clamp may now be placed temporarily on the anterior division of the renal artery and 10 ml of methylene blue injected intravenously in the systemic circulation. This dye will stain the posterior renal segment, thus helping to identify the appropriate line of incision and subsequent dissection into the renal parenchyma. A plastic dam is placed beneath the kidney and wrapped around the pedicle as a reservoir for ice slush. The main renal artery is clamped, and the kidney is packed in ice slush with a goal of obtaining a core temperature of 10°C, as protection from subsequent ischemia. Once the kidney is cooled, a longitudinal

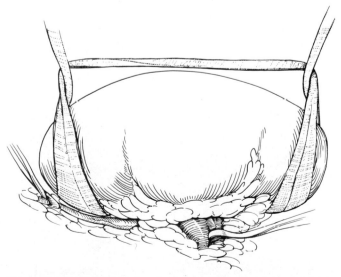

Figure 65–51. The kidney is retracted medially after it is completely mobilized. Vessel loops surround the renal artery and ureter while a sling facilitates handling of the kidney.

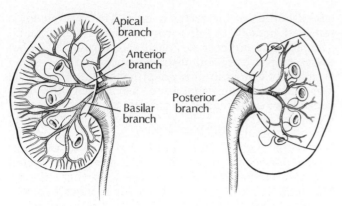

Figure 65–52. The avascular line of incision is defined by the juncture of the anterior and posterior segments of the renal artery. On the surface of the kidney, this avascular plane generally lies on the posterior aspect, approximately two thirds of the distance from the renal hilum to the true lateral border of the kidney.

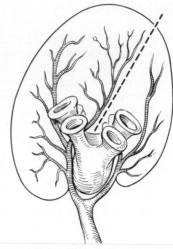

Figure 65–54. The nephrotomy incision is continued in a plane along the line of demarcation between the anterior and posterior arterial segments and extended down toward the renal pelvis. The correct line of dissection generally lies just anterior to the posterior row of infundibula and calyces.

incision is made through the capsule between the anterior and posterior segments, extending to the apical and basilar renal segments (Fig. 65–53). Blunt dissection is used to continue the dissection through the parenchyma. The correct plane is along the line of demarcation between the anterior and posterior arterial segments, down toward the renal pelvis in a plane just anterior to the posterior row of infundibula and calyces (Fig. 65–54). At this time and throughout the subsequent dissection, any venous bleeding is managed by suture ligation with fine chromic sutures. If small arterioles have been cut, they are managed in the same manner. The stone is now usually identified by palpation in one of the involved posterior infundibula or calyces. A longitudinal infundibulotomy is performed and extended down to the renal pelvis (Fig. 65–55). In a similar manner, each posterior infundibulocalyx is opened longitudinally on its anterior aspect, with the infundibulotomy extending out from the renal pelvis toward the calyx.

Upon completion of the longitudinal nephrotomy and exposure of the pelvic and posterior aspect of the stone, the anterior and polar portions are exposed by sequential longitudinal infundibulotomies made on the posterior aspect of the anterior segmental infundibula and on the medial aspects of the polar infundibula (Fig. 65–56A) (Boyce et al., 1979). These infundibulotomies should begin at each infundibulopelvic junction and extend outward toward the calyx as far as necessary to provide adequate exposure for subsequent removal of the calculus. Gradually, the entire staghorn calculus is exposed and is now ready for removal (Fig. 65–56B). During this portion of the procedure, invaluable exposure may be obtained utilizing malleable brain retractors

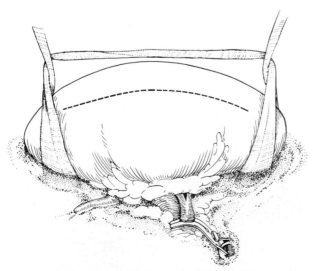

Figure 65–53. After the renal artery has been clamped and the kidney cooled in ice slush, the nephrotomy incision is made through the capsule between the anterior and posterior segments. This nephrotomy incision extends only to the apical and basilar renal segments.

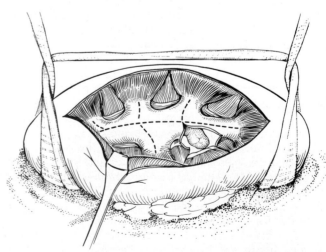

Figure 65–55. A longitudinal infundibulotomy is performed on the anterior aspect of one of the posterior infundibula through which the stone is palpable. The infundibulotomy is extended down to the renal pelvis and the pelvis itself then opened. A longitudinal infundibulotomy is subsequently performed on each posterior infundibulum.

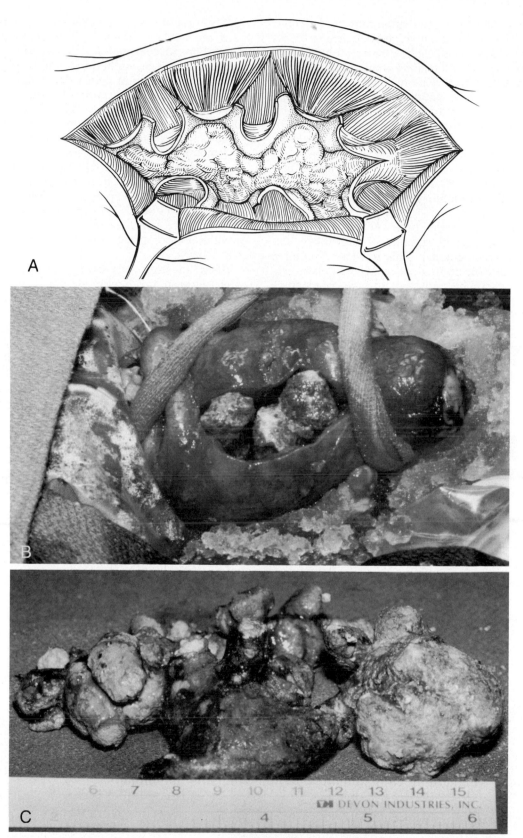

Figure 65–56. *A*, The anterior infundibula and calyces are opened with longitudinal infundibulotomy incisions that are extended from the renal pelvis out toward the calyces. The anterior infundibula are opened on their posterior aspects, and the polar infundibula are opened on their medial aspects. Eventually, the entire stone is exposed.

B, Intraoperative view of a mobilized kidney packed in ice slush. The nephrotomy incision has been made and the stone exposed.

C, Complete staghorn calculus removed with an anatrophic nephrolithotomy.

and nerve hooks. At times, the stone may be delivered intact (Fig. 65–56C). Although a laudable achievement, piecemeal extraction is, in practice, more often the rule as infundibulocalyceal extensions may break off and require separate removal. This may be a result of the relatively soft and friable nature of the stone, or alternatively the entire stone may not have been in continuity to begin with. When infundibulocalyceal extensions of the stone remain, the involved infundibulum should be further incised out toward the calyx. Blunt dissection between the stone and urothelium with a tonsil clamp or similar instrument will help free the stone which, because of a local inflammatory reaction, may be densely adherent.

Following removal of the bulk of the stone, each infundibulocalyceal system should be individually explored for residual fragments. This maneuver requires both visual inspection and palpation. Occasionally, residual fragments can be palpated through thin parenchyma, but the infundibulum leading to the stone cannot be localized. In such a case, the fragment is removed by making a small nephrotomy directly over the stone. The nephrotomy is closed with absorbable sutures in one or two layers, depending on the thickness of the parenchyma. The entire collecting system is now thoroughly lavaged with cold saline, utilizing an appropriate-sized red rubber catheter placed sequentially in each infundibulocalyceal system. During this portion of the procedure, an 8 Fr. catheter should be placed antegrade from within the renal pelvis down the ureter to again help prevent distal migration of stone fragments.

As removal of all stone fragments is an important goal of this operation, intraoperative radiography with "organ films" remains an integral part of the procedure. X-O-mat KS film is ideal, and sterile cassettes should be a routine part of the available instrumentation (Fig. 65–57). When residual stone fragments are noted, intraoperative ultrasonography may allow their localization (Cook and Lytton, 1977). In our experience, however, intraoperative nephroscopy with a flexible neproscope provides a more direct route for rapid localization (Miki et al., 1978).

When all stone has been removed, closure of the collecting system is begun. At this point, the red rubber catheter is withdrawn from the ureter. In selected patients, especially those who may have residual fragments, an internal stent is placed antegrade with the proximal portion positioned in the lower infundibulocalyceal system or renal pelvis. Nephrostomy tubes are rarely employed. Generally, they are placed for those

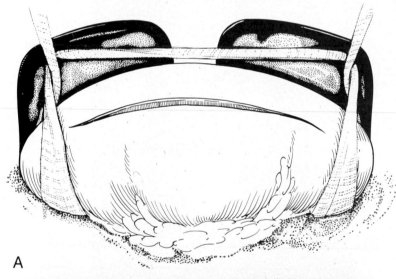

A

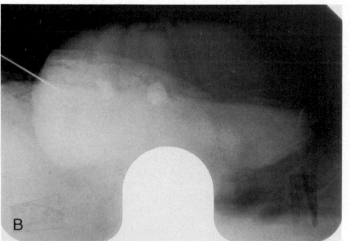

B

Figure 65–57. *A,* Prior to closure of the collecting system an intraoperative organ film is obtained to exclude the presence of residual stones. X-O-mat KS film is ideal for this purpose.

B, Residual calculi are noted on X-O-mat film. Needle localization is a useful adjunct at this time.

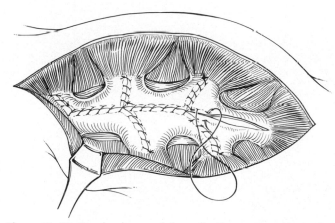

Figure 65-58. Simple closure of the collecting system with running absorbable suture.

patients with severely compromised renal function and very thin parenchyma or for patients with possible residual stones that could be treated with percutaneous extraction or chemolysis.

Separate closure of the collecting system with a running, fine chromic suture is generally recommended. In most cases, this step involves simple closure of each infundibulotomy and the renal pelvis (Fig. 65–58). However, close attention must be paid to areas of significant infundibular stenosis that will require infundibuloplasty. In previous years, infundibular stenosis was considered to be a common sequela of staghorn calculi. However, the success of percutaneous and extracorporeal techniques, alone or in combination for most of these cases, has proved to us that infundibular stenosis is more often apparent than real and is usually not of any functional significance once the stone is removed. As an analogy,

this situation is perhaps best compared to the case of a stone impacted at the ureteropelvic junction. Intravenous or retrograde pyelograms often reveal apparent narrowing just distal to the stone, which can suggest intrinsic ureteropelvic junction obtruction. However, in the majority of cases, such patients can be managed successfully by extracorporeal shock wave lithotripsy or by percutaneous techniques alone, without a concomitant procedure on the ureteropelvic junction. In those patients, follow-up studies will often show complete resolution of the apparent intrinsic obstruction. Occasionally, infundibular stenosis may require reconstruction in the form of infundibuloplasty. In fact, multiple areas of true infundibular stenosis (Fig. 65–59) associated with an extensive staghorn calculus is one of the few primary indications for an anatrophic nephrolithotomy rather than a combined endourologic approach. In such a case, internal reconstruction of the collecting system is an integral part of the operative procedure.

With stenosis of the adjacent infundibula, infundibuloplasty is performed by joining the sides of each to one another, utilizing running fine chromic sutures. These sutures begin at the level of the renal pelvis and are carried out distally to the involved calyx (Fig. 65–60 A).

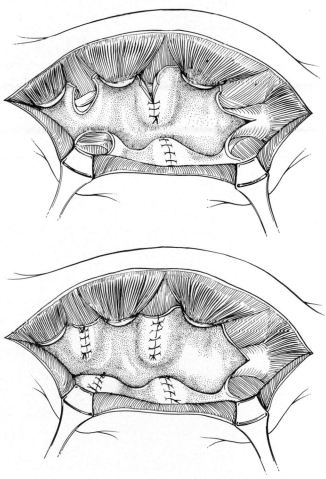

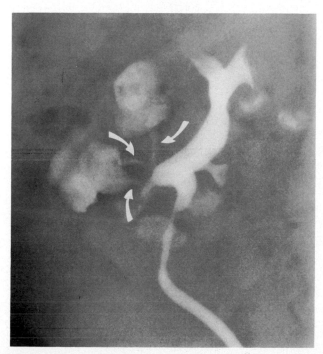

Figure 65-59. Retrograde study in this patient with chronic infection and stones reveals multiple areas of true infundibular stenosis *(arrows)*.

Figure 65-60. *A,* Infundibuloplasty is indicated for repair of stenosis involving two or more adjacent infundibula. Rather than simple closure of the initial longitudinal infundibulotomies, the sides of the adjacent involved infundibula are sutured to each other. The mirroring anterior or posterior infundibula must also be joined. *B,* This maneuver in effect creates a large, well-drained infundibulopelvis.

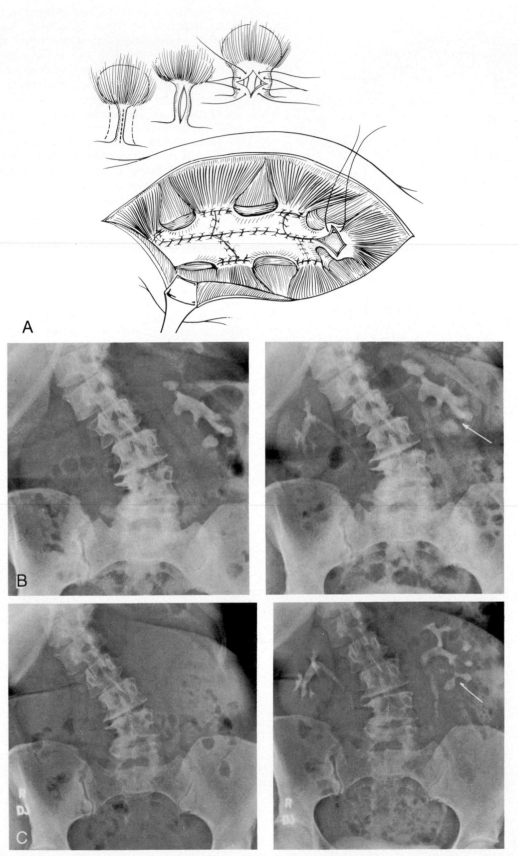

Figure 65–61. *A*, Alternatively, stenosis of isolated infundibula are managed with infundibulorrhaphy. The stenotic infundibulum, which has been opened longitudinally, is closed horizontally in a Heineke-Mikulicz fashion. *B*, Intravenous pyelography (scout and 20-minute film) reveals an extensive left staghorn calculus. Isolated infundibular stenosis of the lower medial infundibulum *(arrow)* is also noted. *C*, Following anatrophic nephrolithotomy and infundibulorrhaphy, the lower medial infundibulum is widely patent and the calyx well drained *(arrow)*.

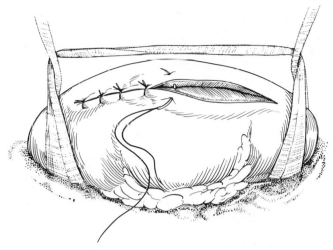

Figure 65–62. Following closure of the collecting system, the renal capsule is approximated with running or interrupted absorbable suture.

In this procedure, the mirroring anterior or posterior infundibula must also be joined. This procedure, in effect, converts two or more stenotic infundibulocalyceal systems to one large portion of the renal pelvis (Fig. 65–60B).

Alternatively, stenosis of isolated infundibula may be managed with infundibulorrhaphy. This involves horizontal closure of the primary vertical infundibulotomy in a Heineke-Mikulicz fashion (Fig. 65–61). This procedure effectively shortens and widens the stenotic infundibulum and brings the renal pelvis closer to the calyx.

Following reconstruction of the collecting system, the renal capsule is approximated with running or interrupted 3-0 chromic suture (Fig. 65–62). At this time, an additional 12 to 15 g of mannitol is given intravenously, and the vascular clamp is removed. Whenever possible, Gerota's fascia and the perirenal fat are reapproximated over the nephrotomy incision. External drainage is accomplished with a Penrose or closed-suction drain placed near, but not directly on, the nephrotomy itself. The wound is thoroughly irrigated and closed in layers in a standard fashion.

Standard Pyelolithotomy

This first use of an incision through the renal pelvis for removal of a stone is credited to Czerny, who performed the procedure in 1880. However, that approach remained controversial for many years, as most surgeons then favored nephrolithotomy. In 1913, Lower, at the Cleveland Clinic, popularized the vertical pyelotomy, which became the preferred method for removal of uncomplicated renal pelvic calculi. In 1965, Gil-Vernet published his studies on the functional anatomy of the renal pelvic musculature. With this work, he advocated a transverse rather than a vertical pyelotomy. This variation of a pyelolithotomy was rapidly accepted for the majority of patients with renal pelvic calculi. Currently, however, almost any patient whose stone could be removed via a pyelotomy incision can and should be managed with either percutaneous or extra-

corporeal shock wave technology. Thus, the role for a pyelolithotomy, once performed routinely as part of every urologic surgeon's armamentarium, is now exceedingly limited.

While a standard pyelolithotomy had been the procedure of choice for most patients with uncomplicated renal pelvic calculi, there are currently only two indications for this procedure. The first is failure of, or contraindication to, both extracorporeal shock wave lithotripsy and percutaneous nephrostolithotomy. The other indication is the presence of an associated anatomic abnormality requiring open operative intervention, such as ureteropelvic junction obstruction.

A pyelolithotomy is generally performed through a standard flank incision, with 12th rib resection, or through a dorsal lumbotomy. Either approach allows rapid access to the renal pelvis posteriorly. With either approach, the retroperitoneum is entered and Gerota's fascia opened posteriorly at the lower pole of the kidney. The proximal ureter is identified and surrounded with a vessel loop to prevent distal migration of the stone during the subsequent dissection. The dissection is carried proximally toward the renal pelvis, along the posterior aspect of the ureter (Fig. 65–63A). In uncomplicated cases, the kidney need not (and should not) be mobilized any more than is necessary to provide adequate exposure of the renal pelvis. Excessive mobilization may result in significant perirenal scarring, which could complicate subsequent interventional procedures.

Once the renal pelvis is adequately exposed posteriorly, stay sutures are placed in preparation for a transverse pyelotomy that should be made well away from the ureteropelvic junction. This pyelotomy is initiated with a curved "banana" blade and extended with Potts scissors as far as necessary to extract the calculus under direct vision (Fig. 65–63B). The stone is removed with standard Randall's forceps (Fig. 65–63C). An 8 Fr. catheter is passed antegrade to the bladder to assure ureteral patency. With the catheter left in place to prevent distal migration of any stone fragments, the renal pelvis is thoroughly irrigated with saline. The pyelotomy is closed in a single layer, utilizing interrupted or running 4-0 chromic sutures through the full thickness of the renal pelvic wall (Fig. 65–63D). If the dissection has been difficult, as may occur in previously operated kidneys, or if the procedure has been performed in the presence of an infection, consideration should be given to placement of an internal stent prior to closure of the pyelotomy. Nephrostomy tubes would be indicated in only the rarest of cases, but could be considered when a question of distal ureteral patency or residual calculi exists. This tube would then allow simpler access in the postoperative period for subsequent antegrade radiographic studies or percutaneous stone extraction. External drainage is routinely provided with a Penrose or closed-suction drain placed near but not on the pyelotomy. The wound is closed in a standard fashion.

Extended Pyelolithotomy

Gil-Vernet, in 1965, advocated the "extended" transverse pyelotomy for management of many patients with

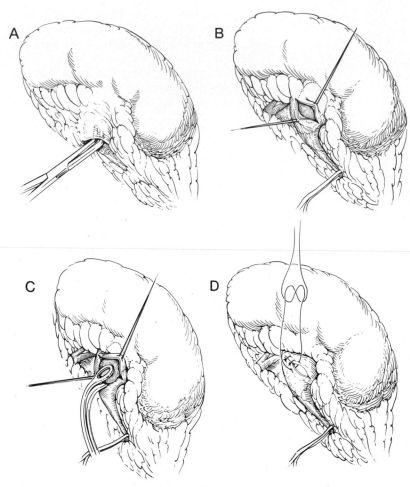

Figure 65–63. *A*, For a standard pyelolithotomy, the proximal ureter and renal pelvis are exposed posteriorly.

B, Stay sutures are placed on the renal pelvis and a horizontal pyelotomy incision performed, well away from the ureteropelvic junction.

C, The stone is extracted with standard Randall's or other stone forceps.

D, Following irrigation of the collecting system, the pyelotomy incision is closed with running or interrupted absorbable suture placed through the full thickness of the renal pelvic wall.

complicated stone disease, including those with extensive staghorn calculi. His approach was based on studies by Henle in 1866 that defined the renal sinus as a rectangular space containing the intrarenal collecting system, vessels, nerves, and lymphatics. Disse, in 1891, described fibrous extensions from the renal capsule to the posterior renal pelvis that normally act to separate the renal sinus from the retroperitoneal space. An extended pyelolithotomy utilizes dissection into the renal sinus to gain access to the intrarenal collecting system.

The extended pyelolithotomy was chosen much more frequently for management of extensive staghorn calculi in Europe than in the United States, where the anatrophic nephrolithotomy was favored. There was general agreement, however, that an extended pyelolithotomy was indicated for relatively large renal pelvic stones, especially those in an intrarenal pelvis, and for partial staghorn calculi that extend into one or more infundibula without multiple dumbbell-shaped calyceal extensions or associated infundibular stenosis. The majority of patients who had been good candidates for extended pyelolithotomy are now managed, however, with extracorporeal shock wave lithotripsy or percutaneous techniques. Thus, a specific indication to use extended pyelolithotomy as a primary approach includes failure of, or contraindication to, both of those less invasive

modalities or an associated anatomic abnormality requiring operative intervention.

The posterior aspect of the renal pelvis is exposed as described for a standard pyelolithotomy. Dissection is carried into the renal sinus by first incising the fibrous tissue between the posterior hilar lip of the renal parenchyma and the pelvis itself, and entering the plane between the renal pelvis and peripelvic fat (Fig. 65–64*A*). Further exposure of the intrarenal collecting system is accomplished utilizing vein retractors or Gil-Vernet renal sinus retractors to elevate the posterior parenchymal lip while dissecting into the sinus with a moist gauze (Fig. 65–64*B*). In selected cases, temporary occlusion of the renal artery, which should be done in conjunction with local hypothermia, softens the renal parenchyma and allows further exposure of the intrarenal collecting system. This maneuver also facilitates palpation of any infundibulocalyceal extensions of the stone (Wulfsohn, 1981).

A transverse pyelotomy is made in a curvilinear fashion between stay sutures, well away from the ureteropelvic junction. The pyelotomy is extended along both the upper and lower infundibula. Thus, a renal pelvic flap is created that affords access for removal of the stone (Fig. 65–64*C*).

If infundibular extensions of the calculus remain after extraction of the pelvic portion, these can generally be

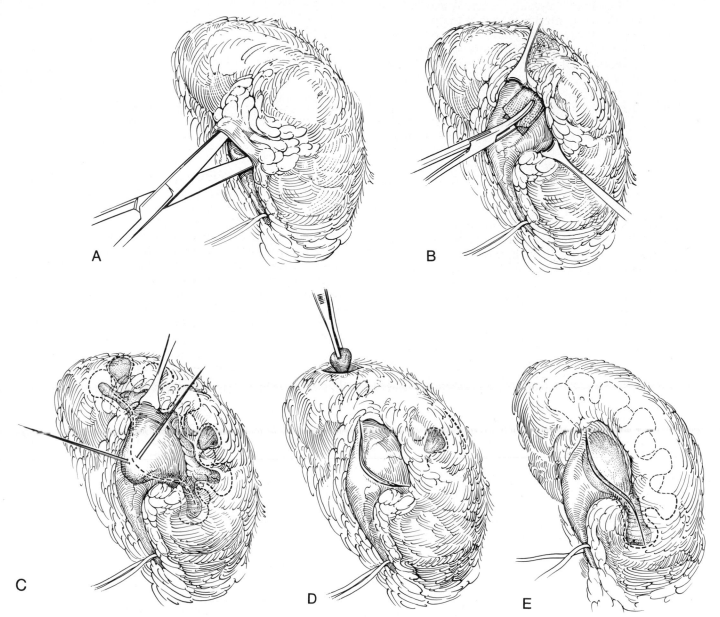

Figure 65–64. *A,* For an extended pyelolithotomy, exposure of the renal pelvis is accomplished initially by dissection into the renal sinus. The correct plane is between the renal pelvis and peripelvic fat.

B, Gil-Vernet or renal vein retractors elevate the posterior parenchymal lip, while dissection into the sinus is continued with a moist gauze.

C, Stay sutures are placed. A curvilinear pyelotomy is performed and extended through the upper and lower infundibula, creating a renal pelvic flap. The stone is then delivered.

D, Dumbbell-shaped calyceal extensions of the stone in the superior pole or midportion of the kidney may be removed with a local nephrotomy made directly over the stone.

E, For lower pole infundibulocalyceal extensions, however, the lower pole indundibulotomy may be extended through the parenchyma itself as an infundibulonephrotomy. This area of the parenchyma is in an avascular plane between the junction of the posterior and basilar arterial segments of the kidney.

removed with Randall's forceps after gentle dilation of the infundibulopelvic junction. However, removal of dumbbell-shaped calyceal extensions near the midportion or superior pole of the kidney may require a local nephrotomy made directly over the stone (Fig. 65–64D). Lower pole infundibulocalyceal extensions may be managed by extending the inferior aspect of the pyeloinfundibulotomy into the posterior parenchyma itself, directly over the lower infundibulum. This infundibulonephrotomy is thus performed in an avascular plane between the junction of the posterior and basilar segments of the kidney (Fig. 65–64E).

When all stone material has been removed, a small catheter is passed antegrade down the ureter and the intrarenal collecting system is thoroughly irrigated. If multiple stones had been present, an intraoperative radiograph should be taken to exclude residual fragments. Flexible nephroscopy may be a valuable adjunctive maneuver at this time.

Nephrostomy tube drainage is rarely indicated. If the dissection was extensive, an internal stent may be left in place. The pyelotomy incision is closed as described for a standard pyelotomy, with external drainage routinely provided by a Penrose or closed-suction drain.

Coagulum Pyelolithotomy

Coagulum pyelolithotomy was first reported by Dees in 1943 who utilized human fibrinogen and clotting globulin to form an extractable cast of the upper collecting system. Since that time, several investigators have reported modifications of the coagulum "recipe" in attempts to both simplify the procedure and to reduce the risk of complications (Kalash et al., 1983; Watson et al., 1984). The technique favored at our institution is that described by Fischer, Sonda, and Diokno in 1980 (Table 65–1). This protocol utilizes cryoprecipitate as the source of fibrinogen, which is converted to fibrin, with thrombin acting as the catalyst. Calcium chloride increases the tensile strength of the coagulum by neutralizing the citrate (an anticoagulant) present in the cryoprecipitate and acts as a co-factor in the conversion of prothrombin to thrombin. In elective cases, autogenous cryoprecipitate can be utilized to eliminate entirely the risk of any viral disease transmission (McVary and O'Conor, 1989).

Classically, the indication for coagulum pyelolithotomy is the presence of multiple stones scattered throughout the collecting system. Stones located in calyces drained by relatively stenotic infundibula will not be extracted with this method because the dumbbell-shaped calyceal extensions of the coagulum will simply break off as the pelvic portion is removed. However, any residual coagulum left this way is of no consequence as it will dissolve within 24 to 48 hours in response to the normally present urokinase.

As is true for all stone procedures described in this section, almost any patient who would have been a candidate for a coagulum pyelolithotomy may now be managed with percutaneous or extracorporeal shock wave technology, either alone or in combination. Cur-

rently, coagulum pyelolithotomy is reserved for patients who fail those techniques or for whom they are contraindicated. Coagulum pyelolithotomy may be indicated as a primary procedure if there is a co-existent anatomic abnormality requiring open operative reconstruction.

The renal pelvis is exposed in the manner described for a standard or extended pyelolithotomy. An occluding vessel loop is placed around the proximal ureter to prevent subsequent distal migration of stone fragments or the coagulum itself. The capacity of the pelviocalyceal system is now estimated by puncturing and draining the renal pelvis with a 14-gauge angiocatheter. The pelvis is refilled to capacity, with a measured amount of saline. The volume of coagulum to be prepared is based on the amount of saline required to gently distend the renal pelvis.

The appropriate amount of cryoprecipitate is drawn up in one large syringe with requisite volumes of thrombin and calcium chloride combined together in a second syringe (Table 65–2). This formulation is based on a ratio of 1 ml cryoprecipitate to 2 units of thrombin to 1 mg calcium chloride.

The angiocatheter, which has been left in place in the renal pelvis, is used to again completely drain the

Table 65–1. PREPARATION OF CONSTITUENTS FOR A COAGULUM PYELOLITHOTOMY

A. Calcium chloride: 1 g/10 ml (Upjohn ampule = 100 mg/ml)
  1. Aspirate contents into a sterile 10-ml syringe and warm to room temperature.
  2. Draw required volume directly into a sterile tuberculin syringe: 0.25 ml = 25 mg of calcium chloride.
B. Topical bovine thrombin: 5000 U/vial (Parke-Davis) plus 5 ml of standard diluent = 1000 U/ml.
  1. Using a sterile 10 ml syringe, draw up 1 ml of thrombin and 9 ml of saline (= 100 U/ml).
C. Cryoprecipitate: Arrives from the blood bank and is thawed to room temperature.
  1. Draw required volume into a sterile syringe.

From Fischer, C. P., Sonda, L. P., III, and Diokno, A. C.: Urology, 15:6, 1980.

Table 65–2. CONSTITUENTS USED IN COAGULUM PYELOLITHOTOMY RELATED TO MEASURED VOLUME OF RENAL COLLECTING SYSTEM

Measured Capacity of Renal Pelvis (ml)	Volume of Cryoprecipitate (ml)*	Calcium Chloride (100 mg/ml)	Thrombin (100 U/ml)
10	9	9 (0.10 ml)	18 (0.20 ml)
15	14	14 (0.15 ml)	28 (0.30 ml)
20	19	19 (0.20 ml)	38 (0.40 ml)
25	24	24 (0.25 ml)	48 (0.50 ml)
30	28	28 (0.30 ml)	56 (0.55 ml)
35	33	33 (0.35 ml)	66 (0.65 ml)
40	38	38 (0.40 ml)	76 (0.75 ml)
45	43	43 (0.45 ml)	86 (0.85 ml)
50	48	48 (0.50 ml)	96 (1.00 ml)

(qs with saline to make 1, 2, or 3 ml)

*Ratio of 1 ml cryoprecipitate to 2 U thrombin to 1 mg calcium chloride is maintained regardless of the volume required to fill the collecting system. qs, sufficient quantity. (From Fischer, C. P., Sonda, L. P., III, and Diokno, A. C.: Urology, 15:6, 1980.)

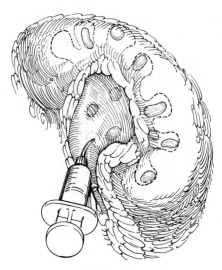

Figure 65–65. The mixture of thrombin, calcium chloride, and cryoprecipitate is injected via a large angiocatheter or red rubber catheter into the renal pelvis. The proximal ureter has been occluded with a vessel loop. The amount of coagulum to be injected has been predetermined as described in the text.

pelviocalyceal system. Additionally, the vessel loop around the proximal ureter can be temporarily loosened to allow complete drainage. This loop is then resecured prior to the injection of the coagulum.

The thrombin and calcium chloride are injected into the syringe with the cryoprecipitate. The mixture, which will clot within 45 seconds, is immediately introduced via the angiocatheter into the pelviocalyceal system (Fig. 65–65).

If the measured capacity was correct, there should be complete filling and gentle distention of the renal pelvis. Care must in fact be taken not to overdistend the collecting system, as this could result in pyelovenous backflow or, rarely, pulmonary embolus (Pence, 1981).

After 5 to 10 minutes, the coagulum is well established. A standard or extended pyelotomy incision is made, and the coagulum is extracted (Fig. 65–66). When performed correctly, the coagulum has formed a cast of the collecting system, with multiple stones trapped within its substance (Fig. 65–67).

Intraoperative radiographs and nephroscopy are performed as necessary to exclude the possibility of residual calculi. If internal stents are placed, they are placed antegrade at this time. The renal pelvis is then closed as previously described. External drainage is routinely provided with a Penrose or closed-suction drain.

Calyceal Diverticulolithotomy

Calyceal diverticula are cavities in the renal parenchyma lined by transitional epithelium. Although communication with a calyx is implied by definition, the communication may not be demonstrable at the time of patient presentation. Failure to demonstrate the area of communication may be the result of localized obstruction from edema or true stricture formation, secondary to chronic inflammation or infection. Because calyceal diverticula are associated with localized urinary stasis, they may be a source of stone formation.

As for any upper tract stone, indications to intervene for calculi in calyceal diverticula include pain, obstruction, or infection associated with it. In properly selected patients, stones in calyceal diverticula can be treated successfully with extracorporeal shock wave lithotripsy (Psihramis and Dretler, 1987). The best candidates for that procedure are those in whom the stone is relatively small and in whom a patent calyceal communication can be demonstrated, by filling of the diverticulum with contrast material by either intravenous or retrograde pyelography. Extracorporeal shock wave lithotripsy remains a controversial treatment for stones in calyceal

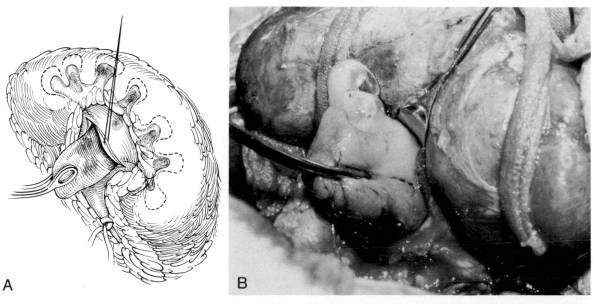

A   **B**

Figure 65–66. A, A standard or extended pyelotomy incision is performed and the coagulum extracted. B, Intraoperative view of the coagulum being extracted through a pyelotomy incision.

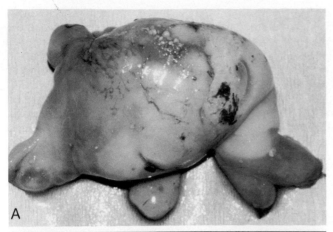

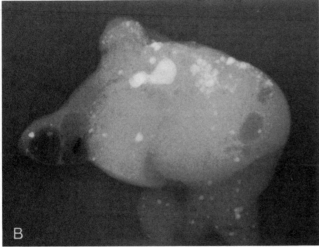

Figure 65–67. *A,* The extracted coagulum forms a cast of the collecting system. Multiple small calculi can be seen near the surface of the coagulum. *B,* A radiograph of the coagulum reveals multiple larger stones trapped within its substance.

diverticula because the source of the stone persists, even when the stone itself has been resolved.

Alternatively, a percutaneous approach may be utilized. Although this is more invasive than extracorporeal shock wave lithotripsy, it does allow the primary problem to be addressed directly with dilatation or with fulguration and obliteration of the diverticular neck (Hulbert et al., 1986). A transureteropyeloscopic approach has also been reported, although experience with the approach has been limited (Clayman, 1989).

Currently, indications for open diverticulolithotomy are still changing. Clearly, failures of, or contraindications to, both extracorporeal shock wave lithotripsy and percutaneous techniques would dictate an open approach. However, open surgery may still be recommended as a primary procedure when the anatomy dictates. In order to determine the feasibility of a percutaneous or open surgical approach, three-dimensional radiographic localization of the diverticulum is required. Oblique and lateral films obtained during intravenous or retrograde pyelography will be helpful and should be a routine part of the evaluation. However, more precise localization will be available through the use of CT scanning (Fig. 65–68*A* to *C*).

Exposure of the kidney is accomplished through a standard flank incision, generally with resection of a lower rib. Upon entering Gerota's fascia, the diverticulum will usually be evident by palpation of a soft or fluctuant area in the parenchyma or by inspection alone (Fig. 65–68*D*). If not, intraoperative radiographs with organ films and needle localization, or intraoperative ultrasonography will be valuable. In all cases, confirmation that a suspicious area represents the diverticulum can be accomplished with a small gauge needle, either by aspiration of urine or by "sounding" of the calculus.

In most cases, the diverticulum may be managed with marsupialization, similar to that performed for a simple renal cyst. To accomplish this effect, the thinned parenchyma overlying the diverticulum is excised and the calculi removed (Fig. 65–68*E*). The diverticular neck should be identified. If this is difficult, injection of methylene blue either intravenously or retrograde via a ureteral catheter placed at the outset of the procedure may prove useful. The neck is then oversewn with absorbable suture, as is the rim of remaining parenchyma (Fig. 65–68*F*). Alternatively, the urothelial lining of the diverticulum may be excised, although this can be associated with bleeding that is difficult to control. Another alternative is simple fulguration of the entire lining and diverticular neck.

A Penrose or closed-suction drain is placed, and the wound irrigated and closed in standard fashion.

Partial Nephrectomy

Percutaneous and extracorporeal shock wave technology have virtually eliminated the role of partial nephrectomy for removal of otherwise uncomplicated infundibular or calyceal calculi. Furthermore, as reviewed by Roth and Findlayson in 1983, partial nephrectomy is no longer accepted as a reliable method of preventing stone recurrences. Currently, partial nephrectomy is considered only when less invasive techniques fail or are contraindicated. In such a case, if the stone is associated with a localized area of irrecoverable renal function, as may occur with chronic obstruction or infection, removal of the diseased portion of the kidney along with the stone may be the best option (Fig. 65–69). In these cases, partial nephrectomy is performed as described previously in this chapter.

Nephrectomy

Nephrectomy is indicated only rarely for management of renal calculi. However, it does have a role in well-defined cases. Specifically, if the stone is associated with a nonfunctioning or poorly functioning kidney that is unlikely to recover adequate function with removal of the stone alone, nephrectomy may be the best option. This possibility is especially true for older patients with significant concomitant medical problems in whom the contralateral kidney is normal. Obviously, however, if overall renal function would be significantly compromised by nephrectomy, every attempt should be made to salvage the kidney instead.

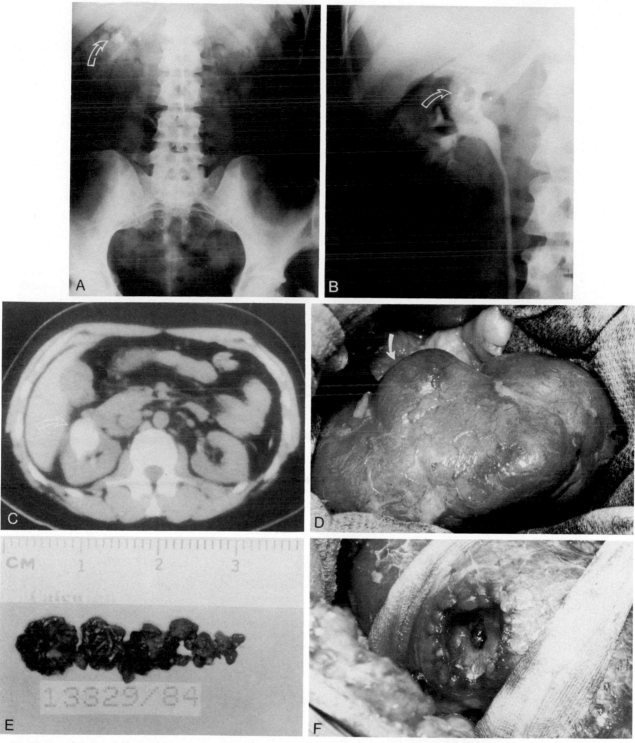

Figure 65–68. *A* and *B*, Scout film and intravenous urogram reveal a cluster of calculi in the mid portion of the right kidney *(arrows)*.

C, Computed tomography (CT) scan in this same patient 1 day following the urogram clearly reveals contrast material remaining in the area surrounding the stones, consistent with a partially obstructed calyceal diverticulum *(arrow)*. The anatomic location of this diverticulum in the anterior midportion of the kidney is well visualized on the CT scan.

D, Intraoperative view of the same patient reveals the calyceal diverticulum bulging from the anterior midportion of the kidney *(arrow)*.

E, Following diverticulotomy, multiple "jackstone" calculi were removed. The configuration of these stones is consistent with urinary stasis as the etiology.

F, The diverticular cavity is marsupialized. In this intraoperative view, the neck is evident at the base of the diverticulum. The diverticular neck is then oversewn or fulgurated.

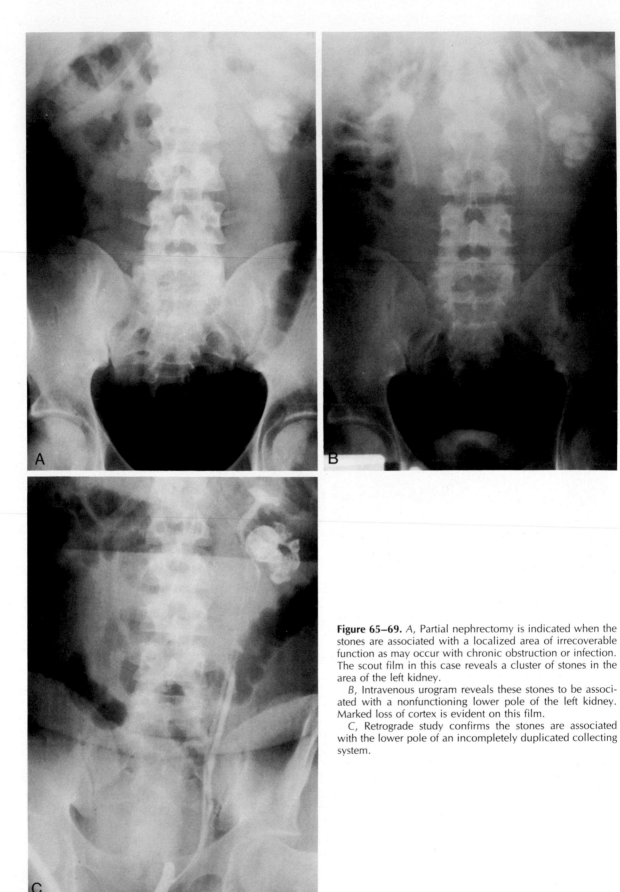

Figure 65–69. *A,* Partial nephrectomy is indicated when the stones are associated with a localized area of irrecoverable function as may occur with chronic obstruction or infection. The scout film in this case reveals a cluster of stones in the area of the left kidney.

B, Intravenous urogram reveals these stones to be associated with a nonfunctioning lower pole of the left kidney. Marked loss of cortex is evident on this film.

C, Retrograde study confirms the stones are associated with the lower pole of an incompletely duplicated collecting system.

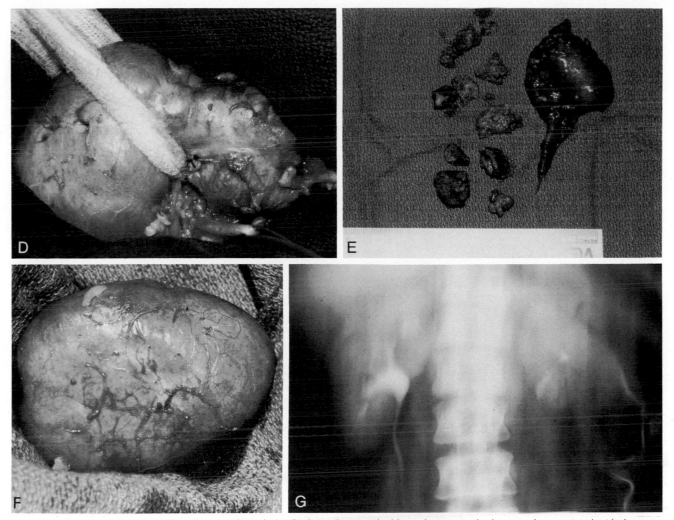

Figure 65–69 *Continued D,* Left renal exploration through the flank confirms marked loss of cortex in the lower pole associated with the stones.
E, Excised lower pole and stones.
F, Intraoperative view of remaining, well-functioning upper pole.
G, Early postoperative study reveals excellent function in the remaining upper pole on the left side.

Salvageability of the kidney is determined preoperatively with a complete radiographic evaluation. The possibility that irrecoverable loss of renal function has occurred is generally suggested first when an intravenous pyelogram reveals nonvisualization of the involved kidney, even on delayed films (Fig. 65–70 *A*). In such cases, neither a pyelogram nor a nephrogram phase is perceived. A CT scan should then be performed to determine the degree of parenchymal atrophy, as significant cortical thinning is also consistent with irrecoverable loss of function from obstruction (Fig. 65–70*B*). A technetium 99-DTPA scan may also be helpful, as it can estimate differential renal function (Fig. 65–70*C*). With a normally functioning contralateral kidney, nephrectomy will be considered a primary option when the scan reveals that less than 10 per cent of overall function is being contributed by the involved kidney (Fig. 65–70*D*).

When there remains any question as to recoverability of function, especially in the presence of obstruction, placement of a percutaneous nephrostomy may provide valuable information. Following the relief of obstruction and the treatment of any associated infection, differen-

tial creatinine clearances may be attained and nuclear scans repeated.

Once the decision for nephrectomy is made, it is performed as described previously in this chapter. Generally, a flank incision is used, although an anterior approach may be preferred in the presence of previous flank surgery.

Complications

Bleeding into the collecting system or the perinephric space generally resolves spontaneously. As such, conservative supportive measures should be the primary treatment. When intervention is required, selective or superselective transcatheter embolization is the treatment of choice. Surgical exploration is reserved only for refractory cases, because it generally results in partial or complete nephrectomy (Assimos et al., 1986).

Persistent fistulas are uncommon and generally imply a devascularized renal segment or distal obstruction. Conservatism is the rule as most fistulas resolve, as long

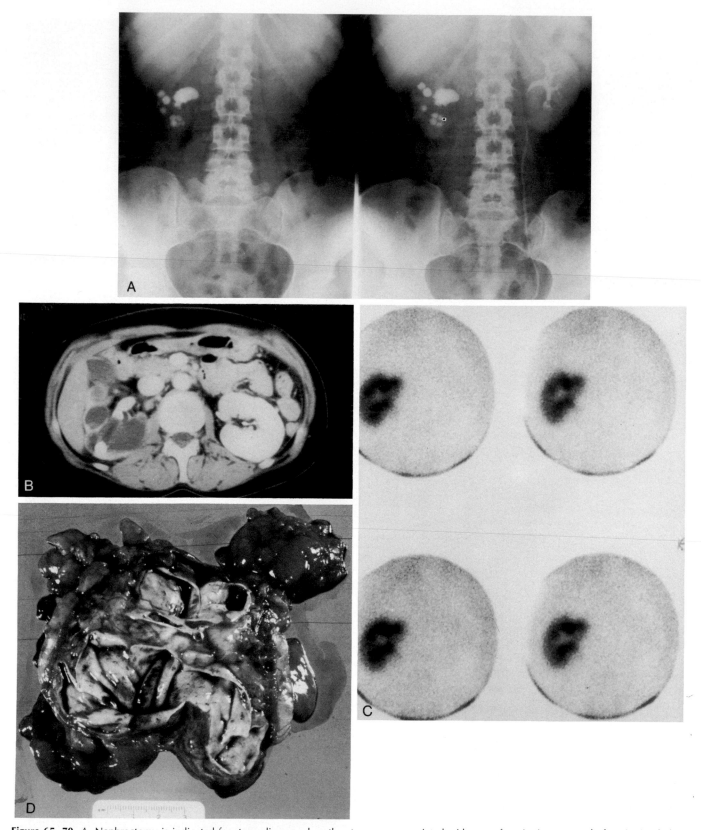

Figure 65–70. *A*, Nephrectomy is indicated for stone disease when the stones are associated with a nonfunctioning or poorly functioning kidney that is unlikely to recover with removal of the stone alone. The contralateral kidney should be normal, otherwise every attempt should be made to salvage the kidney. The scout film in this case reveals multiple right renal calculi. With contrast material injection, there is no discernible uptake in the right kidney. The left kidney appears normal.

B, A computed tomography scan performed with contrast material again reveals the left kidney to be normal. On the right, however, there is only a thin shell of parenchyma. Stones are evident in the renal pelvis and in one of the markedly dilated calyces in this view.

C, A technetium 99-DTPA scan reveals nonfunction of the right kidney. All these studies together suggest clearly that this is a nonsalvageable right kidney.

D, Gross appearance of the right kidney following nephrectomy reveals marked cortical loss and parenchymal thinning confirming that this was a nonsalvageable kidney.

as they are properly drained. If urinary leakage persists after 10 to 14 days, further investigation is indicated. Intravenous or retrograde pyelography are utilized to define the area of extravasation and to rule out distal obstruction. If obstruction is found distal to the level of the fistula, passage of an internal stent will generally allow rapid resolution of the problem.

Retained calculi is a discouraging complication that occurs in up to 20 per cent of patients. Stones associated with obstruction, pain, or chronic infection or active stone growth require further intervention. Currently, all residual calculi may be managed with percutaneous techniques or extracorporeal shock wave lithotripsy. Whenever possible, such treatment should be delayed for at least 4 to 6 weeks following the initial operative intervention.

URETEROPELVIC JUNCTION OBSTRUCTION

The diagnosis of ureteropelvic junction obstruction implies functionally significant impairment of urinary transport from the renal pelvis to the ureter. Although most cases are probably congenital in origin, the problem may not become clinically apparent until much later in life (Jacobs et al., 1979). Patients with acquired conditions, such as stone disease, postoperative or inflammatory stricture, or urothelial neoplasms, may also present clinically with symptoms and signs of obstruction at the level of the ureteropelvic junction. This section of the chapter is limited primarily to a discussion of the diagnosis and treatment of "congenital" ureteropelvic junction obstructions, although at times the treatment may be applied appropriately to the management of some acquired conditions.

Pathogenesis

Congenital ureteropelvic junction obstruction most often results from intrinsic disease. A frequently found defect is the presence of an aperistaltic segment of the ureter, perhaps similar to that found in primary obstructive megaloureter. Histopathologic studies reveal that the normal spiral musculature has been replaced by an abnormal longitudinal muscle bundle or fibrous tissue (Allen, 1970; Foote et al., 1970; Gosling and Dixon, 1978; Hanna et al., 1976). This results in failure to develop a normal peristaltic wave for propagation of urine from the renal pelvis to the ureter. Recognition that this type of segmental defect is often responsible for ureteropelvic junction obstruction is of utmost importance clinically, as such ureters may appear grossly normal at the time of surgery and in fact may often be calibrated to 14 Fr. or greater. A less frequent intrinsic cause of congenital ureteropelvic junction obstruction is true ureteral stricture. Such congenital ureteral strictures are most frequently found at the ureteropelvic junction, although they may be located at multiple sites anywhere along the lumbar ureter. Abnormalities of ureteral musculature are again implicated as electron microscopy has

demonstrated excessive collagen deposition at the site of the stricture (Hanna et al., 1976).

Intrinsic obstruction at the ureteropelvic junction may also result from kinks or valves produced by infoldings of the ureteral mucosa and musculature (Maizels and Stephens, 1980). In these cases, the obstruction may actually be at the level of the most proximal ureter. This phenomenon appears to result from retention or exaggeration of congenital folds normally found in the ureter of developing fetuses. In some of these cases, the defects are bridged by ureteral adventitia. Grossly, this occurrence can appear as external bands or adhesions that seem to be causing the obstruction. In fact, Johnson, in 1977, reported that lysis of external adhesions can at times re-establish nonobstructed flow without formal pyeloplasty. In the majority of cases, however, these bands or adhesions are likely to be a secondary phenomenon associated with intrinsic obstruction, so that formal pyeloplasty would generally be warranted. The presence of these kinks, valves, bands, or adhesions may also produce angulation of the ureter at the lower margin of the renal pelvis in such a manner that as the pelvis dilates anteriorly and inferiorly, the ureteral insertion is carried further proximally. In these cases, the most dependent portion of the pelvis is inadequately drained and the apparent "high insertion" of the ureteral ostium is actually a secondary phenomenon (Kelalis, 1973). In at least some cases, the high insertion itself is likely the primary obstructing lesion because this phenomenon is found more frequently in the presence of renal ectopia or fusion anomalies (Das and Amar, 1984; Zincke et al., 1974).

Controversy persists regarding the potential role of "aberrant" vessels in the etiology of ureteropelvic junction obstruction. Arteries entering directly into the lower pole of the kidney have been noted in up to one third of cases of ureteropelvic junction obstruction, which represents an incidence higher than that of the normal population. In this clinical setting, these lower pole vessels have often been referred to as aberrant. However, these segmental vessels, which may be branches from the main renal artery or may arise directly from the aorta, are in fact usually normal variants (Stephens, 1982). In a minority of patients, these lower pole vessels cross the ureter posteriorly and as such truly have an aberrant course. In any case, as reviewed by Hanna in 1978, it is unlikely that the associated vessel is causing the primary obstruction. Rather, there is probably an intrinsic lesion at the ureteropelvic junction or proximal ureter that causes dilatation and ballooning of the renal pelvis over the polar vessel.

As previously mentioned, ureteropelvic junction obstruction may also result from acquired lesions. In children, vesicoureteral reflux can lead to upper tract dilation with subsequent elongation, tortuosity, and kinking of the ureter. In some cases, these changes may only mimic the radiographic findings of true ureteropelvic junction obstruction. However, true ureteropelvic junction obstruction may definitely co-exist with vesicoureteral reflux, although it may be difficult to determine whether the anomalies are merely coincident or whether the upper tract ureteral obstruction has resulted from the reflux (Lebowitz and Johan, 1982). Other acquired causes of obstruction at the ureteropelvic junction include benign tumors such as fibroepithelial polyps (Berger et al., 1982; Macksood et al., 1985), urothelial malignancy, stone disease, and postinflammatory or postoperative scarring or ischemia. For these acquired diseases, the surgical techniques discussed in this section may be useful adjuncts for management of the obstruction as long as the primary problem is also appropriately addressed.

Patient Presentation and Diagnostic Studies

Ureteropelvic junction obstruction, although generally the result of a congenital problem, can occur at anytime, from prenatally to geriatrically. Classically, the most common presentation in neonates and infants was the finding of a palpable flank mass. However, the current widespread use of maternal ultrasonography has led to a dramatic increase in the number of asymptomatic newborns being diagnosed with hydronephrosis, many of whom are subsequently found to have ureteropelvic junction obstruction (Bernstein et al., 1988; Wolpert et al., 1989). A relatively small number of cases may also be found during evaluation of azotemia, which may result from bilateral obstruction or obstruction in a functionally or anatomically solitary kidney. Ureteropelvic junction obstruction may also be incidentally found during contrast studies performed to evaluate unrelated anomalies, such as congenital heart disease (Roth and Gonzales, 1983). In older children or adults, intermittent abdominal or flank pain, at times associated with nausea or vomiting, is a frequent presenting symptom. Hematuria, either spontaneous or associated with otherwise relatively minor trauma, may also be an initial symptom. Laboratory findings of microhematuria, pyuria, or frank urinary tract infection might also bring an otherwise asymptomatic patient to the attention of a urologist. Rarely, hypertension may be a presenting finding (Riehle and Vaughan, 1981).

Radiographic studies should be performed with the goal of determining both the anatomic site and the functional significance of an apparent obstruction. Excretory urography remains a cornerstone of radiographic diagnosis. Classically, findings on the affected side include delay in function associated with a dilated pelviocalyceal system (Fig. 65–71). If the ureter is visualized, it should be of normal caliber. In some patients, symptoms may be intermittent. Intravenous pyelography between painful episodes may be normal. In such a case, the study should be repeated during an acute episode when the patient is symptomatic (Nesbit, 1956). Alternatively, provocative testing with a diuretic urogram may allow an accurate diagnosis. The patient should be well hydrated, and the study performed by injecting intravenous furosemide, 0.3 to 0.5 mg/kg, at the time of intravenous urography (Fig. 65–72) (Malek, 1983).

Ultrasonography has also maintained an important role in diagnosis. Obviously, it is a valuable initial diagnostic study under any circumstance in which overall

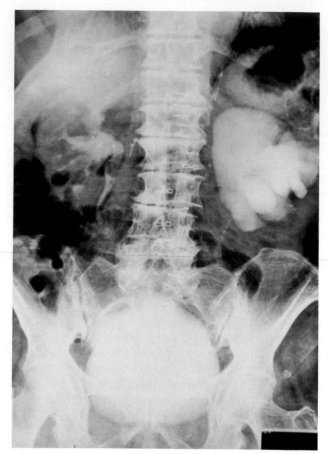

Figure 65–71. Intravenous urogram in this older patient with left flank pain reveals marked hydronephrosis on the left to the level of the ureteropelvic junction consistent with ureteropelvic junction obstruction.

renal function is inadequate to perform intravenous urography. It should also be performed in any patient in whom the initial intravenous urogram revealed nonvisualization of the affected collecting system in order to differentiate obstruction from other causes of nonfunction. In some patients, CT scanning may be performed in addition to or in place of ultrasonography. In general, the information obtained will be similar. Both ultrasonography and CT scanning also have a role in differentiating potential acquired causes of obstruction, such as radiolucent calculi or urothelial tumors.

In neonates and infants, the diagnosis of ureteropelvic junction obstruction has generally been suggested either by routine performance of maternal ultrasonography or by the finding of a flank mass. In either clinical setting, renal ultrasonography will usually be the first radiographic study performed. Ideally, ultrasonography should visualize dilatation of the collecting system, help differentiate ureteropelvic junction obstruction from multicystic kidney, and help determine the level of obstruction. Ureteropelvic junction obstruction and multicystic kidneys should in fact be distinguishable in the majority of cases by ultrasound alone. With ureteropelvic junction obstruction, the pelvis is seen as a large, medial, sonolucent area surrounded by smaller, rounded sonolucent structures representing dilated calyces. At

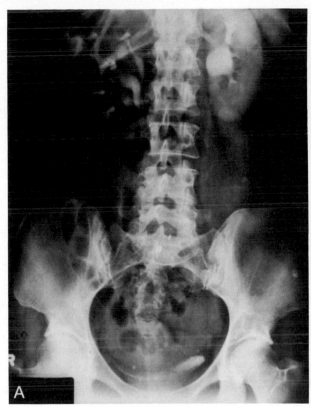

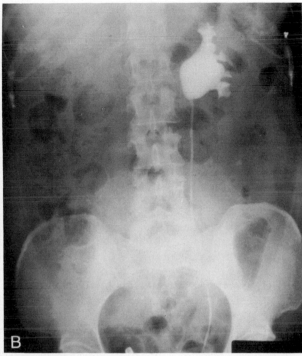

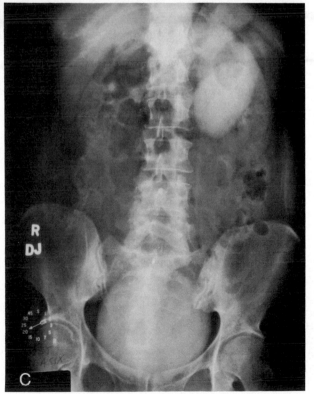

Figure 65–72. *A*, This patient with intermittent left flank pain underwent intravenous urography. The calyces are sharp bilaterally without evidence of obstruction. However, there is a box-shaped pelvis on the left side, which may be associated with intermittent obstruction.

B, Retrograde study confirms sharp calyces, although the presence of an extrarenal, boxed-shaped pelvis is still evident.

C, In the same patient, the intravenous urogram was performed along with injection of intravenous furosemide, which brought out the obvious left-sided ureteropelvic junction obstruction. The patient's symptoms were subsequently relieved with a left pyeloplasty.

times, dilated calyces are seen connecting to the pelvis via dilated infundibula. Occasionally, a solid-appearing renal cortex can be seen surrounding the sonolucent areas or separating the dilated calyces. In contrast, the cysts of multicystic kidneys are visualized as varying sized sonolucent areas in random distribution. Although the cysts may be connected, this is rarely noted sonographically. Furthermore, little solid tissue is seen and that which is present has a random distribution among the cysts.

Rarely, a large centrally located cyst may cause confusion in the diagnosis (King et al., 1984). In this setting, nuclear renography should be performed. Specifically, a technetium 99-DTPA scan allows differentiation of these two entities. Multicystic kidneys rarely reveal concentration of this isotope. When uptake is observed, the areas of functioning tissue are discreet initially and are usually medial to the bulk of the mass, which itself remains a "cold" area. In contrast, neonatal kidneys with ureteropelvic junction obstructions generally exhibit good concentration of the isotope. Furthermore, even with severe obstruction in which only a cortical rim remains, uptake of the isotope is seen peripherally in the cortex, helping to differentiate this condition from multicystic kidney (King et al., 1984). A nuclear scan is also of value in predicting recoverability of function in the cases in which intravenous urography provided nonvisualization. In this clinical setting, a technetium 99-DTPA scan can help predict recoverability of function as essentially all kidneys that function on such scans will improve following relief of obstruction (King et al., 1983). A technetium 99-DTPA scan will also be of value in differentiating dilated, nonobstructed systems from those with functional obstruction by combining the renogram with injection of furosemide, 0.5 mg/kg, to obtain a "diuretic renogram." This study will allow quantification of the degree of obstruction and, if standard studies are equivocal, help differentiate the level of obstruction (Fig. 65–73) (Koff et al., 1979, 1980; O'Reilly, 1978, 1986).

The diagnosis of ureteropelvic junction obstruction can generally be made with a high degree of certainty based on the clinical presentation and the results of any one or more of the relatively noninvasive studies just discussed here. However, retrograde pyelography remains the procedure of choice for confirmation of the diagnosis and demonstration of the exact site and nature of obstruction prior to surgical repair. In most cases, this study is performed at the time of planned operative intervention in order to avoid the risk of introducing infection in the presence of obstruction. However, retrograde pyelography is indicated emergently when ureteropelvic junction obstruction requires acute decompression, such as in cases of infection or compromised renal function. In such cases, an attempt can be made to pass a floppy-tipped guide wire followed by an open-ended ureteral catheter or internal stent to allow decompression of the system and thus better prepare the patient for reconstruction at a later date.

In cases in which cystoscopic retrograde manipulation has been unsuccessful or may be hazardous, such as in male neonates or infants, placement of a percutaneous nephrostomy is an excellent alternative. This method allows the performance of antegrade studies, which will help define the nature and exact anatomic site of obstruction. The nephrostomy also allows decompression of the system in cases of associated infection or compromised renal function and allows assessment of recoverability of renal function following decompression. If some doubt remains as to the clinical significance of a dilated collecting system, placement of percutaneous nephrostomy allows access for pressure perfusion studies. As described and later modified by Whitaker in 1973 and 1978, the renal pelvis is perfused at 10 ml/minute with normal saline. Alternatively, a dilute radiographic contrast material solution may be used and the procedure performed under fluoroscopic control. Renal pelvic pressure is monitored during the infusion, and the pressure gradient across the presumed area of obstruction is determined. During the infusion, the bladder is continuously drained with an indwelling catheter to prevent transmission of intravesical pressures. Renal pelvic pressure ranging up to 12 to 15 cm H_2O during this infusion suggests a nonobstructed system. In contrast, pressure in excess of 15 to 22 cm H_2O is highly suggestive of a functional obstruction. Pressures between these extremes may be nondiagnostic (O'Reilly, 1986).

Although pressure perfusion studies can often provide valuable information on the functional significance of an apparent obstruction, these studies, like any other test currently available for assessing obstruction, can at times be inaccurate because of the variation in renal pelvic anatomy and compliance (Koff et al., 1986). As such, there remains an important role for the urologist as a diagnostician to collate the results of the clinical presentation and the multitude of diagnostic studies in order to appropriately prescribe the timing and nature of subsequent intervention.

Indications and Options For Intervention

Indications for intervention include the presence of symptoms from the obstruction, impairment of renal function, or development of stones or infection. In such cases, the primary goal of intervention is relief of symptoms and preservation or improvement of renal function. In general, such intervention should be a reconstructive procedure aimed at restoring nonobstructed urinary flow. This goal is especially true for neonates, infants, or children in whom early repair is desirable, as these patients will have the best chance for improvement in renal function following relief of obstruction (Bejjani and Belman, 1982; Roth and Gonzales, 1983; Wolpert et al., 1989). Obviously, for any age patient, a reconstructive procedure is always indicated whenever overall renal function is comprised because of involvement in a solitary kidney or bilateral disease (Kumar et al., 1988).

Ureteropelvic junction obstruction may not become apparent until middle age or later (Jacobs et al., 1979). Occasionally, if the patient is asymptomatic and the physiologic significance of the obstruction seems inde-

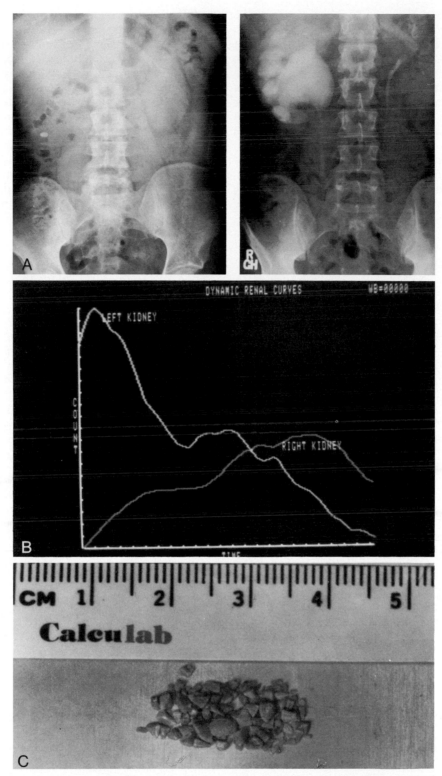

Figure 65–73. *A,* A diuretic renogram can help differentiate dilatation of the collecting system from functional obstruction. This patient had undergone a pyeloplasty as a child several years earlier. The scout film now reveals a 1-cm ovoid calcification in the area of the right lower pole. Following contrast material injection, there is obvious dilatation of the collecting system with a normal caliber ureter. Differentiation of residual dilatation from ongoing obstruction is of utmost importance in this case before recommending definitive treatment.

B, A diuretic renogram reveals a shift to the right in uptake by the right kidney, followed by a rapid fall-off of the radionucleide after injection of furosemide. This occurrence is consistent with dilatation without obstruction.

C, The patient was subsequently treated with extracorporeal shock wave lithotripsy. The multiple fragments passed without difficulty. At 1 month follow-up, the patient was symptom-free and stone-free. The ease with which this patient passed these fragments supports the diagnosis of residual dilatation without obstruction.

terminate, careful observation with serial follow-up studies may be appropriate. However, the majority of affected patients can in fact benefit from reconstructive intervention (Clark and Malek, 1987; Jacobs et al., 1979; O'Reilly, 1989).

When intervention is indicated, the procedure of choice is generally an "open" repair of the ureteropelvic junction, that is, a pyeloplasty. Percutaneous procedures ("endopyelotomies") may also have a role, although long-term follow-up is still unknown. Rarely, nephrectomy may be the procedure of choice. Indications for this ablative approach as primary therapy include nonfunction of the involved renal unit on both radiographic and radionuclide studies. In such cases, ultrasonography or CT scanning should also be performed and should reveal only a thin shell of remaining parenchyma. If the potential for salvage of function is still unclear, an internal stent or percutaneous nephrostomy may be placed for the temporary relief of obstruction and the renal function studies subsequently repeated.

Nephrectomy may also be considered for a patient in whom the obstruction has led to extensive stone disease with chronic infection and significant loss of function in the presence of a normal contralateral kidney (Fig. 65–74). Removal of the kidney may also be chosen over reconstruction for patients in whom repeated attempts at repair have already failed and in whom further intervention would therefore be extremely complicated.

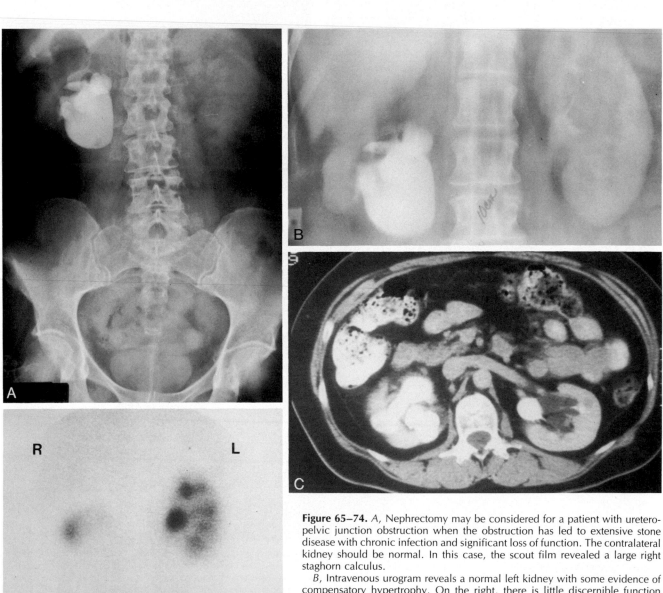

Figure 65–74. *A,* Nephrectomy may be considered for a patient with ureteropelvic junction obstruction when the obstruction has led to extensive stone disease with chronic infection and significant loss of function. The contralateral kidney should be normal. In this case, the scout film revealed a large right staghorn calculus.

B, Intravenous urogram reveals a normal left kidney with some evidence of compensatory hypertrophy. On the right, there is little discernible function and marked parenchymal loss, especially in the midportion and upper pole.

C, Computed tomography scan in this patient confirms the marked parenchymal loss associated with the stones and obstruction on the right side.

D, Technetium 99-DTPA renogram was performed and revealed that less than 10 per cent of overall function was being contributed by the right kidney. The patient subsequently underwent simple right nephrectomy.

This option should be considered only when the contralateral kidney is normal. If the patient's life expectancy is limited either because of advanced age or significant associated medical problems, nephrectomy may be the best option, providing that the contralateral kidney is normal.

General Surgical Principles of Pyeloplasty

A variety of incisions have been described for performance of a pyeloplasty. An anterior extraperitoneal approach is preferred by some, as it allows an "in situ" repair with minimal mobilization of the pelvis and proximal ureter. An anterior transperitoneal approach may also be of value, especially in the presence of previous flank incisions or for repair of bilateral disease. Alternatively, a posterior lumbotomy offers direct exposure to the ureteropelvic junction and allows repair with minimal mobilization of surrounding tissue. Similar to the anterior extraperitoneal approach, this approach is best suited to relatively thin patients in whom there has been no previous ipsilateral surgery. Although a posterior lumbotomy is an attractive approach for an uncomplicated pyeloplasty, its use has been limited, at least in the United States. Our personal preference for most patients who are undergoing primary surgical repair is

an extraperitoneal flank approach. This may be subcostal, although in adults it usually is performed through the bed of the 12th rib or carried anteriorly of its tip. This incision is advantageous in that it is familiar to all urologists and provides excellent exposure without regard to body habitus. In the presence of other renal anomalies associated with the ureteropelvic junction, such as horseshoe or pelvic kidney, alternative incisions may be required as the ureter and pelvis will generally be oriented anteriorly. In such a case, an anterior extraperitoneal approach is preferable (Fig. 65–75).

Preoperative drainage of a kidney with ureteropelvic junction obstruction is recommended only in specific instances. These include infection associated with the obstruction or azotemia resulting from obstruction in a solitary kidney or bilateral disease. In either case, preliminary drainage will result in better healing with less risk of complications. Rarely, the patient will present with severe, unrelenting pain requiring emergent relief of obstruction, and preliminary drainage will be of value. For any of these problems, such drainage can be provided by passage of an internal stent or placement of a percutaneous nephrostomy.

The indications for placement of stents or nephrostomy tubes intraoperatively remain controversial and may be different in pediatric and adult practices. In the past, ureteral stents and nephrostomy tubes were utilized almost routinely in neonates and infants (Perlmutter

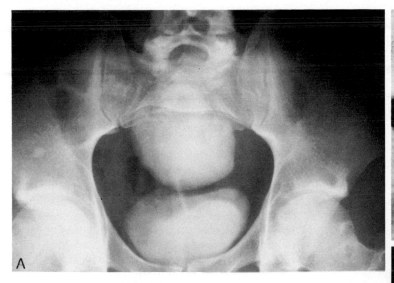
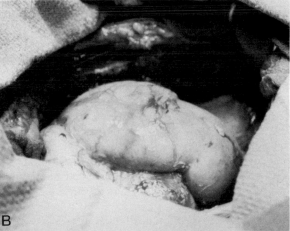
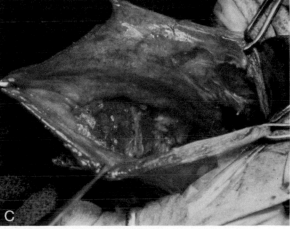

Figure 65–75. *A,* Intravenous urogram in this patient with lower abdominal pain revealed a hydronephrotic left pelvic kidney.

B, Exposure was obtained through an anterior extraperitoneal Gibson incision in the left lower quadrant.

C, This incision provided excellent exposure to the anteriorly located renal pelvis and proximal ureter. This intraoperative view shows the dilated renal pelvis after it has been opened in preparation for reduction pyeloplasty.

et al., 1980). Most pediatric urologists now believe, however, that routine use of stents and nephrostomy tubes is no longer indicated. Rather, such diversion is reserved for complicated cases such as those involving secondary repairs or active inflammation (Bejjani and Belman, 1982; King et al., 1984; Nguyen et al., 1989; Roth and Gonzales, 1983). For adults, however, our preference is for routine placement of a soft, inert, self-retaining internal stent that is removed 4 to 6 weeks postoperatively. In contrast to use in infants and children, such stents in adults are removed simply, in an outpatient setting without the need for general anesthesia and without the risk of urethral injury. Also, the adult-sized ureter accepts these stents without risk of local ischemia. Routine use of internal stents offers several advantages, especially in the early postoperative period. Most importantly, they appear to decrease the amount and length of time of urinary extravasation, thereby reducing the risk of secondary fibrosis. Less extravasation also allows earlier removal of external drains and generally shortens the length of hospital stay. Routine internal stents may also help prevent kinking of the ureter in the early postoperative period, which could lead to secondary obstruction.

For the uncomplicated pyeloplasty in adults, there appears to be no advantage to selecting both a nephrostomy and a stent as these may result in a prolonged hospital stay and higher incidence of infection (Wollin et al., 1989). Rather, nephrostomy tubes are reserved for complicated procedures, such as those required for secondary repairs or those associated with active inflammation. However, if a percutaneous nephrostomy had been placed preoperatively, it should generally remain indwelling to allow proximal diversion and access for antegrade radiographic studies during the postoperative period.

Although the use of internal stents and nephrostomy tubes remains somewhat controversial, provision of external drainage from the line of repair is mandatory. This practice prevents urinoma formation and its possible subsequent disruption of the suture line, scarring, or sepsis. Such external drainage is accomplished with a Penrose or closed-suction drain placed near but not on the suture line and brought out through a separate stab incision.

In the past, proximal diversion was often accomplished with a "slash pyelotomy," made transversely in the renal pelvis above the suture line (Schaeffer and Grayhack, 1986). Theoretically, this vented the suture line and allowed adequate drainage during the period of edema associated with the repair. This practice is now rarely utilized, however, as most reconstructive surgeons believe that the increased extravasation, although perhaps "controlled," leads to excessive fibrosis and scar formation.

Historical Notes

Historical aspects of ureteropelvic junction repair have been reviewed by Kay in 1989 and Schaeffer and Grayhack in 1986. The first reconstructive procedure was performed by Trendelenburg in 1886, although the patient died of postoperative complications. Kuster is credited with the first successful pyeloplasty. In 1891, he divided the ureter and re-anastomosed it to the renal pelvis, thus apparently performing the first dismembered pyeloplasty. His technique, however, was prone to recurrent stricture. In 1892, Fenger applied the Heineke-Mickulicz principle to reconstruction of the ureteropelvic junction. This technique involves transverse closure of a longitudinal incision. Unfortunately, for repair of ureteropelvic junction obstruction, this technique can cause shortening of the suture line on one side of the ureteropelvic junction, thus resulting in buckling or kinking with recurrent obstruction. Flap techniques were introduced by Schwyzer in 1923. His Y-V pyeloplasty was modified successfully by Foley in 1937. This procedure was best applied to high insertions and was essentially unsuitable when the ureteropelvic junction itself was already in a dependent position. Subsequently, flap techniques were developed that were more universally applicable. These included the spiral flap of Culp and DeWeerd in 1951, and the vertical flap of Scardino and Prince reported in 1953. Thompson and associates, in 1969, reported a renal capsular flap for complex cases in which an adequate amount of renal pelvis is not available for repair.

Nesbit, in 1949, modified Kuster's dismembered procedure by utilizing an elliptic anastomosis to decrease the likelihood of stricture formation at the site of repair. Also in 1949, Anderson and Hynes, two English surgeons, described their modification of this technique that involved anastomosis of the spatulated ureter to a projection of the lower aspect of the pelvis after a redundant portion was excised.

A separate issue has been the development of techniques for repair of extensive or multiple strictures of the proximal ureter. These techniques of intubated ureterotomy were popularized by Davis in 1943 but had been previously described by Fiori in 1905, Albarran in 1909, and Keyes in 1915.

Although a variety of procedures have been described for management of the obstructed ureteropelvic junction, several basic principles must always be applied in order to ensure successful repair. For any technique, the resultant anastomosis should be widely patent and performed in a watertight fashion without tension. The reconstructed ureteropelvic junction should allow a funnel-shaped transition between the pelvis and ureter, which is in a position of dependent drainage.

Dismembered Pyeloplasty

Currently, most urologists rely on a variation of a dismembered pyeloplasty for the majority of their patients, as this procedure is almost universally applicable for repair of the ureteropelvic junction. Specifically, it can be employed regardless of whether the ureteral insertion is high on the pelvis or dependent. The procedure also allows reduction of a redundant pelvis if necessary or straightening of a lengthy or tortuous proximal ureter. In addition, anterior or posterior transposition of the ureteropelvic junction can be accomplished when the obstruction is associated with accessory or aberrant lower pole vessels. In contrast to all flap techniques, only a dismembered pyeloplasty allows complete excision of the anatomically or functionally abnormal ureteropelvic junction. A dismembered pyeloplasty is, however, poorly suited to ureteropelvic junction obstruction associated with lengthy or multiple proximal ureteral strictures or to ureteropelvic junction obstruction associated with a small relatively inaccessible intrarenal pelvis.

Exposure to the ureteropelvic junction is obtained by first identifying the proximal ureter in the retroperitoneum. The ureter is dissected cephalad to the renal pelvis, leaving a large amount of periureteral tissue in order to preserve ureteral blood supply. A marking stitch of fine suture is then placed on the lateral aspect of the proximal ureter, below the level of the obstruction, in order to subsequently maintain proper orientation for the repair. In a similar fashion, the medial and lateral aspects of the dependent portion of the renal pelvis are delineated with traction sutures (Fig. 65–76A). The ureteropelvic junction is excised, and the proximal ureter is spatulated on its lateral aspect. The apex of this lateral, spatulated aspect of the ureter is brought to the inferior border of the pelvis, while the medial side of the ureter is brought to the superior edge of the pelvis (Fig. 65–76B). The anastomosis is performed with fine interrupted or running absorbable sutures, placed full thickness through the ureteral and renal pelvic walls, in a watertight fashion (Fig. 65–76C). As previously mentioned, our preference for adult patients is to routinely perform the anastomosis over an internal stent that remains indwelling. Alternatively, the anastomosis can be performed over a ureteral catheter, which is simply removed before the last few sutures are placed.

If the renal pelvis is particularly large or redundant, a "reduction" pyeloplasty is performed by excising the redundant portion of the pelvis (Fig. 65–77A). The cephalad aspect of the pelvis is closed with running absorbable sutures down to the dependent portion that will subsequently be joined to the ureter (Fig. 65–77B).

When aberrant or accessory lower pole vessels are found in association with the ureteropelvic junction obstruction, a dismembered pyeloplasty allows proper repositioning of the ureteropelvic junction in relation to these vessels (Fig. 65–78).

Foley Y-V Plasty

The Foley Y-V plasty was originally designed for reconstruction of a ureteropelvic junction obstruction associated with a high ureteral insertion. As for other flap techniques, however, it has generally been supplanted by the more versatile dismembered pyeloplasty. Similar to other nondismembered flap techniques, the Foley Y-V plasty is specifically contraindicated when the transposition of lower pole vessels is required. The Foley Y-V plasty is also of little value when significant reduction of renal pelvic size is required.

The pelvis and proximal ureter are exposed as previously described. A widely based triangular or V-shaped flap is outlined with methylene blue, some other tissue marker, or fine stay sutures. The base of the V-shaped

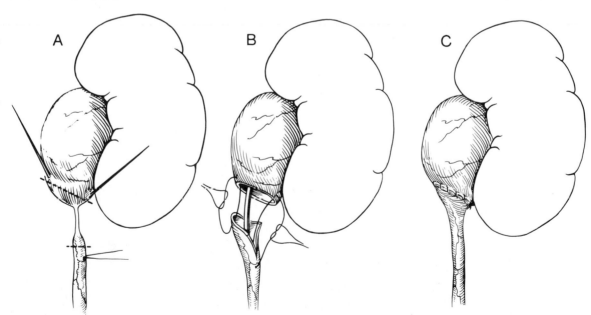

Figure 65–76. *A,* Traction sutures are placed on the medial and lateral aspects of the dependent portion of the renal pelvis in preparation for dismembered pyeloplasty. A traction suture is also placed on the lateral aspect of the proximal ureter, below the level of the obstruction. This suture will help maintain proper orientation for the subsequent repair.

B, The ureteropelvic junction is excised. The proximal ureter is spatulated on its lateral aspect. The apex of this lateral, spatulated aspect of the ureter is then brought to the inferior border of the pelvis while the medial side of the ureter is brought to the superior edge of the pelvis.

C, The anastomosis is performed with fine interrupted or running absorbable sutures placed full thickness through the ureteral and renal pelvic walls in a watertight fashion. In general, we prefer to leave an indwelling internal stent in adult patients. The stent is removed 4 to 6 weeks later.

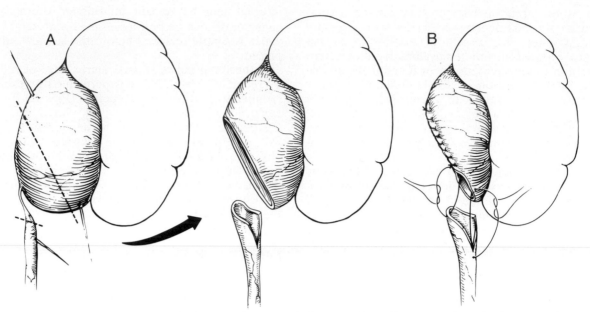

Figure 65–77. *A,* For a large or redundant renal pelves, a reduction pyeloplasty is performed by excising the redundant portion between traction sutures.

B, The cephalad aspect of the pelvis is then closed with running absorbable suture down to the dependent portion. The dependent aspect of the pelvis is anastomosed to the proximal ureter as described in Figure 65–76.

flap is positioned on the dependent, medial aspect of the renal pelvis and the apex at the ureteropelvic junction. The incision from the apex of the flap (the stem of the Y) will be carried out along the lateral aspect of the proximal ureter. The incision in the ureter should be long enough to completely traverse the area of stenosis and to extend for several millimeters into the normal caliber ureter (Fig. 65–79A).

The pelvic flap and ureterotomy are then developed. A fine scalpel blade is utilized for the initial pelvic incision. Potts or fine Metzenbaum scissors completes the flap and ureterotomy (Fig. 65–79B). An internal

stent is now placed and the repair performed over it. The apex of the pelvic flap is brought to the apex (inferior aspect) of the ureterotomy incision, using fine absorbable suture. The posterior walls are approximated employing interrupted or running suture (Fig. 65–79C). As for all pyeloplasty repairs, our preference is generally for interrupted suture technique as we believe this decreases the likelihood of pursing or buckling of the suture line. Interrupted technique is also less likely to cause local ischemia. Anastomosis of the anterior walls is then accomplished, thus completing the repair (Fig. 65–79D).

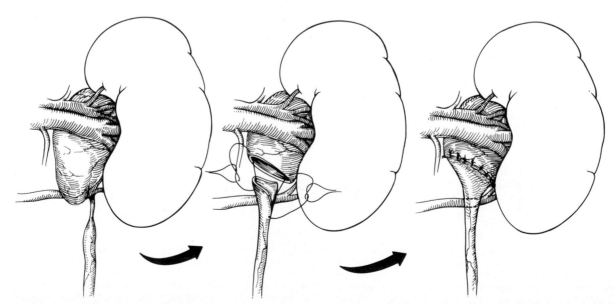

Figure 65–78. When aberrant or accessory lower pole vessels are found in association with the ureteropelvic junction obstruction, a dismembered pyeloplasty allows transposition of the ureteropelvic junction in relation to the vessels.

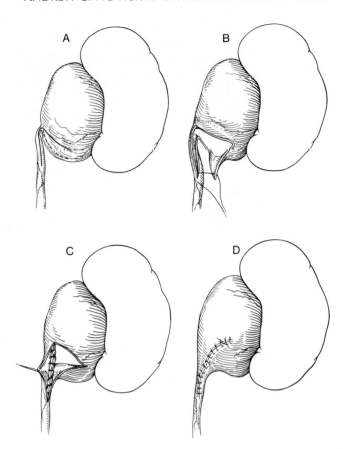

Figure 65–79. *A,* A Foley Y-V plasty is best applied to a ureteropelvic junction obstruction associated with a high insertion of the ureter. The flap is outlined with tissue marker or stay sutures. The base of the V is positioned on the dependent, medial aspect of the renal pelvis and the apex at the ureteropelvic junction. The incision from the apex of the flap, which represents the stem of the Y, is then carried along the lateral aspect of the proximal ureter well into an area of normal caliber.

B, The flap is developed with fine scissors. The apex of the pelvic flap is brought to the inferiormost aspect of the ureterotomy incision.

C, The posterior walls are approximated utilizing interrupted or running fine absorbable suture.

D, The anastomosis is completed with approximation of the anterior walls of the pelvic flap and ureterotomy.

Culp-DeWeerd Spiral Flap Technique

The Culp-DeWeerd spiral flap is best suited to large, readily accessible extrarenal pelves in which the ureteral insertion is already in a dependent, oblique position. Although most patients so affected are generally also good candidates for a standard or reduction dismembered pyeloplasty, the spiral flap may be of particular value when the ureteropelvic junction obstruction is associated with a relatively long segment of proximal ureteral narrowing or stricture.

The spiral flap is outlined with a broad base situated obliquely on the dependent aspect of the renal pelvis. To preserve blood supply to the flap, the base is situated in a position anatomically lateral to the ureteropelvic junction, that is, between the ureteral insertion and the renal parenchyma. The flap itself may be spiralled posteriorly to anteriorly or vice versa. In either case, the anatomically medial line of incision (farthest from the parenchyma) is carried down the ureter, completely through the obstructed segment (Fig. 65–80*A*). Proper placement of the apex of the flap is determined by the length of flap needed. This length is in turn a function of the length of proximal ureter to be bridged. The longer the flap required, the farther away will be the apex from the base. However, to preserve vascular integrity of the flap, the ratio of flap length to width should not exceed 3 to 1. In general, the outline of the flap should be made longer than what may initially be perceived as necessary, because the flap will shrink once the pelvis is incised. If the flap is in fact too long, length

can safely be reduced by trimming back the apex, thus keeping blood supply intact. Once the flap is developed, the apex is rotated down to the most inferior aspect of the ureterotomy (Fig. 65–80*B*). The anastomosis is performed over an internal stent, utilizing fine absorbable sutures (Fig. 65–80*C*).

Scardino-Prince Vertical Flap

The Scardino-Prince vertical flap technique has limited application today. It may appropriately be used only when a dependent ureteropelvic junction is situated at the medial margin of a large, square ("box-shaped") extrarenal pelvis (Fig. 65–81*A*). In most instances, the technique has been supplanted by a standard dismembered pyeloplasty, although the vertical flap may be preferable for relatively long areas of proximal ureteral narrowing. However, while the vertical flap can bridge stenotic areas of average length, the procedure cannot produce as long a flap, and thus bridge as long a stricture, as the spiral flap.

The vertical flap technique itself is similar to the spiral flap procedure except that the base of the flap is situated more horizontally on the dependent aspect of the renal pelvis, between the ureteropelvic junction and the renal parenchyma. The flap itself is formed by straight incisions converging from the base vertically to the apex on either the anterior or posterior aspects of the renal pelvis. The site of the apex, and thus the length of the flap, are determined by the length of proximal ureter to

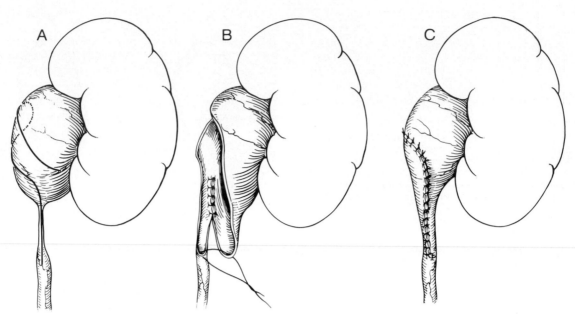

Figure 65–80. *A,* A spiral flap may be indicated for relatively long areas of proximal ureteral obstruction when the ureteropelvic junction is already in a dependent position. The spiral flap is outlined with the base situated obliquely on the dependent aspect of the renal pelvis. The base of the flap is positioned anatomically lateral to the ureteropelvic junction, between the ureteral insertion and the renal parenchyma. The flap is spiralled posteriorly to anteriorly or vice versa. The anatomically medial line of incision is carried down completely through the obstructed proximal ureteral segment into normal caliber ureter. The site of the apex for the flap is determined by length of the flap required to bridge the obstruction. The longer the segment of proximal ureteral obstruction, the farther away is the apex as this will make the flap longer. To preserve vascular integrity to the flap, however, the ratio of flap length to width should not exceed 3 to 1.

B, Once the flap is developed, the apex is rotated down to the most inferior aspect of the ureterotomy.

C, The anastomosis is completed, usually over an internal stent, utilizing fine absorbable sutures.

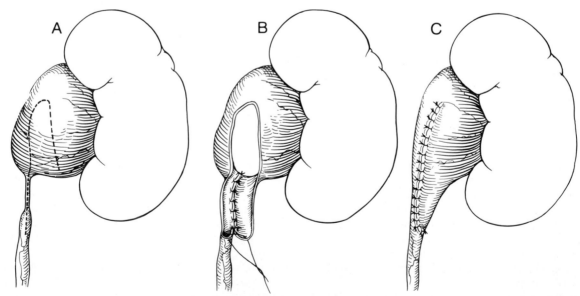

Figure 65–81. *A,* The vertical flap technique may be utilized when a dependent ureteropelvic junction is situated at the medial margin of a large, box-shaped extrarenal pelvis. In contrast to the spiral flap, the base of the vertical flap is situated more horizontally on the dependent aspect of the renal pelvis, between the ureteropelvic junction and the renal parenchyma. The flap itself is formed by two straight incisions converging from the base vertically up to apex on either the anterior or posterior aspects of the renal pelvis. As for the spiral flap, the position of the apex determines the length of the flap, which should be a function of the length of proximal ureter to be bridged. The medial incision of the flap is carried down the proximal ureter completely through the strictured area into normal caliber ureter.

B, The apex of the flap is rotated down to the inferiormost aspect of the ureterotomy.

C, The flap is closed by approximating the edges with interrupted or running fine absorbable sutures.

be bridged. The medial incision is carried down the proximal ureter, completely through the strictured area and into normal caliber ureter (Fig. 65–81*B*). The flap is developed with fine scissors. The apex of the flap is then rotated down and sutured to the inferior most aspect of the ureterotomy. Closure of the flap is completed with interrupted or running fine absorbable sutures (Fig. 65–81*C*).

Intubated Ureterotomy

The intubated ureterotomy, popularized by Davis in 1943, is rarely employed today. Its primary role was for repair of lengthy or multiple ureteral strictures. If these strictures are found in association with ureteropelvic junction obstruction, the intubated ureterotomy may be combined with any of the standard pyeloplasty techniques. At least in principle, however, the Davis intubated ureterotomy would be best combined with a spiral flap procedure. Compared with the vertical flap, the spiral flap can be made longer, thus allowing more of the strictured area to be bridged by a pelvic flap. This leaves a shorter area that relies on healing by "secondary intention." Any flap technique, however, would be preferable to a dismembered repair, at least in regard to preservation of blood supply and subsequent healing.

A flap is outlined as previously described, with the ureterotomy to be carried completely through the long strictured area (Fig. 65–82*A*). The flap is developed, taking care to use minimal dissection of the ureter in order to preserve its blood supply. In contrast to uncomplicated pyeloplasties, nephrostomy tube drainage is routinely accomplished in these cases in order to divert the urine and to prevent subsequent urinoma formation. Nephrostomy drainage in these cases also allows access for antegrade radiographic studies as necessary during the postoperative period. Originally, the ureteral intubation was accomplished with a stenting catheter that was placed across the strictured area to the distal ureter or bladder. Proximally, it was brought out through the cortex alongside a nephrostomy tube. Currently, most urologists would prefer a self-retaining, soft, inert internal ureteral stent instead. The apex of the flap is brought as far down as possible over the stent on the ureterotomy, and the flap is closed with interrupted or running absorbable suture (Fig. 65–82*B*). The distal aspect of the ureterotomy is left open to heal secondarily by ureteral regeneration, although a few fine absorbable sutures may be placed loosely to keep the sides of the ureter in accurate relation to the stent (Fig. 65–82*C*).

A nephrostogram should be obtained after 6 to 8 weeks. If there is no extravasation the internal stent is removed cystoscopically and antegrade radiographic studies are repeated. When adequate ureteral patency has been assured, without evidence of extravasation, the

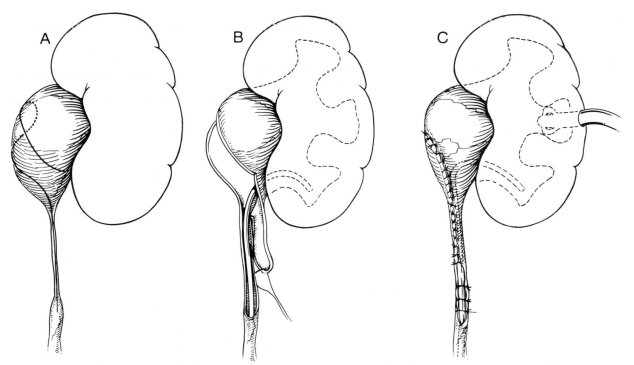

Figure 65–82. *A,* The intubated ureterotomy may be of value when a ureteropelvic junction obstruction is associated with extremely long or multiple ureteral strictures. A spiral flap is outlined and developed as described in Figure 65–80. The ureterotomy incision will be carried completely through the long strictured area or through each of the multiple areas of stricture.

B, The flap is developed, taking care to use minimal dissection of the ureter in order to preserve its blood supply. In contrast to uncomplicated repairs, nephrostomy tube drainage is utilized routinely. A self-retaining, soft, inert internal ureteral stent is placed and positioned proximally in the renal pelvis or lower infundibulum and distally in the bladder. The apex of the flap is brought as far down as possible over the stent on the ureterotomy. The flap is closed with interrupted or running absorbable suture.

C, The distal aspect of the ureterotomy is left open to heal secondarily by ureteral regeneration. A few fine absorbable sutures may be placed loosely to keep the sides of the ureter in apposition to the stent.

nephrostomy tube is clamped and subsequently removed.

"Salvage" Procedures

Management of the "failed pyeloplasty" is a challenging problem. At times, successful reconstruction can be achieved utilizing one of the flap or dismembered techniques already described. In these clinical settings, the secondary reconstruction will be aided by preliminary cystoscopic or antegrade placement of a ureteral catheter to help intraoperative identification and subsequent dissection of the ureter and renal pelvis. Often, a relatively long proximal ureteral stenosis needs repair. As such, in contrast to primary repairs in which dissection of the kidney and ureter is to be minimized, wide mobilization of both is generally a necessity. This maneuver allows the kidney to be displaced downward and the ureter up, thus helping to bridge the area of stenosis and perform the secondary pyeloplasty without tension.

Several other options are available for these secondary and often complex repairs. Many of these surgical alternatives are those generally available for any extensive ureteral problems. The standard options for preserving renal function include an ileoureteral replacement and autotransplantation with a Boari flap pyelovesicostomy. For cases in which function of the involved kidney is already significantly compromised and the contralateral kidney is normal, consideration can be given to nephrectomy, especially when previous attempts at salvage have failed or the repair would be particularly complex for any reason. Other options, more specific for the "failed pyeloplasty," include the renal capsule flap and ureterocalycostomy.

Renal Capsular Flap Technique

The use of a renal capsule flap for repair of complicated or secondary ureteropelvic junction obstruction was described by Thompson and associates in 1969. The kidney itself can be approached anteriorly or posteriorly, depending on local anatomy and type of previous surgery, although a posterior approach through the flank would generally be preferable. In either case, the corresponding surfaces of the kidney, renal pelvis, and ureter are exposed. An inverted V- or U-shaped flap is outlined on the renal capsule, with a wide base oriented medially at the renal sinus. A vertical incision is made through the ureteropelvic junction into normal proximal ureter (Fig. 65–83A). The apex of the flap is brought down to the inferior aspect of the ureterotomy. The edges of the pyeloureterotomy incision are then sutured to the corresponding sides of the flap, with running or interrupted fine absorbable sutures (Fig. 65–83B). These complex repairs generally include routine utilization of both nephrostomy tubes and internal stents.

Ureterocalycostomy

Anastomosis of the proximal ureter directly to the lower calyceal system has become a well-accepted sal-

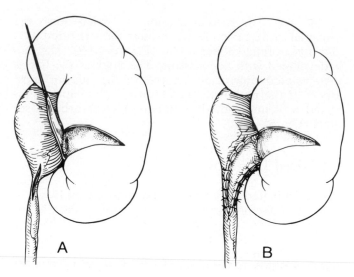

Figure 65–83. *A,* A renal capsule flap may be valuable as a "salvage" procedure in the case of failed previous attempts at repair or inadequate renal pelvis associated with the ureteropelvic junction obstruction. An inverted V- or U-shaped flap is outlined on the renal capsule. The base of this flap is oriented medially at the renal sinus to preserve its blood supply. A vertical ureteropyelotomy is made completely through the ureteropelvic junction into normal caliber, proximal ureter.

B, The renal capsule flap is developed by sharp dissection and the apex brought down to the inferior aspect of the ureterotomy, over an internal stent. Nephrostomy tube drainage will also be of value in these complicated repairs. The edges of the pyeloureterotomy incision are sutured to the corresponding sides of the flap with running or interrupted fine absorbable sutures.

vage technique for the failed pyeloplasty (Ross et al., 1990). Ureterocalycostomy may also be utilized as a primary reconstructive procedure whenever a ureteropelvic junction obstruction or proximal ureteral stricture is associated with a relatively small intrarenal pelvis or whenever the ureteropelvic junction is associated with rotational anomalies, such as horseshoe kidney (Levitt et al., 1981). In those cases, it may be of particular value as it provides completely dependent drainage. Many of the indications for a ureterocalycostomy are illustrated in Figure 65–84.

The ureter is isolated in the retroperitoneum and dissected proximally as far as possible with a large amount of periureteral tissue. For secondary procedures, extensive scarring may preclude identification and dissection of the renal pelvis itself (Fig. 65–85A). The kidney is mobilized as much as necessary to gain access to the lower pole. An important technical point to be emphasized is that the parenchyma overlying the lower pole calyx must be resected rather than simply incised (Couvelaire et al., 1964). The amount of parenchyma to be removed depends on the extent of cortical thinning already present. However, a simple nephrotomy over a calyx will not be adequate, as a secondary stricture may result.

The proximal ureter is spatulated laterally, and the ureterocalyceal anastomosis is performed over an internal stent. Consideration should also be given to leaving a nephrostomy tube. The first suture is placed at the apex of the ureteral spatulation and lateral wall of the calyx; the second one is placed 180 degrees away (Fig. 65–85B). The remainder of the anastomosis is com-

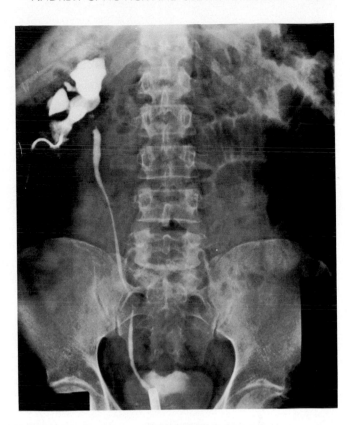

Figure 65–84. This patient was referred with persistent urinary drainage following an open pyelolithotomy and pyeloplasty. A percutaneous nephrostomy was placed. Several indications for ureterocalycostomy are demonstrated by this simultaneous antegrade and retrograde pyelogram. These include the fact that the patient has undergone previous surgery suggesting that there will be a significant amount of peripelvic fibrosis. The obstruction is also associated with an intrarenal pelvis. A relatively long gap occurs between the renal pelvis and nonobstructed proximal ureter. Note, however, that the normal proximal ureter will reach the lower calyx without tension, especially if the kidney is mobilized downward and the ureter dissected distally for additional length.

pleted, utilizing an interrupted, open suture technique, that is, each suture is placed but is left untied until the final one is in place. This practice allows a more accurate anastomosis to be performed under direct vision. When the full set of circumferential sutures has been placed, they are secured down together (Fig. 65–85C and D).

Whenever possible, the renal capsule is closed over the cut surface of the parenchyma but not close enough to the anastomosis itself to compromise its lumen by extrinsic compression. Rather, the anastomosis should be protected by surrounding it with perinephric fat or a peritoneal or omental flap (Fig. 65–85E).

Postoperative Care and Management of Complications

In general, external drains are advanced and removed 24 to 48 hours after urinary drainage has ceased. When internal stents have been placed, our preference is to remove them on an outpatient basis in 4 to 6 weeks. If a nephrostomy tube is present, a nephrostogram is obtained no sooner than 7 to 10 days postoperatively or even later for particularly complicated repairs. When that study demonstrates a patent anastomosis without obstruction or extravasation, the tube is clamped for 12 to 24 hours and removed if no flank pain, fever, or leakage around the tube is noted.

If an indwelling internal stent had not been left and if urinary drainage persists after 7 to 10 days or recurs after the external drain has been removed, retrograde studies should be obtained and an attempt made to pass an internal stent. The problem generally resolves im-

mediately, and the internal stent is removed 1 month later. If an attempt at passing an internal stent is unsuccessful, a percutaneous nephrostomy is placed and managed as if it had been left intraoperatively. If drainage persists despite nephrostomy tube placement, an internal or internal/external stent should be placed in an antegrade fashion. At times, despite appropriate application of stents, drains, and nephrostomy tubes, urinary extravasation will result in urinoma formation. This is best managed with direct percutaneous drainage of the fluid collection, utilizing ultrasound or CT guidance.

Standard follow-up of the functional result is accomplished with a urogram or renogram obtained approximately 4 weeks postoperatively, or after any stents or nephrostomy tubes have been removed. Earlier studies are indicated if the patient becomes symptomatic. Compared with preoperative studies, radiographic evaluation at this time should show a definite improvement in hydronephrosis (Fig. 65–86). If a question remains unanswered as to the functional significance of any residual caliectasis, further evaluation can be done using any of the studies outlined previously in this chapter for ureteropelvic junction obstruction.

MISCELLANEOUS RENAL OPERATIONS

Open Renal Biopsy

Open renal biopsy may be necessary to establish a tissue diagnosis in patients with renal disease; to assess

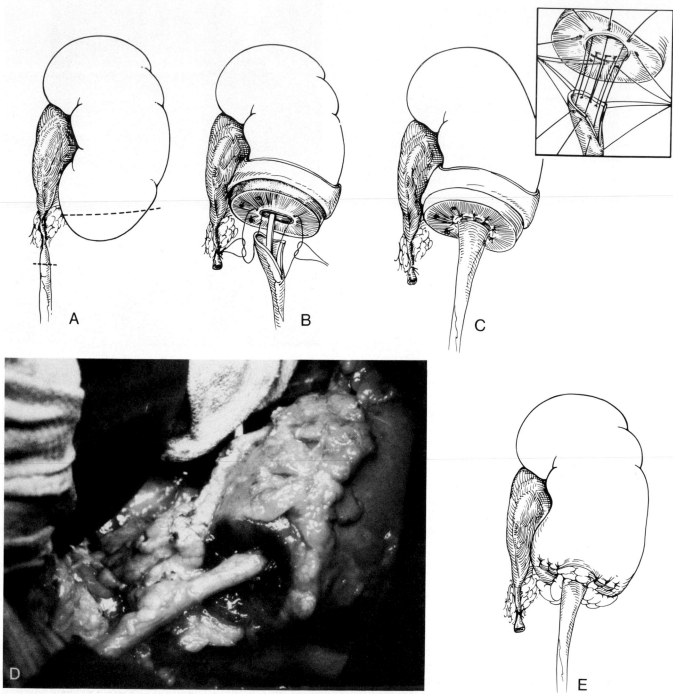

Figure 65–85. *A*, The ureter is identified in the retroperitoneum and dissected proximally as far as possible. The kidney is mobilized as much as necessary to gain access to the lower pole and to subsequently perform the anastomosis without tension. A lower pole nephrectomy is performed, removing as much parenchyma as necessary to widely expose a dilated lower pole calyx.

B, The proximal ureter is spatulated laterally. The anastomosis should subsequently be performed over an internal stent and consideration given to leaving a nephrostomy tube. The initial suture is placed at the apex of the ureteral spatulation and the lateral wall of the calyx, with another suture placed 180 degrees from that.

C, The anastomosis is completed in an open fashion, placing each suture circumferentially but not securing them down until the anastomosis has been completed.

D, Intraoperative view of completed ureterocalycostomy.

E, The renal capsule is closed over the cut surface of the parenchyma whenever possible. However, the capsule should not be closed close to the anastomosis itself as that may compromise the lumen by extrinsic compression. Instead, the anastomosis should be protected with a graft of perinephric fat or with a peritoneal or an omental flap.

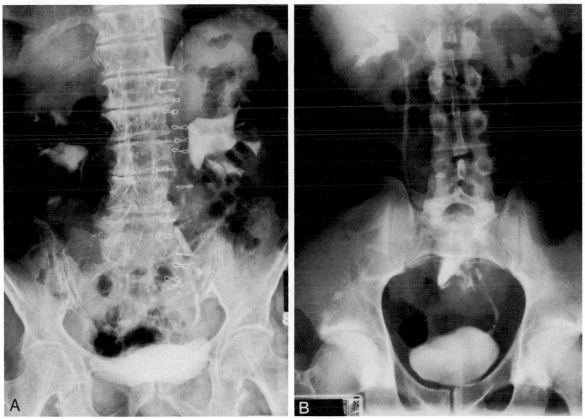

Figure 65–86. *A,* Intravenous urogram 2 months after a left dismembered pyeloplasty reveals sharp calyces without any residual obstruction. Compare this with the patient's preoperative urogram (Fig. 65–71).

B, Intravenous urogram following dismembered pyeloplasty of a left pelvic kidney. Compare this with the patient's preoperative urogram (Fig. 65–75).

the severity of such disease; or to evaluate the potential for salvageable renal function in patients with known correctable disorders, who are also candidates for reconstructive operations. Open biopsy is usually preferred over a percutaneous biopsy technique in a patient with solitary kidney, coagulopathy, atypical anatomy, or other factors that may increase the risk of a closed biopsy. An open biopsy also provides more tissue for study and minimizes the potential for complications, such as arteriovenous fistula, perirenal hematoma, and gross hematuria.

An open renal biopsy may be performed through an extraperitoneal flank or a posterior incision. A general anesthetic agent is preferable. However, in a thin patient who is cooperative, local anesthesia may be employed. The right kidney is usually biopsied preferentially because of its more caudal location.

After making the surgical incision, Gerota's fascia is opened and the lower pole of the kidney is exposed. An elliptic incision is made in the renal capsule, which is usually 1 to 2 cm long and 0.5 to 1.0 cm wide (Fig. 65–87A). The incision is deepened on either side with a scalpel and bevelled so that the final wedge depth (usually 5–8 mm) includes an adequate segment of cortical tissue. Fine Metzenbaum scissors complete the transection of cortex at the bottom of the wedge. The tissue is then gently lifted out, using the slightly spread scissors' blades rather than forceps, which might crush

the specimen (Fig. 65–87B). Suction is avoided during this final maneuver to prevent loss of tissue into the suction tip. This technique of elliptic wedge biopsy is preferred over an open needle biopsy because bleeding is more readily controlled and because more renal tissue is obtained. The renal incision is closed with absorbable 2-0 or 3-0 sutures placed across the defect and gently tied over oxycel (Fig. 65–87C).

Surgery for Simple Renal Cysts

Simple renal cysts usually occur as mass lesions and are often detected during renal imaging studies performed for unrelated reasons. A small number of patients require exploration to distinguish between a cyst and an atypical tumor mass. Large renal cysts causing obstruction may also occasionally require open surgical drainage with unroofing (Stanisic, 1977).

The preferred surgical approach for drainage of a renal cyst is through an extraperitoneal posterior, flank, or anterior incision, according to the number and location of lesions present. Gerota's fascia is opened, and the cystic lesion is exposed by dissection of perirenal fat from the cyst and adjacent parenchyma (Fig. 65–88A). The surrounding area is packed off, and cyst fluid is aspirated for diagnostic study. The cyst wall is entered sharply and resected near its junction with normal

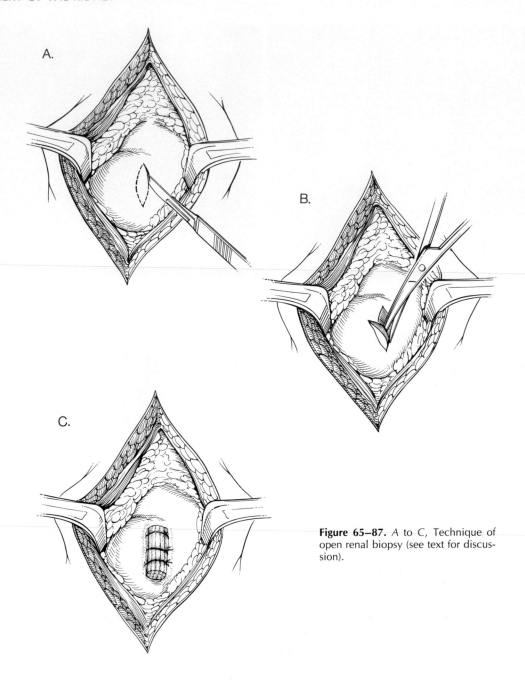

Figure 65–87. *A* to *C,* Technique of open renal biopsy (see text for discussion).

parenchyma (Fig. 65–88*B*). The base of the cyst cavity is inspected, and any suspicious-looking areas are biopsied with immediate frozen-section examination. After unroofing, the perimeter of the cyst wall is oversewn with absorbable 3-0 or 4-0 continuous suture to achieve hemostasis (Fig. 65–88*C*). Alternatively, the edge of the cyst wall may be cauterized and persistent bleeders controlled with interrupted figure-of-eight absorbable sutures. Drainage is not required unless the cyst is infected.

Open Nephrostomy Insertion

Nephrostomy tube drainage is usually achieved by the percutaneous approach. An open operation is occasion-

ally necessary because of difficult anatomy or a minimally dilated upper urinary tract. Open nephrostomy insertion may also be performed at the time of a reconstructive procedure, such as pyeloplasty or ureterocalicostomy.

Primary nephrostomy insertion is usually performed through an extraperitoneal flank incision. After mobilizing the kidney, the renal pelvis is exposed and opened. A Willscher nephrostomy tube, as illustrated in Figure 65–89, is particularly simple to place because of a built-in malleable stylet within a smoothly tapered sheath (Noble, 1989). The stylet of the catheter is passed through the pyelotomy and is used to puncture the cortex from within a calyx (Fig. 65–89*A*). It is important to ensure that the nephrostomy is made near the convex border of the kidney and not in the anterior or posterior

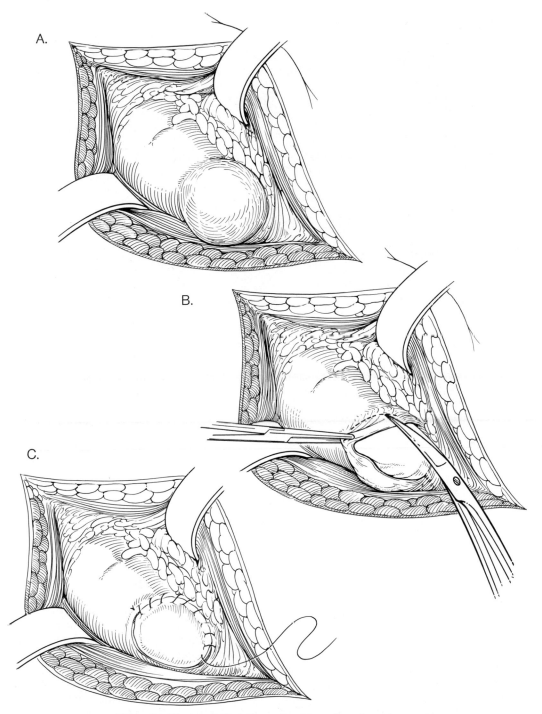

Figure 65–88. *A* to *C*, Technique of excision of renal cyst (see text).

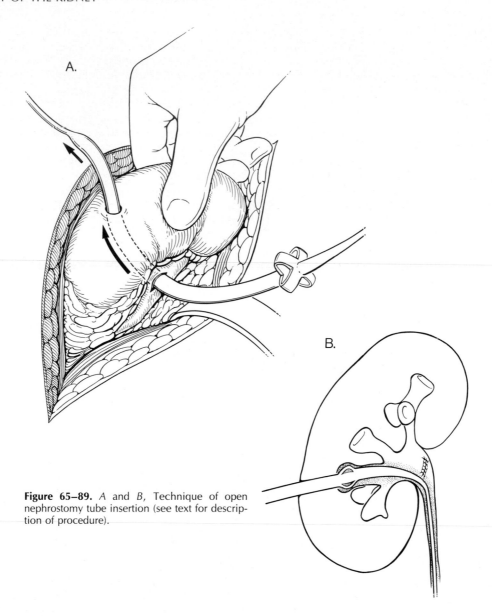

Figure 65–89. *A* and *B*, Technique of open nephrostomy tube insertion (see text for description of procedure).

surface, as this location allows for a better placement of the tube and minimizes the risk of injury to large intrarenal vessels. Usually, a 22 Fr. or 24 Fr. catheter is used. The Willscher tube has a flared portion with wide openings followed by a long tip, which may be utilized as a splint through the ureteropelvic junction, if necessary.

The catheter is pulled through the cortex until the flared portion lies in a good position within the collecting system, usually in the pelvis or a dependent calyx (Fig. 65–89*B*). The nephrostomy tube is secured to the renal capsule with a 3-0 absorbable pursestring suture. The pyelotomy is closed with 3-0 or 4-0 absorbable suture. The stylet of the nephrostomy tube is passed through the flank muscle, subcutaneous tissue, and skin with care taken to ensure proper alignment of the tube as it passes from the kidney to the exterior. Heavy 2-0 skin sutures are inserted to secure the tube near the flank wall exit point to prevent inadvertent dislodgement. A Penrose drain is placed near the pyelotomy site and brought out through a separate stab wound in the flank.

Ongoing care of a nephrostomy tube is important to prevent infection and ensure unobstructed drainage. Periodic urine cultures are obtained, and significant intercurrent urinary infection is appropriately treated. If the tube is dislodged within 7–10 days of its insertion, it may not be possible to replace it through the tract and a secondary procedure may be necessary. Even with the best of care, encrustations will form around the tube and will require periodic tube replacement at 6- to 8-week intervals. This procedure is usually readily performed under fluoroscopic guidance, once a tract has been established.

Surgery for Polycystic Kidney Disease

Bilateral nephrectomy may be necessary in selected patients with end-stage renal failure from polycystic kidney disease who are candidates for renal transplantation. The indication for bilateral nephrectomy in this setting is a history of significant bleeding or renal infection or massively enlarged kidneys, which may interfere with placement of an allograft in the pelvis. This operation is best performed through an anterior bilateral subcostal or midline transperitoneal incision.

Occasionally, unilateral nephrectomy is required before the patient develops end-stage renal failure when the polycystic kidney is a site of complications, such as infection, severe pain due to bleeding or obstruction, and tumor development. Cyst puncture and cyst unroofing may be helpful when the cyst obstructs the collecting system or causes flank pain (Lue, 1966). Punctures of multiple cysts and unroofing of cysts (Rovsing's operation) do not appear to improve renal function or to prevent further deterioration and is not recommended for this purpose (Milam, 1963).

Isthmusectomy for Horseshoe Kidney

Horseshoe kidney occurs in about one in 700 individuals and is frequently associated with other urologic anomalies. The isthmus that joins the kidneys usually lies anterior to the great vessels. Ureteral obstruction with hydronephrosis, stone formation, or infection is the most common associated problem in this condition and may require surgical treatment (Culp, 1955). In patients with ureteral or ureteropelvic junction obstruction, division of the isthmus alone is insufficient. Appropriate correction of the obstruction is required. In such a case,

isthmusectomy may be a helpful adjunctive measure to allow repositioning of the kidney and maintenance of an unobstructed upper urinary tract. Abdominal pain in the absence of any demonstrable renal symptomatology is rarely caused by the presence of polar fusion alone and is not an indication for isthmusectomy.

When performing surgery on a horseshoe kidney, an anterior subcostal extraperitoneal approach is preferred. This provides good access to the isthmus as well as to the pelvis and ureter, which are rotated anteriorly. The isthmus may be fibrous but often consists of parenchymal tissue. Isthmusectomy is performed by mobilizing the isthmus from the great vessels, being careful to avoid injury to any anomalous vessels, and placing mattress sutures of 0 chromic catgut through the parenchyma, about 1 cm on either side of the line of section to control bleeding. The divided ends can subsequently be further oversewn with sutures passed through the capsule of the cut edges. Two or three sutures through the divided isthmus and into the fascia overlying the muscles of the posterior abdominal wall are selected to fix the lower pole, which is rotated outward to allow room for the ureter to lie on the posterior abdominal wall.

Local Excision of Renal Pelvic Tumor

In patients with localized transitional cell carcinoma (TCC) of the renal pelvis, nephroureterectomy with a

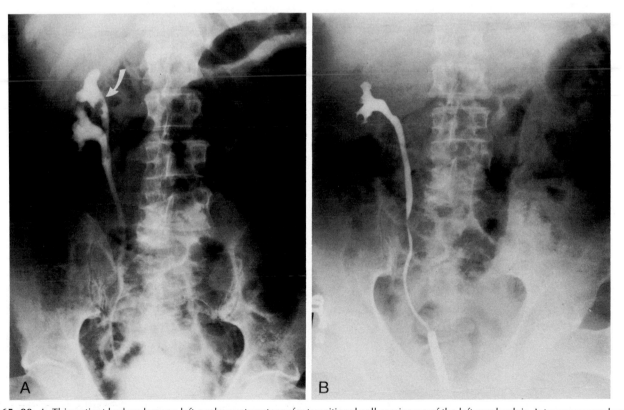

Figure 65–90. *A,* This patient had undergone left nephroureterectomy for transitional cell carcinoma of the left renal pelvis. Intravenous pyelography now suggested a lesion in the upper infundibulum of the remaining right kidney *(arrow).* This finding was confirmed at the time of retrograde pyelography.

B, Upper pole partial nephrectomy was performed, leaving the pelvis and lower infundibulocalyceal system intact, as demonstrated on this postoperative retrograde pyelogram. (From Novick, A. C., Streem, S. B., and Pontes, E. (Eds.): Stewart's Operative Urology, 2nd ed. Baltimore, Williams & Wilkins, 1989.)

bladder cuff is the treatment of choice. A nephron-sparing operation may be indicated in selected patients with low-grade, noninvasive malignancy bilaterally or in a solitary kidney to avoid the need for dialytic renal replacement therapy. A variety of conservative surgical approaches are available in such cases, including open pyelotomy with tumor excision and fulguration, partial nephrectomy (Fig. 65–90), and endourologic techniques with or without adjunctive topical chemotherapy (Huffman, 1985; Smith, 1987; Streem, 1986; Ziegelbaum, 1987; Zincke, 1984). The latter two approaches are reviewed elsewhere in this text.

Open pyelotomy and tumor excision may be employed in patients with noninvasive TCC confined to a portion of the renal pelvis. Occasionally, small lesions involving an infundibulum may be accessible for this approach. This operation is performed through an extraperitoneal flank incision after mobilization of the entire kidney within Gerota's fascia.

The upper ureter and renal pelvis are mobilized along the posterior renal aspect. The renal pelvic dissection is carried into the renal sinus, which often also exposes one or more infundibula. Small vein or Gil-Vernet retractors will maintain this operative exposure (Fig. 65–91A). The renal pelvic incision is made to expose the tumor-bearing portion of the renal pelvis (Fig. 65–91B). This incision may be extended into an infundibulum if necessary.

It is preferable to excise a full-thickness segment of the renal pelvis encompassing the tumor (Fig. 65–91C). Frozen sections are prepared to ensure that the resected margins are free of disease. An alternative approach is to sharply excise the tumor at its base, while preserving the integrity of the renal pelvic wall, and to then fulgurate the base and surrounding area extensively. Following excision of all gross tumor, operative pyeloscopy is employed to examine the intrarenal collecting system for any remaining lesions. The site of renal pelvic

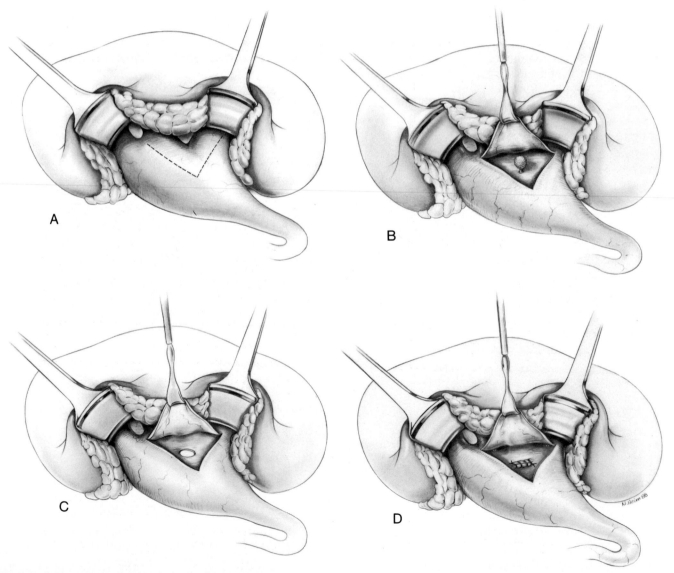

Figure 65–91. *A* to *D*, Technique of open pyelotomy and tumor excision for transitional cell carcinoma of the renal pelvis (see text). (From Novick, A. C., Streem, S. B., and Pontes, E. (Eds.): Stewart's Operative Urology, 2nd ed. Baltimore, Williams & Wilkins, 1989.)

tumor excision is repaired with 4-0 chromic suture (Fig. 65–91D), and the pyelotomy incision is then similarly closed. A Penrose drain is placed near the pyelotomy and brought out through a separate stab wound in the flank.

REFERENCES

Abele, R. P., Novick, A. C., Ishigami, N., et al.: Comparison of flushing solutions for in situ renal preservation. Urology, 18:485, 1981.

Allen, T. D.: Congenital ureteral strictures. J. Urol., 104:196, 1970.

Anderson, B., Hansen, J. B., and Jorgensen, S. J.: Survival after nephrectomy. Scand. J. Urol. Nephrol., 2:91, 1968.

Anderson, J. C., and Hynes, W.: Retrocaval ureter: A case diagnosed preoperatively and treated successfully by a plastic operation. Br. J. Urol., 21:209, 1949.

Aoi, W., Akahoshi, M., Seto, S., Doi, Y., Suzuki, S., Matsumoto, Y., Kuramochi, M., Hashiba, K., and Tsuda, N.: Correction of hypertension by partial nephrectomy in segmental renal artery stenosis and electron microscopic studies of renin. Jpn. Heart J., 22:686, 1981.

Aperia, A., Broberger, O., Wikstad, I., and Witon, P.: Renal growth and function in patients nephrectomized in childhood. Acta Pediatr. Scand., 66:185, 1977.

Askari, A., Novick, A. C., Stewart, B. H., et al.: Surgical treatment of renovascular disease in the solitary kidney: Results in 43 cases. J. Urol., 127:20, 1982.

Assimos, D. G., Boyce, W. H., Harrison, L. H., McCullough, D. L., Kroovand, R. L., and Sweat, K. R.: The role of open stone surgery since extracorporeal shock wave lithotripsy. J. Urol., 142:263, 1989.

Assimos, D. G., Boyce, W. H., Harrison, L. H., Hall, J. A., and McCullough, D. L.: Postoperative anatrophic nephrolithotomy bleeding. J. Urol., 135:1153, 1986.

Bates, R. J., Heaney, J. A., and Kerr, W. S., Jr.: Segmental calculus disease: Potential of partial nephrectomy. Urology, 17:409, 1981.

Bazeed, M. A., Scharfe, T., Becht, E., Jurincic, C., Alken, P., and Thuroff, J. W.: Conservative surgery of renal cell carcinoma. Eur. Urol., 12:238, 1986.

Bejjani, B., and Belman, A. B.: Ureteropelvic junction obstruction in newborns and infants. J. Urol., 128:770, 1982.

Belis, J. A., Pae, W. E., Rohner, T. J., Myers, J. L., Thiele, B. L., Wickey, G. C., and Martin, D. E.: Cardiovascular evaluation before circulatory arrest for removal of vena cava extension of renal carcinoma. J. Urol., 141:1302, 1989.

Berg, A. A.: Malignant hypernephroma of the kidney, its clinical course and diagnosis, with a description of the author's method of radical operative cure. Surg. Gynecol. Obstet., 17:463, 1913.

Berger, R. M., Lebowitz, J. M., and Carroll, P. A.: Ureteral polyps presenting as ureteropelvic junction obstruction in children. J. Urol., 128:805, 1982.

Bernstein, G. T., Mandell, J., Lebowitz, R. L., Bauer, S. B., Colodny, A. H., and Retik, A. B.: Ureteropelvic junction obstruction in the neonate. J. Urol., 140:1216, 1988.

Blandy, J. P., and Singh, M.: The case for a more aggressive approach to staghorn stones. J. Urol., 115:505, 1976.

Bodner, H., and Briskin, H. J.: Subdiaphragmatic renal exposure by resection of the eleventh rib. Urol. Cutan. Rev., 54:272, 1950.

Boyce, W. H., Russell, J. M., and Webb, R.: Management of the papillae during intrarenal surgery. Trans. Am. Assoc. Genitourin. Surg., 71:76, 1979.

Boyce, W. H., and Smith, M. G. V.: Anatrophic nephrotomy and plastic calyrrhaphy. Trans. Am. Assoc. Genitourin. Surg., 59:18, 1967.

Brodel, M.: The intrinsic blood vessels of the kidney and their significance in nephrotomy. Bull. Johns Hopkins Hosp. 12:10, 1901.

Cherrie, R. J., Goldman, D. G., Lindner, A., and deKernion, J. G.: Prognostic implications of vena caval extension of renal cell carcinoma. J. Urol., 128:910, 1982.

Chute, R., Baron, J. A., Jr., and Olsson, C. A.: The transverse upper abdominal "chevron" incision in urological surgery. J. Urol., 99:528, 1968.

Chute, R., Soutter, T., and Kerr, W.: The value of thoracoabdominal incision in the removal of kidney tumors. N. Engl. J. Med., 241:951, 1956.

Clark, C. D.: Survival after excision of a kidney, segmental resection of vena cava, and division of the opposite renal vein. Lancet, 2:1015, 1961.

Clark, W. R., and Malek, R. S.: Ureteropelvic junction obstruction: Observations on the classic type in adults. J. Urol., 138:276, 1987.

Clarke, B. G., Rudy, H. A., and Leadbetter, W. F.: Thoracoabdominal incision for surgery of renal, adrenal and testicular neoplasms. Surg. Gynecol. Obstet., 106:363, 1958.

Clayman, R.: Personal communication, 1989.

Cockett, A. T. K.: The kidney and regional hypothermia. Surgery, 50:905, 1961.

Collins, G. M., Green, R. D., Boyer, D., et al.: Protection of kidneys from warm ischemic injury: Dosage and timing of mannitol administration. Transplantation, 29:83, 1980.

Collins, G. M., Taft, P., Green, R. D., et al.: Adenine nucleotide levels in preserved and ischemically injured canine kidneys. World J. Surg., 1:237, 1977.

Collste, H., et al.: ATP in cortex of canine kidneys undergoing hypothermic storage. Life Science, 10:1201, 1971.

Cook, J. H., and Lytton, B.: Intraoperative localization of calculi during nephrolithotomy by ultrasound scanning. J. Urol., 117:543, 1977.

Couvelair, R., Auvert, J., and Moulonguet, A.: Implantations et anastomoses ureterocalicielles: techniques et indications. J. Urol. Nephrol., 70:437, 1964.

Culp, O. S.: Anterior nephro-ureterectomy: Advantages and limitations of a single incision. J. Urol., 85:193, 1961.

Culp, O. S., and DeWeerd, J. H.: A pelvic flap operation for certain types of ureteropelvic obstruction: Preliminary report. Mayo Clinic Proc., 26:483, 1951.

Culp, O. S., and Winterringen, J. R.: Surgical treatment of horseshoe kidney: Comparison of results after various type of operations. J. Urol., 73:747, 1955.

Cummings, K. B., Li, W. I., Ryan, J. A., Horton, W. G., and Paton, R. R.: Intraoperative management of renal cell carcinoma with supradiaphragmatic caval extension. J. Urol., 122:829, 1979.

Czerny, H. E.: Cited by Herczel, E.: Ueber Nierenextirpation beitr 2. Klin. Chir., 6:485, 1890.

Czerny, V.: Ueber Nierenextripation. Zentralbl. Chir., 6:737, 1897.

Das, S., and Amar, A. D.: Ureteropelvic junction obstruction with associated renal anomolies. J. Urol., 131:872, 1984.

Davis, D. M.: Intubated ureterotomy: A new operation for ureteral and ureteropelvic stricture. Surg. Gynecol. Obstet., 76:513, 1943.

Dees, J. E.: The use of intrapelvic coagulum in pyelolithotomy: Preliminary report. South. Med. J., 36:167, 1943.

Farcon, E. M., Morales, P., and Al-Askari, S.: In vivo hypothermic perfusion during renal surgery. Urology, 3:414, 1974.

Fenger, C.: Operation for the relief of valve formation and stricture of the ureter in hydro- or pyonephrosis. JAMA, 22:335, 1894.

Fischer, C. P., Sonda, L. P., and Diokno, A. C.: Use of cryoprecipitate coagulum in extracting renal calculi. Urology, 15:6, 1980.

Foley, F. E. B.: New plastic operation for stricture at the ureteropelvic junction. J. Urol., 38:643, 1937.

Foote, J. W., Blennerhassett, J. B., Wigglesworth, F. W., and MacKinnon, K. J.: Observations on the ureteropelvic junction. J. Urol., 104:252, 1970.

Foster, R. S., Mahomed, Y., Bihrle, R. R., and Strup, S.: Use of caval-atrial shunt for resection of a caval tumor thrombus in renal cell carcinoma. J. Urol., 140:1370, 1988.

Gardiner, R. A., Naunton-Morgan, T. C., Whitefield, H. N., et al.: The modified lumbotomy versus the oblique loin incision for renal surgery. Br. J. Urol., 51:256, 1979.

Gibbons, R. P., Correa, R. J., Cummings, K. B., et al.: Surgical management of renal lesions using in situ hypothermia and ischemia. J. Urol., 115:12, 1976.

Gibson, S., Kuzmarov, I. W., McClure, D. R., and Morehouse, D. D.: Blunt renal trauma: the value of a conservative approach to major injuries in clinically stable patients. Can. J. Surg., 25:25, 1982.

Gil-Vernet, J.: New surgical concepts in removing renal calculi. Urol. Int., 20:255, 1965.

Goldfarb, D. A., Novick, A. C., Lorig, R., Bretan, P. N., Montie, J. E., Pontes, J. E., Streem, S. B., and Siegel, S. W.: Magnetic resonance imaging for assessment of vena caval tumor thrombi: A comparative study with vena cavography and CT scanning. J. Urol., 144:1110, 1990.

Goldstein, A. E.: Longevity following nephrectomy. J. Urol., 76:31, 1956.

Gosling, J. A., and Dixon, J. S.: Functional obstruction of the ureter and renal pelvis: A histological and electron microscopic study. Br. J. Urol., 50:145, 1978.

Graham, S. D., Jr., and Glenn, J. F.: Enucleation surgery for renal malignancy. J. Urol., 122:546, 1979.

Graves, F. T.: The anatomy of the intrarenal arteries and its application to segmental resection of the kidney. Br. J. Surg., 42:132, 1954.

Hanna, M. K.: Some observations on congenital ureteropelvic junction obstruction. Urology, 12:151, 1978.

Hanna, M. K., Jeffs, R. D., Sturgess, J. M., and Baskin, M.: Ureteral structure and ultrastructure. Part II. Congenital ureteropelvic junction obstruction and primary obstructive megaureter. J. Urol., 116:725, 1976.

Harker, L. A.: Bleeding after cardiopulmonary bypass. N. Engl. J. Med., 314:1446, 1986.

Harvey, R. B.: Effect of temperature on function of isolated dog kidney. Am. J. Physiol., 197:181, 1959.

Hess, E.: Resection of the rib in renal operations. J. Urol., 42:943, 1939.

Huffman, J. L., Bagley, D. H., Lyon, E. S., Morse, M. J., Herr, H. W., and Whitmore, W. F.: Endoscopic diagnosis and treatment of upper tract urothelial tumors. Cancer, 55:1422, 1985.

Hughes, F. A.: Resection of the twelfth rib in surgical approach to the renal fossa. J. Urol., 61:159, 1949.

Hulbert, J. C., Reddy, P. K., Hunter, D. W., Castaneda-Zuniga, W., Amplatz, K., and Lange, P. H.: Percutaneous techniques for the management of calyceal diverticula containing calculi. J. Urol., 135:225, 1986.

Jacobs, J. A., Berger, B. W., Goldman, S. M., Robbins, M. A., and Young, J. D.: Ureteropelvic obstruction in adults with previously normal pyelograms. A report of five cases. J. Urol., 121:242, 1979.

Johnson, J. H., Evans, J. P., Glassberg, K. I., and Shapiro, S. R.: Pelvic hydronephrosis in children: A review of 219 personal cases. J. Urol., 117:97, 1977.

Kahnoski, R. J., Lingeman, J. E., Coury, T. A., Steele, R. E., and Mosbaugh, P. G.: Combined percutaneous and extracorporeal shock wave lithotripsy for staghorn calculi: An alternative to anatrophic nephrolithotomy. J. Urol., 135:679, 1986.

Kalash, S. S., Campbell, E. W., Jr., and Young, J. D., Jr.: Further simplification of cryoprecipitate coagulum pyelolithotomy without thrombin. Urology, 22:483, 1983.

Kay, R.: Procedures for ureteropelvic junction obstruction. In Novick, A. C., Streem, S. B., and Pontes, J. E. (Eds.): Stewart's Operative Urology, 2nd edition. Baltimore, Williams & Wilkins, 1989.

Kelalis, P. P.: Ureteropelvic junction. In Kelalis, P. P., and King, L. R. (Eds.): Clinical Pediatric Urology. Philadelphia, W. B. Saunders Co., 1973.

Khoury, E. N.: Thoraco-abdominal approach in lesions of kidney, adrenal and testis: morbidity studies. J. Urol., 96:631, 1966.

Kimbrough, J. C., and Morse, W. H.: Subcapsular nephrectomy. Surg. Gynecol. Obstet., 96:235, 1953.

King, L. R., Coughlin, P. W. F., Bloch, E. C., Bowie, J. D., Ansong, K., and Hanna, M. K.: The case for immediate pyeloplasty in the neonate with ureteropelvic junction obstruction. J. Urol., 132:725, 1984.

King, L. R., Kozlowski, J. M., and Schacht, M. J.: Ureteroceles in children: A simplified and successful approach to management. JAMA, 249:1461, 1983.

Kittredge, W. E., and Fridge, J. C.: Subcapsular nephrectomy. JAMA, 168:758, 1958.

Kocher, T., and Langham, T.: Ein Nephrotome wegen neirnsarkom. Zugleich ein beitrag zur histologie des nierenkrebses. Deutsch. Z. Chirc. (Leipzig), 9:312–328, 1878.

Koff, S. A., Hayden, L. J., Cirulli, C., and Short, R.: Pathophysiology of ureteropelvic junction obstruction: experimental and clinical observations. J. Urol., 136:336, 1986.

Koff, S. A., Thrall, J. H., and Keyes, J. W., Jr.: Diuretic radionuclide urography: A noninvasive method for evaluating nephroureteral dilatation. J. Urol., 122:451, 1979.

Koff, S. A., Thrall, J. H., and Keyes, J. W., Jr.: Assessment of hydroureteronephrosis in children using diuretic radionuclide urography. J. Urol., 123:531, 1980.

Kretschmer, H. L.: Life after nephrectomy. JAMA, 121:473, 1943.

Kumar, A., Sharma, S. K., and Vaidyanathan, S.: Results of surgical reconstruction in patients with renal failure owing to ureteropelvic junction obstruction. J. Urol., 140:484, 1988.

Kuster: Ein fall von Resection des Ureter. Arch. Klin. Chir., 44:850, 1892.

Kyriakidis, A., Karidis, G., Papachaialambous, A., et al.: Surgical management of renal staghorn calculi by selective hypothermic perfusion. Eur. Urol., 5:173, 1979.

Leach, G. E., and Kieber, M. M.: Partial nephrectomy: Mayo Clinic experience 1957–1977. Urology, 15:219, 1980.

Leary, F. J., Utz, D. C., and Wakim, K. G. P.: Effects of continuous and intermittent ischemia or renal function. Surg. Gynecol. Obstet., 116:311, 1963.

Lebowitz, R. L., and Johan, B. G.: The coexistence of ureteropelvic junction obstruction and reflux. Am. J. Radiol., 140:231, 1982.

Levitt, S. B., Nabizadeh, I., Javaid, M., Barr, M., Kogan, S. J., Hanna, M. K., Milstein, D., and Weiss, R.: Primary calicoureterostomy for pelvioureteral junction obstruction: Indications and results. J. Urol., 126:382, 1981.

Levy, M.: Oxygen consumption and blood flow in the hypothermic perfused kidney. Am. J. Physiol., 197:1111, 1959.

Libertino, J. A., Zinman, L., and Watkins, E.: Long-term results of resection of renal cell cancer with extension into inferior vena cava. J. Urol., 137:21, 1987.

Lower, W. E.: Conservative surgical methods in operating for stone in the kidney. Cleve. Med. J., 12:260, 1913.

Lue, Y. B., Anderson, E. E., and Harrison, J. H.: The surgical management of polycystic renal disease. Gynecol. Obstet., 122:45, 1966.

Luttrop, W., Nelson, C. E., Nilsson, T., et al.: Study of glomerular and tubular function after in situ cooling of the kidney. J. Urol., 115:133, 1976.

Lyon, R. P.: An anterior extraperitoneal incision for kidney surgery. J. Urol., 79:383, 1958.

Maatman, T. J., Novick, A. C., Tanzinco, B. F., et al.: Renal oncocytoma: A diagnostic dilemma. J. Urol., 132:878, 1984.

Macksood, M. J., Roth, D. R., Chang, C. H., and Perlmutter, A. D.: Benign fibroepithelial polyps as a cause of intermittent ureteropelvic junction obstruction in a child: a case report and review of the literature. J. Urol., 134:951, 1985.

Maizels, M., and Stephens, F. D.: Valves of the ureter as a cause of primary obstruction of the ureter: Anatomic, embryologic and clinical aspects. J. Urol., 123:742, 1980.

Malek, R. S.: Intermittent hydronephrosis: The occult ureteropelvic obstruction. J. Urol., 130:863, 1983.

Marberger, M., Georgi, M., Guenther, R., et al.: Simultaneous balloon occlusion of the renal artery and hypothermic perfusion in in situ surgery of the kidney. J. Urol., 119:463, 1978.

Marberger, M., Pugh, R. C. B., Auvert, J., Bertermann, H., Costantini, A., Gammelgaard, P. A., Peterson, S., and Wickham, J. E. A.: Conservative surgery of renal carcinoma: the EIRSS experience. Br. J. Urol., 53:528, 1981.

Marshall, F. F., and Reitz, B. A.: Technique for removal of renal cell carcinoma with suprahepatic vena caval tumor thrombus. Urol. Clin. North Am. 13:551, 1986.

Marshall, F. F., Taxy, J. B., Fishman, E. K., and Chang, R.: The feasibility of surgical enucleation for renal cell carcinoma. J. Urol., 135:231, 1986.

McLaughlin, G. A., Heal, M. R., and Tyrell, I. M.: An evaluation of techniques used for production of temporary renal ischemia. Br. J. Urol., 50:371, 1978.

McVary, K. T., and O'Conor, V. J.: Transmission of non-A non-B hepatitis during coagulum pyelolithotomy. J. Urol., 141:923, 1989.

Metzner, P. J., and Boyce, W. H.: Simplified renal hypothermia: An adjunct to conservative renal surgery. Br. J. Urol., 44:76, 1972.

Middleton, R. G., and Presto, A. J., III: Radical thoracoabdominal nephrectomy for renal cell carcinoma. J. Urol., 110:36, 1973.

Miki, M., Inaba, Y., and Machida, T.: Operative nephroscopy with fiberoptic scope: Preliminary report. J. Urol., 119:166, 1978.

Milam, J. H., Magee, J. H., and Bunts, R. C.: Evaluation of surgical decompression of polycystic kidneys by differential renal clearances. J. Urol., 90:144, 1963.

Mitchell, R. M.: Renal cooling and ischemia. Br. J. Surg., 46:593, 1959.

Morris, H.: A case of nephrolithotomy or the extraction of a calculus from an undilated kidney. Trans. Clin. Soc. (London), 14:31, 1881.

Neely, W. A., and Turner, M. D.: The effect of arterial venous and arteriovenous occlusion on renal blood flow. Surg. Gynecol. Obstet., 108:669, 1959.

Nesbit, R. M.: Diagnosis of intermittent hydronephrosis: Importance of pyelography during episodes of pain. J. Urol., 75:767, 1956.

Nesbit, R. M.: Elliptical anastomosis in urologic surgery. Ann. Surg., 130:796, 1949.

Neves, R. J., and Zincke, H.: Surgical treatment of renal cancer with vena cava extension. Br. J. Urol., 59:390, 1987.

Nguyen, D. H., Aliabadi, H., Ercole, C. J., and Gonzalez, R.: Nonintubated Anderson-Hynes repair of ureteropelvic junction obstruction in 60 patients. J. Urol., 142:704, 1989.

Noble, M.: Miscellaneous renal operations. In Novick, A. C., Streem, S. B., and Pontes, J. E. (Eds.): Stewart's Operative Urology, 2nd ed. Baltimore, Williams & Wilkins, 1989.

Nosowsky, E. E., and Kaufman, J. J.: The protection action of mannitol in renal artery occlusion. J. Urol., 89:295, 1963.

Novick, A. C.: Posterior surgical approach to the kidney and ureter. J. Urol., 124:192, 1980.

Novick, A. C.: Renal hypothermia: In vivo and ex vivo. Urol. Clin. North Am., 10:637, 1983.

Novick, A. C.: Partial nephrectomy for renal cell carcinoma. Urol. Clin. North Am., 14:419, 1987.

Novick, A. C., and Cosgrove, D. M.: Surgical approach for removal of renal cell carcinoma extending into the vena cava and the right atrium. J. Urol., 123:947, 1980.

Novick, A. C., Kaye, M., Cosgrove, D., et al.: Experience with cardiopulmonary bypass and deep hypothermic circulatory arrest in the management of retroperitoneal tumors with large vena caval thrombi. Ann. Surg., 212:472, 1990.

Novick, A. C., Streem, S., Montie, J. E., et al.: Conservative surgery for renal cell carcinoma: A single-center experience with 100 cases. J. Urol., 141:835, 1989.

O'Reilly, P. H.: Diuresis renography eight years later: An update. J. Urol., 136:993, 1986.

O'Reilly, P. H.: Functional outcome of pyeloplasty for ureteropelvic junction obstruction: Prospective study in 30 consecutive cases. J. Urol., 142:273, 1989.

O'Reilly, P. H., Testa, H. J., Lawson, R. S., Farrar, D. J., and Edwards, E. C.: Diuresis renography in equivocal urinary tract obstruction. Br. J. Urol., 50:76, 1978.

Papathanassiadis, S., and Swinney, J.: Results of partial nephrectomy compared with pyelolithotomy and nephrolithotomy. Br. J. Urol., 38:403, 1966.

Parrott, T. S., Woodard, J. R., Trulock, T. S., and Glenn, J. F.: Segmental renal vein renins and partial nephrectomy for hypertension in children. J. Urol., 131:736, 1984.

Pathak, I. C.: Survival after right nephrectomy, excision of infrahepatic vena cava and ligation of left renal vein: A case report. J. Urol., 106:599, 1971.

Pence, J. R., Airhart, R. A., and Novicki, D. E.: Coagulum pyelolithotomy. J. Urol. (Letter), 125:134, 1981.

Perlmutter, A. D., Kroovand, R. L., and Lai, Y. W.: Management of ureteropelvic obstruction in the first year of life. J. Urol., 123:535, 1980.

Petersen, H. K., Moller, B. B., and Iverson, H. J.: Regional hypothermia in renal surgery for severe lithiasis. Scand. J. Urol. Nephrol., 11:27, 1977.

Poutasse, E. F.: Anterior approach to the upper urinary tracts. J. Urol., 85:199, 1961.

Pritchett, T. R., Raval, J. K., Benson, R. C., Lieskovsky, G., Colletti, P. M., Boswell, W. D., and Skinner, D. G.: Preoperative magnetic resonance imaging of vena caval tumor thrombi: Experience with 5 cases. J. Urol., 138:1220, 1987.

Psihramis, K. E., and Dretler, S. P.: Extracorporeal shock wave lithotripsy of calyceal diverticula calculi. J. Urol., 138:707, 1987.

Rehn, R.: Gefasskomplikationem und ihre beherrschung bei dem Hypernephrom. Z. Urol. Chir., 10:326, 1922.

Resnick, M. I.: Evaluation and management of infection stones. Urol. Clin. North Am., 8:265, 1981.

Rezvani, A., Ward, J. N., and Lavengood, R. W., Jr.: Intrarenal aneurysm following partial nephrectomy. Urology, 2:286, 1973.

Riehle, R. A., Jr., and Vaughan, E. D., Jr.: Renin participation in hypertension associated with unilateral hydronephrosis. J. Urol., 126:243, 1981.

Robitalle, P., Mongeau, J. G., Lortie, L., and Sinnassamy, P.: Long-term follow-up of patients who underwent unilateral nephrectomy in childhood. Lancet, 1:1297, 1985.

Robson, C. J., Churchill, B. M., and Anderson, W.: The results of radical nephrectomy for renal cell carcinoma. J. Urol., 101:297, 1969.

Rosenthal, C. L., Kraft, R., and Zingg, E. J.: Organ-preserving surgery in renal cell carcinoma: Tumor enucleation versus partial kidney resection. Eur. Urol., 10:222, 1984.

Ross, J. H., Streem, S. B., Novick, A. C., Kay, R., and Montie, J.: Ureterocalicostomy for reconstruction of complicated pelviureteric junction obstruction. Br. J. Urol., 65:322, 1990.

Roth, D. R., and Gonzales, E. T., Jr.: Management of ureteropelvic junction obstruction in infants. J. Urol., 129:108, 1983.

Roth, R. A., and Findlayson, B.: Partial nephrectomy and nephrectomy for stones. In Roth, R. A., and Findlayson, B. (Eds.): Stones: Clinical Management of Urolithiasis. Baltimore, Williams & Wilkins, 1983.

Rous, S. N., and Turner, W. R.: Retrospective study of 95 patients with staghorn calculus disease. J. Urol., 118:902, 1977.

Scardino, P. L., and Prince, C. L.: Vertical flap ureteropelvioplasty: Preliminary report. South. Med. J., 46:325, 1953.

Schaeffer, A. J., and Grayhack, J. T.: Surgical management of ureteropelvic junction obstruction. In Walsh, P. C., Gittes, R. F., Perlmutter, A. D., and Stamey, T. A. (Eds.): Campbell's Urology, 5th ed. Philadelphia, W. B. Saunders Co., 1986.

Schefft, P., Novick, A. C., Stewart, B. H., et al.: Renal revascularization in patients with total occlusion of the renal artery. J. Urol., 124:184, 1980.

Schefft, P., Novick, A. C., Straffon, R. A., and Stewart, B. H.: Surgery for renal cell carcinoma extending into the vena cava. J. Urol., 120:28, 1978.

Schirmer, H., Taft, J. L., and Scott, W. W.: Renal metabolism after occlusion of the renal artery and after occlusion of the renal artery and vein. J. Urol., 96:136, 1966.

Schulze, H., Hertle, L., Graff, J., Funke, P. J., and Senge, T.: Combined treatment of branched calculi by percutaneous nephrolithotomy and extracorporeal shock wave lithotripsy. J. Urol., 135:1138, 1986.

Schwyzer, A.: New pyeloureteral plastic operation for hydronephrosis. Surg. Clin. North Am., 3:1441, 1923.

Simon, G.: Extirpation einer allere am menschen. Deutsch. Klin., 22:137, 1870.

Skinner, D. G., Colvin, R. B., Vermillion, C. D., Pfister, R. C., and Leadbetter, W. F.: Diagnosis and management of renal cell carcinoma: a clinical and pathological study of 309 cases. Cancer, 28:1165, 1971.

Skinner, D. G., Pritchett, T. R., Lieskovsky, G., Boyd, S. D., and Stiles, Q. R.: Vena caval involvement by renal cell carcinoma: Surgical resection provides meaningful long-term survival. Ann. Surg., 210:387, 1989.

Smith, A. D., Orihada, E., and Crowly, A. R.: Percutaneous management of renal pelvic tumors: A treatment option in selected cases. J. Urol., 137:852, 1987.

Smith, R. B., deKernion, J. B., Ehrlich, R. M., Skinner, D. G., and Kaufman, J. J.: Bilateral renal cell carcinoma and renal cell carcinoma in the solitary kidney. J. Urol., 132:450, 1984.

Snodgrass, W. T., and Robinson, M. J.: Intrarenal arteriovenous fistula: A complication of partial nephrectomy. J. Urol., 91:135, 1964.

Spencer, W. F., Novick, A., Montie, J. E., Streem, S. B., and Levin, H. S.: Surgical treatment of localized renal carcinoma in von Hippel-Lindau's disease. J. Urol., 139:507, 1988.

Spirnak, J. P., Resnick, M. I., and Persky, L.: Cutaneous pancreatic fistula as a complication of left nephrectomy. J. Urol., 132:329, 1984.

Stanisic, T. H., Babcock, J. R., and Grayhack, J. T.: Morbidity and mortality of renal exploration for cyst. Surg. Gynecol. Obstet., 145:733, 1977.

Stephens, F. D.: Ureterovascular hydronephrosis and the "aberrant" renal vessels. J. Urol., 128:984, 1982.

Streem, S. B., Geisinger, M. A., Risius, B., Zelch, M. G., and Siegel, S. W.: Endourologic "sandwich" therapy for extensive staghorn calculi. J. Endourol., 1:253, 1987.

Streem, S. B., and Pontes, J. E.: Percutaneous management of upper tract transitional cell carcinoma. J. Urol., 135:773, 1986.

Stubbs, A. J., Resnick, M. I., and Boyce, W. H.: Anatrophic nephrolithotomy in the solitary kidney. J. Urol., 119:457, 1978.

Swanson, D. A., and Borges, P. M.: Complications of transabdominal radical nephrectomy for renal cell carcinoma. J. Urol., 129:704, 1983.

Tessler, A. N., Yuvienco, F., and Farcon, E.: Paramedian extraperitoneal incision for total nephroureterectomy. Urology, 5:397, 1975.

Thompson, I. M., Baker, J., Robards, V. L., Jr., Kovacsi, L., and Ross, G., Jr.: Clinical experience with renal capsule flap pyeloplasty. J. Urol., 101:487, 1969.

Topley, M., Novick, A. C., and Montie, J. E.: Long-term results following partial nephrectomy for localized renal adenocarcinoma. J. Urol., 131:1050, 1984.

Vargas, A. D., Bragin, S. D., and Mendez, R.: Staghorn calculus: Its clinical presentation, complications and management. J. Urol., 127:860, 1982.

Vermooten, V.: Indications for conservative surgery in certain renal tumors: a study based on the growth pattern of clear cell carcinoma. J. Urol., 64:200, 1950.

Wagenknecht, L. V., Lupe, W., Bucheler, E., et al.: Selective hypothermic perfusion of the kidney for intrarenal surgery. Eur. Urol., 3:62, 1977.

Ward, J. P.: Determination of optimum temperature for regional renal hypothermia during temporary renal ischema. Br. J. Urol., 47:17, 1975.

Watson, G. M., Wickham, J. E. A., and Colvin, B.: Does calcium contribute to the effectiveness of a coagulum pyelolithotomy? Br. J. Urol., 56:131, 1984.

Welch, M., Bazaral, M. G., Schmidt, R., Pontes, J. E., Cosgrove, D. M., Montie, J. E., and Novick, A. C.: Anesthetic management for surgical removal of renal cell carcinoma with caval or atrial tumor thrombus using deep hypothermic circulatory arrest. J. Cardiothoracic. Anesth., 3:580, 1989.

Wells, S.: Successful removal of two solid circum-renal tumors. Br. Med. J., 1:758, 1884.

Whitaker, R. H.: Methods of assessing obstruction in dilated ureters. Br. J. Urol., 45:15, 1973.

Whitaker, R. H.: Clinical assessment of pelvic and ureteral function. Urology, 12:146, 1978.

Wickham, J. E. A., Hanley, H. G., and Joekes, A. M.: Regional renal hypothermia. Br. J. Urol., 39:727, 1967.

Wilson, D. H., Barton, B. B., Parry, W. L., et al.: Effects of intermittent versus continuous renal arterial occlusion on hemodynamics and function of the kidney. Invest. Urol., 8:507, 1971.

Wollin, M., Duffy, P. G., Diamond, D. A., Aguirre, J., Ratta, B. S., and Ransley, P. G.: Priorities in urinary diversion following pyeloplasty. J. Urol., 142:576, 1989.

Wolpert, J. J., Woodard, J. R., and Parrott, T. S.: Pyeloplasty in the young infant. J. Urol., 142:573, 1989.

Woodruff, L. M.: Eleventh rib, extrapleural approach to the kidney. J. Urol., 73:183, 1955.

Wulfsohn, M. A.: Extended pyelolithotomy: the use of renal artery clamping and regional hypothermia. J. Urol., 125:467, 1981.

Zabbo, A., and Novick, A. C.: Digital subtraction angiography for non-invasive imaging of the renal artery. Urol. Clin. North Am., 11:409, 1984.

Zabbo, A., Streem, S. B., Novick, A. C., and Risius, B.: Intravenous digital subtraction angiography for preoperative evaluation of patients with extensive calculus disease. Cleve. Clin. J. Med., 55:263, 1988.

Ziegelbaum, M., Novick, A. C., Streem, S. B., et al.: Conservative surgery for transitional cell carcinoma of the renal pelvis. J. Urol., 138:1146, 1987.

Zincke, H., Engen, D. E., Henning, K. M., and McDonald, M. W.: Treatment of renal cell carcinoma by in situ partial nephrectomy and extracorporeal operation with autotransplantation. Mayo Clin. Proc., 60:651, 1985.

Zincke, H., Kelalis, P. P., and Culp, O. S.: Ureteropelvic obstruction in children. Surg. Gynecol. Obstet., 139:873, 1974.

Zincke, H., and Neves, R. J.: Feasibility of conservative surgery for transitional cell cancer of the upper urinary tract. Urol. Clin. North Am., 11:717, 1984.

Zinner, M. J., Baker, R. R., and Cameron, J. L.: Pancreatic cutaneous fistulas. Surg. Gynecol. Obstet., 138:710, 1974.

66
RENAL TRANSPLANTATION

John M. Barry, M.D.

Why should urologists and urology residents be interested in renal transplantation? Each renal transplant operation is a study of pelvic anatomy, each cadaver nephrectomy is a study of retroperitoneal anatomy, and each living-donor nephrectomy is an operation on a kidney, a procedure that is decreasing in frequency because of nonoperative methods of treating renal stones and obstruction. Nowhere in urology must the principles of urinary tract reconstruction and infection control be more rigorously applied than in the immunosuppressed kidney transplant recipient. Understanding the molecular mechanisms of antigen-lymphocyte interactions in transplantation should provide insights into other disease processes such as cancer and infection. Renal preservation principles are often applied to parenchyma-sparing renal operations and to complex renovascular reconstruction procedures. As more renal transplant operations are performed, more of these patients are apt to present to the practicing urologist for pretransplant urinary tract evaluations and for the care of urologic problems that may or may not be related to the renal transplantation.

INCIDENCE OF END-STAGE RENAL DISEASE

In 1987, the number of patients starting renal replacement therapy for end-stage renal disease (ESRD) in the

Table 66–1. CAUSES OF END-STAGE RENAL DISEASE

Primary Disease	Number	% of Total
Diabetes mellitus	10,025	29.9
Hypertension	8,740	26.0
Glomerulonephritis	4,836	14.4
Cystic kidney disease	1,215	3.6
Other urologic diseases	2,018	6.0
Other identifiable diseases	1,938	5.8
Cause unknown	2,569	7.6
Cause missing	2,237	6.7
Total	33,578	100.0

Adapted from U.S. Renal Data System: USRDS 1989 Annual Data Report. Bethesda, National Institute of Diabetes and Digestive and Kidney Diseases, August 1989.

United States was 130 per million population (U.S. Renal Data System, USRDS 1989 Annual Report). The median age of those new ESRD patients was 60 years, a rise of 6 years during the preceding decade. Both the prevalence and incidence of ESRD are more common in the elderly than in the young, in men than in women, and in black persons than in white. Diabetes is the most frequent cause of ESRD, followed by hypertension and glomerulonephritis (Table 66–1). The incidence rate for hypertension-caused ESRD in black persons is 6.5 times that for white.

Treatment Options

In-center hemodialysis is the predominant form of therapy for ESRD. In 1988, it accounted for 82% of all dialysis patients and 63% of all ESRD patients (USRDS, 1989). Transplantation, however, is the predominant mode of care for the young. In recent years, the proportion of ESRD patients treated with chronic ambulatory peritoneal dialysis and continuous-cycling peritoneal dialysis has increased. Desire for self-care and difficulties with hemodialysis therapy are the most frequent indications for peritoneal dialysis. The estimated medical payment for ESRD in the United States in 1987 was $4.4 billion, and by 1991 this amount will exceed $5 billion. Renal transplantation is the preferred method of therapy for most patients with ESRD because it is more cost-effective (Eggers, 1988) and allows a return to a more normal lifestyle than does maintenance dialysis (Evans et al., 1985). In February, 1990, 16,656 patients were still on the waiting list for cadaver kidney grafts of the United Network for Organ Sharing (UNOS), even though there were 8886 kidney transplants performed in the United States in the preceding year and of those, 7064 were from cadaver donors (UNOS, 1990).

Results of Treatment

The survival probabilities for patients treated with transplantation or dialysis are presented in Figure 66–1.

2501

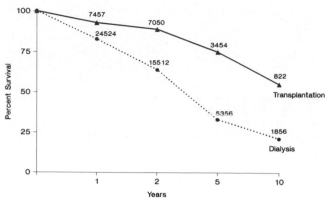

Figure 66–1. The effect of treatment modality on patient survival may reflect selection of better-risk patients for transplantation. (From data in U.S. Renal Data System: USRDS 1989 Annual Data Report. Bethesda, National Institute of Diabetes and Digestive and Kidney Diseases, August 1989.)

Although survival after renal transplantation is significantly better than that for patients treated with dialysis, this result may simply mean that healthier patients are more likely to be transplant recipients. Patients whose diagnosis was diabetes or hypertension had poorer survival than did patients with other causes of ESRD.

Survival of kidney grafts has improved. The 2-year survival of grafts from a living related donor increased from 79 per cent for transplants done in 1982 to 86 per cent for those done in 1986 (USRDS, 1989). For cadaver-donor kidney grafts, the 2-year graft survival increased from 55 to 70 per cent for the same interval. This change corresponds to the introduction of cyclosporine in 1983 and the more widespread use of antilymphocyte antibody preparations such as muromonab CD3 (OKT3) and Minnesota antilymphocyte globulin (MALG).

HISTORY OF HUMAN RENAL TRANSPLANTATION

The history of renal transplantation illustrates the successful combination of the fields of surgery, medicine, immunology, and politics. In 1933, the first human renal allograft was performed by Voronoy in the Ukraine (Hamilton and Reid, 1984). The recipient was a 26-year-old woman who had attempted suicide by ingesting mercuric chloride. The donor was a 60-year-old man whose kidney was removed 6 hours after death. With local anesthesia, the renal vessels were anastomosed to the femoral vessels and a cutaneous ureterostomy was performed. A small amount of blood-stained urine appeared, and the patient died 48 hours after the procedure. The first long-term success with human renal allografting occurred in Boston in 1954 when a kidney from one twin was transplanted into the other who had ESRD (Hamilton, 1988). In 1958, the first histocompatibility antigen was described. Radiation was used for immunosuppression in 1959, azathioprine became available for use in humans in 1961, and prednisolone became part of a standard immunosuppression regimen with

azathioprine in 1962. In the same year, tissue matching to select donor and recipient pairs was first done. The direct cross-match between donor lymphocytes and recipient serum was introduced in 1966, and heterologous antilymphocyte serum was used as an immunosuppressant in human renal transplantation. In the late 1960s, preservation of human kidneys for more than 24 hours became possible with either pulsatile machine perfusion (Belzer et al., 1967) or simple cold storage after flushing with an intracellular electrolyte solution (Collins et al., 1969). The beneficial effect of blood transfusions was described by Opelz and co-workers, in 1973, which led to immunologic conditioning with blood products for both cadaver and living-donor renal transplants. Donor-specific blood transfusions eventually became part of standardized pretransplant immunologic conditioning protocols for living-donor renal transplantation (Salvatierra et al., 1980). Medicare coinsurance for ESRD patients was passed into law in 1972 and was instituted in 1973. This law removed a significant impediment to renal transplantation in the United States. In the mid-1970s, laws concerning brain death were passed, which allowed organ retrieval from beating-heart cadaver donors and reduced warm ischemia time. The first clinical trials with cyclosporine were reported by Calne and colleagues in 1978, and this report was followed 3 years later by accounts of the successful use of monoclonal antibody for the treatment of renal allograft rejection in humans (Cosimi et al., 1981). In 1984, Congress passed the National Transplant Act, which authorized a national organ-sharing system and grants for organ procurement.

PRETRANSPLANT EVALUATION

Overview

The preimmunosuppression evaluation is usually performed well in advance of the renal transplant operation. The objectives of the work-up are diagnosis of the primary disease and its risk of recurrence in the kidney graft, treatment of infections, discovery of occult malignancy, reduction of risk for post-transplant complications, and psychosocial and financial evaluation (Nohr, 1989). Generally accepted contraindications to renal transplantation and immunosuppression are the following: active invasive infection, active malignancy, high probability of operative mortality, unsuitable anatomic situation for technical success, and severe psychosocial or financial problems. Potential sources of dental sepsis must be treated. Immunizations against pneumococcal pneumonia, hepatitis B, and influenza are commonly done before transplantation. Patients with a history of heart disease or diabetes mellitus or who are older than 50 years usually have a cardiac performance evaluation and, if necessary, coronary arteriography. Significant coronary artery lesions are corrected before transplantation. Peptic ulcer disease must be controlled, cholelithiasis must be treated, and patients with a history of diverticulitis usually require segmental colectomy before transplantation. Patients with focal glomerulosclerosis need to be counseled about the high probability of disease recurrence in the kidney graft (Cheigh et al., 1980).

Urologic Evaluation

The purpose of the pretransplant urologic evaluation is to determine the suitability of the urinary bladder or conduit for urinary tract reconstruction and the necessity for pretransplant nephrectomy (Barry and Lemmers, 1989; Reinberg et al., 1990). The urologic evaluation includes determination of a history of urologic disease, especially tumors, stones, obstruction, and infection; physical examination; urinalysis; urine or bladder wash culture; voiding cystourethrography; and imaging of the upper urinary tract, usually by ultrasonography. Voiding cystourethrography is probably unnecessary for a patient with no history of urologic abnormalities, no significant hematuria, a negative urine culture result, and an ultrasound examination that reveals no stones, hydroureteronephrosis, or significant residual bladder urine. If urinary diversion is present, a retrograde contrast study with antibiotic coverage and drainage films will reveal the suitability of the conduit for urinary tract reconstruction during renal transplantation. Many ESRD patients with upper urinary tract diversions have bladders that are acceptable for transplantation, especially if the original reason for diversion was reflux pyelonephritis. These defunctionalized bladders usually regain normal volume within weeks of grafting. It is wise to obtain biopsies of the bladders of patients who have small, contracted bladders after multiple lower urinary tract operations. If bladder fibrosis is extensive on histologic examination and the bladder is not compliant, it may not be salvageable, and intestinal augmentation cystoplasty may be required before renal transplantation (Thomalla et al., 1989). These patients usually require clean, intermittent catheterization after grafting. A bladder wash for cytologic examination is recommended for patients with prior cyclophosphamide treatment because of reports of associated transitional cell carcinoma (Tuttle et al., 1988).

Clean, intermittent catheterization has been used successfully in transplant programs for the past decade in patients with diabetes mellitus, meningomyelocele, or transient bladder outlet obstruction (Shneidman et al., 1984). Continent intestinal pouches have been created before transplantation in patients with surgically absent bladders, and renal transplantation has been successful (Heritier et al., 1989). These pouches require daily irrigation until transplantation for removal of mucus.

Older men with obstructing prostates are managed with pretransplant transurethral prostatectomy or transurethral incision of the bladder neck and prostate (Orandi, 1987). If the patient has oligoanuria, a suprapubic cystostomy done at the time of bladder outlet surgery will allow the patient to instill sterile water and void daily until the operative site has healed, usually within 6 weeks. This procedure prevents scarring or obliteration of the prostatic fossa. An alternative to suprapubic cystostomy and daily bladder instillation is daily intermittent self-catheterization, with bladder filling and then voiding.

The indications for pretransplant nephrectomy are hypertension that is not controlled by dialysis and use of medications, persistent renal infection, renal calculi, renal obstruction, severe proteinuria, and polycystic kidneys with infection, severe bleeding, or massive enlargement. Severe proteinuria can also be managed by renal infarction, with nephrectomy thus avoided. Pretransplant nephrectomy is usually performed 6 weeks before transplantation to allow wound healing and the detection and treatment of surgically associated infection. The use of synthetic erythropoietin has reduced the effects of postnephrectomy anemia while the patient awaits transplantation. Bilateral vertical lumbotomies are well tolerated by patients with small kidneys who undergo nephrectomy (Freed, 1976). This procedure is illustrated in Figure 66–2. The flank approach is used when the patient is quite obese or a kidney is too large to remove via vertical lumbotomy. The abdominal approach is used when both kidneys are removed from a large patient; when the kidneys are too large to remove through the back; or when additional procedures, such as total ureterectomy, intestinal conduit removal, augmentation cystoplasty, or creation of a continent intestinal pouch, are planned at the same time.

Impotence is a significant problem in men with ESRD. Contributing factors are the accelerated arteriosclerosis of dialysis, hyperprolactinemia with secondary testosterone deficiency, side effects from antihypertensive medications, and poor self-image. If penile prosthesis surgery is to be done before renal transplantation, one of the semirigid devices is recommended because the risk of reoperation is less than that for the inflatable devices and because no prevesical reservoir is present to interfere with urinary tract reconstruction. If an inflatable device is selected, one that is self-contained or has a scrotal reservoir is advisable.

Dialysis Access

As patients approach the need for renal replacement therapy, dialysis access is required unless renal graft availability is such that the patient can undergo transplantation without dialysis. Temporary vascular access is more commonly accomplished by percutaneous subclavian catheter placement than by arteriovenous shunt construction (Hefty et al., 1989). Long-term vascular access is obtained by the formation of a native arteriovenous fistula or an interposition graft of synthetic material or treated bovine carotid artery. The nondominant forearm is usually chosen. Figure 66–3 is an algorithm for decision-making in access surgery. The exit site for a chronic ambulatory peritoneal dialysis catheter should be placed well away from any potential kidney transplant incision.

DONOR SURGERY

Whether the kidney graft is removed from a living donor or a brain-dead cadaver donor, the surgical goals

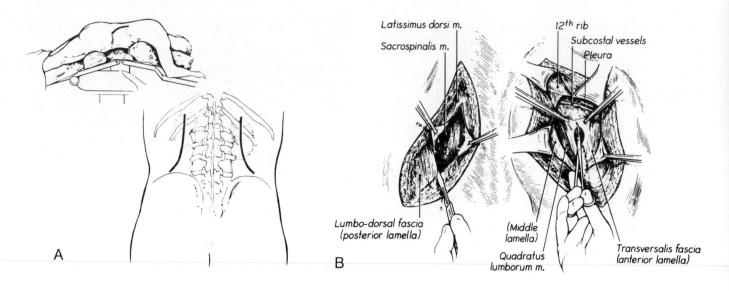

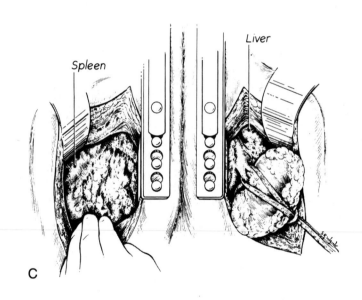

Figure 66–2. *A,* Prone position for bilateral removal of small end-stage kidneys. See text for indications. *B,* Simultaneous bilateral dissection. *C,* Self-retaining retractor with blades reversed facilitates exposure of renal pedicles. The incision can be extended by removing a section of the neck of the 12th rib. (From Freed, S. Z.: The present status of bilateral nephrectomy in transplant recipients. J. Urol., 115:8–11, © by Williams & Wilkins, 1976.)

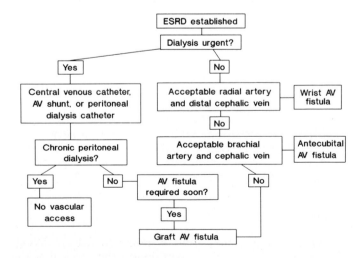

Figure 66–3. Algorithm for decision-making in dialysis access surgery. AV, arteriovenous. (Modified from Hefty, T. R., Hatch, T. R., and Barry, J. M.: Dialysis access surgery. *In* Novick, A. C., Streem, S. B., and Pontes, J. E. (Eds.): Stewart's Operative Urology. Baltimore, Williams & Wilkins Co., 1989, pp. 345–359. © 1989, the Williams & Wilkins Co., Baltimore.)

are the same: minimize warm ischemia time, preserve renal vessels, and preserve ureteral blood supply.

Living Donor

The advantages of renal transplantation with living, related donors are better graft survivals and less recipient morbidity when compared with cadaver kidney transplantation, specific planning of the operation to limit the waiting time on dialysis, and partial alleviation of the insufficient supply of cadaver kidneys. On the basis of a preoperative evaluation, one must be able to assure the donor of nearly normal renal function after unilateral nephrectomy. On evaluation, if one of the potential donor's kidneys is better than the other, the better kidney is left with the donor. Some physicians prefer to use the right kidney from women who may become pregnant because hydronephrosis of pregnancy occurs predominantly in that kidney. The initial evaluation includes a family conference, medical history, determination of ABO blood group compatibility, tissue typing, and microcytotoxicity lymphocyte cross-match. Potential donors then undergo a physical examination; laboratory assays including complete blood count and urinalysis, urine culture and sensitivity, serial serum creatinine levels, fasting blood glucose, serum electrolyte levels, liver function studies, and serologic screening for human immunodeficiency virus (HIV), human T-cell lymphotrophic virus type I (HTLV-I), hepatitis, cytomegalovirus (CMV), and syphilis; chest x-ray; electrocardiography; and intravenous pyelography. If the preceding results are satisfactory, aortography or digital subtraction arteriography is performed.

Living-donor nephrectomy is usually performed through a flank incision with a rib-resecting or supracostal approach (Fig. 66–4). The donor receives 25 g of mannitol in a 1-hour infusion beginning with the skin incision, and intravenous fluids are given to maintain a diuresis. The diuresis is confirmed by transecting the ureter and observing urine flow before interrupting renal circulation. After nephrectomy, the kidney is immediately placed in a pan of ice-cold solution and flushed with Ringer's lactate, Euro-Collins, or University of Wisconsin (UW) solution at 4°C. It is not necessary to administer heparin to the living related donor. The kidney is then taken in an ice bath into the recipient's operating room. The donor's wound is irrigated and is usually closed without drains, and the patient is taken to the recovery room where a chest x-ray film is obtained to exclude the possibility of pneumothorax. The complications are those of a standard flank nephrectomy. Endogenous creatinine clearance rapidly approaches 70 to 80 per cent of the preoperative level, and this level has been shown to be sustained for more than 10 years (Vincenti et al., 1983). The risk of development of late hypertension is nearly the same as that for the general population (Weiland et al., 1984). The short-term and long-term risks of living-donor nephrectomy are low enough, and the probability of successful graft outcome high enough, to make the procedure acceptable for fully informed donors.

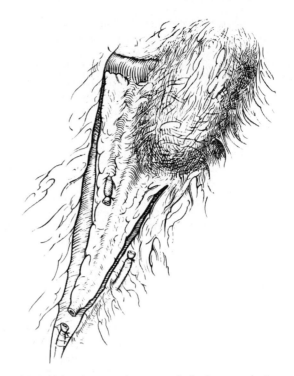

Figure 66–4. Living-donor nephrectomy via flank approach. A generous amount of periureteral tissue remains to preserve the ureteral blood supply. Renal circulation is not interrupted until a diuresis is ensured from the proximal end of the divided ureter. (From Streem, S. B.: Live donor nephrectomy. In Novick, A. C., Streem, S. B., and Pontes, J. E. (Eds.): Stewart's Operative Urology, Baltimore, Williams & Wilkins Co., 1989, pp. 312–323. © 1989, the Williams & Wilkins Co., Baltimore.)

Cadaver Donor

The usual criteria for cadaver kidney donors are ages 18 months to 55 years, no hypertension requiring treatment, no diabetes mellitus, no malignancy other than primary brain tumor or treated skin cancer, no evidence of renal disease, no generalized viral or bacterial infection, normal blood urea nitrogen and serum creatinine levels, acceptable urinalysis results, and negative assay results for syphilis, hepatitis, HIV, and HTLV-I. The lower age limit of 18 months for cadaver renal donors is because of small anatomic parts and the risk of technical problems, although there are reports of kidneys from younger donors functioning satisfactorily (Hudnall et al., 1989; Salvatierra and Belzer, 1975), and en bloc techniques have been used for transplanting small kidneys from pediatric patients into large recipients (Anderson et al., 1974; Goodwin et al., 1963). The upper age limit exists because of nephrosclerosis. An analysis of 13,911 first cadaver kidney transplants revealed that the 1-year graft survival for kidneys from donors between the ages of 55 and 60 years was 12 per cent lower than that for kidneys from donors between the ages of 16 and 30 years and that this survival was 17 per cent lower for kidney grafts from donors older than 60 years (Terasaki et al., 1988). Kidney grafts from 397 donors aged between 3 and 6 years into adult recipients had significantly poorer survival when compared with 10,545 kidney grafts from cadaver donors whose age at death was more than 6 years. Kidney grafts from old or small donors are thus used only when organ shortage is extreme.

The initial goals of resuscitation of the brain-dead cadaver donor are systolic blood pressure of 90 mm Hg and urinary output exceeding 0.5 ml/kg/hour. A central venous line is helpful for intravenous fluid management. Serum electrolyte levels are checked every 2 to 4 hours. If the resuscitation goals cannot be met by a fluid challenge and the central venous pressure is greater than 15 cm H_2O, a vasopressor (dopamine, dobutamine, or isoproterenol) can be infused. If intravascular volume expansion and vasopressors are unsuccessful in promoting a diuresis, furosemide at 1 mg/kg and/or mannitol at 0.5 to 1.0 g/kg can be infused. If diabetes insipidus results in an unmanageable diuresis, vasopressin with chlorobutanol (Pitressin) can be administered. High doses of glucocorticoids may reduce the incidence of delayed graft function when cold storage time is prolonged. Tissue typing and cross-matching can be performed on a peripheral blood sample before organ retrieval. The cadaver donor is maintained in the operating room by the anesthesiology team to ensure ventilation and circulatory support and to administer drugs such as diuretics, heparin, and alpha-adrenergic–blocking agents.

More than three fourths of renal donors are now multiple organ donors, and the classic abdominal midline and cruciate incisions are being abandoned in favor of the total midline approach with median sternotomy (Fig. 66–5A), even when kidneys alone are retrieved (Barry, 1989). The retroperitoneum is entered, much as for a retroperitoneal lymphadenectomy, by incising the posterior peritoneum from the portal triad around the hepatic flexure, right colon, and cecum up to the ligament of Treitz (Fig. 66–5B). The intestines are retracted anteriorly and, if the liver and the pancreas are not to be retrieved, the superior mesenteric artery is divided between secure ligatures. (When the liver and pancreas are also retrieved, the supraceliac aorta must be controlled.) The inferior vena cava and aorta are controlled at their respective bifurcations and above the level of the renal veins and superior mesenteric artery. Heparin is administered to the donor, and the distal aorta and inferior vena cava are cannulated (Fig. 66–5C). An alpha-adrenergic–blocking agent such as chlorpromazine or phentolamine can be administered at this point to prevent or reverse renal vasospasm unless the cardiac or liver retrieval teams request that it not be given. The proximal aorta and inferior vena cava are occluded, the vena cava is vented through its cannula, and in situ flushing with ice-cold preservation solution is begun through the aortic cannula. Bilateral, en bloc, simultaneous radical nephrectomies are then performed. The aorta and inferior vena cava are transected distally, gently elevated with the cannulas, and the lumbar arteries and veins are divided between clips. Care must be taken to avoid injury to the right renal artery as it passes posterior to the inferior vena cava. The aorta and inferior vena cava are transected proximally, and the en bloc specimen is taken to the back table and is flipped over; the kidneys are separated by splitting the aorta

first on its posterior surface (Fig. 66–5D), then on its anterior surface, and finally dividing the left renal vein at its entrance into the inferior vena cava. Splenic tissue and lymph nodes are removed for histocompatibility testing. The in situ flushing technique is preferred to the ex situ flushing technique because the shorter warm ischemia time results in a lower incidence of delayed graft function. The en bloc retrieval technique allows the preservation of multiple or anomalous renal vessels, permits the use of aortic patches for arterial reconstruction, and leaves the inferior vena cava with the right kidney for extension of the right renal vein. It has also allowed the retrieval of horseshoe kidneys for transplantation as a single unit or as two renal units by splitting them at the isthmus (Barry and Fincher, 1984).

KIDNEY PRESERVATION

Warm ischemic injury is due to failure of oxidative phosphorylation and cell death because of ATP depletion. The ability of a cell to resynthesize ATP as measured by ^{31}P magnetic resonance spectroscopy has been used as a measure of the reversibility of ischemic injury (Bretan et al., 1987). ATP is required for the cellular sodium-potassium pump to maintain a high intracellular concentration of potassium and a low intracellular concentration of sodium. When the sodium-potassium pump is impaired, sodium chloride and water passively diffuse into the cells, resulting in cellular swelling and the "no-reflow" phenomenon, with renal revascularization. Cellular potassium and magnesium are lost, calcium is gained, anaerobic glycolosis and acidosis occur, and lysosomal enzymes are activated. Cellular suicide results. During reperfusion, hypoxanthine, a product of ATP degradation, is oxidized to xanthine, with the formation of free radicals that cause further cell damage (Belzer and Southard, 1988).

Cellular energy requirements are significantly reduced by hypothermia, which is accomplished by surface cooling, hypothermic pulsatile perfusion, or flushing with an ice-cold solution followed by cold storage. Making the flush solution slightly hyperosmolar with impermeable solutes such as mannitol will help to prevent endothelial cell swelling and the no-reflow phenomenon. ATP-$MgCl_2$ infusions have been evaluated as an energy source. Calcium channel blockers, xanthine oxidase inhibitors, free radical scavengers, and lysosome stabilizers such as methylprednisolone have all been used to reduce ischemic injury (Marshall et al., 1988).

The basic methods of kidney preservation are pulsatile machine perfusion with a protein-based solution (Belzer et al., 1967) and hypothermic flushing followed by simple cold storage (Collins et al., 1969). After demonstration that the two methods provided equivalent results with ideally harvested dog kidneys after 48 hours of preservation (Halasz and Collins, 1976), simple cold storage became more widely used for human kidney preservation. Machine perfusion has provided reliable human kidney preservation for over 48 hours (Feduska et al., 1978), and there are reports of successfully extending preservation time for 48 to 95 hours with cold

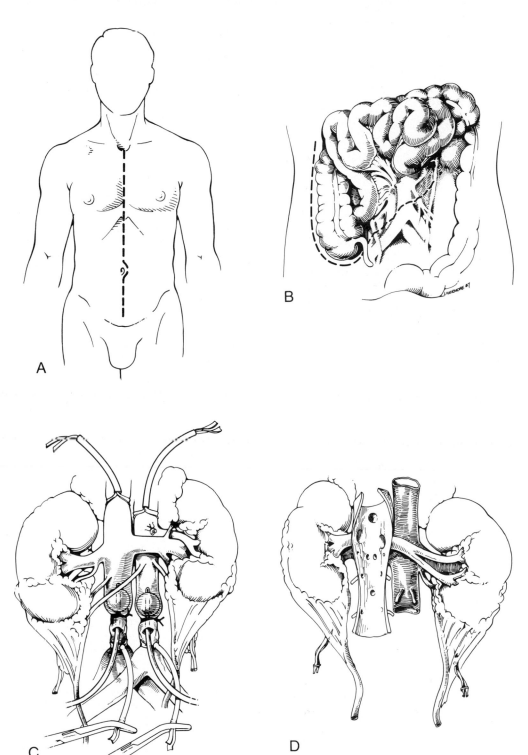

Figure 66–5. *A,* Total midline incision with splitting of sternum and diaphragm exposes all transplantable organs in chest and abdomen. It provides excellent exposure for retrieving only abdominal organs. *B,* The retroperitoneum is exposed as for a retroperitoneal lymphadenectomy. *C,* The aorta and inferior vena cava are controlled above and below the renal vessels, heparin is administered to the donor, and the great vessels are cannulated. *D,* After in situ flushing with preservation solution and bilateral en bloc radical nephrectomies, the specimen is placed "face down" in a pan of slush and is separated, first, by splitting the aorta posteriorly between lumbar arteries to identify all renal arteries, second, by splitting the anterior aortic wall, and third, by dividing the left renal vein where it enters the inferior vena cava. (From Barry, J. M.: Cadaver donor nephrectomy. *In* Novick, A. C., Streem, S. B., and Pontes, J. E. (Eds.): Stewart's Operative Urology. Baltimore, Williams & Wilkins Co., 1989, pp. 294–300. © 1989, the Williams & Wilkins Co., Baltimore.)

A

B

C

D

Table 66–2. COMMONLY USED HYPOTHERMIC RENAL PRESERVATION SOLUTIONS

| UW Solution | | Intracellular Electrolyte Flush Solutions | | |
Substance	Amount in 1 L	Substance	Collins 2	Euro-Collins
Potassium lactobionate	100 mM	KH_2PO_4	15 mM	15 mM
KH_2PO_4	25 mM	$MgSO_4$	30 mM	0
$MgSO_4$	5 mM	KCl	15 mM	15 mM
Raffinose	30 mM	K_2HPO_4	42.5 mM	42.5 mM
Adenosine	5 mM	$NaHCO_3$	10 mM	10 mM
Glutathione	3 mM	Glucose	25 g	35 g
Allopurinol	1 mM			
Hydroxyethyl starch	50 g			
Insulin	40 U			
Dexamethasone	16 mg			
Penicillin	200,000 U			
Osmolarity (mOsm/L)	320		320	340

storage alone or in combination with machine perfusion (Haberal et al., 1984). The commonly used flushing solutions are compared in Table 66–2. The recently introduced University of Wisconsin (UW) solution (Belzer and Southard, 1988) minimizes cellular swelling with the impermeable solutes lactobionate, raffinose, and hydroxyethyl starch. Phosphate is used for its hydrogen ion–buffering qualities, adenosine is for ATP synthesis during reperfusion, glutathione is a free radical scavenger, allopurinol inhibits xanthine oxidase and the generation of free radicals, and magnesium and dexamethasone are membrane-stabilizing agents. A major advantage of this new preservation solution has been its value as a universal preservation solution for all intraabdominal organs. A prospectively randomized study of 257 cadaver kidney grafts preserved with either UW solution or Euro-Collins solution showed that the UW solution resulted in a significantly more rapid reduction in postoperative serum creatinine level and a trend toward a lower postoperative dialysis rate when compared with kidneys preserved with the Euro-Collins solution (Ploeg, 1990). Animal experiments have shown satisfactory kidney preservation for up to 72 hours with the UW solution (Ploeg et al., 1988).

RECIPIENT SELECTION FOR CADAVER KIDNEY TRANSPLANTS

A point system proposed by Starzl and colleagues in 1987 has been modified and adopted in the United States for the selection of cadaver kidney transplant recipients (Table 66–3). Initial screening consists of ABO blood group compatibility testing, negative microcytotoxicity lymphocyte cross-match between donor and recipient, and roughly matching the size of the donor kidney with that of the recipient. Kidneys from donors 10 years old or younger are offered for pediatric recipients 15 years old or younger before being offered for an older recipient. Patients whose serum reacts to a high proportion of lymphocytes on a random or selected panel receive points because the probability of obtaining a cross-match–negative kidney for them is decreased when compared with minimally sensitized potential recipients. Time on the waiting list and histocompatibility between donor and recipient result in additional points. For example, assume that there are 12 potential blood group O adult recipients for a cross-match–negative blood group O adult cadaver kidney graft. Each of the 12 is ranked by the time of waiting on the list. The patient who has been waiting the longest is then given one point, the one who has been most recently added to the list receives 1/12 point, and the others are assigned fractions of a point depending on their time-of-waiting rank. A patient waiting for 2 years receives an additional 2×0.5, or 1 point. If the panel reactive antibody is $\geq$ 80%, 4 more points are added. If there is a 0 human leukocyte antigen (HLA) mismatch of HLA-B, HLA-DR with the cadaver donor, 7 points are added. This patient and each of the other 11 potential recipients now have a total score, and they are then ranked by that score. The patient with the highest score is ranked number one. The kidney graft is then offered in turn to each of the potential recipients by the final rank. If there is no suitable recipient on the local list, the kidney graft is offered to those on the regional list and, if necessary, the national list. Currently, there is mandatory national sharing of a kidney when six HLA-A, HLA-B, and HLA-DR antigens are matched between a cadaver donor and a recipient.

Many programs do not cross the CMV barrier in recipients who are insulin-dependent diabetics or over

Table 66–3. POINT SYSTEM FOR ALLOCATION OF CADAVER KIDNEYS

Parameter			Maximal Points
Time of waiting			1
Time of waiting $\geq$ 1 year			0.5/year
Panel reactive antibody $\geq$ 80% and a negative preliminary cross-match			4
Histocompatibility			10
		Points	
0	A, B, DR mismatch	10	
0	B, DR mismatch	7	
0	A, B mismatch	6	
1	B, DR mismatch	3	
2	B, DR mismatch	2	
3	B, DR mismatch	1	

Adapted from UNOS Articles of Incorporation, By-Laws, and Policies. Policy 3.5 Allocation of Cadaveric Kidneys. UNOS, June 20, 1989.

the age of 50 years because of the morbidity of this infection when CMV-seronegative high-risk recipients receive kidneys from CMV-positive donors (Hennell et al., 1989). Others recommend prophylaxis with immunoglobulin (Steinmuller et al., 1989) or acyclovir (Balfour et al., 1989) when the CMV barrier is crossed or when there is significant risk of reactivation of CMV disease in seropositive recipients.

On urgent admission for cadaver kidney transplantation, the history and the physical examination of the recipient focus on a search for acute invasive infections, interval medical problems such as symptomatic cardiac disease, and the need for an additional cross-matching because of recent blood transfusions.

RECIPIENT OPERATION

A prophylactic antibiotic, usually a second-generation cephalosporin, is administered just before surgery and continued postoperatively until the results of intraoperative cultures are known. Immunosuppression is usually started 1 week before transplantation in the recipient of a living-donor kidney transplant, and just before or during surgery in the cadaver kidney graft recipient.

Technique

After induction of anesthesia and placement of a central venous pressure monitor, the genitalia and skin are prepared, and a Foley catheter is placed in the bladder. The bladder is rinsed with an antibiotic solution and is gravity filled to capacity, and the catheter is clamped until it is time to do the ureteroneocystostomy. A self-retaining ring retractor bolted to the operating table allows the operation to be performed by a surgeon and one assistant. Antibiotic irrigation is used liberally during the procedure. Central venous pressure is maintained between 10 and 15 cm H_2O with intravenous fluids. If the blood pressure cannot be maintained at

>90 mm Hg with that maneuver, a dopamine infusion is started.

In adults and large children, the kidney graft is usually placed extraperitoneally in the contralateral iliac fossa via a Gibson incision so that the renal pelvis and ureter are the most medial structures in case subsequent urinary tract surgery is necessary on the kidney graft. In men, the spermatic cord is mobilized, preserved, and medially retracted. Ligation and division of the spermatic cord resulted in ipsilateral hydrocele, testicular atrophy, testicular necrosis, or recurrent testicular pain in 74.5 per cent of 94 testes at risk in a report by Penn and co-workers (1972). An alternative method of spermatic cord preservation involves performance of the transplant in the potential triangle bounded by the peritoneum, vas deferens, and spermatic vessels (Barry, 1982). In women, the round ligament is divided between ligatures. The recipient's blood vessels are dissected, and lymphatics are divided between ligatures to avoid the development of postoperative lymphocele. Before the use of donor inferior vena cava to provide extension of the right renal vein in cadaver kidney transplants, the left kidney was preferred because of the longer renal vein. Methods of extending the right renal vein are illustrated in Figure 66–6. During the vascular anastomoses, an infusion of mannitol (0.5 to 1.0 g/kg) is begun to scavenge free radicals and to promote a diuresis after revascularization. The renal vein, with or without an extension, is usually anastomosed end to side to the external iliac vein. The renal artery is usually anastomosed end to end to the internal iliac artery (Fig. 66–7). Some prefer to do the renal artery anastomosis first because it is the more critical of the two vascular anastomoses. In the event of significant arteriosclerosis involving the internal iliac artery, the renal artery is anastomosed end to side to the external iliac artery or to the common iliac artery. A male candidate for a second kidney graft whose first transplant was anastomosed to the contralateral internal iliac artery should not have the ipsilateral internal iliac artery used to ensure a blood supply to the corpora cavernosa and to

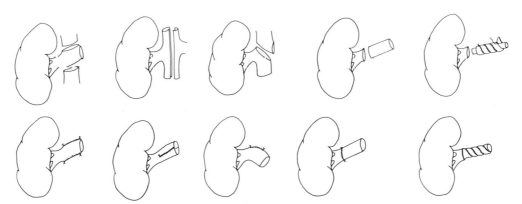

Figure 66–6. Methods of extending the right renal vein include modifications of the inferior vena cava, a free graft of donor external iliac vein, and a spiral graft of recipient gonadal vein. (Adapted from Barry J. M., and Fuchs, E. F.: Arch. Surg., 113:300, 1978, © American Medical Association; Barry, J. M., Hefty, T. R., and Sasaki, T.: Clam-shell technique for right renal vein extension in cadaver kidney transplantation. J. Urol., 140:1479, © by Williams & Wilkins, 1988; Chopin, D. K., Popov, Z., Abbou, C. C., et al.: Use of vena cava to obtain additional length for the right renal vein during transplantation of cadaveric kidneys. J. Urol., 141:1143–1144, © by Williams & Wilkins, 1989; Nghiem, D. D.: Spiral gonadal vein graft extension of right renal vein in living renal transplantation. J. Urol., 142:1525, © by Williams & Wilkins, 1989.)

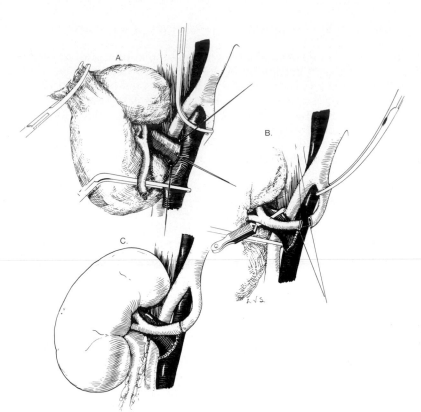

Figure 66–7. *A*, The renal vein is anastomosed to the external iliac vein, usually medial to the external iliac artery. When the recipient has a tortuous external iliac artery, the venous anastomosis is commonly performed lateral to the bowed external iliac artery. *B*, In the absence of significant recipient arteriosclerosis, the renal artery is anastomosed to the internal iliac artery with 5-0 or 6-0 monofilament, nonabsorbable sutures. Some prefer to perform the renal artery anastomosis before the venous anastomosis. *C*, The completed venous and arterial anastomoses. (From Salvatierra, O., Jr.: *In* Glenn, J. F. (Ed.): Urologic Surgery. 3rd ed. Philadelphia, J. B. Lippincott Co., 1983, pp. 362–366.)

reduce the risk of arteriogenic impotence (Gittes and Waters, 1979).

Multiple renal arteries are managed by making a "pair of pants" of two renal arteries and by anastomosing the waist to the recipient's artery, anastomosing the end of a small renal artery to the side of a larger one and then sewing the end of the larger artery to the recipient's artery, separately anastomosing the renal arteries to the recipient's arterial supply, anastomosing a lower-pole segmental artery end to end with the recipient's inferior epigastric artery and the main renal artery to one of the iliac arteries, anastomosing an aortic patch containing the renal arteries to the recipient's artery, or performing ex situ reconstruction with a branched internal iliac artery graft (Hinman, 1989; Novick, 1989). Children weighing less than 20 kg who receive an adult kidney usually have the renal artery and vein anastomosed to the aorta and inferior vena cava, respectively, and the graft placed posterior to the cecum and right colon (Fig. 66–8).

Urinary tract reconstruction is usually by antireflux ureteroneocystostomy. Ureteroureterostomy and pyeloureterostomy are usually reserved for patients with short or ischemic allograft ureters. Many physicians prefer the extravesical rather than the transvesical approach for ureteroneocystostomy because it is faster, a separate cystotomy is not required, and less ureteral length is necessary, thus ensuring the distal ureteral blood supply. The transvesical approach is illustrated in Figure 66–9. The two commonly used extravesical techniques are illustrated in Figure 66–10. Regardless of the technique, ureteral stents are used when there is concern about urinary leakage or obstruction related to a thickened bladder or to edema.

Patients with prior urinary diversions and unaccepta-

ble bladders for transplantation can be transplanted successfully. Standard vascular anastomoses are performed, and the ureter is anastomosed to the base of the urinary conduit over a stent that is left in place for 3 to 6 weeks and is then removed after a retrograde contrast study demonstrates the absence of extravasa-

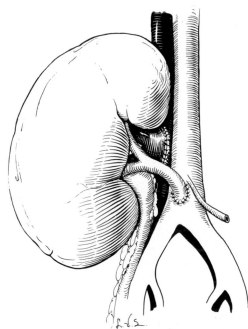

Figure 66–8. Transplantation of an adult kidney into a small child with anastomosis of the renal vein to the inferior vena cava and the renal artery to the aorta. (From Salvatierra, O., Jr.: *In* Glenn, J. F. (Ed.): Urologic Surgery. 3rd ed. Philadelphia, J. B. Lippincott Co., 1983, pp. 362–366.)

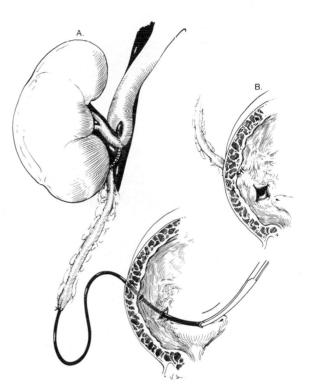

Figure 66–9. Transvesical ureteroneocystostomy. *A*, A No. 8 catheter is passed through the submucosal tunnel and secured to the transplant ureter. *B*, The ureter is drawn into the bladder, transected, spatulated, and secured with interrupted 4-0 or 5-0 absorbable sutures. The distal suture anchors the ureter to the bladder muscularis. (From Salvatierra, O., Jr.: *In* Glenn, J. F. (Ed.): Urologic Surgery. 3rd ed. Philadelphia, J. B. Lippincott Co., 1983, pp. 362–366.)

tion. The technique of ureteral implantation into a continent intestinal pouch is the same as that for ureteroneocystostomy except that it is protected by a stent. The pouch is irrigated free of mucus with an antibiotic solution, such as neomycin-polymyxin B sulfate, and the best site for the stented ureteral implantation is chosen with the pouch filled (Hatch and Hefty, 1990). Ureteral implantation into the afferent limb of a Kock pouch was described by Heritier and colleagues in 1989.

Opinions about wound closure vary. The uncomplicated renal transplant is usually closed without drains. The transverse muscle of the abdomen and the internal oblique muscle can be closed as a single running layer with 0 synthetic absorbable suture. The external oblique muscle and the anterior rectus sheath can be approximated by the same method. Closure of the reoperated iliac fossa is different. The muscle and fascial layers are closed as a single layer with interrupted far-far, near-near sutures of 0 polydioxanone suture. Vertical midline abdominal incisions in small children are closed with interrupted sutures of 2-0 or 3-0 polydioxanone. When a vertical midline incision has been used in an adult, it is closed with interrupted 0 nylon far-far, near-near sutures, especially if a reoperation or a combined kidney and pancreas transplant has been done. When drains are necessary, the closed-suction type are preferred. They are discontinued when the output is less than 30 ml/day.

Postoperative Care

Postoperative fluid and electrolyte management is simple for patients with initial kidney graft function.

Intravenous fluid of 0.45 per cent saline in 0 to 5 per cent dextrose is given at a rate equal to the previous hour's urinary output plus the estimated hourly insensible loss. When the urinary output is high, solutions with a lower dextrose concentration reduce the probability of iatrogenic solute diuresis. Serum electrolyte levels are monitored every 4 to 8 hours and potassium is added to the intravenous solution when the serum potassium level declines to the middle of the normal range. An estimate of the amount of potassium to add is based on a spot check of the urinary potassium concentration. After 24 to 48 hours, the diuresis slows, bowel continuity returns, oral fluids are administered, and the intravenous fluid rate is slowed and then stopped. When delayed graft function occurs, the previously described intravenous fluid is administered at a rate to maintain the central venous pressure at 10 to 15 cm H_2O for 2 to 3 hours, and furosemide is administered. After that, the rate just described is used. The oliguric patient may require urgent treatment of hyperkalemia or fluid overload, which is usually managed by dialysis. High levels of serum potassium can be counteracted by giving intravenous calcium chloride, and the levels then lowered by using intravenous sodium bicarbonate and/or glucose and insulin. These measures drive potassium into cells for 4 to 6 hours.

A baseline radioisotope renogram and ultrasonogram are obtained within 24 to 48 hours to detect the presence or absence of graft blood flow, urinary extravasation, ureteral obstruction, and fluid collections. A urine culture is obtained 24 hours before catheter removal, and antibiotics are started or changed on the basis of the identity of the organism or sensitivity testing. The timing of catheter removal varies from 12 hours in patients who

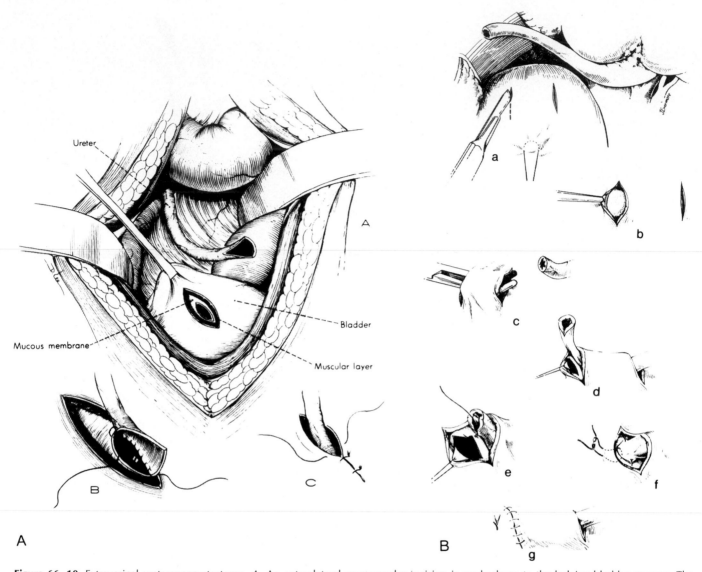

Figure 66–10. Extravesical ureteroneocystostomy. *A*, An anterolateral seromuscular incision is made down to the bulging bladder mucosa. The bladder is drained, the mucosa incised, and the ureter anastomosed to the bladder (as shown) with fine absorbable sutures. The seromuscular layer is loosely closed over the ureter. (From Konnak, J. W., Herwig, K. R., Finkbeiner, A., et al.: Extravesical ureteroneocystostomy in 170 renal transplant patients. J. Urol., 113:299–301, © by Williams & Wilkins, 1975.) *B*, Steps a through c are completed with the bladder full of an antibiotic solution. The anesthesiologist unclamps the catheter before mucosal incision, and steps d through g are completed with fine absorbable sutures. The catheter is removed on the fifth postoperative day after a gravity cystogram has demonstrated no leak. The catheter is removed on the seventh postoperative day in diabetics. (From Barry, J. M.: Unstented extravesical ureteroneocystostomy in kidney transplantation. J. Urol., 129:918–919, © by Williams & Wilkins, 1983.)

had uncomplicated extravesical ureteroneocystostomy (Konnak et al., 1975) to 7 days in diabetic recipients (Barry and Hatch, 1985) to 14 days in recipients of combined cadaver kidney and pancreas transplants with duodenocystostomy. Many physicians prefer to delay catheter removal until a gravity retrograde cystogram documents the absence of extravasation. If a ureteral stent was used to protect the urinary tract reconstruction, it is removed as an outpatient procedure 4 to 6 weeks after operation. Skin sutures or staples are removed 7 to 14 days postoperatively.

RENAL ALLOGRAFT REJECTION

Most kidney graft losses are caused by rejection, and most of those losses occur within 3 months of grafting.

Hyperacute rejection occurs immediately after renal revascularization. It is an irreversible process mediated by preformed circulating cytotoxic antibodies that develop after pregnancy, blood transfusions, or an earlier failed transplant. Accelerated rejection is mediated by humoral and cellular components of the immune response. It occurs within days to weeks and often does not respond to antirejection therapy. Acute rejection occurs within weeks to months after transplantation. The symptoms of acute kidney transplant rejection are those of influenza accompanied by pain over the kidney graft. Fever, increased blood pressure, decreased urinary output, fluid retention, increased blood urea nitrogen and serum creatinine levels, kidney graft enlargement, and decreased renal blood flow, glomerular filtration, and tubular function on radioisotope renography are signs associated with acute rejection. Acute

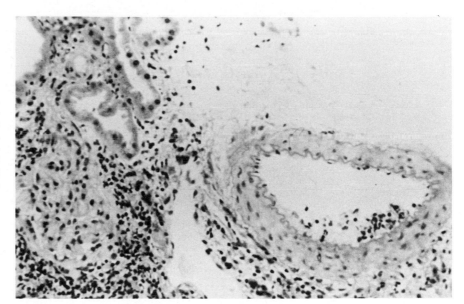

Figure 66–11. Acute renal allograft rejection. Mononuclear cells have infiltrated the interstitium, and there are subendothelial inflammatory cells in the small and medium sized arteries. (From Burdick, J. F., and Strom, T. B.: Immunosuppression in transplantation: The biology and therapeutic modalities. *In* Belzer, F. O. (Ed.): Transplant Surgical Resource Series. Raritan, NJ, Ortho Pharmaceutical Corp., 1988, pp. 2–28.)

pyelonephritis must be ruled out by urinalysis and subsequently negative urine culture results. Ultrasonically guided fine-needle biopsy of the kidney graft is sometimes necessary to confirm the diagnosis of acute rejection. The typical histologic findings are mononuclear cellular infiltration and vasculitis (Fig. 66–11). Chronic rejection is characterized by a gradual decline in renal function associated with interstitial fibrosis, vascular changes, and minimal mononuclear cell infiltration. The incidence and severity of rejection are modified by histocompatibility between donor and recipient, immunosuppression, and pretransplant immunologic conditioning, most commonly with transfusion of blood products.

Histocompatibility

The histocompatibility systems of greatest importance in renal transplantation are the ABO blood group and the HLA systems (Dallman and Morris, 1988). The donor and recipient must be ABO compatible because A and B substances are present on endothelial cells and most individuals have antibodies to the red blood cell antigens they lack. The major histocompatibility antigens are glycoproteins on the cell membrane. They are encoded by major histocompatibility complex (MHC) autosomal genes on the short arm of chromosome 6. These antigens are subdivided into class I and class II antigens. Class I antigens are known as the HLA-A, HLA-B, and HLA-C antigens, and they are present on nearly all nucleated cells. They are detected by serotyping T-lymphocytes. HLA-DR, HLA-DQ, and HLA-DP antigens are class II antigens present on B-lymphocytes, activated T-lymphocytes, monocytes, macrophages, dendritic cells, and some endothelial cells. HLA-DR antigens are detected by serotyping B-lymphocytes. Testing for HLA-DQ and HLA-DP antigens is not routinely done. Incompatibility with these MHC antigens on donor tissue stimulates the immune response (Fig. 66–12 and Table 66–4).

Class I and class II antigens on donor dendritic cells can directly stimulate recipient T-cells and initiate the rejection process (Krensky et al., 1990; Strom, 1990). These MHC antigens are also processed by host macrophages, which present class II antigens to the CD4-positive helper T-cells and class I antigens to the CD8-positive precursor cytotoxic T-cells. These macrophages produce interleukin (IL)-1. IL-1 has been described as a paracrine substance that activates helper T-cells di-

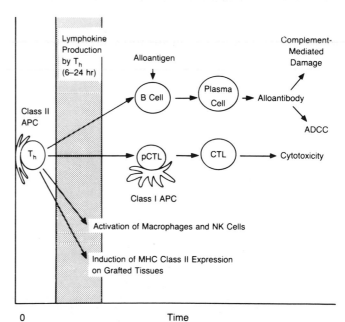

Figure 66–12. Cellular interactions in renal transplant rejection. CD4-positive helper T-cells (T_h) are activated by antigen-presenting cells (APC) expressing incompatible MHC class II antigens. The T_h cells produce lymphokines that promote proliferation of B-cells, maturation of CD8-positive cytotoxic T-cells (CTL), activation of macrophages and natural killer (NK) cells, and induction of MHC class II antigens on renal tissue. ADCC, antibody-dependent cell-mediated cytotoxicity; pCTL, precursor cytotoxic T-cell. (From Krensky, A. M., Weiss, A., Crabtree, G., et al. Reprinted, by permission of the New England Journal of Medicine, 322:510, 1990.)

Table 66-4. MAJOR FACTORS IN THE IMMUNE RESPONSE

Factor	Major Action
Afferent limb	
Major MHC antigens	
Class I	Induction of antibody production by B-cells; cytotoxic T-cell activation
Class II	Helper T-cell activation
Antigen processing and presentation	
Dendritic cells	Class I and II antigen presentation to T- and B-cells
Macrophages	Class I and II antigen presentation to T- and B-cells; interleukin-1 and -6 production
Helper T-cells (CD4 phenotype)	Cytokine production (interleukin-2, -3, -4, -5, -6; interferon-γ)
Cytokines	
Interleukin-1	Induction of interleukin-6 production by macrophages; helper T-cell activation
Interleukin-2	T-cell proliferation; lymphokine release by helper T-cells
Interleukin-3	Stem cell proliferation
Interleukin-4	B-cell growth and differentiation; T-cell proliferation
Interleukin-5	B-cell growth and differentiation
Interleukin-6	Helper T-cell activation; B-cell growth and differentiation
Interferon-γ	Induction of class II molecules on graft tissue; macrophage activation
Efferent limb	
Cytotoxic T-cells (CDC phenotype)	Infiltration and destruction of graft tissue
Natural killer cells	Infiltration and destruction of graft tissue
B-cells	Differentiation into plasma cells, which produce antibodies against graft tissue

Data from Krensky, A. M., Crabtree, G., et al.: N. Engl. J. Med., 322:510, 1990; and Strom, T. B.: Clin. Aspects Autoimmun., 4:8–19, 1990.

rectly and as an autocrine substance that activates transcription of the IL-6 gene in macrophages (Strom, 1990). The macrophage then secretes IL-6, which, in the presence of class II antigen, causes the CD4-positive helper T-cells to secrete the T-cell growth factor IL-2 and to express de novo cell surface IL-2 receptors. IL-2 is necessary for the maturation of CD8-positive cytotoxic T-cell precursors into cytotoxic T-cells. IL-2 also stimulates antigen-activated helper T-cells to release other lymphokines such as IL-3, IL-4, IL-5, IL-6, and interferon-γ. IL-3 is a growth factor for bone marrow stem cells. IL-4, IL-5, and IL-6 enable class I antigen–activated B-cells to mature into plasma cells, which produce cytotoxic antibodies against the class I MHC molecules of the graft. Interferon-γ activates the cytodestructive capabilities of macrophages, augments natural killer cell activity, and induces the expression of MHC class II antigens on kidney graft cells.

Because of the inheritance patterns of the HLA antigens, each potential kidney graft recipient is a "half-match," or haploidentical, with his or her parents and has a 0.25 probability of HLA identity, a 0.50 probability of haploidentity, and a 0.25 probability of a total HLA mismatch with a sibling. HLA identity is usually confirmed by a mixed lymphocyte culture. The importance of histocompatibility in long-term kidney graft survival has been documented by the UCLA Transplant Registry (Cook, 1987). They showed kidney graft half-lives of 22, 12, and 8 years in recipients of HLA-identical sibling, haploidentical parent, and cadaver kidney grafts, respectively. There is a significant beneficial effect of tissue matching in cadaver kidney graft survival (even in the cyclosporine era) when thousands of cases are analyzed (Table 66–5). This effect becomes more significant with time, and it is even more striking in survival of second cadaver kidney grafts (Opelz, 1989). It has been estimated that 74 per cent of cadaver kidney transplant recipients could receive a 0 HLA-B, HLA-DR mismatched kidney graft if all cadaver kidneys were shared on a nationwide basis (Terasaki et al., 1989). More than 100 HLA specificities have been identified, with high agreement among tissue-typing laboratories for the well-defined antigens. Now that the amino acid sequences of HLA antigens are being determined, the results of HLA epitope matching among donor-recipient pairs are being analyzed (Cicciarelli and Corcoran, 1988).

Table 66-5. EFFECT OF HUMAN LEUKOCYTE ANTIGEN INCOMPATIBILITY ON FIRST CADAVER KIDNEY TRANSPLANT SURVIVAL

HLA-A, -B, -DR Mismatches	No.	6-Month Survival (%)	HLA-B, -DR Mismatches	No.	6-Month Survival (%)	HLA-DR Mismatches	No.	6-Month Survival (%)
0	305	87						
1	576	86	0	532	86			
2	1671	82	1	1804	85	0	1278	83
3	2980	83	2	3889	82	1	5383	82
4	3286	81	3	3765	81	2	6087	81
5	2184	80	4	1803	78			
6	784	76						

Modified from Gjertson, D. W.: In Terasaki, P. I. (Ed.): Clinical Transplants 1989. Los Angeles, UCLA Tissue Typing Laboratory, 1989, pp. 353–360.

Blood Transfusions

The association of pretransplant blood transfusions with improved cadaver kidney graft survivals was noted in the mid-1970s (Opelz et al., 1973). This beneficial effect is still present, but reduced in the cyclosporine, antilymphocyte globulin era (Cecka and Toyotome, 1989; USRDS, 1989). One of the most significant advances in living-donor renal transplantation has been the improvement in graft survival associated with donor-specific transfusion protocols, in which blood from a prospective donor is transfused into a recipient (Salvatierra et al., 1980). If donor-specific cytotoxic antibodies do not develop, renal transplantation is usually successful. This has allowed enlargement of the donor pool to include total HLA mismatches, distant relatives, spouses, and close friends of recipients (Sollinger et al., 1984). Transfusions are thought to be beneficial because the recipient's immune system selects the donor antigens to which it will not respond or because blocking antibodies or suppressor T-cells are induced by antigen pretreatment. The undesirable effects of blood transfusions are the development of cytotoxic antibodies and the transmission of viruses such as hepatitis, CMV, and HIV. Reduction of donor-specific cytotoxic antibody production has been achieved by treatment of recipients with azathioprine (Sollinger et al., 1984b) or the use of stored blood (Light et al., 1982).

Unrelated third-party blood transfusions, cyclosporine immunosuppression, and induction immunosuppression with antilymphocyte globulin have replaced donor-specific transfusion protocols and reduced the risk of donor-specific sensitization in many programs, and good graft survival rates have persisted (Flatmark, 1987; Hodge et al., 1989; Sommer et al., 1986).

Immunosuppression

Immunosuppressive drug regimens include a glucocorticoid in combination with other immunosuppressants such as azathioprine, cyclosporine, and antilymphocyte globulin (Strom, 1990). A sample immunosuppression protocol is presented in Table 66–6, and the major mechanisms of action are outlined in Table 66–7. Cyclosporine is usually unnecessary in recipients of HLA-identical sibling transplants. Steroid-resistant rejection is documented by biopsy before OKT3 or antilymphocyte globulin treatment. Some programs taper patients off one of the maintenance immunosuppressants after many months of stable graft function. Glucocorticoids block T-cell proliferation by blocking the production of IL-1 and IL-6. IL-1 was formerly called endogenous pyrogen. This action accounts for the ability of steroids to prevent fever during sepsis. Because IL-2 production and release depend on IL-1 and IL-6, glucocorticoids also indirectly block IL-2, thereby inhibiting the maturation of cytotoxic T-cells, antibody secretion by B-cells, and macrophage activation. Glucocorticoids are usually started at high doses and then are rapidly tapered during the first 6 months after grafting. Conventional treatment for acute renal allograft rejection includes high-dose pulses of glucocorticoids, usually prednisone, 5 mg/kg/day for 5 days, with a taper to maintenance doses. The undesirable side effects of steroids include increased susceptibility to infection, impaired wound healing, growth suppression, aseptic necrosis of bone, glaucoma, psychiatric disturbances, hyperglycemia, fluid retention, increased capillary fragility, and hypertension.

The antimetabolite azathioprine is a derivative of 6-mercaptopurine. It is structurally similar to purine, a base constituent of nucleic acids, and it blocks RNA

Table 66–6. EXAMPLE OF AN IMMUNOSUPPRESSION PROTOCOL

Postoperative Day	Prednisone* (mg/kg)	Azathioprine† (mg/kg)	Cyclosporine‡ (mg/kg)
Prophylactic Immunosuppression			
0	7	2.5	8
1	1.5	2.5	8
2	1.0	2.5	8
3	0.9	2.5	8
4	0.8	2.5	8
5	0.7	2.5	8
6	0.6	2.5	8
7–30	0.5	2.5	8
31–181	Taper	2.5	Taper
181	0.1	2.5	5 (usually)
365	0.1	2.5	5 (usually)

Rejection Crisis Treatment

Prednisone: 5 mg/kg/day × 5 days
Steroid-resistant rejection: OKT3: 5 mg/day IV × 10–14 days
Steroid-resistant rejection: MALG: 15 mg/kg/day central IV × 10–14 days

Prophylactic Anti-Infective Therapy

Broad-spectrum IV antibiotic perioperatively
Trimethoprim-sulfamethoxazole × 3 months
Clotrimazole lozenges × 3 months
Acyclovir as needed for risk of CMV, herpes simplex virus, or varicella-zoster virus infections

*The IV dose is the same as the oral dose.
†The IV dose is the same as the oral dose. Reduce if leukopenia occurs.
‡The IV dose is one third the oral dose. Reduce if nephrotoxicity and high blood levels occur.

Table 66–7. MECHANISMS OF ACTION OF IMMUNOSUPPRESSANTS

Drug	Major Mechanisms of Action
Glucocorticoid	Blocks production of IL-1 by macrophages
Azathioprine	Blocks DNA and RNA synthesis
Cyclosporine	Blocks production of IL-2 by helper T-cells
Antilymphocyte globulins	Lyse lymphocytes, mask T-cell antigens
IL-2 receptor antibodies	Block IL-2 binding by T-cells
FK 506	Blocks production of IL-2 by helper T-cells

Data from Kahan, B. D.: N. Engl. J. Med., 321:1725, 1989; Kirkman, R. L., Shapiro, M. E., Carpenter, C. E., et al.: Transplant. Proc., 21:1766, 1989; Starzl, T. E., and Fung, J. J.: JAMA, 263:2686, 1990; Strom, T. B.: Clin. Aspects Autoimmun., 4:8–19, 1990; and Todd, P. A., and Brogden, R. N.: Drugs, 37:871, 1989.

and DNA synthesis and thus inhibits T-cell proliferation. The potential undesirable side effects of azathioprine are leukopenia, thrombocytopenia, hepatotoxicity, hypersensitivity pancreatitis, increased susceptibility to infection, and an increased risk of neoplasia.

Cyclosporine blocks production and release of IL-2 and other lymphokines that are responsible for proliferation and maturation of cytotoxic T-cells (Kahan, 1989). It prevents interferon-γ release and macrophage activation and prevents the release of B-cell–activating factors such as IL-4. Cyclosporine also inhibits IL-2 receptor expression on helper and cytotoxic T-lymphocytes. The major disadvantage of cyclosporine is nephrotoxicity, which is usually dose related and potentially reversible. Other side effects are hepatotoxicity, hypertension, hirsutism, breast fibroadenomas, gingival hypertrophy, increased susceptibility to infection, and tremors. Drugs that increase cyclosporine levels are ketoconazole, danazol, metoclopramide, glucocorticoids, and diltiazem. Drugs that decrease cyclosporine levels are isoniazid, phenobarbital, phenytoin, and rifampin. Drugs that can cause additive nephrotoxicity are aminoglycosides, amphotericin B, acyclovir, melphalan, and trimethoprim. Determination of cyclosporine blood levels is helpful when toxicity is suspected. The characteristics of cyclosporine toxicity and those of acute rejection are contrasted in Table 66–8.

Triple maintenance immunosuppression with prednisone, azathioprine, and cyclosporine is currently popular

Table 66–8. DIFFERENTIATION OF CYCLOSPORINE TOXICITY FROM ACUTE REJECTION

Characteristic	Cyclosporine Toxicity	Acute Rejection
Fever	No	Yes
Urinary output	Maintained	Decreased
Graft tenderness	No	Yes
Graft size	Stable	Increased
Serum creatinine level rise	Slow	Rapid
Graft blood flow	Maintained	Decreased
Cyclosporine blood level	High	Normal or low
Graft biopsy	May be normal	Cellular infiltration and vasculitis

for cadaver kidney transplantation to reduce the dosage of each drug and to minimize side effects while maintaining immunosuppression.

Polyclonal immune globulins such as Minnesota antilymphoblast globulin are obtained by injecting animals, usually horses, with human lymphoid cells and then harvesting and separating the immune serum to obtain gamma globulin fractions (Strom, 1990). The major mechanisms of action are complement-mediated lysis of lymphocytes, uptake of lymphocytes by the reticuloendothelial system, expansion of suppressor cell populations, and masking of T-cell antigens. Important side effects are thrombocytopenia, granulocytopenia, serum sickness, and increased susceptibility to infection. These preparations are used prophylactically in some cadaver kidney transplant immunosuppressive regimens to allow the graft to recover from acute tubular necrosis before the institution of potentially nephrotoxic cyclosporine maintenance therapy (Sommer et al., 1986). They are also valuable for the treatment of steroid-resistant rejection crises.

The monoclonal antibody Orthoclone OKT3 is an antilymphocyte globulin produced by using a mouse hybridoma technique (Todd and Brogden, 1989). It is administered as an intravenous bolus daily for 10 to 14 days. Concomitant conventional immunosuppression is decreased to prevent excessive immunosuppression. Its principal value is probably the treatment of steroid-resistant rejection. Its immunologic disadvantage is the development of antimouse antibodies, which often prevents subsequent effective courses of the drug. When used prophylactically for cadaver kidney recipients, the mean postoperative day of onset of first rejection was significantly delayed. When used for the treatment of first rejection crises in cadaver kidney transplant recipients, 94 per cent of the rejection episodes were reversed; the corresponding figure for the control group treated with high-dose steroids with or without lymphocyte immune globulin (Atgam) was 75 per cent (P < .05). The major side effects were influenza-like symptoms in most of the patients after the first and second doses, increased susceptibility to infection, and hypotension. Severe pulmonary edema has occurred in fluid-overloaded patients.

When prophylactic antilymphocyte globulin is used in cadaver or non–HLA-identical sibling renal transplantation, it is administered from day 0 for 5 to 14 days, and cyclosporine administration is delayed until recovery from acute tubular necrosis has been ensured.

New Immunosuppressants

Many new monoclonal anti–T-cell antibodies are being evaluated for the prevention and treatment of renal allograft rejection. Because interaction of IL-2 with its T-cell receptor is required for the clonal expansion and continued viability of activated T-cells, antibodies directed at the IL-2 receptor should prevent this unwanted immune response. Two monoclonal anti–IL-2 receptor antibodies, anti-Tac and 33B3.1, which bind to the 55-kilodalton alpha-chain of the IL-2 receptor, have prevented or delayed renal allograft rejection in humans (Cantarovich et al., 1989a; Kirkman et al., 1989). 33B3.1 was shown to be inadequate therapy for treatment of acute rejection (Cantarovich et al., 1989b), and the future of anti–IL-2 receptor antibodies is probably for prophylaxis against rejection.

The immunosuppressants FK 506 and rapamycin are structurally related to the macrolide antibiotic erythromycin. FK 506 has been successfully used as rescue therapy in human liver transplantation and as part of a maintenance regimen with low-dose steroids for kidney, liver, and thoracic organ transplants (Starzl and Fung, 1990).

COMPLICATIONS

Vascular Complications

Immediate vascular complications include kinking of the kidney graft's artery or vein, suture line stenosis, and thrombosis. These problems are more common with transplantation of the right kidney because of the long right renal artery and the short right renal vein, which limits final positioning of the kidney graft. Blood in the kidney graft may clot because of hyperacute rejection or a hypercoagulable state in a recipient with deficiencies of protein C, protein S, or antithrombin III. Renal artery stenosis is usually diagnosed after renal transplantation because of hypertension, with or without impaired renal function. The causes are recipient atheroma, faulty suture technique, trauma, and immunologic mechanisms (Lacombe, 1988). Surgical intervention is difficult, with a significant risk of technical failure, and percutaneous transluminal angioplasty is the initial treatment of choice (DeMeyer et al., 1989).

Renal Allograft Rupture

This complication is rare and requires immediate operation. Most commonly it is due to acute rejection or renal vein thrombosis. If it is due to the former, rejection crisis treatment and operative repair with bolstered mattress sutures, administration of topical thrombotic agents, and use of synthetic glue and polyglactin mesh wrap have resulted in graft salvage (Chopin et al., 1989a). If it is due to renal vein thrombosis, graft salvage with thrombectomy and repair of graft rupture are rare, and allograft nephrectomy is usually necessary (Richardson et al., 1990).

Hematuria

If immediate post-transplant hematuria cannot be controlled with catheter irrigation, endoscopy with fulguration of bleeding sites is necessary. Bleeding is usually at the ureteroneocystostomy or cystotomy site. If that treatment fails, transvesical exploration and control of hemorrhage are necessary. Late hematuria can be due to recurrence of the original renal disease in the kidney graft, infection, calculus, or malignancy. If hematuria persists after treatment of a documented urinary tract infection, a standard hematuria work-up with phase-contrast microscopy for dysmorphic red blood cells should be done, followed, if necessary, by imaging of the native kidneys and kidney transplant, cystoscopy, bladder wash for cytologic examination, and pertinent urothelial biopsies.

Fluid Collections, Including Lymphocele

Most fluid collections after renal transplantation are incidental findings on baseline ultrasound examinations and require no treatment (Pollack et al., 1988). When fluid collections are associated with dilation of the collecting system, pain, fever, or unexplained decline in renal function, ultrasonically guided diagnostic aspiration is necessary. If the fluid is purulent, microscopic examination of the fluid for organisms is done, and antibiotic treatment is initiated. Open surgical drainage is usually necessary for fluid collections showing infection. Lymph, urine, and blood can be differentiated from one another by creatinine and hematocrit determinations. Lymph has a creatinine concentration nearly the same as that of serum, urine has a creatinine concentration higher than that of serum and approaching that of bladder urine, and blood has a high hematocrit level when compared with the other two fluids. If urinary tract obstruction is relieved by aspiration and there is no recurrence of the fluid, no further treatment is required. If blood reaccumulates, exploration and control of bleeding are required. If an uninfected lymphocele recurs, it is usually treated by marsupialization into the peritoneal cavity after ureteral identification (Schweizer et al., 1972), although some have reported success with iodine sclerosis (Gilliand et al., 1989). If the lymphocele is infected, open drainage is usually needed. Urinary extravasation often requires open surgical repair. A retrograde cystogram will document leakage at the cystotomy or ureteroncocystostomy site. If the retrograde cystogram does not show extravasation, excretory urography or percutaneous antegrade pyelography will document the site of extravasation from the ureter or renal pelvis. Some urinary leaks at the ureteroneocystostomy site may be managed simply by bladder catheter drainage, with or without percutaneous nephrostomy, or by performance of another ureteroneocystostomy. At the time of open repair, retrograde pyelography and passage of a ureteral catheter into the native ureter will facilitate identification of that structure if it is needed for ureteroureterostomy or ureteropyelostomy. If the urinary tract repair is extensive, it is often protected with a stent, a small nephrostomy tube, omentum wrap, suction drainage, antibiotics based on culture and sensitivity test results, and reduction of immunosuppression.

Obstruction, Including Calculi

Ureteral obstruction in the immediate postoperative period is due to technical error, edema, or a blood clot.

The first is repaired via another ureteroneocystostomy. Edema resolves within days, and ureteral blood clots pass or are lysed with urokinase.

Other causes of urinary tract obstruction are late periureteral fibrosis, chronic ischemia of the distal ureter, calculi, and, rarely, tumor. Although ureteral stenosis has been managed by ureteral meatotomy (Marchioro and Tremann, 1973) and percutaneous ureteral dilation followed by stent placement (Streem et al., 1986), open surgical repair is frequently necessary. The principles of ureteropyelostomy and ureteroureterostomy were described earlier. If the renal allograft ureteral length is sufficient, a second ureteroneocystostomy will suffice. Vesicopyelostomy (Linstedt et al., 1981), vesicocalycostomy (Ehrlich et al., 1983), and interposition of a small-bowel segment between the renal pelvis and the bladder (Orton and Middleton, 1982) have been used as surgical treatments for an obstructed allograft ureter.

Upper tract calculi are managed via the same techniques as calculi in the normal urinary tract; however, negotiation of the transplanted ureter may be difficult or impossible because of tortuosity, thus favoring percutaneous techniques (Caldwell and Burns, 1988; Hulbert et al., 1985; Locke et al., 1988). Extracorporeal shock-wave lithotripsy has been used successfully with the patient placed prone in the water bath. Bladder calculi are managed by standard techniques.

Reflux

The indications for antireflux surgery of the kidney transplant ureter are the same as those for nontransplant patients (Reinberg et al., 1990). If the reflux is due to high-pressure voiding, relief of bladder outlet obstruction or augmentation cystoplasty with intermittent catheterization must be considered. Ureteral advancement techniques, ureteroureterostomy into the nonrefluxing native ureter, and submucosal injection techniques are all possible surgical therapies.

Impotence

Impotence can be due to the factors described under Recipient Operation. The immunosuppressant cyclosporine can cause hyperprolactinemia, with suppression of testosterone production and loss of libido (Kahan, 1989). Intracorporeal injections of vasoactive drugs and implantation of penile prostheses have successfully treated this problem (Sidi et al., 1987); however, the transplant recipient must be warned of the increased risk of infection from either of these treatment modalities.

Cancer

Immunosuppressed patients are more likely to develop cancer than age-matched control subjects in the general population. The acquisition or liberation of oncogenic viruses is facilitated by impaired cellular immunity, and immunosuppressants may have a mutagenic role in tumorigenesis. Follow-up of nearly 4000 renal transplant patients revealed that the incidence of cancer increased from 3 per cent after 1 year after grafting to 49 per cent 14 years after grafting (Sheil et al., 1985). Skin cancer was the most common malignancy. Rarely, renal malignancy is transplanted with the kidney graft. Treatment is by removal of the transplanted kidney and discontinuation of immunosuppressive therapy. Bacille Calmette-Guérin vaccine should be avoided for the treatment of superficial transitional cell carcinoma of the bladder in immunosuppressed kidney transplant recipients because of the risk of systemic infection and the likelihood of diminished therapeutic response. Absorbed thiotepa may have an additive myelosuppressive effect if the patient is also taking the immunosuppressant azathioprine.

CONCLUSIONS

Renal transplantation is the best therapy for most patients with ESRD. Morbidity and mortality have been significantly reduced by attention to pretransplant evaluations, donor surgery, kidney preservation, recipient selection, recipient surgery, histocompatibility, immunologic conditioning with pretransplant transfusions, immunosuppression, and successful management of complications.

REFERENCES

Anderson, O. S., Jonasson, O., and Merkel, F. K.: En bloc transplantation of pediatric kidneys into adult patients. Arch. Surg., 108:35, 1974.

Balfour, H. H., Jr., Chace, B. A., Stapleton, J. T., et al.: A randomized, placebo-controlled trial of oral acyclovir for the prevention of cytomegalovirus disease in recipients of renal allografts. N. Engl. J. Med., 320:1381, 1989.

Barry, J. M.: Spermatic cord preservation in kidney transplantation. J. Urol., 127:1076, 1982.

Barry, J. M.: Unstented extravesical ureteroneocystostomy in kidney transplantation. J. Urol., 129:918, 1983.

Barry, J. M.: Cadaver donor nephrectomy. In Novick, A. C., Streem, S. B., and Pontes, J. E. (Eds.): Stewart's Operative Urology. Baltimore, Williams & Wilkins, 1989, pp. 294–300.

Barry, J. M., and Fincher, R.: Transplantation of a horseshoe kidney into two recipients. J. Urol., 131:1162, 1984.

Barry, J. M., and Fuchs, E. F.: Right renal vein extension in cadaver kidney transplantation. Arch. Surg., 113:300, 1978.

Barry, J. M., and Hatch, D. A.: Parallel incision unstented extravesical ureteroneocystostomy: Follow-up of 203 kidney transplants. J. Urol., 134:249, 1985.

Barry, J. M., Hefty, T. R., and Sasaki, T.: Clam-shell technique for right renal vein extension in cadaver kidney transplantation. J. Urol., 140:1479, 1988.

Barry, J. M., and Lemmers, M. J.: Update on renal transplantation. In Stamey, T. A. (Ed.): 1989 Monographs in Urology. Princeton, Medical Directions Publishing, 1989, pp. 5–14.

Belzer, F. O., Ashby, B. S., and Dunphy, J. E.: 24- and 72-hour preservation of canine kidneys. Lancet, 2:536, 1967.

Belzer, F. O., and Southard, J. H.: Principles of solid-organ preservation by cold storage. Transplantation, 45:673, 1988.

Bretan, P. N., Jr., Vigneron, D. B., Hricak, H., et al.: Assessment of clinical renal preservation by phosphorus-31 magnetic resonance spectroscopy. J. Urol., 137:146, 1987.

Burdick, J. F., and Strom, T. B.: Immunosuppression in transplantation: The biology and therapeutic modalities. *In* Belzer, F. O. (Ed.): Transplant Surgical Resource Series. Raritan, NJ, Ortho Pharmaceutical Corp., 1988, pp. 2–28.

Caldwell, T. C., and Burns, J. R.: Current operative management of urinary calculi after renal transplantation. J. Urol., 140:1360, 1988

Calne, R. Y., White, D. J. G., Thiru, S., Evans, D. B., McMaster, P., Dunn, D. C., Craddock, G. N., Pentlow, B. D., and Rolles, K.: Cyclosporine A in patients receiving renal allografts from cadaver donors. Lancet, 2:1323, 1978.

Cantarovich, D., Le Mauff, B., Hourmant, M., Giral, M., Denis, M., Jacques, Y., and Souillou, J. P.: Anti-IL2 receptor monoclonal antibody (33B3.1) in prophylaxis of early kidney rejection in humans: A randomized trial versus rabbit antithymocyte globulin. Transplant. Proc., 21:1769, 1989a.

Cantarovich, D., Le Mauff, B., Hourmant, M., et al.: Anti–interleukin-2-receptor MAb in the treatment of ongoing acute rejection episodes of human kidney graft—a pilot study. Transplantation, 47:454, 1989b.

Cecka, J. M., and Toyotome, A.: The transfusion effect. *In* Terasaki, P. I. (Ed.): Clinical Transplants, 1989. Los Angeles, UCLA Tissue Typing Laboratory, 1989.Cheigh, J. S., Mouradian, J., Susin, M., et al.: Kidney transplant nephrotic syndrome: Relationship between allograft histopathology and natural course. Kidney Int., 18:358, 1980.

Chopin, D. K., Abbou, C. C., Lottmann, H. B., Popov, Z., Lang, P. R., Buisson, C. L., Belghiti, D., Colombel, M., and Auvert, J. M.: Conservative treatment of renal allograft rupture with polyglactin 910 mesh and gelatin resorcin formaldehyde glue. J. Urol., 142:363, 1989a.

Chopin, D. K., Popov, Z., Abbou, C. C., et al.: Use of vena cava to obtain additional length for the right renal vein during transplantation of cadaveric kidneys. J. Urol., 141:1143, 1989b.

Cicciarelli, J., and Corcoran, S.: An update on HLA matching, including HLA "epitope" matching: A new approach. *In* Terasaki, P. I. (Ed.): Clinical Transplants, 1988. Los Angeles, UCLA Tissue Typing Laboratory, 1988, pp. 329–338.

Collins, G. M., Bravo-Sugarman, M. B., and Terasaki, P. I.: Kidney preservation for transportation: Initial perfusion and 30 hours ice storage. Lancet, 2:1219, 1969.

Cook, D. J.: Long-term survival of kidney allografts. *In* Terasaki, P. I. (Ed.): Clinical Transplants, 1987. Los Angeles, UCLA Tissue Typing Laboratory, 1987.

Cosimi, A. B., Colvin, R. B., Goldstein, G., et al.: Treatment of acute renal allograft rejection with OKT3 monoclonal antibody. Transplantation, 32:535, 1981.

Dallman, M. J., and Morris, P. J.: The immunology of rejection. *In* Morris, P. J. (Ed.): Kidney Transplantation. 3rd ed. Philadelphia, W. B. Saunders Co., 1988, pp. 15–33.

DeMeyer, M., Pirson, Y., Dautrebande, J., et al.: Treatment of renal graft artery stenosis: Comparison between surgical bypass and percutaneous transluminal angioplasty. Transplantation, 47:784, 1989.

Eggers, P. W.: Effect of transplantation on the Medicare end-stage renal disease program. N. Engl. J. Med., 318:223, 1988.

Ehrlich, R. M., Whitmore, K., and Fine, R. N.: Calycovesicostomy for total ureteral obstruction after renal transplantation. J. Urol., 129:818, 1983.

Evans, R. W., Manninen, D. L., Garrison, L. P., et al.: The quality of life of patients with end-stage renal disease. N. Engl. J. Med., 312:553, 1985.

Feduska, N. J., Belzer, F. O., et al.: A ten-year experience with cadaver kidney preservation using cryoprecipitated plasma. Am. J. Surg., 135:356, 1978.

Flatmark, A.: Optimal use of kidneys from living donors. Transplant. Proc., 19:167, 1987.

Freed, S. Z.: The present status of bilateral nephrectomy in transplant recipients. J. Urol., 115:8, 1976.

Gilliland, J. D., Spies, J. B., Brown, S. B., Yrizarry, J. M., and Greenwood, L. H.: Lymphoceles: Percutaneous treatment with povidone-iodine sclerosis. Radiology, 171:227, 1989.

Gittes, R. F., and Waters, W. B.: Sexual impotence: The overlooked complication of a second renal transplant. J. Urol., 121:719, 1979.

Gjertson, D. W.: Short- and long-term effects of HLA matching. *In* Terasaki, P. I. (Ed.): Clinical Transplants, 1989. Los Angeles, UCLA Tissue Typing Laboratory, 1989, pp. 353–360.

Goodwin, W. E., Kaufman, J. J., Mims, M. M., et al.: Human renal transplantation. I. Clinical experiences with 6 cases of renal homotransplantation. J. Urol., 89:13, 1963.

Haberal, M., Oner, Z., Karamehmetoglu, M., et al.: Cadaver kidney transplantation with cold ischemia time for 48 to 95 hours. Transplant. Proc., 16:1330, 1984.

Halasz, N. A., and Collins, G. M.: Forty-eight hour kidney preservation: A comparison of flushing and ice storage with perfusion. Arch. Surg., 1:175, 1976.

Hamilton, D.: Kidney transplantation: A history. *In* Morris, P. J. (Ed.): Kidney Transplantation. 3rd ed. Philadelphia, W. B. Saunders, Co., 1988, pp. 1–11.

Hamilton, D. N. H., and Reid, W. A.: Yu. Yu. Voronoy and the first human kidney allograft. Surg. Gynecol. Obstet., 159:289, 1984.

Hatch, T., and Hefty, T.: Personal communication, 1990.

Hefty, T., Hatch, T., and Barry, J. M.: Dialysis access surgery. *In* Novick, A. C., Streem, S. B., and Pontes, J. E. (Eds.): Stewart's Operative Urology. Baltimore, Williams & Wilkins, 1989, pp. 345–359.

Henell, K. R., Chou, S., and Norman, D. J.: Use of cytomegalovirus seropositive donor kidneys in seronegative patients: Results of prospective serotesting and matching in one center. Transplant. Proc., 21:2082, 1989.

Heritier, P., Perraud, Y., Relave, M. H., Barral, X., Guerin, C., Genin, C., Gilloz, A., and Berthoux, F.: Renal transplantation and Kock pouch: A case report. J. Urol., 141:595, 1989.

Hinman, F., Jr.: Atlas of Urologic Surgery. Philadelphia, W. B. Saunders Co., 1989, pp. 746–755.

Hodge, E., Banowosky, L., Novick, A., et al.: Alternative immunosuppressive strategies in the management of recipients of living related renal transplants. Transplant. Proc., 21:1609, 1989.

Hudnall, C. H., Hodge, E. E., Centeno, A. S., et al.: Evaluation of pediatric cadaver kidneys transplanted into adult recipients receiving cyclosporine. J. Urol., 142:1181, 1989.

Hulbert, J. C., Reddy, P., Young, A. T., et al.: The percutaneous removal of calculi from transplanted kidneys. J. Urol., 134:324, 1985.

Kahan, B. D.: Cyclosporine. N. Engl. J. Med., 321:1725, 1989.

Kirkman, R. L., Shapiro, M. E., Carpenter, C. B., Milford, E. L., Ramos, E. L., Tilney, N. L., Waldmann, T. A., Zimmerman, C. E., and Strom, T. B.: Early experience with anti-TaC in clinical renal transplantation. Transplant. Proc., 21:1766, 1989.

Konnak, J. W., Herwig, K. R., Finkbeiner, A., et al.: Extravesical ureteroneocystostomy in 170 renal transplant patients. J. Urol., 113:299, 1975.

Krensky, A. M., Weiss, A., Crabtree, G., et al.: T-lymphocyte–antigen interactions in transplant rejection. N. Engl. J. Med., 322:510, 1990.

Lacombe, M.: Renal artery stenosis after renal transplantation. Ann. Vasc. Surg., 2:155, 1988.

Light, J. A., Metz, S., Oddenino, K., et al.: Donor-specific transfusion with diminished sensitization. Transplantation, 34:352, 1982.

Lindstedt, E., Bergentz, S. E., and Lindholm, T.: Long-term clinical follow-up after pyelocystostomy. J. Urol., 126:253, 1981.

Locke, D. R., Steinbock, G., Salomon, D. R., et al.: Combination extracorporeal shock wave lithotripsy and percutaneous extraction of calculi in a renal allograft. J. Urol., 139:575, 1988.

Marchioro, T. L., and Tremann, J. A.: Technique for treating stricture at a ureteroneocystostomy. Surgery, 73:634, 1973.

Marshall, V. C., Jablonski, P., and Scott, D. F.: Renal preservation. *In* Morris, P. J. (Ed.): Kidney Transplantation. 3rd ed. Philadelphia, W. B. Saunders Co., 1988, pp. 151–182.

Nghiem, D. D.: Spiral gonadal vein graft extension of right renal vein in living renal transplantation. J. Urol., 142:1525, 1989.

Nohr, C.: Non-AIDS immunosuppression. *In* Wilmore, D. W., Brennan, M. F., Harken, A. H., Holcroft, J. W., and Meakins, J. L. (Eds.): Care of the Surgical Patient. Vol. 2. New York, Scientific American, 1989, pp. 1–18.

Novick, A. C.: Technique of renal transplantation. *In* Novick, A. C., Streem, S. B., and Pontes, J. E. (Eds.): Stewart's Operative Urology. Baltimore, Williams & Wilkins, 1989, pp. 324–340.

Opelz, G.: Influence of HLA matching on survival of second kidney transplants in cyclosporine-treated recipients. Transplantation, 47:823, 1989.

Opelz, G., Sengar, D. P. S., Mickey, M. R., et al.: Effect of blood transfusions on subsequent kidney transplants. Transplant. Proc., 5:253, 1973.

Orandi, A.: Transurethral incision of prostate compared with trans-urethral resection of prostate in 132 matching cases. J. Urol., 138:810, 1987.

Orton, K. R., and Middleton, R. G.: Ileal substitution of the ureter in renal transplantation. J. Urol., 128:374, 1982.

Penn, I., Mackie, E., Halgrimson, C. G., et al.: Testicular complications following renal transplantation. Ann. Surg., 176:697, 1972.

Ploeg, R. J.: Kidney preservation with the UW and Euro-Collins solutions. Transplantation, 49:281, 1990.

Ploeg, R. J., Goossens, D., McAnulty, J. F., et al.: Successful 72-hour cold storage kidney preservation with UW solution. Transplantation, 46:191, 1988.

Pollak, R., Beremis, S. A., Maddux, M. S., et al.: The natural history of and therapy for peri-renal fluid collections following renal transplantation. J. Urol., 140:716, 1988.

Reinberg, Y., Bumgardner, G. L., and Aliabadi, H.: Urological aspects of renal transplantation. J. Urol., 143:1087, 1990.

Richardson, A. J., Higgins, R. M., Jaskowski, A. J., et al.: Spontaneous rupture of renal allografts: The importance of renal vein thrombosis in the cyclosporine era. Br. J. Surg., 77:558, 1990.

Salvatierra, O., Jr.: Renal transplantation. In Glenn, J. F. (Ed.): Urologic Surgery. 3rd ed. Philadelphia, J. B. Lippincott, 1983, pp. 362–366.

Salvatierra, O., Jr., and Belzer, F. O.: Pediatric cadaver kidneys: Their use in renal transplantation. Arch. Surg., 110:181, 1975.

Salvatierra, O., Jr., Vincenti, F., Amend, W. J. C., et al.: Deliberate donor-specific blood transfusions prior to living related transplantation. Ann. Surg., 192:543, 1980.

Schweizer, R. T., Cho, S., Kountz, S. L., et al.: Lymphoceles following renal transplantation. Arch. Surg., 104:42, 1972.

Sheil, A. G. R., Flavel, S., Disney, A. P. S., et al.: Cancer development in patients progressing to dialysis and renal transplantation. Transplant. Proc., 17:1685, 1985.

Shneidman, R. S., Pulliam, J. P., and Barry, J. M.: Clean, intermittent self-catheterization in renal transplant recipients. Transplantation, 38:312, 1984.

Sidi, A. A., Peng, W., Sanseau, C., et al.: Penile prosthesis surgery in the treatment of impotence in the immunosuppressed man. J. Urol., 137:681, 1987.

Sollinger, H. W., Burlingham, W. J., Sparks, E. M. F., et al.: Donor-specific transfusions in unrelated and related HLA-mismatched donor-recipient combinations. Transplantation, 38:612, 1984a.

Sollinger, H. W., Glass, N. R., et al.: Comparison between DST and DST plus imuran in HLA-nonidentical living-related transplants. Transplant. Proc., 16:8, 1984b.

Sommer, B. G., Henry, M. L., and Ferguson, R. M.: Sequential conventional immunotherapy with maintenance cyclosporine following renal transplantation. Transplant. Proc., 18(Suppl. 1):69, 1986.

Starzl, T. E., and Fung, J. J.: Transplantation. JAMA, 263:2686, 1990.

Starzl, T. E., Hakala, T. R., et al.: A multifactorial system for equitable selection of cadaver kidney recipients. JAMA, 257:3073, 1987.

Steinmuller D.R., Graneto, D., Swift, C., et al.: Use of intravenous immunoglobulin prophylaxis for primary cytomegalovirus infection post living-related-donor renal transplantation. Transplant. Proc., 21:2069, 1989.

Streem, S. B.: Live donor nephrectomy. In Novick, A. C., Streem, S. B., and Pontes, J. E. (Eds.): Stewart's Operative Urology. Baltimore, Williams & Wilkins, 1989, pp. 312–323.

Streem, S. B., Novick, A. C., Steinmuller, D. R., et al.: Percutaneous techniques for the management of urologic renal transplant complications. J. Urol., 135:456, 1986.

Strom, T. B.: Immunosuppressive treatments that thwart transplant rejection. Clin. Aspects Autoimmun., 4:8, 1990.

Terasaki, P. I., Cecka, J. M., Takemoto, S., et al.: Overview. In Terasaki, P. I. (Ed.): Clinical Transplants, 1988. Los Angeles, UCLA Tissue Typing Laboratory, 1988, pp. 409–434.

Terasaki, P. I., Park, M. S., Takemoto, S., et al.: Overview and epitope matching. In Terasaki, P. I. (Ed.): Clinical Transplants, 1989. Los Angeles, UCLA Tissue Typing Laboratory, 1989, pp. 499–516.

Thomalla, J. V., Mitchell, M. E., Leapman, S. B., et al.: Renal transplantation into the reconstructed bladder. J. Urol., 141:265, 1989.

Todd, P. A., and Brogden, R. N.: Muromonab CD3. A review of its pharmacology and therapeutic potential. Drugs, 37:871, 1989.

Tuttle, T. M., Williams, G. M., and Marshall, F. F.: Evidence for cyclophosphamide-induced transitional cell carcinoma in a renal transplant patient. J. Urol., 140:1009, 1988.

United Network for Organ Sharing: Number of patients on UNOS waiting lists by organ need and ABO blood group. UNOS Update, 6(3):11, 1990.

United Network for Organ Sharing: Articles of Incorporation, By-Laws, and Policies: Policy 3.5, Allocation of Cadaveric Kidneys. UNOS, June 20, 1989.

U.S. Renal Data System; USRDS 1989 Annual Data Report. Bethesda, National Institute of Diabetes and Digestive and Kidney Diseases, August 1989.

Vincenti, F., Amend, W. J. C., Jr., Kaysen, G.: Long-term renal function in kidney donors: Sustained compensatory hyperfiltration with no adverse effects. Transplantation, 36:626, 1983.

Weiland, D., Sutherland, D. E. R., Chavers, B., et al.: Information on 628 living-related kidney donors at a single institution, with long-term follow-up in 472 cases. Transplant. Proc., 16:5, 1984.

67
RENOVASCULAR SURGERY*

John A. Libertino, M.D.

The evaluation and treatment of patients with renovascular lesions have changed dramatically as a result of the availability of new diagnostic studies, such as digital subtraction angiography and angiotensin-converting enzyme inhibitor challenge (Wilcox et al., 1988), as well as the advent of new treatment options, such as new antihypertensive drugs (Hollenberg, 1988), balloon angioplasty (Sos et al., 1984; Tegtmeyer et al., 1984), and alternative surgical bypass procedures. These technical advances have resulted in the emergence of a new set of contemporary management principles. These include a more aggressive approach to the diagnosis and treatment of renal arterial atherosclerotic disease and, therefore, to the surgical treatment of older patients; the option of revascularization procedures for total renal artery occlusion as well as for renal failure, with preservation and restoration of renal function; and the bench surgery and autotransplantation techniques for aneurysms, arteriovenous malformations, and segmental or branch disease (Libertino et al., 1988).

Many factors must be considered when attempting to determine whether a patient is a candidate for medical therapy, percutaneous transluminal angioplasty, or surgical treatment. The response of blood pressure to medical therapy, the natural history of the offending renal artery lesion, the general medical condition of the patient, the risk of renal parenchymal loss, and the success rates of various surgical and radiologic techniques are weighed carefully to arrive at the best treatment option for each individual patient.

Although the true incidence of renovascular hypertension is unknown, it is estimated to be present in 5 to 10 per cent of the 60 million hypertensive individuals in the United States (Sosa and Vaughan, 1987). With the advent of more sensitive and specific diagnostic screening tests for renovascular disease, it may become apparent that the true incidence of renal artery conditions has been underestimated.

The devastating ravages of poorly controlled hypertension, such as myocardial infarction, congestive heart failure, stroke, and renal failure, underscore the importance of identifying and treating all correctable forms of hypertension.

RENAL ARTERY LESIONS

The presence of renal artery stenosis in a hypertensive patient does not establish the diagnosis of renovascular hypertension. Functional tests, such as divided renal vein renin assays and other functional studies, must be performed to determine whether the hypertension is due to the stenosis. Complications associated with renal angiography and renal vein renin assays occur but are uncommon. These and other studies are essential in determining the functional significance of a renal artery lesion (see Chapter 55 on the natural history and diagnostic evaluation of patients suspected of having renovascular hypertension).

Various lesions can cause stenosis or total occlusion of the main renal artery or its primary branches. Although the most common lesions are associated with atherosclerosis and fibrous disorders, emboli, traumatic thrombosis, dissection, Takayasu's disease, syphilitic aortitis, thromboangiitis, and periarteritis nodosa have all been described (Kincaid and Davis, 1966).

Atherosclerotic Lesions

Atherosclerotic stenosis or occlusion accounts for approximately two thirds of all renal artery pathologic lesions. This lesion is typically discovered in middle aged or older men but is now being discovered more frequently in older women. Pathologically, the atherosclerotic renal artery lesion is similar to the atherosclerotic lesions found elsewhere in the body. It can be bilateral but when unilateral, more frequently involves the left renal artery. The lesion occurs at or near the origin of the renal artery as either a circumferential atheroma, containing lipid with focal calcification, or an eccentric

*Portions of this chapter are adapted from Libertino J. A., and Zinman L. N.: Surgery for renovascular hypertension. *In* Libertino J. A. (Ed.): Pediatric and Adult Reconstructive Urologic Surgery, 2nd ed. © 1987, Baltimore, Williams & Wilkins, pp. 119–161.

fibrous plaque, composed of collagen and lipid deposits (Fig. 67–1). Thrombosis and dissecting hematomas are complicating features of this lesion.

Nonatherosclerotic Lesions

In 1938 Leadbetter and Burkland reported a case of hypertension due to a renal artery obstruction produced by a cast of smooth muscle attached to the arterial wall. A subsequent report described stenosis produced by fibrous intimal proliferation (Goodman, 1952).

These initial reports led to the investigations of McCormack and associates (1966) who based their classification of renal mural dysplasia on the lesion's predominant mural location and tissue composition. The fibrous dysplasias are now classified as intimal fibroplasia, medial fibroplasia, fibromuscular hyperplasia, and subadventitial fibroplasia. These mural dysplasias are more prevalent in females. When unilateral, these lesions affect the right renal artery more often than the left (Fig. 67–2). The mean age of patients at presentation is 35 years.

Intimal fibroplasia, in addition to causing stenosis, may cause renal artery dissection or aneurysm formation (Fig. 67–3). Pathologically, medial fibroplasia is characterized by the presence of multiple microaneurysms that may be associated with large aneurysms (Fig. 67–4). True fibromuscular hyperplasia is characterized by a concentric, segmental stenotic lesion that is occasionally associated with disruption of the internal elastic membrane, causing dissecting aneurysms. The patient with subadventitial fibroplasia usually presents with a severely stenotic lesion characterized by dense collagen deposition in the outer portion of the media (Fig. 67–5). The natural history of most of the mural dysplasias is that of progressive occlusion associated with dissection or aneurysm formation, mandating some form of interventional treatment.

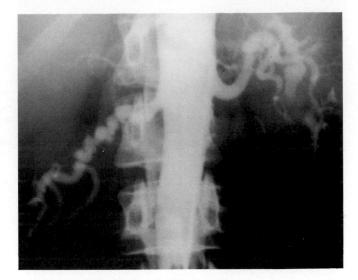

Figure 67–2. Right medial fibroplasia.

Renal Artery Aneurysms

Although they are uncommon, renal artery aneurysms are being diagnosed with greater frequency as a result of the advent of standard and digital subtraction angiography. Their true incidence is unknown but, in one study, were found in 1.5 per cent of potential kidney donors who underwent angiographic evaluation (Harrison et al., 1978). The reported incidence of renal artery aneurysms in patients who are undergoing angiography for evaluation of nonrenal disease has ranged from 0.09 to 0.3 per cent (Hagerman et al., 1978; Stanley et al., 1975).

Renal artery aneurysms are clinically significant because they may cause hypertension, may be associated with local symptoms, or may undergo catastrophic rup-

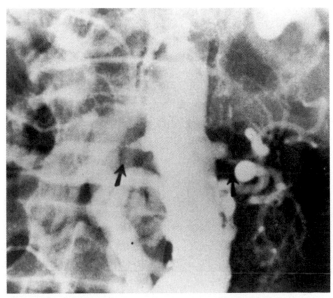

Figure 67–1. Bilateral atherosclerotic renal artery stenosis. Right occlusion, left stenosis.

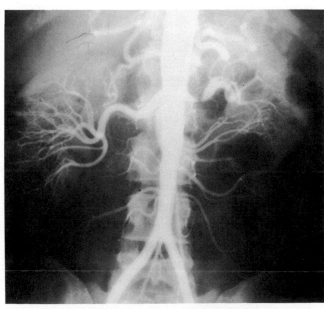

Figure 67–3. Intimal fibroplasia.

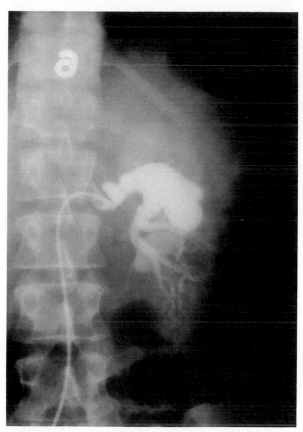

Figure 67–4. Medial fibroplasia with associated aneurysm.

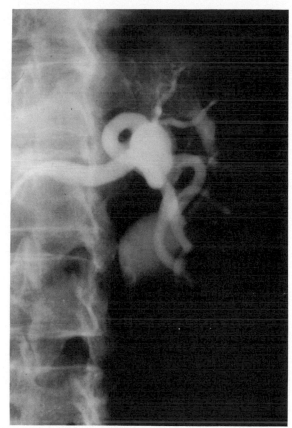

Figure 67–6. Saccular aneurysm in left renal artery (atherosclerotic).

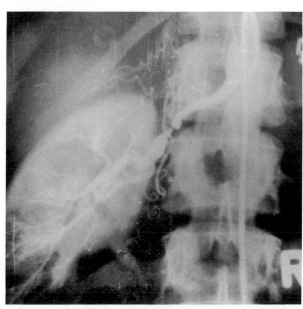

Figure 67–5. Subadventitial fibroplasia.

ture. Four types are known: saccular, fusiform, dissecting, and intrarenal.

Saccular aneurysms usually occur at the bifurcation of the main renal artery or one of its branches (Fig. 67–6), in association with medial fibroplasia and atherosclerosis. In addition to possible spontaneous rupture, these aneurysms may also cause erosion into the renal vein or renal pelvis or mural thrombosis with peripheral embolization.

Fusiform aneurysms are generally not calcified and are found in younger hypertensive persons with fibrous mural dysplasia (Fig. 67–7). The major complication of this lesion is thrombosis of the renal artery.

Dissecting aneurysms result from disruption of the internal elastic membrane (Fig. 67–8). This process may be confined to the main renal artery or may extend into the segmental blood supply. Some dissections re-enter the lumen, and others cause arterial thrombosis with renal infarction or rupture and hemorrhage. Atherosclerosis, intimal fibroplasia, and perimedial fibroplasia are most often associated with dissecting aneurysms of the renal artery. Dissecting aortic aneurysms may also involve the renal vasculature.

Intrarenal aneurysms are caused by atherosclerosis, trauma, congenital vascular malformations, arteritis, fibrous dysplasia, or needle biopsy of the kidney (Fig. 67–9).

Small (<2 cm), well-calcified aneurysms in a nonhypertensive asymptomatic patient do not require surgical treatment. Surgical intervention is indicated when the aneurysm is causing ischemia or clinical symptoms; is dissecting; or is associated with a functionally significant lesion, resulting in decreased renal function or hypertension. Radiologic evidence of expansion or thrombus formation with distal embolization or the clinical presentation of the aneurysm in a woman of childbearing age requires surgical treatment. Various surgical proce-

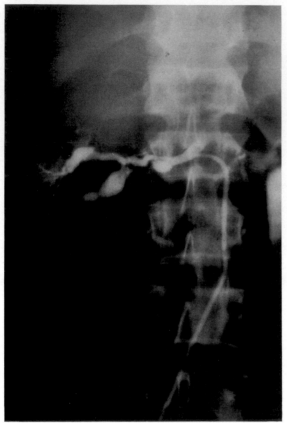

Figure 67–7. Fusiform aneurysms in right renal artery.

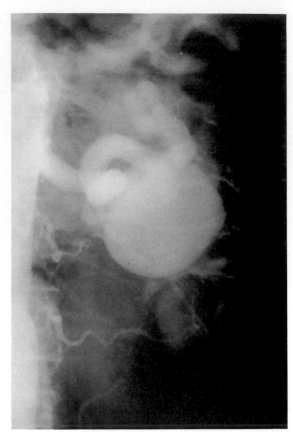

Figure 67–9. Intrarenal aneurysm.

dures are available, ranging from nephrectomy and partial nephrectomy to resection and in situ or bench revascularization procedures with or without a vein

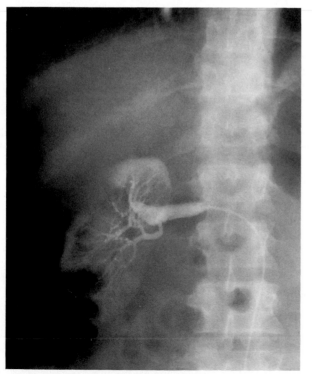

Figure 67–8. Dissecting renal artery lesion.

patch graft. Aneurysmectomy with renal preservation is possible in most patients and is described further in this chapter.

Arteriovenous Fistulas

Arteriovenous fistulas are rare and may be congenital, idiopathic, or acquired (Fig. 67–10). Congenital fistulas (cirsoid) have multiple communications, occur equally in both sexes, and usually become manifest in adulthood. Idiopathic fistulas usually have a single communication, are not cirsoid, and have no apparent cause. It has been postulated that they are due to venous erosion by a large pre-existing renal artery aneurysm. Acquired fistulas are the most frequently encountered, accounting for 75 per cent of all renal arteriovenous fistulas. The most common cause is iatrogenic injury from a percutaneous needle biopsy or percutaneous nephrolithotomy. Other causes are renal surgery, blunt or penetrating trauma, and renal carcinoma.

The treatment of renal arteriovenous fistulas varies with the etiology of the lesion. Nephrectomy is indicated in patients with renal carcinoma. Most fistulas resulting from needle biopsy or other percutaneous procedures and a smaller number resulting from trauma close spontaneously.

Reconstructive surgery or transcatheter occlusion is indicated in patients suffering from hypertension, congestive heart failure, and hematuria. The surgical

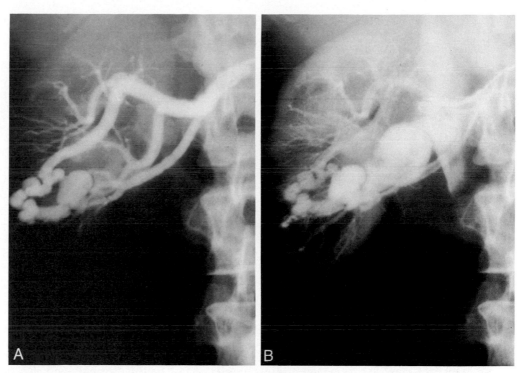

Figure 67–10. *A,* Right renal arteriovenous fistula. *B,* Right arteriovenous malformation with early filling of renal vein and inferior vena cava.

options range from total nephrectomy for huge arteriovenous fistulas to partial nephrectomy for smaller lesions as well as extracorporeal or in situ surgery using microvascular techniques to preserve functioning renal parenchyma (Fig. 67–11 and Fig. 67–12).

Renal Artery Emboli

Renal artery emboli are a result of embolic phenomena from mitral valvular disease; atrial fibrillation; acute myocardial infarction; ventricular aneurysms; subacute bacterial endocarditis; cardiac tumors; and, rarely, a clot originating in the venous system in a patient with an intracardiac septal defect. In addition, atherosclerotic aortic disease, complications of surgical treatment of calcific aortic stenosis or cardiac prosthetic valves, and thrombi originating in renal artery aneurysms are known

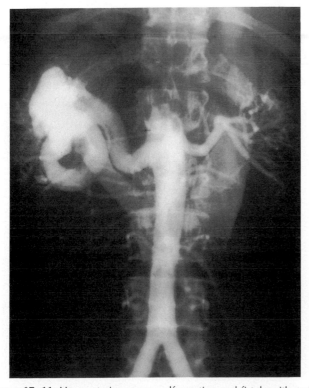

Figure 67–11. Huge arteriovenous malformation and fistula with early filling of renal vein and inferior vena cava before bench surgery.

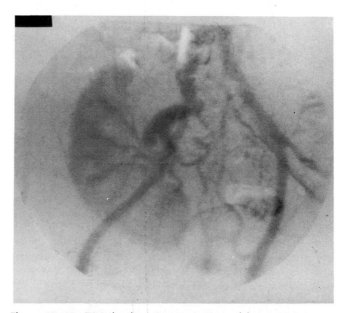

Figure 67–12. Digital subtraction angiogram of huge arteriovenous fistula following bench surgery (resection) and autotransplantation.

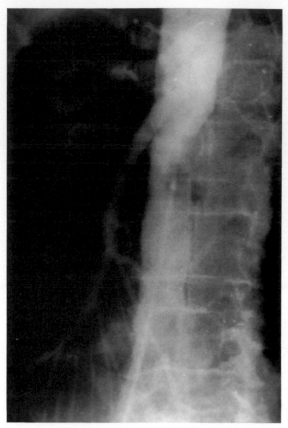

Figure 67–13. Bilateral renal artery emboli with bilateral total renal artery occlusion.

causes of acute emboli and renal artery occlusion (Fig. 67–13).

Renal artery embolization occurs more frequently in the secondary or peripheral vasculature and more commonly affects the left renal artery because of the acute angle that exists between the origin of this artery and the aorta. Iatrogenic emboli to the renal arteries are being seen more frequently with the increasing use of invasive vascular procedures. These emboli may result from angiography or percutaneous transluminal angioplasty.

Operative versus nonoperative treatment for renal artery emboli remains controversial without good guidelines, because the severity and the extent of renal artery embolization vary greatly (Nicholas and DeMuth, 1984). Patients usually have suffered a recent cardiac event and are medically unstable. In general, patients who have unilateral complete renal embolic occlusion are best treated by either nonoperative anticoagulant therapy or percutaneous transcatheter thromboembolectomy (Millan et al., 1978). The patient with bilateral renal artery emboli or an embolus to a solitary kidney may be a candidate for anticoagulant therapy, streptokinase catheter embolectomy, supportive hemodialysis, or surgical treatment as determined by medical status and response to initial conservative therapy. If the patient is a reasonable surgical risk, then preparation for a bypass graft, transection of the renal artery with embolectomy, and reconstruction of the renal circulation by an aortorenal

saphenous vein bypass graft give the surgeon a better chance for salvage.

Renal Trauma

Acute renal artery thrombosis may result from trauma caused by surgical manipulation of a vascular clamp or from external trauma of a blunt or penetrating nature. The left renal artery is more frequently involved in blunt traumatic occlusion, perhaps as a result of deceleration of the mobile kidney with acute angulation of the left renal artery at its aortorenal junction. The more elastic components of the arterial wall, e.g., the adventitia and muscularis, stretch, but the inflexible intima is contused and produces hemorrhage and a propagated thrombus (Fig. 67–14) (Collins and Jacobs, 1961).

The management of traumatic renal artery thrombosis presents the problem of an often irreversible ischemic lesion. In all reported therapeutic successes, the patients have undergone arterial reconstructions within 12 hours of the injury. In one report, only five of 35 patients (14 per cent) with a unilateral traumatically obstructed renal artery who underwent revascularization had return of renal function, all with an ischemia time of less than 12 hours (Spirnak and Resnick, 1987). In general, the patient with a traumatic renal artery thrombosis should undergo an attempt at repair only when a solitary kidney is present or when involvement is bilateral. Repair should not be attempted in the patient who has severe associated injuries and a normal contralateral kidney. The historically poor results of renal revascularization in this situation should lower the surgeon's expectations in any patient with traumatic renal artery thrombosis.

Arteritis (Takayasu's Disease)

Takayasu's arteritis, an inflammatory disease affecting the aorta and its primary branches, is characterized by

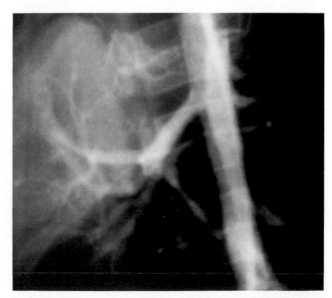

Figure 67–14. Traumatic complete occlusion of dual blood supply to left kidney.

stenosis or aneurysmal dilatation of these vessels (Fig. 67–15) (Ishikawa, 1978). The etiology of this condition is unclear. It is usually progressive and as a result requires treatment. One study of a series of 32 patients with Takayasu's disease treated with balloon angioplasty reported an 86 per cent beneficial response rate at 6 months (Dong et al., 1987). Until longer follow-up studies are available, surgical intervention appears to be the treatment of choice.

Neurofibromatosis

Neurofibromatosis is characterized by café-au-lait spots, cutaneous fibromas, and neurofibromas. A hereditary disorder, it is associated with renovascular lesions and pheochromocytomas. The vascular lesions are characterized by intimal endothelial proliferation with or without aneurysmal formation and cellular nodules in the vessel wall. The aorta is frequently involved, and the renal arteries may demonstrate long areas of stenosis (Grad and Rance, 1972), which are probably best treated by revascularization procedures rather than by angioplasty.

TREATMENT OF RENOVASCULAR LESIONS: GENERAL PRINCIPLES

Medical therapy, percutaneous transluminal angioplasty, and surgery are the three options currently available for patients with renovascular hypertension. In patients with atherosclerosis, the indications for surgical correction are more limited, owing to the older age of the patients and the presence of extrarenal vascular disease. In these patients, treatment with newer more potent antihypertensive drugs is warranted initially and may in fact be preferred, especially in patients with generalized atherosclerosis. Our own poor results with percutaneous transluminal angioplasty for atherosclerotic lesions prevent us from offering this therapeutic option to our patients unless they have a very short mid main renal artery plaque. Surgical treatment is being recommended more frequently in older patients when the hypertension is poorly or inadequately controlled or when the renal function is compromised. This circumstance is especially true in the presence of bilateral, high-grade stenotic disease or stenosis in a solitary kidney. Surgical treatment is recommended in these so-affected patients not only for control of hypertension but also for preservation or restoration of renal function (Libertino et al., 1988).

The choice of treatment in patients with mural dysplasia is determined by the type of the specific dysplastic process and its natural history. Medial fibroplasia is best treated by antihypertensive medication until the patient "breaks through" on this therapeutic regimen. Excellent results have been achieved with percutaneous transluminal renal angioplasty for the treatment of mural dysplasias, with 60 per cent cured, 35 per cent improved, and 7 per cent failed, as reported by Sos and colleagues (1983 and 1984). A review of our results using this technique revealed an 85 per cent overall success rate. Thus, balloon angioplasty is now our first line of treatment in patients with mural dysplasia. Surgical treatment is reserved for those patients who experience failure with percutaneous angioplasty or who develop recurrent disease or who are found to have aneurysmal disease or dissection as a component of the presenting mural lesion. If recurrent disease develops after a successful dilatation, we prefer to proceed with surgical correction rather than redilatation. In our experience, complications following percutaneous balloon angioplasty, such as intimal dissection or rupture, have developed only in those patients who underwent redilatations of mural dysplastic lesions.

Indications for Operation

Generally, corrective surgery for renovascular hypertension or a renal artery pathologic condition should be considered in a patient who has significant diastolic hypertension secondary to a functionally significant renal artery lesion and who is a reasonable surgical risk. Specifically, a patient with the following manifestations of renovascular disease is clearly a candidate for surgical intervention: poor control of hypertension after aggressive, appropriate drug therapy; poor compliance; total renal artery occlusion or dissection; deterioration of renal function as manifested by an elevation of either the blood urea nitrogen or creatinine level; pyelographic evidence of renal parenchymal loss; angiographic evidence of progressive renal artery disease; severely symptomatic or accelerated hypertension; anuria from arterial occlusion to a solitary kidney; failure of percutaneous transluminal angioplasty; and any combination of these factors (Libertino and Zinman, 1987).

As previously mentioned, the pathologic entity and its natural history also influence our judgment about who should or should not undergo surgical treatment. Because of the natural history of atherosclerosis, it

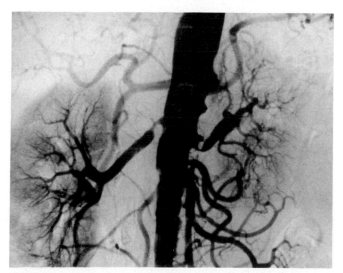

Figure 67–15. Bilateral renal artery stenosis caused by Takayasu's disease.

seems advisable to operate on a patient who is a good risk, with a recent onset of hypertension and a functionally significant unilateral lesion. A patient with long-standing hypertension, evidence of disseminated atherosclerosis, and bilateral disease has a poorer risk. Operation should be advised only when uncontrolled hypertension persists, vascular obstruction progresses, or renal function deteriorates. The mural dysplasias are best treated initially by balloon angioplasty. When this fails, surgical intervention is warranted.

When choosing the proper procedure for a patient with renovascular hypertension, the surgeon should not deal with the complexities of the disease unless nephrectomy, partial nephrectomy, endarterectomy, resection and reanastomosis, bypass grafting, microvascular surgery, and autotransplantation are included in his or her surgical armamentarium. Our large experience with the surgical management of the patients with complex renovascular problems that have been referred to us constitutes the basis for the technical aspects of the renovascular surgery described in this chapter.

Preoperative and Intraoperative Adjunctive Aids

Patients with renovascular hypertension may present with the complex problems of systemic arteriosclerosis and widespread effects on the vasculature of other organs. Careful preoperative recording of all distal arterial pulses and bruits in the extremities and the neck should be noted as baseline values. If cerebrovascular or cardiac disease is suspected in a patient with a history of stroke, transient ischemic episode, or angina, cerebral or coronary angiography should be performed. Significant obstructive lesions are repaired before attempting a major procedure on the renal artery. The reason for this practice is that the perfusion pressure of the heart and brain may be reduced appreciably after successful renal revascularization, with the decreased blood pressure possibly resulting in stroke or myocardial injury (Javid et al., 1971). Antihypertensive drugs that deplete catecholamine stores in the nerve end plates are discontinued 2 weeks before operation. Hypokalemia from secondary hyperaldosteronism or long-term use of diuretics should be corrected before operation to avoid the potentiating effects of anesthetic agents.

To protect the already somewhat impaired renal parenchyma from the effects of ischemia, both mannitol and furosemide (Lasix) are given approximately 2 hours before the renal vessels are clamped. In addition, renal dose dopamine may be required to maintain adequate renal perfusion during the surgical procedure. Central venous pressure and Swan-Ganz catheters are required in the atherosclerotic elderly patient to monitor the intraoperative and postoperative hemodynamic status carefully. If cross-clamping of the aorta is required and prolonged, sodium bicarbonate and colloid plasma expanders are administered. Systemic anticoagulation is routine—3000 to 5000 units of heparin are administered intravenously 30 minutes before the renal vessels or aorta is clamped. Without heparinization, thrombi may form proximal to the vascular clamps, with possible embolization to the kidneys or lower extremities. This possibility is even more critical during microvascular surgery on 2- to 3-mm secondary or tertiary branches, where anastomotic patency is dependent on adequate heparinization. Generally, I do not reverse the heparinization with protamine but, rather, allow the heparin to be metabolized within 4 to 6 hours of administration.

Exposure of the Renal Vessels

The patient is placed in a supine position with the arms at the sides. A Foley catheter is introduced into the bladder to monitor urinary output. The skin of the chest, abdomen, and both legs is prepared and draped so that both legs as well as the abdomen and lower part of the chest are exposed. The feet are wrapped in sterile Lahey intestinal bags so that they can be observed carefully during the procedure. This practice allows access to the lower arterial tree so that the color of the legs and the distal pulses can be assessed during operation if embolization of an atherosclerotic plaque should occur. We have also used Doppler monitoring to evaluate the pedal pulses intraoperatively and postoperatively. This method for draping also provides an operative field for saphenous vein procurement.

The type of incision selected to approach the renal circulation is of great importance in safely facilitating dissection and subsequent technical manuevers. A transverse upper abdominal incision from the lateral border of the contralateral rectus muscle extending across the midline into the ipsilateral flank between the 11th and 12th ribs provides excellent access and greater technical freedom to the high-lying retroperitoneal aortorenal junctions and their covering veins (Fig. 67–16).

The renal vessels are best exposed by reflecting the colon. The right colon is mobilized by entering the retroperitoneal space through an incision in the lateral peritoneal gutter along the white line of Toldt. The peritoneum is incised around the cecum up to the ligament of Treitz. The hepatic flexure and proximal transverse colon are detached from the hepatic peritoneal ligaments.

The avascular space between the colonic mesentery and anterior surface of Gerota's fascia is entered without opening Gerota's fascia. The duodenum is "kocherized," and the right renal vein and inferior vena cava are exposed (Fig. 67–17). The right colon, small bowel, and duodenum are retracted upward and medially, allowing an approach to both renal veins, aorta, and infrahepatic portion of the inferior vena cava (Fig. 67–18).

The left descending colon, the splenic flexure, and the distal half of the transverse colon are mobilized by incising the peritoneal reflection along the lateral descending colon to dissect the left renal vasculature. The spleen is protected by dividing the gastrocolic ligament and extending the incision laterally into the avascular space toward the splenocolic attachments, which are then divided. The splenic flexure is retracted downward and medially, exposing the left renal vein, adrenal gland,

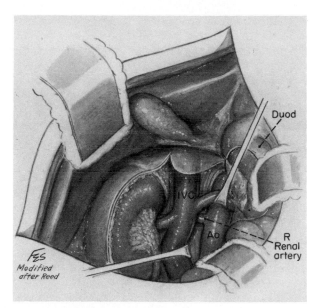

Figure 67–18. Exposure of renal veins and origin of right renal artery. IVC, inferior vena cava; Ao, aorta. (From Libertino, J. A., and Zinman, L.: Surgery for renovascular hypertension. *In* Breslin, D. J., et al. (Eds.): Renovascular Hypertension. © 1982, the Williams & Wilkins Co., Baltimore, p. 170.)

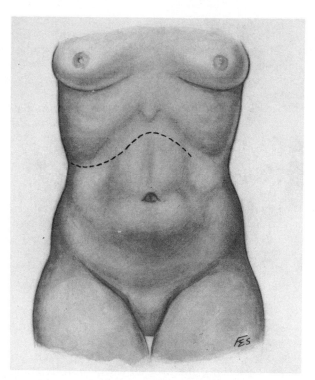

Figure 67–16. Transverse upper abdominal incision. (From Libertino, J. A., and Zinman, L.: Renovascular hypertension. *In* Libertino, J. A. (Ed.): Reconstructive Urologic Surgery: Pediatric and Adult, 2nd ed. © 1987, the Williams & Wilkins Co., Baltimore, p. 122.)

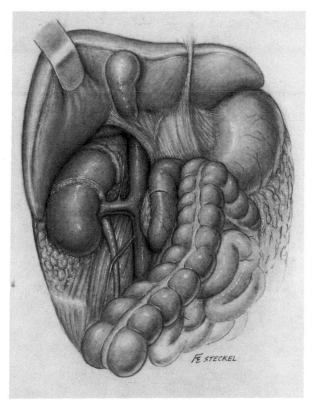

Figure 67–17. Exposure of right renal vein and inferior vena cava. (From Libertino, J. A., and Zinman, L.: Renovascular hypertension. *In* Libertino, J. A. (Ed.): Reconstructive Urologic Surgery: Pediatric and Adult, 2nd ed. © 1987, the Williams & Wilkins Co., Baltimore, p. 122.)

and distal portion of the pancreas (Fig. 67–19). The spleen is retracted with a covering protective abdominal pad. The kidney is not mobilized from its bed so as not to interfere with collateral circulation that may have developed. Great care is taken not to injure the spleen because splenectomy and the attendant rise in platelet count may occasionally produce hypercoagulability. Nevertheless, splenic lacerations do occur and require either splenorrhaphy or splenectomy.

The extent of the vascular dissection depends largely on the type of reconstructive procedure selected. Bypass techniques require less exposure of the suprarenal portion of the aorta, whereas transaortic endarterectomy requires suprarenal aortic control. The vena cava is retracted laterally and the left renal vein upward to expose the origin of the right renal artery (see Fig. 67–18). Vessel loops are placed around the renal veins so that they can be retracted into optimal position for access to the proximal and distal main renal circulation. If renal endarterectomy is planned, the aorta is exposed from just above the superior mesenteric artery to the inferior mesenteric artery. The lumbar arteries are preserved. A space is then developed by careful dissection between the celiac axis and the superior mesenteric arteries. An umbilical tape is placed at this point, marking the site for the proximal aortic clamp. The renal arteries are dissected from their origin to the first major bifurcation of the anterior and posterior divisions. The inferior mesenteric artery should not be divided if occlusive lesions are present in the celiac or superior mesenteric artery, because this may be the major blood supply to the entire small and large bowel.

Another surgical approach to left renal artery stenosis is through a supracostal 11th rib incision. The splenic and renal arteries can then be mobilized by a purely retroperitoneal approach with a direct splenorenal anas-

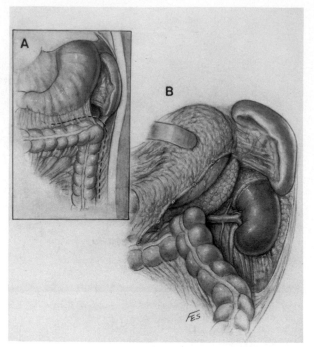

Figure 67–19. Exposure of left renal pedicle. (From Libertino, J. A., and Zinman, L.: Renovascular hypertension. *In* Libertino, J. A. (Ed.): Reconstructive Urologic Surgery: Pediatric and Adult, 2nd ed. © 1987, the Williams & Wilkins Co., Baltimore, p. 125.)

tomosis. We have performed approximately 100 splenorenal bypass procedures and now prefer this surgical approach.

ABLATIVE SURGERY

General Considerations

Nephrectomy or partial nephrectomy is indicated in patients who have renovascular disease that is not technically correctable by revascularization and in patients who have technically correctable lesions but who rate as a poor surgical risk. Renal revascularization is advised in all other clinical situations. The indications and types of procedure vary with the nature and extent of the arterial lesion and are described in some detail in the following sections.

Nephrectomy

Reconstructive surgery is clearly preferable to nephrectomy particularly when the kidney is fundamentally healthy, apart from the abnormality in the renal vasculature and that both atherosclerosis and mural dysplasia are potentially bilateral entities. However, nephrectomy may be indicated in older or patients at high risk when unilateral disease of the segmental vessels is so extensive that reconstruction is not technically feasible (multiple branch lesions), when arterial reconstruction has failed resulting in complete graft occlusion,

when partial nephrectomy has failed, or when subsequent hemorrhage ensues from unilateral renal infarction. Nephrectomy is also indicated for severe unilateral parenchymal disease and for stenosis or poor flow through a previous vascular repair unresponsive to balloon angioplasty.

The totally occluded renal artery with a nonfunctioning kidney has traditionally been treated by nephrectomy. Since the early 1970s, we have performed revascularization procedures on a large number of patients with both total renal artery occlusion and nonfunctioning kidneys, with restoration of function and cure or improvement of the hypertension (Zinman and Libertino, 1973 and 1977). Therefore, not all patients with total renal artery occlusion and a kidney not visible on intravenous pyelography should be treated by nephrectomy. In our experience certain predictive criteria have emerged that are helpful in deciding whether a nephrectomy or revascularization procedure should be carried out.

The kidney with a totally occluded renal artery may be revascularized if the following criteria are fulfilled: demonstration by arteriography of a nephrogram, a visualization of perihilar collaterals, or a retrograde filling of the distal renal arterial circulation by collaterals; back bleeding from the renal arteriotomy distal to the total occlusion during operation; and demonstration by intraoperative frozen-section biopsy of histologically viable glomeruli (Figs. 67–20 to 67–24) (Libertino et al., 1980).

Nephrectomy is best performed through a supracostal 11th or 12th rib incision when operating on the patient at high risk, with multiple branch lesions that are not technically reconstructable, with arterial reconstruction that has failed, with previous partial nephrectomy, and with severe unilateral parenchymal disease or renal infarction. In patients with a stenosed graft, poor flow through a previous vascular repair, or right nonfunctioning or totally occluded renal artery, an anterior approach should be used if revascularization can be accomplished. If nephrectomy is necessary, the renal pedicle that has been isolated is divided and doubly ligated utilizing 0 silk ligatures. If potential microvascular surgery or autotransplantation for peripheral branch lesions is considered, the ureteral segment is deliberately left long.

The nephrectomy for autotransplantation should be performed with the same degree of care taken in a living related donor nephrectomy. The longest lengths of artery and vein possible should be preserved, and injury to the renal pelvic and ureteral blood supply avoided—a delicate procedure (Figs. 67–25 and 67–26).

Partial Nephrectomy

Removal of a portion of the kidney is based on the premise that the disease process is localized and that preservation of the normal remaining nephrons is worth the increased operative time and surgical risk. Patients with branch lesions that produce segmental ischemia and localized overproduction of renin may be treated by arterial bypass, if the segmental branch is large enough (Fig. 67–27); by arteriotomy and dilatation,

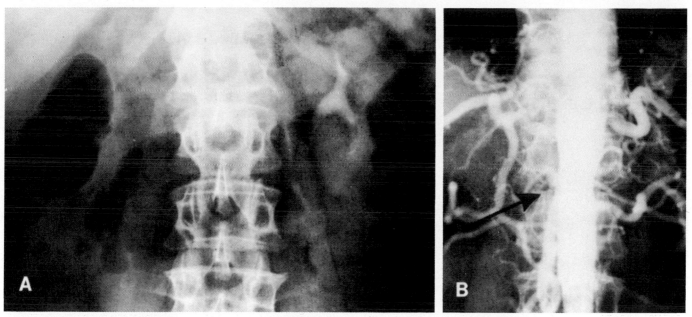

Figure 67–20. *A*, Preoperative intravenous pyelogram. Right nonfunctioning kidney. *B*, Preoperative arteriogram. Total right renal artery occlusion with visualization of perihilar collaterals *(arrow)*. (From Libertino, J. A., and Zinman, L.: Surgery for renovascular hypertension. *In* Breslin, D. J., et al. (Eds.): Renovascular Hypertension. © 1982, the Williams & Wilkins Co., Baltimore, p. 172.)

especially in pediatric patients; or by partial nephrectomy with an upper, lower, or midsegmental renal resection. Knowledge of the segmental blood supply to the kidney is essential for proper performance of partial nephrectomy (Fig. 67–28).

Polar Nephrectomy

In polar nephrectomy, the kidney is dissected from its perirenal attachments and the renal pedicle exposed. The polar vessel with arterial disease is identified, ligated, and injected distally with a dilute solution of methylene blue dye. This maneuver defines the remaining avascular tissue that might lead to subsequent necrosis, poor healing, or ischemic hypertension. The capsule

over the portion of the kidney to be removed is rolled back and preserved for subsequent closure (Fig. 67–29). I prefer not to clamp the main renal artery with instruments or tourniquets to avoid the risk of intimal damage that might result in the thrombosis and loss of the viable portion of the kidney.

The collecting system is closed separately with 5–0 chromic catgut sutures. The cut edges of the parenchyma are closed by bringing forward the previously peeled back capsular flaps and suturing their edges over the repaired collecting system. This procedure helps to avoid the formation of a urinary fistula. The capsular coverings are held in place with separate horizontal mattress sutures. Each suture punctures the capsule eight times before it is tied (Fig. 67–30). A Penrose drain is left

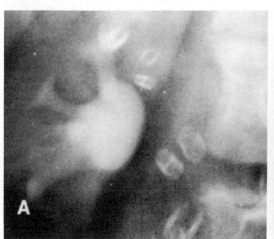
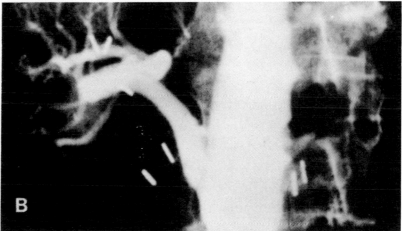

Figure 67–21. *A*, Postoperative intravenous pyelogram. Restoration of right renal function. *B*, Postoperative arteriogram. Patent aortorenal saphenous vein bypass graft. (From Libertino, J. A., and Zinman, L.: Surgery for renovascular hypertension. *In* Breslin, D. J., et al. (Eds.): Renovascular Hypertension. © 1982, the Williams & Wilkins Co., Baltimore, p. 172.)

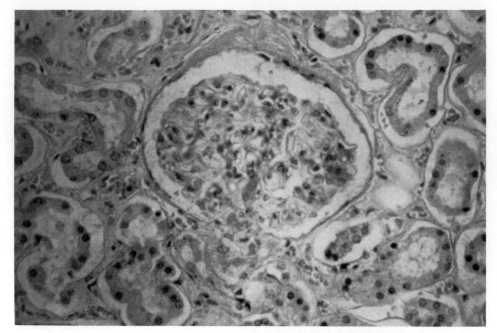

Figure 67–22. Biopsy specimen reveals histologically viable glomeruli. Note evidence of interstitial fibrosis and tubular atrophy. (From Libertino, J. A., and Zinman, L.: Surgery for renovascular hypertension. *In* Breslin, D. J., et al. (Eds.): Renovascular Hypertension. © 1982, the Williams & Wilkins Co., Baltimore, p. 173.)

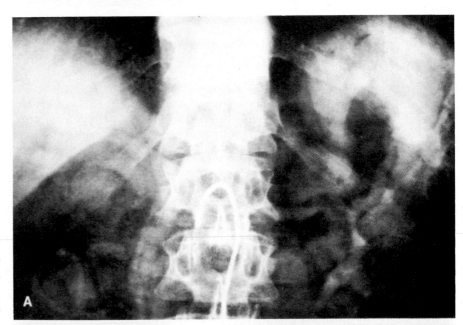

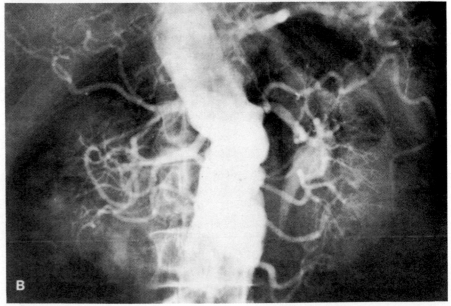

Figure 67–23. *A,* Intravenous pyelogram after angiogram demonstrates right nonfunctioning kidney with faint nephrogram. *B,* Arteriogram. Right renal artery occlusion with retrograde filling of renal circulation via collaterals. Note aortic aneurysm and right renal nonfunction. (From Libertino, J. A., and Zinman, L.: Surgery for renovascular hypertension. *In* Breslin, D. J., et al. (Eds.): Renovascular Hypertension. © 1982, the Williams & Wilkins Co., Baltimore, p. 174.)

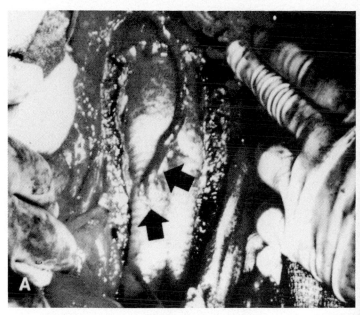

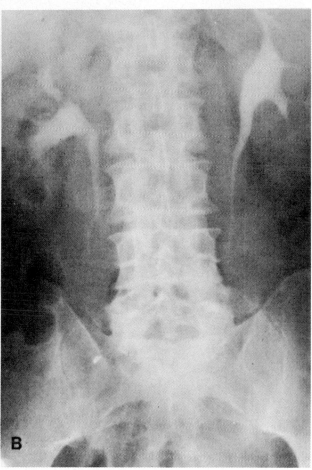

Figure 67–24. *A,* Intraoperative appearance of aortic replacement graft and saphenous vein bypass graft to right renal artery *(arrow). B,* Postoperative intravenous pyelogram. Excellent right renal function after revascularization. (From Libertino, J. A., and Zinman, L.: Surgery for renovascular hypertension. *In* Breslin, D. J., et al. (Eds.): Renovascular Hypertension. © 1982, the Williams & Wilkins Co., Baltimore, p. 175.)

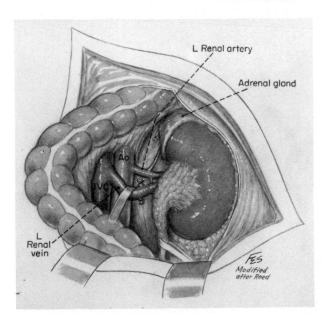

Figure 67–25. Surgical exposure of left renal artery and left renal vein. Note mobilization of left renal vein achieved by ligation of left adrenal and gonadal veins. (From Libertino, J. A., and Zinman, L.: Surgery for renovascular hypertension. *In* Libertino, J. A. (Ed.): Reconstructive Urologic Surgery: Pediatric and Adult, 2nd ed. © 1987, the Williams & Wilkins Co., Baltimore, p. 128.)

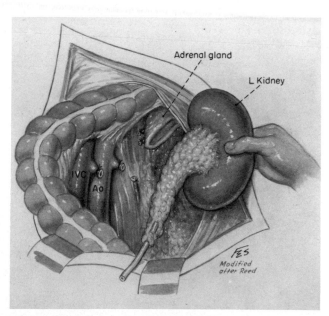

Figure 67–26. Removal of left kidney if autotransplantation or microvascular workbench surgery is indicated. IVC, inferior vena cava; Ao, aorta. (From Libertino, J. A., and Zinman, L.: Surgery for renovascular hypertension. *In* Libertino, J. A. (Ed.): Reconstructive Urologic Surgery: Pediatric and Adult, 2nd ed. © 1987, the Williams & Wilkins Co., Baltimore, p. 129.)

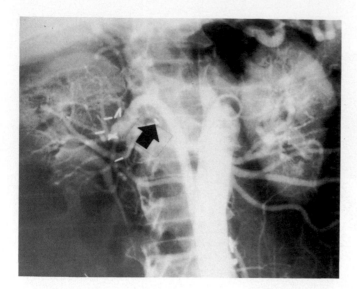

Figure 67–27. Postoperative angiogram. Selective study of aortorenal saphenous vein bypass graft to upper polar artery *(arrow)*. (From Libertino, J. A., and Zinman, L.: Surgery for renovascular hypertension. *In* Breslin, D. J., et al. (Eds.): Renovascular Hypertension. © 1982, the Williams & Wilkins Co., Baltimore, p. 176.)

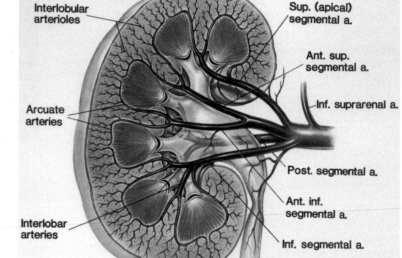

Figure 67–28. Anatomic relationship of cascading intrarenal vessels. (Printed by permission of the Lahey Clinic.)

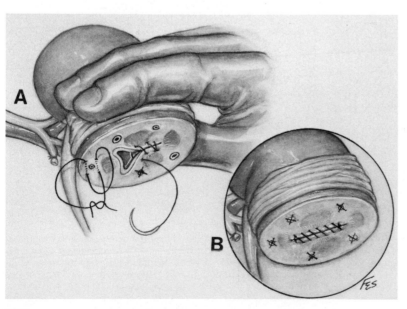

Figure 67–29. Hemostasis of the cut surface is achieved with figure-of-eight shallow sutures. Manual pressure by the assistant controls loss of blood. Intermittent release of pressure identifies pulsatile open vessels for ligation by suture. Note open collecting system and rolled-back cuff of capsular layer. (From Libertino, J. A., and Zinman, L.: Surgery for renovascular hypertension. *In* Libertino, J. A. (Ed.): Reconstructive Urologic Surgery: Pediatric and Adult, 2nd ed. © 1987, the Williams & Wilkins Co., Baltimore, p. 130.)

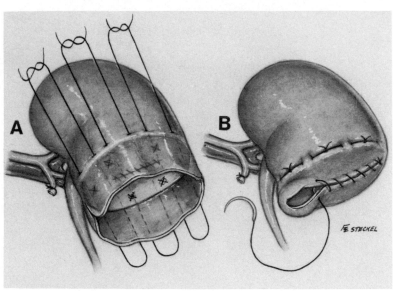

Figure 67–30. Closure of capsular layer over cut edge of renal parenchyma. Horizontal mattress sutures of 3-0 catgut catch the free edges of capsule (inset) after arterial hemostasis has been completed and after the collecting system has been closed. Gentle compression of these sutures and apposition of the capsular tissue against the cut parenchyma complete hemostasis and prevent post-operative fistula formation. (From Libertino, J. A., and Zinman, L.: Surgery for renovascular hypertension. In Libertino, J. A. (Ed.): Reconstructive Urologic Surgery: Pediatric and Adult, 2nd ed. © 1987, the Williams & Wilkins Co., Baltimore, p. 130.)

adjacent to the site of the partial nephrectomy, and Gerota's fascia is closed.

Midpolar Partial Nephrectomy

Midpolar partial nephrectomy represents a sophisticated development in tissue-sparing reconstructive surgery. It may be useful in patients with segmental lesions that affect the superior or inferior branches of the anterior segmental renal artery. Painstaking selective arteriography with oblique views is essential to understand the arrangement and distribution of the anterior and posterior arterial branches. Venography and segmental renal venous renin assays are obtained from the venous branches draining the affected tissue. These are helpful when main renal vein renin levels do not lateralize.

The arterial branches are meticulously identified by exposing the renal hilum, isolating the renal pelvis, and gently cleaning the vascular structures of obscuring fat. Silastic loops are placed around the primary and secondary arterial branches to the segment of parenchyma to be removed. The secondary branches with arterial disease are injected with a dilute solution of methylene blue dye or indigo carmine (Fig. 67–31). If the parenchyma demarcated corresponds to that seen on arteriography, vascular tagging is correct and the appropriate segmental arteries are ligated. The secondary veins are doubly tied and divided in a like manner, and the calyceal infundibulum draining the targeted tissue is transected and ligated (Fig. 67–32). The capsule is incised in a coronal semicircle and is peeled back on each side to expose the wedge of demarcated central parenchyma. With a scalpel, a full-thickness central wedge is excised, enclosing the affected segment. At this point, the surgeon must be assured that no calyceal cavities of the upper or lower pole are left open. The cut surfaces and the hilar branches are checked for significant bleeding.

The collecting system is closed and checked for leaks by injecting dilute methylene blue into the renal pelvis. The capsular apron is draped over the cut edges, and the two poles are approximated with horizontal mattress sutures (Fig. 67–33). Occasionally, partial nephrectomy may be performed judiciously as a component of a bypass procedure. When stenosis of the main renal artery is simply corrected by a bypass procedure, coexisting disease in a branch of the artery may be remedied by simultaneous partial nephrectomy.

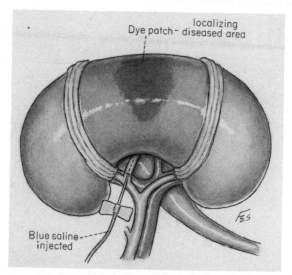

Figure 67–31. Dissection technique in partial nephrectomy of the midsection. Tertiary arterial branches are dissected gently in the renal sinus aided by palpebral retractors of the Gil-Vernet type. Identification of a small blood vessel, such as one that supplies part of the diseased parenchyma, is achieved by injecting a diluted solution of indigo carmine dye into the lumen with a scalp vein needle and correlating the region stained with that seen angiographically. (From Gittes, R. F.: Partial nephrectomy and bench surgery: Techniques and applications. In Libertino, J. A., and Zinman, L. (Eds.): Reconstructive Urologic Surgery: Pediatric and Adult. © 1977, the Williams & Wilkins Co., Baltimore, p. 48.)

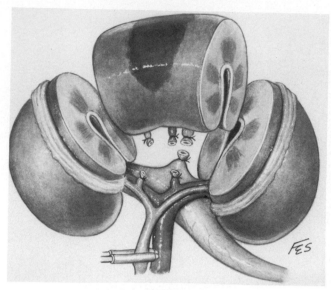

Figure 67–32. Excision is completed by division of tertiary vascular branches and of the infundibulum draining the involved calix. (From Gittes, R. F.: Partial nephrectomy and bench surgery: Techniques and applications. *In* Libertino, J. A., and Zinman, L. (Eds.): Reconstructive Urologic Surgery: Pediatric and Adult. © 1977, the Williams & Wilkins Co., Baltimore, p. 48.)

RECONSTRUCTIVE SURGICAL PROCEDURES

A great variety of revascularization techniques for the surgical treatment of renovascular lesions have been used during the past 2 decades. The two procedures that have emerged as applicable and widely utilized are endarterectomy and aortorenal bypass grafting with synthetic material, autogenous saphenous vein, or splenic or hypogastric artery.

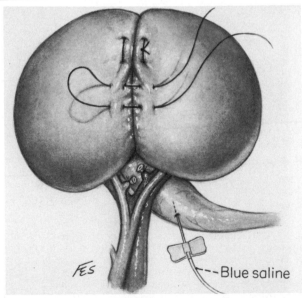

Figure 67–33. Polar remnants are rejoined after releasing the arterial clamp and achieving hemostasis. Closure of the collecting system is tested with blue saline solution. (From Gittes, R. F.: Partial nephrectomy and bench surgery: Techniques and applications. *In* Libertino, J. A., and Zinman, L. (Eds.): Reconstructive Urologic Surgery: Pediatric and Adult. © 1977, the Williams & Wilkins Co., Baltimore, p. 49.)

Endarterectomy

Endarterectomy has been advocated as the procedure of choice for renal artery stenosis secondary to atherosclerosis. The pattern of this disease varies from a focal occlusive plaque at the orifice of the renal artery to extensive involvement of the aorta, renals, and other visceral branches. Dos Santos, who introduced the technique of endarterectomy in 1949, noted that an occlusive plaque could be removed successfully with its adherent intima and media attached and a patent artery achieved. He destroyed the myth that intimal integrity was necessary for preventing thrombosis and achieving luminal patency.

Renal Endarterectomy

Renal endarterectomy has traditionally been accomplished through a renal arteriotomy with extension into the aorta. The aortic wall is partially occluded with a vascular clamp around the orifice of the renal artery (Fig. 67–34). This approach has distinct disadvantages and should be selected only for the management of occlusive atherosclerosis of the renal artery when thrombotic extension involves the distal renal artery and its branches.

The renal artery incision does not afford adequate exposure for the aortic portion of the endarterectomy where the disease originates. It is difficult to continue the point of dissection safely and to obtain a clear demarcation between the renal artery and the aortic lesion. After endarterectomy, the renal artery is often thin-walled and fragile and requires the added complexity of a vein patch angioplasty to avoid narrowing. The incidence of thrombosis secondary to a distal intimal flap and recurrent stenosis with this technique are substantial (Kaufman, 1975). For all of these reasons, I

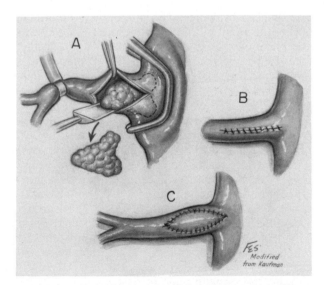

Figure 67–34. Technique for renal endarterectomy with or without vein patch closure. (From Libertino, J. A., and Zinman, L.: Surgery for renovascular hypertension. *In* Breslin, D. J., et al. (Eds.): Renovascular Hypertension. © 1982, the Williams & Wilkins Co., Renovascular Hypertension. Baltimore, p. 180.)

currently find very limited use for this operative technique.

Transaortic Endarterectomy

The transaortic endarterectomy avoids some of the problems inherent in renal endarterectomy. It also allows potential revascularization of a renal artery with multiple lesions, including occluded smaller aberrant vessels, through only one vascular incision.

The surgical technique involves complete mobilization of the aorta from the superior mesenteric to the iliac bifurcation (Fig. 67–35). The lumbar vessels are controlled with microvascular bulldog clamps in the proximal portion of the aorta. Vascular clamps are placed proximal to the superior mesenteric artery and distal to the inferior mesenteric artery. Gentle Swartz microvascular clamps are placed on the distal renal arteries and superior and inferior mesenteric arteries to control back bleeding. Systemic heparinization with 3000 to 5000 units of heparin is administered intravenously, approximately 30 minutes before the clamps are applied.

The aorta is opened through a vertical anterior aortotomy extending from the level of the inferior mesenteric artery cephalad to a point above and to the left of the superior mesenteric artery (Fig. 67–36). Great care must be taken in establishing the initial plane of the endarterectomy. The proper plane is obtained by starting the dissection with a blunt-tipped, slightly curved instrument such as a Schnitt clamp or a no. 3 Penfield dural elevator (Fig. 67–36). This procedure should be performed by the gentlest of manuevers. With the blunt

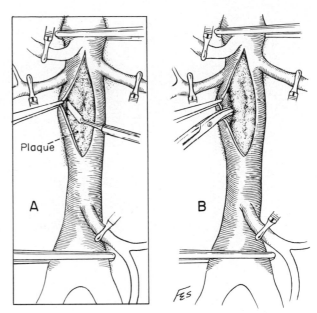

Figure 67–36. Transaortic endarterectomy. Initial dissection between the plaque and the aortic wall with the tip of clamp and dural elevator. (From Libertino, J. A., and Zinman, L.: Surgery for renovascular hypertension. *In* Libertino, J. A. (Ed.): Reconstructive Urologic Surgery: Pediatric and Adult, 2nd ed. © 1987, the Williams & Wilkins Co., Baltimore, p. 134.)

endarterectomy spatula, the plaque is lifted away from the artery, and a plane is developed circumferentially and distal to the lower most portion of the aortotomy. The plaque is lifted anteriorly and away from the posterior wall with a blunt-tipped right-angle clamp and is transected cleanly with Potts scissors.

To prevent dissection, the distal intima is transfixed with four or five mattress sutures of 6–0 polypropylene (Prolene) tied on the outer aortic wall (Fig. 67–37). The divided plaque is lifted up, and the dissection is continued cephalad to the renal orifices where the plaque is carefully dissected into the renal artery. With traction on the aortic plaque, the plane is developed within the lumen of the renal artery until the normal intima appears. Usually, the plaque separates easily from the intimal surface of the normal renal artery and can be delivered into the aortic lumen (Fig. 67–38).

A similar procedure is performed on the contralateral renal artery if it is involved, and the dissection is extended cephalad to the superior mesenteric artery where the plaque is again transected and lifted from the lumen of the aorta. The aortotomy is flushed with a dilute solution of heparin, and the clamps are released momentarily to flush loose plaque or thrombi at their points of coaptation. The intima of the renal artery is inspected through the orifice for residual fragments or any elevated intimal flaps. Gauze pledgets may be used to cleanse the distal renal artery. The renal artery clamps are released momentarily to flush out trapped debris in a retrograde fashion. The aortotomy is closed with continuous 4–0 Prolene sutures. If bleeding from the aortotomy persists, it may be buttressed by wrapping a collar of woven dacron graft around the aorta at the point of the aortotomy. Inspection of the renal artery should reveal a soft wall with no palpable disease and a

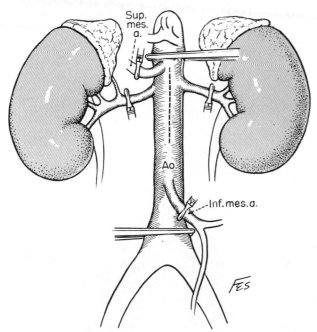

Figure 67–35. The aortotomy for transaortic endarterectomy extends from just above the inferior mesenteric to the level of the superior mesenteric artery. (From Libertino, J. A., and Zinman, L.: Surgery for renovascular hypertension. *In* Libertino, J. A. (Ed.): Reconstructive Urologic Surgery: Pediatric and Adult, 2nd ed. © 1987, the Williams & Wilkins Co., Baltimore, p. 133.)

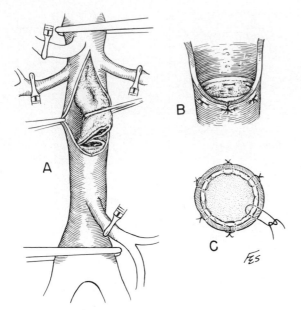

Figure 67–37. Distal intima is transected sharply and tacked to the aortic wall with six mattress sutures to prevent intimal flap dissection. (From Libertino, J. A., and Zinman, L.: Surgery for renovascular hypertension. *In* Libertino, J. A. (Ed.): Reconstructive Urologic Surgery: Pediatric and Adult, 2nd ed. © 1987, the Williams & Wilkins Co., Baltimore, p. 134.)

good pulse. Patency and the absence of an intimal flap can be confirmed by intraoperative angiography.

Endarterectomy should not be undertaken unless the surgeon is experienced and well-versed in the nuances

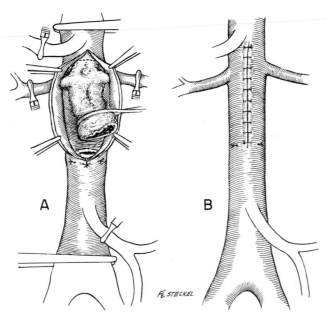

Figure 67–38. *A,* Atherosclerotic plaque is removed from the aorta in continuity with its lateral renal extensions.

B, Simple closure of aortotomy may occasionally require reinforcing interrupted mattress sutures or prosthetic cuff for hemostasis. (From Libertino, J. A., and Zinman, L.: Surgery for renovascular hypertension. *In* Libertino, J. A. (Ed.): Reconstructive Urologic Surgery: Pediatric and Adult, 2nd ed. © 1987, the Williams & Wilkins Co., Baltimore, p. 134.)

of atherosclerotic lesions of the aorta and the renal artery. The procedure has the disadvantage of requiring aortic cross-clamping with bilateral renal ischemia that may be prolonged in a technically difficult situation and may result in renal injury. The denuded medial and intimal surfaces are more prone to early thrombosis, and long-term results in most series reveal a significant incidence of recurrent stenotic disease. The poor results reported in the literature on this procedure as performed by capable surgeons dissuade us from resorting to renal or transaortic endarterectomy as the procedure of choice for atherosclerotic disease of the renal arteries.

Resection and Reanastomosis

Resection and reanastomosis are occasionally suited for patients with mural dysplasia who have a short, well-defined diseased segment. It may be combined with a dacron or saphenous vein interposition graft (Fig. 67–39). The true extent of mural disease is not always appreciated or delineated by its angiographic appearance. For this reason and because mural disease left behind after resection and reanastomosis is prone to restenosis, we prefer an aortorenal bypass procedure.

Aortorenal Bypass Graft

The widespread popularity of the bypass graft for renal artery disease was attained by virtue of its technical ease of insertion and the favorable short- and long-term patency rates achieved. Bypass grafts are applicable to almost any disease process involving the main renal artery or its branches. This procedure also eliminates the more hazardous and tedious dissection of the juxtarenal portion of the aorta required in endarterectomy.

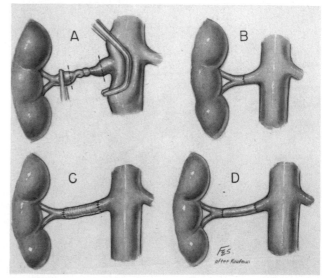

Figure 67–39. *A* to *D,* Resection and reanastomosis with or without interposition grafts of Dacron or saphenous vein. (From Libertino, J. A., and Zinman, L.: Surgery for renovascular hypertension. *In* Breslin, D. J., et al. (Eds.): Renovascular Hypertension. © 1982, the Williams & Wilkins Co., Baltimore, p. 184.)

Bypass grafts are particularly suitable for fibrous lesions that affect long and multiple segments of the renal artery and its branches (Fig. 67–40). Dacron, autogenous artery (hypogastric and splenic), and autogenous saphenous vein may be chosen as aortorenal bypass grafts in properly selected patients.

Dacron has been applied extensively in renal artery reconstruction but has been associated with a relatively high rate of early thrombosis. Excellent long-term patency rates have been reported with a segment of autogenous hypogastric artery. Such a graft matches the size of the renal artery and is sutured more simply than the dacron prosthesis.

Autogenous hypogastric artery is the most favorable graft material for children with renal artery disease because the saphenous vein is usually too small and is more prone to aneurysmal dilatation than in adults. The major disadvantage is that the hypogastric artery is often the first to be involved with generalized atherosclerosis and therefore is not suitable graft material in older patients. It is also a short vessel and, occasionally, technically more difficult to insert between the renal arteries and aorta.

During the past 2 decades the autogenous saphenous vein has emerged as our preferred graft material and is the most common source for restoration of renal blood flow at our hospital (Libertino and Zinman, 1980). Saphenous vein is readily available and closer in size to the lumen of the renal artery than other vascular conduits. Its intima is less thrombogenic than prosthetic material and accommodates the creation of a precise contoured anastomosis with a delicate thin-walled distal renal artery. Patent anastomoses can be achieved with the most challenging 2- to 3-mm lumen branches beyond the major bifurcation. Because of its inherent properties and the favorable surgical results obtained, saphenous vein has become the conduit of choice for aortorenal bypass at most major treatment centers. If the saphenous veins are not available, we use cephalic vein and Gor-Tex graft, in that order, as substitutes.

Procurement of Saphenous Vein

The procurement of an adequate segment of the long saphenous vein is critical to the success of the graft procedure. Meticulous technique in exposure and excision of the vein is essential to prevent mural trauma and ischemia. Improper harvesting of the vein may result in the delayed complications of stenosing intimal hyperplasia and aneurysmal dilatation. Removal of the saphenous vein should be performed by the more experienced surgeon.

The saphenous vein is usually obtained from the thigh opposite the renal lesion so that two surgeons may simultaneously expose the renal vessels and mobilize the graft, shortening the operative time. The vein is mobilized through a single long incision in the upper thigh (Fig. 67–41), which begins parallel to and below the groin crease over the palpable femoral pulses and is extended toward the knee after the junction of the saphenous and femoral veins has been exposed. The incision should be made directly over the vein to avoid producing devascularized skin flaps that can result in necrotic edges and wound sepsis. Finger dissection between the trunk of the vein and the skin is helpful to ensure accurate placement of the incision and, thus, to avoid the development of these flaps (see Fig. 67–41). On the day before operation, the course of the saphenous vein is outlined with an indelible pen while the patient is standing.

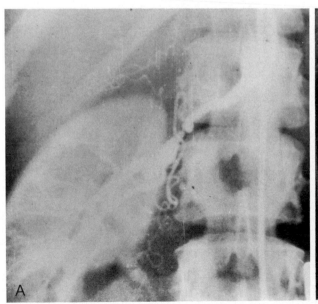 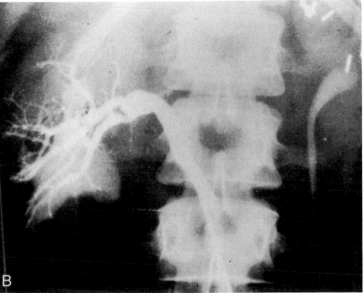

Figure 67–40. *A,* Preoperative arteriogram. Subadventitial disease with involvement of lower segmental artery and small aneurysm at the bifurcation of the renal artery.
B, Postoperative arteriogram. Saphenous vein graft bypassing main stem and segmental lesion. This demonstrates the versatility and ease with which saphenous vein can be contoured to the anatomic situation encountered. (From Libertino, J. A., and Zinman, L.: Surgery for renovascular hypertension. *In* Breslin, D. J., et al. (Eds.): Renovascular Hypertension. © 1982, the Williams & Wilkins Co., Baltimore, p. 185.)

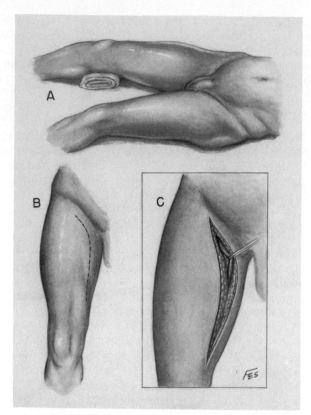

Figure 67–41. Procurement of saphenous vein. (From Libertino, J. A., and Zinman, L.: Surgery for renovascular hypertension. *In* Libertino, J. A. (Ed.): Reconstructive Urologic Surgery: Pediatric and Adult, 2nd ed. © 1987, the Williams & Wilkins Co., Baltimore, p. 138.)

Technique of Insertion of Saphenous Vein Graft

Heparin is initially given systemically after the surgical dissection has been completed and approximately 30 minutes before the arteries are clamped. The saphenous vein graft should be oriented properly to avoid misalignment during implantation. Either an end-to-end or an end-to-side anastomosis can be accomplished, depending on the anatomic situation encountered. An end-to-end anastomosis is preferred under usual circumstances because it permits the best laminar flow.

The aorta, which has already been mobilized and exposed from the renal arteries to the level of the inferior mesenteric artery, is carefully palpated to determine a suitable soft location for the anastomosis that is relatively free of atherosclerotic plaque. A medium-sized DeBakey clamp is placed on the anterolateral portion of the infrarenal aorta in a tangential manner. A vertical 13- to 16-mm aortotomy is made without excising any of the aortic wall or attempting to perform a localized endarterectomy (Fig. 67–43), which may dislodge intimal plaque fragments that can form emboli to the lower extremities when the clamp is released.

Excision of the aortic wall is not necessary because intraluminal aortic pressure spreads the edge of the linear aortotomy to the appropriate dimensions when the clamp is released. The vein graft is anastomosed to the aorta with a continuous 5–0 Prolene suture after it has been satisfactorily spatulated (Fig. 67–44). A micro-

A 20-cm long vein graft with an outside diameter of 4 to 6 mm is usually adequate for reconstruction of the renal artery. Excess vein should always be available for revision of any intraoperative technical problems that may occur during anastomosis. The vein is handled gently without stretching or tearing its branches. The tributaries are tied in continuity with fine silk before they are divided. The areolar tissue is not dissected from the specimen, and the adventitia is left undisturbed.

To decrease transmural ischemia, the vein graft remains in situ until the renal vessels are mobilized and it is ready to be used. If the graft is inadvertently removed prematurely, it is placed in cold Ringer's lactate solution or autologous blood, even if only a short period of time will ensue. The distal end of the vein is transected, cannulated with a Marks needle, and secured with a silk tie (Fig. 67–42). A dilute heparinized solution of autologous blood distends the vein graft before the proximal portion is transected. This step helps to identify any untied tributaries or unrecognized leakage and washes out any residual blood clots. The vein is distended to a minimal diameter of 5 to 6 mm by exerting gentle pressure on the syringe. The proximal end of the vein is transected, and the vein graft is now ready for use. The thigh incision is not closed until the bypass procedure has been completed to ensure that any delayed bleeding due to the heparinized state is identified and controlled.

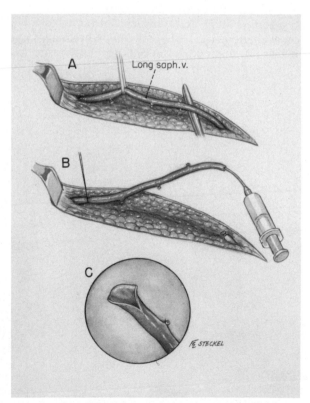

Figure 67–42. Harvesting of saphenous vein. (From Libertino, J. A., and Zinman, L.: Surgery for renovascular hypertension. *In* Libertino, J. A. (Ed.): Reconstructive Urologic Surgery: Pediatric and Adult, 2nd ed. © 1987, the Williams & Wilkins Co., Baltimore, p. 139.)

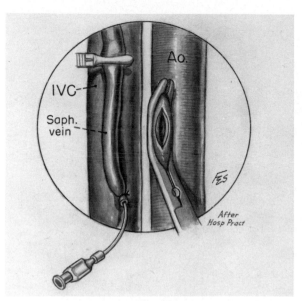

Figure 67–43. An easily accessible segment of the aorta *(Ao)* is partially occluded with a DeBakey exclusion clamp. A 13- to 16-mm aortotomy is made preparatory to constructing the proximal anastomosis. IVC, inferior vena cava; Saph vein, saphenous vein. (From Libertino, J. A., and Zinman, L.: Surgery for renovascular hypertension. *In* Libertino, J. A. (Ed.): Reconstructive Urologic Surgery: Pediatric and Adult, 2nd ed. © 1987, the Williams & Wilkins Co., Baltimore, p. 141.)

vascular Schwartz clamp is placed on the end of the saphenous vein graft, and the aortic clamp is released. The graft is allowed to lie anterior to the vena cava on the right side or anterior to the renal vein on the left side. Although it is preferable to leave the vein too long than too short, it should not be so long as to bend into an acute angle at any point.

The renal artery is secured distally with a smooth-jawed Schwartz microvascular clamp placed on either the distal main renal artery or its branches. The proper site for the arterial anastomosis is selected. An end-to-end anastomosis is performed utilizing a continuous 6–0 Prolene suture or interrupted sutures of the same material, depending on the diameter of the anastomosis (Fig. 67–45). When the saphenous vein graft is being anastomosed with two branches 3 mm or less in size, interrupted sutures are chosen. An interrupted suture line is also selected in children to prevent a pursestring effect with growth of the vessels when the patients become older. This effect may also occur with running synthetic monofilament sutures when too much tension is applied during the creation of the anastomosis. The pursestring effect can be avoided by placing sutures at four quadrants in the arterial wall before beginning the anastomosis. Operating loupe magnification and fiberoptic head lamps are very helpful at this point in the operation to allow precise placement of sutures, particularly when exposure in the renal artery is difficult.

The single most important factor responsible for long-term patency is a wide flawless anastomosis with the renal artery. After completion of the anastomosis, the microvascular bulldog clamps are removed from the distal renal circulation and the saphenous vein graft, permitting reconstitution of the renal circulation (Fig. 67–46).

Alternative Bypass Procedures

When a difficult or troublesome aorta precludes aortorenal revascularization, alternative bypass procedures can be employed for the restoration of renal blood flow (Libertino and Selman, 1982).

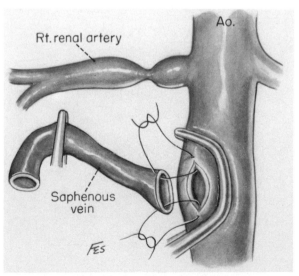

Figure 67–44. Aortic-to-graft anastomosis is carried out before graft-to-renal anastomosis when an end-to-end anastomsis is desired. (From Libertino, J. A., and Zinman, L.: Surgery for renovascular hypertension. *In* Breslin, D. J., et al. (Eds.): Renovascular Hypertension. © 1982, the Williams & Wilkins Co., Baltimore, p. 191.)

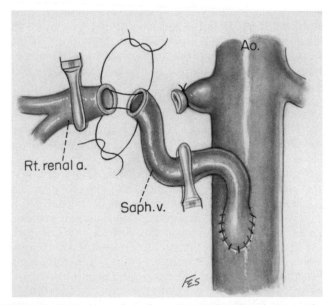

Figure 67–45. End-to-end renal anastomosis is initiated. (From Libertino, J. A., and Zinman, L.: Surgery for renovascular hypertension. *In* Breslin, D. J., et al. (Eds.): Renovascular Hypertension. © 1982, the Williams & Wilkins Co., Baltimore, p. 191.)

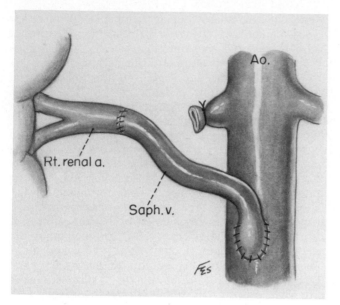

Figure 67–46. Completed end-to-end renal anastomosis. (From Libertino, J. A., and Zinman, L.: Surgery for renovascular hypertension. *In* Breslin, D. J., et al. (Eds.): Renovascular Hypertension. © 1982, the Williams & Wilkins Co., Baltimore, p. 191.)

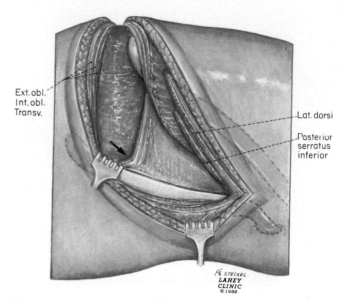

Figure 67–47. Relationship of flank musculature to supracostal area. (Printed by permission of the Lahey Clinic.)

Splenorenal Arterial Bypass

Splenorenal arterial bypass has many desirable features as a substitute for aortorenal bypass in patients with stenosis of the left renal artery. It is particularly suitable for patients who have diffuse atherosclerotic disease or thrombosis of the aortic lumen and for those who have previously undergone difficult aortic reconstructions.

The splenic artery has the advantages of being an autogenous artery that has not been separated from its nutrient vasovasorum, of being exposed without difficulty by a relatively uncomplicated anatomic dissection, and of requiring only one vascular anastomosis. Carefully monitored oblique and lateral angiography of the celiac axis is required to determine the patency of this artery, because atherosclerosis can affect the arterial lumen early in the patient's life. Surgical exploration and intraoperative evaluation by palpation and measurement of splenic blood flow are also helpful in establishing its suitability for renal revascularization. If the blood flow is less than 125 ml per minute, the splenic artery should probably not be utilized for renal artery bypass.

We now prefer to expose the splenic artery through a supracostal 11th rib flank incision (Fig. 67–47). The dissection is continued along the upper border of the rib. The overlying latissimus dorsi, the serratus posterior inferior, and the intercostal muscles are divided. Division of the intercostal ligament permits the rib to move freely. The external, internal oblique, and transversus abdominis muscles are divided in the usual fashion.

The intercostal muscle attachments on the distal 1 inch of the rib are divided carefully until the corresponding intercostal nerve is identified. The investing fascia around the nerve is entered. Dissection in this plane allows an extrapleural approach and generally avoids entry into the pleural cavity. This approach also allows excellent exposure, for the ribs are free to pivot downward in a "bucket-and-handle" fashion (Fig. 67–48).

The plane between Gerota's fascia and the adrenal gland posteriorly and the pancreas anteriorly is entered. The splenic artery is identified at the upper border of the pancreas. Its enveloping fascia is entered, and the splenic artery is mobilized by a purely retroperitoneal approach. Several small pancreatic branches are identified, isolated, ligated, and divided. The splenic artery can usually be mobilized from the splenic hilum to the celiac axis without difficulty, and it provides sufficient length to reach the left renal artery.

After the splenic artery is mobilized, a sponge soaked with papaverine is placed upon it to permit it to dilate.

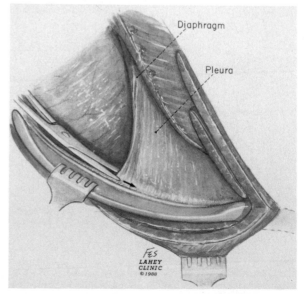

Figure 67–48. Following the intercostal nerve to remain extrapleural back to the intercostal ligament. (Printed by permission of the Lahey Clinic.)

The artery is divided just proximal to its primary bifurcation in the hilum of the spleen, after a suitable vascular clamp has been applied to the origin of the artery. If necessary, the artery may be dilated with a Grunzig balloon or Fogarty catheter intraoperatively to obtain maximum caliber. Removal of the spleen is not necessary because it continues to receive adequate blood flow from the short gastric arteries. The left kidney is approached posteriorly, and the left renal artery is identified and mobilized (Fig. 67–49). The renal artery is ligated at the aorta, and an end-to-end anastomosis between the splenic artery and the distal renal artery is carried out using continuous or interrupted 6–0 Prolene sutures (Fig. 67–49). We have employed this approach in nearly 100 patients and now prefer it to our traditional transabdominal technique.

On rare occasions, a sufficient length of splenic artery cannot be achieved. In this instance, an interposition saphenous vein graft from the splenic artery to the renal artery can be utilized. This manuever enables the creation of a tension-free anastomosis (Fig. 67–50).

Splenic artery disease, the risk of pancreatitis, and the formation of a pancreatic pseudocyst are some of the limitations that have restricted splenorenal bypass as a routine procedure in the management of disease of the left renal artery.

Hepatic, Gastroduodenal, Superior Mesenteric, and Iliac-To-Renal Artery Bypass Grafts

Extensive atherosclerosis, previous aortic surgery, and complete thrombosis of the aorta may preclude the use of the aortorenal bypass procedure for renal artery

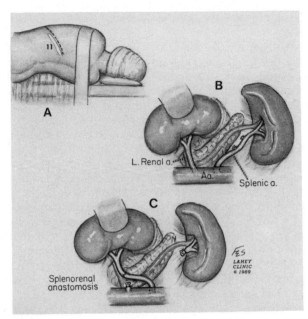

Figure 67–49. *A,* Supracostal eleventh rib flank incision. *B,* Mobilization of splenic and left renal arteries. *C,* Splenorenal bypass procedure. (Printed by permission of the Lahey Clinic.)

reconstruction. When the surgeon is treating a patient with stenosis of the right renal artery in association with these pathologic limitations of the aorta, an hepatic-to-renal artery saphenous vein bypass (Chibaro et al., 1984; Libertino et al., 1976) or gastroduodenal-to-renal artery bypass procedure (Libertino and Lagneau, 1983) can be selected. The value of these alternative procedures, initially described by my colleagues and myself, has

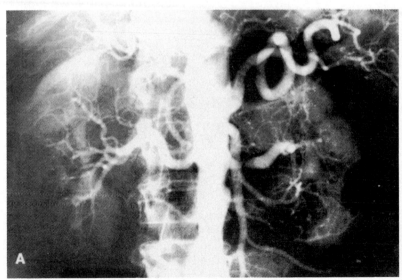
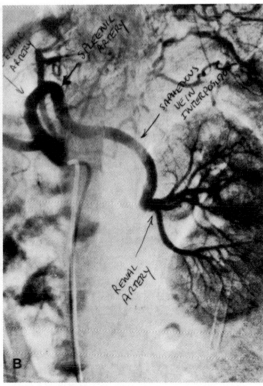

Figure 67–50. *A,* Preoperative angiogram. Left renal artery stenosis. *B,* Postoperative angiogram. End-to-end splenorenal bypass graft with saphenous vein interposition graft. (From Libertino, J. A., and Zinman, L.: Surgery for renovascular hypertension. *In* Breslin, D. J., et al. (Eds.): Renovascular Hypertension. © 1982, the Williams & Wilkins Co., Baltimore, p. 194.)

been confirmed by others (Moncure et al., 1986 and 1988).

Arising from the celiac axis and continuing along the upper border of the pancreas, the hepatic artery reaches the portal vein and divides into an ascending and a descending limb. The ascending limb is a continuation of the main hepatic artery upward within the lesser omentum; it lies in front of the portal vein and to the left of the biliary tree. The descending limb forms the gastroduodenal artery. In the porta hepatis, the hepatic artery ends by dividing into the right and left hepatic branches, which supply the corresponding lobes of the liver (Fig. 67–51). The anatomic variations in the hepatic circulation must be appreciated before this procedure can be utilized. The right hepatic artery is more variable than the left. It may be anterior (24 per cent of patients) or posterior (64 per cent of patients) to the common bile duct, and in 12 per cent, this artery arises from the superior mesenteric artery (Fig. 67–52). The hepatic artery lies anterior (91 per cent of patients) or posterior (9 per cent of patients) to the portal vein. In addition, the left hepatic artery arises from the left gastric artery in 11.5 per cent of patients.

Careful dissection of the porta hepatis is essential; and the common hepatic, gastroduodenal, and right and left hepatic arteries should be identified before an anastomotic procedure is attempted. Vascular elastic loops are placed about these vessels, and the common bile duct and portal vein are identified.

After careful dissection and mobilization of the renal artery, clamps are placed on the proximal portion of the common hepatic artery and its distal branches. The gastroduodenal artery is divided (Fig. 67–53). The inferior surface of the hepatic artery is mobilized from the underlying portal vein and the common bile duct (Fig.

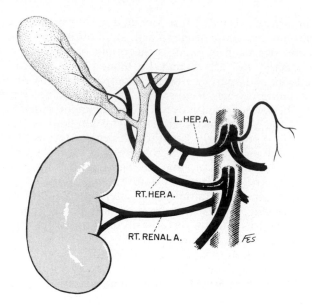

Figure 67–52. The most common variation in the hepatic circulation is to have the right hepatic artery arise from the superior mesenteric artery. (From Libertino, J. A., and Zinman, L: Surgery for renovascular hypertension. *In* Libertino, J. A. (Ed.): Reconstructive Urologic Surgery: Pediatric and Adult, 2nd ed. © 1987, the Williams & Wilkins Co., Baltimore, p. 148.)

67–54). An arteriotomy, 10 to 12 mm in length, is made in the anterior inferior wall of the common hepatic artery, beginning at the ostium of the gastroduodenal artery. A reversed autogenous saphenous vein is inserted with and end-to-side anastomosis between the vein graft and the hepatic artery. This maneuver is usually accomplished with a continuous 6–0 Prolene suture. A microvascular clamp is placed on the vein graft after it has been filled with heparin and after the

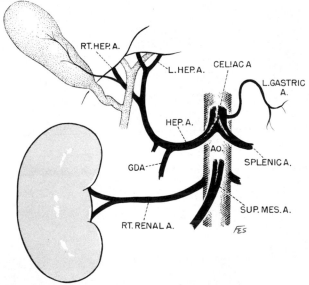

Figure 67–51. Most common pattern of hepatic artery circulation, with the common hepatic dividing into the right and left hepatic arteries, which supply the corresponding lobes of the liver. GDA, gastroduodenal artery. (From Libertino, J. A., and Zinman, L.: Surgery for renovascular hypertension. *In* Libertino, J. A. (Ed.): Reconstructive Urologic Surgery: Pediatric and Adult, 2nd ed. © 1987, the Williams & Wilkins Co., Baltimore, p. 148.)

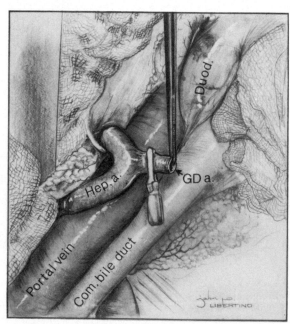

Figure 67–53. Mobilization of the anterior surface of the common hepatic artery. GD a., gastroduodenal artery. (Printed by permission of the Lahey Clinic.)

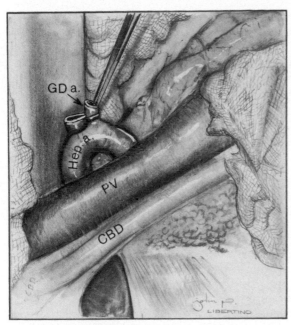

Figure 67–54. Mobilization of the posterior surface of the common hepatic artery. GD a., gastroduodenal artery; PV, portal vein; CBD, common bile duct. (Printed by permission of the Lahey Clinic.)

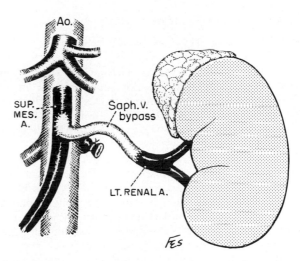

Figure 67–56. Superior mesenteric to renal artery end-to-end anastomosis. (From Libertino, J. A., and Zinman, L.: Surgery for renovascular hypertension. *In* Breslin, D. J., et al. (Eds.): Renovascular Hypertension. © 1982, the Williams & Wilkins Co., Baltimore, p. 200.)

proper alignment and length for the renal artery anastomosis has been determined. The clamps are removed from the hepatic circulation, and a small Schwartz microvascular clamp is placed on the distal renal artery. The vein graft is anastomosed to the right renal artery in an end-to-end fashion (Fig. 67–55). When the gastroduodenal artery is used, it is divided, and an end-to-end anastomosis between the gastroduodenal artery and the renal artery is accomplished.

We have employed this procedure in approximately 50 patients with good results. Postoperative angiography

has demonstrated the absence of a renal-hepatic steal syndrome. Liver function has not been compromised in any of our patients to date. We no longer advocate the use of the gastroduodenal artery in adult patients, but it is a perfectly acceptable bypass procedure in the pediatric patients.

We have also utilized the superior mesenteric-to-renal artery saphenous vein bypass as a "bailout procedure" as well, with good results (Fig. 67–56). An iliac-to-renal bypass graft has been done as an alternative to the aortorenal bypass procedure in ten of our patients, with favorable results (Fig. 67–57).

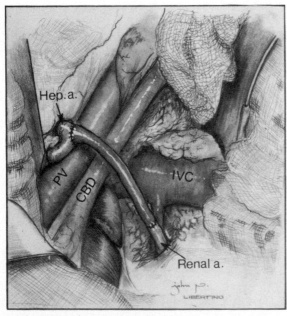

Figure 67–55. Hepatic–to–renal artery saphenous vein bypass graft. PV, portal vein; IVC, inferior vena cava; CBD, common bile duct. (Printed by permission of the Lahey Clinic.)

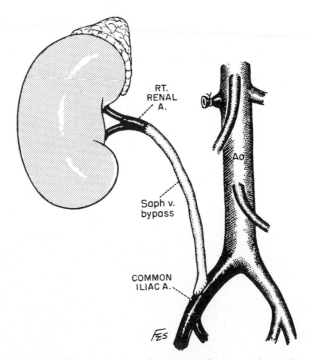

Figure 67–57. Iliac–to–renal saphenous vein bypass graft. An alternative to autotransplantation. (From Libertino, J. A., and Zinman, L.: Surgery for renovascular hypertension. *In* Breslin, D. J., et al. (Eds.): Renovascular Hypertension. © 1982, the Williams & Wilkins Co., Baltimore, p. 201.)

RENAL AUTOTRANSPLANTATION AND EX VIVO BENCH SURGERY

On rare occasions, kidneys with lesions of the renal artery or its branches are not amenable to in situ reconstruction. In these circumstances, temporary removal of the kidney, ex vivo preservation, microvascular repair (workbench surgery), and autotransplantation may permit salvage.

Autotransplantation developed as an outgrowth of the technique in renal transplantation. Early attempts at this procedure were unsuccessful. In 1963, Hardy successfully autotransplanted a kidney into the ipsilateral iliac fossa in a patient with a severe ureteral injury from previous aortic surgery. The simultaneous development of an apparatus that could preserve kidneys extracorporeally for long periods of time and of preservation solutions led to this extracorporeal renal repair (workbench surgery) and subsequent autotransplantation. Ota and co-workers (1967) have been credited with the first successful ex vivo repair and autotransplantation of the kidney. Many other subsequent investigators have reported their experience with these procedures.

Autotransplantation and ex vivo repair should be considered in patients with traumatic arterial injuries, when disease of the major vessels extends beyond the bifurcation of the main renal artery into the segmental branches, and when multiple vessels supplying the affected kidney are involved. Bench surgery may also be required in patients who have very large aneurysms, arteriovenous fistulas, or malformations (Fig. 67–58).

Other indications for autotransplantation that usually do not require ex vivo repair include abdominal aortic aneurysms that involve the origin of the renal arteries and extensive atheromatous aortic disease when an operation on the aorta itself may prove hazardous. In the last case, the patients usually have extensive internal iliac artery disease that precludes utilization of this artery for autotransplantation. However, we have noted that in these instances the external iliac artery is spared extensive atherosclerosis and is suitable for autotransplantation, with an end-to-side renal artery anastomosis or an iliac-to-renal bypass graft (Fig. 67–59).

Techniques for Autotransplantation

Autotransplantation can be accomplished through a large single midline incision or two separate flank and iliac fossa incisions. When the kidney is removed, care is taken to preserve the maximum length of renal vessels and ureter. If the transabdominal approach is selected, ureteral continuity can be retained, necessitating only vascular anastomosis after the kidney is flipped over. If ex vivo surgery requires transection of the ureter, ureteroneocystostomy is necessary in addition to vascular anastomosis.

When ureteral continuity is preserved, autotransplantation is performed as illustrated in Figure 67–60. When the kidney has been excised completely, the standard techniques for renal homotransplantation are used.

During dissection of the iliac vessels, meticulous care is taken to ligate the lymphatics in this area to prevent the development of a lymphocele. The external iliac vein is freed to the point where it is crossed by the internal iliac artery (Fig. 67–61A). The renal vein is anastomosed end-to-side to the external iliac vein using 5–0 Prolene sutures (Fig. 67–61B). If the renal artery is free of atherosclerotic disease, it is then anastomosed end-to-end to the internal iliac artery, employing 6–0 Prolene sutures (Fig. 67–61C and 67–61D). If the internal iliac artery is diseased, the renal artery is anastomosed end-to-side to the external iliac artery.

When the ureter requires reimplantation, we prefer a

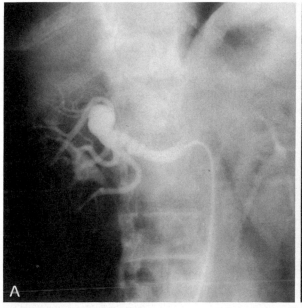 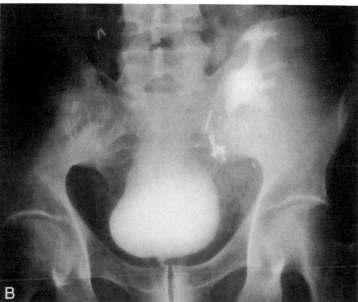

Figure 67–58. A, Mural dysplastic aneurysm with segmental branch involvement. B, Intravenous pyelogram after bench surgery and autotransplantation.

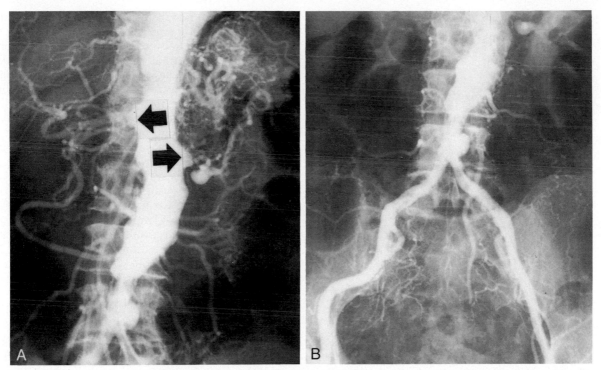

Figure 67–59. *A,* Total right renal artery occlusion *(arrow)*; 95 per cent left renal artery stenosis *(arrow)* with extensive aortic atherosclerosis in an azotemic patient.

B, External iliac arteries are suitable for revascularization. (From Libertino, J. A., and Zinman, L.: Surgery for renovascular hypertension. *In* Breslin, D. J., et al. (Eds.): Renovascular Hypertension. © 1982, the Williams & Wilkins Co., Baltimore, p. 202.)

modification of the Politano-Leadbetter ureteroneocystostomy. Saline solution, 2 to 3 ml, is injected submucosally, raising a mucosal bleb (Fig. 67–62A). A small segment of mucosa is removed from the inferior portion of the bleb (Fig. 67–62B). A right-angle clamp is inserted into this opening, and a 3-cm long submucosal tunnel is created (Fig. 67–63A). At the apex of the tunnel, the right-angle clamp is rotated 180 degrees to pierce the detrusor muscle. The ureter is brought to lie in the submucosal tunnel (Fig. 67–63B). The distal ureter is cut at a 45-degree angle, and the ureter is anastomosed to the bladder with interrupted 4–0 or 5–0 chromic sutures (Fig. 67–63C and 67–63E).

COMPLICATIONS OF RENAL REVASCULARIZATION

Hemorrhage and thrombosis are the two major problems inherent in any vascular procedure. Serious bleeding from a disrupted anastomosis is fortunately a rare event and is usually associated with approximation of diseased vessels or errors in surgical technique. Prolene sutures, in renal and aortic anastomosis, have helped to avoid bleeding at the suture line in the presence of systemic heparinization.

Bleeding may occur during the first 24 hours from periphilar collateral vessels, which attain significant size with high-grade renal artery stenosis. Unrecognized venous bleeding can also be encountered from the adrenal vessels during and after a difficult left renal artery

dissection, because the adrenal gland may be adherent to the anterior portion of the renal vein, renal artery, and perihilar tissue. This bleeding has occurred on two occasions in my experience and demands gentle handling of the adrenal gland with compulsive hemostasis during the dissection.

False aneurysms may occur in any vascular anastomosis including the renal arteries. These occasionally result in intermittent delayed bleeding into the gastrointestinal tract or retroperitoneal space. This complication can be minimized by giving meticulous attention to detail during the anastomosis, by avoiding silk sutures, and by creating a tension-free anastomosis between the graft to a normal undiseased portion of the renal artery.

Late bleeding has been reported to occur from an aortoduodenal erosion after a prosthetic bypass graft (Cerny et al., 1972). Intestinal hemorrhage is more common with prosthetic replacement when silk has been utilized for the anastomosis. Delayed bleeding with erosion of the third portion of the duodenum has accounted for most of these instances and could have been prevented with the use of autogenous graft material, synthetic sutures, and interposition of the peritoneum or omentum between the graft and the duodenum.

Renal artery thrombosis is the most prevalent postoperative complication. This is more common after renal artery bypass with dacron prostheses or renal artery endarterectomy. Thrombosis of this type usually occurs early in the postoperative period and may be difficult to detect, especially when an end-to-side anastomosis has been accomplished and when the kidney is being per-

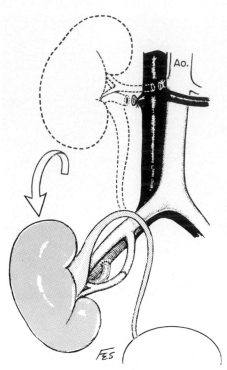

Figure 67–60. Flip-over maneuver for ipsilateral autotransplantation of kidney after workbench surgery with maintenance of ureteral continuity. The renal vessels are turned posteriorly against the recipient vessels, and the pelvis and ureter course unimpeded anteriorly. (From Libertino, J. A., and Zinman, L.: Surgery for renovascular hypertension. *In* Breslin, D. J., et al. (Eds.): Renovascular Hypertension. © 1982, the Williams & Wilkins Co., Baltimore, p. 203.)

fused through its native renal artery as well as the bypass graft. Factors that may predispose the patient to the threat of thrombosis are porous dacron grafts of small caliber, atrophy of the kidneys with a thin-walled diseased main renal artery and high intrarenal resistance, coincidental splenectomy with its hypercoagulable sequelae, and any significant hypotension or hypovolemia in the postoperative period. Normal rapid sequence intravenous pyelography cannot ensure a patent graft. Therefore, when severe unexplained hypertension persists after operation, digital subtraction angiography is performed to determine graft patency.

Aortic thrombosis and distal extremity embolization from aortic plaque dislodgment and cholesterol microembolization are uncommon but extremely ominous complications that may occur at the time of aortic clamping or unclamping. Systemic heparinization aids in preventing this catastrophe, but the groin and lower extremities should be prepared in the operative field so that the color of the lower legs and distal pulses can be assessed after aortic unclamping.

One should be more acutely aware of the possibility of this complication developing in the patient with a diffusely atherosclerotic aorta and a compromised ileofemoral circulation. If this event is suspected, aortic thrombectomy and femoral artery embolectomy should be performed, followed by carefully monitored systemic heparinization. Cholesterol microemboli shower, papaverine, systemic heparinization, and fasciotomy may be

of help. When vessels such as ditigal arteries are involved, amputation may be required.

Aneurysmal dilatation of the autogenous saphenous vein graft and internal iliac artery bypass graft have been shown to occur on late angiographic follow-up studies. Most of these studies demonstrate a uniform increase in the diameter throughout the length of the graft, with a few frank aneurysms noted. We have seen several referred patients with vein graft dilatation. When these patients were re-evaluated with posterior-anterior and oblique angiography, they had narrowing at the distal renal artery anastomosis. It is possible that stenosis of the renal artery suture line caused aneurysmal dilatation of the graft proximal to the stenosis, because of the high-pressure aortic inflow. I can find no reports as yet of an instance of rupture of a dilated vein graft, and patients thus far have remained normotensive with good renal function. Autologous hypogastric artery appears to be superior in this respect, with less dilatation seen on long-term follow-up.

Despite a patent successful renal artery revascularization, persistent hypertension and hypertensive crisis may occur in the early postoperative period. Hypertension can develop from fluid overload during operation,

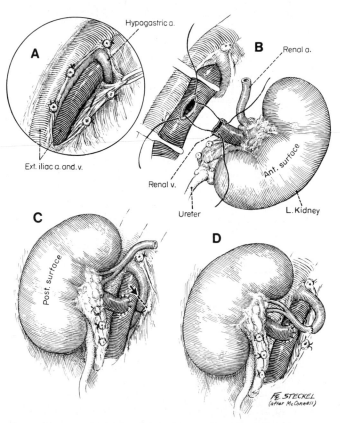

Figure 67–61. *A,* Operative field after exposure of the iliac vessels. *B,* Anastomosis of the renal and external iliac veins. *C,* Preparation of hypogastric artery for vascular anastomosis. *D,* Appearance of transplanted kidney after venous and arterial anastomoses are completed. (From Libertino, J. A., and Zinman, L.: Surgery for renovascular hypertension. *In* Libertino, J. A. (Ed.): Reconstructive Urologic Surgery: Pediatric and Adult, 2nd ed. © 1987, the Williams & Wilkins Co., Baltimore, p. 154.)

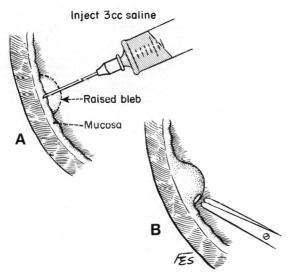

Figure 67–62. *A,* Submucosal injection of saline. *B,* Small ellipse of bladder mucosa is excised to allow creation of submucosal tunnel. (From Libertino, J. A., and Zinman, L.: Surgery for renovascular hypertension. *In* Libertino, J. A. (Ed.): Reconstructive Urologic Surgery: Pediatric and Adult, 2nd ed. © 1987, the Williams & Wilkins Co., Baltimore, p. 156.)

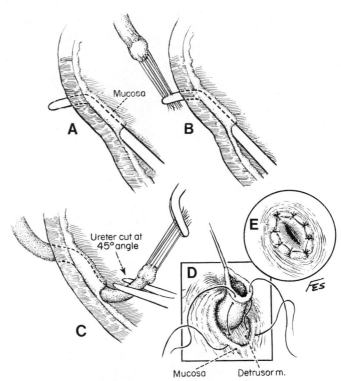

Figure 67–63. *A,* At the apex of the submucosal tunnel, the right-angle clamp is turned 180 degrees so as to pierce the detrusor muscle.

B, The ureter is guided into its new submucosal tunnel.

C, The distal ureter is cut to a 45-degree angle, creating a new ureteral meatus.

D, The ureter is anastomosed to the bladder detrusor muscle at the 5 and 7 o'clock positions.

E, Completion of anastomosis of ureter to bladder mucosa. (From Libertino, J. A., and Zinman, L.: Surgery for renovascular hypertension. *In* Libertino, J. A. (Ed.): Reconstructive Urologic Surgery: Pediatric and Adult, 2nd ed. © 1987, the Williams & Wilkins Co., Baltimore, p. 156.)

vasoconstriction from postoperative total body hypothermia, and excessive poorly controlled incisional pain. When these conditions have been ruled out or when no response to appropriate therapy takes place, control can usually be obtained by intravenous alpha-methyldopa or nitroprusside. Patients may remain moderately hypertensive for weeks or even months following successful renal revascularization and should be treated with appropriate antihypertensive medication that can be gradually withdrawn over an appropriate period of time. In fact, 50 per cent of the patients who are ultimately classified as cured, with successful restoration of blood flow to the kidney, have been discharged from the hospital requiring some antihypertensive medication. An early dramatic drop in blood pressure is not always a sequela to successful revascularization, and blood pressure may take 3 to 4 months to return to normal levels. In contrast, if a patient has unexplained hypertension early in the postoperative period, digital subtraction angiography is performed to rule out graft stenosis or occlusion.

SURGICAL RESULTS

During the past 20 years, I have treated more than 500 patients with renovascular hypertension using the various surgical techniques described in this chapter. The initial 225 patients had the following clinical characteristics: diastolic hypertension greater than 110 mm Hg while receiving triple-drug therapy (70 per cent), significant preoperative cardiac disease (20 per cent), significant preoperative cerebrovascular disease (15 per cent), and azotemia (20 per cent) (Table 67–1). In view of the nature of this high-risk patient population, the mortality rate of 2.1 per cent was acceptable. This result

compares favorably with the overall operative mortality rate of 8 per cent reported by the National Cooperative Study Group (Foster et al., 1975). The blood pressure response at 1 year demonstrated either cure or improvement in 97 per cent of the patients; only 3 per cent failed to demonstrate any beneficial response in blood pressure as a result of the operation (Table 67–2). This result also compares favorably with the results reported by the National Cooperative Study Group, with a 66 per cent cure and improvement rate and a 34 per cent failure rate (Foster et al., 1975).

Table 67–1. PATIENT POPULATION

Clinical Characteristic	Percentage
Diastolic hypertension > 110 mmHg on multiple drugs	70
Cardiac disease	20
Cerebrovascular disease	15
Azotemia—creatinine > 1.5 mg/dl	20

(From Libertino, J. A., and Zinman, L. N.: Surgery for renovascular hypertension. *In* Breslin, D. J., Swinton, N. W., Jr., Libertino, J. A., and Zinman, L. N. (Eds.): Renovascular Hypertension. © 1982, the Williams & Wilkins Co., Baltimore, p. 211.)

Table 67–2. BLOOD PRESSURE RESPONSE TO SURGERY*

	Cured (%)†	Improved (%)†	Failure (%)‡
Atherosclerosis	66	30	4
Mural dysplasia	86	14	0
Miscellaneous	77	23	0
Arteriovenous malformations			
Trauma			
Total	72	25	3

*225 consecutive cases.
†Cured and improved = 97%.
‡Failure = 3%.
(From Libertino, J. A., and Zinman, L. N.: Surgery for renovascular hypertension. In Breslin, D. J., Swinton, N. W., Jr., Libertino, J. A., and Zinman, L. N. (Eds.): Renovascular Hypertension. © 1982, the Williams & Wilkins Co., Baltimore, p. 211.)

Because we are currently being referred more elderly patients with atherosclerotic disease and fewer young patients with mural disease whose lesions are amenable to balloon angioplasty, our patient profile has changed dramatically. In a later series of 123 patients undergoing 152 surgical procedures, the following clinical characteristics were noted: uncontrollable hypertension (55.3 per cent), cardiac disease (60.2 per cent), cerebrovascular disease (31.7 per cent), and azotemia (30.1 per cent). In this second group of higher risk patients, the cure rate was reduced to 43.5 per cent. The improvement rate increased to 51.5 per cent and the failure rate (no beneficial blood pressure response) to 5 per cent. The major reason for the decline in the cure rate with a concomitant increase in the improvement rate is because many of the patients had significant bilateral disease and underwent only unilateral reconstruction for azotemia and renal preservation (Table 67–3).

We have also analyzed another interesting subset of 105 patients who have undergone renal revascularization for preservation of renal function. After a mean follow-up of 2.2 years, a successful outcome was obtained in 85 per cent of the initial 82 patients, with stabilization or improvement of renal function. The rate of graft occlusion in this group was 6.5 per cent and the operative mortality rate, 5.7 per cent. Renal revascularization was a successful method for preservation of renal function with acceptable morbidity and mortality in this high-risk patient population, but the preoperative serum creatinine level was not a predictor of surgical outcome (Table 67–4). Revascularization with visceral artery bypass procedures was very beneficial in reducing the morbidity and mortality in these high-risk patients who had diffuse abdominal aortic atherosclerosis.

Table 67–3. CLINICAL CHARACTERISTICS AND SURGICAL RESULTS IN 123 PATIENTS (152 PROCEDURES)

Patient Population (%)	Cured (%)	Improved (%)	Failure (%)
Uncontrollable hypertension (55.3)			
Cardiac disease (60.2)			
Cerebrovascular disease (31.7)			
Azotemia (30.1)			
Total	43.5	51.5	5.0

Table 67–4. RENAL REVASCULARIZATION FOR PRESERVATION OF RENAL FUNCTION

Outcome	Serum Creatinine Level (mg/dl)				
	<1.7	1.7–2.5	2.6–4.0	>4.0	Total
Improved	NA*	15	19	6	40
Stabilized	16	6	9	0	30
Failure	2	6	2	2	12
% Success	88 (16/18)	78 (21/27)	93 (27/29)	75 (6/8)	85 (70/82)

*NA = not applicable.

The differences in the patient population referred to us have mandated changes in the surgical procedures and have altered the results that can be expected. Blood pressure response is no longer the sole criterion for the success or failure of renal revascularization. Preservation of renal function must also be taken into account when the surgical results of renal revascularization are analyzed. The concept of renal revascularization for preservation of renal function and renal salvage, which we introduced in the early 1970s, has withstood the test of time and has been validated by our surgical experience and that of others (Zinman and Libertino, 1973 and 1977). The predictive criteria to determine whether a kidney is salvageable have also been unaltered by time and subsequent experience (Libertino et al., 1980).

Proper patient selection, performance of an operation individualized to the needs of the patient and the disease, and meticulous surgical technique with adherence to the maneuvers outlined in this chapter are important in achieving a satisfactory result in the treatment of renovascular hypertension.

REFERENCES

Cerny, J. C., Fry, W. J., Gambee, J., and Koyangyi, T.: Aortoduodenal fistula. J. Urol., 107:12, 1972.

Chibaro, E. A., Libertino, J. A., and Novick, A. C.: Use of the hepatic circulation for renal revascularization. Ann. Surg., 199:406, 1984.

Collins, H. A., and Jacobs, J. K.: Acute arterial injuries due to blunt trauma. J. Bone Joint Surg., 43:193, 1961.

Dong, Z. J., Li, S. H., and Lu, X. C.: Percutaneous transluminal angioplasty for renovascular hypertension in arteritis: Experience in China. Radiology, 162:477, 1987.

dos Santos, J. C.: Note sur la désobstruction des anciennes thromboses artérielles. Presse Méd., 57:544, 1949.

Foster, J. H., Maxwell, M. H., Franklin, S. S., et al.: Renovascular occlusive disease: Results of operative treatment. JAMA, 231:1043, 1975.

Goodman, H. L.: Malignant hypertension with unilateral renal-artery occlusion. N. Engl. J. Med., 246:8, 1952.

Grad, E., and Rance, C. P.: Bilateral renal artery stenosis in association with neurofibromatosis (Recklinghausen's disease): Report of two cases. J. Pediatr., 80:804, 1972.

Hagerman, J. H., Smith, R. F., Szilagyi, D. E., and Elliott, J. P.: Aneurysms of the renal artery: Problems of prognosis and surgical management. Surgery, 84:563, 1978.

Hardy, J. D.: High ureteral injuries: Management by autotransplantation of the kidney. JAMA, 184:97, 1963.

Harrison, L. H., Jr., Flye, M. W., and Seigler, H. F.: Incidence of anatomic variants in renal vasculature in the presence of normal renal function. Ann. Surg., 188:83, 1978.

Hollenberg, N. K.: Medical therapy for renovascular hypertension: A review. Am. J. Hypertens., 1(4 pt. 2):338S, 1988.

Ishikawa, K.: Natural history and classification of occlusive thromboaortopathy (Takayasu's disease). Circulation, 57:27, 1978.

Javid, H., Ostermiller, W. E., Hengesh, J. W., et al.: Carotid endarterectomy for asymptomatic patients. Arch. Surg., 102:389, 1971.

Kaufman, J. J.: Renal vascular disorders. In Glenn, J. F. (Ed.): Urologic Surgery, 2nd ed. Hagerstown, Harper and Row, 1975, pp. 874–918.

Kincaid, O. W., and Davis, G. D. (Eds.): Renal Angiography. Chicago, Year Book Medical Publishers, Inc., 1966.

Leadbetter, W. F., and Burkland, C. E.: Hypertension in unilateral disease. J. Urol., 39:611, 1938.

Libertino, J. A., Flam, T. A., Zinman, L. N., et al.: Changing concepts in surgical management of renovascular hypertension. Arch. Intern. Med., 148:357, 1988.

Libertino, J. A., and Lagneau, P.: A new method of revascularization of the right renal artery by the gastroduodenal artery. Surg. Gynecol. Obstet., 156:220, 1983.

Libertino, J. A., and Sinman, F. J., Jr.: Alternatives to aortorenal revascularization. J. Cardiovasc. Surg., 23:318, 1982.

Libertino, J. A., and Zinman, L. N.: Renal revascularization using aortorenal saphenous vein bypass grafting. Surg. Clin. North Am., 60:487, 1980.

Libertino, J. A., and Zinman, L. N.: Surgery for renovascular hypertension. In Libertino, J. A. (Ed.): Pediatric and Adult Reconstructive Urologic Surgery, 2nd ed. Baltimore, Williams & Wilkins Co., 1987, pp. 119–161.

Libertino, J. A., Zinman, L. N., Breslin, D. J., and Swinton, N. W., Jr.: Hepatorenal artery bypass in the management of renovascular hypertension. J. Urol., 115:369, 1976.

Libertino, J. A., Zinman, L. N., Breslin, D. J., Swinton, N. W., Jr., and Legg, M. A.: Renal artery revascularization: Restoration of renal function. JAMA, 244:1340, 1980.

McCormack, L. J., Poutasse, E. F., Meaney, T. F., et al.: A pathologic-arteriographic correlation of renal arterial disease. Am. Heart J., 72:188, 1966.

Millan, V. G., Sher, M. H., Deterling, R. A., Jr., Packard, A., Morton, J. R., and Harrington, J. T.: Transcatheter thromboembolectomy of acute renal artery occlusion. Arch. Surg., 113:1086, 1978.

Moncure, A. C., Brewster, D. C., Darling, R. C., Abbott, W. M., and Cambria, R. P.: Use of the gastroduodenal artery in right renal artery revascularization. J. Vasc. Surg., 8:154, 1988.

Moncure, A. C., Brewster, D. C., Darling, R. C., Atnip, R. G., Newton, W. D., and Abbott, W. M.: Use of the splenic and hepatic arteries for renal revascularization. J. Vasc. Surg., 3:196, 1986.

Nicholas, G. G., and Demuth, W. E., Jr.: Treatment of renal artery embolism. Arch. Surg., 119:278, 1984.

Ota, K., Mori, S., Awane, Y., et al.: Ex situ repair of renal artery for renovascular hypertension. Arch. Surg., 94:370, 1967.

Sos, T. A., Pickering, T. G., Saddekni, S., et al.: The current role of renal angioplasty in the treatment of renovascular hypertension. Urol. Clin. North Am., 11:503, 1984.

Sos, T. A., Pickering, T. G., Sniderman, K., et al.: Percutaneous transluminal renal angioplasty in renovascular hypertension due to atheroma or fibromuscular dysplasia. N. Engl. J. Med., 309:274, 1983.

Sosa, R. E., and Vaughan, E. D., Jr.: Renovascular hypertension. In Gillenwater, J. (Ed.): Adult and Pediatric Urology, Vol. 1. Chicago, Year Book Medical Publishers, Inc., 1987, pp. 752–776.

Spirnak, J. P., and Resnick, M. I.: Revascularization of traumatic thrombosis of the renal artery. Surg. Gynecol. Obstet., 164:22, 1987.

Stanley, J. C., Rhodes, E. L., Gewertz, B. L., et al.: Renal artery aneurysms. Significance of macroaneurysms exclusive of dissections and fibrodysplastic mural dilations. Arch. Surg., 110:1327, 1975.

Tegtmeyer, C. J., Kofler, T. J., and Ayers, C. A.: Renal angioplasty: Current status. AJR, 142:17, 1984.

Wilcox, C. S., Williams, C. M., Smith, T. B., Frederickson, E. D., Wingo, C., and Bucci, C. M.: Diagnostic uses of angiotensin-converting enzyme inhibitors in renovascular hypertension. Am. J. Hypertens., 1(4 pt 2):344S, 1988.

Zinman, L. N., and Libertino, J. A.: Revascularization of the totally occluded renal artery (abstract). Circulation, 48(Suppl. 4):31, 1973.

Zinman, L. N., and Libertino, J. A.: Revascularization of the chronic totally occluded renal artery with restoration of renal function. J. Urol., 118:517, 1977.

68
SURGERY OF THE URETER

Alexander Greenstein, M.D.
M. J. Vernon Smith, M.D., Ph.D.
Warren W. Koontz, Jr., M.D.

The foundation of ureteral surgery was laid in the 19th century, when the first planned operation on the ureter was reported in *Lancet* in 1852 by Sir John Simon (Simon, 1852). As reported, in this operation, he deliberately created a fistula between the ureters and the rectum in a case of bladder extrophy. Until the introduction of roentgenography in 1895, nephrectomy was the end stage of ureteral injuries or neoplasms. Further innovations in surgical approaches, such as the development of the bladder flap technique (first suggested by Boari in 1894) by Ockerblad (1947) and the concept of internal stenting by Davis (1943), have allowed urologists to treat the more complex diseases of the ureter. Advanced techniques, which permit the use of bowel segments and the mobilization of the bladder and the mobilization and/or autotransplantation of the kidney, allow the urologist to operate on any part of the ureter. Nevertheless, re-establishment of urinary continuity remains a challenge that requires a full surgical armamentarium.

SURGICAL ANATOMY

The ureter is a muscular tube that transports urine from the ureteropelvic junction of the kidney to the bladder. It lies loosely in the retroperitoneum in its upper portion, and becomes attached to the parietal peritoneum as it crosses the iliac vessels in its lower portion. The ureter varies in length from 20 to 30 cm, depending on the size of the individual and the anatomic position of the kidney.

Surgically, the ureter is divided into three parts. The ureter courses up and over (anterior) to the psoas muscle and lateral to the transverse processes in its proximal third. The middle third of the ureter passes posterior to the gonadal vessels (spermatic or ovarian). On the right side, the duodenum lies in front of the ureter and more distally the ureter is crossed by the right colic and ileocolic vessels. Sometimes, the appendix may lie on the right ureter. The left ureter is crossed by the left colic vessels and at the level of the pelvic brim by the sigmoid colon. More distally, the ureter crosses the iliac vessels and lies anterior to the sacroiliac joint. The ureter courses posteriorly and laterally, following the course of the hypogastric vessels, in close proximity to the wall of the pelvis. The ureter then turns medially toward the bladder, lying anterior to the hypogastric artery and medial to the obturator nerve and vessels.

In the male, just before the ureter enters the bladder, it is crossed anteriorly by the vas deferens. In the female, the ureter crosses anterior to the internal iliac artery, below the broad ligament, runs behind the uterine artery and vein, and passes within 1 to 2 cm of the uterine cervix, before entering the base of the bladder.

The ureters enter the bladder obliquely, passing through a submucosal tunnel so that, when the bladder is filling, the tunnel prevents vesicoureteral reflux. The ureter in both males and females is crossed by the obliterated umbilical vessels.

The three anatomic points of narrowing of the ureter are the ureteropelvic junction, the area where the ureter passes over the iliac vessels, and the intramural ureter (Motola et al., 1988). The ureter develops its arterial blood supply from branches of the aorta. Branches of the renal artery also supply the upper third of the ureter and the renal pelvis. Branches from the aorta and from the gonadal, iliac, hypogastric, and superior vesical supply the middle third of the ureter. Branches of the uterine, inferior vesical, obturator, gluteal, vaginal, and middle hemorrhoidal arteries supply the lower third of the ureter.

The vessels from these many sources anastomose with each other and create a network in the adventitial tissue of the ureter. This fine capillary network allows interruption of the arterial supply in one area but will not ordinarily affect the vascular integrity of the ureter.

The venous drainage of the ureter arises from the submucosal and muscular layers and courses through the adventitial tissue to drain into veins parallel to the

2552

arterial blood supply (Daniel and Shackman, 1952). The ureter is composed of three anatomic layers: an outer adventitial sheath through which courses its blood supply; a middle layer of smooth muscle arranged in a spiral, circular, or longitudinal fashion; and an inner layer of transitional cells. Ureteral contractions or peristaltic waves propel a bolus of urine from the kidney to the bladder. These contractions normally occur at a frequency of two to six times per minute. Therefore, the urine enters the bladder in spurts. For efficient propulsion of the bolus, the contraction wave must completely coapt the ureteral wall and the urine then passes into the bladder. Any alteration that interferes with the function of this urinary transport mechanism may lead to renal deterioration and eventually to loss of that kidney unit.

URETERAL DISORDERS THAT REQUIRE SURGERY

The indications for ureteral surgery are to manage the presence of disease itself, such as neoplasm of the ureter; to re-establish an unobstructed urine flow from the kidney; and to repair ureteral fistulas. Some disorders may be treated endoscopically, but any disorder that would be inadequately treated endoscopically should be treated with open surgery.

Table 68–1 summarizes the various intrinsic ureteral disorders that require surgery, and Table 68–2 summarizes the various extrinsic ureteral disorders that require surgery.

PRINCIPLES OF URETERAL SURGERY

Preoperative Consideration

The first step in the preoperative planning of a surgical procedure on the ureter is to have as much information about the urinary system as needed. Delineation of the full length of the ureter to be operated on can be accomplished by an intravenous urogram. At that time, information is acquired about the anatomy, position, and function of the kidneys, the contralateral ureter, and the bladder.

Cystoscopy and retrograde bulb occlusive ureteropyelography may be necessary to complete the information about the surgical field. In some patients in whom retrograde urography is not feasible, antegrade pyeloureterography, employing a percutaneous nephrostomy, may be beneficial in delineating the collecting system.

Table 68–1. INTRINSIC URETERAL DISORDERS REQUIRING SURGERY

1. Congenital ureteral abnormalities
2. Urinary calculi
3. Inflammatory conditions (tuberculosis, schistosomiasis)
4. Benign tumors (lipoma, leiomyoma, fibroma, neuroma, endometrioma)
5. Malignant tumors (uroepithelial, sarcoma).

Table 68–2. EXTRINSIC URETERAL DISORDERS REQUIRING SURGERY

1. Vascular (arterial aneurysm, arterial anomalies, retrocaval ureter)
2. Female reproductive system (ovarian cyst, fibroid uterus, tubo-ovarian abscess, pelvic endometriosis, malignant tumors)
3. Gastrointestinal disorders (granulomatous Crohn's disease, appendiceal abscesses, diverticulitis, malignant tumors)
4. Retroperitoneal diseases (idiopathic fibrosis, fibrosis secondary to infection, side effect of medication, abscess, benign tumors, malignant primary or metastatic tumor, lipomatosis)
5. Ureteral injuries (during surgery of adjacent organs, ureter; during urologic endoscopic manipulation; nonsurgical trauma; radiation)

Other imaging modalities such as ultrasound, computer tomography, and magnetic resonance imaging enable cross-section visualization of the ureter and the extra-ureteral and retroperitoneal area. When segments of bowel are to be utilized, evaluation of the alimentary tract may be required regarding factors such as inflammatory bowel diseases, previous surgeries, resections, and radiation therapy involving the bowel in the past. When indicated, evaluation may require barium enema and upper gastrointestinal radiology and/or endoscopy.

Healing and Regeneration of the Ureter

A number of factors affect ureteral healing. Ureteral repair is enhanced because a longitudinal strip of ureter allows bridging of a defect, around which new epithelium can spread to develop a new ureteral lumen. The ureter can close its own defect by regenerating all of its components. The defect is first bridged by transitional cell epithelium, and mucosal healing is complete at 3 weeks with smooth muscle bridging at 6 weeks (Schlossberg, 1987). Prolonged and profuse urinary drainage may lead to abnormal epithelialization. Urinary flow across a repair may promote a lumen and stimulate transitional cell and muscle growth. However, newly formed epithelium may also be distracted and urinary extravasation may lead to a reactive fibrosis with subsequent stenosis and obstruction.

After the bridging of a defect by transitional cell epithelium, fibrous tissue will develop and then contract, pulling already present smooth muscle into the gap. This occurrence stimulates the growth of new smooth muscle to complete the repair. The tissue surrounding the ureter is important in repair. Rigid tissue, such as fascia, produces a disorderly repair, whereas less rigid tissue, such as fat, allows the ureteral walls to renew peristaltic activity. If a repaired ureter is to lie on fascia or bony tissue, the wrapping of the ureter with fatty tissues, such as omentum, may allow improved healing and more rapid return of normal peristaltic activity.

For successful ureteral healing with regeneration of smooth muscle, minimal fibrosis is important for the re-establishment of peristaltic activity. Butcher and Sleator (1956) have shown that a period of 28 days is required for the resumption of the passage of electrical activity across an anastomotic ureteral site. Cineradiographic study after ureteral anastomosis in humans was in accord with this observation (Caine and Hermann, 1970). This finding may account for the occasionally observed delayed pelvic emptying after a dismembered pyeloplasty or ureteroureterostomy. Normally, electrical activity propagates from cell to cell as peristaltic activity is associated with the transport of urine. It is postulated that in the period immediately after anastomosis the electrical event propagates to the anastomotic site and then stops.

Some stasis of urine proximal to the anastomosis occurs, with no urine passing the point of anastomosis until proximal ureteral pressure increases to a critical level and some urine passes beyond the anastomosis. This bolus then stretches the ureteral muscle just distal to the anastomotic site and serves to initiate peristaltic activity distal to the anastomosis (Weiss, 1987).

Stenting

Davis (1943) popularized the placement of stents and stimulated the subsequent investigation and controversy that continue to this day. Proponents of ureteral stenting believe that the stent will (1) immobilize the ureter until healing occurs; (2) inhibit the growth of granulation tissue and allow the orderly regrowth of an intact epithelial layer, followed by its muscular covering; (3) prevent the leakage of urine at the anastomotic site; (4) help maintain an adequate lumen of the ureter during the healing phase; and (5) minimize any tendency to angulation of the ureter (Persky, 1984).

A well-fitting stent provides a mold around which the appropriate healing processes occur (Davis, 1958). The correct size is probably the one that fits comfortably without placing tension on the ureteral wall. Weaver (1957) noted fibrosis and stricture formation with large stents, which was not present with stents that were considerably smaller. Davis (1958) advocated larger stents but not to the size at which blanching of the ureteral wall occurred. Experimental evidence suggests that too large a stent places undue stress on the ureter and particularly on the area of the repair (Persky, 1967).

Some investigators believe that complications may follow the placement of stenting catheters, thus outweighing their possible merits. A frequent complication (Saltzman, 1988), related to the utilization of modern day indwelling internal ureteral stents, is encrustation with deposits of amorphous phosphate material. These cause obstruction with hydroureter and hydronephrosis.

Other common complications are migration of the stent in either direction and erosion that leads to a periureteral collection and fistula formation necessitating further endoscopic or surgical procedures. Care must be taken with these tubes to prevent them from becoming dislodged, obstructed, kinked, or encrusted. Stents may be held in place by suture materials; by holding catheters, such as nephrostomy tubes; or by bladder Foley catheters.

More popular today are the single- or double-ended pigtail catheters that restrict migration up or down the ureter. If prolonged stenting is needed, more frequent changes of the stent may minimize the described complication. Stents placed blindly during open surgery are more likely to malposition.

Vesicoureteral reflux can occur in patients with indwelling stents. This reflux may be used in positioning of the stent during surgery. During surgery, the bladder is filled with indigo carmine dye, and stained fluid will reflux to the proximal end of the stent, verifying the proper position of the distal end of the stent in the bladder.

One of the problems associated with the stent is an inflammatory stricture or calcification at the site of the repair. Stents made of silicone material seem to be the first choice. It is less irritating and resistant to encrustation and at body temperature becomes soft and pliable.

In summary, significant controversy remains over the routine placement of the stent. The surgeon must weigh the advantages of the stent against the disadvantages of this foreign body and the possible related complications.

Urinary Diversion and Drainage

During the healing phase, a ureteral defect may be watertight within 24 to 48 hours. Large defects may take 4 to 6 weeks for complete epithelialization and regeneration of fibrotic tissue and smooth muscle without functional obstruction. Urine flow through an anastomosis does not seem to interfere with the organization of repair; however, with continued urine flow the process requires a longer time.

A longitudinal ureterotomy with drainage for removal of stone or foreign body will allow adequate decompression. After healing, peristalsis will be normal throughout the ureter (Hamm, 1957). In this circumstance, proximal urinary diversion is not necessary for satisfactory ureteral regeneration. If there is a large defect, complete transection of the ureter, severe inflammatory reaction around the ureter, or pooling of extravasated urine, urinary drainage and diversion are applicable. Without adequate drainage a marked fibrous reaction and scarring may result with poor muscular organization, stricture formation, and obstruction.

The type of drain is not as important as the efficiency of the drain. The Penrose drain has been the mainstay for years and can remain indwelling down to the site of any potential extravasation of urine or hemorrhage. It should be left as long as there is a possibility of urinary leakage and should be removed in steps over several days. A self-contained drainage system, such as a sump type (Jackson-Pratt or Hemovac), may also be utilized and can keep the wound cleaner and drier and the patient more satisfied and more comfortable. However, care should be taken to ensure that these devices drain the periureteral area and do not rest on the ureter itself, where they may hold the wound open (wick effect).

Urinary diversion is of benefit to prevent the site of repair from being bathed in urine. This task can be accomplished effectively by means of an internal stent or a nephrostomy. Another form of diversion may be a proximal ureterotomy (with a T-tube) or tube pyelotomy. An important decision is whether or not to divert, and this continues to be a controversy. The guidelines to divert are also variable. Proximal urinary diversion may not be necessary in a well-performed uncomplicated ureteral repair. But in a patient with serious infection, contaminated wound, impaired renal function, or difficult anastomosis, the safety valve or proximal diversion may be an important adjuvant to allow proper healing. The urologic surgeon should be adept at all techniques. The choice of diversion is left to the surgeon's preference, the patient's diagnosis and condition, the type of lesion, and the type of repair.

Suturing and Anastomosis

At the time of the surgical procedure, the delicate and gentle manipulation of ureteral tissue that results in minimal tissue trauma is most important. The ureter should be handled with fingers, fine vascular forceps, or traction sutures and should never be intentionally grasped with a hemostat or other crushing instrument. Scalpel blades (No. 11 and 12) and fine Potts vascular scissors for incisions reduce crush injuries and preserve the blood supply to the operated area. The least amount of ureteral mobilization required to accomplish the operation will prevent vascular compromise. It is the ureteral adventitia that carries the blood supply to the ureter that is to be repaired. Preoperative insertion of an ureteral catheter may allow quick localization of the ureter and prevent inadvertent injury during difficult surgery.

Several factors affect epithelialization of a ureteral defect. These include no tension on the area to be repaired, no urinary leakage, and mucosa-to-mucosa approximation of the defect. Some investigators (Oesterwitz et al., 1988) recommend microsurgery to create a double-layer, end-to-end anastomosis. The advantages of microvascular technique, such as shorter duration of hospitalization and higher success rate, do not justify the use of this technique in every case of reconstructive surgery of the ureter. Laser welding of the ureters has also been recommended for ureteral anastomosis (Merguerian and Rabinowitz, 1986).

The suture material should be absorbable. Silk, Prolene, or other nonabsorbable material may lead to fistula formation, encrustation, and calculi (Silber and Thornbury, 1973). Fine, absorbable sutures, such as 4–0 to 5–0 chromic catgut or synthetic absorbable material, are preferable. Placing the sutures should be atraumatic and should produce a minimal tissue reaction. A tense watertight closure is not recommended because too many sutures placed too closely to each other may cause ischemia of the suture line. The suture should approximate and not strangulate the ureteral wall. No tension should be placed on the suture line.

A circumferential scar of the ureter may contract, causing stricture, hydroureter, hydronephrosis, and possible renal damage. Therefore, spatulation of the ureter before anastomosis is advised. An adequate debridement of devitalized tissue, a mucosa-to-mucosa tensionless approximation of the defect, an internal stent, and

a drain from the periureteral area are helpful in the successful healing of ureteral anastomosis.

ROLE OF URETEROSCOPY IN URETERAL SURGERY

The introduction of ureteroscopy to daily urologic practice has changed the face of ureteral surgery. An operation such as ureterolithotomy, traditionally done by open surgery, is rare and has been replaced by the endoscopic approach. The indicatons for therapeutic ureteroscopy in general are removal of stones, resection of ureteral tumors, treatment of obstruction caused by strictures, and removal of foreign bodies.

The ureteroscope and particularly the newer, smaller, rigid and flexible scope introduced another tool to the diagnosis of ureteral lesions and gradually eliminated the need for "exploratory ureterotomy." Ureteroscopy is used for the diagnosis of radiologic filling defects in the collecting system, unilateral hematuria, abnormal unilateral cytology, and stricture evaluation. However, ureteroscopy may cause ureteral injuries, such as perforation, ureteral avulsion, and strictures; breakage of the endoscope in the ureter will necessitate open surgery (Flam et al., 1988). The urologist practicing endourology must remain familiar with the principles and techniques of ureteral surgery. A full discussion of ureteroscopy is found in Chapter 61.

APPROACHES TO SURGERY OF THE URETER

The incision and approach to the ureter depend on the segment to be operated upon. They also depend on the type of disease that necessitates surgery and its extent, e.g., short upper third stricture and diffuse retroperitoneal fibrosis. On the one hand, an extraperitoneal approach is preferable because of the possibility of urine leakage postoperatively. On the other hand, a transperitoneal approach to the ureter may provide access to the ureter from its insertion in the bladder to its origin at the ureteropelvic junction. Therefore, the transperitoneal approach combined with adequate drainage, stenting, and urinary diversion may be ideal when bowel, omental flap, or transureteroureterotomy is indicated (Fig. 68–1 A).

Surgical approaches to the upper third of the ureter are, in general, the same as those for the kidney. These are detailed in Chapter 65. The subcostal flank incision approaches the upper third of the ureter (Fig. 68–1 C). This approach may require the incision to go through the bed of the 12th rib or above.

A posterior lumbotomy incision may be of help, but the limitations of this incision are a problem if one is treating an upper-third ureteral stone, which then moves to an area that is very difficult to get to through the posterior lumbotomy approach.

For calculi in the middle third of the ureter, a muscle-splitting incision at the appropriate level, sometimes called a Gibson incision (Fig. 68–2A), provides simple

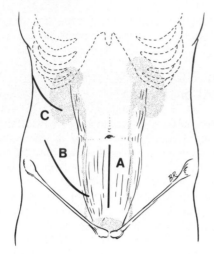

Figure 68–1. Incisions for surgical approaches to the ureter.

access to the ureter, with the possibility of extension of the incision if that is deemed necessary. The fascia and muscle bundles of the external oblique, internal oblique, and transverse abdominis are separated bluntly parallel to their fibers for a distance of 4 to 5 cm (Fig. 68–2B). The underlying peritoneum is mobilized and reflected medially, and as the fat is pulled aside anteriorly, the ureter is located (Fig. 68–2C). Because the ureter is attached to the underside of the parietal peritoneum, it may be displaced medially with the mobilized peritoneum during the dissection and may not be posterior where the surgeon expects it to be.

The lower third of the ureter can be approached through a muscle-splitting, lower quadrant, modified Gibson incision. If necessary, the lower quadrant incision can be extended medially in order to retract the

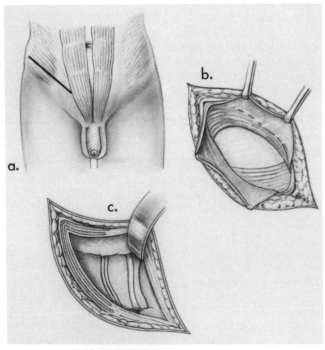

Figure 68–2. Gibson incision.

rectus muscle, or the rectus muscle can be divided for greater access to the lower ureter just before entry into the bladder. Depending on the surgical procedure to be performed on the lower ureter, it may be advantageous to have as much exposure as possible in the area. A transverse, Pfannenstiel, lower midline, or paramedian extraperitoneal approach may be better than a Gibson-type incision (Fig. 68–1B). If special problems arise with scarring around the ureter, a low anterior midline incision, either extraperitoneal or transperitoneal, may be required.

SURGICAL TECHNIQUES

Ureterolysis

Ureterolysis as a primary procedure is indicated whenever there is ureteral entrapment with resultant obstruction and compromise of renal function. Ureteral entrapment or periureteral fibrosis may occur secondary to a number of pathologic processes, including intraperitoneal inflammatory disease, abscess formation from granulomatous bowel disease, pelvic inflammatory disease, endometriosis, neoplasm, previous radiation therapy, periaortic aneurysmal fibrosis, or drugs (methysergide maleate). Retroperitoneal fibrosis may be idiopathic (Ormond's disease) (Ormond, 1948). Initial management and timing of surgical intervention are dictated by the extent of disease and renal compromise. The primary objective of therapy is relief of obstruction, and this frequently can be accomplished by the passage of an indwelling catheter or stent. If the ureters cannot be catheterized and renal insufficiency is present, temporary upper tract diversion by means of a percutaneous nephrostomy is mandatory to stabilize renal function before surgical exploration and definitive ureterolysis is undertaken.

Retroperitoneal fibrosis, whatever the etiology, may manifest itself initially as unilateral disease; however, even with what appears to be a totally normal opposite system, the other ureter may be involved with the process and may require "prophylactic therapy." Thus, a midline transabdominal incision is preferable.

Technique

A generous midline incision gives exposure from the renal pedicles to the level of the ureterovesical junction. Initially, routine abdominal exploration is performed. Ureteral exposure may be achieved in one of two ways: through a single incision in the posterior peritoneum in the midline, between the duodenum and the inferior mesenteric vein, and on each side, by reflecting the colon along the white line of Toldt from the iliac bifurcation to the splenic and hepatic flexure.

Tissue for biopsy and frozen-section examination should be obtained to rule out the presence of malignancy. The ureter is identified either at the level of the iliac vessel or at the ureteropelvic junction above the fibrotic process. Ureterolysis is accomplished from the ureteropelvic junction to below the iliac vessels. Usually

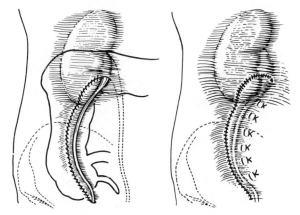

Figure 68–3. *Left,* The right ureter displaced laterally and intraperitonealized from the renal pelvis to the peritoneal reflection. *Right,* Lateral displacement of the right ureter with chromic catgut sutures fixing the parietal peritoneum to the psoas or quadratus lumborum muscle.

the fibrotic process can be stripped from the ureter rather simply with blunt dissection, using a right-angle clamp and finger dissection. If the correct plane is entered, the fibrotic process usually comes off in a peel. If it does not strip off easily, malignancy should be considered. Because the fibrotic process is diffuse and covers the major vessels, vascular injury is rare. After complete lysis, the ureter should promptly fill with urine. If it does not, significant fibrotic material may remain behind and the ureteral wall itself may be involved.

Ureterolysis alone is inadequate treatment to prevent reinvolvement by the fibrotic process. At this point, the ureters may be handled in one of three ways: (1) transplanted to an intraperitoneal position; (2) transposed laterally and anteriorly, with retroperitoneal fat placed between the ureters and the fibrosis; and (3) covered by omental sleeves. In the first method, the parietal peritoneum is sutured with 2–0 absorbable suture posterior to the ureter, from the level of the ureteropelvic junction to the iliac vessels, leaving generous entrance and exit windows to prevent subsequent stenosis and obstruction (Fig. 68–3 *left*). With extensive fibrosis or intraperitoneal involvement, lateral displacement and fixation may offer a better result. For this procedure, interrupted 2–0 chromic catgut sutures are placed between the parietal peritoneum and psoas or quadratus lumborum muscle, fixing it medial to the ureter. The peritoneal defect is then closed (Fig. 68–3 *right*).

To further improve results, Tresidder and co-workers (1972) and Blandy (1986) recommended wrapping the ureters in omentum (Fig. 68–4). If stents can be placed preoperatively, they should remain for at least 3 to 4 days postoperatively to be sure that ureteral obstruction does not recur and to help the ureters remain in the position where they were placed during surgical lysis.

Postoperative steroids are controversial but may be beneficial in helping to resolve fibrosis and in preventing recurrent fibrosis. Renal function should be monitored at monthly intervals for several months, with follow-up upper tract studies at approximately 3 months.

Ureterectomy

Primary ureterectomy is most frequently done in combination with nephrectomy for the treatment of neoplasms of the renal pelvis or ureter. In some selected patients with small, well-differentiated ureteral tumors or in patients with a single kidney, a more conservative resection of only the involved part of the ureter may be chosen. Other indications for ureterectomy, with or without nephrectomy, include cases of tuberculosis, severe hydronephrosis secondary to reflux, pyoureter, hydroureter, stricture, and complete duplication.

When ureterectomy is performed at the time of nephrectomy, either portion of the procedure may be done first. The most important consideration, if tumor is present, is to remove all of the tissue en bloc. If tumor is suspected but not proved, the ureteral exploration should be done first. Whether to do a nephroureterectomy through one flank incision or two separate incisions depends on the patient's body habitus and the need for a ureteral cuff excision for carcinoma. Resection of the upper part of the ureter necessitates pyeloureteral anastomosis or ureterocalicostomy (Robert, 1988; Mesrobian and Kelalis, 1989). Resection of the midportion of the ureter may be completed by a simple end-to-end anastomosis of the resected ureter. With resection of the lower section, the ureter should be reimplanted into the bladder directly or with a bladder flap and/or bladder mobilization. If the ureter is too short to be reimplanted

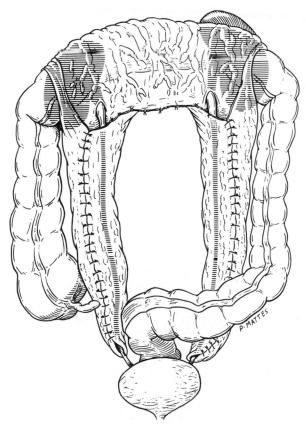

Figure 68–4. Omentum sleeves wrapping both ureters.

into the bladder, a transureteroureterostomy may be done.

Technique

The patient may be placed in the 45-degree oblique position. A flank incision is made, and all renal attachments except the ureter are divided. If a distal ureterectomy with excision of a bladder cuff cannot be performed with adequate exposure, the incision may be extended as a Gibson incision and the ureter freed by blunt dissection to the intramural portion. The distal ureterectomy may be performed in one of two ways: by making a separate anterior incision in the bladder and circumscribing the ureteral orifice with a 1-cm margin (Fig. 68–5) or by staying completely extravesical and placing two right-angle clamps across the ureterovesical junction, with the bladder divided between the clamps.

The bladder is oversewn with 2–0 absorbable suture (Fig. 68–6). If the bladder is opened, the ureteral hiatus as well as the vesicotomy is closed in two layers with 0 or 2–0 absorbable sutures. The major disadvantage for bladder cuff excision without vesicotomy is the inability to identify and prevent an iatrogenic injury to the opposite ureteral orifice.

If a distal ureterectomy is performed first for tumor, a sterile glove can be tied over the end of the ureter to prevent any tumor spillage and then tucked into the retroperitoneum. The remainder of the procedure can be accomplished through the flank. If the ureterectomy is being done for benign disease, it is seldom necessary to remove a bladder cuff.

Secondary Ureterectomy—Excision of Ureteral Stump

Ureteral excision may be done at the time of nephrectomy or may be delayed. Depending on the reason for excision, resection of an adjacent cuff of bladder may be necessary. The indications for secondary ureterec-

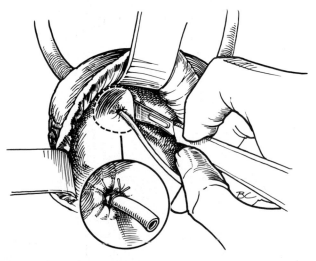

Figure 68–5. Excision of the ureterovesical junction by taking a 1-cm cuff of bladder mucosa and bladder wall with a ureteral catheter in place.

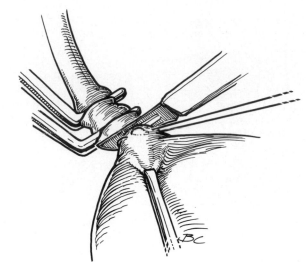

Figure 68–6. Division of the ureter across the ureterovesical junction. A figure-of-eight or pursestring suture is placed distal to the second clamp, and the ureter is excised.

tomy include vesicoureteral reflux into the ureteral stump, pyoureter, tuberculous ureteritis, tumor, ureter with a stricture and calculus above the stricture preventing adequate drainage, and ectopic ureters of dysplastic duplicated kidneys.

Ureterectomy after nephrectomy may be performed through a midline infrapubic incision, a Gibson incision, or a Pfannenstiel incision. Even though dense adhesions may be present from previous surgery, an extraperitoneal approach is usually possible without too much difficulty. Blunt and sharp dissection frees the ureter from its attachments, with care taken not to injure the iliac vessels or overlying intraperitoneal structures. The ureter is freed to the ureterovesical junction and may be excised by placing a right-angle clamp as close as possible to the ureterovesical junction, excising the ureter and oversewing the bladder wall distal to the clamp with a 2–0 absorbable suture. If complete excision with a bladder cuff is required, a cystotomy is done, the ureteral orifice circumscribed, and the stump removed. The ureteral hiatus and cystotomy are closed in a standard two-layer fashion with 2–0 absorbable sutures. In cases in which the bladder was opened, a drain should be left in the ureteral bed.

Ureterolithotomy

With the advent of newer technology and more experience with shock-wave lithotripsy, ureteroscopic lithotripsy, and endoscopic removal of stones, indications for ureterolithotomy are changing. The limiting factors to the aforementioned technology are availability of the instruments, the needed surgical expertise, and some anatomic variations. In selected cases, ureterolithotomy may be indicated with concomitant repair of an ureteral disorder. Ureteral stones can move either down or up the ureter when least expected. Documentation of the exact position of the stone should be made as close as possible to the time of surgery, even on the operating table, employing abdominal radiography before the most appropriate approach for ureterolithotomy is decided.

For upper-third calculi, the extraperitoneal flank approach is preferred. For middle-third calculi, the approach may be extraperitoneal through a subcostal incision or a modified Gibson incision. For lower-third calculi, a midline, Pfannenstiel, or Gibson incision may be utilized. A transvaginal approach may be chosen for a calculus located near the ureterovesical junction. For a stone located in the intramural ureter, the transvesical approach may be employed.

Upper Ureter

For an upper-third calculus, a subcostal flank incision is made. The retroperitoneal space is entered carefully, so as not to open the peritoneum inadvertently. The ureter is gently exposed with blunt and sharp dissection, and care is taken not to dislodge the calculus. After the calculus is located, the ureter is mobilized only enough to allow a ureterotomy directly over the calculus. Fine chromic traction sutures may be placed at the site of the proposed ureterotomy. A longitudinal ureterotomy is made with a hook-blade knife. The ureteral incision begins just above the stone and extends the incision distally so as not to dislodge the stone back to the kidney.

As described by Cohen and Persky (1983), the chance of disrupting ureteral blood supply is less likely with a longitudinal incision than with a transverse incision, because the blood supply travels in the periureteral tissue. They also believed that the muscular sheath that composes the middle layer of the ureter tends to heal better after a longitudinal incision than it does after a transverse incision. The calculus is teased out of the ureter with the end of the knife blade or small forceps.

After the calculus is removed, ureteral patency and urine flow should be established by passing an 8 Fr. ureteral catheter into the bladder and into the renal pelvis, irrigating continuously while withdrawing it. The ureterotomy may be left open and the area drained, but under most circumstances, several 4–0 or 5–0 chromic gut or absorbable sutures may be placed through the adventitia to close the defect. Care must be taken not to narrow the ureter. A Penrose drain is brought out either through a stab wound or through the posterior portion of the incision. The wound is closed in appropriate layers with material of the surgeon's preference.

Calculi located at the level of the transverse process of L3 or L4 may be removed either through a muscle-splitting incision as described by Foley (1935) or through a posterior lumbotomy approach (Gil-Vernet, 1983). Both of these approaches offer the patient the advantages of reduced morbidity, shortened hospital stay, and less postoperative pain. For the Foley muscle-splitting incision, the external oblique, internal oblique, and latissimus dorsi muscles are mobilized but not incised. The oblique muscles are retracted forward and the latissimus dorsi backward, exposing the lumbar fascia. The fascia is opened, the edges retracted, and the retroperitoneal space entered. The posterior layer of

Gerota's fascia is separated from the posterior abdominal wall, and the ureter is located. The calculus is extracted as described previously.

The Gil-Vernet incision is used with the patient in the lateral position, without lumbar support, with the legs flexed to the point of maximal suppression of physiologic lordosis, or in the prone position. A vertical incision is made 2 cm medial to the muscle mass of the lumbosacral muscles, from the 12th rib to the posterosuperior iliac crest. The incision is carried through the posterior layer of the lumbodorsal fascia around the sacral spinalis and quadratus lumborum muscles, which are retracted medially to enter the perinephric space. A self-retaining retractor may then be placed in the wound. Gerota's fascia is entered by incising the thin layer of dorsal fascia that is the posterior extension of the transversalis fascia. With careful blunt dissection, the upper ureter is exposed and the calculus removed as previously described.

Middle Third of Ureter

Calculi at the level of L5 or in the middle ureter are approached through an appropriate level muscle-splitting incision (Gibson). The ureter should be identified, as it clings to the posterior peritoneum at the level of the iliac vessels. The calculus is located and extracted as previously described for a stone in the upper ureter. The ureter is closed with fine absorbable sutures, and the wound is closed in standard fashion leaving a Penrose drain in the ureterotomy area.

Lower Ureter

Lower-third ureteral calculus may be removed through a Gibson incision or with a midline approach, through either a vertical or a Pfannenstiel incision. After incision of the rectus abdominis fascia, the peritoneum is mobilized medially and upward. The ureter is identified at the pelvic brim, where it crosses the iliac vessels and is traced to the level of the calculus. If the stone is located down the ureter toward the bladder, retracting the bladder medially and dividing the superior vesical pedicle allow better visualization of the ureter. A ureterotomy is made, and the calculus is extracted. The ureterotomy is closed, and the site is drained. The drains are left 5 to 7 days or until all drainage ceases. If calculi are present on the opposite side, the midline incision offers the advantage of simultaneous surgical correction without another incision.

For the special instance in which the calculus is impacted in or near the intramural ureter, a transvesical approach may prove efficacious. The bladder is opened in the midline, a meatotomy done, and the calculus extracted by forceps or by being milked out by means of extravesical palpation. Occasionally, when a calculus is impacted, ureteroneocystostomy may be necessary. If a calculus is dislodged at any time and not located or retrieved without difficulty, a basket extractor or Fogarty catheter may be passed up the ureter and, with intraoperative fluoroscopy, the calculus is then located and retrieved. A flexible ureteroscope may be passed up the ureter to allow visual extraction of the calculus.

Complications

The most common complication following a ureterolithotomy is persistent urinary leakage. In general, if drainage persists for longer than 5 to 7 days, an excretory urography or a retrograde study should be performed to rule out distal obstruction and an indwelling ureteral catheter or a stent placed for a period of 24 to 48 hours. Rarely will leakage continue longer; however, as is the case with intubated ureterotomies, stents and drains may be left for a period of 6 weeks. The patient is discharged, and removal of stents and drains is done on an outpatient basis in an office setting. Sepsis and infection may occur in any type of urologic surgery. If a specific organism has been cultured from the urine or blood preoperatively, appropriate antibiotic coverage should be employed. The judicious and appropriate administration of prophylactic antibiotics usually prevents significant complications. Although the exact incidence of ureteral stricture and urinoma following ureterolithotomy is unknown, these complications are uncommon. A follow-up upper tract study should be obtained about 3 months after surgery.

Transvaginal Approach to Ureter

Transvaginal approaches to the ureter now are rarely needed. The ureteroscope has made this operation virtually unnecessary. Occasionally, a female patient with a large lower ureteral stone that is impacted is treated. Therefore, the transvaginal approach to ureteral lithotomy may be worth consideration. The advantage of this approach is that it is rapid to perform and involves a minimum of tissue dissection and trauma. It eliminates the complications of transabdominal surgery and the hospitalization and recovery period is short.

The disadvantages of this approach include the minimal ureteral exposure, the lack of control of the proximal ureter, and the risk of postoperative ureterovaginal fistula. If the stone is dislodged and migrates proximally, retrieval may be difficult. Attempts at recovery can be made with a stone basket or a Fogarty catheter assisted by intraoperative fluoroscopy. Because little tissue exists between the ureter and vagina, the suture lines may be in proximity. If infection, hematoma, distal obstruction, vascular compromise, or prolonged drainage occurs, the risk of fistula is high. An internal double-J stent after such an approach may help to prevent fistula formation.

Technique

The basic technique is shown in Figure 68–7 (Persky et al., 1979). With the patient in the lithotomy position, a weighted speculum is placed deep in the vagina. The cervix is grasped with tenaculum forceps and traction applied down and to the side opposite the calculus. It is extremely important to be able to palpate the stone

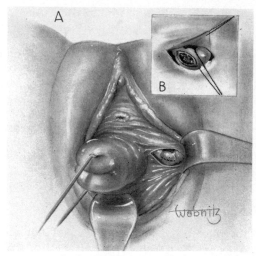

Figure 68–7. Vaginal ureterolithotomy. *A,* The cervix is drawn forward and laterally toward the opposite side. In inset *B,* the ureter has been incised over the calculus after placement of holding sutures immediately above the obstruction.

before making the incision. The incision is made overlying the calculus with a No. 15 blade. The ureter is mobilized above and below the stone with blunt and sharp dissection, and the ureterotomy is made. The calculus is extracted and the ureteral incision is closed with 5.0 chromic catgut suture; the vaginal incision is closed with a running 4.0 chromic catgut suture (Koontz et al., 1986).

It is best not to attempt this operation unless the stone can be palpated. If the stone is not palpable, Walsh (1984) suggested that the patient be placed in an exaggerated lithothomy position as for radical perineal prostatectomy and the bladder filled in order to push the lower ureteral segment and the stone to a position where the stone can be found.

Ureteroureterostomy

Ureteroureterostomy is defined as the end-to-end anastomosis of any two ureteral segments, including ipsilateral duplicated ureters. Ureteroureterostomy may be performed in the case of resection of short postoperative fibrotic strictures, intraoperative injury, infection, blunt or penetrating trauma, short segments of periureteral inflammation, short segments of radiation injury, obstruction or reflux in an ectopic or a duplicated ureter, congenital stricture, vascular obstruction from a retrocaval ureter or crossing blood vessels, or segmental resection for a localized carcinoma. The primary contraindication to ureteroureterostomy is inadequate length to assure a tension-free anastomosis. Relative contraindications include the presence of abscess, hematoma, or urinoma; vascular compromise of the ureter from dissection or mobilization; previous ureteral injury; and previous therapeutic irradiation.

To rationally discuss the surgical approach, the ureter should be considered as being divided into upper-, middle-, and lower-third segments. The reason for repair is also discussed as either a primary elective repair or a repair at the time of exploration for another problem (e.g., intraoperative ureteral injury). As stated by Young (1983), various factors are evaluated to determine if ureteroureterostomy is appropriate. In some cases the decision about ureteroureterostomy can be made only during the surgery itself. Once it is determined that ureteroureterostomy is feasible and there is enough length for a tension-free anastomosis, one may proceed with the surgery.

Technique

In the case of intraoperative ureteral injury, repair can usually be made through the incision at hand. In the case of upper-third injury, the best approach is via the flank or 12th rib. For middle-third exposure, a Gibson incision is appropriate, because it can be extended upward to the 12th rib for better exposure of the kidney or across the midline for better exposure of the distal ureter, if necessary. The lower-third approach is best made through a midline infraumbilical incision.

The upper-third ureter or middle-third ureter should be located through the aforementioned incisions by dissecting posteriorly along the psoas muscle and reflecting the peritoneum medially. The ureter comes into view anteriorly, attached to the peritoneum. The area of pathology is isolated, the ureter dissected free, only to obtain adequate length for a tension-free anastomosis, and the edges are prepared for anastomosis.

For lower-third exposure, the midline approach is preferred. The rectus muscles are separated and the retropubic space entered by careful blunt dissection. This dissection is continued around the bladder on the side of the diseased area, exposing the ureter at the level of the iliac vessels. Exposure may be expedited by dividing the obliterated umbilical artery. Injuries in this area are best handled by ureteroneocystostomy, often requiring a psoas hitch or bladder flap. Ureteroureterostomy may be indicated in injuries at a site 5 cm or more proximal to the bladder. If the ureteral injury is discovered at the time of an intra-abdominal or a retroperitoneal procedure, access to the ureter may be sufficient by the exposure previously done during the surgery. If not, additional exposure may be obtained in one of two ways: by reflecting the colon along its lateral gutter or by incising the posterior peritoneum medial to the inferior mesenteric artery from the ligament of Treitz to the sacral promontory.

Once dissection is performed, anastomosis is deemed possible, and any devitalized ureteral ends are debrided, a number of anastomotic techniques are available. It is imperative that no distal obstruction is present. Several techniques of anastomosis are shown in Figure 68–8. The ends may be spatulated and sutured obliquely as a fish mouth, with running or interrupted suture, or by Z-plasty and interrupted suture.

The most common anastomotic technique is spatulation, with sutures of 4–0 or 5–0 absorbable material, placed at the right angle of each cut end into the angle of the spatulating incision on the opposing ureteral cut end. After the first suture is tied, the second and third sutures are placed 1 to 2 mm apart and tied. If a stent is placed it should be done at this point. The remainder of the sutures are then placed and tied.

As much as possible, the repair should be retroperitonealized. Stents can be a valuable aid to ureteroureterostomy if any question exists of ureteral wall tissue trauma or tension anastomosis. Drainage of the anastomosis area is necessary. A Penrose drain or a suction catheter may be brought out through a separate stab incision or through the incision itself. Drains are usually removed by the 5th to 7th postoperative day, or when there is no evidence of any further leakage. Stents should be left in place for at least 4 weeks and removed only after appropriate postoperative healing is demonstrated on intravenous urography.

Ureteroureterostomy of duplicated ureters on the same side are performed for reflux or ectopia, or whenever there is one abnormal or damaged ureter and one normal ureter. This anastomosis is usually performed end-to-side with care being taken not to damage the recipient ureter (Fig. 68–9). Likewise, to assure a successful anastomosis, as little dissection as possible should be done of the recipient ureter in order to maintain the best possible blood supply. The incision in the recipient ureter should be parallel to its long axis and the exact length of the obliquely cut end of the donor ureter. The end-to-side anastomosis is performed with 4–0 or 5–0 absorbable interrupted sutures, 1 to 2 mm apart. Whether or not to stent this anastomosis and to use a diverting nephrostomy remains controversial. If there is a large discrepancy in size, stenting and diversion may

Figure 68–8. Ureteroureterostomy techniques of anastomosis. *A,* Oblique. *B,* Z-plasty. *C,* Spatulated. (Modified from Young, J. D., Jr.: In Glenn J. F. (Ed.): Urologic Surgery, 3rd ed. Philadelphia, J. B. Lippincott Co., 1983.)

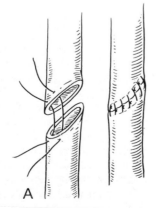

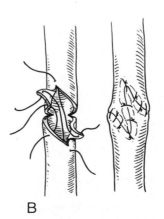

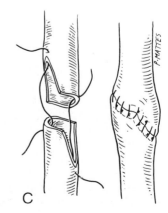

A   B   C

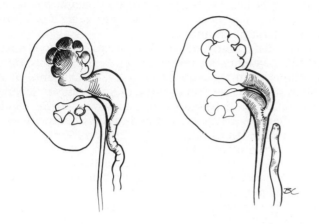

Figure 68–9. Ureteroureterostomy of duplicated ureters. The refluxing upper pole segment is sutured end-to-side to the normal lower pole segment.

be indicated. Extraureteral drains should be placed in the same manner as previously described. The results of properly performed ureteroureterostomies are excellent (Carlton, et al. 1971; Rober, 1990). Carlton reported 92 per cent satisfactory results when this technique was utilized in 25 patients with watertight anastomoses.

Complications

Complications are usually rare and include prolonged drainage of urine from the drain or the incision and anastomosal stricture. If urine leakage persists more than 5 to 7 days, evaluation should be made as described for leakage following ureterolithotomy.

Transureteroureterostomy

Transureteroureterostomy was first reported as an experimental technique by Sharpe (1906). The first successful clinical application was by Higgins (1934). Initial reluctance to use the procedure was based on the anastomosis of a diseased nephroureteral unit to a clinically normal unit. Since 1934, clinical experience with this technique has been considerable. Results reported by Pearse (1985) show that there is little risk to the recipient ureter if the patient is selected properly and adherence to surgical technique is strict.

Clinically, transureteroureterostomy may be applied when it is necessary to reconstruct a lower-third or, occasionally, a middle-third defect. For the operation to succeed, there must be sufficient length for the ureter to cross the midline for a tension-free anastomosis to its mate on the opposite side. A gentle sweeping path without kinking is desired. The more proximal the end of the donor ureter, the more acute the sweep and the greater the possibility of mechanical obstruction. The optimal point for crossing the midline is at the level of the bifurcation of the aorta, where the ureters lie closest to one another.

Contraindications to transureteroureterostomy include inadequate length to permit a tension-free anastomosis, previous dissection or ureteral mobilization, previous ureter injury, previous ureter exposure to therapeutic radiation, ureteral or renal tuberculosis, recurrent stones in either or both kidneys, uroepithelial tumors, retroperitoneal fibrosis, chronic pyelonephritis in either kidney, or reflux of the recipient ureterovesical unit (unless corrected).

Technique

Transureteroureterostomy is best performed through an anterior midline transperitoneal incision. If previous cystoscopy and passage of ureteral catheters were possible, localization and dissection of the ureter may be facilitated. In most situations, however, they are not needed. The intestines are reflected upward and packed out of the way. Each ureter is identified, and the overlying posterior peritoneum is incised for a length of several centimeters. The donor ureter is freed from its area of involvement proximally and transected. The distal end is ligated with a 0 or 2–0 chromic catgut ligature.

The proximal end of the ureter may be tagged with a fine suture to mark the anterior surface and to facilitate later manipulation and traction, when the ureter is drawn to the opposite side. The area of the recipient ureter for anastomosis is isolated with minimal mobilization in an attempt to preserve as much blood supply as possible. After the donor ureter is sufficiently free proximally to allow a gentle sweep across the retroperitoneal space, a tunnel is created bluntly beneath the sigmoid and preferably above the inferior mesenteric artery.

If the inferior mesenteric artery is a barrier to mobilization, it may be divided provided that the remainder of the left colon vascular supply is intact. The suture on the donor ureter is grasped. With gentle tension, the ureter is drawn through the tunnel to the opposite side. Care is taken to avoid any inadvertent rotation.

The donor ureter is spatulated on its antimesenteric border to a length of about 1.5 cm. An incision, of equal length, is made on the anteromedial surface of the recipient ureter. The anastomosis is performed with interrupted 4–0 or 5–0 absorbable sutures placed approximately 2 mm apart. The first suture is placed from the apex of the spatulated ureter to the proximal apex of the ureterostomy in the recipient ureter, with the knot tied extraluminally. The remaining sutures are placed in the posterior and anterior walls in a stepwise fashion (Fig. 68–10). Continuous sutures can be placed on the posterior and anterior walls. The area should be drained extraperitoneally.

The posterior peritoneal incision is reapproximated with 3–0 absorbable sutures and the incision closed according to the surgeon's preference. Stenting the anastomosis is optional but should not be required in a technically well-performed anastomosis in which the ureters are well vascularized. If a stent is used, one end should lie in the donor renal pelvis and traverse the recipient ureter into the bladder. If the recipient ureter is large enough, a second stent may be passed from the recipient renal pelvis into the bladder. Drains should remain until all leakage has stopped; stents can remain

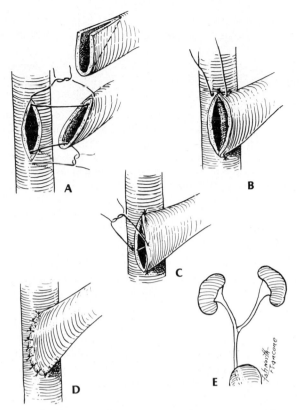

Figure 68–10. Transureteroureterostomy. The ureteroureteral anastomosis is done end-to-side using an uninterrupted or a running layer of 4–0 chromic catgut suture for the posterior layer. The anterior layer is approximated with interrupted sutures of the same material. (From Young, J. D., Jr.: *In* Glenn J. F. (Ed.): Urologic Surgery, 3rd ed. Philadelphia, J. B. Lippincott Co., 1983.)

until an intravenous urography shows no leakage or obstruction and then can be removed cystoscopically.

Results

Reports of transureteroureterostomy have been favorable, with few complications (Van Arsdalen and Hackler, 1983). Ehrlich and Skinner (1975) reported six cases of severe complications. Four patients had damage to the recipient unit, necessitating ileal substitution in two. One had persistent mild ureteral stricture, and one required an extensive vesicopsoas hitch. Three donor kidneys required subsequent nephrectomy.

Sandoz and associates (1977) reported on four patients of 23 who had injuries to the recipient ureters. Of these, three eventually had good results after reoperation, and one died secondary to operative complications.

Good results from transureteroureterostomy have been reported by Pearse and associates (1985) and by Udall and associates (1973), who had good results in 61 of 67 patients. Of the six patients who had unsatisfactory results, three required cutaneous diversion secondary to reflux, one developed stenosis of the diseased donor ureter at the anastomosis site, one developed obstruction by tumor growth of both ureters at the anastomosis site, and one had progression of pre-existing pyelonephritis leading to donor nephrectomy.

Brannan (1975) reported on 17 patients with no com-

plications or renal deterioration. Hendren and Hensle (1980) reported on 112 patients, mostly children, who underwent transureteroureterostomy for reflux or undiversion. No deaths, leaks, or nephrectomies were reported in their series; however, three patients required reoperation for technical reasons.

Hodges and associates (1980) reported 25 years experience with 100 transureteroureterostomies done primarily for ureteral stricture, injury, or lower ureteral tumor. They did state a 97 per cent success rate, with no damage to the recipient ureter. At least 92 per cent of the patients had excellent results of both renal units. Two deaths were reported, one due to myocardial infarction and one due to mycotic sepsis. A total of 23 complications were reported—three involved the recipient ureter and were secondary to the development of tumor and subsequent obstruction at the anastomotic site. The investigators believed that these complications could have been prevented by the use of frozen sections at the time of surgery. One anastomotic leak subsequently led to nephrectomy. Two nephrectomies secondary to persistent pyelonephritis were reported. Two patients required reoperations for inferior mesenteric artery syndrome.

In summary, transureteroureterostomy is a successful procedure with a low complication rate if strict attention is paid to technique and proper patient selection. Urologic surgeons should be familiar with this procedure and be able to perform it, when the situation dictates.

Intubated Ureterotomy

The intubated ureterotomy arose from the classic work of Davis, reported in 1943. The technique is based on the ability of the uroepithelial outgrowth to cover a ureteral defect in 4 to 7 days. This occurrence is followed by the slower ingrowth of muscular tissue into the granulation tissue that covers the defect. For this type of regeneration or healing to occur, normal uroepithelial mucosa must be present without abnormal folds, pockets, or diverticula. The lumen must be patent and distensible and offer a low resistance, such that the flow of urine is unimpeded from the renal pelvis to the bladder. Likewise, the surrounding muscularis must show normal amounts of smooth muscle bundles with appropriate vascular and nerve supply. The surrounding adventitia should also be free of inflammation, foreign bodies, necrotic debris, and periureteral adhesions. If not, the healing process may be incomplete and normal ureteral architecture may not be formed. Under these circumstances, false passages, diverticula, and strictures can develop. With the addition of periureteral fatty coverage, adherence to surrounding muscle may be prevented as well as fixation, angulation, traction, and dense encapsulation.

The primary indication for intubated ureterotomy is a long, strictured ureteral segment or a long ureteral gap that is not amenable to conventional repair. This technique is readily applicable to strictures of the ureter as long as 10 to 12 cm.

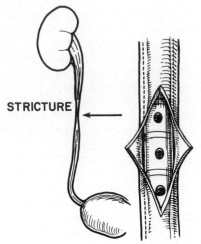

Figure 68–11. For the intubated ureterotomy, the ureteral defect is left to close spontaneously around a catheter.

Technique

After the involved segment of the ureter is exposed, a longitudinal ureterotomy is performed through the desired area. Care should be taken not to spiral the incision (Fig. 68–11). A posterior incision has been advocated by some workers (Persky, 1967; Persky, 1979; Smart, 1961). All intubated ureterotomies should have proximal urinary diversion by means of nephrostomy.

After the ureterotomy has been performed, a stent is chosen and placed. The stent catheter may be a double-J, running from the renal pelvis to the bladder; or polyethelene tubing, bridging the defect and brought out as a nephrostomy tube (Fig. 68–12). To assure optimal healing, the stent and ureter should be in close proximity, which can be achieved by wrapping the ureter with fat or omentum.

Drainage of the periureteral and renal bed area is accomplished by drains. Postoperatively, the drains are left until drainage subsides. The stent should remain for a minimum of 6 to 8 weeks. A nephrostogram is performed before the stent is removed. Long-term follow-up should include intravenous urography in 3 months.

Renal Descensus

The addition of renal descensus to the techniques of ureteral surgery was originally made by Popescu in 1964 for the management of the pelvic ureter in postoperative ureterovaginal fistula. This maneuver, however, can be applied whenever extra ureteral length is needed to bridge a gap or to relieve tension on a ureteral anastomosis.

Technique

Through a transperitoneal approach, the colon on the affected side is reflected medially from the colonic flexure to the level of the diseased ureteral area in the pelvis. Gerota's fascia is incised anteriorly and, using blunt and sharp dissection, the kidney is completely mobilized. After the kidney is completely free, the vessels and the proximal ureter are displaced downward and inward by pressure exerted on the upper pole. With constant pressure holding the kidney in this position, the lower pole is fixed to the iliac fossa with three or four 2–0 absorbable sutures (Fig. 68–13). The redundant ureter is freed from the peritoneum with care to preserve as much periureteral tissue as possible in order to decrease the possibility of postoperative vascular injury. After primary ureteral repair, the peritoneum is reapproximated and the retroperitoneum drained. As much as an 8-cm section of ureter may be replaced with this technique. In selected cases, more right kidney inferior displacement can be achieved by transection of the right renal vein and reanastomosis on the vena cava in a lower position (Gil-Vernet, 1978).

PSOAS HITCH. Psoas hitch is indicated whenever there is a gap in the distal ureter, which prevents the direct reimplantation of the ureter into the bladder. A

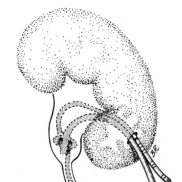

Figure 68–12. Pyelotomy for placement of nephrostomy tube and splint.

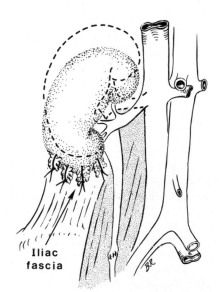

Iliac fascia

Figure 68–13. Suture placement in renal descensus.

successful operation should prevent reflux; thus, fixation of the ureter to the bladder wall with adequate ureteral backing is essential. Paquin, in 1959, mentioned the bladder hitch procedure to reduce anastomotic tension. This procedure was popularized in the United States by Harrow (1968) and in Europe by Turner-Warwick (1969), who gave it its name.

The technique itself is simple and is based on the fact that distortion of the bladder does not usually interfere with function and gains the surgeon between 3 and 5 cm of additional length. The relative contraindication to this procedure is a contracted scarred bladder or previous pelvic surgery in which the blood supply to the bladder was compromised.

Prior to attempting this adjunctive technique, the mobility of the bladder can be assessed by means of a preoperative cystogram. If this modality is not available to the surgeon intraoperatively, passage of a semirigid catheter into the bladder and tenting of the appropriate wing will facilitate the decision as to whether a psoas hitch is possible. This maneuver becomes particularly important if the surgeon intends a concomitant bladder flap procedure, because the base of the flap and its blood supply should not be compromised by the immobilizing sutures. Additional mobility of the bladder can be obtained (at the discretion of the surgeon) by mobilizing the contralateral bladder pedicle after division of all the umbilical ligaments.

Technique

The lateral walls of the bladder are mobilized and the peritoneum stripped from the dome and the posterior wall. Through a small and appropriately placed vesicotomy, the index finger is inserted, directing a bladder horn toward the proximal ureter. Some surgeons anchor the bladder at this point. Others create the submucosal tunnel and then anchor the bladder. Ideally, the bladder is sutured to the tendon of the psoas minor muscle with several 2–0 absorbable sutures (Fig. 68–14). Frequently, this tendon is absent. In this case, it is important to ensure that large bites of the muscle are taken with the

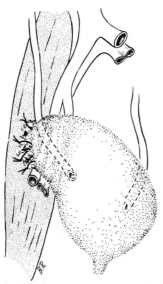

Figure 68–14. Suture placement in psoas bladder hitch.

suture, being careful to avoid the genitofemoral nerve. Once the bladder has been fixed to the psoas muscle above the iliac vessels, the ureter can be reimplanted, either by an antireflux anastomosis with a submucosal tunnel or by a direct anastomosis if adequate length is not present. The bladder is closed in two layers, and ureteral stents may be left at the discretion of the surgeon.

Prout and Koontz (1970) pointed out that occasionally it is possible to fix the bladder to the lateral pelvic wall. No kinking of the ureter can be occasioned by this hitch maneuver. This procedure is quite satisfactory for short defects and has gained popularity by allowing tension-free anastomoses in the operation of ureteroneocystostomy (Middleton, 1980).

BOARI FLAP PROCEDURE. A bladder tube to bridge large ureteral defects in dogs was successfully demonstrated in 1894 by Boari (Spies et al., 1933). It was not until 1947, when Ockerblad (1947) reported his 10-year follow-up of the bladder flap technique to bridge defects of 10 to 15 cm on a single patient, that this technique assumed its present popularity. This standard urologic procedure of creating a pedicle tube graft from the bladder has stood the test of time.

Benson and colleagues (1990) have reported good results in the follow-up of patients who have undergone this surgery and thus reinforced the confidence of most surgeons in this maneuver. For successful results, an adequate vascular supply to the vesical pedicle and the ureter is obtained by a tension-free anastomosis. The surgeon should carefully identify the superior vesical artery or one of its major branches and base the pedicle upon this. Principles of plastic surgery usually require graft length-to-width ratio of 3:2, and one must keep in mind that the tubularized flap is, in essence, an artificially created diverticulum of the bladder and has no functional activity as a tube. Therefore, the tube opening must always be widemouthed to drain satisfactorily.

Technique

The bladder flap operation can be performed through a variety of incisions, selecting whichever is appropriate to approach and resect the distal and damaged ureter. Once the diseased ureter has been resected back to normal tissue, implantation can be undertaken. The bladder should be fully mobilized, particularly on its lateral and medial-posterior aspects. This maneuver always involves dividing all of the umbilical ligaments, so that bladder mobility is maximal. It is helpful to distend the bladder with normal saline, following which the previously placed Foley catheter is clamped.

A bladder flap is created from the posterior wall with a base of at least 4 cm and an apex of approximately 3 cm. This trapezoid-shaped pedicle should be marked, supported with sutures, and based on the superior vesical artery or one of its major branches. Under most circumstances, up to 12 cm of bladder tube can be created in this manner. If increased length is required, a spiral flap placed across the anterior surface of the bladder may be helpful (Fig. 68–15).

The flap should be handled mainly by means of supporting stay sutures and not instruments. Minimal trauma should occur, because edema of the bladder mucosa may lead to partial obstruction during the post-

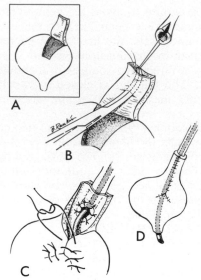

Figure 68–15. Bladder flap procedure for ureteral replacement.

operative period. The vesical flap should be closed with interrupted sutures of 0 or 2–0 absorbable sutures. The ureter may be sutured to the end of the flap or tunnelled submucosally as an antirefluxing anastomosis. This antireflux anastomosis should not be established at the sacrifice of a tension-free suture line.

Stents should be left for 10 to 14 days. Adequate drainage of the anastomosis and closure site must be maintained for at least 5 days postoperatively. A suprapubic catheter placement is at the surgeon's discretion.

Results

Results are usually satisfactory, especially when a Boari flap is combined with a psoas hitch (Olsson and Norlen, 1986).

CUTANEOUS URETEROSTOMY

Cutaneous ureterostomy was the common form of urinary diversion until the 1950s, when the Bricker conduit was introduced. The main advantage of this procedure is that it is simple to perform with minimal exposure and operative trauma. To be effective, both ureters should be brought to the skin to a single stoma so that they can be fitted with a single collection device without intubation (Fig. 68–16). The various forms of temporary ureterostomies, frequently used in children, are discussed elsewhere.

In the adult, ureterostomy has been replaced either by more complex forms of urinary diversion employing bowel segments or by percutaneous nephrostomy (MacGregor et al., 1987). Cutaneous ureterostomy should be considered whenever intraoperative problems necessitate urinary diversion on the one hand and rapid termination of the operation on the other hand. There are three major disadvantages to cutaneous ureterostomy as follows:

1. *The problem of two stomas.* Many techniques have been advanced to surmount this problem. Swenson and Smyth (1959) described a double-barrelled stoma placed in an infraumbilical position over which a single appliance could be worn. Straffon and colleagues (1970) described several methods, whereby both ureters could be joined on their medial borders and combined with a Z-plasty technique. The skin is interposed to prevent stenosis of the stoma. The technique of transureteroureterostomy and end cutaneous urctcrostomy has been advocated by Young and Aledia (1966).

2. *The problem of stricture formation.* The relatively poor ureteral blood supply frequently leads to a distal ureteral slough, recession of the stoma, or stomal stricture.

3. *The problem of urinary collection.* The presence of an enterostomal therapist has made handling of the collection device and educational support simpler for the patient and the physician.

Technique

The ureters may be approached peritoneally or extraperitoneally, depending on the circumstances of the cutaneous diversion. For the transperitoneal technique, the posterior parietal peritoneum overlying the right ureter is opened, usually at the level of the iliac vessels. The ureter is mobilized very carefully as far down as feasible. During the mobilization, it is essential that the periureteral tissue be preserved and that no cautery be applied. Prior to transection of the ureter, a stay suture should be placed on the ureter so as to facilitate mobilization and allow greater handling of the ureter. The suture also serves to identify anterior and posterior relationships, thus preventing twisting of the ureter when it is brought out through the abdominal tissues. The ureter should be mobilized in a cranial direction as far as necessary to make sure that there is a smooth, gentle curve of the ureter to reach the skin with a protrusion of at least 2 cm without tension.

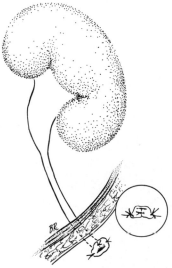

Figure 68–16. Cutaneous ureterostomy with a single stoma.

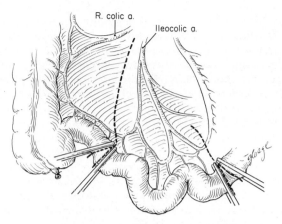

Figure 68–17. Isolation of a suitable segment of distal ileum for ureteral replacement. Note long division of distal mesentery.

Transperitoneal mobilization of the left ureter is always best accomplished by mobilization lateral to the sigmoid colon. In the obese individual, ureteral length may become a particular problem, and the ureter may be brought transperitoneally. Ideally, the site for the emergence of the ureteral stoma has been selected preoperatively. The site should be selected so that the patient will be able to see and manage the stoma in a position below the belt line. The site of the stoma should be assessed in the sitting, standing, and supine positions. The body habitus of the patient and the avoidance of skin creases play significant roles in planning the site of the stoma. The muscular backing of the stoma must be able to support the filled collection device. Thus, the ideal site is at or on the lateral border of the rectus muscle, about one third of the way down a line from the umbilicus to the anterior superior iliac spine.

Once the stomal site has been selected and an incision made, a very liberal opening must be made in the muscle and fascial layers, utilizing a cruciate incision with excision of the fascial components. Very careful attention must be paid to preventing angulation or rotation of the ureter, because the shuttering effect of various muscle layers can compromise the ureteral blood supply. The distal 1 to 2 cm of ureter is then spatulated and a V flap of skin sewn into the spatulated area, with four to six interrupted 4–0 absorbable sutures.

Fixation of the ureter to the internal oblique may result in compromise of the blood supply and probably should not be done. Temporary catheter drainage of the cutaneous ureterostomy is a matter of individual preference. A small No. 8 Fr. indwelling catheter may be selected so that it will not occlude the ureteral lumen. This catheter should be left indwelling for the first 7 to 10 days postoperatively. All catheters should have an open distal end so that a guide wire may be passed, if and when a new catheter has to be placed (particularly if satisfactory union between the skin and the ureter does not occur).

Results and Complications

The most significant early complication is stoma necrosis. Compromised blood supply during mobilization, tight opening in the abdominal wall, and eversion of the stoma from the skin contribute to stoma necrosis. Late complication includes stomal stenosis or retraction. Interpositioning of the skin flap into the stoma decreases the incidence of stomal stenosis.

Feminella and Lattimer (1971) reported long-term follow-up of cutaneous ureterostomies with a stomal stricture rate of 64 per cent in 70 patients. They related this stricture formation to three factors: (1) a ureter with a radiographic diameter of greater than 8 mm had a lower stricture rate than a normal caliber ureter; (2) an everted stoma had a stricture rate of 56 per cent, whereas a flush stoma had a stricture rate of 92 per cent; and (3) patients with preoperative irradiated ureters and skin were predisposed to stomal stenosis.

Holden and Whitmore (1981) reported experience with 135 patients with elective bilateral cutaneous ureterostomies. Almost two thirds of the patients developed unilateral or bilateral ureteral strictures. The overall

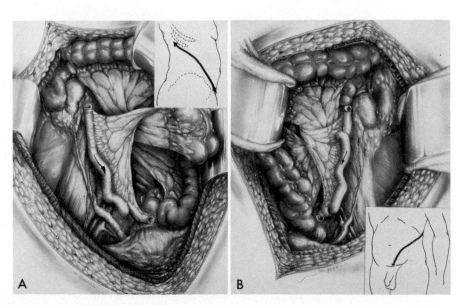

Figure 68–18. Isolated ileal segment has been passed through an opening in the colonic mesentery and rotated 180 degrees to lie on the iliopsoas muscle in an isoperistaltic direction. *A,* Right side. *B,* Left side. (From Goodwin, W. E.: *In* Riches, E. (Ed.): Modern Trends in Urology [Second Series]. London, Butterworth and Co., Ltd., 1960, p. 172. Illustrator, Mary P. Goodwin.)

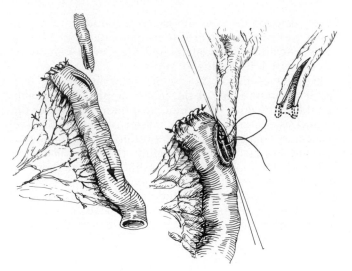

Figure 68–19. The ileal ureter is used with the proximal ureter still patent. Note medial spatulation of the ureter with an end-to-side ureteroileal anastomosis. (From Goodwin, W. E.: *In* Riches, E. (Ed.): Modern Trends in Urology [Second Series]. London, Butterworth and Co., Ltd., 1960, p. 172. Illustrator, Mary P. Goodwin.)

long-term results of patients with permanent cutaneous ureterostomies are not satisfying. More than half required conversion of their ureterostomy to intestinal conduit within 7 years of the original ureterostomy (Eckstein, 1983).

Ileoureteral Substitution

The intact isolated ileal segment provides the only reliable replacement for ureter. In 1906, Shoemaker performed the first human ureteral repair employing an isolated segment of ileum in a patient with inflamed ureters (Thorne and Resnick, 1986). Other bowel segments such as the appendix were also utilized. Because of its limited length, the appendix was used only for bridging gaps between the renal pelvis and the ureter

(Mesrobian, 1989). An ileal segment is reserved for a patient with an extensive loss of the ureter due to trauma, previous surgery, tuberculosis, uncontrollable urinary stone disease, ureteral carcinoma in a single kidney, or undiversion (Boxer et al., 1979). Bladder outlet obstruction, if uncorrected before surgery, is a relative contraindication to surgery. Patients with compromised renal functions may deteriorate to overt renal failure because of the absorption of urine across the ileal ureter. In patients with diffuse malignant diseases in the retroperitoneum, this procedure is also contraindicated. The evaluation, preparation, anastomotic techniques, and the preoperative and postoperative management of these patients are described elsewhere in this book.

Technique

The peritoneal cavity is entered through a generous midline or paramedian incision that allows access to the renal pelvis and to the bladder. The terminal ileum is identified and an ileum segment 20 to 25 cm in length is isolated between two clamps (Fig. 68–17). In isolating the segment, it is important to create a long distal mesenteric incision so that the segment can reach to the bladder. Continuity of the intestine is restored by an end-to-end ileal anastomosis anterior to the isolated segment. The isolated segment should be irrigated at this point with saline and antibiotic solution to clear any bowel contents that were left after the bowel preparation.

The mesocolon on the right or left side is opened, and the ileal segment is passed through this opening. The segment is rotated 180 degrees, so that the isoperistaltic ileum is now retroperitoneal in position (Fig. 68–18). The mesenteric defects are closed to prevent internal herniation. If a segment of the ureter can be used, the ureteral segment should be spatulated and an end-to-end or an end-to-side ansastomosis performed, with interrupted absorbable full-thickness sutures (Fig. 68–19).

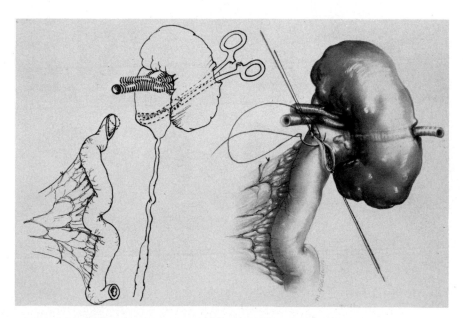

Figure 68–20. Stone-searching forceps is inserted through a pre-existing nephrostomy site to facilitate dissection of renal pelvis. (From Goodwin, W. E.: *In* Riches, E. (Ed.): Modern Trends in Urology [Second Series]. London, Butterworth and Co., Ltd., 1960, p. 172. Illustrator, Mary P. Goodwin.)

When the anastomosis is between the renal pelvis and the ileum segment, the kidney should be mobilized and the renal pelvis should be opened widely. The proximal end of the segment is anastomosed directly to the pelvis, utilizing interrupted absorbable full-thickness sutures. This anastomosis should be wide and tension-free. The back wall of the anastomosis should be completed first, with the knots placed on the outer side of the anastomosis.

Placement of a nephrostomy tube should be done before completely closing the anastomosis of the upper tract (Fig. 68–20). The anastomosis of the distal end to the bladder should be on the posterior wall or near the base of the bladder. A bladder psoas hitch may allow a better ileal position with a shorter segment and may eliminate kinking and angulation of the ileal segment and its mesentery (Fig. 68–21).

Usually, a direct refluxing anastomosis is done with interrupted, absorbable, full-thickness sutures. A suprapubic tube is left in the bladder for the drainage of the urine and the large amount of mucus produced by the intestine. Penrose drains are placed near each anastomosis. The abdominal wall is closed in the usual manner. Bilateral replacement can be done, using the same ileal segment by running the proximal end from one pelvis to the other and down to the bladder. Another method for bilateral replacement is the terminal ileum on one side and the colon on the other (Boxer et al., 1979).

RESULTS. Results are satisfactory in adequately selected patients, with stabilization of renal function and symptomatic improvement (Benson et al., 1990).

COMPLICATIONS. Plugging of the drainage tubes by mucus may occur during the postoperative period. Renal function deterioration has been described by Tanagho. Although reflux is present, the natural peristalsis of the ileal segment may protect or eliminate the transfer of bladder pressure to the kidney. Postoperative urinary tract infection may occur in about 60 per cent of the patients (Benson et al., 1990).

REFERENCES

Andreas, B. F., and Oosting, M.: Primary amyloidosis of the ureter. J. Urol., 79:929, 1958.

Benson, M. C., Ring, K. S., and Olsson, C. A.: Ureteral reconstruction and bypass: Experience with ileal interposition, the Boari flap-psoas hitch and renal autotransplantation. J. Urol., 143:20, 1990.

Blandy, J.: The ureter. In Blandy, J. (Ed.): Operative Urology, 2nd ed. Oxford, Blackwell Scientific Publications, 1986, pp. 89–114.

Boxer, R. J., Fritzsche, P., Skinner, D. G., Kaufman, J. J., Belt, E., Smith, R. B., and Goodwin, W. E.: Replacement of the ureter by small intestine: clinical application and results of the ileal ureter in 89 patients. J. Urol., 121:728, 1979.

Boyarsky, S., and Duque, O.: Ureteral regeneration in dogs: An experimental study bearing on the Davis intubated ureterotomy. J. Urol., 73:53, 1955.

Boyarsky, S., Labay, P., and Teague, N.: Aperistaltic ureter in upper urinary tract infection—cause or effect? Urology, 12:134, 1978.

Brannan, W.: Useful applications of transureteroureterostomy in adults and children. J. Urol., 113:460, 1975.

Butcher, H. R., Jr., and Sleator, W., Jr.: The effect of ureteral anastomosis upon conduction of peristaltic waves: An electro-ureterographic study. J. Urol., 75:650, 1956.

Caine, M., and Hermann, G.: The return of peristalsis in the anastomosed ureter: a cine-radiographic study. Br. J. Urol., 42:164, 1970.

Carlton, C. E., Jr., Guthrie, A. G., and Scott, R., Jr.: Surgical correction of ureteral injury. J. Trauma, 9:457, 1969.

Carlton, C. E., Jr., Scott, R., Jr., and Guthrie, A. G.: The initial management of ureteral injuries: A report of 78 cases. J. Urol., 105:335, 1971.

Cohen, J. D., and Persky, L.: Ureteral stones. Urol. Clin. North Am., 10:699, 1983.

Daniel, O., and Shackman, R.: Blood supply of human ureter in relation to ureterocolic anastomosis. Br. J. Urol., 24:334, 1952.

Davis, D. M.: Intubated ureterotomy: A new operation for ureteral and ureteropelvic stricture. Surg. Gynecol. Obstet., 76:513, 1943.

Davis, D. M.: Intubated ureterotomy. J. Urol., 66:77, 1951.

Davis, D. M.: The process of ureteral repair: A recapitulation of the splinting question. J. Urol., 79:215, 1958.

Eckstein, H. B.: Ureteral diversion. In Glenn, J. F. (Ed.): Urologic Surgery, 3rd ed. Philadelphia, J. B. Lippincott Co., 1983, pp. 491–499.

Ehrlich, R. M., and Skinner, D. G.: Complications of transureteroureterostomy. J. Urol., 113:467, 1975.

Feminella, J. G., Jr., and Lattimer, J. K.: A retrospective analysis of 70 cases of cutaneous ureterostomy. J. Urol., 106:538, 1971.

Flam, T. A., Malone, M. J., and Roth, R. A.: Complications of ureteroscopy. Urol. Clin. North Am., 15:167, 1988.

Foley, F. E. B.: Management of ureteral stone. JAMA, 104:1314, 1935.

Gil-Vernet, J. M.: Pyelolithotomy. In Glenn, J. F. (Ed.): Urologic Surgery, 3rd ed., Philadelphia, J. B. Lippincott Co., 1983, pp. 159–175.

Gregory, J. G., Starkloff, E. B., Miyai, K., and Schoenberg, H. W.: Urologic complications of ileal bypass operation for morbid obesity. J. Urol., 113:521, 1975.

Hamm, F. C., and Weinberg, S. R.: Management of the severed ureter. J. Urol., 77:407, 1957.

Harrow, B. R.: A neglected maneuver for ureterovesical reimplantation following injury at gynecologic operations. J. Urol., 100:280, 1968.

Hendren, W. H., and Hensle, T. W.: Transureteroureterostomy: experience with 75 cases. J. Urol., 123:826, 1980.

Higgins, C. C.: Transuretero-ureteral anastomosis; report of clinical case. Trans. Am. Assoc. Genitourin. Surg., 27:279, 1934.

Hinman, F., Jr.: Ureteral repair and the splint. J. Urol., 78:376, 1957.

Hodges, C. V., Barry, J. M., Fuchs, E. F., Pearse, H. D., and Tank, E. S.: Transureteroureterostomy: 25-year experience with 100 patients. J. Urol., 123:834, 1980.

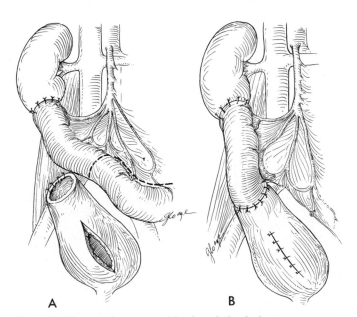

Figure 68–21. Use of vesicopsoas hitch with the ileal ureter operation. Redundant ileum is dissected (A), and an ileovesical anastomosis is performed (B) with interrupted 3–0 absorbable sutures.

A   B

Hofmann, A. F., Thomas, P. J., Smith, L. H., and McCall, J. T.: Pathogenesis of secondary hyperoxaluria in patients with ileal resection and diarrhea. Gastroenterology, 58:960, 1970.

Holden, S., and Whitmore, W. F., Jr.: Ureteral diversion. *In* Bergman, H. (Ed.): The Ureter, 2nd ed. New York, Springer-Verlag, 1981, pp. 717–754.

Johnson, H. W., and Ankenman, G. J.: Bilateral ureteral primary amyloidosis. J. Urol., 92:275, 1964.

Kearney, G. P., Mahoney, E. M., Sciammas, F. D., Colpoys, F. L., Norton, A. T., Swinney, J., and Harrison, J. H.: Venacavography, corticosteroids and surgery in the management of idiopathic retroperitoneal fibrosis. J. Urol., 115:32, 1976.

Koontz, W. W., Jr., Klein, F. A., and Vernon Smith, M. J.: Surgery of the ureter. *In* Walsh, P. C., Gittes, R. F., Perlmutter, A. D., and Stamey, T. A. (Eds): Campbell's Urology, 5th ed. Philadelphia, W. B. Saunders Co., 1986, pp. 2580–2600.

Lapides, J., and Caffrey, E. L.: Observation on healing of ureteral muscle: relationship to intubated ureterotomy. J. Urol., 73:47, 1955.

MacGregor, P. S., Montie, J. E., and Straffon, R. A.: Cutaneous ureterostomy as palliative diversion in adults with malignancy. Urology, 30:31, 1987.

Makker, S. P., Tucker, A. S., Izant, R. J., Jr., and Heymann, W.: Nonobstructive hydronephrosis and hydroureter associated with peritonitis. N. Engl. J. Med., 287:535, 1972.

Merguerian, P. A., and Rabinowitz, R.: Dismembered nonstented ureteroureterostomy using the carbon dioxide laser in the rabbit: comparison with suture anastomosis. J. Urol., 136:229, 1986.

Mesrobian, H-G. J., and Azizkhan, R. G.: Pyeloureterostomy with appendiceal interposition. J. Urol., 142:1288, 1989.

Mesrobian, H-G. J., and Kelalis, P. P.: Ureterocalicostomy: indications and results in 21 patients. J. Urol., 142:1285, 1989.

Middleton, R. G.: Routine use of the psoas hitch in ureteral reimplantation. J. Urol., 123:352, 1980.

Motola, J. A., Shahon, R. S., and Smith, A. D.: Anatomy of the ureter. Urol. Clin. North Am., 15:295, 1988.

Ockerblad, N. F.: Reimplantation of the ureter into the bladder by a flap method. J. Urol., 57:845, 1947.

Ockerblad, N. F., and Carlson, H. E.: Surgical treatment of ureterovaginal fistula. J. Urol., 42:263, 1939.

Oesterwitz, H., Bick, C., Muller, P., Hengst, E.: Reconstructive microsurgery of the upper urinary tract. Int. Urol. Nephrol., 20:453, 1988.

Olsson, C. A., and Norlen, L. J.: Combined Boari bladder flap-psoas hitch procedure in ureteral replacement. Scand. J. Urol. Nephrol., 20:279, 1986.

Ormond, J. K.: Bilateral ureteral obstruction due to envelopment and compression by an inflammatory retroperitoneal process. J. Urol., 59:1072, 1948.

Paquin, A. J., Jr.: Ureterovesical anastomosis: the description and evaluation of a technique. J. Urol., 82:573, 1959.

Pearse, H. D., Barry, J. M., and Fuchs, E. F.: Intraoperative consultation for the ureter. Urol. Clin. North Am., 12:423, 1985.

Persky, L.: Splinting vs. nonsplinting in ureteral surgery. *In* Bergman, H. (Ed.): The Ureter. New York, Harper & Row, 1967, pp. 566–575.

Persky, L., and Carlton, C. E., Jr.: Urinary diversion in ureteral repair. *In* Scott, R., Jr. (Ed.): Current Controversies in Urologic Management. Philadelphia, W. B. Saunders Co., 1972, pp. 169–175.

Persky, L., and Hoch, W. H.: Iatrogenic ureteral and vesical injuries. *In* Kendall, A. R., and Karafin, L. (Eds.): Goldsmith Practice of Surgery (Urology). New York, Harper & Row, 1984, vol. 2, chap. 5, pp. 1–56.

Persky, L., Hoch, W. H., and Kursh, E. D.: Surgical management of the ureter. *In* Harrison, J. H., Gittes, R. F., Perlmutter, A. D., Stamey, T. A., and Walsh, P. C. (Eds.): Campbell's Urology. Philadelphia, W. B. Saunders Co., 1979, pp. 2188–2210.

Popescu, C.: The surgical management of postoperative ureteral fistulas. Surg. Gynecol. Obstet., 119:1079, 1964.

Prout, G. R., Jr., and Koontz, W. W., Jr.: Partial vesical immobilization: an important adjunct to ureteroneocystostomy. J. Urol., 103:147, 1970.

Rober, P. E., Smith, J. B., and Pierce, J. M., Jr.: Gunshot injuries of the ureter. J. Trauma, 30:83, 1990.

Robert, K.: Ureterocalicostomy. Urol. Clin. North Am., 15:129, 1988.

Saltzman, B.: Ureteral stents. Urol. Clin. North Am., 15:481, 1988.

Sandoz, I. L., Paull, D. P., and MacFarlane, C. A.: Complications with transureteroureterostomy. J. Urol., 117:39, 1977.

Schlossberg, S. M.: Ureteral healing. Semin. Urol., 5:197, 1987.

Schmidt, J. D., Flocks, R. H., and Arduino, L.: Transureteroureterostomy in the management of distal ureteral disease. J. Urol., 108:240, 1972.

Scott, F. B.: Submucosal bladder flap ureteroplasty: experimental study. J. Urol., 88:42, 1962.

Sharpe, N. W.: Transuretero-ureteral anastomosis. Ann. Surg., 44:687, 1906.

Silber, S. J., and Thornbury, J.: The fate of non-absorbable intraureteral suture. J. Urol., 110:40, 1973.

Simon, J.: Ectropia vesicae. Lancet, 2:568, 1852.

Smart, W. R.: An evaluation of intubation ureterotomy with a description of surgical technique. J. Urol., 85:512, 1961.

Spies, J. W., Johnson, C. E., and Wilson, C. S.: Reconstruction of the ureter by means of bladder flaps. Proc. Soc. Exp. Biol. Med., 30:425, 1933.

Straffon, R. A., Kyle, K., and Corvalan, J.: Techniques of cutaneous ureterostomy and results in 51 patients. J. Urol., 103:138, 1970.

Swenson, O., and Smyth, B. T.: Aperistaltic megaloureter: treatment by bilateral cutaneous ureterostomy using a new technique. Preliminary communication. J. Urol., 82:62, 1959.

Thompson, I. M., and Ross, G., Jr.: Long-term results of bladder flap repair of ureteral injuries. J. Urol., 111:483, 1974.

Thorne, I. D., and Resnick, M. I.: The use of bowel in urologic surgery: An historical perspective. Urol. Clin. North Am., 13:179, 1986.

Tresidder, G. C., Blandy, J. P., and Singh, M.: Omental sleeve to prevent retroperitoneal fibrosis around the ureter. Urol. Int., 27:144, 1972.

Turner-Warwick, R. T., and Worth, P. H. L.: The psoas bladder-hitch procedure for the replacement of the lower third of the ureter. Br. J. Urol., 41:701, 1969.

Udall, D. A., Hodges, C. V., Pearse, H. M., and Burns, A. B.: Transureteroureterostomy: a neglected procedure. J. Urol., 109:817, 1973.

Van Arsdalen, K. N., and Hackler, R. H.: Transureteroureterostomy in spinal cord injury patients for persistent vesicoureteral reflux: 6- to 14-year followup. J. Urol., 129:1117, 1983.

Walsh, P. C.: Personal communication, 1984.

Weaver, R. G.: Ureteral regeneration: experimental and clinical: Part II. J. Urol., 77:164, 1957.

Weinberg, S. R.: Injuries of the ureter. *In* Bergman, H. (Ed.): The Ureter. New York, Harper & Row, 1967, pp. 355–393.

Weinberg, S. R., Hamm, F. C., and Berman, B.: The management and repair of lesions of the ureter and fistula. Surg. Gynecol. Obstet., 110:575, 1960.

Weiss, R. M.: Physiology of the upper urinary tract. Semin. Urol., 5:148, 1987.

Young, J. D., Jr.: Ureteroureterostomy and transureteroureterostomy. *In* Glenn, J. F. (Ed.): Urologic Surgery. Philadelphia, J. B. Lippincott Co., 1983, pp. 427–434.

Young, J. D., Jr., and Aledia, F. T.: Further observations on flank ureterostomy and cutaneous transureteroureterostomy. J. Urol., 95:327, 1966.

69
GENITOURINARY TRAUMA

Paul C. Peters, M.D.
Arthur I. Sagalowsky, M.D.

With the exception of the external genitalia in the male, the genitourinary tract is well protected from external violence and penetrating trauma, because of the surrounding viscera and musculoskeletal structures and because of its inherent mobility. Patients with genitourinary injuries may be immediately placed into two groups for purposes of triage and management: (1) those suffering from penetrating injuries who must undergo exploration and (2) those suffering from blunt external trauma who, uncommonly, need immediate surgery. Management of those in the second group often taxes surgical judgment and clinical skill application.

ADRENAL TRAUMA

Isolated adrenal trauma is indeed rare. No cases have been recorded from the Parkland Memorial Hospital (Dallas, Texas) emergency trauma service for the past 7 years, during which time more than 16,100 patients were seen with varying problems of penetrating and blunt trauma. Iatrogenic trauma has been reported by Skinner and colleagues (1990), and we have observed similar cases (Peters and Sagalowsky, 1986). The medulla is very susceptible to hemorrhage from trauma, as observed during adrenal harvest for transplantation and during breech extraction for delivery. No cases of adrenal hemorrhage following breech delivery have been reported or occurred in more than 28,000 normal deliveries at Parkland Memorial Hospital. Bilateral adrenal trauma during breech extraction, a rare injury, has been made even more rare because of the recent tendency of the obstetrician to perform cesarean section for persistent breech presentation.

GENERAL ASSESSMENT OF THE PATIENT SUSPECTED OF GENITOURINARY INJURY

History of the Injury

The history is invaluable in planning treatment, seeking to verify the integrity of specific portions of the urinary tract, and in classification, i.e., penetrating or blunt injury. The conscious patient will usually be able to provide details of the injury, such as a fall from a height, an auto or a pedestrian accident, a bullet or stab wound, or a sudden deceleration. Especially sought is a history of shock (defined as a systolic pressure <80 mm Hg) or a history of gross hematuria, in predicting the need for radiographic studies to assess the magnitude of injury. The conscious patient can provide or has usually provided a urine sample for analysis. The patient should be asked for this sample, except for the male patient with a known straddle injury in which case urethrography should be carried out prior to catheterization or voiding.

In the unconscious patient, there is usually some history available from witnesses or from attendants who have brought the patient to the emergency care area. Lacking this information, inspection of the flanks for hemorrhage; bruises over the lower abdomen; fall in hematocrit; abdominal findings, such as distention or infraumbilical midline mass; enlargement of the scrotum or flank; or discoloration of the external genitalia may give a clue to the presence of genitourinary injury.

Retrograde urethrography should be considered if there is blood at the meatus, or a history of such; discoloration in the perineum; or pelvic fracture, such as a Malgaigne fracture, making one suspect urethral injury. If there is no information, urethrography is probably safer to perform first with sterile water-soluble contrast material. Lacking this procedure or lacking facilities for retrograde urethrography, a small (16 to 18 Fr.) retention catheter may be passed in the unconscious patient. Passage of the catheter may give a clue as to the presence of hematuria or the rupture of the urethra or bladder and allows cystography and measurement of urine output, as one guide to effective replacement therapy of blood and extracellular and intracellular fluids.

Priorities in system care should be observed. Although urologists are concentrating on the urinary tract injury, they should be certain that (1) an adequate airway has been established, (2) an access to the vascular system for fluid replacement is accomplished, (3) bleeding points have been controlled, (4) catheter drainage is secure, and (5) nasogastric intubation, especially in the unconscious patient, has been carried out.

After priorities in care and system resuscitation have been carried out, one must choose between ultrasonography and radiographic contrast studies to further define the lesions present. In general, bladder and urethral injuries are best evaluated by retrograde cystography and urethrography with postvoiding or postdrainage films. Upper tract injuries are evaluated by computed tomography (CT) if available.

CT has largely replaced the arteriogram and the excretory urogram in the diagnostic work-up and management of the patient with abdominal and/or genitourinary trauma. The tendency of the trauma surgeon to use abdominal CT for evaluation of an abdomen after blunt trauma has decreased the need for both arteriography and excretory urography at our institution and other major trauma centers (Carroll and McAninch, 1989). The presence of a distended abdomen; absence of bowel sounds; a history of a deceleration injury; presence of abdominal or flank mass; suspicion of injury to the pancreas, liver, or spleen; high blood leukocyte count (>20,000); or injury to the bowel is an indication to the examining surgeon for CT of the abdomen. Renal and other abdominal visceral outlines are more clearly seen on CT. Minimal urinary extravasation not seen on an intravenous pyelography (IVP) may be discerned by CT with contrast material.

The patient with penetrating trauma has a high incidence of associated injuries and needs contrast radiographic studies to pinpoint the multiple injuries present. In the series reported by Mee and McAninch (1989), at the University of California, all patients with penetrating trauma (stab or gunshot wounds) to the abdomen underwent complete radiographic staging except for those few so severely injured (hemodynamically unstable) that they were subjected to immediate exploratory laparotomy. This parallels the Parkland Memorial Hospital experience.

In the past, one caveat has been that if even a nephrogram showed on an excretory urogram, one could state with some assurance that there was a 95 to 97 per cent chance that no surgically correctable renal arterial injury was present. This is not true of the patient undergoing CT. The CT scan is so sensitive as to visualize contrast material in a kidney with severe vascular injury. Even a parasitized (collateralized) intercostal or capsular vessel may show a cortical rim sign, and a kidney-threatening main renal artery injury may be present. In such a case, it is well advised to complement CT with selective renal arteriography before deciding on observation and nonoperative intervention (Fig. 69–1) (Cass and Luxenberg, 1987).

A trend is developing to be more selective in deciding to order radiographic contrast studies in victims of blunt renal trauma. Mee and McAninch (1989) have suggested limiting intravenous contrast studies, such as IVP and abdominal CT with contrast, to individuals (1) with a history of shock (systolic blood pressure <80 mm Hg) and/or gross hematuria and (2) with a history of microhematuria and shock. Such a limitation would eliminate a large group of patients with microhematuria (<500

red blood cells/high power field) and no shock. Combining their data with those of Cass and associates (1987), and with a study from our institution by Hardeman and associates (1987), Mee and McAninch (1989) found only one of 1671 (0.05 per cent) would have had serious renal injury not detectable utilizing the aforementioned indications for study in *blunt* trauma patients.

Another caveat states that the nature of the injury must not be overlooked. A rare patient who exhibits no gross hematuria and has no history of shock occasionally will have serious renal injury. Seven such patients were reported by Cass and colleagues (1985) in a retrospective study of 494 patients with blunt renal trauma and one such patient (severe deceleration injury) of 506 patients in another series (Kennedy et al., 1988). An accurate history indicating a severe blow or fall from a great height may in itself be an indication for CT.

Radionuclide studies may be helpful (e.g., technetium-99 DPTA or DMSA and ^{131}I Hippuran). Extravasation of contrast material may be seen. Pre-existing disease, such as hydronephrosis or ureteropelvic junction obstruction (UPJ), may be detected, and an estimate of the differential function of the two kidneys may be obtained. Poor or absent renal function and the presence of ectopia may be determined. The differential diagnosis can be made of acute torsion from testicular trauma or tumor by isotope studies. However, they are often not available, and this should not delay alternatives to diagnosis and treatment, especially during the hours from 8 P.M. to 8 A.M., when a number of trauma patients are seen.

Differential isotope scans have been of most value in evaluating results of vascular repair, in evaluating collecting system emptying after ureteral or renal pelvis reconstruction, or in helping to decide the salvageability of repaired kidneys and collecting systems. Isotope scan studies have their greatest use in trauma management when they are located near the trauma center and are staffed on a 24-hour basis by a radiologist with expertise in isotope techniques. We do not delay exploration for acute torsion of the spermatic cord unless the isotope scan is immediately available!

Trauma Work-up

For the urologist who, for varying reasons, has no access to CT scanning, the trauma work-up consisting of an IVP and a cystogram performed concomitantly gives valuable information for assessing injury and planning treatment (Fig. 69–2). The trauma work-up is done by obtaining a kidney, ureter, bladder (KUB) study, and then injecting (after obtaining a negative history of allergy to iodine or contrast material) a bolus of 50 to 60 ml of 30 per cent iodine-containing contrast material. At the time of the 5-minute abdominal film, the bladder is filled with contrast material and a film taken. Films are made at 10, 15, and 30 minutes. The bladder is then evacuated, and postevacuation or oblique voiding and postvoiding films are made. In this manner, preoperative integrity of the urinary tract can be established, or the necessity to intervene determined. In diagnosis of uri-

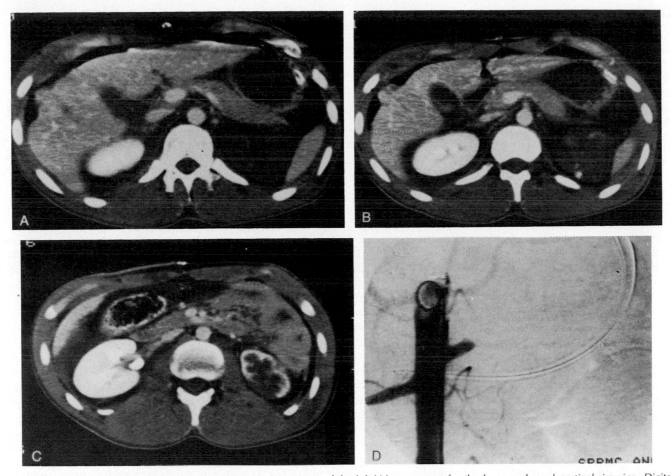

Figure 69–1. Computed tomography (CT) showing nonenhancement of the left kidney, except for the lower pole and *cortical rim sign*. Digital subtraction arteriogram shows total occlusion of the left renal artery in a kidney in which the cortex is visualized by CT. Such a kidney would have been nonfunctioning by intravenous pyelography. This case shows the need for occasional arteriography to complement CT findings. (Adapted from Cass, A. S., and Luxenberg, M.: Management of renal artery injuries from external trauma. J. Urol., 138:266, 1987. © Williams & Wilkins.)

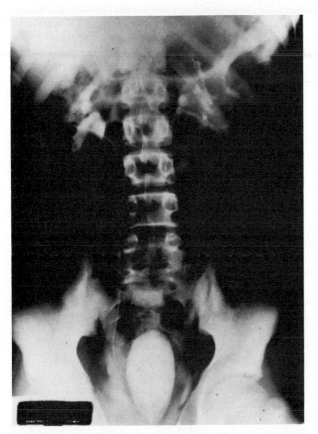

Figure 69–2. A 5-minute film illustrating trauma work-up in which the bladder is filled with contrast material 5 minutes after injection of the contrast material and after taking a plain film. Such a survey film may give the urologist who is working with the general surgeon in a trauma center valuable information.

Extraperitoneal rupture of the bladder is seen in this film. The typical "sunburst" appearance of the extravasated contrast material is seen. Note that the bladder shadow descends to the level of the symphysis.

nary tract injuries in our experience, less than 5 per cent of blunt trauma cases were classified as major renal injury, whereas 70 per cent of penetrating genitourinary injuries were of major significance in a separate experience at the University of California (Carrol and McAninch, 1989).

RENAL INJURIES

Introduction and Classification

Renal injuries may be classified, for management purposes, as penetrating or blunt. Penetrating injuries must be explored. A rare stab wound not entering the pleural or peritoneal cavity may be observed as an exception. Patients with blunt renal injuries do well under observation in our experience 96 per cent of the time. Renal injuries may be classified as major or minor (Fig. 69–3). A major renal injury includes pedicle avulsions (in which there may be no hematuria) and lacerations of the parenchyma, such as polar avulsions or lacerations extending *through* the parenchyma into the collecting system associated with gross hematuria. Except for the rare exception in which the nature of the injury alone, e.g., severe deceleration, demands study, individuals presenting with blunt trauma, no shock, and only microhematuria may be safely excluded from complete radiographic staging. When studied in the past, such individuals were found to have renal contusion as the cause of delay in function and *microhematuria*. Such

Table 69–1. RELATIVE FREQUENCY OF PENETRATING VS. BLUNT RENAL INJURY

Institution	Number	Penetrating	Blunt
Parkland Memorial (Peters, 1989)	272	202	70
University of California (Mee, 1989)	1146	1007	139

patients are often excluded from further study in major trauma centers today. Sonography and urinalysis might be considered as a screening procedure.

In most trauma centers, the ratio of blunt renal trauma to penetrating trauma is in the range of eight to nine blunt to one penetrating (Table 69–1). The Parkland Memorial Hospital experience is nearly the opposite, because of a predominance of gunshot wounds.

Diagnosis

With the advent and subsequent improvement in CT, the diagnosis of renal lesions no larger than 1 cm is possible. A renal lesion may be suspected in an individual with gross or microscopic hematuria, a history of injury to the flank or abdomen, a bruise over the flank, and fractured ribs posteriorly on the chest radiography or plain abdominal film (usually ribs 10, 11, 12) or in an individual with a penetrating missile injury and gross or microscopic hematuria. For the physician who has no access to CT or who sees only three or four cases a year of renal injury, the performance of an excretory urogram, a renal sonography, a differential isotope excretion ([131]I Hippuran or technetium-99 DMSA), with urinalysis may allow a more secure position when electing to follow blunt renal trauma victims.

In large trauma centers with dozens of patients monthly, considerable cost effectiveness is achieved by excluding patients from radiographic staging, except in cases of gross hematuria with or without shock (systolic pressure <80 mm Hg) or of microhematuria and shock. Of the radiographic studies available, CT scan of the abdomen is preferred. It defines associated visceral organ injuries more precisely than excretory urography; it shows minute extravasations of contrast material from the urinary tract or bowel that might be missed by excretion urography. Abdominal CT scan gives the same or more precise idea of blood flow to the renal parenchyma than excretion urography (with the caveat regarding the inability to predict main renal artery injury as well as the excretion urogram). CT scan also gives a more accurate portrayal of the ectopic or the absent kidney than other tests. It defines precisely small (<1.5 cm) areas of infarction in the kidney. CT of the pelvis most accurately depicts injuries to and defines the anatomy of the pelvis and urogenital outlet anatomy of any radiographic study available.

Arteriography for the diagnosis of renal injury is decreasing in our experience. One use for it remains— when one wishes to see the arterial pattern in a case in which the CT scan suggests that major injury may be

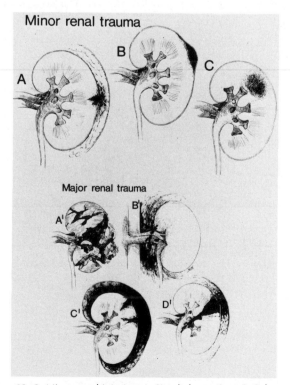

Figure 69–3. Minor renal injuries. *A*, Simple laceration. *B*, Subcapsular hematoma. *C*, Renal contusion. Major renal injuries: *A'*, Renal rupture. *B'*, Laceration of renal artery and vein. *C'*, Perirenal hematoma. *D'*, Laceration through collecting system. (From Peters, P. C., and Bright, T. C., III: Urol. Clin. North Am., 4:19, 1977.)

present, i.e., cortical rim sign. Certainly, nonenhancement of parenchyma on CT scan or nonvisualization on excretory urography suggests major arterial intimal disruption. Arteriography may complement CT when congenital UPJ obstruction or associated neoplasm is suspected. One thinks of this possibility when hematuria occurs that seems disproportionate to the magnitude of the trauma. When disproportionate hematuria or proteinuria is found in a renal injury case, think in terms of *pre-existing disease* (Fig. 69–4).

Many comparisons may be made between blunt and penetrating renal injuries. Associated injuries are more numerous and often more severe in penetrating trauma cases, particularly those caused by gunshot wounds (Table 69–2).

Blunt renal trauma is usually associated with sudden deceleration and is commonly suspected when gross hematuria appears. Two unique injuries are associated with sudden deceleration and are seen in children as well as adults. These are arterial intimal tear and UPJ disruption (see Fig. 69–4). The arterial intimal tear is associated with greater mobility of the renal pedicle in the child and more sparse perirenal fat. The disruption of the UPJ occurs in hyperextension injuries and is associated with greater mobility of the spine in the child. Arterial intimal disruption occurs, however, in the victim of penetrating injuries as well.

Of 96 patients diagnosed to have renal pedicle injuries, 94 were surgically explored at Parkland Memorial Hospital, in the period from 1960 to 1979. A total of 68 per cent (64) had suffered penetrating trauma. Of 12 arterial repairs attempted, four were successful. Trauma surgeons at the University of California had reported 30 attempted repairs with ten patencies. None of the kidneys in this group was thought capable of supporting life on its own (Peters and Sagalowsky, 1986).

The arterial intimal disruption remains one of the imperfectly solved problems in the diagnosis and management of the trauma victim. Early diagnosis and early intervention, coupled with existing vascular expertise, may improve results in the next decade. At Parkland Memorial Hospital, the mortality rate was 37 per cent in the renal pedicle group (nephrectomy rate was 44 per cent) and was related more to severe associated injuries. Only two of 11 were thought to have bled to death from the pedicle injury alone. By contrast, in 115 patients hospitalized at Parkland Memorial Hospital with blunt

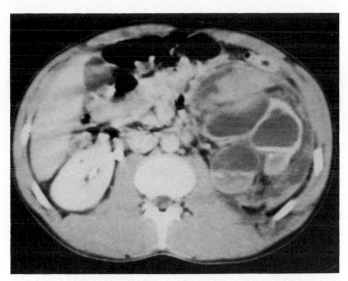

Figure 69–4. Patient had hematuria out of proportion to magnitude of flank injury incurred during spring football practice. Computed tomography suggests pre-existing hydronephrosis. Note the cortical rim sign. Arteriography may provide further information.

renal trauma and associated injuries, death occurred in 12 patients (10 per cent).

In contrast to the policy of surgically exploring patients with penetrating renal injuries, most patients with blunt trauma can be observed. In this group are the patients who suffer parenchymal fractures with preservation of the blood supply to the separated fragments (Fig. 69–5). We prefer observation and follow-up with CT. Others have advocated the use of collagen nets to surround the disrupted fragments. In our experience, attempts to mobilize such kidneys and place them in nets results in more blood loss and more renal loss than observation of the kidney tamponaded by Gerota's fascia.

One subset of blunt trauma patients that does profit from early exploration and repair has been defined by Husmann and Morris (1990). This group is the small subset with devascularized polar avulsion. In reviewing our data at Parkland Memorial Hospital, Husmann found that 83 per cent of these patients required delayed surgery, greatly prolonging total hospitalization time. We are currently advocating early operation and repair in this group (Table 69–3) (Fig. 69–6). These patients

Table 69–2. COMPARISON OF ABDOMINAL INJURIES IN PATIENTS SUSTAINING PENETRATING RENAL INJURIES VS. BLUNT RENAL INJURIES

Penetrating Renal Injuries, 122 Cases Associated Non-Renal Injuries		Blunt Renal Injuries, 84 Cases Associated Non-Renal Injuries	
Liver	58	Spleen	57
Small intestine	47	Liver	22
Stomach	45	Pancreas	4
Colon	43	Chest	4
Spleen	28	Colon	2
Pancreas	25	Small intestine	1
Chest	12		
Vena cava	9		
Aorta	5		
Ureter	3		

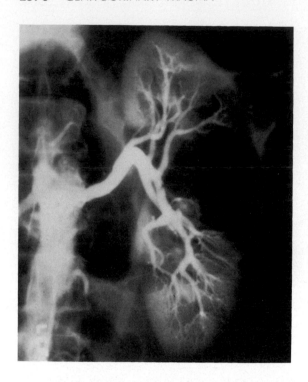

Figure 69–5. Major renal injury with complete parenchymal fracture and preservation of segmental blood supply.

Table 69–3. UNSTABLE (BLOOD PRESSURE <90 mm Hg) AND STABLE (BLOOD PRESSURE >90 mm Hg) PATIENTS WITH MAJOR RENAL LACERATIONS

	Number of Unstable (%)	Number of Stable	
		With Vascularized Renal Fragments (%)	*With Avascular Renal Fragments (%)*
Method of injury			
Motor vehicle accident	5 (55)	15 (50)	7 (64)
Pedestrian-motor vehicle accident	4 (45)	6 (20)	3 (27)
Fall		4 (13.5)	1 (9)
Aggravated assault		4 (13.5)	
Athletic activity		1 (3)	
Totals	9 (18)	30 (60)	11 (22)

Adapted from Husmann, D.A., and Morris, J.S.: Attempted nonoperative management of blunt renal lacerations extending through the corticomedullary junction: the short-term and long-term sequelae. J. Urol., 143:682, 1990. © By Williams & Wilkins, 1992.

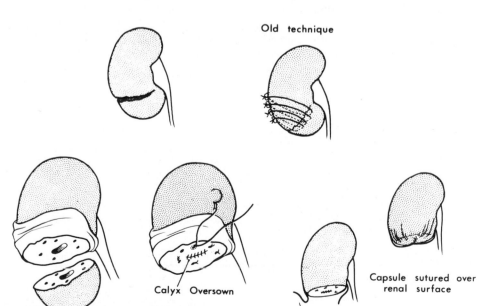

Old technique

Calyx Oversown

Capsule sutured over renal surface

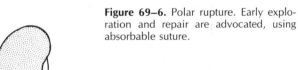

Figure 69–6. Polar rupture. Early exploration and repair are advocated, using absorbable suture.

are commonly diagnosed using CT scan, because of failure of the injured parenchyma to enhance after the injection of contrast material. Selective arteriography can be utilized to further define indeterminate cases.

Carlton (1978) has stated that about 85 per cent of blunt renal injuries require no surgery, 5 to 10 per cent require judgment and surgical exploration, and 5 per cent are nonsalvageable and require nephrectomy.

TECHNIQUES OF REPAIR AND AVOIDANCE OF COMPLICATIONS

We prefer to open most trauma patients requiring exploration through a midline incision from the xiphoid to the pubis. This is the incision generally used by the general surgeons with whom we work. A complete exploration of all abdominal organs is best accomplished through this incision. The pedicle must be secured before exposing the kidney! This may be accomplished by reflecting the colon and securing the renal pedicle before opening Gerota's fascia, approaching through the root of the mesentery (Peters and Sagalowsky, 1986), or by making an incision around the cecum and through the root of the mesentery, sacrificing the IMA and IMV if necessary to expose the renal pedicles (Figs. 69–7 and 69–8). One must consider the effects carefully before dividing the IMA in infants less than 2 years of age and in older patients (more than 70 years), with marked atherosclerosis. It usually is not necessary.

Once the vessels are secured, the colon is reflected to expose the kidney. Vascular clamps may be necessary at any moment, if brisk bleeding occurs when Gerota's fascia is opened. Medial mobilization of the duodenum (Kocher maneuver) is helpful to expose the renal pelvis

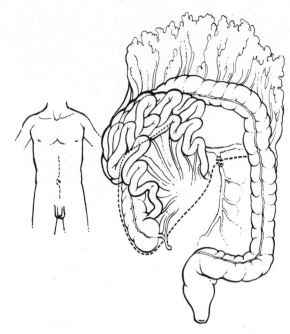

Figure 69–7. A long vertical midline incision allows rapid exposure in renal trauma cases. The entire small bowel and ascending colon may be rapidly mobilized by incising the posterior peritoneum, as shown. The inferior mesenteric vein may be ligated and divided to increase exposure to the renal vessels. (From Sagalowsky, A. I.: In Ehrlich, R. M. (Ed.): Modern Technics in Surgery. Mount Kisco, N.Y., Futura Publishing Co., 1984.)

and hilar area on the right. Once the renal artery is clamped, the vein may be left open to identify vessels needing ligation or repair. The kidney may be cooled, and repairs carried out in situ. This practice is preferable to bench surgery in most cases.

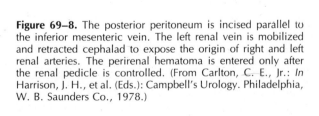

Figure 69–8. The posterior peritoneum is incised parallel to the inferior mesenteric vein. The left renal vein is mobilized and retracted cephalad to expose the origin of right and left renal arteries. The perirenal hematoma is entered only after the renal pedicle is controlled. (From Carlton, C. E., Jr.: In Harrison, J. H., et al. (Eds.): Campbell's Urology. Philadelphia, W. B. Saunders Co., 1978.)

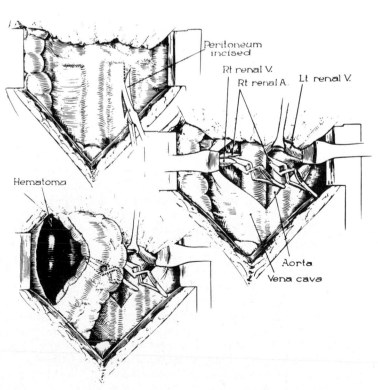

One should remember certain principles—reflect the capsule over devascularized polar ruptures and use it to cover bare areas of parenchyma (preferable to omental pedicle or fascial free graft). Always select absorbable suture to repair the collecting system—we prefer 4–0 chromic catgut. Similar suture is employed to ligate exposed parenchymal vessels on the cut surface of the kidney, as in Figure 69–6.

When repairing a polar rupture, move the lower pole of the kidney away from the UPJ area and interpose fat (Deming procedure), when possible. This maneuver prevents adherence of the ureter to the healing kidney and secondary UPJ obstruction. We prefer to do a nephropexy of the kidney to the muscle fascia after partial nephrectomy, to avoid a postoperative torsion of the pedicle with resulting Dietl's crisis (vomiting and abdominal pain), or, worse, renal infarction.

Renal artery and vein lacerations are repaired with interrupted 5–0 Prolene sutures on a C-1 needle or as a continuous suture, indicated by the size and length of the defect. For UPJ disruptions, we prefer a spatulated repair over a double-J stent with interrupted 4–0 or 5–0 chromic catgut suture.

Drainage for leaking urine should be provided after repairing disruptions of the kidney and its collecting system. A Jackson-Pratt 7- to 10-mm drain is placed near the site of repair and brought out the flank through a *separate* stab wound, with an indwelling double-J ureteral stent for lacerations more than 2 cm in length. Perioperative broad-spectrum antibiotics, with inclusion of coverage for anaerobic organisms in those individuals with bowel leak or disruption, are provided for renal trauma victims who are undergoing surgery.

Pertinent to this discussion are suggestions of how to prevent complications in trauma victims undergoing urologic surgery (Table 69–4).

URETERAL INJURIES

Diagnosis

Ureteral injury must be suspected in any patient who is suffering abdominal trauma. UPJ avulsions occur in thin children with acute hyperextension of the spine and blunt trauma. A penetrating missile may injure the ureter at any point from the UPJ to the intramural portion. An iatrogenic injury not recognized at the time usually causes flank pain within 4 to 9 days and fever higher than 100° F. Tenderness to palpation of the kidney is nearly always present. The presence or absence of hematuria cannot be relied on for diagnosis. In a series of surgical patients sustaining ureteral injury reviewed by Carlton (1978), only 11 per cent exhibited hematuria, whereas 90 per cent in a series of his patients sustaining external violence exhibited hematuria.

The ureter is rarely injured. It is well protected by its mobility and its location. A direct hit by a penetrating missile is a rare event. Only 19 isolated injuries of the ureter were reported in United States forces in World War I and 24 in World War II. At Parkland Memorial

Table 69–4. PREVENTION OF COMPLICATIONS OF SURGERY FOR GENITOURINARY INJURIES

Operation	Complication of GU Trauma Surgery	Prevention
Partial nephrectomy for polar rupture	Stricture of upper ureter adherent to lower pole of surgical kidney	Nephropexy Deming maneuver
Partial nephrectomy for polar rupture (late)	Abscess perirenal urinoma (extravasation)	Early operation and removal of devascularized fragments
Ureteroureterostomy	Fistula, extravasation infected urine	Thorough debridement Proximal diversion of urine
Suprapubic cystostomy	Pelvic abscess	Pelvic drains Repeated sonography for fluid collection
Arterial repair	Renal artery thrombosis	Early angiography Early exploration Fix intima to vessel wall distally Remove fragmented intima completely
Urethral reanastomosis		
Posterior	Incontinence Stricture Abscess	Exact epithelial approximation Adequate mobilization of proximal and distal urethra
Anterior	Stricture Fistula	Fix proximal portion of anastomosis to underlying fascia

GU, genitourinary.

Hospital, we were able to find 59 cases in a 10-year period (Bright and Peters, 1977).

Four major considerations apply in deciding the given management of a ureteral injury:

1. Site of the injury, i.e., upper, middle, or lower third of the ureter.

2. Nature of the injury, i.e., blunt trauma with avulsion or penetrating injury, when there is a high incidence of associated organ injury. The presence of high-velocity missile injury (>2200 ft/sec) with extensive coagulation necrosis of the ureter introduces lesions not noted in the more common low-velocity missile injury (<2200 ft/sec) from 22-caliber (700 ft/sec) or 38-caliber (745 ft/sec) bullets.

3. Time of recognition, i.e., repair, proximal diversion, plus stenting for immediately recognized injuries. This is in contrast to drainage and diversion with later reconstruction in cases associated with extensive abscess formation, urinoma, and ureteral necrosis recognized later.

4. Associated injuries and their presence modifying the standard treatment, i.e., nephrectomy becoming the operation of choice in certain elderly patients who require vascular graft and diverting colostomy at the same time because of perforation. Desire to have absolutely no urine leaks in patients (elderly) requiring simultaneous aortic or iliac artery graft may make nephrectomy preferable to ureterostomy or ureteral ligation and delayed repair in such circumstances.

In addition to ureteral injury secondary to external violence, e.g., penetrating missiles and blunt trauma, operative ureteral injuries continue to account for a significant percentage of ureteral injuries. These injuries are secondary to gynecologic, urologic, and vascular surgical procedures and rarely to orthopedic or neurosurgical injury during laminectomy. A study of such cases reveals the interesting fact that it is the part of the ureter at the pelvic brim that is most commonly injured rather than the lower ureter that bears intimate relationship to the uterine artery, bladder, hypogastric vessels, external iliac vein, broad ligament, and so forth. Injury to the ureter occurred 16 times in a series of 1093 extensive abdominal gynecologic operations reported by Daly and Higgins (1988). Twelve of the 16 ureteral injuries occurred at the pelvic brim, ten on the right side; eight of the patients had undergone previous hysterectomies. No patient in their series had injury to the ureter during a vaginal procedure. The incidence of ureteral injury in gynecologic surgery continues to be about ten cases during abdominal surgery for one case during vaginal surgery.

Spirnak and colleagues (1989), in a small series of eight patients incurring iatrogenic ureteral injury during placement or revision of a vascular graft, have recommended ureteral repair rather than nephrectomy in this circumstance. This was their recommendation even though three of the eight patients ultimately required nephrectomy—two with persistent extravasation. No graft complications occurred.

This series would differ, however, from the situation in which a penetrating missile caused concomitant colon, aorta, common iliac artery injury, and ureteral perforation or avulsion in an elderly patient. Following the course of the ureter through the pelvis may be difficult or impossible when extensive scar or neoplasm surrounds it. Identification of the ureter at the pelvic brim where it crosses the common iliac artery on either side with placement of a small vascular tape around the ureter for periodic identification and/or elevation during pelvic dissection is an important step in preventing iatrogenic ureteral complication at a point where the ureter has been most commonly injured!

We perform the definitive ureteroureterostomy in a spatulated fashion, with a minimal number (5 to 6) of 5–0 chromic sutures. In addition, we provide urinary diversion by means of a Silastic ureteral stent (Fig. 69–9). An alternate method is to divert the urine by means of a double-J stent and to put a drain down near the site of repair, as illustrated in Figure 69–10. Most surgeons prefer a 10-mm, flat Jackson-Pratt drain (see Fig. 69–10). Carlton (1978) has reported a 47 per cent early and 54 per cent late failure rate of nonwatertight anastomoses with stenting. In our series, the complication rate is 19 per cent. Carlton recommends a watertight, continuous suture line without a stent and reports a 100 per cent success rate. Because of the high complication rates of other forms of mid-ureteral management, ureteroureterostomy is the preferred method of closure for the injured ureter in the upper and middle thirds.

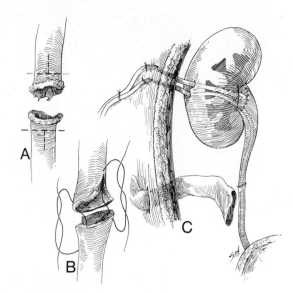

Figure 69–9. Ureteroureterostomy. *A*, The ureteral edges are debrided to viable bleeding tissue, and the ureter is longitudinally spatulated on opposite sides to prevent twisting.

B, The apex of one spatulated side is sutured to the nonspatulated edge of the other ureteral end, with care taken to exclude the suture from the ureteral lumen.

C, The anastomosis is completed with interrupted sutures. Urinary diversion is accomplished by nephrostomy drainage in connection with a Silastic ureteral stent placed through the anastomosis. (From Peters, P. C., and Bright, T. C., III: *In* Longmire, W. P., Jr. (Ed.): Advances in Surgery. Chicago, Year Book Medical Publishers, 1976.)

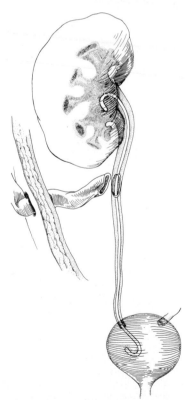

Figure 69–10. Alternate method to that depicted in Figure 69–9. Currently favored by most young trauma surgeons. P.C.P. prefers the technique shown in Figure 69–9.

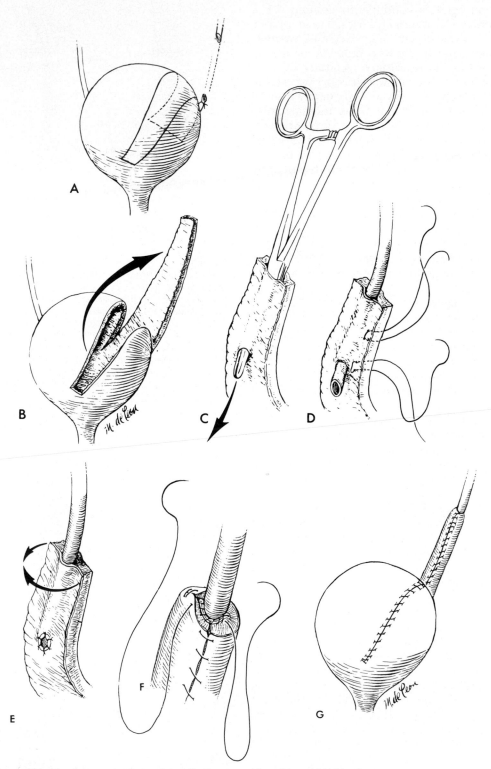

Figure 69–11. Technique of bladder flap ureteroplasty. *A* and *B*, Creation of broad-based bladder flap.
C, Submucosal tunnel created for antireflux reimplantation of the ureter.
D, Submucosal reimplantation of the ureter. Sutures in the posterior aspect of the flap rigidly fix the flap to the psoas muscle.
E, Bladder flap rolled into tube.
F, Ureter fixed to proximal flap.
G, Completed bladder flap ureteroplasty. (From Carlton, C. E., Jr.: *In* Harrison, J. H., et al. (Eds.): Campbell's Urology, 4th ed. Philadelphia, W. B. Saunders Co., 1978.)

For intramural or lower ureteral defects, we employ ureteral reimplantation with a tunneled technique (Politano-Leadbetter) and have had no complications in more than 15 cases.

With both ureteroureterostomy and ureteral reimplantation, over 90 per cent of ureteral defects may be adequately managed immediately following injury. If there have been more than 7 cm of destruction, the mobilization of the kidney and bladder allows the ends to be reapproximated. A psoas-bladder hitch may be employed for extraureteral mobility and to decrease the tension on the suture line. To bridge a longer ureteral gap, a submucosal ureteral reimplantation into the Boari bladder flap is employed (Fig. 69–11). If there is massive destruction of the lower ureter, a transureteroureterostomy provides adequate results. For total destruction of the ureter, a segment of ileum may be utilized as a substitute. The bowel segment is tapered and placed submucosally through the bladder wall (see Figure 69–12 for variable indications and techniques of ureteral repair).

RUPTURE OF THE URINARY BLADDER

Rupture of the urinary bladder can be divided conveniently into the categories of extraperitoneal and intraperitoneal ruptures. Intraperitoneal rupture often occurs when there is blunt external force applied to the urinary bladder. Common cause are a motor vehicle accident, a fall from a height, and an injury by penetrating missile. Often alcoholic beverage intake preceded the motor vehicle accident, and the patient had a full bladder prior to the rupture. Corriere and Sandler (1986) have pointed out that intraperitoneal rupture, as well as extraperitoneal rupture, may be associated with pelvic fracture with or without *laceration* by a fractured pelvic bone, usually a pelvic ramus.

Intraperitoneal rupture should be suspected in patients with sudden deceleration injury, with lower abdominal tenderness not well localized (no point tenderness) who have hematuria and occasionally inability to void. A cystogram with evacuation films will usually establish the diagnosis (Fig. 69–13). One must be sure to instill at least 250 ml of sterile contrast material into the bladder in order to distend the bladder. Otherwise, one may see what appears to be an intact small bladder as the constraction of the bladder muscle may seal off the area of disruption (Fig. 69–14). Intraperitoneal rupture is commonly associated with other intraperitoneal injuries.

It is our policy to recommend exploratory laparotomy at the time of suprapubic cystostomy to look for these injuries. A thorough search of the peritoneal cavity is indicated if bloody fluid is encountered when the peritoneal cavity is opened. If exploration findings are negative, the bladder wall is closed in three layers with chromic catgut or Vicryl and a suprapubic tube. This 20 Fr. Malecot catheter is brought out through a separate stab wound in the bladder. Extraperitoneal drainage with a Jackson-Pratt drain is accomplished.

After 10 to 14 days, a cystogram is performed through the suprapubic tube with a postevacuation film. If no extravasation is seen and it is determined that the patient can void without residual urine, the suprapubic tube is removed. The suprapubic tube may be left in longer when necessary, e.g., with an associated urethral disruption; with a need for immobilization of the patient in a cast; to make urinary nursing care less difficult; and to avoid complications of urethritis, epididymitis, epididymo-orchitis, and urethral stricture seen in male patients on long-term catheter drainage. In a woman with intraperitoneal rupture, the healing occurs promptly when the suprapubic tube is removed if voiding function is normal.

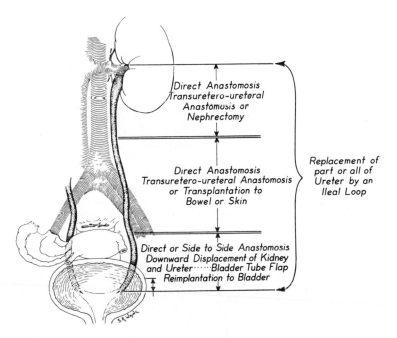

Figure 69–12. Management of ureteral injury, depending on location. (Reprinted and modified from Orkin, 1964.)

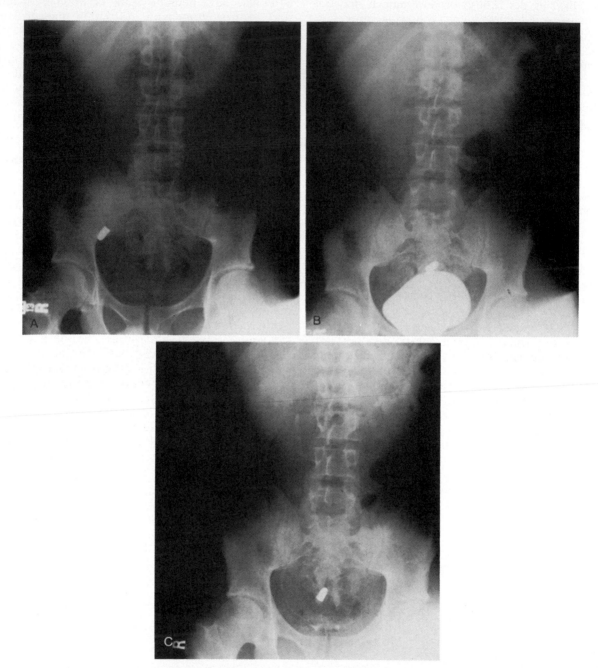

Figure 69–13. Pitfall in the diagnosis of penetrating intraperitoneal rupture of the bladder. *A,* Scout film in a patient with a 38-caliber gunshot wound of the abdomen and gross hematuria. *B,* Cystogram with intravenous urogram injection at the same time. No extravasation is seen. *C,* Drainage film 5 minutes later shows normal kidneys and ureters bilaterally and no evidence of extravasation.

At exploration, two through-and-through holes were found in the bladder dome. Missile was lying free in the peritoneal cavity. All penetrating wounds should be explored because of the high incidence of associated injuries. (From Peters, P. C.: Urol. Clin. North Am., 16:279, 1989.)

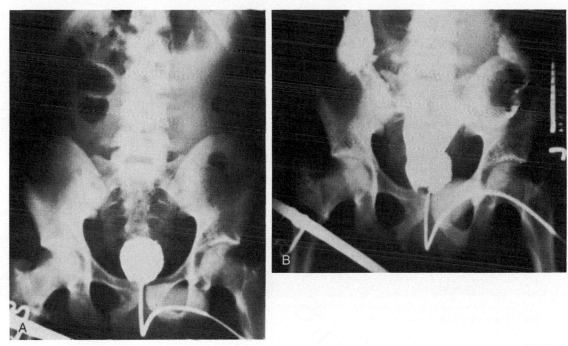

Figure 69–14. Danger of cystogram with inadequate volume of contrast material. *A*, Cystogram shows an apparently intact bladder when only 50 ml of contrast material had been instilled via catheter in a patient complaining of severe, but not well-localized, lower abdominal pain after an auto accident.

B, Same patient a few moments later after 250 ml of contrast material had been instilled via the urethral catheter; evidence of previously undetected rupture of the bladder with intraperitoneal extravasation. Exploratory laparotomy is indicated. (From Peters, P. C.: Urol. Clin. North Am., 16:279, 1989.)

Extraperitoneal rupture of the bladder (see Fig. 69–2) is more commonly associated with pelvic fracture when the patient is seen by a urologist. When a patient with a pelvic fracture is managed by an orthopedic surgeon, only about 5 or 6 per cent are seen to have urinary extravasation. Herzog reviewed 512 consecutive pelvic fractures at Parkland Memorial Hospital and found 25 ruptured bladders (4.8 per cent) and 12 ruptured urethras (1.3 per cent). Thus, the orthopedic surgeon is less apt to think of bladder or urethral rupture in the patient with a pelvic fracture, unless a Malgaigne fracture is present.

RUPTURE OF THE POSTERIOR URETHRA

Rupture of the posterior urethra is a serious injury often associated with a severe external force delivered to the lower abdomen and pelvis. It is not uncommonly associated with pelvic fracture, particularly the vertical fracture through ilium and one or more pubic rami (the Malgaigne fracture) (Fig. 69–15). It may be associated with those fractures that have severe disruptions of the pelvic ring, with displacement of the symphysis pubis. One may obtain a history of seeing blood at the meatus, carried there by a spasm of the bulbocavernosus muscle at the time of the injury.

One should perform urethrography with water-soluble contrast material prior to instrumentation. The bladder is often palpable above the symphysis and distended

with urine because the normal vesical neck is competent. When radiographic studies are done, the bladder silhouette is seen to be floating above the symphysis full of contrast material. This finding compares with the radiographic findings in a patient with extraperitoneal rupture of the bladder, in which the contrast material in the deformed bladder (teardrop or light-bulb shaped) descends to the level of the symphysis. The radiographic view of posterior urethral rupture with the intact vesical neck and bladder distended with contrast material well above the symphysis has been referred to as "pie in the sky" by Turner-Warwick (1989).

Rectal examination of a patient with a complete posterior urethral disruption may reveal that the prostate has been lifted from its usual position just inside the anal canal to a much higher and more difficult to reach position in the true pelvis. This finding was reported by Vermooten in 1946, who referred to the "high riding" prostate. Voiding in such patients is difficult or impossible, if it has been attempted prior to urologic consultation. One of us (P.C.P.) saw a patient who had been in a hospital for 37 days on the orthopedic service who could not void at all but who had been found to have a large residual each time the catheter was passed by a medical student. Urethrography confirmed the diagnosis (Fig. 69–16).

Some debate exists about the initial management of this condition. We prefer to perform suprapubic cystostomy at the time the patient presents and to accept an inevitable stricture, which is excised during reconstruction (Fig. 69–17). Reconstruction is delayed until the

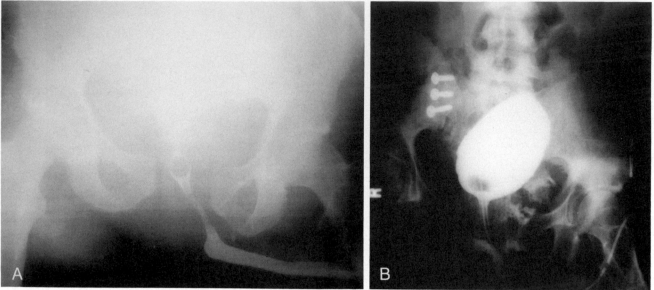

Figure 69–15. *A,* Malgaigne fracture and urethral disruption. The catheter passed and was left indwelling. *B,* Same patient. Malgaigne fracture was repaired and catheter removed. Extravasation from necrotic posterior urethra is seen. Suprapubic cystostomy is indicated that should have been done initially.

tissues are healed, often 3 months or longer. Reconstruction will be discussed in the section on urethroplasty (see Chapter 83), but a few points are germane here. The three major complications of posterior urethral injury are stricture, urinary incontinence, and impotence. In our experience, these are minimized by initial cystostomy and delayed repair compared with the results obtained with these three problem areas by attempted restoration of alignment over catheters or kissing sounds the night of injury in a pelvis full of hematoma, bone fragments, and external debris (Peters and Sagalowsky, 1986).

Morehouse (1990) has a similar opinion based on results after adopting this method of initial cystostomy and delayed repair as a suggestion from Bengt Johansen (Table 69–5).

The importance of proximal epithelial to distal epithelial apposition was brought out in the experimental studies of McRoberts and Rajde (1970), who showed in dogs that strictures inevitably resulted in healing of posterior disruptions treated by catheter traction alone but did not occur when complete epithelial apposition was accomplished by a suture technique. In these animals, the disruptions were accomplished with the knife and if repair was to be done it was accomplished immediately. These experimental results may vary from

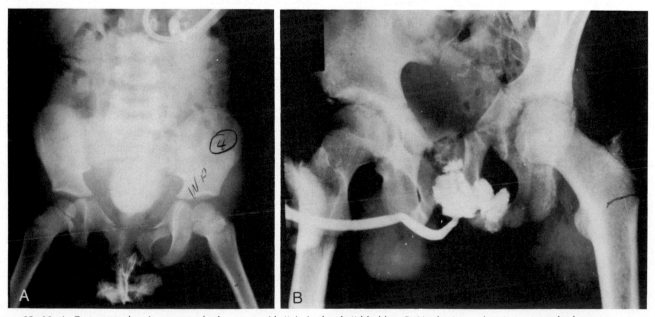

Figure 69–16. *A,* Cystogram showing posturethral rupture with "pie-in-the-sky" bladder. *B,* Urethrogram showing posturethral rupture.

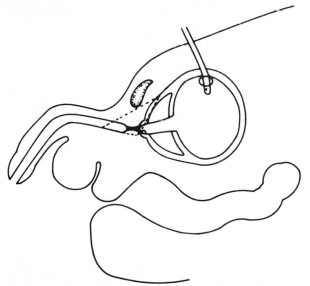

Figure 69–17. Initial cystostomy as advocated. The inevitable stricture, occurring in 95 per cent of the cases, is depicted and was subsequently corrected by reconstructive surgery.

those obtained by operating on disrupted, bruised tissue from deceleration injuries, but the principle of epithelial apposition remains. When epithelial apposition is not accomplished, one often obtains the history that the voided well once or twice but then began to have progressive difficulty and within 36 hours could not void at all. Inevitably, endoscopy shows the presence of a stricture and the lack of epithelial apposition.

Posterior urethral injuries vary greatly in magnitude as to the extent of urethra involved and magnitude of disruption. In all, however, we believe that the initial step is the cystostomy, delaying the repair until the traumatized tissues have healed and have the strength to hold suture materials without disruption.

Certainly, variations of this approach are being carried out. When disruption is mild, hematoma minimal, and prostate descended, Witherington has advocated immediate repair and realignment over indwelling catheter with good initial results. Devine and co-workers (1989) have reported early intervention, particularly when puboprostatic ligaments were restricting descent of prostate (Fig. 69–18).

The prostate should descend to the pelvic outlet to minimize the length of stricture. In some patients, descent to the pelvic floor is impeded by bone fragments, clots, or tissue debris. In these cases, cystostomy alone

may still be done at the time of injury, particularly in patients with severe associated injuries and vasomotor instability. Elective debridement to remove impediments to prostate descent, i.e., bone fragments, can be carried out 3 or 5 days later when the patient's condition has stabilized. Devine has advocated early surgical exploration and division of the puboprostatic ligaments when the prostate has been carried high or otherwise displaced in the pelvis by intact puboprostatic ligaments attached to a displaced bone fragment. Alignment of the prostatourethral junction may be accomplished at the same time. Details of reconstructive methods are given in Chapter 83.

Vesicostomy is preferable in an infant as an alternative to suprapubic cystostomy. Of posterior urethral disruptions, 95 per cent are complete in our experience and reconstruction of the accepted strictured area will be necesssary. About 5 per cent are minimal disruptions and may heal without stricture following cystostomy or vesicostomy alone (Fig. 69–19).

RUPTURE OF THE ANTERIOR (BULBOUS AND PENDULOUS) URETHRA

Anterior urethral injuries are more common than posterior urethral injuries and result, most commonly, from straddle injuries (e.g., fall from a bicycle). They may result from direct blows to the perineum, as is common in Texas if the patient is kicked with the toe of a boot. The urethra may be partially or completely severed. If the integrity of Buck's fascia, which has attachments near the suspensory ligament of the penis, is not destroyed, the extravasation of urine and blood from urethral or cavernosal injury will follow the distribution of the shaft of the penis, a "sleeve" of the penis (Fig. 69–20). If Buck's fascia is ruptured, the attachments of Colles' fascia become the limiting factors (Fig. 69–21).

Extravasations do not extend down the thigh as a rule, because of the fusion of Colles' fascia with the fascia lata of the thigh. Extensions along or above the clavicle from urethral rupture are limited by fusion of Scarpa's fascia with the coracoclavicular fascia (Fig. 69–22). If there is any question regarding the integrity of the urethra, especially if severe contusion of the anterior or posterior urethra is present, cystostomy and delayed reconstruction of the urethra are preferred to Foley catheter *urethral* drainage (Fig. 69–23). Partial or com-

Table 69–5. RESULTS OF IMMEDIATE REPAIR VS. INITIAL CYSTOSTOMY AND DELAYED REPAIR

	Immediate Repair				Initial Cystostomy & Delayed Repair (Johansen Technique)			
	Points	*Impotence*	*Incontinence*	*Stricture*	*Points*	*Impotence*	*Incontinence*	*Stricture*
Wilson and Husmann (Parkland Memorial Hospital)	17	8	2	16	64	33	8	4
Morehouse (Royal Victoria)	128	33	21	14	119	10	6	6

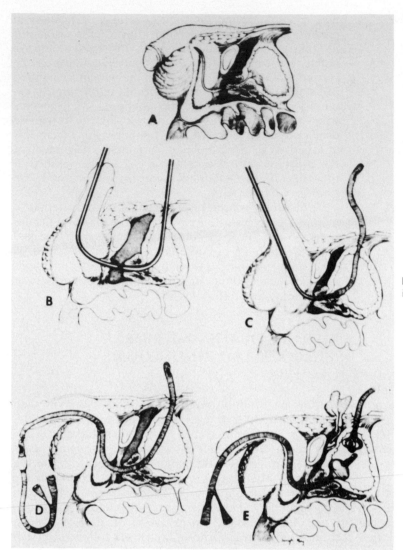

Figure 69–18. *A to E*, Technique of immediate realignment of indwelling catheter.

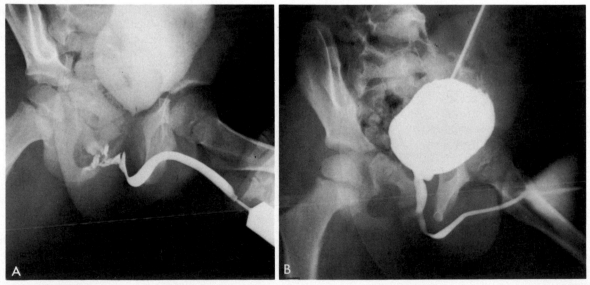

Figure 69–19. *A*, Retrograde urethrogram in a child with urethral rupture in the posterior portion. *B*, Voiding cystourethrogram: 1-month postoperative appearance of urethra after treatment with a cutaneous vesicostomy alone. No urethral reconstruction was necessary. (Courtesy of Dr. Dymis Lawrence, Compton, California.)

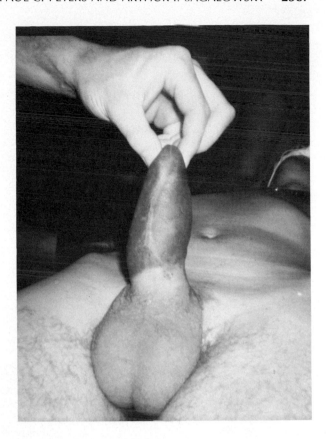

Figure 69–20. Typical "sleeve" of the penis injury caused by rupture of the corpus cavernosum. Buck's fascia is intact. Also, note the normal scrotum.

plete severance of the urethra by stab wound or knife wound or a blow to the perineum may be treated by exploration through a perineal or low scrotal incision and oblique spatulated reanastomosis of the urethra. This procedure is accomplished using fine 5-0 or 6-0 chromic catgut suture. In such instances, it is important to fix the proximal urethra, open and spatulated, to the underlying fascia to immobilize the proximal anasto-

motic site and to minimize the occurrence of postoperative urethral stricture (Fig. 69–24). When an oblique spatulated urethral anastomosis is done, a urethral catheter is left in from 10 days to 2 weeks. A stent and voiding cystourethrogram is done at the time of removal.

Devastating blow-out injuries of the perineum may occur from shotgun blast or power machine injuries. Initial management consists of hemostasis and careful

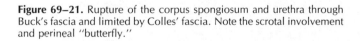

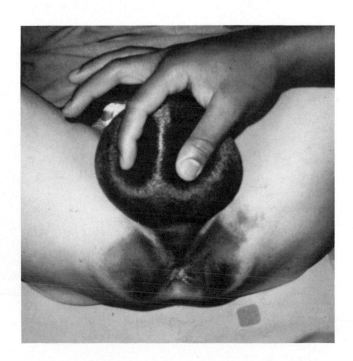

Figure 69–21. Rupture of the corpus spongiosum and urethra through Buck's fascia and limited by Colles' fascia. Note the scrotal involvement and perineal "butterfly."

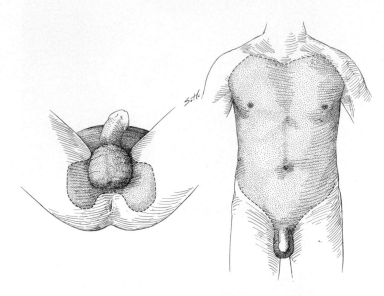

Figure 69–22. Areas of potential urinary extravasation in rupture of the urethra confined to Colles' fascia attachment. Note the fusion of Colles' fascia with coracoclavicular fascia superiorly and peritoneal limits of Colles' fascia.

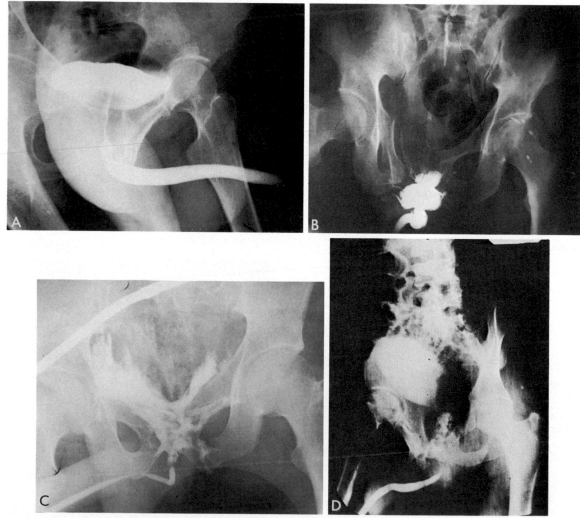

Figure 69–23. *A,* Normal retrograde urethrogram. Note that the contrast material has been injected *during* the exposure to ensure delineation of deep bulbar, membranous, and prostatic urethra. *B* to *D,* Rupture of urethra superior to urogenital diaphragm in male.

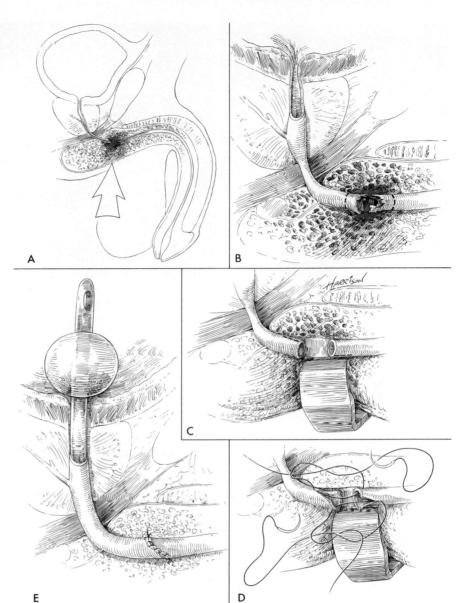

Figure 69–24. Technique of primary urethral repair with end-to-end anastomosis of rupture of the anterior urethra. *A*, Appearance of injury. *B*, Urethral ends excised transversely to viable bleeding tissue. *C*, Urethral ends spatulated 1 to 2 cm. *D* and *E*, Interrupted suture line with Silastic catheter in place.

debridement to preserve any viable tissue, including the testis on each side. Proximal diversion, cystostomy, and colostomy for associated urethral and rectal injuries are common. Proctoscopy is mandatory in bullet wounds of the suprapubic area and perineum, whether or not the missile can be seen on plain radiography. The hope is to accomplish at least a decent perineal urethrostomy on completion of the initial repair, which can be handled subsequently as a posterior or anterior staged urethroplasty. Vascularized musculocutaneous flaps may be transferred to the perineum to compensate for large tissue defects.

INJURIES TO THE PENIS

Buck's fascia tightly surrounds the erectile bodies, including the corpora spongiosum of the urethra. Injuries to the erectile bodies may result in extravasation of blood, corresponding to the extent of Buck's fascia. Such lesions may occur from a penetrating wound, such as a bullet wound or a stab wound, or may result from rupture of the corpora by blunt trauma, such as occurs from sexual intercourse when the corpus is impacted against the pubic bone of the partner (see Fig. 69–20). Ruptures through Buck's fascia result in a distribution of extravasation of blood or urine corresponding to the attachment limits of Colles' fascia. Usually, the defect in the corpus can be palpated and repaired using local or general anesthesia, with inverted knot, nonabsorbable sutures.

Prompt repair tends to minimize deviations from scar formation, which may cause problems, especially during erection, mimicking the deformities of Peyronie's disease. Strangulating lesions of the penis may occur when objects are placed about its circumference for purposes of deviate sexual practices or masturbation. When these cannot be removed by the patient, as was the case with

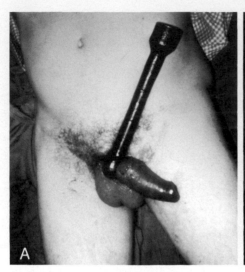

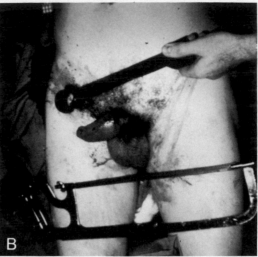

Figure 69–25. Large metal objects used for masturbation may require metal cutting tools and anesthesia for their removal.

the tire tool in Figure 69–25, general anesthesia and metal-cutting tools solve the problem. One may decrease penile edema and allow the offending object to slip off the penis distally by applying liquid soap to the penile skin or by wrapping a string circumferentially around the distal penis, starting at the meatus, to compress the penis and diminish its diameter relative to the offending agent.

Penile Amputations

Penile amputations, either partial or complete, may occur by accident or as a result of a personal attack, either by an assailant or by a self-inflicted wound. An epidemic of penile amputation, reported in the *American Journal of Surgery* in 1983, allowed surgeons in Thailand to treat a large number of penile amputations in a short period of time and to elucidate a number of principles that are important in salvage:

1. The amputated part should be cleansed with sterile saline and placed on ice or in a sterile salt solution surrounded by ice as soon as possible, for the subsequent reimplantation or transportion to a regional center. A tourniquet should be applied to the proximal penile part to arrest hemorrhage.

2. The patient should be transported to a facility where microsurgery is regularly done, if time permits (<8 hours).

3. If microsurgery cannot be done to repair the dorsal penile arteries and dorsal veins or the urethral cavernous artery with 10-0 or 11-0 nonabsorbable suture, a minimum of repair can be accomplished by re-establishing venous continuity with an 8-0 to 10-0 nonabsorbable suture. Approximation of the proximal corpora to the distal part can be carried out. Often, the distal member will survive if venous drainage can be established (Fig. 69–26).

4. Urethral continuity can be established by a running or an interrupted fine 5-0 or 6-0 chromic catgut or Vicryl suture material. Icing down of the dismembered portion

as soon as possible after injury is the most important factor in subsequent survival of the amputated tissues.

Degloving Injuries of the Penis

In degloving injuries of the penis, as often occurs when the penis and clothing are caught in machinery, such as garden or farming tools, one should remember to debride the distal penile skin and extirpate it to the level of the coronal sulcus, if split-thickness grafting is necessary, and to graft proximally from the coronal

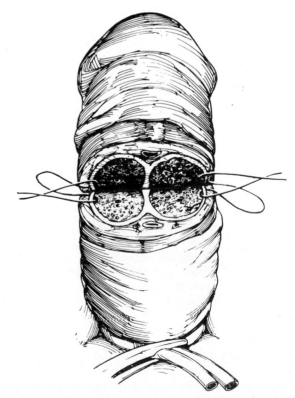

Figure 69–26. Closure of corpora. One should attempt to restore continuity of the dorsal veins. Dorsal penile artery reanastomosis requires microsurgical training and equipment.

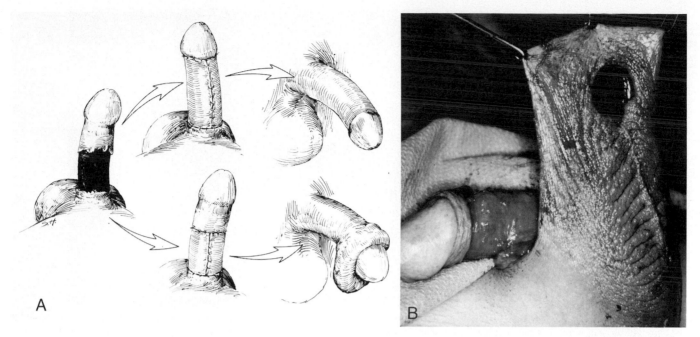

Figure 69–27. *A*, Use of split-thickness skin graft *to the level of coronal sulcus*. *B*, Scrotal flap may be utilized as an immediate pedicle flap in repair of many genital injuries.

sulcus to the intact body skin. One should use split-thickness skin grafts of approximately 0.15-mm thickness to allow for normal expansion of the healed penis during erection. Thin split-thickness grafts less than 0.15 cm to the shaft of the penis sometimes do not permit proper corporal expansion during erection and become a source of discomfort to the patient (Fig. 69–27).

SCROTAL INJURIES

When loss of the scrotum covering the testis occurs (Fig. 69–28), only a few principles need be remembered. First, positioning of the testis and the adjacent superficial thigh is preferable to subcutaneous abdominal placement, as the temperature is about 10° lower in the superficial thigh position and favors spermatogenesis. When only a small amount of scrotum remains, flaps can be mobilized employing perineal skin, as outlined by McDougal (1983), to cover the testis (Fig. 69–29). In patients suffering multiple injuries, particularly with fear of wound contamination or anticipated need for repeated debridement the testis may be left in place and treated with daily applications of warm saline or .25 per cent acetic acid soaks, until scrotal granulations are adequate to permit the application of a skin mesh or thickness graft. Orchiectomy is usually not needed in such cases.

When a laceration through the tunica albuginea of the testis occurs and contamination of the testis parenchyma is obvious, as by a penetrating close-range gunshot wound or a violent external injury, the testis parenchyma should be treated with meticulous debridement of foreign materials (dirt, shotgun pellets, shotgun wadding, clothing) and with thorough irrigation of the affected area with tepid saline. Then, primary closure

of the tunica albuginea with fine running chromic catgut suture is accomplished.

Scrotal drains may be placed, but they should not be placed beneath the tunica albuginea of the testis, as they will merely provide an exit for the tubules (Fig. 69–30). Broad-spectrum antibiotic coverage is indicated. Orchiectomy is rarely needed. The possibility of reimplantation of the amputated testis and cord must be

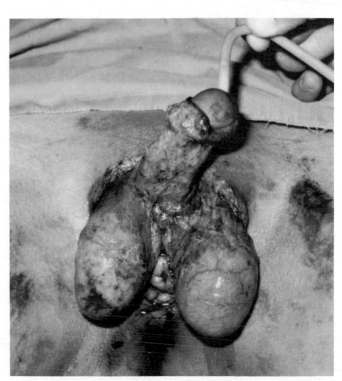

Figure 69–28. Degloving injury with complete loss of scrotum.

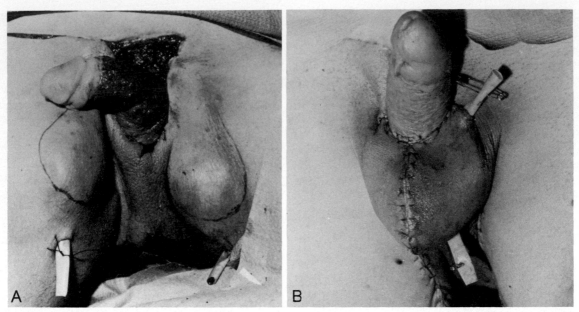

Figure 69–29. *A*, Penis and perineum are covered with split-thickness skin. Scrotal reconstruction is begun 4 to 6 weeks after thigh implantation of testes. All wounds should be healed before this stage is undertaken. Proposed flaps are outlined. *B*, Closure of thigh defects and drainage of reconstructed scrotum complete procedure. (From McDougal, W. S.: J. Urol., 129:757, 1983. © By Williams & Wilkins, 1983.)

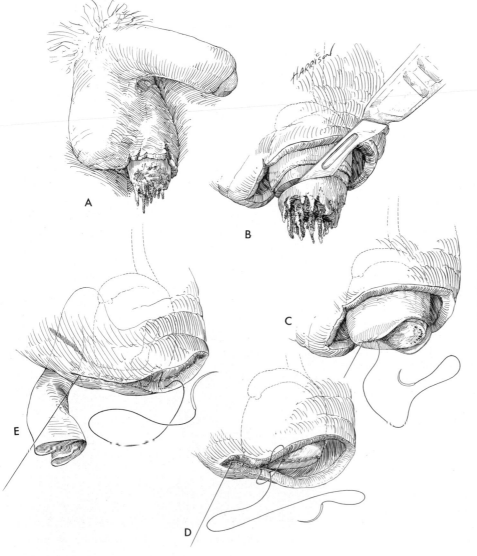

Figure 69–30. Technique of closure of traumatic scrotal and testicular defect. *A*, Appearance of injury. *B*, Sharp debridement of seminiferous tubules. *C*, Closure of tunica albuginea. *D*, Closure of dartos layer—important in prevention of scrotal hematoma. *E*, Skin closure, with drain in tunica vaginalis.

considered in cases seen within 8 hours of injury. Microvascular techniques exist today for successful revascularization, although most have been done as elective procedures.

TRAUMA IN PREGNANCY

In general, the health of the mother takes precedence over the health of the fetus. In considering penetrating wounds of the abdomen, exploration is indicated when perforation of the peritoneal cavity or the uterus has been determined. Doppler ultrasound may be decided on to monitor the fetus. Ultrasonography is of great value as well to aid in determining the anatomic changes that may be present. The location of the placenta, the status of the fetus, including monitoring of the fetal heartbeats, are possible by ultrasonography and should be the study of choice, particularly in early pregnancy when radiation exposure is to be minimized.

Sakala and Kort (1988) have suggested an algorithm for triage of the patient suffering an abdominal stab wound in pregnancy, including the indications for immediate cesarean section (Fig. 69–31). Measures undertaken in the male trauma victim, thus, may be altered in the pregnant female by a desire to minimize irradiation exposure, particularly in early pregnancy. Fortunately, ultrasound will allow painless assessment of the integrity of the renal parenchyma, the status of the fetus and uterus, as well as suggesting the possibility of displacement of the kidneys by hematoma or extravasation following penetrating injuries.

Renal parenchymal lacerations in the pregnant female should be managed with the health of the mother taking precedence over that of the fetus, as mentioned. Angioinfarction may be considered for branched lesions of the renal artery, which are diagnosed by arteriography, but open surgery is indicated for the majority of penetrating renal injuries and renal artery lacerations. Location of the placenta and evidence of placental injury may be determined by ultrasound, and fetal survey may be done as well.

Conservative management is most commonly indicated in patients with no history of gross hematuria or microhematuria and shock. Upper abdominal penetrating trauma is especially serious in the pregnant female, as the gravid uterus has forced most of the bowel into the upper quadrants of the abdomen, making it more vulnerable to injury. In the absence of placental injury, there is only rarely a need for delivery of the fetus. The indication for cesarean section would be a fetus demonstrated to be alive by ultrasonography having a gestational age of 26 to 35 weeks and suffering distress. Usually, no problem occurs in operating on the pregnant woman, even within a few days of term, if there is an injury to the kidney, collecting system, or bladder. Nephrectomy and/or urinary drainage may be performed following the usual indications, as indicated in the nonpregnant female.

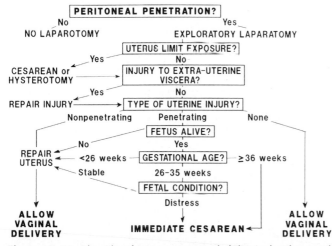

Figure 69–31. Algorithm for management of abdominal stab wounds in pregnancy. (From Sakala, E. P., and Kort, D. D.: Management of stab wounds to the pregnant uterus: a case report and a review of the literature. Obstet. Gynecol. Surv., 43:319, 1988. © By Williams & Wilkins, 1988.)

REFERENCES

Bright, T. C., III, and Peters, P. C.: Ureteral injuries due to external violence: 10 years' experience with 59 cases. J. Trauma, 17:616, 1977.

Carlton, C. E., Jr.: Injuries of the kidney and ureter. In Harrison, J. H., Gittes, R. F., Perlmutter, A. D., Stamey, T. A., and Walsh, P. C. (Eds.) Campbell's Urology, 4th ed. Philadelphia, W. B. Saunders Co., 1978.

Carroll, P. R., and McAninch, J. W.: Staging of renal trauma. Urol. Clin. North Am., 16:193, 1989.

Cass, A. S., Bubrick, M., Luxenberg, M., et al.: Renal trauma found during laparotomy for intra-abdominal injury. J. Trauma, 25:997, 1985.

Cass, A. S., and Luxenberg, M.: Management of renal artery injuries from external trauma. J. Urol., 138:1987.

Cass, A. S., Luxenberg, M., Gleinch, P., et al.: Clinical indications for radiographic evaluation of blunt renal trauma. J. Urol., 136:370, 1987.

Corriere, J. N., Jr., and Sandler, C. N.: Management of the ruptured bladder: 7 years of experience with 111 cases. J. Trauma, 26:830, 1986.

Daly, J. W., and Higgins, K. A.: Injury to the ureter during gynecologic surgical procedures. Surg. Gynecol. Obstet., 167:19, 1988.

Devine, C. J., Jordan, G. H., and Devine, P. C.: Primary realignment of the disrupted prostatomembranous urethra. Urol. Clin. North Am., 16:291, 1989.

Glenn, J. F.: Trauma to the kidney. Trauma, 3:82, 1961.

Hardeman, S., Husmann, D. A., Chinn, H. K. W., et al.: Blunt urinary tract trauma: identifying those patients who require radiological studies. J. Urol., 138:99, 1987.

Husmann, D. A., and Morris, J. S.: Attempted non-operative management of blunt renal lacerations extending through the corticomedullary junction: the short-term and long-term sequelae. J. Urol., 143:682, 1990.

Kennedy, T. J., McConnell, J. D., and Thal, E. R.: Urine dipstick vs. microscopic urinalysis in the evaluation of abdominal trauma. J. Trauma, 28:615, 1988.

McAninch, J. W., and Carroll, P. R.: Renal exploration after trauma—indications and reconstructive techniques. Urol. Clin. North Am., 16:203, 1989.

McDougal, W. S.: Scrotal reconstruction using thigh pedicle flaps. J. Urol., 129:757, 1983.

McRoberts, J. W., and Rajde, H.: Severed canine posterior urethra: a study of two distinct methods of repair. J. Urol., 104:724, 1970.

Mee, S. L., and McAninch, J. W.: Indications for radiographic assessment in suspected renal trauma. Urol. Clin. North Am., 16:187, 1989.

Morehouse, D.: Personal communication, 1990.

Peters, P. C.: Editorial comment. J. Urol., 144:838, 1990.

Peters, P. C., and Sagalowsky, A. I.: Genitourinary trauma. *In* Walsh, P. E., Gittes, R. F., Perlmutter, A. D., and Stamey, T. A. (Eds.): Campbell's Urology, 5th ed. Philadelphia, W. B. Saunders Co., 1986, pp. 1192–1246.

Sakala, E. P., and Kort, D. D.: Management of stab wounds to the pregnant uterus: a case report and a review of the literature. Obst. Gynecol. Surv., 43:319, 1988.

Skinner, E. C., Boyd, S. D., and Apuzzo, M. L. J.: Technique of left adrenalectomy for autotransplantation to the caudate nucleus in Parkinson's disease. J. Urol., 144:838, 1990.

Spirnak, J. P., Hampel, N., and Resnick, M. I.: Ureteral injuries complicating vascular surgery: Is repair indicated? J. Urol., 141:13, 1989.

Turner-Warwick, R. T.: Prevention of complications resulting from pelvic fracture urethral injuries and from their surgical management. Urol. Clin. North Am., 16:335, 1989.

Vermooten, V.: Rupture of the urethra: a new diagnostic sign. J. Urol., 56:228, 1946.

70

USE OF INTESTINAL SEGMENTS IN THE URINARY TRACT: BASIC PRINCIPLES

W. Scott McDougal, M.D.

Bowel is frequently used in reconstructive urologic surgery for ureteral substitutes, bladder augmentations, and bladder replacements. Less commonly, it may be employed as a urethral or vaginal substitute. The stomach, jejunum, ileum, and colon have all been utilized in these various procedures. The appropriate use of these intestinal segments requires a thorough knowledge of their surgical anatomy, methods of preparing the intestine for an operative event, techniques of isolating segments of the intestine and reconstituting continuity of the enteric tract, problems and techniques of anastomosing the urinary tract to the intestine, and complications that may occur. With this knowledge, reconstruction of the urinary tract may be performed with the proper segment of intestine in the least morbid way.

This chapter reviews the technical aspects involved in the use of intestine in urologic surgery that are germane to all types of reconstructive procedures; the difficulties and complications encountered, and the problems that may arise, both acutely and chronically, following their placement in the urinary tract.

SURGICAL ANATOMY

The segments of bowel with which urologists frequently deal include the ileum, the colon, and the rectum. Less commonly, the jejunum and stomach may be utilized for reconstructive procedures. As mentioned, a thorough knowledge of the surgical anatomy of these structures is necessary in order to properly mobilize and fashion them according to the requirements of the often complex reconstructive procedures being performed.

Stomach

The stomach is a very vascular organ that receives its blood supply primarily from the celiac axis (Fig. 70–1). Three branches of the celiac axis give rise to the majority of the arterial supply of the stomach: (1) the left gastric (coronary) artery arises directly from the celiac axis and supplies the lesser curvature; (2) the hepatic artery after arising from the celiac axis gives off the right gastric artery, which also supplies the lesser curve of the stomach and the gastroduodenal artery, which supplies the antrum and duodenum before giving off the right gastroepiploic artery; (3) the splenic artery arises from the celiac axis giving off the vasa brevia, which supply the fundus and cardia, and the left gastroepiploic artery.

The right gastroepiploic artery anastomoses with the left gastroepiploic artery and both supply the greater curve of the stomach. Utilizing the gastroepiploic vessels, a pedicle of stomach may be mobilized to the pelvis. The pedicle may consist of the entire antrum/pylorus or a wedge of the fundus. The blood supply for these segments is based either on the left or right gastroepiploic artery, depending on the portion of stomach. Occasionally, the left gastroepiploic artery will be atretic at some point in its course and will not provide an adequate blood supply. Under these circumstances, the right gastroepiploic artery must be employed. When a wedge of fundus is used, it should not include a significant portion of the antrum and should never extend to the pylorus or all the way to the lesser curve of the stomach. When based on the left gastroepiploic artery, the short gastric vessels that course from the gastroepiploic artery to the stomach are ligated along the greater curve, proximal to the pedicle to the origin of the gastroepiploic artery.

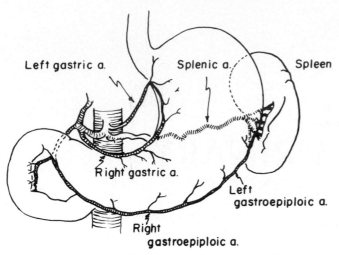

Figure 70–1. The arterial supply of the stomach.

jejunum or ileum, the mesentery should be transected in such a way that the isolated intestinal segment receives its blood supply from an arcade supplied by a palpable artery of substance, which courses through the base of the mesenteric pedicle.

Two portions of the small bowel may lie within the confines of the pelvis and as such may be exposed to pelvic irradiation and/or pelvic disease. These two portions are (1) the last 2 inches of the terminal ileum and (2) the 5 feet of small bowel beginning approximately 6 feet from the ligament of Treitz. The former is often fixed in the pelvis by ligamentous attachments. The mesentery of the latter is the longest of the entire small bowel and as such this portion of the small bowel can descend into the pelvis. In a patient who has undergone radiation therapy, one should try to avoid using these two segments of the small intestine in any reconstructive procedure.

The omentum is left attached to the gastroepiploic vessels and helps secure and support them. It may be necessary for proper pedicle mobility to detach the omentum from the colon along the avascular plane located at the point of its attachment to the transverse colon. If an antrectomy is performed, a Billroth I anastomosis reconstitutes gastrointestinal continuity. The stomach has a thick seromuscular layer that can be simply separated from the mucosa should a submucosal ureteral reimplantation be necessary.

Small Bowel

The small bowel is about 22 feet long; however, it may vary from 15 to 30 feet. Its largest diameter is in the duodenum, and the lumen becomes smaller in the more distal portions, reaching its smallest diameter in the ileum approximately 12 inches from the ileocecal valve. About two fifths of the small bowel is jejunum, whereas the distal three fifths is ileum. No definite demarcation occurs between the two; however, each possesses several unique properties that allow distinction of one from the other intraoperatively. The ileum being more distal in location has a smaller diameter. It has multiple arterial arcades, and the vessels in the arcades are smaller than those in the jejunum. The ileal mesentery is also thicker than the jejunal mesentery. In contrast, the jejunal diameter is larger, and the arterial arcades are usually single. The vessels composing them are larger in diameter.

The arcades anastomose one with another and give off straight vessels, which enter the bowel and form an anastomotic network within the bowel wall. It has been shown experimentally that up to 15 cm of small bowel can survive lateral to a straight vessel. Thus, theoretically, the mesentery could be cleaned from the small bowel for a length of 15 cm without necrosis of the end. Generally, however, it is unwise to assume that more than 8 cm of small bowel will survive away from a straight vessel. The arcades receive their blood from the superior mesenteric artery. When isolating segments of

Colon

The large bowel is divided into the cecum, ascending colon, transverse colon, left colon, sigmoid colon, and rectum. Portions of the large bowel are fixed and/or retroperitoneal and other segments lie free within the peritoneal cavity. The cecum, on rare occasion, may lie free within the abdominal cavity and therefore has great mobility. Generally, however, it is fixed in the right lower quadrant.

Two accessory peritoneal bands bind the cecum and distal ileum to the retroperitoneum and lateral abdominal wall. One band arises from the distal ileum, attaches to the cecum, and is fixed to the retroperitoneum. A second band arises from the cecum and fixes the cecum to the posterior abdominal wall laterally. The remainder of the ascending colon is fixed to the right posterior abdominal wall to the level of the hepatic flexure, at which point the hepatocolic ligament secures this portion of the colon to the liver. The transverse colon lies free within the abdominal cavity and is fixed in the left upper quadrant at the splenic flexure by the phrenicocolic ligament.

The transverse colon is attached to the stomach by the gastrocolic omentum. The descending colon is fixed to the lateral abdominal wall; however, the sigmoid colon may or may not lie free within the abdominal cavity. The rectosigmoid colon's most cephalad portion is intraperitoneal and as its more distal caudad portions are approached, it becomes retroperitoneal and, finally, subperitoneal. The colon receives its blood supply from the superior mesenteric artery, the inferior mesenteric artery, and the internal iliac arteries (Fig. 70–2).

The major arteries supplying the colon and rectum include the ileocolic, right colic, middle colic, left colic, sigmoid, superior hemorrhoidal, middle hemorrhoidal, and inferior hemorrhoidal arteries. These arteries anastomose one with the other to form the arc of Drummond and allow for considerable leeway in mobilizing the colon. The middle colic artery arises from the first portion of the superior mesenteric artery and generally ascends the transverse mesocolon to the right of midline.

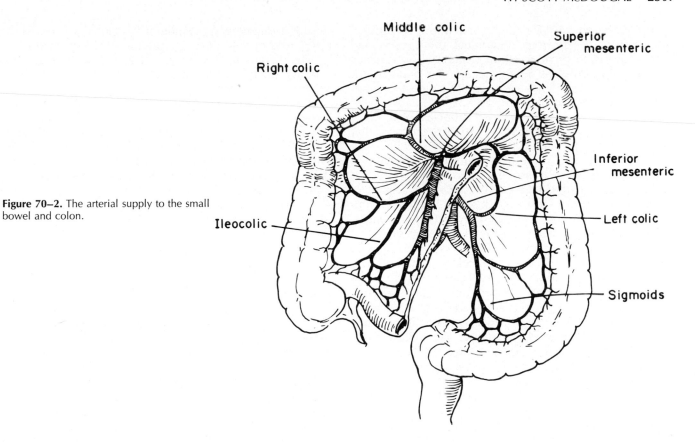

Figure 70–2. The arterial supply to the small bowel and colon.

The right colic artery usually arises just below the middle colic artery from the superior mesenteric artery and courses to the right colon. However, it may arise from the ileocolic or directly from the middle colic artery. If it arises from the ileocolic artery, mobilization of the distal ascending colon is facilitated so that this portion of the colon can be brought into the deep pelvis without difficulty. On occasion, however, it is necessary to sever the right colic artery at its origin in order to mobilize the distal portion of the ascending colon to the pelvis. This is particularly true if the right colic artery originates from the middle colic artery.

The ileocolic artery is the terminal portion of the superior mesenteric artery and supplies the last 6 inches of ileum and ascending colon. The left colic artery arises from the interior mesenteric artery. The inferior mesenteric artery gives off four to six sigmoid branches, the last of which becomes the superior hemorrhoidal artery. This anastomoses with the middle hemorrhoidal artery, a branch of the internal iliac artery which in turn anastomoses with the inferior hemorrhoidal artery, i.e., the terminal branch of the internal pudendal artery. The middle sacral artery, which originates directly from the aorta, may supply the posterior aspect of the rectum.

Three weak points involving the vascular supply to the colon have been described. Sudeck's critical point, which is located between the junction of the sigmoid and superior hemorrhoidal arteries, was thought to be a particularly tenuous anastomotic area such that if the colon were transected in this region, the anastomosis would heal with difficulty because the blood supply might be compromised. Similarly, the mid points be-

tween the middle colic and right colic arteries and between the middle colic and left colic arteries also have somewhat tenuous anastomotic communications. Although anastomoses in these areas generally heal very well provided the principles of proper technique are adhered to, it is usually wise to choose an area for the anastomosis to one side of these points.

The ascending colon is mobilized first by transecting the cecal and distal ileal fibrous attachments to the lateral abdominal wall and retroperitoneum just described and then detaching it from the lateral abdominal wall along the avascular line of Toldt. This is a bloodless plane provided the colonic mesentery is not violated. The transverse colon is mobilized by detaching the gastrocolic omentum along the avascular plane of its attachment to the colon; the hepatocolic ligament, which may have some small vessels coursing through it; and the phrenicocolic ligament. The descending colon is mobilized much as the right colon by incising the avascular line of Toldt lateral to the colon. When these attachments are taken down, considerable mobility of the colon is achieved. Further mobility is gained by isolating a pedicle of intestine, which should be based on one of the major arterial vessels previously described.

SELECTING THE SEGMENT OF INTESTINE

The stomach, jejunum, ileum, and colon have unique properties that give each special advantages and disadvantages. The selection of the proper intestinal segment should be based on the patient's condition, renal function, history of previous abdominal procedures, and type of diversion or substitution required. The stomach has been employed as a replacement for bladder, for augmentation cystoplasty, as a conduit, and for continent diversions (Adams et al., 1988; Bihrle et al., 1989; Leong, 1978). The advantage of stomach over other intestinal segments for urinary intestinal diversion is that it is less permeable to urinary solutes, it acidifies the urine, it has a net excretion of chloride rather than a net absorption, and it produces less mucus. Urodynamically, stomach behaves as other intestinal segments.

When used in urinary reconstruction, electrolyte imbalance rarely ensues, although a hypochloremic metabolic alkalosis has been described. The incidence of bacteriuria is 25 per cent, much less than the 60 to 80 per cent reported for ileal and colon segments. The acidic urine which usually has a pH of 5 to 7 does not result in a greater incidence of peristomal skin problems.

Generally, serum gastrin levels are normal or minimally elevated, depending on what portion of stomach and how much are used (Adams et al., 1988; Leong, 1978). Although excluding the antrum from the gastrointestinal tract has not resulted in elevated serum gastrin levels or an ulcer diathesis clinically (Lim et al., 1983), experimentally, antral exclusion results in elevated gastrin levels and causes major intestinal ulcerative problems in the postoperative period (Tiffany et al., 1986).

No severe ulcerative complications have been reported thus far in the small series that have employed stomach for urinary reconstruction. When the antral portion of stomach is employed, reconstitution is generally by a Billroth I anastomosis. Complications with Billroth I gastroduodenostomy are well documented. Early complications include gastric retention due to atony of the stomach or edema of the anastomosis, hemorrhage most commonly originating from the anastomotic site, hiccups secondary to gastric distention, and pancreatitis due to intraoperative injury and duodenal leakage.

Delayed complications include dumping syndrome, steatorrhea, small stomach syndrome, increased intestinal transit time, bilious vomiting, afferent loop syndrome, hypoproteinemia, and megaloblastic and/or iron deficiency anemia. Postoperative bowel obstruction occurs with an incidence of 10 per cent (2/21) (Leong, 1978). Gastrourethral and gastroureteral leaks have also been reported, occasionally resulting in a fatal outcome (Leong, 1978).

Stomach for urinary intestinal diversion may be considered when other segments in a patient with a decreased amount of intestine will result in serious nutritional problems and when extensive renal dysfunction is present. One advantage of stomach in the patient with severe abdominal adhesions is that, generally, the area of the stomach is adhesion-free and simply mobilized.

The jejunum is usually not employed for reconstruction of the urinary system because this often results in severe electrolyte imbalance. Generally, diseases that would make the ileum inappropriate to use would also make the jejunum inappropriate to use. Rarely, it is the only segment available. Under these circumstances, as

distal a segment of jejunum as possible should be employed to minimize electrolyte-related problems.

The ileum and colon are selected most often for urinary tract reconstruction and have been used in all types of reconstructive procedures. The ileum is mobile, has a small diameter and a constant blood supply, and serves well for ureteral replacement and formation of conduits. Loss of significant portions of the ileum results in nutritional problems caused by lack of vitamin B_{12} absorption, diarrhea due to lack of bile salt reabsorption, and fat malabsorption. On occasion, the mesenteric fat is excessive making mobility and anastomoses difficult. Also, the mesentery may be so short that it is difficult to mobilize the ileum into the deep pelvis. Postoperative bowel obstruction occurs in about 10 per cent of patients who have segments isolated from the ileum for urinary tract reconstruction. One half of the obstructions occur in the early postoperative period (Jaffe et al., 1968).

The colon requires mobilization from its fixed positions for urinary reconstruction. The colon has a larger diameter than the ileum and is usually mobilized without difficulty into any portion of the abdomen or pelvis. In patients who have received pelvic irradiation, portions of the right, transverse, and descending colon may be utilized confidently, with the knowledge that they have not been exposed to radiation. Removing segments of colon from the enteric tract results in fewer nutritional problems than removing segments of ileum, provided the ileocecal valve is not violated. Alternatively, should the ileocecal valve be utilized, diarrhea, excessive bacterial colonization of the ileum with malabsorption, and fluid and bicarbonate loss may occur. The incidence of postoperative bowel obstruction is 4 per cent—less than that with ileum.

Both ileal and colon segments result in the same type of electrolyte imbalance with similar frequency. An antireflux ureterointestinal anastomosis by the submucosal tunnel technique is less difficult to perform with colon. In general, ileum and colon are comparable and have few differences, which would strongly argue for the selection for one over the other except under very special circumstances.

Bowel Preparation

Urologic operations in which the bowel is utilized for genitourinary reconstruction are usually elective and as such bowel preparation is appropriate. Although the bacterial population in the stomach is relatively low, the remainder of the bowel including jejunum and ileum have high bacterial population counts and therefore require mechanical and antibiotic preparation. The need for appropriate bowel preparation is evident from studies that compare bowel anastomoses in unprepared bowel with prepared. Patients who have intestinal procedures on unprepared bowels have an increased wound infection rate, incidence of intraperitoneal abscess, and anastomotic dehiscence rate when compared with patients who have had a proper bowel preparation prior to surgery (Dion et al., 1980; Irvin and Goligher, 1973).

A good mechanical preparation results in collapsed bowel at the time of surgery, which has been shown to reduce the incidence of anastomotic leaks (Christensen and Kronborg, 1981). In experimental animals, it has been shown that an anastomosis that has vascular compromise at the anastomotic line, which would normally result in perforation, heals if the bowel has been properly prepared with antibiotics. Also, solid feces place a strain on the anastomosis in the early phase of healing and result in ischemia with subsequent perforation.

Complications that occur as a result of bacterial contamination are a major cause of morbidity and mortality in patients undergoing urologic procedures. Infectious complications following radical cystectomy that are a direct result of fecal contamination occur in 18 to 20 per cent of patients who undergo cystectomies and include wound infections, peritonitis, intra-abdominal abscesses, wound dehiscence, anastomotic dehiscence, and systemic sepsis (Bracken et al., 1981).

There are two aspects of bowel preparation: mechanical and antibiotic. Both methods attempt to reduce the complication rate from intestinal surgery. The mechanical preparation reduces the amount of feces, whereas the antibiotic preparation reduces the bacterial count. The bacterial flora in the bowel consist of aerobic organisms, the most common of which are *Escherichia coli* and *Streptococcus faecalis*, and anaerobic organisms, the most common of which are *Bacteroides sp.* and *Clostridium sp.* The bacterial concentration in the jejunum ranges from 10^0 to 10^5, in the distal ileum from 10^5 to 10^7, in the ascending colon from 10^6 to 10^8, and in the descending colon from 10^{10} to 10^{12} organisms per gram of fecal content.

MECHANICAL BOWEL PREPARATION. A mechanical bowel preparation reduces the total number of bacteria but not their concentration. Thus, the same number of organisms are present per gram of fecal content (Nichols et al., 1972). Therefore, the spilling of enteric contents during the procedure is less likely to occur with the mechanically prepared bowel because there is less of it to spill; however, once spilled, milliliter for milliliter, the inoculum is the same as if the bowel had not been prepared.

Conventional bowel preparations may exhaust the patient and exacerbate nutritional depletion because they generally require a 3-day preparation period of suboptimal calorie intake (Table 70–1). Elemental diets have been advocated to clean the colon of feces while not compromising the nutritional status of the patient. Unfortunately, they have not proven useful because elemental diets do not empty the colon of feces or reduce the bacterial flora (Arabi et al., 1978).

In an attempt to reduce the time required for intestinal preparation, to obviate low calorie intakes, and to contain cost by reducing hospitalization prior to surgery, whole-gut irrigation has gained popularity. Originally, whole-gut irrigation was performed by placing a nasogastric tube into the stomach and infusing 9 to 12 L of lactated Ringer's solution or normal saline over a several hour period. These fluids were subsequently replaced with 10 per cent mannitol, which was equally successful in ridding the bowel of its fecal content; however, the mannitol served as a bacterial nutrient and thereby facilitated microbial growth (Hares and Alexander-Williams, 1982).

These solutions have largely been replaced by a polyethylene glycol electrolyte solution. Whole-gut irrigation may be exhausting to the patient and may in fact result in a fluid gain, particularly when either saline or mannitol is utilized. It is contraindicated in patients with unstable cardiovascular systems and patients with cirrhosis, severe renal disease, congestive failure, or obstructed bowel. Whole-gut irrigation has been found to be no more effective in reducing wound infections and septic complications than conventional preparations (Christensen and Kronborg, 1981), even though a reduction of aerobic flora is noted when compared with the conventional preparation (van den Bogaard et al., 1981).

The advantages of the whole-gut irrigation are dietary freedom, short preparation time, and elimination of the enema. Its disadvantages are that it may result in exhaustion, is rather rigorous, and does result on occasion in fluid overload.

A polyethylene glycol electrolyte lavage solution (GoLYTELY) has shown considerable promise as an effective lavage agent in preparing the gut for both elective colon and rectal surgery as well as urologic surgery in which bowel is utilized. For the adult, 20 to 30 ml per minute or approximately 1 L per hour for 5

Table 70–1. MECHANICAL BOWEL PREPARATION

Preoperative Day	Conventional			Whole Gut Irrigation (Polyethylene Glycol Electrolyte Solution)	
	Diet	Cathartic	Enema	Diet	Irrigation
3	Low residue plus supplements	250 ml citrate of magnesia at 6 P.M.		Regular plus supplements	
2	Clear liquids	250 ml citrate of magnesia at 10 A.M. and 6 P.M.	SSE*	Low residue plus supplements	
1	Clear liquids	250 ml citrate of magnesia at 10 A.M. and 2 P.M.	SSE until clear	Clear liquids	20 to 30 ml/min (adults) or 25 mg/kg/hour (children) × 5 hours or until rectal effluent clear (not to exceed 10 L in adults)

*SSE, soap suds enema.

hours is given either orally or through a small caliber nasogastric tube placed into the stomach. If taken by mouth, it is better tolerated if the solution is chilled. The administration of GoLYTELY is stopped when the rectal effluent is clear and there is no particulate matter in it or when 10 L of fluid have been given.

This preparation, in the adult, has been as effective as conventional ones. The septic complications with its use are approximately 4 per cent. An inadequate preparation occurs in 5 per cent of the patients (Wolff et al., 1988). For children, even those under the age of 1 year, GoLYTELY may be given at a rate of 25 ml/kg/hour and given until the rectal effluent is clear and free of particulate matter (Tuggle et al., 1987). Metoclopramide (Reglan), 10 mg, is often given simultaneously to control nausea.

ANTIBIOTIC BOWEL PREPARATION. Considerable controversy existed as to whether the addition of antibiotics in elective colon and small bowel surgery reduced mortality and morbidity significantly. The wealth of evidence, however, would suggest that an antimicrobial bowel preparation is advantageous in reducing postoperative complications.

In one study, the septic complication rate was reduced from 68 per cent in the control group to 8 per cent in the group given antibiotics (Washington et al., 1974). Most series, however, report a lesser incidence of reduction in wound infection, generally from 35 per cent without antibiotics to 9 per cent with them (Clarke et al., 1977). Others have suggested that the mortality rate drops from 9 to 3 per cent with the administration of antibiotics (Baum et al., 1981). Antibiotics protect vulnerable bowel—they may allow the tenuous anastomosis to survive. Other studies, however, have shown that without antibiotics in mechanically prepared bowel in elective surgery, the septic complication rate is 6 per cent—comparable to studies utilizing antibiotics (Menaker et al., 1981). In the presence of a bowel obstruction, however, oral antibiotics are of little value because they do little good in sterilizing the bowel.

The disadvantages of antibiotics include a postoperative increase in the incidence of diarrhea and pseudomembranous enterocolitis and a theoretical increase in the incidence of tumor implantation at the suture line, which is not germane to urologic surgery; monilial overgrowth resulting in stomatitis, thrush, and diarrhea; and, when prolonged, malabsorption of protein, carbohydrate, and fat. The antibiotics that are most commonly provided for bowel preparation include kanamycin, which is the best single agent, neomycin and erythromycin base, and neomycin and metronidazole (Table 70–2). With an appropriate antibiotic preparation, enteric organisms are reduced to 10^2 organisms per gram feces (Nichols et al., 1972).

Perioperative intravenous antibiotic administration is exceedingly controversial. Systemic antibiotics must be given before the procedure, if they are to be effective. They appear to be most effective against the anaerobic flora and apparently reduce the complications caused by these organisms (Dion et al., 1980). Perioperative systemic antibiotics, when added to the oral regimen, reduced the septic complication rate of 15 to 20 per cent to half that in several series (Gottrup et al., 1985; Hares and Alexander-Williams, 1982). Other studies, however, have shown no effect of systemic cephalosporin, for example, in reducing septic complications (Wolff et al., 1988). If perioperative antibiotics are given, they should be effective against anaerobes as it is complications from these organisms against which perioperative antibiotics appear to be particularly effective.

DIARRHEA AND PSEUDOMEMBRANOUS ENTEROCOLITIS. Antibiotic bowel preparations may result in diarrhea and pseudomembranous enterocolitis. Clinically, this problem occurs following a bowel preparation in the postoperative period and is heralded by abdominal pain and diarrhea, usually in the absence of fever or chills. As the symptoms and infection become more severe, systemic toxicity supervenes. The patient can develop a toxic megacolon, and if this occurs mortality may exceed 15 to 20 per cent.

Historically, pseudomembranous enterocolitis was thought to be due to *Staphylococcus*, but there was in fact little evidence to support this organism as the etiologic agent. *Clostridium difficile* plays a significant role in the majority of cases. *C. difficile* elaborates at least two toxins that cause diarrhea and enterocolitis. *C. difficile* does not invade the bowel nor is it normally a significant inhabitant of the fecal flora. Its growth is inhibited by other bacteria. Thus, antibiotics, when given, destroy the bacteria that inhibit the growth of *C. difficile* and thereby allow it to flourish. The toxin produces a diffuse inflammatory response with cream-colored plaque formation, erythema, and edema of the bowel wall. Microscopically, the villi appear to be intact and there is a polymorphonuclear leukocyte infiltrate of the submucosa.

As the disease progresses, large areas of mucosa may slough and areas of the bowel are thereby denuded. The lesions may involve the colon, in which case it is called pseudomembranous colitis, or the small bowel, in which case it is called pseudomembranous enteritis, or they may involve both, pseudomembranous enterocolitis.

Table 70–2. ANTIBIOTIC BOWEL PREPARATION

Preoperative Day	Kanamycin	Neomycin plus Erythromycin Base	Neomycin plus Metronidazole
3	1 g kanamycin p.o. q 1 hr × 4, then q.i.d.	—	—
2	1 g kanamycin p.o. q.i.d.	—	1 g neomycin q.i.d. plus 750 mg metronidazole q.i.d.
1	1 g kanamycin p.o. q.i.d.	1 g erythromycin base plus 1 g neomycin at 1 P.M., 2 P.M., 11 P.M.	1 g neomycin q.i.d. plus 750 mg metronidazole q.i.d.

q, each, every; p.o., orally; q.i.d., four times a day.

The diagnosis is suspected by the symptomatology and endoscopy and is confirmed by the culture of the organism or identification of its toxin. Since culture takes a prolonged period of time, it is more expeditious and therefore clinically useful to confirm the diagnosis by identifying the toxin produced by *C. difficile* through tissue culture techniques. Once diagnosed, the treatment involves the administration of vancomycin and the discontinuance of the other antibiotics, which the patient is receiving. Vancomycin is very effective in most cases. Rarely, toxic megacolon supervenes that requires subtotal colectomy as a life-saving procedure (Chang, 1985).

INTESTINAL ANASTOMOSES

Irrespective of the type of anastomosis or the methods utilized to perform it, certain fundamental principles must be observed in order to minimize morbidity and mortality from intestinal surgery. In urologic procedures in which gut is utilized, the most common cause of mortality and morbidity within the immediate postoperative period is related to complications involving the bowel: either with the enteroenterostomy or with the segment interposed in the urinary tract. Therefore, great care must be taken and proper techniques employed in handling bowel in urologic procedures. Unfortunately, the portion of the procedure that involves mobilization of the intestine and reanastomosis often follows a rather lengthy urologic endeavor and is performed at a time when the surgical team is not fresh. Therefore, the following principles should be so firmly ingrained in the surgeon that they are performed without the need to specifically recall each one.

The first principle of proper technique for intestinal anastomoses is adequate exposure. The intestine should be mobilized sufficiently so that the anastomosis may be performed without struggling for exposure. If possible, it is preferable to mobilize the intestine sufficiently so that the anastomosis can be performed on the anterior abdominal wall. The area of the anastomosis should be walled off from the rest of the abdominal cavity with Mikulicz pads. This maneuver is important so that any inadvertent enteric spills will not be distributed throughout the abdominal cavity. The mesentery must be cleaned from the bowel segments to be anastomosed for a suitable distance (usually 0.5 cm) from the intestinal clamps at the severed ends, so that good serosal apposition may be achieved without interposed mesentery. Sufficient serosa must be exposed so that the seromuscular sutures can be placed directly in the serosa without traversing the mesentery.

The second principle of performing a proper anastomosis is to maintain a good blood supply to the severed ends of the bowel. The blood supply may be compromised by creating anastomosis under tension, excessive dissection or mobilization of the bowel, excessive use of the electrocautery, and tying the sutures so tight that the intervening tissue is strangulated. A cut margin of bowel that is pink and bleeds freely suggests that the blood supply has not been compromised; however, hemostasis must be assured before beginning the anastomosis. The site of transection is selected at a point where the blood supply is adequate to both segments. The mesentery should be transilluminated so that the blood supply may be defined prior to transection of the bowel segment. In urologic surgery, the location of the transection is elective so that an area may be selected in which excellent arcades supply both sections of the transected segment. The area must be selected with an eye to how deep the mesenteric transection must be for proper segment mobility. After locating the appropriate area where the mesentery is to be transected, it is cleaned from the serosa, severed between mosquito clamps, and tied with 4–0 silk sutures.

The third principle involves preventing local spillage of enteric contents. The best way of preventing spills is to operate on properly prepared bowel, i.e., devoid of feces and collapsed. By stripping the enteric contents between the fingers both cephalad and caudad from the proposed transection site and by applying a noncrushing occlusive clamp across the bowel, a spill is made even less likely. This clamp should prevent the enteric contents from exiting the cut ends of the bowel without interference with the mesenteric blood supply. After applying linen shod clamps and walling off the area, Allen clamps are applied to the bowel. The bowel is transected between the Allen clamps. An anastomotic staple device may be utilized to transect the bowel at this point in place of Allen clamps (see following discussion). Local spills and local sepsis have an adverse effect on the healing anastomosis. For this reason, noncrushing occlusion clamps, in addition to an adequate bowel preparation, are advisable. If a spill does occur, it should be caught in the Mikulicz pads if the bowel has been properly walled off as described. The isolated segment that is to be used in the reconstructive procedure should be irrigated through and through with a solution containing 2 ampules of neomycin sulfate—polymyxin B sulfate solution (GU Irrigant) in 1 L of normal saline. The segment should be walled off. The irrigant is placed in one end of the segment and caught in a kidney basin, as it exits the other end. This procedure should be continued until the efflux is clear. This will prevent local spills during the ureterointestinal anastomosis and other aspects of reconstruction.

The fourth principle, germane to all intestinal anastomoses, is that there should be an accurate apposition of serosa to serosa of the two segments of bowel to be anastomosed. The anastomosis should be watertight and performed without tension. The bowel must be handled gently with noncrushing forceps. The anastomotic line should be inverted and not everted. Considerable controversy exists with regard to this issue in that an everted anastomosis has been shown to heal with few complications. When marginal conditions occur, an inverted anastomosis is more likely to remain intact than is an everted anastomosis.

The fifth principle is not to tie the sutures so tight that the tissue is strangulated. Obviously, the sutures must bring the serosa of the two segments firmly together. Nonabsorbable sutures utilized for the anastomosis result in a stronger anastomotic line in the early healing phase when compared with reabsorbable sutures. The difference is minimal and probably not particularly significant.

The final principle involves realignment of the mesentery of the two segments of bowel to be joined. These should be parallel to each other and will assure no twist upon completion of the anastomosis.

Those factors that significantly contribute to anastomotic breakdown include a poor blood supply, local sepsis induced by fecal spillage, drains placed on an intra-abdominal anastomosis, and anastomosis performed in radiated bowel. Poor blood supply and local sepsis cause ischemia. Drains placed on the anastomosis increase the likelihood of a leak, and an anastomosis performed in irradiated bowel is more likely to result in failure than that performed in nonirradiated bowel. The importance of careful technique and adherence to the aforementioned principles is emphasized by the fact that, in one series of urinary intestinal diversion, 75 per cent of the lethal complications that occurred in the postoperative period were related to the bowel. Of these patients, 80 per cent had received radiation prior to the intestinal surgery (Mansson et al., 1979).

Types of Anastomoses

Intestinal anastomoses may be performed with sutures or staples. Properly performed, both have similar complication rates. In selected circumstances, however, one method may have advantages over the other. In general, sutured anastomoses are preferable for intestinal segments which will be exposed to urine, i.e., suturing intestine to renal pelvis or bladder, closing the butt end of a conduit (Costello and Johnson, 1984), and forming an intestinal pouch for urine.

ENTEROENTEROSTOMY BY A TWO-LAYER SUTURE ANASTOMOSIS (Fig. 70–3). A 3–0 silk holding suture is placed on the mesenteric border just beneath the Allen clamps traversing both segments to be anastomosed. A second suture is similarly placed on the antimesenteric border just beneath the Allen clamps. It is important that the mesentery is cleaned sufficiently so that these sutures are placed in the serosa under direct vision. A row of silk sutures is placed 2 mm apart between the two holding sutures. This maneuver is accomplished by rotating the two Allen clamps away from each other, thus opposing the serosal surfaces. Sutures must traverse the muscularis but should not traverse the full thickness of the bowel. After all sutures have been placed, each is tied and the tails of all the sutures cut except those at each end. These are used as holding sutures.

The Allen clamps are removed and hemostasis is achieved, if necessary, with the light application of electrocautery. A 3–0 double-ended chromic intestinal suture is placed in the posterior suture line through all layers and tied to itself. Each end of the suture is then run in a locking fashion away from the midpoint until the mesenteric and antimesenteric borders are approached. As the lateral aspects of the bowel are approached, the suture is converted to a Connell suture (Fig. 70–4), which proceeds onto the anterior bowel wall.

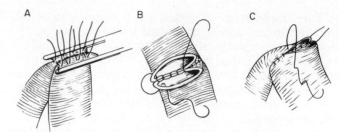

Figure 70–3. Two layer suture anastomosis. *A,* Two holding sutures of 3–0 silk have been placed at the mesenteric and antimesenteric borders, and the posterior wall is approximated with seromuscular sutures of 3–0 silk.

B, A 3–0 intestinal chromic suture is placed through the full thickness of the bowel posteriorly, tied to itself, and run to the lateral borders with a continuous locking suture. At the lateral borders, it is converted to a Connell suture.

C, The Connell suture brings the anterior margins together inverting the suture line. The anastomosis is completed by placing horizontal mattress seromuscular sutures of 3–0 silk over the anterior suture line (not depicted).

The sutures meet anteriorly in the midline and are tied together. The anterior serosa is then opposed with interrupted 3–0 silk sutures. The noncrushing occlusive clamps are removed, and the mesentery is closed with interrupted 3–0 silk sutures. Patency of the anastomosis is assured by palpating the anastomosis with the thumb and forefinger and feeling an annulus of tissue around the fingers. This anastomotic technique is employed when the antrum/pylorus is removed and intestinal continuity is restored by a Billroth I procedure. It is also the most secure of all the anastomoses and should be used when one is forced to do an anastomosis under less than ideal circumstances.

ENTEROENTEROSTOMY BY A SINGLE-LAYER SUTURE ANASTOMOSIS. The mesenteries of the two segments of bowel to be anastomosed are aligned, and a 3–0 silk suture is passed through the seromuscular layers of both segments on the mesenteric side and a second suture is similarly placed on the antimesenteric side. The mesenteric suture is tied, and

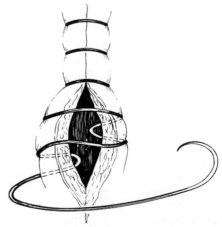

Figure 70–4. Connell suture. The suture traverses the bowel from serosa to mucosa followed by mucosa to serosa on the same side of the anastomosis. The suture is placed on the opposite side of the anastomosis "outside in/inside out." The sequence is repeated until the two segments are approximated.

the antimesenteric suture is left untied. The Allen clamps are removed, and hemostasis is achieved with light electrocautery. The critical point of the anastomosis, where most leaks occur, is at the mesenteric border. This problem generally occurs because the sutures are placed carelessly or the serosa has not been cleaned of mesentery sufficiently so that the sutures are placed through it under direct vision.

Because this mesenteric border is the critical area, it is approached first. Two 3–0 silk sutures are placed through the full thickness of the bowel on either side of the mesenteric holding suture. These sutures are placed in such a way as to include more serosa than mucosa, thus causing inversion of the suture line (Fig. 70–5A). Some prefer to utilize a Gambee stitch at this point, which involves placing the suture through the full thickness of the bowel followed by traversing a small segment of mucosa of each segment of bowel before exiting through the full thickness of the bowel of the other segment (Fig. 70–5B). The two sutures on the mesenteric border are tied, being careful to invert the suture line, thus opposing serosa. Next, 3–0 silk sutures are placed 2 mm apart, both on the anterior and posterior wall, inverting the suture line, thus opposing the serosa of the two bowel segments to each other. Upon approaching the antimesenteric holding suture, several sutures are placed before all are tied. A patent anastomosis is confirmed by feeling the annulus with the thumb and forefinger as previously described.

END-TO-SIDE ILEOCOLIC SUTURED ANASTOMOSIS. The butt end of the colon is closed in the following manner (Fig. 70–6). A 3–0 silk suture is placed beneath the Allen clamp on the mesenteric border and a second suture on the antimesenteric border. These are tied. A 3–0 chromic suture is placed beneath the clamp in a horizontal mattress fashion. Beginning at the mesenteric border, it is tied to itself, the horizontal mattress suture is placed until the antimesenteric border is

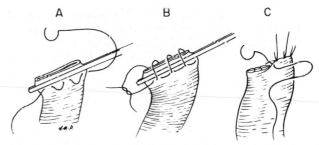

Figure 70–6. Closure of the butt end of intestine. *A*, A 3–0 chromic suture is tied to itself at the antimesenteric border and placed proximal to the intestinal clamp in a horizontal mattress fashion until the mesenteric border is reached. The suture is then tied to itself at this point.

B, The intestinal clamp is removed, and an over-and-over suture through the full thickness of the bowel returns the chromic suture to its point of origin, where it is again tied to itself.

C, Interrupted horizontal mattress seromuscular sutures of 3–0 silk invert the chromic suture line.

reached at which point the suture is again tied to itself. The clamp is removed and an over-and-over suture is performed utilizing the same chromic suture through the full thickness of the bowel, until returning to the point of origin, i.e., the mesenteric border is approached. At this point, the suture is again tied to itself. The suture line is buried by approximating the serosa on each side with interrupted 3–0 silk sutures placed 2 mm apart.

The mesenteries are aligned and the ileal serosa is sutured with interrupted 3–0 silk sutures to the colonic serosa 2 mm below a tinea (Fig. 70–7). The tinea is incised the length of the diameter of the ileum adjacent to it. As previously described, for the two layer anastomosis, a 3–0 double-ended intestinal chromic suture is placed through all layers of the colon and ileum in the midpoint of the posterior wall and run in a locking fashion laterally to either side of the incision in the

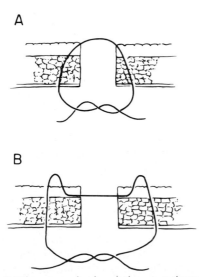

Figure 70–5. *A*, When properly placed, the suture through the intestine should include more serosa than mucosa. *B*, The Gambee stitch. The suture is placed through the full thickness of the bowel following which the mucosa is traversed before the mirror image is performed on the segment to be anastomosed.

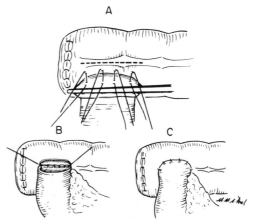

Figure 70–7. End-to-side anastomosis. *A*, The serosa of the ileum is sutured to the serosa of the colon, 2 to 3 mm below a tinea.

B, The tinea is opened for a distance sufficient to accommodate the diameter of the ileum. A 3–0 chromic suture is placed through all layers on the posterior wall, tied to itself, run in a locking fashion to both borders, and converted to a Connell suture laterally completing the inversion anteriorly.

C, The anterior margin of serosa is reapproximated with interrupted horizontal mattress sutures of 3–0 silk.

tinea. At the lateralmost border, the suture is converted to a Connell suture and the anterior wall is closed. Seromuscular sutures of 3–0 silk placed from ileum to colon bury the anterior suture line. The mesentery is reapproximated.

ILEOCOLONIC END-TO-END SUTURED ANASTOMOSIS WITH DISCREPANT BOWEL SIZES (Fig. 70–8). A 3–0 silk suture is placed on the mesenteric border of the ileum and colon; a second 3–0 silk suture is placed on the antimesenteric border of the colon, immediately beneath the Allen clamp. The other end of the suture is placed on the antimesenteric border of the ileum at a distance proximal to the Allen clamp, such that the serosal lengths between the two sutures of both ileal and colon segments are equal. Thus, an equal amount of ileal serosa is applied to the length of colonic serosa bordering the severed end of bowel.

Next, 3–0 silk sutures are placed 2 mm apart in the seromuscular layers of ileum and colon, thus opposing the serosa of the ileum to the colon. The Allen clamps are removed. Hemostasis is achieved, and the antimesenteric border of the ileum incised to the level of the most proximal suture in the ileum. Thus, the bowel lumens now are of identical size. Using a 3–0 chromic double-ended intestinal suture, the posterior row is run in a locking fashion, laterally converting to a Connell suture and the anterior row completed. Seromuscular sutures of 3–0 silk bury the anterior suture line.

Stapled Anastomoses

The theoretical benefits of a stapled anastomosis are that it provides for (1) better blood supply to the healing

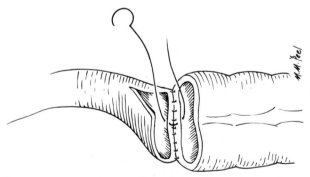

Figure 70–8. Anastomosis of discrepant-sized bowel. A seromuscular suture of 3–0 silk is placed adjacent to each end of the lumen on the mesenteric side. A second 3–0 silk seromuscular suture is placed adjacent to the lumen on the colon and on the antimesenteric border, proximal to the cut end of the small bowel at a distance sufficient so that when the antimesenteric border is incised, the lumens will be of the same size. Interrupted seromuscular sutures of 3–0 silk are then placed at 2-mm intervals between the two holding sutures. The small bowel is opened on its antimesenteric border, until the opening in the small bowel is of the same size as the opening in the colon. A 3–0 chromic suture is placed through all layers, tied to itself, and run laterally in a running locking fashion. At the borders, it is converted to a Connell suture, thus inverting the anterior margin. The anastomosis is completed with interrupted horizontal mattress 3–0 silk sutures that bring the seromuscular layers together anteriorly. This is similar to the closure depicted in Figure 70–3.

margin, (2) reduced tissue manipulation, (3) minimal edema with uniformity of suture placement, (4) wider lumen, (5) greater ease and less time involved in performing the anastomosis, and (6) reduced length of postoperative paralytic ileus. When placed in the intestine through which urine traverses, however, they not infrequently cause stone formation (Bisson et al., 1979; Costello and Johnson, 1984).

Stapled anastomoses evert the suture line. Because staples close in a "B" and do not crush the tissue, theoretically they prevent ischemia at the suture line. This effect may be obvious when a staple line is used to transect the bowel and bleeding continues to occur. The bleeding points may be lightly electrocoagulated or tied off with fine absorbable suture. Stapled bowel anastomoses have been shown to be as efficacious as a hand sewn anastomosis because both have similar complication rates. They usually require less time to perform when the techniques are properly learned. For prolonged procedures, they save little, if any, time when the length of the whole procedure is taken into account.

In a large prospective randomized trial in which a two-layer closure was compared with a staple closure, the complication rate was the same but the time required to complete the stapled anastomosis was 10 minutes less than the hand sewn anastomoses, and when the total operative time was compared between the two, it was the same (Didolkar et al., 1986).

A comparison of complications between sutured and stapled anastomoses reveals a leak and fistula rate of 2.8 per cent for stapled and 3.0 per cent for sutured anastomoses (Chassin et al., 1978). The clinically significant leak rate, however, is only 0.9 per cent (Fazio et al., 1985). A 4.5 per cent incidence of stapled anastomotic leakage has been reported during ileal conduit construction (Costello and Johnson, 1984). Thus, the use of staples is dependent on the preference of the surgeon. A stapled anastomosis appears to be superior to the hand sewn anastomosis in an esophageal-intestinal anastomosis and a low rectal anastomosis. In these two areas, the circular stapler allows for a more precise anastomosis than is often possible utilizing hand sewn techniques. Because these are not problems of urologic surgery, staples are used at the discretion of the surgeon.

The one area in urology in which I believe the stapling device is superior is in the ileocolonic end-to-side anastomosis. Utilizing the circular stapling device, a widely patent anastomosis can be achieved. Three staple instruments are commonly employed in urinary intestinal reconstruction: the linear stapler, the anastomotic stapler, and the circular stapler.

The linear stapler places a double row of staggered staples in a straight line. Depending on the cartridge and instrument chosen, various lengths of staple lines and heights of the closed staples may be chosen. The length is selected depending on how long one wishes the staple line to be. The height of the staple is selected according to the tissue to be stapled. Vascular and pulmonary tissues require staples with a closed height of 1 mm (open height of 2.5 mm). Most intestinal anastomoses are performed with medium staples that have a closed height of approximately 1.5 mm (open height of 3.5 mm). Occasionally, for very thick tissues, large staples are required that have a closed height of 2 mm (open height of 4.8 mm). If there is any doubt in selecting the staple size, the tissue thickness may be measured with a special instrument for this purpose. In general, tissues less than 1 mm or greater than 3 mm in thickness are not amenable to staples.

The anastomotic stapler places two linear double rows of staggered staples. When the knife is advanced, the staple line is divided. The height of the staples is chosen depending on the tissue to be transected.

The circular stapler places two concentric staggered circular staple rows and cuts the tissue within the circle completely from the surrounding tissue. It may be selected in various diameters and with various heights of staples. The diameter and height are selected according to the tissue to be anastomosed. The diameter is determined by the diameter of the tissue to be stapled. Special sizers are available for this maneuver. In most intestinal anastomoses in urology, the height of the closed staple is 1.5 to 2.0 mm. The following is a description of various types of stapled anastomoses.

ILEOCOLONIC ANASTOMOSIS UTILIZING THE CIRCULAR STAPLING DEVICE (Fig. 70–9).
The mesenteric borders are cleared for a distance of 1.5 cm from the cut end of both the colon and the ileum. Holding sutures of 3–0 silk are placed on the mesenteric and antimesenteric borders of the colon. Two other holding sutures are placed on the medial and lateral wall of the colon, midway between the mesenteric and antimesenteric sutures. A pursestring suture of 2–0 Prolene is placed around the ileum no more than 2 mm from the cut end. It is important to take small bites of serosa to avoid bunching the tissue. Sutures must be placed evenly to avoid a gap. A pursestring instrument

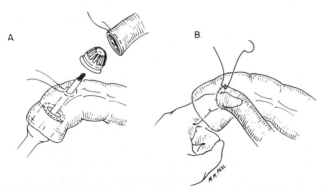

Figure 70–9. Stapled circular anastomosis. *A,* A pursestring suture of 2–0 Prolene is placed around the circumference of the small bowel, and a second pursestring suture 1 cm in diameter is placed on a medial tenia 5 to 6 cm from the open end of the colon. The anvil is removed. A stab wound in the center of the pursestring suture in the colon is made, and the circular stapler is introduced through the end of the colon, with its post thrust through the stab wound made in the center of the pursestring suture.
B, The anvil is placed on the post and introduced into the end of the small bowel. The pursestring sutures in the small bowel and colon are tied snugly around the post. The circular stapler is approximated with a gap of 1.5 to 2 mm, being careful not to include any mesentery in the gap. The anastomosis is completed by placing interrupted silk sutures around its circumference.

is available for this step, if preferred. The ileal diameter is determined with sizers so that the correct circular stapler diameter instrument may be chosen. A pursestring suture is also placed in a circle, 1 cm in diameter, through which a tinea traverses on the medial aspect of the colon. A stab wound is made in the center of the colonic pursestring suture. The distal anvil of the circular stapler is removed, and the instrument is placed through the open end of the colon with its post passed out the stab wound made in the center of the pursestring on the medial wall of the colon. The pursestring is tied tight. The top anvil is then secured to the post and the ileum is placed over it. The ileal pursestring suture is tied. Care must be taken to align the mesenteries at this point. The instrument is approximated with a staple gap of 1.5 to 2.0 mm. Care must be taken not to catch fat or mesentery in the gap. The instrument is fired and is removed by rotatory movement from the colon.

Two "doughnuts" of tissue should be identified on the instrument, and they should have their complete circumference intact with no gaps. With a finger in the open end of the colon and through the anastomosis, seromuscular sutures of 3–0 silk are placed 3 to 4 mm apart, around the circumference of the anastomotic line. The butt end of the colon may be closed by the suture technique or by staples. If the end is to be closed with sutures, a 3–0 chromic suture is brought out the mesenteric and a second 3–0 chromic suture is brought out the antimesenteric border. Both are tied to themselves with the knots on the inside of the bowel. The two sutures are run to each other using a Connell suture until they meet at which point they are tied to each other. The suture line is inverted by placing a second row of 3–0 silk seromuscular sutures. If staples are preferred, the holding sutures are held cephalad and a linear stapler is applied across the open end. Excess tissue is trimmed and the stapler removed.

By holding the holding sutures up, one is secure in applying the staple line to the serosa and mucosa circumferentially around the bowel. Some surgeons invert the staple line with seromuscular sutures of 3–0 silk. However, this step is not necessary. The mesentery between the two segments is now approximated with interrupted 3–0 silk sutures.

END-TO-END STAPLED ANASTOMOSIS: ILEAL-ILEAL OR ILEOCOLONIC ANASTOMOSIS
(Fig. 70–10). The antimesenteric border of the two bowel segments to be joined is approximated with a 3–0 silk suture 5 to 6 cm from the cut ends of the bowel. A holding suture is placed through both segments of bowel at their cut ends at the midpoint of the antimesenteric borders. Stay sutures are placed at the mesenteric border of each bowel segment, and two other sutures midway between the mesenteric and antimesenteric border on the lateral aspects of the bowel are also placed.

The anastomotic stapler is positioned in the lumens of both segments of bowel along the antimesenteric border. The antimesenteric holding suture is pulled up adjacent to the stapler. The anastomotic stapler is locked in place, the staples fired, and the knife advanced. The staple lines are inspected for bleeders, which if persistent

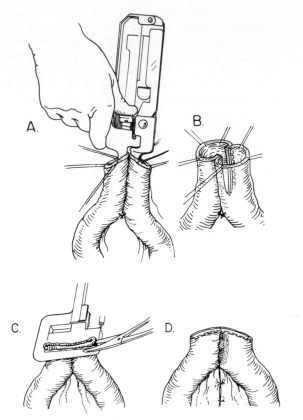

Figure 70–10. Stapled end-to-end anastomosis. *A*, A 3–0 silk suture is placed 5 to 6 cm from the cut ends of the intestine on the antimesenteric borders of both intestinal segments and tied. Holding sutures are placed around the circumference of both intestinal lumens, one securing the antimesenteric borders of both intestinal segments together. The linear anastomotic stapler is placed into the lumens. It is then secured and locked in placed and fired. The knife is then advanced.

B, The appearance of the intestinal anastomosis is indicated after firing the staple device.

C, The open end of the two intestinal segments is closed with a linear stapler by holding the holding sutures up while applying the linear stapler so that the circumference of the mucosa and serosa are incorporated in the staple margin.

D, The anastomosis is completed by closing the mesentery with interrupted 3–0 silk sutures.

should be ligated with absorbable suture. Several 3–0 silk sutures are placed at the apex of the stapled and cut antimesenteric incision. It is at this point that slight tension on the anastomotic line can place undue stress on the staple margin and cause a leak.

The holding sutures are held up, and a linear stapler is placed across the open end of bowel and fired. Care must be taken so that the staples include the serosa in its entire circumference. Excess bowel tissue is excised flush with the instrument before it is disengaged. The mesentery is then reapproximated.

POSTOPERATIVE CARE

The patient should not begin oral alimentation for a minimum of 4 days following surgery. Coordinated small bowel activity begins within hours after the operative event, and stomach activity may return as early as 24

hours. Colonic activity, however, does not return for 2 to 4 days (Woods et al., 1978). Clear liquids may be begun when the paralytic ileus resolves and bowel activity resumes. If clear liquids are tolerated, the diet may be advanced after the patient has a bowel movement. This sequence of events generally takes 4 to 7 days.

If the nutritional condition of the patient is impaired preoperatively, there is a complication postoperatively that will delay feeding or, if paralytic ileus is still present on the 6th postoperative day, intravenous nutrition that supplies the total caloric requirement (hyperalimentation) should begin. It is preferable to begin hyperalimentation the day following surgery if any of these complications are anticipated.

We routinely start all of our patients with intestinal anastomoses on total parenteral hyperalimentation the day following surgery. Once started, it is discontinued only when oral caloric intake is sufficient to satisfy the body's requirements. A jejunal feeding tube for the early institution of intestinal feeding has been advocated by some workers but has not been shown to have any significant advantage over hyperalimentation as outlined.

Nasogastric or gastrostomy decompression during the postoperative period of ileus is somewhat controversial. A prospective study of elective intestinal anastomoses in which 274 patients had postoperative gastric decompression and 261 patients had "nothing by mouth" (NPO) until bowel activity resumed demonstrated no significant difference in major intestinal complications between the two groups. However, those who did not have gastric decompression showed a much greater incidence of abdominal distention, nausea, and vomiting.

Only otherwise healthy patients who had no complications were entered into the study. At least 60 per cent of the patients initially entered were excluded. Specific exclusion criteria included emergency surgery with peritonitis, extensive fibrous adhesions, enterotomies, previous pelvic irradiation, intra-abdominal infection, pancreatitis, chronic obstruction, prolonged operating time, and difficult endotracheal intubation (Wolff et al., 1989). It is therefore prudent to decompress all patients but the most medically fit, because vomiting in the postoperative period increases the risk of aspiration and morbidity. Moreover, tube decompression allows for the administration of ice chips by mouth before enteric activity resumes, thus enhancing patient comfort.

If the patient has severe pulmonary disease, decompression by placing a gastric tube at the time of surgery facilitates pulmonary toilet and also enhances patient comfort. During the period of ileus, the patient should receive an H_2 blocker and be given an antacid via the stomach tube every 2 hours as necessary to keep the gastric pH above 5.0. By keeping the gastric contents alkaline in the postoperative period, the incidence of stress ulceration is markedly reduced.

COMPLICATIONS AFTER ANASTOMOSES

The complications following anastomoses include leakage of fecal contents, sepsis, wound infections, abdominal abscesses, hemorrhage, anastomotic stenosis, pseudo-obstruction of the colon (Ogilvie's syndrome), and intestinal obstruction. These untoward events increase morbidity and are frequently major contributors to mortality. The complication rate for elective colocolonic and ileocolonic anastomoses performed in prepared bowel are: intestinal leak, 2 per cent; hemorrhage, 1 per cent; and stenosis or obstruction, 4 per cent. These complications require reoperations in 1 per cent of the patients and result in death in 0.2 per cent of patients (Jex et al., 1987).

FISTULAS. Fistulas in the postoperative period are of two types: fecal and urinary. These generally occur within the first several weeks following the operative event. They frequently result in sepsis and markedly increase patient morbidity and mortality. Fecal fistulas occur in 4 to 5 per cent of patients (Beckley et al., 1982; Sullivan et al., 1980). Sepsis is a common complication of these untoward events and carries with it a mortality of (1/47) 2 per cent (Hill and Ransley, 1983).

SEPSIS AND OTHER INFECTIOUS COMPLICATIONS. Wound infections, pelvic abscesses, and wound dehiscences all may complicate the immediate postoperative period. Although wound dehiscences and pelvic abscesses are very rare complications, morbid wound infections occur with an incidence of 5 per cent (3/62) (Loening et al., 1982). Many of these complications may be averted by operating on a properly prepared bowel, by walling off the intestine with Mikulicz pads while the anastomosis is being completed, and by irrigating the intestinal segment to be utilized in the reconstruction until it is free of any residual enteric contents before it is manipulated and its contents are spilled in the abdomen and pelvis.

BOWEL OBSTRUCTIONS. The incidence of intestinal obstruction following abdominal procedures for urinary intestinal diversion differs depending on whether the stomach, ileum, or colon is used for the diversion. In a patient who has had a segment of stomach or ileum removed for the diversion, there is a 10 per cent incidence of postoperative bowel obstruction requiring treatment. When the colon is utilized, the incidence of postoperative obstruction requiring an operation is 4 per cent (Table 70–3).

Half the bowel obstructions occur in the early postoperative period. In one series, following radical cystectomy and ileal conduit, 15 per cent of the patients had mild obstructions in the first 6 months, which responded to conservative management. Some 3 per cent required an operation to relieve the obstruction during this period. The occurrence of obstruction following this 6-month period was much less frequent (Sullivan et al., 1980). Bowel obstruction can be a morbid event because 21 per cent of patients who develop obstructions following ileal conduits and require operations die.

The most common cause of obstruction is adhesions followed by recurrent cancer. These two causes account for the majority of cases. Volvulus and internal hernia account for far fewer cases (Jaffe et al., 1968).

The incidence of postoperative bowel obstruction may

Table 70–3. COMPLICATIONS OF URINARY INTESTINAL DIVERSION*

Complication	Type of Diversion	Number of Patients (Complication/Total Number)	Incidence (%)
Bowel obstruction	Ileal conduit	124/1289	10
	Colon conduit	9/230	4
	Gastric conduit	2/21	10
	Continent diversion	9/250	4
Ureteral intestinal obstruction	Ileal conduit	90/1142	8
	Antireflux colon conduit	25/122	20
	Colon conduit	8/92	9
	Continent diversion	16/461	4
Urine leak	Ileal conduit	23/886	3
	Colon conduit	6/130	5
	Continent diversion		
	Ileum	104/629	17
	Colon	5/123	4
Stomal stenosis/hernia	Ileal conduit	196/806	24
	Colon conduit	45/227	20
	Continent diversion	28/310	9
Renal calculi	Ileal conduit	70/964	7
	Antireflux colon conduit	9/56	16
Pouch calculi	Continent diversion	42/317	13
Acidosis requiring treatment	Ileal conduit	46/296	16
	Antireflux colon conduit	5/94	5
	Gastric conduit	0/21	0
	Continent diversion		
	Ileum	21/263	8
	Colon/colon-ileum	17/63	27
Pyelonephritis	Ileal conduit	132/1142	12
	Antireflux colon conduit	13/96	13
	Continent diversion	15/296	5
Renal deterioration	Ileal conduit	146/808	18
	Antireflux colon conduit	15/103	15

*Composite from the literature. Follow-up averages 5 years for ileal conduits, 3 years for colon conduits, 2 years for gastric conduits, and 2 years for continent diversions.

be reduced by using nonirradiated bowel, closing all apertures, reperitonealizing the isolated segment, decompressing the gastrointestinal (GI) tract for an adequate period of time, placing omentum over the anastomosis, and reconstituting the pelvic floor following exenterative surgery. The isolated segment is reperitonealized by tacking its antimesenteric border to the lateral abdominal side wall peritoneum. The proximal mesenteric border should be tacked to the posterior parietal peritoneum, because failure to obliterate this potential space has resulted in entrapment of bowel resulting in a bowel obstruction. The pelvic space left following an anterior exenteration may be closed by placing the sigmoid colon in the area. This maneuver will effectively prevent small bowel from herniating into the raw pelvis. Omentum may also be mobilized and used to fill any space the sigmoid colon does not fill.

In a total exenteration, sufficient sigmoid colon is not available and often the omentum is not bulky enough to fill the pelvis and thus prevent small bowel from filling the denuded pelvis. This problem is of particular concern in a patient who must receive postoperative pelvic irradiation. The bowel may be kept out of the pelvis by reconstructing the pelvic floor with polyglactin mesh. The mesh is sutured along the posterior pelvic brim to the sacral promontory and presacral fascia and sutured laterally to the adventitia of the iliac vessels. Laterally and anteriorly, it is sewn to the peritoneum, two thirds of the distance between the pubis and umbilicus. Omentum is then brought down, placed over the mesh, and sutured in position. This maneuver will effectively exclude the bowel from the pelvis for 4 to 6 weeks while postoperative irradiation is being administered (Sener et al., 1989).

HEMORRHAGE. Hemorrhage is a rare complication of intestinal anastomoses. It is much more likely to occur when stomach is utilized and a Billroth I anastomoses is created. Hemorrhage is usually due to failure to secure bleeding at the time of anastomosis or to anastomotic ulcers that develop on the suture line.

INTESTINAL STENOSIS. Intestinal stenosis occurs at two distinct times: in the immediate postoperative period and over the long term. Intestinal stenosis in the immediate postoperative period is due to technical misadventures or edema. Edema resolves by continuing the intestinal decompression, whereas a technical problem requires a reoperation.

PSEUDO-OBSTRUCTIONS. Pseudo-obstructions of the colon or Ogilvie's syndrome on rare occasion may complicate the early postoperative period. The etiology is not understood. Pseudo-obstruction usually occurs within the first 3 days postoperatively in patients with multiple medical illnesses. The patient complains of severe abdominal pain and a roentgenogram of the abdomen reveals a dilated cecum. A gentle, water-soluble contrast enema will eliminate the possibility of a mechanical obstruction. In the presence of a rising leukocyte count or cecum that is increasing in size and exceeds 12 to 15 cm in diameter, rupture may be imminent. Under these circumstances, an emergency cecostomy should be performed (Clayman et al., 1981). In less acute circumstances, an attempt at endoscopic decompression may be tried.

COMPLICATIONS OF THE ISOLATED INTESTINAL SEGMENT

INTESTINAL STRICTURE. Strictures of intestinal segments are usually late complications primarily occurring in conduits, although they have been described in ileal ureters as well. The stricture is thought to be a consequence of lymphoid depletion of the intestine exposed to urine. The lymphoid depletion contributes to persistent infection, which may result in mid-loop stricture, bacterial seeding of the upper tracts, and renal deterioration (Tapper and Folkman, 1976). Because of the persistent infection and lack of intestinal resistance to the detrimental action of bacteria, submucosal edema with fibrosis and stricture formation occurs. The intestinal segment may also be blocked by encroachment of hypertrophied mesenteric lymph nodes. Hypertrophied mesenteric lymph nodes, submucosal lymphoid depletion, edema, and fibrosis are commonly found when intestinal segments that have been chronically exposed to urine are examined pathologically.

Elongation of the Segment

Another complication of the intestinal segment is elongation—occasionally resulting in massive enlargement. When this occurs in conduits or ureteral substitutes, there is usually a distal obstruction. In continent diversions, it may signal failure to intermittently catheterize the pouch frequently enough. If allowed to persist, the increased pressure may result in deterioration of renal function. Enlargement and elongation of the intestine may also result in a volvulus of the segment (Fig. 70–11).

ABDOMINAL STOMAS

Two types of stomas may be created on the anterior abdominal wall, those that are flush and those that protrude. The former are preferable for the continent type of diversion in which intermittent catheterization will be carried out and over which a small dressing will be placed. The latter are preferable when a collection device is worn. A properly protruding stoma worn with an appliance results in a lesser incidence of stomal stenosis with epithelial overgrowth and a better appliance fit with fewer peristomal skin problems. There are two types of protruding stomas: the end stoma and the loop end ileostomy. Most complications of stomas are the result of technical errors in their creation. Therefore, specific technical points must be rigidly adhered to, to minimize such complications.

The site of the stoma should be selected preoperatively. This is performed by marking the stomal site with the patient in the sitting position as well as the supine position, care being taken to place the site over the rectus muscle at least 5 cm away from the planned incision line. The point chosen should be well away from skin creases, scars, umbilicus, belt lines, and bony prominences. A site in which radiotherapy has previ-

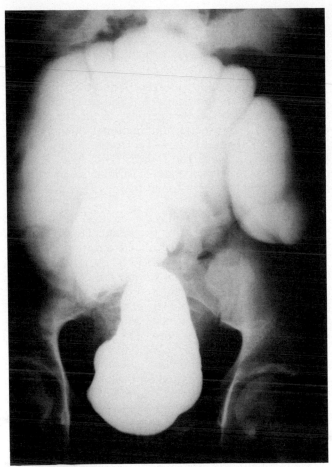

Figure 70–11. Volvulus of an orthotopic right colon bladder. This segment is enlarged markedly owing to the lack of adherence to a frequent regimen of intermittent catheterization.

ously injured the area should be avoided. All stomas should be placed through the belly of the rectus muscle and should be located at the peak of the infraumbilical fat roll. If the stoma is placed lateral to the rectus sheath, a parastomal hernia is likely to occur. The bowel should traverse the abdominal wall perpendicular to the peritoneal lining, i.e., it should come straight out. One should avoid trimming fat or epiploic appendages from around the margin of the stoma, and the appliances should be applied in the operating room.

A circular incision is made at the predetermined site. A perfectly circular opening in the skin may be created by placing the finger hole of a Kelly clamp at the desired point and grasping the skin in the center of the hole with a Kocher clamp. By pulling up on the Kocher clamp and pushing the handle of the Kelly clamp against the abdominal wall, a small button of skin may be removed with a single pass of the knife. This maneuver creates a perfectly circular opening in the skin. The tendency to remove too much skin is great, resulting in a circular opening that is too large. In order to avoid this complication, one should not cut the skin flush with the Kelly clamp but rather immediately beneath the Kocher clamp. The subcutaneous tissue is left intact. This is spread, not excising any fat, for the fat will fall back adjacent to the bowel and eliminate any dead space. Kocher clamps are placed on the fascia in the

incision and pulled medially, so that when the fascia and peritoneum are incised, they are incised directly over the skin line and thus do not result in angulation of the gut when the abdominal incision is closed. The fascia is incised in a cruciate manner and the rectus muscles spread. The peritoneum is incised. The opening should accommodate two fingers snugly.

NIPPLE STOMA ("ROSEBUD") (Fig. 70–12). A Babcock clamp is placed through the opening, and the bowel grasped and brought out for a distance of 5 to 6 cm in order to create a nipple of about 2 to 3 cm in length. Sutures of 3–0 chromic are placed through the seromuscular layer of the bowel and the peritoneum on the anterior abdominal wall. The mesentery is aligned in its normal anatomic direction prior to suturing the serosa to the peritoneal wall. Usually, the ileum will be curved concave toward the mesentery. If this curvature is severe, the mesentery may be partially incised but not all the way to the bowel wall. Thus, a portion of mesentery is preserved along the entire length of the bowel. This should straighten the curve in the bowel significantly if not completely. Chromic sutures of 3–0 are placed in quadrants through the full thickness of the bowel edge and through the seromuscular layer of the bowel, 3 cm from the cut edge and then through the subcuticular skin layer. Sutures should not pass through the full thickness of the skin but through the subcuticular and subdermal layers only. When the sutures are tied, the bowel is everted and forms a nipple. A more secure nipple may be formed by performing multiple myotomies through the seromuscular layer of the bowel above the skin line prior to creation of the nipple. This maneuver causes serosa-to-serosa adherence and reduces the risk of stomal retraction. This step is particularly appropriate for patients who are obese.

FLUSH STOMA. Quadrant sutures of 3–0 chromic are placed through the full thickness of the bowel and subsequently passed through the subdermal layer and tied. Several sutures are placed between the quadrant sutures from bowel to subdermal skin. This maneuver creates a flush stoma, which has a 1-mm raised margin.

LOOP END ILEOSTOMY (Fig. 70–13). Obese patients have a thick abdominal wall and often a thick, short ileal mesentery. This makes creation of an end ileal stoma extremely difficult. The loop-end ileostomy

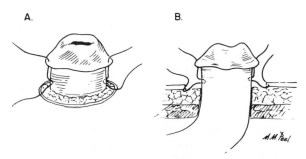

Figure 70–12. A and B, Nipple stoma. About 5 to 6 cm of intestine are brought through the abdominal wall. The serosa is scarified, and quadrant sutures of 3–0 chromic are placed through the entire thickness of the distal end of the intestine. Each suture is placed in the seromuscular layer 3 cm proximal and then secured to the dermis before it is tied.

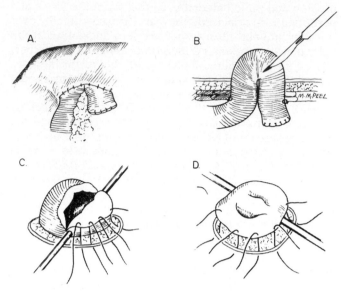

Figure 70–13. Loop end ileostomy. *A,* After closing the distal end of the loop and drawing the bowel through the rent in the abdominal wall, it is held in place by a rod passed through the mesentery. The mesentery is realigned, and the peritoneum is sutured to the serosa of the bowel circumferentially.

B, A transverse incision is made in the bowel four fifths of the loop's distance, cephalad.

C, The cephalad portion of the stoma is simply sutured to the dermal layer of skin with interrupted 3–0 chromic sutures.

D, On the inferior aspect of the incision, sutures of 3–0 chromic are placed through the full thickness of the cut edge and then through the seromuscular layer followed by the dermis. This maneuver everts the caudal portion of the stoma.

obviates some of these problems and is usually simpler to perform than the ileal-end stoma in the obese patient. To create this type of stoma, the distal end of the ileum is closed as previously described for closing the butt end of an intestinal segment. A loop is brought up through the belly of the rectus muscle and onto the anterior abdominal wall. This maneuver avoids bringing the mesenteric border onto the abdominal wall and eliminates one side of the ileostomy being involved with mesentery. A slightly larger skin opening is required than that for the end stoma. A 3-cm disc of skin is removed. The subcutaneous tissue is spread, the fascia incised, the rectus spread, and the peritoneum incised as previously described. The opening should admit two fingers comfortably.

The loop may be pulled through the opening in the abdominal wall by passing an umbilical tape through a small opening in the mesentery at a distance from the distal end sufficient to leave that end in the abdomen, when the loop has been pulled through the abdominal wall. By gentle traction on the umbilical tape, the loop is brought onto the abdomen. The distal portion of the bowel is brought through the opening, such that the closed end lies cephalad to the body of the segment. When a sufficient amount of loop protrudes beyond the skin edge, a small rod is placed through the hole in the mesentery at the apex of the loop and holds the bowel on the anterior abdominal wall during suturing.

If the rent in the rectus muscle is too large, it may be closed with interrupted 0 chromic sutures from within

the abdomen. The serosa is sutured to the peritoneum on the anterior abdominal wall. The bowel wall is opened in a transverse direction at a point four fifths the distance cephalad to the caudal most portion of the loop.

Utilizing 3–0 chromic sutures, the full thickness of the caudal incision in the bowel is sutured back to itself (serosa) and then to the dermis, as in the rosebud technique. The cephalad nonfunctional opening is sutured directly to the dermis. The rod is sutured to the skin and left in place for 7 days. This type of stoma results in a lesser incidence of stomal stenosis but a higher incidence of parastomal hernias (Emmott et al., 1985).

Stomas for the colon may be created in much the same way as end stomas for the ileum. However, their suturing is usually more flush than everted.

COMPLICATIONS OF INTESTINAL STOMAS. Complications of abdominal stomas are the single most common problems encountered in the postoperative period of urinary intestinal diversion. Early complications of abdominal stomas include bowel necrosis, bleeding, and irritative skin lesions. Later complications include bleeding, dermatitis, parastomal hernia, prolapse, obstruction, stomal retraction, and stomal stenosis. At some point, virtually every patient will have one of these complications. Many of these complications can be reduced by proper construction of the stoma. If periodic visitations with the enterostomal therapist are made, products for skin care are appropriately used, nonirritative stomal adhesives are used, urine in the collection device is maintained acidic, and properly fitting collection devices are used, most of the stomal complications can be significantly reduced and many eliminated.

Parastomal skin lesions may be classified as (1) irritative, which are manifested by hypopigmentation, hyperpigmentation, and skin atrophy; (2) erythematous and erosive, which appear as macular and scaly with loss of the epidermis; and (3) pseudoverrucous, which are wart-like (Borglund et al., 1988).

Stomal stenosis has been reported, on average, in 20 to 24 per cent of patients with ileal conduits and 10 to 20 per cent of patients with colon conduits (see Table 70–3). This incidence has been considerably reduced by better attention to stomal care and better-fitting appliances. Stomal stenosis is less for loop stomas than for end stomas. Parastomal hernias occur rarely (1 to 4 per cent) with end stomas, but are more likely with loop stomas, with reported incidences ranging from 4 to 20 per cent.

Bleeding, stomal stenosis, and dermatitis can be markedly reduced by attention to parastomal skin care and by a properly fitting appliance around a protruding stoma. The other complications are minimized by correct surgical technique.

URETEROINTESTINAL ANASTOMOSES

The ureter may be anastomosed to the colon or small bowel in such a manner as to produce a refluxing or nonrefluxing anastomosis. Considerable controversy exists as to whether a nonrefluxing or refluxing anastomosis is desirable in urinary tract reconstruction. Deterioration of the upper tracts for ileal and colon conduits has been reported in 10 to 60 per cent of patients. In one series, 49 per cent of the upper tracts showed changes after conduit diversion, 16 per cent of which had an increase of the blood urea nitrogen of 10 mg/dl or more (Schwarz and Jeffs, 1975).

Deterioration of the upper tracts is usually a consequence of infection or stones or less commonly of obstruction at the ureteral intestinal anastomosis. Because bacteriuria occurs in almost all conduits and because the intestine certainly does not inhibit and may, in fact, promote bacterial colonization, many have suggested that a nonrefluxing anastomosis would minimize the incidence of renal deterioration.

The evidence that would suggest that a nonrefluxing system in urinary intestinal diversions is desirable comes from several observations. In a group of patients who had nonrefluxing colon conduits constructed, those whose anastomoses remained nonrefluxing had a lesser incidence of renal deterioration than those whose antireflux anastomoses failed. Follow-up for 9 to 20 years revealed that 79 per cent (22/28) of the refluxing renal units deteriorated, whereas only 22 per cent (11/51) of the nonrefluxing units deteriorated (Elder et al., 1979; Husmann et al., 1989). Others have reported that in continent diversions, the majority of patients who experienced reflux showed upper tract dilation and deterioration, whereas few experienced deterioration when a nonrefluxing anastomosis was present (Kock et al., 1978).

Similar findings have been reported in experimental animals. If a nonrefluxing ureteral colonic conduit diversion is constructed, only 7 per cent of the renal units show evidence of pyelonephritic scarring after 3 months, whereas if a refluxing anastomosis is constructed, 83 per cent of the renal units show scarring. Half of the conduits in both groups have significant bacteriuria (Richie and Skinner, 1975).

Other workers have not found the same high incidence of renal deterioration associated with ureteral intestinal reflux. One group of investigators studying colon conduits noted no difference in the incidence of renal deterioration, irrespective of whether the colon conduit refluxed or not: 17 per cent (5/29) of nonrefluxing renal units showed deterioration compared with 18 per cent (5/27) of refluxing units (Hill and Ransley, 1983). In another series, only three of 135 renal units with refluxing ureteral intestinal anastomoses that were unobstructed showed evidence of renal deterioration (Shapiro et al., 1975).

It does not appear that conduit pressures are transmitted to the renal pelvis. The pressure within the renal pelvis in refluxing conduit diversions is not elevated above normal nor is it dependent on the segment of bowel, i.e. ileum or colon (Hayashi et al., 1986; Kamizaki and Cass, 1978; Magnus, 1977). Peristaltic ureteral contractions apparently dampen pressure transmission from intestine to renal pelvis, attesting to the importance of normal ureters. When bowel is substituted for the ureter, it does not appear that it makes any difference whether there is reflux at the bladder. The voiding pressure is blunted by the distensible bowel segment. Moreover, there is no difference in ileal and colon conduits between those that reflux and those that do not in renal function measured 2 to 5 years postoperatively (Mansson et al., 1984).

Also, the successful creation of an antirefluxing anastomosis does not prevent bacterial colonization of the renal pelvis. In six of eight patients with nonrefluxing enterocystoplasties and 1 patient with a nonrefluxing colon conduit in whom the absence of reflux was documented by loopogram, percutaneous renal pelvic aspiration revealed positive culture findings (Gonzalez and Reinberg, 1987). One advantage of a refluxing anastomosis in the patient who has urothelia which is prone to malignancy is that the upper tracts may be followed by periodically introducing contrast material into the conduit.

From these studies, it appears that reflux associated with impaired ureteral peristalsis in the presence of bacteriuria and/or obstruction results in renal deterioration. It has not been established that for either conduit or continent diversions, reflux associated with the normal ureter in the absence of obstruction is detrimental to the adult kidney.

Although many techniques have been described for creating the various types of ureterointestinal anastomoses, certain basic surgical principles are germane to all the anastomoses, irrespective of type. Only as much ureter as needed should be mobilized so that there is no redundancy or tension on the anastomosis. Mobilization should not strip the ureter of its periadventitial tissue because it is in this tissue that the ureter's blood supply courses. The ureter should be cleaned of its adventitial tissue only for 2 to 3 mm at its distal most portion, where the ureter to intestinal mucosa anastomosis will be performed.

The ureterointestinal anastomosis must be performed with fine absorbable sutures, which are placed in such a manner so that a watertight mucosa-to-mucosa apposition is created. The bowel should be brought to the ureter. The ureter should not be extensively mobilized so that it can be brought into the wound to the bowel lying on the anterior abdominal wall.

At the completion of the anastomosis, the bowel should be fixed to the abdominal cavity preferably adjacent to the site of the ureterointestinal anastomosis. If possible, the anastomosis should be retroperitonealized or a pedicle flap of peritoneum should be placed over the anastomosis.

In those diversions in which the intestinal stoma will be brought to the abdomen and the proximal end of the bowel fixed to the retroperitoneum, there are two places where the bowel may be conveniently fixed to the retroperitoneum, without jeopardizing mesenteric blood supply. The most convenient point of fixation is below the root of the small bowel mesentery at the level of the pelvic brim. Thus, the ureterointestinal anastomosis may be retroperitonealized at the level of the pelvic brim, thus fixing the bowel segment to the posterior body wall. In those cases in which the ureters are short, a more cephalad fixation to the posterior peritoneum may be accomplished by placing the proximal end in the right upper quadrant cephalad to the origin of the right colic artery and immediately below the duodenum. This is a relatively avascular area and places the intestine fairly close to the right and left kidney, thus reducing the length of ureter required to reach the intestinal segment.

Perhaps one of the most difficult complications of ureterointestinal anastomoses to manage is a stricture. This is generally caused by ischemia, urine leak, radiation, or infection. The incidence of urine leak for all types of ureterointestinal anastomoses is 3 to 5 per cent (see Table 70–3). This incidence of leak can be reduced to near zero, if soft Silastic stents are utilized. In one series of ureterointestinal anastomoses done at the same institution, the nonstented patient group had a 2 per cent anastomotic leak and a 4 per cent stricture rate. When non-Silastic rigid stents were used, there was a 10 per cent incidence of stricture. However, when a soft Silastic stent was utilized, there were no strictures or leaks (Regan and Barrett, 1985).

In a similar series in which colon conduits were created following gynecologic exenterative operations, the nonstented group had an 18 per cent leak rate and an 18 per cent stricture rate, whereas those who had been stented had a 3 per cent leak rate and an 8 per cent stricture rate (Beddoe et al., 1987). Thus, with the advent of soft Silastic stents, the evidence indicates that they are effective in reducing the leak rate and subsequent stricture formation.

In creating a submucosal tunnel in those procedures in which a nonrefluxing anastomosis is made, it is often helpful to inject saline with a 25-gauge needle, submucosally, to raise the mucosa away from the seromuscular layer. This maneuver makes dissection considerably simpler (Menon et al., 1982).

These principles of surgical technique are common to all ureterointestinal anastomoses. Each type of ureterointestinal anastomosis, however, has specific technical points unique to its creation. Techniques involving ureterocolonic anastomoses are discussed next, followed by the ureteral small bowel anastomoses.

URETEROCOLONIC ANASTOMOSES

COMBINED TECHNIQUE OF LEADBETTER AND CLARKE (Fig. 70–14). This method establishes a nonrefluxing ureterocolonic anastomosis by employing a submucosal tunnel. The technique combines the ureterocolonic anastomosis of Nesbitt, which is a refluxing elliptic anastomosis to the intestine, with the tunneled technique of Coffey (Leadbetter and Clarke, 1954).

The anterior tenia is incised obliquely for 2.5 to 3 cm as close to the mesenteric border as possible. The mucosa is dissected off the muscularis for the entire length of the incision. At the distal end of the incision in the tenia, the mucosa is picked up with a fine Adson forceps and a small button is excised. The ureter is spatulated for 5 to 7 mm, such that an elliptic anastomosis may be created. The ureter is sewn mucosa to mucosa with 5–0 polydioxanone suture (PDS) utilizing interrupted sutures with the knots tied on the outside or a running suture.

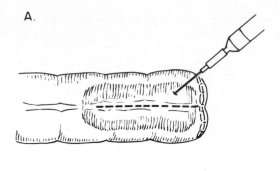

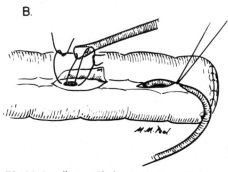

Figure 70–14. Leadbetter-Clarke ureterointestinal anastomosis. *A,* Injection of the submucosal tissues with saline facilitates the dissection.

B, A linear incision is made in the tinea, the tinea raised, and the mucosa identified. A small button of mucosa is removed, the ureter is spatulated and then is sutured to the mucosa with 5–0 polydioxanone suture. The seromuscular layer is sutured over the ureter, being careful not to compromise or occlude the ureter.

If the suture line is to be run, it is well to begin the anastomosis at the apex of the ureter. This suture is tied, and the posterior row is run to the distal most portion of the ureter and is subsequently tied. A second running suture completes the anterior aspect. The seromuscular layer is then reapproximated loosely over the ureter in such a way as to allow ". . . the ureter [to] lie in the bowel as a hammock without being compressed" (Leadbetter and Clarke, 1954). The bowel should be fixed to the peritoneum so that there is no tension on the ureters. The complications reported with this procedure include a leak rate of 2.5 per cent, a deterioration of the upper tracts that varies between 4.3 and 25 per cent, and a stricture rate that varies between 8 and 14 per cent (Table 70–4).

TRANSCOLONIC TECHNIQUE OF GOODWIN (Fig. 70–15). This method establishes a nonrefluxing ureterocolonic anastomosis by creating a submucosal tunnel. Utilizing this technique, the anastomosis is performed from within the bowel (Goodwin et al., 1953). If it is performed in bowel in continuity with the GI tract, a noncrushing occlusive clamp is applied across the bowel, cephalad to the desired point of the ureterointestinal anastomosis. This clamp is loosely placed about the bowel in such a way as not to occlude the arterial supply in the mesentery. A vertical incision is made in the bowel anteriorly and the desired point of entrance of the ureter into the bowel identified. A 0.5-cm incision is made in the posterior mucosa. Utilizing a curved hemostat, the mucosa is dissected from the submucosa layer in an oblique fashion, coursing from

Table 70–4. COMPLICATIONS OF URETEROINTESTINAL ANASTOMOSES

Procedure*	Number of Patients	Stricture	Leakage	Reflux
COLON				
Leadbetter-Clarke[1–4]	127	14%	3%	4%
Strickler[5]	28	14%	—	—
Pagano[6]	63	7%	—	6%
SMALL BOWEL				
Bricker[7, 8]	1809	7%	4%	—
Wallace-Y[9–11]	129	3%	2%	—
Nipple[8]	37	8%	—	17%
Serosal tunnel[12]	10	10%	—	0%
LeDuc[13–16]	82	5%	2%	13%

*Literature cited: 1. Hagen-Cook and Althausen, 1979; 2. Leadbetter and Clarke, 1954; 3. Hill and Ransley, 1983; 4. King, 1987; 5. Jacobs and Young, 1980; 6. Pagano et al., 1984; 7. Clark, 1979; 8. Patil et al., 1976; 9. Clark, 1979; 10. Beckley et al., 1982; 11. Wendel et al., 1969; 12. Starr et al., 1975; 13. Hautmann et al., 1988; 14. LeDuc et al., 1987; 15. Klein et al., 1986; 16. Lockhart and Bejany, 1987.

medial to lateral. The hemostat is passed beneath the mucosa for a distance of approximately 3 to 4 cm and then brought through the serosa.

A traction suture that has been placed on the ureter is then grasped with the hemostat and the ureter brought into the colon. Both ureters should be brought into the bowel before suturing them to the mucosa. The ureters should lie without tension or angulation. A No. 5 feeding tube is passed through the ureter to be sure that there is no kinking, as it passes through the bowel wall. The redundant ureter is excised—its end spatulated and sewn with interrupted 5–0 PDS to the mucosa. Care is taken to include with the mucosa some muscularis so that the ureter is securely fixed in place. Silastic stents are placed up both ureters.

As the ureters come through the serosa from without

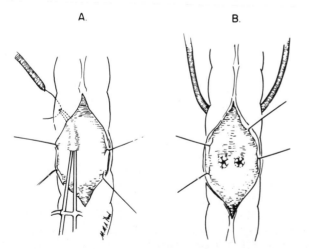

Figure 70–15. Transcolonic technique of Goodwin. *A*, The bowel is opened on its anterior surface, a small rent in the mucosa made. Utilizing a mosquito hemostat, the mucosa is raised from the submucosa extending laterally. A 3- to 4-cm tunnel is created before the clamp exits the serosal wall. The ureter is grasped and pulled into the submucosal tunnel.

B, Both ureters have been drawn into the bowel through their submucosal tunnels before each is spatulated and circumferentially sutured to the mucosa. These sutures should also incorporate a portion of the muscularis for security. Where the ureter enters the colonic sidewall adjacent to the mesentery, the adventitia of the ureter is secured to the colonic serosa with interrupted 5–0 polydioxanone sutures.

the bowel, the adventitia of the ureter is sutured to the serosa of the colon with two 4–0 PDSs. The anterior bowel wall is closed in two layers. The reported results with this technique appear to be quite satisfactory; however, specific reliable data on the complication rate are not available.

STRICKLER TECHNIQUE (Fig. 70–16). This method establishes a nonrefluxing ureterocolonic anastomosis by creating a submucosal tunnel (Jacobs and Young, 1980; Strickler, 1965). A 1-cm incision is made on the margin of the tenia. Originally, the technique described removal of a 2-mm button of seromuscular tissue. A 2-cm tunnel is formed laterally beneath the seromuscular layer with a hemostat. The seromuscular layer is incised, with care being taken not to tent up the mucosa and inadvertently incise it. The holding suture in the ureter is grasped and drawn through the submucosal tunnel. The ureter is spatulated for 0.5 cm. A button of mucosa is removed, and the full thickness of the ureter is sewn to the mucosa of the bowel with either interrupted or running 5–0 PDS.

The serosa is reapproximated over the ureter with 4–0 silk sutures. The serosal suture line is perpendicular

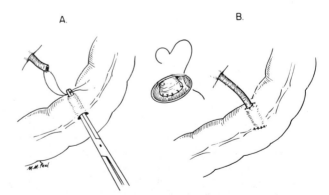

Figure 70–16. Strickler ureterointestinal anastomosis. *A*, A small linear incision is made in the tinea and the submucosa dissected from the mucosa laterally. After a distance of 3 to 4 cm is achieved, a small hole is made in the serosa and the ureter then drawn through.

B, A button of mucosa is excised, and the ureter is spatulated and sutured to the mucosa with 5–0 polydioxanone suture. The rent in the tinea is closed with interrupted sutures, and an adventitial suture at the ureter's entrance point into the colon secures it to the serosa of the colon.

to the course of the ureter. Where the ureters enter the serosa, they are also fixed with interrupted 4–0 PDSs. A lateral peritoneal flap is placed over the anastomosis. The advantage of this anastomosis is that because the tenia do not need to be aligned, one can form the tunnel according to the normal course of the ureter, thus avoiding angulation. This technique reliably prevents reflux but results in a stricture rate of approximately 14 per cent (see Table 70–4).

PAGANO TECHNIQUE (Fig. 70–17). This method establishes a nonrefluxing ureterointestinal anastomosis by creating a submucosal tunnel (Pagano, 1980). The tenia is incised for a length of 4 to 5 cm, and the seromuscular layer is separated from the mucosa on both sides of the tinea laterally as far as the mesenteric border. The ureter is brought in one end, i.e., the distal end, laterally and laid in the 4- to 5-cm tunnel parallelling the mesenteric border. A button of mucosa is excised; the ureters are spatulated and sutured to the mucosa with either interrupted or running 5–0 PDS. The seromuscular layer is then closed loosely with silk sutures in the midline. Each suture includes the seromuscular layer of the tenia and the mucosa in the midline. This technique has a reported complication rate that is very low. The leakage rate is approximately 3 per cent, the stricture rate is 6 per cent, and the reflux rate is approximately 6 per cent (see Table 70–4) (Pagano et al., 1984).

CORDONNIER AND NESBITT TECHNIQUES. These techniques utilize no tunnel and are direct refluxing anastomoses of the ureter to the colon (Cordonnier, 1950; Nesbitt, 1949). They are not desirable for ureterosigmoidostomies, and perhaps their only role lies in creating a refluxing ureterocolonic conduit anastomosis. They are performed in much the same way a Bricker anastomosis would be performed for the small bowel (see next section).

Ureteral Small Bowel Anastomoses

A number of ureteral small bowel anastomoses are possible, which are of two basic types: end-to-side and

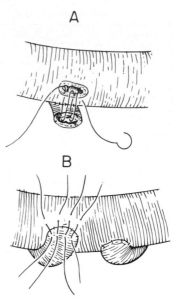

Figure 70–18. Bricker ureterointestinal anastomosis. *A,* The adventitia of the ureter is sutured to the serosa of the bowel. A small full-thickness serosa and mucosal plug is removed. Interrupted 5–0 polydioxanone suture approximates the ureter to the full thickness of the mucosa and serosa. *B,* The anterior layer is completed by interrupted sutures placed through the adventitia of the ureter and the serosa of the small bowel.

end-to-end. The end-to-side anastomoses may be constructed in a refluxing or nonrefluxing manner.

BRICKER ANASTOMOSIS (Fig. 70–18). The Bricker anastomosis is a refluxing end-to-side ureteral small bowel anastomosis that is simple to perform and has a low complication rate (Bricker, 1950). Although originally described for the small bowel, it may be employed in any suitable intestinal segment. The original description involved suturing the adventitia of the ureter with interrupted silk sutures to the serosa of the bowel. The mucosa and serosa were incised, a small mucosa plug removed, and using fine reabsorbable chromic sutures, the full thickness of the ureter was sewn to the mucosa of the bowel. The anterior layer of ureteral adventitia was then sewn with interrupted silk sutures to the serosa of the bowel. A less cumbersome method of performing this anastomosis is to excise a small button of seromuscular tissue and mucosa, spatulate the ureter for 0.5 cm, and suture the full thickness of the ureter to the full thickness of the bowel, i.e., mucosa and seromuscular layer to ureteral wall with either interrupted or running 5–0 PDS. The anastomosis is stented with a soft Silastic catheter. The stricture rate for this anastomosis varies between 4 and 22 per cent (average of 6 per cent), with a leak rate of approximately 3 per cent in the absence of stents (see Table 70–4).

WALLACE TECHNIQUE (Fig. 70–19). A frequently employed anastomotic technique is that of Wallace in which the end of the intestine is sutured to the end of the ureter (Albert and Persky, 1971; Wallace, 1970). This is a refluxing anastomosis. The intestinal segment employed may be either small bowel or colon. There are three basic types of anastomoses as follows:

1. The end of one ureter is sutured to the end of the

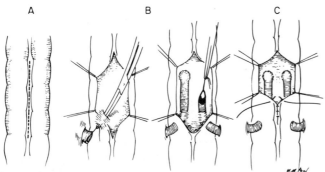

Figure 70–17. Pagano ureterointestinal anastomosis. *A,* A linear incision is made in the tinea between 4 and 5 cm in length.
B, The submucosa is dissected from the mucosa laterally on both sides to the level of the mesentery. The ureters are drawn into the submucosal tunnel distally and sutured to the mucosa with 5–0 polydioxanone suture proximally. *C,* The serosa is reapproximated, incorporating the mucosa in the midline.

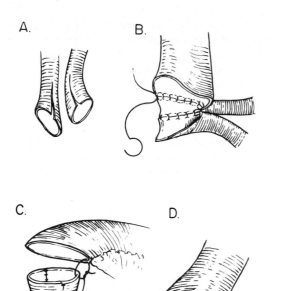

Figure 70–19. Wallace ureterointestinal anastomosis. *A,* Both ureters are spatulated and are laid adjacent to each other.

B, The apex of one ureter is sutured to the apex of the other ureter with 5–0 polydioxanone suture (PDS). The posterior medial walls of both ureters are then sutured together with interrupted or running 5–0 PDS—the knots tied to the outside. Upon completion of this step, the lateral ureteral walls are sutured to the intestine.

C, A Y-type of anastomosis is formed by completing the anterior row of the anterior lateral ureteral walls of *D* and then suturing the end of the ureters directly to the intestine.

D, The head-to-tail anastomosis involves suturing the apex of one ureter to the end of the other. The posterior medial walls are sewn together following which the ends and lateral walls are sewn to the intestine.

other ureter. This composite anastomosis is sutured to the end of the bowel.

2. A Y anastomosis of the ureters is created, which is sutured to the end of the bowel.

3. A head-to-tail ureteroureteral anastomosis is formed, which is then sutured to the end of the bowel.

The ureters are spatulated for 1.5 to 2 cms, and fine 5–0 PDS is utilized for each anastomosis. For the first anastomosis, a fine suture is placed at the apex of each ureter with the knot tied to the outside. The posterior medial ureteral walls are sutured together, and the anterior lateral walls are sutured directly to the bowel with interrupted 5–0 PDS. Where the suture line of the end of the ureters comes to the bowel, a horizontal mattress suture is placed to make the anastomosis watertight.

If a Y-type of anastomosis is desired, after suturing the posterior ureteral walls together as previously described, the anterior walls of the ureters are sutured together and the end of the composite anastomosis is sutured to the bowel. Again, where the suture lines meet the bowel, a horizontal mattress suture is placed so that the anastomosis is watertight.

The head-to-tail anastomosis involves suturing the end

of one ureter to the apex of the other. The posterior medial walls of the two ureters are approximated. The anterior lateral walls are sutured to the bowel. The Wallace anastomosis has the lowest complication rate of any of the ureteral intestinal anastomotic techniques. Stricture formation is approximately 3 per cent, deterioration of the upper tracts is about 4 per cent, and leakage is about 2 per cent (see Table 70–4). The Wallace technique is not recommended for a patient who has extensive carcinoma in situ or a high likelihood of recurrent tumor in the ureter. A recurrent tumor at the anastomotic line in one ureter would block both ureters causing uremia from bilateral obstruction.

The two small bowel ureterointestinal anastomoses as described are refluxing in type. The following techniques describe nonrefluxing anastomoses.

TUNNELED SMALL BOWEL ANASTOMOSIS (Fig. 70–20). This method attempts to establish a nonrefluxing anastomosis by creating a submucosal tunnel (Starr et al., 1975). Two 0.5-cm incisions are made in the serosa on the antimesenteric border 2.5 cm apart, at right angles to the long axis of the bowel. The seromuscular layer is then gently separated from the mucosa with a blunt hemostat. The ureter is pulled through one incision, a button of mucosa removed over the other incision, and the ureter spatulated and sutured to the mucosa with interrupted 5–0 PDS. The serosa is closed with interrupted 4–0 silk, and the adventitia of the ureter is sutured at its entrance through the serosa of the bowel to the serosa. Good results have been reported, but this technique has not been widely used, therefore long-term follow-up is not available.

SPLIT NIPPLE (Fig. 70–21). This method attempts to establish a nonrefluxing anastomosis by employing a nipple mechanism. This technique was described by Griffiths and involves forming a nipple in the ureter and implanting it into the small bowel (Turner-Warwick and Ashken, 1967). A 0.5-cm longitudinal incision in the ureter is made and the ureteral wall turned back on

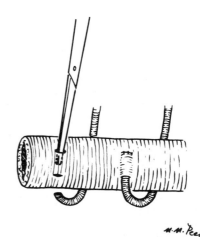

Figure 70–20. Tunneled small bowel anastomosis. A small transverse incision is made in the small bowel and a second transverse incision 3 cm lateral to it is also made. The submucosal tunnel is created, and a button of mucosa is removed. The ureter is drawn through the tunnel and sutured directly to the mucosa. The rent in the serosa is closed. An adventitial ureteral suture is placed and secured to the serosa at the ureter's entrance to the small bowel.

A   B

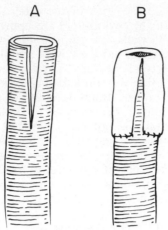

Figure 70–21. *A* and *B*, Split nipple technique. The ureter is spatulated and turned back on itself. The end of the ureter is secured to the adventitia of the ureter with interrupted 5–0 polydioxanone suture.

itself, creating a nipple at least twice as long as its width. The cuff is stabilized at the corners with sutures. A button of seromuscular and mucosal tissue is removed, the ureter is then placed into the bowel such that it protrudes through the mucosa.

The adventitia just proximal to the point where the ureter has been sewn to itself is sutured to the full thickness of the bowel wall with interrupted 5–0 PDS. The anastomosis is stented. In one series, this type of anastomosis prevented reflux in greater than 50 per cent of the patients and in other subsequent series, approximately 80 per cent of patients had a nonrefluxing anastomosis with an acceptably low incidence of stenosis (see Table 70–4).

LEDUC METHOD (Fig. 70–22). This method establishes a nonrefluxing anastomosis by laying the ureter onto the interior of the bowel wall—eventually resulting in a submucosal tunnel when it is reepithelialized

A.   B.   C.

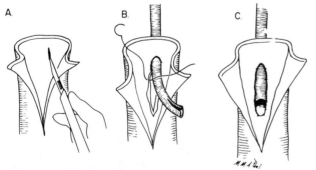

Figure 70–22. LeDuc ureterointestinal anastomosis. *A,* The small bowel is opened for approximately 4 to 5 cm. A longitudinal rent in the mucosa is made and the mucosa raised.

B, At the distal end of the mucosal rent, a hole is made in the serosa. The ureter is then drawn through. The entrance of the ureter through the serosa should be at least 2 cm proximal to the cut end of the bowel to allow for sufficient bowel length to close the end.

C, The ureter is spatulated and sutured to the mucosa and muscular layers. The mucosa is not reapproximated over the top of the ureter but rather sutured to the side of it.

(LeDuc et al., 1987). This technique has been utilized to prevent reflux in the ureteral small intestinal anastomosis. Excellent exposure is required; therefore, the small bowel needs to be opened along its antimesenteric border for a length of approximately 5 cm. The mucosa is incised for a length of 3 cm, beginning 2 cm proximal to the cut edge of the bowel. It is important to begin the mucosal tunnel away from the cut edge of the bowel to allow enough distal bowel for closure without jeopardizing the entrance point of the ureter. The ureter is brought through the serosa at the distal most portion of the mucosal sulcus, laid in the trough, spatulated, and sutured to the proximal end of the sulcus with interrupted 5–0 PDS utilizing the full thickness of ureteral wall and anchored to the muscularis and mucosal layers of the bowel.

The mucosa of the sulcus of the bowel is then sutured to the adventitia of the ureter. The mucosa of the bowel should not be sutured over the ureter but rather to its lateral aspect. The mucosa will eventually grow over the top of the ureter. Where the ureter enters the small bowel, its adventitia is sutured to the bowel serosa with 4–0 silk suture.

Stents are placed in the ureter, and their passage must be unimpeded to assure that there is no angulation. The bowel should be fixed to the body wall near the site of the ureteral implantation so that the ureters do not angulate. The complication rate for this technique is relatively low, although the follow-up is also relatively short. It carries with it an 87 per cent incidence of maintaining an antireflux valve, with a 5 per cent incidence of stricture and a 2 per cent incidence of leak (see Table 70–4).

Several other types of ureteral small intestinal anastomoses mainly involve buried ureter in the small bowel serosa and/or dissection of mucosa in a funnel-type valve. Neither of these techniques over the long-term have proved to be useful. However, a slight modification of these techniques does show promise.

HAMMOCK ANASTOMOSIS. This type of anastomosis has been described and involves conjoining the ureters and implanting them into the small bowel in a nonrefluxing manner. The small bowel is closed at its proximal end, and three 10-cm longitudinal incisions, separated by 1 to 2 mm, are made through the seromuscular layer to the mucosa. These incisions are crosshatched by multiple incisions. This effect serves as a hammock.

The ureters are conjoined as per the Wallace technique and sutured to the intestinal mucosa. The ureters are buried by closing the intestinal wall over the top of them with seromuscular sutures of 3–0 polyglycolic acid suture (Hirdes et al., 1988). With this technique there is a 6 per cent incidence of ureteroileal stenosis and approximately a 20 per cent incidence of reflux. At this time, follow-up, however, is relatively short.

INTESTINAL ANTIREFLUX VALVES

Another technique of preventing reflux into the ureter involves creation of an antireflux mechanism with the bowel distal to the ureterointestinal anastomosis. The ureter is sutured either by the technique of Bricker or Wallace as previously described to the end of the bowel, and the bowel is utilized to create a one-way valve. Three basic types of antireflux mechanisms are commonly employed utilizing the bowel: (1) ileocecal intussusception, (2) ileoileal intussusception, and (3) ileal nipple valve placed into colon.

INTUSSUSCEPTED ILEOCECAL VALVE (Fig. 70–23). The mesentery is cleaned from the ileum for a length of 8 cm beginning at the cecum and coursing proximal. At least 5 cm of ileum proximal to the detached mesentery must be intact to ensure intestinal viability. Thus, the ileum should not be transected less than 13 cm from the ileocecal junction. A No. 22 Fr. catheter is placed through the ileum into the cecum. The ileal serosa is scarified either by multiple cross incisions with a knife or by the electrocautery unit.

The 8-cm segment is intussuscepted over the catheter into the cecum. The intussuscepted ileum is secured to the cecal wall with 3–0 silk sutures placed circumferentially 2 mm apart. The valve has a moderate tendency to fail as the intussusception has a significant chance of reducing. In one series, the antireflux mechanism remained intact in 55 per cent of the patients over the long-term (Hensle and Burbige, 1985).

The intussusception may be made more secure by employing a modification described by King. The mes-

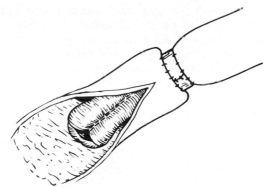

Figure 70–24. Intussuscepted ileal nipple valve. About 8 cm of ileal mesentery is cleaned from the serosa. Through an avascular place adjacent to the rent in the mesentery, a second rent is made. A polyglycolic acid mesh cuff of 2.5 cm width is placed but not secured. The ileum distally is opened within 2 to 3 cm of the rent in the mesentery. A total of 5 cm of ileum is intussuscepted and secured by placing staples in quadrants.

The ileal mucosa is incised adjacent to an incision in the intussuscepted segment, and the two muscularis are sutured together with interrupted 3–0 chromic. The polyglycolic acid mesh cuff is then sutured together snugly, a No. 24 Fr. catheter having been placed to make sure that the collar is not too snug. The cuff is then sutured to the intussuscepted segment distally and proximally to the base of the ileum, into which the proximal segment is intussuscepted with interrupted chromic suture.

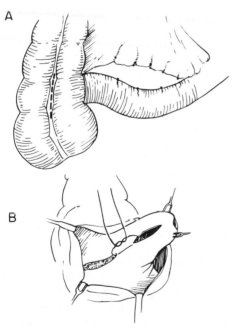

Figure 70–23. Ileocecal intussusception. *A,* An 8-cm segment of ileal mesentery is cleaned from the serosa beginning at the ileocecal junction. At least 5 cm of mesentery remains attached to the proximal ileum. An incision is made along a tinea at the level of the ileocecal valve.

B, The ileum is intussuscepted over a No. 22 Fr. catheter into the cecum under direct vision. The mucosa of the intussuscepted segment is incised, and the mucosa of the cecum adjacent to it is also incised. The muscularis of both segments are sutured together. The serosa of the ileum is secured to the serosa of the cecum with interrupted 3–0 silk sutures placed circumferentially (not depicted).

entery is cleaned as previously discussed. The cecum is opened along a tinea and the ileum intussuscepted over the catheter under direct vision. Where the intussusception lies adjacent to the cecal wall, mucosa of the intussuscepted ileum and the cecal mucosa adjacent to it are incised down to muscle. The muscles are sewn to each other with interrupted 3–0 chromic suture. Long-term follow-up in 8 patients reveals maintenance of the antireflux valve in seven, using the modified technique (King, 1987).

INTUSSUSCEPTED ILEAL VALVE (Fig. 70–24). The mesentery is cleaned from an 8-cm segment of ileal serosa. There must be 5 cm of ileal mesentery proximal and distal to the cleared segment to ensure proper blood supply. A 2.5-cm wide strip of polyglycolic mesh is placed through an avascular area in the mesentery, adjacent to the serosa proximal to the mesenteric rent. It is left alone until the intussusception is secured. The ureters will be sewn to the proximal end of ileum. The distal end of ileum is opened along its antimesenteric boarder to within 2 to 3 cm of the cleared mesentery to provide adequate exposure and direct visualization of the intussuscepted segment. A Babcock clamp is placed into the lumen of the bowel and a portion of bowel wall grasped by invaginating it into the clamp with a finger. The ileal segment is intussuscepted by pulling on the Babcock clamp with gentle constant traction. If there is resistance, the mesentery is generally too bulky. It must be defatted carefully before trying again to intussuscept the segment. When intussuscepted, the polyglycolic mesh should lie at the base of the intussuscepted segment. A 5-cm intussuscepted segment should protrude.

Using the gastrointestinal stapler without the knife or the linear stapler (from both of which the distal 5 to 8 staples have been removed), three rows with the former or four rows with the latter are placed in quadrants to secure the intussusception in place. The staple size should be 4.8 mm. The proximal staples are important in securing the intussusception and preventing its reduction. The distal staples are less effective and more prone to be exposed to urine, thus facilitating stone formation. It is for this reason that the distal staples are removed from the staple cartridge before being placed in the stapler and before stapling the intussusception.

Using the cautery unit, the mucosa of the intussusception is incised along its length. Adjacent to this incision, another is made in the mucosa of the ileum. The muscularis of both are exposed and sewn together with interrupted 3–0 chromic suture. With a finger inside the intussuscepted segment, the polyglycolic mesh is formed into a collar and secured firmly and sutured to itself. It is then sutured proximally to the intussuscepted segment circumferentially and distally to the serosa of the ileum circumferentially, into which the segment was intussuscepted with 3–0 chromic sutures. This maneuver is meant to secure the intussusception and prevent its reduction with failure of the antireflux mechanism. The valve is successful in preventing reflux 90 per cent of the time (Kock et al., 1982; Skinner et al., 1989).

NIPPLE VALVE (Fig. 70–25). The simplest intestinal antireflux valve to create is the nipple valve utilizing ileum. The mesentery is cleared from the last 8 cm of the cut end of the ileum. The distal 6 cm of serosa is scarified by multiple cross striations and then turned back on itself to form a nipple. The nipple should be at least 4 to 4.5 cm in length. The end of the inverted ileum is sutured to itself with interrupted 4–0 PDS. An incision on the tinea, which is large enough to accommodate the segment, is made. A No. 22 Fr. catheter is placed through the segment, and its serosa is sutured to the colon serosa circumferentially with interrupted 3–0

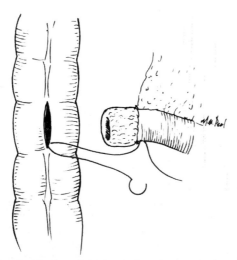

Figure 70–25. Nipple valve. Approximately 8 cm of mesentery is cleaned from the distal end of the ileum. The serosa is scarified and turned back on itself to form a nipple of approximately 4 cm in length. The end of the ileum is sutured to itself with interrupted 4–0 polydioxanone suture (PDS). A rent is made in the colon through a tinea. The nipple valve is placed through the rent and secured in place with circumferential interrupted 4–0 PDS, placed through the full thickness of the colon and the seromuscular layer of the ileum.

silk sutures placed 2 mm apart. The long-term success rate for this type of valve is unknown but would appear to be less than that for the other two methods as described.

COMPLICATIONS OF URETEROINTESTINAL ANASTOMOSES

The complications that occur with ureterointestinal anastomoses include leakage, stricture, and reflux in those anastomoses that were performed to prevent reflux and pyelonephritis. In reviewing the various types of procedures, it appears that of the colonic antirefluxing procedures, i.e., the Pagano technique, offers the lowest incidence of stricture with an acceptable incidence of reflux. With respect to small bowel antireflux procedures, the LeDuc procedure seems to offer the lowest incidence of stricture with the highest success rate in preventing reflux. With respect to stricture formation and leakage, it appears the Wallace technique has the best results. However, in a comparison of the Bricker, the open technique, the Wallace, and the nipple valve in one series, there was no difference in complication rate among any of the procedures. All had an incidence of approximately 29 per cent of some form of obstruction over the long-term (Mansson et al., 1979).

URINARY FISTULAS. Urinary fistulas invariably occur within the first 7 to 10 days postoperative, with an incidence of 3 to 9 per cent (Beckley et al., 1982; Loening et al., 1982) (see Table 70–4). The incidence of urinary intestinal leak is markedly reduced by the use of soft Silastic stents (see previous discussion). A urinary intestinal leak may cause periureteral fibrosis and scarring, with subsequent stricture formation.

STRICTURES. In general, antirefluxing techniques have a slightly higher incidence of strictures. A patient is at risk for ureterointestinal stricture for the life of the anastomosis and must be followed on a scheduled, periodic basis. A stricture has been reported to develop 13 years following the procedure (Shapiro et al., 1975). Ureteral strictures also occur away from the ureterointestinal anastomosis. These are most common in the left ureter and are usually found as the ureter crosses over the aorta, beneath the inferior mesenteric artery. It has been suggested that this finding is due to too aggressive stripping of adventitia and angulation of the ureter at the inferior mesenteric artery.

Once a stricture has developed, various techniques may be utilized to rectify the situation. The most successful is re-exploration—removing the stenotic segment and reanastomosing the ureter to the bowel by one of the aforementioned techniques. In a study that compared open surgical correction of ureterointestinal anastomotic strictures with endourologic methods, it was found that the open procedure resulted in an approximately 90 per cent success rate, whereas endourologic methods resulted in a 70 per cent early success rate. As follow-up increased, a significant number of those treated endourologically failed. The morbidity, of course, with the endourologic procedures was less (Kramolowsky et al., 1988).

Open surgical methods may be morbid and very difficult procedures. Endourologic procedures employing balloon dilatation and/or incision of the stricture have a lesser morbidity. When several series employing endourologic methods are combined, there is a 50 per cent success rate over the short-term. At this juncture, there are no long-term studies that would indicate that the 50 per cent success rate will be long lasting (Kramolowsky et al., 1987).

PYELONEPHRITIS. Acute pyelonephritis occurs both in the early postoperative period and over the long-term. Its incidence is approximately 12 per cent in patients who underwent diversion with ileal conduits and 9 per cent in those who underwent diversion with antirefluxing colon conduits (see Table 70–3). These complications cause considerable morbidity and, in fact, are associated with significant mortality. In one series of intestinal segments in the urinary tract, eight of 178 patients died of sepsis (Schmidt et al., 1973). The fact that these complications may result in delayed mortality is indicated by the fact that two of 115 children and three of 127 adults died of septic complications, five to 14 years following intestinal diversion (Pitts and Muecke, 1979). When sepsis is associated with decreasing renal function and uremia, the morbidity and mortality are markedly increased.

Table 70–4 summarizes the complications and success rates for the various types of anastomoses. The information is derived from composite reports in the literature in which specific anastomoses were discussed and from which data could be accurately analyzed. Because of these two requirements, it is not possible to comment, for example, on the incidences of reflux or leakage among various anastomotic types inclusively. These complications can be minimized by adhering to the principles of ureterointestinal surgery as discussed.

RENAL DETERIORATION

The incidence of renal deterioration following conduit urinary intestinal diversion has varied from 10 to 60 per cent. This is perhaps due to the fact that many reports include both renal units that were abnormal as well as those that were normal prior to diversion. When analyzing abnormal renal units prior to diversion and documenting progressive disease, it is difficult to be sure whether the urinary diversion caused the progression or whether the progression is due to the intrinsic abnormality for which the diversion was created. When the incidence of renal deterioration is determined by comparing renal units that were normal prediversion and then deteriorated postdiversion, 18 per cent of patients who have ileal conduits will show progressive deterioration vs. 13 per cent who have nonrefluxing colon conduits (see Table 70–3).

Of patients with nonrefluxing continent ileal cecal bladders, 20 per cent show some evidence of deterioration of the upper tracts when followed over the long-term (Benchekroun, 1987). This deterioration leads to a 10 per cent (8/96) incidence of azotemia in children

with ileal conduits (Schwarz and Jeffs, 1975) and a 12 per cent (5/41) incidence of renal failure in patients with colon conduits constructed for benign disease (Elder et al., 1979).

The incidence of both sepsis and renal failure is greater in patients with ureterosigmoidostomy than in those with conduits. Sepsis and renal failure may occur in the immediate postoperative period or many years later. The most common cause of death in a patient who has had a ureterosigmoidostomy for more than 15 years is acquired renal disease, i.e., sepsis or renal failure. In this group of patients, approximately 10 to 22 per cent succumb to these disorders (Zabbo and Kay, 1986), some as late as 4 to 27 years after the diversion (Mesrobian et al., 1988). In patients with ileal conduits, about 6 per cent will ultimately die of renal failure (Richie, 1974).

Renal Function Necessary for Urinary Intestinal Diversion

The amount of renal function required to effectively blunt the reabsorption of urinary solutes by the intestinal segment and prevent serious metabolic side effects is dependent on the type of urinary intestinal diversion created—the amount of bowel to be used and the length of time the urine will be exposed to the intestinal mucosa. Thus, a greater degree of renal function is necessary for retentive (continent) diversions than for short conduit diversions.

It is beyond the scope of this chapter to discuss all the ramifications of renal function, but several points must be understood if patients are to be properly evaluated. There are five components of renal function: renal blood flow, glomerular filtration, tubule transport, concentration and dilution, and glomerular permeability. Those aspects of renal function that must be specifically addressed are glomerular filtration rate, best determined by an inulin clearance, ability of the tubule to acidify as determined by ammonium chloride loading, concentrating ability as determined by water deprivation, and glomerular permeability as determined by urinary protein concentrations.

In general, patients with normal urinary protein content who have a serum creatinine level below 2.0 mg/dl will do well with intestine interposed in the urinary tract. At a level of serum creatinine below 2.0 mg/dl, renal blood flow, glomerular filtration rate, tubule transport, and concentrating and diluting ability are relatively well preserved. In a patient with a serum creatinine level that exceeds 2.0 mg/dl who is being considered for retentive diversion or in whom long segments of intestine will be used, a more detailed analysis of renal function is necessary. If the patient has a urine pH of 5.8 or less following an ammonium chloride load, a urine osmolality of 600 mOsm/kg or greater in response to water deprivation, a glomerular filtration rate that exceeds 35 ml/min, and minimal protein in the urine, he or she may be considered for a retentive diversion.

METABOLIC AND NEUROMECHANICAL PROBLEMS OF URINARY INTESTINAL DIVERSION

Problems that occur as a result of interposing intestine in the urinary tract may be conveniently divided into three areas for the purposes of discussion: (1) metabolic, (2) neuromechanical, and (3) technical/surgical. Metabolic complications are the result of altered solute reabsorption by the intestine of the urine which it contains. Neuromechanical aspects involve the configuration of the gut that affects storage volume and contraction of the intestine that may lead to difficulties in storage. Finally, technical/surgical complications involve those aspects of the procedure that result in surgical morbidity. The last of these has been discussed following each section on the technical aspects of urinary intestinal diversion. The following is a discussion of metabolic and neuromechanical problems.

METABOLIC COMPLICATIONS. Metabolic complications include (1) electrolyte abnormalities, (2) altered sensorium, (3) abnormal drug metabolism, (4) osteomalacia, (5) growth retardation, (6) persistent and recurrent infections, (7) formation of renal and reservoir calculi, (8) problems ensuing from removal of portions of the gut from the intestinal tract, and (9) development of urothelial/intestinal cancer. Many of these complications are a consequence of altered solute absorption across the intestinal segment. The factors that influence the amount of solute and type of absorption are the segment of bowel utilized, the surface area of the bowel, the amount of time the urine is exposed to the bowel, the concentration of solutes in the urine, the renal function, and the pH of the fluid.

ELECTROLYTE ABNORMALITIES. Serum electrolyte complications and the type of electrolyte abnormalities that occur are different, depending on the segment of bowel utilized. If stomach is employed, a hypochloremic metabolic alkalosis may occur. If jejunum is the segment used, hyponatremia, hyperkalemia, and metabolic acidosis occur. If the ileum or colon is utilized, a hyperchloremic metabolic acidosis ensues. Other electrolyte abnormalities that have been described include hypokalemia, hypomagnesemia, hypocalcemia, hyperammonemia, and elevated blood urea and creatinine levels. The subsequent discussion details specific abnormalities for each segment of intestine.

Electrolyte disorders that occur when jejunum is utilized for urinary intestinal diversion, particularly proximal jejunum, include hyponatremia, hypochloremia, hyperkalemia, azotemia, and acidosis. These result from an increased secretion of sodium and chloride with an increased reabsorption of potassium and hydrogen ions. This excessive loss of sodium chloride carries with it water, and thus the patient becomes dehydrated. The dehydration results in hypovolemia that increases renin secretion and thereby aldosterone production (Golimbu and Morales, 1975). Aldosterone production may also be stimulated by hyperkalemia. The high levels of renin aldosterone facilitate sodium reabsorption by the kidney and potassium loss, which produces a urine low in sodium and high in potassium. This urine, when presented to the jejunum, results in a favorable concentration gradient for loss of sodium by the jejunum and an increased reabsorption of potassium, thus perpetuating the abnormalities.

These electrolyte abnormalities result in lethargy, nausea, vomiting, dehydration, muscular weakness, and elevated temperature. If allowed to persist, the patient may become moribund and finally succumb. This syndrome may be exacerbated by administering hyperalimentation solutions. The mechanism by which hyperalimentation solutions exacerbate this syndrome in a patient with jejunal intestine interposed in the urinary tract is unclear (Bonnheim et al., 1984). The severity of the syndrome depends on the location of the segment of jejunum which is used. The more proximal the segment, the more likely the syndrome is to develop. Its incidence varies from 25 per cent of patients (Klein et al., 1986) to the majority of patients demonstrating significant abnormalities. The treatment for the disorder is rehydration with sodium chloride and correction of the acidosis with sodium bicarbonate. Provided renal function is normal, the hyperkalemia will be corrected by renal secretion. After restoration of normal electrolyte balance, long-term therapy involves oral supplements with sodium chloride.

The electrolyte abnormality that occurs with the ileum and colon is a hyperchloremic metabolic acidosis. This acidosis develops to some degree in most patients who have ileum or colon interposed in the urinary tract but is generally of a minor degree. Its clinical significance when it is of a minor degree, at this time, is unknown. Hyperchloremic acidosis has been reported with a frequency of 68 per cent (19/28)—ten of the 19 cases were severe enough to require treatment—in patients with ileal conduits (Castro and Ram, 1970).

In another study, 70 per cent of patients with ileal conduits followed for 4 years or more had decreased bicarbonate levels (Malek et al., 1971). A severe electrolyte disturbance occurs to a much lesser degree; severe electrolyte disturbances have been reported to be a major problem in 18 per cent (8/45) of patients with intestinal cystoplasties (Whitmore and Gittes, 1983); in 10 per cent (17/178) of patients with ileal conduits (Schmidt et al., 1973); and in 80 per cent (112/141) of patients with ureterosigmoidostomies (Ferris and Odel, 1950). In continent diversions involving ileum and cecum or cecum alone, the majority of patients have elevated serum chloride and depressed serum bicarbonate levels (Ashken, 1987; McDougal, 1986). Of the patients with MAINZ pouches, 65 per cent require alkali therapy to maintain a normal acid-base balance (Thuroff et al., 1987). Early reports of patients with continent diversions made of ileum have a much lower incidence of electrolyte problems in the range of 10 to 15 per cent (Allen, 1985; Boyd et al., 1989) (see Table 70–3). Symptoms in those in whom the syndrome is severe include fatigability, anorexia, weight loss, polydipsia, and lethargy. Those with ureterosigmoidostomies also have exacerbation of their diarrhea.

These electrolyte abnormalities, if significant and allowed to persist, result in major metabolic abnormalities discussed subsequently. In and of themselves, however, they may be lethal to the patient. Severe electrolyte abnormalities have contributed to patient death (Heidler et al., 1979).

The treatment of hyperchloremic metabolic acidosis involves administering alkalizing agents and/or blockers of chloride transport. Alkalinization with oral sodium bicarbonate is very effective in restoring normal acid-base balance. Oral administration of bicarbonate, however, may not be tolerated particularly well because it can produce considerable intestinal gas. Bicitra or Shohl's Solution (sodium citrate and citric acid) is an effective alternative; however, many patients do not care for the taste. Polycitra (potassium citrate, sodium citrate, citric acid) may be used instead, if excessive sodium administration is a problem due to cardiac or renal disease and if potassium supplementation is desirable or at least not harmful.

In those patients in whom persistent hyperchloremic metabolic acidosis occurs and in whom excessive sodium loads are undesirable, chlorpromazine or nicotinic acid may be given to limit the degree of acidosis. These agents used alone do not correct acidosis, but they limit its development and thus reduce the need for alkalinizing agents. Chlorpromazine and nicotinic acid inhibit cyclic AMP and thereby impede chloride transport. Chlorpromazine may be given in a dose of 25 mg three times a day (t.i.d.). Occasionally, as much as 50 mg t.i.d. may be necessary, but at such doses side effects are not uncommon. Chlorpromazine should be used with care in adults because there are many untoward side effects, including tardive dyskinesia. Nicotinic acid may be given in a dose of 400 mg three to four times a day. The drug should not be administered to patients with peptic ulcer disease or significant hepatic insufficiency. Those side effects that may be observed include exacerbation of liver dysfunction, exacerbation of peptic ulcer disease, headaches, and double vision. Flushing and dermatitis are not uncommon and generally disappear as the patient becomes adapted to the drug.

Hypokalemia and total body depletion of potassium may occur in patients with urinary intestinal diversion. These side effects are more common in patients with ureterosigmoidostomies than those with other types of urinary intestinal diversion (Geist and Ansell, 1961). In one study, patients with ureterocolonic diversions had a 30 per cent reduction in total body potassium, whereas those with ileal conduits had, as a group, no significant alteration in total body potassium. However, individually, some had as much as a 14 per cent reduction in total body potassium (Williams et al., 1967). The depletion is probably due to renal potassium wasting as a consequence of renal damage, and osmotic diuresis and of gut loss through intestinal secretion. The last, probably quantitatively, plays a relatively minor role.

Ileal segments when exposed to high concentrations of potassium in the urine reabsorb some of the potassium, whereas colon is less likely to do so (Koch et al., 1990). Thus, ileum interposed in the urinary tract likely blunts the potassium loss by the kidney, whereas colon does not, thus explaining why patients with ureterosigmoidostomies and ureterocolonic diversions are more likely to be total body potassium depleted. When the depletion is severe, the patient may develop a flaccid paralysis. If the hypokalemia is associated with severe hyperchloremic metabolic acidosis, treatment must involve replacement of potassium as well as correcting acidosis with bicarbonate. If the acidosis is corrected without attention to potassium replacement, severe hypokalemia may occur, marked flaccid paralysis may develop, and significant morbidity may ensue (Koff, 1975).

Because the bowel transports solutes and because its membrane is not particularly watertight, osmolality generally re-equilibrates across the bowel wall. Thus, attempts to deprive a patient of water and determine osmolality as a reflection of renal function are inappropriate because the bowel alters the osmotic content. The bowel also makes the contents more alkaline; therefore, it is impossible to determine the ability of the kidney to acidify simply by measuring urinary pH in patients with urinary intestinal diversion. Because urea and creatinine are reabsorbed by both the ileum and colon, serum concentrations of urea and creatinine do not necessarily reflect accurately the renal function (Koch and McDougal, 1985; McDougal and Koch, 1986).

Histologic alterations of the intestine may take place over time when urine is chronically exposed to the mucosa. Villous atrophy and pseudocrypt formation may occur, particularly in the ileum. These changes are patchy because normal ileal mucosa is interspersed between these abnormalities. Submucosal inflammatory infiltrates may also be observed. There appears to be fewer changes in the colonic mucosa over the long term. In the colon, a decrease in the size of goblet cells has been described. Over time, some transport processes may be altered. Some solutes are less actively transported. At the same time, other processes of solute transport remain active (Philipson et al., 1983). However, the ability to establish hyperchloremic metabolic acidosis appears to be retained by most segments of ileum and colon over time.

ALTERED SENSORIUM. Alteration of the sensorium may occur as a consequence of magnesium deficiency, drug intoxication, or ammonia metabolism abnormalities. Patients who develop magnesium deficiency do so either secondary to nutritional depletion or in relation to magnesium wasting by the kidney, in much the same way that calcium wasting occurs (see subsequent discussion). Alterations in the sensorium have also occurred because of diabetic hyperglycemia; however, this is not a consequence of the intestinal diversion. In such patients, however, reabsorption of urinary glucose can result in hyperglycemia without demonstrable glucosuria (Onwubalili, 1982).

Perhaps the more common cause of altered sensorium is a consequence of altered ammonia metabolism. Ammoniagenic coma in patients with urinary intestinal diversion has been reported in those with cirrhosis (Silberman, 1958), in those with altered liver function without underlying chronic liver disease (McDermott, 1957), and in those with normal hepatic function as determined by serum enzyme studies (Kaufman, 1984; Mounger and Branson, 1972). The syndrome, however, is most commonly associated with decreased liver function. Even in those cases in which normal liver function has been reported, the crude methods by which it was assessed has not confirmed that subtle alterations in liver function are not present. The syndrome is most commonly reported in patients with ureterosigmoidostomies but has been reported in those with ileal conduits as well (McDermott, 1957).

The treatment of ammoniagenic coma involves draining the urinary intestinal diversion with either a rectal tube in the case of ureterosigmoidostomy or a Foley catheter in the case of continent diversion, so that the urine does not remain exposed to the intestine for extended periods of time. Neomycin is administered orally to reduce the ammonia load from the enteric tract. Protein consumption is curtailed, thus limiting the nitrogen load until serum ammonium levels return to normal. In severe circumstances, arginine glutamate, 50 g in 1000 ml of 5 per cent dextrose in water (D5W), may be given intravenously. This solution complexes the ammonia by providing substrate for the formation of glutamine (Silberman, 1958). Lactulose may be given orally or rectally (Edwards, 1984) and will complex the ammonia in the gut and prevent its absorption.

ABNORMAL DRUG ABSORPTION. Drug intoxication has been reported in patients with urinary intestinal diversions. Drugs that are more likely to be a problem are those that are absorbed by the gastrointestinal tract and excreted unchanged by the kidney. Thus, the excreted drug is re-exposed to the intestinal segment that then reabsorbs it, and thus toxic serum levels develop. This finding has been reported for phenytoin (Dilantin) (Savarirayan and Dixey, 1969) and has been observed for certain antibiotics that are excreted unchanged.

Although chemotherapy is generally well tolerated by patients with conduits, methotrexate toxicity has been documented in a patient with an ileal conduit (Bowyer and Davies, 1986). In those patients who are receiving antimetabolites, one must carefully monitor those toxic antimetabolites that are excreted in the urine and are capable of intestinal absorption less lethal toxic serum levels develop. Moreover, in patients with continent diversions who are receiving chemotherapy, consideration should be given to draining the pouch during the period of time the toxic drugs are being administered.

OSTEOMALACIA. Osteomalacia or renal rickets occurs when mineralized bone is reduced and the osteoid component becomes excessive. Osteomalacia has been reported in patients with colocystoplasty (Hassain, 1970), ileal ureters (Salahudeen et al., 1984), and colon and ileal conduits, and most commonly in patients with ureterosigmoidostomies (Harrison, 1958; Specht, 1967). The etiology of osteomalacia may be multifactorial but commonly involves significant acidosis. With persistent acidosis, the excess protons are buffered by the bone with release of bone calcium. With its release, calcium is excreted by the kidney. Support for chronic acidosis being the cause of the osteomalacia comes from those cases in which the correction of the acidosis results in remineralization of the bone (Richards et al., 1972; Siklos et al., 1980). However, major alterations in serum

bicarbonate are not necessary in order for the syndrome to develop (Koch and McDougal, 1988; McDougal et al., 1988).

Moreover, some patients with osteomalacia secondary to urinary intestinal diversion do not experience corrections of bony demineralization with restoration of normal acid-base balance. These patients have been found to manifest vitamin D resistance, which is independent of the acidosis. It is likely that this resistance is of renal origin. Resistance can be overcome by supplying 1α-hydroxycholecalciferol, a vitamin D metabolite that is much more potent than vitamin D_2. By providing this substrate in an excess amount, remineralization of bone occurs (Perry et al., 1977).

Reabsorption of urinary solutes may play a role in increasing calcium excretion by the kidney. Sulfate filtered by the kidney inhibits calcium reabsorption and results in both calcium and magnesium loss by the kidney. Thus, if the gut increases its sulfate reabsorption and requires the kidney to increase its sulfate excretion, hypercalciuria and hypermagnesuria will result (McDougal and Koch, 1989).

In summary, osteomalacia in urinary intestinal diversion may be due to persistent acidosis, vitamin D resistance, and excessive calcium loss by the kidney. The degree to which each of these contributes to the syndrome may vary from patient to patient.

Those patients who develop osteomalacia generally complain of lethargy; joint pain, especially in the weight bearing joints; and proximal myopathy. Analysis of serum chemistry results reveals that the calcium is either low or normal. The alkaline phosphatase level is elevated, and the phosphate level is low or normal (Harrison, 1958). The treatment as previously indicated involves correcting the acidosis and providing dietary supplements of calcium. If this therapy does not result in remineralization of the bone, the active form of vitamin D may be administered. If this is not successful, the more active metabolite of vitamin D_3, 1α-hydroxycholecalciferol should be administered.

GROWTH AND DEVELOPMENT. Considerable evidence suggests that urinary intestinal diversion has a detrimental effect on growth and development. In a study of 93 myelodysplasia patients followed for 17 to 23 years, significant aberrations in growth were noted when morphometric parameters were analyzed. Anthropometric measurements in those with urinary intestinal diversions showed a decrease in linear growth in all indices measured with a statistically significant decrease in biacromial span and in elbow-hand length. More patients with urinary intestinal diversions fell below the 10th percentile than did patients with intermittent catheterizations. There was in fact no difference in height and weight between the two groups studied (McDougal and Koch, 1991). There is also experimental evidence for impaired linear growth in urinary intestinal diversion. Rats with unilateral ureterosigmoidostomies, when followed over the long-term, demonstrate significantly decreased femoral bone length when compared with controls (Koch and McDougal, 1988). Although obvious alterations in growth and development are not usually noticed, when carefully studied, patients who have urinary intestinal diversions created in childhood that were maintained for more than 10 years have significant changes in linear growth.

INFECTION. Increased incidences are noted of bacteriuria and bacteremia and septic episodes, in patients with bowel interposition. A significant number of patients with intestinal cystoplasty develop pyelonephritis, and 13 per cent have septic and major infectious complications (Kuss et al., 1970). The episodes are more frequent following colocystoplasty than ileocystoplasty (Kuss et al., 1970). Acute pyelonephritis occurs in 10 to 17 per cent of patients with colon and ileal conduits (Hagen-Cook and Althausen, 1979; Schmidt et al., 1973; Schwarz and Jeffs, 1975). Approximately 4 per cent (8/178) of patients with ileal conduits die of sepsis (Schmidt et al., 1973).

Patients with conduits have a high incidence of bacteriuria. Indeed, approximately three fourths of ileal conduit urine samples are infected (Elder et al., 1979; Guinan et al., 1972; Middleton and Hendren, 1976). Some cases are merely colonized at the distal ends of the conduits because the incidence of positive findings can be markedly diminished by culturing the proximal portion of the loop by a double catheter technique (Smith, 1972). Many of the patients so affected, however, show no untoward effects and seem to do quite well even with chronic bacteriuria.

Deterioration of the upper tracts is more likely when the culture becomes dominant for *Proteus* or *Pseudomonas*. Thus, patients with relatively pure cultures of these organisms should be treated, whereas those with mixed cultures may generally be observed provided they are not symptomatic.

Patients with continent diversions also have a significant incidence of bacteriuria and septic episodes (McDougal, 1986). Indeed, two thirds of patients with Kock continent diversions have positive culture findings (Kock, 1987). The reasons for the increased incidence of bacteriuria and sepsis are unclear, but it is likely that the intestine is incapable of inhibiting bacterial proliferation unlike the urothelium. Thus, bacteria that normally live symbiotically in the intestine serve as a source for ascending infection and septic complications when these segments are interposed in the urinary tract. Moreover, the intestine may make the urine less bacteriostatic and thereby promote the growth of bacteria.

STONES. One of the consequences of persistent infection is the development of magnesium ammonium phosphate stones. Indeed, the majority of stones formed in patients with urinary intestinal diversions are composed of calcium, magnesium, and ammonium phosphate. Those most prone to develop renal calculi are patients who have hyperchloremic metabolic acidosis, pre-existing pyelonephritis, and urinary tract infection with a urea-splitting organism (Dretler, 1973). The incidence of renal stones in patients with colon conduits is 3 to 4 per cent (Althausen et al., 1978; Hagen-Cook and Althausen, 1979) and in those with ileal conduits, 10 to 12 per cent (Schmidt et al., 1973).

In those with continent cecal reservoirs, there is a 20 per cent incidence of calculi within the reservoir (Ashken, 1987). The stones may be due to persistent infection

with alkalinization of the urine, persistent hypercalciuria for reasons previously described, and alteration of urinary excretion products by the intestine. A major cause in conduits and pouches of calculus formation is a foreign body, such as staples or nonabsorbable sutures, on which concretions form.

SHORT BOWEL AND NUTRITIONAL PROBLEMS. Many nutritional problems may occur as the result of a loss of significant intestinal absorptive surface due to the removal of substantial portions of the gut for construction of urinary intestinal diversions. In a patient with a significant loss of ileum, vitamin B_{12} malabsorption has been reported and results in anemia and neurologic abnormalities. Vitamin B_{12} deficiency has been shown to occur in ten of 41 patients who received radiotherapy prior to radical cystectomy and ileal ureterostomy (Kinn and Lantz, 1984).

Loss of significant portions of the ileum also results in malabsorption of bile salts. Because the ileum is the major site of bile salt reabsorption, the lack of their reabsorption allows them entry into the colon, which causes mucosal irritation and diarrhea. Also, loss of the ileum results in the loss of the "ileal break." The ileal break is a mechanism whereby when lipids come in contact with the ileal mucosa, gut motility is reduced so that increased absorption can occur. With the loss of ileum, the lipid does not result in decreased motility and is presented unmetabolized to the colon, which may result in fatty diarrhea.

Loss of the ileal cecal valve may have a number of untoward effects. Because of the loss of the valve, reflux of large concentrations of bacteria into the ileum may occur that will result in small intestinal bacterial overgrowth. This may result in nutritional abnormalities that involve interference with fatty acid reabsorption and bile salt interaction. With the lack of absorption of fats and bile salts, these are presented to the colon and result in diarrhea. Moreover, reflux of bacteria into the small bowel may result in bacterial metabolism of vitamin B_{12}, which may result in its deficiency. The lack of fat absorption may produce deficiencies of the fat-soluble vitamins, which may lead to visual disturbances due to the lack of vitamin A and osteomalacia due to the lack of vitamin D and the complexing of calcium with the fats to form soaps and thus lack of its absorption. The ileal cecal valve also serves as a break, and an intact valve prolongs transit time of the small bowel and enhances absorption. Thus, its loss may contribute to nutritional abnormalities.

Loss of the jejunum to a significant degree may result in malabsorption of fat, calcium, and folic acid; however, it is rare that significant portions of jejunum are utilized for urologic reconstructive procedures. Loss of the colon may result in (1) diarrhea due to lack of fluid and electrolyte absorption, (2) loss of bicarbonate due to its increased secretion in the ileum and lack of reabsorption, and (3) dehydration due to the loss of fluids.

CANCER. The incidence of cancer developing in a patient with ureterosigmoidostomy varies between 6 and 29 per cent, with a mean of 11 per cent (Schipper and Decter, 1981; Stewart et al., 1982; Zabbo and Kay,

1986). Generally, a 10- to 20-year delay occurs before the cancer becomes manifest. Histologically, the tumors include adenocarcinomas, adenomatous polyps, sarcomas, and transitional cell carcinomas. Case reports of tumors developing in patients with ileal conduits, colon conduits, and bladder augmentation have been described. Anaplastic carcinomas and adenomatous polyps have been reported in patients with ileal conduits. Adenocarcinoma has developed in patients with colon conduits. Bladder augmentations, using both ileum and colon, have developed adenocarcinomas, undifferentiated carcinomas, sarcomas, and transitional cell carcinomas (Filmer, 1986).

The etiologic mechanism of the development of the carcinoma is not understood. Whether the tumor arises from transitional epithelium or colonic epithelium is unclear. Because most of the tumors are adenocarcinomas, it has been assumed that the tumor arises from the intestinal epithelium. Adenocarcinomas have been shown to arise from transitional cell epithelium exposed to the fecal stream in the experimental animal (Aaronson et al., 1987). Furthermore, studies show that the ureters in patients with ureterosigmoidostomies have an exceedingly high incidence of dysplasia (Aaronson and Sinclair-Smith, 1984). Moreover, if the transitional epithelium is removed from the enteric tract, patients do not develop adenocarcinomas.

However, if the urothelium is left in contact with the intestinal mucosa, even though the diversion is defunctionalized and the area is not bathed in urine, adenocarcinoma may still develop. This is illustrated by a case report in which a patient developed cancer who had a ureterosigmoidostomy that was defunctionalized 9 months following its creation with a conduit. The distal ureters at the sigmoid were left in situ. The patient developed cancer at the site of the ureterointestinal anastomosis 22 years later (Schipper and Decter, 1981). This suggests that when ureterointestinal anastomoses are defunctionalized, they should be excised rather than merely ligated and left in situ. Other evidence including cell-staining techniques suggest that the colon is the primary organ of origin (Mundy, 1991). Whether the urothelium or intestine is the primary site of origin, it seems likely that tumors can arise from both tissues. The highest incidence of cancer occurs when the transitional epithelium is juxtaposed to the colonic epithelium and both are bathed by feces and urine (Shands et al., 1989).

Nitrosamines, known mutagens, are produced in rats with ureterosigmoidostomy (Cohen et al., 1987), but there appears at least at this juncture no convincing evidence to support a primary role for them in the genesis of the tumor. An abnormal pattern of colonic mucin secretion has been demonstrated in patients with ureterosigmoidostomies, but its significance is unclear (Iannoni et al., 1986). Induction of specific enzymes associated with carcinoma have also been demonstrated. Ornithine decarboxylase, an enzyme that has been found to be elevated in malignant colonic mucosa is also elevated in experimental animals with vesicosigmoidostomy (Weber et al., 1988). The role epidermal growth factor plays is currently being investigated. At this time, the etiology of the genesis of cancer in urinary intestinal diversion is not known. Because its incidence is significant in patients with ureterosigmoidostomies, they should have routine colonoscopies on a frequent periodic basis.

NEUROMECHANICAL ASPECTS OF INTESTINAL SEGMENTS

Both small bowel and colon contract to propel luminal contents in an aboral direction. The ability to propel luminal contents is a consequence of muscular activity as well as coordinated nerve activity. Both the small bowel and colon have an outer longitudinal layer of muscle and an inner circular layer. A muscularis mucosa is immediately beneath the mucosa and may extend into the villi. The outer and inner layers of muscle, however, play the major role in peristalsis. In the colon, the outer longitudinal layer of muscle condenses to form three tenia coli. The bowel receives its parasympathetic innervation from the vagus. It is also innervated by the sympathetic nervous system. The nerves lie between the circular and longitudinal layers of muscle. The enteral nervous system operates autonomously and therefore one can denervate the intestine and not effect the coordinated contractions. These contractions are termed activity fronts and may be stimulated by feeding, or they may be inhibited by exposing the lumen to various substances, e.g., lipid in the ileum decreases ileal motility. Two aspects of neuromechanical properties are particularly germane to urinary intestinal diversion: volume-pressure relationships and motor activity.

VOLUME-PRESSURE CONSIDERATIONS. The volume-pressure relationships are dependent on the configuration of the bowel. If one splits the bowel segment and turns it back on itself, the volume may be doubled if the ends aren't closed (Fig. 70–26). However, in reconstructing intestinal segments for the urinary tract, one must close the ends. Thus, the limit of doubling the volume is never quite reached. Indeed, the greater the ratio of length to diameter, the greater the volume change when the ends are closed. If the ends are closed when a ratio of 1:3.5 diameter to length is reached, splitting the segment no longer increases the volume. By splitting most segments, one is in fact increasing the volume by about 50 per cent. The goal in reconfiguration of the bowel is to achieve a spherical storage vessel. This configuration has the most volume for the least surface area. By increasing the volume, it has been suggested that pressure relationships within the confines of the intestine are reduced. This effect is based on Laplace's law, which states that for a sphere, the tension in its wall is proportional to the product of the radius and pressure. Thus, theoretically, for a given wall tension, the larger the radius, the smaller the generated pressure. This situation is desirable in an attempt to prevent deterioration of the upper tracts. However, this relationship (Laplace's law) may not be accurately reflected for intestinal segments. They are not perfectly spherical, and the intestinal wall does not conform to Hooke's law. Rather, the intestine demon-

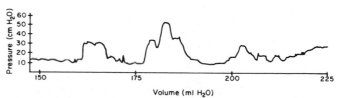

$$C_1 = 2\pi r_1$$
$$V_1 = \pi r_1^2 L$$

$$C_2 = 2\pi r_2 = 2(2\pi r_1)$$
$$r_2 = 2r_1$$
$$V_2 = \pi r_2^2 (1/2\ L) = 2\pi r_1^2 L$$

To close the cylinder's ends
area required $= 2\pi r_2^2$

$$2\pi r_2^2 = 2\pi r_2 L_2$$
$$r_2 = L_2$$
$$V_3 = \pi r_2^2 (1/2\ L - r_2)$$

Figure 70–26. Effect of "detubularization." The bowel is split on its antimesenteric border and divided in two. By placing the two segments together, the circumference is doubled, thus doubling the volume. Closing the ends of the cylinder requires a reduction in its length equal to the radius of the end, limiting the increase in volume that occurs by reconfiguration.

strates viscoelastic properties, which tend to distort the relationship between pressure applied at the wall and tension generated in it. In any event, it does seem desirable to make an attempt to create as spherical a container as possible, if one is attempting to create a reservoir.

Over time, the volume capacity of segments will increase, if they are frequently filled. Their volume will decrease with time if they are nonfunctional (Kock et al., 1978). A marked accommodation in volume of pouches created from intestine can be demonstrated with time. For ileal pouches, the capacity increases sevenfold after 1 year (Berglund et al., 1987). As the reservoirs increase in volume, there is a significant increase in smooth muscle thickness of the bowel wall (Philipson et al., 1985).

MOTOR ACTIVITY. Splitting the bowel on its antimesenteric border discoordinates motor activity and thereby creates a lesser intraluminal pressure. Clearly, the ideal situation is to provide the patient with a spherical vessel, which has few or ineffective contractions of its walls. It can be demonstrated in the experimental animal that by splitting the bowel wall on its antimesenteric border and reconfiguring it, a marked acute interruption of coordinated activity fronts occurs. Over a period of 3 months, they return to their normal coordinated state (Concepcion et al., 1988). This finding has also been demonstrated clinically. Initially after reconfiguring the bowel ("detubularization"), coordinated activity fronts have been shown to decrease. However, over extended periods of time, many of the "peristaltic waves" (activity fronts) reappear and can be readily demonstrated (Fig. 70–27).

The literature is contradictory with respect to the effect of detubularization on segments of ileum and colon used to construct storage vessels for continent diversions. Pressure within the lumen of bowel which has both ends closed may be increased by adding volume or by reducing the size of the bowel through contractions of its wall. Because the bowel wall is freely permeable to water, the higher osmotic content of urine obligates movement of water into the bowel lumen. Most patients

with continent diversions excrete 2 to 4 L per day (McDougal, 1986). In evaluating whether motor activity is the primary determinant of intravesical pressure, one must be cognizant of fluid volume changes. Also, as previously indicated, early reports of detubularized segments would be expected to differ from later reports, when coordinated activity fronts in these segments return. These facts are often forgotten, and because pressure measurements are employed to infer motor activity rather than directly measuring it, as reflected by changes in bowel wall tension, it is not difficult to understand why there are so many contradictions reported in the literature.

Detubularization of ileal segments has been reported by some to decrease motor activity at a year compared with immediately postoperative (Berglund et al., 1987). Others have noted increased motor activity at 1 year. Involuntary pressure waves occur in 25 per cent of patients with Kock pouches. Maximum intravesical pressures average 41 cm H_2O in these pouches (Chen et al., 1989). Ileum has also been shown to have less activity fronts per unit period of time than cecum (Berglund et al., 1986). Cecum has been observed to have the same number of activity fronts 1 year postoperatively, but the amplitude of the pressure waves has been observed to decrease over time (Hedlund et al., 1984). Maximum pressures in normal cecum have been shown to range from 18 to 100 cm H_2O (Jakobsen et al., 1987). In comparison, detubularized cecum has been shown to

Figure 70–27. Pressure waves recorded 1 year postoperatively in a patient with a continent diversion created from detubularized ileum and right colon. Notice the coordinated pressure waves that are of similar magnitude and frequency to those found in a normal colon or ileal segment.

have pressures that range between 5 and 25 cm H_2O 1 year postoperatively (Hedlund et al., 1984). Others, comparing ileum with cecum, find no difference in pressure generated after a year (Hedlund et al., 1984).

The MAINZ pouch that employs both ileum and cecum has an average pressure at capacity of 39 cm H_2O, with a maximum pressure of 63 cm H_2O (Thuroff et al., 1987). Thus, reconfiguring bowel usually increases the volume but its effect on motor activity and wall tension over the long-term is unclear at this time.

SUMMARY

This chapter has addressed complications that are both independent and dependent on the specific type of urinary intestinal diversion. Each unique type of diversion has its own set of individual complications, which must be added to those previously outlined. Moreover, the procedure preceding the urinary intestinal diversion also has a set of complications that must be added to those described. With current modalities of urinary intestinal diversion, long-term complications significantly contribute to patient mortality and morbidity. However, many patients who undergo intestinal diversions following extirpative procedures for cancer, will in fact die of cancer rather than these long-term complications. It is those for whom a urinary intestinal diversion has been created for benign disease and those who are cured of cancer who are most likely to realize one of the long-term morbid complications. The knowledge of the frequency of these complications and the correct performance of preoperative preparation, surgical technique, and postoperative care, as outlined in this chapter, should provide the best chance for the least mortality and morbidity in patients undergoing urinary intestinal diversions.

REFERENCES

Aaronson, I. A., Constantinides, C. G., Sallie, L. P., Sinclair-Smith, C. C.: Pathogenesis of adenocarcinoma complicating ureterosigmoidostomy. Experimental observations. Urology, 29:538–543, 1987.

Aaronson, I. A., and Sinclair-Smith, C. C.: Dysplasia of ureteric epithelium: a source of adenocarcinoma in ureterosigmoidostomy? Z. Kinderchir., 39:364–367, 1984.

Adams, M. C., Mitchell, M. E., and Rink, R. C.: Gastrocystoplasty: an alternative solution to the problem of urological reconstruction in the severely compromised patient. J. Urol., 140:1152–1156, 1988.

Albert, D. J., and Persky, L.: Conjoined end-to-end uretero-intestinal anastomosis. J. Urol., 105:201–204, 1971.

Allen, T., Peters, P. C., and Sagalowsky, A.: The Camey procedure: preliminary results in 11 patients. World J. Urol., 3:167, 1985.

Althausen, A. F., Hagen-Cook, K., and Hendren, W. H., III.: Nonrefluxing colon conduit: experience with 70 cases. J. Urol., 120:35–39, 1978.

Arabi, Y., Dimock, F., Burdon, D. W., Alexander-Williams, J., and Keighley, M. R. B.: Influence of bowel preparation and antimicrobials on colonic microflora. Br. J. Surg., 65:555–559, 1978.

Armstrong, W. M.: Cellular mechanisms of ion transport in the small intestine. In Johnson, L. R. (Ed.): Physiology of the Gastrointestinal Tract. New York, Raven Press, 1987, p. 1251.

Ashken, M. H.: Urinary cecal reservoir. In King, L. R., Stone, A. R., and Webster, G. D. (Eds.): Bladder Reconstruction and Continent Urinary Diversion. Chicago, Year Book Medical Publishers, 1987, pp. 238–251.

Bartlett, J. G., Condon, R. E., Gorback, S. L., Clarke, J. S., Nichols, R. L., and Ochi, S.: Veterans Administration Cooperative Study on bowel preparation for elective colorectal operations: Impact of oral antibiotic regimen on colonic flora, wound irrigation cultures, and bacteriology of septic complications. Ann. Surg., 188:249–254, 1978.

Baum, M. L., Anish, D. S., Chalmers, T. C., Sacks, H. S., Smith, H., Jr., and Fagerstrom, R. M.: A survey of clinical trials of antibiotic prophylaxis in colon surgery: evidence against further use of no-treatment controls. N. Engl. J. Med., 305:795–799, 1981.

Beckley, S., Wajsman, Z., Pontes, J. E., and Murphy, G.: Transverse colon conduit: a method of urinary diversion after pelvic irradiation. J. Urol., 128:464–468, 1982.

Beddoe, A. M., Boyce, J. G., Remy, J. C., Fruchter, R. G., and Nelson, J. H., Jr.: Stented versus nonstented transverse colon conduits: a comparative report. Gynecol. Oncol., 27:305–313, 1987.

Benchekroun, A.: The ileocecal continent bladder. In King, L. R., Stone, A. R., and Webster, G. D. (Eds.): Bladder Reconstruction and Continent Urinary Diversion. Year Book Medical Publishers, Chicago, 1987, pp. 224–237.

Berglund, B., Kock, N. G., and Myrvold, H. E.: Volume capacity and pressure characteristics of the continent cecal reservoir. Surg. Gynecol. Obstet., 163:42–48, 1986.

Berglund, B., Kock, N. G., Norlen, L., and Philipson, B. M.: Volume capacity and pressure characteristics of the continent ileal reservoir used for urinary diversion. J. Urol., 137:29–34, 1987.

Bihrle, R., Foster, R. S., Steidle, C. P., Adams, M. C., Woodbury, P. W., Sutton, G. P., and McNulty, A.: Creation of a transverse colon-gastric composite reservoir: A new technique. J. Urol., 141:1217–1220, 1989.

Binder, H. J., and Sandle, G. I.: Electrolyte absorption and secretion in the mammalian colon. In Johnson, L. R. (Ed.): Physiology of the Gastrointestinal Tract. New York, Raven Press, 1987, p. 1389.

Bisson, J. M., Vinson, R. K., and Leadbetter, G. W.: Urolithiasis from stapler anastomosis. Am. J. Surg. 137:280–282, 1979.

Bonnheim, D. C., Petrelli, N. J., Steinberg, A., and Mittelman, A.: The pathophysiology of the jejunal conduit syndrome and its exacerbation by parenteral hyperalimentation. J. Surg. Oncol., 26:172–175, 1984.

Borglund, E., Nordstrom, G., and Nyman, C. R.: Classification of peristomal skin changes in patients with urostomy. J. Am. Acad. Dermatol., 19:623–628, 1988.

Bowyer, G. W., and Davies, T. W.: Methotrexate toxicity associated with an ileal conduit. Br. J. Urol., 60:592, 1986.

Boyd, S. D., Schiff, W. M., Skinner, D. G., Lieskovsky, G., Kanellos, A. W., and Klimaszewski, A. D.: Prospective study of metabolic abnormalities in patients with continent Kock pouch urinary diversion. Urology, 33:85–88, 1989.

Bracken, R. B., McDonald, M. W., and Johnson, D. E.: Cystectomy for superficial bladder cancer. Urology, 18:459–463, 1981.

Bricker, E. M.: Bladder substitution after pelvic evisceration. Surg. Clin. North Am. 30:1511–1521, 1950.

Camey, M., Richard, F., and Botto, H.: Bladder replacement by ileocystoplasty. In King, L. R., Stone, A. R., and Webster, G. D. (Eds.): Bladder Reconstruction and Continent Urinary Diversion. Chicago, Year Book Medical Publishers, 1987, pp. 336–359.

Castro, J. E., and Ram, M. D.: Electrolyte imbalance following ileal urinary diversion. Br. J. Urol., 42:29–32, 1970.

Chang, T. W.: Antibiotic-associated injury to the gut. In Berk, J. E. (Ed.): Gastroenterology. Philadelphia, W. B. Saunders Co., 1985, pp. 2585–2590.

Chassin, J. L., Rifkind, K. M., Sussman, B., Kassel, B., Fingaret, A., Drager, S., and Chassin, P. S.: The stapled gastrointestinal tract anastomosis: incidence of postoperative complications compared with the sutured anastomoses. Ann. Surg. 188:689–696, 1978.

Chen, K. K., Chang, L. S., and Chen, M. T.: Urodynamic and clinical outcome of Kock pouch continent urinary diversion. J. Urol. 141:94–97, 1989.

Christensen, P. B., and Kronborg, O.: Whole-gut irrigation versus enema in elective colorectal surgery: a prospective, randomized study. Dis. Colon Rectum, 24:592–595, 1981.

Clark, P. B.: End-to-end ureteroileal anastomoses for ileal conduits. Br. J. Urol., 51:105–109, 1979.

Clarke, J. S., Condon, R. E., Barlett, J. G., et al.: Preoperative oral antibiotics reduce septic complications of colon operations. Ann. Surg., 186:251–259, 1977.

Clayman, R. V., Reddy, P., and Nivatvongs, S.: Acute pseudo-obstruction of the colon: a serious consequence of urologic surgery. J. Urol., 126:415–417, 1981.

Cohen, M. S., Hilz, M. E., Davis, C. P., and Anderson, M. D.: Urinary carcinogen (nitrosamine) production in a rat animal model for ureterosigmoidostomy. J. Urol., 138:449–452, 1987.

Concepcion, R. S., Koch, M. O., McDougal, W. S., and Richards, W. O.: Detubularized intestinal segments in urinary tract reconstruction: why do they work? Abst. Am. Urol. Assoc., 592, 1988.

Cordonnier, J. J.: Ureterosigmoid anastomosis. J. Urol., 63:276–285, 1950.

Costello, A. J., and Johnson, D. E.: Modified autosuture technique for ileal conduit construction in urinary diversion. Aust. N. Z. J. Surg., 54:477–482, 1984.

Dekleck, J. N., Lambrechts, W., and Viljoen, I.: The bowel as substitute for the bladder. J. Urol., 121:22–24, 1979.

Didolkar, M. S., Reed, W. P., Elias, E. G., Schnaper, L. A., Brown, S. D., and Chaudhary, S. M.: A prospective randomized study of sutured versus stapled bowel anastomoses in patients with cancer. Cancer, 57:456–460, 1986.

Dion, Y. M., Richards, G. K., Prentis, J. J., and Hinchey, E. J.: The influence of oral versus parenteral preoperative metronidazole on sepsis following colon surgery. Ann. Surg., 192:221–226, 1980.

Dretler, S. P.: The pathogenesis of urinary tract calculi occurring after conduit diversion. I. Clinical study; II. Conduit study; III. Prevention. J. Urol., 109:204–209, 1973.

Edwards, R. H.: Hyperammonemic encephalopathy related to ureterosigmoidostomy. Arch. Neurol., 41:1211–1212, 1984.

Elder, D. D., Moisey, C. U., and Rees, R. W. M.: A long-term follow-up of the colonic conduit operation in children. Br. J. Urol., 51:462–465, 1979.

Emmott, D., Noble, M. J., and Mebust, W. K.: A comparison of end versus loop stomas for ileal conduit urinary diversion. J. Urol., 133:588–590, 1985.

Fall, M., and Anderstrom, C.: Funneled ureteroileal anastomosis. J. Urol., 128:249–251, 1982.

Fazio, V. W., Jagelman, A. G., Lavery, I. C., and McGonagle, B. A.: Evaluation of the Proximate-ILS circular stapler. A prospective study. Ann. Surg., 201:108–114, 1985.

Ferris, D. O., and Odel, H. M.: Electrolyte pattern of blood after ureterosigmoidostomy. JAMA, 142:634–641, 1950.

Filmer, R. B.: Malignant tumors arising in bladder augmentations and ileal and colon conduits. Soc. Pediatr. Urol. Newsletter, December 9, 1986.

Flanigan, R. C., Kursh, E. D., and Persky, L.: Thirteen-year experience with ileal loop diversion in children with myelodysplasia. Am. J. Surg., 130:535–538, 1975.

Geist, R. W., and Ansell, J. S.: Total body potassium in patients after ureteroileostomy. Surg. Gynecol. Obstet., 113:585–590, 1961.

Golimbu, M., and Morales, P.: Jejunal conduits: technique and complications. J. Urol., 113:787–795, 1975.

Gonzalez, R., and Reinberg, Y.: Localization of bacteriuria in patients with enterocystoplasty and nonrefluxing conduits. J. Urol., 138:1104–1105, 1987.

Goodwin, W. E., Harris, A. P., Kaufman, J. J., and Beal, J. M.: Open, transcolonic ureterointestinal anastomosis. Surg. Gynecol. Obstet., 97:295–300, 1953.

Gottrup, F., Diederich, P., Sorensen, K., Nielsen, S. V., Ornsholt, J., and Brandsborg, O.: Prophylaxis with whole gut irrigation and antimicrobials in colorectal surgery. A prospective randomized double-blind clinical trial. Am. J. Surg., 149:317–322, 1985.

Guinan, P. D., Moore, R. H., Neter, E., and Murphy, G. P.: The bacteriology of ileal conduit urine in man. Surg. Gynecol. Obstet., 134:78–82, 1972.

Hagen-Cook, K., and Althausen, A. F.: Early observations on 31 adults with non-refluxing colon conduits. J. Urol., 121:13–16, 1979.

Hardy, B. E., Lebowitz, R. L., Baez, A., and Colodny, A. A.: Strictures of the ileal loop. J. Urol., 117:358–361, 1977.

Hares, M. M., and Alexander-Williams, J.: The effect of bowel preparation on colonic surgery. World J. Surg., 6:175–181, 1982.

Harrison, A. R.: Clinical and metabolic observations on osteomalacia following ureterosigmoidostomy. Br. J. Urol., 30:455–461, 1958.

Hassain, M.: The osteomalacia syndrome after colocystoplasty: a cure with sodium bicarbonate alone. Br. J. Urol. 42:243–245, 1970.

Hautmann, R. E., Egghart, G., Frohneberg, D., and Miller, K.: The ileal neobladder. J. Urol., 139:39–42, 1988.

Hayashi, T., Ikai, K., Kiriyama, T., Taki, Y., and Hiura, M.: Percutaneous intrapelvic pressure registration in patients with ureterointestinal urinary diversion. Urology, 28:176–178, 1986.

Hedlund, H., Lindstrom, K., and Mansson, W.: Dynamics of a continent caecal reservoir for urinary diversion. Br. J. Urol., 56:366–372, 1984.

Heidler, H., Marberger, M., and Hohenfellner, R.: The metabolic situation in ureterosigmoidostomy. Eur. Urol., 5:39–44, 1979.

Hensle, T. W., and Burbige, K. A.: Bladder replacement in children and young adults. J. Urol., 133:1004–1010, 1985.

Hill, J. T., and Ransley, P. G.: The colonic conduit: a better method of urinary diversion? Br. J. Urol., 55:629–631, 1983.

Hirdes, W. H., Hoekstra, I., and Vlietstra, H. P.: Hammock anastomoses: a nonrefluxing ureteroileal anastomoses. J. Urol., 139:517–518, 1988.

Husmann, D. A., McLorie, G. A., and Churchill, B. M.: Nonrefluxing colonic conduits: a long-term life-table analysis. J. Urol., 142:1201–1203, 1989.

Iannoni, C., Marcheggiano, A., Pallone, F., Frieri, G., Gallucci, M., DiSilverio, F., and Caprilli, R.: Abnormal patterns of colorectal mucin secretion after urinary diversion of different types: histochemical and lectin binding studies. Hum. Pathol., 17:834–840, 1986.

Irvin, T. T., and Goligher, J. C.: Aetiology of disruption of intestinal anastomosis. Br. J. Surg., 60:461, 1973.

Jacobs, J. A., and Young, J. D., Jr.: The Strickler technique of ureterosigmoidostomy. J. Urol., 124:451–454, 1980.

Jaffe, B. M., Bricker, E. M., and Butcher, H. R., Jr.: Surgical complications of ileal segment urinary diversion. Ann. Surg., 167:367–376, 1968.

Jakobsen, H., Steven, K., Stigsby, B., Klarskov, P., and Hald, T.: Pathogenesis of nocturnal urinary incontinence after ileocaecal bladder replacement. Continuous measurement of urethral closure pressure during sleep. Br. J. Urol., 59:148–152, 1987.

Jex, R. K., van Heerden, J. A., Wolff, B. G., Ready, R. L., and Illstrup, D. M.: Gastrointestinal anastomoses. Factors affecting early complications. Ann. Surg., 206:138–141, 1987.

Kamizaki, H., and Cass, A. S.: Conduit and renal pelvic pressure after ileal and colonic urinary diversion in dogs. Invest. Urol., 16:27–32, 1978.

Kaufman, J. J.: Ammoniagenic coma following ureterosigmoidostomy. J. Urol., 131:743–745, 1984.

King, L. R.: Protection of the upper tracts in undiversion. In King, L. R., Stone, A. R., and Webster, G. D. (Eds.): Bladder Reconstruction and Continent Urinary Diversion. Chicago, Year Book Medical Publishers, 1987, pp. 127–153.

Kinn, A., and Lantz, B.: Vitamin B_{12} deficiency after irradiation for bladder carcinoma. J. Urol., 131:888–890, 1984.

Klein, E. A., Montie, J. E., Montague, D. K., Kay, R., and Straffon, R. A.: Jejunal conduit urinary diversion. J. Urol., 135:244–246, 1986.

Koch, M. O., and McDougal, W. S.: Chlorpromazine: adjuvant therapy for the metabolic derangements created by urinary diversion through intestinal segments. J. Urol., 134:165–169, 1985.

Koch, M. O., and McDougal, W. S.: Determination of renal function following urinary diversion through intestinal segments. J. Urol., 133:517–520, 1985.

Koch, M. O., and McDougal, W. S.: Nicotinic acid: treatment for the hyperchloremic metabolic acidosis following urinary diversion through intestinal segments. J. Urol., 134:162–164, 1985.

Koch, M. O., and McDougal, W. S.: The pathophysiology of hyperchloremic metabolic acidosis after urinary diversion through intestinal segments. Surgery, 98:561–570, 1985.

Koch, M. O., and McDougal, W. S.: Bone demineralization following ureterosigmoid anastomosis: an experimental study in rats. J. Urol., 140:856–859, 1988.

Koch, M. O., Gurevitch, E., Hill, D. E., and McDougal, W. S.: Urinary solute transport by intestinal segments: a comparative study of ileum and colon in rats. J. Urol., 143:1275–1279, 1990.

Kock, N. G.: The development of the continent ileal reservoir (Kock pouch) and application in patients requiring urinary diversion. In King, L. R., Stone, A. R., and Webster, G. D. (Eds.): Bladder Reconstruction and Continent Urinary Diversion. Chicago, Year Book Medical Publishers, 1987, pp. 269–290.

Kock, N. G., Nilson, A. E., Nilsson, L. O., Norlen, L. J., and

Philipson, B. M.: Urinary diversion via a continent ileal reservoir: clinical results in 12 patients. J. Urol., 128:469–475, 1982.

Kock, N. G., Nilson, A. E., Norlen, L., Sundin, T., and Trasti, H.: Changes in renal parenchyma and the upper urinary tract following urinary diversion via a continent ileum reservoir. An experimental study in dogs. Scand. J. Urol. Nephrol. (Suppl.), 49:11–22, 1978.

Koff, S. A.: Mechanisms of electrolyte imbalance following urointestinal anastomoses. Urology, 5:109–114, 1975.

Kramolowsky, E. V., Clayman, R. V., and Weyman, P. J.: Endourological management of ureteroileal anastomotic strictures: Is it effective? J. Urol., 137:390–394, 1987.

Kramolowsky, E. V., Clayman, R. V., and Weyman, P. J.: Management of ureterointestinal anastomotic strictures: comparison of open surgical and endourological repair. J. Urol., 139:1195–1198, 1988.

Kuss, R., Bitker, M., Camey, M., Chatelain, C., and Lassau, J. P.: Indications and early and late results of intestinocystoplasty: a review of 185 cases. J. Urol., 103:53–63, 1970.

Leadbetter, W. F., and Clarke, B. G.: Five years' experience with uretero-enterostomy by the "combined" technique. J. Urol., 73:67–82, 1954.

LeDuc, A., Camey, M., and Teillac, P.: An original antireflux ureteroileal implantation technique: Long-term follow-up. J. Urol., 137:1156–1158, 1987.

Leong, C. H.: Use of stomach for bladder replacement and urinary diversion. Ann. R. Coll. Surg. Engl., 60:283–289, 1978.

Lim, S. T. K., Lam, S. K., Lee, N. W., Wong, J., and Ong, G. B.: Effects of gastrocystoplasty on serum gastrin levels and gastric acid secretion. Br. J. Surg., 70:275–277, 1983.

Lockhart, J. L., and Bejany, D. E.: The antireflux ureteroileal reimplantation in children and adults. J. Urol., 135:576–579, 1986.

Lockhart, J. L., and Bejany, D. E.: Antireflux ureteroileal reimplantation: an alternative for urinary diversion. J. Urol., 137:867–870, 1987.

Loening, S. A., Navarre, R. J., Narayana, A. S., and Culp, D. A.: Transverse colon conduit urinary diversion. J. Urol., 127:37–39, 1982.

Magnus, R. V.: Pressure studies and dynamics of ileal conduits in children. J. Urol., 118:406–407, 1977.

Malek, R. S., Burke, E. C., and DeWeerd, J. H.: Ileal conduit urinary diversion in children. J. Urol., 105:892–900, 1971.

Mansson, W.: The continent cecal urinary reservoir. In King, L. R., Stone, A. R., and Webster, G. D. (Eds.): Bladder Reconstruction and Continent Urinary Diversion. Chicago, Year Book Medical Publishers, 1987, p. 209.

Mansson, W., Colleen, S., Forsberg, L., Larsson, I., Sundin, T., and White, T.: Renal function after urinary diversion. A study of continent caecal reservoir, ileal conduit, and colonic conduit. Scand. J. Urol. Nephrol., 18:307–315, 1984.

Mansson, W., Colleen, S., and Stigsson, L.: Four methods of ureterointestinal anastomoses in urinary conduit diversion. Scand. J. Urol. Nephrol., 13:191–199, 1979.

McDermott, W. V., Jr.: Diversion of urine to the intestines as a factor in ammoniagenic coma. N. Engl. J. Med., 256:460–462, 1957.

McDougal, W. S.: Bladder reconstruction following cystectomy by uretero-ileo-colourethrostomy. J. Urol., 135:698–701, 1986.

McDougal, W. S.: Mechanics and neurophysiology of intestinal segments as bowel substitutes. J. Urol., 138:1438–1439, 1987.

McDougal, W. S., and Koch, M. O.: Accurate determination of renal function in patients with intestinal urinary diversion. J. Urol., 135:1175–1178, 1986.

McDougal, W. S., and Koch, M. O.: Effect of sulfate on calcium and magnesium homeostasis following urinary diversion. Kidney Int., 35:105–115, 1989.

McDougal, W. S., and Koch, M. O.: Impaired growth and development and urinary intestinal interposition. Abst. Am. Assoc. GU Surg., 105:3, 1991.

McDougal, W. S., Koch, M. O., and Flora, M. D.: Ammonium metabolism in urinary intestinal diversion. Abst. Am. Assoc. GU Surg., p. 45, 1989.

McDougal, W. S., Koch, M. O., Shands, C., III, and Price, R. R.: Bony demineralization following urinary intestinal diversion. J. Urol., 140:853–855, 1988.

Menaker, G. J., Litvak, S., Bendix, R., Michel, A., and Kerstein, M. D.: Operations on the colon without preoperative oral antibiotic therapy. Surg. Gynecol. Obstet., 152:36–38, 1981.

Menon, M., Yu, G. W., and Jeffs, R. D.: Technique for antirefluxing ureterocolonic anastomosis. J. Urol., 127:236–237, 1982.

Merricks, J. W.: A continent substitute bladder and urethra. In King, L. R., Stone, A. R., and Webster, G. D. (Eds.): Bladder Reconstruction and Continent Urinary Diversion. Chicago, Year Book Medical Publishers, 1987, pp. 179–203.

Mesrobian, H. J., Kelalis, P. P., and Kramer, S. A.: Long-term follow-up of 103 patients with bladder exstrophy. J. Urol., 139:719–722, 1988.

Middleton, A. W., Jr., and Hendren, W. H.: Ileal conduits in children at the Massachusetts General Hospital from 1955 to 1970. J. Urol., 115:591–595, 1976.

Mitchell, M. E., and Hensle, T. W.: Total bladder replacement in children. In King, L. R., Stone, A. R., and Webster, G. D. (Eds.): Bladder Reconstruction and Continent Urinary Diversion. Chicago, Year Book Medical Publishers, 1987, pp. 312–320.

Mounger, E. J., and Branson, A. D.: Ammonia encephalopathy secondary to ureterosigmoidostomy: a case report. J. Urol., 108:411–412, 1972.

Mount, B. M., Susset, J. G., Campbell, J., et al.: Ureteral implantation into ileal conduits. J. Urol., 100:605–609, 1968.

Mundy, A. R.: Personal communication, 1991.

Nesbitt, R. M.: Ureterosigmoid anastomosis by direct elliptical connection: a preliminary report. J. Urol., 61:728–734, 1949.

Nichols, R. L., Condon, R. E., Gorback, S. L., and Nyhus, L. M.: Efficacy of preoperative antimicrobial preparation of the bowel. Ann. Surg., 176:227–232, 1972.

Norlen, L., and Trasti, H.: Functional behavior of the continent ileum reservoir for urinary diversion. An experimental and clinical study. Scand. J. Urol. Nephrol. (Suppl.), 49:33–42, 1978.

Nurmi, M., and Puntala, P.: Antireflux ureteroileal anastomosis in ileal conduit urinary diversion and in ileocystoplasty following cystoprostatectomy. Scand. J. Urol. Nephrol., 22:271–273, 1988.

Onwubalili, J. K.: Overt diabetes mellitus without glycosuria in a patient with cutaneous ureteroileostomy. Br. Med. J., 284:1836–1837, 1982.

Pagano, F.: Ureterocolonic anastomoses: description of a technique. J. Urol., 123:355–356, 1980.

Pagano, F., Cosciani-Cunico, S., Dal Bianco, M., and Zattoni, F.: Five years of experience with a modified technique of ureterocolonic anastomosis. J. Urol., 132:17–18, 1984.

Patil, U., Glassberg, K. I., and Waterhouse, K.: Ileal conduit surgery with a nippled ureteroileal anastomoses. Urology, 7:594–597, 1976.

Perry, W., Allen, L. N., Stamp, T. C. B., and Walker, P. G.: Vitamin D resistance in osteomalacia after ureterosigmoidostomy. N. Engl. J. Med., 297:1110–1112, 1977.

Philipson, B. M., Kock, N. G., Jagenburg, R., Ahren, C., Norlen, L., Robinson, J. W. L., and Menge, H.: Functional and structural studies of ileal reservoir used for continent urostomy and ileostomy. Gut, 24:392–398, 1983.

Philipson, B. M., Leth, R., and Kock, N. G.: Hypertrophy of ileal smooth muscle after construction of ileal reservoir in the rat. Virchows Arch., 406:417–424, 1985.

Pitts, W. R., Jr., and Muecke, E. C.: A 20-year experience with ileal conduits: the fate of the kidneys. J. Urol., 122:154–157, 1979.

Regan, J. B., and Barrett, D. M.: Stented versus nonstented ureteroileal anastomoses: is there a difference with regard to leak and stricture? J. Urol., 134:1101–1103, 1985.

Richards, P., Chamberlain, M. J., and Wrong, O. M.: Treatment of osteomalacia of renal tubular acidosis by sodium bicarbonate alone. Lancet, 2:994–997, 1972.

Richie, J. P.: Intestinal loop urinary diversion in children. J. Urol., 111:687–689, 1974.

Richie, J. P., Skinner, D. G.: Urinary diversion: The physiological rationale for non-refluxing colonic conduits. Br. J. Urol., 47:269–275, 1975.

Rowland, R. G., Mitchell, M. E., Bihrle, R., Kahnoski, R. J., and Piser, J. E.: Indiana continent urinary reservoir. J. Urol., 137:1136–1139, 1987.

Salahudeen, A. K., Elliott, R. W., and Ellis, H. A.: Osteomalacia due to ileal replacement of ureters: report of 2 cases. J. Urol., 131:335–337, 1984.

Savarirayan, F., and Dixey, G. M.: Syncope following ureterosigmoidostomy. J. Urol., 101:844–845, 1969.

Scher, K. S., Scott-Conner, C., Jones, C. W., and Leach, M.: A comparison of stapled and sutured anastomoses in colonic operations. Surg. Gynecol. Obstet., 155:489–493, 1982.

Schipper, H., and Decter, A.: Carcinoma of the colon arising at ureteral implant sites despite early external diversion: pathogenetic and clinical implications. Cancer, 47:2062–2065, 1981.

Schmidt, J. D., Bucksbaum, H. J., and Nachtsheim, D. A.: Long-term follow-up, further experience with and modifications of the transverse colon conduit in urinary tract diversion. Br. J. Urol., 57:284–288, 1985.

Schmidt, J. D., Hawtrey, C. E., Flocks, R. H., and Culp, D. A.: Complications, results, and problems of ileal conduit diversions. J. Urol., 109:210–216, 1973.

Schwarz, G. R., and Jeffs, R. D.: Ileal conduit urinary diversion in children: computer analysis of follow-up from 2 to 16 years. J. Urol., 114:285–288, 1975.

Sener, S. F., Imperato, J. P., Blum, M. D., Ignatoff, J. M., Soper, T. G., Winchester, D. P., and Meiselman, M.: Technique and complications of reconstruction of the pelvic floor with polyglactin mesh. Surg. Gynecol. Obstet., 168:475–480, 1989.

Shands, C., III, McDougal, W. S., and Wright, E. P.: Prevention of cancer at the urothelial enteric anastomotic site. J. Urol., 141:178–181, 1989.

Shapiro, S. R., Lebowitz, R., and Colodny, A. H.: Fate of 90 children with ileal conduit urinary diversions a decade later: analysis of complications, pyelography, renal function, and bacteriology. J. Urol., 114:289–295, 1975.

Siklos, P., Davie, M., Jung, R. J., and Chalmers, T. M.: Osteomalacia in ureterosigmoidostomy: healing by correction of the acidosis. Br. J. Urol., 52:61–62, 1980.

Silberman, R.: Ammonia intoxication following ureterosigmoidostomy in a patient with liver disease. Lancet, 2:937–939, 1958.

Skinner, D. G., Lieskovsky, G., and Boyd, S.: Continent urinary diversion. J. Urol., 141:1323–1327, 1989.

Smith, E. D.: Follow-up studies on 150 ileal conduits in children. J. Pediatr. Surg. 7:1–10, 1972.

Specht, E. E.: Rickets following ureterosigmoidostomy and chronic hyperchloremia. J. Bone Joint Surg., 49:1422–1430, 1967.

Starr, A., Rose, D. H., and Cooper, J. F.: Antireflux ureteroileal anastomosis in humans. J. Urol., 113:170–174, 1975.

Stewart, M., Macrae, F. A., and Williams, C. B.: Neoplasia and ureterosigmoidostomy: a colonoscopy survey. Br. J. Surg., 69:414–416, 1982.

Stewart, W. W., Cass, A. S., and Matsen, J. M.: Bacteriuria with intestinal loop urinary diversion in children. J. Urol., 122:528–531, 1979.

Stone, A. R., and MacDermott, J. P. A.: The split-cuff ureteral nipple reimplantation technique: reliable reflux prevention from bowel segments. J. Urol., 142:707–709, 1989.

Strickler, W. L.: A modification of the combined ureterosigmoidostomy. J. Urol., 93:370–373, 1965.

Sullivan, J. W., Grabstald, H., and Whitmore, W. F., Jr.: Complications of ureteroileal conduit with radical cystectomy: review of 336 cases. J. Urol., 124:797–801, 1980.

Tapper, D., and Folkman, J.: Lymphoid depletion in ileal loops: mechanism and clinical implication. J. Pediatr. Surg., 11:871–880, 1976.

Thuroff, J. W., Alken, P., and Hohenfellner, R.: The MAINZ pouch (mixed augmentation with ileum 'n' zecum) for bladder augmentation and continent diversion. In King, L. R., Stone, A. R., and Webster, G. D. (Eds.): Bladder Reconstruction and Continent Urinary Diversion. Chicago, Year Book Medical Publishers, 1987, p. 252.

Tiffany, P., Vaughan, E. D., Marion, D., and Amberson, J.: Hypergastrinemia following antral gastrocystoplasty. J. Urol., 136:692, 1986.

Tuggle, D. W., Hoelzer, D. J., Tunell, W. P., and Smith, E. I.: The safety and cost-effectiveness of polyethylene glycol electrolyte solution bowel preparation in infants and children. J. Pediatr. Surg., 22:513–515, 1987.

Turner-Warwick, R. T., and Ashken, M. H.: The functional results of partial, subtotal, and total cystoplasty with special reference to ureterocaecocystoplasty, selective sphincterotomy and cystocystoplasty. Br. J. Urol., 39:3–12, 1967.

van den Bogaard, A. E. J. M., Weidema, W., Hazen, M. J., and Wesdorp, R. I. C.: A bacteriological evaluation of three methods of bowel preparation for elective colorectal surgery. Antonie van Leewenhoek, 47:86–88, 1981.

Wallace, D. M.: Uretero-ileostomy. Br. J. Urol., 42:529–534, 1970.

Washington, J. A., Dearing, W. H., Judd, E. S., and Elveback, L. R.: Effect of preoperative antibiotic regimen in development of infection after intestinal surgery: prospective, randomized double-blind study. Ann. Surg., 180:567–572, 1974.

Weber, T. R., Westfall, S. H., Steinhardt, G. F., Webb, L., Sotelo-Avila, C., and Connors, R. H.: Malignancy associated with ureterosigmoidostomy: detection by ornithine decarboxylase. J. Pediatr. Surg., 23:1091–1094, 1988.

Wendel, R. G., Henning, D. C., and Evans, A. T.: End-to-end ureteroileal anastomosis for iliac conduits: preliminary report. J. Urol., 102:42–43, 1969.

Whitmore, W. F., III, and Gittes, R. F.: Reconstruction of the urinary tract by cecal and ileocecal cystoplasty: review of a 15-year experience. J. Urol., 129:494–498, 1983.

Williams, R. E., Davenport, T. J., Burkinshaw, L., and Hughes, D.: Changes in whole body potassium associated with uretero-intestinal anastomoses. Br. J. Urol., 39:676–680, 1967.

Wolff, B. G., Beart, R. W., Jr., Dozois, R. R., Pemberton, J. H., Zinsmeister, A. R., Ready, R. L., Farnell, M. B., Washington, J. A., and Heppell, J.: A new bowel preparation for elective colon and rectal surgery. A prospective, randomized clinical trial. Arch. Surg., 123:895–900, 1988.

Wolff, B. G., Pemberton, J. H., van Heerden, J. A., Beart, R. W., Nivatvongs, S., Devine, R. M., Dozois, R. R., and Ilstrup, D. M.: Elective colon and rectal surgery without nasogastric decompression. A prospective, randomized trial. Ann. Surg., 209:670–675, 1989.

Woods, J. H., Erickson, L. W., Condon, R. E., Schulte, W. J., and Sillin, L. F.: Postoperative ileus: a colonic problem? Surgery, 84:527–533, 1978.

Zabbo, A., and Kay, R.: Ureterosigmoidostomy and bladder exstrophy: A long-term follow-up. J. Urol., 136:396–398, 1986.

71

AUGMENTATION CYSTOPLASTY IMPLANTATION OF ARTIFICIAL URINARY SPHINCTER IN MEN AND WOMEN AND RECONSTRUCTION OF THE DYSFUNCTIONAL URINARY TRACT

Michael E. Mitchell, M.D.
Richard C. Rink, M.D.
Mark C. Adams, M.D.

This chapter covers the salient aspects of reconstructing the dysfunctional lower urinary tract to achieve dryness and preserve renal function. It is our goal to focus on the principles of some very important reconstruction techniques, specifically, augmentation cystoplasty and artificial urinary sphincter. Every patient is unique. The formula that works for one patient may not work for another patient, even though both present with the same basic problem. For example, the artificial sphincter may be ideally suited to one patient, yet, in another patient with *similar* physiology it may prove to be totally inappropriate, possibly because of the patient's attitude and commitment or lack of manual dexterity.

With the reconstruction of the dysfunctional urinary tract in the pursuit of dryness comes a tremendous responsibility. Successfully meeting the challenge of this responsibility rests not only on the absolute cooperation and effort of the patient, but also on the support system, not the least of which is the physician and his or her staff. The best of surgical techniques and principles applied inappropriately or applied to a patient not committed to following postoperative protocol and self-care will ultimately lead to a disastrous outcome. Patient evaluation and selection, skillful execution of planned surgery, and careful meticulous follow-up are all *equally* important to a successful outcome.

Every positive surgical and medical treatment is balanced with some negative consequences. For example, augmentation cystoplasty can create a larger bladder and one with better compliance (Mitchell and Piser, 1987). The price paid, however, is reduced emptying efficiency, infection potential, chronic retention, and reduced bladder wall strength as shown by Gleason and co-workers (1972). If these limitations are not respected, retention, or as Elder and associates (1988) and Sheiner and Kaplan (1988) have reported, spontaneous bladder rupture may result. Therefore, before the specifics of augmentation and reconstruction of the urinary tract and the use of the artificial sphincter are discussed, the general principles of lower tract reconstruction and patient selection are now considered.

GENERAL PRINCIPLES OF LOWER TRACT RECONSTRUCTION

A variety of techniques have been developed that have facilitated reconstruction of the lower urinary tract. All are described in detail elsewhere, but to mention a few would be implantation of the ureter into the bowel or bladder to prevent reflux, techniques for ureteral tapering to facilitate ureteral implantation, techniques for augmentation of the bladder with bowel segments (small bowel, large bowel, even stomach), and techniques for improving urethral resistance. Perhaps, however, the most significant of all is nonsurgical, clean intermittent catheterization (CIC), a development due largely to the efforts of Lapides and colleagues (1972). Many patients with bladder dysfunction who are unable to void to completion may now be treated with CIC, preventing the need for urinary diversion. CIC is a simple, long-term, nonsurgical solution for urinary retention.

However, CIC has also facilitated reconstruction of the lower urinary tract, enabling techniques previously not possible. For example, Goodwin and co-workers (1958) and Kuss and co-workers (1970) showed bladder augmentation could be performed as the treatment of choice for patients with interstitial cystitis and with tuberculous cystitis. Augmentation, however, was *not* applied to patients with neurogenic bladder dysfunction because augmentation clearly made any retention state worse.

Gleason and associates (1972) focused on the dynamic changes of augmentation in "normal" patients, particularly relating to the problem with bladder emptying. With CIC these concerns with periodic emptying became much less significant, and, therefore, as reported by Mitchell and co-workers (1986), CIC has enabled surgical reconstruction in patients who previously were treatable only with urinary diversion.

Patients with bladder augmentation who also require CIC, in general, do as well as patients on CIC who have not had augmentation (Mitchell et al., 1986). Crooks and Emile (1983) have shown that these patients do better than patients who previously underwent diversion with an ileal conduit. Periodic urinary infection in all groups is to be expected, but, in the absence of reflux, is not generally associated with pyelonephritis or systemic illness (Lapides et al., 1976; Mitchell et al., 1986).

The requirements of CIC in the augmented bladder, however, are somewhat different from those of the nonaugmented bladder. Most notable is that in the presence of augmentation mucus production can sometimes result in obstruction of catheters with retention. Often this problem occurs without patient cognizance and can lead to spontaneous bladder rupture. The problem is particularly significant in younger patients in whom intermittent catheterization is done with smaller lumen catheters and in patients who are less aware of bladder distention (i.e., in myelodysplasia).

Intermittent catheterization in combination with augmentation cystoplasty will usually also require periodic irrigation of the bladder with 3 Normal saline solution or as Gillon and Mundy (1989) have shown with muco-lytic agents to prevent build-up of mucus and to provide a mechanical cleansing of the bladder. This irrigation may not be indicated if the catheter size is larger than 16 Fr. but is definitely indicated if the catheter size is smaller than 14 Fr.

Patient Selection

Patient selection for augmentation cystoplasty follows the same logic as patient selection for reconstruction of the lower urinary tract. Careful consideration should be given to pathophysiology of the entire urinary tract, including renal function, ureteral dynamics, and bladder urethral dynamics. Furthermore, as much attention directed to pathology should also be directed to the psychosocial aspects of the patient.

Physiologic considerations encompass the entire urinary tract. Renal function can be critical, and abnormalities in renal function may become magnified with the use of intestine in the lower urinary tract. As shown by Koch and McDougal (1985) and Demos (1962), solutes, particularly chloride, are resorbed from urine. In a patient with renal acidosis, placement of large or small bowel in the lower urinary tract will result in an increase in base demand. From clinical experience, augmentation with large or small bowel and ureterosigmoidostomy cause a metabolic acidosis to intensify (Mitchell and Piser, 1987). In contrast, however, a patient with salt-losing nephropathy, with stomach utilized to reconstruct the lower urinary tract, may develop a severe state that would require salt replacement (Rink et al., 1988).

Because of reduced urine output, patients with renal failure and oliguria have a greater potential for problems with viscous mucus, particularly if large bowel is used in the lower urinary tract. In the absence of urine to wash out mucus, a patient with anuria and augmentation has great potential for collection of inspissated mucus and requires frequent bladder irrigations. Bladder augmentation with stomach in such a patient results in less of a problem with mucus, but the acid produced by the gastric segment is *unbuffered* and potential exists for painful irritation or even ulcer formation in the bladder. This complication can be prevented by blocking gastric acid secretion.

If the concentrating ability of the kidneys is lost (as would commonly occur in many patients with congenital and acquired hydronephrosis), careful consideration to bladder volume must be given. Clearly, failure of other organ systems produces an impact on outcome, particularly when bowel is placed in the urinary tract. For example, in the patient with hepatic failure the net resorption of ammonia by large or small intestine in contact with urine could lead to hepatic coma (Koch and McDougal, 1985). Savauagen and Dixey (1969) have reported syncope related to resorption of medication excreted intact in the urine and resorbed by bowel.

It is, therefore, wise to carefully consider and evaluate the *total* patient prior to reconstruction with intestine. Prior to augmentation, serum electrolyte, blood urea nitrogen (BUN), creatinine, and 24-hour urine for volume and creatinine clearance determinations should be obtained on every patient. Liver function tests and arterial blood gas studies would be considered in selected patients.

The dynamics of the ureters are sometimes mistakenly ignored in patients considered for augmentations. The normal ureter, undilated and with normal peristalsis, will facilitate successful lower tract reconstruction. Dilated ureters, however, should never be completely trusted, and they require evaluation for peristalsis. Ureters in patients with refluxing diversions (ileal conduits), multiple previous surgeries (chronic recurrent reflux), or altered dynamics for other reasons (urethral valves, chronic obstruction, prune-belly syndrome, and so forth) have the potential for transmural scarring and may have little or no effective peristalsis. Such ureters behave as "stiff pipes." Reimplantation techniques for such ureters should have minimal resistance to flow because in the absence of a "peristaltic pump," flow is dependent on the pressure gradient between the kidney and the bladder. In patients with dilated ureters, it is very helpful to fluoroscopically observe the ureters when filled with contrast material.

Assessment of bladder dynamics is critical in all patients who undergo augmentation cystoplasty. Urodynamics, preferably with fluoroscopy, should define a bladder of insufficient volume and/or poor compliance. Urethral and bladder neck function must also be accurately evaluated. As shown by McGuire and co-workers (1981), a leak point pressure of greater than 40 cm H_2O is necessary for dryness in most patients. It is presumed that CIC will be necessary; therefore, an intact catheterizable urethra is absolutely necessary. Any urethral abnormality, such as diverticula, tortuosity, or an elevated bladder neck, which would make CIC more difficult, must *not* be taken lightly. A patient who is difficult to catheterize during the process of urodynamic testing is to be considered a *poor* candidate for bladder augmentation, unless a catheterizable stoma is also planned. This is true even when spontaneous voiding is anticipated. The need for intermittent catheterization is assumed. Any patient considered for augmentation cystoplasty or lower urinary tract reconstruction who cannot do or have done intermittent catheterization is *not* a surgical candidate.

In our attempt to create a catheterizable reservoir or fully functioning continent lower urinary tract we cannot ignore the limitations determined by the patient. A cutaneous diversion in an elderly patient who has great difficulty with personal care is sometimes far better than an internal diversion or a reconstruction. The same rationale may apply to the very young, to the severely handicapped (mental or physical), and those with limited prognoses or progressive neurologic lesions.

As important as these physical limitations may be, consideration of the psychologic and social situation of the patient is more important and is unfortunately often slighted or ignored. Although this issue is probably truer for the younger patient and the chronically disabled patient, considerations in this regard remain appropriate even for the older patient seeking reconstruction after cancer surgery. If a patient is emotionally uncommitted to reconstructive surgery and/or is unwilling to perform intermittent catheterization, that patient is *not* a candidate for surgery. Likewise, patients willing, but incapable of performing intermittent self-catheterization, must have support systems that will ensure long-term regular assistance with care. The major determinant of *success* rests with the patient and the patient's support system. The best engineered and executed procedure will invariably fail if the patient is not committed to its success. Unlike urinary diversion with an external appliance in which a patient can play a rather *passive* role, internal diversion demands active and continuous patient and family participation. If this is not the case, renal function and the patient's general health is jeopardized. As simple and as obvious as they may seem, these principles are equal to, if not more important than, the surgical procedure itself.

Fitting the Right Operation to the Patient

This section relates, in very simplistic terms, concepts of lower urinary tract (LUT) function employed to achieve dryness in the patient. The two functions of the LUT are urine *storage* and evacuation or *emptying*. The importance of CIC is that it solves the problem of emptying. Any patient incapable of "normal" voiding may potentially be treated with intermittent catheterization. The problems, therefore, that the surgeon must address are (1) establishing a dependable channel with the ability to catheterize and (2) storage. In most patients a catheterizable channel, usually the urethra, is a given. Mitrofanoff (1980) has reported the appendix and Duckett and Snyder (1986) and Mitchell and co-workers (1988) the distal ureter, or even a tapered segment of small intestine, may be tunneled into the bladder wall and brought to the abdominal wall or perineum as a dry catheterizable stoma.

Establishing effective urine storage is the most challenging problem and the essence of urinary continence. To do this, a favorable dynamic balance between urethral (bladder/reservoir outlet) *resistance* and bladder (reservoir) *volume/compliance* is established. Both parameters are usually assessed with urodynamics. Volume and compliance can usually be measured with a water or gas cystometrogram, which gives a reasonably accurate assessment of the fibroelastic character of the bladder. Usually a bladder pressure study with fluoroscopy and slow filling provides maximal information.

It is worthwhile to note (1) the integrity of the ureterovesical valve and (2) the bladder neck. The appearance of the bladder can be confusing. Trabeculations do not necessarily equate with poor compliance, and a smooth bladder wall does *not* guarantee compliance.

In general, it is the slope of the pressure (P) versus volume (V) curve during filling, not the curve near capacity, that is most critical. If there is a constant increment in P to capacity, the slope of the P versus V curve may have meaning and would ideally be greater than 10 ml V increase per cm H_2O P ($\Delta V/\Delta P \geq 10$ ml/

cm H_2O). Small bladders or even moderately sized ones that have significant loss of elastic character (e.g., after multiple surgeries or infections) may have relatively flat P versus V curves, with acute upsweep at capacity (i.e., V/P is high until near capacity).

This type of bladder cannot be distinguished very well from a small potentially normal bladder in a patient with a previous diversion or with a very low outflow resistance. A previously diverted normal bladder with a flat P versus V curve during filling does have the potential to enlarge with cycling. However, an abnormal (e.g., neurogenic or scarred) and small bladder with upward slope to the P versus V curve (V/P is < 10 ml/ cm H_2O) will probably not distend with preoperative cycling. If a small bladder does not change with preoperative cycling, presume that it will not after diversion.

In general, any patient with marginal bladder compliance or capacity after maximal anticholinergic therapy should have bladder augmentation, particularly if urethral resistance is to be increased. It is much safer to make the bladder of greater compliance (ideally, a V/P > 20 ml per cm H_2O) with augmentation than to risk both continence and the upper tracts in an effort to avoid augmentation. In the neurogenic bladder (patient incontinent with frequent CIC) and in congenital low urethral resistance (patient with exstrophy/epispadias or bilateral ectopic ureter), it should be presumed that an augmentation will be necessary unless the urodynamics demonstrate a flat P versus V (high $\Delta V/\Delta P$) and good capacity. In general, to preserve upper tracts and urinary continence, bladder or reservoir pressure should be *minimized,* preferably always well below 40 cm H_2O.

Urethral resistance is much more difficult to assess, particularly in patients with small, poorly compliant bladders. Measurement of the urethral pressure profile may help to define urethral resistance, but McGuire and colleagues (1981) have found leak point pressure to be the most simple to define and utilize. Ideally, urethral resistance is defined with a dynamic study performed with no catheter in the urethra because, in the small patient, even a 5 or an 8 Fr. urethral catheter can change urethral resistance measurement.

In general, in the wet patient without normal voiding and sensation (on CIC) a urethral pressure of greater than 40 cm H_2O may be necessary to achieve dryness in a patient who has good bladder compliance. Obviously, the poorer the bladder compliance (V/P < 10 ml/cm H_2O) the greater the urethral resistance required to achieve dryness and the greater the risk for upper tract damage. High urethral resistance, as can be achieved by the Kropp and Angwafo (1986) procedure or the artificial urinary sphincter, in the patient with poor or no sensation of fullness may also raise the risk of spontaneous bladder rupture, particularly with bladder augmentation.

Urinary dryness dependent on intermittent catheterization is a state of retention with a proper balance between urethral resistance and bladder compliance. It is incorrect to increase urethral resistance without careful regard to bladder compliance in a wet patient. Dryness may result with loss of renal function. High urethral resistance *demands* good bladder compliance

(high $\Delta V/\Delta P$). A patient with low compliance is safe only with *low* urethral resistance. Increasing bladder compliance with augmentation in a patient with low urethral resistance may not result in dryness, but renal function should not be at risk. With careful consideration of the physiologic considerations previously mentioned and proper patient selection, more than 90 per cent of previously wet patients can be made dry (Rink and Mitchell, 1984). These are the simple principles. What follows are a few of the techniques selected to improve both bladder compliance and urethral resistance.

Patient Preparation

Augmentation cystoplasty is a major intra-abdominal operation that necessitates the optimization of the patient's hemodynamic fluid and electrolyte status. It is imperative that the patient or the parents in the case of children understand the operative procedure and its potential risks. They should also be made aware of alternatives. The patient should be informed of the preoperative bowel preparation and should also have knowledge of the usual postoperative course.

Is the patient mentally prepared for the operation? Any patient who may need CIC to empty must demonstrate the ability and the willingness to do so prior to intestinocystoplasty. Many patients considered for augmentation cystoplasty have a small-capacity defunctionalized bladder from prior urinary diversion. Perlmutter (1980) and Kogan and Levitt (1977) have shown that bladder cycling (e.g., intermittent instillation of saline solution to distend the bladder) may allow recuperation of most of the lost capacity. This cycling may be done through a suprapubic tube or CIC. However, the patient can practice and understand the demands of CIC prior to the operation if bladder cycling is done by urethral catheterization. Increasing volumes of normal saline solution may be instilled for 20 minutes to 1 hour, three times daily. In this process, the urethral resistance and the ability to store the instilled saline solution may also be assessed.

The segment of bowel used for augmentation or bladder replacement is not nearly as important as its size and configuration (Mitchell and Piser, 1987; Smith et al., 1977). Furthermore, Hinman (1989) has noted that there is no objective data that one segment is superior to another. After clinical consideration, therefore, the segment utilized is based primarily on the surgeon's preference. The patient's medical history may direct the surgeon toward a particular bowel segment. A history of ulcerative colitis or diverticulitis may preclude colon. Likewise, a history of ulcers should warn against stomach. The patient with prior pelvic irradiation would be better served by tissues outside the field of exposure (e.g., transverse colon or stomach). Intractable diarrhea may occur with ileocecal valves in patients with neurogenic bladders. Its use in patients with spinal dysraphism is to be avoided when possible. Gonzalez and Cabral (1987) have reported a child with myelomeningocele who developed severe diarrhea following the use of the ileocecal valve in urinary reconstruction. Control was obtained only after reincorporation of the valve into the intestinal tract.

Patients undergoing gastrocystoplasty or ileocystoplasty may require little or no bowel preparation. However, because one cannot predict the needs at the time of surgery, it is the best policy that all patients having bladder augmentation have full bowel preparations. Clear liquids are begun 2 days prior to surgery. One day before, a GoLYTELY preparation is initiated. Frequently, this must be given per nasogastric tube in children and usually requires admission to the hospital. In the patient with neurogenic bladder, it is occasionally necessary to evacuate the fluid from the bowel with a bisacodyl (Dulcolax) suppository after the GoLYTELY has been stopped. Adequate hydration is maintained by intravenous fluids overnight.

Antiembolism stockings or sequential compression devices are placed on the lower extremities of adults prior to surgery. The enterostomal therapist should mark the proposed stoma site where the abdominal wall stoma is to be constructed with a continent urinary reservoir.

SURGICAL TECHNIQUE FOR BLADDER AUGMENTATION

There are two separate components to any bladder augmentation. The first is management of the bladder and the second is the type and configuration of the intestinal segment. Each component can be handled by varying means and each has its own proponents.

Bladder Treatment

Various artificial substitutes for total bladder replacement or augmentation have been attempted as noted by Olsson (1988), but none has met with success because of either unsuccessful anastomosis or calculus formation. Intestine remains the primary bladder replacement tissue. Other options are available, however, for improving bladder compliance and increasing bladder capacity.

Cartwright and Snow (1989) have described such an alternative. They excise the detrusor muscle over the entire dome of the bladder, leaving the underlying epithelium to bulge as a wide-mouthed diverticulum to increase storage capacity. This procedure has been termed "autoaugmentation" (Fig. 71–1). The preserved detrusor muscle remains open by securing the bladder to the psoas muscles bilaterally. The initial experience noted improved compliance in four of the five patients studied and improved capacity in three of the five. One technical failure was reported. This "augmentation" would eliminate many of the problems associated with bowel in the urinary tract. However, long-term compliance is of concern when studies in dogs have shown collagen deposition overlying the epithelium after 6 weeks. Hinman (1989) notes that only rarely will this procedure provide adequate capacity and compliance.

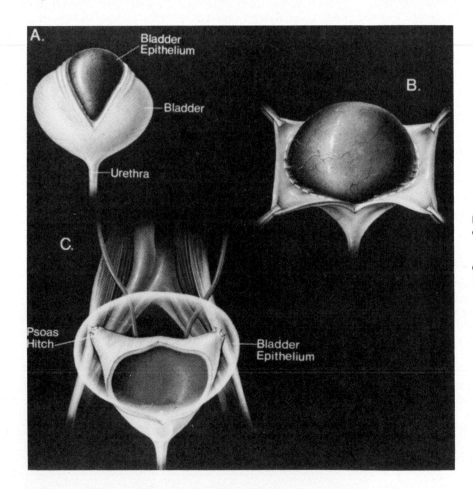

Figure 71–1. Autoaugmentation. *A,* Detrusor incised.
B, Detrusor stripped and excised from mucosa.
C, Bulging mucosa with bladder filling. (From Cartwright, P. C., and Snow, B. W.: J. Urol., 142:505, 1989.)

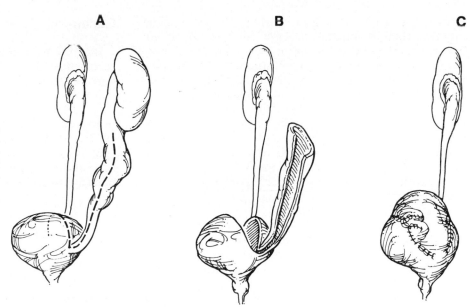

Figure 71–2. Ureteral augmentation. *A,* Proposed bladder incision transversely, with extension up the ureteral wall. *B,* Nephrectomy for nonfunctioning kidney with ureter and bladder opened. *C,* Ureteral bladder augmentation complete.

Alternatively, bladder capacity and compliance may be improved by using a massively dilated ureter from a nonfunctioning kidney (Fig. 71–2). This technique may be applied in the patient with a nonfunctioning hydronephrotic kidney secondary to poor vesical compliance, such as the child with the VURD (valves, unilateral reflux, dysplasia) syndrome (Rink and Salvas, 1991).

The initial incision for bladder augmentation, regardless of anticipated procedure, should be midline. The peritoneum is not opened until completion of any bladder neck surgery or ureteral reimplantation into the native bladder, to minimize third space fluid loss. A number of important principles should be followed no matter which bowel segment is selected. These would include the following:

1. The proposed segment of bowel for augmentation should be long enough to achieve the desired bladder capacity.
2. Vesicoureteral reflux, if present, should be corrected.
3. The tissues should be handled with care, and the procedure done with meticulous attention to detail.

Controversy has existed with regard to the management of the native bladder. Couvelaire (1950), Kerr and associates (1969), Gil-Vernet (1965), Turner-Warwick and Ashkem (1967), and Zinman and associates (1980) have recommended excision of the entire supratrigonal bladder. A cuff of bladder surrounding the trigone is left intact in order not to disturb the ureterovesical junction. This maneuver has been recommended for two reasons. First, to resect the diseased bladder when the etiology for bladder contraction is tuberculous cystitis, schistosomiasis, or interstitial cystitis. Second, to prevent the augmentation from forming a diverticulum. The second was a particularly important consideration, when normal voiding was anticipated. Conversely, many workers have not considered the importance of bladder excision, as long as the bladder is widely opened for a large-mouthed anastomosis (Abel and Gow, 1978; Goodwin et al., 1959; Hinman, 1989; Kay, 1986; Lieskovsky and Skinner, 1986; Mitchell and Rink, 1985). This practice prevents diverticulum formation and can be achieved by resecting the dome of the bladder, as described by Abel (1978) and Goodwin (1959), or by incising the bladder widely in the sagittal plane ("clam shell") as described by Bramble (1982) and Mitchell and Rink (1985) (Fig. 71–3).

Fall and Nilsson (1982) have noted that urgency may persist in some patients with interstitial cystitis even with supratrigonal cystectomy and enterocystoplasty. It is technically simpler to anastomose the bowel to an opened, bivalved bladder than to a small trigone or bladder neck. Further, the opened, native bladder adds to the overall capacity.

Ileal Cystoplasty

Tizzoni and Foggi (1888) selected ileum as the first segment of bowel for experimental augmentation. Ileum

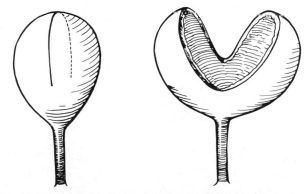

Figure 71–3. Sagittal incision of the bladder from bladder neck anteriorly to the trigone posteriorly, in preparation for augmentation ("clam shell").

was also chosen by Mikulicz to perform the first bladder augmentation in humans in 1898 (Orr et al., 1958). Experimental work in the early 1900s was directed more toward total bladder replacement with bowel rather than augmentation of the bladder. By the 1950s, numerous reports in the world literature on various techniques for ileocystoplasty had appeared (Cibert, 1953; Goodwin et al., 1959; Pyrah and Raper, 1955; Scheele, 1923; Tasker, 1953).

The ileum is opened along its antimesenteric border and is most commonly employed today for augmentation in one of three forms: Tasker's (1953) patch, Goodwin's (1959) cup patch, or as a hemi-Kock pouch (Weinberg, 1988) (Figs. 71–4 and 71–5).

A segment of ileum 20 to 40 cm in length is selected, such that it will easily reach the bladder. The segment is resected, taking all precautions necessary to preserve the blood supply. A two-layer ileoileostomy is performed. The bowel clamps on the isolated ileal segment are removed, and the ileum is irrigated with neomycin in saline solution until clear. The ileum is opened its entire length on the antimesenteric border with electrocautery and may be folded in a U-shape, anastomosing the margins in two layers (Fig. 71–6). A common suture technique is a two-layer closure: an inner layer of running interlocking 3-0 chromic and outer layer of running 3-0 Vicryl suture. This reconfigured ileum may be placed on the bladder or further folded to create a cup patch prior to anastomosis to the bladder.

If vesicoureteral reflux exists and implantation into the native bladder is not possible, ileum may still be chosen for augmentation and reflux prevented by creating an ileal nipple valve. The hemi-Kock pouch meets these requirements but requires nearly 60 cm of small intestine (see Fig. 71–5). A 7-cm afferent segment is left as a tube and the remainder is opened as previously described. The nonrefluxing nipple valve is fashioned by stripping 8 cm of mesentery from the afferent limb adjacent to the pouch. The ileum is then intussuscepted and stapled in three parallel rows. The nipple is anchored to the pouch with a fourth row of staples, and a mesh strip is sewn circumferentially around the afferent limb to prevent slippage. The pouch is completed by folding the augmentation portion on itself and anastomosing this to the native bladder. The ureters are anastomosed to the afferent limb, end-to-side. Of the first seven patients reported by Weinberg and co-workers (1988), two did require surgical revision for valve problems.

Cecum

In 1950 Couvelaire first reported the utilization of cecum to augment the urinary bladder. Numerous reports of cecocystoplasty have appeared since Couvelaire's report (Chau et al., 1980; Dounis et al., 1980; Kass and Koff, 1983; Menville et al., 1958; Shirley and Mirelman, 1978; Skinner, 1982; Whitmore and Gittes, 1983), but Gil-Vernet (1965), Turner-Warwick and Ashkem (1967), and Zinman and co-workers (1987) have been the main proponents. The three basic configurations are as follows:

1. A simple cecocystoplasty used as a cap.
2. An ileocecal cystoplasty with the cecum reconfigured and the ileum anastomosed to the ureters.
3. An ileocecal cystoplasty with the cecum opened and reconfigured, incorporating the opened terminal ileum into the augmenting segment.

Many variations have been described, but in all the technique begins similarly. The ileum, cecum, and ascending colon are mobilized. For augmentation, the segment is based on the ileocolic artery, but if more bowel is needed for extensive bladder replacement, the right colic artery may be included with this segment. The colon is divided close to the right colic artery and approximately 15 cm proximal to the ileocecal valve (i.e., that segment of ileum supplied by the ileocolic artery). For a simple cap cecoplasty, a very short segment of ileum is resected and discarded after division of its blood supply near the cecum. The stump of ileum is turned into the cecum or closed in two layers.

An appendectomy is usually performed; however, the proximal appendix may be tunneled into the cecum along a taenia and the distal end brought through the abdominal wall as a catheterizable stoma (Mitrofanoff, 1980). The cecum is now opened between the taeniae on the antimesenteric border and folded into a cap to anastomose to the bladder in two layers as noted for ileocystoplasty (Fig. 70–7).

Ureters can be reimplanted into the cecum by either a tunnel or nipple technique. However, Robertson and King (1986) had to revise 23 per cent of their ureterocecal anastomoses, a much greater proportion than in their ureterosigmoid anastomoses. Simple cecocystoplasty *without* reconfiguration is not now commonly performed. Part of the attraction of the cecum is the ileum and ileocecal valve. Ileum can be opened and used to patch the cecum to prevent unit contractions and to

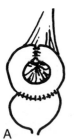
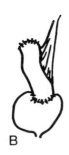
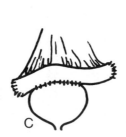
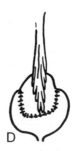
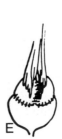

A   B   C   D   E

Figure 71–4. Ileocystoplasty types.
A, Ring plastik (Scheele).
B, "Rat tail" (Cibert).
C, U-shaped tube (Pyrah).
D, Flap or patch (Tasker).
E, Cup-patch (Goodwin). (From Goodwin, W. E., Winter, C. C., and Barker, W. F.: Surg. Gynecol. Obstet., 108:240, 1959. By permission of Surgery, Gynecology and Obstetrics.)

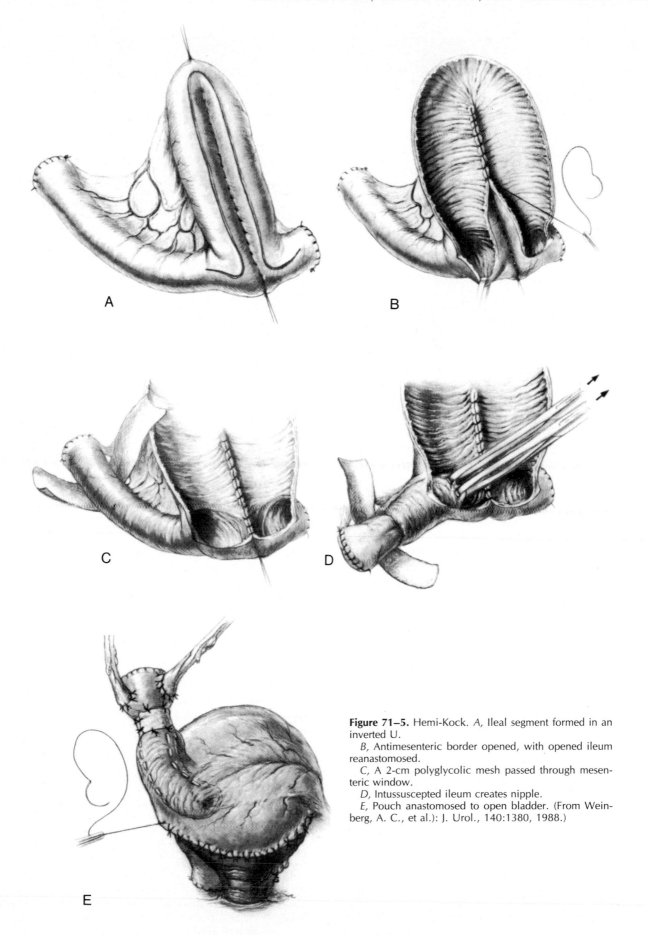

Figure 71–5. Hemi-Kock. *A,* Ileal segment formed in an inverted U.

B, Antimesenteric border opened, with opened ileum reanastomosed.

C, A 2-cm polyglycolic mesh passed through mesenteric window.

D, Intussuscepted ileum creates nipple.

E, Pouch anastomosed to open bladder. (From Weinberg, A. C., et al.): J. Urol., 140:1380, 1988.)

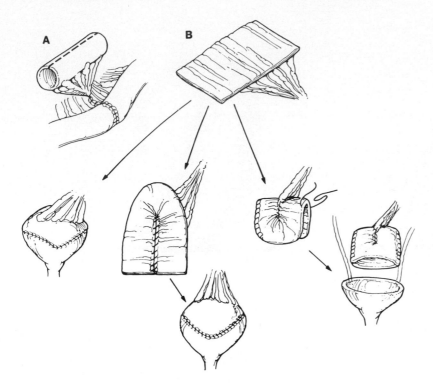

Figure 71–6. Ileal augmentation. *A,* Ileal segment selected. *B,* Ileum segment opened on antimesenteric border. Options include patch augmentation, reconfigured and placed on bivalved bladder, or reconfigured as cup on bladder, after the dome is excised.

create a larger reservoir. The incorporation of the ileum into the cecum may be done in a variety of ways but is most commonly done in the manner proposed by Light and Scardino (1986) and Light and Engelman (1986)— "Le Bag,"—or the "MAINZ pouch" by Thuroff and co-workers (1985 and 1987) (Figs. 71–7 and 71–8).

In both techniques, the entire ileocecal segment is opened along the antimesenteric border. In the Le Bag technique, the opened ileum is anastomosed to the opened cecum to create a cup, which is sutured to the opened bladder. The MAINZ pouch differs in that the ileum is first folded into two segments of equal length; the opened cecum and the two ileal segments are then sutured side-to-side. Thuroff and co-workers (1987) recommend a subtotal cystectomy. With a longer ileal segment either method may be chosen for total bladder replacement.

Good reasons for the utilization of the ileocecal segment in urinary reconstruction are that the ileocecal valve may be used to prevent ureteral reflux and the ileum may be used for ureteral replacement. Unfortunately, prevention of reflux with the intussuscepted ileocecal valve has been successful in only 50 per cent of our cases, and similar results were noted by Hensle and Burbige (1985).

A variety of techniques aimed at the reinforcement of the ileocecal valve have been developed. Hendren (1980) recommended the division of the mesentery from the terminal ileum for 6 to 8 cm, to allow intussusception of the ileum into the cecum. Fixation by suturing serosal surfaces together, stapling the intussuscepted nipple, or scarifying the serosa have all been attempted to improve results.

Currently, Robertson and King's (1986) modification of Hendren's technique seems promising (Fig. 71–9). In this technique, the full-thickness outer wall of the nipple is incised with cautery for 2.5 cm. The opposing cecal mucosa is incised, and the incisions are sutured together

with chromic catgut. Reflux was prevented in seven of eight patients by this method. The ileal segment is left as long as necessary to bridge the gap to the ureters, which are sutured to the ileum end-to-side or end-to-end. This form of augmentation is very appealing when the ureters are short.

Sigmoid Colon

In 1912, Lemoine first reported colocystoplasty in humans (Charghi et al., 1967). Bisgard and Kerr first reported sigmoid colon for augmentation cystoplasty in the United States in 1949. Reports of larger series by Mathisen (1955), Winter and Goodwin (1958), and Kuss (1958) appeared by the mid 1950s. Since that time, many reports support colocystoplasty (Charghi et al., 1967; Dounis and Gow, 1979; Krarstein and Mathisoen, 1981). Similar to other bowel segments, but even more so with sigmoid, the cystoplasty must be constructed as a patch rather than a tube to prevent high pressure unit contractions (Mitchell and Piser, 1987).

Sigmoid colon does have some advantages over other bowel segments, including its thick muscular wall, large lumen, and bladder proximity. Further, reliable antirefluxing ureteral reimplantation into the taenia is possible. Disadvantages to the use of sigmoid colon are the strong unit contractions; mucus production; diverticular formation; and, as noted by Sheiner and Kaplan (1988) and Elder and associates (1988), perhaps a higher incidence of spontaneous perforation than other bowel for augmentation.

A minimal length of 15 to 20 cm sigmoid colon segment is selected. The mesentery can be divided for a relatively short distance at either end of the segment because of the proximity of the bladder. The sigmoid segment is irrigated with neomycin until clear. The rest of the abdominal cavity is packed to prevent possible

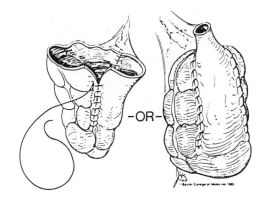

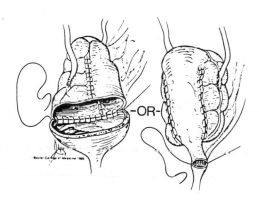

Figure 71–7. "Le Bag." *A*, Ileocecal segment outlined.
B, Ileocecal segment opened on antimesenteric border with ileocolic anastomosis.
C, Ileocolonic segment anastomosed to native bladder. (From Light, J. D., Scardino, P. T.: Urol. Clin. North Am., 13:261, 1986.)

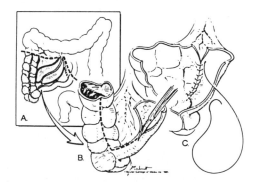

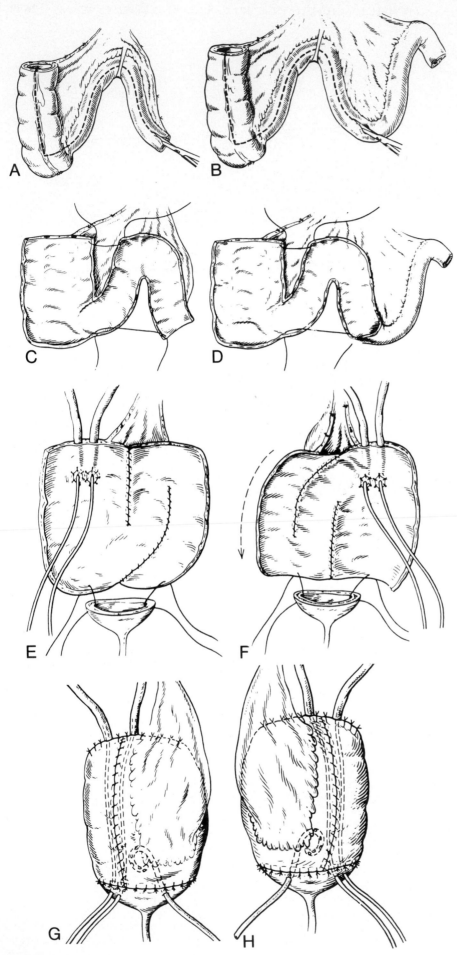

Figure 71–8. MAINZ (augmentation/pouch). *A,* Opening resected segment of terminal ileum and cecum.

B, Same in preparation for pouch.

C and *D,* Closure to form large reservoir.

E and *F,* Alternative techniques of augmentation and reimplantation of ureters.

G and *H,* Completed alternative augmentations. (From Thuroff, J. W., et al.: *In* King, L. R., et al. (Eds.). Bladder Reconstruction and Continent Urinary Diversion. Chicago, Year Book Medical Publishers, 1987.)

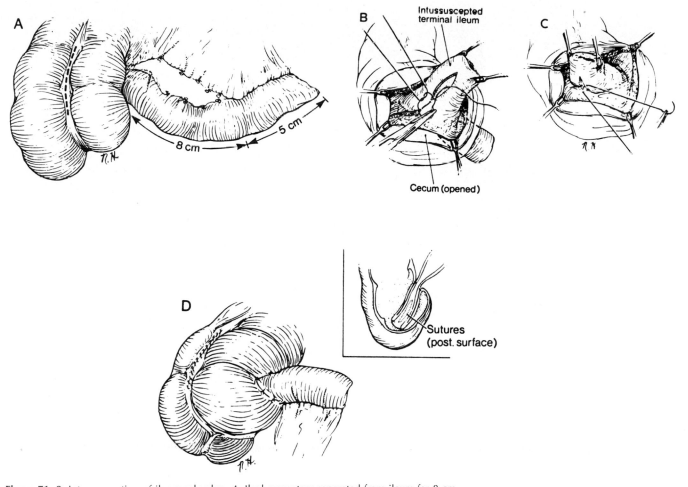

Figure 71–9. Intussusception of ileocecal valve. *A,* Ileal mesentery separated from ileum for 8 cm.
  B, Ileum intussuscepted, 2- to 3-cm incision through outer layer of intussusception with equal-sized mucosal incision.
  C, Cut edges anastomosed.
  D, Interrupted seromuscular sutures placed. (From Robertson, C. N., and King, L. R.: Urol. Clin. North Am., 13:333, 1986.)

contamination. If a sphincter is to be implanted at the time of augmentation the plane around the bladder neck is dissected prior to augmentation, but the sphincter placed *after* augmentation is completed. The sigmoid colon is opened along the antimesenteric border. Tubular sigmoid colon must *never* be utilized for augmentation. The sigmoid segment may be folded on itself and the edges approximated in two layers of chromic and Vicryl sutures. The resultant cup fits well on the bladder following subtotal bladder excision. Alternatively, as described by Mitchell (1986), both ends of the isolated sigmoid segment may be closed and antimesenteric border opened. This bowel segment can now be placed on the bivalved bladder in either the transverse or the sagittal plane (Fig. 71–10). The anastomosis is completed in two layers. As in all augmentations of the bladder, a suprapubic tube is placed through the native bladder wall.

Stomach

Searching for a bladder substitute that would obviate the hyperchloremic acidosis associated with bowel seg-

ments, Sinaiko (1956) created a gastric urinary reservoir in dogs. This was a large Heidenhain pouch from gastric fundus and corpus. In 1956, this same procedure was performed in a 38-year-old woman with bladder cancer (Sinaiko, 1957).

Since Sinaiko's original work, stomach has been employed for bladder augmentation and total bladder replacement and as a cutaneous conduit and catheterizable urethra (Adams et al., 1988; Leong, 1988; Rink, 1988; Ruddick et al., 1977). Two separate techniques have emerged for bladder augmentation or replacement. Leong and Ong (1972) and Leong (1988) have championed the use of the entire antrum with the blood supply maintained by the left gastroepiploic artery. Continuity of the gastrointestinal tract is obtained by a Bilroth I anastomosis (Fig. 71–11).

Ruddick and colleagues (1977) chose a gastric wedge from the greater curvature to create a gastric reservoir. A similar technique for bladder augmentation has been popularized by Mitchell, Rink, and Adams (Adams et al., 1988; Kennedy et al., 1988; Piser et al., 1987; Rink, 1988). Stomach offers the advantages over bowel segments of less mucus production; net *chloride excretion,* as demonstrated by Piser (1987); ease of ureteral reim-

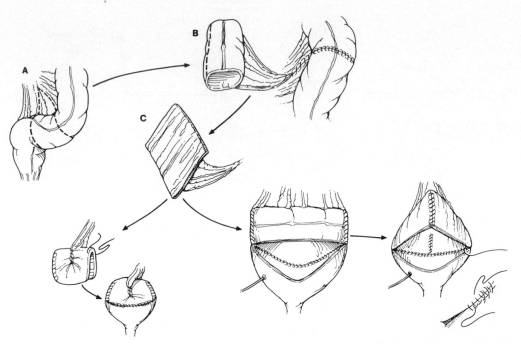

Figure 71–10. Sigmoid augmentation. *A,* Sigmoid segment selected. *B* and *C,* Proposed incision antimesenteric border with patch options of cup-patch on bladder after dome excision or ends closed and placed on bivalved bladder.

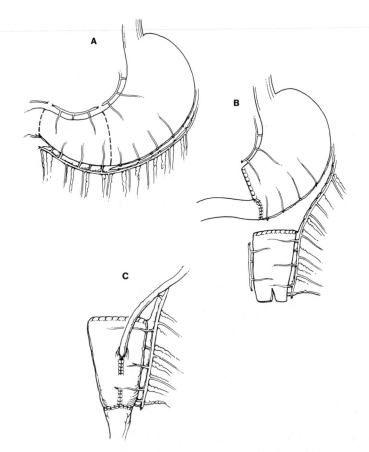

Figure 71–11. Antral gastrocystoplasty. *A,* Antral segment selected. Gastric arteries and right gastroepiploic artery divided.

B, Antrectomy with Bilroth I anastomosis. Antrum supplied left gastroepiploic.

C, Ureteral reimplantation into antral pouch, which is anastomosed to urethra (Leong technique).

plantation (similar to native bladder); and tissue that is readily available and only rarely in the field of radiation. Furthermore, stomach will not tend to further compromise the patient with short gut syndrome.

The gastric wedge flap for augmentation may be based on either the right or the left gastroepiploic artery. The right, however, is most constant. The wedge is outlined with a skin scribe, with the length along the greater curvature being 10 to 20 cm, depending on patient size. The radii extend almost to the lesser curvature and usually measure 7 to 15 cm. The vasa brevia are ligated, leaving only the blood supply to the gastric wedge. When utilizing the right gastroepiploic artery, the short gastrics may be divided to give greater motility to the left side of the stomach. This triangular segment is excised with the apex stopping just short of the lesser curvature using the GIA stapler. After the removal of the staples, the stomach is closed in two layers—outer, interrupted silk, and inner, running Vicryl. The gastric flap may now be passed through the transverse mesocolon and the small bowel mesentery such that the pedicle is in the retroperitoneum. The opened wedge fits well on the bivalved bladder. This anastomosis is accomplished with two running layers of chromic and Vicryl suture (Fig. 71–12). Nasogastric decompression is all that is necessary.

EARLY POSTOPERATIVE MANAGEMENT

Care of the patient following augmentation cystoplasty is similar, regardless of gastrointestinal segment. These procedures are lengthy, with significant fluid losses and shifts. Strict attention to fluid and electrolyte management is mandatory. The patients are routinely monitored in the intensive care unit for 24 hours. Nasogastric suction is maintained until bowel function recovers.

All patients are maintained on suprapubic drainage. Mucus production can be excessive early and may occlude the suprapubic tube. Suprapubic tube irrigation should be performed at least three times daily within the immediate postoperative period, particularly with sigmoid, cecal, and ileal augmentations.

At 1 week following augmentation, a cystogram is obtained. If no urinary leak is noted, the patient may be discharged from the hospital while on suprapubic tube drainage. Intermittent irrigation must continue at home with frequency dependent on mucus production. At 3 weeks postoperatively, *all* patients are started on intermittent catheterization every 2 to 3 hours during the day and one to two times during the night. The catheterization is modified, depending on individual patient requirements. Patients without neurologic impairment may spontaneously void, obviating the need for catheterization. Any patient with significant post void residual volumes must be maintained on CIC.

Routine evaluation of the upper urinary tract (renal ultrasound, intravenous pyelography, or renal scan) is obtained at 6 weeks, 6 months, and 1 year following the intestinocystoplasty. If clinical conditions warrant, more frequent studies may be necessary. Electrolytes, BUN, and creatinine determinations along with urine cultures are routinely performed at 3-month intervals during the 1st operative year. A cystogram is obtained at 6 months. Antibiotics are usually continued for 2 months after surgery. Yearly evaluation by ultrasound and serum chemistry studies continues for the long-term.

COMPLICATIONS OF CYSTOPLASTY

Although complications of bowel in the urinary tract are discussed elsewhere, a few problems unique to augmentation cystoplasty should be mentioned here.

Spontaneous bladder perforation after intestinocystoplasty has now been reported by a number of groups for all segments of bowel and stomach (Elder et al., 1988; Rink et al., 1988; Rushton et al., 1988; Sheiner and Kaplan, 1988). This perforation is a potentially life-threatening occurrence, and diagnosis can be elusive. In 231 patients with augmentations, Rink and associates (1988) have identified 14 patients with 16 ruptures. These occurred equally in males and females. Importantly, the interval to rupture ranged from 2 to 75 months. Unfortunately, delay in diagnosis is common.

Nausea and vomiting are most commonly noted (88 per cent). Only 50 per cent of patients with ruptures have abdominal pain. Cystogram frequently does not identify the perforation. Computed tomography scanning is usually diagnostic. By history, one elicits a prolonged interval between catheterizations. The exact cause is also often difficult to assign. Usually, the patients are noted to have high urethral resistance and impaired sensation due to spinal dysraphism. Sheldon and co-workers (1990) propose that high intravesical pressures result in ischemia of the augmenting segment, resulting in perforation. A high index of suspicion of bladder perforation is mandatory following augmentation cystoplasty.

A review article by Filmer and Spencer (1990) noted 14 cases of primary malignancies in bladders following augmentation. Currently, research is centered on carcinogenic substances, most notably nitrosamines, but the exact etiology is unknown.

Klee and associates (1990) stated that papillomas did occur in five of 15 rats studied that underwent gastrocystoplasty. These workers found histologic changes in both the transplanted gastric patch and the native bladder, including squamous hyperplasia and cystic dilatation of the glands. The significance of these findings in humans is unknown. However, patients undergoing bladder augmentations need long-term surveillance. Because malignancy may arise within 10 years following augmentations, yearly cystoscopy should begin at that time (Filmer and Spencer, 1990). Perhaps in the future, flow cystometry or cytology will prove beneficial.

Hyperchloremic metabolic acidosis is a well-recognized complication of intestinocystoplasty. Stomach has prevented this complication, because there is an energy-dependent chloride pump, which results in a net urinary loss of chloride. Rarely, this chloride pump has led to significant metabolic alkalosis (Adams et al., 1988). This

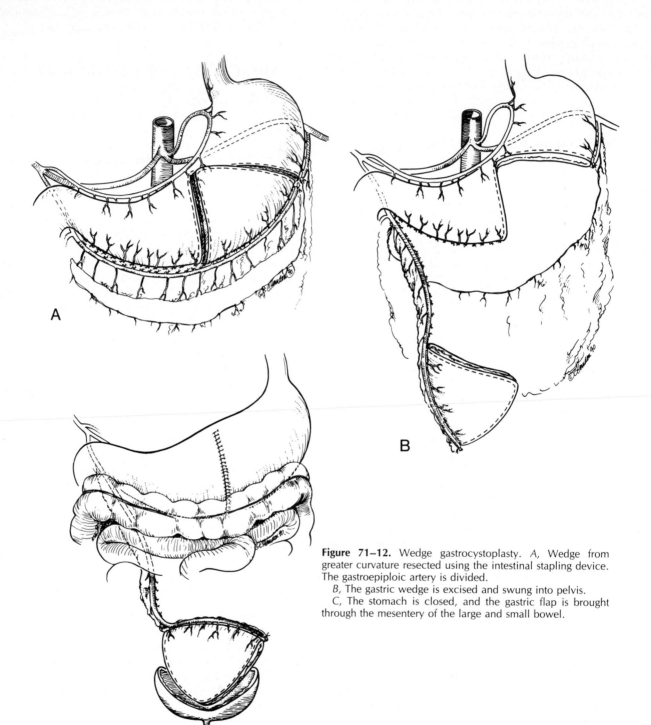

Figure 71–12. Wedge gastrocystoplasty. *A,* Wedge from greater curvature resected using the intestinal stapling device. The gastroepiploic artery is divided.

B, The gastric wedge is excised and swung into pelvis.

C, The stomach is closed, and the gastric flap is brought through the mesentery of the large and small bowel.

problem occurred in two patients with renal insufficiency who had significant tubular concentrating defect and increased salt-wasting. Both episodes followed severe viral gastroenteritis with nausea, vomiting, diarrhea, and poor fluid intake, and both were relieved with intravenous salt replacement.

Bladder calculus formation is not a rare event following augmentation cystoplasty. This finding is a consequence of poor bladder emptying, frequent infection, and mucus. Because of the potential for bladder stone formation, an annual KUB should be obtained.

ALTERNATIVE CONSIDERATIONS

One group of patients continues to be excluded from reconstruction with bladder augmentation. These are primarily females who are unable to routinely catheterize the native urethra. Often these patients are wheelchair bound. A catheterizable abdominal wall stoma, employing the Mitrofanoff principle (1980), is a highly successful option. Any supple tube (appendix, ureter, ileum, stomach) may be tunneled into the native bladder or bowel and brought out the abdominal wall as a catheterizable stoma. The umbilicus has been a particularly attractive site, providing excellent cosmesis and ease of catheterization.

Improving Urethral Resistance

In the reconstruction of the lower urinary tract, an important goal is to keep bladder pressure lower than urethral resistance most of the time. As discussed previously, when medical therapy fails, a compliant reservoir can generally be achieved in a reliable fashion with bladder augmentation. Achievement of adequate urethral resistance is often a more difficult task and is accompanied by its own side effects and potential complications. A logical first step in attempting to improve urethral resistance is medical manipulation. Alpha-adrenergic agonists produce smooth muscle contraction of the bladder neck and proximal urethra and, theoretically at least, increase maximum urethral closure pressure. Beta-adrenergic antagonists may potentiate alpha-adrenergic effects and increase outlet resistance. Such medications may produce clinical improvement but rarely are adequate alone, in cases of significant impairment of urethral resistance.

The physiologic bases of surgical attempts to improve urethral resistance vary greatly and depend on the anticipated mechanism of emptying, normal voiding, or CIC. Reconstruction of the bladder neck anticipating normal voiding usually is an attempt to enhance the inherent function of local musculature. Tubularization of the bladder neck and trigone, as described by Young and modified by Dees and Leadbetter (Leadbetter, 1964), has a success rate approaching 70 per cent in the best of hands (Lepor and Jeffs, 1983). Tanagho (1981) reports a similar success rate employing the anterior bladder neck. Kropp's (1986) procedure of urethral lengthening and reimplantation anticipates CIC and, therefore, is basically a form of orthotopic diversion.

Continence is based on submucosal tunneling of the tubular urethra into the bladder as a flap-valve mechanism. Mechanical compression of the bladder neck and urethra may be achieved with a fascial sling, a periurethral injection of various materials, or an artificial urinary sphincter. This compression is fixed with a sling or an injection and is intermittent with an artificial sphincter.

The artificial urinary sphincter usually assumes "normal" voiding and in a sense mimics the normal functioning sphincter mechanism and is quite physiologic. A properly functioning artificial sphincter provides effective outflow resistance that can be readily reduced to allow voiding much as the native sphincter. The artificial sphincter does so, however, utilizing prosthetic material that is totally foreign to the body. In addition, this prosthetic sphincter will not grow with the patient.

The incontinent patient who potentially benefits the most from an artificial urinary sphincter has a *compliant bladder* with *poor outflow resistance* and can empty the bladder. Figure 71–13 illustrates such a case—a 6-year-old boy with myelodysplasia. When first evaluated for neurogenic dysfunction and urinary incontinence, the urodynamics revealed a small, noncompliant bladder and marginal urethral resistance with a leak point pressure of 30 cm H_2O. The patient was able to void to completion by Valsalva's maneuver. The upper tract was normal. This patient initially underwent bladder augmentation using ileum. However, he continued to wet after dry intervals of only 2 hours. Repeat urodynamics demonstrated a compliant reservoir but leakage at pressures of 20 to 30 cm H_2O. With effort, the patient was still able to completely empty the bladder spontaneously by Valsalva's maneuver. An American Medical Systems model 800 artificial urinary sphincter was placed, which resulted in the patient being dry for intervals of 4 to 5 hours between voiding.

With follow-up of 4 years, this boy remains dry, has normal upper tracts, and has been free of urinary tract infection. No other procedure to enhance bladder outlet resistance could be expected to be effective yet result in continued spontaneous voiding in this clinical setting.

History

The first attempted prosthetic augmentation of urethral resistance was made by Berry in 1961. An acrylic prosthesis was placed between the urethra and bulbocavernosus muscle. Kaufman (1973) then developed a silicone prosthesis that was strapped against the bulbar urethra.

The first attempt at a true artificial urinary sphincter was made by Scott and associates in 1973: the AS-721 prosthesis (Fig. 71–14). This silicone prosthesis consisted of an inflatable cuff for placement around the urethra or bladder neck, separate inflation and deflation pumps, and a reservoir. Cuff pressure was maintained by a valve in the deflation limb. This valve tended to fail with time. A pressure-regulating balloon was added to the deflation limb in the AS-761 model. The balloon helped regulate and maintain cuff pressure at an acceptable level. How-

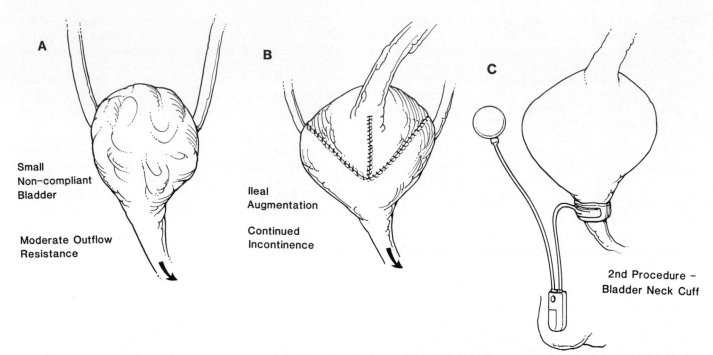

Figure 71–13. *A,* Six-year-old boy with myelodysplasia and urinary incontinence based on neurogenic bladder dysfunction and marginal bladder outflow resistance.
B, The bladder was augmented using ileum; however, the patient remained wet after 2 hour–dry intervals.
C, An artificial urinary sphincter was placed at a second procedure. The patient is dry and able to void spontaneously by Valsalva's maneuver.

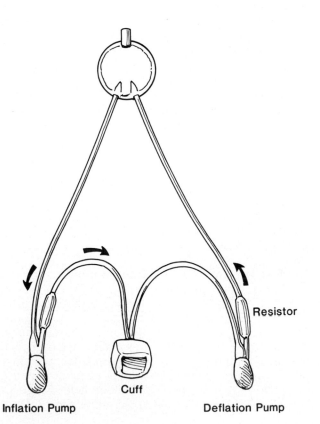

Figure 71–14. The AS 721 prosthesis with separate inflation and deflation pumps.

ever, the large number of components made this device susceptible to mechanical failure.

The AS-742 model was the first to have a pressure-regulating balloon as a reservoir for cuff fluid. The reservoir itself generated and exerted a predetermined pressure on the cuff. This pressure was dependent on the thickness of the balloon. This mechanism allowed for automatic refill of the cuff after voiding. A resistor between the balloon and cuff slowed return filling of the cuff to allow adequate time for voiding.

The AS-791/792 prosthesis further consolidated the components by placing the valves and resistor of the AS-742 model in a single control assembly.

Improvements continued, and in 1982 the current AS-800 prosthesis was introduced (Fig. 71–15). The valve and resistor were moved into the pump mechanism. The pump also included a new deactivation mechanism that allowed external deactivation and artificial sphincter activation. Thus, the sphincter cuff could be left in a deflated state immediately following placement and activated later. Delayed primary activation of previous models had required a second operation for connection of the parts. Subsequent modifications included improvements in the dip-coated cuff, which decreased wear and the potential for cuff leaks. New reinforced tubing was less prone to kinking.

Technique

As previously discussed, the primary objective in any patient who is undergoing reconstruction for urinary

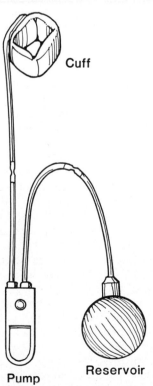

Figure 71–15. The AS 800 prosthesis with pump, valve, and resistor within the pump mechanism.

incontinence is a compliant bladder. Therefore, patients with small, noncompliant bladders should undergo correction prior to or at the time of any procedure to increase outflow resistance. In patients with very poor urethral resistance, early leakage around the urodynamic catheter may make it difficult to truly estimate bladder capacity even with good compliance. A catheter with the balloon seated at the neck may prevent leakage and may better predict bladder volume. This technique may also unmask uninhibited contractions, particularly in the patient with neurogenic dysfunction.

Very poor urethral resistance and constant leakage of urine may provide little stimuli for the bladder to expand to its full capacity. As mentioned previously, this problem may be reflected on cystometrogram by a bladder that is smaller in capacity than expected but compliant until full. Such a bladder will often stretch and function well with increased urethral resistance alone, although failure to do so threatens the upper urinary tract. Close follow-up care in this clinical setting is imperative to ensure that such a bladder responds as expected.

Ideally, an ability to adequately empty the bladder should be demonstrated. Furthermore, a properly functioning artificial urinary sphincter alone should *not* adversely affect such emptying. Intermittent catheterization can be practiced in conjunction with an artificial sphincter, and a well-placed cuff should provide no difficulty during catheterization.

The patients who benefit the most from artificial sphincters, however, are those who can empty and who do not require CIC. For those patients already committed to catheterization (e.g., cannot empty), adequate outflow resistance can usually be obtained with the previously mentioned procedures (fascial sling, Kropp, Young-Dees-Leadbetter) rather than with artificial sphincters.

The dynamics and physiology of the entire urinary tract must be considered prior to placement of an artificial urinary sphincter. Upper urinary tract obstruction and vesicoureteral reflux should be corrected if present. The patient must be willing and able to empty the bladder reliably. Failure to address these issues can create problems much worse than urinary incontinence. High urethral resistance, in an improper clinical setting, places the upper tracts and overall renal function at risk, often in a patient who is newly dry. As previously discussed, such concerns are particularly valid for any patient with underlying impairment of renal function. Such a patient often has a defect in renal concentrating ability and produces very large volumes of urine. Failure to appreciate the magnitude of this volume can result in further renal damage and progress to renal failure.

The artificial urinary sphincter works best in a motivated and committed patient. To ultimately achieve a good result, the bladder must be emptied completely on a timely basis. This commitment is seldom a problem in adults. However, in younger patients, cooperation and commitment can be *very* limiting. Support systems must be involved and include family, school nurses and officials, and local health officials. A passive noncompliant patient will overstress such a system, usually remain wet, and risk renal function. The appropriate age for sphincter placement depends more on emotional maturity than chronologic age. The sphincter can work well in a 5- or 6-year-old patient and be totally inappropriate in an uncooperative or a rebellious 15-year-old one.

Children grow, and the artificial sphincter will not. This problem can slowly create a situation of unrecognized urinary retention, particularly in the pubescent male. Furthermore, the dynamics of the urinary tract may change with time, particularly in a child with cord tethering. Thus, the child being considered for an artificial sphincter and his or her family must be committed to a lifetime of close follow-up care. The onset of wetting in the patient with a normally functioning sphincter is an important and ominous sign.

Clearly, everyone involved with placement of the artificial sphincter, including the surgeon, the patient, and the family, must understand its mechanical nature. This means recognizing and accepting the likelihood of future surgery to revise and repair the device. Constant modifications have improved the artificial sphincter; however, mechanical breakdowns still may occur.

As with all reconstructive surgery, proper patient preparation for surgery is important. *Sterile urine* should be documented preoperatively. Patients should receive preoperative prophylactic antibiotics to achieve the appropriate serum and tissue levels of the drugs at the time of sphincter placement. When the urine is sterile, the skin is the most likely source of potential contamination. *Staphylococcus epidermidis* is the predominant pathogen and should be susceptible to the antibiotic chosen.

All patients need a light bowel preparation, to ensure an empty rectum. Any patient who has had previous major reconstructive surgery of the bladder or surgery at the bladder neck, such that dissection may be difficult, should have a full mechanical and antibiotic bowel preparation. Females should have a complete vaginal preparation. A sterile pack in the rectum in the male or in the vagina in the female aids immensely in dissection of the bladder and proximal urethra.

The artificial sphincter cuff can be placed around the bladder neck in males and females or the bulbar urethra in males after puberty. Cuff placement at the bladder neck is generally more effective (Scott, 1989). In routine cases the patient may be placed in the supine position and a midline or transverse lower abdominal incision made. In difficult reoperative cases access to the perineum may, at times, be beneficial, and the patient should be in the low lithotomy position. In such a case, a lower midline incision is preferable. Exposure of the bladder neck and proximal urethra may be difficult in a patient after multiple previous surgeries.

Palpation of a Foley catheter balloon is very helpful in identifying the bladder neck. Do not hesitate to enter the bladder cephalad to the area of anticipated cuff placement. Entry into the bladder facilitates tremendously the dissection around the bladder neck and the location of the ureteral orifices. If the bladder is entered, it is our preference to place a suprapubic tube rather than a urethral catheter for postoperative drainage.

Incision of the endopelvic fascia on either side of the urethra helps to visualize the proper plane posterior to the bladder neck and urethra. Great care must be taken to avoid injury to adjacent organs or the urethra itself. Palpation of the previously placed sponge in the vagina in females or rectum in males will help prevent inadvertent entry into these organs.

After the plane posterior to the urethra has been developed, the sphincter sizer is placed around the urethra and pulled gently. This maneuver will determine the appropriate cuff size (length) and assure that the width of dissection is appropriate to prevent folding of the cuff. The cuff is placed *deflated* and should fit snugly, never tightly (Fig. 71–16). In adults, the majority of cuffs placed at the bladder neck range from 7 to 8.5 cm in length (Scott, 1989). Appropriate cuff length in children will vary greatly, and the tendency probably should be to err toward a larger cuff size. Tubing from the bladder neck cuff should be passed through the abdominal wall to the subcutaneous space anterior to the rectus fascia.

Exposure for a bulbous cuff can be obtained by a midline perineal incision and separation of the bulbo-cavernosus muscle. The urethra within the corpus spongiosum can be freed, circumferentially away from the overlying corpora. Cuff length will be much shorter with bulbous urethral placement, generally 4.5 cm in adults (Fig. 71–17) (Scott, 1989). From the bulbar cuff, the tubing can be tunneled subcutaneously up to the lower abdominal wall for connection. Never attempt bulbar placement in the prepubescent male, because the tissues of the immature bulb are thin and the risk of cuff erosion is high.

The sphincter pump is placed in the dependent scrotum or labia. Approximation of dartos or subcutaneous tissue between the tubing exiting the pump may help keep it dependent (Fig. 71–18). The balloon reservoir is placed intra-abdominally or in the paravesical space, if there is adequate space to avoid compression of the reservoir. Occasionally, the reservoir must be placed intraperitoneally, particularly after bladder augmentation. In either case, the tubing is again passed through the rectus muscle and fascia to the subcutaneous space. Care should be taken that the reservoir does not lie on the sphincter cuff or tubing to avoid wear.

In general, a medium pressure (P = 61 to 70 cm H_2O) reservoir is appropriate and should provide adequate urethral resistance. Higher reservoir pressure does not necessarily result in more dryness and significantly increases the likelihood of sphincter cuff erosion (Bosco et al., 1990; Kil et al., 1989; Scott, 1989). The tubing from cuff, reservoir, and pump are connected in the subcutaneous space. Once the sphincter is totally in place and connected, the device should be tested to make sure it functions properly. It should then be left in the *deactivated* state from *four* to *six weeks* to allow healing and development of collateral vascular supply of the tissue within the sphincter cuff. Scott (1989), however, feels that the sphincter can be activated much sooner in routine cases.

Urinary retention is the norm due to edema of the bladder neck and posterior urethra for the first 5 to 7 days. This situation can be managed until the edema resolves by CIC through a *small* indwelling urethral

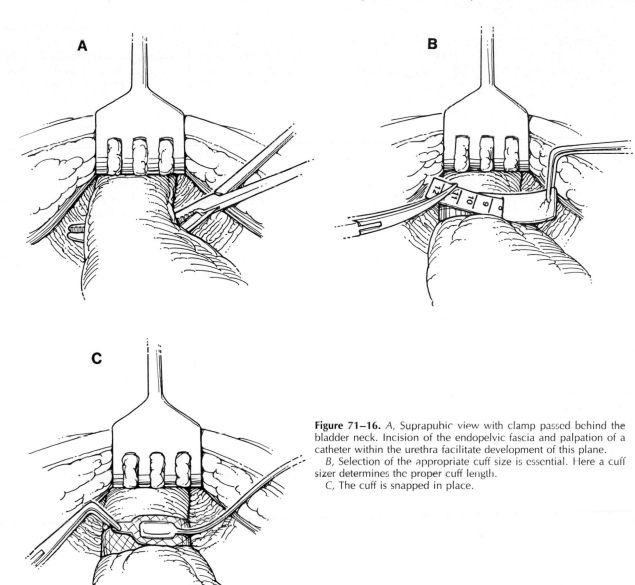

A

B

C

Figure 71–16. *A,* Suprapubic view with clamp passed behind the bladder neck. Incision of the endopelvic fascia and palpation of a catheter within the urethra facilitate development of this plane.

B, Selection of the appropriate cuff size is essential. Here a cuff sizer determines the proper cuff length.

C, The cuff is snapped in place.

Figure 71–17. Exposure to the bulbar urethra is obtained by a midline perineal incision. A cuff is passed around the urethra within corpus spongiosum.

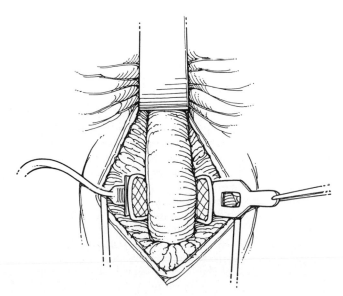

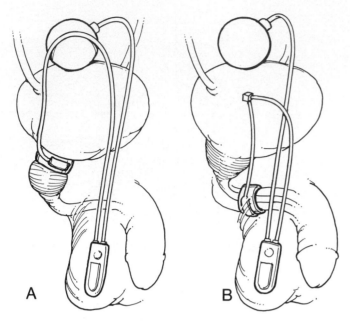

Figure 71–18. The connected sphincter in place with (A) cuff at the bladder neck and (B) cuff around the bulbar urethra.

catheter or suprapubic tube. In general, indwelling urethral catheters should be avoided to decrease the chance of cuff erosion. Suprapubic cystotomy tubes are potential tracts for sphincter contamination and should be located away from the device and tubing. Drains are usually avoided for the same reason.

Results

A properly functioning, well-placed artificial sphincter will reliably provide adequate outflow resistance (usually 61 to 70 cm H_2O). In adults, initial satisfactory urinary continence is achieved in up to 95 per cent of cases after sphincter placement (Fishman et al., 1989; Gundian et al., 1989; Marks and Light, 1989). Scott (1989), however, has noted some decline in acceptable continence rates with longer follow-up, particularly when the cuff is placed around the bulbar urethra. He suggests that atrophy of tissue within the cuff may cause such a lack of sustained control.

Improvements in design and construction of the sphincter have decreased the frequency of mechanical breakdowns. Mechanical malfunctions, such as a cuff leak or pump malfunction, and surgical problems, such as tubing kink, pump migration, or improper cuff size, still occur in 20 to 35 per cent of adult patients after placement of newer models, requiring reoperation and sphincter revision (Fishman et al., 1989; Gundian et al., 1989; Diokno et al., 1987). This percentage will surely increase with longer follow-up data.

In general, bladder dynamics are usually stable in adult patients, and the development of hydronephrosis or the need for secondary bladder augmentation after sphincter placement is rare. Severe complications requiring removal of the device, such as sphincter erosion or infection, are, unfortunately, not rare. With early

sphincter models, such complications occurred in up to 40 per cent of patients (Scott, 1989). With later models (AMS 791, AMS 800) sphincter erosion and/or infection occurred in only 8 to 13 per cent of adults (Fishman et al., 1989; Gundian et al., 1989; Marks and Light, 1989; Scott, 1989).

In properly selected children with a functioning artificial sphincter, satisfactory continence will be achieved in up to 95 per cent of cases (Adams et al., 1989; Barrett and Parulkar, 1989; Gonzalez et al., 1989). Bosco and co-workers (1990), Adams and co-workers (1989), Gonzalez et al. (1989), and Barrett and Parulkar (1989) have reported revision of the sphincter in 25 to 50 per cent of their pediatric patients, as in adults. Because of longer life expectancy and physical growth, it is anticipated that all pediatric patients will ultimately require reoperation at some point to maintain a properly functioning artificial sphincter. Because of potential changes in upper tract and bladder function after sphincter placement, particularly in patients with neurogenic dysfunction, secondary ureteral surgery or bladder augmentation is necessary much more frequently than in adults.

Despite careful preoperative urodynamic evaluation, *secondary bladder augmentation* in the neurogenic patient population has been necessary in up to *30 per cent* of those not previously augmented (Adams et al., 1989; Bosco et al., 1990; Gonzalez et al., 1989). In some of these cases, reasonably compliant, but small capacity bladders, have simply failed to expand with increased outflow resistance. Occasionally, a pediatric patient with neurogenic dysfunction demonstrates marked deterioration in bladder function after sphincter placement with decreased compliance and/or uninhibited contractions (Adams et al., 1989; Bosco et al., 1990; Roth et al., 1986). These patients often suffer not only persistent incontinence, but also new hydronephrosis. It is not clear whether this change in bladder function is a secondary response to the natural progression of disease, a further neurologic insult such as cord tethering, or an exaggerated response of the neurogenic bladder to bladder outlet obstruction.

Hydronephrosis, rarely seen in adults after sphincter placement, does occasionally occur in children. Frequent, thorough, follow-up care is thus essential for young patients, particularly those with neurogenic dysfunction, even when they are dry and apparently doing well. The appearance of wetting in a previously dry patient with a functioning sphincter should be presumed to represent a change in bladder dynamics until proved otherwise.

Artificial sphincter erosion or infection apparently occurs more frequently in pediatric patients than in adults. Such complications requiring removal of the device have occurred in 13 to 25 per cent of pediatric cases (Adams et al., 1989; Bosco et al., 1990; Decter et al., 1988; Gonzalez et al., 1989). In most series, patients with previous bladder neck and urethral surgery, particularly those with exstrophy/epispadias, have been at slightly higher risk for erosion. However, as reported by Adams et al. (1989) and Aliabadi and Gonzalez (1990), reimplantations of a sphincter cuff at the site of a previous erosion have almost invariably failed, owing to recurrent erosion.

Not infrequently, pediatric patients require both bladder augmentation and sphincter implantation or some other procedure to increase outflow resistance in order to achieve continence. The artificial sphincter has been effective with bladder augmentation in many such patients. Simultaneous utilization of the two procedures has been reported by several workers (Adams et al., 1989; Gonzalez et al., 1989; Strawbridge et al., 1989). When the need for both is apparent preoperatively, it is probably worthwhile doing both procedures in the same operation. The theoretical concern is that contamination of the sphincter with bowel contents may cause sphincter infection or erosion. Clinical experience to date, however, suggests that bladder augmentation and placement of the artificial sphincter can be accomplished simultaneously with good results and with no significant increase in the rate of erosion and infection, when performed with good bowel preparation, prophylactic antibiotics, and meticulous surgical technique.

SUMMARY

A few of the significant principles and procedures that have been used to achieve dryness in patients, young and old, when the usual medical modalities fail are discussed. The importance of patient evaluation and selection and of achieving good bladder compliance are emphasized. The techniques described are not to be considered exhaustive, but they are current. However, surgery for continence is still in its early stages. With research and expanding clinical experience, it should develop wonderful and exciting advances in patient care.

REFERENCES

Abel, B. J., and Gow, J. G.: Results of caecocystoplasty for tuberculosis bladder contracture. Br. J. Urol., 50:511, 1978.

Adams, M. C., Mitchell, M. E., and Rink, R. C.: Gastrocystoplasty: An alternative solution to the problem of urological reconstruction in the severely compromised patient. J. Urol., 140:1152, 1988.

Adams, M. C., Mitchell, M. E., and Rink, R. C.: Artificial urinary sphincters in the pediatric population. Presented at the Meeting of the American Urological Association. Dallas, Texas, May, 1989.

Aliabadi, H., and Gonzalez, R.: Success of the artificial urinary sphincter after failed surgery for incontinence. J. Urol., 143:987, 1990.

Barrett, D. M., and Parulkar, B. G.: The artificial sphincter (AS 800): Experience in children and young adults. Urol. Clin. North Am., 16:119, 1989.

Berry, J. L.: A new procedure for correction of urinary incontinence: Preliminary report. J. Urol., 85:771, 1961.

Bisgard, J. D., and Kerr, H. H.: Substitution of urinary bladder with an isolated segment of sigmoid colon. AMA Arch. Surg., 49:588, 1949.

Bosco, P. J., Bower, S. B., Colodny, A. M., Mandell, J., and Retik, A. B.: The long-term results of artificial sphincters in children. Presented at the Meeting of the American Urological Association. New Orleans, Louisiana, May, 1990.

Bramble, F. J.: The treatment of adult enuresis and urge incontinence by enterocystoplasty. Br. J. Urol., 54:693, 1982.

Cartwright, P. C., and Snow, B. W.: Bladder augmentation: Partial detrusor excision to augment the bladder without use of bowel. J. Urol., 142:1050, 1989.

Cartwright, P. C., and Snow, B. W.: Bladder autoaugmentation: Early clinical experience. J. Urol., 142:505, 1989.

Charghi, A., Charbonneau, J., and Gauthier, G.: Colocystoplasty for

bladder enlargement and bladder substitution: A study of late results in 31 cases. J. Urol., 97:849, 1967.

Chau, S. L., Ankenman, G. J., Wright, J. E., et al.: Cecocystoplasty in the surgical management of the small contracted bladder. J. Urol., 124:338, 1980.

Cibert, J.: Ileocystoplasty for contracted bladder of tuberculosis: Report of a case. Br. J. Urol., 25:99, 1953.

Couvelaire, R.: La "Petite Vessie" des tuberculeux genitourinaires. Essai de classification place et variantes des cysto-intestinoplasties. J. d'Urol., 56:381, 1950.

Crooks, K. K., and Emile, B. G.: Comparison of the ileal conduit and clean intermittent catheterization for myelomeningocele. Pediatrics, 72:203, 1983.

Decter, R. M., Roth, D. R., Fishman, I. J., Shabsigh, R., Scott, F. B., and Gonzalez, E. T., Jr.: Use of the AS 800 device in exstrophy and epispadias. J. Urol., 140:1202, 1988.

Demos, M. P.: Radioactive electrolyte absorption studies of small bowel, comparison of different segments for use in urinary diversion. J. Urol., 88:638, 1962.

Diokno, A. C., Hollander, J. B., and Anderson, T. P.: Artificial urinary sphincter for recurrent female urinary incontinence: Indications and results. J. Urol., 138:778, 1987.

Dounis, A., Abel, B. J., and Gow, J. G.: Cecocystoplasty for bladder augmentation. J. Urol., 123:164, 1980.

Dounis, A., and Gow, J. G.: Bladder augmentation: A long-term review. Br. J. Urol., 51:264, 1979.

Duckett, J. W., and Snyder, H. M., III: Continent urinary diversion: Variations on the Mitrofanoff principle. J. Urol., 136:58, 1986.

Elder, J. S., Snyder, H. M., Hulbert, W. C., and Duckett, J. W.: Perforation of the augmented bladder in patients undergoing clean intermittent catheterization. J. Urol., 140:1159, 1988.

Fall, M., and Nilsson, S.: Volume augmentation cystoplasty and persistent urgency. Scand. J. Urol., 16:125, 1982.

Filmer, R. B., and Spencer, J. A.: Malignancies in bladder augmentation and intestinal conduits. J. Urol., 143:671, 1990.

Fishman, I. J., Shabsigh, R., and Scott, F. B.: Experience with the artificial urinary sphincter model AS 800 in 148 patients. J. Urol., 141:307, 1989.

Gil-Vernet, J. M., Jr.: The ileocolic segment in urologic surgery. J. Urol., 94:418, 1965.

Gillon, G., and Mundy, A. R.: The dissolution of urinary mucus after cystoplasty. Br. J. Urol., 63:372, 1989.

Gleason, D. M., Gittes, R. F., and Bottaccini, M. R.: Energy balance of voiding after cecal cystoplasty. J. Urol., 108:259, 1972.

Gonzalez, R., and Cabral, B. H. P.: Rectal continence after enterocystoplasty. Dialogues in Pediatric Urology, Vol. 10, No. 12, December, 1987.

Gonzalez, R., Koleilat, N., Austin, C., and Sidi, A. A.: The artificial sphincter AS 800 in congenital urinary incontinence. J. Urol., 142:512, 1989.

Gonzalez, R., Nguyen, D. H., Koleilat, N., and Sidi, A. A.: Compatibility of enterocystoplasty and the artificial urinary sphincter. J. Urol., 142:502, 1989.

Goodwin, W. E., Turner, R. D., and Winter, C. C.: Results of ileocystoplasty. J. Urol., 80:461, 1958.

Goodwin, W. E., Winter, C. C., and Barker, W. F.: "Cup-patch" technique of ileocystoplasty for bladder enlargement or partial substitution. Surg. Gynecol. Obstet., 108:240, 1959.

Gundian, J. C., Barrett, D. M., and Parulkar, B. G.: Mayo Clinic experience with use of the AMS 800 artificial urinary sphincter for urinary incontinence following radical prostatectomy. J. Urol., 142:1459, 1989.

Hendren, W. H.: Reoperative ureteral reimplantation: Management of the difficult case. J. Pediatr. Surg., 15:770, 1980.

Hensle, T. W., and Burbige, K. A.: Bladder replacement in children and young adults. J. Urol., 133:1004, 1985.

Hinman, F., Jr.: Bladder augmentation. In Hinman, F., Jr. (Ed.): Atlas of Urologic Surgery. Philadelphia, W. B. Saunders Co., 1989, p. 534.

Kass, E. J., and Koff, S. A.: Bladder augmentation in the pediatric neuropathic bladder. J. Urol., 129:552, 1983.

Kaufman, J. J.: Treatment of postprostatectomy urinary incontinence using a silicone gel prosthesis. Br. J. Urol., 45:646, 1973.

Kay, R., and Straffon, R.: Augmentation cystoplasty. Urol. Clin. North Am., 13:295, 1986.

Kennedy, H. A., Adams, M. C., Mitchell, M. E., and Rink, R. C.:

Chronic renal failure and bladder augmentation: Stomach vs. sigmoid colon in the canine model. J. Urol., 140:1152, 1988.

Kerr, W. K., Gale, G. L., and Peterson, K. S. S.: Reconstructive surgery for genitourinary tuberculosis. J. Urol., 101:254, 1969.

Kil, P. J. M., DeVries, J. D. M., VanKerrebroeck, P. E. V. A., Zwiers, W., and Debruyne, F. M. J.: Factors determining the outcome following implantation of the AMS 800 artificial urinary sphincter. Br. J. Urol., 64:586, 1989.

Klee, L. W., Hoover, D. M., Mitchell, M. E., and Rink, R. C.: Long-term effects of gastrocystoplasty in rats. J. Urol., 144:1283, 1990.

Koch, M. O., and McDougal, W. S.: The pathophysiology of hyperchloremic metabolic acidosis after urinary diversion through intestinal segments. Surgery, 98:561, 1985.

Kogan, S. J., and Levitt, S. B.: Bladder evaluation in pediatric patients before undiversion in previously diverted urinary tracts. J. Urol., 118:443, 1977.

Krarstein, B., and Mathisoen, W.: Sigmoid cystoplasty in adults with enuresis. Surg. Gynecol. Obstet., 153:65, 1981.

Kropp, K. A., and Angwafo, F. F.: Urethral lengthening and reimplantation for neurogenic incontinence in children. J. Urol., 135:533, 1986.

Kuss, R.: Colocystoplasty rather than ileocystoplasty. J. Urol., 80:467, 1958.

Kuss, R., Bitker, M., Camey, M., et al.: Indications and early and late results of intestinocystoplasty: A review of 185 cases. J. Urol., 103:53, 1970.

Lapides, J., Dileno, A. C., Gould, F. R., et al.: Further observations on self-catheterization. J. Urol., 116:169, 1976.

Lapides, J., Diokno, A. C., Silber, S. J., and Lowe, B. S.: Clean intermittent self-catheterization in the treatment of urinary tract disease. J. Urol., 107:458, 1972.

Leadbetter, G. W., Jr.: Surgical correction of total urinary incontinence. J. Urol., 91:261, 1964.

Leong, C. H.: The use of gastrocystoplasty. Dialogues in Pediatric Urology, Vol. 2, No. 9, September, 1988.

Leong, C. H., and Ong, G. B.: Gastrocystoplasty in dogs. Aust. NZ J. Surg., 41:272, 1972.

Lepor, M., and Jeffs, R. D.: Primary bladder closure and bladder neck reconstruction in classical bladder exstrophy. J. Urol., 130:1142, 1983.

Lieskovsky, G., and Skinner, D. G.: Use of intestinal segments in the urinary tract. In Walsh, P. C., Gilles, R. F., Perlmutter, A. D., and Stamey, T. A. (Eds.): Campbell's Urology, 5th ed. Philadelphia, W. B. Saunders Co., 1986, p. 2620.

Light, J. K., and Engelman, U. H.: Le Bag: Total replacement of the bladder using an ileocolonic pouch. J. Urol., 136:27, 1986.

Light, J. K., and Scardino, P. T.: Radical cystectomy with preservation of sexual and urinary function. Use of the ileocolonic pouch ("Le Bag"). Urol. Clin. North Am., 13:261, 1986.

Marks, J. L., and Light, J. K.: Management of urinary incontinence after prostatectomy with the artificial urinary sphincter. J. Urol., 142:302, 1989.

Mathisen, W.: Open loop sigmoid cystoplasty. Acta Chir. Scand., 110:227, 1955.

McGuire, E. J., Woodside, J. R., Borden, T. A., and Weiss, R. M.: Prognostic value of urodynamics testing in myelodysplastic patients. J. Urol., 126:205, 1981.

Menville, J. G., Nix, J. T., and Pratt, A. M.: Cecocystoplasty. J. Urol., 79:78, 1958.

Mitchell, M. E.: Use of bowel in undiversion. Urol. Clin. North Am., 13:349, 1986.

Mitchell, M. E., Adams, M. C., and Rink, R. C.: Urethral replacement with ureter. J. Urol., 139:1282, 1988.

Mitchell, M. E., Kulb, T. B., and Backes, D. J.: Intestinocystoplasty in combination with clean intermittent catheterization in the management of vesical dysfunction. J. Urol., 136:228, 1986.

Mitchell, M. E., and Piser, J. A.: Intestinocystoplasty and total bladder replacement in children and young adults: Follow-up in 129 cases. J. Urol., 138:579–584, 1987.

Mitchell, M. E., and Rink, R. C.: Urinary diversion and undiversion. Urol. Clin. North Am., 12:111, 1985.

Mitrofanoff, P.: Cystostomie continente trans-appendiculaire dans le traitement des vessies neurologiques. Chir. Pediatr., 21:297, 1980.

Olsson, C. A., Benson, M. C., Sawzuk, I. S., and Blaivas, J. G.: Bladder substitution. In Resnick, M. I. (Ed.): Current Trends in Urology. Baltimore, Williams & Wilkins, 1988, p. 4–149.

Orr, L. M., Thomley, M. W., and Campbell, M. F.: Ileocystoplasty for bladder enlargement. J. Urol., 79:250, 1958.

Perlmutter, A. D.: Urinary tract reconstruction and the abnormal bladder. Urol. Clin. North Am., 7:379, 1980.

Piser, J. A., Mitchell, M. E., Kulb, T. B., Rink, R. C., et al.: Gastrocystoplasty and colocystoplasty in canines: The metabolic consequences of acute saline and acid loading. J. Urol., 138:1009, 1987.

Pyrah, L. N., and Raper, F. P.: Some uses of an isolated loop of ileum in genitourinary surgery. Br. J. Surg., 42:337, 1955.

Rink, R. C.: The use of gastrocystoplasty. Dialogues in Pediatric Urology, Vol. 2, No. 9, September, 1988.

Rink, R. C., Leong, C. H., Vaughan, E. D., Tiffany, P., and Mitchell, M. E.: The use of gastrocystoplasty. Dialogues in Pediatric Urology, 11:9, 1988.

Rink, R. C., and Mitchell, M. E.: Surgical correction of urinary incontinence. J. Pediatr. Surg., 19:637, 1984.

Rink, R. C., and Salvas, D.: Ureteral augmentation in preparation for transplantation. Submitted for publication, 1991.

Rink, R. C., Woodbury, P. W., and Mitchell, M. E.: Bladder perforation following enterocystoplasty. J. Urol., 139:234A (Abstract 285), 1988.

Robertson, C. N., and King, L. R.: Bladder substitution in children. Urol. Clin. North Am., 13:333, 1986.

Roth, D. R., Vyas, P. R., Kroavard, R. L., and Perlmutter, A. D.: Urinary tract deterioration associated with the artificial urinary sphincter. J. Urol., 125:528, 1986.

Ruddick, J., Schonholz, S., and Weber, H. N.: The gastric bladder: A continent reservoir for urinary diversion. Surgery, 82:1, 1977.

Rushton, H. G., Woodard, J. R., Parrott, T. S., et al.: Delayed bladder rupture following augmentation enterocystoplasty. J. Urol., 140:344, 1988.

Savauagen, F., and Dixey, G. M.: Syncope following ureterosigmoidostomy. J. Urol., 101:844, 1969.

Scheele, K.: Ueber gosseringplastik der narbigen schrumpfblase. Beitr. Klin. Chir., 129:414, 1923.

Scott, F. B.: The artificial urinary sphincter: Experience in adults. Urol. Clin. North Am., 16:105, 1989.

Scott, F. B., Bradley, W. E., and Timm, G. W.: Treatment of urinary incontinence by implantable prosthetic sphincter. Urology, 1:252, 1973.

Sheiner, J. R., and Kaplan, G. W.: Spontaneous bladder rupture following enterocystoplasty. J. Urol., 140:1157, 1988.

Sheldon, C. A., Essig, K. A., Wacksman, J., et al.: Intravesical pressure dependent ischemia—A cause of spontaneous rupture in colocystoplasty? Presented at the American Academy of Pediatrics—Urology Section, Boston, October 6, 1990.

Shirley, S. W., and Mirelman, S.: Experiences with colocystoplasties, cecocystoplasties and ileocystoplasties in urologic surgery: 40 patients. J. Urol., 120:165, 1978.

Sinaiko, E. S.: Artificial bladder from segment of stomach and study effect of urine on gastric secretion. Surg. Gynecol. Obstet., 102:433, 1956.

Sinaiko, E. S.: Artificial bladder in man from segment of stomach. Surg. Forum, 8:635, 1957.

Skinner, D. G.: Further experience with the ileocecal segment in urinary reconstruction. J. Urol., 128:252, 1982.

Smith, R. B., Van Cangh, P., Skinner, P. G., Kauffman, J. J., and Goodwin, W. E.: Augmentation enterocystoplasty: A critical review. J. Urol., 118:799, 1977.

Strawbridge, L. R., Kramer, S. A., Castillo, O. A., and Barrett, D. M.: Augmentation cystoplasty and the artificial genitourinary sphincter. J. Urol., 142:297, 1989.

Tanagho, E. A.: Bladder neck reconstruction for total urinary incontinence: Ten years of experience. J. Urol., 125:321, 1981.

Tasker, J. H.: Ileocystoplasty: A new technique (an experimental study with report of a case). Br. J. Urol., 25:349, 1953.

Thuroff, J. W., Aiken, P., Engleman, U., et al.: The MAINZ pouch (Mixed Augmentation Ileum 'n' Zecum) for bladder augmentation and continent urinary diversion. Eur. Urol., 11:152, 1985.

Thuroff, J. W., Alken, P., and Hohenfellner, R.: The MAINZ pouch (Mixed Augmentation with Ileum 'n' Zecum) for bladder augmentation and continent diversion. In King, L. R., Stone, A. R., and

Webster, G. D. (Eds.): Bladder Reconstruction and Continent Urinary Diversion. Chicago, Year Book Medical Publishers, 1987, p. 252.

Tizzoni, G., and Foggi, A.: Die wiederherstellung der harnblase. Zentralbl. Chir., 15:921, 1888.

Turner-Warwick, R. T., and Ashkem, M. H.: The functional results of partial, subtotal and total cystoplasty with special reference to urcterocaecocystoplasty, selective sphincterotomy and cystoplasty. Br. J. Urol., 39:3, 1967.

Weinberg, A. C., Boyd, S. D., Lieskovsky, G., Ahlering, T. E., and Skinner, D. G.: The hemi-Kock augmentation ileocystoplasty: A low pressure antirefluxing system. J. Urol., 140:1380, 1988.

Whitmore, W. F., III, and Gittes, R. F.: Reconstruction of the urinary tract by cecal and ileocecal cystoplasty: Review of 15 year experience. J. Urol., 129:494, 1983.

Winter, C. C., and Goodwin, W. E.: Results of sigmoid cystoplasty. J. Urol., 80:467, 1958.

Zinman, L., and Libertino, J. A.: Technique of augmentation ceco-cystoplasty. Surg. Clin. North Am., 60:703, 1980.

Zinman, L., Libertino, J. A., and Flava, T. A.: Ileocecocystoplasty for bladder augmentation and replacement. *In* Libertino, J. A. (Ed.): Pediatric and Adult Reconstructive Urology. Baltimore, Williams & Wilkins, 1987, p. 357.

72
URINARY DIVERSION

Mitchell C. Benson, M.D.
Carl A. Olsson, M.D.

This chapter reviews all permanent forms of urinary diversion utilized in the adult and pediatric patient populations. Temporary urinary diversion, as often required in pediatric surgery, is discussed elsewhere.

Many of the principles and techniques of bowel surgery, as well as bowel surgery complications, have been reviewed in Chapter 69. Techniques of ureterointestinal anastomoses and complications resulting from these anastomoses have also been presented in that chapter. These features are not repeated here, except where essential to the appropriate description of the operative procedures reviewed. Intubated urinary diversion procedures, such as nephrostomy, are not included in this chapter, which deals entirely with open operative permanent urinary diversion procedures.

HISTORY

The purpose of a historical review of standard and continent urinary diversion is twofold. First, it should lead to a new respect for the innovative procedures developed by our predecessors. The second reason is best summarized in a treatise published by Hinman and Weyrauch (1936). In referring to historical reviews, they state, "Such an analysis leaves something to be desired because the historical material is of importance to the surgeon of today only insofar as it teaches the way to implant ureters more successfully than it has been done in the past and in what particulars even the most successful methods are at fault." Stated otherwise, we can learn from the successes and mistakes of others.

At the time of the Hinman and Weyrauch review, most urinary diversion was performed into the intact intestinal tract, because collecting devices were imperfect at best and " . . . implantations to the skin, which perhaps do not seriously endanger the life of the patient at the time of operation, permanently place a burden of care and discomfort because of incontinence." Thus, continent urinary diversion into the intact fecal stream

was the standard of the day. However, one group of surgeons advocated either complete or partial diversion of the fecal stream so as to diminish ascending infection.

Continent urinary diversion was first reported by Simon (1852). Operating on a patient with bladder exstrophy, Simon performed a ureterorectal anastomosis. However, the earliest attempt to fashion an artificial bladder was made in a dog by Tizzoni and Foggi (1888). They created an isolated closed loop of intact ileum and re-established bowel continuity. One month later, they anastomosed the ureters into the blind ileal loop and sutured the loop to the bladder neck. The dog survived. The operation was performed in one stage in a second dog and the dog survived only 8 days. The experimental model, remarkably like the Camey I operation, represented the first time that an intestinal neobladder was directed to the control of the vesical sphincter.

The first clinical use of small intestine to fashion a continent urinary reservoir was performed by Cuneo in 1911 (Marion, 1912). He staged the procedure that was done in three patients with exstrophy. At the first stage, an 18- to 20-cm segment of intact ileum was isolated at a point 20 cm from the ileocecal valve. Intestinal continuity was re-established end to end. Through a simultaneous perineal approach, the rectal mucosa was dissected free anteriorly for 4 to 5 cm. Through this opening, a Kocher clamp was utilized to grasp the intestinal segment. The edges of the ileal reservoir were sutured to the anal mucosa. Each patient was allowed to rest from this stage. At a second procedure 6 weeks later, the ureters were implanted to the peritoneal end. Two of three patients survived, although both experienced transient urinary fistulas.

Mauclaire (1895) described the isolated rectosigmoid colon as a urinary reservoir. The ureters were implanted into the cranial end of the rectosigmoid colon. The divided end of the sigmoid was brought to the iliac region as an end colostomy. This procedure had the advantage of avoiding an intra-abdominal fecal anastomosis. Although Mauclaire successfully performed this operation in dogs, it was left to Remedi (1906), to attempt this procedure clinically in 1905. The procedure was also utilized by Kronig (1907) and Rovsing (1916).

As means of a urinary diversion for the treatment of bladder cancer, Mauclaire's procedure was first done by Schmieden (1923). He performed the operation in three stages: 1) sigmoid colostomy, 2) ureteral rectal anastomosis, and 3) cystectomy. This procedure, which was performed in eight patients, was successful in six.

Warbasse, in 1899, reported Gersuny's technique for utilizing the isolated rectum as a urinary reservoir (Hinman and Weyrauch, 1936). Gersuny developed an operation at the turn of the century that was intended to maintain fecal as well as urinary continence. He implanted the trigone into the lumen of the isolated rectum. The sigmoid was then brought through an opening made along the anterior of the anus. The anal sphincter controlled both the bladder (old rectum) and the new rectum (old sigmoid).

Heitz-Boyer and Hovelacque (1912) developed a modification of Gersuny's technique in 1910. They resected the coccyx and brought the sigmoid through an opening made posterior to the rectum. They implanted the ureters directly into the rectum, not utilizing the trigone as described by Maydl (1894) and performed by Gersuny and others of their day. At the time of the review by Hinman and Weyrauch, five cases had been reported utilizing the Gersuny and Heitz-Boyer procedures. Two surgical deaths were reported, a 40 per cent mortality rate.

The first true clinical application of an intestinal neobladder was reported by Lemoine (1913). Following a radical cystectomy for carcinoma of the bladder, he isolated the rectum and joined it to the urethral stump. The ureters were anastomosed directly. Unfortunately, the patient did not survive long enough for the merits of the operation to be assessed. The patient expired 18 days postoperatively from renal infection and fecal leak.

Verhoogan (1908) utilized the ileal cecal segment and the appendix to create the first catheterizable continent reservoir in two patients with bladder cancer. The ileum was anastomosed to the hepatic flexure and the appendix was brought out to the skin as a stoma. Verhoogan performed the operation in two cases of bladder carcinoma. Both patients expired. The first successful report of this procedure was made by Makkas (1910). He modified the procedure by implanting the trigone (Maydl reimplantation, 1894) into the cecum at a second stage and merely isolated the reservoir at the first stage. Lengemann (1912) further modified the Verhoogan-Makkas procedure by isolating the distal 30 cm of ileum with the cecum and by utilizing the ileum to reimplant the ureters. Lengemann believed that the long terminal ileum afforded a tension-free retroperitoneal anastomosis to the left ureter and that the isoperistaltic ileum would be a good defense against obstruction. The overall operative mortality of the Verhoogan-Makkas-Lengemann procedure was 67 per cent—eight of the initial 12 patients died.

The high operative mortality (approximately 50 per cent) experienced, regardless of which of the aforementioned procedures was performed, led to the temporary abandonment of attempts to create continent urinary reservoirs or conduits separate from the fecal stream. However, during the same time period, other surgeons were developing procedures in which the ureters were implanted into the intestinal tract. Reluctance to place the ureters in direct contact with the fecal stream was again noted. These operations utilized various segments, but the concept behind them all was the same. The urine was directed to the fecal stream via an intervening segment, and continence was dependent on the intact anal sphincter.

Borelius (1903) performed a side-to-side anastomosis at the base of an intact folded loop of sigmoid colon. This bypass, suggested by his assistant Erglund, resulted in a functional exclusion of feces from the bypassed loop. The trigone was anastomosed to the apex of the loop. Muller (1903) modified Borelius's procedure by dividing the upper sigmoid and sewing the divided end to the side of the lower sigmoid. The ureters were still implanted with the trigone. Muscatello (1905) performed the same operation except the lower sigmoid was anastomosed to the side of the rectum, resulting in a larger Y limb.

Goldenberg (1904) employed an ileal segment, which was reimplanted into the cecum in an antiperistaltic fashion. The trigone was anastomosed to the distal end. Berg (1907) isolated a segment of ileum and anastomosed it Roux-en-y to the rectum. The trigone was anastomosed to the transposed ileal segment at a second procedure. Moskowicz (1909) performed an operation similar to Goldenberg's, utilizing the transverse colon.

Intervening intestinal segments anastomosed to the fecal stream also resulted in a high operative mortality—41 per cent. Thus, in the preantibiotic era, intestinal surgery to reconstruct the urinary tract was extremely hazardous. In attempts to minimize the mortality and complication rates, procedures were developed to directly anastomose the ureter to the intact colon.

Numerous methods of ureteral implantation were described in the late 19th and early 20th centuries. Many of these procedures, which were described as new, represented subtle permutations of existing concepts. In general, these various procedures were designed to decrease the risk of peritonitis. Bacterial peritonitis in the preantibiotic era was associated with a high mortality rate and, when accompanied by a failed surgical anastomosis, was almost universally fatal, representing the major cause of postoperative mortality (Hinman and Weyrauch, 1936).

Hinman and Weyrauch (1936) recognized and described 11 unique surgical principles, which evolved into their concept of the perfect ureterointestinal anastomosis. Some of these principles would later be discarded. A review of these "breakthroughs" in urinary diversion allows for an understanding of the evolution of thought that has brought us to where we are today.

PRINCIPLE 1. FORMATION OF A FISTULOUS TRACT BETWEEN THE URETER AND A BOWEL SEGMENT

Sir John Simon (1852) passed two sutures from each ureter of an exstrophic bladder to the rectum. The rectal ends were tied. At 3 weeks, the patient began passing large quantities of urine per rectum, but the native orifice could never be successfully closed. The patient later expired from pelvic peritonitis. At autopsy, the fistulas were patent.

PRINCIPLE 2. DIRECT ANASTOMOSIS OF THE URETER AND BOWEL

The first actual clinical implantation of the ureters into the bowel of a human was performed by T. Smith in 1878 (Smith, 1879). The method was later attributed to Chaput in 1892 (Chaput, 1905). Smith created a full-thickness slit in the large intestine and performed an end-to-side, mucosa-to-mucosa anastomosis. The anastomosis was completed by closing the serosa and muscularis over the ureter.

PRINCIPLE 3. CREATION OF A MUSCULAR CANAL AROUND THE URETER

The creation of a muscular canal was not initially intended to prevent reflux but to prevent leakage of intestinal contents. Although thought to arise from Witzel's gastrostomy technique, Bardenheuer (1887) utilized the concept 5 years earlier, in 1886. However, he was unsuccessful. It was not until 1905 that Tichoff developed a technique that was a modification of the Witzel gastrostomy (Belawenetz, 1910).

PRINCIPLE 4. PRESERVATION OF THE URETEROVESICAL ORIFICE

Maydl (1894) first proposed transplantation of the entire trigone from exstrophied bladders in 1892. This modification decreased both the incidence of ureteral obstruction and peritonitis by allowing for more secure suturing of the ureteral implantation. Unfortunately, the incidence of peritonitis was still significant, because of contaminated sutures and long suture lines.

Bergenhem (1895) suggested a retroperitoneal implantation of each ureter and a surrounding rosette of bladder urothelium in 1894. Unfortunately, leakage still developed.

PRINCIPLE 5. TEMPORARY DIVERSION OF URINE UNTIL HEALING

The first record of a ureteral catheter to afford temporary urinary diversion was by Giordano (1894). Ureteral catheters did not gain popularity until Coffey (1925) employed them in a one-stage bilateral submucosal transplantation. Unfortunately, the catheters of the day tended to obstruct easily. They sometimes caused as many problems as they prevented.

Temporary urinary diversion by nephrostomy tube was first suggested by Heitz-Boyer and Hovelacque (1912). Hinman (1926) stressed the value of preliminary nephrostomy tube placement, particularly in the patient with hydronephrosis secondary to obstruction.

PRINCIPLE 6. FLAP ACTS AS AN ANTIREFLUXING VALVE

Vignoni (1895) employed the principle of an antirefluxing flap fashioned after the structure found in animals possessing ureters that emptied into cloacas. A flap to prevent ascending infection failed because it tended to slough after the operation.

PRINCIPLE 7. MECHANICAL DEVICES TO PREVENT DEVELOPMENT OF ANASTOMOTIC STENOSIS

Boari (1897) described the development of mechanical buttons of various sizes that he utilized to create a ureterointestinal anastomosis. The button was actually a "sandwich" of two spring-loaded discs that were secured on either side of the anastomosis. The button would eventually slough into the bowel. Unfortunately, this device did little to prevent the development of urinary and fecal extravasation.

PRINCIPLE 8. URETERAL IMPLANTATION INTO STRUCTURES THAT NORMALLY ENTER INTO THE GASTROINTESTINAL TRACT

In an attempt to prevent fecal spillage and ascending infection, the major causes of morbidity and mortality, attempts were made to implant the ureters into structures already communicating with the gastrointestinal (GI) tract. Roux implanted a ureter into the appendix using a Boari button (Hinman and Weyrauch, 1936). Similar procedures were independently performed by Eaton (1910) and Babcock (1914) in 1910. Baird and co-workers (1917) attempted ureteral anastomosis to the pancreatic duct, and Dardel (1922) attempted ureterocholecystostomy. These procedures were both performed in dogs with little success.

PRINCIPLE 9. CONSTRUCTION OF A SUBMUCOSAL TUNNEL TO CREATE AN ANTIREFLUXING MECHANISM

Krynski (1896) was the first to attempt to create an antirefluxing mechanism via a submucosal tunnel. Beck (1899) combined the submucosal tunnel with the muscular canal of Witzel. This procedure was very similar to what we today call a Leadbetter implant (Leadbetter and Clark, 1954).

PRINCIPLE 10. TEMPORARY DIVERTING COLOSTOMY

The first temporary colostomy was performed to allow for direct inspection of the site of ureteral reimplant and not for diversion of stool (Barber, 1915). This operation was successful in seven of eight dogs. Higgins (1934) performed a temporary diverting colostomy, also in dogs, and then irrigated the distal limb with boric acid and merbromine (Mercurochrome). Ureteral implantation was performed 1 week later.

PRINCIPLE 11. STAGED URETERAL ANASTOMOSIS AND INTACT URETER

Because all attempts at creating direct one-stage anastomosis between the ureters were accompanied by high failure and mortality rates, procedures were developed that allowed for staged ureterointestinal anastomosis while preventing spillage and extravasation. At the first stage, an intact ureter was embedded in a submucosal tunnel created in the muscle layers of the bowel, usually the rectum, while not attempting to direct the urine into the fecal stream. The urine continued to drain into the bladder. At the second stage, the lumina of the ureter and the bowel were connected by inserting a fulguration tip into the ureter just below its point of egress from the submucosal tunnel (Ferguson, 1931; Higgins, 1933; Nesbitt, 1935; Winsbury-White, 1933).

MODERN APPROACHES

The introduction of effective antibiotic therapy after World War II resulted in a significant decrease in postoperative mortality, but urologic surgeons were, for the most part, dissatisfied with the techniques available for urinary diversion. The combination of improved patient survival from major surgery and the lack of socially and medically accepted forms of urinary diversion was responsible for the wave of enthusiasm that greeted Bricker's (1950) report on his technique for ileal conduit. In actuality, Seiffert (1935) reported on the construction of the ileal conduit 15 years earlier. However, he lacked an effective means of collecting and storing urine so that his technique was not so heralded.

Bricker utilized Rutzen's bag, which was attached to the anterior abdominal wall with adhesive. It was this breakthrough that allowed for socially acceptable nonfecal urinary diversion. The ease of construction and the low incidence of complications led to the Bricker ileal conduit becoming the "gold standard" of urinary diversion.

However, some urologic surgeons were still not satisfied with conduit diversion. Among these was Gilchrist (1950), who utilized a 9-inch segment of the ileum and the right colon to fashion a continent urinary reservoir. The anti-incontinence mechanism was the peristaltic ileum proximal to the ileocecal valve and in some instances the valve itself. The right colon served as the reservoir. Unfortunately, the ileocecal valve was not always competent. The isoperistaltic segment was not sufficient to ensure continence, when faced with the pressure generated by the nondetubularized colon. Thus, although the first of the modern day reservoirs, the Gilchrist substitute bladder did not gain acceptance.

Maurice Camey (1979) reintroduced the reservoir anastomosed to the urethral stump and renewed interest in the fashioning of a functional bladder substitute. Similar to Gilchrist's right colon pouch, Camey's enterocystoplasty utilized a nondetubularized intestinal segment. However, the enterocystoplasty was created from ileum, not colon, and therefore was more compliant. Additionally, the Camey procedure relied on a functional sphincteric mechanism. Although the failure to utilize a detubularized ileal segment increased the likelihood of both daytime and nighttime incontinence, the operation initiated a concerted effort throughout the world toward the search for the ideal bladder substitute.

The subsequent operative descriptions detail the means by which modern urologic surgeons have learned from these pioneers and the novel techniques that have developed in the search for the perfect bladder substitute. As indicated by the numerous techniques currently employed, the perfect solution still remains elusive.

OPERATIONS REQUIRING APPLIANCES

Despite considerable enthusiasm for continent urinary diversion operations, those requiring external urinary collecting appliances remain the most common. Many reasons exist for this observation. First, there is no unanimity relative to the "best" form of continent urinary diversion (Olsson, 1984). Second, although continent urinary diversions are certainly appropriate in

selected patients, the procedures are technically more challenging and potentially fraught with higher complication rates than those that involve collecting devices. These last procedures, with all of their shortcomings, have stood the test of time. They have become part of every urologic surgeon's armamentarium, in contrast to continent diversion procedures, which are newer and involve technologic demands not yet incorporated into everyone's armamentarium.

Because stoma care is essential to the patient undergoing surgery that requires an appliance, the patient must be assessed for his or her ability to care for this appliance. The interaction of an enterostomal therapist with the patient and the urologist is extremely helpful in this regard. Certain categories of patients may not be able to care for an appliance by themselves. Patients with severe multiple sclerosis, quadriplegic patients, and very frail or mentally impaired patients require that appliances be cared for by members of the family or visiting nurses. Usually, a collecting appliance can simply be emptied when full; nighttime bedside drainage can be attached to the collecting appliance in order that long periods of uninterrupted sleep may be experienced. Usually, the entire apparatus must be removed and replaced after cleansing the peristomal area on a 4-day schedule.

Prior to the operation, the site for the external stoma should be selected with extreme care. In general, the location must be free from fat creases in both the standing and sitting position. It should not be close to prior abdominal scars that might interfere with proper adherence of the appliance. The aid of an enterostomal therapist is extremely helpful in this regard. In general, the stoma should be brought through the right or left lower quadrant of the abdomen, on a line extending between the umbilicus and the anterosuperior iliac spine. The stoma should be as far lateral from the midline as possible but should *always* be selected so as to require the ureter or bowel composing the stoma to traverse the rectus muscle. Failure to adhere to this feature promotes the incidence of parastomal hernias. The selected site for the stoma should be marked with an X scratched on the skin of anterior abdominal wall. Marking the stoma site with ink should be avoided, as the ink may be washed away during the antiseptic preparation of the skin.

All operations described require a long midline incision, skirting the umbilicus to the side opposite the selected stoma site. As an alternative, a paramedian incision may be utilized opposite the side of the anticipated stoma.

After abdominal exploration, urinary diversion operations proceed by the isolation, transection, and direction of the ureters to an appropriate place for subsequent diversion. The right retroperitoneum is opened over the iliac artery to expose the right ureter. In the typical circumstance of bowel diversion, the ureter may be transected at the level of the iliac artery or slightly below this level. The sigmoid colon is freed from its lateral peritoneal attachments by incising along the line of Toldt. After the colon is medially reflected, the left ureter can be identified and dissected somewhat more distally than the right. A wide tunnel is created by blunt finger dissection beneath the inferior mesenteric artery to gain access to the previously incised right retroperitoneum. When the surgeon is assured of appropriate length, the ureter can be transected. In cases of uroepithelial malignancy, a small portion of the distal most ureter on each side should be sent for frozen-section analysis for determination of a possible ureteral neoplasm. The left ureter is directed to the right retroperitoneum through the tunnel beneath the inferior mesenteric artery.

In carrying out sigmoid colon conduit diversion, the procedures are reversed with longer segments of right ureter transected and directed to the left retroperitoneum. In cutaneous ureterostomy, jejunal and transverse colon conduits, the dissection and direction of the ureteral stumps vary somewhat and are described individually.

All sutures utilized in the urinary tract should be absorbable. The individual surgeon's preference dictates the caliber and type of suture material utilized, i.e., simple chromic catgut or synthetic absorbable materials. In general, when carrying out bowel surgery for those urinary diversions requiring bowel, we prefer a stapled bowel segment division as well as a stapled reconstruction of bowel continuity. We believe that this shortens the operative time greatly and affords safe bowel anastomoses. Suturing is not necessary, except to take one or two silk Lembert sutures at the apex of side-to-side stapled bowel anastomoses. In order to avoid stone formation on the stapled butts of conduits, the simple expedient of either oversewing the stapled end of the conduits with absorbable material or the single application of an absorbable staple distal to the metal stapled margin suffices.

In constructing the urinary diversion stoma, a skin button matching the diameter of the structure to be utilized in the diversion is circumcised. Cutaneous tissues are separated down to the level of the anterior rectus fascia and a similar diameter circle is excised from this fascia or the fascia is opened in cruciate fashion (Fig. 72–1). In carrying out this maneuver, the surgeon should take care that the fascia and skin are properly aligned, so that angulation does not occur. Rectus muscle fibers are separated bluntly and an instrument passed through to the posterior peritoneum and fascia. A similar size circle of posterior fascia and peritoneum are removed or these tissues incised, taking care to ensure proper alignment of all layers of the abdominal wall.

Our preference is to utilize diverting stents in all cases of urinary diversion, regardless of whether standard diversion or continent diversion is selected. We also utilize stents that will drain externally, ensuring that the urine is safely diverted beyond any anastomotic site during the early healing interval. Stents are utilized that can be replaced, if needed. Therefore, any number of end-hole single J–type of long ureteral diverting stent is preferred. The proximal end of the J-stent should be patent to allow replacement of the stent, if necessary, by means of guide wire exchange.

Suction drain catheters are advocated by us in all cases of urinary diversion in which anastomotic leaks may be experienced. Soft silicone rubber suction drains are preferred because they have less potential for tissue damage with migration into conduits and pouches.

Abdominal closure is performed according to the surgeon's preference. A single layer closure, utilizing No. 2 nylon or Prolene, taken through all layers of fascia and muscle, provides a secure abdominal closure quickly in the majority of patients. In obese patients or those with tissues of poor quality or nutritional depletion, through-and-through stay sutures are also placed. Subcutaneous sutures are utilized to close dead space, and skin is closed with staples. Ureteral stents are always sutured to the anterior abdominal wall near the edge of the stoma site, and they are directed into the temporary urinary appliance, which is applied in the operating theater.

Postoperative Care and Comments

Paralytic ileus is nearly always experienced after all forms of urinary diversion procedures. Therefore, gastric decompression is always achieved by means of either nasogastric intubation or gastrostomy at the time of the operation. We maintain this gastric decompression until the patient experiences the passage of flatus. Nasogastric tubes suffice in the majority of patients. However, certain patients may best be managed by formal gastrostomy decompression. These include individuals in whom multiple prior abdominal procedures have been performed and prolonged ileus may be anticipated. In addition, patients with chronic pulmonary disease may benefit from the improved pulmonary toilet that can be achieved in the absence of a nasogastric tube.

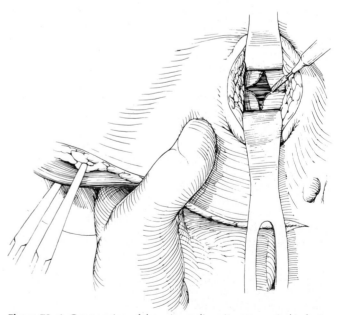

Figure 72–1. Construction of the urinary diversion stoma. A skin button matching the diameter of the structure to be utilized is circumcised and cutaneous tissues are separated down to the level of the anterior rectus fascia. A similar diameter circle excised from this fascia is opened in cruciate fashion as shown. (From Hinman, F., Jr.: Atlas of Urologic Surgery. Philadelphia, W. B. Saunders Co., 1989.)

If formal gastrostomy is carried out, this is achieved by means of puncturing the anterior wall of the stomach and inserting a Malecot catheter. A purse string suture is taken to ensure against gastric content leakage. A small stab wound is made in the left upper quadrant through which the Malecot catheter can be directed. The stomach wall is sutured around the margins of the tube exit site to the posterior fascia to prevent intraperitoneal leakage of gastric contents after tube removal. When gastrostomy tubes are applied, they may be clamped upon resolution of the ileus. If gastric residuals are small, they can simply be removed and the stoma site will heal within 1 day. If the duration of paralytic ileus is projected to be in excess of 4 to 5 days, intravenous hyperalimentation is initiated on the 2nd postoperative day. If the patient is nutritionally depleted preoperatively, hyperalimentation has been suggested to be of value if initiated before surgery (Askanazi et al., 1985; Hensle, 1983).

In conduit urinary diversions, ureteral stents are generally removed 1 week following surgery. At the time of removal, however, radiologic contrast studies are carried out to ensure against any anastomotic leakage. If there is any question of extravasation, the stents are left in situ for an additional 5 days and repeat studies are carried out. Upon removal of the stents, drainage films are taken to observe that the upper tracts are able to drain without significant dilatation.

CUTANEOUS URETEROSTOMY

Urinary diversion by means of cutaneous ureterostomy offers the distinct advantage of being able to achieve the goals of the procedure without the need for bowel surgery. Therefore, many of the complications associated with bowel anastomoses can be avoided and one need not be concerned at all about reabsorption of urinary constituents by the bowel mucosa (Chute and Sallade, 1961).

The major disadvantages of cutaneous ureterostomy relate to the conditions of the ureters themselves. If normal caliber ureters are brought through the skin, even with V-flap techniques designed to widen the stoma, the incidence of stomal stenosis is considerable (Chute and Sallade, 1961). Furthermore, the length of ureter that must be freed from its blood supply in order to traverse the distance from the retroperitoneum to the anterior abdominal skin necessitates that the ureter be dependent on collateral circulation for its survival (Mingledorf et al., 1964). A reasonable degree of ureteral peristaltic power is required for the ureter to propel urine through the relatively obstructing posterior rectus sheath and rectus muscle. In all regards, a moderately dilated ureter is superior. Its thickened muscularis is generally efficient in peristaltic propulsion and is usually generously vascularized by collaterals (Rinker and Blanchard, 1966). Furthermore, the diameter of the moderately dilated ureter is such that cutaneous stomal stenosis is less likely. If both ureters are dilated, they can be brought to the anterior abdominal wall as a double-barreled stoma site. If one ureter is dilated and the other of normal caliber, the dilated ureter should be brought out as a single-barreled stoma and the normal caliber ureter managed by proximal transureteroureterostomy (Straffon et al., 1970).

Every attempt should be made to avoid two separate stoma sites with the attendant requirement for wearing separate urinary appliances. The severely dilated ureter with thin muscularis does not accommodate to cutaneous ureterostomy well (Straffon et al., 1970).

Procedure

In cutaneous ureterostomy, the stoma site should be marked on the side of the dilated ureter. If both ureters are dilated and a double-barreled cutaneous ureterostomy is planned, the stoma should be on the side contralateral to the longer of the two ureters. A considerably longer length of ureter will be necessary to traverse the distance from the contralateral retroperitoneum to the stoma site. In cutaneous ureterostomy, the ureter must be dissected retroperitoneally, nearly to the urinary bladder. Umbilical tape should be used to measure the distance from the retroperitoneum to the anterior abdominal skin. With this measurement as a guide, the surgeon should ensure that sufficient ureter distal to the iliac artery region has been freed prior to transecting the ureter.

Similar attention is directed to the ureter traversing the retroperitoneum. Before transecting the ureter, a piece of umbilical tape is taken to measure the length of ureter that will be required to traverse the tunnel beneath the inferior mesenteric artery and to reach the anterior abdominal skin. When the surgeon is assured of appropriate ureteral length, the ureter can be transected. When freeing the ureters for cutaneous ureterostomy, special care is required to ensure that collateral circulation remains intact. Therefore, the freed ureteral length should include as much of the periureteral adventitial tissue as possible. The ureter is directed to the appropriate retroperitoneum through a tunnel beneath the inferior mesenteric artery. The medial aspects of both ureters are spatulated for a distance of 2 cm or more (Fig. 72–2A). The ureters are then joined by interrupted or running sutures of absorbable material.

In the case of markedly dilated ureters, a simple circular stoma can be created on the anterior abdominal skin at the previously selected site, as described. The double-barreled ureterostomies are brought through this stoma site, and the stoma is fashioned by one of two techniques. A flush stoma can be created by simply suturing the double-barreled ureterostomy to the circumference of the stoma skin. This procedure can be carried out with interrupted absorbable sutures without difficulty. Preferentially, if there is sufficient ureteral length, double-barreled ureterostomy can be averted upon itself to create a projecting ureterostomy nipple (Fig. 72–2B) (Chute and Sallade, 1961).

When both ureters are dilated, there is often no reason for V-flap widening of the cutaneous stoma. However, if the degree of dilation is marginal, double V-flap skin inserts are needed (Fig. 72–3) (Straffon et

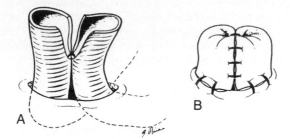

Figure 72–2. *A,* The medial aspects of both ureters are spatulated and joined by interrupted or running sutures of absorbable material. (From Eckstein, H. B.: *In* Glenn, J. F. (Ed.): Urologic Surgery. Philadelphia, J. B. Lippincott Co., 1983.) *B,* Double-barrel ureterostomy everted upon itself to create a projecting ureterostomy nipple. (From Eckstein, H. B.: *In* Glenn, J. F. (Ed.): Urologic Surgery. Philadelphia, J. B. Lippincott Co., 1983.)

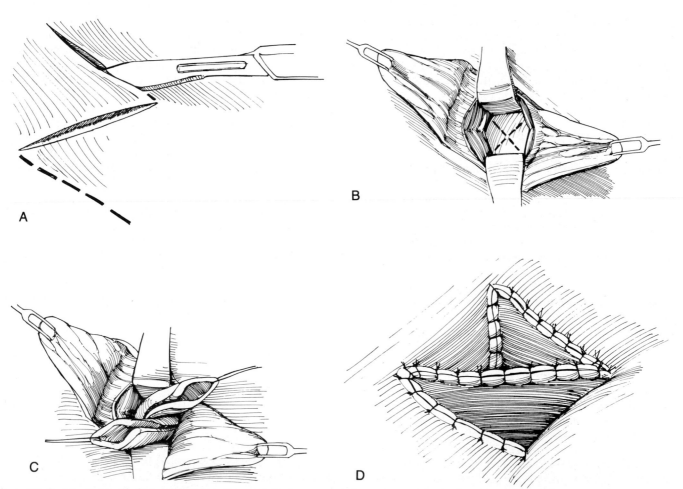

Figure 72–3. *A* to *D,* Double V-flap skin inserts are needed when ureteral diameter is marginal. The ureters are brought through the abdominal wall and spatulated at opposite poles. The resultant stoma is larger than could otherwise have been accomplished. (From Hinman, F., Jr.: Atlas of Urologic Surgery. Philadelphia, W. B. Saunders Co., 1989.)

al., 1970). Similarly, if only a single ureter is dilated and a single-barreled ureterostomy will be selected, the surgeon is well advised to use a V-flap technique to widen the stoma (Fig. 72–4).

Proximal transureteroureterostomy can be conducted in the usual fashion. A linear incision is made in the medial aspect of the recipient ureter, and the normal caliber ureter is spatulated on its medial aspect. The length of these two incisions should be 2.5 to 3 cm. The anastomosis between the ureters is conducted by means of two to four separate running sutures of adsorbable material (Fig. 72–5A). Just prior to closing the transureteroureterostomy, both indwelling stents should be directed to the renal pelves and led through the stoma site (Fig. 72–5B). Similarly, in double-barreled ureterostomies, each ureter can be catheterized at the termination of the procedure, with ureteral stents of the surgeon's choice.

Some surgeons advocate "retroperitonealizing" the transperitoneal course of the ureters. This effect can be achieved by suturing the posterior and anterior peritoneum together to form a covering for the entire intraperitoneal course of the ureters (Straffon et al., 1970).

In those cases in which a transureteroureterostomy has been performed, a suction drain catheter is placed at the anastomotic site and brought through a separate stab incision on the side opposite to the stoma site. In double-barreled ureterostomies, this preventive drain is not mandated.

Postoperative Care and Comments

The most common early complications associated with cutaneous ureterostomy are necrosis of the portion of ureters utilized to create the stoma site and leakage from a transureteroureterostomy anastomosis when employed (Eckstein, 1983). The routine utilization of perioperative ureteral stents has greatly decreased the impact of the second complication. The development of necrosis of the ureterostomy stoma is a calamitous complication. Ureteral length is usually insufficient to allow for standard stoma revision by exteriorization principles. The patient requires reoperation and the formation of a bowel conduit.

The commonest late complication of cutaneous ureterostomy is stomal stenosis (Feminella and Lattimer, 1971). This may occur in as many as 50 per cent of cases, particularly when patients are not appropriately selected. The dilated ureters tend to approach normal caliber in the postoperative interval, so that standard stoma revision surgery is usually insufficient to relieve the cutaneous obstruction. Conversion to a bowel conduit is the preferential mode of therapy.

If the ureteral complication is early or late and bowel diversion is necessitated, our preference is to employ the ileal conduit. A sigmoid colon conduit could be used alternatively. Some workers have suggested that colon conduit is necessitated for a failed left-sided ureteral stoma; An ileal conduit is favored for salvage of a right-

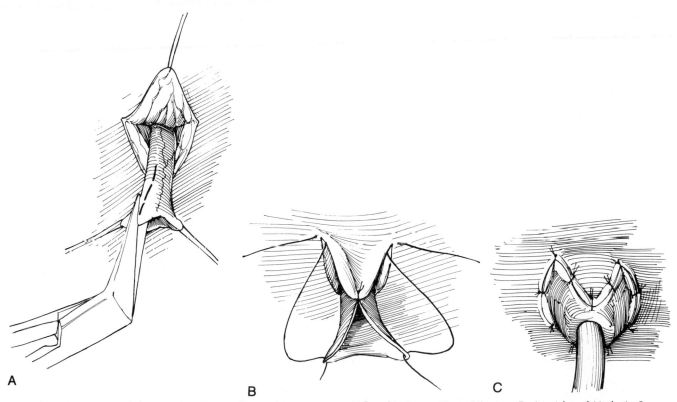

Figure 72–4. *A* to *C, A* single dilated ureter can be used to construct a V-flap skin insert. (From Hinman, F., Jr.: Atlas of Urologic Surgery. Philadelphia, W. B. Saunders Co., 1989.)

A   B   C

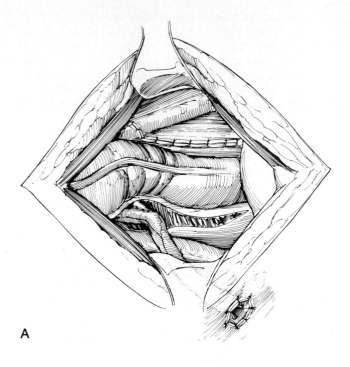

A

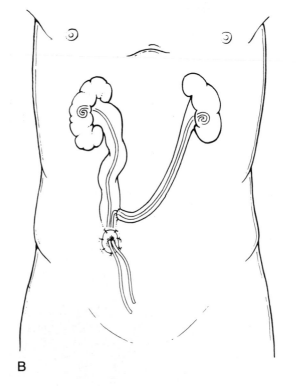

B

Figure 72–5. *A,* Proximal transureteroureterostomy is performed by a linear incision in the medial aspect of the recipient ureter, and the normal caliber ureter is spatulated on its medial aspect. (From Hinman, F., Jr.: Atlas of Urologic Surgery. Philadelphia, W. B. Saunders Co., 1989.) *B,* Prior to closing the transureteroureterostomy, both indwelling stents should be directed to the renal pelves and led through the stoma site.

sided failure (Eckstein, 1983). However, we have found that either portion of bowel can be utilized to salvage either right-sided or left-sided ureterostomy failures.

ILEAL CONDUIT

Urinary diversion by ileal conduit consists of diverting the urine to a short ileal segment that is directed to the anterior abdominal wall. Urinary diversion by means of an isolated ileal segment has become the most common surgical option in the patient who requires removal of the bladder for malignancy or who lacks functional or anatomic integrity of the urinary bladder.

As with all operations for urinary diversion requiring the interruption of bowel continuity, bowel preparation is essential to ileal conduit diversion. The principles of bowel preparation have been discussed in Chapter 69. They will not be re-emphasized except to note that our preference is a mechanical bowel cleansing along with a systemic antibiotic administration, in the perioperative interval. The preoperative bowel preparation should consist of a gradually diminishing dietary load, along with a balanced electrolyte solution cleansing of the bowel. Since the trend to shorten the preoperative stay of patients undergoing major surgery has taken place, patients are advised to limit intake to a full liquid diet 2 days prior to hospital admission, changing to a clear liquid diet in the 24-hour interval before hospital admission. Upon hospital admission (usually 18 hours before surgery), a clear liquid diet is maintained and administration of 5 liters of balanced electrolyte solution by mouth is initiated. Systemic intravenous antibiotics are initiated as well during this period.

These systemic antibiotics are maintained for a total duration of 4 days, extending 3 days into the postoperative period. Shortening the total administration time of broad-spectrum systemic antibiotics decreases the incidence of complications, such as moniliasis, and, more importantly, overgrowth of bowel flora by *Clostridium difficile*.

In ileal conduit urinary diversion, the condition of the ureters, except for the totally aperistaltic ureter, is not a particular concern. Either dilated or normal caliber ureters can be diverted to an isolated ileal segment without fear of damage. In general, ureteroileal anastomoses do not afford an antirefluxing valvular mechanism. However, even though some workers have stipulated that an antireflux mechanism is essential in the maintenance of upper urinary tract integrity, others have found no difference between refluxing and antirefluxing ureterointestinal anastomoses (Elder et al., 1979; Hill and Ransley, 1983; Husmann et al., 1989).

Because the majority of patients with ureterointestinal urinary diversions suffer from bacteriuria and because bacteriuria in the presence of renal reflux is generally considered to be of adverse prognostic potential, our preference is ureterointestinal diversions that afford antireflux ureterointestinal anastomoses. However, this preference is imposed most often in the young surgical candidate rather than in the more typical older candidate whose bladder must be removed for purposes of cure of uroepithelial malignancy.

The ileal conduit can be adapted to simple diversion of the distal ureters to the anterior abdominal wall or, in the case of totally defective transmission of urine along the ureters, may be adapted to the diversion of urine from each renal pelvis directly.

In general, the selected stoma site is in the right lower quadrant, as described previously. However, the ileum may be directed by rotation on its long axis to the left lower quadrant. This is particularly true if both renal pelves are to be diverted directly.

In patients with regional enteritis or extensive irradiation with subsequent damage to the distal ileum, ileal conduit diversion is relatively contraindicated. In these circumstances, a more healthy piece of bowel and a more healthy portion of ureter should be selected for the urinary diversion. In cases of regional enteritis, the proximal bowel (jejunum) may be selected. Alternatively, the sigmoid colon or transverse colon may be utilized. In patients who have been heavily irradiated, a transverse colon or jejunal conduit may also be indicated.

In any patient who will have an interposed portion of intact bowel between the kidneys and abdominal urinary appliance, there will be the potential for reabsorption of urinary constituents. In the ordinary patient with normal renal function, this should not constitute a clinically significant problem. However, in the patient who has pre-existing damage to renal function, great care should be taken to select the shortest portion of bowel that will be capable of diverting the urine from the ureters or renal pelves to the abdominal surface.

Procedure

After the ureters have been directed to the right retroperitoneum, isolation of the selected ileal segment and bowel reanastomosis is carried out (Fig. 72–6A to C). Although some have suggested retroperitonealizing the entire ileal conduit, our preference is to utilize a segment of ileum that is sufficiently long to be directed to the anterior abdominal wall directly from the right retroperitoneum. This preference allows for the construction of a considerably shorter ileal conduit, thus decreasing the potential for reabsorption of urinary constituents in the postoperative period. Only the base of the ileal conduit is retroperitonealized, and the remaining ileum traverses the peritoneal cavity directly.

When selecting an appropriate bowel segment for division from bowel continuity, it is helpful to transilluminate to bowel mesentery. When surgeons are selecting the appropriate segment, they should bear in mind the potential of a long-term circulatory disturbance of the bowel ("pipe-stem" conduit) and attempt to ensure the very best vascular supply to the conduit possible. In order to achieve this result, the mesenteric attachments of the isolated conduit should be as broad as possible. In general, the length of the mesenteric windows need not be more than 5 to 6 cm, in order to

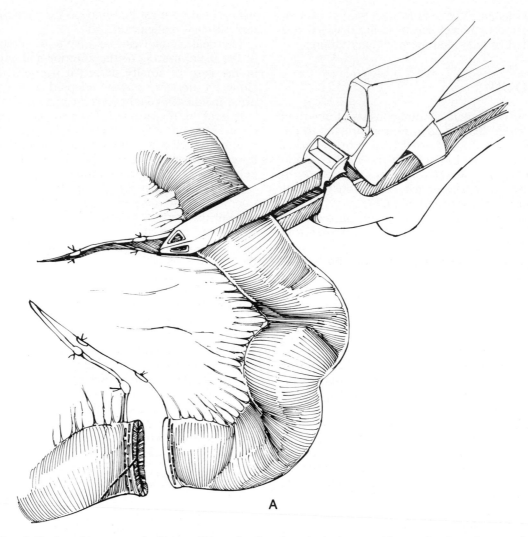

Figure 72–6. *A* to *C*, The bowel is transected utilizing a GIA stapler. Bowel continuity is restored by opening the antimesenteric corner of the two ileal ends and sliding an arm of the GIA down each limb. Prior to firing, proper orientation is assured. The opening is closed with a TA-55 stapler. (From Hinman, F., Jr.: Atlas of Urologic Surgery. Philadelphia, W. B. Saunders Co., 1989.) *D*, The ileal segment is dropped caudally so as to lie below the area of selected ileoileal anastomosis. The mesenteric trap is closed with interrupted nonabsorbable sutures. (From Hinman, F., Jr.: Atlas of Urologic Surgery. Philadelphia, W. B. Saunders Co., 1989.)

isolate an appropriately long ileal segment and to conduct enteroenteral anastomosis. The base of the mesenteric segment supplying blood to the isolated ileal segment should contain at least two major vascular supplies, ensuring adequate arterialization of the isolated segment as well as adequate venous and lymphatic return from the segment.

In constructing the windows of Deaver in the mesentery, we prefer mechanical stapling devices (ligating and dividing stapler, LDS). If these are not available, electrocautery is utilized to fashion the mesenteric windows. The cautery can be adjusted to cutting current in order to incise the peritoneum overlying the mesentery. Thereafter, coagulating current can be utilized to divide the mesentery proper and to coagulate the mesenteric blood supply. On occasion, it will be necessary to separately clamp and ligate mesenteric blood vessels.

After the ileal segment is isolated, it is dropped down caudally, to lie below the area of selected ileoileal anastomosis. The mesenteric trap is closed with interrupted nonabsorbable sutures in this operation, as well as in all procedures wherein bowel segments are isolated, to avoid postoperative internal herniation of bowel loops (Fig. 72–6*D*).

A Kocher clamp is directed through the prepared stoma site, which is usually sufficiently capacious to allow the insertion of the surgeon's first two fingers. The Kocher clamp grasps the distal portion of the ileal conduit on the stapled resection line and directs it out to the abdominal skin. The surgeon usually sees that the orientation of the mesenteric margin of the isolated segment is best directed toward the left shoulder in order to reduce any tethering effect of the mesentery. The distal staple line can then be transected, and a "rosebudding" suture technique is employed to create a protruding stoma. Sutures of absorbable material are taken from skin edge to proximal serosa of bowel and then directed to full thickness of the end of the ileal

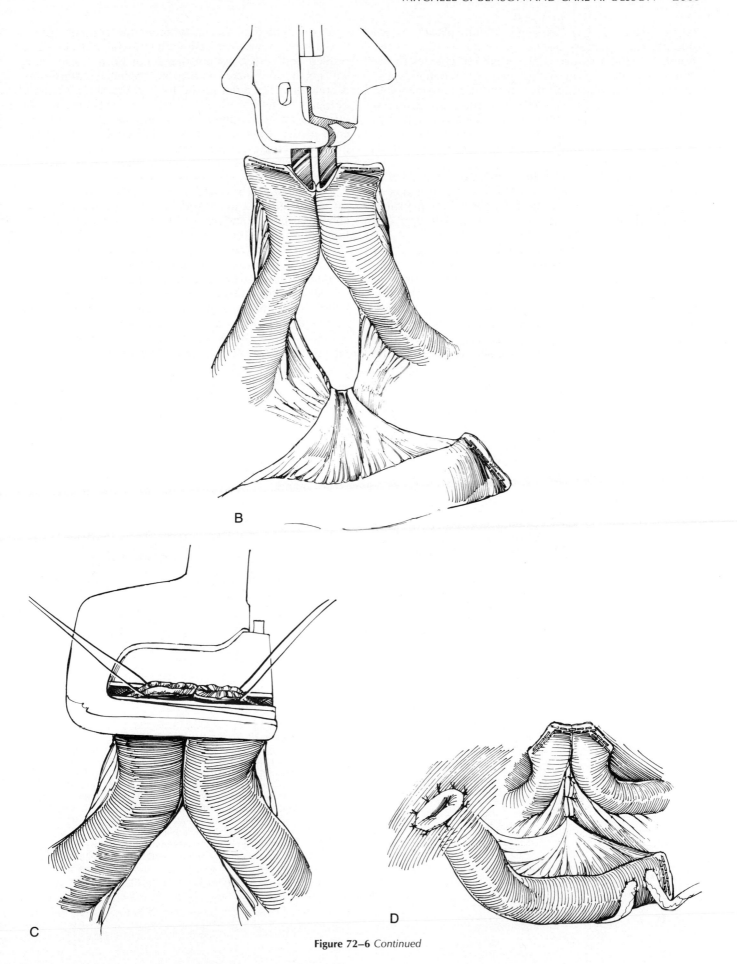

B

C

D

Figure 72–6 Continued

segment (Fig. 72–7*A*). These are initially placed to each side of the mesentery at the upper left portion of the stoma. A similar suture is placed at 180 degrees to the initial two sutures. Thereafter, two or three interrupted sutures are taken to each side of the stoma to complete the ileal rosebud (Fig. 72–7*B*). No suturing is required at the fascia level; no suturing technique is required at the peritoneal level, provided the construction of the peritoneal and posterior fascial opening has not been overly generous.

In markedly obese individuals, it is extremely difficult to create a rosebud appearance when the terminus of the ileum is employed. Sufficient tethering by the small bowel mesentery is evident, so that an appropriately elevated stoma cannot be achieved.

In this circumstance, a modified Turnbull stoma should be created (Turnbull and Hewitt, 1978). The surgeon determines the distance from anterior fascia to the skin level and applies this measurement to the ileal terminus. At that point, a Babcock clamp or Penrose drain is placed. The folded ileal segment is advanced to the level of the abdominal surface (Fig. 72–7*C*). The folded, blind-ending terminus will simply extend to the

anterior abdominal fascia, whereas the conduit proper is the only bowel traversing the fascial buttons. The stapled end of the conduit need not be resected, as it will not be in contact with urine. A linear enterotomy is created at the point of the fold on the antimesenteric border of the bowel. The length of the enterotomy incision can be estimated to be one-half the circumference of the stoma site. Hereafter, budding sutures are placed to create a protruding stoma. After the stoma has been completely constructed, attention is directed to the ureteroileal anastomoses.

The base of the conduit is directed to the right retroperitoneum and tucked beneath the inferior mesenteric artery. Standard end-to-side ureteroileal anastomoses can then be conducted as described in another chapter. Our preference is to spatulate each ureter and excise a small button of full-thickness ileal wall on its antimesenteric border. Two separate running absorbable sutures are taken from the apex of the ureteral spatulation to full thickness of bowel, and these are run along each edge of the spatulated ureter and tied to one another. No need exists to buttress the anastomosis by means of additional seromuscular sutures. Just prior to

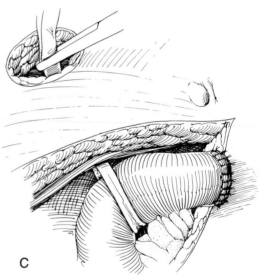

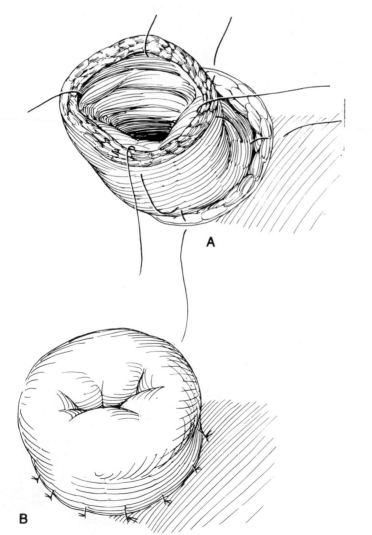

Figure 72–7. *A* and *B*, The distal staple line is transected, and a "rosebudding" suture technique is employed to create a protruding stoma. Sutures are taken from skin edge to proximal serosa of bowel and are then directed to full thickness of the end of the ileal segment. *C*, Modified Turnbull stoma. A Babcock clamp or Penrose drain is placed, and the folded ileal segment is advanced to the level of the abdominal surface. The blind-ending terminus will extend to the anterior abdominal fascia. The conduit proper is the only bowel traversing the fascial buttons. (From Hinman, F., Jr.: Atlas of Urologic Surgery. Philadelphia, W. B. Saunders Co., 1989.)

completion of each ureteral anastomosis, stents should be directed to each renal pelvis. A Yankauer suction instrument with the end tip removed is helpful in directing these stents to the appropriate ureter (Fig. 72–8).

The remainder of the base of the conduit is thoroughly retroperitonealized by bringing the excess right-sided retroperitoneum anteriorly to cover the region of the ureteroileal anastomoses. A suction drain is placed beneath this recreated peritoneal leaflet and directed through the left lower quadrant.

Variations on the ileal conduit include the circumstance in which the ureters are dilated bilaterally and other circumstances in which ureteral function is poor. When both ureters are dilated, they may be individually spatulated and sewn to one another in preparation for anastomosis to the proximal end of the isolated ileal segment (Wallace, 1970). Obviously, if such a technique is employed, the proximal stapled resection line is transected prior to creating the ureterointestinal anastomosis. In general, the Wallace technique is not as adaptable to normal caliber ureters as it is to somewhat dilated ureters (Skinner et al., 1987a). Additionally, the surgeon must keep in mind that, if there ever develops a reason for removal of one kidney and ureter, the contralateral ureteral anastomosis will be in some jeopardy. Therefore, in an individual with multifocal urothelial malignancy, it may not be appropriate to utilize the Wallace anastomosis.

When both ureters are sufficiently diseased or damaged so as to necessitate direct diversion of urine from the renal pelves bilaterally, a longer ileal segment is required. After the ileal segment is isolated, it is dropped caudal to the site of intestinal anastomosis and then rotated cephalad so that its proximal end is directed toward the left renal pelvis. The line of Toldt, lateral to the right colon and the posterior peritoneum along the root of the mesentery, is incised. With blunt dissection the right colon and entire small bowel can be reflected cephalad and draped over the superior edge of the wound, affording excellent access to the retroperitoneum (Fig. 72–9A). A generous tunnel is created bluntly by digital dissection between the right and left retroperitoneum in the space between the superior and inferior

mesenteric arteries. The remaining conduit is then directed to the region of the right renal pelvis and its distal most extent is directed to the selected right lower quadrant stoma site.

The entire left colon is mobilized. After appropriate mobilization and medial reflection, the proximal extent of the isolated ileal segment can be identified, its stapled line of resection resected, and direct anastomosis to the left renal pelvis conducted with interrupted or running absorbable suture technique (Fig. 72–9B). When this anastomosis has been completed, the left colon is reflected back to its normal position and attention is directed to the region of the right renal pelvis. A retroperitoneal anastomosis is carried out in an end-to-side fashion, utilizing absorbable suture material. The right colon and small bowel are allowed to be replaced in the abdominal cavity, and the stoma is finally created. Because the pelvoileal anastomoses are a considerable distance apart, separate suction drains are employed, bringing the drains through the flank region bilaterally.

Postoperative Care and Comments

A review of serious complications associated with ileal conduit urinary diversion has been completed (Benson et al., 1990). It is surprising to see how often a second operation is required for this operation, either in the early postoperative period (15 to 23 per cent) or later, with longer follow-up (17 to 23 per cent) (Neal, 1985; Pernet and Jonas, 1985; Svare et al., 1985). In the pediatric population, the predominant feature of stomal stenosis (38 per cent of cases) adds to the requirement for reoperation (Shapiro et al., 1975).

Many of the complications of bowel conduit urinary diversion have been reviewed in Chapter 69. However, one of the most highly morbid complications resulting from this procedure is related to the intestinal anastomosis and the need for reoperation to repair problems in this area. Anastomotic leakage and bowel obstruction, if they require surgery, carry nearly a 20 per cent mortality (Sullivan, 1980). Therefore, the surgeon is well advised to become thoroughly familiar with a technique of a hand-sewn or stapling-device intestinal anas-

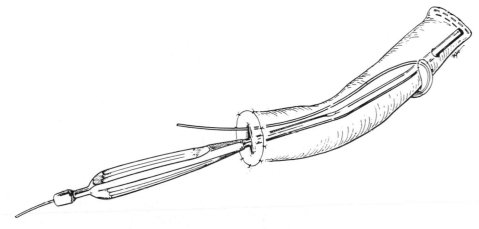

Figure 72–8. Prior to completion of each ureteral anastomosis, stents should be directed to each renal pelvis. A Yankauer suction instrument with the end tip removed is helpful in directing these stents to the appropriate ureter.

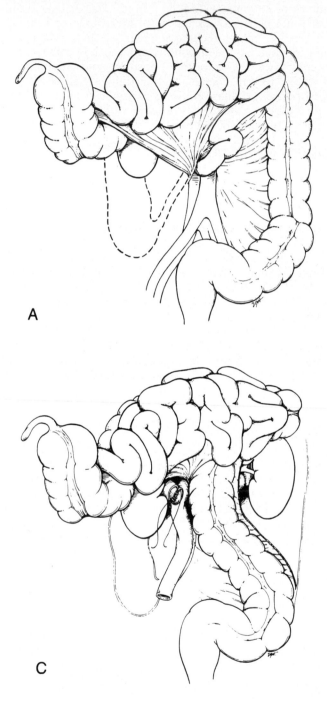

A

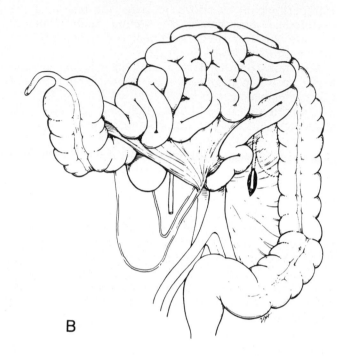

B

C

Figure 72–9. *A*, The line of Toldt lateral to the right colon and the posterior peritoneum along the root of the mesentery are incised. With blunt dissection the right colon and entire small bowel can be reflected cephalad.

B, The right and left ureters are identified, or the colon can be mobilized.

C, The entire left colon is mobilized. The proximal extent of the isolated ileal segment is anastomosed to the left renal pelvis, as conducted with interrupted or running absorbable suture technique.

tomosis that is dependable in all circumstances. In general, with normal bowel, our preference is to utilize a stapled anastomosis solely. If the bowel is damaged by irradiation, an additional layer of seromuscular silk sutures can be placed to strengthen the anastomotic site.

The incidence of ureteroileal extravasation has been greatly decreased by the routine utilization of ureteral stents directed to the collecting appliance. Many operative series have been published indicating that these stents reduce the incidence of urinary extravasation to 1 to 3 per cent of cases (Bedoe et al., 1987; Regan and Barrett, 1985). Similarly, the consequences of urinary extravasation, such as subsequent ureteroileal stenosis, have been greatly ameliorated by indwelling stents. Urinoma formation is rarely, if ever, seen.

Long-term complications of ileal conduit urinary diversion include delayed sequelae of intestinal surgery, ureteroileal stenosis, elongation and subsequent failure of the ileal conduit to appropriately propel urine, and upper urinary tract deterioration from other causes.

As many as 5 to 10 per cent of individuals who undergo ileal conduit urinary diversion experience bowel complications at some time in the future (Sullivan et al., 1980). These may be temporary episodes of surgical ileus, which may respond to intervals of gastrointestinal decompression. In contrast, they may require reoperative surgery to repair bowel obstruction consequent to anastomotic stenoses or adhesions causing intestinal obstruction.

Ureterointestinal stenosis may occur at any time in the patient with any bowel conduit. This sequela should be regarded with considerable concern in the individual who has undergone cystectomy for uroepithelial malignancy, because one of the reasons for ureteral obstruction would be a primary ureteral neoplasm. Any patient with cancer who develops ureteral obstruction should be thoroughly investigated by means of urinary cytology, imaging, and endoscopy of the conduit to rule out neoplastic causes.

Ureterointestinal anastomotic stenosis can also occur without the influence of uroepithelial malignancy. This is particularly true on the left side, where the necessity to free a portion of ureter from its blood supply is considerably longer. Additionally, ureteroileal anastomotic failure because of angulation beneath the inferior mesenteric artery is more likely in the left ureter. When ureteroileal anastomotic stenosis has been discovered, an attempt may be made to solve the problem by endoscopic technology (Kramolowsky et al., 1987). The region of the anastomotic stricture may be dilated with a balloon catheter, which can be either directed from the ileal stoma or percutaneously placed to traverse the stenotic segment. After balloon dilation has been accomplished, ureteroileal intubation is required for a period of 6 to 8 weeks in order to ensure patency. This technique is successful in approximately 50 per cent of ureteroileal strictures, although the long-term outcome of the patients managed in this fashion is not yet known. In contrast, open reoperation to revise the ureteroileal anastomosis is somewhat more dependable, although it is associated with all of the complications of a major operative intervention (Kramolowsky et al., 1988). If

ureteroileal stenosis requires intraluminal stenting over a long time period, instances have occurred wherein the stent has eroded through the ureter and the adjacent common iliac artery, resulting in considerable conduit hemorrhage.

The preservation of a wide-based mesenteric supply to the isolated ileal segment is usually sufficient guard against "pipe-stem" loop formation. This complication seems to be a consequence of insufficient vascular ingress or return. It is associated with isolated strictured areas along the course of the conduit and a generally thin, noncompliant conduit throughout its entire length. Obviously, peristalsis is impaired and proximal upper tract deterioration results. The only appropriate management for pipe-stem loop is replacement of the entire conduit (Knapp et al., 1987). Attempts to dilate portions of the conduit have been met with failure uniformly.

Upper urinary tract deterioration is not inconsiderable in the patient undergoing ileal conduit urinary diversion. The reviews of large series of patients long-term suggest that, overall, at least one third of renal units experience some degree of deterioration with time (Middleton and Hendren, 1976; Schwarz and Jeffs, 1975; Shapiro et al., 1975). This finding may be a consequence of a variety of influences, including those already described, such as ureteroileal stenosis and pipe-stem loop. However, the simple presence of chronic bacteriuria in association with a free refluxing conduit may be at fault in other instances. Therefore, even though the ileal conduit is a "gold standard" against which all other urinary diversions should be compared, it is not a panacea. This is particularly relevant in the more youthful individual who requires urinary diversion rather than in the elderly patient who requires removal of the urinary bladder for malignancy. Serious electrolyte abnormalities should not occur in the individual with normal renal function and a well-fashioned short ileal or colonic conduit. Although one series suggests that alkali therapy is needed in more than a third of patients (Castro and Ram, 1970), most modern experience suggests that treatment is rarely needed.

Stoma complications are seen in almost every patient with an external urinary appliance device. Urea dermatitis of the surrounding skin is experienced at intervals by nearly every patient. Stomal stenosis is a pertinent feature, particularly in the younger individual whose bowel is of somewhat smaller diameter than in the adult (Schwarz and Jeffs, 1975; Shapiro et al., 1975). All patients with ileal conduit stomas experience a gradual contraction of the sites. Frequent attention to this aspect of postoperative care must be directed by either the surgeon or the enterostomal therapist. Most patients require the alteration of an appliance faceplate size at least once. If the stoma becomes sufficiently stenotic, stoma revision is necessitated. This can usually be achieved by simple circumcision of the stoma site, freeing up of the distal most ileal segment through to the fascial or peritoneal level and refashioning of a wider diameter rosebud stoma.

Parastomal hernia is another long-term postoperative complication of ileal conduit urinary diversion. Although not as frequently encountered as in colonic urinary diversions, wherein the fascial windows are much broader in diameter, parastomal herniation can still occur after ileal conduit diversion (Hampel et al., 1986). We have often thought that one of the major reasons for these hernias is the necessity to open the internal rectus fascia and peritoneum sufficiently to allow the mesentery to progress through the inner abdominal opening. The simple expedient of "defatting" the mesentery to be directed through the stoma obviates the need to create a larger internal stoma and, as a consequence, decreases the incidence of parastomal herniation. Similarly, the additional expedient of devascularizing the terminal 1 to 2 cm of the ileal stoma results in the same prevention against parastomal hernia formation.

JEJUNAL CONDUIT

The use of jejunum as a bowel segment to divert the urine to the anterior abdominal wall has many potential benefits. In general, it allows the avoidance of areas of pelvic irradiation that might be utilized in patients with bladder, cervix, uterine, or rectal malignancy who have the need for subsequent urinary diversion. However, the physiologic consequences of jejunal conduits are such that this procedure should be selected only when other alternatives are less attractive.

The longer the length of contact of urine with the jejunal mucosa, the more likely a tendency for the patient to experience hyponatremic, hypochloremic acidosis. The incidence of this electrolyte complication is sufficiently high to warrant salt replacement in nearly half the patients (Golimbu and Morales, 1975). Alternative forms of urinary diversion, utilizing the transverse colon, should be considered by the surgeon who is to perform a jejunal conduit.

Patients who have radiation damage to the distal bowel also have radiation damage to the distal ureters. Therefore, when conducting urinary diversion in patients who have severe radiation injury, the principle of utilizing nonirradiated bowel is no more important than the principle of utilizing nonirradiated ureter for the urinary diversion procedure. Because, in most instances, the radiation damage is confined to the true anatomic pelvis, ureters should be transected at a point above their entry into the pelvic cavity. This procedure generally necessitates that the left ureteroenteric anastomosis is conducted above the level of the inferior mesenteric artery.

If jejunum is selected as the bowel segment to be employed, the length of the segment should be as short as possible to minimize metabolic complications. In order to achieve this end, the surgeon should work in cooperation with the enterostomal therapist during the preoperative preparation, because it is less likely that the stoma can be directed to the lower abdominal quadrants. Positioning the stoma somewhat above the umbilicus may be necessitated, in order to achieve a short jejunal length.

The isolation of the jejunal conduit is carried out precisely in the same fashion as the isolation of an ileal segment. As much as possible, the surgeon should attempt to utilize the proximal ileum in contrast to the preferred jejunum proper. After the isolated segment is created, the enteroenteral anastomosis is performed, and the mesenteric trap is closed, the proximal end of the conduit is directed to a tunnel created between the left and right retroperitoneal regions in the space bounded by the superior and inferior mesenteric arteries.

The entire right colon should be mobilized to expose the more proximal extent of the left ureter, as in performing a high ileal conduit (see Fig. 72–9A). By mobilizing the entire right colon and small bowel mesentery along its root, the right colon and entire small bowel can be delivered from the wound cephalad. Additionally, the right ureter in its proximal extent can be exposed and prepared for ureterointestinal anastomosis. The remainder of the procedure is identical to that employed for ileal conduit urinary diversion, with ureterointestinal anastomoses conducted according to the surgeon's preference. The placement of stents is of value in patients with jejunal conduits. By diverting the urine from contact with jejunal mucosa, early postoperative electrolyte alterations may be avoided.

Postoperative Care and Comments

Many features of postoperative care and complications associated with jejunal conduits are identical to those with ileal conduit urinary diversions. The single difference is the prevalence of electrolyte disturbances following removal of diverting stents. Many patients experience the development of hyponatremic hypochloremic acidosis (Golimbu and Morales, 1975; Klein et al., 1986). The degree of hyponatremia is substantial, leading to the development of secondary hyperaldosteronism in some. This syndrome may worsen when conditions resulting in salt loss are experienced (e.g., perspiration during hot weather).

Therefore, the electrolyte status of each patient undergoing jejunal conduit urinary diversion must be monitored at frequent intervals. Each patient must be evaluated relative to the demand for salt replacement, which can be administered in the form of NaCl tablets. The patient should be advised to take additional NaCl replacement in hotter months or when traveling in hotter climates.

Little has been reported regarding the long-term effects of jejunal conduit diversion on renal function (Golimbu and Morales, 1975). Because the jejunal conduit is a freely refluxing diversion and because the incidence of urinary tract infection is similar to the ileal conduit, it would be anticipated that long-term renal deterioration would be experienced at a similar rate to that in an ileal conduit. Left ureteral obstruction may be somewhat less common, particularly if the surgeon employs a high ureteral anastomosis. The space between the superior and inferior mesenteric arteries is usually quite generous, and the opportunity for angulation or compression of the ureter beneath the inferior mesenteric artery as in ileal conduit is avoided.

COLON CONDUIT

Two forms of colon conduit are possible, one employs the sigmoid colon as first reported by Mogg (1967) and the other the transverse colon. Both share the theoretical advantage of affording a nonrefluxing ureterointestinal anastomosis, a feature that some workers have suggested as advantageous in the avoidance of upper urinary tract deterioration (Husman et al., 1989; Richie and Skinner, 1975). However, the advantages of antireflux ureterointestinal anastomoses have not been experienced by all patients (Hill and Ransley, 1983).

Tunneled anastomoses are not appropriate in those individuals with dilated ureters (Haltiwanger, 1983). If a ureter is significantly dilated, creating a colonic tunnel will result in an accentuated hydronephrosis. Therefore, if the ureters are dilated, other portions of bowel should be selected for the urinary diversion, or a classic end-to-side, direct ureteral colonic anastomosis may be utilized. However, Hendren (1975) has successfully tapered and implanted dilated ureters in children.

The sigmoid conduit should be avoided in the heavily irradiated pelvis (Richie, 1986). Because the superior hemorrhoidal artery is often sacrificed, the distal colon and rectum have insufficient blood supply if there has been any radiation damage to the smaller collateral vessels. Similarly, sigmoid should be avoided in cystectomy cases because, if the internal pudendal artery is damaged, blood supply to the rectum is compromised (Skinner, 1987a). In contrast, however, when carrying out total pelvic exenteration, it is extremely useful to create a sigmoid conduit, because there is no need for any intestinal anastomosis.

In cases of total pelvic exenteration in which sigmoid conduits are employed, urinary conduits are directed to stoma sites previously selected in the right lower quadrant. The permanent colostomy is created in a site marked in the left lower quadrant. In contrast, when a sigmoid conduit is constructed for urinary diversion alone, the preferred stoma site is on the left.

The transverse colon conduit is utilized in patients with heavily irradiated pelves. The transverse colon affords the opportunity to complete the urinary diversion, utilizing nonirradiated segments of both bowel and ureter. Stoma location for a transverse colon conduit is generally in the left lower quadrant.

Because both the number and frequency of diseases affecting the large bowel are greater than those affecting the small bowel, it is our prejudice that preoperative barium studies and/or colonoscopy be carried out, whenever the large bowel has been selected to perform urinary diversion (continent or conduit).

Procedure

When carrying out a sigmoid conduit, the line of Toldt lateral to the left colon is incised along its entire length. Mobilizing considerable length of the entire left colon will facilitate colocolostomy after isolating the sigmoid segment. An appropriate length of sigmoid colon is marked and prepared for isolation (Fig. 72–10A). Mesenteric windows are cut in the process of which the superior hemorrhoidal artery may be ligated. In the large bowel as well as in the small bowel, it is advisable to avoid a narrow base to the mesenteric supply of the isolated segment.

Colocolostomy is carried out by either suture or staple technique (Fig. 72–10B). We prefer to utilize the EEA circular stapling device. Side-to-side anastomosis with the GIA and TA devices may also be used, if colonic length is generous. After restoring bowel continuity and closing the mesenteric trap, the base of the conduit is directed to the retroperitoneum just lateral to the colocolostomy. The ureters are identified and transected as in other urinary diversion procedures. However, the surgeon should keep in mind that longer ureteral segments are required, in order to provide the antireflux ureterointestinal anastomoses. Both the stoma construction and ureterointestinal anastomoses differ in the colon conduit versus the ileal or jejunal conduit. Tunneled anastomoses of ureters to the isolated colon can be performed by means of one of numerous techniques described in Chapter 69. We utilize the Leadbetter technique of ureterocolonic anastomosis. In order to accommodate the somewhat larger diameter of the colon, the stoma site requires the excision of a larger skin button as well as larger anterior and posterior fascia and peritoneum buttons.

The typical rosebud technique is utilized at the cutaneous level, employing interrupted suture of absorbable material. Although it is not necessary in all cases, in the very obese patient we sometimes suture the circumference of the posterior fascial stoma to the bowel with interrupted absorbable or nonabsorbable suture (taken through the seromuscular layer of bowel only), as an additional guard against parastomal herniation.

In these conduits as well as others described previously, bilateral ureteral stents are directed to each renal pelvis and through the stoma (Fig. 72–10C). The suction drain is placed at the point of ureteral anastomoses and brought through the abdomen on the contralateral side.

The technique of transverse colon conduit is not very different from that of sigmoid conduit. However, a few features need description. First, the length of colon necessary in transverse colon conduit is somewhat longer than that in sigmoid conduit. A high ureteral anastomosis is carried out at the base of the mesentery, and yet the left lower quadrant stoma site is the same.

Second, because a generous length of transverse colon is removed, either the right or left colon requires mobilization, in order to allow for colocolostomy without undue tension (Fig. 72–11). We mobilize the entire right colon, avoiding the potential pitfalls of splenic injury in the dissection of the splenocolic ligament. Many workers suggest directing the ureters through the small bowel mesentery just to the right of the ligament of Treitz (Loening et al., 1982; Schmidt, 1985).

However, mobilizing the entire right colon and incising the posterior peritoneum along the base of the mesentery and reflecting bowel contents cephalad affords excellent exposure in the region of ureteral anastomoses (see Fig. 72–9A). If this technique is employed, the only additional task is finding the left ureter in its

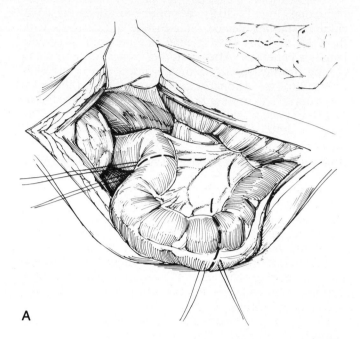

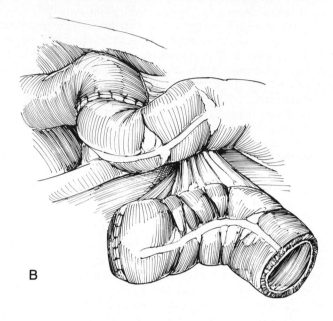

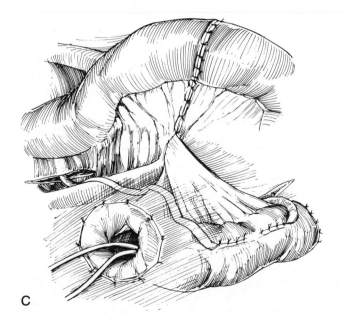

Figure 72–10. *A,* An appropriate length of sigmoid colon is marked and prepared for isolation.

B, Bowel continuity is restored and the mesenteric trap closed. The base of the conduit is directed to the retroperitoneum lateral to the colocolostomy.

C, Bilateral ureteral stents are directed to each renal pelvis and through the stoma. (From Hinman, F., Jr.: Atlas of Urologic Surgery. Philadelphia, W. B. Saunders Co., 1989.)

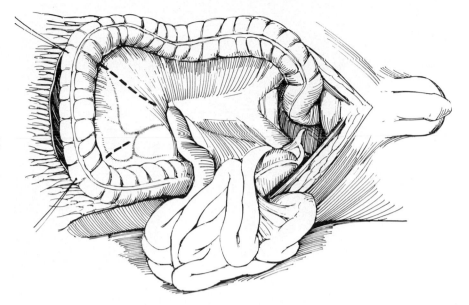

Figure 72–11. Transverse colon conduit with development of lesser sac and delineation of conduit and middle colic artery. (From Hinman, F., Jr.: Atlas of Urologic Surgery. Philadelphia, W. B. Saunders Co., 1989.)

midpoint. This can be accomplished by reflecting the left colon medially or by incising the left colon mesentery somewhat lateral to the midline. Once the left ureter has been isolated, it can be transected and a generous tunnel created between the superior and inferior mesenteric arteries. The left ureter is directed through this tunnel to the right retroperitoneum. Hereafter, the operation is precisely the same as that described for sigmoid conduit.

Postoperative Care and Comments

No substantial differences are noted in the postoperative care of the patient undergoing colon conduit diversion compared with other forms of bowel diversion. Complications are similar as well, with the exception of a slightly higher incidence of ureterointestinal stenosis (13 per cent) as well as a higher incidence of parastomal herniation or stomal prolapse (13 per cent) and a lower incidence of stomal stenosis, when using large bowel as a conduit (Golimbu and Morales, 1975; Richie, 1986).

Although one might anticipate a higher incidence of electrolyte disturbances utilizing colon, careful animal studies have not confirmed any statistically significant differences (Richie and Skinner, 1975). As previously mentioned, controversy exists relative to the improved preservation of upper tracts in nonrefluxing colon conduits versus ileal conduits. Some groups report significant advantages (Althausen et al., 1978; Elder et al., 1979; Husman et al., 1989), whereas others report no differences (Hill and Ransley, 1983). A reoperation rate of 16 per cent has been reported, primarily for ureterocolonic stenosis (Althausen et al., 1978).

ILEOCECAL CONDUIT

The ileocecal conduit was proposed by Libertino and Zinman (1986), as an alternative means of diverting the

urine, utilizing an antireflux technique. In this procedure, the ileocecal segment is employed for construction of the conduit. Ureters are anastomosed to the ileum in the standard freely refluxing fashion, and the cecal diameter brought to the abdominal wall as the stoma. This operation, therefore, depends on the integrity of the ileocecal valve to prevent upper tract reflux. Preferably, the ileocecal valve is buttressed by means of a novel technique to ensure against reflux.

Procedure

The ileocecal segment is resected, basing its blood supply on ileocolic artery branches (Fig. 72–12A). The segment is dropped inferior to the ileocolic anastomosis. A larger button of abdominal skin and anterior and posterior fascia are excised in a previously marked right lower quadrant site. After performing routine appendectomy and buttressing the ileocecal valve, the cecum is directed through the stoma and a projecting stoma is created with typical rosebud sutures. The base of the ileum is directed to the right retroperitoneum, where both ureters are led. Typical ureteroileal anastomosis can be carried out according to the surgeon's preference.

As described by Libertino and Zinman (1986), the ileocecal valve should be augmented (Fig. 72–12B and C). Multiple windows are created in the ileal mesentery, close to the border of the bowel and between blood vessels. The ileal segment, if folded inferolaterally along the foot of cecum, is then wrapped around the distal ileum. Seromuscular sutures are taken through the mesenteric windows to secure the cecal wrap.

Postoperative Care and Comments

No substantial differences are noted in the postoperative management of the patients undergoing ileocecal urinary diversions compared with patients undergoing

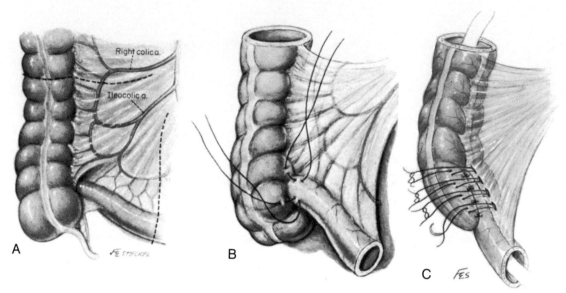

Figure 72–12. *A,* The ileocecal segment bases its blood supply on ileocolic artery branches.
B and *C,* The ileocecal valve should be augmented by creating multiple windows in the ileal mesentery. The ileal segment is folded inferolaterally along the foot of cecum, which is then wrapped around the distal ileum with seromuscular sutures. (From Libertino, J. A., and Zinman, L.: Ileocecal segment for temporary and permanent urinary diversion. Urol. Clin. North Am., 13:241–250, 1986.)

other bowel conduits. No variations exist in the incidence and management of complications compared with other conduit diversions, although the creation of a dependable antireflux mechanism may arguably protect against renal deterioration. Indeed, Libertino and Zinman (1986) reported no episodes of nonobstructive pyelonephritis in 62 patients and measured the competence of the buttressed ileocecal valve to withstand 55 to 75 cm H_2O without reflux, in 36 of 38 patients studied. However, additional surgery was required in 16 of 150 patients undergoing either ileocecal conduit or ileocecalcystoplasty. Interestingly, nine operations were for stomal prolapse or parastomal herniation.

CONTINENT URINARY DIVERSION

Continent urinary diversion can be divided into three major categories. First, ureterosigmoidostomy and its variations, such as ileocecal sigmoidostomy, rectal bladder, and sigmoid hemi-Kock operation with proximal colonic intussusception are discussed. These techniques allow for excretion of urine by means of evacuation. Second are orthotopic voiding pouches that are suitable, particularly in the male patient with an intact sphincteric apparatus. The third large category of continent diversions requires clean intermittent catheterization for emptying urine at intervals from the constructed pouch.

An acceleration of interest in the continent diversion of the upper urinary tract has occurred. For example, the concept of refashioning bowel so that it serves as a urinary reservoir rather than a conduit has become universally accepted, based on original pioneering observations by Goodwin and others (1958) in the development of the cystoplasty augmentation procedure. The destruction of peristaltic integrity and the refashioning of bowel so that peristaltic forces oppose one another have led to the development of many innovative urinary reservoirs constructed from bowel. Antireflux principles are utilized as are additional surgical techniques to provide for urinary continence.

An excess of 40 variants of continent urinary diversions are utilized worldwide. Obviously, a complete review of all operative techniques is beyond the scope of this chapter. However, many of the procedures are simple variants of parent procedures, and this chapter addresses each parent operation as well as major modifications in detail. Because so many continent urinary diversion procedures are described reveals an obvious corresponding fact—the "best" continent diversion has yet to be devised. No unanimity of opinion indicates that one continent diversion is superior to date.

In particular, controversy continues to exist as to which bowel segment should be appropriately fashioned into a urinary reservoir. Additional points of controversy are related to the many different techniques utilized for achieving urinary continence and the prevention of reflux of urine into the diverted upper urinary tract.

All continent diversions allow for substantial reabsorption of urinary constituents. This effect necessitates an increasing work load on the kidneys. No patient with substantial renal impairment should be considered for these procedures. In general, the preoperative serum creatinine level must be less than 2.0 mg/dl.

The long-term sequelae of conduit urinary diversion are well understood and, unfortunately, involve a considerable degree of damage to renal units. The absence of reflux to the upper urinary tract (in catheterizing pouches) and the relative absence of bacteriuria in orthotopic voiding pouches as well as the absence of reflux in most may greatly reduce the long-term impact of the newer continent diversion procedures on renal function. However, long-term data have yet to be achieved in these newer operations.

Many studies have suggested an improved psychosocial adjustment in the patient with continent urinary and fecal diversion compared with the patient with diversion requiring collecting appliances (Boyd et al., 1987; Gerber, 1980; McLeod and Fazio, 1984). Although this is indeed true and is best exemplified by the individual with a conduit who desires to undergo conversion to a continent procedure, it is also true that many individuals seem to adjust rather well to the wearing of appliances. The sense of body image is a remarkably personal and subjective parameter that is considerably variable from patient to patient. For this reason, each patient undergoing urinary diversion should be interviewed separately by the urologist and the enterostomal therapist. The patient is then made aware of the impact of wearing a urinary appliance as well as the price that must be exacted in order to opt for an alternate form of urinary diversion.

The process of patient counseling that we employ always refers to conduit urinary diversion as the gold standard against which other operations must be compared. The patient is well advised that long-term data are not yet available for continent diversion procedures and that continent diversion, in general, is associated with a longer hospital stay, higher complication rate, and greater potential for reoperative surgery, all other considerations being equal.

However, an extensive review from our institution has demonstrated no statistically significant difference in reoperation, hospital stay, or mortality in patients undergoing continent diversions versus conduit diversions, by the same three surgeons over a 3-year period (Benson et al., 1990). Analysis of the two patient groups, on the other hand, showed that, in general, those selected for continent diversions were 12 years younger and four times less likely to have significant intercurrent illnesses. What this review seems to indicate is that, with proper patient selection, continent diversion operations can be conducted at the same cost to the patient and to society as conduit diversions.

URETEROSIGMOIDOSTOMY

Ureterosigmoidostomy can be regarded as the original continent urinary diversion—reports of this procedure can be found in the medical literature dating back to the 1870s (Smith, 1879). The operation has vacillated in its appeal to the urologic surgeon owing to the considerable complications associated with transplantation of the ureters directly to the intact fecal stream. Complications, including hyperchloremic acidosis, hypokalemia with nephropathy, pyelonephritis, and development of colonic malignancy, have been reviewed elsewhere.

Nevertheless, some workers believe that despite its pitfalls, ureterosigmoidostomy continues to offer a form of continent urinary diversion that is rather simple in comparison to the newer operative techniques devised for creating urinary reservoirs by means of complex refashioning of bowel segments.

The selection of the patient for continent diversion by ureterosigmoidostomy is most important. Because the potentially adverse long-term sequelae of this operation are so severe, most urologists would utilize the procedure only for older individuals. The operation is not very suitable for the patient with neurogenic bladder, as there may be associated bowel or anal sphincter dysfunction. Individuals with dilated ureters are not candidates for ureterosigmoidostomy, for reasons similar to those recounted in the section on colon conduits (Ambrose, 1983; Richie, 1986). The patient with established renal impairment is a poor candidate for ureterosigmoidostomy or any continent diversion. The patient who has undergone extensive pelvic irradiation is also not a good candidate for ureterosigmoidostomy, because of the condition of the irradiated bowel as well as the irradiated distal ureters (Ambrose, 1983; Spirnak and Caldamone, 1986). Patients with hepatic dysfunction should not undergo ureterosigmoidostomy (or perhaps any continent diversion), because of the possibility of ammonia intoxication (Silberman, 1958).

Preoperative evaluation of the patient selected for ureterosigmoidostomy should include studies for bowel disease that might contraindicate the operation. The presence of diverticulitis and/or colon polyps may be investigated by means of barium studies of the large bowel and/or by colonoscopy. By no means should any patient undergo ureterosigmoidostomy without having an adequate test of anal sphincter integrity. Incontinence of the mixture of stool and urine is a calamitous complication that can be avoided by a simple assessment. Various tests have been proposed to assess sphincter integrity; the most useful are those that require the patient to retain an enema solution of solid and liquid material for a specified time in the upright and ambulating position without soilage. A thin mixture of oatmeal and water serves well in this regard (Spirnak and Caldamone, 1986). The patient should retain 400 to 500 ml for 1 hour in the upright position.

Procedure

Immediately prior to surgery, a multiperforate 28 Fr. rectal tube is advanced through the anus and sutured in place to the perianal skin. This tube should be advanced sufficiently far so that it can be reached at the time of surgery.

A longitudinal incision in the posterior peritoneum overlying the right ureter is made, so that the distal most ureter can be retrieved (Fig. 72–13A). A submucosal tunnel requires additional ureteral length. The line of Toldt is incised along its course deep into the pelvis and the sigmoid colon reflected medially. The left ureter is identified and similarly transected at a low level (Fig. 72–13B).

Because it is our opinion that all urinary diversion procedures should be protected by means of indwelling ureteral stents bilaterally, the open colotomy approach is preferred for ureterosigmoidostomy (Fig. 72–13C). These stents can be directed to the outside through the lumen of the rectal tube (Fig. 72–13D). The open

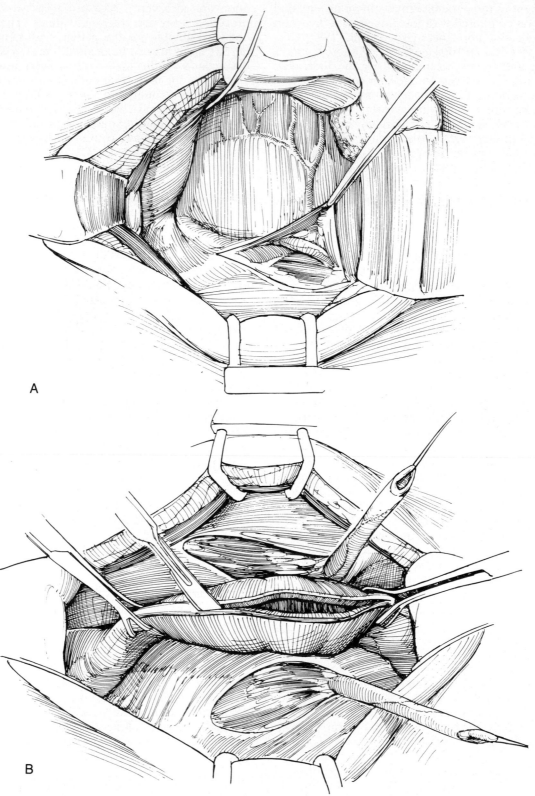

A

B

Figure 72–13. *A*, A longitudinal incision is made in the posterior peritoneum overlying the right ureter. *B*, The sigmoid colon is reflected medially, and the left ureter identified and transected.

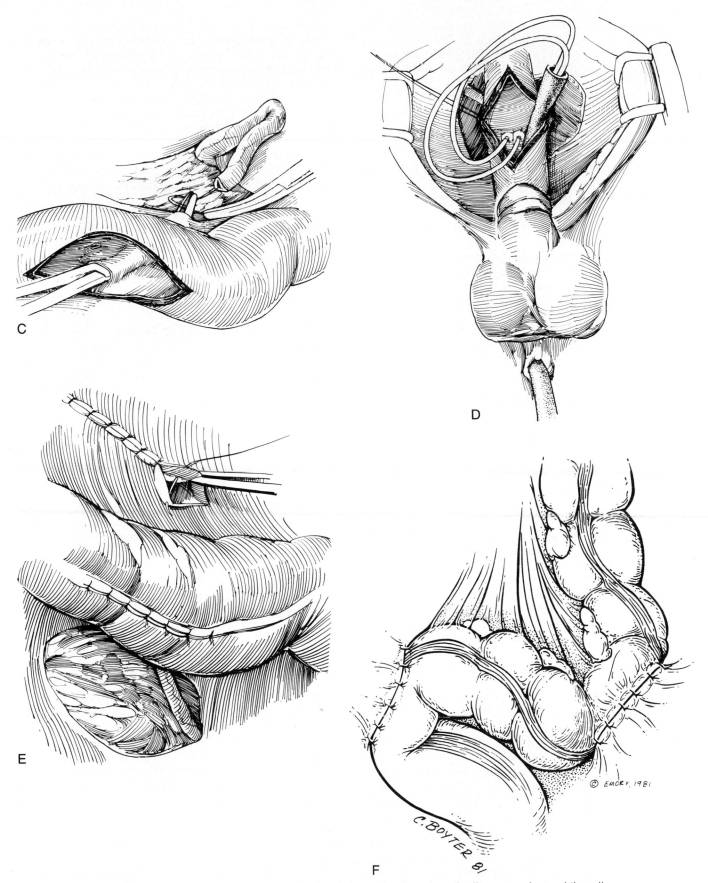

Figure 72–13 *Continued C,* The open colotomy approach is preferred because it allows for indwelling ureteral stents bilaterally.
   D, The stents are directed to the outside through the lumen of the rectal tube.
   E, The colon is closed with a simple two-layer technique. The retroperitoneal windows are closed with a running suture.
   F, The ureteral colonic anastomoses are retroperitonealized if possible. (From Hinman, F., Jr.: Atlas of Urologic Surgery. Philadelphia, W. B. Saunders Co., 1989.)

colotomy approach affords greater ease in achieving this maneuver, although the intubation of the ureters and the direction of the stent through the rectal tube can be accomplished, somewhat awkwardly, using the Leadbetter technique of implantation.

The various techniques of ureterocolostomy have been described in another chapter. If the open colon technique is utilized, an anterior colotomy is made in the region of the appropriate taenia selected for the ureteral transplantation sites. After completing ureteral anastomosis and intubation, the colon can be closed with a simple two-layer technique (Fig. 72–13E). The inner layer should be closed with a running suture of absorbable material taken through all layers of intestine, whereas the outer layer is closed with seromuscular nonabsorbable material.

At the surgeon's preference, an attempt at retroperitonealizing the ureterocolonic anastomoses may be made. On the right side, this is somewhat easier to achieve, because the peritoneal incision can simply be closed. On the left side, the colon can be rotated toward the left so that the lateral peritoneal incision utilized to expose the ureter can be sutured in place to the anterior sigmoid wall (Fig. 72–13F).

Postoperative Care and Comments

The ureteral stents are placed within the lumen of a urinary drainage device, which can then be directly fitted to the rectal tube. The total diversion of urine in this operation serves the additional function of decreasing postoperative electrolyte disturbances.

Radiologic studies of the stents are carried out on the 6th or 7th postoperative day. Prior to conducting these studies, an enema (Gastrografin) may be given through the rectal tube itself, in order to assure that the region of ureterocolonic anastomoses is intact. Follow-up films are taken to observe that prompt drainage of the upper urinary tracts into the rectosigmoid region is taking place. The rectal tube may be removed at this point, but usually it is advisable to have the tube reinserted for evening drainage, over the forthcoming week. The patient can be instructed in this function so that he or she may be discharged from the hospital early. The patient is instructed to empty the colon at intervals of no more than every 2 hours, particularly in the early postoperative period.

When the rectal tube is removed, the patient must be closely monitored for the development of hyperchloremic acidosis. This problem will occur in the majority of cases, and it is wise to initiate a bicarbonate replacement program at the outset. Because hypokalemia is also a feature of ureterosigmoidostomy, replacement of base along with potassium may be achieved with potassium citrate. Routine nightly insertion of a rectal tube is advocated in the long-term care of the patient. However, many patients reject this practice as uncomfortable and unappealing. Nighttime urinary drainage must be mandated in any patient who is not experiencing electrolyte homeostasis with oral medication.

Obviously, all patients have exposure of the urinary

tract to fecal flora. Most investigators would advocate long-term antibacterial therapy in all patients (Duckett and Gazak, 1983; Spirnak and Caldamone, 1986). Ureteral strictures require reoperative surgery, and these are experienced in 26 to 35 per cent of cases, over time (Duckett and Gazak, 1983; Williams et al., 1969).

Because of the definite concern for the occurrence of rectal cancer after ureterosigmoidostomy (some 5 to 50 years, average 21 years) (Ambrose, 1983), it is suggested that a patient with long-term ureterosigmoidostomy be subjected to annual colonoscopy (Filmer and Spencer, 1990). According to Williams, barium enemas are relatively contraindicated, as reflux of this material into the kidneys (if the antireflux procedure fails) has resulted in dire consequences. A further test that might be utilized for colon carcinoma is the monitoring for blood in the stool and the attempted cytologic examination of the mixed urine and feces specimen (Filmer and Spencer, 1990).

ILEOCECAL SIGMOIDOSTOMY

Early animal experimentation had suggested that the reason for the development of bowel malignancy after ureterosigmoidostomy is related to the presence of a fecal carcinogen in contact with juxtaposed transitional and colonic epithelium (Crissey et al., 1980). In an effort to avoid this phenomenon, the technique of ileocecal sigmoidostomy was developed (Kim et al., 1988; Rink and Retik, 1987). This operation is really a hybrid procedure, incorporating a modified ileocecal segment as in ileocecal conduit construction and anastomosing the resected cecal margin to the antimesenteric border of the sigmoid colon. In this fashion, contact between transitional and colonic epithelium is totally avoided. As in ureterosigmoidostomy, the colon should be assessed for disease and anal sphincter competence judged intact preoperatively. Similar to the ileocecal conduit, the native ileocecal valve may not be totally reliable in preventing reflux of the fecal stream to the upper urinary tract.

Procedure

At the time of surgery a 28 Fr. multiperforate rectal tube is inserted and sewn to the skin around the anus. An ileocecal segment of bowel, based on the ileocolic artery blood supply, is isolated (Fig. 72–14A). This segment consists of 12 to 13 cm of distal ileum and sufficient cecum to support an intussuscepted nipple valve. After ileoascending colostomy and closure of the mesenteric trap, King describes the intussusception of the distal ileum into the ileocecal valve (q.v. Duke pouch) in order to produce reliable separation of urinary and fecal streams (Fig. 72–14B) (Webster and King, 1987).

In the Rink and Retik (1987) variant of the procedure, the intussuscepted ileum is stabilized by applying staples. The bowel segment is directed externally as an ileocecal conduit, and cecosigmoidostomy is performed at a sep-

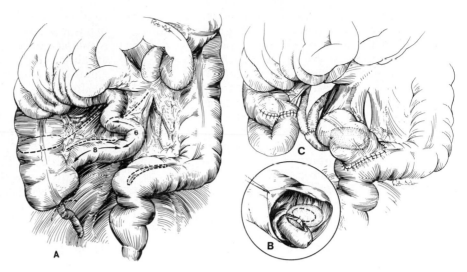

Figure 72–14. *A,* The ileocecal segment consisting of 12 to 13 cm of distal ileum and sufficient cecum to support an intussuscepted nipple valve are isolated.
B, The mucosa of the intussuscepted ileum and the cecum is incised, and the muscularis of ileum is sutured to the muscularis of cecum with nonabsorbable material.
C, Ureteroileal anastomoses are performed to the tail of ileum. An end-to-side cecosigmoidostomy completes the procedure. (From Kim, K. S., Susskind, M. R., and King, L. L.: Ileocecal ureterosigmoidostomy: An alternative to conventional ureterosigmoidostomy. J. Urol., 140:1494–1498, 1988. © By Williams & Wilkins, 1988.)

arate stage. In the Duke variant, the bowel segment is rotated 180 degrees laterally to appose the cecal margin to the sigmoid colon. Ureteroileal anastomoses are performed, and end-to-side cecosigmoidostomy completes the procedure (Fig. 72–14C). Ureteral stents may be directed through the intussusception and led out through the rectal tube.

Postoperative Care and Comments

The postoperative care and management of complications of the ileocecal sigmoidostomy are precisely the same as those in ureterosigmoidostomy. Insufficient data are available at this writing to evaluate either the protection of the upper tracts that might result from the antireflux valves or the proposed decreased incidence of colon cancer.

RECTAL BLADDER URINARY DIVERSION

Various innovative surgical techniques have been advocated for separating the fecal and urinary streams, yet still employing ureterosigmoidostomy principles. These operations can generally be discussed together as rectal bladder urinary diversions. In each of these operations, ureters are transplanted to the rectal stump. The proximal sigmoid colon is managed by terminal sigmoid colostomy or, more commonly, by bringing the sigmoid to the perineum. The anal sphincter is utilized in an effort to achieve both bowel and urinary control.

Although these operations continue to have some popularity abroad, they have never been well accepted in the United States, for a variety of reasons. The principal reason is the calamitous complication of combined urinary and fecal incontinence, presumably occurring as a consequence of damage to the anal sphincter mechanism during the dissection processes (Culp, 1984).

If the urologist selects one of these procedures, the

preoperative evaluations should include all of the caveats of ureterosigmoidostomy. Dilated ureters are not acceptable. The patient with extensive pelvic irradiation is not a candidate. Existing renal insufficiency will disqualify a patient from this type of surgery. Anal sphincteric tone must be judged competent before electing these operations. Finally, colonoscopy should be carried out to ensure against pre-existing colorectal disease.

Procedures

In addition to the Mauclaire (1895) technique, in which a terminal sigmoid colostomy is created, the three more common operations are those described by Gersuny (Hinman and Weyrauch, 1936), Duhamel (1957), and Heitz-Boyer and Hovelacque (1912). In each of these three procedures, a combined abdominoperineal approach is required. Each of these operations is difficult to achieve in the patient who has not undergone cystoprostatectomy, as exposure in the region of the rectal sphincteric mechanism is achieved more simply when these structures have been removed. Possible threats to rectal vasculature in cystectomy cases have been discussed, and the surgeon should recognize them. Similarly, in the female, the presence of the vagina serves as a potential barrier to appropriate surgical exposure. A multiperforate rectal tube is sutured in place, as in ureterosigmoidostomy.

After the abdomen has been entered, the ureters and sigmoid colon are freed, essentially in the same fashion as they would be for ureterosigmoidostomy. In addition, the entire right colon is separated from its attachment to the lateral peritoneum (line of Toldt) to the splenocolic ligament. This structure may be divided in order to gain additional bowel mobility. The inferior mesenteric artery may be found at its origin and may be clamped with a temporary vascular clamp to ensure that the marginal artery of Drummond is adequate to maintain sigmoid colon viability. After this factor has been ascertained, the marginal artery is compressed to ensure that the rectal stump appears viable as well. After vascular integrity is apparent, the rectosigmoid can be transected at the level of the sacral promontory. The inferior mesenteric artery or its branches can then be ligated to further free the sigmoid colon.

Ureterocolonic anastomosis into the distal rectal stump is carried out according to the surgeon's preference (Fig. 72–15A). If a stapled resection has been employed, a single layer of absorbable staples may be placed across the end of the rectal stump to avoid metal contact with urine. Ureteral stents, reaching the renal pelves bilaterally, are directed through the rectal tube.

Attention is then directed to the perineum. The approach involves a semicircular transverse perineal incision situated 1 to 2 cm anterior to the anal verge, extending from one ischial tuberosity to the other. This is the classic incision utilized for radical perineal prostatectomy. However, instead of dividing the central tendon anterior to the sphincteric region, the anterior wall of the rectum is immediately identified and separated from the deep and superficial external anal sphincters. Further dissection along this plane will lead the surgeon to the prerectal space previously occupied by the removed bladder. A wide-bore tunnel is created through which the proximal stump of the sigmoid colon may be directed. The sigmoid stump is led through this tunnel from above and advanced beyond the cutaneous incision level by approximately 4 inches in order to ensure against sigmoid retraction in the postoperative period (Fig. 72–15B). Nonabsorbable sutures are taken between the margins of the skin incision and the seromuscular layers of sigmoid, such that a redundant stump projects through the perineal incision for a period of 1 week. At this point, scar tissue is reasonably well formed so that further sigmoid retraction will not occur and the redundant stump may be divided and permanently sutured to the incision margins in a second formal operative procedure (Fig. 72–15B).

Because stenosis of the perineal sigmoidostomy is a common complication, some workers have advised a cruciate incision in the perineum to allow the interposition of flaps of cutaneous skin. These may be utilized to create a plastic perineosigmoidostomy (Fig. 72–15C).

If the posterior pull-through procedure of Duhamel is selected, the operation is precisely the same except that an incision is made posterior to the anus and the pull through as well as perineosigmoidostomy is created posterior to the anus proper. When the Heitz-Boyer technique is employed, the perineal incision is made actually within the anal verge, and blunt dissection of the rectal mucosa is carried out for a distance of 5 to 8 cm. At this point, the posterior wall of the rectum is perforated dorsally and the retrorectal space is widened bluntly to accommodate the sigmoid pull through. In this procedure, injury to the sphincteric mechanism is less common, because the rectal wall is left adherent to the deep and superficial anal sphincters (Fig. 72–15D).

Postoperative Care and Comments

Each of the sigmoid pull-through operations requires a second operation. Because sigmoid retraction is so common in the early postoperative period, it is advised that a week pass before the second operative procedure is completed, resecting the redundant sigmoid colon and anchoring it to the perineal incision situated either anterior or posterior to the anal verge (Garske et al., 1960).

To prevent early fecal soilage of the operative site, the redundant perineal sigmoid stump may remain closed for 2 to 3 days following surgery. At this point, the stapled resection line may be transected with cautery at the bedside. The management of the rectal bladder and ureteral stents is precisely the same as that for ureterosigmoidostomy. However, once radiographic studies of the rectal stump have shown integrity of the ureterocolonic anastomosis and stent studies have shown good drainage from the upper urinary tract to the rectal stump, the patient is advised to evacuate urinary contents on an hourly basis rather than every 2 hours, in order that overdistention of the rectal stump is not experienced in the early postoperative interval.

Because patients undergoing rectal bladder urinary diversion are subject to all of the electrolyte aberrations associated with ureterosigmoidostomy, management necessitates sodium bicarbonate or, preferentially, potassium citrate therapy, as soon as the ureteral stents are removed. Rectal stump drainage by means of a rectal tube is advocated for at least the first week or two, following removal of the rectal tube. Nighttime rectal tube drainage is advised in all patients.

In addition to complications mentioned earlier, those particularly associated with rectal bladder urinary diversion include stenosis of the perineosigmoidostomy. This can be ameliorated in the patient who has a cruciate perineal incision allowing for interposition of perineal skin flaps in the perineal sigmoidostomy. However, continued observation of the patient with rectal bladder urinary diversion is necessary to observe for the future development of this problem. If this stenosis does occur, revision of the perineal sigmoidostomy will be required.

In the Heitz-Boyer technique, retraction of the anterior segment of the pull through is not at all uncommon. When this retraction advances cephalad to only a few centimeters, the anterior limit of the rectal bladder and posterior limit of the sigmoid pull through are both situated above the external anal sphincter such that intermingling of bowel and urinary contents has been allowed. This complication obviously defeats the entire purpose of the operation, which is to separate the fecal and urinary streams. In such cases, patients are advised to undergo alternate forms of urinary diversion.

Because of the added risk of sphincteric incontinence of both urine and feces in all rectal bladder procedures, many workers believe these procedures should be relegated to operations of historical interest only (Culp, 1984; Hinman, 1984). Furthermore, with the advent of newer operations that provide better reservoirs and that result in more dependable continence, traditional rectal bladders are anachronistic.

AUGMENTED VALVED RECTUM

Kock developed this technique to be utilized in certain underdeveloped countries, where stoma appliances were

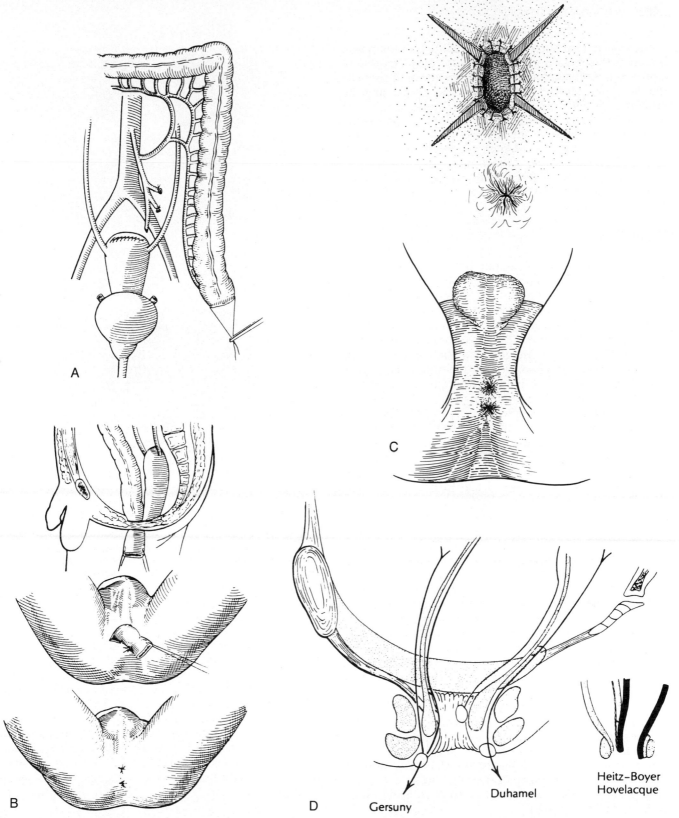

Figure 72–15. *A*, The branches of the inferior mesenteric artery have been divided to increase the mobility of the left colon and the sigmoid colon. The ureters have been anastomosed to the rectal stump. (From de Campos Freire, G.: *In* Glenn, J. F. (Ed.): Urologic Surgery. Philadelphia, J. B. Lippincott Co., 1983.)

B, A semicircular transverse perineal incision is situated 1 to 2 cm anterior to the anal verge and extends from one ischial tuberosity to the other. The anterior wall of the rectum is immediately identified and separated from the deep and superficial external anal sphincters. A wide-bore tunnel is created through which the proximal stump of the sigmoid colon is directed for approximately 4 inches. (From de Campos Freire, G.: *In* Glenn, J. F. (Ed.): Urologic Surgery. Philadelphia, J. B. Lippincott Co., 1983.)

C, Nonabsorbable sutures are taken between the margins of the skin incision and the seromuscular layers of sigmoid, such that a redundant stump projects through the perineal incision. The redundant stump is divided and permanently sutured to the incision margins. A cruciate incision in the perineum as shown may be utilized to create a plastic perineosigmoidostomy. (From Garske, G. L., Sherman, L. A., Twidwell, J. E., and Tenner, R. J.: *In* Whitehead, E. D., and Leiter, E. (Eds.): Current Operative Urology. New York, Harper and Row, 1984.)

D, The anatomic relationships between the various pull through procedures and the rectum are shown. (From de Campos Freire, G.: *In* Glenn, J. F. (Ed.): Urologic Surgery. Philadelphia, J. B. Lippincott Co., 1983.)

not readily available (Kock et al., 1988). This operation is similar to standard ureterosigmoidostomy except that a proximal intussusception of the sigmoid colon confines the urine to a smaller surface area, thus minimizing the problems of electrolyte imbalance. Additionally, the rectum was patched with ileum to improve its urodynamic properties as a urinary reservoir. Preoperative evaluation is similar to that in ureterosigmoidostomy. The large bowel must be studied for pre-existing disease, and anal sphincteric integrity must be tested before surgery.

Procedure

The left colon and sigmoid are freed from their attachments to the line of Toldt. The anterior wall of the rectum is opened from the rectosigmoid junction inferiorly for a distance of 10 cm. A 6- to 8-cm portion of distal sigmoid is cleared of its mesenteric attachments and appendices epiploicae by means of electrocautery. A Babcock clamp is directed into the sigmoid lumen through the rectal opening and the full thickness of sigmoid grasped. This is pulled down into the rectum as an intussuscipiens, which is then stapled with four applications of the TA55 stapler (Fig. 72–16A). The distal four to five staples are removed from the cartridge before firing to ensure that no staples reside at the tip of the nipple valve. If the stabilizing pin is utilized in order to obtain proper alignment of the staples and anvil, resulting pin holes are closed with figure-of-eight absorbable sutures. The opposing faces of the nipple valve and rectum are cauterized to denude the mucosa. A fifth staple line is placed from the outside to fix the intussuscipiens to the rectal wall. This maneuver is performed by sliding the anvil of the stapling device between the leaves of the intussuscipiens.

The ureters are anastomosed to the rectum by leading them down between the leaves of the intussuscipiens to button holes created bluntly at the summit of the nipple valve (Fig. 72–16A). The ureters are sewn to the buttonholes with absorbable sutures. The nipple valve is further stabilized by attaching the rectum to the intussuscepted sigmoid with interrupted seromuscular sutures.

A 20-cm segment of ileum is isolated and ileoileostomy employed to reconstruct the bowel. After closing the mesenteric trap, the ileal segment is opened on its antimesenteric border and folded in the shape of an upside-down U where adjacent borders are sutured together with absorbable material. This broad ileal plate is employed to close the rectal incision by patch graft technique (Fig. 72–16B).

Postoperative Care and Comments

No substantial differences occur in the postoperative care of these patients compared with those undergoing standard ureterosigmoidostomy. The patched rectal pouch has been studied urodynamically by Kock and associates (1988) and was found to expand in volume

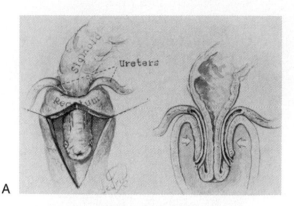

A

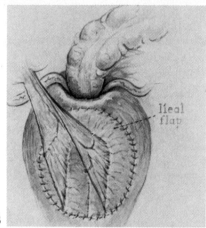

B

Figure 72–16. *A,* The anterior wall of the rectum is opened from the rectosigmoid junction inferiorly for a distance of 10 cm. A 6- to 8-cm portion of distal sigmoid is cleared of its mesenteric attachments and directed into the sigmoid lumen through the rectal opening and secured with a TA-55 stapler. The ureters are anastomosed to the rectum.

B, A 20-cm segment of ileum is opened on its antimesenteric border and folded in the shape of an upside-down U. This ileal plate is used to close the rectal incision. (From Kock, N. G., Ghoneim, M. A., Lycke, K. G., and Mahran, M. R.: Urinary diversion to the augmented and valved rectum: Preliminary results with a novel surgical procedure. J. Urol., 140:1375–1379, 1988. © By Williams & Wilkins, 1988.)

from 200 ml perioperatively to 700 ml at 6 months postoperatively. Basal pressures increased gradually to only 30 cm H_2O at capacity. All patients reported excellent day and nighttime control. Reoperation for bowel obstruction was reported in one of 19 patients.

Because of the limited surface area bathed by urine, no metabolic disturbances were reported and no patient required sodium bicarbonate or potassium citrate therapy. No episodes of large bowel obstructions were reported, despite the presence of a sigmoid intussusception.

HEMI-KOCK PROCEDURE WITH VALVED RECTUM

In the description of the augmented valved rectum procedure, Kock and colleagues (1988) described a foreshortened hemi-Kock pouch to be utilized as a rectal patch when the ureters were too dilated to bring down between the leaves of the intussuscepted sigmoid. Skinner and co-workers (1989) modified this procedure slightly, utilizing an entire hemi-Koch segment to augment the rectum after sigmoid intussusception.

The surgery consists of the construction of a hemi-Koch pouch employing doubly folded, marsupialized ileum and a proximal intussusception to prevent pouch-ureteral reflux. This hemi-Koch pouch is then anastomosed to the rectum. Contact of urine with the proximal colon is avoided by the intussusception of the sigmoid colon proximal to the anastomotic site. Because the competence of the intussuscepted ileocecal valve is approximately the same as that of the ileal intussusception achieved with the hemi-Koch operation, this last feature of confining the urinary absorption area to a smaller portion of bowel remains the most compelling reason for conducting this complicated surgery in comparison to simple ileocecal sigmoidostomy.

Many of the same caveats are applicable to this procedure as in other colonic diversions. The anal sphincteric integrity must be ensured to be intact prior to selecting this operation. The patient must have a reasonable degree of renal function in order to undergo this form of urinary diversion. The large bowel should be ascertained to be free of disease prior to surgery as evidenced by colonoscopy and/or barium studies. In contrast to direct ureterocolonic anastomotic procedures, however, dilated ureters may be accommodated by this operation.

Procedure

After abdominal incision, the ureters are transected and led to the right retroperitoneum in the fashion described for ileal conduit diversion. A 55-cm segment of ileum is selected, preserving the distal 10 to 20 cm of ileum. The distal ileal resection margin should be selected at the avascular plane of Treves, which separates the segment of ileum supplied by the ileocolic artery from that segment dependent on a more proximal vascular supply. At the proximal ileal resection margin, a small triangular wedge of mesentery is resected along with approximately 5 cm of ileum in order to achieve appropriate hemi-Koch mobility while preserving adequate blood supply (Skinner et al., 1987b).

The lower 40 cm of ileum is then marsupialized along its antimesenteric border, using electrocautery, and the opened ileum is fashioned in the shape of a U (Fig. 72–17A). The posterior plate is formed by sewing together the medial limbs of the U with multiple running sutures of absorbable material (Fig. 72–17B). Once the posterior plate has been created, an intussusception of the proximal limb is required. Measuring approximately 3 cm from the end of the plate, the intact ileal limb is freed from its mesenteric attachments by means of electrocautery over a distance of 6 to 8 cm. Freeing the mesenteric attachments from the middle portions of the intussuscipiens will prevent the potential of mesenteric tension disrupting the intussusception. A Babcock clamp is directed inside the intact proximal ileal limb. While grasping a full thickness of ileum, intussusception is carried out, creating at least a 5-cm intussuscipiens. This

is stapled in two or three quadrants with the TA55 stapling device from which four or five inner staples have been removed (Fig. 72–17C). This simple maneuver avoids the deposition of staples at the distal aspect of the nipple valve (Skinner et al., 1984). More proximal staples are usually well covered by mucosa and not available to the urine to act as a nidus for stone formation. A fourth stapled line is taken in an additional quadrant so as to attach the intussuscipiens to the side wall of the reservoir (Fig. 72–17D). This effect can be achieved in one of two fashions (q.v. Kock pouch). Pinholes from the stabilizing pin of the stapling device must be oversewn. After the proximal intussusception is completed, stented ureteroileal anastomoses can be conducted in the right lower quadrant as in ileal conduit urinary diversion. The caudal margin of the posterior plate may then be brought cephalad to close half the pouch (Fig. 72–17E). This closure is accomplished with running absorbable sutures that are interrupted frequently at distances of 8 to 10 cm. The remaining inferior portion of the pouch is left patent for anastomosis to the rectum.

A 10-cm linear enterotomy is made on the anterior rectal surface, after freeing the entire sigmoid colon from the line of Toldt. A 6- to 8-cm segment of distal sigmoid colon is freed from its mesenteric blood supply and sigmoid intussusception performed as in the augmented valved rectum procedure.

When completed, the rectal enterotomy receives the inferior hemi-Koch pouch margin. Anastomosis of these two structures is carried out by the interval running absorbable suture technique (Fig. 72–17F). Prior to closing the entire anastomosis, the ureteral stents are directed to a rectal tube previously placed at the initiation of the procedure.

Postoperative Care and Comments

Postoperative management and complications associated with this operation are very similar to those experienced with ileocecal sigmoidostomy and need not be recounted. As in the augmented valved rectum, there is potentially less of a tendency to hyperchloremic acidosis, because the ability of urine to contact larger portions of colonic epithelium is impeded by the proximal intussusception. Nevertheless, attention should be paid to electrolyte levels after removal of stents and rectal tubes. Reoperation rates distinctly attributable to this procedure have been reported.

ORTHOTOPIC VOIDING DIVERSIONS

A variety of operative procedures have been developed for the provision of a urinary pouch of low pressure and high capacity that will accommodate to the collection of urine and allow the male patient to initiate voiding by Valsalva's maneuver, following cystoprostatectomy. These operations have been popularized by the singular work of Maurice Camey (1979), whose

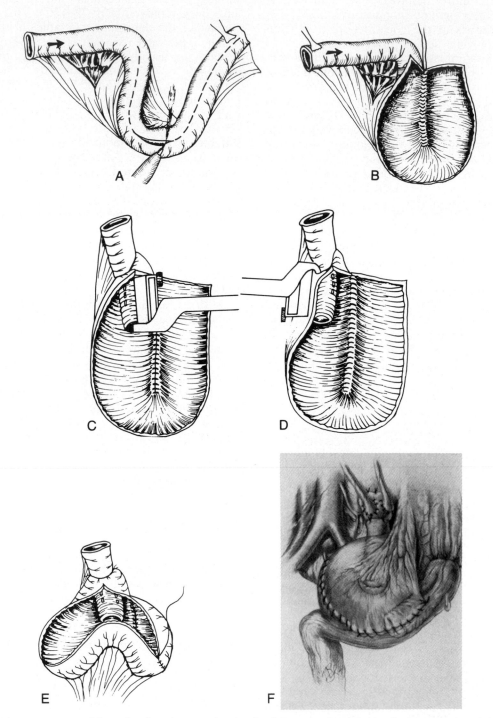

Figure 72–17. *A,* A 55-cm segment of ileum is selected, preserving the distal 10 to 20 cm of ileum. The lower 40 cm of ileum is marsupialized along its antimesenteric border.

B, The posterior plate is formed by sewing together the medial limbs of the U with running sutures.

C, A 5-cm intussusception is secured in two or three quadrants with the TA stapling device.

D, An additional staple line is taken to attach the intussuscipiens to the side wall of the reservoir.

E, The caudal margin of the posterior plate may be brought cephalad to close one half of the pouch. The inferior portion of the pouch is left patent for anastomosis to the rectum. (*A* to *E* from Ghoneim, M. A., Kock, N. G., Kycke, G., and Shehab El-Din, A. B.: An appliance-free, sphincter-controlled bladder substitute: the urethral Kock pouch. J. Urol., 138:1150–1154, 1987.)

F, A 10-cm linear enterotomy is made on the anterior rectal surface. A 6- to 8-cm segment of distal sigmoid colon is freed from its mesenteric blood supply and sigmoid intussusception performed as in the augmented valved rectum procedure. The rectal enterotomy receives the inferior hemi-Kock pouch margin. (From Skinner, D. G., Lieskovsky, G., and Boyd, S.: Continent urinary diversion. J. Urol., 141:1323–1327, 1989. © By Williams & Wilkins, 1989.)

Camey I operation was a pioneer step in this form of urinary diversion. The original Camey operation utilized intact ileum as the reservoir. However, since the concepts of bowel refashioning and interruption of peristaltic integrity are later developments, only the Camey II operation is described in this section, along with the other reconfigured operative techniques that are commonly utilized today. Other procedures using intact bowel are also omitted.

All the orthotopic voiding operations share similar features. First, they are not adaptable to the female patient, for the most part. Typically, in carrying out cystectomy for malignancy in the female, the entire urethra is removed along with the bladder. Of course, variations of the procedure may be adapted to a female with benign disease, wherein the entire urethra with a button of vesical neck may be safely retained.

Continence is dependent on the preservation of the external sphincteric apparatus in the male. One of the additional benefits of the Walsh technique of nerve-sparing prostatectomy is the improved identification of the prostatic apex with the better preservation of the sphincteric apparatus (Walsh et al., 1983; Schlegel and Walsh, 1987). The preserved male sphincter results in a daytime continence rate in orthotopic voiding operations well in excess of 95 per cent.

Nocturnal enuresis is common to all orthotopic voiding procedures. The reason for enuresis in these operations, as contrasted with radical prostatectomy in which enuresis is rare, is that in radical prostatectomy the native bladder and its reflexes remain intact. During bladder filling, a spinal reflex arc ensures the continued recruitment of external sphincteric contraction. Because the bladder has been removed in the patient undergoing orthotopic voiding diversion, this reflex is ablated and external sphincteric recruitment does not occur except under voluntary conscious control (Jakobsen et al., 1987).

The incidence of enuresis and the degree of wetting vary remarkably from series to series and appear independent of the type of bowel utilized to construct the voiding pouch. The lowest incidence of nocturnal wetting has been reported from Johns Hopkins Hospital, suggesting that added experience with the Walsh technique results in improved sphincteric integrity (Marshall, 1988; Marshall et al., 1990). Nevertheless, most series suggest that at least some patients are bothered by nocturnal wetting (Kock et al., 1989; Melchior et al., 1988; Schreiter and Noll, 1989; Studer et al., 1989; Thuroff et al., 1988; Wenderoth et al., 1990). Means of managing this wetting vary remarkably as well. In the usual patient, the simple technique of waking two or three times per night results in a dry sleep period. If this does not suffice, the patient can undergo various sphincter operations, as suggested by others (Lange, 1991; Skinner et al., 1989). In patients who may not wish to undergo sphincter placements, they may be suitably managed by condom catheter drainage or by the simple wearing of a penile incontinence clamp during sleeping hours.

The additional feature shared by all of the orthotopic voiding procedures, when they are utilized for treatment of bladder cancer, is the risk of urethral cancer recurrence. The incidence of anterior urethral recurrence in bladder cancer patients is approximately 4 to 5 per cent overall (Cordonnier and Spjut, 1961). This is obviously too low a percentage to warrant routine urethrectomy in all patients. The recurrence frequency is higher in certain patients. Certainly, a patient who has transitional cell cancer of the prostatic urethra is at high risk for distal urethral recurrence (Schellhammer and Whitmore, 1976). Others have suggested that diffuse intravesical carcinoma in situ warrants distal urethrectomy as well.

If distal urethrectomy is required, the patient is not a candidate for continent voiding diversion. In order to ensure the proper selection of a patient for this operation, we conduct prostatic urethral biopsy in all individuals being considered. We agree with others and have not routinely disqualified patients with in situ carcinoma from continent voiding diversions (Hickey et al., 1986). However, we advocate formal transurethral resection of the prostatic urethra in these instances, mandating that all the transitional epithelium in the prostate is free of disease prior to suggesting that a orthotopic voiding procedure is safe. Only long-term experience will clarify the exclusion criteria appropriately, and these have not yet been developed, however.

Another feature in regard to urethral recurrence in the patient undergoing continent voiding diversion is that monitoring for potential of urethral recurrence is greatly simplified. In the individual with an alternate form of urinary diversion wherein the urethra remains after cystoprostatectomy for cancer, urethral washings are required at intervals to monitor for malignant change in the urethral stump. In the patient undergoing continent diversion, simple voided urine may be utilized in this respect for cytologic examination.

Whatever the risk of urethral recurrence or enuresis, the continent voiding diversion appears to be the most popular among male candidates undergoing cystoprostatectomy. Patients can be restored to micturition that is nearly normal and, if nerve-sparing technique is appropriately utilized, may preserve sexual function as well (Marshall et al., 1990). All patients should be advised, however, of the occasional need for clean intermittent catheterization. A rare patient will be unable to void by Valsalva's maneuver (Marshall et al., 1990). Furthermore, there have been reports of greatly distended pouches occurring with the passage of time after continent voiding diversion (Camey et al., 1987). Such patients will necessarily be assigned to permanent clean intermittent catheterization in order to achieve urinary emptying. In an effort to obviate the silent development of this complication, we advise patients to self-catheterize at least monthly in order to measure post-void residual volume.

The literature is replete with opinion relative to the bowel segment that is best to employ in orthotopic voiding diversion. Most procedures utilize the small bowel in whole or in part and there does appear to be somewhat less contractility in the reformed small bowel compared with large bowel. Furthermore, there is evidence that mucosal atrophy, with resultant decrease in reabsorption of urinary constituents, is more dependable in small bowel than in large bowel (Norlen and Trasti, 1978). However, those continent voiding diversion procedures employing large bowel in part (MAINZ pouch) or in whole (sigmoid pouch) appear to work equally well in all regards. Similar degrees of daytime and nocturnal incontinence are reported; similar metabolic complications have been experienced (Thuroff et al., 1988; Reddy, 1987).

Common to the operative and postoperative care of all voiding pouches is the management of tubes and drains. Long single-J end-hole stents drain the kidneys externally. A Foley catheter can be placed transurethrally, and if there is a small urethral capacity it may be preferable to direct the stents through a suprapubic site. A suprapubic tube is optional. Pouch integrity should always be tested intraoperatively by saline insufflation. A suction drain is placed in the region of the ureteral anastomosis, draped across the membranous urethral region, and led out through a lower quadrant stab wound.

If stents or a suprapubic tube are led through the bowel wall it is advised to secure the bowel puncture sites with purse string sutures to prevent urinary leakage. It is also helpful to secure the pouch to the posterior abdominal wall at the suprapubic tube exit site to prevent urinary pooling following tube removal.

Postoperatively the urethral catheter or suprapubic tube must be irrigated at 4- to 6-hour intervals to ensure that the tube remains clear of mucous plugs. As soon as practical, the patient can be taught to carry out this process on his or her own. Before removing the stents, a radiographic pouch study is performed at about 10 days postoperatively. If the pouch shows no leakage of contrast material, the stents are removed with radiologic control to ensure that the kidneys drain promptly. If a suprapubic tube has been used, it may be removed at this time as well along with the suction drains. By 14 days, the urethral catheter can be taken out and a voiding trial initiated. Patients are usually catheterized once daily for irrigation of mucous debris during the subsequent 2 weeks and monthly thereafter. If there is only a small amount of mucus remaining after voiding, catheterizing intervals can be lengthened appropriately. In the early postoperative period, capacities may be quite small, especially with small bowel pouches. In order to afford restful overnight sleep, Foley or condom catheter drainage may be helpful.

CAMEY II OPERATION

The Camey I operation, utilizing a U-shaped intact ileal reservoir is no longer being utilized and is not described in this chapter. In contrast, the Camey II operation is a modification of the original technique developed by Camey to accommodate the principle of refashioning of bowel so that peristaltic integrity is abrogated (Camey, 1990). A length of ileum measuring 65 cm is selected for its ability to reach the region of the membranous urethral anastomosis without tension (Fig. 72–18A). This point is marked, and the ileal segment is isolated from the bowel (Fig. 72–18B). After ileoileostomy has been utilized to restore bowel integrity and the mesenteric trap is closed, the ileum is opened along its antimesenteric border throughout its entire length, with the exception of the region previously marked for ileourethral anastomosis.

At this point, the spatulation curves toward the mesenteric border (Fig. 71–18C). The totally spatulated ileum is folded over itself in the form of a transverse U, with the medial borders of the U sutured to one another with running absorbable material (Fig. 72–18D). A fingertip opening is made in the ileal wall at the site selected for ileourethral anastomosis. The entire broad, wide plate of ileum is advanced into the pelvis for ileourethral and ureteral anastomosis. Eight urethral sutures, previously placed from inside to outside the urethra, are completed by taking full thickness of ileum at the posterior margin of the ileourethral anastomosis. As the ileum is advanced into the pelvis, these sutures are tied so that the knots lie within the lumen of the anastomosis.

Ureteral anastomoses are carried out by the LeDuc technique (1987), described in another chapter. The remaining ileum is closed by folding the plate to complete the pouch construction (Fig. 72–18E). At these points, the ileal plate is sutured to the pelvic fascia to reduce tension on the anastomoses. Closure is achieved with running sutures of absorbable material (Fig. 72–18F).

Postoperative Care and Comments

Daytime continence rates of 96 per cent are reported by Camey (1990). However, there is a time lag to the development of total daytime continence. Sphincter exercises are utilized uniformly and can be initiated preoperatively among most patients. More than 75 per cent of men have achieved nocturnal continence as a consequence of the simple expedient of voiding at two or three planned awakenings.

Baseline pouch pressures of 10 cm H_2O have been reported, and minimal contractility averaging 32 cm H_2O has been observed during pouch fillings. Full pouch pressures averaged 30 cm H_2O and mean pouch capacity is 434 ml. In an unselected series of 57 patients, Camey described the need for reoperation in ten (17 per cent). However, none of the complications requiring reoperation was related to the urinary pouch construction (Camey, 1990).

No substantial differences are noted in the postoperative care of patients with voiding pouches and other procedures. The sphincteric exercises and ensuring that the patient recognizes the sense of pelvic fullness associated with the need to void are two exceptions.

VESICA ILEALE PADOVANA (VIP) POUCH

A technique of ileal bladder replacement very similar to the Camey II procedure was developed by a group

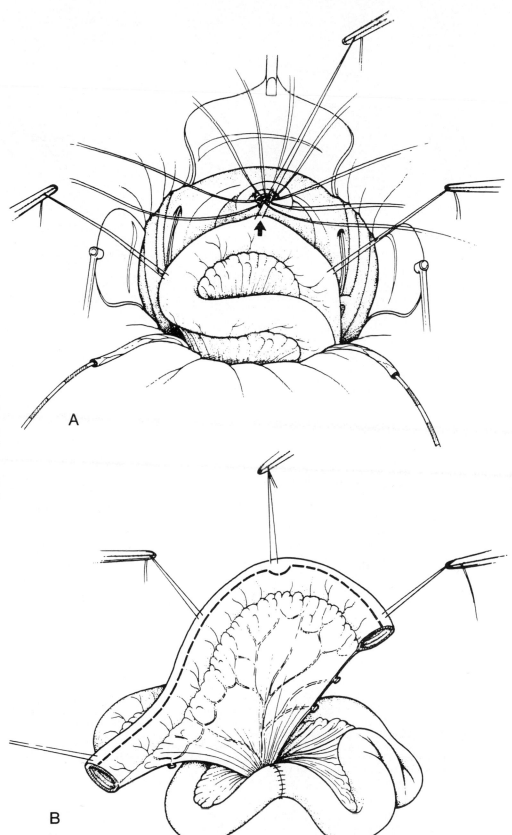

Figure 72–18. *A*, A length of ileum measuring 65 cm is selected for its ability to reach the region of the membranous urethra.

B, The ileal segment is isolated and opened along its antimesenteric border throughout its length.

*Illustration continued
on following page*

A

B

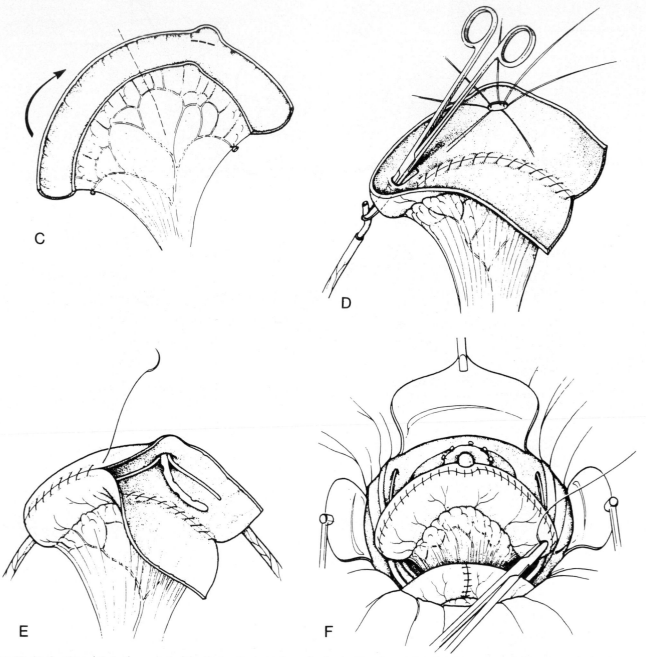

Figure 72–18 *Continued C,* In the region of the ileourethral anastomosis, the incision is spatulated to curve toward the mesenteric border.

D, The ileum is folded in the form of a transverse U with the medial borders of the U sutured to one another. A fingertip opening is made in the ileal wall at the site selected for ileourethral anastomosis. The ureters are reimplanted by the LeDuc technique. Eight urethral sutures are tied so that the knots lie within the lumen of the anastomosis.

E, The ileum is closed by folding the plate to complete the pouch construction.

F, The ileum is sutured to the pelvic fascia to reduce tension on the anastomoses. (From Camey, M.: Detubularized U-shaped cystoplasty (Camey 2). Curr. Surg. Tech. Urol., 3:1–8, 1990.)

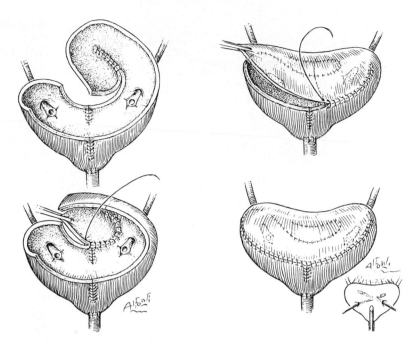

Figure 72–19. *A* and *B*, A 60-cm length of ileum is employed, and ileourethral anastomosis is carried out. LeDuc ureteral implants are performed. The spatulated bowel is refashioned in a "jelly roll" to produce the posterior plate, which is then closed anteriorly. (From Pagano, F., Artibani, W., Ligato, P., Piazza, R., Garbeglio, A., and Passerini, G.: Vesica Ileale Padovana: a technique for total bladder replacement. Eur. Urol., 17:149–154, 1990.)

in Padova, Italy (Pagano et al., 1990) called the Vesica Ileale Padovana or VIP pouch. The operation is precisely the same in many regards. Approximately a 60-cm length of ileum is employed, and ileourethral anastomosis is carried out in a very similar fashion. LeDuc ureteral implants are similarly performed. The only difference is in the way the spatulated bowel is refashioned. In the VIP pouch, the spatulated ileum is rolled on itself, as in a jelly roll to produce the posterior plate, which is then closed anteriorly (Fig. 72–19).

Postoperative Care and Management

No substantial differences are reported in the postoperative care of these patients compared with the patients undergoing Camey II orthotopic diversions. The Padova group reports a 92 per cent daytime continence rate. An 87 per cent incidence of "dry sleep" is noted. Ultimate bladder capacities have ranged from 400 to 650 ml, and basal pouch pressures of 3 to 5 cm H_2O and capacity pressures of 10 to 30 cm H_2O have been reported.

OTHER DETUBULARIZED ILEAL VOIDING POUCHES

Other groups have described reconfigurations of the ileum for anastomosis to the urethra. These are probably too numerous to mention, and many represent only minor variations of one another. Reddy (1987) described a technique of near total detubularization with the dependent portion of a U-shaped segment of ileum remaining intact and the upper limbs spatulated and reconfigured into a cup cystoplasty configuration (Fig.

72–20). Schreiter and Noll (1989) described a technique of total spatulation of an ileal segment, which is refashioned into a broad plate by means of an S or incomplete W configuration (Fig. 72–21). In both instances, LeDuc ureteral anastomoses were carried out.

ILEAL NEOBLADDER

This operation, devised at the University of Ulm in Germany, is an extension of the Camey principle, incorporating Goodwin's cup cystoplasty principles (Hautmann et al., 1988 and Wenderoth et al., 1990).

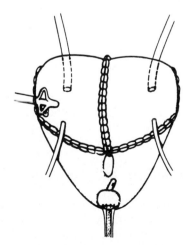

Figure 72–20. The Reddy configuration where the dependent portion of ileum is left intact while the upper portion is reconfigured. (From Reddy, P. K.: Non-stomal continent reservoir: use of detubularized ileal segment for bladder replacement. World J. Urol., 5:190–193, 1987.)

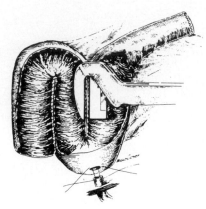

Figure 72–21. The ileum is reconfigured in an S or a W shape. (From Schreiter, F., and Noll, F.: Kock pouch and S bladder: two different ways of lower urinary tract reconstruction. J. Urol., 142:1197–1200, 1989. © By Williams & Wilkins, 1989.)

Procedure

A segment of ileum 70 cm in length is chosen while preserving the distal 15 cm of terminal ileum (Fig. 72–22A). The distal resection margin is at the junction of ileocolic and superior mesenteric blood supplies. After reconstituting the bowel and closing the mesenteric trap, the isolated ileum is spatulated at its antimesenteric border except for the area selected for ileourethral anastomosis. This is where the incision is made at the anterior mesenteric border, creating a U-shaped flap (as in the Camey II operation), which will serve as the new bladder neck. The bowel is arranged in an M or a W configuration, and the four limbs are sutured one to another with running absorbable material to form a broad ileal plate (Fig. 72–22B).

A button of tissue is removed from the previously selected ileourethral anastomotic site. This button is approximately the size of a fingertip. Six separate absorbable sutures are placed from the inside of the ileal plate to the urethra, with the ends brought back into the ileourethral aperture. A Foley catheter is placed through the urethra into the ileal aperture, and all six sutures are tied on the inside of the pouch while traction on the catheter directs the ileal plate to the urethral stump. LeDuc ureteral implants are carried out in the posterior margin of the ileal plate, and the plate itself is closed into a pouch (Fig. 72–22C).

Postoperative Care and Comments

The University of Ulm group recommends that ureteral stent studies be carried out at 12 days and that urethral catheter drainage be maintained for 3 weeks. In our experience, these are not necessary, although we utilize nighttime Foley or condom catheter drainage for a few weeks while the pouch is expanding. The patient then has the ability to sleep soundly in the early postoperative period.

Bladder capacities averaging 755 ml are reported with the mean intravesical pressure at a capacity of 26 cm H_2O and a half capacity intravesical pressure of 10 cm H_2O. Of patients, 82 per cent are totally continent day and night. An additional 11 per cent of patients experience only occasional enuresis or else have mild stress urinary incontinence in the daytime. Early reoperations were required in five of 113 patients (4 per cent). None were related to the pouch construction, although five additional patients required percutaneous nephrostomy to relieve temporary ureteral obstruction. Complications led to late corrective surgery in 8 per cent—half of which were related to the pouch.

ORTHOTOPIC HEMI-KOCK POUCH

This operation was designed by Ghoneim and Kock (Ghoneim et al., 1987) to accommodate the male patient needing cystectomy. In this instance, prevention against reflux is dependent on the construction of a nipple valve. As previously described, nipple valve construction usually requires staples to stabilize the intussusception of the bowel. Thus, this form of voiding pouch has some potential for the development of urinary calculi within the pouch, a feature not shared by the other orthotopic voiding operations.

Procedure

The operative procedure is carried out precisely as that described for the hemi-Kock with sigmoid intussusception. The sole difference is that the closure of the inferior portion of the pouch leaves a smaller aperture patent to be utilized for the urethral anastomosis. Alternatively, the entire pouch may be closed and a buttonhole opening used (Fig. 72–23). It is our practice to fashion this opening such that it will accept a size 24 Fr. catheter without resistance. Ileourethral anastomosis is carried out in the usual fashion, employing four to eight interrupted absorbable sutures, previously placed in the urethral stump.

Some workers advocate double J-stents in which the lower portions reside within the pouch after traversing the nipple valve. We utilize open-end single J-stents to divert the urine from the entire pouch.

Postoperative Care and Comments

The postoperative management of this voiding pouch is precisely that of the others. The only specific complication of this procedure relative to the others is the development of stones on any exposed staples in the urinary tract. If stones are found at a small enough size, they can usually be managed cystoscopically by forceps extraction, along with the offending staple. If somewhat larger stones are found, electrohydraulic or ultrasound lithotripsy may be used to fracture the stones. The fragments and staple are removed by a combination of forceps and irrigating techniques.

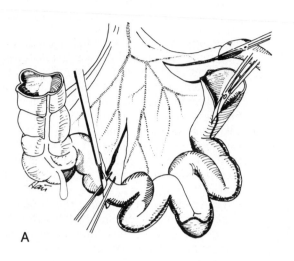

A

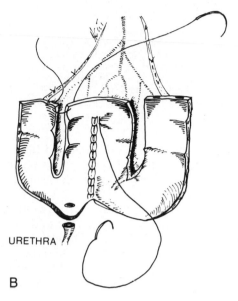

URETHRA

B

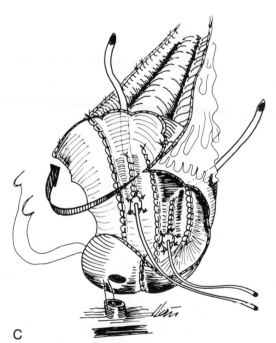

C

Figure 72–22. *A,* A segment of ileum 70 cm in length is chosen while preserving the distal 15 cm.

B, The isolated ileum is spatulated at its antimesenteric border except for the area selected for ileourethral anastomosis. The segment is arranged in an M or a W configuration, and the four limbs are sutured one to another with running absorbable suture material.

C, A button of tissue is removed from the selected ileourethral anastomotic site. Six separate absorbable sutures are placed from the inside of the ileal plate to the urethra, with the ends brought back into the ileourethral aperture. LeDuc ureteral implants are performed, and the plate itself is closed into a pouch. (From Wenderoth, U. K., Bachor, R., Egghart, G., Frohneberg, D., Miller, K., and Hautman, R. E.: The ileal neobladder: Experience and results of more than 100 consecutive cases. J. Urol., 143:492–497, 1990. © By Williams & Wilkins, 1990.)

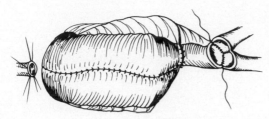

Figure 72–23. The operative procedure is carried out precisely as described (see Fig. 72–17). The closure of the inferior portion of the pouch leaves a small aperture patent to be utilized for the urethral anastomosis. (From Ghoneim, M. A., Kock, N. G., Kycke, G., and Shehab El-Din, A. B.: An appliance-free, sphincter-controlled bladder substitute: the urethral Kock pouch. J. Urol., 138:1150–1154, 1987. © By Williams & Wilkins, 1987.)

Ghonheim and associates (1987) reported 100 per cent daytime continence. Nocturnal control or mild spotting was seen in 12 of the first 16 patients studied. At 3 months, pouch capacity was 300 ml on average and expanded to 750 ml by 11 months. Urodynamic evaluation showed pressures below 20 cm H_2O until reservoir capacity was reached. In a later article, reporting results in 34 evaluable patients (Kock et al., 1989), 30 patients (88 per cent) are continent day and night. One patient required reoperation early for bowel obstruction. Nearly half the patients required surgery to correct slipped antireflux valves.

LOW-PRESSURE BLADDER SUBSTITUTE

A variation of the orthotopic hemi-Kock procedure which avoids the need for a nipple valve is the pouch described by Studer and co-workers (1988).

Procedure

An ileal segment measuring 60 to 65 cm in length is isolated, leaving the distal 25 cm of ileum intact. After reconstituting the bowel and closing the mesenteric trap the ileum is rotated 180 degrees on its mesentery so that its proximal end lies in the right retroperitoneum (Fig. 72–24A). Both ileal ends are oversewn with absorbable material, or else they may be managed by application of absorbable staples. The distal 40 to 45 cm is opened along the antimesenteric border and folded in the configuration of a U, facing the patient's right side. The posterior plate is completed by joining the limbs of the U with running absorbable sutures. Standard ureteroileal (refluxing) anastomoses are carried out at the apex of the intact limb of ileum (Fig. 72–24B). Anastomosis of the posterior plate of ileum to the urethra is completed with six previously placed urethral sutures. The left side of the ileal plate is brought to the patient's right, and the plate is closed in a cup cystoplasty configuration with running absorbable suture material (Fig. 72–24C). Ureteral stents are brought through a separate abdominal incision, and suction drainage is achieved. Studer et al. (1989) describe the use of a

suprapubic tube, but we have performed this operation with urethral drainage only.

Postoperative Care and Comments

The immediate postoperative capacity after catheter removal is 150 ml. Within a few weeks, capacities exceeding 300 ml are reached. By 6 months, mean pouch volume is 450 ml and pressures at capacity vary from 20 to 35 cm H_2O (Studer, personal communication). Daytime continence was total when Studer utilized the Walsh nerve sparing technique; however, enuresis is experienced by 50 per cent of men (Studer et al., 1989). Two complications (one relating to the pouch) requiring reoperation were reported in Studer's original 18 patients. In over 60 patients, there has been no need for bicarbonate replacement (Studer, personal communication).

The concept of utilizing the intact 20-cm proximal ileal limb for prevention of deleterious effects of reflux is novel. Indeed, the maintenance of the peristaltic integrity of the proximal limb serves to dampen the effects of any but the most overfilled reservoir, according to Studer's radiographic studies. Since patients with voiding pouches can often maintain a sterile urine, more definitive techniques to avoid reflux into the upper urinary tract may not be important.

ORTHOTOPIC MAINZ POUCH

The MAINZ pouch is actually done in two separate operations, sharing the common principle of employing the cecum and two portions of the distal ileum to create a broad intestinal plate, which can then be closed in a spherical fashion (Thuroff et al., 1985 and 1987). One variation of the MAINZ pouch is a catheterized version, which is described later in this chapter. The MAINZ pouch variant that allows for orthotopic voiding will be described here.

Procedure

A segment of bowel, utilizing 10 to 15 cm of cecum as well as 20 to 30 cm of ileum, is isolated from the bowel. Ileoascending colostomy is utilized to re-establish intestinal continuity (Fig. 72–25A). After closing the mesenteric trap, the entire bowel segment is marsupialized along its antimesenteric border, sacrificing the ileocecal valve (Fig. 72–25B). The bowel is then fashioned in the shape of an incomplete W, with the first limb of the W represented by cecum and the middle two limbs of the W represented by marsupialized ileum. A broad posterior plate of one-third cecum and two-thirds ileum is created by suturing the apposing margins of the three limbs of the incomplete W with running absorbable material (Fig. 72–25C).

At the apex of the cecal portion of the posterior plate,

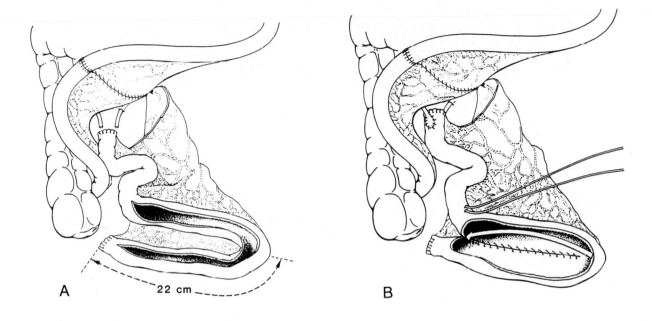

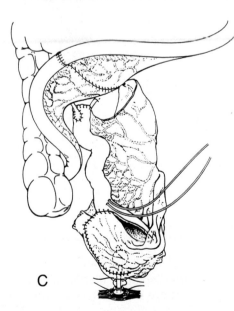

Figure 72–24. *A,* An ileal segment measuring 60 to 65 cm in length is isolated, leaving the distal 22 cm of ileum intact. The distal 40 to 45 cm is opened along the antimesenteric border and folded in the configuration of a U.

B, The posterior plate is completed by joining the limbs of the U with running absorbable sutures. Standard ureteroileal (refluxing) anastomoses are performed. Stents are brought out through separate stab wounds.

C, Anastomosis of the posterior plate of ileum to the urethra is carried out with six urethral sutures. The left side of the ileal plate is brought to the patient's right, and the plate is closed in a cup cystoplasty configuration. (From Studer, U., et al: Br. J. Urol., 124:797–801, 1988.)

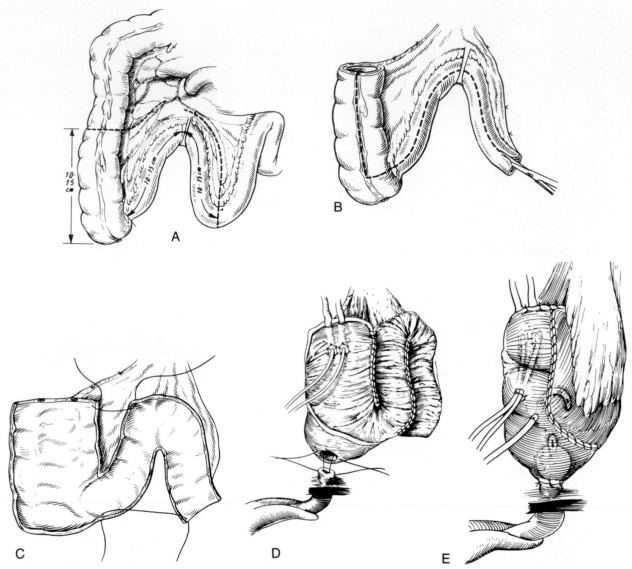

Figure 72–25. *A,* Shown is 10 to 15 cm of cecum in continuity with 20 to 30 cm of ileum is isolated.
B, The entire segment is marsupialized along its antimesenteric border.
C, A broad posterior plate is created by suturing the apposing margins of the three limbs of the incomplete W.
D, At the apex of the cecal portion of the posterior plate, tunneled ureterocolonic anastomoses are performed. Appendectomy is routinely performed. A buttonhole incision is made at the base of the cecal portion of the reservoir, serving as the site for urethrointestinal anastomosis.
E, The ileal portions of the faceplate are brought anteriorly and to the right side to close the pouch. (From Thuroff, J. W., Alken, P., and Hohenfellner, R.: The MAINZ pouch (mixed augmentation with ileum 'n zecum) for bladder augmentation and continent diversion. *In* King, L. R., Stone, A. R., and Webster, G. D. (Eds.): Bladder Reconstruction and Continent Urinary Diversion. Chicago, Year Book Medical Publishers, 1987.)

tunneled ureterocolonic anastomoses can be carried out. Long ureteral stents are placed into the renal pelves bilaterally. These will be led out through the urethra or a separate suprapubic site, depending on the capacity of the urethra.

Appendectomy is routinely performed, and a buttonhole incision is made at the base of the cecal portion of the reservoir (Fig. 72–25*D*). Urethrointestinal anastomosis is carried out as previously described. Gentle traction on a Foley catheter balloon reduces tension on the sutures until the anastomosis is complete. The ileal portions of the faceplate are then brought anteriorly and to the right side in order to close the pouch (Fig. 72–25*E*). This is accomplished by running sutures of absorbable material.

Postoperative Care and Comments

The postoperative care of orthotopic MAINZ pouch is identical to other voiding diversions. Mean pouch capacities of 510 ml are reported. Pressures range from 33 cm H_2O at 50 per cent capacity to 41 cm H_2O at 100 per cent capacity. Daytime continence is reported in 93 per cent of patients. Dry sleep is reported in 75 per cent of patients if they wake 2 to 3 times to void.

Late complications of incontinence or urethral anastomotic stricture required endoscopic or open surgery in four of 34 cases undergoing orthotopic MAINZ pouch. Combining the 34 patients with orthotopic MAINZ pouch with the 66 treated by other variants, reoperations were required in only four cases.

ILEOCOLONIC POUCH (LE BAG)

The group at Baylor University (Light and Scardino, 1986) has developed a modification of the MAINZ pouch that utilizes a single segment of ileum along with cecum.

Procedure

About 20 cm of ascending colon and cecum are isolated along with an equal length of distal ileum. After reconstituting bowel integrity and closing the mesenteric trap, the entire antimesenteric-mesenteric border of the large and small bowel segments is split to create two flat sheets, which are then sewn to one another posteriorly. The Baylor group believes that metal stapling techniques can be utilized in this regard (Fig. 72–26A). When the first variant of this operation was described, the proximal most few centimeters of ileum were left intact, and the pouch was rotated 180 degrees cephalad to caudad so that the ileal stump could be utilized for ileourethral anastomosis (Fig. 72–26B). With increasing experience, suggesting that the intact ileal segment was peristaltic and promoted urinary wetting, the technique was modified to spatulate the entire bowel (Light and Marks, 1990). The urethra is anastomosed end to side to the cecum in the modern variant, and ureterocolonic anastomoses are carried out by the surgeon's preference (Fig. 72–26C).

Postoperative Care and Comments

No alterations in postoperative care pertain. Pouch capacities vary from 400 to 700 ml, and cystometry 6 weeks after surgery shows low pressure contractions. End pressures of 20 to 58 cm H_2O are reported. Continence rates have improved since completely detubularizing the bowel but overall are lower than in other series.

DETUBULARIZED RIGHT COLON POUCH

Utilizing the right colon exclusively has been reported by two groups. Goldwasser and Benson (1986) described a technique of replacing bladder employing a partly detubularized right colon.

Procedure

The entire right colon is isolated on a pedicle fed by the ileocolic and right colic arteries (Fig. 72–27). Ileocolonic anastomosis is utilized to restore bowel continuity, and the mesenteric trap is closed. The ileal stump at the ileocecal valve is closed by a running suture of absorbable material. The colon segment is opened along the anterior taenia, leaving the proximal 2 to 3 inches of cecum intact. Appendectomy is performed, and ure-

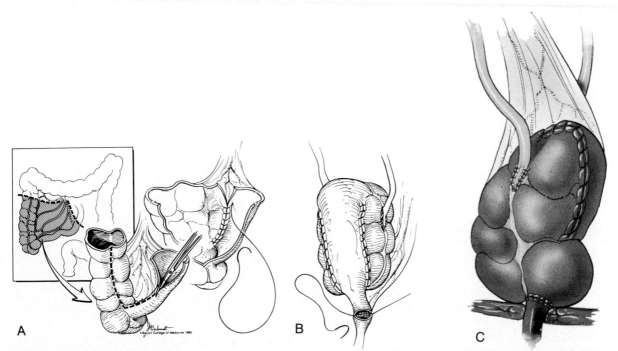

Figure 72–26. *A*, A total of 20 cm of ascending colon and cecum are isolated along with an equal length of distal ileum. The entire antimesenteric border of the large and small bowel segments is split to create two flat sheets, which are sewn to one another posteriorly.

B, The first variant of this operation left intact the proximal ileum.

C, The entire bowel segment is spatulated. (From Light, J. K., and Marks, J. L.: Total bladder replacement in the male and female using the ileocolonic segment (Le Bag). Br. J. Urol., 65:467–472, 1990.)

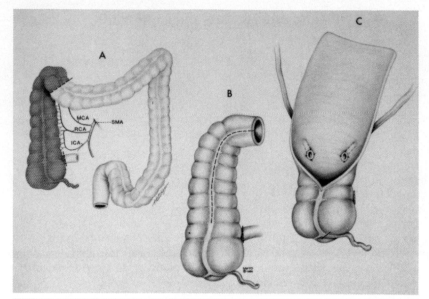

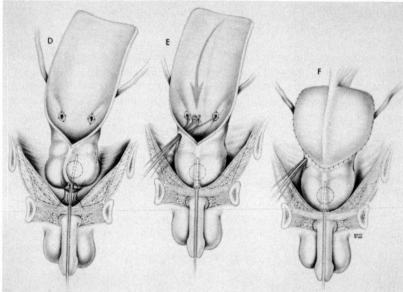

Figure 72–27. The entire right colon is isolated on a pedicle fed by the ileocolic and right colic arteries. The ileal stump at the ileocecal valve is closed by a running suture of absorbable material, and the colon segment is opened along the anterior taenia leaving the proximal 2 to 3 inches of cecum intact. Appendectomy is performed, and ureters are implanted by standard antireflux technique. Urethrocecal anastomosis is performed over a ureteral catheter. (From Goldwasser, B., Barrett, D. M., and Benson, R. C., Jr.: Complete bladder replacement using the detubularized right colon. *In* King, L. R., Stone, A. R., and Webster, G. D. [Eds.]: Bladder Reconstruction and Continent Urinary Diversion. Chicago, Year Book Medical Publishers, 1987.)

ters are implanted by standard antireflux technique. Urethrocecal anastomosis is performed over a ureteral catheter.

Postoperative Care and Comments

Although this procedure is presented as utilizing detubularized right colon, the original description of the procedure allowed for the cecum to remain intact. We believe that this would be problematic and suggest that the entire right colon be spatulated and reconfigured in a Heinecke-Mikulicz fashion.

Too few procedures have been reported to allow for evaluation of day and night continence. The urodynamic studies performed so far suggest good compliance at low volumes. However, contractions of 44 cm H_2O are below capacity levels.

MANSSON POUCH

The Mansson pouch (Mansson and Colleen, 1990) is a variant on the Goldwasser pouch in which the entire colon is spatulated. This principle of complete detubularization appears to offer advantages over the Goldwasser technique, wherein the proximal cecum remains intact (Fig. 72–28). All patients were continent in the daytime. Nocturnal continence was not reported. Pouch capacities varied from 320 to 600 ml. Measuring at high-level pouch filling, low basal pressures were recorded (11 to 22 cm H_2O).

SIGMOID POUCH

The use of the sigmoid colon for creation of a voiding reservoir has been popularized both in the United States, at the University of Minnesota, and in Egypt. Originally employing a nonreconfigured, U-shaped por-

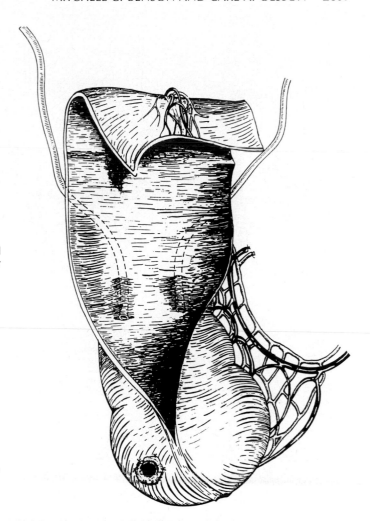

Figure 72–28. The entire colon is spatulated. (From Mansson, W., and Colleen, S.: Experience with a detubularized right colonic segment for bladder replacement. Scand. J. Urol. Nephrol., In press, 1990.)

tion of colon (similar to the Camey I operation), the Minnesota group soon abandoned that technique because of high pressure contractions in the nonreconfigured pouch. A partially detubularized segment was then reported, and it improved the urodynamic characteristics of the pouch (Reddy, 1987). Fully reconfigured sigmoid is now utilized (Lange, personal communication). The group at Al-Azhar University in Cairo has reviewed a series of totally reconfigured sigmoid pouches as well (Khakaf, personal communication).

The sigmoid colon as a continent voiding pouch offers a few potential advantages as well as disadvantages. For example, the sigmoid colon is often affected by diverticulosis and/or malignancy. For this reason it might not be a suitable bowel segment for long-term urinary diversion. However, the facility with which the sigmoid colon can be brought to the membranous urethral region and the simplicity with which it can be reconfigured by Heinecke-Mikulicz maneuver afford distinct advantages over other bowel segments. Furthermore, the loss of the sigmoid colon has little if any impact on the nutritional status or bowel habits of the patient.

Procedure

As described by Reddy (1987), a portion of sigmoid and descending colon measuring 35 cm is isolated and folded in the shape of a U, with the curve of the U oriented to the pelvis (Fig. 72–29A). The medial taenia of the U is incised down to a point a few centimeters cephalad to the site of the urethral anastomosis (Fig. 72–29B). Medial limbs of the U are sutured together with running absorbable material (Fig. 72–29C). Tunneled ureteral implantation is carried out with stents through separate stab wounds. A small button of tissue is removed from the inferior most portion of the pouch, and urethral anastomosis is carried out with previously placed urethral stump sutures (Fig. 72–29D). Foley catheter drainage is achieved transurethrally. The pouch is closed by rotating each side of the pouch medially, utilizing running absorbable suture material. The pouch is, therefore, only partially detubularized, with its inferior aspect (shaped like the bottom half of a doughnut) intact.

A theoretically more advantageous bowel reconfiguration would involve the total marsupialization of the sigmoid segment. This has been reported by the group in Cairo and has been utilized in our own experience with considerable success. The entire sigmoid colon is opened on its antimesenteric border and reconfigured by either a Heinecke-Mikulicz procedure or by classic Goodwin cup principles. The remaining portions of the operative procedure are identical.

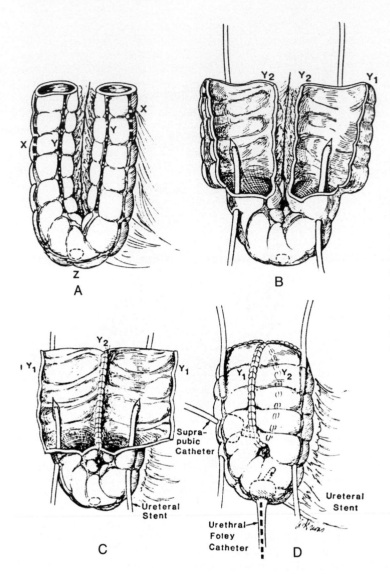

Figure 72–29. *A*, A portion of sigmoid and descending colon measuring 35 cm is isolated and folded in the shape of a U.

B, The curve of the U is oriented to the pelvis. The medial taenia of the U is incised down to a point a few centimeters cephalad to the site of the urethral anastomosis.

C, The medial limbs of the U are sutured together, and a tunneled ureteral implantation is performed (Y-2 to Y-2).

D, A button of tissue is removed from the inferior most portion of the pouch, and urethral anastomosis is performed. The pouch is closed by rotating each side of the pouch medially and suturing Y-1 to Y-1. (From Reddy, P. K.: Detubularized sigmoid reservoir for bladder replacement after cystoprostatectomy. Urology, 29:625–628, 1987.)

Postoperative Care and Comments

In the single case study reported by Reddy (1987), the partially detubularized sigmoid resulted in a capacity of 760 ml and pressures less than 20 cm H_2O until capacity was reached. The Cairo group report excellent urodynamic characteristics with total bowel reconfiguration in a large series. Data relating to the need for reoperation are not reported yet.

CONTINENT CATHETERIZING POUCHES

Numerous operative techniques have been developed for continent diversion of urine, wherein urine is emptied at intervals by clean self-catheterization. The majority of operations are described in this chapter, although certain pioneering procedures, such as those of Gilchrist (1950), Ashken (1987), Mansson (1984, 1987), Benchekroun (1987), and others, are not described because intact bowel was utilized. The chapter focuses on those pouches that incorporate the principles of attempted spherical configuration and disruption of peristaltic integrity.

A few initial comments about self-catheterizing pouches are appropriate. First, it is mandatory that patients undergoing these procedures have sufficient hand-eye coordination to perform clean intermittent catheterization. All quadriplegic patients and some individuals with multiple sclerosis would not be candidates for this operation. Furthermore, patients with any degree of dementia that would interfere with their understanding of the catheterizing process would not be appropriate candidates.

The location of the catheterizing portal is different according to the individual surgeon's preference. The two favorite sites for stomal location are at the umbilicus and in the lower quadrant of the abdomen, through the rectus bulge and below the "bikini" line. This latter location is often preferred by female patients, in particular, because it affords them the opportunity to wear bathing suits without the unsightly presence of an abdominal stoma. Some men may also prefer this location for the same reasons. The umbilicus is a preferred location for the individual confined to a wheelchair. This location makes it far easier for the paraplegic individual to catheterize without the need for chair transfer and disrobing. The umbilical stoma location is actually preferred by some surgeons, even in those patients who are not confined to wheelchairs. The umbilical location of a stoma is barely perceptible from a normal umbilical dimple, particularly in an individual with a recessed umbilicus. Generally, the stoma site is covered with gauze or a square Band-Aid between catheterizations to avoid mucus soiling of clothing.

Orthotopic location of a catheterizing portal has been carried out in certain patients. Particularly in the female, the construction of a neourethra to the introitus is attractive, provided there is no substantial difficulty in the catheterizing process. Because it can be so difficult to direct a catheter through the "chimney" of an intussuscepted nipple valve, particularly if there is a long portion of bowel leading to the chimney, those continent diversions employing nipple valves are not particularly adaptable to orthotopic location although they have been performed with success in a small number of patients (Olsson, 1987). In contrast, however, the imbricated and tapered ileal segment leading to an Indiana pouch is relatively simpler to catheterize and can be utilized for orthotopic catheterizing diversion (Rowland et al., 1987).

A comment should be made about the relative surgical complexity required in the construction of various of the catheterizing pouches. Perhaps the single most demanding technical feature of each pouch is the construction of the continence mechanism. Furthermore, it is the success or failure of this mechanism that assures the success or failure of the diversion.

Some general techniques have been employed to create a dependable, catheterizable continence zone. Appendiceal tunneling techniques are probably the simplest of all to perform in that they utilize already established techniques that are in the urologist's armamentarium. In these techniques, the appendix is tunneled into the cecum in a fashion similar to ureterocolonic anastomosis. Appendiceal continence mechanisms have been criticized, however. The appendix may be absent in some patients because of prior appendectomy. The appendiceal stump may be too short to reach the anterior abdominal wall or umbilicus while still maintaining sufficient length for tunneling. This criticism has been addressed by an operative variation described by Mitchell, wherein the appendiceal stump can be lengthened by the inclusion of a tubular portion of proximal cecum (Burns and Mitchell, 1990). Instead of simply removing the appendix with a button of cecum before preparing it for tunneling, the entire base of the cecum leading to the appendix can be resected in continuity with the appendix by the application of the GIA stapler (Figs. 72–30A and 72–30B).

Appendiceal continence mechanisms share the feature of allowing for only small diameter catheters to be utilized for intermittent catheterization. The large amount of mucus produced by an intestinal reservoir is emptied much more simply by using a catheter of 20 to 22 Fr., rather than the typical 14 Fr. catheter, which would be admitted by an appendiceal stump.

Two techniques of appendiceal continence mechanisms have been reported. Mitrofanoff reported excising the appendix with a button of cecum and reversing it upon itself before doing the tunneled reimplant (Duckett and Snyder, 1986). Riedmiller and colleagues (1990) have left the appendix attached to the cecum and have buried it into the adjacent cecum, by rolling it back onto itself. A wide tunnel is created in the tenia, extending 5 to 6 cm from the base of the appendix (Fig. 72–31A). Windows are created in the mesoappendix between blood vessels. The appendix is folded cephalad into the tunnel, and seromuscular sutures are placed

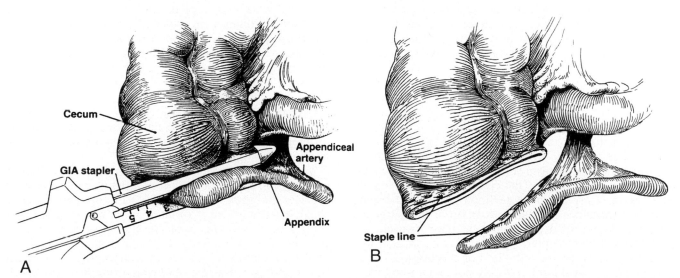

Figure 72–30. *A,* The appendiceal stump is lengthened by the inclusion of a tubular portion of proximal cecum and by the application of the GIA stapler to the terminal cecum.

B, The added length is demonstrated. (From Burns, M. W., and Mitchell, M. E.: Tips on constructing the Mitrofanoff appendiceal stoma. Contemp. Urol., May 1990, pp. 10–12.)

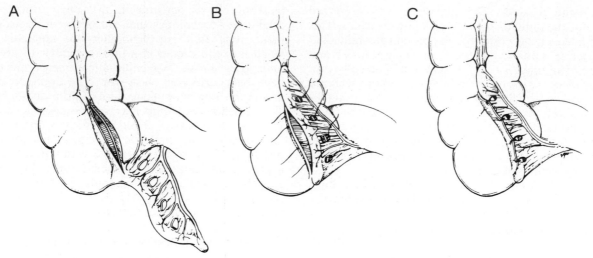

Figure 72–31. *A* to *C,* The appendix is left attached to the cecum and buried into the adjacent cecal tenia by rolling it back onto itself. A wide tunnel is created that extends 5 to 6 cm from the base of the appendix. Windows are created in the mesoappendix between blood vessels. The appendix is folded cephalad into the tunnel, and seromuscular sutures are placed through the mesoappendix.

through the mesoappendix windows to complete the tunneling (Fig. 72–31*B* and *C*). The tip of the appendix is amputated and brought to the selected stoma site.

Another major type of continence mechanism is the tapered and imbricated terminal ileum and ileocecal valve, adaptable to right colon conduits. The surgical technology is rather simple, with imbrication or plication of the ileocecal valve region along with tapering of the more proximal ileum in the fashion of a neourethra (Bejany and Politano, 1988; Lochhart, 1987; Rowland, 1985). These techniques afford a reliable continence mechanism. The only apparent fault is the potential of the ileal neourethra becoming lengthened with time. This is a consequence of the catheter meeting resistance at the imbricated ileocecal valve during each catheterization. The other feature of ileocecal plication and proximal ileal tapering that has been criticized is the loss of the ileocecal valve. Although this does result in frequent bowel movements in a number of patients, at least in the short term, the majority of patients experience bowel regularity given simple pharmacologic therapy. Some patients have developed rather severe diarrhea following the loss of the ileocecal valve. This may be particularly true in the pediatric patient with neurogenic bowel dysfunction (e.g., myelomeningocele) (Mitchell, personal communication).

A further surgical principle utilized in constructing the continence mechanism is the application of an intussuscepted nipple valve. The creation of these nipple valves is certainly the most technologically demanding of all the continence mechanisms. In order that surgeons achieve a degree of dependability in their own clinical results with intussuscepted valves, a significant learning curve must be overcome initially. For this reason, nipple valve construction should probably not be chosen by the surgeon carrying out occasional construction of continent pouches. Furthermore, many modifications of the original technique of Kock for construction of a stable

nipple valve have been introduced. The single reason for all of these modifications is the rather disappointing long-term stability of nipple valves in some patients.

One of the major advances in nipple valve construction has been the removal of mesenteric attachments from the middle 6 to 8 cm of bowel to be utilized (Hendren, 1980). This maneuver reduces the tethering effect of the mesentery that serves to evert the intussusception. The next major advance has been the attachment of the nipple valve to the reservoir wall itself. This has been achieved by two or three different stapling techniques as well as by a suturing technique described by Hendren, King, and others (Hendren, 1976; King, 1987; Skinner et al., 1984). Nevertheless, nipple valve failure can be anticipated in 10 to 15 per cent of cases despite the very best of operative techniques.

A final feature of stapled nipple valves is the potential for stone formation on exposed staples. Although this has been greatly lessened by the omission of staples at the tip of the intussuscepted nipple valve, as suggested by Skinner and co-workers (1984), occasionally, more proximal staples erode into the pouch and serve as a nidus for stone formation. These stones are usually managed with endoscopy with forceps extraction of the stones and staples or with electrohydraulic or ultrasonic disintegration of the stones with subsequent staple extraction with forceps.

The final major technique of continence mechanism construction is the provision of a hydraulic valve as in the Benchekroun nipple (1987). In this procedure, a small bowel segment is isolated and a reversed intussusception is carried out, apposing the mucosal surfaces of the small bowel. Tacking sutures are taken to a portion of the circumference of the intussusception to stabilize the nipple valve while allowing urine to flow freely between the leaves of apposed ileal mucosa so that, as the pouch fills, hydraulic pressure closes the intussuscipiens, assuring continence. Although we have no personal experience with these types of hydraulic valves, clinical reports have suggested their long-term success. However, destabilization of nipples, in general, remains a concern.

Certain features of all continent catheterizable pouches are constant. As mentioned, we prefer long ureteral stents placed to each renal pelvis and diverted beyond the pouch itself to avoid urinary contact with the pouch in the early postoperative period. These stents may be led out through the continence mechanism, if it is sufficiently capacious as in nipple valves. Alternatively, in appendiceal or plicated ileocecal valve continence mechanisms, they are brought out through a separate stab wound with or without an additional suprapubic tube. Purse string sutures should be utilized around the bowel stab wounds and the bowel is fixed to the anterior abdominal wall at the tube sites to prevent urinary leakage after tube removal. In general, the continence mechanism is catheterized by an appropriately sized tube. Soft silicone rubber suction drains are placed and brought through the lower quadrant contralateral to the stoma.

During construction of the pouch intraoperative testing for pouch integrity is always performed. The continence mechanism is also tested for ease of catheterization as well as for continence, after the pouch construction has been completed. The pouch is filled with saline, the continence mechanism catheter is removed, and the pouch can be compressed slightly to look for points of leakage as well as to test the continence mechanism for its ability to contain urine. Thereafter, the continence mechanism is catheterized to ensure ease of catheter passage.

Postoperatively, certain principles must be adhered to in all catheterizing pouches. The larger bore catheter utilized for drainage of the pouch should be irrigated at frequent intervals in order to ensure against mucus obstruction. This procedure can be performed at 4-hour intervals by simple irrigation with 45 to 50 ml of saline. Less frequent intervals of irrigation can be employed when the urine is totally diverted from the kidneys by means of long indwelling stents. As soon as possible, patients are instructed in how to conduct their own irrigation programs, both to familiarize themselves with the process as well as to reduce the burden on the nursing staff.

At about the 10th to 12th postoperative day, a contrast study is done to ensure that there is no pouch leakage. Thereafter, ureteral stents may be removed, with radiologic control. If a separate suprapubic tube is employed, it may be removed at this juncture, and after healing of the suprapubic site intermittent catheterization can be taught to the patient. After it has been ascertained that the pouch and ureteral anastomoses are intact, the suction drain is removed.

In the case of gastric or Kock pouches, capacity will initially be low (150 ml). Therefore, the frequency of catheterization will be significantly different compared with right colon pouches, in which initial comfortable capacities well in excess of 300 ml are experienced. In order to ensure restful sleeping hours, the smaller capacity pouches may best be managed by indwelling catheterization during those sleeping hours. The patient is instructed in irrigation of mucous debris on a 2 to 3 times daily basis initially, with increasing intervals as mucous production decreases with time.

Because all patients with catheterized pouches have chronic bacteriuria, antibiotic management should be discussed. Most investigators would suggest that bacteriuria in the absence of symptomatology does not warrant antibiotic treatment (Skinner, 1987a). The construction of an effective reflux mechanism in all of these pouches may ensure against clinical episodes of pyelonephritis, in contrast to diversions by means of free refluxing conduits. Obviously, if pyelonephritis does occur clinically, antibiotic treatment should be instituted. In one other circumstance, antibiotics should be administered. A condition has been described manifested by pain in the region of the pouch along with increased pouch contractility ("pouchitis"). Although infrequent, this condition may result in temporary failure of the continence mechanism, because of the hypercontractility of the bowel segment employed for construction of the pouch. The patient typically presents with a history of sudden explosive discharge of urine through the continence mechanism rather than dribbling incontinence, along with discomfort in the region of the pouch.

Urinary retention is an infrequent occurrence in catheterizable pouches. It is most commonly seen in the pouch where the continence mechanism consists of a nipple valve. In these circumstances, if the chimney of the nipple valve is not near the abdominal surface, the catheter can be directed into folds of bowel rather than into the nipple valve proper, such that urinary retention results. This complication is a true emergency, and the patient must seek immediate attention so that catheterization by experienced individuals can be achieved promptly.

After the immediate problem has been resolved by emptying the pouch, the patient should be kept under observation for the ability to successfully catheterize on a number of occasions. Sometimes a coudé-tipped catheter is helpful in this regard. Rarely, a flexible cystoscope will be necessary. The appropriate angle of entry can be taught to patients until they are comfortable with the new catheter. In fact, our preference is to utilize such coudé catheters on a regular basis, even with nonnipple valve pouches.

Intraperitoneal rupture of catheterizable pouches has been reported. In general, these episodes are more common in the neurologic patient in whom the sensation of pouch fullness may be less distinct (Hensle, personal communication; Mitchell, personal communication). Oftentimes, associated mild abdominal trauma, such as a fall, is antecedent to the rupture. In general, the patient requires immediate pouch decompression and abdominal exploration with drainage of infected urine. If the amount of urinary extravasation is small, and the patient does not have a surgical abdomen, occasionally catheter drainage and antibiotic administration suffice in treating intraperitoneal rupture of a pouch. We have successfully employed this nonoperative approach in one patient, with a right colon pouch.

CONTINENT ILEAL RESERVOIR (KOCK POUCH)

This operation, first reported by Kock (1982), for urinary diversion in 1982, was singularly responsible for the reawakened interest in continent diversion procedures. An outgrowth of the Kock procedure for continent ileostomy (1971), the Kock pouch combined reasonably dependable techniques for securing continence of urine and preventing reflux to the upper urinary tracts (nipple valves), along with a carefully refashioned bowel that provided a low pressure urinary reservoir. Skinner and co-workers (1989) have carefully studied and improved the technique over the years, while amassing a prodigious experience with the operations and its variants. It is Skinner's operative description that will be followed closely in this chapter.

Procedure

Approximately 70 to 80 cm of small bowel is isolated from a point at the avascular plane of Treves cephalad. If the patient has a pre-existing ileal conduit and is undergoing conversion to a Kock pouch, the previous small bowel anastomosis should be resected and the length of ileum measured cephalad from this point. A 5-cm segment of proximal ileum and mesentery is sacrificed to provide added mobility to the isolated segment.

The middle portion of the ileum is folded in the shape of a U, with each limb of the U measuring 20 to 22 cm in length (Fig. 72–32A). The medial borders of the U may be sutured to one another on the serosal surface before opening the bowel. Alternatively, the bowel may be opened along its antimesenteric border, extending into each ileal terminus for a few centimeters prior to closing the posterior wall of the ileal plate with running absorbable material (Figs. 72–32B and 72–32C). A 10-cm length of ileum is selected on both the afferent and efferent ileal termini for creating the intussuscepted nipple valves. The middle 6 to 8 cm of the 10-cm segment is denuded of mesentery by electrocoagulation. An Allis or Babcock clamp is advanced into the ileal terminus, grasping the full thickness of the intussuscipiens and inverting the ileum into the pouch (Fig. 72–32D).

With the TA55 stapler, three rows of 4.8-mm staples are applied to the intussuscepted nipple valve (Fig. 72–32E). The distal six staples from each cartridge are removed prior to staple application to ensure that the tip of the valve is free of the staples. Most workers suggest that the pin of the stapling instrument should always be kept in place so that staple misalignment does not occur. A pinhole puncture site at the base of the nipple valve should be oversewn, to prevent fistula formation after staple application is complete.

The nipple valve is then fixed by one of two stapling techniques to the back wall of the reservoir (Skinner et al., 1984). A small buttonhole may be made in the back wall of the ileal plate so that the anvil of the stapler can be passed through the buttonhole and advanced into the nipple valve before application of the fourth row of staples (Fig. 72–32F). If this maneuver is carried out, the buttonhole is oversewn afterward with absorbable material. Alternatively, the anvil of the stapler can be directed between the two leaves of the intussuscipiens and the fourth row of staples utilized to fix the inner leaf of the nipple valve to the pouch wall (Fig. 72–32G). The pinhole puncture sites are oversewn.

Some investigators, including Skinner et al. (1989), suggest the application of absorbable mesh collars to subsequently anchor the base of the nipple valve. If collars are utilized, 2.5-cm wide strips of absorbable mesh are placed through additional windows of Deaver at the base of each nipple valve. The mesh strips are fashioned into collars and sewn both to the base of the pouch as well as to the ileal terminus with seromuscular sutures of absorbable material (Figs. 72–32H and 72–32I). The posterior plate is then closed to create the pouch by folding the ileum in a cup cystoplasty fashion (Figs. 72–32J and 72–32K). The closure is completed by running absorbable suture material.

The pouch can then be inverted on its own mesentery to achieve proper anterior-posterior alignment of the ileal termini. The proximal terminus is prepared for ureteroileal anastomosis, which can be conducted according to the surgeon's preference. A Yankauer suction tip is useful to traverse the two nipple valves and to direct long ureteral stents, from the renal pelves out through the distal valve. The distal ileal terminus is directed to the previously selected stoma site. A small button of skin is removed with small-sized plugs of anterior and posterior fascia. If a collar has been employed, separate heavy absorbable sutures are taken from anterior fascia in a horizontal mattress fashion to the cuff to anchor the cuff to the anterior fascia (Figs. 72–32L and 72–32M). This assures a short "chimney". Alternatively, the base of the pouch may be fixed to the posterior fascia or peritoneal margins with interrupted heavy absorbable sutures.

A bulky mesentery at the cephalad extent of the stoma invites parastomal herniation. Our preference in avoiding this problem is either to "defat" the mesentery before it is led through the stoma site or to actually remove some of the mesentery from the ileal terminus. Alternatively, Skinner and co-workers (1984) suggest a Marlex sling, which is passed through the window of Deaver used for the collar and sutured to each side of the stoma site to prevent parastomal herniation (Figs. 72–32L and 72–32M).

Excess ileum is transected at the skin level and a flush stoma is created by suturing the ileum to the skin with interrupted absorbable material. A 30-Fr. Medina catheter is advocated by Skinner for postoperative drainage. Our practice has been to utilize a 24 Fr. multiperforate rubber tube, which is sutured to the anterior abdominal wall along with ureteral stents.

Postoperative Care and Comments

General comments have been made regarding the postoperative care of all catheterizable pouches. Specific

Text continued on page 2707

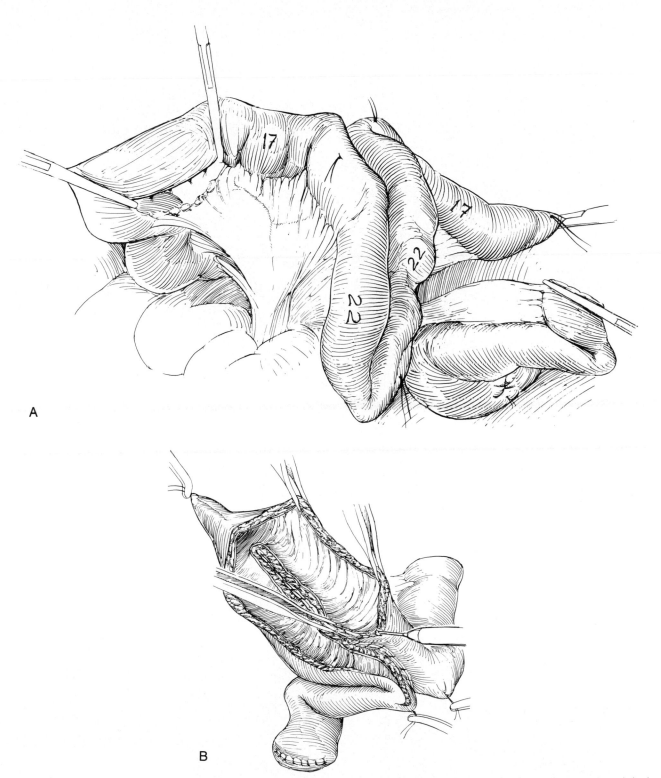

A

B

Figure 72–32. *A,* From 70 to 80 cm of small bowel are isolated. The middle portion of the ileum is folded in the shape of a U, with each limb of the U measuring 22 cm in length.
   B, The medial borders of the U may be sutured on the serosal surface before opening the bowel.

Illustration continued on following page

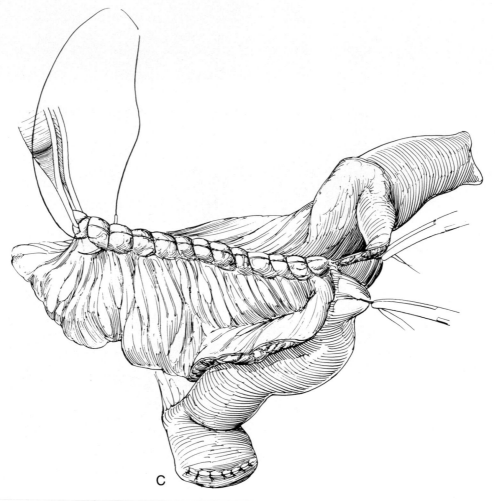

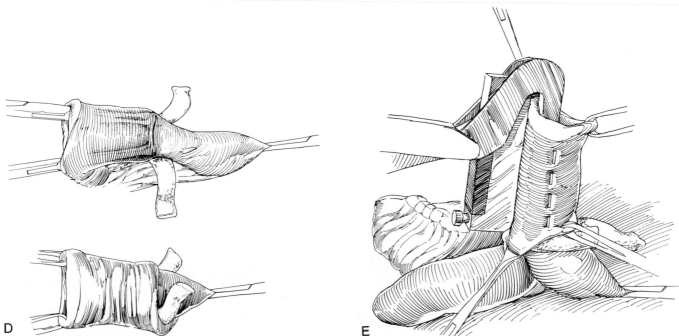

Figure 72–32 *Continued C*, This figure demonstrates the bowel being opened along its antimesenteric border prior to closing the posterior wall of the ileal plate.

D, An Allis or Babcock clamp is advanced into the ileal terminus. The full thickness of the intussuscipiens is grasped, and it is prolapsed into the pouch.

E, Three rows of 4.8-mm staples are applied to the intussuscepted nipple valve using the TA-55 stapler.

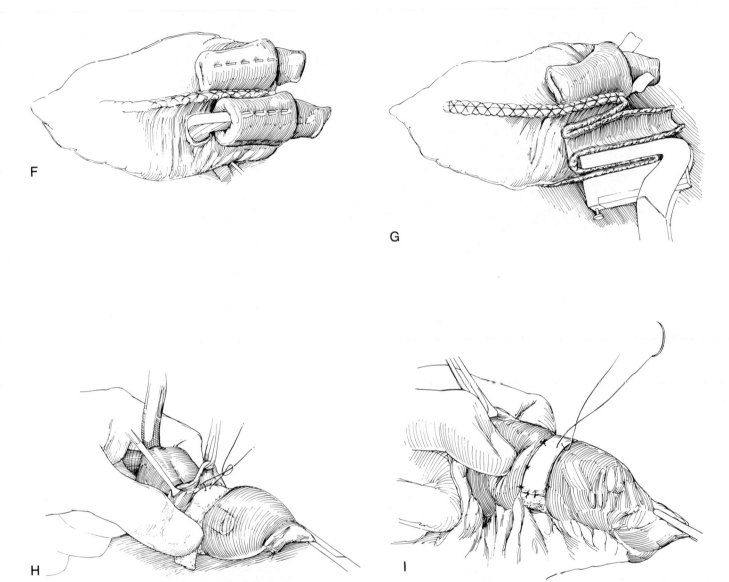

F

G

H

I

Figure 72–32 *Continued F,* A small buttonhole is made in the back wall of the ileal plate to allow the anvil of the TA-55 stapler to be passed through and advanced into the nipple valve. A fourth row of staples is applied.

G, The anvil of the stapler can be directed between the two leaves of the intussuscipiens and the fourth row of staples applied in this manner.

H, A 2.5-cm wide strip of absorbable mesh is placed through additional windows of Deaver at the base of each nipple valve. The mesh strips are fashioned into collars.

I, The collars are sewn to the base of the pouch as well as to the ileal terminus with seromuscular sutures.

Illustration continued on following page

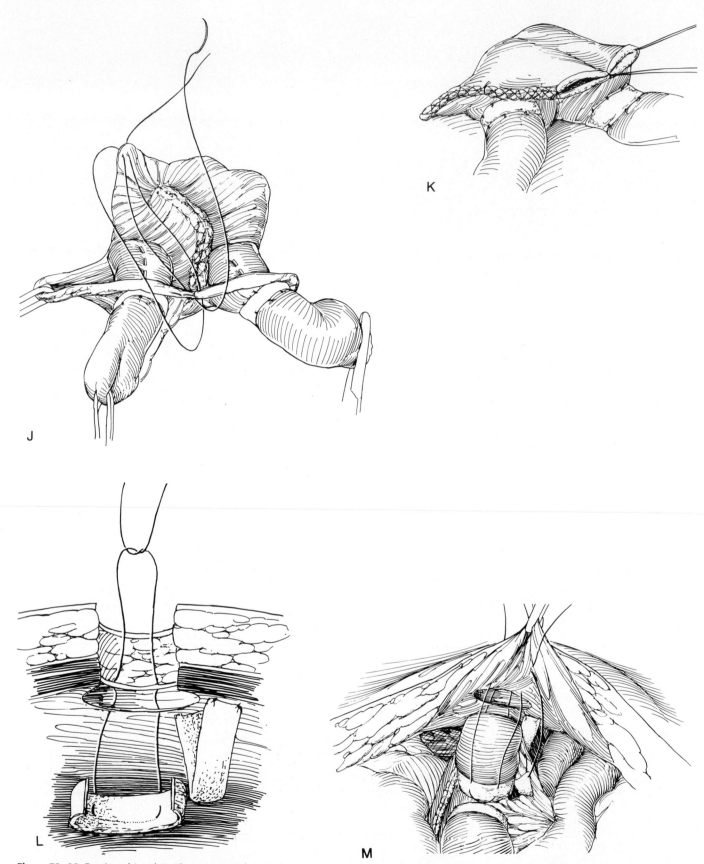

Figure 72–32 *Continued J* and *K*, The posterior plate is closed to create the pouch by folding the ileum in a cup cystoplasty fashion.
L and *M*, A button of skin is removed with small-sized plugs of anterior and posterior fascia. If a collar has been employed separate heavy absorbable sutures are taken from anterior fascia in a horizontal mattress fashion to the cuff, to anchor the cuff to the anterior fascia. (From Hinman, F., Jr.: Atlas of Urologic Surgery. Philadelphia, W. B. Saunders Co., 1989.)

to the Kock pouch is the small initial capacity. Skinner and colleagues (1989) advise leaving the Medina tube in place for 3 weeks. Kock and associates (1982) have suggested that the patient clamp the tube until a point of discomfort before releasing after the second week. If double J-stents remain in the pouch, the pouch is examined endoscopically with a cystoscope upon tube removal. Stents are removed. Patients are trained in intermittent catheterization. Catheterization intervals are increased by 1 hour weekly.

Average pouch capacities exceeding 500 ml are achieved by 3 to 6 months. Overall the Kock pouch affords average capacities of 700 ml or more, and urodynamic evaluations suggest pouch pressures averaging 4 to 8 cm H_2O in the long-term (at two-thirds pouch capacity) (Chen et al., 1989).

Management of the complications of stone formation has been discussed. Managing a failed nipple valve is considerably more complicated. Three general reasons for failure can be cited. Pinhole fistulas at the base of the nipple are a consequence of setting the aligning pin of the staple instrument. Such fistulas can be simply oversewn during formal re-exploration. Nipple valve prolapse may occur, in which case bowel can be intussuscepted once more, restapled, and fixed to the reservoir wall with a suture or stapling technique. Shortening of the nipple length beneath the 2.5 to 3 cm necessary for urinary continence probably occurs as a consequence of ischemia. Repair necessitates the isolation of 15 cm of ileum, which is utilized to create a new nipple valve (Lieskovsky et al., 1987). One end of this ileum is fashioned into a new stoma, and the other is spatulated and sewn onto the established pouch.

Nipple valve failure of one sort or another may occur at any time following surgery to create pouches of any type that utilize intussusception principles. Even in the best of hands a failure rate of 15 per cent or higher is experienced. In regard to an individual surgeon's initial experience in constructing nipple valves, the failure rate is higher still. Excluding the original patients in Kock's own series in which a reoperation rate exceeding 80 per cent was noted (Berglund et al., 1987), other workers have reported the need for reoperation in approximately one third of patients (deKernion et al., 1985; Waters et al., 1987).

MAINZ POUCH

The catheterizable MAINZ pouch has undergone considerable modification over the years (Thuroff et al., 1985). Problems in stabilizing the stapled nipple valve represented the primary reasons for modifications to be carried out. The operative technique has now been modified so as to utilize the intact ileocecal valve as a means of further stabilizing the intussusception (Thuroff et al., 1988). This procedure is described here without further reference to earlier prototypes.

Procedure

The catheterizable MAINZ pouch varies somewhat from the orthotopic voiding MAINZ pouch. A longer segment of bowel is utilized. A 10- to 15-cm portion of cecum and ascending colon is isolated along with two separate, equal-sized limbs of distal ileum and an additional portion of ileum, measuring 20 cm (Fig. 72–33A). The entire colon and distal segments of ileum are spatulated, taking care to preserve the ileocecal valve. These three bowel segments are folded in the form of an incomplete W, and their posterior aspects are sutured to one another to form a broad posterior plate (Fig. 72–33B). A portion of the intact proximal ileal terminus is freed of its mesentery for a distance of 6 to 8 cm, and intussusception of the segment is achieved. Two rows of staples are taken on the intussuscipiens itself (Fig. 72–33C). Thereafter, the intussuscipiens is led through the intact ileocecal valve and a third row of staples is taken to stabilize the nipple valve to the ileocecal valve (Fig. 72–33D). A fourth row of staples is then taken inferiorly, securing the inner leaf of the intussusception to the ileal wall (Fig. 72–33E).

Ureterocolonic anastomoses are created at the apex of the reservoir, which is then folded on itself in a side-to-side fashion to complete the pouch construction. The entire pouch is rotated cephalad to bring the ileal terminus to the region of the umbilicus. A small button of skin is removed from the depth of the umbilical funnel, and the ileal terminus is directed through this buttonhole (Fig. 72–33F). The pouch is secured to the posterior fascia with interrupted absorbable sutures, and the ileal terminus is sewn similarly to anterior fascia. Excess ileal length is resected, and ileum is sutured at the depth of the umbilical funnel with interrupted absorbable sutures.

Postoperative Care and Comments

No specific differences in postoperative care or complications associated with the MAINZ pouch are addressed. Initial capacities are higher than in the Kock pouch. Final mean capacity averaging over 600 ml has been reported. Pouch pressures are 23 cm H_2O at half capacity and 31 cm H_2O when the pouch is full. Contraction waves, beginning at 50 per cent pouch fullness can be recorded at an amplitude of 12 cm H_2O. Thus, this pouch seems to produce a reasonably fine low pressure urinary reservoir, although the pressure is not as low as that achieved with small bowel alone.

Ultimately, a 96 per cent day and night continence rate was reported. Before stabilizing the nipple valve through the intact ileocecal valve there was a need for surgical revision in one third of cases. In a short follow-up of subsequent cases utilizing the ileocecal stabilization, there has been no need for reoperation (Thuroff et al., 1988).

RIGHT COLON POUCHES WITH INTUSSUSCEPTED TERMINAL ILEUM

Additional pouches utilizing nipple valve technology for the continence mechanism include those right colon pouches in which intussusception of the terminal ileum and ileal cecal valve is employed. As such, they are

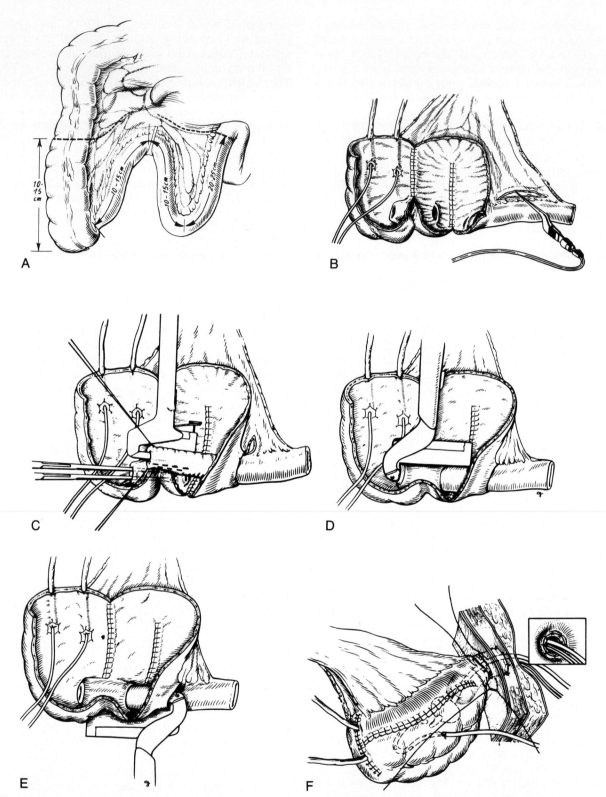

Figure 72–33. *A,* A 10- to 15-cm portion of cecum and ascending colon is isolated along with two separate, equal-sized limbs of distal ileum and an additional portion of ileum measuring 20 cm.

B, A portion of the intact proximal ileal terminus is freed of its mesentery for a distance of 6 to 8 cm.

C, The intact ileum is intussuscepted and two rows of staples are taken on the intussuscipiens itself.

D, The intussuscipiens is led through the intact ileocecal valve, and a third row of staples is taken to stabilize the nipple valve to the ileocecal valve.

E, A fourth row of staples is taken inferiorly, securing the inner leaf of the intussusception to the ileal wall.

F, A button of skin is removed from the depth of the umbilical funnel, and the ileal terminus is directed through this buttonhole. Excess ileal length is resected, and ileum is sutured at the depth of the umbilical funnel. (From Thuroff, J. W., Alken, P., Riedmiller, H., Jacobi, G. H., and Hohenfellner, R.: 100 cases of MAINZ pouch: Continuing experience and evolution. J. Urol., 140:283–288, 1988.)

variations on the continent cecal reservoir initially described by Mansson (1987), employing an intact cecal segment. These three pouches are the UCLA pouch (Raz, personal communication), the Duke pouch (Webster and King, 1987), and LeBag (Light and Scardino, 1987). These operations differ from one another with only a few features, predominantly the technique employed for stabilizing the nipple valve.

Procedures

The UCLA pouch is created by isolating the entire right colon along with 15 cm of distal ileum (Fig. 72–34A). The entire colon segment is incised along the anterior taenia (Fig. 72–34B). Our preference would be to incise along the antimesenteric border, preserving all possible taenial sites for ureteral reimplantation.

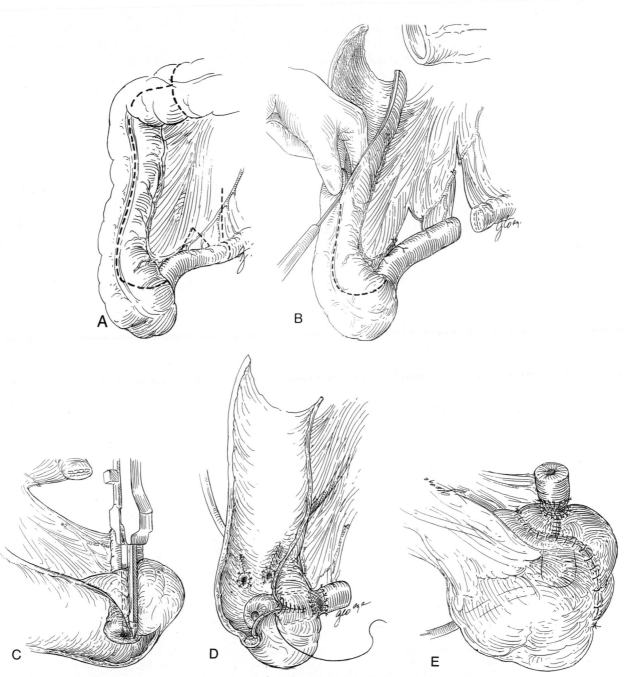

Figure 72–34. *A,* The entire right colon along with 15 cm of distal ileum is isolated.
   B, The entire colon segment is incised along the anterior taenia. About 6 to 8 cm of ileum are cleared of mesenteric attachments.
   C, The ileum is intussuscepted through the ileocecal valve and staples stabilize the nipple valve.
   D, The nipple is also anchored to the sidewall of the pouch with continuous absorbable sutures. An absorbable mesh collar is placed at the base of the nipple valve.
   E, The pouch is closed by folding the colon in a Heineke-Mikulicz configuration. (Courtesy of S. Raz.)

Measuring from the tip of the projected intussusception, 6 to 8 cm of ileum are cleared of mesenteric attachment and the ileum is intussuscepted through the ileocecal valve into the cecum. Staples are applied to stabilize the nipple valve. Two rows of staples are placed employing the bladeless GIA device. The anvil of the device is then directed between the leaves of the intussuscipiens so that the inner leaf of the nipple valve can be stapled to the anterior and inferior walls of the marsupialized cecal pouch (Fig. 72–34C). Further anchoring of the nipple to the sidewall of the pouch is achieved by multiple runs of continuous absorbable suture material sewing the nipple to the pouch (Fig. 72–34D). An absorbable mesh collar is advocated at the base of the nipple valve.

Ureterocolonic anastomosis is carried out by typical tunneling technique, and the pouch is closed by folding the colon in a Heineke-Mikulicz configuration with multiple running absorbable sutures (Fig. 72–34E). The stoma construction proceeds as in the Kock pouch.

The Duke pouch consists of the isolation of a similar segment of distal ileum and cecum with ascending colon. The cecum and ascending colon are detubularized by incising the antimesenteric border (Fig. 72–35A). Ureterocolonic anastomoses are carried out in the usual tunneled fashion.

A length of 6 to 8 cm of mesentery is freed from the middle portion of the planned intussusception. The ileum is intussuscepted through the ileocecal valve (Fig. 72–35B). Stabilization of the intussusception is carried out by suture technique rather than stapling technique. A broad patch of mucosa is excised from the posterior

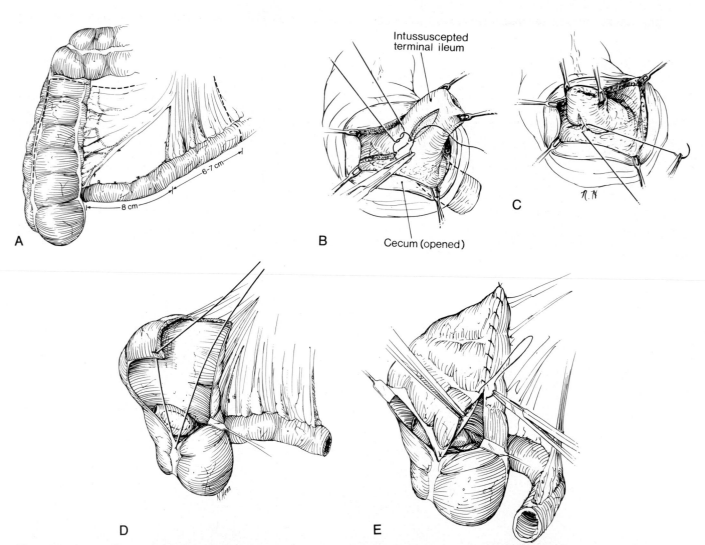

Figure 72–35. *A,* Fifteen-cm segments of distal ileum and cecum with ascending colon are isolated. (From Webster, G. D., and King, L. R.: Further commentary: Cecal bladder. *In* King, L. R., Stone, A. R., and Webster, G. D. (Eds.): Bladder Reconstruction and Continent Urinary Diversion. Chicago, Year Book Medical Publishers, 1987, pp. 206–208.)

B, The ileum is intussuscepted through the ileocecal valve and stabilized with sutures. A patch of mucosa is excised from the posterior cecal plate. One entire thickness of the intussuscipiens is incised to reveal the serosa of the inner leaf of the intussuscipiens. Seromuscular sutures taken in this structure are placed into the muscularis of the back wall of the cecum. (From Robertson, C. M., and King, L. L.: Bladder substitution in children. Urol. Clin. North Am., 13:333–344, 1986.)

C, Mucosal sutures connect the edge of the outer leaf to the mucosal edge of the cecal denudation. (From Robertson, C. M., and King, L. L.: Bladder substitution in children. Urol. Clin. North Am., 13:333–344, 1986.)

D and *E,* The pouch is closed with running sutures in a Heineke-Mikulicz configuration. (From Webster, G. D., and King, L. R.: Further commentary: Cecal bladder. *In* King, L. R., Stone, A. R., and Webster, G. D. (Eds.): Bladder Reconstruction and Continent Urinary Diversion. Chicago, Year Book Medical Publishers, 1987, pp. 206–208.)

cecal plate. One entire thickness of the intussuscipiens is incised to reveal the serosa of the inner leaf of the intussuscipiens. Seromuscular sutures taken in this structure are placed into the muscularis of the back wall of the cecum, and mucosal sutures connect the edge of the outer leaf to the edge of the cecal denudation (Fig. 72–35C). The pouch is closed by serial applications of running absorbable sutures taken to close an angled Heineke-Mikulicz configuration into the form of a pouch (Figs. 72–35D and 72–35E).

This pouch has the advantage of requiring no staples in its construction. We have found that the stabilization achieved by this suturing technique is as dependable as affixing the nipple valve to the sidewall utilizing staples. In fact, we prefer to combine the two techniques using both staple fixation and suture fixation to the reservoir sidewall (variant of the Hendren, 1976 concept).

A final adaptation utilizing an ileocecal bowel segment and an intussuscepted nipple valve is the variation of LeBag, previously described in the section on orthotopic voiding diversions. In this variation, a somewhat longer length of distal ileum is taken and remains intact for construction of the nipple valve in the usual fashion, after removing mesentery from the mid portion of the intussuscipiens. The nipple valve is stapled to itself in three quadrants, and the fourth quadrant staple line attaches the nipple valve to the posterior reservoir wall. The completely marsupialized colon and ileum are sewn to one another with running absorbable suture material (Fig. 72–36). In the catheterizing LeBag pouch, further nipple valve stabilization by means of absorbable mesh collars is not needed. The stoma is brought flush to the umbilical funnel so that the reservoir wall lies immediately beneath the skin level.

Postoperative Care and Comments

No substantive differences exist in the management of the patients undergoing these procedures compared with those patients undergoing MAINZ pouch diver-

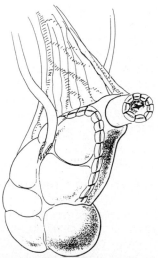

Figure 72–36. A completely marsupialized colon and ileum are sewn to one another with running absorbable suture material. (Courtesy of J. Keith Light.)

sions. The UCLA group has not reported urodynamic data. Pouch capacities have varied between 600 and 700 ml. Altogether, 30 of 34 patients were dry night and day, and only one operation for a fistula at the base of a nipple valve was required. One additional reoperation is planned. The outcomes of the Duke and LeBag pouches are unknown as of this writing.

INDIANA POUCH

The concept of using the buttressed ileocecal valve as a dependable continence mechanism that can withstand the trauma of intermittent catheterization was first reported from Indiana University by Rowland and coworkers (1987). This modification along with the original partial spatulation of the cecal segment and attachment of an ileal patch represented major contributions over the ileocecal reservoir described by Gilchrist (1950), wherein the intact bowel reservoir was employed and no attempt was made to strengthen the ileocecal valve.

Originally, strengthening the ileocecal valve consisted of a double row of imbricating sutures taken to the entire ileal segment (Rowland et al., 1985 and 1987). It soon became apparent that this step was necessary only in the region of the ileocecal valve. "Neourethral" pressure profiles showed that the continence zone was confined to the region of the reconfigured ileocecal valve (Bejany and Politano, 1988). The remaining "neourethra" could be tapered and brought through an abdominal or a perineal stoma. At Indiana University as well as other institutions, the concept of marsupializing only a portion of the ascending colon segment left sufficient peristaltic integrity in the cecal region to generate pressures sufficiently high to overcome the continence mechanism, in some patients. A number of groups contributed to the concept of utilizing the entire right colon or more, marsupializing the entire structure and refashioning it in a Heineke-Mikulicz configuration (Bejany and Politano, 1988; Benson, et al., 1988; Lockhart, 1987; Rowland, personal communication).

Procedure

The Indiana pouch, in its present form, involves isolating a segment of terminal ileum approximately 10 cm in length along with the entire right colon (Fig. 72–37A). After bowel continuity is achieved, appendectomy is performed and the appendiceal fat pad obscuring the inferior margin of the ileocecal junction is removed by cautery (Fig. 72–37B). The entire right colon is opened along its antimesenteric border, and ureteral implants are fashioned (Fig. 72–37C). The ileocecal junction is buttressed according to different techniques, depending on the investigator. Interrupted Lembert sutures are taken over a short distance (3 to 4 cm) in two rows for the double imbrication of the ileocecal valve as described at Indiana (Fig. 72–37D). Nonabsorbable material is utilized, and the second row of sutures is an attempt to bring the opposite mesenteric edges of ileum together, usually over a 12 to 14 Fr. catheter. These two rows of sutures should be placed approximately 8 mm from one

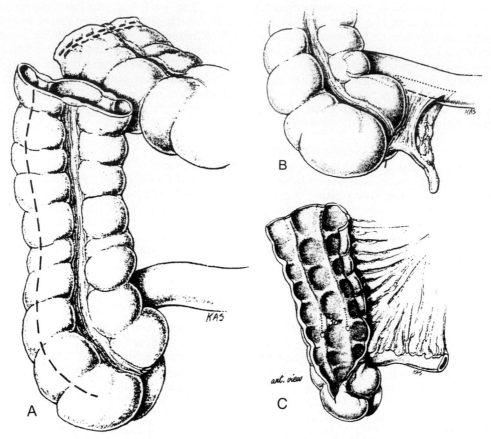

Figure 72–37. *A,* A segment of terminal ileum approximately 10 cm in length along with the entire right colon is isolated.
B, Appendectomy is performed, and the appendiceal fat pad obscuring the inferior margin of the ileocecal junction is removed by cautery.
C, The entire right colon is opened along its antimesenteric border. (*A* to *C* from Benson, M. C., Sawczuk, I. S., Hensle, T. W., Haus, T., and Olsson, C. A.: Modified Indiana University continent diversion. Curr. Surg. Tech. Urol., 1:1–8, 1988.)

another, and the initial suture in each row may be taken in a purse string fashion around the cecal margin as well.

Alternatively, the University of Miami group suggests purse string sutures being taken in the ileum in the same region (Bejany and Politano, 1988). Lockhart suggests the application of apposing Lembert sutures being taken on each side of the terminal ileum (Fig. 72–37*E*). The remaining ileum can be tapered over the catheter and excess ileum removed by stapling technique (Fig. 72–37*F*).

It is important to carry out the imbrication while the cecal reservoir is still open (Rowland, personal communication). In this fashion, one can observe the gradual closure of the ileal cecal valve. The pouch is then closed in a Heineke-Mikulicz configuration with running absorbable suture material. Ureteral stents and a suprapubic tube are taken through the lower abdominal quadrant. The pouch is rotated so as to bring the ileal neourethra as close as possible to the selected stoma site. A fingerbreadth-width skin button is transected along with a similar button from the anterior and posterior fascia. The ileal neourethra is advanced between bundles of the rectus muscle through the stoma, and excess ileum is transected. The ileal edges are sewn to skin with interrupted sutures, to create a flush stoma.

In addition to the differences in the technique of ileocecal valve imbrication, both the University of Miami and the Florida pouch described by Lockhart (1987) differ in the amount of colon utilized and the manner in which it is reconfigured. The entire ascending colon and the right third or half of the transverse colon is isolated, along with 10 to 12 cm of ileum. The entire upper extremity of the large bowel is mobilized laterally in the fashion of an inverted U (Fig. 72–38*A*). The medial limbs of the U are sutured to one another after the bowel is spatulated (Fig. 72–38*B*). The bowel plate is then closed side to side (Fig. 72–38*C*). In this fashion it is noted that the reconfiguration of bowel is perhaps not as advantageous as that with the Heineke-Mikulicz reconfiguration, because the bowel has been refashioned in a neotubular form.

Postoperative Care and Comments

The postoperative care of the patient with an Indiana pouch or a variant is not substantially different from that for other right colon catheterizable diversions. Rowland recommends the patient be discharged from the hospital with the cecostomy tube in place. On

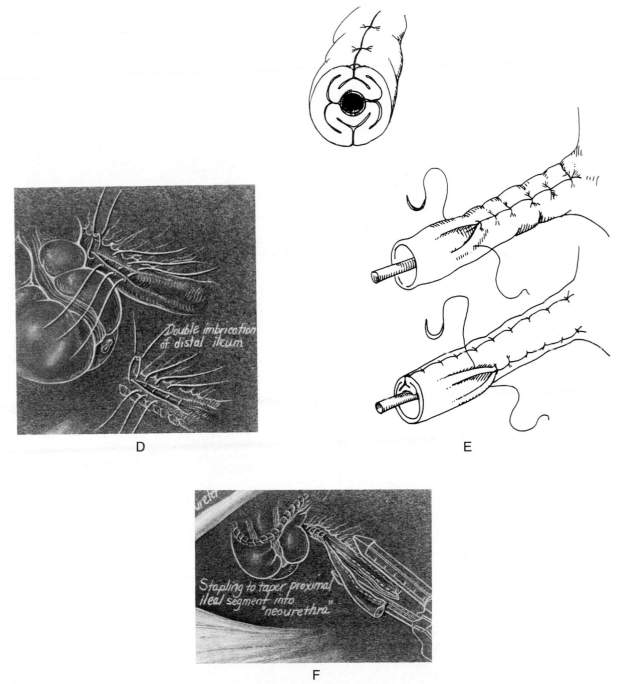

Figure 72–37 *Continued D,* Interrupted Lembert sutures are taken over a short distance (3 to 4 cm) in two rows for the double imbrication of the ileocecal valve as described at Indiana University. (From Olsson, C. A.: Contemporary Urology. September, 1989.)

E, Application of opposing Lembert sutures on each side of the terminal ileum. (Courtesy of J. Lockhart.)

F, Excess ileum can be tapered by stapling technique. (From Olsson, C. A.: Contemporary Urology. September, 1989.)

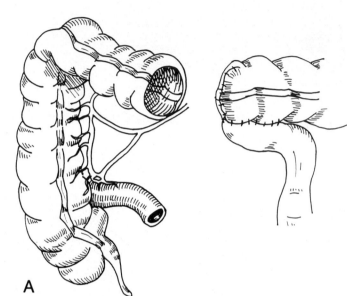

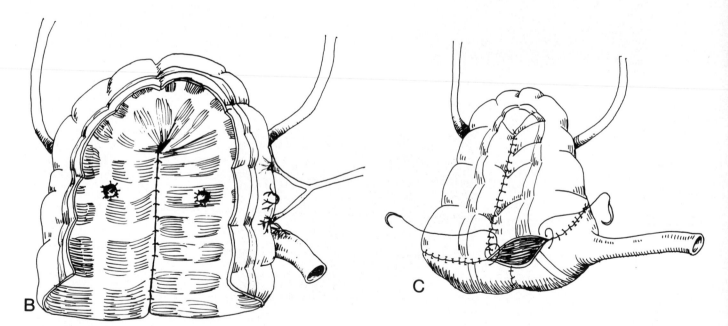

Figure 72–38. *A,* The entire ascending colon and the right third or half of the transverse colon are isolated along with 10 to 12 cm of ileum.

B, The entire upper extremity of the large bowel is mobilized laterally in the fashion of an inverted U. The medial limbs of the U are sutured after the bowel is spatulated.

C, The bowel plate is closed side to side. (Courtesy of J. Lockhart.)

A

B

C

readmission to the hospital 3 weeks later, tube removal and instruction in self-catheterization are completed.

Average pouch capacities of 400 to 500 ml have been reported by the Indiana group (Rowland et al., 1987). Combining the partially and totally spatulated bowel procedures, this group reports a reoperation rate of 26 per cent, although overall continence rates of 93 per cent were achieved (Schiedler et al., 1989). Very elegant urodynamic studies were conducted in Indiana pouch variants by Carroll and co-workers (1989). They found only 86 per cent of patients totally continent in a small series. However, pouch capacities exceeded 650 ml. Peak contractions of 47 cm H_2O were recorded at capacity.

The University of Miami group (Bejany and Politano, 1988) report total continence in all of a small group of patients. One ureteral obstruction treated by balloon dilation was experienced; no other reoperations were necessary. Average pouch capacities were 750 ml or higher. End-filling pressures of 20 cm H_2O were reported. No patient required alkali therapy.

The Florida pouch has been performed in over 100 patients (Lockhart, 1987). Overall, a 7.2 per cent reoperation rate was reported. Although hyperchloremia was noted in 70 per cent of patients, only four patients, including those who had pre-existing renal disease, required treatment. Reservoir capacities ranged from 400 to 1200 ml, and maximal reservoir pressures at capacity ranged from 18 to 55 cm H_2O (Lockhart, 1987).

PENN POUCH

The Penn pouch is the first continent diversion employing the Mitrofanoff principle (1980) wherein the appendix serves as the continence mechanism. This operation has the singular feature of affording a catheterizable continent diversion that can be performed utilizing techniques already in the urologic armamentarium.

As described by Duckett and Snyder (1986), an ileocecal pouch is created by isolating a segment of cecum up to the junction of the ileocolic and middle colic blood supplies along with a similar length of terminal ileum. These two structures are marsupialized on the antimesenteric borders and sutured to one another in the form of a neotubularized pouch. The superior margin of the pouch is sutured in a transverse fashion—all sutures being of absorbable material. A button of cecum surrounding the origin of the appendix is circumcised, and the resulting cecal aperture is closed with running absorbable suture. The mesentery of the appendix is dissected carefully from the base of the cecum, preserving its blood supply. The appendix is reversed on itself, so that the cecal button can reach the anterior abdominal wall and the tail of the appendix can be directed to the taenia of the colon (Fig. 72–39). As previously described, if additional appendiceal length is required the variation proposed by Burns and Mitchell (1990), creating a tube of the base of the cecum, may be employed. A button of appendix is cut from the appendiceal tip, and tunneled reimplantation is carried out. These inves-

tigators have found that spatulating the distal tip of the appendix until a catheter of at least 12 to 14 Fr. can be passed is helpful.

Postoperative Care and Comments

Although not shown in Duckett's surgical drawings, we would suggest that a large bore suprapubic tube be utilized to drain the pouch in the early postoperative interval. The size of the catheter admitted by the appendiceal stump is insufficient to allow for the passage of ureteral stents along with the 12 to 14 Fr. catheter. In addition, safe irrigation of mucus debris is best managed by a larger bore catheter.

Data are not available on pouch capacities, urodynamic measurements, or reoperation rates. In our own small experience, however, we have found the appendix to provide a very dependable continence mechanism, able to withstand the pressures generated by reconfigured colon.

GASTRIC POUCHES

Pioneering animal experimentation demonstrated the feasibility of employing stomach as a bladder patch or urinary reservoir (Rudick et al., 1977; Sinaiko, 1956). The use of the stomach to create a urinary reservoir has theoretical and real advantages (Adams et al., 1988). Electrolyte reabsorption is greatly diminished, utilizing stomach in the reservoir. This would potentially make the stomach the selected reservoir for individuals with pre-existing renal insufficiency. Hyperchloremic acidosis would not be a problem. In fact, in addition to presenting a barrier against the absorption of chloride and ammonium, the gastric mucosa secretes chloride ions (Piser et al., 1987). In patients in whom shortening of the bowel may be expected to lead to degrees of malabsorption, stomach is an attractive alternative. When the entire lower bowel has been irradiated, stomach may be an intact segment to consider for performing

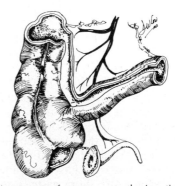

Figure 72–39. A segment of cecum up to the junction of the ileocolic and middle colic blood supplies, along with a similar length of terminal ileum, is isolated and marsupialized on the antimesenteric borders. A button of cecum surrounding the origin of the appendix is circumcised. The mesentery of the appendix is dissected carefully from the base of the cecum, preserving its blood supply. (From Duckett, J. W., and Snyder, H. M., III: The Mitrofanoff principle in continent urinary reservoirs. Semin. Urol., 5:55–62, 1987.)

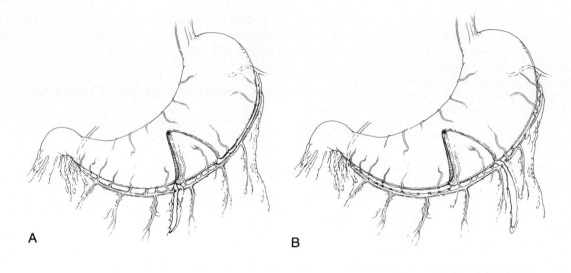

A   B

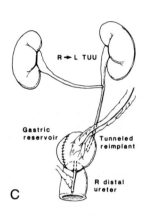

R → L TUU

Gastric
reservoir   Tunneled
reimplant

R distal
ureter

C

Figure 72–40. *A* and *B,* A wedge-shaped segment of stomach with the greatest width of 7 to 10 cm is fashioned from the greater curvature. The left gastroepiploic artery is preferentially utilized as the blood supply for the isolated gastric wedge, by dividing the short gastric vessels up to the gastric fundus. Alternatively, if there is a problem with the left artery, the right gastroepiploic vessel may be employed.

C, The isolated wedge is refashioned into nearly a sphere by folding it back on itself and suturing the edges together with running absorbable material. One ureter is tunneled into the reservoir. A proximal transureteroureterostomy (TUU) is performed. The ipsilateral distal ureter is tunneled into the reservoir with its distal extent brought to the introitus to serve as a catheterization portal. (From Adams, M. C., Mitchell, M. E., and Rink, R. C.: Gastrocystoplasty: an alternative solution to the problem of urological reconstruction in the severely compromised patient. J. Urol., 140:1152–1156, 1988. © By Williams & Wilkins, 1988.)

continent diversion. Given these theoretical advantages, a number of groups have initiated trials with gastric pouches, particularly in the pediatric population (Adams et al., 1988).

Procedure

A wedge-shaped segment of stomach in which the greatest width is 7 to 10 cm is fashioned from the greater curvature. Care is taken not to extend the wedge through to the lesser curvature in order to preserve vagal innervation and normal gastric emptying. The left gastroepiploic artery is preferentially utilized as the blood supply for the isolated gastric wedge, dividing the short gastric vessels from the more proximal artery up to the gastric fundus. Alternatively, if there is a problem with the left artery, the right gastroepiploic vessel may be employed, dividing the short gastrics to the level of the pylorus (Figs. 72–40*A* and 72–40*B*). The stomach is then closed according to the surgeon's preference.

Gastroduodenostomy or gastrojejunostomy is not mandatory unless the antrum of the stomach has been utilized. The isolated wedge is refashioned into nearly a sphere by folding it back on itself and by suturing the edges together with running absorbable material. Before pouch closure, one ureter is tunneled into the reservoir in the surgeon's preferred antireflux fashion. A proximal transureteroureterostomy is performed, and the ipsilateral distal ureter is also tunneled into the reservoir with its distal extent brought to the introitus to serve as a catheterization portal (Fig. 72–40*C*).

Postoperative Care and Comments

Adams and colleagues (1988) report mean pouch capacities of 245 ml and end-filling pressures averaging 35 cm H_2O in a small patient sample. Combining their experience of gastric continent diversion with gastrocystoplasty, they report minimal mucus production—only three of 13 patients required any irrigation and the majority maintained sterile urine. Urine pH values have ranged from 4 to 7. No introital ulceration from acid urine is reported. Three patients had minor elevations of serum gastrin levels. None of the continent diversions required reoperations. Leong (1978) has utilized similar concepts in gastric pouch construction and has alluded to the creation of a voiding pouch created from stomach as well. Although experience with stomach is small to date, its various intrinsic advantages as a reservoir suggest that its popularity may certainly increase.

REFERENCES

Adams, M. C., Mitchell, M. E., and Rink, R. C.: Gastrocystoplasty: an alternative solution to the problem of urological reconstruction in the severely compromised patient. J. Urol., 140:1152–1156, 1988.

Althausen, A. F., Hagen-Cook, K., and Hendren, W. H., III: Nonrefluxing colon conduit: experience with 70 cases. J. Urol., 120:35–39, 1978.

Ambrose, S. S.: Ureterosigmoidostomy. In Glenn, J. F. (Ed.): Urologic Surgery. Philadelphia, J. B. Lippincott Co., 1983, pp. 511–520.

Ashken, M. H.: Urinary cecal reservoir. In King, L. R., Stone, A. R., and Webster, G. D. (Ed.): Bladder Reconstruction and Continent Diversion. Chicago, Year Book Medical Publishers, 1987, p. 238–251.

Askanazi, J., Hensle, T. W., Starker, P., Lockhart, S. H., LaSala, P. A., Olsson, C. A., and Kinney, J. M.: Effect of immediate postoperative nutritional support on length of hospitalization. J. Urol., 134:1032–1036, 1985.

Babcock, W.: A note as to the recognition of the ureter. Report of a case of anastomosis of the ureter into the appendix. Surg. Gynecol. Obstet., 18:119–120, 1914.

Baird, J. S., Scott, R. L., and Spencer, R. D.: Studies on the transplantation of the ureters into the intestines. Surg. Gynecol. Obstet., 24:482–484, 1917.

Barber, W. H.: Uretero-enteric anastomosis. A new enteroureteral operation. An inductive study based on surgical physiology. Ann. Surg., 61:273–275, 1915.

Bardenheuer: Extraperitonealer Explorativschnitt. Stuttgart, 1887, p. 273.

Beck, C.: Implantation of both ureters into sigmoid flexure. Chicago Medical Recorder, 17:303–305, 1899.

Beddoe, A. M., Boyce, J. G., Remy, J. C., Fruchter, R. G., and Nelson, J. H., Jr.: Stented versus nonstented transverse colon conduits: a comparative report. Gynecol. Oncol., 27:305–313, 1987.

Bejany, D. E., and Politano, V. A.: Stapled and nonstapled tapered distal ileum for construction of a continent colonic urinary reservoir. J. Urol., 140:491–494, 1988.

Belawenetz, P. P.: Ein Fall von Harnleitertransplantation in den Darm. (Prof. P. J. Tichoff's operation.) Zentralbl. f. Chir., 37:457, 1910.

Benchekroun, A.: The ileocecal continent bladder. In King, L. R., Stone, A. R., and Webster, G. D. (Eds.): Bladder Reconstruction and Continent Urinary Diversion. Chicago, Year Book Medical Publishers, 1987, p. 224–237.

Benson, M. C., Sawczuk, I. S., Hensle, T. W., Haus, T., and Olsson, C. A.: Modified Indiana University continent diversion. Curr. Surg. Tech. Urol., 1:1–8, 1988.

Benson, M. C., Slawin, K. M., Wechsler, M. H., and Olsson, C. A.: Analysis of continent versus standard urinary diversion. Br. J. Urol., Submitted, 1990.

Berg, J.: Ueber die Behandlung der Ectopia vesicae. Nord. Med. Arkiv. Abt. I, Nr. 4, 1907.

Bergenhem, B.: Ectopia vesicae et adenoma destruens vesicae; exstirpation of blasen; implantation of ureterena i rectum. Eira, 19:265–273, 1895.

Berglund, B., Kock, N. G., Norlen, L., and Philipson, B. M.: Volume capacity and pressure characteristics of the continent ileal reservoir used for urinary diversion. J. Urol., 137:29–34, 1987.

Boari, A.: An easy and rapid method of fixing the ureters in the intestines without sutures by the aid of a special button; with experimental researches. Columbus Med. J., 19:1–20, 1897.

Borelius: Eine neue Modifikation der Maydl'schen Operations-methode bei angeborener Blasenektopie. Zentralbl. f. Chir., 30:780–782, 1903.

Boyd, S. D., Feinberg, S. M., Skinner, D. G., et al.: Quality of life survey of urinary diversion patients: Comparison of ileal conduits versus continent Kock ileal reservoirs. J. Urol., 138:1386–1389, 1987.

Bricker, E. M.: Bladder substitution after pelvic evisceration. Surg. Clin. North Am., 30:1511–1521, 1950.

Burns, M. W., and Mitchell, M. E.: Tips on constructing the Mitrofanoff appendiceal stoma. Contemp. Urol., May 1990, pp. 10–12.

Camey, M.: Detubularized U-shaped cystoplasty (Camey 2). Curr. Surg. Tech. Urol., 3:1–8, 1990.

Camey, M., and LeDuc, A.: L'enetrocystoplastie avec cystoprostatectomie totale pour cancer de la vessie. Ann. Urol., 13:114, 1979.

Camey, M., Richard, F., and Botto, H.: Bladder replacement by ileocystoplasty. In King, L. R., Stone, A. R., and Webster, G. D.: (Eds.): Bladder Reconstruction and Continent Urinary Diversion. Chicago, Year Book Medical Publishers, 1987, pp. 336–359.

Carrol, P. R., Presti, J. C., Jr., McAninch, J. W., and Tanagho, E. A.: Functional characteristics of the continent ileocecal urinary reservoir: Mechanisms of urinary continence. J. Urol., 142:1032–1036, 1989.

Castro, J. E., and Ram, M. D.: Electrolyte imbalance following ileal urinary diversion. Br. J. Urol., 42:29–32, 1970.

Chaput. Guerison d'une fistule ureterale elevee par l'abouchement dans le rectum. Ann. Des. Mal. Des Org. Gen. Ur., 26:466–471, 1905.

Chen, K. K., Chang, L. S., and Chen, M. T.: Urodynamic and clinical outcome of Kock pouch continent urinary diversion. J. Urol., 141:94–97, 1989.

Chute, R., and Sallade, R. L.: Bilateral side-to-side cutaneous urethrostomy in the midline for urinary diversion. J. Urol., 85:280–283, 1961.

Coffey, R. C.: A technique for simultaneous implantation of the right and left ureters into the pelvic colon which does not obstruct the ureters or disturb kidney function. Northwest Med., 24:211–215, 1925.

Cordonnier, J. J., and Spjut, H. J.: Urethral occurrence of bladder carcinoma following cystectomy. Trans. Am. Assoc. Genitourin. Surg., 53:13, 1961.

Crissey, M. M., Steele, G. D., and Gittes, R. F.: Rat model for carcinogenesis in ureterosigmoidostomy. Science, 207:1079, 1980.

Culp, D. A.: Commentary: Heitz-Boyer-Havelacque procedure: Not the procedure of choice. In Whitehead, E. D., and Leiter, E. (Eds.): Current Operative Urology, 2nd ed. New York, Harper and Row, 1984, pp. 782–783.

Dardel: Un nouveau procede de greffe de ureteres, l'ureterocholecystoneostomy. Ztlorg. f. d. ges. Chir. u. Grenzgeb., 15:193, 1922.

de Campos Freire, G.: In Glenn, J. F. (Ed.): Urologic Surgery. Philadelphia, J. B. Lippincott Co., 1983.

deKernion, J. B., Den Besten, L., Kaufman, J., and Ehrlich, R.: The Kock pouch as a urinary reservoir: pitfalls and perspectives. Am. J. Surg., 150:83, 1985.

Duckett, J. W., and Gazak, J. M.: Complications of ureterosigmoidostomy. Urol. Clin. North Am., 10:473–481, 1983.

Duckett, J. W., and Snyder, H. M., III: Use of the Mitrofanoff principle in urinary reconstruction. Urol. Clin. North Am., 13:271–274, 1986.

Duckett, J. W., and Snyder, H. M., III: The Mitrofanoff principle in continent urinary reservoirs. Semin. Urol., 5:55–62, 1987.

Duhamel, M. B. H.: Creation d'une nouvelle vessie par exclusion du rectum et abaissement retro-rectale et transanal du colon. J. Urol. Med. Chir., 63:925, 1957.

Eaton, G. L.: Transplantation of right ureter into appendix. Am. J. Urol., 6:230–232, 1910.

Eckstein, H. B.: Ureteral diversion. In Glenn, J. F. (Ed.): Urologic Surgery. Philadelphia, J. B. Lippincott Co., 1983, pp. 491–499.

Elder, D. D., Moisey, C. U., and Rees, R. W. M.: A long-term follow-up of the colonic conduit operation in children. Br. J. Urol., 51:462–465, 1979.

Feminella, J. G., and Lattimer, J. K.: A retrospective analysis of 70 cases of cutaneous ureterostomy. J. Urol., 106:538, 1971.

Ferguson, C.: Experimental transplantation of the ureters in the bowel by a two-stage operation. The Military Surgeon, 69:181–187, 1931.

Filmer, R. B., and Spencer, J. R.: Malignancies in bladder augmentations and intestinal conduits. J. Urol., 143:671–678, 1990.

Garske, G. L., Sherman, L. A., Twidwell, J. E., and Tenner, R. J.: Urinary diversion: Ureterosigmoidostomy with continent pre-anal colostomy. J. Urol., 84:322–333, 1960.

Garske, G. L., Sherman, L. A., Twidwell, J. E., and Tenner, R. J.: In Whitehead, E. D., and Leiter, E. (Eds.): Current Operative Urology. New York, Harper and Row, 1984.

Gerber, A.: Improved quality of life following a Kock continent ileostomy. West. J. Med., 133:95, 1980.

Ghoneim, M. A., Kock, N. G., Kycke, G., and Shehab El-Din, A. B.: An appliance-free, sphincter-controlled bladder substitute: the urethral Kock pouch. J. Urol., 138:1150–1154, 1987.

Gilchrist, R. K., Merricks, J. W., Hamlin, H. H., and Rieger, I. T.: Construction of a substitute bladder and urethra. Surg. Gynecol. Obstet., 90:752–760, 1950.

Giordano, D.: Sulla questione se si possano trapiantare gli ureteri nel retto. Clin. Chir. Milano, 2:80–91, 1894.

Goldenberg, T.: Ueber die Totalexstirpation der Harnblase und die Versorgung der Ureteren. Beitr. z. Klin. Chir., 44:627–649, 1904.

Goldwasser, B., and Benson, R. C., Jr.: Continent urinary diversion. Mayo Clin. Proc., 61:615–621, 1986.

Goldwasser, B., Barrett, D. M., and Benson, R. C., Jr.: Complete bladder replacement using the detubularized right colon. In King, L. R., Stone, A. R., and Webster, G. D. (Eds.): Bladder Reconstruction and Continent Urinary Diversion. Chicago, Year Book Medical Publishers, 1987.

Golimbu, M., and Morales, P.: Jejunal conduits: technique and complications. J. Urol., 113:787–795, 1975.

Goodwin, W. E., Turner, R. D., and Winter, C. C.: Results of ileocystoplasty. J. Urol., 80:461–466, 1958.

Haltiwanger, E.: Sigmoid conduit. In Glenn, J. F. (Ed.): Urologic Surgery. Philadelphia, J. B. Lippincott Co., 1983, pp. 509–510.

Hampel, N., Bodner, D. R., and Persky, L.: Ileal and jejunal conduit diversion. Urol. Clin. North Am., 13:207–224, 1986.

Hautmann, R. E., Egghart, G., Frohneberg, D., and Miller, K.: The ileal neobladder. J. Urol., 139:39–42, 1988.

Heitz-Boyer, M., and Hovelacque, A.: Creation d'une nouvelle vessie et d'un nouvel uretre. J. d'Urol., 1:237–258, 1912.

Hendren, W. H.: Non-refluxing colon conduit for temporary or permanent urinary diversion in children. J. Pediatr. Surg., 10:381, 1975.

Hendren, W. H.: Urinary diversion and undiversion in children. Surg. Clin. North Am., 56:425, 1976.

Hendren, W. H.: Reoperative ureteral reimplantation: Management of the difficult case. J. Pediatr. Surg., 15:770–786, 1980.

Hensle, T. W.: Nutritional support of the surgical patient. Urol. Clin. North Am., 10:109, 1983.

Hickey, D. P., Soloway, M. S., and Murphy, W. M.: Selective urethrectomy following cystoprostatectomy for bladder cancer. J. Urol., 136:828–833, 1986.

Higgins, C. C.: Aseptic uretero-intestinal anastomosis. Surg. Gynecol. Obstet., 57:359–361, 1933.

Higgins, C. C.: Aseptic uretero-intestinal anastomosis. J. Urol., 31:791–802, 1934.

Hill, J. T., and Ransley, P. G.: The colonic conduit: a better method of urinary diversion? Br. J. Urol., 55:629–631, 1983.

Hinman, F.: The indication of nephrostomy preliminary to uretero-rectoneostomy. J.A.M.A., 86:921–926, 1926.

Hinman, F., and Weyrauch, H. M., Jr.: A critical study of the different principles of surgery which have been used in ureterointestinal implantation. Trans. Am. Assn. G.U. Surgeons, 29:15–156, 1936.

Hinman, F., Jr.: Overview: The choice between ureterosigmoidostomy with perineal (Gersuny, Heitz-Boyer) or abdominal (Mauclaire) colostomy. In Whitehead, E. D., and Leiter, E. (Eds.): Whitehead Operative Urology, 2nd ed. New York, Harper and Row, 1984, pp. 782–783.

Hinman, F., Jr.: Atlas of Urologic Surgery. Philadelphia, W. B. Saunders Co., 1989.

Husmann, D. A., McLorie, G. A., and Churchill, B. M.: Nonrefluxing colonic conduits: a long-term life-table analysis. J. Urol., 142:1201–1203, 1989.

Jakobsen, H., Steven, K., Stigsby, B., Larskov, P., and Hald, T.: Pathogenesis of nocturnal urinary incontinence after ileocaecal bladder replacement. Continuous measurement of urethral closure pressure during sleep. Br. J. Urol., 59:148–152, 1987.

Kim, K. S., Susskind, M. R., and King, L. R.: Ileocecal ureterosigmoidostomy: an alternative to conventional ureterosigmoidostomy. J. Urol., 140:1494–1498, 1988.

King, L. R.: Protection of the upper tracts in undiversion. In King, L. R., Stone, A. R., and Webster, G. D. (Eds.): Bladder Reconstruction and Continent Urinary Diversion. Chicago, Year Book Medical Publishers, 1987, pp. 127–153.

Klein, E. A., Montie, J. E., Montague, D. K., Kay, R., and Straffon, R. A.: Jejunal conduit urinary diversion. J. Urol., 135:244–246, 1986.

Knapp, P. M., Jr., Konnak, J. W., McGuire, E. J., and Savastano, J. A.: Urodynamic evaluation of ileal conduit function. J. Urol., 137:929–932, 1987.

Kock, N. G.: Ileostomy without external appliance: A survey of 25 patients provided with intestinal reservoir. Ann. Surg., 173:545, 1971.

Kock, N. G., Ghoneim, M. A., Lycke, K. G., and Mahran, M. R.: Urinary diversion to the augmented and valved rectum: Preliminary results with a novel surgical procedure. J. Urol., 140:1375–1379, 1988.

Kock, N. G., Ghoneim, M. A., Lycke, K. G., and Mahran, M. R.: Replacement of the bladder by the urethral Kock pouch: Functional results, urodynamics and radiological features. J. Urol., 141:1111–1116, 1989.

Kock, N. G., Nilson, A. E., Nilsson, L. O., et al.: Urinary diversion via a continent ileal reservoir: Clinical results in 12 patients. J. Urol., 128:469, 1982.

Kramolowsky, E. V., Clayman, R. V., and Weyman, P. J.: Endourological management of ureteroileal anastomotic strictures: Is it effective? J. Urol., 137:390–394, 1987.

Kramolowsky, E. V., Clayman, R. V., and Weyman, P. J.: Management of ureterointestinal anastomotic strictures: comparison of open surgical and endourological repair. J. Urol., 139:1195–1198, 1988.

Kronig: Die Anglegung eines Anus praeternaturalis zur Vermeidung der Colipyelitis bei Einpflanzung der Ureteren ins Rectum. Zentralbl. f. Gynak, 31:559–561, 1907.

Krynski, L.: Zur Technik der Ureterimplantation in den Mastdarm. Centralbl. i. Chir., 23:73–75, 1896.

Leadbetter, W. F., and Clarke, B. G.: Five years' experience with uretero-enterostomy by the "combined" technique. J. Urol., 73:67, 1954.

LeDuc, A., Camey, M., and Teillac, P.: An original antireflux ureteroileal implantation technique: Long-term follow-up. J. Urol., 137:1156–1158, 1987.

Lemoine, G.: Creation d'une vessie nouvelle par un procede personnel apres cystectomie totale pour cancer. J. d'Urol., 4:367–372, 1913.

Lengemann, P.: Ersatz der exstirpierten Harnblase durch das Coecum. Zentralbl. f. Chir., 40:14–15, 1913.

Leong, C. H.: Use of stomach for bladder replacement and urinary diversion. Ann. Roy. Coll. Surg., 60:283–289, 1978.

Libertino, J. A., and Zinman, L.: Ileocecal segment for temporary and permanent urinary diversion. Urol. Clin. North Am., 13:241–250, 1986.

Lieskovsky, G., Boyd, S. D., and Skinner, D. G.: Management of late complications of the Kock pouch form of urinary diversion. J. Urol., 137:1146, 1987.

Light, J. K., and Marks, J. L.: Total bladder replacement in the male and female using the ileocolonic segment (LeBag). Br. J. Urol., 65:467–472, 1990.

Light, J. K., and Scardino, P. T.: Radical cystectomy with preservation of sexual and urinary function: Use of the ileocolonic pouch ("LeBag"). Urol. Clin. North Am., 13:261–270, 1986.

Lockhart, J. L.: Remodeled right colon: an alternative urinary reservoir. J. Urol., 138:730–734, 1987.

Loening, S. A., Navarre, R. J., Narayana, A. S., and Culp, D. A.: Transverse colon conduit urinary diversion. J. Urol., 127:37–39, 1982.

Makkas, M.: Zur Behandlung der Blasenektopie Umwandlung der ausgeschalteten Coecum zur Blase und der Appendix zur Urethra. Zentralbl. f. Chir., 37:1073–1076, 1910.

Mansson, W.: The continent cecal urinary reservoir. In King, L. R., Stone, A. R., and Webster, G. D. (Eds.): Bladder Reconstruction and Continent Urinary Diversion. Chicago, Year Book Medical Publishers, 1987, p. 209.

Mansson, W., and Colleen, S.: Experience with a detubularized right colonic segment for bladder replacement. Scand. J. Urol. Nephrol., In press, 1990.

Mansson, W., Colleen, S., Forsberg, L., Larsson, I., Sundin, T., and White, T.: Renal function after urinary diversion. A study of continent caecal reservoir, ileal conduit, and colonic conduit. Scand. J. Urol. Nephrol., 18:307–315, 1984.

Marion: Exstrophie de la vessie. Creation d'une vessie nouvelle. Observations et. procedes operatoires, de MM. Cuneo, Heitz-Boyer et Hovelacque. Bull. et Mem. Soc. de Chir., 38:2–24, 1912.

Marshall, F. F.: Creation of an ileocolic bladder after cystectomy. J. Urol., 139:1264–1268, 1988.

Marshall, F. F., Mostwin, J. C., Radebaugh, L. C., Walsh, P. C., and Brendler, C. B.: Ileocolic neobladder post cystectomy: Continence and potency. J. Urol., In press, 1990.

Mauclaire: De quelques essais de Chirurgie experimentale applicables au traitement (a) de lexstrophie de la vessie; (b) des abouchements anormaux du rectum; (c) des anus contre nature complexes. Congres Francais de Chirurgie, pp. 546–552, 1895.

Maydl, K.: Ueber die radikaltherapie der Ectopia vesicae urinariae. Wien. Med. Wchnschr., 44:1113–1115, 1894.

McLeod, R. S., and Fazio, V. W.: Quality of life with the continent ileostomy. World J. Surg., 8:90, 1984.

Melchior, H., Spehr, C., Knop-Wagemann, I., Persson, M. C., and Juenemann, K. P.: The continent ileal bladder for urinary tract reconstruction after cystectomy: A survey of 44 patients. J. Urol., 139:714–718, 1988.

Middleton, A. W., Jr., and Hendren, W. H.: Ileal conduits in children at the Massachusetts General Hospital from 1955 to 1970. J. Urol., 115:591–595, 1976.

Mingledorf, W. E., Rinker, J. R., and Owen, G.: Experimental study of the blood supply of the distal ureter with reference to cutaneous ureterostomy. J. Urol., 92:424, 1964.

Mogg, R. A.: The treatment of urinary incontinence using the colonic conduit. J. Urol., 97:684–692, 1967.

Moskowicz: Verhand. Deut. Gesell. f. Chir., 38:32, 1909.

Muller, P. A.: Abanderung der Borelius'schen Modifikation der Maydl'schen Operationsmethode bei kongenitaler Blasenektopie. Zentralbl. f. Chir., 30:886, 1903.

Muscatello, G.: Zur Radicalbehandlung der Blasenektopie. Arch. f. klin. Chir., 76:1066–1077, 1905.

Neal, D. E.: Complications of ileal conduit diversion in adults with cancer followed up for at least five years. Br. Med. J., 290:1695, 1985.

Nesbit, R. M.: Total cystectomy and ureteral transplantations in malignant conditions of the bladder with a description of a new operative procedure. J.A.M.A., 105:852–854, 1935.

Norlen, L., and Trasti, H.: Functional behavior of the continent ileum reservoir for urinary diversion. An experimental and clinical study. Scand. J. Urol. Nephrol. (Suppl.), 49:33–42, 1978.

Olsson, C. A.: Continent urinary diversion. J. Urol., 132:1157–1158, 1984.

Olsson, C. A.: Kock continent ileal reservoir for urinary diversion. In King, L. R., Stone, A. R., and Webster, G. D. (Eds.): Bladder Reconstruction and Continent Urinary Diversion. Chicago, Year Book Medical Publishers, 1987, pp. 291–310.

Pagano, F., Artibani, W., Ligato, P., Piazza, R., Garbeglio, A., and Passerini, G.: Vesica Ileale Padovana: a technique for total bladder replacement. Eur. Urol., 17:149–154, 1990.

Pernet, F. P. P. M., and Jonas, U.: Ileal conduit urinary diversion: early and late results of 132 cases in a 25-year period. World J. Urol., 3:140, 1985.

Piser, J. A., Mitchell, M. E., Kulb, T. B., et al.: Gastrocystoplasty and colocystoplasty in canines: the metabolic consequences of acute saline and acid loading. J. Urol., 138:1009, 1987.

Reddy, P. K.: Detubularized sigmoid reservoir for bladder replacement after cystoprostatectomy. Urology, 29:625–628, 1987.

Reddy, P. K.: Non-stomal continent reservoir: use of detubularized ileal segment for bladder replacement. World J. Urol., 5:190–193, 1987.

Regan, J. B., and Barrett, D. M.: Stented versus nonstented ureteroileal anastomoses: Is there a difference with regard to leak and stricture? J. Urol., 134:1101–1103, 1985.

Remedi, V.: Un caso di estrofia della vescica. La Clinica Chirurgica, 14:608–640, 1906.

Richie, J. P.: Sigmoid conduit urinary diversion. Urol. Clin. North Am., 13:225–232, 1986.

Richie, J. P., and Skinner, D. G.: Urinary diversion: The physiological rationale for non-refluxing colonic conduits. Br. J. Urol., 47:269–275, 1975.

Riedmiller, H., Steinbach, F., Thuroff, J., and Hohenfellner, R.: Continent appendix stoma—A modification of the MAINZ pouch technique. Presented E.A.U. Congress, Amsterdam, June 1990.

Rink, R. C., and Retik, A. B.: Ureteroileocecalsigmoidostomy and avoidance of carcinoma of the colon. In King, L. R., Stone, A. R., and Webster, G. D. (Eds.): Bladder Reconstruction and Continent Urinary Diversion. Chicago, Year Book Medical Publishers, 1987, pp. 172–178.

Rinker, J. R., and Blanchard, T. W.: Improvement of the circulation of the ureter prior to cutaneous ureterostomy: a clinical study. J. Urol., 96:44, 1966.

Rovsing, T.: En ny Metode til Helbredelse af Ektopia vesicae. Hospitalstidende, 59:1109–1121, 1916.

Rowland, R. G., Mitchell, M. E., and Bihrle, R.: The cecoileal continent urinary reservoir. World J. Urol., 3:185–190, 1985.

Rowland, R. G., Mitchell, M. E., Bihrle, R., Kahnoski, R. J., and Piser, J. E.: Indiana continent urinary reservoir. J. Urol., 137:1136–1139, 1987.

Rudick, J., Schonholz, S., and Weber, H. N.: The gastric bladder: a continent reservoir for urinary diversion. Surgery, 82:1, 1977.

Schellhammer, P. F., and Whitmore, W. F., Jr.: Transitional cell carcinoma of the urethra in men having cystectomy for bladder cancer. J. Urol., 115:56, 1976.

Scheidler, D. M., Klee, L. W., Rowland, R. G., et al.: Update on the Indiana continent urinary reservoir. J. Urol., 141:302A, 1989.

Schlegel, P. N., and Walsh, P. C.: Neuroanatomical approach to radical cystoprostatectomy with preservation of sexual function. J. Urol., 138:1402, 1987.

Schmidt, J. D., Bucksbaum, H. J., and Nachtsheim, D. A.: Long-term follow-up, further experience with, and modifications of the transverse colon conduit in urinary tract diversion. Br. J. Urol., 57:284–288, 1985.

Schmieden, V.: Erfahrungen bei zwei Totalexstirpationen der karzinomatosen Harnblase. Ztschr. f. Urol., 17:1–4, 1923.

Schreiter, F., and Noll, F.: Kock pouch and S bladder: two different ways of lower urinary tract reconstruction. J. Urol., 142:1197–1200, 1989.

Schwarz, G. R., and Jeffs, R. D.: Ileal conduit urinary diversion in children: computer analysis of follow-up from 2 to 16 years. J. Urol., 114:285–288, 1975.

Seiffert, L.: Die "Darm-siphonblase." Arch. f. klin. Chir., 183:569–574, 1935.

Shapiro, S. R., Lebowitz, R., and Colodny, A. H.: Fate of 90 children with ileal conduit urinary diversions a decade later: analysis of complications, pyelography, renal function, and bacteriology. J. Urol., 114:289–295, 1975.

Silberman, R.: Ammonia intoxication following ureterosigmoidostomy in a patient with liver disease. Lancet, 2:937–939, 1958.

Simon, J.: Ectropia vesicae (absence of the anterior wall of the bladder and pubic abdominal parietes); operation for directing the orifices of the ureters into the rectum; temporary success; subsequent death; autopsy. Lancet, 2:568–570, 1852.

Sinaiko, E.: Artificial bladder segment of stomach and study of effect of urine on gastric secretion. Surg. Gynecol. Obstet., 102:433, 1956.

Skinner, D. G., Boyd, S., and Lieskovsky, G.: Clinical experience with the Kock continent ileal reservoir for urinary diversion. J. Urol., 132:1101–1107, 1984.

Skinner, D. G., Lieskovsky, G., Skinner, E., and Boyd, S.: Urinary diversion. Curr. Probl. Surg., 24:401–471, 1987a.

Skinner, D. G., Lieskovsky, G., and Boyd, S.: Continuing experience with the continent ileal reservoir (Kock pouch) as an alternative to cutaneous urinary diversion: an update after 250 cases. J. Urol., 141:1140–1145, 1987b.

Skinner, D. G., Lieskovsky, G., and Boyd, S.: Continent urinary diversion. J. Urol., 141:1323–1327, 1989.

Smith, T.: An account of an unsuccessful attempt to treat extroversion of the bladder by a new operation. St. Barth. Hosp. Rep., 15:29–35, 1879.

Spirnak, J. P., and Caldamone, A. A.: Ureterosigmoidostomy. Urol. Clin. North Am., 13:285–294, 1986.

Straffon, R. A., Kyle, K., and Corvalan, J.: Techniques of cutaneous ureterostomy and results in 51 patients. J. Urol., 143:138–146, 1970.

Studer, U., Ackermann, D., Casanova, G. A., and Zingg, E. J.: A newer form of bladder substitute based on historical perspectives. Semin. Urol., 6:57–65, 1988.

Studer, U., Ackermann, D., Casanova, G. A., and Zingg, E. J.: Three years' experience with an ileal low pressure bladder substitute. Br. J. Urol., 63:43–52, 1989.

Sullivan, J. W., Grabstald, H., and Whitmore, W. F., Jr.: Complications of ureteroileal conduit with radical cystectomy: review of 336 cases. J. Urol., 124:797–801, 1980.

Svare, J., Walter, S., Kristensen, J. K., and Lund, F.: Ileal conduit urinary diversion—Early and late complications. Eur. Urol., 11:83, 1985.

Thuroff, J. W., Alken, P., and Hohenfellner, R.: The MAINZ pouch (mixed augmentation with ileum 'n zecum) for bladder augmentation and continent diversion. *In* King, L. R., Stone, A. R., and Webster, G. D. (Eds.): Bladder Reconstruction and Continent Urinary Diversion. Chicago, Year Book Medical Publishers, 1987, p. 252.

Thuroff, J. W., Alken, P., Riedmiller, H., et al.: The MAINZ pouch (mixed augmentation ileum 'n zecum) for bladder augmentation and continent diversion. World J. Urol., 3:179, 1985.

Thuroff, J. W., Alken, P., Riedmiller, H., Jacobi, G. H., and Hohenfellner, R.: 100 cases of MAINZ pouch: Continuing experience and evolution. J. Urol., 140:283–288, 1988.

Tizzoni, and Foggi: Die Wiederherstellung der Harnblase. Centralbl. f. Chir., 15:921–924, 1888.

Turnbull, R. B., Jr., and Hewitt, C. R.: Loop-end myotomy ileostomy in the obese patient. Urol. Clin. North Am., 5:423–429, 1978.

Verhoogen, J.: Neostomie uretero-cecale. Formation d'une nouvelle poche vesicale et d'un nouvel uretre. Assoc. Franc. d'Urol., 12:352–365, 1908.

Vignoni, E.: Del trapiamento degli ureteri nell'intestimo. Gazz. Med. di Torino, 46:17–28, 1895.

Wallace, D. M.: Uretero-ileostomy. Br. J. Urol., 42:529–534, 1970.

Walsh, P. C., Lepor, H., and Eggleston, J. C.: Radical prostatectomy with preservation of sexual function: anatomical and pathological considerations. Prostate, 4:473, 1983.

Waters, W. B., Vaughan, D. J., Harris, R. G., and Brady, S. M.: The Kock pouch: initial experience and complications. J. Urol., 137:1151, 1987.

Webster, G. D., and King, L. R.: Further commentary: Cecal bladder. *In* King, L. R., Stone, A. R., and Webster, G. D. (Eds.): Bladder Reconstruction and Continent Urinary Diversion. Chicago, Year Book Medical Publishers, 1987, pp. 206–208.

Wenderoth, U. K., Bachor, R., Egghart, G., Frohneberg, D., Miller, K., and Hautmann, R. E.: The ileal neobladder: Experience and results of more than 100 consecutive cases. J. Urol., 143:492–497, 1990.

Williams, D. F., Burkholder, G. V., and Goodwin, W. E.: Uretero-sigmoidostomy: A 15-year experience. J. Urol., 101:168–170, 1969.

Winsburg-White, H. P.: A new method of implanting ureters into the bowel. Proc. Roy. Soc. Med., 26:1214–1216, 1933.

73
URINARY UNDIVERSION: REFUNCTIONALIZATION OF THE PREVIOUSLY DIVERTED URINARY TRACT

W. Hardy Hendren, M.D.

Diversion of the urinary tract by a variety of means has been used in treating certain urologic problems in infants and children (Hendren, 1976; Johnston, 1963; Mitchell and Rink, 1987b; Mitchell, 1981a and b; Perlmutter and Patil, 1972; Retik et al., 1967; Zinman and Libertino, 1975). A good example is the child with myelomeningocele and neuropathic bladder. In the 1950s, many of the children so treated were maintained on long-term urethral or suprapubic catheter drainage to make them dry and to relieve pressure on the upper tracts, if there was hydronephrosis. This treatment provided a poor quality of life because of recurrent infections, stones, and complications from inlying tubes.

It was considered to be a major advance when the ileal loop urinary diversion could be chosen for many of the children (Bricker, 1950). However, it was clear, in time, that the ileal loop urinary diversion also had many complications, including recurring infection because of reflux, stones, and stricture of the stoma or the bowel segment itself (Middleton and Hendren, 1976; Pitts and Muecke, 1979; Richie et al., 1974; Smith, 1972; Shapiro et al., 1975). This diversion also required living with a bag on the abdomen to collect urine.

Today, the majority of children with neuropathic bladders can be managed by intermittent catheterization, popularized by Lapides and colleagues (1976), or by various reconstructive operations, depending on the state of continence, the presence or absence of vesicoureteral reflux, the size and innervation of the bladder, and other factors. Intermittent catheterization has made it possible to reverse prior urinary diversions in myelodysplastic bladders (Perlmutter, 1980).

Progress has been made in managing various obstructive uropathies, such as boys with urethral valves (Bauer et al., 1974; Campaiola et al., 1985; Duckett, 1974; Glassberg, 1985; Hendren, 1970, 1971, 1974); children with ureteroceles (Hendren and Mitchell, 1979); and children with major malformations, such as epispadias and exstrophy of the bladder (Jeffs, 1986). Many advances have allowed the repair of these problems instead of resorting to urinary diversions, which in the past provided an "easy way out" for the surgeon but not a good long-term solution for the patient.

Continent urinary diversion (Gilchrist et al., 1950; King et al., 1987a and b; Kock et al., 1982; Mitrofanoff, 1980; Skinner et al., 1984; Thuroff et al., 1988), which entails construction of an internal reservoir or pouch of bowel for storage of urine that can be intermittently catheterized by the patient, has come into use in the past several years, much like the ileal loop in the 1950s and 60s. *It is my hope that the continent diversion does not become overused instead of performing appropriate reconstructive surgery for those complex problems that can be repaired.*

This chapter summarizes a 20-year experience in reconstructing the previously diverted urinary tract of 182 patients. Figure 73–1 shows the types of urinary diversions present in these patients. Many reasons were given for the original diversions, such as complex anatomy, thought to be unsalvageable except by diversions; failed ureteral reimplantation surgery; urinary incontinence; and hydronephrosis, thought to be too severe to be corrected. In most such cases today, diversions can be avoided (Hendren, 1978a and 1980a). The majority of the patients had diversions originally planned as permanent measures. Others had undergone diversions as temporary measures, such as loop ureterostomy, nephrostomy, and vesicostomy. However, in many instances, the "temporary" diversion had been present for many years.

URINARY UNDIVERSION
1969 - 1990   182 CASES

66	ILEAL LOOP (14 pyelo-ileal)	127	permanent diversions
14	COLON CONDUIT (3 had been ileal loops)	55	temporary diversions
39	LOOP URETEROSTOMY or PYELOSTOMY	70	females
		112	males
17	END URETEROSTOMY	46	pts. had one kidney (2 a transplant)
38	CYSTOSTOMY or VESICOSTOMY	1	patient anephric (later transplanted)
7	NEPHROSTOMY		
1	URETEROSIGMOIDOSTOMIES		

12 personal diversions; 170 had been diverted elsewhere

Figure 73–1. Undiversion case data.

A total of 46 of the patients had only one kidney—in two of them, a renal transplant, one into an ileal loop and one into the bladder with a continuing vesicostomy. Another patient had no kidneys at all, having been on hemodialysis after two failed transplants. He also had the same poor, noncompliant bladder that had initially led to renal deterioration. The lower urinary tract was reconstructed and augmented, and a third transplant was performed successfully with a living related donor, his mother.

Figure 73–2 shows the ages of the patients. Any patient with a urinary diversion, regardless of age, should be thought of as a possible candidate for undiversion. Indeed, a series of undiversions in adults has been reported (Goldstein and Hensle, 1981).

Figure 73–3 shows the duration of urinary diversion. The longest was an ileal loop that had been done 27 years previously, when the patient was only 4 years old. Thus, a long duration of a urinary diversion is not a contraindication to eventual repair.

GENERAL CONSIDERATIONS

When considering an individual patient for possible refunctionalization of the diverted urinary tract, a number of factors must be weighed. Every patient differs in some respect from all of the others that one may have treated. It is important to examine why the patient's urinary tract was previously diverted. The most common causes encountered include severe obstructive uropathy from urethral valves, prune-belly syndrome, failed ureteral reimplantation, failed megaureter repair, failed surgery for urinary incontinence, stricture of the urethra, and myelodysplasia causing neurogenic bladder.

If the patient was originally incontinent, obviously undiversion will require not only joining the upper tract to the bladder but also correcting that problem. Correction may involve revising the bladder outlet, creating a urethra (Hendren, 1980b), increasing the size and compliance of the bladder, or all of these. Bladder augmentation can be done by a variety of techniques.

Renal Function

Many patients with diverted urinary tracts have reduced renal function. About a third of those for whom I have performed undiversions had such severe upper tract damage at the outset that it could be predicted that transplantation would be necessary in the future. To date, 23 of the patients have undergone renal transplantations (three antedated reconstruction). Approximately 40 others from the group will likely need transplantations as they grow older, judging from the present creatinine clearance rates and the state of the upper tracts. It is common to see a steady rise in serum creatinine levels as young patients grow, especially at adolescence when the body mass increases to a size greater than poor kidneys can support.

In a patient with borderline renal function, undiversion has invariably improved the quality of life between the time of reconstruction and the time when dialysis or transplantation was needed. Many patients with diver-

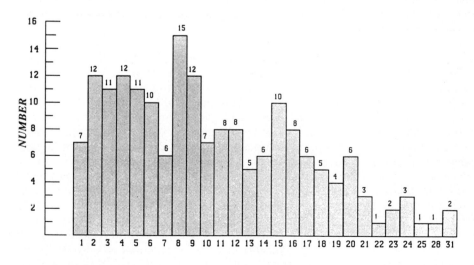

AGE, YEARS

Figure 73–2. Age in 182 patients with undiversions.

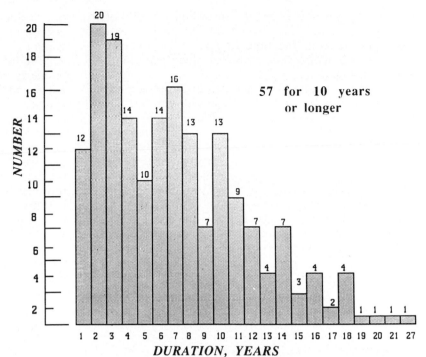

Figure 73–3. Duration of diversion in 182 patients with undiversions.

sions have chronic bacilluria. It is often possible to maintain a sterile urinary tract after undiversion. When transplantation is necessary in these patients, it is much better done into a functioning lower urinary tract than into a urinary diversion that imposes additional possible complications.

If bowel is to be utilized in the urinary tract, one should anticipate solute reabsorption through the bowel surface (Ferris and Odel, 1950; Koch and McDougal, 1985). The patient so treated must be followed closely. All patients with diminished renal function are managed collaboratively with a nephrologist. This collaborative monitoring is of great help in maintaining metabolic homeostasis when there is declining renal function. This practice has provided a smooth transition to dialysis and transplantation for the patient who has reached that stage.

Psychologic Factors

A patient with a long-term urinary diversion has grown accustomed to it as a way of life. If undiversion should require temporary or permanent intermittent self-catheterization postoperatively to empty the bladder, such as in neuropathic bladder, the patient must be fully prepared to cooperate and to do this. Failure to comply with this regimen is one of the factors that can lead to spontaneous rupture of the bladder, if augmentation cystoplasty has been performed (Elder et al., 1981; Rushton et al., 1988; Sheiner and Kaplan, 1988).

Anesthesia

Undiversion operations are long and complicated— seldom do they last less than 5 to 6 hours. The most

difficult one I have performed lasted 20 hours. The child had undergone 13 prior operations. Undiversion required repair of ureters, bladder neck, urethra, and vagina and simultaneous repositioning of a previously pulled through rectum. Obviously, expert anesthesia management is mandatory. Constant monitoring of acid-base balance and blood gases should be in effect along with replacement of blood and fluids. These patients cannot withstand inadequate fluid replacement, which can cause renal tubular necrosis. Fluid replacement for ordinary intra-abdominal pediatric surgical operations is in the range of 5 ml per kilogram of body weight per hour.

In my experience, these patients generally require four to five times that volume, i.e., 20 to 25 ml per kilogram per hour, to maintain a satisfactory urinary output intraoperatively. These amounts are reduced appropriately for older adult patients. Wide retroperitoneal dissection and exposure of the intestines create enormous fluid losses and "third spacing."

If only parameters of blood pressure and hematocrit are followed to estimate fluid requirements, replacement will fall behind. We routinely measure urinary output intraoperatively as a guide for the anesthesiologist. Even when the urinary tract has been taken apart, by securing a catheter within each ureter while working, a timed output can be obtained for each kidney, draining the end of the catheter into a small receptacle in the operative field. This gives a very good guide to speeding up or slowing down fluid administration during these long cases. Invariably, the anesthesiologist who has not been involved in these major cases will fall behind in replacement of fluid and blood. Renal shutdown from inadequate volume replacement is a preventable complication and its importance cannot be overemphasized. Many patients with renal failure and inability to concentrate urine have an obligatory high output. Preoperatively, they are not placed on an ordinary "NPO after midnight regimen." They are maintained on intravenous fluid therapy from the time oral intake is stopped in order to be adequately hydrated when entering the operating room.

Nitrous oxide should be avoided in these long cases. It diffuses into the gut and creates distention, which makes intraoperative exposure and later wound closure significantly more difficult. Not only should nitrous oxide be avoided during these cases, but also during the induction of anesthesia. I have opened many bellies containing bowel filled with gas, which required milking the gas up to the stomach to evacuate it. This is a poor way to start a major operation. Continuous epidural analgesia has proved very helpful in the last several years, reducing the amount of anesthesia required intraoperatively, and providing pain relief postoperatively. This analgesia will give reduced sensation to the legs and feet. Safeguards must be taken against compression of the lower extremities by tightly fitting bandages, which can cause pressure sores.

Assessment of Bladder Function

Urodynamic evaluation of the lower urinary tract is an important tool in modern day urology and can help in some cases (Bauer et al., 1980). Nevertheless, it has not been the keystone for predicting how a long defunctionalized bladder will function when urine flow is reestablished. Cystography will demonstrate bladder size and sensation as well as the presence of diverticula, urethral valves, and reflux into ureteral stumps. Cystoscopy can provide additional information. Usually, the long diverted bladder is small and has a smooth lining, which bleeds readily when filled with irrigating solution under pressure. It is important not to overfill the bladder, which can cause it to rupture, a complication we have encountered on four occasions when attempting to stretch a bladder preoperatively using anesthesia.

Preoperative "bladder cycling" can help (Kogan, 1976 and 1977). A small Silastic catheter is introduced during cystoscopy. The patient is taught to fill the bladder with saline to test continence, ability to empty, and stretch. Some bladder capacities increase rapidly in just a week or two from a very small initial capacity of 2 or 3 ounces, to a normal or near-normal capacity—others will not. This finding may signify the need for augmentation during undiversion. The length of time spent doing bladder cycling may vary from a few days to several months, depending on the findings, the degree of cooperation of the patient, and other factors. Optimally, the patient should fill the bladder by rapid drip from a reservoir bottle about 3 to 4 feet above the level of the bladder. This is done as many times during the day as possible. The irrigating fluid is tap water to which 2 teaspoons of salt per quart were added. (Boiled to sterilize it and cooled before use.) A few milliliters of 0.5 per cent neomycin or other antibiotic solution are added to this solution to reduce the likelihood of contamination and infection.

Occasionally, the catheter will pass through the bladder neck into the urethra so that irrigation will not fill

the bladder. In this instance, it can be pulled back an appropriate distance to remedy the problem. If the patient's original problem was urinary incontinence, it will be of no avail to attempt cycling the bladder. Similarly, if it is a tiny scarred bladder that leaks after a few milliliters are introduced into it, cycling will prove fruitless. In point of fact, I cycle bladders today preoperatively much less often than 10 years ago. In part, this change is from being more willing to augment the small bladder with intestine when it is too small, and in part, perhaps, from having a selectively poorer group of patients on whom to do undiversions compared with those earlier in my experience.

When urethral valves are encountered at cystoscopy in a patient whose bladder is diverted, they can be destroyed by fulguration if bladder cycling is to commence immediately. Conversely, urethral valves should never be fulgurated in a "dry urethra" that will remain dry postoperatively. In several cases, I have seen that fulguration leads to impermeable strictures (Crooks, 1982), creating a need for an additional reconstructive operation.

SURGICAL PRINCIPLES

The bowel is cleansed thoroughly preoperatively. Clear liquids are taken by mouth for 2 days preoperatively. Gastrointestinal lavage takes place the night before using GoLYTELY. This polyethylene glycol electrolyte gastrointestinal lavage solution is a powder that is diluted with tap water and administered orally. It passes rapidly through the gastrointestinal tract, cleaning it well. An adult patient drinks 4 liters of this solution, taking one 8-ounce glass by mouth every 10 minutes until the entire 4 liters is consumed. By the time the fourth or fifth glass is swallowed, the first begins passing by rectum, washing out the gastrointestinal tract effectively. A reduced amount is given to children. Pediatric patients are usually given the solution by tube, because most will not voluntarily drink a large volume of fluid. It has a slightly salty taste. Rapid administration is essential for it to be effective. It is my impression that a GoLYTELY bowel preparation may dehydrate the patient somewhat, an added point to bear in mind, especially in the patient with high output renal failure as mentioned earlier. Preoperative and intraoperative broad-spectrum antibiotic administration is given in these cases.

Wide Transabdominal Exposure

This is essential. Although some patients will have had previous urologic surgery through a transverse lower abdominal incision, a long midline incision is preferred, usually from the pubis to the xiphoid. This incision will give access to all levels of the urinary tract. A large ring retractor is desirable. To expose the kidneys and ureters, the right and left colon are mobilized and reflected medially. When the ureter is mobilized, all of its periureteral tissue should be kept with it, skeletonizing the other structures in the retroperitoneum, not the ureter

(Fig. 73–4). The gonadal vessels should be maintained with the ureter for collateral blood supply. We have done this many times without loss of a testis or an ovary. Similarly, the kidney can be mobilized and moved downward and medially to facilitate obtaining sufficient length for a foreshortened ureter, whether it is to be joined to the bladder or to the contralateral renal pelvis or ureter.

Psoas Hitch

This is a most helpful adjunct (Fig. 73–5). It can compensate for some shortness of the ureter, which must be implanted without tension. It can also allow a super-long tunnel to be obtained, which is necessary if reflux is to be prevented when reimplanting a bowel segment or a slightly dilated and scarred ureter. Obtaining a tunnel length-to-ureter diameter ratio of 5:1 may mandate having a tunnel 5 to 10 cm long. Fixation to the psoas muscle will allow that—it anchors the ureteral hiatus, and when the bladder fills no angulation and obstruction of the ureter occur. The hitch is done with monofilament nonabsorbable sutures (Prolene), taking care not to enter the bladder lumen. Note that the reimplant is performed before the bladder psoas hitch.

Transureteroureterostomy or Transureteropyelostomy

This is another extremely useful adjunct in these cases (Hendren and Hensle, 1980; Hodges et al., 1963) (Fig. 73–6). It is rarely feasible to join two ureters to the bladder in reoperative cases. Most often, the better ureter is implanted, draining the other across into it. This maneuver must be done without tension. It is important to avoid angulation of a ureter beneath a mesenteric vessel, especially the inferior mesenteric artery. When mobilizing a ureter to be swung over to the opposite side, the same principle should be employed as shown in Figure 73–4, i.e., mobilizing it with all of its periureteral tissue and the gonadal vessels, so that its blood supply will be well maintained.

The contralateral ureter to receive it is not mobilized and is not brought over to meet the end of the ureter to be drained into it. Both ureters are routinely drained by a soft, 5 Fr. plastic catheter, passed through the abdominal wall, the side wall of the bladder, and up the common ureter, threading one to each kidney before the anastomosis is completed. These catheters provide individual drainage of each kidney and are also useful to determine differential function. A contrast study is performed 10 to 12 days postoperatively to exclude a leak. (None has been encountered in more than 150 transureteroureterostomies.) The catheters are removed one at a time, a day apart.

Bladder Augmentation

This is an indispensable part of the urologic armamentarium (Courvelaire, 1950; Goldwasser and Webster, 1986; Goodwin et al., 1958 and 1959; Kass and Koff, 1983; Linder et al., 1983; Mitchell, 1981a; Mitchell et al., 1986 and 1987; Sidi et al., 1986 and 1987; Smith et al., 1977; Stephenson and Mundy, 1985; Turner-Warwick, 1979; Whitmore and Gittes, 1983). In 62 of our 182 undiversion cases augmentation was needed. Whereas bladder augmentation was at one time used principally in adult patients with bladder tuberculosis, interstitial cystitis, and carcinoma, in later years it has become a mainstay of urologic reconstructive surgery. My own experience with augmentation includes 146 cases with a wide variety of indications, but the need in all was to enlarge the capacity of the bladder (Hendren

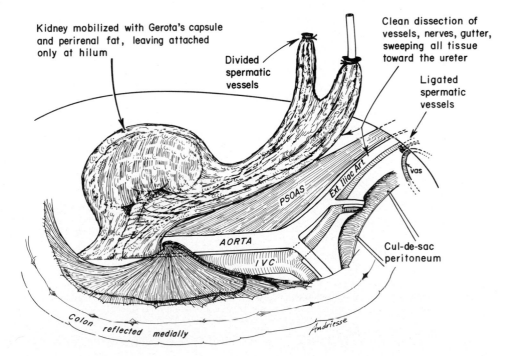

Figure 73–4. Technique for mobilizing kidney and ureter to gain additional length by wide dissection of structures, while preserving periureteral tissue for blood supply, including gonadal vessels (IVC, inferior vena cava; vas, vas deferens).

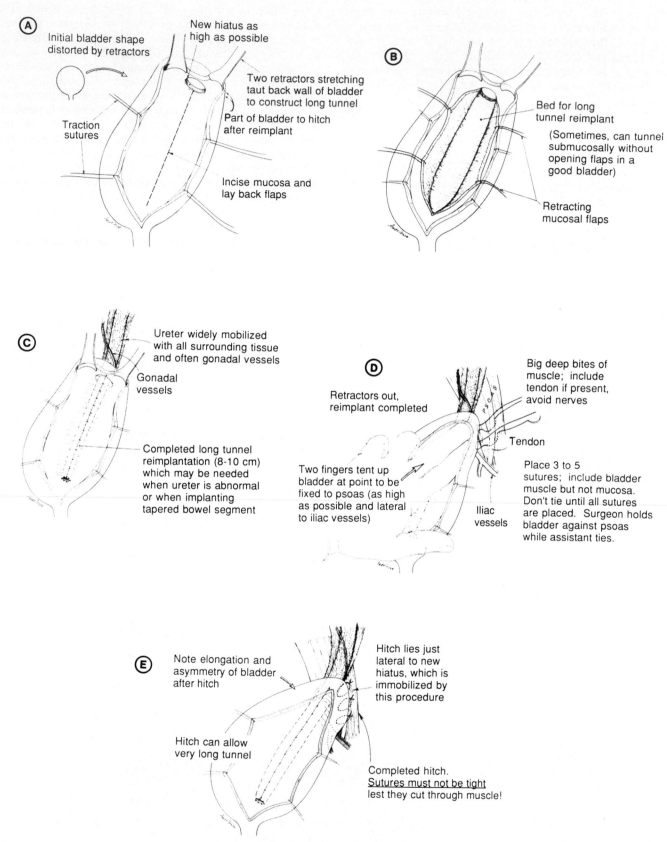

Figure 73–5. *A* to *E*, Technique for psoas hitch, which allows the creation of a very long reimplantation tunnel and prevents angulation of the ureter or tapered bowel segment when the bladder fills. Monofilament nonabsorbable suture material is used to fix bladder to psoas muscle. Care must be taken to avoid entering the bladder to avoid stone formation on a suture.

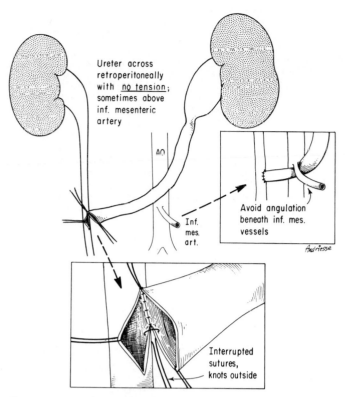

Figure 73–6. Technique for transureteroureterostomy (AO, aorta; inf. mes. art., inferior mesenteric artery).

and Hendren, 1990). The segments were cecum, 65; sigmoid, 34; small intestine, 27; stomach, 19; and left colon, 1. Experience has shown that whatever segment is added to the bladder, it should be "detubularized" so that the bowel cannot exert peristaltic waves, which may excede in amplitude the resistance of the bladder neck and cause incontinence.

In some patients, the surgeon may have a wide choice of bowel segment. In others, this choice may be restricted, such as with cloacal exstrophy in which there is little or no colon. The small bowel may be short, making gastrocystoplasty the only reasonable choice. The stomach has some outstanding advantages as a means for augmentation (Adams et al., 1988; Kennedy et al., 1988; Leong, 1978). Stomach is metabolically better than bowel or colon regarding chloride absorption and base loss, which occur in segments of small bowel and colon. The small bowel segments tend to lose bicarbonate and potassium and to a lesser extent sodium, while reabsorbing chloride. However, gastric mucosa secretes chloride ion and is, therefore, better in patients with poor renal function who cannot tolerate an increase in solute resorption, which can aggrevate acidosis. Furthermore, the urine is more often sterile after gastrocystoplasty because it is less alkaline.

In regard to ureteral drainage in patients undergoing bladder augmentations, we prefer to place one or both ureters into the bladder if that is possible. However, frequently, the ureters are too short or the bladder is too scarred to accomplish even one good ureteral reimplantation. Therefore, it may be necessary to implant the ureter into the augmentation. A good ureter (not too wide, not too scarred, adequate length) can be implanted with a tunnel in the colon, cecum, or stomach. We prefer the technique in which the ureter is tunneled beneath the mucosa from inside the bowel (Goodwin et al., 1953). If the ureters are too short or dilated to reimplant, they can be joined to the terminal ileum of a cecal cystoplasty, making an antireflux nipple of the intussuscepted terminal ileum (Fig. 73–7). An antireflux nipple will not stand the test of time unless it is sewn to the adjacent wall of the cecum to prevent its popping out of the cecum and allowing reflux. When there is no ureter, an inadequate terminal ileum, or a failed antireflux nipple, the technique shown in Figure 73–8 can be employed to drain the upper tracts into the cecum in order to prevent reflux.

When small bowel or sigmoid is chosen to augment the bladder, it is opened longitudinally, sewing the edges to one another to produce a cup-like dome to join to the bladder. A simple patch of bowel is utilized less often.

Although stomach provides an excellent source of tissue for increasing the size of the bladder, I believe it is technically more difficult and hazardous because of the long vascular pedicle required to bring the middle third of the stomach down to the pelvis. In sigmoid colon, the mesentery is adjacent to the bladder. Little danger exists of compromising the vascular pedicle. Similarly, the ileal mesentery or ileocecal mesentery seldom presents a problem in reaching the pelvis without tension. When stomach is to be used, the right gastroepiploic pedicle is best, although alternative techniques have been described (Leong, 1978).

The many small branches running from the right gastroepiploic artery to the greater curvature of the gastric antrum are divided in a meticulous manner. The length of this mobilization depends on the distance to which the stomach must be brought. Resecting the middle third of the stomach, while maintaining intact the lesser curvature, yields a large diamond-shaped patch with excellent blood supply. This patch is brought through the transverse mesocolon, usually to the right of the middle colic vessels. A generous tunnel is made beneath the small bowel mesentery, emerging at the terminal ileum to bring the patch and its pedicle to the bladder. The part of stomach most distant from the pedicle is sewn to the lowest part of the bladder opening, lastly closing the upper part of the opening near the vascular pedicle. It is important to avoid tension on the vascular pedicle.

In any type of augmentation the bladder is doubly drained, utilizing one catheter through the urethra and the other as a suprapubic tube through the augmentation and out the abdominal wall. The suprapubic tube remains postoperatively until the patient can void or self-catheterize. It can take a great deal of time and patience to teach a patient to catheterize, especially when an extensive narrowing of the urethra and bladder neck has been performed, such as in myelodysplasia or exstrophy-epispadias. Catheterization is not attempted until 2 weeks postoperatively. It often requires endoscopy using anesthesia to locate the passage and to dilate it to make catheterization possible. If the passage is not

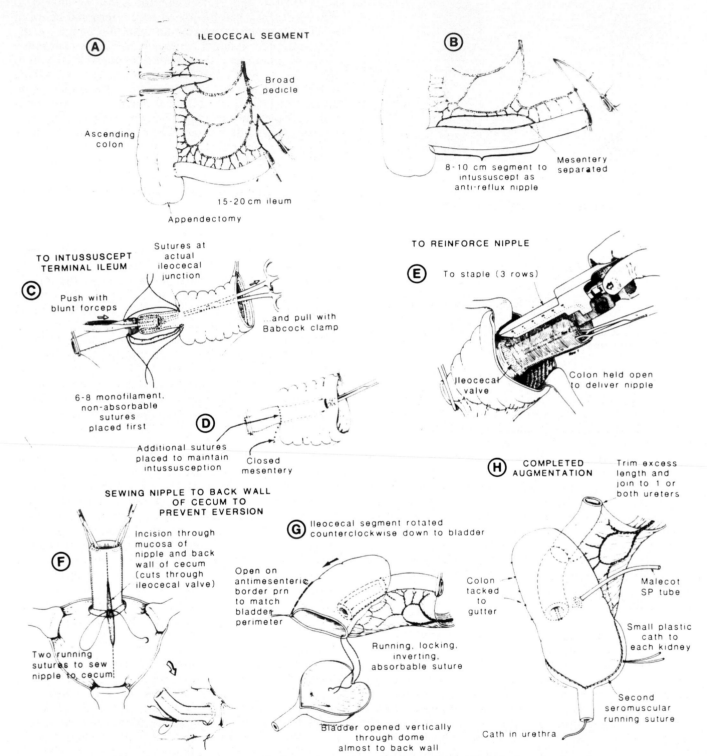

Figure 73–7. *A* to *H*, Technique for ileocecal cystoplasty with intussuscepted ileal nipple to prevent reflux.

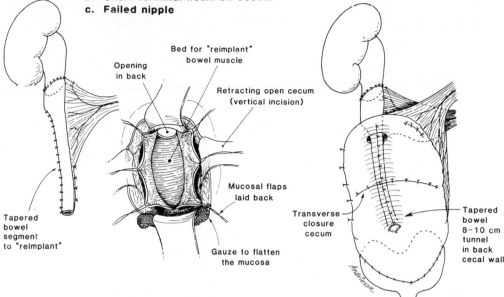

CECAL AUGMENTATION:
Preventing reflux when:
a. No ureter
b. Short terminal ileum on cecum
c. Failed nipple

Figure 73–8. "Ureter" from tapered small bowel.

visualized because of postoperative edema and the presence of sutures in the reconstructed bladder outlet, a ureteral catheter is passed upward, following it with the endoscope, just as one might negotiate a urethral stricture.

Blind dilatation is not safe, because it risks making a false passage. Catheterization can be done with a straight catheter, a coudé tipped catheter, or a catheterizing sound, depending on what is simplest in a given patient. The suprapubic tube is never removed until it is evident that the bladder can be emptied by either voiding or catheterization. Emptying should be done on a regular schedule, about every 4 hours, to avoid overfilling an augmentation. In young males whose urethras will accept only small catheters, saline irrigation and syringe aspiration may be necessary. Mucus can block a small catheter. Production of mucus seems to decrease in time when colon or small bowel is used. Mucus is less of a problem when stomach augments the bladder.

A cardinal principle in reconstructing previously diverted urinary tracts is to lay out all of the anatomic structures at the operating table, listing the various options available and choosing the one that has the greatest likelihood of success. In my experience, failure is much more likely when the surgeon attempts to get by with a minor procedure, with the aim of avoiding a major one. Generally, most of the more extensive procedures will succeed if they are well conceived and skillfully executed. The patient cannot tolerate a major complication, such as leakage from an anastomosis under tension, ureteral obstruction, or devascularization of a part of the urinary tract.

SELECTED CASES

The following cases, and others that have been described previously, illustrate some of the technical de-

tails to be encountered in undiversion surgery (Hendren, 1973, 1974b, 1987, and 1990). Because the ileal loop is the most common type of previous diversion extant, it is emphasized here. The same principles apply, however, with undiversions in patients with long-standing diversions by vesicostomy, end ureterostomy, loop ureterostomy, pyelostomy, or nephrostomy.

The principal options available in reconstructions of the urinary tract in patients with ileal loop diversions are shown in Figure 73–9. Autotransplantation will be indicated only rarely. Whenever the bowel loop can be discarded, using one or both ureters to drain the upper tracts into the bladder, that is preferred. Often this is not possible, however.

Case 1 (Figs. 73–10 and 73–11)

An 11-year-old boy was referred in 1974 with an ileal loop done at age 3 years. His original pathologic condition was urethral valves with hydronephrosis, infection, and stones. Prior surgery included suprapubic cystoscopy at age 3 months, bilateral pyelolithotomies at age 2 years, urinary diversion at age 3 years, and later a second left pyelolithotomy. The ileal loop was tapered and reimplanted with a long tunnel to prevent reflux. The patient is now 28 years of age, more than 17 years after undiversion. He is well, free from urinary infection or stones. Originally a scrawny youngster, with a bag on his abdomen and chronic urinary infection, he is now a robust adult (6 feet 3.5 inches tall). Creatinine clearance level is 48 $L/m^2/(BSA)$ per day, i.e., about 50 per cent of normal.

COMMENT. In tapering an ileal loop that is to serve as a substitute ureter, several important points must be respected. Mobilization of the ileal loop from the abdominal wall should be done with great care, because it may be necessary to use the full length of the bowel

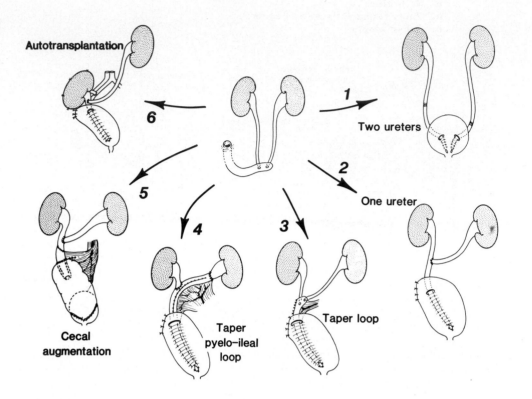

Figure 73–9. Principal options available for undiversion of an ileal loop.

Figure 73–10. Case 1 before *(A)* and after *(B)* reconstruction (TUR, transurethral).

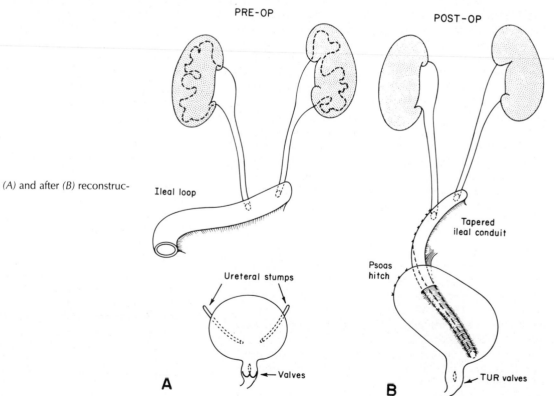

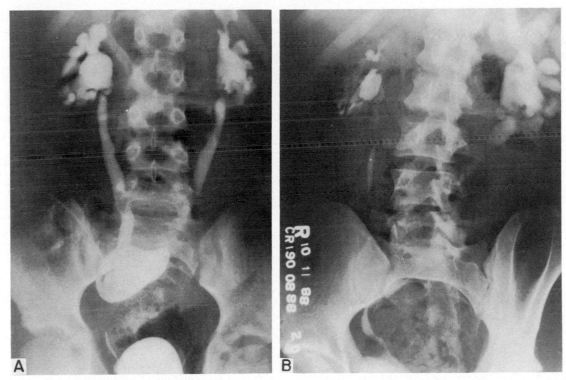

Figure 73–11. Case 1 roentgenograms. *A*, Preoperative simultaneous loopogram and cystogram. Note small bladder and short unusable ureteral stumps. *B*, Intravenous pyelogram 14 years after undiversion. Bladder size was normal.

segment. In dissecting free the intra-abdominal part of the loop, catheters through the loop and up the ureters can prove helpful. This dissection can be facilitated by gently distending the system with saline with a ligature occluding the end of the loop around the catheters. It is often necessary to incise the mesentery to straighten the loop, taking care not to devascularize the bowel.

The strip of bowel to be removed on its antimesenteric border should be marked with a skin pencil to ensure accuracy, resecting not more than one third of the circumference of the bowel. A two-layer inverting closure with catgut sutures requires several additional millimeters of bowel circumference. The first layer is running, inverting sutures. The second layer is interrupted sutures. It is important to create a nonrefluxing anastomosis of the tapered bowel to the bladder.

Because the bowel loop, even when tapered, will be 1 to 1.5 cm in diameter, the tunnel must be very long (5 to 10 cm). Obviously, this length will be possible only in a favorable bladder of good size. It is fruitless to attempt reimplantation of a tapered small bowel segment into a small, scarred, contracted bladder. The optimal method for making a long tunnel is shown in Figure 73–5.

Mucosal flaps are dissected sharply to prepare a bed for the tapered bowel. The tapered bowel is tacked to the muscle of the back wall of the bladder, with its suture line lying posteriorly, not adjacent to the mucosa to be closed over it in order to avert fistula formation. Psoas hitch is essential to immobilize the hiatus through which the tapered bowel segment enters the bladder wall. This practice will prevent angulation when the bladder fills.

In tapering 28 ileal loops and reimplanting them into the bladder, 19 attempts were completely successful, as in this patient. Nine patients required reoperations because of reflux. In six patients, it was possible to make a longer tunnel, which stopped the reflux. The bladders were basically good—in which a longer tunnel could be made. Three were poor bladders, indicating that it had been an error in judgment to attempt implantation of a tapered loop in the first place. Ileocecal cystoplasty solved the problem in these small, noncompliant bladders. Avoiding the pitfalls learned from experience, which have been mentioned previously, should lead to a high success rate when implantating a tapered bowel segment is necessary.

Patients with intestine in the urinary tract will notice mucus in the urine. Occasionally, a blob of mucus temporarily obstructs the urethra in a male during micturition. The amount of mucus, and the patient's awareness of it, seems to diminish in time. Late stricture is a well-known complication of ileal loop urinary diversions. Late stricture of a tapered bowel segment has been noted in three cases as well as in two other cases that were referred, with untapered bowel serving as ureter (Hendren and McLorie, 1983). This problem underscores the need to maintain long-term, continuing surveillance of all patients with bowel in the urinary tract, especially when it has been utilized as a substitute ureter. When bowel has been used as a ureter, it is easy to pass up from below with a straight endoscope. In two cases in which narrowing occurred later from a mucosal web, it was incised with a cutting electrode, dilated, and injected with triamcinolone diacetate, to help prevent future scar formation.

Case 2 (Figs. 73–12 and 73–13)

A 15-year-old boy with prune-belly syndrome was referred in 1973 for possible undiversion. Bilateral nephrostomies had been done at birth. Later, an ileal loop was done, but it had never drained. The left ureter was obstructed by the left colic artery; the right kidney was blocked by ureteropelvic junction obstruction. An extensive reconstruction was performed, converting the conduit to a pyeloileal conduit to correct obstruction of both ureters. The conduit was then tapered and implanted with a long tunnel to prevent reflux. Creatinine clearance at that time was 30 L/m²/BSA. The patient's clinical status was excellent during the next 9 years.

At age 25 years, after treatment of a duodenal ulcer with cimetidine, the serum creatinine level rose to 12 mg/dl. Dialysis was begun, and he received a kidney transplant from his brother. Now, at age 32 years, and 7 years after transplantation, the patient is in good general health and works full time as a stockbroker.

COMMENT. There were 14 patients with pyeloileal conduits among the 66 patients with ileal loops for undiversion. It is well recognized that patients with pyeloileal loops have the greatest degree of long-term deterioration when the loop drains into a bag on the abdominal wall. Thus, these patients in particular can benefit from eliminating the bags and diverting the drainage into the bladder, provided it is done in a manner that averts reflux. Bladder cycling was not used in 1975, but the bladder, which had been defunctioned since birth, increased in size and functioned well nevertheless. Nephritis is a rare complication of cimetidine therapy. Evidently, this tipped a precarious balance with renal function, which had been stable for several years. Considering the very bad state of the kidneys at birth, this patient represents a striking example of how careful metabolic management by an excellent nephrologist prevented the need for renal transplantation until age 25 years.

Case 3 (Figs. 73–14 and 73–15)

A 16-year-old boy was referred in 1982 with an ileal loop performed 8 years previously, after failed ureteral reimplantation surgery elsewhere two times. Hydrostatic stretching preoperatively increased the bladder size from about 50 to 250 ml. The boy was able to retain saline instilled into the bladder, and he could void it at will. At operation, both previously reimplanted lower ureters were too short to be useful. The strictured ileal loop also was unusable. Because the two kidneys and upper ureters were nearly normal, and this was a favorable bladder in which reimplantation of a ureter would be relatively simple, autotransplantation of the right kidney was done, draining the left kidney by transureteropyelostomy. The patient convalesced uneventfully following this lengthy operation. He is now age 25 years, works full time as a mechanic, has a child, and is free from urologic problems.

COMMENT. Autotransplantation is an operation that can be considered in selected cases. I have considered it the best choice in only two patients to date. Both had strictured ileal loops, raising the possibility that a bowel segment to be employed as a ureter might become strictured. Both had two good kidneys, lending a margin of safety in case the transplanted kidney should sustain a serious complication, although that is a low risk. It is vital to consider all possible methods in each case. Generally, the best choice will be clear when all factors are taken into account—renal function, length of the ureters, state of the bladder, and so on.

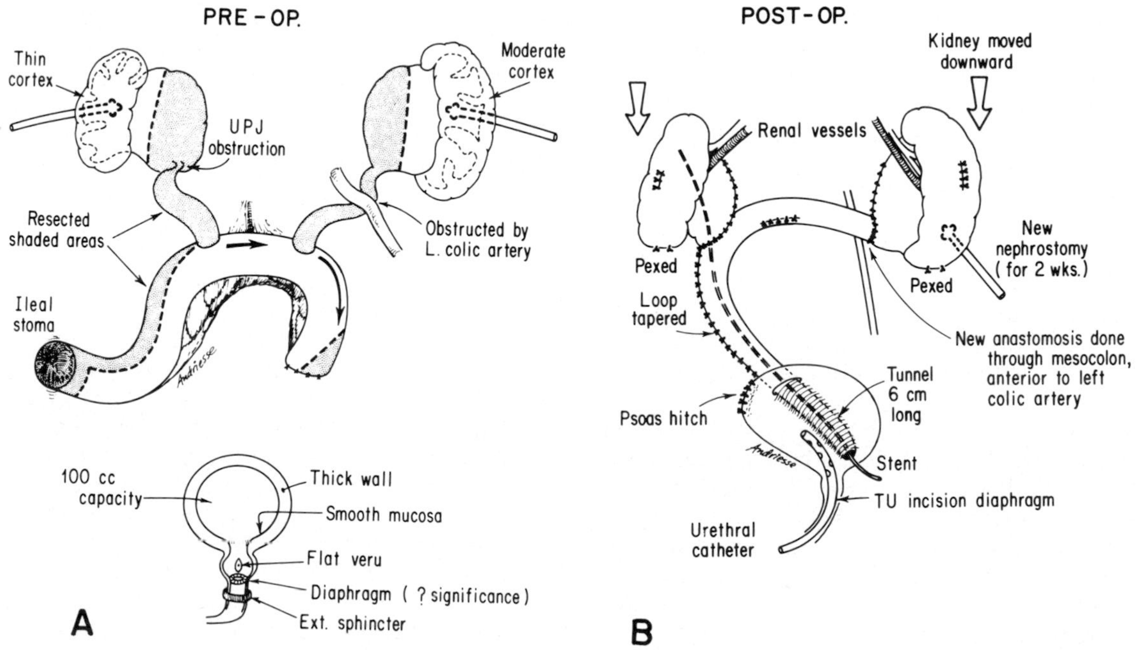

Figure 73–12. Case 2. Before *(A)* and after *(B)* reconstruction.

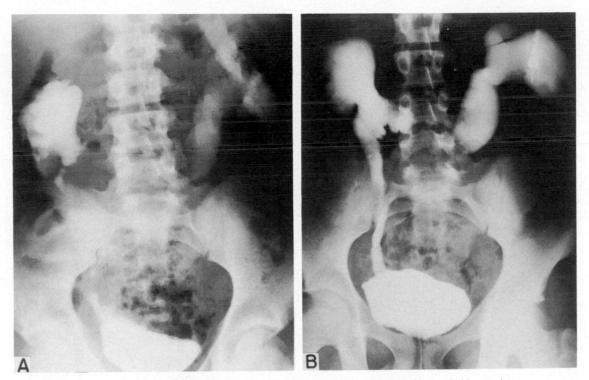

Figure 73–13. Case 2. Antegrade perfusion pyelography 8 years postoperatively. *A,* Bladder on drainage. *B,* Bladder being allowed to fill during the study. Note needle in left kidney.

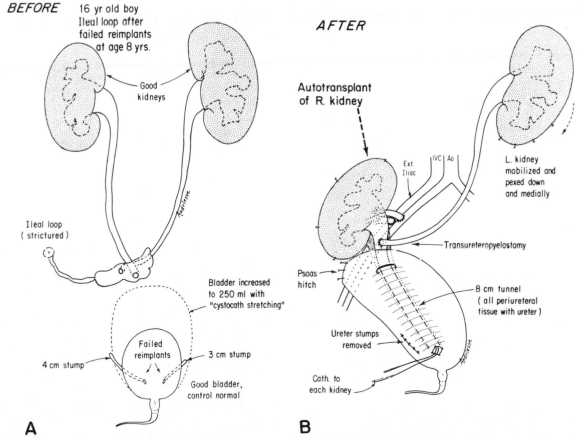

BEFORE   16 yr old boy
Ileal loop after
failed reimplants
at age 8 yrs.

Good kidneys

AFTER

Autotransplant of R. kidney

Ext. Iliac   IVC | Ao

L. kidney mobilized and pexed down and medially

Transureteropyelostomy

Ileal loop (strictured)

Bladder increased to 250 ml with "cystocath stretching"

Psoas hitch

8 cm tunnel (all periureteral tissue with ureter)

Ureter stumps removed

4 cm stump   Failed reimplants   3 cm stump

Good bladder, control normal

Cath. to each kidney

A   **B**

Figure 73–14. Case 3. Before *(A)* and after *(B)* reconstruction.

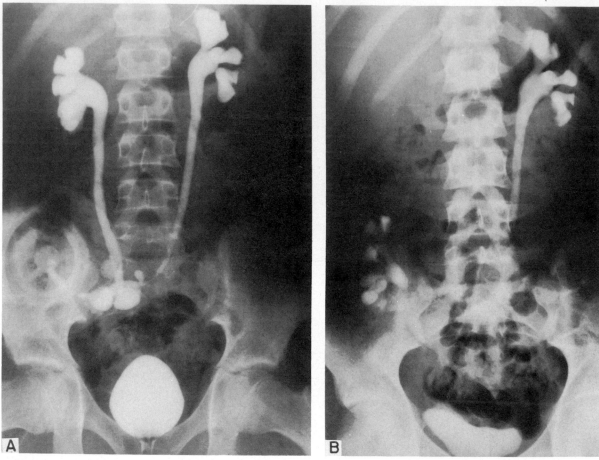

Figure 73–15. Case 3 roentgenograms. *A,* Preoperative simultaneous cystogram and loopogram. Note relatively small bladder and severely strictured ileal loop.

B, Intravenous pyelogram 1 year postoperatively. Note autotransplanted right kidney in right lower quadrant.

Case 4 (Figs. 73–16 and 73–17)

A 15-year-old girl was referred in 1982 with an ileal loop that had been present for 10 years. The underlying problem was a neurogenic bladder secondary to sacral agenesis. YV plasty had been performed to the bladder neck at age 2 years for inability to empty the bladder. Ileal loop was elected later because she was incontinent. Hydrostatic "cycling" of the bladder for 3 months showed that there was small capacity and complete incontinence. It could be predicted, therefore, that undiversion would require increasing outlet resistance as well as augmenting the bladder to provide a low-pressure reservoir of good size.

The patient's neurologic deficit showed that she must be prepared to do intermittent self-catheterization. Undiversion consisted of narrowing the bladder neck and urethra to increase outlet resistance and augmenting the bladder with cecum. The ureters were not satisfactory for reimplantation into the bladder or into the cecal wall. An antireflux mechanism was constructed by intussuscepting the terminal ileum to make a nipple, stapling the nipple, and sewing it to the back wall of the cecum. The right ureter was joined end to end and the left ureter end to side into the terminal ileum.

Postoperative urodynamic study showed urethral resistance of 85 cm H_2O, with a functional urethral length of 3.5 cm. The bladder capacity was 400 ml. The cecum did not exhibit uninhibited contraction waves. She has done well during the 9 years since undiversion. She empties the bladder without difficulty by self-catheterization, using a metal hollow sound. She is dry, free from urinary infection, and the kidneys have remained stable.

COMMENT. If an ileocecal nipple is made for prevention of reflux, it must be sewn to the back wall of the cecum or the nipple will pop out of the cecum and allow reflux. A report has been made in which ileocecal augmentation was performed in a patient with myelodysplasia, which resulted in diarrhea and required putting the ileal cecal valve back into the gastrointestinal tract (Gonzalez et al., 1986). Many patients with spina bifida and neurogenic bladder have alternating constipation and overflow diarrhea. Therefore, it may be better to retain the ileocecal valve in that group of patients if another method of augmentation and reflux prevention can be done.

I have found staples more reliable than simple sutures in approximating the walls of an intussuscepted nipple. Whenever staples are used, endoscopy should be performed several months later. Most become covered by mucosa. However, if some are still exposed, stones form on them. They can be plucked out by alligator forceps, through a panendoscope. However, if they are not

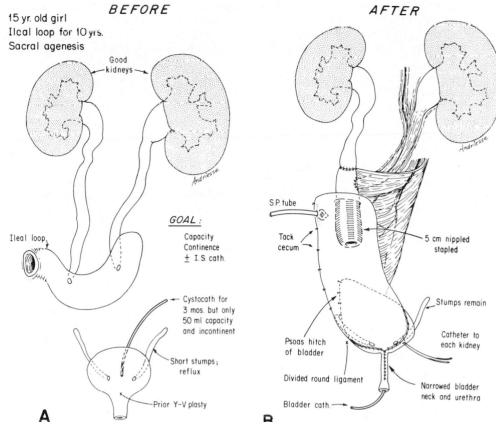

Figure 73–16. Case 4. Before *(A)* and after *(B)* reconstruction.

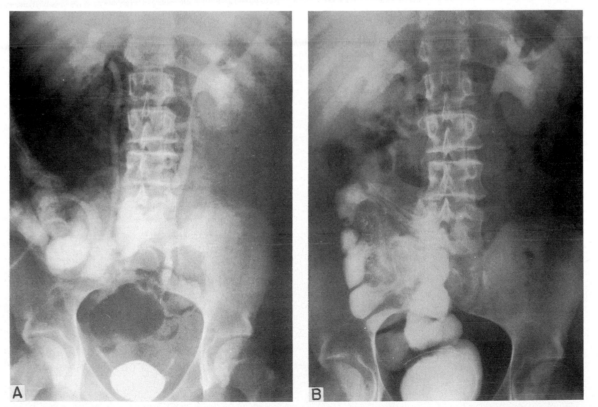

Figure 73–17. Case 4 roentgenograms. *A,* Simultaneous loopogram and cystogram preoperatively. Note small bladder and sacral agenesis.
B, Intravenous pyelogram 9 months postoperatively. Note the cecal augmentation of the small bladder and the filling defect in the cecum, which is intussuscepted terminal ileum. Note the staples in the nipple.

removed, the stones can become large and difficult to remove. In my opinion, staples should never be applied in the urinary tract in a location that is not easily accessible with a straight endoscope and an alligator forceps.

Artificial sphincters are utilized today in some medical centers to create continence in patients with these problems (Light and Engelmann, 1985; Mitchell and Rink, 1983; Scott et al., 1974). In my opinion, however, increasing outlet resistance and resorting to intermittent catheterization may prove safer and more satisfactory in the long term for most patients. There is still a substantial long-term failure rate with prosthetic devices. Narrowing the bladder neck does not "burn any bridges." If sphincter technology advances to a point at which there is no failure rate from erosion or mechanical malfunction, it would be relatively simple to open the previously narrowed bladder neck by endoscopic resection, creating incontinence, and subsequently implanting an artificial sphincter to control it.

Case 5 (Figs. 73–18 and 73–19)

A 3-year-old boy was referred in 1977 with bilateral loop cutaneous ureterostomies, suprapubic cystostomy, and complete stricture of the membranous urethra. Imperforate anus had been treated by colostomy when he was a newborn. Subsequent urinary tract evaluation at 6 months disclosed urethral valves and hydronephrosis. Cutaneous vesicostomy was performed, but the bladder prolapsed, causing increasing hydronephrosis.

Bilateral skin ureterostomies were performed. Later, the valves were resected, and a rectal pull through was done. The vesicostomy was closed and converted into a suprapubic cystostomy. Pyocystis was treated by antibiotic irrigation. Ileal loop urinary diversion was recommended but was declined by the parents, who then sought further advice.

Hydrostatic testing of the bladder showed good function despite previous diversion and pyocystis. At the first operation, the urethral stricture was resected and continuity was re-established by primary anastomosis. Undiversion was accomplished 8 weeks later. This included removing the nonfunctional right kidney, closing the left ureterostomy, reimplanting the left ureter, and excising the suprapubic cystostomy site. Today the patient is age 17 years, is 6 feet 1 inch tall and weighs 190 pounds. He has normal urinary control and normal bowel control. Recent blood chemical values disclosed blood urea nitrogen (BUN), 13 mg/dl; creatinine, 1.5 mg/dl; and creatinine clearance, 60 L/m²/BSA, which is about 60 per cent of normal. This clinical picture likely bodes well for the future because he has already attained full adult growth.

COMMENT. This case illustrates several points. First, cutaneous vesicostomy was a simple procedure to perform, but it set the stage for a series of major complications. It failed to drain the bladder adequately because of prolapse, following which ureterostomies were performed. It would have been better to resect the valves in the first place, probably followed by left ureteral reimplantation and right nephroureterectomy. Second, it is probable that complete stricture of the

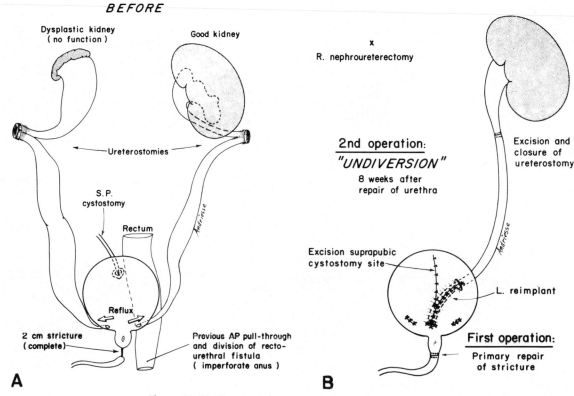

BEFORE

Figure 73–18. Case 5. Before (A) and after (B) reconstruction.

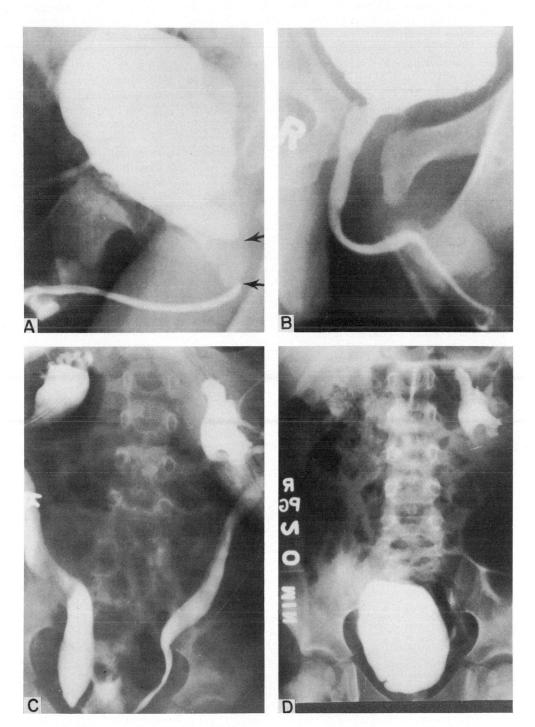

Figure 73–19. Case 5 roentgenograms. *A*, Preoperative cystourethrogram showing long stricture *(arrows).*

B, Cystourethrogram after repair of stricture by excision and anastomosis.

C, Preoperative ureterograms via the bilateral cutaneous loopureterostomies; right kidney was nonfunctional.

D, Intravenous pyelography 1 year after undiversion. Note the normal bladder and normal left ureter.

membranous urethra was caused by endoscopic resection of valves when there was a "dry urethra," i.e., supravesical diversion of the urine.

Rectal pull through with division of the rectourethral fistula may also have contributed to that complication, however. Ileal loop diversion was suggested elsewhere as being the best alternative, ". . . since reconstruction would be difficult and might be fraught with some uncertainties."

It has been my experience, however, that worse results come from a lesser procedure, as compared with a major reconstructive procedure that is well planned and skillfully performed. In performing reconstructive surgery in the patient who has undergone loop ureterostomy, I have found that it is best to do the entire reconstruction at one procedure—repair the obstructive problem and close the ureterostomies simultaneously (Hendren, 1978b).

Case 6 (Figs. 73–20 and 73–21)

This 17-year-old girl was referred in 1987 for urinary tract reconstruction. During infancy she had closure of a meningocele and ventricular peritoneal shunt for hydrocephalus. At age 2 years, an ileal loop was performed for urinary incontinence of the myelodysplastic bladder. During the next 15 years, there were many episodes of infection. Progressive dilatation of the upper tract and multiple strictures of the ileal loop were noted. Bladder cycling was not performed because the bladder was completely incontinent when filled with saline.

At operation, the urethra was lengthened and narrowed to increase outlet resistance. It was possible to reimplant the left ureter, with a psoas hitch, draining the right ureter by transureteroureterostomy. A 30-cm long segment of sigmoid colon was detubularized and reconfigured to augment the bladder. She tolerated this 16-hour operation well. Now 4 years later, the patient is well and free from urinary infection, being maintained on prophylactic medication. Unexpectedly, she is able to void by abdominal effort and Credé's maneuver, which she does every 3 to 4 hours to empty the bladder. She has been instructed, however, to catheterize at least twice daily in the morning and evening to make certain that the bladder is being emptied completely. Urodynamic study postoperatively showed the bladder capacity to be 550 ml, with very little rise in pressure during filling. At capacity, there were contraction waves from 10 to 30 cm H_2O, but they caused no leakage. Resistance at the repaired bladder neck measured 60 cm H_2O.

COMMENT. This patient was an ideal candidate for undiversion, being an intelligent and a highly motivated teenager who was anxious to get rid of the bag on her abdomen and end the recurrent episodes of infection. She and one other female are the only ones of the 18

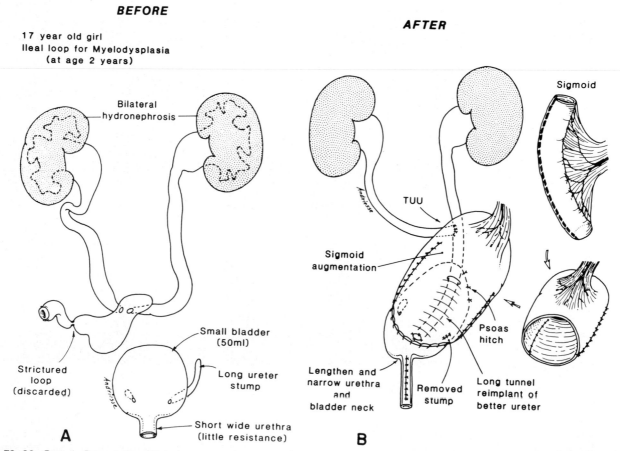

BEFORE

17 year old girl
Ileal loop for Myelodysplasia
(at age 2 years)

Bilateral hydronephrosis

Strictured loop (discarded)

Small bladder (50ml)

Long ureter stump

Short wide urethra (little resistance)

A

AFTER

Sigmoid

TUU

Sigmoid augmentation

Lengthen and narrow urethra and bladder neck

Removed stump

Psoas hitch

Long tunnel reimplant of better ureter

B

Figure 73–20. Case 6. Preoperative (A) and postoperative (B) anatomy. Note the reconfiguration of bowel augmentation, which dampens its peristalsis and increases its volume (TUU, transureteroureterostomy).

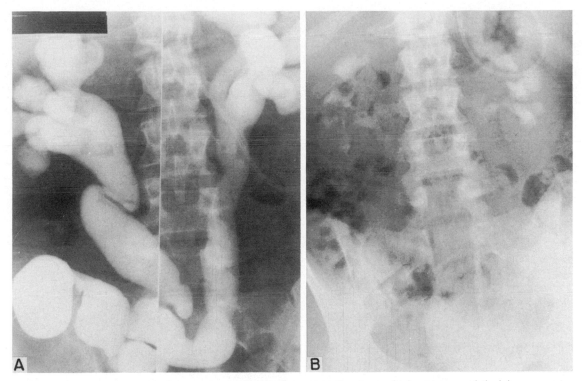

Figure 73–21. Case 6 roentgenograms. *A*, Preoperative retrograde loopogram showing multiple strictures of ileal loop, massive reflux, and hydronephrosis. The patient had long-term recurring urinary infections.
B, Postoperative intravenous pyelography that showed relatively delicate upper tracts that are draining well into bladder augmented with sigmoid. Cystogram showed no reflux. Unexpectedly, this patient does not require intermittent catheterization to empty the bladder.

neurogenic bladder cases in this series who have been able to void most of the urine without self-catheterization. It is, nevertheless, important to check the residual at least twice daily, to avert overdistention and possible spontaneous perforation of the bowel segment in a patient with myelodysplasia and diminished sensation. Urinary diversion was a very common operation for this type of patient 10 to 20 years ago. There are, therefore, many like this patient who could undergo undiversion today. Her long-term outlook will be greatly improved not only from the standpoint of stopping recurrent infection from reflux, but from the standpoint of her greatly improved social status. The upper urinary tract is now much more delicate in appearance than it was originally with hydronephrosis (see Fig. 73–21).

Case 7 (Figs. 73–22 and 73–23)

This 19-year-old young man was referred in 1986 for urologic reconstruction. Urinary infection had occurred, and study showed a very large bladder with massive reflux. At age 9 years, ureteral reimplantation and 50 per cent cystectomy were performed. He continued to have severe infection with deteriorating upper tracts and so ileal loop was performed at age 14 years.

Magnetic resonance imaging of the lumbosacral spine was performed to rule out a spinal cord malformation, because the etiology of the bladder problem was not clear. The study results were normal. Bladder cycling

was not attempted because much of the bladder had been surgically removed. The bladder was augmented with cecum. The right ureter was implanted, employing a submucosal tunnel in the back wall of the cecum. The terminal ileum was too short to make a nipple to prevent reflux, but that did not matter because the right ureter was very satisfactory for a tunneling reimplantation, which is the preferred method. The terminal ileum was opened and placed on the anterior wall of the cecum to render it incapable of producing strong peristaltic waves. Transureteroureterostomy was performed.

The patient's preoperative urodynamic study showed normal urethral sphincter function. As expected, he proved able to empty the bladder without difficulty postoperatively and is clinically well. BUN measures 20 mg/dl, and the serum creatinine level, 1.3 mg/dl (normal is 0.5 to 0.8 mg/dl). Creatinine clearance measures 54 L/m²/BSA. The patient's postoperative status has been good, except for one episode of epididymitis and traumatic small bowel perforation in an industrial accident.

COMMENT. Early detection of urinary infection and technically successful ureteral reimplantation would have almost certainly prevented the severe scarring with which this patient presented, in which very little function remained in the left kidney. Enlargement of the bladder is common with massive reflux. That enlargement would probably have disappeared with technically successful antireflux surgery. Thus, partial cystectomy was probably not necessary at age 9 years, and it made necessary augmentation of the bladder as part of the reconstructive surgery.

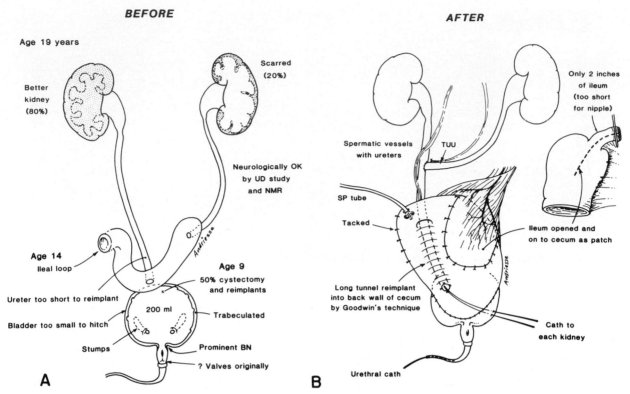

Figure 73–22. Case 7. Preoperative *(A)* and postoperative *(B)* anatomy.

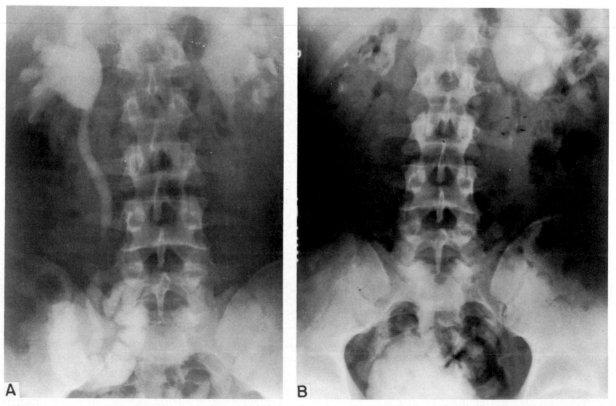

Figure 73–23. Case 7 roentgenograms. *A,* Preoperative intravenous pyelography (IVP). *B,* Postoperative IVP. Upper tract stable.

Case 8 (Figs. 73–24 and 73–25)

This 12-year-old boy was referred in 1975 with a strictured ileal loop and a parastomal hernia. Previous surgery had included nephrostomies and suprapubic cystostomy at age 1 month, resection of urethral valves at age 6 weeks, resection of the bladder neck at age 6 months, two operations for urinary incontinence, and an ileal loop at age 8.5 years. There was a good right ureteral stump without reflux. The right ureter of the horseshoe kidney was joined to it, and the left side of the horseshoe was drained by left-to-right ureteropyelostomy.

By splitting the pubic symphysis for exposure, the urethra and bladder neck were narrowed extensively to provide more outlet resistance. The bladder increased gradually in size. Urinary wetting occurred initially, but it disappeared during the next 2 years. The patient is now age 27 years, has full-time employment, and is in good general health. However, he has psychologic problems secondary to multiple hospitalizations as a young child.

COMMENT. Endoscopic resection of the urethral valves during infancy would have likely sufficed in this patient who first had tube diversion, and then open resection of valves, which left him incontinent, followed by failed surgery for incontinence, and finally an ileal loop for permanent urinary diversion. Modern fiberoptic infant panendoscopes have greatly changed the treat-

ment of urethral valves during infancy in recent years. I have found that splitting the symphysis pubis has proved key in achieving urinary continence in the patient who requires narrowing of the urethra and bladder neck to increase outlet resistance (Peters and Hendren, 1990). A high pressure, small volume, noncompliant "valve bladder" develops in some boys with urethral valves. Augmentation is needed to prevent back pressure on the upper tracts.

Case 9 (Figs. 73–26 to 73–29)

This 9-year-old boy was referred in 1976 with a strictured ileal loop and hydronephrosis and a small, scarred bladder following chemotherapy and radiation therapy for sarcoma of the prostate 4 years earlier. A nonrefluxing colon conduit was constructed because this is far better than the ileal loop that allows reflux (Althausen et al., 1982; Hendren, 1975; Kelalis, 1974; Richie and Skinner, 1975; Skinner et al., 1975). The bladder was extremely fibrotic, and so it was decided to defer undiversion. Meanwhile, drainage was converted to a nonrefluxing colon conduit (see Fig. 73–26). Five years later, total obstruction of the membranous urethra and secondary pyocystis developed. The stricture was repaired (see Fig. 73–27). The bladder was still small, but the bladder neck was no longer densely fibrotic as

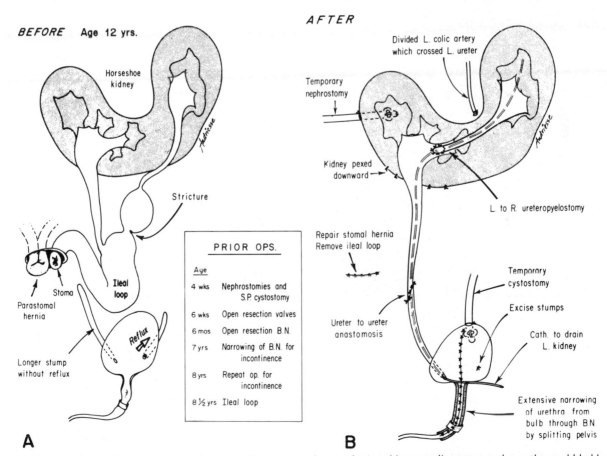

Figure 73–24. Case 8. Preoperative (A) and postoperative (B) anatomy. The symphysis pubis was split to narrow the urethra and bladder neck.

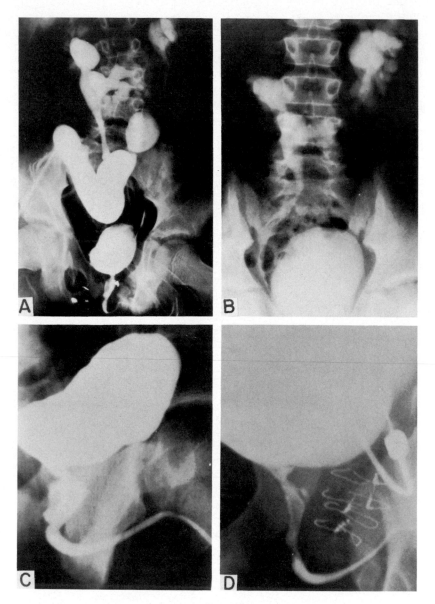

Figure 73–25. Case 8 roentgenograms. *A,* Preoperative loopogram and cystogram.

B, Postoperative intravenous pyelography (IVP). It has remained stable for 16 years.

C, Preoperative cystogram of defunctionalized bladder. Note the wide prostatic urethra, despite two previous attempts to narrow the bladder outlet.

D, Postoperative cystogram (note needle in bladder) showing narrowed prostatic urethra and higher bladder neck. The patient is now continent. Splitting the symphysis pubis was key in this repair.

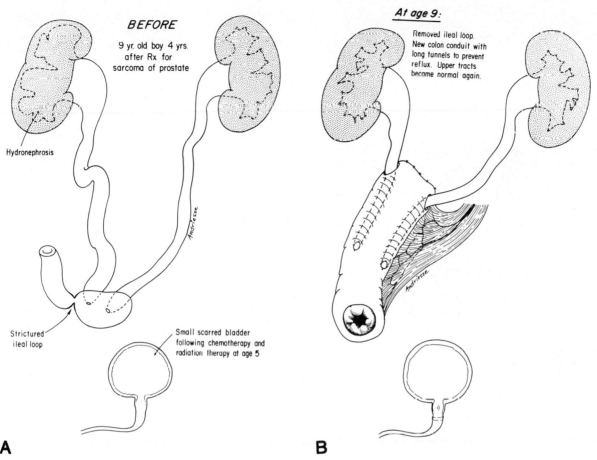

Figure 73–26. Case 9. Preoperative anatomy *(A)* and anatomy following nonrefluxing colon conduit *(B)*. Upper tracts then improved dramatically by roentgen follow-up.

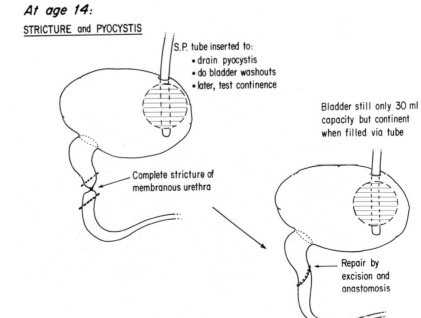

Figure 73–27. Case 9. Urethral stricture and its repair at age 14 years when pyocystis developed.

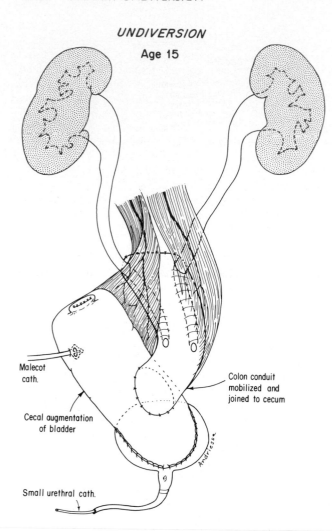

UNDIVERSION
Age 15

Malecot cath.

Cecal augmentation of bladder

Colon conduit mobilized and joined to cecum

Small urethral cath.

Andriesse

Figure 73–28. Case 9. Anatomy using composite augmentations.

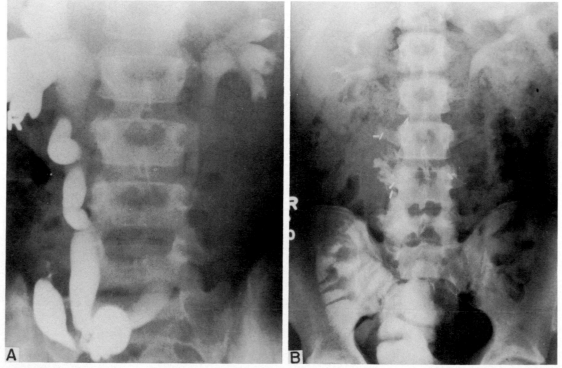

Figure 73–29. Case 9 roentgenograms. *A,* Preoperative loopogram. Note severe ileal loop stricture and dilated upper tracts. The patient had recurrent urinary infections.

B, Postoperative intravenous pyelography showing excellent upper tracts, which have remained stable.

it had been 5 years earlier. After the stricture repair, the patient could hold saline instilled into the bladder.

Undiversion was performed by adding the cecum to the bladder and by joining the nonrefluxing colon conduit to it (see Fig. 73–28). The patient is now 24 years old. He voids well by abdominal effort. He is dry and sexually active and has excellent renal function and stable upper tracts. He was recently found to have a bladder stone, which will be removed.

COMMENT. This patient is one of 13 patients who had a nonrefluxing colon conduit made with the plan to later consider undiversion. He demonstrates how radiation therapy and chemotherapy can cure some genitourinary rhabdomyosarcomas but result in a badly scarred urinary tract, which requires major reconstructive surgery. He is continent despite stricture resection at the site of the membranous urethra because the bladder neck is intact. Voiding is accomplished by abdominal effort, which raises intravesical pressure, while simultaneously voluntarily opening the bladder neck. The finding of a bladder stone recently, a decade later, illustrates that these patients can never be discharged from medical supervision.

Case 10 (Figs. 73–30 to 73–32)

This 3-year-old girl was referred in 1988 for reconstructive surgery. Born with severe bilateral obstructive megaureters and hydronephrosis, bilateral end ureterostomies had been performed at age 1 month. The ureterostomies did not drain well. Therefore, bilateral loop cutaneous ureterostomies were performed at age 1

year. Hydronephrosis improved. The ureterostomies were later closed, but severe hydronephrosis recurred.

Preoperative assessment showed the bladder volume to be only 10 ml. When contrast material was introduced through the end ureterostomy stomas, the ureters drained well, but the contrast material remained in the kidneys, indicating functional ureteropelvic junction obstruction on both sides. At operation, the better ureter was reimplanted with as long a tunnel as possible in her tiny bladder, together with psoas hitch. Transureteroureterostomy drained the opposite ureter. Both upper ureters were obstructed from angulation at the site of the ureterostomy closures. Therefore, bilateral dismembered pyeloplasties were performed, maintaining ureteral blood supply in the surrounding periureteral tissues.

The bladder was augmented with stomach, based on the right gastroepiploic artery. The patient tolerated this 13-hour operation well. Bladder emptying was performed initially by intermittent catheterization by her mother. The child gradually learned to void to completion and catheterization was stopped.

Postoperative evaluation showed reflux. Subureteric injection of Teflon paste beneath the ureteral orifice stopped the reflux (O'Donnell and Puri, 1988; Puri and O'Donnell, 1987). Now 3 years postoperatively, the patient voids normally, is dry, and is free from urinary infection.

Blood chemical values are remarkably normal considering the degree of hydronephrosis originally present: BUN, 10 mg/dl; serum creatinine, 0.3 mg/per cent; and creatinine clearance, 121 L/m²/BSA. Postoperative urodynamic study showed bladder capacity to be 275 ml,

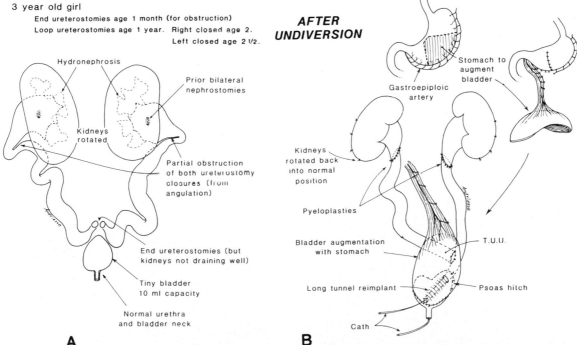

BEFORE

3 year old girl
End ureterostomies age 1 month (for obstruction)
Loop ureterostomies age 1 year. Right closed age 2.
Left closed age 2½.

Hydronephrosis

Prior bilateral nephrostomies

Kidneys rotated

Partial obstruction of both ureterostomy closures (from angulation)

End ureterostomies (but kidneys not draining well)

Tiny bladder 10 ml capacity

Normal urethra and bladder neck

A

AFTER UNDIVERSION

Stomach to augment bladder

Gastroepiploic artery

Kidneys rotated back into normal position

Pyeloplasties

Bladder augmentation with stomach

Long tunnel reimplant

T.U.U.

Psoas hitch

Cath

B

Figure 73–30. Case 10 preoperative and postoperative anatomy (T.U.U., transureteroureterostomy).

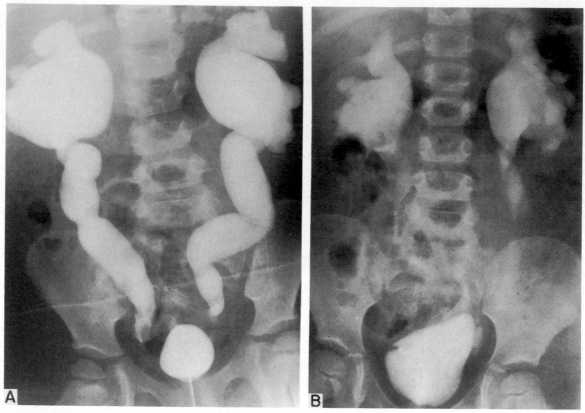

Figure 73–31. Case 10 roentgenograms. *A,* Preoperative simultaneous retrograde ureterograms and cystogram. Ureters emptied quickly, but contrast material remained in the renal pelvis on both sides, each being partially obstructed from angulation at closure of former ureterostomies. Note the very small bladder.

B, Intravenous pyelography 1 year later. Upper tracts draining well, with less hydronephrosis.

with no uninhibited contractions and normal sphincter function.

COMMENT. The stomach for bladder augmentation has some outstanding advantages over small bowel and colon. It is metabolically superior regarding the chloride absorption and base loss that are seen with segments of small bowel and especially of colon. Those segments tend to lose bicarbonate and potassium and, to a lesser extent, sodium while resorbing chloride.

If potassium loss is replaced as potassium chloride, bicarbonate loss can be accelerated, aggravating aci-

dosis. In comparison, gastric mucosa secretes chloride ion and is, therefore, preferred in patients with poor renal function who cannot tolerate increased solute resorption and resulting acidosis.

The urine is more often sterile after operation because it is not so alkaline in pH. Ureters can be tunneled and implanted without difficulty into gastric wall. Stomach is very durable, yet quite compliant.

The stomach may be the only reasonable means for reconstructing certain cases of cloacal exstrophy, with little or no colon and a short small bowel. The stomach's

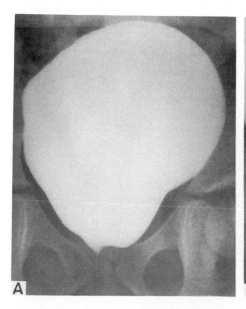

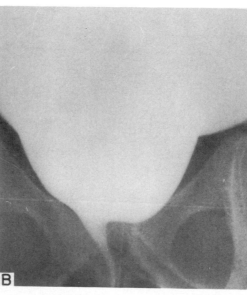

Figure 73–32. Case 10 roentgenograms. *A,* Bladder filled to 275 ml. Most of the bladder wall is gastric augmentation.

B, Voiding film showing normal bladder neck and urethra. Patient empties completely by abdominal effort, while voluntarily opening the bladder neck and sphincter.

metabolic superiority probably makes it the augmentation of choice in patients with very poor renal functions. Three of the 31 patients for whom I have used gastrocystoplasty had pain in the region of the bladder, which was relieved by cimetidine. Only seven of the 31 were undiversion patients, because I began utilizing stomach wall for bladder augmentation only recently. These patients do not have excess mucus in the urine, which is an added advantage, because mucus provides a nidus for stones. Because gastrocystoplasty has been employed only recently in children, as compared with intestine and colon, long-term observations are needed. Cutaneous ureterostomy was a common type of temporary diversion in infants several years ago. It can cause many complications, however, as shown in this case.

RESULTS AND COMPLICATIONS

No early postoperative deaths occurred, indicating that these global reconstructions can be performed with safety if meticulous attention is paid to avoid ureteral obstruction, anastomotic leakage, and so on. Eight late deaths (1 to 14 years after operation) were recorded, the causes for which were trauma (2), septicemia during hemodialysis (1), massive stroke (1), varicella infection after renal transplantation (1), acute leukemia (1), anaphylactic reaction during intravenous pyelogram examination (1), and failure to take prescribed immunosuppressive drugs (1).

Renal transplantation was performed, to date, in 23 patients. These included two patients who had undergone transplantations before undiversion and one patient who was anephric at the time of bladder reconstruction. Approximately 42 more of the 182 cases will probably require renal transplantations within the coming decade, judging from the original and current renal function values. Renal function did not fail in any patient soon after undiversion from an obstruction or other complication. In most patients it was the expected decline in creatinine clearance, which occurs with growth, in which the body weight increases, resulting in relative renal insufficiency. For example, our third undiversion patient underwent reconstruction at age 6 years in 1969. Creatinine clearance was then only 24 L/m^2/BSA, about 20 per cent of normal. Renal transplantation was performed 20 years later at age 26 years in 1989.

Some 23 patients required reoperations for persisting reflux. Sites of reflux included the ureter (9), bowel ureter (6), and ileocecal nipple (8). Longer tunnels were made for the ureters. Longer tunnels were made in three of the bowel ureters, and three were converted to ileocecal conduits. The nipples were revised by sewing them to the cecal wall or by substituting a tapered and tunneled bowel segment. Two patients had perforations of bladder augmentations, one from a karate kick and the other from a spontaneous event. This is a known risk of bladder augmentation. Both perforations were successfully closed surgically.

Eight patients required reoperation for partial obstruction. The partial obstructions were in the ureter in

three. Late stricture of a bowel ureter occurred in three, each very localized.

An endoscope can be passed up a bowel ureter (1) to incise a web, (2) to inject a steroid solution, or (3) to dilate. Urinary tract stones developed in 12 patients and required removal. Most of the stones had a staple nidus. When staples have been used, I always perform a cystoscopy several months later to remove any staples not covered by mucosa. Otherwise, they can form stones on the nipple or drop off into the bladder and grow larger, which occurred in two patients who did not return soon for follow-up examination.

Three patients had postoperative leaks and each closed spontaneously. Two patients had pigment gallstones on follow-up, presumably from a large intraoperative transfusion requirement during undiversion. Cholecystectomy was done in each of these patients. One patient had a traumatic urethralvaginal fistula that required closure. Ten patients required secondary operations for persistent wetting.

One patient had an artificial sphincter (Rosen type) placed. It worked well, but later eroded the urethra and was removed. Many successes have been reported with the use of artificial sphincters; however, I prefer to avoid them, opting to surgically narrow the outlet and catheterize to empty, if necessary.

CONCLUSION

Urinary undiversion should be considered for patients who have undergone diversion in the past. Reconstructions of this magnitude require meticulous attention to all technical surgical details. Many of these patients have poor renal function. However, this is not a contraindication to undiversion, because restoration of bladder function gives a much better quality of life. Furthermore, it is ultimately better to transplant a kidney into a bladder than into a cutaneous diversion. Undiversion may reduce urinary infection and prolong the time before transplantation is needed.

REFERENCES

Adams, M. C., Mitchell, M. E., and Rink, R. C.: Gastrocystoplasty: an alternative solution to the problem of urological reconstruction in the severely compromised patient. J. Urol., 140;1152, 1988.

Althausen, A. F., Hagen-Cook, K., and Hendren, W. H.: Nonrefluxing colon conduit: Experience with 70 cases. J. Urol., 120:35, 1982.

Bauer, S. B., Dieppa, R. A., Labib, K. K., and Retik, A. B.: The bladder in boys with posterior urethral valves, a urodynamic assessment. J. Urol., 121:769, 1974.

Bauer, S. B., Colodny, A. H., Hallet, M., et al.: Urinary undiversion in myelodysplasia criteria for selection and predictive value of urodynamics. J. Urol., 124:87, 1980.

Bricker, E. M.: Bladder substitution after pelvic evisceration. Surg. Clin. North Am., 30:1511, 1950.

Campaiola, J. M., Perlmutter, A. D., and Steinhardt, G. F.: Noncompliant bladder resulting from posterior urethral valves. J. Urol., 134:708, 1985.

Courvelaire, R.: La "petite vessie" des tuberculeaux genitourinaires. Essai de classification place et variantes des cysto-intestino-plasties. J. d'Urol., 56:381, 1950.

Crooks, K. K.: Urethral strictures following transurethral resection of posterior urethral valves. J. Urol., 127:1153, 1982.

Duckett, J. W., Jr.: Current management of posterior urethral valves. Urol. Clin. North Am., 1:471, 1974.

Elder, J. S., Snyder, H. M., Hulbert, W. C., and Duckett, J. W.: Perforation of the augmented bladder in patients undergoing clean intermittent catheterization. J. Urol., 140:1159, 1981.

Ferris, D. O., and Odel, H. M.: Electrolyte pattern of the blood after bilateral ureterosigmoidostomy. JAMA, 142:634, 1950.

Gilchrist, R. K., Merricks, J. W., Hamlin, H. H., et al.: Construction of a substitute bladder and urethra. Surg. Gynecol. Obstet., 90:752, 1950.

Glassberg, K. I.: Current issues regarding posterior urethral valves. Urol. Clin. North Am., 12:175, 1985.

Goldstein, H. R., and Hensle, T. W.: Urinary undiversion in adults. J. Urol., 128:143, 1981.

Goldwasser, B., and Webster, G. D.: Augmentation and substitution enterocystoplasty. J. Urol., 135:215, 1986.

Gonzalez, R., Sidi, A., and Zhang, G.: Urinary undiversion: indications, technique and results in 50 cases. J. Urol., 136:13, 1986.

Goodwin, W. E., Harris, A. P., Kaufman, J. J., and Beal, J. M.: Open transcolonic ureterointestinal anastomosis; a new approach. Surg. Gynecol. Obstet., 97:295, 1953.

Goodwin, W. E., Turner, R. D., and Winter, C. C.: Results of ileocystoplasty. J. Urol., 80:461, 1958.

Goodwin, W. E., Winter, C. C., and Barker, W. F.: "Cup-patch" technique of ileocystoplasty for bladder enlargement or partial substitution. Surg. Gynecol. Obstet., 108:240, 1959.

Hendren, W. H.: A new approach to infants with severe obstructive uropathy: early complete reconstruction. J. Pediatr. Surg., 5:184, 1970.

Hendren, W. H.: Posterior urethral valves in boys: A broad clinical spectrum. J. Urol., 106:298, 1971.

Hendren, W. H.: Reconstruction of previously diverted urinary tracts in children. J. Pediatr. Surg., 8:135, 1973.

Hendren, W. H.: Urethral Valves: Diagnosis and Endoscopic Resection. Eaton Film Library, 1974a.

Hendren, W. H.: Urinary tract refunctionalization after prior diversion in children. Ann. Surg., 180:494, 1974b.

Hendren, W. H.: Non-refluxing colon conduit for temporary or permanent urinary diversion in children. J. Pediatr. Surg., 10:381, 1975.

Hendren, W. H.: Urinary diversion and undiversion in children. Surg. Clin. North Am., 56:425, 1976.

Hendren, W. H.: Some alternatives to urinary diversion in children. J. Urol., 119:652, 1978a.

Hendren, W. H.: Complications of ureterostomy. J. Urol., 120:269, 1978b.

Hendren, W. H., and Mitchell, M. E.: Surgical correction of ureteroceles. J. Urol., 121:590, 1979.

Hendren, W. H.: Reoperative ureteral reimplantation: Management of the difficult case. J. Pediatr. Surg., 15:770, 1980a.

Hendren, W. H.: Construction of female urethra from vaginal wall and a perineal flap. J. Urol., 123:657, 1980b.

Hendren, W. H., and Hensle, T. W.: Transureteroureterostomy: Experience with 75 cases. J. Urol., 123:826, 1980c.

Hendren, W. H., and McLorie, G. A.: Late stricture of intestinal ureter. J. Urol., 129:584, 1983.

Hendren, W. H.: Techniques for urinary undiversion: In King, L. R., Stone, A. R., and Webster, G. D. (Eds.): Reconstruction and Continent Urinary Diversion. Chicago, Year Book Medical Publishers, 1987, p. 101.

Hendren, W. H., and Hendren, R. B.: Bladder augmentation: experience with 129 cases in children and young adults. J. Urol., 144:445, 1990a.

Hendren, W. H.: Urinary tract refunctionalization after long-term diversion. A 20-year experience with 177 patients. Ann. Surg., 212:478, 1990b.

Hodges, C. V., Moore, R. J., Lehman, T. H., and Behnam, A. M.: Clinical experiences with transureteroureterostomy. J. Urol., 90:552, 1963.

Jeffs, R.: Exstrophy of the urinary bladder. In Welch, K. J., et al. (Eds.): Pediatric Surgery. Chicago, Year Book Medical Publishers, 1986.

Johnston, J. H.: Temporary cutaneous ureterostomy in the manage-

ment of advanced congenital urinary obstruction. Arch. Dis. Child., 38:161, 1963.

Kass, E. J., and Koff, S. A.: Bladder augmentation in the pediatric neuropathic bladder. J. Urol., 129:552, 1983.

Kelalis, P.: Urinary diversion in children by sigmoid conduits: its advantages and limitations. J. Urol., 112:666, 1974.

Kennedy, H. A., Adams, M. C., Mitchell, M. E., et al.: Chronic renal failure and bladder augmentation: stomach versus sigmoid colon in the canine model. J. Urol., 140:1138, 1988.

King, L. R., Webster, G. D., and Bertram, R. A.: Experience with bladder reconstruction in children. J. Urol., 138:1002, 1987a.

King, L. R., Stone, A. R., and Webster, G. D. (Eds.): Bladder Reconstruction and Continent Urinary Diversion. Chicago, Year Book Medical Publishers, 1987b.

Koch, M. O., and McDougal, W. S.: The pathophysiology of hyperchloremic metabolic acidosis after urinary diversion through intestinal segments. Surgery, 98:561, 1985.

Kock, N. G., Nilson, A. E., Nilsson, L. O., et al.: Urinary diversion via a continent ileal reservoir: Clinical results in 12 patients. J. Urol., 128:469, 1982.

Kogan, S. J., Kim, K., and Levitt, S. B.: Preoperative evaluation of bladder function prior to renal transplantation or urinary tract reconstruction in children: Description of a method. J. Pediatr. Surg., 11:1007, 1976.

Kogan, S. J., and Levitt, S. B.: Bladder evaluation in pediatric patients before undiversion in previously diverted urinary tracts. J. Urol., 118:443, 1977.

Lapides, J., Diokno, A. C., Gould, F. R., and Low, B. S.: Further observations on self-catheterization. J. Urol., 116:169, 1976.

Leong, C. H.: Use of the stomach for bladder replacement and urinary diversion. Ann. Roy. Col. Surg., 60:283, 1978.

Light, J. K., and Engelmann, U. H.: Reconstruction of the lower urinary tract: observations on bowel dynamics and the artificial urinary sphincter. J. Urol., 133:594, 1985.

Linder, A., Leach, G. E., and Raz, S.: Augmentation cystoplasty in the treatment of neurogenic bladder dysfunction. J. Urol., 129:491, 1983.

Middleton, A. W., Jr., and Hendren, W. H.: Ileal conduits in children at the Massachusetts General Hospital from 1955 to 1970. J. Urol., 115:591, 1976.

Mitchell, M. E.: The role of bladder augmentation in undiversion. J. Pediatr. Surg., 16:790, 1981a.

Mitchell, M. E.: Urinary tract diversion and undiversion in the pediatric age group. Surg. Clin. North Am., 61:1147, 1981b.

Mitchell, M. E., and Rink, R. C.: Experience with the artificial urinary sphincter in children and young adults. J. Pediatr. Surg., 18:700, 1983.

Mitchell, M. E., Kulb, T. B., and Backes, D. J.: Intestinocystoplasty in combination with clean intermittent catheterization in the management of vesical dysfunction. J. Urol., 136:288, 1986.

Mitchell, M. E., and Piser, J. A.: Intestinocystoplasty and total bladder replacement in children and young adults: Follow-up in 129 cases. J. Urol., 138:579, 1987a.

Mitchell, M. E., and Rink, R. C.: Pediatric urinary diversion and undiversion. Pediatr. Clin. North Am., 34:1319, 1987b.

Mitrofanoff, P.: Cystostomie continente trans-appendiculaire dans le traitement des vessies neruologiques. Chir. Pediatr., 21:297, 1980.

O'Donnell, B., and Puri, P.: Technical refinements in endoscopic correction of vesicoureteral reflux. J. Urol., 140:1101, 1988.

Perlmutter, A. D., and Patil, J.: Loop cutaneous ureterostomy in infants and young children: Late results in 32 cases. J. Urol., 107:655, 1972.

Perlmutter, A. D.: Experiences with urinary undiversion in children with neurogenic bladder. J. Urol., 123:402, 1980.

Peters, C. A., and Hendren, W. H.: Splitting the pubis for exposure in difficult reconstructions for incontinence. Urol. Clin. North Am., 17:37, 1990.

Pitts, W. R., Jr., and Muecke, E. C.: A 20-year experience with ileal conduits: The fate of the kidneys. J. Urol., 122:154, 1979.

Puri, P., and O'Donnell, B.: Endoscopic correction of grades IV and V primary vesicoureteric reflux: six to 30 month follow-up in 42 ureters. J. Pediatr. Surg., 22:1087, 1987.

Retik, A. B., Perlmutter, A. D., and Gross, R. E.: Cutaneous ureteroileostomy in children. N. Engl. J. Med., 277:217, 1967.

Richie, J. P., Skinner, D. G., and Waisman, J.: The effect of reflux on the development of pyelonephritis in urinary diversion: An experimental study. J. Surg. Res., 16:256, 1974.

Richie, J. P., and Skinner, D. G.: Urinary diversion: The physiological rationale for non-refluxing colonic conduits. Br. J. Urol., 47:269, 1975.

Rushton, H. G., Woodward, J. R., Parrott, T. S., Jeffs, R. D., and Gearhart, J. P.: Delayed bladder rupture after augmentation enterocystoplasty. J. Urol., 140:344, 1988.

Scott, F. B., Bradley, W. E., and Tumm, G. W.: Treatment of urinary incontinence by an implantable prosthetic urinary sphincter. J. Urol., 112:75, 1974.

Shapiro, S. R., Lebowitz, R., and Colodny, A. H.: Fate of 90 children with ileal conduit urinary diversion a decade later: analysis of complications, pyelography, renal function and bacteriology. J. Urol., 114:289, 1975.

Sheiner, J. R., and Kaplan, G. W.: Spontaneous bladder rupture following enterocystoplasty. J. Urol., 140:1157, 1988.

Sidi, A. A., Reinberg, Y., and Gonzalez, R.: Influence of intestinal segment and configuration on the outcome of augmentation enterocystoplasty. J. Urol., 136:1201, 1986.

Sidi, A. A., Aliabadi, H., and Gonzalez, R.: Enterocystoplasty in the management and reconstruction of the pediatric neurogenic bladder. J. Pediatr. Surg., 22:153, 1987.

Skinner, D. G., Gottesman, J. E., and Richie, J. P.: The isolated sigmoid segment: Its value in temporary urinary diversion and reconstruction. J. Urol., 113:614, 1975.

Skinner, D. G., Boyd, S. D., and Lieskovsky, G.: Clinical experience with the Kock continent ileal reservoir for urinary diversion. J. Urol., 132:1101, 1984.

Smith, E. D.: Follow-up studies on 150 ileal conduits in children. J. Pediatr. Surg., 7:1, 1972.

Smith, R. B., VanCangh, P., Skinner, D. G., Kaufman, J. J., and Goodwin, W. E.: Augmentation enterocystoplasty: a critical review. J. Urol., 118:35, 1977.

Stephenson, T. P., and Mundy, A. R.: Treatment of the neuropathic bladder by enterocystoplasty and selective sphincterotomy or sphincter ablation and replacement. Br. J. Urol., 57:27, 1985.

Thuroff, J. W., Alken, P., Riedmiller, H., Jacobi, G. H., and Hohenfellner, R.: 100 cases of MAINZ pouch continuing experience and evolution. J. Urol., 140:283, 1988.

Turner-Warwick, R.: Cystoplasty. Urol. Clin. North Am., 6:259, 1979.

Whitmore, W. F., III, and Gittes, R. F.: Reconstruction of the urinary tract by cecal and ileocecal cystoplasty: review of a 15-year experience. J. Urol., 129:494, 1983.

Zinman, L., and Libertino, J. A.: Ileocecal conduit for temporary and permanent diversion. J. Urol., 113:317, 1975.

74
OPEN BLADDER SURGERY

Fuad S. Freiha, M.D.

Open bladder operations are commonly performed procedures that account for approximately 15 per cent of all urologic surgery done in a university hospital. The most common is radical cystectomy for treatment of invasive bladder cancer.

The urinary bladder is a forgiving organ. Its rich blood supply and its power of "regeneration" make it withstand major and repeated surgical trauma. Large segments of its wall can be excised, and it will expand to regain good functional capacity. The urinary bladder can be extensively mobilized and the majority of its blood supply interrupted without major untoward effects on its function or capacity. The bladder can also be augmented or totally replaced.

Because of its rich blood supply and compliance, bleeding into its lumen can be profuse and unabatable because of lack of tamponade. Attention to complete hemostasis, therefore, is of the utmost importance. The close proximity of the bladder to and association with a number of pelvic organs, and its position deep in the pelvic cavity where adequate exposure may not always be possible, compels the surgeon to be cautious and to be fully aware of the variations in anatomic relationships.

The surgical approach to the bladder may be through a midline, a transverse Pfannenstiel, or a Cherney incision; it may be extraperitoneal or intraperitoneal. The choice of incision and approach is dictated by the type of operation, the patient's habitus, and, sometimes, the surgeon's personal preference.

Similar to elsewhere in the urinary tract, nonabsorbable suture material should never be used in the bladder because of possible stone formation and creation of a focus of infection.

The bladder may be drained with either a urethral catheter or a suprapubic tube. Suprapubic tube drainage should be avoided in bladder cancer to prevent tumor implantation along the tube tract. Long-term urethral catheter drainage should also be avoided in men to prevent urethral strictures and erosions. The length of bladder drainage depends on the extent and complexity of the open bladder operation and on whether or not the bladder had been previously irradiated. The bladder

should be drained for a minimum of 4 to 5 days after simple cystotomy and for as long as 3 weeks after bladder augmentation.

The majority of this part of the chapter is devoted to the detailed description of radical cystectomy in both the male and the female. [Discussion of urethrectomy is presented last.] A description of some of the more commonly performed open bladder operations, namely, simple cystectomy, partial cystectomy, bladder diverticulectomy, suprapubic cystotomy, and Y-V plasty of the bladder neck, and the surgical treatment of enterovesical fistula are included. Bladder augmentation is described in Chapter 71, and bladder operations to correct incontinence are described in Chapters 75 and 76.

RADICAL CYSTECTOMY

Over the past 40 years, the treatment of invasive bladder cancer has undergone many changes and modifications: from cystectomy, to radiation therapy, to the combination of both, and back again to cystectomy.

Being discouraged by the results of the earlier series of total and radical cystectomy (Table 74–1) and by the significant morbidity and mortality, which was as high as 15 per cent, urologists started searching for alternatives to cystectomy. External beam radiation therapy was the natural alternative; however, the results were as discouraging (Table 74–2). Combination therapy then emerged, using different doses of preoperative irradiation followed by cystectomy. The results of the combined modality approach were better than those of any

Table 74–1. RESULTS OF EARLIER SERIES OF TOTAL AND RADICAL CYSTECTOMY FOR INVASIVE BLADDER CANCER

Authors	Year	Per Cent Survival		
		P2	P3a	P3b
Brice et al.	1956	—	— 9	
Jewett et al.	1964	50	16	12
Poole-Wilson and Barnard	1971	— 25	—	12
Long et al.	1972	— 36	—	24
Morabito et al.	1979	— 17	—	6

Table 74–2. RESULTS OF RADIATION THERAPY FOR INVASIVE BLADDER CANCER

Authors	Year	T2(B1) (%)	T2(B1) and T3a(B2) (%)	T3a(B2) (%)	T3b(C) (%)
Sagerman et al.	1965	33		25	25
Frank	1970	57		31	—
Edsmyr et al.	1971	34		25	—
Goffinet et al.	1975	—	35	—	20
Rider and Evans	1976	50		18	—

one treatment alone (Table 74–3). During the same period, however, more recent series of cystectomy were reported showing better results than ever before, often better than the combined approach (Table 74–4). This indicated that the survival benefit derived from preoperative irradiation was due to a better cystectomy, with a much lower rate of morality, rather than to the combined modality treatment.

Potency sparing techniques that were developed for radical prostatectomy (Walsh et al., 1983), which can be successfully applied to cystectomy, bladder substitution operations, or continent diversions to the urethra that eliminate the need for a urostomy (Freiha, 1990), and the excellent results achieved with modern day cystectomy (see Table 74–4) have all combined to rejuvenate interest in radical cystectomy. Over the past decade, this procedure has become the treatment of choice for the patient with invasive bladder cancer.

In the Male

Radical cystectomy in the male implies the en bloc removal of the bladder with its peritoneal covering and urachal remnant up to the umbilicus, perivesical adipose tissue, lower ureters, prostate gland and seminal vesicles, pelvic vas deferens and its ampulla, and pelvic lymph nodes. Removal of the urethra in continuity with the radical cystectomy specimen is indicated in patients with multicentric, primary carcinoma in situ and in patients with involvement of the bladder neck and/or prostatic urethra and ducts with transitional cell carcinoma.

Because of the high propensity of transitional cells to implant on raw surfaces, it is extremely important to avoid opening the bladder during the operation and spilling its contents into the pelvic cavity. If spillage occurs, thorough irrigation with liters of distilled water or normal saline solution should be done.

Table 74–3. RESULTS OF PREOPERATIVE IRRADIATION FOLLOWED BY CYSTECTOMY FOR INVASIVE BLADDER CANCER

Authors	Year	Dose (rad)	Per Cent Survival T2(B1)		T3a(B2)	T3b(C)
Miller and Johnson	1972	5000	—		— 53	—
van der Werf Messing	1973	4000	43		— 40	—
Reid et al.	1976	2000	—		— 34	—
Whitmore et al.	1977	4000	50		34	33
		2000	45		42	33
Boileau et al.	1980	5000	38		51	57
Freiha	1990	2000		57	—	57

Table 74–4. RESULTS OF MORE RECENT SERIES OF CYSTECTOMY FOR INVASIVE BLADDER CANCER

Author	Year	Per Cent Survival P2	P2 and P3a	P3a	P3b
Bredael et al.	1980	53		36	11
Mathur et al.	1981	88		57	40
Montie et al.	1982	50		63	29
Skinner and Lieskovsky	1988	83		69	29
Freiha	1990	—	83	—	47

Preoperative Preparation

The aims of preoperative preparation are to ensure a sterile urinary tract and a sterile intestinal tract and to determine and mark the most optimal site for the stoma. A urine culture is taken on hospital admission and checked the next morning. If results are positive, the proper parenteral antibiotic is started the day before the operation and continued for 24 to 48 hours after.

Different protocols exist for the preparation of the intestinal tract. The one described here has been used successfully by me for the past 20 years and is very effective in reducing the incidence of postoperative wound infection (Freiha, 1977).

Patients are usually admitted 2 days before the operation, started immediately on a clear liquid diet, and given 30 g of magnesium citrate and 2 tablets of bisacodyl. In the evening of the day of admission, cleansing soap suds enemas are administered, until the colonic returns are clear. Oral antibiotics are started on the 2nd day of admission: 1 g neomycin sulfate hourly for 4 hours, and then 1 g every 4 hours for a total of 7 g, and 1 g erythromycin base 4 times that day. Intravenous fluids with either lactated Ringer's solution or with 5 per cent dextrose in half normal saline are started the day before the operation and continued, at a rate of 120 ml per hour, until the operation. If a colonic segment is to be utilized for the conduit or for bladder substitution, a neomycin sulfate enema (500 mg neomycin sulfate in 500 ml normal saline) is given on the evening before the day of operation. Gentamycin (80 mg) or any parenteral broad-spectrum antibiotic is given on call to the operating room and continued postoperatively for a total of 3 doses.

With increasing restraints on hospital admissions, patients are often denied two preoperative hospital days; therefore, the protocol as described is often modified. Patients are started on a clear liquid diet at home 2 days before the operation and are given 30 g of magnesium citrate and 2 tablets of bisacodyl to take that afternoon. They are instructed to give themselves a Fleet enema that evening. They are admitted to the hospital as early as possible on the day prior to surgery and are given oral antibiotics, according to what was described. The rest of the protocol is the same.

Patients with histories of thromboembolic disease or with varicose veins begin prophylactic doses of heparin, 5000 units subcutaneously, the night before the operation and every 12 hours thereafter, until full ambulation. Antiembolic stockings and/or sequential compression boots are recommended for all patients.

The most optimal site for the stoma is determined and marked the day before the operation by the stoma therapist and agreed to by the surgeon. This determination is done by examining the patients in a standing, sitting, and supine position with their clothes on and off, in order to prevent interference with the stoma and appliance by skin creases, folds, or scars, and by belts and garments. The patients are given preliminary instructions on how to manage a urostomy. Even if bladder substitution (continent diversion to the urethra) is planned, a site for a stoma is always determined in case the substitution cannot be performed.

Position

In men, and unless a urethrectomy is planned, the patient is placed in a supine position with gentle hyperextension and legs apart (Fig. 74–1). This allows for adequate preparation of the genitalia, which will be in the surgical field for easy access to the penis for urethral catheterization. The arms can be either along the sides or on arm boards at 90 degrees to the table, depending on the preference of the anesthesiologist.

If a urethrectomy is planned and in a woman, the patient is placed in a gentle lithotomy position for access to the perineum. The anus is draped outside the surgical field, or an O'Conor drape is placed to isolate and allow for access to the rectum. A Foley catheter is inserted after the draping.

Surgical Technique

INCISION. A midline skin incision is made from the mid-epigastrium to the symphysis pubis, curving around the umbilicus opposite the side of the stoma mark. This incision is carried down through subcutaneous tissues and through the linea alba to the preperitoneal space. The peritoneal cavity is entered by incising the peritoneum above the umbilicus. The peritoneal incision is carried inferiorly on either side of the urachal remnant and slightly, laterally in order to include with it all the adipose tissue covering it. The urachal remnant is dissected off its attachment with the umbilicus and clamped, to be removed later en bloc with the bladder (Fig. 74–2). The peritoneal cavity is now carefully inspected.

Adequate exposure is essential. In my experience, the Bookwalter retractor with its versatile attachments gives excellent exposure (Fig. 74–3). Before placing the retractor, the anterior and lateral walls of the bladder are bluntly dissected free from the undersurface of the rectus muscles, the pubic bones, and the lateral pelvic walls (Fig. 74–4), carefully preserving the inferior epigastric vessels. This maneuver, when done early, allows for palpation and visual inspection of the pelvic nodes and perivesical tissues and for adequate placement of the retractor. It also gives the dome and posterior wall of the bladder more mobility.

After the retractor is placed to spread the abdominal incision apart, the intestines and omentum are covered with moist pads or towels, packed in the upper abdomen, and held in place by the curved maleable and deep retractors of the Bookwalter retractor, thus freeing the pelvic cavity of all bowel loops except for the rectum (Fig. 74–5).

EXTENT OF PELVIC LYMPHADENECTOMY. Pelvic lymphadenectomy may be performed either at this stage or after the removal of the bladder. If palpation and visual inspection reveal no gross abnormalities in the pelvic lymph nodes, I prefer to delay the pelvic lymphadenectomy until after the cystectomy is completed, for two reasons: (1) less retraction and manipulation of the bladder, the cancerous organ, may take place and (2) lymphadenectomy may be achieved more simply and more completely, if the bladder is out of the way.

The extent of pelvic lymphadenectomy is a matter of preference. Some surgeons start as high as 2 cm above the aortic bifurcation and perform an extensive lymphadenectomy, skeletonizing the common, internal, and external iliac vessels circumferentially (Skinner, 1990). Others prefer a limited dissection, extending from the common iliac bifurcation along the medial aspect of the external iliac artery, moving distally to the beginning of the femoral canal, where the node of Cloquet is located, and along the internal iliac artery medially and posteriorly to the deep pelvic vein. All lymphatic and adipose tissues within these boundaries are excised, including all tissues between the external iliac artery and vein and lateral and posterior to the obturator nerve (Fig. 74–6).

The generous utilization of ties, hemoclips, and electrocautery is recommended during lymphadenectomy in order to secure even the smallest of lymphatics and to prevent leakage of lymph, which may lead to the formation of lymphoceles or to excessive postoperative drainage and loss of protein.

INCISION OF PERITONEAL REFLECTIONS. The lateral reflections of the parietal peritoneum between the bladder and the lateral abdominal wall are incised on either side. The incision is carried posteriorly

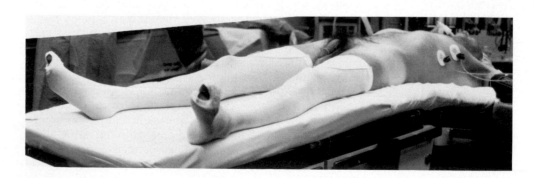

Figure 74–1. Supine position with gentle back extension and legs apart of a man about to undergo radical cystectomy without urethrectomy.

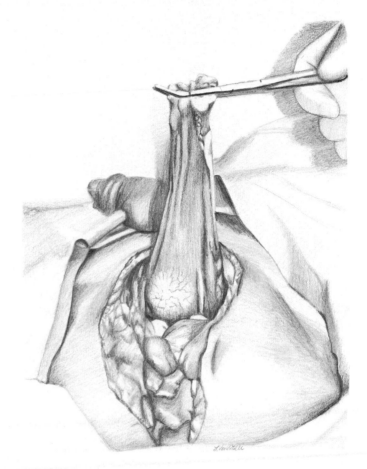

Figure 74–2. The urachal remnant excised with a wide margin and in continuity with the bladder.

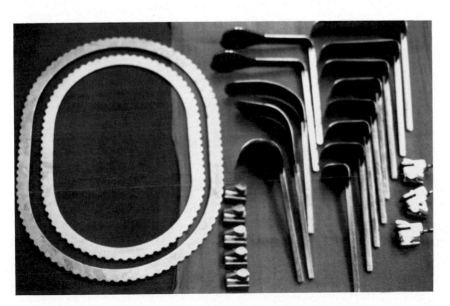

Figure 74–3. Display of the Bookwalter retractor with two different ring sizes and many different retractors.

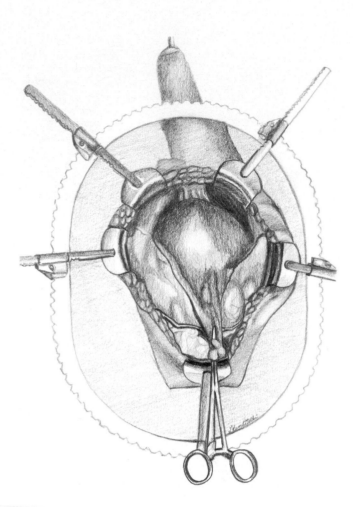

Figure 74–4. The bladder is bluntly dissected off the lateral pelvic walls for placement of the Bookwalter retractor.

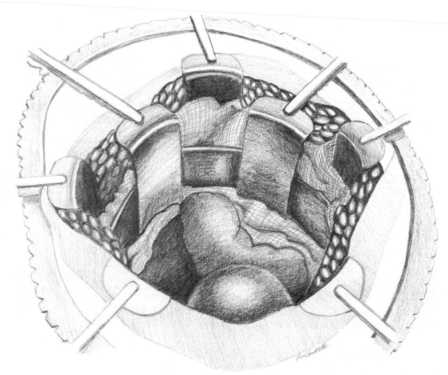

Figure 74–5. The bowels are packed in the upper abdominal cavity with moist laps and held there with a curved malleable retractor, which is kept in place by the deep retractors of the Bookwalter.

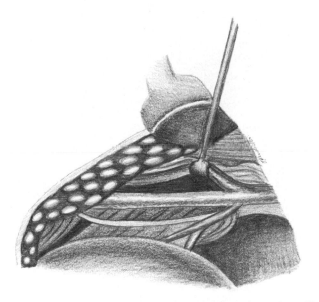

Figure 74–6. Extent of pelvic lymphadenectomy from the common iliac bifurcation to the beginning of the femoral canal, excising all lymphatic tissues medial to the external iliac artery, around the external iliac vein, and around the obturator nerve and vessels.

and caudally toward the most dependent point of the pouch of Douglas and then across the midline anterior and very close to the rectum. Thus, the visceral peritoneum covering the posterior wall of the bladder is separated from that covering the anterior rectal wall, in preparation for developing the proper plane between the bladder and rectum (Fig. 74–7).

The first structure encountered during the incision of the lateral peritoneum is the vas deferens, which is cross clamped, cut, and tied. By continuing the incision posteriorly, the second structure encountered is the superior vesical artery. This is followed proximally, all the way to its origin at the internal iliac artery, where it is cross clamped, cut, and tied with nonabsorbable material, such as silk.

If the superior vesical artery cannot be identified on the posterolateral wall of the bladder while incising the peritoneal reflections, the following technique may be applied: The internal iliac artery (hypogastric artery) is identified beyond the common iliac bifurcation and followed toward the bladder. The first anterior branch is usually the superior vesical artery, which can be cross clamped and tied at its origin. The obturator and other smaller arteries may arise from the internal iliac or from the superior vesical artery at this site. They can be cross clamped and tied. The continuation of the internal iliac artery becomes the inferior vesical artery, which can be cross clamped and tied beyond the origin of the superior vesical artery. Care must be taken to avoid tying the superior gluteal artery, which arises from the internal iliac close to the origin of the superior vesical and dips posterolaterally. Tying the superior gluteal may cause gluteal claudications.

DISSECTION AND TRANSECTION OF PELVIC URETERS. Incisions are made in the posterior peritoneum over the ureters where they cross the iliac vessels. These incisions are continued distally over the course of the ureters, until they connect with the incisions of the

lateral peritoneal reflections. The ureters, with their periureteral tissues and vessels are dissected free down to a few centimeters from their entry into the bladder, where they are cross clamped, cut, and ligated. The small vessels supplying the distal ureters should be clipped or ligated as far away from the ureter as possible, in order not to compromise the ureteral artery and vein that run within the adventitia along the course of the ureter.

A segment of ureter, 2 to 3 mm in length, is taken from the proximal cut ends and sent for frozen-section examination, asking the pathologist to look for dysplasia and carcinoma in situ. If the ureteral mucosa shows any pathologic abnormality, a more proximal segment is submitted until a free proximal margin is reached. If, at the time of urinary diversion, excess ureter needs to be excised, another proximal margin may be checked to ensure the presence of a normal mucosa for the ureterointestinal anastomosis, because dysplasia and carcinoma in situ may be multicentric and "skip areas" may exist.

Two points need to be emphasized. The first is the gentle handling and dissection of the ureter in order not to compromise its blood supply, resulting in a nonviable ureter, which will lead to stricture formation. The second is the early ligation of the proximal ureters that allows them to dilate during the rest of the procedure, making the ureterointestinal anastomosis less difficult to perform.

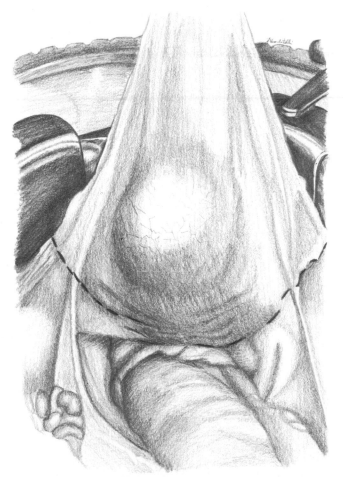

Figure 74–7. Site of incision of peritoneal reflections laterally and across the anterior rectal wall deep in the pouch of Douglas.

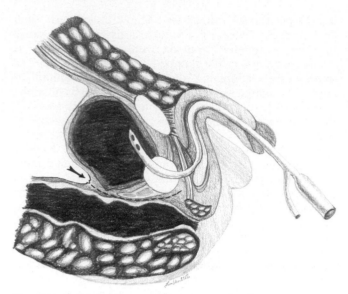

Figure 74–8. Site of separation of anterior rectal wall from the posterior bladder wall, seminal vesicles, and prostate.

DISSECTION OF BLADDER OFF ANTERIOR RECTAL WALL. Developing the plane between the anterior rectal wall and the bladder starts at the previously made incision separating the visceral peritoneum covering the posterior wall of the bladder from that covering the anterior rectal wall in the pouch of Douglas (Fig. 74–8). In most patients, this plane is developed in the midline, by lifting the bladder off the rectum by blunt dissection with the fingers (Fig. 74–9), until the

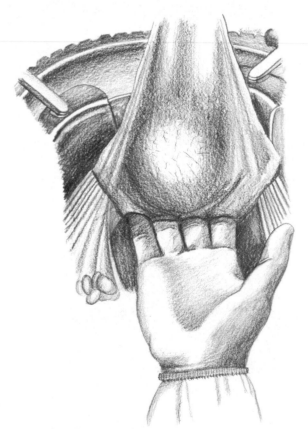

Figure 74–9. Blunt finger dissection of the plane between the anterior rectal wall and the bladder.

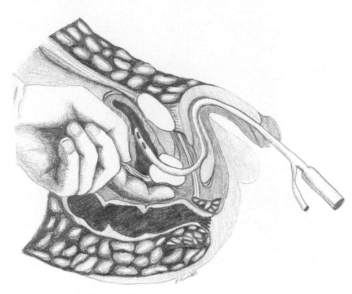

Figure 74–10. Lateral view of the plane of dissection between the anterior rectal wall and the bladder.

ampullae of the vas deferens are completely separated from the anterior rectal wall. If this plane is difficult to find and develop in the midline, the next maneuver is to identify the vas deferens on the back wall of the bladder and to follow it posteriorly with blunt dissection, lifting it off the rectum on either side until the ampullae are reached. Once the rectal wall is identified, the plane in the midline can be developed with sharp dissection.

When this plane is correctly developed, the blunt dissection can be carried distally—all the way to the apex of the prostate between the rectum and Denonvilliers's fascia, which should remain adherent to the posterior surface of the prostate (Fig. 74–10). It is therefore imperative to start this plane of dissection as close to the rectum as possible, in order to avoid creating false planes between the bladder and seminal vesicles and between the prostate and Denonvilliers's fascia, thereby risking a positive margin.

CONTROL OF LATERAL PEDICLES. Once the bladder, the seminal vesicles, the vas deferens and ampullae, and the prostate gland are lifted off the rectum, the lateral pedicles become identifiable. They should be separated medially from the lateral rectal surface by blunt dissection in order to avoid rectal injury while clamping them and, more importantly, to take them as far posteriorly as possible for a better surgical margin. By placing the pedicle between the index and middle fingers and the bladder in the palm of one hand and lifting (Fig. 74–11), the pedicles can now be transected between hemoclips or cross clamped, cut, and tied under direct vision. This maneuver can be carried distally to the apex of the prostate except when a nerve-sparing cystectomy is planned. In that case, control of the lateral pedicles should stop at the superior pedicle of the prostate until the neurovascular bundles are freed and allowed to drop laterally (see Nerve-Sparing Radical Cystectomy).

INCISION OF ENDOPELVIC FASCIA AND DIVISION OF PUBOPROSTATIC LIGAMENTS. The endopelvic fascia is incised on either side with a scalpel or electrocautery, starting at the puboprostatic ligaments

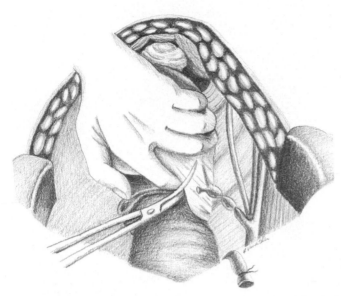

Figure 74–11. Holding the lateral pedicle between the index and middle fingers of one hand and the bladder in the palm of the hand and lifting allows for better visualization of the pedicles and simpler control. The index finger protects the rectum.

anteriorly. One then continues posteriorly along the junction of its parietal leaf, covering the levator ani muscle, and its visceral leaf, covering the lateral aspect of the prostate, bladder, and rectum. This incision is curved superiorly along the lateral wall of the rectum until it ends at the transected lateral pedicles. The levator ani muscle is bluntly dissected off the prostate and membranous urethra, until the Foley catheter is felt in the membranous urethra beyond the apex of the prostate (Fig. 74–12).

The puboprostatic ligaments are identified and freed of all adipose tissue and of the superficial branch of the dorsal vein of the penis, which runs between the two ligaments toward the bladder neck. The ligaments are transected with scissors as close to the undersurface of the symphysis pubis as is safe, without impinging on the dorsal vein complex (Fig. 74–13). These cuts should be made with the tip of the scissors under direct vision. Transecting the puboprostatic ligaments allows the prostatic apex to drop posteriorly and makes access to the dorsal vein complex possible.

LIGATION OF DORSAL VEIN COMPLEX. Control of the dorsal vein complex is the most critical part of the operation because the volume of lost blood is determined during this maneuver. Ligation of the dorsal vein can be accomplished by either (a) passing a right-angle clamp between the urethra and dorsal vein complex distal to the prostatic apex (Fig. 74–14) and tying it with a heavy ligature (0 polyglycolic acid, polyglactin 910, or silk) and then placing a figure-of-eight suture ligature distal to the tie to ensure control should the first ligature slip *or* (b) placing a suture ligature as far distally as possible without the use of a clamp. If bladder substitution is planned, I recommend against the use of the clamp in order to avoid injury to the anterior fibers of the external sphincter, which may lead to postoperative incontinence.

Once the dorsal vein complex is secured, it is transected just beyond the apex of the prostate cephalad to the ligatures. Should bleeding occur following transection it can be controlled with suture ligatures placed under direct vision. Back bleeding is minimal because all of the bladder and prostatic pedicles should have already been tied and transected.

Occasionally, while placing the clamp between the dorsal vein complex and urethra or while placing suture ligatures in the dorsal vein complex, excessive bleeding is encountered owing to tears in the vein. A suture ligature of 0 chromic on a 5/8 needle placed as far

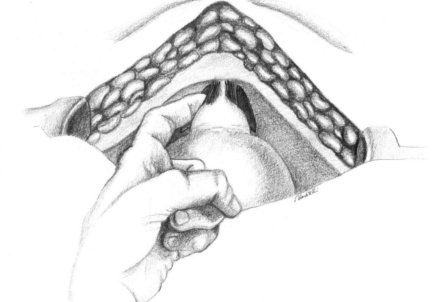

Figure 74–12. Incision of endopelvic fascia on either side of the prostate with blunt finger dissection of the levator ani muscle off the lateral aspect of the prostate and urethra.

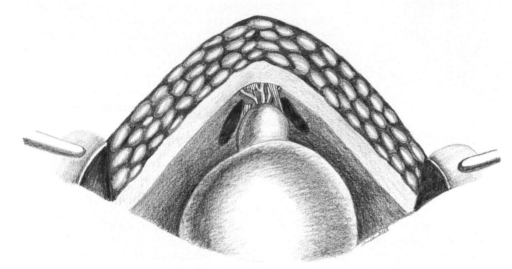

Figure 74–13. Incision of puboprostatic ligaments close to the undersurface of the symphysis pubis.

Figure 74–14. Clamp placed between the dorsal vein complex and the urethra to pass a ligature and secure the vein.

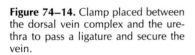

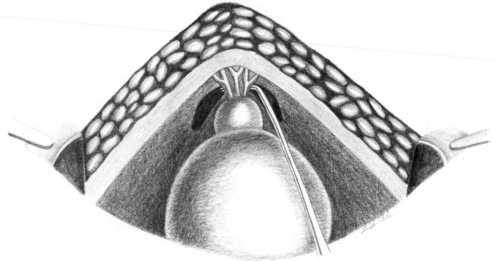

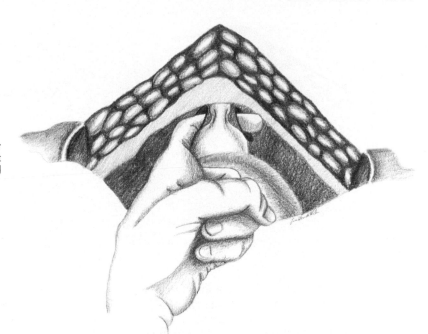

Figure 74–15. The urethra is dissected free off the anterior rectal wall and the finger is wrapped around it to protect the rectum while transecting the dorsal vein complex and urethra distal to the prostatic apex.

distally as possible usually controls the bleeding. However, if bleeding continues and instead of attempting to place more suture ligatures and risk more injury and blood loss, the following maneuver is recommended: The membranous urethra is dissected off the anterior rectal wall by blunt finger dissection. Keeping the finger behind the urethra (Fig. 74–15), the Foley catheter is withdrawn and the dorsal vein complex and urethra are transected just distal to the apex of the prostate, protecting the rectum with the finger. The apex of the prostate is lifted superiorly, and a 24 Fr. Foley catheter with a 30-cc balloon is introduced per urethra into the pelvic cavity; the balloon is inflated to 30 to 60 cc, and traction on the catheter is applied (Fig. 74–16). The balloon tamponades the dorsal vein, and bleeding ceases immediately. If bladder substitution is not planned, the

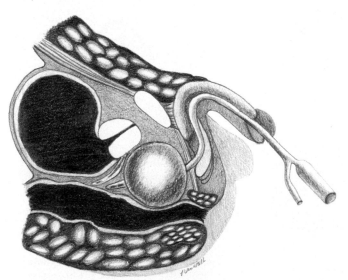

Figure 74–16. Lateral view of the pelvic cavity following transection of the dorsal vein complex and urethra. The apex of the prostate is lifted and a Foley catheter with its balloon inflated to tamponade bleeding from the dorsal vein of the penis.

Foley catheter can remain on traction for 24 to 48 hours. In the meantime, the catheter may be used as a pelvic drain. If the membranous urethra is going to be utilized for bladder substitution, traction on the Foley catheter is maintained for 10 to 15 minutes while the surgical specimen is being removed. If not done previously, pelvic lymphadenectomy is performed.

Once the bladder and prostate are removed, better visualization of and access to the pelvic floor become possible. Traction on the Foley catheter is released and the catheter pulled away from the pelvic floor. A suture ligature can now be placed anterior to the urethra and around the dorsal vein complex. Sometimes, a longer period of traction on the catheter is needed before the bleeding stops and visualization is clear enough to place adequate sutures.

DISSECTION OF MEMBRANOUS URETHRA. Transection of the dorsal vein complex beyond the prostatic apex brings into view the anterior wall of the urethra and, on either side, the prostato-ischial ligaments of Mueller, commonly referred to as urethral pillars.

If bladder substitution is not planned, the prostato-ischial ligaments are dissected off the urethra and transected distal to the apex of the prostate. The urethra is lifted off the rectal wall behind Denonvilliers's plate by finger dissection, which is carried all the way behind the prostate to meet the previously established plane between the bladder and anterior rectal wall. At this stage, the only structure keeping the surgical specimen attached is the urethra. By gentle cephalad traction on the bladder, the urethra can be circumferentially dissected off distally, for 2 to 3 inches beyond the apex of the prostate. If a total urethrectomy is not planned, the Foley catheter is removed and the urethra is transected sharply as far distally as possible (Fig. 74–17). The surgical specimen is removed. If a total en bloc urethrectomy is planned, the dissection from within the pelvic cavity is terminated at this point, until the perineal

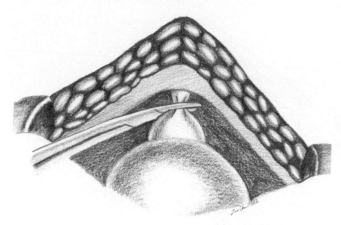

Figure 74–17. Transection of the membranous urethra beyond the prostatic apex.

dissection of the urethra is accomplished. (See section on Urethrectomy at the end of this chapter.)

If bladder substitution is planned, the membranous urethra should be carefully dissected. Following transection of the dorsal vein complex as outlined here, the anterior half of the urethra with the prostato-ischial ligaments is sharply cut with a scalpel just beyond the apex of the prostate over the Foley catheter. Sutures are placed through the full thickness of the urethral wall at 2 o'clock and 10 o'clock, including the prostato-ischial ligaments. These sutures will be needed later for the anastamosis between the bladder substitution reservoir and the membranous urethra. The Foley catheter is removed, and the posterior half of the urethra and Denonvilliers's plate are transected. The surgical specimen is removed. Sutures are placed at 5 o'clock and 7 o'clock, including Denonvilliers's plate. These sutures will also be utilized for the anastamosis with the reservoir. The type of suture material selected for the anastamosis is a matter of personal preference. I use 3–0 polyglactin sutures on a gastrointestinal needle.

If a pelvic lymphadenectomy was not done earlier, it is performed at this stage, followed by urinary diversion or bladder substitution (see Chapter 72).

Nerve-Sparing Radical Cystectomy

The first stages of the radical cystectomy should proceed in a fashion similar to that described previously, until the step to control the lateral pedicles is reached. At this stage, only the most superior of the lateral pedicles should be transected, leaving the rest until after the neurovascular bundles are freed.

The neurovascular bundles run posterolateral to the prostate and membranous urethra and are covered by the lateral prostatic fascia, which keeps them in close proximity to the prostatic capsule. The endopelvic fascia is incised and the puboprostatic ligaments transected, as described previously. I prefer to secure the dorsal vein complex after the neurovascular bundle is freed, in case the bleeding that may occur during control of the dorsal vein interferes with adequate visualization and neurovascular bundle dissection.

Incising the endopelvic fascia and dropping the prostate by transecting the puboprostatic ligaments brings into view the lateral surface of the prostate, which is covered by the lateral fascia. This fascia is lifted off the prostatic capsule with a pair of fine forceps and sharply and bluntly dissected off the prostatic capsule all along the lateral surface of the prostate. By following this plane between the lateral prostatic fascia and the prostatic capsule posteriorly, the neurovascular bundle is dissected free of the prostate (Fig. 74–18). With blunt finger dissection, the neurovascular bundle can now be freed and pushed laterally, all the way from the membranous urethra up to the superior prostatic pedicle. Although the neurovascular bundle is now free from the prostate, it is still attached to Denonvilliers's fascia posteriorly. To free the neurovascular bundle completely, Denonvilliers's fascia has to be incised along

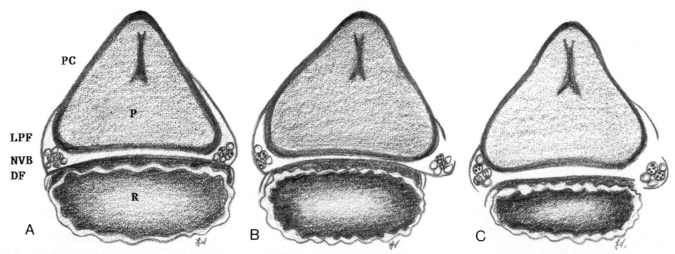

Figure 74–18. Schematic cross-sectional representation of the relationships among the prostate, the neurovascular bundle, the lateral prostatic fascia, and Denonvilliers' fascia, and the planes of dissection to follow to separate the neurovascular bundle off the prostate. *A*, Cross-section at the level of the mid-prostate where the separation of the neurovascular bundle should start (P, prostate; PC, prostatic capsule; LPF, lateral prostatic fascia; NVB, neurovascular bundle; DF, Denonvilliers' fascia; R, rectum). *B*, Incision in lateral prostatic fascia is made, and the NVB is bluntly separated off the prostatic capsule. *C*, Incision is made in Denonvilliers' fascia to completely separate the NVB, which comes to lie lateral to the prostate and away from the planes of dissection to complete the cystectomy.

the medial border of the neurovascular bundle. This maneuver can be aided by placing the finger in the plane previously created between Denonvilliers's fascia and the rectal wall. Once Denonvilliers's fascia is incised, the neurovascular bundle is now completely free and tends to lie laterally and away from the planes of dissection.

Often, veins leave the neurovascular bundle and pierce the prostatic capsule along this plane. These veins must be clipped or tied. Avoid electrocautery to control bleeding from these veins in order to minimize damage to the nerves.

Once the neurovascular bundle is freed, the superior prostatic pedicle and the remaining lateral bladder pedicles can now be cross clamped, cut, and tied. The dorsal vein complex and the membranous urethra can now be handled as previously described. For a nerve-sparing urethrectomy, see the last part of this chapter.

Drainage and Closure

The pelvic cavity is thoroughly irrigated and complete hemostasis secured. Careful inspection of the anterior rectal wall should be done to identify any unrecognized rectal injury. Because of the large raw surface area created by removal of the bladder and prostate, a significant volume of tissue fluid tends to collect in the pelvic cavity and needs to be drained, especially in patients on heparin. The choice of drains is a matter of personal preference. I prefer a closed-suction drain left deep in the pelvic cavity and brought out through a separate skin incision. If a Foley catheter has to be left in for control of bleeding from the dorsal vein, it may also serve as a pelvic drain. Drains are left until draining stops, which is usually 3 to 5 days postoperatively.

The rectosigmoid is dropped into the pelvic cavity. The omentum is draped over the intestines, and its free edge is directed into the pelvic cavity.

The method of abdominal closure is also a matter of personal preference. I employ a running fascial suture of 1–0 polyglycolic acid material with several interrupted reinforcing sutures of the same material, placed 1 to 2 inches apart. If the patient is obese, a subcutaneous closed-suction drain is left for 2 to 3 days to prevent seromas. Staples are utilized to approximate the skin edges. Retention sutures are used routinely in debilitated, poorly nourished patients and in those on a long-term steroid regimen.

Postoperative Management

Over the past few years, I have come to prefer tube gastrostomy over nasogastric drainage. A tube gastrostomy, placed just before abdominal closure, is less irritating to the patient, does not interfere with pulmonary hygiene, and allows immediate clear liquids orally. Gastrointestinal drainage with either nasogastric or gastrostomy tubes is continued until normal bowel activity returns, as evidenced by the passage of flatus. In the meantime, the patient is maintained on intravenous fluids and, if needed, parenteral nutrition.

Epidural or patient-controlled analgesia has become a routine practice at Stanford University and is preferred by the patient as well as by the medical and nursing staff. This analgesic is continued for as long as the patient needs it and is gradually discontinued and replaced with oral analgesics when bowel activity returns.

Ambulation is started on the evening of the day of surgery and is continued with increasing frequency thereafter. Once the patient is fully ambulatory, the heparin, if started preoperatively, is discontinued.

The teaching of stoma care or catheter irrigation if the patient has a continent diversion to the urethra begins on the 4th or 5th postoperative day and continues until the time of discharge.

Drains are removed when drainage ceases. Skin staples are removed and replaced with Steri-Strips on the day of discharge.

The patient is discharged when on a regular diet and having normal bowel function.

Complications

Modern day anesthesia, complete and careful preoperative preparation, good surgical technique, and intensive postoperative care have significantly reduced the morbidity and mortality from radical cystectomy. Table 74–5 lists the complications in the last 100 radical cystectomies I have performed and serves to identify the complications that may be encountered during or after the operation—19 complications and two deaths occurred in 16 patients.

The two major intraoperative complications are excessive blood loss and rectal injury. The average blood loss during radical cystectomy is about 600 ml, and transfusions are seldom needed. Occasionally, bleeding from the dorsal vein complex may be excessive and may require transfusions. Autotransfusion and cell savers have significantly reduced the need for donor blood and, therefore, the risk of hepatitis and transfusion reaction. Patients are usually asked to donate 2 to 3 units of blood prior to the operation if their general health allows. Intraoperative autotransfusion and the cell saver in cancer surgery are controversial; however, if the bladder is not opened during the operation and if spillage of cancer cells does not occur, the cell saver should be safe (Hart et al., 1989).

Table 74–5. MORBIDITY AND MORTALITY IN 100 CONSECUTIVE RADICAL CYSTECTOMIES

Complications	Number
Intraoperative	
Rectal perforation	1
More than 4 units transfusion needed	2
Immediate postoperative	
Wound infection	7
Pelvic abscess	1
Sepsis	1
Deep venous thrombosis	3
Non-fatal pulmonary embolus	2
Pneumonia	1
Late postoperative	
Intestinal obstruction	1
Mortality	2
Total	21*

*Nineteen complications and two deaths occurred in 16 patients.

Rectal injury is rare and occurs while developing the plane between the bladder and prostate and the anterior rectal wall. Careful inspection of the anterior rectal wall should always take place after the surgical specimen is removed in case an unrecognized injury had occurred. Most rectal injuries are small and can be corrected with a two layer closure, a through-and-through layer of absorbable suture, and an inbricating muscular layer of silk.

It is recommended that, if rectal injury had occurred and was corrected, the anal sphincter be dilated at the end of the operation in order to decrease the intraluminal rectal pressure and tension on the suture line in the immediate postoperative period, during the healing process.

If rectal injury occurs during salvage cystectomy or in a previously irradiated rectum, consideration should be given to a temporary diverting colostomy over and above closure of the perforation (Freiha and Faysal, 1983).

Other less commonly encountered intraoperative complications include injury to the iliac vessels and transection of the obturator nerve.

The immediate postoperative complications are the most common and are those encountered with any major intra-abdominal procedure (see Table 74–5). Late postoperative complications are rare and usually secondary to the urinary diversion itself.

The mortality from cystectomy is low—2 per cent or less. One of the two deaths reported in Table 74–1 occurred in a 77-year-old woman with steroid-dependent, severe and chronic obstructive pulmonary disease in whom the cystectomy had to be performed because of a bladder capacity of 30 ml and the need to void every 15 to 30 minutes, day and night, giving her no rest. She developed pneumonia and pelvic abscess and died of pulmonary failure.

The other death occurred in a 67-year-old man who, on the day of operation, developed anterior chest pain. The operation was cancelled after he had received a full bowel preparation. The chest pain was later found not to be secondary to any significant abnormality, and he was readmitted 2 weeks later and underwent another bowel preparation and was operated on. On the 7th postoperative day he developed fever and sepsis secondary to candidemia and died, despite the use of intravenous amphotericin. It was assumed that the administration of antibiotics for two bowel preparations 2 weeks apart caused an overgrowth of *Candida*, which led to sepsis and death. It is, therefore, recommended that when such a condition prevails, the operation should be delayed until the bowels recover normal flora, which takes at least 3 to 4 weeks. Alternatively, the second bowel preparation should be only mechanical—without antibiotics. In either case, the patient may benefit from preoperative oral antifungal agents.

In the Female

Radical cystectomy in the female implies the en bloc removal of the bladder with its peritoneal coverings and the urachal remnant up to the umbilicus; the entire urethra including the external meatus; the uterus, fallopian tubes, and ovaries; the anterior vaginal wall; and the pelvic lymph nodes. This procedure is also known as anterior pelvic exenteration.

In most cases, only the anterior third of the vagina is resected, leaving enough wall to reconstruct a functional vagina. However, loss of a functional vagina is possible and every patient should be appraised of that possibility prior to the operation. In young, sexually active women whose tumors are located on the anterior wall or dome of the bladder and whose biopsy samples of the trigone and floor show no carcinoma, resection of the anterior vaginal wall may be avoided.

Women should be carefully counseled regarding the loss of the uterus and ovaries and the possible need for the future use of estrogens, the possible loss of a functional vagina, dyspareunia, and diminished sexual sensations due to complete urethrectomy, and the possible need for postoperative vaginal dilation.

Surgical Technique

The incision, exposure, timing, and extent of pelvic lymphadenectomy and the initial steps of the operation are the same as those described for radical cystectomy in the male.

The first structure encountered during incision of the lateral peritoneal reflection is the round ligament, which is cross clamped, cut, and tied. Its medial end can be utilized for traction to pull up on the uterus for better exposure. The next structures are the superior vesical artery and just behind are the uterine vessels, which cross over the ureter. These vessels are also cross clamped, cut, and tied. Both the superior vesical and the uterine arteries are branches of the hypogastric artery. If isolating these arteries separately is technically difficult, isolating the hypogastric artery and tying it distal to the posterior superior gluteal artery achieve the same result. Care should be taken to keep the posterior superior gluteal artery intact in order to prevent postoperative gluteal claudications.

Once the uterine arteries are transected, the distal ureter comes into view and can now be isolated, cross clamped, cut, and tied. The ureter is handled in the same manner as described in the male, as far as surgical margins are concerned. The incision made for the peritoneal reflections is carried superiorly along the course of the ureter, reflecting the broad ligament, ovary, and fallopian tubes medially, until the ovarian vessels are reached. The ureter is separated from the ovarian vessels, which are cross clamped, cut, and suture ligated. Proximal dissection of the ureter is continued for as long as needed.

The broad ligament, which is now free laterally, is incised posterior to the ovary and fallopian tube, toward and all the way to the posterior fornix of the vagina, at the junction of the vagina and rectum in the pouch of Douglas.

A sponge on a sponge forceps is inserted into the vagina, all the way to the posterior fornix and gently pushed cephalad, stretching the vaginal wall (Fig. 74–19). This maneuver facilitates the exposure and dissec-

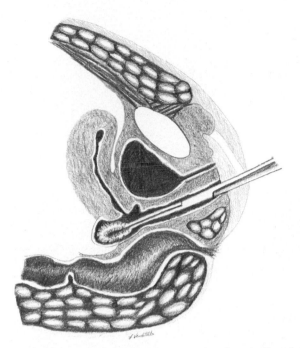

Figure 74–19. A sponge on a forceps is introduced vaginally, all the way to the posterior fornix.

tion of the lateral pedicles of the bladder, which should take place along the lateral surface of the vaginal wall, exposing the lateral vaginal wall just above its junctions with the rectum. Control of the lateral pedicles is continued distally to the junction of the parietal and visceral reflections of the endopelvic fascia deep in the pelvic cavity. The endopelvic fascia is incised along this junction in order to expose the most distal portion of the vaginal wall.

Following control of the lateral bladder pedicles bilaterally, a transverse incision is made in the posterior fornix of the vagina just above its junction with the rectum, thus entering the vaginal cavity. This maneuver is facilitated by upward retraction of the uterus and by the sponge on the forceps placed in the vagina with cephalad retraction (Fig. 74–20). Once the vaginal cavity is entered, the sponge and forceps are removed (Fig. 74–21). The lateral vaginal wall is now placed between the middle and index fingers of the hand. With the uterus and bladder in the palm of the hand (Fig. 74–22), upward traction is applied and the lateral vaginal wall incised on either side all the way to the entroitus. During this maneuver, large venous sinuses, which run along and in the vaginal wall, are unroofed. Bleeding may be profuse. Suture ligating these sinuses, as they are transected, decreases blood loss.

The pubourethral ligaments are incised under direct vision. The venous plexus is suture ligated, as close to the symphysis pubis as possible, and transected. Through a vaginal approach, the vaginal entroitus is now incised around the anterior lip of the external urethral meatus. The surgical specimen is delivered out of the pelvic cavity.

The pelvic cavity is thoroughly irrigated and hemostasis completed. The vaginal wall is sutured in the midline along its longitudinal axis, employing a running heavy absorbable suture material with frequent interruptions. Sometimes, in order to be able to approximate the lateral vaginal wall in the midline and achieve an adequate vaginal cavity, the vagina has to be partially freed

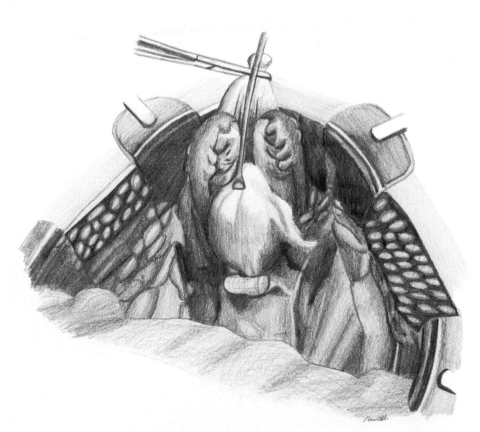

Figure 74–20. With the uterus, ovaries, tubes, and bladder lifted upward, the sponge in the vagina can be palpated and a transverse incision made in the vaginal wall, exposing the sponge.

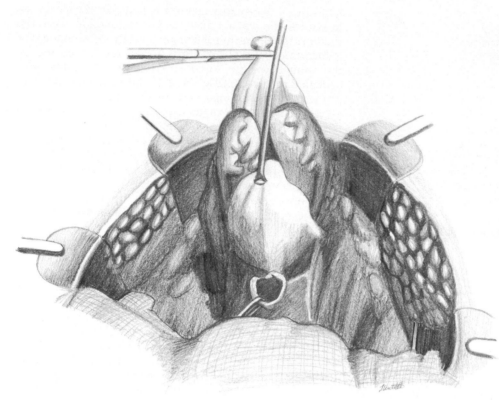

Figure 74–21. The sponge and forceps are removed out of the vagina, and the edges of the vaginal incision are held open with Ellis clamps.

Figure 74–22. With the index finger in the vaginal cavity and the uterus and bladder in the palm of the hand, upward traction will bring to view the lateral vaginal wall, which is incised all the way to the introitus.

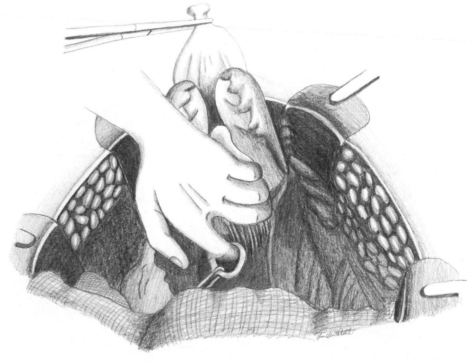

off the anterior rectal wall. The vaginal introitus at the site of the excised external urethral meatus is closed from the vaginal side with absorbable 3–0 chromic or polyglactin suture material. A vaginal packing is left in for 24 hours.

In a patient who has had a prior hysterectomy, the normal anatomy of the pouch of Douglas and of the normal planes and demarcations between the vaginal vault and the rectum posteriorly and the bladder anteriorly have been disturbed. Extreme caution should be exercised while trying to enter at the vaginal vault. This is where rectal injury occurs and where inadvertent entry into the bladder is most common. The sponge on a forceps in the vagina is of great help in dissecting and finding the vaginal vault and in preventing rectal and bladder injury. Otherwise, the operation should proceed in the same manner as already described.

In women in whom the anterior vaginal wall is not to be resected, the operation should proceed as described, until the step of opening the vagina at the posterior fornix or vault. Following control of the lateral pedicles and incision of the endopelvic fascia, the pubourethral ligaments are incised and the venous plexus suture ligated. The next step is performed vaginally. With the Foley catheter in place, the external urethral meatus is circumscribed and a plane is developed between the anterior vaginal wall and the urethra along with the base of the bladder. The urethra is freed circumferentially as far proximally as is possible with the vaginal approach. The urethra and Foley catheter are then placed into the pelvic cavity.

The operation is now continued from within the pelvic cavity. With cephalad traction on the Foley catheter and packing in the vagina, the plane between the anterior vaginal wall and bladder can be sharply dissected under direct vision, suture ligating venous sinuses as the dissection is carried cephalad until the bladder is completely separated from the vagina.

The surgical specimen is delivered off the field and the pelvic cavity thoroughly irrigated. Hemostasis is completed. The incision in the vaginal introitus at the site of the excised external urethral meatus is approximated with fine absorbable sutures, such as 3–0 chromic or polyglactin. The vaginal packing is left for 24 hours.

It is possible to perform the cystectomy without a vaginal approach; however, the risks of urethral tear and incomplete resection of the external urethral meatus are higher. Following transection of the pubourethral ligaments and suture ligation of the venous plexus, a large Foley catheter is inserted into the bladder. The plane between the urethra and anterior vaginal wall is developed by blunt finger dissection as far distally as possible, until the urethra is completely encircled. The dissection is carried distally until the vaginal introitus from within the pelvic cavity is reached. The Foley catheter is removed. With cephalad traction on the urethra, the external urethral meatus is pulled into the pelvic cavity. A right-angle clamp is placed as far distally as possible, with the hope that it is beyond the external urethral meatus. The urethra is transected. A suture ligature of heavy absorbable material is placed around the right-angle clamp, and the clamp is removed. The

Foley catheter is reinserted into the urethra and bladder, which are retracted cephalad. The plane between the urethra and bladder and the anterior vaginal wall is developed under direct vision, until the bladder is removed.

The only possible advantage of avoiding the combined pelvic and vaginal approach is the diminished risk of contamination and, therefore, infection.

If a pelvic lymphadenectomy was not performed in continuity or before removal of the bladder, it is performed now, followed by urinary diversion (see Chapter 72).

Drainage and postoperative management are basically the same as those for men. The vaginal packing is removed on the 1st postoperative day. Vaginal hygiene, with sitz baths and gentle douches, is started on the 3rd to 4th postoperative day, if needed.

Complications

The complications listed in Table 74–1 are encountered in both men and women. Complications specific to women include vaginal infections and prolonged vaginal drainage, vaginal bleeding from the suture line, vaginal contracture, and total loss of a functional vagina. Patients who develop vaginal contracture or shortening can be successfully managed with vaginal dilation. Reconstruction with skin grafts, flaps, or bowel segments is rarely needed. Dyspareunia and some loss of sexual sensations have been encountered and are usually caused by scarring and urethral meatal resection, respectively, conditions that are hard to avoid or guard against.

Comment

A single stage radical cystectomy and urinary diversion or bladder substitution is a well-tolerated major operation with acceptable morbidity and mortality. Alone, or in combination with radiation therapy and/or chemotherapy, it constitutes the optimal treatment for patients with invasive or multifocal bladder cancer and offers effective palliation for those with locally advanced disease. Careful selection, preoperative preparation, attention to good surgical technique, and postoperative management significantly reduce morbidity. Radical cystectomy is thus a much more acceptable operation.

SIMPLE CYSTECTOMY

Simple cystectomy is the total excision of the bladder without removal of any of the surrounding structures and organs. In sexually potent men, in the absence of prostatic disease, removal of the prostate gland and the seminal vesicles should be avoided in order to preserve potency. Otherwise, removing the prostate and seminal vesicles in continuity with the bladder simplifies the operation.

In women, removing the anterior vaginal wall and external urethral meatus is not necessary except when the simple cystectomy is being performed for interstitial cystitis. In this case, leaving the external urethral meatus may not totally alleviate the symptoms of the disease.

The indications for simple cystectomy are benign problems, such as pyocystis, small contracted bladders from radiation cystitis, tuberculosis, schistosomiasis, cyclophosphamide (Cytoxan) cystitis and interstitial cystitis, uncontrollable bleeding from either radiation or Cytoxan cystitis, and severe unmanageable vesical fistulas and incontinence. It is also performed for palliation from locally advanced bladder cancer in patients with metastatic disease.

Surgical Technique

Preoperative preparation, position, and exposure are the same as those described for radical cystectomy. In patients who have undergone previous supravesical urinary diversions, the simple cystectomy may be performed through a lower abdominal, extraperitoneal approach. This eliminates the possible need for lysis of intestinal adhesions which, in previously irradiated patients, may be extensive.

Irrespective of the approach, every attempt should be made to preserve the pelvic peritoneum covering the bladder in order to use it later as a shield to separate the peritoneal cavity from the extraperitoneal pelvic cavity and to prevent loops of intestine from dropping down and adhering to raw surfaces.

Following entry into the peritoneal cavity or into the retropubic space in case of an extraperitoneal approach, and after achieving adequate exposure, the pelvic peritoneum is stripped off the dome and posterior wall of the bladder by sharp and blunt dissection, cauterizing or tying all bleeders. This maneuver is facilitated by filling and distending the bladder through the indwelling Foley catheter. If tears in the peritoneum occur while dissecting it off the bladder they should be closed with fine sutures of 3–0 or 4–0 chromic, polyglycolic acid, or silk material.

In a man, dissection of the peritoneum off the bladder should proceed posteriorly until the junction of the bladder and anterior rectal wall. During this dissection, the vas deferens is encountered. If resection of the seminal vesicles and prostate is to be performed in continuity with the bladder, the vas deferens is cut between clamps and tied. Its medial end is followed posteriorly, lifting it off the anterior rectal wall as described for radical cystectomy. If the seminal vesicles and prostate are not to be resected, the vas deferens is left intact and is separated off the wall of the bladder all the way posteriorly, thus creating a plane between the bladder and anterior surface of the seminal vesicles and ampulla of the vas. While dissecting the vas off the bladder wall, the superior vesical artery comes into the field and is cross clamped, cut, and tied as close to the bladder as possible.

Following the bilateral control of the superior vesical artery and dissection of the vas deferens, the ureters can now be identified, dissected circumferentially, and followed proximally and extraperitoneally as far as is necessary. If the patient had had prior supravesical diversion, the ureters are followed proximally until the site where they were previously transected, in order to ensure complete excision of the distal ureters. If a urinary diversion is part of the simple cystectomy, the ureters are transected close to the bladder and freed proximally off the iliac vessels to be brought later intraperitoneally through small incisions in the posterior peritoneum in preparation for the urinary diversion.

If the prostate gland and the seminal vesicles are to be resected with the bladder the operation from this point on should proceed according to that described for radical cystectomy. If only the bladder is to be removed, it is now separated from the prostate at the prostatovesical junction or bladder neck anteriorly and laterally until the posterior bladder neck is reached. The electrocautery is a good instrument to use for this separation to minimize blood loss. If the patient has significant benign prostatic hypertrophy, which will interfere with the adequate closure of the distal bladder neck or prostatic capsule, a suprapubic enucleation of the adenoma is performed at this stage (see Chapter 77).

Hemostasis in the prostatic fossa should be meticulous and complete because a Foley catheter cannot be used postoperatively to help with control of bleeding. The posterior bladder neck is now incised from within the bladder going through the full thickness of the bladder wall until the ampullae of the vasa are seen. The trigone and base of the bladder are bluntly dissected off the ampullae of the vasa and seminal vesicles until the plane started previously by freeing the vas deferens off the bladder wall is reached and both planes become one. The lateral pedicles are now in view and can be clamped and tied or clipped as close to the bladder as possible in order to avoid injury to the neurovascular bundle. The bladder is now completely free and is delivered out of the pelvic cavity.

The distal bladder neck is now closed by approximating the prostatic capsule with interrupted figure-of-eight or horizontal mattress sutures, using heavy absorbable material such as 0 chromic or 0 polyglactin sutures.

In women, dissection of the peritoneum off the bladder should proceed posteriorly and should be continued between the uterus and bladder until the anterior vaginal fornix is reached. In a patient who had had a previous hysterectomy, the dissection ends at the vaginal vault. With the aid of a sponge on a forceps placed in the vagina with cephalad retraction, the plane between the bladder and anterior vaginal wall can now be started and carried distally, lifting the bladder off the vagina.

Lateral dissection will identify the superior vesical arteries, which are ligated close to the bladder and transected. The ureters are freed and handled in the same manner as previously described, depending on whether or not the patient had had a prior supravesical diversion. While dissecting the ureters proximally, care should be taken to avoid injury to the uterine vessels if the patient had not undergone a hysterectomy.

Once the ureters and superior vesical arteries are controlled, dissection of the plane between the bladder and anterior vaginal wall is continued distally, transecting the lateral bladder pedicles as they develop. Once the urethra is reached, the Foley catheter is removed, and the urethra is transected between clamps and tied. If the simple cystectomy is being performed for interstitial cystitis, the whole urethra and external urethral meatus have to be excised. The technique will be the same as that described for radical cystectomy in the female without resection of the anterior vaginal wall.

After the surgical specimen is removed the pelvic cavity is thoroughly irrigated and hemostasis completed. A closed-suction drain is left in the pelvic cavity and brought out through a separate skin incision.

Urinary diversion is now performed (see Chapter 72).

During closure of the abdominal incision, the anterior free edge of the pelvic peritoneum has to be incorporated into the closure in order to completely isolate the pelvic from the peritoneal cavity and to prevent herniation of intestinal loops between the edge of the peritoneum and the anterior abdominal wall.

The postoperative management and complications of simple cystectomy are the same as those of radical cystectomy.

PARTIAL CYSTECTOMY

Partial cystectomy, also known as segmental cystectomy, is the resection of a segment of bladder wall. It is the ideal operation for localized benign lesions of the bladder, such as leiomyomas, fibromas, and Hunner's ulcers that cannot be completely eliminated by transurethral resection alone, and for invasion of the bladder wall by tumors arising from adjacent organs, such as the colon, cervix, uterus, and ovaries. Such lesions are extremely rare, and the majority of partial cystectomies are being performed for invasive bladder cancer.

Partial cystectomy for bladder cancer is controversial. The multicentric or field change nature of transitional cell carcinoma and the high propensity of transitional cells to implant on any raw surface cause a significant incidence of recurrence both in the bladder and outside. However, a patient with a solitary tumor in the dome or posterior wall of the bladder who is elderly or who poses a significant surgical risk or a patient who refuses total cystectomy, partial cystectomy for invasive bladder cancer is an acceptable operation. It can also be applied to palliate symptoms of local disease in a patient with metastasis.

The two major situations to guard against while performing a partial cystectomy are (1) too generous a resection, which may result in a functionally useless, small capacity bladder, and (2) tumor cell spillage, which may lead to recurrences in the pelvis and abdominal wall. A short course of 2000 R of external beam irradiation given immediately preoperatively may reduce the incidence of tumor cell implantation (van der Werf Messing, 1969).

It is imperative that multiple bladder biopsy specimens be taken from elsewhere in the bladder at the time of initial resection of the primary bladder tumor. Patients with carcinoma in situ or mucosal dysplasia found on random biopsy samples should be advised against partial cystectomy.

Surgical Technique

A cystoscopy is performed immediately before partial cystectomy. With the bladder partially distended, the tumor is encircled with the coagulating electrode about 2 cm around its base—the site of the open resection.

The patient is placed in a supine position with gentle extension. Partial cystectomy may be performed through an extraperitoneal approach. However, if the tumor is located in an area where the overlying peritoneum has to be excised with the bladder wall, the peritoneal cavity will have to be entered. The anterior and lateral walls of the bladder are freed to give as much mobility to the bladder as possible and to aid later in a tension-free closure. A pelvic lymphadenectomy, if indicated, may be performed at this stage.

The operative field is carefully isolated. All raw surfaces, except for the planned site of resection, are packed off with moist towels in order to minimize tumor cell seeding. The bladder wall is incised with the electrocautery for a distance of 1 to 2 inches and away from the tumor but as close to the midline as possible in order to avoid injury to the major vessels and to simplify closure (Fig. 74–23). For example, if the tumor is located in the dome, the incision is made longitudinally in the anterior bladder wall close to the bladder neck. The edges of the incision are grasped with Allis or Babcock clamps. The inside of the bladder is inspected to visualize the tumor and the already marked site of resection by the coagulating electrode. The incision is then extended to the marked site of resection (Fig. 74–24). A full-thickness segment of bladder wall around the base of the tumor is resected with its overlying perivesical fat and/or peritoneum. Electrocautery minimizes bleeding.

Histologic examination of the margins of resection is performed by frozen-section techniques to determine either a free margin or a need for a wider resection. Once the margins are determined to be free of tumor,

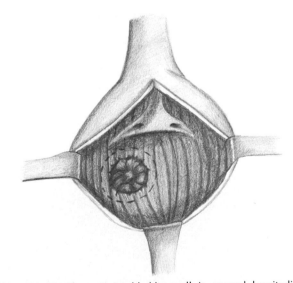

Figure 74–23. The anterior bladder wall is opened longitudinally, exposing a posteriorly located tumor with electrocautery marks surrounding it and made cystoscopically just prior to the open operation.

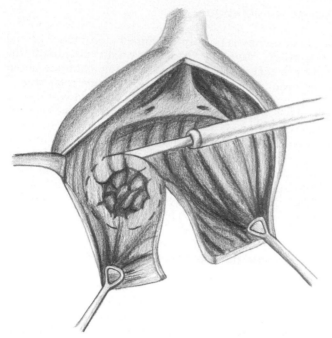

Figure 74–24. The incision in the bladder wall is extended to meet the previously marked site of resection, and a full-thickness segment of bladder wall is resected with the tumor.

the bladder wall is closed in two layers, a full-thickness layer of running sutures (Fig. 74–25) and an inverting muscular layer, using 0 or 2–0 absorbable material, such as chromic or polyglactin suture. Closure can also be accomplished equally well with a mucosal and submucosal layer of running 3–0 absorbable sutures and a muscular layer of running or interrupted 0 or 2–0 absorbable sutures.

The packings are removed, and the operative field is thoroughly irrigated with sterile water. A drain is left in the retropubic space and brought out through a separate stab wound skin incision. The abdominal incision is closed.

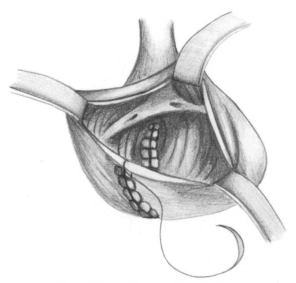

Figure 74–25. Closure of the bladder.

Bladder drainage is provided by a urethral Foley catheter. Suprapubic tubes should be avoided, especially if the partial cystectomy is being performed for transitional cell carcinoma for fear of tumor cell implantation along the suprapubic tube tract. Bladder drainage is continued postoperatively for 5 to 7 days or longer, if the patient had had prior irradiation. A cystogram may be performed just prior to removing the catheter to ensure adequate healing. I prefer to leave the retropubic space drain until the urethral catheter is removed and the patient has had good voiding trials without evidence of extravasation.

Complications

The immediate complications of partial cystectomy are bleeding, extravasation, and infection. The late and the more serious and disturbing complications are a resultant small capacity bladder and pelvic and abdominal wall recurrences from tumor cell spillage. If the tumor to be treated by partial cystectomy is not very large and if the resection is just enough to ensure a free margin, a resultant small capacity bladder is extremely rare. Treatment of small capacity bladders that are associated with very frequent voiding is augmentation cystoplasty.

Preoperative irradiation, careful patient selection, and isolation of the operative field prior to opening the bladder have reduced the incidence of pelvic and abdominal wall recurrences.

SUPRAPUBIC CYSTOTOMY

Indications

Suprapubic cystotomy is indicated for the following reasons:

1. For placement of a large-caliber drainage tube when urethral catheterization is impossible or contraindicated, such as in traumatic rupture of the membranous urethra.
2. For removal of large bladder stones, which cannot be crushed and removed transurethrally.
3. For open resection of papillary bladder tumors, which cannot be resected transurethrally because of size or location.
4. For bladder diverticulectomy.

Surgical Technique

Suprapubic cystotomy may be performed through either a midline or a Pfannenstiel incision. The anterior wall and dome of the bladder are identified and cleared of all adipose tissue. The wall of the bladder is grasped on either side with Allis or Babcock clamps and incised between the clamps in the midline with the electrocautery. The site and extent of the cystotomy depend on the condition for which it is being performed.

For placement of a large-caliber drainage tube, a small cystotomy to accommodate a 22 or 24 Fr. tube is made in the dome of the bladder, and a tube is placed. The cystotomy is closed around the tube with a purse string suture of heavy absorbable material. The tube is brought out through a separate stab wound skin incision.

For removal of large bladder stones, a 1- to 2-inch cystotomy is made in the anterior wall of the bladder and the inside of the bladder carefully inspected. The stones are grasped with forceps and removed. The bladder is reinspected to ensure that all stones were removed. The cystotomy is closed with running, full-thickness sutures of 2–0 absorbable material and an inverting muscular layer of the same.

For open resection of bladder tumors, a cystoscopy is performed just prior to the cystotomy to identify the site and number of tumors. The abdominal incision is carefully packed to minimize tumor cell spillage onto raw surfaces. A generous cystotomy is made away from the tumor, and the edges are kept apart with Allis or Babcock clamps or with stay sutures. Tumors are resected with the loop electrode, taking deep tissues for adequate staging. The resected sites are fulgurated with the ball or roller electrode, until complete hemostasis is secured. The cystotomy is closed as previously described, the packing is removed, and the pelvic cavity is thoroughly irrigated with water.

For bladder diverticulectomy, the cystotomy is started at the dome and extended into the anterior wall for 3 to 4 inches to ensure adequate exposure and space, because most of the dissection to excise the diverticulum will be performed from within the bladder (see subsequent discussion).

BLADDER DIVERTICULECTOMY

Diverticula of the bladder are either congenital or secondary to bladder outlet obstruction. The majority do not require treatment. However, large diverticula that interfere with normal voiding or carry a large residual, which predisposes the patient to stone formation or difficult to treat infection, require excision. Superficial transitional cell carcinoma in a bladder diverticulum that cannot be safely or completely resected transurethrally requires a partial cystectomy rather than a diverticulectomy only. A full-thickness segment of the bladder wall is excised, including the diverticulum with its overlying tissues.

Treatment of bladder diverticula that are secondary to bladder outlet obstruction should always be preceded or accompanied by correcting the cause of obstruction: transurethral resection or incision of the prostate or bladder neck, suprapubic prostatectomy or Y-V plasty of the bladder neck.

Surgical Technique

A cystoscopy is performed just prior to the open procedure in order to evaluate for bladder outlet obstruction, if any, and to decide whether or not a transurethral or a suprapubic prostatectomy, transurethral incision or Y-V plasty of the bladder neck is needed. Also, one needs to identify the neck of the diverticulum and, if the open operation is being performed for a tumor in the diverticulum, to identify and resect other tumors.

The patient is placed in a supine position with gentle extension. The retropubic space may be approached through a midline or Pfannenstiel extraperitoneal incision. If the diverticulectomy is being performed for a benign condition, the anterior wall of the bladder is identified and cleaned of all adipose tissues. A cystotomy is performed as described under Suprapubic Cystotomy. The edges of the cystotomy can be kept apart by stay sutures or a self-retaining retractor. The inside of the bladder is carefully inspected and the mouth of the diverticulum identified. For smaller diverticula, a circumferential mucosal incision is made around the mouth

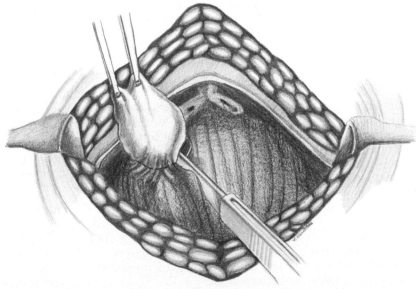

Figure 74–26. The diverticulum is inverted into the lumen of the bladder and its neck is transected.

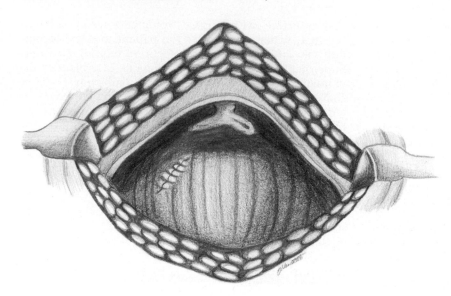

Figure 74–27. Closing the mouth of the diverticulum from within the bladder.

of the diverticulum and the mucosa is dissected off the fibrous sac of the diverticulum, which does not usually require excision except for tumors. Dissection of the mucosa can be facilitated by everting it into the lumen of the bladder (Fig. 74–26). This is done by grasping the mucosa at the most dependent site in the diverticulum and pulling it into the bladder lumen. Once the mucosa is excised, the mouth of the diverticulum is closed (Fig. 74–27), with either interrupted or continuous 2–0 absorbable full-thickness sutures, including the mucosa.

For larger diverticula, a combined extravesical and intravesical approach is usually needed to avoid injury to surrounding structures, namely, the ureters. Following the anterior cystotomy and inspection of the bladder, a 5 or 6 Fr. ureteral catheter is placed in the ureter on the side of the diverticulum. The bladder wall on the side of the diverticulum is freed. The fibrous sac of the diverticulum is dissected free from the surrounding tissues. Occasionally, the superior vesicle pedicle may have to be transected inorder to facilitate this dissection. The ureteral catheter helps in identifying the ureter and dissecting it off the diverticulum. Once the diverticulum is completely freed, it is inverted into the bladder and its neck amputated. The defect is closed with absorbable sutures as previously described.

If the diverticulectomy is being performed for tumor, the bladder wall on the side of the diverticulum is dissected free from the lateral pelvic wall before opening the bladder. Filling the bladder through the Foley catheter will aid in identifying the diverticulum, which is dissected all around with all the overlying fibroadipose tissue kept attached to it, until its neck becomes apparent at its junction with the bladder. The pelvic cavity is now carefully packed with moist pads to minimize tumor cell seeding when the bladder is opened. An anterior cystotomy is performed and the mouth of the diverticulum identified. A full-thickness bladder wall is excised, 1 to 2 cm around the mouth of the diverticulum. The surgical specimen is removed. Careful inspection of the ureter is carried out. The defect is closed with absorbable material as already described.

The anterior cystotomy is closed with a running, full-thickness suture of 2–0 absorbable material and an inverting muscular layer of the same. The packing is removed, and the pelvic cavity is thoroughly irrigated. A drain is left in the retropubic space, and the abdominal wall incision is closed.

A Foley catheter left indwelling for 5 to 7 days is usually adequate for bladder drainage. Suprapubic tubes may also be needed, except in the case of bladder tumors. If, during the dissection of the diverticulum, the ureter or its orifice is compromised, a ureteral stent or catheter may be left in for the necessary period of time.

The major complication of bladder diverticulectomy is injury to the ureter, which can be avoided by catheterizing the ureter and freeing it off and away from the diverticulum before excising the latter. Bleeding and extravasation are rare.

Y-V PLASTY OF THE BLADDER NECK

Y-V plasty is the last resort for the treatment of recalcitrant bladder neck contractures, following transurethral or open prostatectomy. Every attempt should be made to correct the contracture transurethrally before subjecting the patient to an open operation. Transurethral incisions in the contracted bladder neck at multiple sites, preferable with a cold knife followed by circumferential injection of triamcinolone diacetate into the bladder neck tissues, followed by a series of dilations, in the majority of cases, will eliminate the contracture and prevent recurrence. Fortunately, only a small number of cases of contracture require open correction by the following technique.

Surgical Technique

Every attempt should be made to resect residual prostatic tissue several weeks prior to the planned Y-V plasty and allow re-epithelialization of the prostatic urethra and bladder neck.

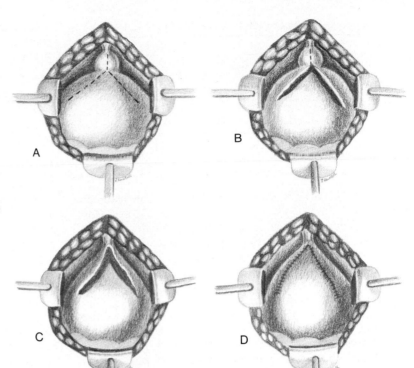

Figure 74–28. *A* to *D*, Y-V plasty of the bladder neck (see text for details).

The patient is placed in the supine position with gentle extension and the retropubic space entered through either a midline or Pfannenstiel extraperitoneal incision. The anterior bladder wall and prostate are cleared of all adipose tissues and the landmarks, namely, prostatovesical junction and puboprostatic ligaments are identified. Occasionally, and if the anterior surface of the prostate is adherent to the undersurface of the symphysis pubis from multiple prior resections, it has to be sharply freed and the puboprostatic ligaments transected in order to drop the prostate posteriorly and allow more room for the Y-V plasty.

The site of the Y-V plasty is carefully planned (Fig. 74–28 *A*). A full-thickness, wide inverted V incision is made in the anterior bladder wall, with its apex at the prostatovesical junction in the midline (Fig. 74–28*B*). Electrocautery will reduce bleeding. The incision is extended distally from the apex of the inverted V at the prostatovesical junction to almost the apex of the prostate, opening the prostatic urethra in the midline, anteriorly (Fig. 74–28*C*). Care should be taken not to extend this incision too far distally, in order to avoid injury to the external sphincter and dorsal veins of the penis. Hemostasis is secured with the electrocautery or with suture ligatures of fine absorbable material.

The apex of the inverted V flap is now approximated to the tip of the distal incision at the apex of the prostate and sutured in place, with heavy absorbable sutures, such as 0 or 2–0 chromic or polyglactin in two layers—a continuous full-thickness layer and an inverting muscular layer (Fig. 74–28*D*).

The bladder is drained with an indwelling Foley catheter, which is usually left in for 5 to 7 days, and the retropubic space drained with a negative pressure drain.

Y-V plasty of the bladder neck is a simple, effective procedure with minimal complications. The rate of recurrent contracture is almost nil.

SURGICAL TREATMENT OF ENTEROVESICAL FISTULA

Etiology and Diagnosis

Enterovesical fistulas are not uncommon. They account for one of every 3000 surgical hospital admissions (Pugh, 1964). These fistulas are more common in males, with the ratio being almost 2:1. It is believed that the uterus acts as a barrier between the intestines and the bladder, thus protecting the bladder from diseases of the bowel.

Colovesical fistulas are the most common of the enterovesical fistulas, and diverticular disease accounts for almost two thirds of its causes. Colon cancer causes about 20 per cent of colovesical fistulas. Other etiologies include Crohn's disease, radiation enteritis, trauma, bladder cancer, appendicitis, gynecologic tumors, tuberculosis, and actinomycosis (Table 74–6).

The classic symptoms of pneumaturia and fecaluria occur in about 63 per cent and 43 per cent of patients, respectively. Irritable bladder symptoms are common, occurring in up to two thirds of patients. These are usually caused by a urinary tract infection, which occurs in 95 per cent of patients (Carson et al., 1978). Infections with more than one organism, however, are not very common, occurring in only one third of patients. Urine per rectum is rare, occurring in less than 10 per cent of

Table 74–6. CAUSES OF COLOVESICAL FISTULAS

Causes*	Prevalence
Diverticular disease	67
Colon cancer	20
Crohn's disease	8
Radiation enteritis	7
Trauma	5
Bladder cancer	4

*Other common causes included appendicitis, gynecologic cancers, tuberculosis, and actinomycosis.

patients and is usually a manifestation of a large fistulous tract.

Enterovesical fistulas are suspected clinically, and the diagnosis is confirmed both radiologically and endoscopically. Although none of the tests alone are extremely accurate, a combination of procedures allows the diagnosis of enterovesical fistula, its origin, and its underlying cause in the majority of cases.

Intravenous urogram is not helpful. Review of the literature indicates only a 10 per cent accuracy in diagnosis. Cystograms, although better than intravenous urograms, allow the diagnosis in only 34 per cent of cases, which is the same as that for barium enema studies. Although sigmoidoscopy or colonoscopy with or without biopsy is essential in every case of suspected colovesical fistula, its accuracy in diagnosis is only about 10 per cent. Cystoscopy, however, is much more accurate, showing changes suggestive of fistula in 77 per cent and allowing a definite diagnosis in 44 per cent of cases (Karamchandani et al., 1984; Shatila et al., 1976).

Computed tomography (CT) scans of the abdomen and pelvis have been the most accurate of all other imaging modalities (Goldman et al., 1985; Labs et al., 1988; Narumi et al., 1988). The typical CT findings in enterovesical fistulas are air in the bladder; focal bladder wall and bowel thickening and apposition; extravesical soft tissue mass, with or without contrast material and with or without air; and contrast material in the bladder. CT scans are also good for staging in case the fistula is secondary to cancer.

Once the diagnosis of fistula and its underlying cause are determined, a one-stage resection of the diseased organs and repair of the fistula are the treatment of choice.

Preoperative Preparation

It is of utmost importance to accurately identify the site of fistula both in the bladder and in the intestine and to diagnose the underlying cause in order to adequately prepare for the operation and plan the nature, site, and extent of resection. Transurethral biopsy of the fistulous tract and the mucosa surrounding it, as well as endoscopic biopsy of any colonic lesion, is an important and essential part of the work-up. Gastrointestinal imaging studies are essential to outline the extent of the diseased segment and to determine whether or not fecal diversion is necessary.

Sterilization of the urinary tract and the intestinal tract is started on hospital admission as described for preoperative preparation for radical cystectomy.

Surgical Technique

A cystoscopy is performed just prior to the open procedure in order to identify the site of fistula. If possible, a ureteral catheter is cystoscopically placed into the fistula to help with its identification when the bladder is opened.

The patient is placed in a supine position, in gentle extension. The peritoneal cavity is entered through a midline incision. Careful exploration of the abdominal cavity is carried out. The segment of bowel communicating with the bladder is identified (Fig. 74–29), and the rest of the intestines are packed out of the pelvic cavity. The site of the fistula is identified and dissected circumferentially as close to the bladder as possible, until the fistulous tract is freed all around (Fig. 74–30). A Penrose drain or umbilical tape is placed around it to help with gentle traction on the wall of the bladder, as the bladder is being opened.

If it had been previously determined that the fistula is malignant, a partial cystectomy is performed, as described previously. At least 1 to 2 cm of normal bladder wall is left around the fistula and tumor. If the

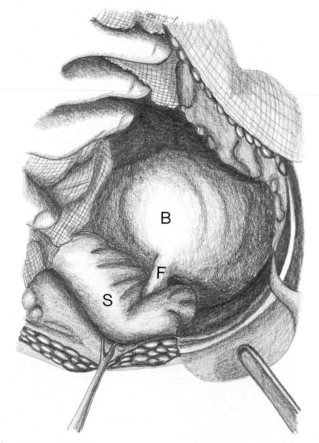

Figure 74–29. Colovesical fistula between the sigmoid colon and dome of the bladder (B, bladder; S, sigmoid; F, fistula).

fistula is inflammatory in origin, the bladder wall immediately around the fistulous tract is excised until normal, healthy-appearing mucosa and muscle are reached (Fig. 74–31). The fistulous tract, which is now separated from the bladder, is carefully covered with moist pack to prevent spillage. The inside of the bladder is carefully inspected. Hemostasis is secured. The bladder wall is closed in two layers, a continuous full-thickness and an inverting muscular layer, using 2–0 chromic or polyglactin suture material.

The segment of diseased bowel is now resected, and the extent of resection depends on the underlying cause of the fistula. If the fistula is secondary to colon cancer, the appropriate colectomy is performed, resecting the mesentery and the lymph node drainage. If the fistula is secondary to diverticulitis, the segment of colon containing the majority of the diverticula is resected together with any adjacent inflammatory masses. The continuity of the bowel is then re-established with an enteroenterostomy. The peritoneal cavity is thoroughly irrigated. Omentum is placed between the bladder and the intestines and then sutured to the bladder with a few interrupted 3–0 chromic sutures to create a barrier between the two suture lines. This maneuver helps with healing and preventing adhesions and recurrences. The bladder is drained with a Foley catheter, which is left indwelling for 5 to 7 days. The abdominal cavity is closed.

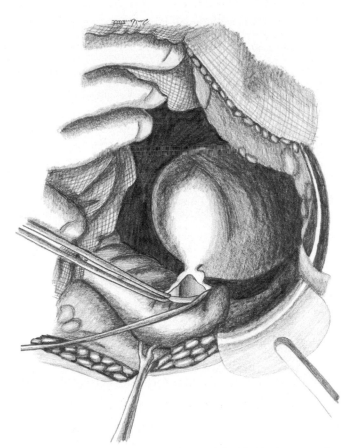

Figure 74–31. The fistula is opened toward the bladder in preparation for circumferentially resecting its origin in the bladder.

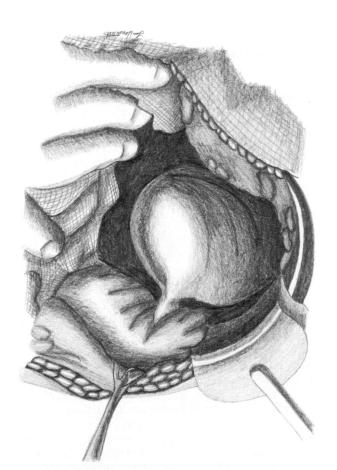

Figure 74–30. The bladder and sigmoid colon are separated to better define and encircle the fistulous tract.

One-stage resection of enterovesical fistula is a well-tolerated and effective operation with complications that are the same as those for any major abdominal operation involving bowel resection. If the disease causing the enterovesical fistula is completely resected and the bowel is separated from the bladder by an omental interposition, the rate of recurrence of the fistula is almost nil. Although the one-stage repair of enterovesical fistula is my choice, other strategies may be very effectively utilized.

REFERENCES

Boileau, M. A., Johnson, D. E., Chan, R. C., and Gonzalez, M. O.: Bladder carcinoma. Results with preoperative radiation therapy and radical cystectomy. Urology, 16:569, 1980.

Bredael, J. J., Crocker, B. P., and Glenn, J. F.: The curability of invasive bladder cancer treated by radical cystectomy. Eur. Urol. 6:206, 1980.

Brice, M., Marshall, V. F., Green, J. L., and Whitmore, W. F., Jr.: Simple total cystectomy for carcinoma of the bladder: One hundred fifty-six consecutive cases—Five years later. Cancer, 9:576, 1956.

Carson, C. C., Malek, R. S., and Remine, W. H.: Urologic aspects of vesicoenteric fistulas. J. Urol., 119:744, 1978.

Edsmyr, F., Jacobsson, F., Dahl, O., and Walstam, R.: Cobalt 60 teletherapy of carcinoma of the bladder. Acta Radiol., 6:81, 1967.

Frank, H. G.: Policy and results of treatment by radiotherapy of carcinoma of the bladder in Leeds. Clin. Radiol., 21:425, 1970.

Freiha, F. S.: Treatment options for patients with invasive bladder cancer. Monogr. Urol., 11:34–47, 1990.

Freiha, F. S.: Continent diversion to the urethra (bladder substitution). *In* Crawford, E. D., and Das, S. (Eds.): Current Genitourinary Cancer Surgery. Philadelphia, Lea & Febiger, 1990, pp. 294–304.

Freiha, F. S.: Preoperative bowel preparation in urologic surgery. J. Urol., 118:955, 1977.

Freiha, F. S., and Faysal, M. H.: Salvage cystectomy. Urology, 22:496, 1983.

Goffinet, D. R., Schneider, M. J., Glatstein, E. J., Ludwig, H., Ray, G. R., Dunnick, N. R., and Bagshaw, M. A.: Bladder cancer: Results of radiation therapy in 384 patients. Radiology, 117:149, 1975.

Goldman, S. M., Fishman, E. K., Gatewood, O. M. D., Jones, B., and Siegelman, S. S.: CT in the diagnosis of enterovesical fistulae. Am. J. Radiol., 144:1229, 1985.

Hart, O. J., and Baker, J.: Intraoperative autotransfusion in radical cystectomy for bladder cancer. Surg. Gynecol. Obstet. 168:302, 1989.

Jewett, H. J., King, L. R., and Shelley, W.: A study of 365 cases of infiltrating bladder cancer: Relation of certain pathological characteristics to prognosis after extirpation. J. Urol., 92:668, 1964.

Karamchandani, M. C., and West, C. F.: Vesicoenteric fistulas. Am. J. Surg., 147:681, 1984.

Labs, J. D., Sarr, M. G., Fishman, E. K., Siegelman, S. S., and Cameron, J. L.: Complications of acute diverticulitis of the colon: and Cameron, J. L.: Complications of acute diverticulitis of the colon: Improved early diagnosis with computerized tomography. Am. J. Surg., 155:331, 1988.

Long, R. T. L., Grummon, R. A., Spratt, J. S., Jr., and Perez-Mesa, C.: Carcinoma of the urinary bladder (comparison with radical, simple and partial cystectomy and intravesical formalin). Cancer, 29:98, 1972.

Mathur, V. K., Krahn, H. P., and Ramsey, E. W.: Total cystectomy for bladder cancer. J. Urol., 125:784, 1981.

Miller, L. S., and Johnson, D. E.: Megavolts irradiation for bladder cancer: Alone, postoperative, or preoperative? *In* Proceedings, 7th National Cancer Conference, Los Angeles, 1972. Philadelphia, J. B. Lippincott Co., 1973, p. 783.

Montie, J., Straffon, R. A., and Stewart, B. H.: Cystectomy with or without radiation therapy: A 20-year analysis. Presented at the 77th Annual Meeting of the AUA, Kansas City, Missouri, May 20, 1982.

Morabito, R. A., Kandzari, S. J., and Milam, D. F.: Invasive bladder carcinoma treated by radical cystectomy. Urology, 14:478, 1979.

Narumi, Y., Sato, T., Kuriyama, K., Fujita, M., Mitani, T., Kemeyama, M., Fukuda, I., Kuroda, M., and Kotake, T.: Computed tomographic diagnosis of enterovesical fistulae: Barium evacuation method. Gastrointest. Radiol., 13:233, 1988.

Poole-Wilson, D. S., and Barnard, R. J.: Total cystectomy for bladder tumours. Br. J. Urol., 43:16, 1971.

Pugh, J. I.: On the pathology and behaviour of acquired non-traumatic vesico-intestinal fistula. Br. J. Surg., 51:644, 1964.

Reid, E. C., Oliver, J. A., and Fishman, I. J.: Preoperative irradiation and cystectomy in 135 cases of bladder cancer. Urology, 8:247, 1976.

Rider, W. D., and Evans, D. H.: Radiotherapy in the treatment of recurrent bladder cancer. Br. J. Urol., 48:595, 1976.

Sagerman, R. H., Bagshaw, M. A., and Kaplan, H. S.: Linear accelerator supervoltage radiation therapy: Carcinoma of the bladder. Am. J. Radiol., 93:122, 1965.

Shatila, A. H., and Ackerman, N. B.: Diagnosis and management of colovesical fistulas. Surg. Gynecol. Obstet., 143:71, 1976.

Skinner, D. G.: Cystectomy for bladder cancer. *In* Crawford, E. D., and Das, S. (Eds.): Current Genitourinary Cancer Surgery. Philadelphia, Lea & Febiger, 1990, pp. 235–246.

Skinner, D. G., and Lieskovsky, G.: Management of invasive and high-grade bladder cancer. *In* Skinner, D. G., and Lieskovsky, G. (Eds.): Diagnosis and Management of Genitourinary Cancer. Philadelphia, W. B. Saunders Co., 1988, pp. 295–312.

van def Werf Messing, B.: Carcinoma of the bladder treated by suprapubic radium implants. The value of additional external irradiation. Eur. J. Cancer Clin. Oncol., 5:277, 1969.

van der Werf Messing, B.: Carcinoma of the bladder treated by preoperative irradiation followed by cystectomy. Cancer, 32:1084, 1973.

Walsh, P. C., Lepor, H., and Eggleston, J. C.: Radical prostatectomy with preservation of sexual function: Anatomical and pathological considerations. Prostate, 4:473, 1983.

Whitmore, W. F., Jr., Batata, M. A., Hilaris, B. S., Reddy, G. N., Unal, A., Ghoneim, M. A., Grabstald, H., and Chu, F.: A comparative study of two preoperative radiation regimens with bladder cancer. Cancer, 40:1077, 1977.

URETHRECTOMY

Charles B. Brendler, M.D.

INDICATIONS

The indications for urethrectomy have been clarified. Previously, indications for urethrectomy included (1) multifocal tumors, (2) bladder neck tumors, (3) diffuse flat carcinoma in situ, and (4) prostatic urethra involvement. Several studies, have shown that the major risk factor for urethral recurrence following radical cystoprostatectomy is extension of tumor into the prostatic urethra, particularly when tumor involves the prostatic stroma. In a series of 124 men undergoing cystoprostatectomy and followed for a mean of 67 months, urethrectomy was required in no patient who presented with a solitary tumor at the bladder neck, in only 1.5 per cent with multifocal tumors, and in only 4.5 per cent with diffuse flat carcinoma in situ. Urethrectomy was required, however, in 17 per cent of men who presented with disease extending into the prostate, including 30 per cent with stromal invasion (Levinson et al., 1990). Thus, prostatic urethral involvement appears to be the most compelling indication for simultaneous urethrec-

tomy. Patients with multifocal tumors and flat carcinoma in situ are candidates for orthotopic reconstruction of the bladder to the urethra, provided they are followed closely with urethral washing cytology (Hickey et al., 1986).

ANATOMY

The anatomic relationship of the cavernous nerves to the prostate and bladder was described by Lepor and associates (1985) and by Schlegel and Walsh (1987). Anatomic dissections of the prostate and membranous urethra have indicated that the cavernous nerves travel posterolateral to the membranous urethra, as they traverse the urogenital diaphragm. Distal to the membranous urethra, the cavernous nerves are difficult to dissect from within the surrounding muscle but appear to diverge laterally into the crura of the corpora cavernosa. Injury to the cavernous nerves with resultant loss of potency after urethrectomy most likely results from intraoperative mobilization of the membranous urethra.

It is possible to preserve potency after urethrectomy by dissecting the membranous urethra from the urogenital diaphragm through a retropubic approach (Brendler et al., 1990). Even in a patient in whom preservation of potency is not an issue, liberation of the membranous urethra during cystoprostatectomy greatly facilitates the remaining perineal dissection of the urethra.

TECHNIQUE

The patient is placed in the supine position. The table is broken at the umbilicus and tilted into Trendelenburg's position until the patient's legs are parallel to the floor (Fig. 74–32). Radical cystoprostatectomy with preservation of the cavernous nerves is performed as described by Schlegel and Walsh (1987). After ligation and division of the dorsal vein of the penis, a 1-0 silk ligature is passed around the urethra and ligated to prevent spillage of urine around the urethral catheter (Fig. 74–33A). An umbilical tape is passed around the urethra, and gentle traction is exerted cephalad. Using a Kitner dissector, the urethra is dissected from the urogenital diaphragm removing only urethral mucosa and smooth muscle, leaving the striated muscle of the urogenital diaphragm (Fig. 74–33B). As the dissection continues, the neurovascular bundles lying immediately posterolateral to the membranous urethra are gently pushed away (Fig. 74–33C and D). This dissection continues until the membranous urethra has been liberated completely from the urogenital diaphragm. The urethra is transected, and the catheter is drawn cephalad into the wound (Fig. 74–33E). The remaining pedicles

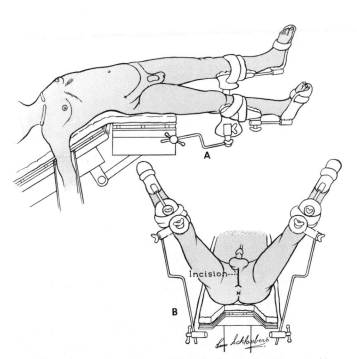

Figure 74–32. *A,* Patient position for radical cystoprostatectomy. Umbilicus is placed over break of table, and table is fully flexed and tilted into Trendelenburg's position, until legs are parallel to floor. *B,* Patient position for urethrectomy. Leg braces are elevated until hips are flexed 60 degrees and knees are fully extended.

to the prostate and bladder are divided, and the specimen is removed.

If a frozen-section examination of the membranous urethra has negative findings, but subsequent urethrectomy is planned, we prefer to delay the urethrectomy at least 2 weeks to avoid excessive mobilization of the cavernous nerves simultaneously from the pelvis and through the perineum. However, if frozen-section examination findings of the membranous urethra are positive, simultaneous urethrectomy is performed. The patient is placed for the urethrectomy in the exaggerated lithotomy position, simply by raising the leg braces until the hips are flexed 60 degrees and the knees are fully extended (Fig. 74–32B). The extra few minutes it takes to change position are worthwhile, because this step facilitates dissection of the remaining urethra through the perineum. It is much more difficult to do this procedure with the patient in a low lithotomy position.

The perineum is prepared and draped as a sterile field. A 24 Fr. Van Buren sound is passed through the urethra to the level of the urogenital diaphragm. Either a vertical or U-shaped incision may be used. Alternatively, an inverted Y incision with the midpoint over the base of the scrotum provides excellent exposure of the bulbar urethra (see Fig. 74–32B). Once the perineal skin and subcutaneous tissue have been incised, the Turner-Warwick perineal ring retractor is positioned, which provides excellent exposure. The bulbocavernosus muscle is divided sharply in the midline posteriorly to the level of the central perineal tendon to expose the bulbar urethra (Fig. 74–34). Palpation of the Van Buren sound in the urethra and incision of the tissues directly over it facilitate this initial dissection.

The sound is removed and replaced with a 20 Fr. red rubber catheter, which is passed to the level of the urogenital diaphragm. The catheter is sutured to the glans penis to maintain it in position until the penile urethra has been liberated. The urethra is dissected from the penis by sharply incising Buck's fascia bilaterally to liberate the urethra from the corpora cavernosa (Fig. 74–35). Care must be taken not to injure the corpora cavernosa—this can result in venous bleeding that is sometimes difficult to control.

The penis is inverted and the urethral dissection continued to the level of the glans penis, at which point the penis is restored to its normal anatomic position. The urethral meatus is circumscribed sharply, and a T-incision is made on the ventral surface to the level of the corona (Fig. 74–36). Placing a tourniquet around the base of the penis reduces bleeding during dissection. The urethra is then dissected free from the glans penis. The entire penile urethra is then brought out through the perineal incision. A drain is placed along the bed of the penile urethra, and the glans penis is reconstructed with 4–0 absorbable sutures. The penile tourniquet is removed.

Dissection of the bulbar urethra begins. The relatively avascular tissues anterior to the bulbar urethra directly beneath the symphysis pubis are dissected first, which allows the urethra to be displaced anteriorly, facilitating exposure of the posterolateral bulbar urethral arteries and decreasing the chance of inadvertent injury to these

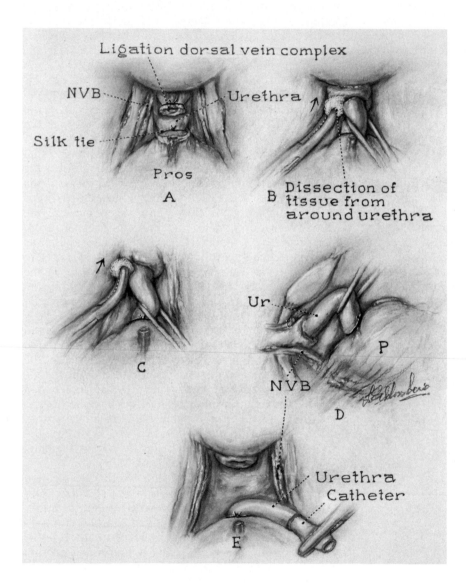

Figure 74–33. *A,* Urethra is ligated with 1-0 silk suture to prevent spillage of urine around catheter (NVB, neurovascular bundle; Pros, prostate).

B, Mobilization of membranous urethra from urogenital diaphragm with Kitner dissector.

C, Further mobilization of membranous urethra.

D, Lateral view shows membranous urethra (Ur) fully mobilized with neurovascular bundles displaced posterolaterally.

E, Urethra is transected, and catheter is drawn cephalad into wound. Neurovascular bundles are seen intact, lateral to the urethra.

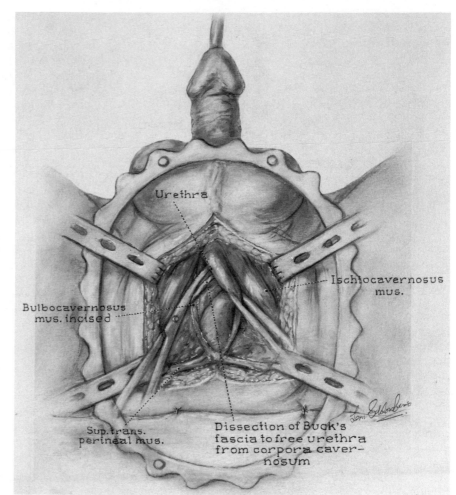

Figure 74–34. Turner-Warwick ring retractor positioned and bulbocavernosus muscle incised to expose bulbar urethra.

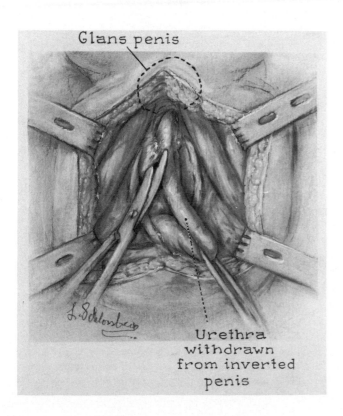

Figure 74–35. Incision in Buck's fascia to liberate urethra from corpora cavernosa.

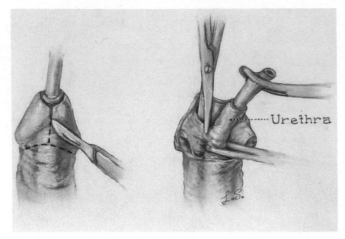

Figure 74–36. Inverted T-incision on glans penis and dissection of glanular urethra.

vessels (Fig. 74–37). The bulbar urethral arteries should be controlled with hemoclips (Fig. 74–38 A and B) rather than fulgurated to avoid injury to the internal pudendal arteries, from which the bulbar urethral arteries arise and which provide arterial supply to the corpora cavernosa (Fig. 74–38C). Having dissected the membranous urethra from above through the pelvis, the perineal dissection is usually completed without difficulty (Fig. 74–39).

In all cases, the dissection must be continued proximally until the entire remaining urethra has been removed. This step is important, because the bulbomembranous urethra adjacent to the prostate is the segment of urethra most likely to be involved with recurrent tumor. It is usually not difficult to dissect the bulbomembranous urethra when the urethrectomy is done concurrently with cystoprostatectomy, especially if the membranous urethra is liberated from above. However, it may be considerably more difficult when the two procedures are separated by more than several weeks. If the urethrectomy is done within 2 weeks of the cystectomy, it is possible to pass a catheter through the urethral lumen proximally into the pelvis. Exposure of the end of the catheter ensures that the dissection has been carried to the urethral stump. In a urethrectomy delayed by more than 2 weeks, it is usually not possible to pass a catheter into the pelvis. The membranous urethra is often encased in fibrous tissue, and it is possible to avulse the urethra by exerting excess traction, leaving a segment behind. Thus, the dissection should be done slowly and methodically, to assure the removal of all of the urethra.

After the urethra has been removed, bleeding is usually minimal, provided the bulbar urethral arteries have been properly controlled. Several small veins usually need to be fulgurated or suture ligated. A flat Jackson-Pratt drain is placed along the bed of the proximal urethra, brought out through a separate stab wound, and sutured in place. The bulbocavernosus muscle and superficial perineal fascia are reapproximated in the midline with continuous 3–0 absorbable

suture, and the skin is closed with a continuous 4–0 absorbable suture (Fig. 74–40). It is difficult to apply a dressing, and a topical spray dressing is usually sufficient. If there is bleeding from the perineal wound, a padded T-binder can be applied. A gauze bandage is wrapped loosely around the penis for mild compression. This bandage should not be placed too tightly to avoid penile ischemia. The glans penis should be kept exposed so that the color can be observed periodically.

POSTOPERATIVE CARE

Postoperatively, the penile and perineal drains can usually be removed after 24 to 48 hours. Perioperative antibiotics are unnecessary unless an abdominal procedure is done concurrently. In an isolated urethrectomy, it is unnecessary to restrict the patient's diet. Normal activity usually is resumed within 1 or 2 days after surgery. The patient is discharged from the hospital by about the 5th postoperative day. He is instructed not to bathe the incision for 1 week postoperatively.

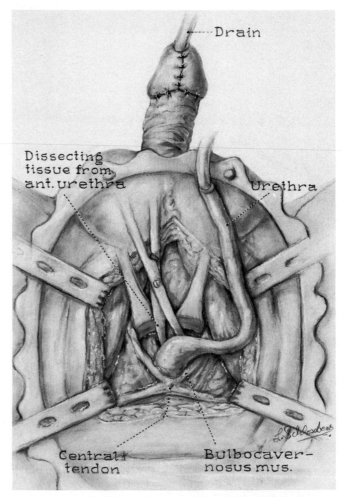

Figure 74–37. Initial dissection of tissue anterior to bulbar urethra to facilitate subsequent exposure and control of posterolateral bulbar urethral arteries.

Figure 74–38. *A* and *B*, Ligation of the bulbar urethral arteries with hemoclips.

C, Lateral view shows the relationship between the internal pudendal and bulbar arteries and the ischium and inferior ramus of the pubis. The bulbar arteries should not be fulgurated to prevent injury to the internal pudendal arteries, from which they arise and which provide arterial supply to corpora cavernosa (NVB, neurovascular bundle).

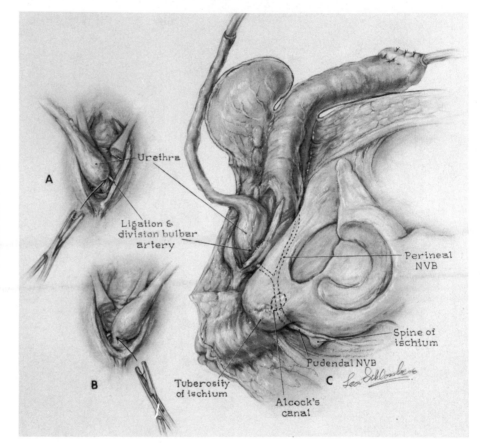

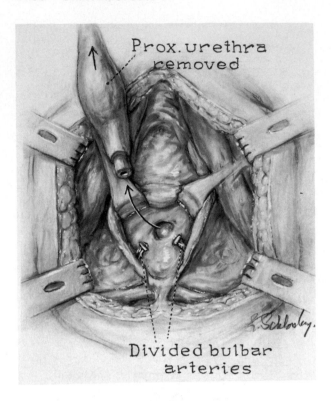

Figure 74–39. Completed urethrectomy. Dissection of bulbar urethra is completed without difficulty, because the membranous urethra has previously been mobilized through the pelvis.

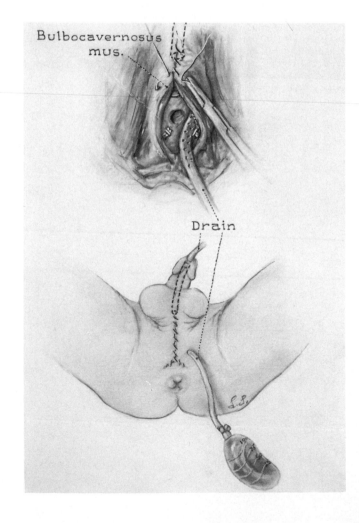

Figure 74–40. Closure of the perineal incision and placement of the Jackson-Pratt drain.

REFERENCES

Brendler, C. B., Schlegel, P. N., and Walsh, P. C.: Urethrectomy with preservation of potency. J. Urol., 144:270, 1990.

Hickey, D. P., Soloway, M. S., and Murphy, W. M.: Selective urethrectomy following cystoprostatectomy for bladder cancer. J. Urol., 136:828, 1986.

Levinson, A. K., Johnson, D. E., and Wishnow, K. I.: Indications for urethrectomy in an era of continent urinary diversion. J. Urol., 144:73, 1990.

Lepor, H., Gregerman, M., Crosby, R., et al.: Precise localization of the autonomic nerves from the pelvic plexus to the corpora cavernosa: a detailed anatomical study of the adult male pelvis. J. Urol., 133:207, 1985.

Schlegel, P. N., and Walsh, P. C.: Neuroanatomical approach to radical cystoprostatectomy with preservation of sexual function. J. Urol., 138:1402, 1987.

75

FEMALE UROLOGY

Shlomo Raz, M.D.
Nancy A. Little, M.D.
Saad Juma, M.D.

URINARY INCONTINENCE

Clinical, urodynamic, radiologic, and endoscopic evaluations as well as operative experience on over 800 cases of female stress incontinence have led us to a better understanding of its pathophysiology. We correlate these concepts with anatomic dissections obtained from whole-mount and step sections of the female pelvis as well as from magnetic resonance images of the female pelvis, the paraurethral and bladder neck areas of females with known stress incontinence, and of normal control females.

Normal continence in the female results from the delicate balance of several forces, including the closing pressure of the urethra, the critical functional and anatomic urethral length, the ability of the pelvic floor to increase urethral pressure at the time of stress, and the proper anatomic location of the sphincteric unit. Normally, anatomic support of the bladder neck and proximal urethra allows for proper transmission of intra-abdominal pressure increases to this area of continence. Together with an intrinsically intact urethra, with its coapting mucosal surface and the reflex pelvic contraction at the time of cough or strain, a leak proof mechanism is achieved. Failure of one of the components of this delicate balance will not invariably produce stress incontinence because of the compensatory effect of the other components. This may explain why a patient with a very short urethra, such as after distal excision or incision, is continent if the bladder neck and urethra are in good anatomic position and the remaining urethra preserves good closing pressures. However, if this short urethra is hypermobile and prolapsed, incontinence occurs. This balance also may explain the phenomenon whereby many patients with urethral and bladder prolapse can be totally asymptomatic and only a small percentage have stress incontinence.

Obstetric trauma and resulting anatomic displacements usually occur at the age of 20 to 30, but "anatomic incontinence" is found mainly at the age of menopause,
suggesting that hormonal changes (e.g., atrophy of urethral tissue) are superimposed on the anatomic displacements producing the resultant leakage.

Anatomy of Pelvic Support

The bony pelvis is the framework that provides support to all pelvic structures. If the pelvic bone is the scaffolding, it is the pelvic diaphragm and perineal musculature that attach to this scaffolding, providing the floor upon which the pelvic organs rest (Fig. 75–1).

PELVIC DIAPHRAGM. The pelvic diaphragm includes the levator ani and coccygeus muscles. The levator ani with its component parts (pubococcygeus, iliococcygeus, and ischiococcygeus) provides the major inferior support of the urethra, vagina, and rectum (Fig. 75–2). Standard anatomy texts describe the muscle together with its surrounding fascia as a broad thin sheet, extending from the pelvic portion of the pubic bone

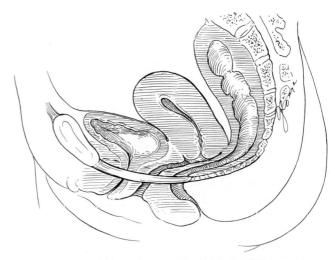

Figure 75–1. Sagittal view through the pelvis.

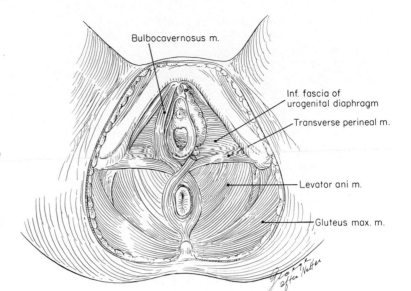

Figure 75-2. View of the perineum in the female. Note the relation of the levator ani to the perineal muscles.

lateral to the symphysis anteriorly and to the inner surface of the ischial spine posteriorly. Between these points it takes origin by the "arcuate line" of the obturator fascia (tendinous arc) (Fig. 75–3). From these origins, the fibers extend back medially to unite with the fibers from the opposite side. In their anterior portion, the levators form a U-shaped hiatus through which the vagina, rectum, and urethra exit the abdominal cavity. Fibers of the pubococcygeus muscle send a number of muscle "fingers" into these structures. Around the urethra they form its external sphincter. The fibers fuse laterally and anteriorly to the rectum, forming part of the perineal support. The proximal half of the vagina lies horizontally over the levator plate.

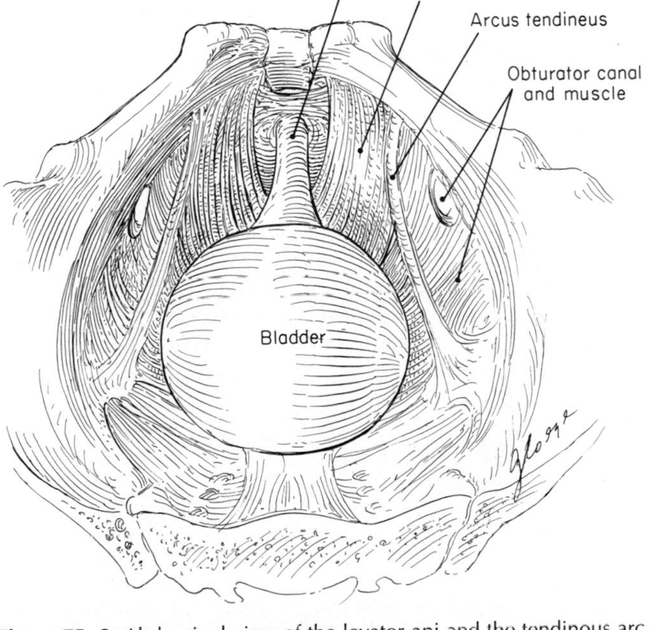

Figure 75-3. Abdominal view of the levator ani and the tendinous arc. Note the relation of the bladder and urethra.

Thus, the levator ani holds the intrapelvic organs like a hammock, providing support as well as stabilization during increases in intra-abdominal pressure. The fascial layer covering the levator muscle (endopelvic fascia) at the level of the urethra and bladder neck has two distinct areas (Fig. 75–4) (Delancey, 1989)—the pubourethral and the urethropelvic ligaments (fusion of endopelvic and periurethral fascia) (Klutke et al., 1990).

PUBOURETHRAL LIGAMENTS. The pubourethral ligaments connect the inner surface of the pubic bone with the mid-urethra (Fig. 75–5). This ligament helps to support and stabilize the urethra and anterior vaginal wall to the inferior aspect of the pubic bone but does not contribute significant support to the bladder neck. Weakness of this ligament permits posterior and inferior movement of the mid-urethra. Just distal to this ligament, the skeletal muscle fibers (external sphincter of the urethra) are located. The pubourethral ligaments divide the urethra into two halves. The proximal half, intra-abdominal, responsible for passive continence and the distal half, extra-abdominal, responsible for active continence.

URETHROPELVIC LIGAMENTS (Figs. 75–5 and 75–6). Another "specialized" group of fibers of more functional significance are the musculofascial attachments of the urethra and bladder neck to the lateral pelvic wall. These attachments formed by the endopelvic fascia fuse to the periurethral fascia (see next part), like two wings that hold the urethra to the tendinous arc (insertion of the levators on the obturator fascia). We have named this musculofascial complex the urethropelvic ligament, and it is the major support to the bladder neck and proximal urethra.

The pubourethral and urethropelvic ligaments are condensations of the levator fascial sheet, as it attaches to the urethra and bladder neck. As described later, it is the urethropelvic ligament, however, that is most important in surgical cure of anatomic stress incontinence because it is ultimately responsible for bladder neck support.

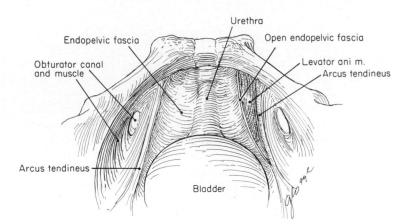

Figure 75–4. Same view as in Figure 75–3, with the endopelvic fascia in place.

PERIURETHRAL FASCIA. If one now examines the anterior vagina after an incision is made in the midline and after the vaginal wall is reflected laterally, one encounters a distinct anatomy. At the level of the urethra, from the meatus to the bladder neck, a glistening fascia is present—the periurethral fascia (Fig. 75–7). While dissecting this fascia laterally toward the pubic bone, as it fuses with the endopelvic fascia, one is stopped by a fibrous structure—the attachment of the urethropelvic ligament to the tendinous arc. The periurethral fascia can be conceptualized as the spinal side of the urethropelvic ligaments.

In the normal female, the vaginal wall ascends laterally and superiorly and attaches very loosely to the urethropelvic fascia in its anchor to the lateral pelvic floor, thereby giving the characteristic H shape of the vaginal lumen cross-sectional imaging.

PUBOCERVICAL FASCIA. When lateral dissection of the vagina is carried out at the level of the bladder base, one encounters the pubocervical fascia just beneath the vaginal wall (Fig. 75–7) (Staskin et al., 1986). This fascia supports the bladder to the lateral pelvic wall superior to the levator plate.

Trauma of delivery, hormonal deficiency, and pelvic floor relaxation may produce one of three types of abnormalities of the bladder support: (1) central defect, (2) lateral defect (paravaginal), and (3) a combination of both. In a patient with a central defect, the bladder is herniated in the midline, through the attenuated pubocervical fascia, whereas the lateral support of the bladder is preserved. In a patient with a lateral defect, the attachment of the bladder to the lateral pelvic wall is defective, resulting in a sliding hernia of the bladder and pubocervical fascia.

CARDINAL LIGAMENTS. The cardinal ligaments are important structures supporting the uterus to the lateral pelvic wall (Fig. 75–8) and play an important role in bladder support. The cardinal ligaments are the base of a rectangle formed by the periurethral fascia and each pubocervical fascia. The fibers of the pubocervical fascia fuse with the anterior extension of cardinal ligaments. When the cervix is well supported, the cardinal ligaments are centrally located and the defect between the pubocervical fasciae is small (Fig. 75–9). When the cardinal ligaments are lax (uterine prolapse), the base of this rectangle is wider and the pubocervical fascia is laterally displaced, facilitating the formation of a cystocele (Fig. 75–10).

Clinical Correlates

We can now make clinical correlates between the different anatomic defects of the anterior vaginal wall. We must first highlight the importance of the insertion of the urethropelvic ligament into the lateral pelvic wall (tendinous arc and obturator fascia). The urethra is seen to be suspended from the lateral pelvic wall and enclosed like a sandwich (between endopelvic and periurethral fascia) by this fascial extension with both strength and elasticity (Fig. 75–11).

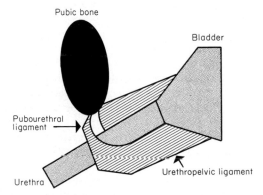

Figure 75–5. Schematic representation of urethral support. Note the relation of the pubourethral and urethropelvic ligaments to the urethra and the pubic bone.

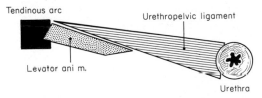

Figure 75–6. Schematic representation of lateral support of the urethra. Note the relationship among the urethropelvic ligament, the tendinous arc, and the levator ani muscle.

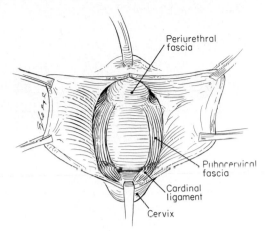

Figure 75–7. Vaginal view of the periurethral fascia and its relation to the pubocervical fascia, the cardinal ligaments, and the cervix.

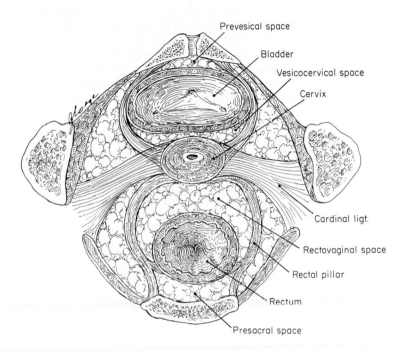

Figure 75–8. Cross-section of the female pelvis at the level of the cervix. Note the relation of the pubocervical and cardinal ligaments to the bladder and the cervix.

Figure 75–9. Schematic representation of the support of the bladder floor. Note the proximity of the pubocervical ligaments to each other and the narrow space in between. The cardinal ligaments meet in the middle at the cervix.

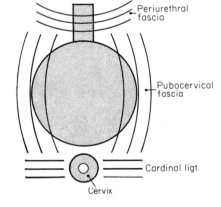

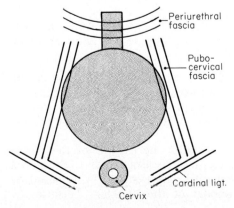

Figure 75–10. Schematic representation of the support of the bladder floor in a patient with cystocele. Note the separation of the pubocervical ligaments and the wide space in between (central defect) where bladder prolapse (cystocele) occurs.

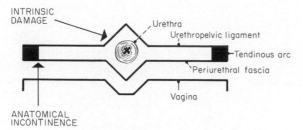

Figure 75–11. Schematic representation of urethral support as seen in a coronal plane. Note the sandwich-like support of the urethra by the endopelvic fascia from above and the periurethral fascia from below with the urethropelvic ligaments in between.

The pubourethral ligaments divide the urethra into two areas of continence. The proximal half, intrapelvic and intra-abdominal, which is responsible for passive continence, and the distal half, responsible for active continence. Passive continence (resting involuntary control) will depend on the integrity, coaptation, and support of this proximal half of the urethra. The area just distal to the pubourethral ligaments is outside the realm of the intra-abdominal forces, is covered by the extension of the levator muscles, and is the area of "high closure pressures" when urethral pressures studies are performed.

Passive continence in an otherwise healthy female is provided by the coaptation and support of the proximal half of the urethra. The spongy tissue surrounded by a thin musculofascial layer creates an effective seal. The tensile forces of the urethropelvic ligaments and indirectly the levator musculature provide further coaptation to the proximal urethra. Of no less importance is the true valvular effect created by the high retropubic fixation of the bladder neck, with the bladder base being in the most dependent position. The basic tone of the skeletal musculature in the mid-urethral area provides further compression (pressure) of the spongy urethra.

In the normal continent patient, during any stress maneuvers such as coughing, straining, or walking, a complex compensatory mechanism is standing by to improve the seal effect of the urethra. A mild posterior bladder rotation during stress against a well-supported urethra will increase the valvular effect of the bladder neck. A sudden change in abdominal pressure will produce a reflex contraction of the levator muscle and an increase of mid-urethral pressure. These two mechanisms are enhanced by voluntary or reflex contraction of the levator and obturator muscles, which increase tension on the urethropelvic ligaments thereby elevating and compressing the proximal urethra. A direct transmission of intra-abdominal pressure to the well-supported proximal urethra increases its closing mechanism.

In patients with incontinence, pelvic floor relaxation and weakening of the urethropelvic and pubourethral ligaments produces posterior and downward rotation of the proximal urethra and bladder neck. As a result, the seal effect and the compensatory mechanism of the proximal urethra are lost.

Urethral hypermobility will transfer the bladder neck area to a dependent position in the pelvis, where sudden elevations in intra-abdominal pressures facilitate its funneling and opening. The valvular effect is lost. A weak levator will not increase mid-urethral pressures efficiently. The urethropelvic ligaments are stretched and weak, diminishing the increase in coaptation of the proximal urethra during stress. The intra-abdominal forces are not transmitted efficiently to the proximal urethra because loss of the "backboard effect" of the strong normal support. Failure of all the compensatory mechanisms results in incontinence.

Surgical transfer of the proximal urethra in a high supported position will restore some of the urethral compensatory mechanisms. The bladder neck is moved away from the disadvantaged position to a more protected one, in which the bladder base is now in the most dependent position, and the valvular effect is restored.

Bladder neck and urethral fixation restores the backboard effect needed for efficient transmission of intra-abdominal forces. Restoring tension on the urethropelvic ligaments improves the seal effect of the proximal urethra, but the increase in mid-urethral pressure during cough is probably not restored.

Surgical Correlates

Armed with a better understanding of the anatomy of stress incontinence, what clinical correlates can be drawn?

With a concept of the structures involved in support of the bladder neck and proximal urethra, the clinician gains a better understanding of what actually occurs when surgical therapy is employed. The various types of bladder neck suspensions are all attempts to replace the bladder neck and proximal urethra into a high fixed retropubic position. Patients with stress incontinence and minimal cystocele have, in general, hypermobility of the bladder neck and urethra due to attenuated levator plate and urethropelvic ligaments. Patients with moderate cystocele have, in addition, attenuation of the pubocervical fascia. Patients with severe pelvic floor relaxation and anterior vaginal prolapse have a combination of anatomic abnormalities, which include urethral hypermobility due to attenuated urethropelvic ligament and cystocele due to weak cardinal ligaments and pubocervical fascia (lateral and/or central defects).

In cases of bladder neck and urethral hypermobility, corrective surgery should restore the normal anatomy by creating a strong anchor of the urethropelvic ligaments and vaginal wall. In patients with severe cystocele, the supporting rectangle of the bladder (the base formed by the cardinal ligaments, the sides by pubocervical fasciae, and the top side by the periurethral fascia) is damaged. Two defects may be found and should be repaired accordingly:

1. The central defect of the rectangle should be repaired by medial approximation of the laterally retracted cardinal ligaments together with medial approximation of the pubocervical fascia (formal cystocele repair).

2. The downward, sliding herniation of the whole bladder as a unit because of lax attachment to the lateral pelvic wall (paravaginal hernia) should be repaired by suspension and support of the bladder. This can be

accomplished by an abdominal approach, such as the Burch or paravaginal colposuspension, or by a transvaginal approach using a bladder neck and bladder suspension technique.

In patients with moderate cystocele, the classic approach has been similar to that for repair of a large cystocele. Nevertheless, in selected cases with mainly lateral (paravaginal) herniation of the bladder, we perform a transvaginal suspension of the bladder neck (urethropelvic ligaments) and bladder base (pubocervical and cardinal complex), calling this operation the four-corner bladder neck and bladder suspension (see subsequent discussion).

Intrinsic Urethral Mechanism

The urethra consists largely of a rich vascular "sponge," lined by a moist mucosal layer and surrounded by a coat of smooth muscle and fibroelastic tissue (Staskin et al., 1985). The mucosa provides coaptation. Made of very loosely woven connective tissue scattered throughout by tiny smooth muscle bundles and an elaborate vascular plexus, the submucosa creates the "washer effect" for the continence mechanism. Functionally, the surrounding smooth muscle coat maintains this mechanism by directing submucosal expansile pressures inward toward the mucosa. This highly efficient "seal" we believe is a major contributor to the normal urinary continence mechanism. The plasticity of this structure normally allows perfect continence even when a grooved sound is inserted into the urethra. This "sphincter" is under hormonal control, and lack of estrogen (menopause) leads to atrophy of the mucosa and substitution of the vascular submucosa by fibrous tissue. Multiple surgery, trauma, radiation, and neurogenic disease also can affect the ability to achieve a perfect seal. When this mechanism is lost, stress incontinence of intrinsic damage results. Simple bladder neck and proximal urethral suspension in this case will be insufficient to achieve continence.

Effective means of evaluating this aspect of continence have not in the past been readily available. Urethral pressure profilometry, although commonly used, has been found to be nonspecific, poorly reproducible, and fraught with artifact. Our findings help us to distinguish genuine stress urinary incontinence into (1) that due to anatomic malposition of an intact sphincteric unit and (2) incontinence secondary to insufficiency of the urethral closing mechanism due to intrinsic urethral dysfunction or damage (see Fig. 75–11).

Although the goal of surgery for anatomic incontinence is to elevate and support the bladder neck in a high, fixed, retropubic position by resuspension of the urethropelvic ligaments, the goal of surgery for intrinsic damage is to provide coaptation and compression of the urethra, in order to restore its sealing function.

Posterior Vaginal Support

A complex fascial and muscular arrangement provides support to the vagina, rectum, perineum, and anal sphincter. Although the fascial support includes the prerectal and pararectal fasciae, there are two levels of muscular support: (1) the pelvic floor (levator sling, in particular its pubococcygeus portion) and (2) the urogenital diaphragm (bulbocavernosus, superficial and deep transverse perineal muscles, external anal sphincter, and central tendon of the perineum) (Huisman, 1983; Joseph, 1986).

In the normally supported patient in the erect position, two vaginal angles can be described. In its midportion the vagina forms a posterior angle of approximately 110 degrees (see Fig. 75–1). This angulation indicates the point where the vagina crosses the pelvic floor. The proximal half of the vagina is practically in a horizontal plane resting over this levator plate. The second angle defines the relationship between the distal half of the vagina and the vertical line. This angle is approximately 45 degrees reflecting the degree of support of the levators and urogenital diaphragm.

In patients with pelvic floor relaxation, both angles are lost. The levator plate relaxes (convex instead of horizontal), the levator hiatus enlarges, and the normal mid-vaginal angulation of 110 degrees disappears (Fig. 75–12). The distal half of the vagina is no longer 45 degrees from the vertical. The vagina is now rotated downward and posteriorly and is no longer in a high supported horizontal position. Herniation of the rectum may ensue.

In a patient with damage to the second level of muscular support (the perineal or urogenital diaphragm), the vaginal outlet (introitus) is wider and the distance between the urethra and posterior fourchette is greater (Figs. 75–13 and 75–14). Different degrees of perineal tear may be seen—minimal, when only a small separation of the perineum occurs, to a severe degree, when the perineal structures have disappeared and the vaginal wall reaches the anterior rectal wall.

Corrective surgery of the posterior vaginal wall should include the following:

1. Correction of the rectocele by reinforcement of the attenuated prerectal and pararectal fasciae.
2. Repair of the defect of the levator muscles by narrowing the size of the levator hiatus and providing a

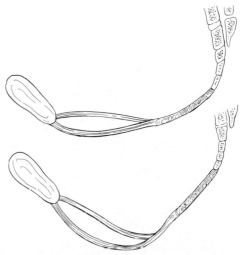

Figure 75–12. The levator hiatus in a normal female *(top)* and in a patient with pelvic floor relaxation *(bottom)*.

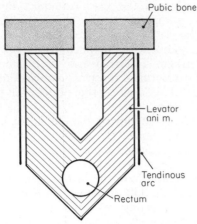

Figure 75–13. Schematic representation of the levator ani muscles. Posteriorly, they unite with each other around the rectum. The U-shaped space represents the hiatus through which the urethra and vagina pass.

horizontal supporting plate for the proximal half of the vagina.

3. Repair of the urogenital diaphragm (musculature of the perineum) providing normal introital size and improved vaginal support.

Vaginal Dome and Uterine Support

A detailed description can be found in a standard textbook of anatomy (see Last, 1978). The most important supporting structures of the uterus are the sacrouterine—the broad and the cardinal ligaments. The sacrouterine ligaments are posteriorly located and run from the cervix to the side of the sacrum. At the level of the cervix they fuse with the posterior aspect of the cardinal ligaments. The broad ligaments are two superiorly located folds of peritoneum attaching the lateral walls of the uterus to the lateral pelvic wall. The ligaments contain the fallopian tubes, round ligaments, ovarian ligaments, uterine arteries, and ovarian vessels.

The cardinal ligaments are described in more detail, not only because of their importance on uterine support,

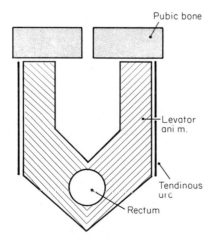

Figure 75–14. Same diagram as Figure 75–13, in a patient with a pelvic floor relaxation.

but because of their significant impact on bladder support, incontinence, bladder prolapse, and vaginal reconstructive surgery. The cardinal ligaments extend from the uterine isthmus to the lateral pelvic wall (obturator and levator fascia). The ligaments are thick and triangular, and contain the uterine arteries. Posteriorly they are fused with the sacrouterine ligaments, whereas superiorly they merge with the endopelvic fascia, covering the bladder and vagina. The anterior extensions of the cardinal ligaments fuse, as previously described, with the pubocervical fascia. These form the base of the bladder rectangle (periurethral, pubocervical, and cardinals) responsible for bladder support (see Fig. 75–9).

URINARY INCONTINENCE IN THE FEMALE

Urinary incontinence, defined as the involuntary loss of urine through the urethra severe enough to be of social or hygienic consequence, is a very common and frequently underreported disorder. At least 10 million Americans suffer from urinary incontinence, including 37 per cent of elderly females and 50 per cent of nursing home residents, at an annual cost of 10 billion dollars (NIH Consensus Report, 1988).

Classification of Incontinence

Urinary incontinence may result from bladder or sphincter dysfunction (Table 75–1). Bladder-related (urge) incontinence may be due to instability, poor compliance, small capacity, or incomplete emptying (overflow incontinence). Sphincter-related (stress) incontinence may be caused by anatomic malposition of an intact sphincter unit (anatomic incontinence) or by intrinsic sphincteric dysfunction with or without associated anatomic abnormality. In the female patient, a mixed type of stress urinary incontinence (SUI) and urge incontinence (UI) is the most common and constitutes approximately 55.5 per cent; pure SUI is seen in 26.7 per cent of incontinent patients (Diokino et al., 1985).

SUI is defined as the involuntary loss of urine per urethra, with a sudden increase in intra-abdominal pressure. Several classifications of SUI are described in the literature (Table 75–2) mostly based on anatomic, urodynamic, and radiologic features. We prefer a simpler classification and divide stress incontinence into anatomic incontinence and intrinsic sphincter dysfunction incontinence.

Table 75–1. ETIOLOGY OF INCONTINENCE

Bladder-related (urge incontinence)
  Instability
  Poor compliance
  Small capacity
  Noncontractile (overflow incontinence)
Sphincter-related (stress incontinence)
  Anatomic incontinence
  Intrinsic sphincteric dysfunction

Table 75–2. CLASSIFICATION OF STRESS URINARY INCONTINENCE (SUI)

Blaivas	McGuire	Raz
Type O h/o SUI but no objective SUI. Bladder neck and urethra open during stress.	Type O No true SUI.	Anatomic—due to malposition of intact sphincter unit.
Type I Bladder neck and urethra open and descend < 2 cm during stress with minimal or no cystocele.	Type I SUI, minimal hypermobility, with/without cystocele, UCP > 20 cm H_2O pressure in supine position at rest.	
Type IIA Bladder neck and urethra open and descend > 2 cm during stress with cystocele.	Type II SUI, marked hypermobility with rotational descent and horizontal position of the urethra at peak abdominal pressure. UCP > 20 cm H_2O pressure in supine position at rest.	
Type IIB Bladder neck and urethra below symphysis at rest. During stress may/may not descend.		
Type III Bladder neck and urethra are open at rest in the absence of detrusor contraction.	Type III Prior failed bladder neck suspension or UCP < 20 cm H_2O.	Intrinsic sphincter dysfunction—due to malfunction of the sphincter with/without hypermobility.

h/o, history of; UCP, urethral closing pressure.

Anatomic incontinence is the most common type and constitutes 90 to 95 per cent of SUI. It results from loss of the pelvic support of the bladder and urethra, from the trauma of delivery, hysterectomy, hormonal changes (menopause), pelvic denervation, or congenital weakness. With loss of urethral support, the urethral compensatory mechanisms are absent during stress maneuvers and urinary leakage results.

Intrinsic sphincteric dysfunction, in comparison, results from damage to the sphincter due to multiple prior operations, trauma, radiation, and neurogenic disorders. The hallmark of this type of incontinence is that the bladder neck and the proximal urethra are open at rest and in the absence of detrusor contractions, thus the proximal urethra no longer functions as a sphincter. This type of incontinence corresponds to type III incontinence in the McGuire and Blaivas classifications (Blaivas and Olsson, 1988). No pathognomonic features distinguish this type of incontinence. However, the diagnosis is based on the entire clinical picture in combination with urodynamic, endoscopic, and radiologic features. Results of urethral pressure profilometry alone have been disappointing. The need to differentiate this type of SUI from anatomic incontinence is of utmost importance, because the therapeutic options are different.

Evaluation of Urinary Incontinence

In addition to history and physical examination, stress test, basic laboratory tests, cystourethroscopy, and urodynamics identify the cause and type of incontinence in all but few patients (Blaivas, 1987; McGuire, 1988). Because normal continence depends on the integrity of pelvic support as much as the intrinsic urethral mechanism, evaluation of the incontinent patient should include identifying the type of incontinence (anatomic versus intrinsic sphincter dysfunction); the degree of cystocele (I to IV); and the presence of any associated anatomic abnormalities of the pelvic floor, such as enterocele, uterine hypermobility and prolapse, rectocele, and perineal laxity.

History

The initial evaluation of the female with urinary incontinence should begin with a thorough history, as this will dictate the direction of further evaluation and, quite often, will define the problem. The history should include the pattern, frequency, and severity of incontinence and the association of other symptoms with incontinence, such as urinary frequency, nocturia, urgency, hesitancy, and slow stream. A voiding diary is very helpful and provides a reference for future evaluation of response to treatment.

Urinary incontinence in association with physical activity is characteristic of SUI. However, 30 per cent of patients with SUI may also have associated urgency. Some patients may give a history of incontinence with minimal activity or at rest and without urgency. A history of frequency, urgency, and nocturia with incontinence is characteristic of bladder instability even though urodynamic studies may not demonstrate uninhibited detrusor contractions (McGuire, 1988).

Because SUI and UI may coexist (mixed incontinence), some patients may have a mixed symptom pattern that is impossible to categorize only by the history. In these cases, urodynamic evaluation is indicated to delineate the type of incontinence. Vaginal mass, fullness and pressure sensation in the vagina, and obstructive voiding symptoms with or without incontinence may be the first clues to the presence of cystocele with or without enterocele, uterine hypermobility, or rectocele.

In addition to urinary symptoms, the patient should be questioned about bowel habits. The anorectal region and the lower urinary tract share common support by the pelvic floor and common nerve supply by the same spinal segment (S2–4). Dysfunction of one system may be associated with dysfunction of the other.

Neurologic symptoms are very important, because neurogenic bladder is a common cause of incontinence and not uncommonly is a part of a more generalized neurologic disorder. Past urologic, obstetric (number of pregnancies, vaginal deliveries, and any difficulties during partum), gynecologic (prior hysterectomy, anterior and posterior repair and so forth), medical, and neurologic problems should be sought as well as any history of prior operations, in particular pelvic procedures.

Diabetes mellitus and prior pelvic operations may be associated with overflow incontinence due to acontractile bladder. Any medication taken should be recorded, particularly in the elderly, as medication may play a role in incontinence. A brief social and sexual history, particularly in the young sexually active woman, is very helpful.

Physical Examination

A complete physical examination with special emphasis on abdominal examination, pelvic and rectal examination, and spine and neurologic assessment is essential. The pelvic examination should be done in every case and must include the assessment of the degree of urethral mobility and the integrity of the support of the urethra, bladder, and other pelvic organs. Anatomic abnormalities secondary to multiple vaginal deliveries, hormonal changes of menopause, and hysterectomy are common in asymptomatic patients. However, only a small subset of patients with anatomic abnormalities will have stress incontinence. Although genital prolapse, cystocele, enterocele, and rectocele are not causally related to SUI, the majority of patients suffering from urinary stress incontinence have other anatomic abnormalities that must be repaired at the time of stress incontinence surgery. These may be important even in the absence of SUI. Further, the degree of cystocele should be defined as this will dictate the type of surgery needed. If urethral hypermobility is seen without SUI but in the presence of cystocele, it should be repaired in conjunction with the cystocele to prevent de novo SUI postoperatively (McGuire, 1988).

In addition, during the vaginal examination, the degree of uterine hypermobility, enterocele, and rectocele should be evaluated. Rectal examination should include evaluation of the sphincter tone and the bulbocavernosus reflex, which reflects the integrity of the sacral arc. Although the absence of this reflex in men is almost always associated with neurologic lesion, up to 30 per cent of otherwise normal women may not demonstrate this reflex (Blaivas, 1989). Neurogenic bladder is a common cause of urinary incontinence and is not uncommonly associated with neurologic disorders. Thus, neurologic assessment with special emphasis on perineal and perianal sensation, motor activity, and deep tendon reflexes of the lower extremities should be included. Patients with neurologic disorders, such as multiple sclerosis, may present initially with voiding symptoms. More commonly, voiding symptoms follow the onset of other neurologic symptoms.

Stress Test

The bladder is filled with fluid and the patient is asked to cough or strain while the urethra is observed for urine leak (Marchetti et al., 1957). The bladder neck is elevated without obstructing the urethra, observing the disappearing of stress incontinence. This objective demonstration of SUI and the potential effect of a bladder neck suspension surgery are important; however, SUI may still exist in spite of negative test results. SUI is a disease that is evidenced in the standing position, and for that reason the test should be done in the supine and standing positions in doubtful cases. Occasionally, cough-induced instability may precipitate incontinence that simulates SUI and it should be differentiated from it.

Caution should be exercised in the presence of cystocele. If the cystocele is not elevated during coughing or straining, the stress test results may be negative, despite the presence of SUI and urethral hypermobility.

Q-Tip Test

This simple test helps to grossly define the degree of urethral hypermobility (Crystle et al., 1971). With the patient in the supine position, the meatus is cleansed and the Q-Tip is lubricated and introduced into the bladder per urethra. The Q-Tip is then pulled back until some resistance is encountered at the urethrovesical junction. The patient is then asked to strain while the angle of the Q-Tip is observed. A change of the Q-Tip angle of more than 35 degrees with straining indicates poor support of the bladder and urethra. Although this test is very simple, it is very subjective and nonspecific, with high false-positive results.

Urinalysis

In addition to the routine laboratory work-up, urine cultures with sensitivity should be done in all cases, in order to rule out infections. This step is important, because 60 per cent of women with urodynamically stable bladders may demonstrate temporary instability at the time of acute cystitis. More specific tests, such as urine cytology, may be done as dictated by the history of hematuria, frequency with urgency, and cystoscopic findings of suspicious-looking velvety red mucosa.

Cystourethroscopy

This is an important part of the evaluation and should be done in all recurrent cases. We recommend a 0-degree lens in the urethra. It allows for the visual assessment of the coaptation of the urethral mucosa, the mobility of the bladder neck, and the presence of diverticulum or any other urethral pathology. Hypermobility and funneling of the bladder neck on straining are hallmarks of SUI; however, not all patients with SUI have hypermobility, and not all patients with hypermobility have SUI. A persistently open bladder neck and proximal urethra are clues to the presence of dysfunction of the intrinsic urethral mechanism. The bladder should be inspected for trabeculation; diverticula; fistula; ectopic ureter; ureterocele; unsuspected tumor; or mucosal changes, like carcinoma in situ. Trabeculation in the absence of obstruction may be indirect evidence of detrusor instability. A patient with carcinoma in situ may present with frequency and urgency of recent onset, simulating a urinary infection (UI).

Cystogram

The physical examination of the bladder with the patient in the supine position is sometimes inaccurate and often subjective. A simple, standing cystogram, with a small catheter in the bladder and with anteroposterior, oblique, and lateral films in both relaxing and straining modes, is an important adjuvant to the diagnostic evaluation. The cystogram provides an excellent tool to objectively assess anatomic defects (Shapiro and Raz, 1983).

Normally, the bladder base is above the inferior ramus of the pubis symphysis and, with stress maneuvers, should not descend more than 1 cm. When the bladder base is hypermobile and descends below the inferior margin of the pubis, a cystocele exists (Fig. 75–15). In the normal continent female, the bladder neck is closed at rest and with straining, as demonstrated in the true lateral cystogram at a urethrotrigonal angle of 90 degrees. When this angle is greater than 90 degrees, it signifies funneling of the bladder neck.

Funneling is a common finding in patients with anatomic incontinence but is often found in patients with instability, bladder fibrosis, and vaginal prolapse without incontinence as well. Thus, the presence of an obtuse urethrotrigonal angle should be interpreted with caution. The angle of inclination of the urethra to the vertical axis with the patient in the standing position is normally less than 35 degrees. When this angle is greater than 35 degrees, this usually indicates urethral hypermobility (urethrocele).

The catheter is removed when the bladder is full. In a 30-degree oblique position, the patient is asked to rest, strain, and void. This test may objectively show stress incontinence, urethral abnormalities, continence level, and post-void residual. In patients with anatomic stress incontinence, the bladder neck funnels and opens on stress (Fig. 75–16). In patients with intrinsic sphincter

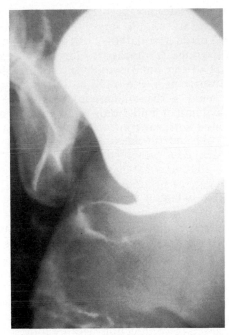

Figure 75–16. Cystogram of a patient with stress urinary incontinence. Note the funneling of the bladder neck and urinary leakage.

dysfunction, the bladder neck is fixed and always open. As previously mentioned the changes in the bladder neck should be interpreted very cautiously when the changes in intravesical pressures are not known.

Urodynamics

The symptom complex in incontinence allows for an index of suspicion about the nature of the problem, but it is not consistently reliable; urodynamics are sometimes necessary to define the problem objectively (Bottaccini and Gleason, 1980; Hilton, 1989; Kuzmarov, 1984; Shepard et al., 1982; Tanagho, 1979). If the history, physical findings, and cystourethroscopy are all consistent with genuine SUI, urodynamics may be unnecessary. However, if the history is not clear, or in the presence of mixed incontinence, urgency, UI, overflow, and total incontinence, urodynamic evaluation is essential (McGuire et al., 1980; Ouslander et al., 1987). Urodynamically, genuine stress incontinence is defined as the loss of urine per urethra during an elevation in intra-abdominal pressure without a true detrusor contraction. This is demonstrated on the cystometrogram in which rectal and intravesical pressures are simultaneously monitored (Stephenson et al., 1984). Urodynamics are particularly helpful when intrinsic sphincteric dysfunction is suspected. In addition to its diagnostic value, this demonstration provides a future reference for the assessment of the efficacy of any therapeutic modality (Juma et al., in press).

Bedside Urodynamics

A simple urodynamic test can be done in most clinical settings at the bedside. After the patient empties her bladder, she is placed on the examining table. A 14 F.

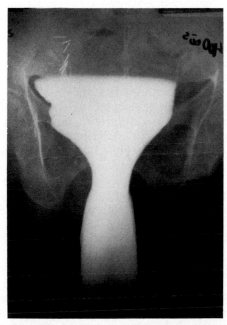

Figure 75–15. Cystogram of a grade IV cystocele.

catheter is inserted into the bladder, and the post-void residual is measured. A large residual is a sign of acontractile bladder or outflow obstruction. The cylinder of a 50-ml syringe is attached to the catheter and held at the level of the pubis symphysis, as the bladder is filled with water at a rate of 50 to 100 ml/minute. The column of fluid in the cylinder is observed. A sudden rise in the column of fluid during filling may be indicative of uninhibited detrusor contraction. The volume at first desire to void and the maximum bladder capacity are also recorded. The catheter is removed. The patient is examined—supine and standing—for continence during stress. Leakage of urine during stress only is typical of genuine SUI, whereas leakage beyond the cough or strain maneuver is a sign of instability. This simple test serves as a screen and may provide preliminary information as to when further urodynamic testing is needed.

Uroflowmetry

Free noninvasive testing of the urinary flow is not diagnostic; however, it is inexpensive and simple and should be done in conjunction with cystometry. With a full bladder, the patient is asked to cough or strain while sitting in the flow chair. Patients with SUI may exhibit urinary loss only at the time of cough. SUI and UI are usually associated with a normal flow or superflow pattern unless obstruction is present. Primary female urethral obstruction is a very rare condition in the non-neurogenic female. It is more common after surgery, because of fibrosis, scarring, and urethral fixation, and in the case of a large cystocele.

Cystometry

This is the most important urodynamic test and involves studying the different phases of bladder function: (1) filling cystometry tests the ability of the bladder to fill and to store urine and (2) voiding cystometry tests the ability of the bladder to empty. The intra-abdominal pressures are recorded simultaneously, and the true detrusor pressures are electronically subtracted (Ask, 1990; Blaivas, 1983 and 1988).

During filling cystometry, we test bladder capacity, sensation, compliance, and involuntary contraction (instability). In the normal patient during filling cystometry, no changes or minimal changes in detrusor pressures should be recorded. Any change in detrusor pressure may be abnormal, in particular if it reproduces the patient's symptoms. Many patients with symptoms of frequency, urgency, and urgency incontinence may be urodynamically stable but still clinically suffering from detrusor instability. Cystometric instability in an otherwise asymptomatic patient does not indicate a pathologic condition.

During filling cystometry, the bladder is filled to capacity. Functional capacity (voided volumes plus residual of urine) may be totally different from cystometric capacity. The rapid bladder filling, the passage of catheters, and the artificial environment of the testing conditions may affect cystometric capacity. Great caution should be exerted in the interpretation of the results.

The patient with a full bladder is asked to cough and strain. Leakage of urine without a change in detrusor pressures will aid in the final diagnosis of stress incontinence. Very often, because of the aforementioned similar reasons, stress incontinence cannot be reproduced in spite of being present under other circumstances.

SUI is usually associated with normal filling cystometry and urine leak during increased intra-abdominal pressure. However, 30 per cent of patients also demonstrate uninhibited detrusor contractions (mixed SUI and UI) (McGuire, 1988). Patients with SUI due to intrinsic sphincteric dysfunction demonstrate urine leak with minimal or no increase in intra-abdominal pressure and in the absence of detrusor contraction.

UI is characterized by the presence of uninhibited detrusor contractions, with urine leak during filling associated with the sense of urgency. Some patients with UI may not demonstrate uninhibited detrusor contractions during urodynamic studies (Cardozo, 1988). Whether these patients are similar to those with sensory urgency is unclear (Coolsaet et al., 1988). We believe that all patients with definite histories of UI should be treated as though they have detrusor instability, whether urodynamic study findings reveal instability or not. In SUI, UI, and mixed incontinence, voiding cystometry is usually normal. In the presence of intrinsic sphincter dysfunction, voiding may be accomplished without any recorded detrusor contraction because the lack of outlet resistance may dissipate any intravesical pressure. Acontractile bladder (e.g., diabetes; spinal cord injury; myelodysplasia; pelvic surgery, such as abdominoperineal resection) will demonstrate low voiding pressure, and the pattern of voiding will be of straining.

Urethral Pressure Profiles

Although urethral pressure profile recordings are a good research tool, their value in the clinical evaluation of urinary incontinence is limited (Massey and Abrams, 1985). No direct correlation exists among urethral pressure profiles, continence, incontinence, and urinary retention except in very rare circumstances.

Continence of the proximal urethra (the area of passive continence) is not the area of highest urethral pressure. Blind recording of urethral pressures without fluoroscopic location of the recording sensor makes the test more difficult to interpret (Constantinou, 1988). Patients with open proximal urethras and relative good levator may show high pressures in the mid-urethra despite severe incontinence. In comparison, patients with low pressures in the mid-urethral area can coapt the proximal half of the urethra perfectly with excellent passive continence. The rotational changes in pressure profile recordings add more confusion. In the normal, supported patient the pressures in the anterior urethra are similar to those in the posterior urethra. In patients with stress incontinence, a reduction in posterior pressures was found.

Urethral closure pressure and functional length tend to be lower in patients with anatomic SUI; however, much overlap with normal values exist (Kaufman, 1979).

A very high urethral pressure recording (> 80 cm H_2O) is rare in stress incontinence but may still be seen. Patients with intrinsic sphincter dysfunction have in general very low pressures in the urethra (< 15 cm H_2O). However, this is not conclusive evidence of intrinsic sphincteric damage, and many patients with similar pressures may be perfectly continent.

Electromyogram

Electromyogram (EMG) studies in SUI are done only in very selected cases (Barnick and Cardozo, 1989). The main use is in patients suspected of having neurologic disorders (e.g., multiple sclerosis, myelodysplasia, and spinal cord injury). Neurologic disorders may show detrusor-sphincter dyssynergia or involuntary sphincter relaxation with detrusor instability (unstable urethra). Sacral evoked responses assess the conductivity of nerve impulse and offer a more quantitative means of evaluating the sacral reflex arc. Needle EMG is very helpful in the diagnosis of denervation potentials of the sacral output, including polyphasic, fibrillation, and positive sharp waves.

Videourodynamics

Videourodynamics represent the ultimate test for the incontinent patient. Filling and voiding cystometry is performed under fluroscopic control. The radiographic image of the bladder neck and urethra are simultaneously observed and correlated with the changes in true detrusor pressure. Videourodynamics help to define the anatomic changes of bladder and urethral support and the coaptation and closure of the urethra during rest and straining. They are of utmost importance in the diagnosis of obstruction (high pressure, low flow), poor bladder contractility (low pressure, low flow), and acontractile bladder (no pressure, interrupted flow by straining). Videourodynamics are helpful in differentiating the various types of incontinence, including intrinsic sphincteric dysfunction.

Patients with anatomic stress incontinence show a closed urethra in the resting position and an open urethra and urinary incontinence during stress, without a change in detrusor pressure. Patients with sphincteric dysfunction have an open urethra all the time (rest and stress), and leakage of urine occurs without a change in detrusor pressures and sometimes without any stress. However, in view of the complexity of videourodynamics and difficulty of interpretation, we believe that they should be limited to specialized medical centers and only in selected cases, because the majority of patients with incontinence can be diagnosed accurately with simpler urodynamic measures.

In summary, the goals of evaluation of the female patient with SUI should include the following:

1. Objective demonstration of SUI by stress test, cystogram, or videourodynamics

2. Demonstration or ruling out of detrusor instability preoperatively because of prognostic implications postoperatively

3. Identification of the type of SUI (anatomic versus intrinsic sphincter dysfunction)

4. Identification and assessment of the degree of cystocele (I to IV)

5. Identification of associated pelvic floor abnormalities, such as enterocele, uterine prolapse, rectocele, and perineal weakness.

TREATMENT OF STRESS INCONTINENCE

Before we discuss the different options in the treatment of SUI, we should address the important question—Who should be treated and why? The medical, psychologic, hygienic, economic, and social consequences of urinary incontinence are immense and should not be underestimated. With the current available therapeutic options, we believe every patient should be offered a treatment option with the intent of cure. Once the criteria for objective stress urinary incontinence have been satisfied and the need for treatment has been established, important factors for deciding on the type of treatment to be performed remain to be evaluated.

As seen in Table 75–3, treatment of stress incontinence can be divided into medical and surgical. Medical treatment should be considered the first line of therapy when possible. However, the long-term side effects of any medical therapy should be weighed against the benefits.

Pelvic Floor Exercise (Kegel)

The use of exercise involving muscles of the pelvic floor is not new and was initially described by Kegel (Kegel, 1948). The rationale is that repetitive voluntary contraction of these skeletal muscles will improve their resting tone as well as their reflex contraction during increased intra-abdominal pressure, such as that which occurs with coughing and straining. This exercise will improve urethral support and closure mechanism, particularly during stress maneuvers, such as coughing, and ultimately will reduce urinary leakage with such maneuvers.

Success rates of these exercises in SUI depend primarily on the severity of incontinence. Patients with

Table 75–3. TREATMENT OPTIONS FOR STRESS URINARY INCONTINENCE

Anatomic incontinence
  Kegel exercise
  Biofeedback
  Estrogen
  Alpha sympathomimetics
  Bladder neck suspension (MMK, Burch, Stamey, Raz, Gittes)
  Periurethral injections (Teflon, collagen, fat, genisphere)
Intrinsic sphincter dysfunction
  Sling procedures (vaginal wall, pubovaginal, mesh)
  Artificial urinary sphincter (AMS-800)
  Periurethral injections (Teflon, collagen, fat, genisphere)

mild symptoms are likely to improve the most; however, to obtain continued benefit, exercises need to be continued. Because not all women will readily identify this group of muscles, it is important to provide patients with educational sessions on how to do the exercises.

These exercises should be done 10 times over 30 seconds every hour. The utilization of weighted vaginal cones may improve the compliance and facilitate the awareness of the pelvic floor muscles. Further, because the anticipated benefit is not immediate, the patient should perform these exercises for 8 to 12 weeks before she experiences any significant benefit. We recommend these exercises in very mild cases of SUI and as adjuncts to other treatment modalities. These exercises rarely cure significant SUI. In mild cases, they will improve the symptoms enough that no further therapy is needed.

Biofeedback

Biofeedback is a behavior modification technique. It is designed to help the patient gain sphincteric control as well as to strengthen the pelvic floor and perineal muscles. Several techniques are available, the principle of which involves an instrument that returns visual or auditory signals that relay to the patient the status of the muscles concerned, whether perineal or otherwise. The person can then be taught to contract or relax these muscles so as to improve the continence mechanism. This is a more objective and quantitative method of pelvic floor exercises, and in fact can be utilized with them to enhance results. The rate of improvement is variable, ranging from 20 to 55 per cent depending on the severity of incontinence and the status of pelvic floor and perineal muscles.

Estrogen

Available evidence suggests that the female urethra is sensitive to estrogen as shown by the cytologic appearance of urethral epithelium that parallels the cytologic changes in the vagina (Smith, 1972). Estrogen stimulates mucosal proliferation, improving mucosal coaptation and enhancing urethral smooth muscle response to alpha-adrenergic stimulation, thus improving the urethral sphincter mechanism (Raz et al., 1973).

At menopause or following removal of the ovaries, there commences a decline in estrogen activity, although some women maintain adequate estrogen levels in the absence of the menstrual cycle. The decline in estrogen is associated with a relative decline in volume of striated muscle and blood vessels and an increase in connective tissue of the urethra. These translate clinically into a decrease in the urethral closure mechanism leading to urinary problems, particularly incontinence. Estrogen supplements in postmenopausal women theoretically improve urethral closure, thus increasing storage capacity primarily by increasing urethral coaptation and outlet resistance. These changes are not reflected by changes in the measured urethral pressure profile. In postmenopausal patients and in those who underwent hysterec-

tomies and in whom there is no absolute contraindication to estrogens, the supplements can be administered by mouth, dermal patch, or injection. We provide Premarin (estrogen) in mild cases of SUI or as an adjunct to other treatment modalities, particularly with cholinolytic agents. In the case of a contraindication for oral estrogen, vaginal cream is a good alternative. Vaginal cream of Premarin has only mild local estrogenic effect until after it is absorbed and the conjugated estrogens are metabolized by the liver.

Alpha-Adrenergic Agonists

These agents are known to enhance urethral closure mechanisms by their direct action on the alpha receptors in the bladder neck. The most common agents are phenylpropanolamine, ephedrine, and pseudoephedrine. No large prospective controlled trials on the results of these medications in SUI are available. However, in the presence of mild degrees of SUI or when surgical intervention is contraindicated, these agents may be considered in conjunction with other nonsurgical modalities. Alpha-agonist medications may have significant side effects, such as hypertension, tachycardia, and arrhythmia. They should be given with great caution.

Bladder Relaxants

Anticholinergic medication, tricyclic antidepressants, and prostaglandin inhibitors in the treatment of pure SUI have no physiologic basis. Further, no prospective controlled clinical trials have assessed the effects of these medications in SUI. Under these circumstances, these drugs should be considered only in the presence of urgency and urge incontinence with SUI or in some cases in which the history, physical findings, and urodynamic testing results are inconclusive as to the exact type of incontinence. Under these circumstances, a diagnostic and therapeutic trial with one of these medications can be tried in deciding the major component responsible for incontinence (stress versus urge).

SURGERY FOR STRESS INCONTINENCE

Surgery for stress incontinence is indicated in motivated patients with significant loss of urine, creating a social and/or hygienic problem. Several options for the treatment of SUI are available. The choice will depend on the severity of SUI, personal preference of the surgeon, and the general medical condition of the patient. When interpreting the success rate of any particular treatment modality for SUI, we should bear in mind that a rare episode of urinary leakage per urethra with straining or coughing in women who are otherwise considered healthy is not uncommon (Iosif et al., 1988). However, this problem is not considered SUI. SUI is urinary leakage under similar circumstances that has social or hygienic consequences.

Table 75–4. CLASSIFICATION OF CYSTOCELE

Grade	Definition	Therapy
I	Bladder neck hypermobility	Bladder neck suspension
II	Bladder base reaching introitus with strain	Four-corner bladder and bladder neck suspension
III	Bladder neck bulging through introitus with strain	Four-corner bladder and bladder neck suspension
IV	Bladder base outside introitus at rest	Bladder neck suspension and formal cystocele repair

There is not one surgery that corrects all types of incontinence. The choice of therapy depends primarily on three factors: (1) type of stress incontinence (see Table 75–2); (2) degree of cystocele (Table 75–4); and (3) presence of other pelvic floor abnormalities, such as enterocele, uterine hypermobility, and rectocele that must be corrected at the time of the stress incontinence surgery.

Type of Incontinence

As previously discussed, we distinguish stress incontinence into two types: (1) anatomic incontinence in which there is malposition of a normal sphincteric unit and (2) incontinence due to intrinsic sphincter dysfunction in which there is damage or paralysis of the sphincteric unit. The goal of surgery for anatomic incontinence is repositioning of the bladder neck and urethra to a high retropubic position, whereas the goal of surgery for intrinsic dysfunction is coaptation, support, and compression of the damaged sphincteric unit.

Surgeries for anatomical incontinence include the abdominal approach, like the Marshall-Marchetti and Burch suspension (Fig. 75 17), vaginal approach, like the anterior colporraphy (Kelly plication) (Fig. 75–18), and needle suspensions, like the Stamey, Gittes, or our own Raz suspensions (Fig. 75–19). With the current advances in the techniques of bladder neck suspension, this procedure can be done with minimal pain, morbidity, and cost, and a success rate of 85 to 95 per cent (Green et al., 1986; Spencer et al., 1987). Thus, we believe that bladder neck suspension should be offered as the standard treatment for anatomic SUI, except in very selected cases in which surgery is absolutely contraindicated. Options for intrinsic sphincter dysfunction include periurethral injections of collagen or Teflon and artificial sphincter and sling procedures.

ANTERIOR REPAIR

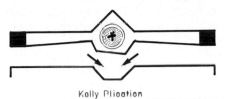

Kelly Plication

Figure 75–18. Diagram of Kelly's plication. Note the principle of plication of the periurethral tissue to support the urethra.

Degree of Anterior Vaginal Wall Prolapse

Most operations for incontinence are done to restore the bladder neck and urethra to a high, supported retropubic position. When cystocele is present, the mere elevation of the bladder neck may create urethral obstruction and exacerbate the cystocele. Cystocele must be corrected at the time of bladder neck suspension. The Marshall-Marchetti operation corrects urethra hypermobility, but the Burch suspension corrects cystocele as well. The anterior colporraphy (Kelly plication) utilized in the treatment of cystocele should be abandoned in the treatment of stress incontinence because of its inability to support and elevate the bladder neck and urethra in a high supported retropubic position. The Stamey and Gittes suspensions relieve only bladder neck hypermobility, without correcting the cystocele.

We have designed three vaginal operations for anatomic incontinence, depending on the degree of anterior vaginal wall prolapse. For minimal cystocele, we perform a simple needle bladder neck suspension. For selected cases of moderate cystocele, we perform a suspension of the bladder base (cardinal ligaments, pubocervical fasciae, and vaginal wall) and bladder neck (vaginal wall and urethropelvic) ligament. We call this operation the four-corner bladder and bladder neck suspension. For severe cystocele, when the bladder is outside the introitus all the time, we repair the central hernia of the bladder by approximating the pubocervical fascia and include suspension of the bladder neck and bladder base by anchoring the cardinal ligaments, pubocervical fascia, and urethropelvic ligaments.

ABDOMINAL SUSPENSIONS

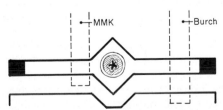

Figure 75–17. Diagram of abdominal approaches to bladder neck suspension procedures. Note the relation of the suspending sutures to the urethra.

TRANSVAGINAL SUSPENSIONS

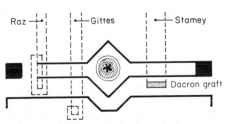

Figure 75–19. Various transvaginal bladder neck suspension procedures. Note the relation of the suspension sutures to the urethra.

Historical Perspective

It was recognized approximately half a century ago that the treatment of SUI due to hypermobility of the proximal urethra and bladder neck is based on the repositioning of these structures into a high, supported position behind the pubic bone. Since Howard Kelly (1914) described the Kelly plication, there have been numerous innovations and advancements in the understanding of the pathophysiology, diagnosis, and treatment of stress urinary incontinence. In 1949, Marshall and colleagues described the retropubic suspension operation for the treatment of stress incontinence. This procedure proved to be very effective and is still considered by some workers as the gold standard when describing results of any new surgery for stress urinary incontinence. A distinct disadvantage is that because the sutures are placed in a periurethral fashion, the potential for obstruction exists. Other disadvantages are the inability to correct a cystocele from this approach and the potential occurrence of osteitis pubis, because of suture placement in the pubic periosteum.

In 1961, John Burch described a retropubic suspension procedure in which chromic sutures are utilized to tack the perivaginal fascia and vaginal wall, excluding the epithelium, to Cooper's ligament. Advantages of the Burch colposuspension include lateral placement of the suspension sutures, thus obviating urethral obstruction: ability to correct mild cystocele; and reliability of Cooper's ligament as a strong anchoring tissue compared with the periosteum of the pubis.

Since its introduction (Pereyra, 1959 and 1967), the transvaginal bladder neck suspension has undergone significant modifications (Cobb, 1978; Harer et al., 1965; Jeffcoate, 1965; Raz, 1981; Stamey, 1973; Tauber et al., 1967; Winter, 1976) and has now become the standard procedure for anatomic SUI. In 1973, Stamey contributed several concepts to needle suspension. He introduced the cystoscopic control of needle placement at the vesical neck and visualization of the bladder neck closure with elevation of the suspension sutures. In addition, Stamey also contributed the concept of bolsters to support the bladder neck.

In 1981 and 1985, Raz introduced another modification of the needle suspension technique. Several principles were introduced with this modification. The inverted U, vaginal epithelial incision as devised to allow for dissection to be lateral to the urethra and bladder neck, thus avoiding dissection directly beneath the urethra and bladder neck. This maneuver avoids the need for mobilization of a vaginal flap, facilitating entrance into the retropubic space. The urethropelvic ligament and the pubocervical and endopelvic fasciae are conveniently approached from the limbs of the inverted U. This principle is similar to that of the Burch suspension in that the sutures are placed laterally, obviating obstruction.

We believe that it is important to enter the retropubic space not merely to facilitate fingertip control of the ligature carrier, but to sufficiently mobilize the urethra and vesical neck from adhesions and scars prior to performing the suspension. In a patient who had prior failure of bladder neck suspension, the scarring and fibrosis from prior suspension prevents adequate repositioning of the bladder neck and the urethra. Thus, repeat transvaginal suspension should be combined with urethrolysis to avoid urethral obstruction and to improve the success rate of the second suspension (McGuire et al., 1989; Zimmern et al., 1987).

The success of surgery depends on the creation of a strong anchor of the bladder neck and urethra. A distinct advantage of this approach is that the anchor can be precisely placed just lateral to the bladder neck. Most important, this anchor can be tested for its strength by pulling from the sutures.

In 1987, Gittes and Loughlin described a "no-incision" modification of the Pereyra technique. This procedure relies on the suspension suture breaking through the vaginal epithelium and becoming incorporated (Morales and VanCott, 1988).

Marshall-Marchetti-Krantz Procedure

This procedure remains to be offered as the standard treatment of SUI in many medical centers in the United States. Since its original description until today, it has undergone several modifications; however, the basic principle of retropubic urethropexy remains the same. We rarely employ this procedure today.

TECHNIQUE. With the patient in the supine frog-leg position, the lower abdomen and external genitalia, including the vagina, are prepared and draped to include the vagina within the operative field. A Foley catheter is inserted into the bladder per urethra. Through a lower midline or Pfannenstiel incision, the retropubic extraperitoneal space of Retzius is entered. A Belfour retractor is utilized to retract the recti muscles apart. With a sponge on a ring forceps, the bladder neck and proximal urethra are separated from the posterior surface of the pubic bone, using very gentle pressure to avoid tearing of the veins. When this surgery is done following a prior failed suspension procedure, a sharper dissection is necessary to free up the bladder neck and proximal urethra. Three 2–0 chromic catgut sutures are inserted equidistant into the vaginal wall on either side, near the urethra. With gentle traction on the Foley catheter and a finger in the vagina, the level of the bladder neck is identified. A similar suture is inserted at the level of the bladder neck on either side. The free ends of these sutures are then passed through the cartilage and the periosteum of the pubic bone to reposition the bladder neck and proximal urethra into a high retropubic position. The sutures are tied while an assistant places a finger in the vagina to aid in the elevation of the vaginal wall, avoiding tension on the sutures.

A Penrose drain is placed into the retropubic space through a separate suprapubic stab wound. The incision is closed in layers after adequate hemostasis is confirmed. The Foley catheter and the drain are removed in 3 to 5 days. The patient is usually discharged from the hospital on the 4th or 5th postoperative day.

The reported success rate with this procedure is 57 to

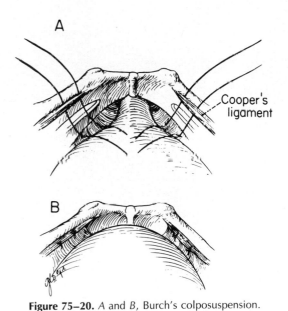

Figure 75–20. *A* and *B*, Burch's colposuspension.

95 per cent (Green et al., 1986; Spencer et al., 1987). Disadvantages include the potential for creating urethral obstruction because of the proximity of the suture to the urethra and the inability to simultaneously correct cystocele.

Burch Colposuspension

This procedure is our preferred abdominal approach to bladder neck suspension. We utilize this procedure when the abdomen is already opened for a different indication, such as abdominal hysterectomy. The lateral placement of the sutures offers the advantage of avoiding urethral obstruction and the ability to repair minimal-to-moderate cystocele. The success rate is comparable to other suspension procedures (Gillon et al., 1984; Van Gleen et al., 1988).

TECHNIQUE (Fig. 75–20). The patient position, preparation, and draping are similar to those of the Marshall-Marchetti-Krantz procedure. A Foley catheter is inserted in the bladder as previously described, and the retropubic space of Retzius is entered through a lower midline or Pfannenstiel incision. A Balfour retractor separates the recti muscles. The bladder neck and proximal urethra are separated from the posterior surface of the pubic bone, employing gentle dissection with a sponge on a ring forceps. Sharp and blunt dissection exposes the retropubic space and the lateral and superior pubic surface, which is covered by the ileopectineal (Cooper) ligament.

The bladder neck is identified and elevated through the vagina as previously described. A 2–0 chromic catgut suture is inserted into the vaginal wall, excluding epithelium, and the paravaginal tissue at the level of the bladder neck. Each suture is passed through the ipsilateral ileopectineal ligament at a point where the vaginal wall and ileopectineal ligament can be brought together without tension. The sutures are then tied. Adequate hemostasis is confirmed, a suprapubic catheter is put

through a separate stab, and the incision is closed in layers. The Foley catheter is removed on the 3rd to 5th postoperative day, and the suprapubic catheter is removed when bladder emptying is confirmed with a low post-void residual.

Stamey Transvaginal Bladder Neck Suspension

This technique is discussed in detail in Chapter 76 (Stamey, 1973 and 1980).

No-Incision (Gittes) Transvaginal Bladder Neck Suspension

TECHNIQUE (Fig. 75–21). After placement of a Foley catheter and a weighted vaginal speculum, a small puncture is made with the tip of a No. 15 scalpel blade into the suprapubic fat pad, about 5 cm lateral to the midline just above the hairline. The transferring needle is passed through the rectus fascia, and the tip is advanced carefully down the posterior aspect of the pubic bone. The anterior vaginal wall at the level of the bladder neck is simultaneously elevated with the operator's second hand pressing upward just lateral to the Foley catheter balloon. The needle is directed from above, toward the intravaginal fingertip. Once the needle tip is palpable by the intravaginal fingertip, the needle is popped through the wall and on out through the introitus.

The suspension suture (0 hydroxypropylene monofil-

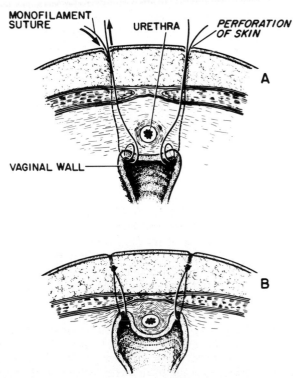

Figure 75–21. *A* and *B*, No-incision (Gittes) transvaginal bladder neck suspension.

ament or 0 monofilament nylon is recommended) is threaded into the eye at the tip of the needle. The needle is pulled back out the suprapubic wound, transferring one end of the suspension suture suprapubically, where it is secured with a hemostat. The second pass of the needle is then made through the same suprapubic skin incision, passing through the rectus fascia 1 or 2 cm, laterally or medially to the first pass. This provides a base of strong fascial support for the suspension.

The point of the transferring needle is again advanced as before, so that the second perforation site on the vaginal wall is selected 1.5 to 2 cm away (cephalad or caudad) from the first puncture site. Prior to suprapubic transfer of the free vaginal end of the suspending suture, it is threaded temporarily on a stout half-circle surgical needle (Mayo type), two to three anchoring, full-thickness helical bites are taken with the suspending sutures through the portion of the vaginal wall that stretches between the first and second vaginal perforations. The half-circle surgical needle is then unthreaded. The free end of the suture is passed through the eye of the long needle already placed. The needle is drawn up to the suprapubic field and secured for later tying of the mattress suture into the small skin perforation. The same procedure is carried out on the opposite side.

Cystourethroscopy is done to rule out injury to the bladder wall by the suspending sutures and to place a percutaneous suprapubic cystostomy under endoscopic control. Both suspending sutures are tied down into their respective suprapubic puncture holes. Multiple knots are made to avoid postoperative loosening, typical of nylon sutures. Knot tension is equivalent to that for fascial stitches elsewhere. Sutures are cut just slightly above the knots, so that no sutures are visible outside the stab wound; the skin holes are covered with an adhesive bandage after umbilication of the skin is eliminated by pulling the puncture site up with small tooth forceps (Gittes et al., 1987; Morales et al., 1988).

This procedure represents one of the most recent modifications of the transvaginal bladder neck suspension procedure. The main advantage of this procedure is its simplicity. However, the site of placement of the suspension sutures are less controlled. The reported success rate is 85 to 90 per cent.

Raz Transvaginal Needle Bladder Neck Suspension

This operation is chosen for patients with anatomic incontinence due to urethral and bladder neck hypermobility, with minimal or no cystocele.

TECHNIQUE. After general or spinal anesthesia is induced, the patient is placed in the dorsal lithotomy position. A weighted speculum is placed in the vagina, and the labia are retracted laterally with stay sutures. A suprapubic catheter is inserted via an intraurethral Lowsley retractor and a stab incision suprapubically, and another Foley catheter is placed into the bladder per urethra (Zeidman et al., 1988). The bladder is drained of urine, and the intraurethral Foley catheter is placed on gentle traction to help locate the bladder neck

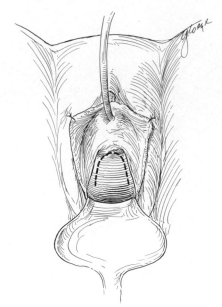

Figure 75–22. U-shaped incision in the anterior vaginal wall.

by palpation of the anterior vaginal wall. Saline is injected in the anterior vaginal wall to develop tissue planes for better dissection. An inverted U-shaped incision is made in the anterior vaginal wall, with the base of the U at a point midway between the bladder neck and the external urethral meatus and the legs of the U extending just proximal to the bladder neck (Fig. 75–22).

The vaginal wall on either side is dissected off the shiny surface of the periurethral fascia toward the pubic bone. At the level of the bladder neck, the retropubic space is entered by detaching the urethropelvic ligament from its attachment to the lateral pelvic wall at the tendinous arc, using curved Mayo scissors (Fig. 75–23).

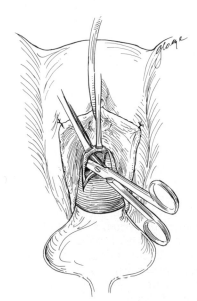

Figure 75–23. The vaginal wall is dissected off the glistening surface of the periurethral fascia, and the retropubic space is entered by detaching the urethropelvic ligament of the lateral pelvic wall.

The scissors should point toward the patient's shoulder on entering the retropubic space. Once the retropubic space has been opened, the operator's index finger is inserted, and all adhesions along the proximal urethra and the bladder neck are bluntly released. With Russian forceps, with the jaws separated as a retractor, the detached edges of the urethropelvic ligaments are retracted medially to allow placement of the suspension sutures. A No. 1 Prolene suture on a Mayo needle is employed to incorporate the urethropelvic ligament, found at the medial edge of the window created in the retropubic space, together with pubocervical fascia and anterior vaginal wall, excluding the epithelium (Fig. 75–24). Three or four helical passes through these structures are made. The strength of the sutures is tested by pulling.

A small, 1-inch incision is made transversely just above the superior margin of the pubic bone and carried down to the level of the underlying rectus fascia. The double-pronged ligature carrier is placed in the suprapubic wound, just cephalad to the pubic bone (Fig. 75–25). With the surgeon's index finger in the retropubic space and under direct digital control, the needle is passed through the vaginal incision. The suspending sutures are transferred suprapubically via the ligature carrier (Fig. 75–26). With the suspending sutures pulled upward, the vaginal examination should now reveal anterior vaginal wall and urethra to be lifted to a high retropubic position.

Cystoscopy is performed to ensure that no bladder perforation occurred, that the suprapubic catheter is in position, and that the ureteric efflux of indigo carmine previously injected intravenously is present bilaterally. With the zero-degree lens at the level of the proximal urethra, the suspending sutures are pulled up and the bladder neck and proximal urethral replacement to a high retropubic position is confirmed.

The anterior vaginal wall incision is closed with running, locking 2–0 Vicryl suture (Fig. 75–27). A vaginal packing, impregnated with antibiotic cream, is inserted

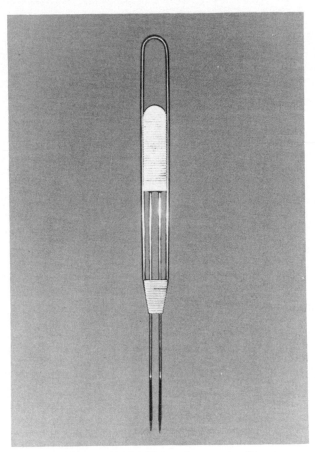

Figure 75–25. Double-needle suture carrier.

into the vagina. The suspending sutures are tied independently with multiple knots snug onto the underlying rectus fascia without tension and across the midline with the sutures from the opposite side. The suprapubic wound is irrigated, and the skin is closed with 4–0 Vicryl in a subcuticular fashion; Steri-Strips are applied (Hadley et al., 1986; Schmidbauer et al., 1986).

The advantages of this approach include accurate placement of the suspending sutures at the level of the bladder neck, finger control of the suture carrier needle to avoid injury to the bladder during suture transfer, and ability to correct simultaneously any degree of vaginal wall prolapse (see further discussion). In a preliminary review of the records of over 400 cases, our success rate based on objective and subjective postoperative evaluations of our patients is 94 per cent (85 per cent cured; 9 per cent have very rare episodes of incontinence).

STRESS INCONTINENCE AND CYSTOCELE (ANTERIOR VAGINAL WALL PROLAPSE)

As previously described, the degree of anterior vaginal wall prolapse can be divided into different grades. In grade I, there is minimal hypermobility of the bladder base; in grade II, the bladder base reaches the introitus but not the outside; and in grade III, the bladder base

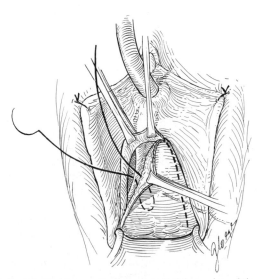

Figure 75–24. The suspending suture in the free edge of the urethropelvic ligament.

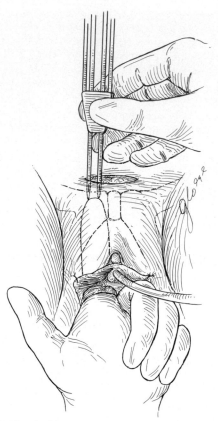

Figure 75–26. The double-needle suture carrier is transfered retropubically under direct finger control to avoid bladder injury.

reaches and comes out the introitus on straining. Severe vaginal prolapse or grade IV cystocele involves herniation of the bladder base outside the introitus at rest (see Fig. 75–15).

Cystocele is generally present with concomitant bladder neck and urethral hypermobility (urethrocele).

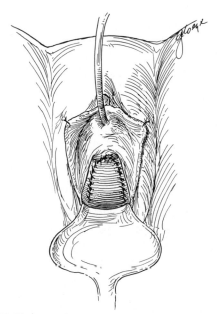

Figure 75–27. The vaginal incision is closed prior to tying the suspension sutures.

Rarely, after a prior bladder neck suspension, cystocele may occur without urethral prolapse. We describe our approach to cystocele with concomitant urethral hypermobility, because this is the most commonly seen entity in anterior vaginal wall prolapse.

Large cystoceles result from weakness of the levator hiatus and pubocervical fascia with a resulting herniation of the bladder neck and bladder base. Three types of cystocele may be described based on the anatomic defect encountered. The first involves a central defect of the pubocervical fascia with the urethropelvic ligament and pubocervical fascia still attached to the pelvic sidewall. In the second type, the pubocervical fascia and urethropelvic ligament have a weak anchor or are detached from the lateral pelvic wall, resulting in a sliding hernia or cystocele. The third and most common cystocele is a combination of these two types.

The classic approach to correction of severe cystocele entails plication of the pubocervical fascia (Kelly) and bladder neck. This maneuver results in poor support of the bladder neck area in a patient with stress incontinence and may lead to de novo incontinence when undertaken for correction of cystocele without stress incontinence. Our transvaginal technique simultaneously repairs the prolapsed bladder neck, the central hernia defect, and the lateral sliding hernia. This repair is accomplished by support of the bladder neck (urethropelvic ligament) and bladder base (pubocervical and cardinal ligaments) utilizing nonabsorbable sutures. Repair of a large cystocele extending outside the introitus at rest requires simultaneous formal cystocele repair and bladder neck suspension, whether or not preoperative incontinence exists. If only cystocele repair is performed de novo stress incontinence may occur by changing the anatomic relation of the bladder and urethra.

Severe cystocele is often associated with other vaginal prolapse, including uterine prolapse, enterocele (previous hysterectomy), rectocele, and vaginal vault prolapse. These conditions require simultaneous correction for total pelvic floor support.

DIAGNOSIS. The patient will usually describe a bulging mass through the introitus, with or without stress incontinence. They may also have a history of obstructive voiding symptoms, with a sensation of incomplete bladder emptying. Recurrent urinary tract infections may be related to high residual urines.

On physical examination in the lithotomy position, the herniation may be less prominent and may be provoked by Valsalva's maneuver or coughing. If this still does not reproduce the symptoms of introital mass, the patient may be placed in the erect position. Physical examination or voiding cystourethrogram in this position will then demonstrate the herniated bladder base.

Voiding cystourethrogram shows the descended bladder base with or without change in the urethral axis. The bladder neck may be funneled with stress-induced urinary leakage. During straining, the cystocele further enlarges. An elevated post-void residual is often seen in the prolapsed bladder base.

Cystourethroscopy confirms the descent of the bladder base and trigone and allows assessment of urethral hypermobility. Urodynamic evaluation aids in the evaluation of the type of stress incontinence and detrusor function and dysfunction.

An intravenous urogram or renal ultrasound may be indicated in a case in which involvement of the distal ureters in the herniated bladder is suspected, to rule out partial ureteral obstruction or hydronephrosis.

Four-Corner Bladder and Bladder Neck Suspension for Moderate Cystocele

Traditionally, the approach to cystourethrocele repair involves reapproximation of the lax pubocervical fascia through the anterior vaginal wall, with narrowing of the bladder neck and proximal urethra by the Kelly-type plication. This procedure corrects the prolapse but may have a high failure rate when utilized for the treatment of incontinence. We developed a transvaginal needle suspension operation that repositions the bladder neck in a high, retropubic position and repairs moderate anterior vaginal wall prolapse with excellent support of the bladder base. Our success rate for the correction of cystocele with this procedure is 98 per cent and for the correction of stress urinary incontinence, 94 per cent. This operation provides a simple vaginal approach for the correction of cystocele with bladder neck suspension with minimal morbidity and short hospital stay (Raz et al., 1989).

TECHNIQUE. The patient is placed in the dorsal lithotomy position. A weighted speculum is placed in the vagina, and the labia are retracted laterally with stay sutures. A suprapubic catheter is inserted via an intraurethral Lowsley tractor, and another catheter is inserted through the urethra. The bladder neck is identified by placing gentle traction on the urethral catheter and by palpating the balloon through the anterior vaginal wall.

An inverted U incision is made in the anterior vaginal wall with the apex located midway between the urethral meatus and bladder neck. The base of the inverted U incision extends farther posteriorly beyond the bladder neck to the base of the bladder, where the anterior extension of the cardinal ligaments is located. If the uterus is still present, the incision is extended lateral to the cervix but not beyond it.

Lateral dissection toward the pubic bone at the level of the bladder neck is performed over the glistening surface of the periurethral fascia, which guides the plane of dissection. The dissection is carried laterally between the levators and the urethropelvic ligaments. The retropubic space is entered at the tendinous arc, the adhesions are freed, and the urethropelvic ligament is detached sharply or bluntly from its attachment to the tendinous arc.

Two pairs of monofilament nonabsorbable sutures (No. 1 polypropylene on a Mayo 5 or 6 needle) are placed on each side. The distal sutures are placed at the level of the bladder neck as in the standard Raz-type bladder neck suspension. Sutures include the vaginal wall minus epithelium; the underlying pubocervical fascia; and the most important anchoring component, the medial edge of the urethropelvic ligament. The proximal sutures are placed at the base of the inverted U incision.

These sutures incorporate the entire vaginal wall minus epithelium, pubocervical fascia, and anterior extension of the cardinal ligaments. Two to three passes are performed with each suture. The strength of the anchoring tissues is tested by pulling. The four sets of sutures are transferred to the anterior abdominal wall with a double-pronged ligature carrier through a small suprapubic incision.

Endoscopic visualization of the bladder neck with lifting of the sutures confirms the proper coaptation of the bladder neck and elevation of the bladder base. Indigo carmine injected intravenously is seen effluxing from the ureteral orifices, ruling out ureteral injury.

After closure of the anterior vaginal wall, the four sutures are tied independently over the anterior rectus fascia without tension; then to each other on each side; and then across the midline. An antibiotic-coated vaginal pack is placed. The suprapubic incision is closed with a 4–0 Dexon subcuticular suture.

The vaginal packing and urethral catheter are removed the morning following surgery, and the suprapubic catheter is left in place for measurement of postvoid residuals.

Raz Transvaginal Repair of Severe Cystocele

The principles for repair of severe cystocele combine bladder neck suspension, repair of the central defect in the pubocervical fascia, and support of the lateral sliding cystocele hernia of pubocervical fascia with permanent sutures. The surgery is done entirely through the vagina (Leach et al., 1986).

TECHNIQUE. The patient is placed in the dorsal lithotomy position. A weighted speculum is placed in the vagina, and the labia are retracted laterally with stay sutures. A percutaneous cystostomy tube is placed utilizing the Lowsley tractor. A urethral catheter is inserted; the bladder is emptied. A Scott retractor is positioned and secured to the vaginal sidewalls with hooks.

While placing gentle traction on the urethral catheter, the bladder neck is identified by palpating the catheter balloon. An Allis clamp grasps the anterior vaginal wall at the level of the mid-urethra. Saline is injected into the anterior vaginal wall to facilitate dissection of the underlying tissues. A vertical midline incision is made in the anterior vaginal wall, which extends from the area of the bladder neck to the posterior edge of the cystocele (Fig. 75–28).

The dissection is carried out laterally in the avascular plane between the vaginal wall and the pubocervical fascia to free the herniated part of the bladder from the anterior vaginal wall. The pubocervical fascia is thin medially and becomes thicker laterally, toward the levator ani muscles (Fig. 75–29). Posteriorly, the dissection will reach the peritoneal fold. At the level of the bladder neck, dissection is carried over the periurethral fascia and urethropelvic ligament to the tendinous arc.

After adequate mobilization of the herniated part of the bladder is accomplished, a gauze is placed to reduce and protect the bladder during the next step of the operation—the needle bladder neck suspension.

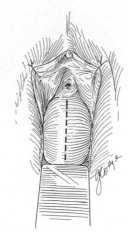

Figure 75–28. Longitudinal incision in the vaginal wall.

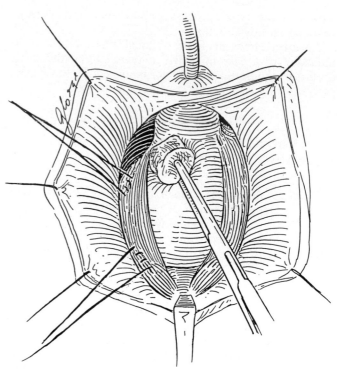

Figure 75–30. Prolene sutures in the anterior extension of the cardinal ligaments and in the pubocervical fascia.

At the level of the bladder neck, the retropubic space is entered by bluntly and sharply dividing the urethropelvic fascia at its insertion to the tendinous arc. All adherent tissue is dissected free from the posterior aspect of the pubic symphysis to completely free the urethra. Placement and transfer of the suspension sutures are then carried out as previously described. Two modifications are introduced for this repair. First, and most important, the permanent Prolene sutures incorporate the anterior extension of the cardinal ligaments as well as the pubocervical fascia (Fig. 75–30). This step repairs the sliding hernia. Second, the permanent sutures incorporate the inner part of the vaginal wall from its medial side through the incision, instead of placing it from its lateral aspect through the U-shaped incision (Fig. 75–31). The suspension sutures are left untied temporarily in the suprapubic region.

To repair the central cystocele defect, 2–0 Vicryl interrupted sutures are placed to approximate the lateral edges of the pubocervical fascia (Fig. 75–32). The sutures are placed in a distal-to-proximal fashion, toward the bladder base, and are left untied until all sutures have been placed (Fig. 75–33).

After indigo carmine is administered intravenously, cystoscopy is performed to confirm the adequate support of the bladder neck and proximal urethra upon gentle traction on the suspension sutures and the proper positioning of the suprapubic tube, and to verify the adequate efflux of dye from the ureteral orifices. In addition, it is confirmed that no sutures have entered the bladder.

The excess vaginal wall is trimmed. The vaginal incision is closed with a running 2–0 Vicryl suture, incorporating the underlying pubocervical fascia in the closure to eliminate the "dead space." A pack coated with antibiotic cream is placed in the vagina. The suspension sutures are tied individually in the suprapubic area and across the midline, without undue tension. The suprapubic incision is closed with a running subcuticular 4–0 Dexon suture.

Postoperative care is not different from that for other vaginal surgeries. The urethral catheter and vaginal packing are removed the morning following surgery. The suprapubic catheter is left in place for measurement of post-void residuals. The patient is discharged from the hospital the second postoperative day, after instruction in measurement of post-void residual. The patient is told to resume activities as tolerated.

The suprapubic catheter is generally removed within 2 weeks of surgery. The patient is seen in follow-up for physical examination at 2 weeks and 6 months and then yearly thereafter. We have had successful results with this technique in the correction of severe anterior vaginal wall prolapse in 94 per cent of cases.

With such a multitude of different procedures to choose from, what is a reasonable approach for the clinician? Is a vaginal approach superior to a retropubic

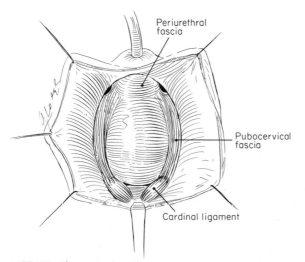

Periurethral
fascia

Pubocervical
fascia

Cardinal ligament

Figure 75–29. The vaginal wall is dissected off the bladder base to expose the pubocervical and periurethral fasciae.

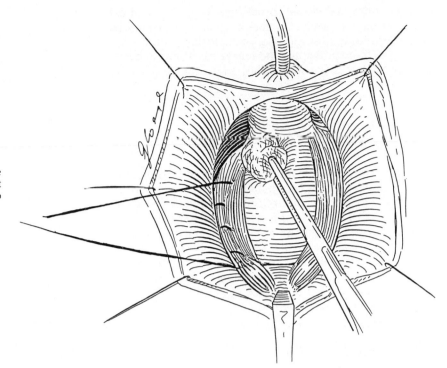

Figure 75–31. When the defect is narrow, only one suture that incorporates both the cardinal ligament and the pubocervical fascia is used rather than two sutures.

approach? Is a no-incision technique better than a technique that requires a vaginal incision? Is there a limitation on the maxim that simpler is better? The answers to these questions can be decided by a comparative analysis of the results and by the advantages and disadvantages of the individual techniques.

The transabdominal suspension procedures, such as the Marshall-Marchetti-Krantz and the Burch, have success rates equal to those of transvaginal suspension procedures. Clearly, if similar results can be achieved

with retropubic and vaginal approaches, it would be in the best interest of the patient to select the procedure that results in the least pain, morbidity, and risk and that results in the shortest hospital stay and most rapid return to a productive lifestyle (Siegel et al., 1988). Further, other anatomic abnormalities, such as cystocele, enterocele, and rectocele, can be dealt with simultaneously.

Occasionally, the transabdominal approach may be preferred, such as when the suspension is done with

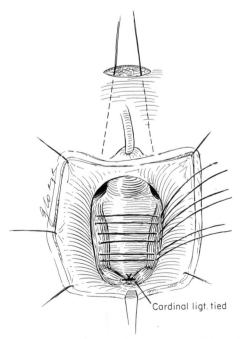

Figure 75–32. Sutures that incorporate the edges of the pubocervical fascia.

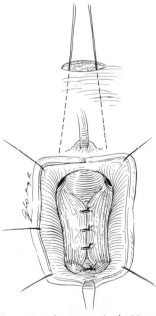

Figure 75–33. The cystocele is repaired. Note the bladder neck suspension sutures and the pubocervical and the cardinal ligaments approximated in the midline.

another intra-abdominal procedure (e.g., abdominal hysterectomy) or when the patient cannot be positioned in the lithotomy position (e.g., ankylosing spondylitis). As long as basic principles and tenets are strictly adhered to, the choice of a particular technique is of little importance.

Surgery for Intrinsic Sphincter Dysfunction

In the presence of intrinsic sphincter dysfunction, simple suspension of the bladder neck is unlikely to correct the problem, and urethral compression becomes necessary to achieve continence. In this situation, the goal of surgery is restoration of the mucosal seal by means of a coapting sling (Aldrige, 1942; Kaufman, 1982; McGuire, 1978; Raz et al., 1989) or an intraurethral injection of a distending substance, such as Teflon (Politano et al., 1974) or collagen (Dairiki et al., 1989), or an artificial urinary sphincter.

Periurethral Injection

The role of periurethral injections in the treatment of SUI is currently being evaluated at several medical centers in this country, employing a multitude of substances, including fat, Teflon, collagen as well as the use of expandable spheres. With the exception of Teflon, long-term follow-up on the results of these injections are not yet available. However, short-term results are very encouraging. Available data indicate that the success rate with periurethral Teflon injection is 62 per cent (Politano et al., 1974). The advantages of periurethral injection include simplicity and the fact that it can be done on outpatient basis.

Urethral Slings

The status of the sling procedure is more established in the treatment of this type of SUI. Several sling procedures have been described in the literature using vaginal wall, rectus fascia, fascia lata, and synthetic material (Fig. 75–34). Our preference is the vaginal wall sling procedure, utilizing an island of well-vascularized vaginal wall to create urethral compression. However, because the results of the various sling procedures are comparable, the choice of a particular procedure depends on personal preference.

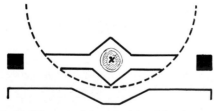

SLING PROCEDURES

Figure 75–34. Diagram of the principle of the sling procedures.

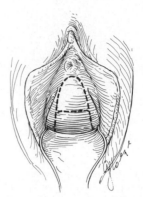

Figure 75–35. A-shaped incision in the anterior vaginal wall.

The function of the sling is to coapt the urethra so that it resists increased intra-abdominal pressure rather than intrinsic detrusor pressure. Urodynamic studies indicate that urethral relaxation associated with decreased urethral pressure precedes detrusor contraction despite the sling. However, during stress, the sling exerts considerable increase of pressure on the urethra to maintain continence (McGuire, 1978 and 1987). Thus, contrary to general belief, the majority of patients are eventually able to void spontaneously and completely.

VAGINAL WALL SLING

Technique. The perineum and vagina are prepared as in the previous procedures after spinal or general anesthesia has been administered. Saline is used to infiltrate the anterior vaginal wall. An A incision is made with its apex just proximal to the urethral meatus. The two arms of the A are extended several centimeters distal to the bladder neck (Fig. 75–35).

Lateral dissection is performed as previously described along the shiny white periurethral fascia to the pubic bone. Blunt and sharp dissection is then carried out along the undersurface of the pubic bone until the urethropelvic ligament is reached. This is then detached from its lateral attachment to the pelvic sidewall at the tendinous arc, with curved Mayo scissors. The urethra is freed of any restraining fascial bands. A transverse incision at the level of the bladder neck joins the two longitudinal arms of the A incision. Dissection is carried from this point cephalad, thus creating a flap cephalad to an island of tissue in the anterior vaginal wall at the level of the proximal urethra (Fig. 75–36).

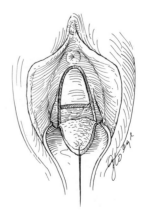

Figure 75–36. An island of vaginal wall is created over the urethra, and an advancement flap of vaginal wall is created over the bladder base.

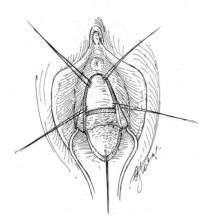

Figure 75–37. The four suspension sutures, two in the distal edges of the sling and two in the proximal edges of the sling.

The four corners of the island are anchored with four individual Prolene sutures—grasping vaginal wall, pubocervical fascia, urethropelvic ligament plus periurethral fascia at the level of the bladder neck, and vaginal wall plus periurethral fascia at the level of the proximal urethra (Fig. 75–37). The four Prolene sutures are transferred through a suprapubic incision via the double-pronged ligature carrier as described in the two previous procedures. Indigo carmine is given intravenously. Cystoscopy is performed to confirm ureteral efflux and to ensure that the urethra and bladder neck are compressed and suspended effectively, when minimal tension is placed on the suspending sutures.

The proximal vaginal wall flap is advanced to cover the island of vaginal wall (Fig. 75–38). A 2–0 Vicryl suture puts the flap in place, thus obliterating any anterior vaginal wall defect. Suspending sutures are tied snugly, onto the underlying rectus sheath without tension through the suprapubic wound: first individually, then with the sutures on the same side, and finally, across the midline. The suprapubic wound is irrigated and approximated with 4–0 Vicryl. A pack impregnated with antibiotic cream is inserted into the vagina. The two catheters (suprapubic and urethral) are connected to closed-bag drainage.

Our success rate with this procedure is 93 per cent, at a mean follow-up of 2 years. In the absence of neurogenic dysfunction and augmentation cystoplasty,

only 5.5 per cent of patients needed intermittent catheterizations on a long-term basis. Further, the simplicity and the reliance on vaginal tissue only make this procedure our preferred approach.

PUBOVAGINAL SLING PROCEDURE

Technique. With the patient in a modified lithotomy position, a transverse Pfannenstiel incision is made two fingerbreadths above the symphysis pubis. Blunt dissection is carried down to the rectus fascia, which is incised and lifted off the underlying musculature. The rectus muscles are split, and the retropubic space is developed by pushing the bladder and urethra posteriorly off the back of the pubic symphysis. A midline vertical incision is made in the anterior vaginal wall from the bladder neck to the proximal urethra. Dissection is carried out laterally, toward the retropubic space. A tunnel is created by advancing an instrument from the suprapubic wound to the vaginal incision. Inadvertent bladder penetration is avoided by directing the advancing instrument parallel to the pubic bone, hugging its inner surface. A palpating finger in the vaginal wound allows greater control of this step of the procedure.

A sling measuring 12 cm by 1 cm is cut as a single strip from the lower leaf of the rectus fascial incision. The sling is applied as a free graft and passed through the tunnel to the vaginal operator and then back from the vaginal operator to the retropubic operator on the other side of the urethra. The sling is then passed through the belly of the rectus muscle on both sides, through the rectus fascia, to which it is sutured in place with monofilament nonabsorbable material.

For convenience, the vaginal incision should be closed prior to suturing the sling in place on the rectus fascia. Firm but not tight sling tension is desirable.

A urethral catheter is left in place for 5 to 7 days and then removed. The patient is cautioned not to attempt voiding by straining but to try to relax as much as possible and to void by detrusor contraction. Intermittent catheterization is performed at regular 4-hour intervals and whenever the patient feels urgency or fullness but is unable to void even if 4 hours have not elapsed. Every patient should be instructed in intermittent self-catheterization at this point, so that inability to empty the bladder completely need not delay discharge from the hospital. The reported success rate with this procedure is 90 to 95 per cent.

Artificial Urinary Sphincter

The artificial urinary sphincter (AMS-800) in the treatment of SUI in the female is limited to only a few medical centers in the United States. Our indications are similar to those for sling procedures. However, the artificial sphincter is selected only when the sling procedure failed to correct the problem. The technique of insertion of artificial urinary sphincter is discussed elsewhere in this text.

POSTOPERATIVE CARE. In addition to standard postoperative care, it is important to develop a routine postoperative regimen for patients who are undergoing vaginal surgery for stress incontinence, including management of diet, catheters, vaginal packing, activity, and follow-up.

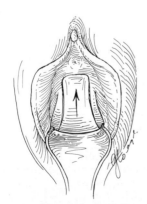

Figure 75–38. The vaginal flap is advanced to cover the island of vaginal wall sling.

The patient is permitted to take food and medication orally as soon as they are tolerated. Antibiotics are continued intravenously for one or two doses and then changed to oral agents for prophylaxis during the period of indwelling catheters. In uncomplicated surgery for incontinence, the Foley catheter and vaginal packing are removed on the 1st postoperative day. The suprapubic catheter is left in place for measurement and emptying of post-void residuals. The patient is discharged from the hospital on the 2nd or 3rd postoperative day and is seen for the first postoperative visit in the clinic in 10 days to 2 weeks. If, at this time, the measured post-void residual is less than 2 ounces, the suprapubic catheter is removed and antibiotics are stopped. If, however, the post-void residual at the first postoperative visit is greater than 2 ounces, the patient is instructed in intermittent self-catheterization. The suprapubic catheter is removed once the patient shows proficiency.

Activity after surgery is advanced steadily from walking and climbing stairs within the 1st week, returning to work and driving at 3 weeks, and sexual activity as well as exercise at 6 weeks. Further follow-up consists of an office visit with physical examination at 1 month, 3 months, 6 months, and thereafter on a yearly basis.

Complications of Vaginal Surgery

Meaningful preoperative diagnostic methods and timely recognition of complications and their management can prevent the untoward late sequelae or serious consequences (Schmidbauer et al., 1986). Satisfactory results are much more likely to be obtained if complications are dealt with at the time of occurrence. Potential complications of vaginal surgery follow.

BLEEDING. A careful history and an adequate preoperative screening should uncover all but the rarest bleeding diathesis. Intraoperative bleeding most commonly occurs in the retropubic space and is best controlled with packing of the retropubic space. An alternative is intravaginal inflation of the balloon of a Foley catheter with 50 to 60 ml of water or more. Hypovolemic shock in the absence of obvious source of blood loss may indicate an extraperitoneal or a retroperitoneal blood loss. Re-exploration may be indicated under these circumstances.

INFECTION. The vagina is a potentially contaminated space, and every effort should be made preoperatively to cleanse the vagina (douche with antibacterial soaps). Perioperative antibiotic therapy (gram-positive, gram-negative, and anerobic coverage) is an important step in the prevention of infection. Urinary tract infections remain the most common type of infections in vaginal surgery. Pelvic infection and pelvic abscess are rare. They should be treated with broad-spectrum antibiotics and surgical drainage (vaginal or abdominal), when necessary.

INJURIES AND FISTULA. Urethral and bladder injuries should be repaired primarily, if recognized intraoperatively. However, delayed recognition of these injuries warrants an attempt at conservative treatment, with catheter drainage initially. If this approach is un-

successful, operative repair is indicated. Ureteric injuries may be due to partial or complete tears or ligature around the ureter. Ligature should be removed. Partial tear is best treated with internal drainage utilizing an indwelling stent or percutaneous method. If this attempt is unsuccessful or if complete tears are encountered, operative exploration and primary repair may be indicated.

Bowel injuries are very rare. The potential for injury with rectocele repair can be avoided by meticulous dissection and by a rectal pack, which aids in the identification of the rectal wall during the dissection. Preoperative stool softeners and liquid diet allow primary closure of a minor perforation; however, in the unlikely event of a major tear, primary closure with proximal colostomy may be indicated.

INCONTINENCE. The occurrence of stress urinary incontinence after vaginal surgery should be evaluated and treated along the same guidelines as previously discussed.

URINARY RETENTION. This may occur particularly with procedures that involve the bladder and urethra; however, retention may follow any vaginal surgery. This problem may be due to transient postoperative edema of the bladder neck and urethra, which will resolve with catheter drainage. Occasionally, urinary retention may be due to denervation or true obstruction by a misplaced suture. We usually leave the suprapubic catheter in place for 1 to 2 weeks and then teach the patient intermittent self-catheterization. If retention persists beyond 3 months, repeat urodynamics are indicated.

PAIN. Low-grade infection and suture granuloma may be the sources of chronic persistent pain. Nerve entrapment and vaginal stenosis are other potential sources of pain.

VAGINAL STENOSIS. This is a serious complication and an important cause of dyspareunia in sexually active women. It is best prevented by avoiding excessive excision of the vaginal wall. In the presence of vaginal ridge, a relaxing incision will correct the problem. Alternative options for correction of stenosis include a longitudinal relaxing incision with horizontal closure and free skin graft.

VAGINAL SHORTENING. This is a potential complication when excessive vaginal tissue is excised at the dome and obviously is best avoided. Vaginal enlargement with bowel segment may be indicated if the shortening is severe.

POSTERIOR VAGINAL WALL PROLAPSE—RECTOCELE AND PERINEAL REPAIR

Pathophysiology

Stretching, weakening, and tearing of the fascia and muscles of the female pelvic floor are often caused by the trauma from the descent of the baby's head through the pelvic diaphragm. Prolonged pressure of the head between the muscles of the pelvic floor weakens the

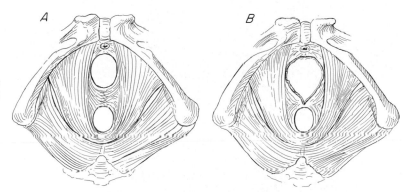

Figure 75–39. Pelvis from above with *A*, normal levator hiatus and fascial attachments and *B*, widened levator hiatus and attenuated fascial attachments.

rectovaginal and vesicovaginal fasciae. The loss of estrogen (due to age), strenuous work, straining at stool, and multiparity, and the pressure of viscera against the pelvic floor are other elements that may produce weakening of the musculofascial supports. This leads to the formation of rectocele and enterocele (see discussion of vaginal anatomy at beginning of the chapter).

Below the level of the cul-de-sac of Douglas, the vagina and rectum are separated by the rectovaginal fascia, an attenuated layer of endopelvic fascia (Kuhn et al., 1982). Weakening of the levator muscle attachment occurs in this area, allowing descent of the rectum through the widened levator hiatus, thus making the posterior vagina prone to rectocele formation (Mattingly et al., 1985). When one looks at the pelvis from above, widening of the levator hiatus and attenuation of the fascial attachments are seen (Fig. 75–39).

Basically, a rectocele is a hernia that develops when the prerectal and pararectal fasciae (pillars of the rectum) are insufficient to support the anterior rectal wall and the rectum prolapses through the levator sling. The posterior vaginal wall lacks sufficient strength to prevent prolapse of the anterior rectal wall into the vaginal vault (Nichols et al., 1970). Correction of the prolapse with restoration of the normal vaginal axis not only restores normal sexual function but also provides for better transmission of intra-abdominal pressure. This prevents the complication of enterocele and rectocele formation after bladder neck suspension.

The perineum is formed by the coalescence of the levator ani muscles with the bulbocavernosus and superficial transverse perineal muscles, forming the perineal body. If an episiotomy or a perineal laceration is not repaired properly, the posterior part of the urogenital diaphragm remains separated.

Diagnosis

The diagnosis of a rectocele is made when the patient complains of a bulging mass through the vagina, mostly with straining. The rectocele may produce no symptoms or may produce the symptoms of a bulging vaginal mass, which is causing discomfort. Occasionally, the patient may have constipation or difficult bowel movements and needs to manually compress the prolapsed rectal wall to obtain proper evacuation of the rectum.

On pelvic examination, the rectocele appears as a bulge in the posterior vaginal wall. Occasionally, a coexistent enterocele appears as a bulge higher in the posterior vaginal wall or at the vaginal apex. The preoperative appreciation of both of these types of herniation is essential so that proper surgical correction is performed.

On rectal examination, the anterior rectal wall is palpated. The extent of the rectal herniation into the posterior vagina is readily demonstrated. When a large symptomatic rectocele is present, laxity and attenuation of the perineum are usually associated, which result in a large, gaping introitus.

Repair of the perineal laxity is described in conjunction with the technique of rectocele repair, because these procedures are usually performed concomitantly (Jeffcoate, 1959; Ward, 1929). The decision to correct a rectocele must be made prior to surgery, because all structures may appear relaxed during anesthesia, making the rectocele difficult to appreciate.

Surgical Treatment

Because perineal body laxity, caused by attenuation of the perineal muscles, usually accompanies a rectocele, reconstruction of the posterior fourchette is also carried out simultaneously. Posterior repair is performed in conjunction with perineorrhaphy to correct a rectocele and to reconstruct a lax vaginal outlet (Moschcowitz, 1912). Some 48 hours prior to surgery, the patient begins a clear liquid diet combined with laxatives. On admission to the hospital, tap water enemas and intravenous antibiotics are administered.

TECHNIQUE. The patient is placed in the dorsal lithotomy position. The lower abdomen and vagina are prepared and draped in a sterile fashion. The rectum is packed with a povidone-iodine (betadine)–impregnated lubricated gauze and then isolated from the operative field with double draping. The labia are retracted laterally with stay sutures. A urethral Foley catheter is inserted, and the bladder is drained.

The introitus is inspected. If significant perineal and introital weakness is present, as is usually the case, two Allis clamps are applied to the mucocutaneous junction at the 5- and 7-o'clock positions of the posterior introitus. These clamps are placed so that when they are

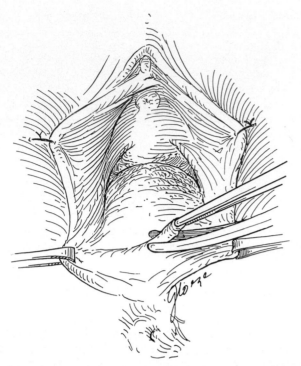

Figure 75–40. Excision of skin triangle of the vaginal perineal margin.

brought together in the midline, the introitus readily admits two large fingers. The mucocutaneous junction is then excised in a triangular fashion between these two clamps, utilizing curved Mayo scissors (Fig. 75–40). A Scott retractor is positioned and affixed with skin hooks.

Two Allis clamps are applied in a longitudinal fashion to the posterior vaginal wall, overlying the rectocele. The vaginal wall is infiltrated with normal saline to facilitate the dissection of tissue planes. A triangular incision is made in the posterior vaginal wall with the apex of the triangle at the apex of the rectocele and the base of the triangle along the previously made perineal incision (Fig. 75–41).

A plane is developed between the herniated rectal wall (attenuated prerectal fascia) and the vaginal epithelium with careful sharp dissection, employing Metzenbaum scissors on the vaginal wall itself. The dissection must stay as close to the vaginal epithelium as possible

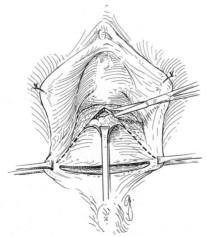

Figure 75–41. Triangular incision in posterior vaginal wall. A plane is developed between the vaginal wall and the prerectal fascia.

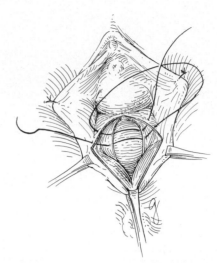

Figure 75–42. Repair of rectocele by reapproximation of vaginal epithelium and prerectal and pararectal fasciae in midline.

to avoid any injury to the rectal wall. Sharp dissection is continued laterally to expose the prerectal and pararectal fascia laterally. Palpation of the previously placed gauze in the rectum during the dissection facilitates identification of the rectum and helps to avoid injury. The isolated triangle of vaginal epithelium is excised.

Obliteration of the rectocele defect in the posterior vaginal wall is carried out after careful protection of the rectum is assured. This is achieved by means of retracting the bulging rectal wall downward with a narrow Deaver or Heaney retractor. The rectocele repair is done in a single layer with running, locking 2–0 Vicryl sutures, starting at the apex of the rectocele. The sutures incorporate the edge of the vaginal epithelium and a generous bite of the prerectal and pararectal fasciae, which is approximated in the midline over the rectocele (Fig. 75–42). At the mid to distal third of the vaginal canal, the levator muscles (pubococcygeus) are included in the suture line (Fig. 75–43A). The closure is carried down to the transverse perineal incision (Fig. 75–44).

The approximation of the fascia creates a strong support for the posterior vaginal wall and prevents bulging of the rectum into the vagina. The approximation of the levators restores the pelvic floor and the posterior angle of the vagina. The perineal laxity is corrected by placing two or three 2–0 Vicryl sutures in a horizontal mattress fashion to reapproximate in the midline the weakened and separated superficial and deep transverse perineal muscles, bulbocavernosus muscle and levator complex, thus recreating the perineal floor and central tendon (Fig. 75–43B). The defect in the perineal skin is closed with a running 4–0 Vicryl suture (Fig. 75–45).

A vaginal packing coated with an antibiotic cream and a periped are placed. The Foley catheter is connected to a closed-bag drainage.

Postoperative Care

The Foley catheter and vaginal packing are removed the morning following surgery. Intravenous antibiotics are administered for 24 hours, followed by oral anti-

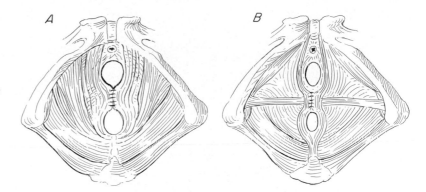

Figure 75–43. *A,* Levator muscles are included in suture line. *B,* Central tendon is reconstructed.

biotics for several days. Stool softeners are prescribed as needed.

Rectal injury is the major complication that can accompany rectocele repair and is prevented by careful development of the plane between the vaginal wall and the rectum. Proper preoperative preparation of the rectum allows primary closure of an injury in multiple layers. Pain and vaginal stenosis or shortening may also be complications of rectocele or enterocele repair.

ENTEROCELE

Pathophysiology

The upper posterior portion of the vagina is adjacent to the cul-de-sac of Douglas. If the peritoneal sac herniates into the rectovaginal space, an enterocele is formed with small bowel protruding into the vagina (Fig. 75–46). An enterocele is defined as a true hernia, at the vaginal dome area, of the peritoneum and its content (small bowel in general), through a defect created by the wide separation of the uterosacral and cardinal ligaments. Widening of the levator hiatus contributes to deepening of the cul-de-sac of Douglas, causing the size of the peritoneal sac to increase (Moschcowitz, 1912).

Enterocele formation may be facilitated by the same factors that lead to rectocele formation. Weakening of the musculofascial supports is caused by the trauma of childbirth, strenuous work, straining at stool, loss of estrogen with age, and pressure of the viscera on the pelvic floor.

Bladder neck suspension (abdominal or vaginal) without repair of the pelvic floor defect may lead to the formation of an enterocele in 5 to 17 per cent of cases (Stanton, 1976; Symmonds et al., 1981). The transfer of the anterior vaginal wall to a high supported position will make the vaginal dome and posterior vaginal wall the most dependent structures in the pelvis, facilitating the formation of an enterocele.

Although a congenital enterocele may be present in the female without a previous history of vaginal surgery, most enteroceles are acquired as a result of the defect created at the vaginal apex between the widely separated uterosacral ligaments after hysterectomy (pulsion enterocele) (Zacharin, 1980; Zacharin et al., 1980). This tissue weakness may also result from ischemia at the distal ends of the excised ligaments, which are tied en masse at hysterectomy (Mattingly et al., 1985).

Many patients have had previous rectocele repairs. Severe uterine and vaginal vault prolapse may facilitate herniation of the peritoneal contents, especially with elevations in intra-abdominal pressure. The uterine de-

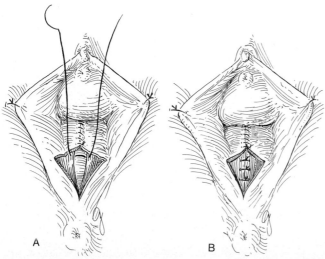

Figure 75–44. *A* and *B,* Repair carried to transverse perineal incision.

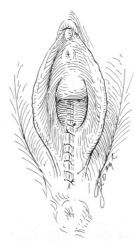

Figure 75–45. Completed repair (see Figs. 75–42 to 75–44).

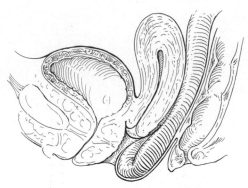

Figure 75–46. Small bowel protruding through widened levator hiatus into vagina.

scent draws the cul-de-sac through the levator hiatus, into the vaginal vault (Birnbaum, 1973; Cruikshank, 1987 and 1988; Hawksworth et al., 1959; McCall, 1957). In general, this "traction" enterocele is posterior to the uterus (rectouterine space). Rarely, it can be present anteriorly in the vesicouterine space.

Surgery is performed in conjunction with repair of rectocele, cystocele, or sacrospinalis fixation and when the prolapse of the enterocele sac creates social or physical discomfort, changes in bowel movement, or inability to reduce the mass. In spite of its size, an enterocele rarely can lead to bowel incarceration.

Diagnosis

The patient may complain of changes in bowel habits or of a bulging mass from the introitus, which disappears when supine. On physical examination, the enterocele appears as a bulge high in the vagina, either posterior to the cervix (if it is present) or at the apex of the vaginal vault after hysterectomy, which is most common.

Because an enterocele is frequently associated with a rectocele, the enterocele bulge may appear as a high continuation of the bulge in the posterior vaginal wall. Inspection will reveal a division between the enterocele and rectocele as a transverse furrow just above the rectocele. The enterocele sac may contain bowel visible through the attenuated vaginal wall.

When performing a bimanual rectal-vaginal examination, the impulse of the enterocele hernia sac may be felt against the fingertip during coughing (analogous to the impulse felt during examination for an inguinal hernia). An increased thickness of the rectal-vaginal septum occurs high in the vagina at the level of the enterocele. Bimanual examination demonstrates the rectocele as distinct from the bulge higher in the vaginal vault. In doubtful cases, the physical examination is done in the sitting or standing position. A cystogram will rule out that the bladder is not part of the bulging mass.

Surgical Treatment

In general, enterocele repair is performed as part of a comprehensive vaginal or abdominal repair of pelvic floor relaxation (e.g., cystocele, rectocele, and so forth).

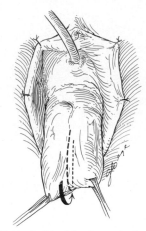

Figure 75–47. Vertical incision in vaginal wall over bowel.

At the time of abdominal repair of bladder prolapse, the peritoneum may be opened and the cul-de-sac herniation repaired (Beecham et al., 1973). If no other reason for a laparotomy is required, we prefer the vaginal approach.

Vaginal Repair of Enterocele

Technique. After general or spinal anesthesia is induced, the patient is placed in the dorsal lithotomy position. The lower abdomen and vagina are prepared and draped in a sterile fashion. The rectum is packed with a povidone-iodine (Betadine)–impregnated lubricated gauze and isolated from the surgical field. A weighted posterior retractor is placed in the vagina, and the labia are retracted laterally with stay sutures. A Scott retractor is positioned and secured with hooks. A Foley catheter is inserted to empty the bladder.

The enterocele bulge is grasped with two Allis clamps, and normal saline is injected to facilitate dissection. A vertical incision is made in the vaginal wall over the bulge (Fig. 75–47).

After the vaginal wall is incised and dissected laterally, the peritoneal hernia sac is defined and separated from the vaginal wall, bladder, and rectum with blunt and sharp dissection. The sac is opened and its contents reduced to facilitate definition of the peritoneal sac and neck of the sac (Fig. 75–48). A small, moist laparotomy pad is inserted into the peritoneal cavity to protect the bowel during obliteration of the enterocele.

Two pursestring sutures of No. 1 Vicryl are placed, incorporating prerectal fascia posteriorly, the sacrouter-

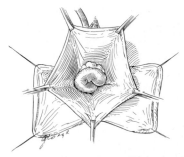

Figure 75–48. Vaginal wall is dissected laterally, and peritoneal sac is identified and opened.

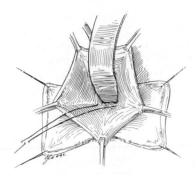

Figure 75–49. Pursestring suture is placed, and bowel and trigone are protected by retractor.

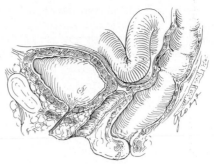

Figure 75–51. Completed repair (see Figs. 75–47 to 75–50).

ine and cardinal ligaments laterally, and the pubocervical fascia over the bladder wall anteriorly. The edge of the vaginal wall is incorporated in each side of the pursestring sutures. With proper retraction of the trigone, care is taken to avoid injury to the ureters (Fig. 75–49). Each pursestring suture is separately tightened, and the two sutures are then tied (Fig. 75–50). The enterocele sac is excised, and the cardinal and pubocervical fasciae reapproximated with interrupted sutures.

The redundant vaginal epithelium is trimmed. If a rectocele is present it should be repaired simultaneously. The vaginal wall is closed with a running 2–0 Vicryl suture, incorporating the area of underlying repair in order to eliminate any dead space (Fig. 75–51). A vaginal packing is placed for 24 hours.

Potential immediate complications include bleeding, ureteral injury, bladder or rectal perforation, and damage to the small bowel. Excessive bleeding may occur but is very rare. Urinary tract bleeding during surgery requires cystoscopy to rule out bladder injury. Ureteric injury may occur. In selected cases, indigo carmine should be given prior to cystoscopy to assure patency of the ureters. Surgery for enterocele must be done after proper bowel preparation, so that in a case of rectal injury, primary repair may be performed, using multiple layers.

Postoperative Care

The Foley catheter and vaginal packing are removed the morning following surgery. Intravenous antibiotics are administered for 24 hours, followed by oral antibiotics for several days. Otherwise, the instructions are identical to those for any vaginal surgery.

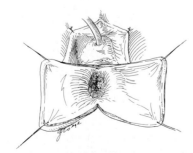

Figure 75–50. Pursestring sutures are tied.

Late complications include vaginal shortening and recurrent enterocele. If the patient is sexually active and severe vaginal vault prolapse is present, we prefer to perform sacrospinalis fixation with minimal excision of the vaginal wall. In older sexually inactive patients, partial colpocleisis can be performed. Recurrent enterocele is very rare.

Abdominal Repair of Enterocele

Abdominal repair of an enterocele may be performed when other intra-abdominal procedures are required.

TECHNIQUE. The patient is placed in the supine position, and laparotomy is performed. If the uterus is present, it is grasped and pulled forward. If the uterus is absent, the posterior wall of the vagina is grasped with Allis clamps and held anteriorly under traction. Starting at the base of the sac, pursestring sutures of 2–0 Vicryl are placed to close the cul-de-sac of Douglas. Included in the suture are the serosal surface of the rectum and the lateral sidewalls and serosal surface of the vagina. When the uterosacral ligaments are reached, they are included in the sutures. Special care is taken to avoid ureteral injury. The sutures are successively tied, without excessive tension.

UTERINE PROLAPSE

Pathophysiology

Uterine prolapse is caused by stretching of the ligamentous support system of the uterus. This may result from childbearing, lack of estrogen with aging, strenuous physical activity, and pressure of the viscera. The uterus is primarily supported by the cardinal and uterosacral ligaments. These are reflections of the endopelvic fascia. The cardinal ligaments are a component of the pubocervical fascia, which surrounds the cervix and base of the bladder and extends to the pelvic sidewall. These ligaments provide the major support to the uterus above the pelvic diaphragm. The posterior reflection of the endopelvic fascia forms the uterosacral ligaments. They form the lateral border of the cul-de-sac of Douglas and pass laterally to the rectum to insert on the fourth sacral vertebra.

These ligaments pull the cervix backward and maintain the uterus in an antiflexed position. The round ligament arises from the anterior surface of the uterus, runs beneath the anterior leaf of the broad ligament, and enters the internal inguinal ring to insert into the labia majora.

Uterine prolapse is one of the many anatomic abnormalities seen with pelvic floor relaxation (Richardson et al., 1989). It may be seen as an isolated defect but more often is seen with simultaneous cystocele, urethral hypermobility, and rectocele.

Diagnosis

The degree of uterine hypermobility can be classified in a manner similar to cystocele. Grade I is minimal mobility, grade II is moderate hypermobility (descends with strain to the mid-vagina), grade III is descencus to the introitus, and grade IV is prolapse outside the introitus at all times (procidentia).

The patient may have a history of vaginal mass. Uterine prolapse may be associated with pelvic discomfort or dyspareunia and may contribute to displacement of the bladder neck and base, aggravating anatomic stress incontinence.

Many surgical alternatives to hysterectomy are well described in the gynecologic literature, and we refer the reader to the proper sources (Copenhaver, 1962 and 1980; Heaney, 1940 and 1942; TeLinde, et al., 1943; Mattingly et al., 1985). Hysterectomy is indicated for medical reasons (e.g., bleeding, fibroids, and so forth) or because of significant prolapse (Bonnar et al., 1970; Porges, 1980).

The vaginal approach is the procedure of choice for significant uterine prolapse, allowing simultaneous correction of other vaginal abnormalities, such as cystocele and rectocele (Pitkin, 1976 and 1977). At the time of surgical correction of cystocele or stress incontinence, the presence of significant uterine prolapse requires a simultaneous hysterectomy. But, if at the time of surgical correction of cystocele or incontinence, minimal or no uterine prolapse is found, hysterectomy is not indicated. The uterus has no impact on the outcome of stress incontinence surgery and should not be routinely removed.

Vaginal Hysterectomy

We modify our surgical technique for hysterectomy, depending on the degree of bladder prolapse. When significant uterine prolapse is present with minimal cystocele (I), we perform the vaginal hysterectomy, close the vaginal cuff, and follow with a simple bladder neck suspension (see previous description). For severe uterine prolapse and moderate cystocele (II to III), we perform the hysterectomy, close the vaginal cuff, and perform a four-corner bladder and bladder neck suspension (see previous description). For patients with grade IV cystocele and uterine prolapse, we perform a vertical incision in the anterior vaginal wall, dissect laterally over

the pubocervical fascia to free the bladder from the cervix, and proceed with hysterectomy. This maneuver allows elevation of the bladder base, facilitating hysterectomy and closure of the cul de sac.

Technique. A posterior weighted vaginal speculum with a glove at the end and a ring retractor with multiple hooks are inserted. The cervix is grasped with two single-toothed tenacula, and the mobility of the uterus is once more assessed.

The cervix is circumscribed. Blunt and sharp dissection is carried out in the plane between the anterior vaginal wall and the uterine corpus beneath. Special care is taken to remain immediately adjacent to the body of the uterus to avoid injury to the bladder. A retractor is placed under the anterior vagina wall to separate the bladder and urethra from the area of dissection. This maneuver also elevates the trigone and distal ureters. Dissection continues in an anterior direction until the vesicouterine fold of peritoneum (anterior cul-de-sac) is reached. Care is taken to avoid dissection laterally, which would result in injury of the uterine vessels. Similar dissection is now carried out posteriorly, separating the posterior vaginal wall with underlying rectum from uterine cervix and body. After the rectum has been dissected away from the posterior cervical wall, the posterior peritoneal fold (cul-de-sac of Douglas) becomes visible (Fig. 75–52). The thin, semilunar folds of peritoneum can now be visualized, attaching to the uterine fundus. These folds are held with forceps, incised with scissors, and opened. The cut edge opposite the uterus is marked with a suture to aid in later identification and closure. A Deaver or Heaney retractor is inserted posteriorly.

Next, the lateral vaginal wall is carefully dissected away from the cardinal and sacrouterine ligaments (Fig. 75–53). These lateral attachments are placed on stretch by means of traction on the cervical tenacula, and they are individually clamped, divided, and ligated with the suture ends left long. The uterine artery and vein are identified and ligated individually (Fig. 75–54). Further parametrial ligation and division are carried out on either side to the level of the peritoneal folds.

The cervix is pulled anteriorly, and the fundus presents itself posteriorly (Fig. 75–55). The fundus is grasped with a tenaculum and partially pulled outside

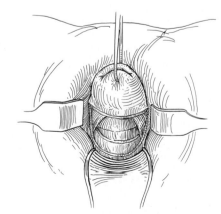

Figure 75–52. Cervix is circumscribed, and a plane between anterior vaginal wall and uterine body is developed.

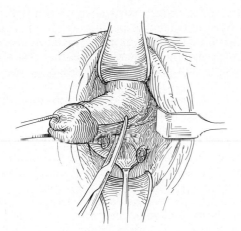

Figure 75–53. Sacrouterine and cardinal ligaments are divided.

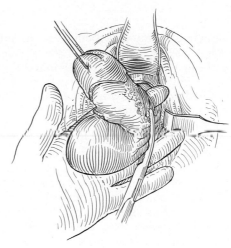

Figure 75–55. Cervix is drawn anteriorly, and fundus presents itself posteriorly; broad ligament is divided.

the introitus. If the adnexa are to remain, their attachments must now be ligated and divided at the uterine insertions. The side chosen to divide first is best exposed by traction on the uterus in the opposite direction. The utero-ovarian ligament, the fallopian tube, and the round ligament are visible in succession from anterior to posterior and can be clamped, divided, and ligated with 0 Vicryl suture in one pedicle.

All remaining fascial attachments to the uterus are divided and it is removed. The peritoneal opening is closed using the previously placed tagging sutures to identify the peritoneal edges. The remaining parametrium together with the tagged ends of the cardinal and sacrouterine ligaments is reapproximated. Inclusion of these ligamentous ends is extremely important in averting later enterocele formation as well as in the plastic reconstruction of the pelvic supports (Symmonds et al., 1960).

The vaginal mucosa is closed with running 2–0 Vicryl suture. A vaginal packing coated with antibiotic cream is inserted. If simultaneous vaginal surgery is planned, such as transvaginal needle bladder neck suspension, it is performed now.

Postoperative Care

Intravenous antibiotics are administered for 24 hours, followed by a course of oral antibiotics. The vaginal packing and urethral catheter are removed the morning following surgery. Patients are discharged from the hospital on the 2nd postoperative day.

URETHRAL DIVERTICULUM

The occurrence of female urethral diverticulum was first described by Hey in 1805. This was a rarely recognized entity until the 1930s. A handful of cases were reported in the literature before 1935. Prior to 1950, just over 100 cases total had been noted in the historical records of three major medical centers: Johns Hopkins, Mayo Clinic, and Cleveland Clinic (Moore, 1952). Since 1950, with the advent of positive pressure urethrography, the general awareness and recognition of this disorder has heightened. In 1958, Davis and Telinde reported as many cases as had been recognized in the previous 60 years.

Incidence

The incidence of female urethral diverticulum is estimated to be between 1 and 6 per cent of all adult females. It generally occurs between the ages of 20 and 60, with the average age being approximately 40 years. A definite racial predilection is noted, with blacks to whites in a ratio of 3.5 to 6:1 (Benjamin et al., 1974).

This condition probably occurs more frequently than it is diagnosed. In 1964, Adams obtained positive pressure urethrograms on 129 consecutive female patients without active urinary tract symptoms and found the incidence of diverticula to be 4.7 per cent (Adams, 1964). Anderson noted an incidence of 3 per cent in a group of 300 women undergoing treatment for cervical carcinoma (Andersen, 1967).

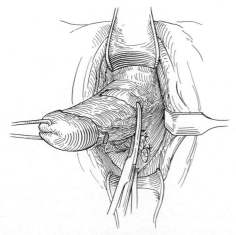

Figure 75–54. Uterine artery and vein are ligated.

Etiology

Even though urethral diverticula are found in the usual location of the periurethral glands, cause and pathogenesis have been vigorously debated throughout this century. The theories of the origin of urethral diverticula chiefly relate to whether they are congenital or acquired, and, if acquired, whether they are secondary to infection or parturition or are iatrogenic.

The arguments for a congenital origin have been weakened by the fact that urethral diverticula are rarely found in children (Davis et al., 1970 and 1958). In the study of 121 female patients with urethral diverticula by Davis and Telinde, no diagnoses were made prior to the age of 20 years. Only 6.5 per cent of these patients dated the onset of symptoms prior to the age of 20 years. Some reported cases, however, point to a congenital origin in certain instances. A urethral diverticulum has been reported at the site where an ectopic ureter emptied into the urethra (Moore, 1952). Urethral diverticula have been located in areas containing remnants of Gartner's ducts (Hinman et al., 1960). These have been noticed when finding Gartner's duct carcinomas within the diverticula.

Several patients have also been treated for diverticula containing cloacogenic rests (Benjamin et al., 1974). In a case cited by Silk and Lebowitz (1969), an anterior diverticulum was postulated to represent an aborted attempt at urethral duplication.

Various theories to explain the development of female urethral diverticulum have been advanced. Although female urethral diverticulum has been described in young infants, presumably occurring as a congenital diverticulum, the majority certainly appear to be acquired.

Earlier in this century, the origin was usually attributed to the trauma of childbirth (McNally, 1935). It was postulated that pressure from the fetal head or delivery forceps would rupture the intrinsic musculature of the urethra, with consequent herniation of the mucosa and diverticular formation. However, studies since then have shown that urethral diverticula are just as likely to arise in nulliparous patients, and this earlier hypothesis has generally been rejected. More readily accepted now is the explanation offered by Routh, who in 1890 postulated that repeated infection and obstruction of the periurethral glands resulted in the formation of suburethral cysts. These cysts would eventually rupture and drain back into the urethral lumen. The continued irritation of pooled urine retained during each voiding in these abscess cavities would then lead to eventual epithelialization and formation of a permanent diverticulum. The acceptance of this explanation now causes most investigators to consider urethral diverticula as representing acquired lesions of infectious etiology.

Two of the most probable causes are gonococcal infection and infection of the periurethral glands from normal vaginal flora (TeLinde, 1953). The most commonly cultured organisms are *Escherichia coli* and other gram-negative bacilli as well as *Staphylococcus aureus* and *Streptococcus fecalis*. In a study by Peters and Vaughan (1976) of 32 patients, they either had proven gonorrhea or a history suggestive of gonorrhea. Other studies have not been so persuasive, and it is generally concluded now that any urethral infection involving the periurethral glands can lead to eventual diverticula formation, although gonorrhea may often be the etiologic factor.

Many other possible etiologies for urethral diverticula have been suggested, including the trauma from childbirth, high intravesical pressures on voiding against a closed or spastic external sphincter in neurogenic cases, instrumentation, urethral calculus, urethral stricture, and any urethral or anterior vaginal surgery complicated by inadequate wound closure or infection.

Congenital factors, including Gartner's duct, faulty union of the primal folds, cell nests, and wolffian ducts or vaginal cysts that rupture into the urethra, may be involved.

Huffman (1948) constructed wax models of infected urethra and found periurethral openings. His experiments support the concept of suburethral infection developing into an abscess that becomes lined with epithelium. The periurethral glands become infected and obstructed and rupture into the urethra to form a communication site between the diverticulum and the urethra itself. Microscopic studies have shown that periurethral glands can be found along much of the length of the urethra (Huffman, 1948). These glands are located primarily posterolaterally, and the majority open into the distal third of the urethra. They constitute a complex system of tubuloalveolar structures that can number more than 30. Skene's glands, the largest of these periurethral glands, empty at the external meatus and are often considered separately.

Diverticula develop beneath the well-defined periurethral fascia. The periurethral glands are tubuloalveolar structures that predominate throughout the distal two thirds of the urethra and mainly open into the distal one third of the urethra. Up to 90 per cent of diverticula open into the mid or distal urethra (Lang and Davis, 1959). Their morphology ranges from simple saccular structures to complex branching sinus tracts. When these glands become infected with the associated obstruction of drainage of the gland into the urethra, a urethral diverticulum that is located in the distal two thirds of the urethra may result. Occasionally, the female urethral diverticulum may be extremely proximal and extend beneath the bladder neck and trigonal area, as well as anteriorly in location (Dretler et al., 1972; Silk and Lebowitz, 1969).

Clinical Presentation

The female patient with urethral diverticulum will sometimes present with a tender, cystic suburethral swelling from which retained urine or purulent material can be milked through the meatus by digital pressure. Patients often more typically present with a myriad of symptoms associated with most common lower urinary tract disorders (Davis and TeLinde, 1958 and 1970; Leach and Bavendam, 1987; Peters and Vaughan, 1976). The patient frequently notes signs of lower urinary tract irritation. Dysuria, frequency, urgency, and hematuria occur in the majority of cases. The complaint most characteristic of urethral diverticulum, however, appears to be postmicturition dribbling. Dribbling accompanied by dyspareunia and dysuria seems to constitute a classic triad for urethral diverticula. A history of recurrent urinary tract infections refractory to antibiotic therapy may be a clue. Other symptoms include dyspareunia, swelling in the vagina, and urethral discharge and pain with ambulation. Pyuria and cystitis may also occur, depending on the location of the diverticular orifice.

The rare finding of urinary retention usually is on the basis of large proximal diverticula that impinge on and obstruct the bladder neck or is subsequent to stricture formation secondary to repeated infections. The finding of hematuria is also usually secondary to active infection; however, Palagiri (1978) reported a diverticular case in which the sac, after excision, was found to contain endometrial stroma and blood clots.

None of the symptoms routinely appear to be proportional to the size of the diverticulum. A large diverticulum may often go unnoticed to the patient, whereas a small sac, when actively infected, may be extremely symptomatic. The chronicity of the complaint is not a uniform finding. Prolonged periods of spontaneous remission are not uncommon.

Over 30 cases of carcinomas have been reported within female urethral diverticula. The patient may be totally asymptomatic, and the diverticulum itself may be detected only on physical examination.

Diagnosis

The diagnosis of urethral diverticulum can be made by a combination of history taking, physical examination, cystourethroscopy, and urethrography. However, the diagnosis of female urethral diverticulum is mainly based on a high index of suspicion that this entity occurs with an incidence that is not insignificant (Bretland, 1973; Moore, 1952). The history may be quite suggestive, although the patient may be asymptomatic.

Routine urologic evaluation, including urologic history, physical examination, urinalysis, cystourethroscopy, and excretory urogram showing the upper tracts and bladder, often is not diagnostic for urethral diverticulum. The presentation of this disorder is rarely typical, and these tests are not sufficiently specific. The history of irritative symptoms is common for most lower urinary tract disorders.

On physical examination, it is extremely important to specifically examine the suburethral area in the female. The urethra is generally tender, and a suburethral mass may be palpated. Manual compression may lead to the expression of purulent material from the external meatus. The diverticulum may also appear as a stony hard mass, especially if the sac contains a calculus or, infrequently, a malignancy.

While examining the urethra, it is also important to determine the position of the proximal urethra and bladder base, assessing hypermobility. The preoperative diagnosis of anatomic stress incontinence may warrant a combined operation to correct the diverticulum and the stress incontinence. When the diagnosis of female urethral diverticulum is suggested on the basis of the history and physical examination, further studies are helpful to delineate the size and location of the diverticulum.

Urethroscopy should be performed using a zero-degree lens and a sheath with a very short beak, allowing the entire urethra to be distended for adequate visualization of the entire urethral lumen. Constant water flow and bladder neck compression at the time of urethroscopy may force the contents of the diverticulum into the urethra, allowing visualization of the orifice. Inflammatory edema may prevent visualization of the orifice. At the time of endoscopy, the urethra is compressed to determine the presence of any active drainage of pus from the mouth of the diverticulum.

The post-void film of an intravenous pyelogram often reveals a collection of contrast material in the subvesical area. The voiding cystogram under fluoroscopic control in the standing, oblique position is the most reliable diagnostic tool and best defines the location, size, and number of diverticula. Frequently, any irregularity of the urethra will be demonstrated during the voiding phase of the vesicoureterogram (VCUG). Should the VCUG not fill a suburethral mass that is clinically suggestive of a urethral diverticulum, other radiographic studies may be helpful.

If a post-void film from a voiding cystourethrogram does not demonstrate the diverticulum, positive pressure urethrography should be performed. In 1959, Lang and Davis introduced their method of positive pressure urethrography. Today, this study, when coupled with voiding cystourethrogram, constitutes the optimal method for detection of urethral diverticula in women.

Positive pressure urethrography is accomplished utilizing a double-balloon catheter. Today in the United States, a single unit model, usually either Davis-Telinde or Trattner catheter, is used (Greenberg, 1981). A double-balloon catheter blocks the urethra proximally and distally. The proximal and distal balloons have separate inflation conduits, and a third conduit opens to a slit between the balloons to be positioned in the urethra (Fig. 75-56).

Following a scout film, the catheter is inserted into the bladder. The proximal balloon is inflated with 20 ml of saline or dilute contrast medium. The distal balloon is then inflated with approximately 30 ml to ensure a snug fit at the meatus and to seal the proximal balloon against the bladder neck. The urethra is filled with 4 to 8 ml of contrast medium. During injection, fluoroscopy is used and anteroposterior and oblique radiographs are obtained. The proximal balloon is deflated, and the catheter is removed. Next, a voiding cystourethrogram is performed. A Robinson catheter is inserted per urethra, and the bladder is filled. With the catheter in place, upright anteroposterior and lateral films are obtained during rest and during straining maneuvers. After this catheter is removed, the important voiding films are taken in the oblique position. The post-void film is obtained in the anteroposterior projection.

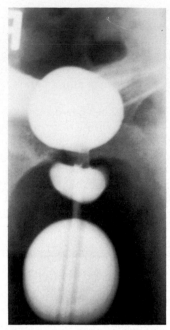

Figure 75–56. Double balloon showing urethral diverticulum.

During radiographic examinations, it was noted that if a patient had a diverticulum, the double-balloon catheter study could maximally outline its sac. The diverticulum would appear as a large, rounded, or lobulated collection of contrast material. However, the relationship of the diverticulum to the urethra and the presence of multiple diverticula were often obscured by the catheter. This problem was overcome by obtaining the voiding cystourethrograms after the double-balloon catheter was removed. The collections of contrast material in the diverticulum were usually retained on the post-void films. The voiding studies also allow evaluation of other genitourinary pathology, such as cystourethroceles and fistulas.

An alternative diagnostic scheme has been devised by Borski and Stutzman (1965). The patient is instructed to empty her bladder. The anterior vaginal wall is compressed and milked to empty any diverticula. A Foley catheter is inserted, and a solution containing 5 ml of indigo carmine, 60 ml of radiopaque contrast medium, and 100 ml of water is instilled into the bladder. The catheter is removed, and the patient is instructed to void while occluding the urethral meatus with one finger. Radiographs are obtained in the anteroposterior and oblique projections. Urethroscopy with urethral compression is performed to identify diverticular orifices from which the blue dye is ejecting.

Coupling positive pressure urethrography with cystourethroscopy thus provides the basis for diagnostic evaluation of this disorder. Other studies that have been proposed to aid in the diagnosis of female urethral diverticulum include ultrasound examination of the pelvis to demonstrate the fluid collection in the diverticulum and the appearance of bladder base elevation of the excretory urogram, signifying a large fluid collection in a diverticulum located in the proximal third of the urethra beneath the bladder (Lee et al., 1977). Urethral

pressure profilmetry has also been recommended. A characteristic biphasic shape of the urethral pressure profile has been noted in women with urethral diverticula. The central depression of this biphasic profile is thought to correspond to the weakened urethral wall at the site of communication with the diverticulum.

Differential Diagnosis

Although a patient may present with a history and physical examination quite suggestive of a suburethral diverticulum, other clinical entities may mimic this condition. Simple bacterial cystitis should be considered; the lower urinary irritative symptoms that usually accompany interstitial cystitis should also be considered. Other intravaginal and suburethral masses that may mimic female urethral diverticulum include Skene's gland abscesses located in the distal urethra without diverticulum formation. These are usually lateral to the midline. An ectopic ureter may extend to the suburethral area. Occasionally, a urethral neoplasm may appear as a suburethral palpable mass (Peters and Vaughan, 1976). Gartner's duct cysts of the anterior vaginal wall may be confused with urethral diverticulum, although these cysts usually arise more laterally in the anterior vaginal wall (Drieger et al., 1954). A hyperreflexic neurogenic bladder, bladder calculus, or bladder neoplasm may also occur with irritative urinary symptoms.

Thorough urologic evaluation with urinalysis, cystourethroscopy, urography, and biopsy may be required to differentiate among them (Spence and Duckett, 1970). The differential diagnosis must also include any lesion manifesting as a suburethral mass. Cystourethroceles are best evaluated with voiding cystourethrograms. An ectopic ureter that opens with a cystic dilatation into the urethra can be excluded by excretory urograms, voiding cystourethrograms, and cystourethroscopy. Gartner's duct cysts are usually found lateral to the urethra and do not communicate with it. Periurethral cysts likewise have no demonstrable urethral communication but are very likely remnants of diverticula with closed orifices.

Indications for Surgery

Surgery is indicated in a patient with significant symptoms related to the presence of a urethral diverticulum. They include recurrent urinary tract infections, severe pain, dyspareunia, frequency, urgency, and post-void dribbling.

Preoperative Care

Once the diagnosis of urethral diverticulum is confirmed, various preoperative factors are worthy of consideration. Should the patient have significant documented genuine SUI and a low, poorly supported, hypermobile urethra and bladder neck, it is advisable to consider the option of initial transvaginal needle suspension of the bladder neck and proximal urethra, followed by urethral diverticulectomy during the same operative procedure. The simultaneous performance of both procedures provides the optimal chance of obtaining adequate postoperative continence.

If both procedures are indicated, it is important to perform the needle suspension as the initial procedure to avoid the risk of contaminating the retropubic space after the diverticulum is manipulated. The technique of transvaginal needle suspension of the bladder neck and proximal urethra is described in detail previously in this chapter, with stress urinary incontinence. We have performed the combined technique of simultaneous transvaginal needle suspension of the proximal urethra and bladder neck and urethral diverticulectomy in numerous females with excellent results.

The surgeon should be especially alert when a preoperative history of severe urinary urgency and frequency is present. When preoperative cystometric evaluation reveals a significant component of detrusor instability, and if this is not treated appropriately during the postoperative period, the high intravesical pressures may certainly increase the risk of postoperative breakdown at the urethral reconstruction site and subsequent formation of a urethral-vaginal fistula or recurrent urethral diverticulum. When significant detrusor instability is documented, we consider anticholinergic therapy to help decrease the risk of postoperative failure. After the diagnosis of female urethral diverticulum is confirmed and the various preoperative surgical considerations have been thoroughly examined, surgical intervention may then be embarked upon.

Prior to surgery, proper antibiotic therapy is mandatory. Reconstructive surgery in a patient with active urinary and diverticular infection may lead to fistula formation and recurrent diverticulum. A suprapubic catheter should be inserted at the time of surgery for safe and uninterrupted bladder drainage. This suprapubic catheter is placed to function as a safety valve during the postoperative period, should the urethral catheter become occluded, and to facilitate the performance of a voiding cystourethrogram with filling of the bladder through the suprapubic catheter. The patient is administered povidone-iodine (Betadine) douches the night before surgery.

Basically, except for the small, noninfected, benign diverticulum, optimal therapy is obliteration or surgical extirpation of the intact sac. Very small diverticula can probably be handled by transurethral incision (widening the orifice intraluminally). In the patient whose surgery must be delayed, the urethra can be stripped intravaginally after each urination (keeping the diverticulum empty), and antibiotics provided prophylactically. Otherwise, surgical excision is the goal.

Historical Perspective

The reported surgical treatments have had several different approaches to diverticula during the past. Furniss (1935) incised the diverticulum transvaginally and packed its sac with gauze. Later, a second stage was employed to excise the resultant urethrovaginal fistula and the granulated sac. Hunner (1938) and Young (1938) both passed a sound per urethra, which was kept in place while the diverticulum was excised transvaginally. Hunner then created a vaginal flap to cover the incision line so that the suture lines were not superimposed. Hyams and Hyams (1939) packed the diverticulum transurethrally with gauze to facilitate transvaginal excision. Cook and Pool (1949) suggested passing a urethral catheter transurethrally into the diverticulum and allowing it to coil up as an aid to transvaginal excision. Moore (1952) exposed the diverticulum transvaginally, incised it, and inserted a Foley catheter with its tip removed into the sac. He inflated the Foley catheter balloon to fill the diverticulum and secured it with a pursestring suture before excision. Moore thought that this better outlined the sac and permitted traction on it to ease the dissection.

Edwards and Beebe (1955) incised the urethra and vaginal wall up to and including the diverticulum. A urethroplasty was then performed to repair the incision. Ellik (1957) devised a technique for incising diverticula near the bladder neck. He incised the sac transvaginally, packed the cavity with oxycel, and oversewed the incision. Subsequently, the surrounding tissues healed by fibrosis. Hirschhorn (1964) injected a liquid Silastic material into the diverticulum prior to its excision. O'Connor and Kropp (1969) utilized firm fibrin that was formed from human fibrinogen clotted with thrombin to fill the diverticular sac.

Spence and Duckett (1970) saucerized the diverticulum and the distal urethra to the external meatus and sutured the edges to the surrounding incised vaginal mucosa. This maneuver created, in effect, a generous meatotomy. They reported no problem with incontinence if the diverticulum was in the distal two thirds of the urethra, stating that the sphincteric control resided in the region bounded by the bladder neck and the proximal one third of the urethra. Flocks and Culp (1975) emphasized that in a transvaginal excision a multilayer closure with no overlapping suture lines was required. Sasnett and co-workers (1978) advocated the jackknife position instead of the lithotomy, to maximize exposure and to permit a downward perspective on the operative field.

Excision Treatment

At UCLA, the technique most commonly used is similar to that described by Busch and Carter (1973) and illustrated by Benjamin and co-workers (1974), but with important modifications. It is based on optimizing the exposure, totally excising the diverticulum, and obtaining a watertight supported closure.

TECHNIQUE. The procedure preferred by us for the treatment of female urethral diverticulum is that of transvaginal excision, utilizing a vaginal flap technique (Leach et al., 1986). The patient is placed in the dorsal lithotomy position and draped, with careful isolation of the rectum from the operative field.

After insertion of a posterior weighted vaginal retrac-

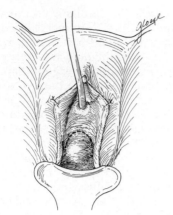

Figure 75–57. Inverted U-incision in anterior vaginal wall with apex distal to urethral diverticulum and proximal to meatus.

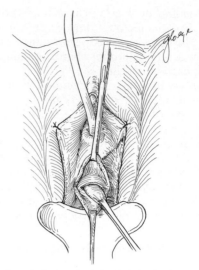

Figure 75–59. Periurethral fascia is incised transversely.

tor and urethral and suprapubic catheters, an inverted U incision is made with the apex distal to the diverticulum and proximal to the urethral meatus (Fig. 75–57). An anterior vaginal wall flap is reflected posteriorly from the urethral meatus to the bladder neck, exposing the periurethral fascia (Fig. 75–58). Care is taken to avoid any perforation or entry into this fascia or the diverticulum by dissection directly on the vaginal wall flap itself. This flap is raised as proximal as necessary to allow complete exposure of the diverticulum and to avoid any overlapping suture lines after the urethral reconstruction is completed.

The periurethral fascia is a distinct layer that surrounds the urethral diverticulum and should be preserved to allow a second layer for reconstruction after the diverticulectomy is completed. The periurethral fascia is incised transversely, and dissection is performed between the periurethral fascia and the diverticulum itself (Fig. 75–59). This fascia may be found to be very attenuated in cases of large diverticulas.

Two flaps are created by dissection of the periurethral fascia proximal and distal to the incision. Thus, the periurethral fascia is opened in an anterior and a posterior direction similar to opening the leaves of a book

to completely expose the urethral diverticulum. With sharp dissection, the wall of the diverticular sac is freed from the surrounding structures. The wall of the diverticulum should be left intact until dissection has reached the neck of the sac. Should there be a significant degree of scarring and fibrosis in this area because of chronic inflammation, the diverticulum itself can be opened to define more clearly the extent of the diverticulum and the location of the communication between the diverticulum and the urethra. It is possible that the diverticulum may extend in a circumferential fashion around the urethra, and complete excision of all diverticular tissue is extremely important so as to minimize the risk of any recurrent diverticulum formation. The communication to the urethral lumen is isolated and excised flush with the urethral wall (Fig. 75–60). All abnormal tissue at this junction is totally excised to decrease the risk of any recurrent diverticulum formation. The lumen of the urethra and the indwelling catheter must be seen.

The mucosa and submucosa layers of the urethra are closed longitudinally with a running 3–0 absorbable suture over a 12 Fr. catheter (Fig. 75–61). No patient has developed urethral stenosis when the urethra has

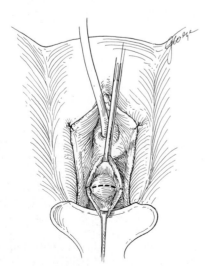

Figure 75–58. Anterior vaginal wall flap is reflected posteriorly, exposing the periurethral fascia.

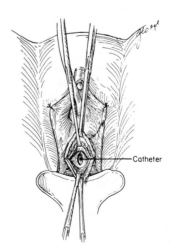

Catheter

Figure 75–60. Communication of diverticulum to urethral lumen is excised flush with urethral wall.

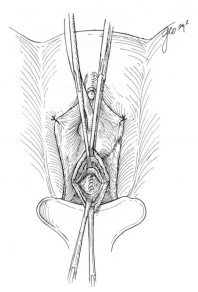

Figure 75–61. Urethra is closed longitudinally with a running 3–0 absorbable suture.

been closed over this size catheter. The closure should be watertight and tension-free. This step will minimize the risk of postoperative extravasation and urethral-vaginal fistula formation. The periurethral fascia is trimmed and closed horizontally, utilizing a 3–0 absorbable suture (Fig. 75–62). This second layer of closure runs in a perpendicular direction with the first and provides a strong second layer of tissue to aid in the reconstruction of the urethra. The anterior vaginal wall flap is advanced well distally over the suture line of the periurethral fascia and trimmed if necessary. This layer is closed with a running locking 2–0 absorbable suture (Fig. 75–63). The flap advancement brings fresh tissue to cover the reconstruction in a third layer and prevents overlapping lines of sutures.

After the procedure is completed, an antibiotic-soaked vaginal pack is placed. Both the suprapubic and the urethral catheter are left to gravity drainage.

Identification of the diverticulum at the time of surgical removal has not presented any particular difficulty.

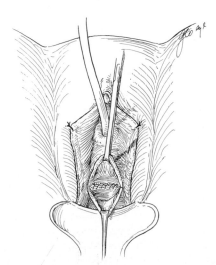

Figure 75–62. Periurethral fascia is closed horizontally with running 3–0 absorbable suture.

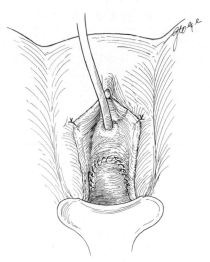

Figure 75–63. Anterior vaginal wall flap is advanced over suture line in periurethral fascia.

Various techniques have been suggested to aid in the identification of the diverticulum, including injection of a coagulum into the diverticulum intraoperatively, as well as coiling a catheter within the diverticulum to facilitate its identification (Mueller et al., 1989). In general, we have found that once the periurethral fascia is opened, the site of the diverticulum is quite obvious and these further maneuvers are usually not indicated. Should it be difficult to identify the communication site between the diverticulum and the urethra, intraoperative urethroscopy can be performed. A pediatric sound can be passed through the communication site into the diverticulum to help facilitate its identification, although this has rarely been necessary.

Endoscopic Treatment

Urethrotomy is performed by splitting the floor of the urethra from the meatus proximally to the diverticular orifice (Miskowiak et al., 1989; Spencer et al., 1987). This maneuver allows better visibility of the diverticular sac during dissection. This technique requires closure and healing of the floor of the urethra along its entire length, which may be tenuous with an infected diverticulum.

Spence Marsupialization Treatment

In 1970, Spence and Duckett suggested marsupialization of the diverticulum to prevent recurrence, minimize operating time, and reduce blood loss (Roehrborn, 1988). This procedure is useful for diverticula in the distal third of the urethra, away from the intrinsic and external sphincter.

Postoperative Care

After the procedure is completed, a vaginal pack is placed and the suprapubic and urethral catheters are connected to a drainage bag. Intravenous antiobiotics are administered as indicated. The patient may be discharged from the hospital 1 to 2 days after surgery. Patients are routinely placed on anticholinergic therapy after the operative procedure to decrease the risk of any bladder spasms related to the catheter drainage. Thus, it is hoped that the urethral reconstruction site is protected from high intravesical pressures. Anticholinergic medication is discontinued 24 hours before a postoperative voiding cystourethrogram is obtained. About 10 to 14 days after surgery, the urethral catheter is removed and a voiding cystogram is performed through the suprapubic catheter. This radiographic examination is performed in the standing position. When the patient experiences the first urge to urinate, voiding is allowed while fluoroscopically monitoring the urethra and obtaining spot radiographs as indicated. Three potential results are possible at the time of voiding cystourethrography. First, the patient may void to completion with no extravasation at the urethral reconstruction site. In this situation, all catheters are removed. Second, the patient may void without extravasation but without complete bladder emptying. The suprapubic catheter is left in place and opened three times daily to monitor post-void residual urine. When the residuals are consistently less than 100 ml, the suprapubic catheter is removed. Third, the patient may have a small degree of extravasation at the urethral reconstruction site. The urethral catheter is not reinserted, but the suprapubic catheter is placed to drainage. The radiographic study is repeated in 1 week. No patient in our series has had persistent extravasation when the voiding cystourethrogram has been repeated.

Intraoperative Complications

Bleeding in the form of profuse oozing is not uncommon, particularly in patients with active infection and abscess formation. A vaginal packing should well control this oozing.

If it is difficult to close the urethral mucosa because of the large defect created during the excision of the diverticulum, it may be necessary to further expose the urethral wall and close over a 5 to 8 Fr. feeding tube. We have not encountered urethral strictures following this procedure.

In cases of difficult closure due to severe inflamed or poor quality tissue, a fibrofatty labial (Martius) flap can be utilized between the periurethral fascia and the vaginal wall. A watertight closure is critical in avoiding postoperative extravasation and fistula formation. Precise anatomic dissection and closure of the urethral layers avoiding overlapping suture lines are crucial.

The finding of a large periurethral abscess may require a staged procedure in which the abscess is drained and the excision of the diverticulum performed as a secondary procedure.

Large proximal urethral diverticula may extend into the trigone. It is possible that, should dissection proceed in an improper plane when the diverticulum extends beneath the trigonal area, bladder or ureteric injury could occur. Instillation of indigo carmine into the bladder will demonstrate bladder and ureteral integrity, and cystoscopy may then be performed in selected cases.

Postoperative Complications

The usual complications of postoperative pain, bleeding, infection, and bladder spasm related to catheters are noteworthy. We believe that appropriate preoperative preparation and perioperative antibiotic therapy, as well as postoperative anticholinergics, are essential.

The new onset of incontinence after the diverticulectomy, as well as the potential exacerbation of pre-existing incontinence, is a complication worthy of consideration. The adequate evaluation of the postion of the urethra, bladder neck, and bladder base, as well as evaluation of the possibility of SUI prior to diverticulectomy, is of the utmost importance if this complication is to be avoided.

Urethral stricture may result if too much urethral wall is removed in the dissection of a large diverticulum. Urethrovaginal fistula formation is the most important complication of the surgery and should be treated after a period of healing. Anterior vaginal wall infection is rare and responds well to antibiotic therapy. Infection may cause the urethral mucosa to become friable. If an abscess is formed, surgical drainage is required in spite of the potential damage to the repair.

Recurrent urethral diverticula may occur in particular in a patient with active urethral infection, difficult dissection, and suture line tension and when postoperative difficulties with catheter drainage are encountered. Secondary surgery should be performed after a prudent period of observation.

Stress incontinence prior to surgery should be well-documented and could be corrected in selected cases at the time of excision of the diverticulum. Secondary urinary stress incontinence not present prior to surgery is rare and may develop in a patient with anatomic defects due to dissection of the urethral support. Severe incontinence due to intrinsic sphincteric dysfunction may occur because of the extensive dissection of the urethral support. Surgery for this condition may require a sling procedure or periurethral injection.

VESICOVAGINAL FISTULA

The appearance of a urinary fistula to the vagina is one of the most devastating complications after surgery. The emotional distress of the patient and the surgeon are high, because conservative therapy offers little hope for cure. In the majority of patients, a second operation is required to correct the problem.

The most important steps in limiting the incidence of fistula is prevention by proper surgical dissection and recognition at initial injury so that immediate repair can be undertaken. In a difficult dissection, indigo carmine can be instilled within the bladder so that any injury will be immediately recognized.

In the United States, gynecologic surgery is the most

common cause of vesicovaginal fistulas. The incidence of bladder injury has increased since the advent of abdominal hysterectomy in the 1940s, occurring in 0.5 to 1 per cent of patients who undergo total abdominal hysterectomy. An increase has occurred in the number of fistulas related to vaginal hysterectomy, with its greater utilization (Everett et al., 1956).

Etiology

In developed countries, the most common cause of vesicovaginal fistula is gynecologic surgery, specifically hysterectomy. Other causes include urologic surgery, gastrointestinal surgery, trauma, and radiation therapy for pelvic malignancies. Obstetric trauma resulting in fistula is more common in underdeveloped nations.

In 1956, Everett and Mattingly reported on 149 cases of bladder fistulas, with 44 per cent resulting from gynecologic surgery, 32 per cent related to cervical cancer and radiation therapy, 20 per cent from obstetric injury, and 4 per cent from other causes. Since that time, a marked decrease in the number of fistula related to obstetric trauma has occurred. In 1985, a report from Grady Memorial Hospital related no fistulas in 150,000 obstetric deliveries. Currently, about 75 per cent of vesicovaginal fistulas are related to abdominal hysterectomy for benign disease (Everett et al., 1956).

In 1980, Goodwin and Scardino reported on their experience with vesicovaginal and ureterovaginal fistulas. They studied 43 patients with vesicovaginal fistulas. The causes included 74 per cent from gynecologic surgery, 14 per cent from urologic surgery, and 5 per cent directly and 16 per cent indirectly related to radiation therapy and only rarely related to obstetrics. Hadley (personal communication) reported on 16 patients with simple vesicovaginal fistulas: 81 per cent resulted from hysterectomy, 13 per cent from trauma, and 6 per cent from partial colectomy (Lawson, 1978).

Factors that appear to predispose the patient to the development of fistulas include infection, ischemia, arteriosclerosis, diabetes mellitus, radiation therapy, pelvic inflammatory disease, and tumor.

Symptoms and Presentation

Most vesicovaginal fistulas classically occur as continuous day-and-night incontinence following a recent pelvic operation. An unaccounted for increase in drainage or the occurrence of bloody urine may be suggestive of fistula formation. However, a watery vaginal discharge accompanied by normal voiding may be the only sign of a small fistula. Fistulas related to radiation therapy may develop months and up to 20 years after therapy, and recurrent tumor must be considered.

Diagnosis

The suspicion of a fistula should lead one to diagnostic maneuvers to confirm or deny its presence. The first step is to confirm that the watery drainage per vagina is indeed urine. Excessive vaginal discharge after pelvic surgery may simulate a urinary fistula. Tablets of phenazopyridine (Pyridium) 100 mg, t.i.d. or the intravenous injection of indigo carmine may confirm the diagnosis of urinary fistula.

The second step is to confirm the diagnosis of urinary fistula and differentiate it from urinary incontinence. This goal is achieved by physical examination with a full bladder and by confirming that the loss of urine is per vagina and not per urethra.

The third step is to diagnose the source of the fistula. The bladder may be distended with saline dyed with methylene blue or indigo carmine and the site of leakage identified in the vagina. If leakage of dyed saline is seen, the diagnosis of vesicovaginal fistula is made. When the vaginal examination shows continuous leakage of urine without dye, a ureteric or uterine fistula must be suspected.

Cystoscopy and vaginoscopy may demonstrate the size, location, and relation to the ureteric orifices as well as the collateral fistulas. A biopsy of the site is mandatory in any patient with a history of pelvic neoplasm. Performing these studies using anesthesia may aid in diagnosis.

Intravenous pyelogram may demonstrate partial or complete obstruction, suggesting a ureterovaginal fistula but many times no obstruction is seen. Retrograde pyelograms are more likely to demonstrate the exact location of a ureterovaginal fistula.

Cystogram or voiding cystourethrogram is very helpful in demonstrating the extent of the fistula, the presence of vesicoureteral reflux, and the associated urethral or vesical prolapse or stress incontinence that may require simultaneous repair.

Principles of Surgical Repair

As soon as the diagnosis of fistula is made, a trial of conservative therapy should be instituted. Measures include proper and undisturbed bladder drainage and antibiotics when indicated (O'Connor, 1980). In small fistulas an attempt to fulgurate the area may be made (Benson and Olsson, 1984). When these conservative measures have failed and most of the urine continues to leak per vagina in spite of good bladder drainage, surgical correction of the fistula is necessary.

Sound surgical principles should be employed in the treatment of this condition. The tissues must be in optimal condition, with adequate blood supply to the area to support the repair—tissues should be free of infection, excessive inflammation, and cancer. A layered closure should be utilized, with avoidance of overlapping suture lines. Suture material must be absorbable and cause little tissue reaction. Continuous uninterrupted postoperative urinary drainage is critical to prevent extravasation and distention with breakdown of suture lines. Urethral and suprapubic catheter drainage are highly recommended.

In planning the treatment of vesicovaginal fistula, several specific issues should be addressed: (1) use of estrogens or antibiotics; (2) timing of surgery; (3) surgical approach (abdominal, vaginal, or combined); (4) whether or not to excise fistulous tract; and (5) use of adjuvant surgical measures to improve the fistula repair, such as Martius fibrofatty flaps from the labia or vaginal flaps.

Use of Estrogens and Antibiotics

The improved turgor and vascular supply of the vaginal wall after estrogen replacement in the postmenopausal or posthysterectomy patient may aid in healing of the vagina, and its early use is strongly recommended (Barnes et al., 1977; Jonas et al., 1984). Broad-spectrum antibiotics are required in any fistula repair, particularly if an early approach is utilized. We, in general, provide a combination of an aminoglycoside and cephalosporin, beginning 24 hours prior to surgery. Because the vaginal area is usually contaminated and infected from the constant urinary drainage, we utilize an iodine solution to scrub and douche the vaginal area the night before and the day of surgery.

Timing of Surgery

The timing of surgery remains a controversial issue. It is obvious that infection of the vaginal cuff or pelvic infection after abdominal hysterectomy requires prolonged antibiotic therapy before any attempted repair is made. The classic opinion regarding timing of repair is to wait 3 to 6 months to allow the surgical inflammatory reaction to subside. This is particularly important if an abdominal approach is contemplated and the etiology of the fistula was a complicated abdominal hysterectomy.

Shortening the waiting period would be of great social and psychologic significance in these distressed patients. However, one should not trade social convenience for a compromise in the surgical success. In the past 10 years, we have prospectively done early transvaginal repair of vesicovaginal fistula and compared our results with others using the "long-wait" abdominal or vaginal approach. We do not believe that the shorter waiting period (2 to 3 weeks after the initial injury) has added any extra risks to the surgical result. Our results were no different from the long-wait approach, regardless of the route of repair. The patients are very satisfied by this early transvaginal repair because it avoids the emotional distress of a month of constant wetting (Goodwin and Scardino, 1980; Hadley et al., 1986; Leach and Raz, 1983; Martius, 1928; Persky et al., 1979; Zimmern et al., 1984).

Abdominal or Vaginal Approach

The best operation for repair of vesicovaginal fistula is the first operation. The selected route of repair depends mostly on the surgeon's training and experience. The best approach is probably the one with which the surgeon feels most comfortable and has had the most experience. We personally favor the vaginal approach because we can avoid laparotomy and opening of the bladder and can provide a quicker recovery with less morbidity.

We reserve the abdominal approach only in rare cases when intra-abdominal pathology requires simultaneous care. The most common case is radiation cystitis and fistula with a small contracted bladder capacity requiring cystoplasty and fistula repair. Radiation fistula per se does not preclude the vaginal approach, if the bladder capacity is adequate.

Excision of the Fistulous Tract

The classic approach to the repair of vesicovaginal fistula or any other fistula occurrence includes the wide excision of the fistulous tract in order to freshen the margins and provide a better repair (Leach et al., 1983, Martius, 1928; Steg et al., 1977; Zimmern et al., 1985). We have challenged this dogma, and in the last 65 cases of early transvaginal repair of vesicovaginal fistula have not excised the fistulous tract and have not seen any apparent adverse effects (Persky et al., 1979; Zimmern et al., 1986).

In our view, many advantages to leaving the fistulous tract undisturbed exist. During repair, a small fistula remains small if not excised, but as soon as a fistulous tract is excised this small opening becomes very large. Bleeding of the freshly excised margins may require coagulation of the edges and compromise the closure. The fistulous tract provides a ring of protection against postsurgical bladder spasms that, if severe, may compromise the healing. In cases in which the fistulous tract is removed, this protective ring is lost. The fresh repair may be at higher risk if severe bladder spasms occur after surgery. We found the greatest advantage of not excising the fistulous tract is in cases in which the fistula is very close to the ureteric orifices. In this situation, excision of the fistula will necessitate open surgery and reimplantation of the ureters. If the fistula is not excised, the ureter can be catheterized with a stent. Under direct vision of the ureteric catheter, a safe transvaginal closure of the fistula can be performed, avoiding ureteric reimplantation.

Adjuvant Measures

In the majority of cases of uncomplicated vesicovaginal fistula, correction requires only multilayer tension-free repair of the fistula. Complicating factors, such as prior radiation, prior failed surgery, or poor quality of tissues, require adjuvant measures.

When the repair is done by an abdominal approach, omentum is commonly used. It is an excellent source of reinforcement and protection of a tenuous closure. Some surgeons employ the omentum routinely, when obtainable (Benson and Olsson, 1984). In selected cases, we have interposed the pericolonic or mesenteric fat.

Our technique of transvaginal repair of vesicovaginal

fistula is described further in detail but in brief includes no excision of the fistulous tract, multilayer tension-free closure of the fistula, and advancement of a vaginal flap, covering the area of repair with healthy tissue. However, very often it is desirable or necessary to reinforce a routine closure. Several measures are available in this case: (1) fibrofatty tissue from the labia (Martius flap), (2) rotation flaps of the entire labia and/or gluteal skin, (3) myocutaneous gracilis muscle flaps (Obrink and Bunne, 1978), and (4) peritoneal flaps in the repair of high fistulas.

Vaginal Approach for Repair of Vesicovaginal Fistulas

The patient is placed in the lithotomy position. An inverted J incision is made in the anterior vaginal wall (Fig. 75–64). The long end of the J should extend toward the apex of the vagina. The convex portion of the incision extends to and circumscribes the fistulous tract. This assymetric incision allows for the later advancement and rotation of the posterior flap over the fistula repair. Two flaps are created on the anterior and posterior side of the fistula (Fig. 75–65). Creation of the posterior flap begins in healthy tissue away from the fistulous tract, which aids in dissection of proper tissue planes. The overlying bladder is well-mobilized to ensure a tension-free closure. Without excision or debridement of its edges, the fistulous tract is closed with 3–0 Dexon or Vicryl suture (Fig. 75–66). Included in this suture line is partial thickness of the bladder and full-thickness vaginal wall, which has remained connected to the fistulous tract.

A second layer of interrupted 3–0 Dexon or Vicryl inverts and closes the perivesical fascia. The axis of this second suture line should be at right angles to the first. The previously raised anterior (distal) flap is now resected (Fig. 75–67). This allows the posterior (proximal) flap to rotate and extend beyond the closure of the fistula in order to cover the fistulous tract with fresh vaginal tissue and to avoid adjacent and overlapping suture lines (Fig. 75–68).

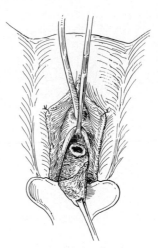

Figure 75–65. Creation of two flaps on either side of the fistula. The posterior flap is started in healthy tissue away from the fistulous tract.

If the patient has a hypermobile or prolapsed urethra and bladder neck, a transvaginal needle bladder neck suspension is performed prior to the repair of the fistula. If the fistula lies near the apex of the vagina, the anterior flap is created with its base toward the introitus of the vagina. The fistula is closed in two layers as described. The raised vaginal wall flap is advanced posteriorly toward the apex of the vagina, avoiding overlapping suture lines.

In the difficult transvaginal repair or, if for any reason the closure of the fistula is tenuous, one can interpose between bladder and vagina a segment of vascularized labial fibrofatty tissue (Martius flap). This tissue is mobilized through a separate vertical incision in the area of the labia majora. Following a subcutaneous tunnel developed in the lateral vaginal wall, this tissue is brought into the vaginal incision where it is interposed between the bladder and vagina.

One of the problems of the Martius flap is the difficulty encountered in some cases in obtaining adequate length to reach the vaginal apex. To circumvent this problem we have employed, in selected cases, a peritoneal flap. The dissection of the posterior vaginal flap is

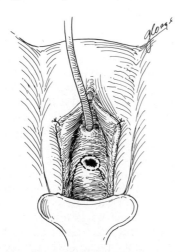

Figure 75–64. Inverted J-shaped incision in the anterior vaginal wall circumscribing the fistula.

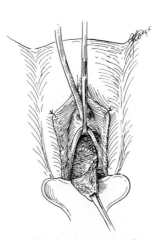

Figure 75–66. Closure of the fistulous tract without excision or debridement of its edges.

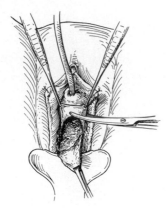

Figure 75–67. Resection of the previously raised anterior vaginal flap.

extended to the peritoneal reflexion. The closed peritoneum is freed from adhesions to the posterior bladder wall and advanced forward to cover the fistula repair. After completion of the two initial layers of closure (fistula and perivesical fascia), the peritoneum is advanced to cover the repair. The last layer will be the advancement of the vaginal wall flap to cover the entire area.

Postoperatively, the patient receives antibiotics until the Foley catheter is removed and anticholinergics to avoid bladder spasms. The most important aspect of postoperative care is uninterrupted catheter drainage. The urethral catheter is removed on the 5th to 7th postoperative day. If the outpatient cystogram performed 2 weeks after operation documents vesical integrity, the suprapubic catheter is removed.

The results of the aforementioned technique for uncomplicated vesicovaginal fistula repair have been very gratifying. Of 69 cases (42/69 or 60 per cent with one to three prior failed repairs), the fistula was cured in the first operation in 64/69 cases (93 per cent). The follow-up was 6 months to 12 years (median 5 years). Three patients required a second vaginal repair and one a third transabdominal repair. One patient underwent urinary diversion, and one has a very small output (one pad a day) residual fistula. The transvaginal approach of simple vesicovaginal fistula offers several advantages: excellent exposure, no opening of the bladder or abdomen

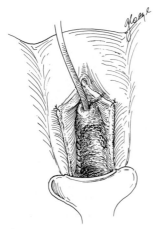

Figure 75–68. The posterior flap is rotated and advanced to cover the underlying suture lines with fresh tissue.

resulting in reduced postoperative discomfort, reduced dissection resulting in minimal blood loss, interposition of viable tissue if needed, multilayer closure, possible correction of associated stress urinary incontinence, and shorter hospital stay.

Nonradiated Complex Vesicovaginal Fistulas

Complex vesicovaginal fistulas include giant fistulas, commonly of obstetric origin, fistulas associated with loss of the urethra, multiple fistulas, and those with severe scarring after multiple previous attempts at repair. Giant fistulas are more than 5 cm in size and involve complete destruction of the trigone, bladder neck, and urethra. Interposition of a Martius flap, gracilis muscle, or partial colpocleisis are techniques that may be utilized. A viable gracilis muscle flap may support the repair of a complex fistula. A long skin incision extends over the course of the muscle from the medial condyle of the femur to the inferior border of the symphysis pubis. Between the adductor longus laterally and the adductor magnus posteromedially, the tendinous part of the muscle is identified, divided, and held with stay sutures. During muscle dissection, it is important to preserve the blood and nerve supply entering the muscle along its lateral border. After adequate mobilization, the gracilis muscle is tunneled through the upper thigh and the labia and into the vagina, where it is fixed with 2–0 Dexon or Vicryl sutures around the fistula.

Partial colpocleisis (Latzko operation) (Latzko, 1942) is particularly advisable in a patient with a deep vagina and a vault fistula. The operation consists of denudation of the vaginal mucosa surrounding the fistula. The colpocleisis is then accomplished in three layers without sutures entering the bladder wall. It is never necessary to transplant the ureter because the procedure does not include excision of the fistulous tract or mobilization of the bladder. Sexual function does not seem to be impaired despite some shortening of the vagina.

Radiation Fistulas

Radiation vesicovaginal fistulas occur following radiation of neoplasia of the uterus and cervix, with an incidence of 1 to 5 per cent. A subsequent surgical procedure, such as Wertheim's hysterectomy, makes fistula formation more likely. Because of radiation-induced obliterative endarteritis, the area around the defect is poorly vascularized, thereby reducing the chances of spontaneous as well as postsurgical healing (Twombly et al., 1946). Therefore, a waiting period of 12 months is recommended before attempt at surgical repair (Wein et al., 1980). During this time, recurrence of cancer can be detected. The edges of the fistula and surrounding tissue must be examined and biopsied preoperatively to rule out residual or recurrent cancer.

Time-honored principles, such as lack of tension, separated sutures lines, and preservation of blood supply, are not always sufficient to obtain successful closure.

Interposition of viable tissue may help in revascularizing the ischemic fistula region. The use of tissues in the immediate vicinity, such as peritoneal flap, omentum, bulbocavernosus muscle, and Martius flap, has frequently been reported, but the likelihood of their exposure to some radiation renders them less than ideal for this purpose. Instead, many workers advocate gracilis muscle brought from one or both sides. The approach depends on the exact site of the fistula, the involvement of the ureteric orifices, the presence of collateral fistulas, the extent of the radiation field, the number of previous attempts at surgical repair, the sexual activity of the patient, and the experience of the surgeon.

In the presence of small contracted bladder capacity due to radiation cystitis, an enlargement cystoplasty is required. In these cases, together with omentum, the augmented segment of small or large bowel is selected to cover the area of the repair.

If the bladder capacity is adequate, we prefer the vaginal approach for radiation fistula. The advantages of the vaginal approach include multilayer closure, advancement of vaginal flap, interposition of labial fibrofatty tissue or gracilis muscle flap, avoidance of bowel manipulation in a previously irradiated field, decreased blood loss, and decreased postoperative discomfort.

In selected cases, it is desirable during the repair of radiation-related fistula to improve urinary drainage. Together with the placement of suprapubic and urethral catheters, bilateral ureteral single J-stents can be inserted for 5 to 7 days. These allow prolonged dryness of the bladder, enhancing the chances for healing.

Abdominal Approach for Vesicovaginal Fistulas

The abdominal or abdominovaginal approach may be utilized for the repair of any type of vesicovaginal fistula but is particularly indicated in the patient who requires ureteric reimplantation or who suffers radiation fistula with small bladder capacity and combined ureteric fistula.

O'Connor has pioneered the suprapubic transvesical approach. The bladder is bivalved to the level of the fistula. The fistulous tract is excised on both the bladder and vaginal sides. The bladder is mobilized away from the vagina, and the two are closed in separate layers.

A midline abdominal approach allows for mobilization of an omental pedicle graft to place between the suture lines. The omentum has abundant blood supply and lymphatic drainage, providing a vascular graft, replacement of tissue, and reabsorption of debris (Turner-Warwick, 1979). After healing, the omentum regains its suppleness and allows a simple separation of tissue planes should reoperation be necessary. The blood supply to the omentum comes from the gastroepiploic arch on the greater curvature of the stomach. The right component is larger than the left, so that the omental graft should be based on the right gastroepiploic artery. In addition, the right pedicle arises lower than the left, closer to the pelvis. First the omentum is mobilized

from the transverse colon. The splenic origin of the left gastroepiploic vessel is divided. If this does not provide adequate length, the short gastric branches are ligated and divided. This maneuver should be accomplished with absorbable sutures—nonabsorbable sutures may lead to formation of urinary stones, if the omentum comes into contact with urine in the area of the fistula. All of the short gastric branches should be ligated to avoid traction on the pedicle, which could cause tearing of any remaining branches. The pedicle graft is brought into the pelvis and may be secured with a few absorbable sutures between the bladder and vagina.

Postoperative Care

Whether a vaginal or an abdominal approach is chosen, the postoperative care is very similar. The vaginal pack is removed on the 1st postoperative day. Intravenous antibiotics are continued for 24 to 48 hours followed by oral antibiotics. Early ambulation is encouraged. The suprapubic and urethral catheters are left to gravity drainage. It is critical that uninterrupted urinary drainage be maintained in the postoperative period. The urethral catheter is removed on the 5th postoperative day.

Most patients are discharged on the 7th postoperative day still on suprapubic catheter drainage. A cystogram is obtained via the suprapubic tube on the 10th to 14th postoperative day. If no urinary extravasation is seen, the suprapubic catheter is removed. Vaginal estrogens in the postmenopausal patient promote vaginal healing. Sexual intercourse is discouraged for 2 to 3 months to allow adequate healing of the suture lines.

REFERENCES

Adams, W. E.: Urethrography. Bull. Tulane Med. Fac., 23:107, 1964.

Aldridge, A. H.: Transplantation of fascia for relief of urinary stress incontinence. Am. J. Obstet. Gynecol., 44:398–411, 1942.

Andersen, M. J. F.: The incidence of diverticula in the female urethra. J. Urol., 98:96, 1967.

Ask, P., and Hok, B.: Pressure measurement techniques in urodynamic investigation. Neurourol. Urodyn., 9:1–15, 1990.

Barnes, R., Hadley, H., and Johnston, O.: Transvaginal repair of vesicovaginal fistulas. Urology, 10:258, 1977.

Barnick, C. G., and Cardozo, L.: Electromyography of the urethral sphincter in genuine stress incontinence. A useless test? Neurourol. Urodyn., 8:318–319, 1989.

Beecham, C. T., and Beecham, J. B.: Correction of prolapsed vagina or enterocele with fascia lata. Obstet. Gynecol., 42:542, 1973.

Benjamin, J., Elliot, L., Cooper, J. F., and Bjornson, L.: Urethral diverticulum in adult female. Clinical aspects, operative procedures, and pathology. Urology, 3:1, 1974.

Benson, M., and Olsson, C. A.: Vesicovaginal fistula. In Paulson, D. F. (Ed.). Genitourinary Surgery. New York, Churchill Livingstone, 1984, pp. 229–236.

Birnbaum, S. J.: Rational therapy for the prolapsed vagina. Am. J. Obstet. Gynecol., 115:414, 1973.

Blaivas, J. G.: Urodynamic testing. In Raz, S. (Ed.): Female Urology. Philadelphia, W. B. Saunders Co., 1983, pp. 79–103.

Blaivas, J. G.: Sphincteric incontinence in the female. Pathophysiology, classification and choice of corrective surgical procedure. AUA Update Series, 25:1–7, 1987.

Blaivas, J. G.: Techniques of evaluation. In Yalla, S. V., McGuire, E. J., Elbadawi, A., and Blaivas, J. G. (Eds.): Neurourology and

Urodynamics. Principles and Practice. New York, Macmillan Publishing Co., 1988, pp. 155–198.

Blaivas, J. G.: Diagnostic evaluation. Semin. Urol., 7:65–77, 1989.

Blaivas, J. G., and Olsson, C. A.: Stress incontinence: Classification and surgical approach. J. Urol., 139:727, 1988.

Bonnar, J., Kraszewski, A., and Davis, W.: Incidental pathology at vaginal hysterectomy for genital prolapse. J. Obstet. Gynecol. Br. Comm., 100:1137, 1970.

Borski, A. A., and Stutzman, R. E.: Diverticulum of female urethra: A simplified diagnostic aid. J. Urol., 93:60, 1965.

Bottaccini, M. R., and Gleason, D. M.: Urodynamic norms in women. I. Normals versus stress incontinent. J. Urol., 124:659–662, 1980.

Bretland, P. M.: A device and technique for urethrography in the female. Br. J. Radiol., 46:311, 1973.

Burch, J. C.: Urethrovaginal fixation to Cooper's ligament for the correction of stress incontinence, cystocele and prolapse. Am. J. Obstet. Gynecol., 81:281, 1961.

Busch, F. M., and Carter, F. H.: Vaginal flap incision for urethral diverticula. Western Section Meeting, American Urological Association, Honolulu, June 29, 1973.

Butler, W. J.: The diagnosis of urethral diverticula in women. J. Urol., 95:63, 1966.

Cobb, O. E., and Ragde, H.: Simplified correction of female stress incontinence. J. Urol., 120:418–420, 1978.

Constantinou, C. E.: Urethrometry: Considerations of static, dynamic, and stability characteristics of the female urethra. Neurourol. Urodyn., 7:521–539, 1988.

Cook, E. N., and Pool, T. L.: Urethral diverticulum in the female. J. Urol., 62:495, 1949.

Coolsaet, B. L. R. A., Blok, C., van Vanrooji, G. E. P. M., and Tan, B.: Subthreshold detrusor instability. Neurourol. Urodyn., 4:309, 1985.

Coolsaet, B. L. R. A., and Elhilali, M. M.: Detrusor overactivity. Neurourol. Urodyn., 7:541–561, 1988.

Copenhaver, E. H.: Vaginal hysterectomy: An analysis of indications and complications among 1000 operations. Am. J. Obstet. Gynecol., 84:123, 1962.

Copenhaver, E. H.: Vaginal hysterectomy: past, present and future. Surg. Clin. North Am., 60:437, 1980.

Cruikshank, S. H.: Preventing posthysterectomy vaginal vault prolapse and enterocele during vaginal hysterectomy. Am. J. Obstet. Gynecol., 156:1433, 1987.

Cruikshank, S. H.: Preventing vault prolapse and enterocele after vaginal hysterectomy. Southern Med. J., 81:594, 1988.

Crystle, C. D., Charme, L. S., and Copeland, W. E.: Q-Tip test in stress urinary incontinence. Obstet. Gynecol., 38:313–316, 1971.

Davis, B. L., and Robinson, D. G.: Diverticula of the female urethra: Assay of 120 cases. J. Urol., 104:850, 1970.

Davis, H. J., and Cian, L. G.: Positive pressure urethrography: A new diagnostic method. J. Urol., 75:753, 1956.

Davis, H. J., and TeLinde, R. W.: Urethral diverticula: An assay of 121 cases. J. Urol., 80:34, 1958.

Delancey, J. O. L.: Pubovaginal ligament: A separate structure from the urethral supports ("pubo-urethral ligament"). Neurol. Urodyn., 8:53–61, 1989.

Delancey, J. O. L.: Anatomy and embryology of the lower urinary tract. Obstet. Gynecol. Clin. North Am., 16:717, 1989.

Diokno, A. C., Brock, B. M., Herzog, A. R., et al.: Prevalence of urologic symptoms in the noninstitutionalized elderly. J. Urol., 133:179, 1985.

Dretler, S. P., Vermillion, C. D., and McCollough, D. L.: The roentgenographic diagnosis of female urethral diverticula. J. Urol., 107:72, 1972.

Drieger, J. S., and Poutasse, E. F.: Diverticulum of the female urethra. Am. J. Obstet. Gynecol., 68:706, 1954.

Edwards, E. A., and Beebe, R. A.: Diverticula of the female urethra. Obstet. Gynecol., 5:729, 1955.

Ellik, M.: Diverticulum of the female urethra: A new method of ablation. J. Urol., 77:234, 1957.

Everett, H. S., and Mattingly, R. F.: Urinary tract injuries resulting from pelvic surgery. Am. J. Obstet. Gynecol., 71:502–514, 1956.

Faysal, M. H., Constantinou, C. E., Rother, L. F., and Govan, D. E.: The impact of bladder neck suspension on the resting and stress urethral pressure profile: A prospective study comparing controls with incontinent patients preoperatively and postoperatively. J. Urol., 125:55, 1981.

Firlit, C.: Urethral abnormalities. Urol. Clin. North Am., 5:41, 1978.

Flocks, R. H., and Culp, D. A.: Surgical Urology, 4th ed. Chicago, Year Book Medical Publishers, 1975, p. 428.

Furniss, H. D.: Suburethral abscesses and diverticula in female urethra. J. Urol., 33:498, 1935.

Gillon, G., and Stanton, S. L.: Long-term follow-up of surgery for urinary incontinence in elderly women. Br. J. Urol., 56:478, 1984.

Gittes, R. F., and Loughlin, K. R.: No-incision pubovaginal suspension for stress incontinence. J. Urol., 138:568, 1987.

Goodwin, W. E., and Scardino, P. T.: Vesicovaginal and ureterovaginal fistulas: a summary of 25 years of experience. J. Urol., 123:370–374, 1980.

Gray, O. A.: Urethrovaginal fistulas. Am. J. Obstet. Gynecol., 101:28, 1968.

Green, D. F., McGuire, E. J., and Lytton, B.: A comparison of endoscopic suspension of the vesical neck versus anterior urethropexy for the treatment of stress urinary incontinence. J. Urol., 136:1205–1207, 1986.

Greenberg, M., Stone, D., Cochran, S. T., Bruskewitz, R., Pagan, J. J., Raz, S., and Barbaric, Z. M.: Female urethral diverticula: Double-balloon catheter study. Am. J. Radiol., 136:259, 1981.

Hadley, H. R.: Personal communication.

Hadley, H. R., Staskin, D. R., Schmidbauer, C. P., Zimmern, P., Leach, G., and Raz, S.: Operative correction for female urethral incompetence. Semin. Urol., 4:13–23, 1986.

Hadley, H. R., Zimmern, P. E., and Raz, S.: Transvaginal repair of vesicovaginal fistulae. Proceedings of the Western Section, American Urological Association, Reno, Nevada, Abstract No. 102, 1984.

Hadley, H. R., Zimmern, P. E., Staskin, D. R., and Raz, S.: Transvaginal needle bladder neck suspension. Urol. Clin. North Am., 12:291–303, 1985.

Harer, W. B., and Gunther, R. E.: Simplified urethrovesical suspension and urethroplasty. Am. J. Obstet. Gynecol., 91:1017–1021, 1965.

Hawksworth, W., and Roux, J.: Vaginal hysterectomy. J. Obstet. Gynecol. Br. Comm., 65:214, 1958.

Heaney, N. S.: Vaginal hysterectomy: Its indications and technic. Am. J. Surg., 48:284, 1940.

Heaney, N. S.: Techniques of vaginal hysterectomy. Surg. Clin. North Am., 22:73, 1942.

Herman, L., and Greene, L. B.: Diverticulum of the female urethra. J. Urol., 52:599, 1944.

Hilton, P., and Laor, D.: Voiding symptoms in the female: The correlation with urodynamic voiding characteristics. Neurourol. Urodyn., 8:308–310, 1989.

Hinman, F., Jr., and Cohlan, W. R.: Gartner's duct carcinoma in a urethral diverticulum. J. Urol., 83:414, 1960.

Hirschhorn, R. C.: A new surgical technique for removal of urethral diverticula in the female patient. J. Urol., 92:206, 1964.

Houser, L. M., and VonEschenbach, A. C.: Diverticula of female urethra. Diagnostic importance of postvoiding film. Urology, 3:453, 1974.

Huffman, J. W.: The detailed anatomy of the paraurethral ducts in the adult human female. Am. J. Obstet. Gynecol., 55:86, 1948.

Huisman, A. B.: Aspects on the anatomy of the female urethra with special relation to urinary continence. Contr. Gynecol. Obstet., 10:1–31, 1983.

Hunner, G. L.: Calculus formation in a urethral diverticulum in women. Report of 3 cases. Urol. Cutan. Rev., 42:336, 1938.

Hyams, J. A., and Hyams, M. N.: New operative procedures for treatment of diverticulum of female urethra. Urol. Cutan. Rev., 43:573, 1939.

Iosif, C. S., Bekassy, Z., and Rydhstrom, H.: Prevalence of urinary incontinence in middle-aged women. Int. J. Gynecol. Obstet. 26:255, 1988.

Jacobo, E., and Greene, L. F.: Diseases of the urethra. In Buchsbaum, H. J., and Schmidt, J. D. (Eds.): Gynecologic and Obstetric Urology, 2nd ed. Philadelphia, W. B. Saunders Co., 1982, p. 445.

Jeffcoate, T. N. A.: Posterior colporrhaphy. Am. J. Obstet. Gynecol., 77:490, 1959.

Jeffcoate, T. N. A.: The principles governing the treatment of stress incontinence of urine in the female. Br. J. Urol., 37:633–643, 1965.

Jeffcoate, T. N. A., and Roberts, H.: Observation of stress incontinence of urine. Am. J. Obstet. Gynecol., 64:721, 1952.

Johnson, C. M.: Diverticula and cyst of the female urethra. J. Urol., 39:506, 1938.

Jonas, U., and Petri, E.: Genito-urinary fistulae. In Stanton, S. L.

(Ed.): Clinical Gynecologic Urology. St. Louis, C. V. Mosby Co., 1984, pp. 238–255.

Joseph, J.: Female genital structure and function. The bones, joints and ligaments of the female pelvis. In Philipp, E., Barnes, J., and Newton, M. (Eds.): Scientific Foundations of Obstetrics and Gynecology. Chicago, Year Book Medical Publisher, 1986, pp. 86–94.

Juma, S., Little, N. A., and Raz, S.: Basic evaluation of urinary incontinence. Am. J. Kid. Dis. (In press).

Kaufman, J. M.: Urodynamics in stress urinary incontinence. J. Urol., 122:778–782, 1972.

Kaufman, J. M.: Fascial sling for stress urinary incontinence. South Med. J., 75:555, 1982.

Kegel, A. H.: Aggressive resistance exercise in the functional restoration of the perineal muscle. Am. J. Obstet. Gynecol., 56:238, 1948.

Kelly, H. A., and Dumm, W. M.: Urinary incontinence in women, without manifest injury to the bladder. Surg. Gynecol. Obstet., 18:444–450, 1914.

Kirby, E. W., Jr., and Reynolds, C. J.: Diverticula of the female urethra: Report of four cases, one containing a calculus. J. Urol., 62:498, 1949.

Klutke, C., Golomb, J., Barbaric, Z., and Raz, S.: The anatomy of stress incontinence: magnetic resonance imaging of the female bladder neck and urethra. J. Urol., 143:563, 1990.

Kuhn, R. J. P., and Hollyock, V. E.: Observations on the anatomy of the rectovaginal pouch and septum. Obstet. Gynecol., 59:445, 1982.

Kuzmarov, I. W.: Urodynamic assessment and chain cystogram in women with stress urinary incontinence. Urology, 24:236–238, 1984.

Lang, E. K., and Davis, H. J.: Positive pressure urethrography: A roentgenographic diagnostic method for urethral diverticula in the female. Radiology, 72:401, 1959.

Last, R. J.: The pelvic floor. In Last, R. J. (Ed.): Anatomy: Regional and Applied. New York, Churchill Livingstone, 1978, pp. 324–326.

Latzko, W.: Postoperative vesicovaginal fistulas. Am. J. Surg., 58:211–228, 1942.

Lawson, J.: The management of genitourinary fistulae. Clin. Obstet. Gynecol. North Am., 5:209–236, 1978.

Leach, G. E., and Bavendam, T. G.: Female urethral diverticula. Urology, 30:110, 1987.

Leach, G. E., and Raz, S.: Vaginal flap technique: A method of transvaginal vesicovaginal fistula repair. In Raz, S. (Ed.): Female Urology. Philadelphia, W. B. Saunders Co., 1983, pp. 372–377.

Leach, G. E., Schmidbauer, H., Hadley, H. R., Staskin, D. R., Zimmern, P., and Raz, S.: Surgical treatment of female urethral diverticulum. Semin. Urol., 4:33, 1986.

Leach, G. E., Zimmern, P., Staskin, D., Schmidbauer, C. P., Hadley, H. R., and Raz, S.: Surgery for pelvic prolapse. Semin. Urol., 4:43–50, 1986.

Lee, T. G., and Keller, F. S.: Urethral diverticulum: Diagnosis by ultrasound. Am. J. Roentgenol., 128:690, 1977.

Loughlin, K. R., Gittes, R. F., Klein, L. A., and Whitmore, W. F.: The comparative medical costs of 2 major procedures available for the treatment of stress urinary incontinence. J. Urol., 127:436, 1982.

Marchetti, A. A., Marshall, V. F., and Shultis, L. D.: Simple vesicourethral suspension. A survey. Am. J. Obstet. Gynecol., 74:57–63, 1957.

Marshall, S., and Hirsch, K.: Carcinoma within urethral diverticula. Urology, 10:161, 1977.

Marshall, V. F., Marchetti, A. A., and Krantz, K. E.: The correction of stress incontinence by simple vesicourethral suspension. Surg. Gynecol. Obstet., 88:509–518, 1949.

Martius, H.: Die operative Wiederherstellung der volkommen fehlenden Harnrohre und des Schiessmuskels derselben. Zentralbl. Gynak., 52:480, 1928.

Massey, A., and Abrams, P.: Urodynamics of the female lower urinary tract. Urol. Clin. North Am. 12:231–246, 1985.

Mattingly, R. F., and Borkowf, H. I.: Acute operative injury to the lower urinary tract. Clin. Obstet. Gynecol., 5:123, 1978.

Mattingly, R. F., and Thompson, J. D.: Relaxed vaginal outlet, rectocele, and enterocele. In Mattingly, R. F., and Thompson, J. D., (Eds.): TeLinde's Operative Gynecology. Philadelphia, J. B. Lippincott Co., 1985, pp. 569–594.

Mattingly, R. F., and Thompson, J. D.: Malpositions of the uterus. In Mattingly, R. F., and Thompson, J. D. (Eds.): TeLinde's Operative Gynecology. Philadelphia, J. B. Lippincott Co., 1985, pp. 541–567.

McCall, M. L.: Posterior culdeplasty: surgical correction of enterocele during vaginal hysterectomy: a preliminary report. Obstet. Gynecol., 10:595, 1957.

McGuire, E. J., Leston, W., and Wang, S.: Transvaginal urethrolysis after obstructive urethral suspension procedures. J. Urol., 142:1037–1039, 1989.

McGuire, E. J.: Bladder instability and stress incontinence. Neurourol. Urodyn., 7:563–567, 1988.

McGuire, E. J.: Adult female urology. In Yalla, S. V., McGuire, E. J., Elbadawi, A., and Blaivas, J. G. (Eds.): Neurourology and Urodynamics, Principles and Practice. New York, Macmillan Publishing Co., 1988, pp. 264–273.

McGuire, E. J., and Lytton, B.: The pubovaginal sling in stress urinary incontinence. J. Urol., 119:82, 1978.

McGuire, E. J., Lytton, B., Kohorn, E. I., and Pepe, V.: The value of urodynamic testing in stress urinary incontinence. J. Urol., 124:256–258, 1980.

McNally, A.: Diverticula of the female urethra. Am. J. Surg., 28:177, 1935.

Miskowiak, J., and Honnens de Lichtenberg, M.: Transurethral incision of urethral diverticulum in the female. Scand. J. Urol. Nephrol., 23:235, 1989.

Moore, T. D.: Diverticulum of female urethra: An improved technique of surgical excision. J. Urol., 68:611, 1952.

Morales, A., and VanCott, G. F.: The Gittes procedure as an improved simplification of current techniques for vesical neck suspensions. Surg. Gynecol. Obstet., 167:243, 1988.

Moschcowitz, A. V.: The pathogenesis, anatomy and cure of prolapse of the rectum. Surg., Gynecol., Obstet., 15:7, 1912.

Muellner, S. R.: Etiology of stress incontinence. Surg. Gynecol. Obstet., 88:237, 1949.

Mueller, E. J., and Drake, G. L.: A new surgical procedure for the removal of the wide-mouthed urethral diverticulum in females. Surg. Gynecol. Obstet., 168:269, 1989.

National Institute of Health Consensus Development Conference Statement. Urinary incontinence in adults. Volume 7, Number 5, 1988.

Nichols, D. H., Milley, P. S., and Randall, C. L.: Significance of restoration of normal vaginal depth and axis. Obstet. Gynecol., 36:251, 1970.

Obrink, A., and Bunne, G.: Gracilis interposition in fistulas following radiotherapy for cervical cancer: A retrospective study. Urol. Int., 33:370–376, 1978.

O'Connor, J. R.: Review of experience with vesicovaginal fistula repair. J. Urol., 123:367–369, 1980.

O'Connor, V. J., Jr., and Kropp, K. A.: Surgery of the female urethra. In Glenn, J. F., and Boyce, W. H. (Eds.): Urologic Surgery. New York, Harper & Row, 1969.

Ouslander, J., Staskin, D., Raz, S., et al.: Clinical versus urodynamic diagnosis in an incontinent geriatric female population. J. Urol., 137:68–71, 1987.

Palagiri, A.: Urethral diverticulum with endometriosis. Urology, 11:271, 1978.

Pereyra, A. J.: Simplified surgical procedure for the correction of stress urinary incontinence in women. West. J. Surg., 67:223, 1959.

Pereyra, A. J., and Lebherz, T. B.: Combined urethrovesical suspension and vaginourethroplasty for the correction of urinary stress incontinence. Obstet. Gynecol., 30:537–546, 1967.

Persky, L., Herman, G., and Guerrier, K.: Non-delay in vesicovaginal fistula repair. Urology, 13:273–275, 1979.

Peters, W. H., and Vaughan, E. D., Jr.: Urethral diverticulum in the female. Obstet. Gynecol., 47:549, 1976.

Pitkin, R. M.: Abdominal hysterectomy in the obese woman. Surg. Gynecol. Obstet., 142:532, 1976.

Pitkin, R. M.: Vaginal hysterectomy in the obese woman. Obstet. Gynecol., 49:567, 1977.

Politano, V. A., Small, M. P., Harper, J. M., and Lynne, C. M.: Periurethral Teflon injection for urinary incontinence. J. Urol., 111:180, 1974.

Porges, R. F.: Changing indications for vaginal hysterectomy. Am. J. Obstet. Gynecol., 136:153, 1980.

Presman, D., Rolnick, D., and Zumerchek, J.: Calculus formation within a diverticulum of the female urethra. J. Urol., 91:376, 1964.

Raz, S.: Modified bladder neck suspension for female stress incontinence. Urology, 17:82–85, 1981.

Raz, S., Golomb, J., and Klutke, C.: Four corner bladder and urethral suspension for moderate cystocele. J. Urol., 142:712–715, 1989.

Raz, S., Siegel, A. L., Short, J. L., and Snyder, J. A.: Vaginal wall sling. J. Urol., 141:43–46, 1989.

Raz, S., Ziegler, M., and Caine, M.: The role of female hormones in stress incontinence. Proceedings of 16th Congress of Societe International d'Urologie. Amsterdam, Paris, Dion, vol. 2, 1973, pp. 397–402.

Richardson, D. A., Scotti, R. J., and Ostergard, D. R.: Surgical management of uterine prolapse in young women. J. Reprod. Med., 34:388, 1989.

Roehrborn, C. G.: Long-term follow-up of the marsupialization technique for urethral diverticula in women. Surg. Gynecol. Obstet., 167:191, 1988.

Routh, A.: Urethral diverticulum. Br. Med. J., 1:361, 1890.

Sasnett, R. B., Mins, W. W., and Witherington, R.: Jackknife prone position for urethral diverticulectomy in women. Urology, 11:183, 1978.

Schmidbauer, C. P., Chiang, H., and Raz, S.: Surgical treatment for female geriatric incontinence. Clin. Geriatr. Med., 2:759–776, 1986.

Schmidbauer, C. P., Hadley, H. R., Staskin, D. R., Zimmern, P., Leach, G. E., and Raz, S.: Complications of vaginal surgery. Semin. Urol., 4:51, 1986.

Shapiro, R. A., and Raz, S.: Clinical applications of the radiologic evaluation of female incontinence. In Raz, S. (Ed.): Female Urology. Philadelphia, W. B. Saunders Co., 1983, pp. 123–136.

Shepard, A. M., Powell, P. H., and Ball, A. J.: The place of urodynamic studies in the investigation and treatment of female urinary tract symptoms. J. Obstet. Gynecol., 3:123–125, 1982.

Sholem, S. L., Wechsler, M., and Roberts, M.: Management of the urethral diverticulum in women: A modified operative technique. J. Urol., 112:485, 1974.

Shortliffe, L. M., Freiha, F. S., Kessler, R., Stamey, T. A., and Constantinou, C. E.: Treatment of urinary incontinence by the periurethral implantation of glutaraldehyde crosslinked collagen. J. Urol., 141:538–541, 1989.

Siegel, A. L., and Raz, S.: Surgical treatment of anatomical stress urinary incontinence. Neurourol. Urodyn., 7:569–583, 1988.

Silk, M. R., and Lebowitz, J. M.: Anterior urethral diverticulum. J. Urol., 101:66, 1969.

Smith, P.: Age changes in the female urethra. Br. J. Urol., 44:667–675, 1972.

Spence, H. M., and Duckett, J. W.: Diverticulum of the female urethra: Clinical aspects and presentation of a simple operative technique for cure. J. Urol., 104:432, 1970.

Spencer, J. R., O'Connor, V. J., and Schaeffer, A. J.: A comparison of endoscopic suspension of the vesical neck with suprapubic vesicourethropexy for treatment of stress urinary incontinence. J. Urol., 137:411, 1987.

Spencer, W. F., and Streem, S. B.: Diverticulum of the female urethral roof managed endoscopically. J. Urol., 138:147, 1987.

Spraitz, A. F., and Welch, J. S.: Diverticulum of the female urethra. Am. J. Obstet. Gynecol., 91:1013, 1965.

Stamey, T. A.: Endoscopic suspension of the vesical neck for urinary incontinence. Surg. Gynecol. Obstet., 136:547–554, 1973.

Stamey, T. A.: Endoscopic suspension of the vesical neck for urinary incontinence in females. Ann. Surg., 192:465–471, 1980.

Stanton, S. L.: The colposuspension operation for urinary incontinence. Br. J. Obstet. Gynecol., 83:890, 1976.

Staskin, D. R., Hadley, H. R., Leach, G. E., Schmidbauer, C. P., Zimmern, P., and Raz, S.: Anatomy for vaginal surgery. Semin. Urol., 4:2–6, 1986.

Staskin, D. R., Zimmern, P. E., Hadley, H. R., and Raz, S.: The pathophysiology of stress incontinence. Urol. Clin. North Am., 12:271–278, 1985.

Steg, A., Vialatte, P., and Olier, C.: Le traitement des fistules vesicovaginales par la technique de Chassar-Moir. Ann. Urol., 11:103–107, 1977.

Stephenson, T., and Wein, A. J.: The interpretation of urodynamics. In Mundy, A. R., Stephenson, T. P., and Wein, A. (Eds.): Urodynamics: Principles, Practice, and Application. New York, Churchill Livingstone, 1984, pp. 93–115.

Symmonds, R. E., and Pratt, J. E.: Vaginal prolapse following hysterectomy. Am. J. Obstet. Gynecol., 79:899, 1960.

Symmonds, R. E., Williams, T. J., Lee, R. A., et al.: Posthysterectomy, enterocele, and vaginal vault prolapse. Obstet. Gynecol., 140:852, 1981.

Tanagho, E.: Urodynamics of female urinary incontinence with emphasis on stress incontinence. J. Urol., 122:200–204, 1979.

Tauber, R., and Wapner, P.: Surgical repair of severe and recurrent urinary incontinence. Obstet. Gynecol., 30:741, 1967.

TeLinde, R. W.: Operative Gynecology. Philadelphia, J. B. Lippincott Co., 1953, p. 777.

TeLinde, R. W., and Richardson, E. H., Jr.: End results of the Richardson composite operation for uterine prolapse. Am. J. Obstet. Gynecol., 45:29, 1943.

Turner-Warwick, R.: Urinary fistulae in the female. In Harrison, J. H., Gittes, R. F., Perlmutter, A. D., et al. (Eds.): Campbell's Urology, 4th edition. Philadelphia, W. B. Saunders Co., 1979.

Twombly, G. H., and Marshall, V. F.: Repair of vesicovaginal fistula caused by radiation. Surg. Gynecol. Obstet., 83:348–354, 1946.

Van Gleen, J. M., Theeuwes, A. G. M., Eskes, T. K. A. B., and Martin, C. B., Jr.: The clinical and urodynamic effects of anterior vaginal repair and Burch colposuspension. Am. J. Obstet. Gynecol., 159:137, 1988.

Ward, G. G.: Operative technique for repair of rectocele and injury to the pelvic floor. Surg. Gynecol. Obstet., 48:399, 1929.

Ward, J. N., Draper, J. W., and Tovell, H. M. M.: Diagnosis and treatment of urethral diverticula in the female. Surg. Gynecol. Obstet., 125:1293, 1967.

Wein, A. J., Malloy, T. R., Carpiniello, V. L., Greenberg, S. H., and Murphy, J. J.: Repair of vesicovaginal fistula by a suprapubic transvesical approach. Surg. Gynecol. Obstet., 150:57–60, 1980.

Wharton, L. R., and Kearns, W.: Diverticula of the female urethra. J. Urol., 63:1063, 1950.

Wharton, L. R., and TeLinde, R. W.: Urethral diverticulum. Obstet. Gynecol., 7:503, 1956.

Winter, C. C.: Unilateral and bilateral bladder neck suspension operation for stress urinary incontinence. J. Urol., 116:47–48, 1976.

Young, H. H.: Treatment of urethral diverticulum. South. Med. J., 31:1043, 1938.

Zacharin, R. F.: Pulsion enterocele: Review of the functional anatomy of the pelvic floor. Obstet. Gynecol., 55:135, 1980.

Zacharin, R. F., and Hamilton, N. T.: Pulsion enterocele: Long-term results of an abdominoperineal technique. Obstet. Gynecol., 55:141, 1980.

Zeidman, E. J., Chiang, H., Alarcon, A., and Raz, S.: Suprapubic cystostomy using Lowsley retractor. Urology, 32:54–55, 1988.

Zimmern, P. E., Hadley, H. R., Leach, G. E., and Raz, S.: Female urethral obstruction after Marshall-Marchetti-Krantz operation. J. Urol., 138:517–520, 1987.

Zimmern, P. E., Hadley, H. R., and Raz, S.: La voie vaginale dans le traitement des fistules vesicovaginales non irradiees. J. Urologie, 90:355–359, 1984.

Zimmern, P. E., Hadley, H. R., Staskin, D. R., and Raz, S.: Genitourinary fistulae: Vaginal approach for repair of vesicovaginal fistulae. Urol. Clin. North Am., 12:361–367, 1985.

Zimmern, P. E., Schmidbauer, C. P., Leach, G. E., Staskin, D. R., Hadley, H. R., and Raz, S.: Vesicovaginal and urethrovaginal fistulae. Semin. Urol., 4:24–29, 1986.

76

URINARY INCONTINENCE IN THE FEMALE: THE STAMEY ENDOSCOPIC SUSPENSION OF THE VESICAL NECK FOR STRESS URINARY INCONTINENCE

Thomas A. Stamey, M.D.

Most of what we know about urinary continence in the normal female is from what we have learned about stress urinary incontinence (SUI). For this reason, plus the fact that SUI is very common, most of the emphasis in this chapter is on SUI, but the urologist should remember that much of the information is applicable to patients with total urinary incontinence from widely diverse causes, such as pelvic fractures, radiation incontinence, and iatrogenic surgical incontinence. The various causes of urinary incontinence are best classified on an anatomic basis; the list in Table 76–1 is based on our experience at Stanford University.

The most common causes of urinary incontinence in the female are SUI and nonobstructive, detrusor instability (spontaneous, unsuppressible contractions of the detrusor muscle). Three female patients with obstructive instability of the bladder have been treated here. Retention was a greater component of the condition than incontinence. Women can, of course, have urinary incontinence from more than one cause (see Table 76–1), for example, SUI and detrusor instability. Some women exist in whom neither SUI nor detrusor abnormalities can be demonstrated, despite the most careful examinations. Patients with SUI and iatrogenic and pelvic

trauma represent the majority of surgically curable patients. Surgical correction in these women requires restoration of the vesical neck from a dependent position in the pelvis to one high behind the symphysis pubis.

DEFINITION, HISTORY, AND PHYSICAL EXAMINATION

Definition

SUI is the most common cause of involuntary loss of urine in women. Indeed, several investigators have shown, from careful interviews with normal women, that about 50 per cent of nulliparous women occasionally experience SUI; however, the occurrence is neither frequent enough nor in sufficient quantity to be socially embarrassing. Precisely because SUI is so common, it is best defined as the involuntary loss of urine through the intact urethra, which is caused by an increase in intra-abdominal pressure and is of sufficient quantity to be socially embarrassing. It is nearly always worse when the patient is in the erect position, it is aggravated by any action or disease that increases abdominal pressure, it is never caused by contraction of the detrusor muscle, and, most important, it can be diagnosed on physical examination.

Some of the text and a few figures in this chapter have been reproduced or adapted from Stamey, T. A.: Endoscopic suspension of the vesical neck for surgically curable urinary incontinence in the female. Monogr. Urol., 2:65, 1981.

Table 76–1. CAUSES OF URINARY INCONTINENCE
IN THE FEMALE

Urethral
Stress urinary incontinence (SUI)*
Iatrogenic trauma
    Transurethral resection
    Vesical neck Y-V plasty
    Urethral diverticulectomy
    Operations for SUI
    Radiation
Pelvic trauma
Congenital anomalies
    Ectopic ureterocele
    Congenitally defective "sphincter" (short urethra)
    Epispadias with or without exstrophy

Bladder (Detrusor)
Involuntary contractions (instability)
    Nonobstructive*
    Obstructive
Acontractile detrusor (overflow)
Vesicovaginal fistulae
Functional (psychiatric)

Ureteral
Ureterovaginal fistulae
Ectopic ureter

Unknown
Women who have neither SUI nor detrusor instability*

---

*SUI, nonobstructive detrusor instability, and women who lose urine in whom neither detrusor instability nor SUI can be demonstrated account for 95 per cent or more of all incontinent women.

History

The history is important. It should exclude at least overt neuromuscular disease; it should emphasize any associated cause if the onset of incontinence was abrupt, such as pelvic surgery, and it should include a careful analysis of the physical forces producing SUI. The classic patient will lose urine with sudden increases in abdominal pressure but never in bed at night (grade I). As the incontinence worsens, lesser degrees of physical stress, such as walking, standing erect from a sitting position, or sitting up in bed, will produce incontinence (grade II). In the severest problems, especially after operative failures or severe pelvic fractures, total incontinence occurs, and urine is lost without any relation to physical activity or to position (grade III). It is important to note the grade of incontinence and even to estimate the amount of urine loss (1 to 10 sanitary napkins per day), because many basically inadequate operations will cure grade I incontinence but not grade II or III.

The history obtained from the patient depends in substantial part on the severity of the urinary incontinence. Although the historic circumstances of urinary loss are important, in surgically curable incontinence these circumstances are helpful only in grade I incontinence and may be misleading in grades II and III. For example, it is helpful to know if the patient is dry in the recumbent position, especially at night when movement is minimal, but a patient with grade II incontinence can be wet at night, whereas one with grade III incontinence is wet all of the time. The distinction between the loss of urine in small spurts from a sharp rise in abdominal pressure and the loss of urine in large amounts from a detrusor contraction that has emptied the bladder is obviously useful in suspecting a neuropathic bladder.

The introductory questions represent an attempt to characterize the degree and circumstances of urinary leakage and are listed in Table 76–2 as the first set of questions. The next set of questions represents an attempt to characterize urgency incontinence. Patients who present solely with urgency incontinence, that is, loss of urine that occurs only after they sense a desire to urinate, cannot be cured by surgery. The difficulty, however, is that at least one third to two thirds of patients with surgically curable incontinence also have urgency incontinence, and they can be cured of both problems by surgical elevation of the vesical neck. It is possible that the urgency component in patients with surgically curable incontinence is due to the well-recognized funneling and low pressure of the internal vesical neck; as detrusor pressure starts to rise, urine flows immediately into the proximal urethra, causing an uncontrollable desire to urinate. With restoration of the vesical neck from a dependent position in the pelvis to one high behind the symphysis pubis, urine presumably cannot enter the proximal urethra during the early rise in pressure just prior to voiding.

In the 1975 series of 44 patients with SUI, the preoperative and postoperative interrelationships of urgency incontinence were carefully analyzed (Stamey et al., 1975). Preoperatively, 27 of the 44 patients had some degree of urgency incontinence, and in five patients it was so marked that it accounted for most of the urinary loss. Postoperatively, 18 patients had some urgency incontinence, a group that included some who had no preoperative urgency, but the problem disappeared within 6 months in all except for two patients. One lost the sensation of urgency at 18 months, and the other's condition was controlled with anticholinergic drugs at 10 months after surgery.

In half of the 27 patients with urgency incontinence, there was a diminution or complete disappearance of preoperative urgency incontinence in the postoperative period, whereas several patients who had no preoperative urgency incontinence experienced some for a short period postoperatively. The second section of the questionnaire in Table 76–2 is designed to determine if urgency incontinence is present and, if so, how much of a problem it is to the patient; it also attempts to quantitate how much of the total urinary leakage is attributable to the urgency component. In general, our impression is that those patients with demonstrable stress incontinence on physical examination who also have a strong component of urgency incontinence often have some problems with a sensation of urgency for the first few months after surgery, even though they no longer have stress incontinence. This finding is particularly true of those patients older than 65 years of age. In the 1980 series of 203 patients, 69 patients had some component of urgency incontinence in the immediate postoperative period, but little remained after 6 months (Stamey, 1980a).

The third group of questions shown in Table 76–2 relates to characterization of voiding habits. An affirmative answer to the first question concerning suprapubic pain when the bladder is full may suggest interstitial

Table 76–2. STANFORD INCONTINENCE QUESTIONNAIRE

History
Characterization of Urinary Leakage

	Always	Sometimes	Never	Comments
Do you lose urine with any of the following?				
Coughing or sneezing..................................				
Laughing..				
Lifting..				
Active exercise (running, and so on)				
Minimal exercise (walking, light housework)				
Sleeping..				
Nervousness or increased anxiety.....................				
Leakage unrelated to any specific cause				

Is your clothing damp _____ , wet _____ , or soaking wet _____ ?
Do you use sanitary napkins _____ , tissue paper _____ , or diapers _____ for protection?
  How many protective pads do you change per day _____ ?
  Are they damp _____ , wet _____ , or saturated _____ at each change?

	YES	NO
Do you leave puddles of urine on the floor?...		
Do you lose urine by continuous dribbling?...		
Do you lose urine in small spurts?...		
If yes, is the loss of urine related to physical activity?......................................		
Do you lose urine in sudden, large amounts as if your whole bladder has emptied uncontrollably?......................		

Characterization of Urgency Incontinence

When you have the desire to urinate, do you lose urine before you can get to the bathroom or toilet seat?.................		

If yes, please indicate which of the following most accurately describes how often you lose urine before you can get to
the toilet: Everytime I have a strong desire to pass urine _____ ; half of the time
I pass urine _____ ; only occasionally when I pass urine _____ .
Does this urgency leakage represent a small amount _____ , a moderate amount _____ , or most of the total urine you
lose in a 24-hour period _____ ?

Characterization of Voiding Habits

	YES	NO
Do you have pain over your bladder when it is full?...		

How often do you pass urine during the day? Every hour or less _____ ; 1 to 2 hours _____ ;
  2 to 3 hours _____ ; 3 to 4 hours _____ ; greater than 4 hours _____ .
How often do you pass urine after going to bed? Every hour or less _____ ; 1 to 2 hours _____ ;
  2 to 3 hours _____ ; 3 to 4 hours _____ ; greater than 4 hours _____ .
Is the volume of urine you usually pass large _____ , average _____ , small _____ ,
  or very small _____ ?
Do you empty your bladder frequently, before you experience the desire to pass urine just so you
  can stay dry?
  Yes _____ , No _____ .

Miscellaneous

	YES	NO
Have you had your uterus removed (a hysterectomy)?..		
Have you had orthopedic or neurosurgical operations on your back or spinal cord?................		
Have you have previous abdominal _____ or vaginal _____ operations to cure your urinary leakage?		

cystitis. Several patients in our series had surgically curable urinary incontinence and interstitial cystitis. The latter disease, of course, is not helped by preventing urinary incontinence.

These, then, are the questions found helpful in evaluating the history of patients who present with urinary incontinence. Many other questions are found in some questionnaires (e.g., queries relating to childhood history, sensations of losing urine, sight or sound of running water causing urinary incontinence, and so on), but such questions were not useful. One of the advantages to the questionnaire presented in Table 76–2 is that the nurse or office assistant can fill it out with the patient before the patient sees the urologist.

Physical Examination

DETERMINATION OF MAXIMUM VOIDED VOLUME AND RESIDUAL URINE. While the patient's history is being taken, she is asked to force fluids until her bladder is very full and she has a strong desire to urinate. Once the bladder is filled to capacity from oral hydration, she is asked first to empty her bladder in the privacy of a bathroom using a standard toilet with a measuring pan beneath the seat. This gives the surgeon an objective measurement of maximal functional volume. Immediately after the voided volume is measured, the patient is placed on an examining table, and the bladder is catheterized with a 14 Fr. straight polyethylene catheter. The residual urine is recorded, and a specimen for urinalysis and urine culture is obtained from the catheter. Significant residual urine is often a sign of a neuropathic bladder. The absence of residual urine, however, does not exclude neurologic disease. Large residuals of several hundred milliliters are usually caused by acontractile bladders. If the patient also has surgically curable incontinence, she invariably requires intermittent catheterization after the vesical neck is suspended behind the symphysis pubis because she will be unable to void, probably for a lifetime.

FILLING THE BLADDER. The open barrel of a

50-ml syringe is attached to the end of the catheter and the bladder filled by gravity flow to a comfortable volume, usually somewhat less than the amount the patient voided. Using the simple technique of holding the catheter vertically with the attached open syringe, the filling rate is about 60 to 100 ml per minute. When the syringe is filled to the 50-ml mark, the water height is about 40 cm above the urethra. This column of water in the syringe and catheter should fall steadily throughout bladder filling until the bladder is comfortably full. At this time, the column of water in the catheter neither falls nor rises and should be less than 15 cm H_2O above the urethral meatus. Bladder instability is often defined as uninhibited spontaneous bladder contractions of 15 cm H_2O or greater; therefore, if the open syringe and catheter are carefully observed during filling, a spontaneous contraction of this magnitude is usually detected as a cessation of the constantly falling water level or sudden rise in the column of the water, which had been falling during bladder filling. This observation represents a crude analysis of bladder instability, at best.

The primary purpose of the catheter, however, is to determine the amount of the patient's residual urine and, even more importantly, to fill the bladder with a known amount of fluid at a volume comfortable to the patient. This purpose needs to be emphasized because though these observations on the presence or absence of spontaneous detrusor contractions as well as the final filling pressure are interesting and represent "free" information without increasing the time or expense of the procedure, they are rarely helpful in patients with surgically curable incontinence and are only occasionally contributory in patients with nonsurgically curable incontinence.

DEMONSTRATION OF SURGICALLY CURABLE INCONTINENCE. With the bladder comfortably full, the catheter removed, and the patient in the lithotomy position, the urologist is ready for the only critical diagnostic step: demonstration of urinary incontinence directly related to coughing. So critical is this observation that we believe surgically curable urinary incontinence in females should be defined literally, as the visual demonstration of a simultaneous loss of urine with the rise and fall of abdominal pressure during coughing. Without this simple demonstration, no patient should be operated on for urinary incontinence. With the exception of grade III total urinary incontinence, the surgeon must be wary when any patient loses urine unrelated to increased abdominal pressure.

Four of the 19 failures in the 1980 series of 203 patients (Stamey, 1980a) were operated on because of a highly suggestive history, even though loss of urine could not be demonstrated on physical examination. Not one of these patients was helped even partially. The patient's history of urinary incontinence can be unreliable, even when the highly focused and selected questionnaire presented in Table 76–2 is used. With this questionnaire, I have often entered the examining room convinced I would be dealing with uncomplicated, surgically curable urinary incontinence, only to find that incontinence could not be demonstrated with sudden elevations in abdominal pressure. However, it is also true that I have often expected nonsurgical incontinence based on the questionnaire findings only to discover gross leakage of urine with coughing. The estimate is that the questionnaire is misleading at least 20 per cent of the time, which is why the surgeon must personally examine the patient with a full bladder.

If the patient does not lose urine when examined in the lithotomy position, she is then tilted to a 45-degree upright position on the cystoscopy table to raise the resting pressure of the bladder by adding the weight of some of the abdominal contents. In the 45-degree tilted position, the surgeon can still observe the urethral meatus by spreading the labia while the patient is coughing. About 80 per cent of patients with surgically curable incontinence lose urine in the lithotomy position with coughing. Another 10 per cent require tilting to the 45-degree position. The last 10 per cent demonstrate loss of urine directly related to coughing only when examined in the standing position. In the erect position, the full weight of the abdominal contents (about 35 cm H_2O) is exerted on the bladder and becomes additive to the pressure generated by the cough.

The urologist, however, must be very careful and perservering when examining the subject in the erect position. The urethral meatus can no longer be seen when the patient coughs. Because the labia cover the urethra somewhat like a dam, leakage of urine may appear a second or so after coughing and even continue to drip after the rise in pressure from coughing has returned to normal. Furthermore, the examiner must be careful also because 90 per cent of patients with surgically curable incontinence have already been eliminated by failure to observe leakage in the lithotomy or tilted position. Thus, there is a greater chance that nonsurgical urinary incontinence or even an overt neuropathic bladder is the problem.

Most of our patients with nonsurgical urinary incontinence simply fail to demonstrate urinary leakage with coughing in the standing position. A few, however, have a cough that causes a spontaneous detrusor contraction, and 5 to 15 seconds after the cough they begin to pass a small volume of water. Because this loss of urine requires a detrusor contraction, it is clearly evident on physical examination that urinary leakage is not simultaneous with cough pressure. Moreover, the urinary loss is usually a stream of urine that slowly ceases after several ounces have been voided.

Hodgkinson (1965), who was the first to recognize these patients, called this condition "idiopathic detrusor dyssynergia." This is not common in the patients we examine with urinary incontinence, but the phenomenon is fascinating to observe and is astonishingly reproducible; most patients with nonsurgical incontinence simply fail to lose urine in any of the three positions in which we examine them.

Those patients who lose urine exactly coincident with the rise and fall of abdominal pressure have been referred to as having surgically curable urinary incontinence (Stamey, 1980a). We prefer this term to SUI because patients with total urinary incontinence (grade III), and even some with grade II incontinence, do not recognize the stress component of the incontinence.

Surgically curable incontinence is also a better term than anatomic incontinence or a number of other terms reviewed by Hodgkinson (1965), because it emphasizes that these patients can be cured of incontinence. Thus, I would propose that surgically curable urinary incontinence be defined on the basis of physical examination and that the definition be confined to those patients in whom the surgeon has visually demonstrated loss of urine exactly coinciding with the rise in abdominal pressure. All other types of incontinence, except for that in a few selected patients with neuropathic bladders and severe spontaneous detrusor contraction in whom cystolysis (Freiha and Stamey, 1979) or vaginal resection of the inferior hypogastric plexus (Hodgkinson and Drukker, 1977) can successfully denervate the bladder, have surgically incurable incontinence, at least at the present state of knowledge.

PRESENCE OF RECTOCELE OR CYSTOCELE. Every patient who is a potential candidate for endoscopic suspension of the vesical neck should be examined for the presence of a rectocele or cystocele. Endoscopic suspension corrects mild and even moderate relaxation of the anterior vaginal wall but, of course, does nothing for rectoceles. In the first 100 of our patients, three of them returned in the early postoperative course with symptomatic rectoceles protruding from the vaginal introitus; these had not been observed by the patient preoperatively. Presumably, counterpressure from the cystocele buttressed against the rectocele prevented prolapse of the rectocele from the introitus. Whatever the reason, we soon learned to recognize significant rectoceles and to repair them after suspending the bladder neck. If very large cystoceles that protrude from the introitus upon straining or standing are present, the anterior vaginal incision is simply extended to the vaginal vault or the cervix, and the cystocele is fixed before suspending the vesical neck. Mild-to-moderate cystoceles never require an extension of the routine incision and are readily corrected by the suspending bolster of dacron at the urethrovesical junction (see the discussion of the operative technique further in this chapter).

The simple right-angle blade, created by separating the usual bivalve vaginal speculum into two halves, is used for assessment of the degree of anterior or posterior vaginal wall relaxation. By lifting the cystocele or depressing the rectocele with the half blade in the midline, and then having the patient perform Valsalva's maneuver, the degree of anterior or posterior relaxation can be determined. The bivalve vaginal speculum is required, of course, to evaluate an enterocele and a vaginal vault prolapse, both of which should be excluded during the physical examination.

ROLE OF URETHROSCOPY. In summary, the instruments needed to diagnose surgically curable urinary incontinence in the urologist's office include an inexpensive urethral catheter, a 50-ml syringe, and a bottle of water (Table 76–3). Observe that cystoscopes, urethroscopes, cystometry, urethral pressure profiles, electromyography recordings, cystograms, and videotape cystourethrography are not only unnecessary but also add needless expense to the evaluation of these patients.

Table 76–3. INSTRUMENTS USED TO DIAGNOSE STRESS URINARY INCONTINENCE

1. Urethral catheter
2. Syringe
3. Bottle of water

Note: Unnecessary Measures
Urethroscope
Cystometrogram
Urethral pressure profile
EMG

Preoperative urethroscopy, with or without gas cystometry to measure the opening pressure of the urethra as advocated by an increasing number of gynecologists, is even more useless than cystometry and should not be tolerated in a health system already overburdened by skyrocketing costs. Urethroscopy often shows an open, lax urethra in the proximal two thirds, but this observation contributes nothing to the diagnosis already made by simple physical examination. Some proponents of urethroscopy attempt to justify its use for observing "trigonitis," "urethritis," and urethral polyps. None of these conditions has anything to do with surgically curable urinary incontinence. Indeed, it is highly doubtful if any of these diagnoses has anything to do with any symptomatic diseases in the female. For example, "trigonitis" does not even exist; the cystoscopic findings of a "cobblestone" or "furry-appearing" trigone actually represent congenital inclusion of normal vaginal epithelium within the bladder, which occurs in all women (Cifuentes, 1947). True "urethritis" in the female cannot be documented bacteriologically (Stamey, 1980b) and has no endoscopic hallmarks, even in the presence of overt, proven bacterial cystitis. Urethral "polyps" are secondary to chronic bacteriuria, but they usually disappear with sterilization of the infection and long-term prophylaxis to prevent reinfection. An incidental urethral diverticulum may be seen on urethroscopy, but it has no pathologic significance unless it occurs as a symptomatic urethral mass. Thus, although it is almost impossible to justify urethroscopy in the female in terms of true urethral disease, the medical profession has experienced a surge of interest among gynecologists based on the false premise that the female urethroscope offers important diagnostic information in SUI.

MARSHALL-MARCHETTI OR BONNEY TEST. We routinely perform the Marshall-Marchetti or Bonney test of elevating the internal vesical neck while the patient coughs, thereby preventing loss of urine that would otherwise appear at the urethral meatus. The test is not discriminatory in a diagnostic sense, because it is inappropriate and cannot be done in the case of urinary loss from a neuropathic bladder (i.e., there is no leakage to stop with coughing). In surgically curable urinary incontinence, the test is almost always positive. It is also technically difficult to elevate the vesical neck with the index finger and not cause direct finger pressure on the urethra. Even the slightest pressure of the finger on even the distal urethra prevents loss of urine with coughing. We have seen only one patient with surgically curable incontinence in whom urinary leakage with coughing could not be stopped by elevating the internal vesical neck. This patient had a skin graft of the anterior vaginal wall that was so thick that we could not put pressure on the vesical neck. At surgery, however, the vesical neck was elevated to a position of continence once the anterior vaginal wall was dissected free. Thus, although the Marshall-Marchetti or Bonney test is non-discriminating for diagnostic evaluation, it is psychologically comforting to the surgeon to see the urinary leakage cease with elevation of the vesical neck. Moreover, the ease of the surgical repair is usually proportional to the mobility and ease with which the tissues lateral to the vesical neck can be elevated behind the symphysis pubis. For this reason, even if the Marshall-Marchetti test is not done to prevent leakage of urine while coughing, the pliability of these tissues around the vesical neck should always be examined by the surgeon.

Before the patient is removed from the lithotomy position, a bimanual pelvic examination is performed to complete the physical examination, the rectum is examined for any masses, and the S_2, S_3, and S_4 dermatomes on the perineum are checked for sensory loss by using a sharp, broken cotton stick. Because the patient has been catheterized and may have been infected by the catheter, she is given 24 hours of an oral antimicrobial agent prophylactically, usually nitrofurantoin or trimethoprim sulfamethoxazole.

Our practice is to record these few crucial observations from the physical examination on the form presented in Table 76–4. The last entry in this table assigns a grade to the degree of urinary incontinence.

ROLE OF URINARY TRACT INFECTIONS IN INCONTINENCE. Although urinary tract infection is commonly mentioned in the literature as a cause of urinary incontinence, and patients with acute cystitis often have urgency incontinence, we have never helped a patient with stress incontinence by clearing the bacteriuria. In fact, urodynamic studies have amply shown that most patients with asymptomatic urinary tract infections have stable bladders.

RADIOLOGIC STUDIES TO DETERMINE THE ANATOMIC POSITION OF THE VESICAL NECK IN RELATION TO THE SYMPHYSIS PUBIS

Every successful operation for SUI is dependent on moving the vesical neck to a higher position behind the symphysis pubis; failure to move the vesical neck is tantamount to surgical failure. Thus, there is a practical reason—at least in surgically difficult cases—for knowing the position of the vesical neck in relation to the symphysis pubis. If the patient remains incontinent after surgery, and the surgeon has not moved the vesical neck, one does not need to look elsewhere for the cause of failure.

Although we never perform radiologic studies today in our evaluation of SUI, they are of historic interest because pre- and postoperative radiologic studies on the anatomy of SUI have done more to add to the understanding of curable incontinence in the female than has any other investigative technique. The credit belongs to Jeffcoate and Roberts (1952), who introduced the lateral urethrocystogram and to Hodgkinson (1953), who introduced and popularized the metallic bead chain urethrocystogram. Whether a catheter (Jeffcoate and Roberts, 1952) or a chain is employed to visualize the urethrovesical junction in relation to the symphysis pubis, the radiographs must be carefully done with the patient straining (but not voiding) in the erect position,

---

Table 76–4. RECORD OF IMPORTANT OBSERVATIONS FROM PHYSICAL EXAMINATION

Volume of urine voided before examination: _____ ml.
    Residual urine: _____ ml.

Volume of water used to fill bladder by gravity (should be less than volume voided before examination): _____ ml.
    Intravesical pressure at final bladder volume: _____ cm H_2O.

How much leakage occurs when the patient coughs hard?
    None _____ ; Minimal (barely dribbles out the urethra) _____ ; Moderate (water spurts 2 or 3 inches beyond the urethral meatus) _____ ; Large (water spurts 6 inches or more beyond the urethral meatus) _____ .

Was it necessary to tilt the patient to a partial upright position (30 to 45 degrees) to demonstrate loss of urine with coughing? Yes _____ ; No _____ .

Did patient have to stand in the erect position to demonstrate stress incontinence with coughing? Yes _____ ; No _____ .

Is sensation to pin prick at S_2, S_3, and S_4 dermatomes normal: Yes _____ ; No _____ .
    If no, describe abnormality: _____

Is anal sphincter tone normal? Yes _____ ; No _____ .

Rectocele: None _____ ; Slight _____ ; Moderate _____ ; Marked (protrudes through vaginal introitus) _____ .

Cystocele: None _____ ; Slight _____ ; Moderate _____ ; Marked (protrudes through vaginal introitus) _____ .

Enterocele: None _____ ; Slight _____ ; Moderate _____ ; Marked (protrudes through vaginal introitus) _____ .

Uterine-vault descent: None _____ ; Slight _____ ; Moderate _____ ; Marked (protrudes through vaginal introitus) _____ .

Grade the degree of incontinence:
    Grade I: Leakage with severe stress only (coughing, sneezing, lifting). _____

    Grade II: Leakage with minimal stress only (walking, standing, shopping). _____

    Grade III: Leakage all the time regardless of activity or position. _____

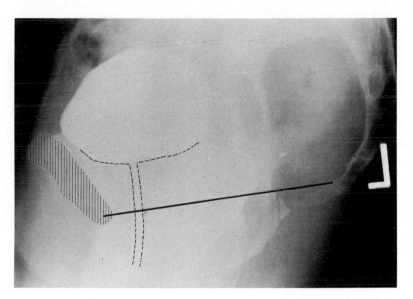

Figure 76–1. A normal, direct lateral urethrocystogram taken in the straining position from a continent female who was not operated upon. Note the high position of the urethrovesical junction behind the symphysis pubis, the flat and posteriorly directed baseplate, and the definite but slight posterior direction of the proximal urethra.

and the radiograph must be taken in a true lateral view across both hips.

The relationship of the urethrovesical junction to the symphysis pubis in the young, normal, nonparous female is shown in Figure 76–1 and is diagrammatically represented in Figure 76–2. The "normal" anatomic position (Fig. 76–2A) is compared with two types of Valsalva urethrocystograms seen in women with SUI (Fig. 76–2B and C). In both of these incontinent configurations, the urethrovesical junction tends to be cone-shaped and is located at the lowest bladder level. Typical lateral urethrocystograms in an incontinent patient before and after endoscopic suspension of the vesical neck are shown in Figures 76–3 and 76–4. Note that the position of the urethrovesical junction has been moved from below the symphyseal fifth sacral vertebral line to several centimeters above it. I reported on the pre- and postoperative lateral radiographs in 44 consecutive patients undergoing endoscopic suspension of the vesical neck (Stamey et al., 1975). In those patients operated on for the first time, the average preoperative position of the urethrovesical junction was almost 2 cm below the symphyseal-S_5 line compared with a postoperative position of 3.5 cm above the line, making the average movement of the urethrovesical junction nearly 5.5 cm (Fig. 76–5). To appreciate this movement of the urethrovesical junction fully, the surgeon should remember that the maximal movement achieved by anterior col-

porrhaphy (Kelly plication) is only 1 cm (Low, 1967; Hodgkinson, 1970).

The configuration of these radiographs does not correspond with either the incidence or the severity of the urinary incontinence, an observation recognized by both Jeffcoate and Hodgkinson. Moreover, if one measures the various angles of these radiographs in relation to the urethrovesical junction—for example, the posterior urethrovesical angle (see Fig. 76–2 A)—there is a substantial overlap between continent and incontinent women (Ala-Ketola, 1973; Greenwald et al., 1967). Despite this radiographic overlap in bladder base configuration in continent and incontinent women, the unique place of the lateral urethrocystogram lies in evaluating the efficacy of the surgery designed to restore the urethrovesical junction to a position of continence behind the symphysis pubis.

In addition to performing lateral urethrocystograms in the 44 consecutive patients we reported in 1975, we continued this routine for another 100 patients. Our observations, as well as those reported in the literature when these radiographs were consistently performed, are absolutely convincing that every successful operative procedure is always accompanied by a forward and upward displacement of the urethrovesical junction. Unsuccessful operations are usually characterized by failure to move the urethrovesical junction.

Indeed, in those few patients in whom we continue

Figure 76–2. A, Relationship of the baseplate of the bladder (directed inferiorly and slightly posteriorly toward the sacrum) in the normal continent female who has not had surgery. Note the posterior urethrovesical angle (PUV) of 90 degrees, indicating a flat baseplate with the proximal urethra; the proximal urethra is directed somewhat posteriorly.

B, Downward and backward displacement with funneling of the urethrovesical junction, characteristic of the Green type I anatomic configuration in stress urinary incontinence.

C, Further downward and backward displacement of the urethrovesical junction (Green type II).

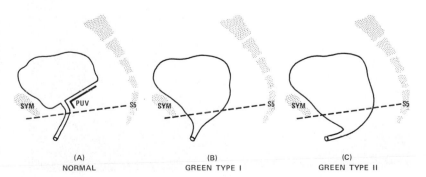

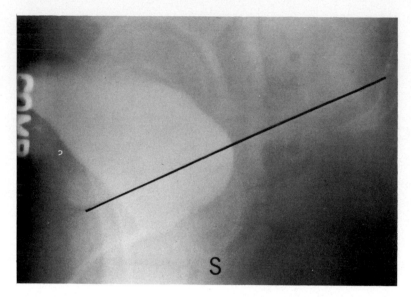

Figure 76–3. Typical preoperative lateral cystourethrogram with straining in a patient with stress urinary incontinence (Green type II). Note complete loss of posterior urethrovesical angle (180 degrees) and, more important, the fact that the urethrovesical junction is far below the inferior border of the symphysis, marked by the symphyseal-S_5 line. (From Stamey, T. A., et al.: Surg. Gynecol. Obstet., 140:355, 1975. By permission of Surgery, Gynecology & Obstetrics.)

to obtain preoperative lateral urethrocystograms to check for postoperative movement of the urethrovesical junction in case of failure, we do not measure any "angles" but rely instead on the position of the urethrovesical junction in relation to the symphysis pubis and its subsequent postoperative movement upward behind the symphysis pubis. Tanagho (1974) has also emphasized the relationship of the urethrovesical junction to the fixed bony structures of the pelvis. In this way, surgeons can answer the crucial question in an operative failure: Did they successfully move the urethrovesical junction with the operation? If they did not achieve upward and forward displacement, they do not need to blame the failure on some hypothetic functional mechanism such as an "unstable bladder."

For these reasons, we reserve preoperative radiographs of the urethrovesical junction for those patients with very complicated cases, having had multiple previous surgeries or radiation fibrosis and in whom we expect substantial difficulty in elevating the internal vesical neck. In the last several years, at the suggestion of Dr. Kenneth Wishnow, we have placed several small surgical clips on one end of the dacron buttress. This maneuver allows postoperative identification of the position of the urethrovesical junction with only a plain film lateral radiograph, thereby avoiding urethral catheterization and the use of contrast medium. Without preoperative assessment, one cannot be certain of the net change, but one of the reasons we ceased these radiologic measurements is that following endoscopic suspension, the urethrovesical junction was virtually always elevated to a position halfway up and behind the symphysis pubis (see Fig. 76–4). Simple surgical clips placed on the end of the dacron tube (see discussion of the surgical procedure), positioned away from the urethra, allow the postoperative observation to be made with a single uncomplicated radiographic study.

At times, this is surprisingly useful. For example, one patient was as incontinent in the immediate postoperative period as she was before surgery. SUI was demonstrable on physical examination. Since the surgeon had expected some difficulty because of several previous operations, he had obtained a preoperative lateral chain urethrocystogram. The operation seemed uneventful;

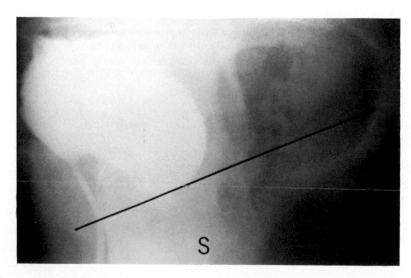

Figure 76–4. Postoperative studies in the same patient as Figure 76–3 but following endoscopic suspension with permanent cure of urinary incontinence (15-year follow-up). Observe that the urethrovesical junction is now at the upper to middle third of the symphysis pubis and that the posterior baseplate forms an acute angle with the urethrovesical junction. (From Stamey, T. A., et al.: Surg. Gynecol. Obstet., 140:355, 1975. By permission of Surgery, Gynecology & Obstetrics.)

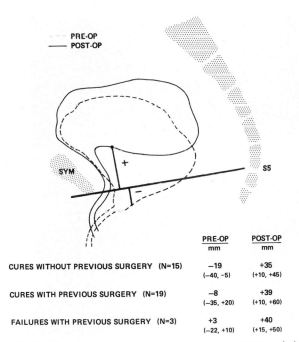

Figure 76–5. The preoperative and postoperative positions of the posterior baseplate of the bladder, 1 cm from the posterior urethrovesical junction during straining. The mean of the three patient groups, together with the minimal and maximal values observed, is presented for each category. The plus sign (+) indicates those positions above the symphyseal (SYM)-fifth sacral vertebral (S₅) line, and the minus sign (−) those below the line. (From Stamey, T. A., et al.: Surg. Gynecol. Obstet., 140:355, 1975. By permission of Surgery, Gynecology & Obstetrics.)

	PRE-OP mm	POST-OP mm
CURES WITHOUT PREVIOUS SURGERY (N=15)	−19 (−40, −5)	+35 (+10, +45)
CURES WITH PREVIOUS SURGERY (N=19)	−8 (−35, +20)	+39 (+10, +60)
FAILURES WITH PREVIOUS SURGERY (N=3)	+3 (−22, +10)	+40 (+15, +50)

the fasical levels and to be resting beneath the rectus muscle above the symphysis pubis!

This finding was not appreciated by the surgeon when he tied the suspending sutures, and we have not seen this complication before. Single buttresses on one side have pulled through in a few radiated patients, but this occurrence has always been recognized at the time of surgery. Perhaps this incident serves as a reminder that these suspending sutures must not be tied tightly and that the technique described later in this chapter should be carefully followed.

Preoperative radiographs that show normal bladder base configuration with a flat base plate and a good posterior urethrovesical angle in patients who have had previous retropubic procedures should not be disconcerting to the surgeon. We have observed and reported several patients with such normal-appearing anatomy who were cured by surgical movement of the urethrovesical junction farther upward behind the symphysis pubis, as illustrated in Figure 76–7.

From an investigative viewpoint, radiographic evaluation of the lateral urethrocystogram represents the only objective way to compare the efficacy of different operations proposed to restore the vesical neck to a higher position behind the symphysis pubis. As seen in Figure 76–5, the mean elevation of the posterior bladder base at a point 1 cm from the urethrovesical junction, achieved by endoscopic suspension of the vesical neck, is about 5 cm. A well-performed Marshall-Marchetti operation (Marshall et al., 1949), or colposuspension of the anterior vaginal wall to the iliopectineal ligament at the pelvic brim (Burch, 1961), probably gives this much elevation, but we are unaware of any substantial series in which consecutive patients have undergone pre- and postoperative radiography.

Anterior colporrhaphy, even in the best of hands, achieves only about 1 cm of elevation. In a careful radiologic study of pre- and postoperative lateral urethrocystograms in all patients undergoing anterior colporrhaphy for SUI, Low (1967) noted a 1-cm "upward and forward elevation of the bladder neck" in 50 per cent of the patients who were cured by surgery.

excellent anatomic and functional closure of the vesical neck was observed by lifting the suspending sutures singularly and in unison (see operative description). The postoperative lateral chain cystogram not only showed no change in the position of the urethrovesical junction, but also, as can be observed in Figure 76–6, the metallic clips marking the dacron buttresses (indicated by the two arrows) showed them to have pulled through all of

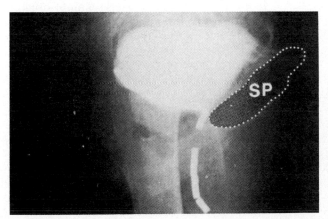
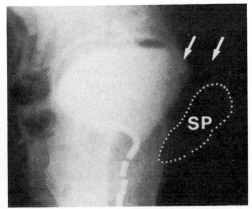

Figure 76–6. Preoperative (left) and postoperative (right) lateral chain cystourethrograms in a patient whose incontinence was not changed by uneventful endoscopic suspension of the vesical neck. Observe that the position of the urethrovesical junction in relation to the symphysis pubis is essentially unchanged, allowing for the slight difference in laterality of the radiograph. Also observe the metallic clips, placed on the end of the dacron buttress at the time of surgery. These clips (arrows) are clearly in the space of Retzius beneath the symphysis pubis and had pulled through the pubocervical and endopelvic fasciae, unknown to the surgeon. (From Stamey, T. A.: Monogr. Urol., 2:65, 1981.)

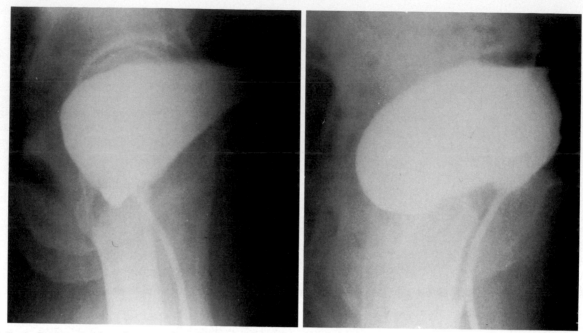

Figure 76–7. *A,* Preoperative lateral cystourethrogram with straining in patient with total urinary incontinence (grade III) who had previously undergone multiple suprapubic and vaginal operations. Note that the baseplate is not funneled in relation to the urethra; indeed, it is flat (90 degrees). Position of the urethrovesical junction is at the lower third of the symphysis pubis, which is not seen well in this radiograph. *B,* Postoperative lateral cystourethrogram during straining. Following endoscopic suspension of the vesical neck, this patient was cured of incontinence (12-year follow-up). Note that the urethrovesical junction has been moved farther upward and forward behind the symphysis pubis, despite previously normal position of the vesical neck. (From Stamey, T. A.: Monogr. Urol., 2:65, 1981.)

Because of these generally poor results when all patients with surgically curable urinary incontinence are treated by anterior colporrhaphy, Green (1968) divided urinary incontinence into type I and type II, based on the lateral urethrocystogram. He believed that although type I (Fig. 76–2B) could be successfully treated by the vaginal route, type II (Fig. 76–2C) required retropubic urethropexy. One of the advantages to endoscopic suspension of the vesical neck is that it makes no difference whether Green's type I or type II bladder configuration is present.

Most anterior colporrhaphy surgery does little to restore the urethrovesical junction. The 1-cm elevation achieved by this surgery in the best of hands can help only the mildest form of urinary incontinence. If the patient requires a vaginal hysterectomy for uterine prolapse and has mild stress incontinence, attempted plication of the internal vesical neck is clearly worthwhile. The danger, however, of overcorrection of the accompanying cystocele is that urinary incontinence can be created or stress incontinence can be made worse. This distressing complication of cystocele repair, apparently caused by creating a funnel at the vesical neck by extensive elevation of the bladder base, is recognized by most gynecologists but was emphasized by Green (1968). These difficulties have often caused the well-informed gynecologist to perform vaginal hysterectomy and retropubic exploration to suspend the vesical neck. Vaginal hysterectomy combined with endoscopic suspension of the vesical neck through the same vaginal incision offers substantial advantages to the patient. The fear of postoperative incontinence from overcorrection of a cystocele would be removed completely.

In our opinion, there is no place for micturition cystography—either single-shot static or cineradiographs—in the diagnosis and practical management of surgically curable urinary incontinence in the female. As interesting and useful as these radiologic observations have been, we have not found it necessary to perform any of these studies in our last 1000 cases.

THE ROLE OF INFLOW CYSTOMETRY, PRESSURE FLOW STUDIES OF VOIDING, AND URETHRAL CLOSURE MEASUREMENTS

If the surgeon follows these simple office evaluation procedures and demonstrates SUI on physical examination, there is usually no reason to perform routine cystometrograms with voiding and urethral pressure studies. We have performed cystometrograms with urethral closure profiles in a number of consecutive, unselected patients in our department's urodynamics laboratory: They do *not* add to the practical decision of whether or not to operate. Indeed, they have not predicted such aspects of the patient's postoperative course as how long postoperative residual urine may persist and whether urgency will continue, subside, or develop anew. In short, cystometry and urethral closure studies, like cystoscopy, are procedures that do not add to the evaluation of women with straightforward SUI, and, therefore, most patients can be spared this medical expense.

There are, however, women in whom these measurements may be useful. Rare patients (less than 1 per cent) with SUI and large post-void residual urine volumes preoperatively, who can be shown by pressure-flow studies during voiding to have acontractile bladders, can still be treated with surgical elevation of the vesical neck. This must be combined with a permanent program of intermittent catheterization. The even rarer patient (we have seen 10 in some 1000 cases), who leaks urine continuously when examined in the lithotomy position, can be shown to have a "stovepipe" urethra with virtually no closure pressure on urethral pressure studies.

Although endoscopic suspension and urethral plication cured all 10, our series is too small to show whether the simple urethral plication we added to the endoscopic suspension of the vesical neck is necessary. The urodynamic information gained in these studies of severely damaged urethras—which may be predicted by a good physical examination—probably does not justify routine urodynamic evaluation of patients with demonstrable SUI. Indeed, Dr. S. Raz has pointed out that the reason we do not need to distinguish patients with SUI, who also have incompetent urethral closure in our studies, is that the dacron buttress, in addition to preventing movement of the nylon suture, also compresses the urethra.

Constantinou, Govan, and Stamey (1986) have performed urodynamics on 151 consecutive unselected women seen in consultation for urinary incontinence. On physical examination, 84 demonstrated SUI (56 per cent), and 67 did not (44 per cent). Upon urodynamic evaluation, 62 per cent of the 84 patients with SUI had stable detrusors when examined in the upright (sitting) position. Some 30 per cent were unstable (8 per cent showed marginal instability but are not considered further). Of those patients without demonstrable SUI, 51 per cent were stable, and 43 per cent were unstable (6 per cent were marginal). Excluding the marginal insta-

bility groups (11 patients), 140 consecutive patients were available for analysis—77 with SUI and 63 without (Table 76–5).

After their maximum urinary flow rate and voided volume were measured, a 10 Fr. double-lumen urethral catheter was passed into the bladder and the residual volume was recorded. With the patient in the upright position, the bladder was filled with warm water at about 20 ml per minute. The bladder volume at first sensation and at urgency to void, the maximum detrusor pressure and urine flow rate during voiding, and the bladder capacity and residual volume after voiding were recorded. Simultaneous recordings of rectal and bladder pressures (accompanied by electronic subtraction), urine flow rates, and electromyography (EMG) tracings were made, as seen in a copy of the original tracing in Figure 76–8. Upon refilling the bladder, isometric pressures were measured in the sitting position by acutely obstructing the vesical neck with a Foley catheter balloon after the initiation of urine flow by a detrusor contraction (Constantinou et al., 1984).

Recognizing the substantial controversy over the meaning of unstable (Turner-Warwick, 1979), we defined unstable as an involuntary, unsuppressible detrusor contraction—spontaneous or evoked—during bladder filling that leads to loss of urine. Marginal instability was defined as an unsuppressible detrusor contraction with a pressure greater than 15 cm H_2O during bladder filling for which urine loss, if it occurs, cannot be determined to be voluntary or involuntary.

The data in Table 76–5 show no single characteristic of the detrusor response that distinguishes an incontinent patient with SUI from one without SUI. We believe it is best to compare stable SUI with stable non-SUI. It is true that patients with non-SUI have a significantly higher maximum detrusor pressure during voiding (p <.001) and that the unstable non-SUI women void at

Table 76–5. URODYNAMIC EVALUATION OF 140 CONSECUTIVE, UNSELECTED, INCONTINENT WOMEN WITH AND WITHOUT STRESS URINARY INCONTINENCE (SUI)

Detrusor Function	SUI (77)		Non-SUI (63)	
	Stable	*Unstable*	*Stable*	*Unstable*
N = Number of patients	52	25	34	29
Age	56 ± 13	60 ± 11	50 ± 16	43 ± 18
Catheter-free voiding				
Max. flow rate (ml/sec)	22 ± 13	21 ± 16	21 ± 15	21 ± 16
Vol. voided (ml)	260 ± 186	182 ± 117	289 ± 231	168 ± 122
Residual vol. (ml)	39 ± 71	30 ± 41	146 ± 163	84 ± 92
Cystometrograms				
Vol. at first sensation (ml)	211 ± 94	179 ± 95**	190 ± 165	144 + 77*
Vol. at urgency (ml)	410 ± 145	337 ± 179	436 ± 211	214 ± 101
Max. detrusor pressure (cm H_2O)	20 ± 13†	26 ± 15*	28 ± 15†	56 ± 26*
Max. flow rate (ml/sec)	21 ± 11	28 ± 19††	19 ± 9	20 ± 17††
Capacity (ml)	531 ± 165	384 ± 201	534 ± 204	283 ± 177
Residual vol. (ml)	40 ± 71	30 ± 41	210 ± 191	195 ± 190
Isometric tests				
Max. isometric pressure	52 ± 65	52 ± 22	46 ± 22	46 ± 21
	(N =35)	(N = 17)	(N = 9)	(N = 4)
Vol. at Max. isometric pressure	430 ± 185	284 ± 205*	494 ± 152	407 ± 127*

* = p < .001 between the two values indicated by *
** = p < .05 between the two values indicated by **
† = p < .001 between the two values indicated by †
†† = p < .01 between the two values indicated by ††
Unstable = Involuntary unsuppressible, spontaneous or provoked, detrusor contraction(s) during bladder filling that leads to loss of urine.

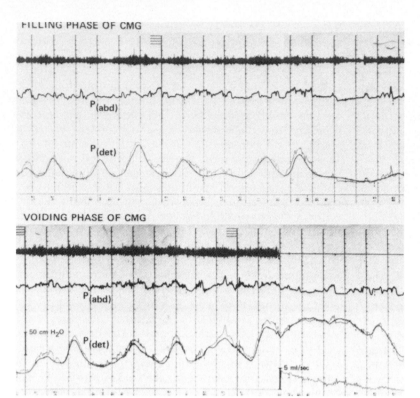

FILLING PHASE OF CMG

VOIDING PHASE OF CMG

Figure 76–8. A cystometrogram (CMG) tracing from a healthy control volunteer woman, without urinary symptoms, representative of the five-channel recording used to obtain the data in Table 76–5 during filling and voiding phases. The top line represents electromyographic activity of the external sphincter; $P_{(abd)}$, the abdominal pressure recorded from a rectal balloon; and $P_{(det)}$, the detrusor pressure from an intravesical catheter.

The solid line along the $P_{(det)}$ tracing is an electronic subtraction of $P_{(det)}$ minus $P_{(abd)}$ and therefore represents true intravesical pressure.

The declining tracing in the right lower corner illustrates urine flow rate caused by the detrusor contraction shown just above it; note the sharp diminution in CMG activity during contraction of the detrusor muscle. The spontaneous detrusor contractions of 50 cm H_2O or more are readily apparent in this healthy volunteer control. Although 25 per cent of the normal volunteers showed unstable bladders, this example of such severe instability was rare.

slower flow rates than unstable SUI women ($p < .01$). These characteristics, however, are compatible with the accepted observation that women with SUI have less urethral resistance and therefore demonstrate a smaller rise in maximum detrusor pressure, often accompanied by a faster urine flow rate.

The maximum isometric pressures (the maximum detrusor pressure in the presence of complete bladder outlet obstruction) are the same in SUI and non-SUI (see Table 76–5), indicating that the detrusor of the SUI patient is capable of generating a normal pressure in the presence of increased urethral resistance. These cystometry data reflect accepted differences in urethral resistance between women with SUI and non-SUI—differences that are more easily recognized during the physical examination by directly observing the patient to lose urine through the urethra simultaneously with a cough-induced rise in abdominal pressure (SUI).

Even at a p-value difference of $< .001$ for maximum detrusor pressures during voiding, the standard deviations are such that these parameters do not differentiate between incontinent individuals with SUI or non-SUI.

Lastly, the residual volumes in Table 76–5, measured both after the initial voiding before the urethral catheterization and after the later voiding around the catheter, are obviously larger in non-SUI women than those with SUI. Whether this finding reflects a component of even greater urethral resistance in women with non-SUI induced by the study conditions per se, we do not know. These non-SUI patients did not show a significant residual when first seen in the outpatient setting, where they were examined in less stressful circumstances.

Because we knew that endoscopic suspension of the vesical neck consistently elevated the urethrovesical junction upward and forward behind the symphysis pubis (Stamey et al., 1975), and that such elevation was curative in 90 to 95 per cent of patients operated upon, we were interested in measuring urethral closure after endoscopic suspension. These urethral closure profiles were measured in the lithotomy position with a specially made 11 Fr. catheter that contained two microtip transducers equally spaced 180 degrees apart at the tip.

This allowed us to evaluate static urethral closure profiles in the anterior and posterior urethra. As can be seen in Table 76–6, the maximum urethral closures are very much lower in women with SUI than in healthy controls without incontinence, an observation well documented in the literature (Enhörning, 1961; Toews, 1967).

Urethral closure is known to decline dramatically with age, and the controls here are less than half the age of the patients, accentuating the difference in urethral closures. Observe, however, that the anterior and posterior maximum closures are approximately equal in the controls and in the non-SUI women, but that the SUI patients demonstrate significantly decreased closures in the posterior urethra in comparison with closures observed in the anterior urethra.

Endoscopic suspension of the vesical neck does not change closure in the anterior urethra but doubles it in the posterior urethra, making it approach the closure of the anterior quadrant. Thus, the maximum impact of endoscopic suspension on resting urethral closure appears to be in restoring the posterior urethral closure to equal that of the anterior urethra. Hilton and Stanton (1983) were among the first to point out that rotational variations in the urethral closure profile may not be as artifactual as observers thought earlier.

Table 76–6. ANTERIOR AND POSTERIOR MAXIMUM URETHRAL CLOSURE IN INCONTINENT WOMEN WITH AND WITHOUT SUI IN COMPARISON WITH VOLUNTEER CONTROLS

	Volunteer Controls		Women With SUI				Women Without SUI	
			Stable Bladders		*Unstable Bladders*			
	Stable	*Unstable*	*Pre-operative*	*Post-operative*	*Pre-operative*	*Post-operative*	*Stable Bladders*	*Unstable Bladders*
Number of subjects	17	4	52	47	25	18	34	29
Age	24 ± 4	27 ± 6	56 ± 13	55 ± 15	60 ± 11	63 ± 10	50 ± 16	43 ± 18
Maximum anterior closure pressure (cm H_2O)	119 ± 25	116 ± 27	60 ± 33	45 ± 43	47 ± 38*	45 ± 43	51 ± 29	82 ± 29*
Maximum posterior closure pressure (cm H_2O)	113 ± 17	107 ± 23	44 ± 25**	58 ± 42	33 ± 20†	51 ± 34	60 ± 42**	82 ± 42†

* = $p < .01$ between the two values indicated by *
** = $p < .01$ between the two values indicated by **
† = $p < .001$ between the two values indicated by †

The resting urethral closure profiles do not afford a complete picture of urethral competence because they are static studies. Enhörning (1961) was the first to measure differential pressures between the bladder and urethra at rest and during cough-induced increases in abdominal pressure. He demonstrated that while cough-induced increases in abdominal pressure added to the closure pressure measured in the continent urethra, they were not as efficiently transferred to the incontinent urethra, thereby allowing leakage of urine with coughing because the bladder pressure exceeded the urethral pressure.

Dynamic urethral closure profiles performed at Stanford University (Constantinou et al., 1981; Constantinou and Govan, 1982) have shown that the cough-induced rise in urethral closure pressure measured in the distal urethra of control volunteers is significantly attenuated in patients with SUI. After endoscopic suspension of the vesical neck, transmission of pressure is enhanced in the distal, as well as in the proximal, urethra. Constantinou (personal communication, 1985), using a four-quadrant microtip transducer, found that these cough-induced increases in urethral pressure appear to localize to the anterior region of the urethra. This finding is contrary to the static studies, which clearly demonstrated a posterior urethral weakness that was corrected with endoscopic suspension. The explanation of these various urethral responses must await further research.

The gynecologic literature, and much of the European urologic literature as well, often warns against operating upon women with SUI who also have urgency incontinence (presumably unstable bladders). Indeed, urgency incontinence is the usual reason given for referral of patients with SUI for urodynamic evaluation. We have repeatedly emphasized, however (see references), that the presence of urgency incontinence—as long as it is clearly and demonstrably accompanied by loss of urine through the urethra exactly coinciding with the cough-induced rise in abdominal pressure—is *not* a contraindication to surgery. Neither does it appear to have an adverse influence on the ultimate course of the patient's incontinence. In fact, about two thirds of our patients operated upon for SUI have some degree of urgency incontinence by history. Moreover, our consecutive un-

selected series of 151 incontinent patients increases insight into the role of urgency incontinence.

Because 30 per cent of those with SUI showed unstable bladders at cystometry, and 51 per cent of patients with non-SUI (despite a history of urgency incontinence) failed to show detrusor instability, the presence of instability on cystometry clearly does not separate SUI from non-SUI patients. More important, the presence of preoperative instability in SUI patients is not predictive of a poor outcome following endoscopic suspension of the vesical neck.

We contacted 38 patients who were operated on for SUI who also had urgency incontinence by history. Twenty-five patients (mean follow-up 11 ± 9 months) had stable preoperative cystometry; 68 per cent of them were cured of urgency, 25 per cent were improved, and only one was worse. Of the 13 patients with SUI and instability on preoperative cystometry, 31 per cent were cured of urgency, 54 per cent said they were better, 15 per cent were the same, and none was worse (mean follow-up 12 ± 6 months).

Although the numbers of patients are small, they support a strong clinical impression that the presence of urgency incontinence—in a patient with demonstrable SUI regardless of whether instability is present on preoperative cystometry—is not a contraindication to endoscopic suspension of the vesical neck. Surgical elevation of the vesical neck for pure-urgency incontinence will not benefit the patient and may make her worse. The surgeon should recognize that to suspend the vesical neck of a patient who claims to lose urine only when she has the urge to urinate and in whom only a drop or two of urine (if any) can be demonstrated with severe coughing in the standing position is a mistake.

Although these research data are interesting from the physiologic view of characterizing continence and incontinence, they are of little practical importance in determining who will benefit from surgery. Why, then, have urodynamic investigations become so popular as a part of the evaluation of patients with urinary incontinence, especially stress urinary incontinence?

One reason is the failure of the surgeon to identify loss of urine with coughing on physical examination. Many physicians fail to make this important observation while knowing how much water is in the bladder and while looking directly at the urethra when the patient coughs. It is interesting that four major investigators in a text on this subject did not even mention this aspect of the physical examination in the preoperative evaluation of their patients with urinary incontinence. Others have gone so far as to *define* stress incontinence on the basis of cystometrographic criteria, even dismissing the validity of directly observing the physical loss of urine on coughing. In such studies there was a poor correlation between all parameters that were measured. If the surgeon does not examine the patient for urinary loss directly related to coughing, referral to a urodynamic unit with videocystourethrographic capability will probably help determine the diagnosis, but this is an expensive way to determine that a patient leaks urine simultaneously with coughing.

Another reason for excessive usage of urodynamic studies in patients with urinary incontinence may relate to surgical techniques that inconsistently elevate the urethrovesical junction to a permanent position of urinary continence. If surgeons do not recognize the anatomic reason for operative failure, they may look for a physiologic explanation. It is the use of an operation that consistently and reliably elevates the vesical neck (in this case, endoscopic suspension) that has allowed us to simplify the evaluation of women with SUI.

ENDOSCOPIC SUSPENSION OF THE VESICAL NECK (STAMEY PROCEDURE)

Endoscopic suspension of the vesical neck was first described in 1973 (Stamey, 1973). It has advantages over open retropubic urethrovesical suspensions, such as the Marshall-Marchetti-Krantz or Burch procedures. The incision is superficial, the bladder and bladder neck are not dissected, and the paraurethral tissues that suspend the vesical neck are buttressed vaginally with knitted dacron. Furthermore, this is the first incontinence operation to utilize the cystoscope to place the sutures precisely at the vesical neck. The operation is still performed as originally described. Because of the distinct advantages and relative simplicity of this operation, this technique is discussed in detail. The reader should see Chapter 75 for alternative procedures.

Preoperative Management

On admission to the hospital, the patient undergoes routine preparations, including soap suds enemas, povidone-iodine douche, and perineal and suprapubic shaving and scrubbing. Urinalysis and urine culture are obtained. Blood is not cross-matched for this procedure. Although any known urinary infection should be treated before the patient enters the hospital, a parenteral aminoglycoside (tobramycin or gentamicin, 80 mg) is given an hour before the operation is started. This dose produces a tissue level of antimicrobial agent during the

operation, which reduces the risk of postoperative pelvic infection. Since 1990, all of these patients are operated on the day of their admission to the hospital.

Anesthesia

The operation can usually be performed using a spinal block with a sensory level of anesthesia to at least T_{10}; however, the patient should be given the form of anesthesia that is best suited to her general health. At least 90 to 120 minutes of anesthetic time should be planned.

Operation

The surgeon can perform the operation from either the standing or sitting position, although I much prefer the standing position with the vagina and urethra at eye level. The patient's legs are extended laterally in the modified lithotomy position, and the knees are bent slightly to ensure a flat lower abdomen. The patient's buttocks should be placed well below the edge of the table in order to place the weighted posterior vaginal retractor.

After careful shaving and scrubbing of the entire perineum, vagina, and suprapubic area, a half towel covered by a sticky plastic drape is sutured across the perineum to exclude the rectum from the surgical field. The central sutures should include the posterior vaginal mucosa. Both labia minora are sutured laterally to expose the vaginal introitus. The legs and abdomen are draped, but the pubis and 4 to 5 cm of the suprapubic area and perineum are kept within the operative field. The cystoscopic fiberoptic cord and water tubing are draped over one leg, and the suction tubing and electrocautery are draped over the other leg.

Two symmetric transverse 2- to 3-cm skin incisions are made to the left and right of midline at the upper border of the symphysis pubis. A Mayo clamp bluntly spreads the subcutaneous tissue down to the anterior rectus fascia (Fig. 76–9). A dry 4 × 4 gauze sponge is packed into each incision while the vaginal portion of the operation is continued.

The urethral length is measured by inserting a catheter into the bladder and inflating the balloon with air. The catheter balloon is placed at the internal vesical neck without traction while the urethral meatus is marked on the catheter with a hemostat. When the catheter is withdrawn, the balloon is reinflated so that the urethral length, from balloon to hemostat, can be measured. The catheter is reinserted into the bladder, and the balloon is inflated with 10 cc of air. The weighted posterior vaginal retractor is placed.

The anterior vaginal mucosa is incised transversely below the urethral meatus, if the urethra is short (<2 cm), but deeper in the vagina nearer the vesical neck, if the urethra is long (2 cm or more). Often, a convenient vaginal fold of tissue between the vesical neck and urethral meatus can be grasped and utilized for this transverse incision. The lateral edges are cut deeper into the vagina to create a U-shaped flap (not shown in

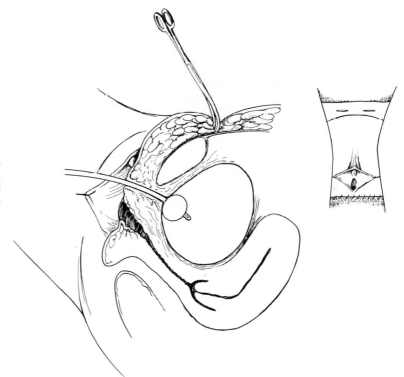

Figure 76–9. A urethral catheter is in place to aid palpation of the urethrovesical junction. Two small skin incisions are made just lateral to midline at the upper border of the pubic symphysis *(inset)*. A Mayo clamp is used to bluntly spread the subcutaneous tissue down to the anterior rectus fascia in each incision. (From Shortliffe, L. M. D., and Stamey, T. A.: In McDougal, W. S. (Ed.): Operative Urology. Kent, England, Butterworth, 1985.)

Figure 76–10, where the older, and sometimes useful, T incision is illustrated).

This transverse incision is started with the scalpel and should be 2 to 2.5 cm. The anterior vaginal wall is separated from the urethra by gently spreading the blunt, curved scissors in the plane between these tissues (Fig. 76–10*B*). The scissors must be kept parallel to the floor with the tips pointed down to prevent inadvertent entry into the bladder or urethra. The tissues alongside the vesical neck and urethra should be left undisturbed, because dissection in this area would weaken the pubocervical fascia that forms part of the suspending tissue. When the vaginal incision permits the tip of the index finger to rest against the bladder neck on each side of the catheter, it is complete.

The long, blunt, steel Stamey needles are specially designed for this procedure.* The straight needle is used in 90 per cent of cases. The needles with the tips angled 15 or 30 degrees are useful when the patient has had earlier open retropubic surgery for urinary incontinence, which may cause the bladder to be stuck to the symphysis pubis.

After the weighted retractor is removed, both the surgeon's hands are used to insert the Stamey needle into the medial edge of one of the suprapubic incisions and through the rectus fascia just above the symphysis pubis (Fig. 76–11). The superior edge of the symphysis is probed with the tip of the needle to find the undersurface of the symphysis, and the needle is now passed

---

*These needles are available from the Greenwald Surgical Company, Inc., 2688 DeKalb Street, Lake Station, Indiana 46405-1519.

Figure 76–10. *A,* The vaginal mucosal incision is made in the shape of a U or T. The transverse portion of the incision is started near the urethral meatus if the urethra is short (<2.0 cm), if it is longer, this incision is made deeper in the vagina. *B,* The anterior vaginal wall is separated from the overlying urethra. If the U-incision is used, rather than the T incision (as shown in c), the lateral edges of the transverse incision at the tip of the scissors shown in b, are cut into the vagina for about 1 cm. *C,* Once the mucosal incision is complete, dissection is continued until the incision permits the tip of the index finger to rest against the bladder neck on each side of the catheter. (From Stamey, T. A.: Surg. Gynecol. Obstet., 136:547, 1973. By permission of Surgery, Gynecology & Obstetrics.)

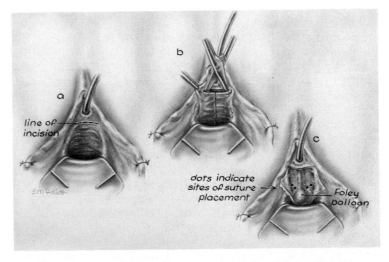

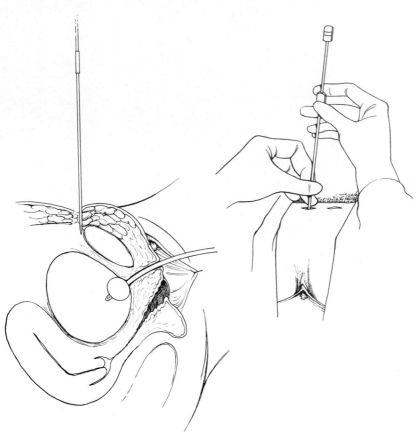

Figure 76–11. Both hands are used to direct the Stamey needle into the medial edge of one of the suprapubic incisions and through the rectus fascia just above the pubic symphysis. (From Shortliffe, L. M. D., and Stamey, T. A.: In McDougal, W. S. (Ed.): Operative Urology. Kent, England, Butterworth, 1985.)

about 1 to 2 cm parallel to the posterior surface of the symphysis pubis but immediately adjacent to the periosteum. At this point, it is important to return the needle to a more vertical position before inserting the index finger into the vaginal incision.

The left (nondominant) index finger is now placed in the vaginal incision at the ipsilateral bladder neck while the right (dominant) hand moves the needle onto the tip of this finger (Fig. 76–12). A more vertical angle of the needle is much more useful than the extreme slanting of the needle shown. Sometimes bouncing the needle vertically in the retropubic space without advancing it helps to locate the point of the needle by the left index finger. The needle is then guided alongside the vesical neck, through the endopelvic and pubocervical fasciae, and into the periurethral tissues adjacent to the bladder neck while controlled by the surgeon's left (nondominant) index finger, which is still on the needle point.

During this maneuver, the urethral catheter is held without tension in the left hand's palm, so that the catheter balloon can be felt at the bladder neck. The urethral catheter must not be tugged on because this would "telescope" the urethra and cause the surgeon to misjudge the natural position of the vesical neck.

The right-angle (70 or 110 degree lens) cystoscope is now passed into the bladder facing the 3-o'clock or 9-o'clock position of the needle, immediately lateral to the vesical neck. The cystoscope is withdrawn to the urethrovesical junction (half in the urethra and half in the bladder) to make sure that the needle has been positioned precisely outside the urethrovesical junction.

If the needle is in the correct position it will indent the ipsilateral vesical neck when the suprapubic end is moved slowly from right to left (Fig. 76–13). A vertical up-and-down motion of the needle is also helpful in identifying precise movement of the vesical neck only.

The dome and ipsilateral bladder wall are also examined to ensure that the needle did not pass into the bladder. The course of the needle outside the bladder is seen by pushing the entire needle medially, which indents the side of the bladder. In some bladders, it can be difficult to visualize the 2 or 3 cm immediately anterolateral to the corner of the vesical neck. It is important to see this area, if possible, with indentation by pushing the needle downward and medially. Otherwise a short perforation of the area can go undetected. If the needle is intramural rather than outside the bladder muscle, the same bladder indentation or fold is seen without pushing the needle medially. In such cases, especially when the fold is seen at volumes less than 250 ml, the needle should be removed and passed again more laterally. If the needle passes into the bladder or if its position is incorrect, it is removed and passed again. The posterior weighted retractor must be removed when the needles are passed so that the tissues are not distorted by posterior pressure. The bladder is carefully emptied through the cystoscope before removing it.

Once the surgeon is satisfied with the needle placement, the posterior vaginal speculum is replaced, a No. 2 monofilament nylon suture is threaded through the eye of the needle, and the needle is pulled suprapubi-

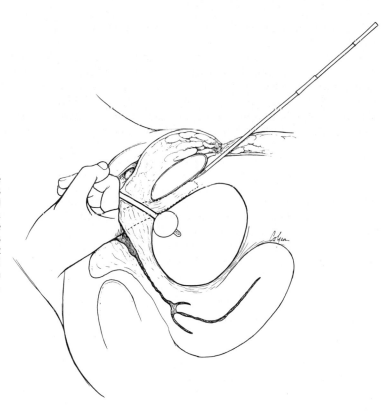

Figure 76–12. After passing through the rectus fascia, the needle is then passed along the posterior surface of the symphysis pubis for 1 to 2 cm, and then the surgeon's left index finger is placed into the vaginal incision at the bladder neck until the retropubic needle can be felt. The index finger guides the needle into the vaginal incision. The severe slanting of the needle in this illustration is somewhat misleading. It should be held almost vertically in order to properly align the vesical neck, the vaginal incision, and the upper border of the symphysis pubis. (From Shortliffe, L. M. D., and Stamey, T. A.: In McDougal, W. S. (Ed.): Operative Urology. Kent, England, Butterworth, 1985.)

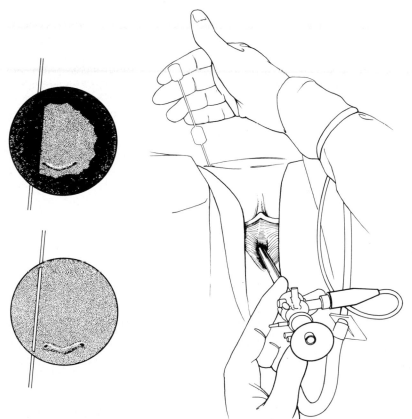

Figure 76–13. Once the needle is in place, the right angle cystoscope is passed into the bladder and withdrawn to the urethrovesical junction to make sure that the needle is placed exactly at the urethrovesical junction. If the needle is in the correct position it will indent the ipsilateral vesical neck when moved medially by the surgeon, as shown in the upper inset. Should the needle penetrate the bladder, as shown in the lower inset, the needle must be removed and repassed. (From Shortliffe, L. M. D., and Stamey, T. A.: In McDougal, W. S. (Ed.): Operative Urology. Kent, England, Butterworth, 1985.)

cally. Hemostats are placed on both the suprapubic and vaginal ends of the nylon suture.

The vaginal speculum is removed, and the needle is passed a second time 1 cm lateral to the first time, as described previously. While this pass is made, the nylon suture is put on tension by placing two additional Mayo clamps on the dangling vaginal suture. This weighted suture helps the surgeon to guide the needle 1 cm laterally. Once passed, the needle position is checked cystoscopically as before. After the vaginal speculum is replaced, the vaginal end of the nylon suture is passed through a 1-cm tube of 5-mm knitted dacron arterial graft, to buttress the vaginal tissues and to add resistance to the vesical neck, and then through the eye of the needle (Fig. 76–14). If the dacron tube is grasped lengthwise with an Allis clamp while the needle is pulled suprapubically, the two ends of the nylon suture can be balanced in the suprapubic incision, and the dacron tube can be visually guided into the area of the urethrovesical junction. The periurethral tissues on one side of the urethra are now suspended at the vesical neck. The same steps are repeated on the other side of the bladder neck.

Now for the first time the foroblique (30 or 150 degree) lens is put in the distal urethra to evaluate closure of the bladder neck when either one or both of the suspending nylon sutures is lifted (Fig. 76–15). Functional closure of the vesical neck is tested by filling the bladder with 300 to 500 ml of irrigating solution and removing the cystoscope while gently pushing down to remove the suspending tension of the dacron tubes. A stream of fluid will immediately leak from the urethral meatus but will stop promptly with gentle elevation of either or both suspending nylon sutures.

It is of physiologic interest that once the nylon sutures have been pulled upward and the flow of water out the urethra stopped, the sutures can be released without the vesical neck returning to its incontinent position of losing water out the meatus. This observation suggests that the resting position of the dacron buttresses, when placed

precisely at the vesical neck between the urethra and the puboischial arch, creates enough resistance to restore continence by itself. This observation at the least means that these suspending nylon sutures should never be tied tightly.

In an occasional person with severe periurethral scarring, unusual suture positions can cause the vesical neck to close when an individual suture is suspended but to open paradoxically when both periurethral sutures are suspended. In such instances, the suspending sutures are replaced to avoid paradoxical opening of the vesical neck, or one suture is removed and the operation is concluded with only one suspending suture at the vesical neck.

When placement of both sutures is satisfactory, the vaginal incision is irrigated with an aminoglycoside solution (usually 80 mg of tobramycin or gentamicin in 200 to 300 ml sterile water) and is closed with a continuous 2–0 chromic suture. Both pieces of dacron graft should be buried well beneath this suture line. The vaginal incision should be closed before tying the suprapubic nylon sutures, because the elevation of the bladder neck and periurethral tissues that accompanies suspension makes the incision difficult or impossible to reach afterward. We employ copious syringe irrigation with the aminoglycoside solution, because the dacron tubes represent foreign bodies and can be potentially infected by a nonsterile vaginal mucosa. A dry vaginal pack is left in the vagina overnight.

While the bladder is still full, a percutaneous polyethylene 10 to 14 Fr. suprapubic Malecot or loop (Stamey suprapubic catheters) or other percutaneous catheter may be placed. Position of the bladder is confirmed by aspirating bladder fluid with a 21-gauge spinal needle. A 3- to 4-mm incision is made 3 to 4 cm above the suprapubic incision. The polyethylene catheter with its obturator locked in position is then passed into the bladder, with the needle entering the skin at a 30-degree angle above the vertical position. The obturator is removed, and the catheter is taped into position when

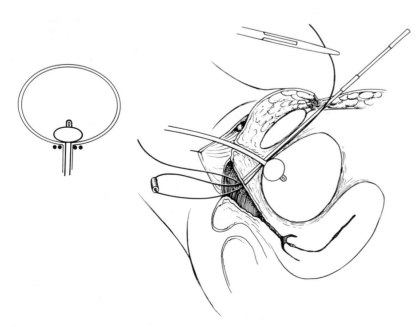

Figure 76–14. When the needle is passed the second time, 1 cm lateral to the first pass, the vaginal end of the nylon suture is passed through a 1-cm tube of 5-mm dacron arterial graft before it is pulled suprapubically. This buttresses the periurethral tissue, which holds up the suspending suture. Importantly, the dacron buttress, trapped between the vesical neck and the puboischial arch, substantially increases urethral resistance. (From Shortliffe, L. M. D., and Stamey, T. A.: In McDougal, W. S. (Ed.): Operative Urology. Kent, England, Butterworth, 1985.)

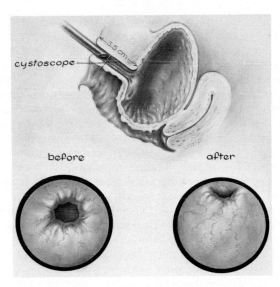

Figure 76–15. When sutures have been placed on both sides of the bladder neck, the panendoscope is put into the distal urethra to evaluate closure of the bladder neck when either or both suspending sutures are lifted. The cystoscopic views of the bladder neck before and after elevation of the sutures are shown in the insets. (From Stamey, T. A.: Surg. Gynecol. Obstet., 136:1547, 1973. By permission of Surgery, Gynecology & Obstetrics.)

the operation is finished. The final position of the catheter in the bladder can be examined with the cystoscope. If the patient has had previous low abdominal surgery and there is concern that low-lying bowel may be punctured, or if the patient is so obese that her pannus interferes with the suprapubic tube, a 16 Fr. urethral catheter can drain the bladder. In fact, this option is important. Many patients are served best by leaving a Foley catheter in the bladder overnight and then removing it along with the vaginal packing the morning after surgery.

They are then taught intermittent self-catheterization and are discharged as soon as they are confident of the technique. Of our patients, 80 per cent are discharged from the hospital the same day the Foley catheter is removed. Their hospitalization is thus limited to the single night following surgery.

Before the two suprapubic suspending sutures are tied, the incisions are irrigated with an aminoglycoside solution, and the weighted vaginal retractor is removed. The bladder is emptied with the cystoscope sheath. The two suprapubic suspending sutures are gently lifted until the loops are taut. Occasionally, it is necessary to press a finger onto the rectus fascia to remove extra slack. The tension is now released and both sutures are tied without tension so that the knot lies flat on the rectus fascia with at least five to six additional throws placed on the knot (Fig. 76–16).

As the surgeon can see with the panendoscope and the physiologic tests to stop bladder leakage, only minimal lifting of the suspending loops closes the neck and prevents incontinence; therefore, *no tension is needed.* Skin and subcutaneous tissue are closed in one layer with several interrupted vertical mattress stitches of 3–0 nylon. If the rectus fascia is shredded and weak from previous surgery or lax musculature, two flat silicone

bolsters may be made and placed on the sutures so that the knot is tied over them.

The suprapubic tube is taped onto the abdomen with waterproof adhesive tape with benzoin placed on the catheter and skin before adhesion. A mesentery on the tape extending from the catheter to the abdomen helps prevent the catheter from being dislodged. In addition, the taping of the Malecot catheter should start from the point where the tube exits from the abdomen. If the Stamey suprapubic Loop catheter is used,* taping is not required, even in massively obese women, since the loop in the dome of the bladder securely holds the catheter within the bladder. No gauze needs to be placed around the base of the catheter. A dry gauze dressing may be placed over the two suprapubic incisions.

Postoperative Management

Each patient receives only two or three additional doses of gentamicin at 8-hour intervals after surgery; then all antimicrobial therapy is stopped until the suprapubic tube is removed. The patient is discharged the day following surgery. Whether she is sent home with a suprapubic tube in place or on intermittent self-catheterization, we emphasize the following regimen: She must wait for a fairly strong urgency to urinate before attempting to do so. Each effort must always be followed by complete emptying of all residual urine, with either the suprapubic tube or self-catheterization.

We explain that Valsalva's maneuver will not help her to urinate so she must rely on detrusor contraction. Once the urgency occurs, however, if the patient is unsuccessful in voiding (always the case at first), she need not prolong suprapubic discomfort for more than a full minute while attempting to initiate urination. She is taught to measure and record the amount she voids and the amount of residual urine. A plastic disposable catch pan, placed below the toilet rim, is useful to measure both the voided and residual urine.

---

*Cook Urological, P.O. Box 227, Spencer, Indiana 47460.

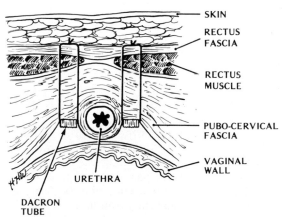

Figure 76–16. The two suprapubic suspending sutures should be tied on the rectus fascia without tension, so that the knot lies flat. (From Stamey, T. A.: Surgery, 192:465, 1980.)

Unlike patients with retropubic operations for incontinence, very few of these patients can void by the 2nd or 3rd postoperative day, even when the nylon sutures are tied without any tension whatsoever. The patients should be told that everyone ultimately voids satisfactorily without residual urine. The percutaneous suprapubic tubes are removed postoperatively or self-catheterization is terminated when the patient is able to consistently void about 75 per cent of total bladder volume. The time required for patients to achieve this degree of bladder emptying varies between 1 and 120 days; in half of the 203 patients in the 1980 series (Stamey, 1980a), the tube was removed by the 7th postsurgical day. In 14 of the 203 patients, more than 30 days were required to establish satisfactory voiding.

It is very important not to remove the supra-pubic tube or to stop self-catheterization when voided volumes are accompanied by equal residual urines, for example, 200 ml voided and 200 ml residual. Such premature action is accompanied by so much frequency and urgency that self-catheterization has to be restarted.

Oral antibiotics are started only when the suprapubic tube is removed or when intermittent self-catheterization is terminated. However, 50 mg of nitrofurantion twice a day may avoid the inevitable bacteriuria that accompanies indwelling catheters or intermittent catheterization (Stamey, 1980b).

The important culture, as always with any urinary tract infection, is that done 2 weeks after stopping all antimicrobial therapy in order to be sure that the patient has sterile urine. This can be determined along with the residual urine at one of the postoperative visits, but catheterization should be followed by 24 hours of oral antimicrobial prophylaxis to prevent reinfection of the bladder.

Postoperative Complications

Few complications have occurred (Stamey, 1981). If a suspending suture has been tied inadvertently too tightly, it can be loosened using local anesthesia and tied again (Araki et al., 1990). As I have emphasized, the nylon sutures should not be tied with tension. A spring scale has been recommended to measure the tension directly (Kondo et al., 1989), but we continue to simply tie the sutures without any discernible tension. Moreover, Yamada and associates (1991), using intraoperative ultrasound for control of vesical neck elevation, observed that suspensions of the same tension resulted in vastly different angulations of the urethrovesical junction.

While the procedure was being developed, silk and braided nylon were used for the suspending sutures, and several suprapubic wound infections occurred with both these materials. Since monofilament nylon has been used, only one patient has developed a suprapubic wound infection that forced removal of both the sutures. This occurred in a diabetic woman in whom a small periurethral abscess was discovered intraoperatively. She developed suprapubic and vaginal *Staphylococcus aureus* wound infections postoperatively.

Another complication from the suture occurred in a patient 7 years after surgery, when the suture and bolster eroded into the bladder. This complication was discovered when the patient developed irritative bladder symptoms without infection and was cystoscoped. The intravesical suture and bolster were excised flush with the mucosa endoscopically. The patient is asymptomatic and continent with only one intact suture. In fact, in one to two per cent of patients who have had this procedure, one suprapubic suture has been removed using local anesthesia for either infection or pain. When infection occurs in the suprapubic incision, it is usually from the dacron tube that has tracked along the nylon. The dacron should be removed vaginally when one suture is removed for infection. The patients have always remained continent from the other suspending suture. Osteitis pubis has not been and should not be a complication with this operation.

Vaginal dacron bolsters became a routine part of the operation after several of the initial patients had the nylon suture pull through the pubocervical and endopelvic fascia within 6 months of surgery. Since the bolsters have been used, only three patients of 1000, to our knowledge, have had the dacron buttress erode into the bladder. In another three patients, the anterior vaginal incision failed to heal completely, resulting in an exposed dacron tube. In each case, the exposed tube and suture were removed, and the patient remained continent with the single remaining suture. The important technique of tying the nylon suspension sutures without tension should eliminate this complication.

Dacron Sling Procedure for Selected Difficult Cases

In the rare patient whose periurethral fascia is too weak to hold even the dacron buttress, a simple sling procedure can be performed by placing the dacron tube beneath the urethra, as illustrated in Figure 76–17. This maneuver has been especially helpful in the very elderly woman (80 plus years), whose tissues will not hold. This dacron sling should be anchored precisely at the internal vesical neck, with a 4–0 Prolene suture. Only one needle pass is required on either side of the urethra. We have treated only four patients in this manner, with all experiencing excellent results.

Surgical Results

The results of this procedure have been reported (Stamey, 1973; Stamey et al., 1975; Stamey, 1980a). This method of elevating the bladder neck has cured 91 per cent of 203 consecutive patients. All have had at least 6 months of follow-up and 47 have had longer than 4 years. Cure was defined by absence of urinary incontinence 6 months after surgery. Nearly all failures occurred early in the postoperative period, and there was only one failure after 1 year.

Of these 203 patients, 188 had had previous surgical attempts to correct SUI, so few of these patients had

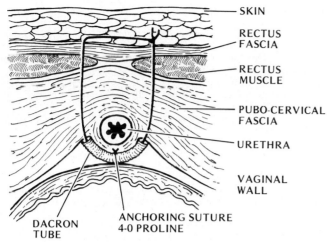

Figure 76–17. In a patient whose periurethral and pubocervical fasciae will not hold the dacron suspension lateral to the urethra at the vesical neck, a dacron sling can be applied with the tube beneath the urethra. As with all sling procedures, the support must be placed precisely at the vesical neck. To make sure the dacron tube does not slip, a 4–0 Prolene suture anchors the center of the tube at the middle of the posterior vesical neck. The Stamey needle needs to be passed only once on each side of the vesical neck.

Labels: SKIN, RECTUS FASCIA, RECTUS MUSCLE, PUBO-CERVICAL FASCIA, URETHRA, VAGINAL WALL, DACRON TUBE, ANCHORING SUTURE 4-0 PROLINE

simple grade I stress incontinence (Stamey, 1980a). In fact 20 per cent (41 of these patients) had total urinary incontinence, that is, they could hold no more than 30 ml in their bladder when standing, and 32 of these women were cured by this operation (Stamey, 1980a). These figures reveal that even women with total urinary incontinence should undergo an endoscopic suspension of the vesical neck prior to more complicated procedures or attempts at implantation of artificial sphincters.

The long-term results from this operation have not been reported since 1980 (Stamey, 1980a). My strong impression after 1000 cases is that the overall results and indications for surgery have not changed in the past 12 years. A few reoperations have been done between the 7th and 12th postoperative years, but not many. At reoperation, the old dacron buttresses should be left in place. In fact, if the needle is passed to either side of the original buttress, it can be used to reinforce the tissues with the new dacron tubes placed just below the old dacron tubes.

The presence or absence of a uterus has not affected the success of this operation. Of the 203 patients evaluated in 1980, 65 had not had hysterectomy, and the surgical result was independent of this factor (Stamey, 1980a). Indeed, in the absence of uterine prolapse, a hysterectomy for urinary incontinence alone is difficult to justify.

Ashken (1990) has also reported his results on 100 Stamey operations.

The most comprehensive follow-up (192 patients) has been reported by Walker and Texter (1992); the overall success rate was 73 per cent.

Conclusion

This method of elevating the urethrovesical neck with two permanent heavy nylon sutures is a successful means of correcting female SUI and even total urinary incontinence. It avoids the current distinction between vesical neck displacement (type I) and primary urethral failure (type II) in SUI because the *dacron* suspension cures both forms of surgically correctable incontinence. The cystoscope guides placement of the nylon sutures at the vesical neck, and the dacron buttress strengthens the suspending tissues in a way that is not accomplished in other open retropubic urethropexies.

This technique is less invasive and causes less blood loss and postoperative discomfort than many others. As a result, blood transfusion may be avoided and hospitalization shortened. It may be utilized in women who have undergone other procedures unsuccessfully and may be combined with other abdominal or vaginal procedures with good results. Furthermore, the operation is no more difficult in obese women than in thin women. Endoscopic suspension of the vesical neck is the ideal operation for the patient who has already had multiple pelvic operations, previous trauma with pelvic fractures, or prior pelvic irradiation for carcinoma. Because it has been so successful in these surgically difficult cases, it is an excellent choice for the routine case. Finally, it is a reversible operation for the occasional, dissatisfied patient who can be returned to her preoperative state by simple removal of the suprapubic nylon suture using local anesthesia in the urologist's office.

REFERENCES

Ala-Ketola, L.: Roentgen diagnosis of female stress urinary incontinence: roentgenological and clinical study. Acta Obstet. Gynecol. Scand. (Suppl.), 23:1, 1973.
Araki, T., Takamoto, H., Hara, T., Fujimoto, H., Yoshida, M., and Katayama, Y.: The loop-loosening procedure for urination difficulties after Stamey suspension of the vesical neck. J. Urol., 144:319, 1990.
Ashken, M. H.: Follow-up results with Stamey operation for stress incontinence of urine. Br. J. Urol., 65:168, 1990.
Burch, J. C.: Urethrovaginal fixation to Cooper's ligament for correction of stress incontinence, cystocele, and prolapse. Am. J. Obstet. Gynecol., 81:281, 1961.
Cifuentes, L.: Epithelium of vaginal type in the female trigone: the clinical problem of trigonitis. J. Urol., 57:1028, 1947.
Constantinou, C. E., and Govan, D. E.: Spatial distribution and timing of transmitted and reflexly generated urethral pressures in healthy women. J. Urol., 127:964, 1982.
Constantinou, C. E., Djurhuus, J. C., Silverman, D. E., et al.: Isometric detrusor pressure during bladder filling and its dependence on bladder volume and interruption to flow in control subjects. J. Urol., 131:87, 1984.
Constantinou, C. E., Faysal, M. H., Rother, L., et al.: The impact of bladder neck suspension on the mode of distribution of abdominal pressure along the female urethra. In Zinner, N. R., and Sterling, A. M. (Eds.): Female Incontinence. New York, Alan R. Liss, 1981, p. 121.
Constantinou, C. E., Govan, D. E., and Stamey, T. A.: Correlation of the physical examination with urodynamic parameters in the diagnosis of female urinary incontinence. Proceedings of the Third Joint Meeting of Urodynamics Society and International Continence Society, Boston, 1986, p. 379.
Drutz, H. P., et al.: Do static cystourethrograms have a role in the investigation of female incontinence? Am. J. Obstet. Gynecol., 130:516, 1978.
Enhörning, G.: Simultaneous recording of intravesical and intraurethral pressure. Acta Chir. Scand., 276:3, 1961.
Freiha, F. S., and Stamey, T. A.: Cystolysis: a procedure for the selective denervation of the bladder. Trans. Am. Assoc. Genitourin. Surg., 71:50, 1979.

Green, T. H., Jr.: The problem of urinary stress incontinence in the female: an appraisal of its current status. Obstet. Gynecol. Surv., 23:603, 1968.

Greenwald, S. W., Thornbury, J. R., and Dunn, L. J.: Cystourethrography as a diagnostic aid in stress incontinence. An evaluation. Obstet. Gynecol., 29:324, 1967.

Hilton, P., Stanton, S. L.: Urethral pressure measurements by microtransducer: the results in symptom-free women and in those with genuine stress incontinence. Br. J. Obstet. Gynaecol., 90:919, 1983.

Hodgkinson, C. P.: Relationships of the female urethra and bladder in urinary stress incontinence. Am. J. Obstet. Gynecol., 65:560, 1953.

Hodgkinson, C. P.: Stress urinary incontinence in the female. Surg. Gynecol. Obstet., 120:595, 1965.

Hodgkinson, C. P.: Stress urinary incontinence—1970. Am. J. Obstet. Gynecol., 108:1141, 1970.

Hodgkinson, C. P., and Drukker, B. H.: Infravesical nerve resection for detrusor dyssynergia. The Ingelman-Sandberg operation. Acta Obstet. Gynecol. Scand., 56:401, 1977.

Jeffcoate, T. N. A., and Roberts, H.: Stress incontinence of urine. J. Obstet. Gynecol. Br. Commonw., 59:685, 1952.

Kondo, A., Kato, K., Gotoh, M., Takaba, H., Tanaka, K., Kinjo, T., and Saito, M.: Quantifying thread tension is of clinical use in Stamey bladder neck suspension: analysis of clinical parameters. J. Urol., 141:38, 1989.

Low, J. A.: Management of anatomic urinary incontinence by vaginal repair. Am. J. Obstet. Gynecol., 97:308, 1967.

Marshall, V. F., Marchetti, A. A., and Krantz, K. E.: The correction of stress incontinence by simple vesicourethral suspension. Surg. Gynecol. Obstet., 88:590, 1949.

Shortliffe, L. M. D., and Stamey, T. A.: Endoscopic suspension of the vesical neck for the correction of urinary stress incontinence in the female. In McDougal, W. S. (Ed.): Operative Urology, London, Butterworth, 1985.

Stamey, T. A.: Endoscopic suspension of the vesical neck for urinary incontinence. Surg. Gynecol. Obstet., 136:547, 1973.

Stamey, T. A.: Urinary incontinence in the female: stress urinary incontinence. In Harrison, J. H., Gittes, R. F., Perlmutter, A. D., et al. (Eds.): Campbell's Urology. Vol. 3. Philadelphia, W. B. Saunders Co., p. 2282, 1979.

Stamey, T. A.: Endoscopic suspension of the vesical neck for urinary incontinence in females: Report of 203 consecutive patients. Ann. Surg., 192:465, 1980a.

Stamey, T. A.: Pathogenesis and Treatment of Urinary Tract Infections. Baltimore, The Williams & Wilkins Co., 1980b.

Stamey, T. A.: Endoscopic suspension of the vesical neck for surgically curable urinary incontinence in the female. Monogr. Urol., 2:65, 1981.

Stamey, T. A., Schaeffer, A. J., and Condy, M.: Clinical and roentgenographic evaluation of endoscopic suspension of the vesical neck for urinary incontinence. Surg. Gynecol. Obstet., 140:355, 1975.

Stanton, S. L., and Tanagho, E. A. (Eds.): Surgery of Female Incontinence. Chaps. 3, 5, 6, and 8. New York, Springer-Verlag, 1980.

Tanagho, E. A.: Simplified cystography in stress urinary incontinence. Br. J. Urol., 46:295, 1974.

Toews, H. A.: Intraurethral and intravesical pressures in normal and stress-incontinent women. J. Obstet. Gynecol., 29:613, 1967.

Turner-Warwick, R.: Observations on the function and dysfunction of the sphincter and detrusor mechanisms. Urol. Clin. North Am., 6:(1)13, 1979.

Walker, G. T., and Texter, J. H., Jr.: Success and patient satisfaction following the Stamey procedure for stress urinary incontinence. J. Urol., In press.

Yamada, T., Masuda, H., Kawakami, S., Kura, N., Watanabe, T., Nibuya, T., Negishi, T., Mizuo, T., and Oshima, H.: Application of transrectal ultrasonography in modified Stamey procedure for stress urinary incontinence. J. Urol., in press, 1991.

77
SUPRAPUBIC AND RETROPUBIC PROSTATECTOMY

Ray E. Stutzman, M.D.
Patrick C. Walsh, M.D.

INDICATIONS

The indications for prostatectomy include acute urinary retention; recurrent or persistent urinary tract infection; significant or intractable symptoms from bladder outlet obstruction; recurrent gross hematuria caused by prostatic enlargement; pathophysiologic changes of the kidneys, ureters, or bladder secondary to prostatic obstruction; and bladder calculi secondary to obstruction and decreased urine flow rate, with or without high intravesical pressures.

Over 90 per cent of prostatectomies for benign hyperplasia are performed by transurethral resection of the prostate (TURP). When the obstructive tissue is estimated to weigh more than 50 g, consideration should be given to an open (suprapubic or retropubic) procedure. If there are sizeable diverticula of the bladder that justify removal, suprapubic enucleation of the prostate and diverticulectomy may be performed. Large bladder calculi, which are not amenable to fragmentation, may also be removed during an open procedure.

Coexisting urethral disease precluding simple transurethral instrumentation is another indication for open surgery. Ankylosis of the hip preventing proper positioning for transurethral resection must also be considered. The presence of an inguinal hernia with an enlarged prostate may lead to an open procedure, because the hernia may be repaired via the same incision using a preperitoneal approach (Schlegel and Walsh, 1987).

The contraindications for an open prostatectomy include a small, fibrous gland; carcinoma of the prostate; and prior prostatectomy in which most of the gland has previously been resected or removed and in which the planes are obliterated.

PREOPERATIVE PREPARATION

The average age of patients who undergo prostatectomy is approximately 70 years. Many patients have a history of cardiovascular disease, chronic obstructive pulmonary disease, diabetes, or hypertension. A thorough evaluation of the patient is essential because this is an elective procedure, and the bladder outlet symptoms could be managed by intermittent catheterization, indwelling Foley catheter, or suprapubic cystostomy. None of these are good alternatives, however, if the patient has a reasonable surgical risk.

If the patient presents with urinary retention and an elevated serum creatinine level, one should delay surgery until renal function has stabilized. If the patient has a documented urinary tract infection, treatment should be initiated prior to planned elective surgery. Catheter drainage may be necessary.

Preoperatively, the upper urinary tract should be evaluated to provide a baseline examination and to identify any lesions or unusual anatomic variations. An intravenous urogram with a post-void film may be done, if the renal function is normal. A noninvasive and often more informative study is a sonogram. Sonography of the upper urinary tract provides an excellent screening method for hydronephrosis and other suspected masses. In addition, sonograms provide a better estimate of residual urine and prostatic size than routine intravenous pyelography (IVP). If the patient has hematuria, an IVP or a CT scan should be performed. Cystoscopy should be performed on all patients to rule out unsuspected bladder tumor, bladder stone, or large diverticulum. However, in most cases, cystoscopy should be delayed until the patient is under anesthesia just prior to surgery.

2851

Imaging of the prostate by transrectal ultrasound or magnetic resonance imaging (MRI) is not routinely performed but aids in assessing size and possible lesions.

As with any other major surgical procedure, the general health of the patient is evaluated with careful history, physical examination, and laboratory studies. The patient should be asked specifically about potential bleeding problems, e.g., those during prior surgery, dental procedures, or relatively minor injuries. He should be advised to discontinue aspirin 7 to 10 days in advance of surgery.

In addition to routine laboratory studies and an electrocardiogram, there should be a full evaluation of coagulation parameters, including prothrombin time, partial thromboplastin time, and platelet measurement. Urinalysis and urine culture are performed. Antibiotics are given to patients with established urinary tract infections and with long-term catheter drainage. An enema is given on the night prior to surgery.

At the time informed consent is obtained, the patient should be told that it is likely that he will have retrograde ejaculation and that he may become impotent postoperatively. The risks of incontinence, bleeding, urinary tract infection, and pulmonary emboli should be discussed.

Most patients can be evaluated on an outpatient basis and admitted to the hospital on the day of surgery. This practice is cost-effective and reduces the time of hospitalization.

Spinal or epidural anesthesia is preferred in all prostatectomy procedures. If regional anesthesia is contraindicated, general anesthesia with adequate relaxation may be utilized.

The transfusion of blood is required in approximately 15 per cent of patients who are undergoing open prostatectomy. It is prudent to have 2 or 3 units of blood available when contemplating an open prostatectomy. The safest transfusion is autologous blood—individual units can be drawn a week apart while the patient is on oral iron medication.

SUPRAPUBIC PROSTATECTOMY

Suprapubic or transvesical prostatectomy is the enucleation of the hyperplastic adenomatous growth of the prostate performed through an extraperitoneal incision of the anterior bladder wall. This procedure does not involve total removal of the prostate because a tissue plane exists between the adenoma and the compressed true prostate, which is left intact.

History

Eugene Fuller of New York is credited with performing the first complete suprapubic removal of a prostatic adenoma in 1894. This was a blind procedure with digital enucleation of the gland. Suprapubic and perineal drainage tubes were placed to wash out clots and control bleeding (Fuller, 1905).

Peter Freyer of London in 1900 popularized the operation and subsequently published his results of over 1600 cases (Freyer, 1900 and 1912), with a mortality rate of just over 5 per cent.

The entire operation was usually a 15-minute procedure. A 2- to 3-inch midline suprapubic incision was made, and the bladder was opened without opening the lateral tissue spaces or entering the space of Retzius.

Digital enucleation of the prostate was then performed. One or two fingers were placed in the rectum for counterpressure, while the suprapubic enucleation was accomplished. The prostatic fossa was left alone. Freyer believed that the capsule and surrounding tissues at the bladder neck would contract enough to control bleeding, somewhat after the fashion of a parturient uterus immediately after childbirth. He left an indwelling urethral catheter and a large suprapubic tube to evacuate clots (Freyer, 1900). The low mortality and morbidity rates are remarkable considering that no blood transfusions or antibiotics were available at that time. This blind enucleation procedure remained popular for over 50 years.

The low transvesical suprapubic prostatectomy with visualization of the bladder neck and prostatic fossa with placement of hemostatic sutures has supplanted the blind procedure (Harvard, 1954; Nanninga and O'Connor, 1986). This operation is presented here in more detail.

Surgical Considerations

Suprapubic prostatectomy should accomplish the following:

1. Surgical access to the bladder neck and prostate with minimal disturbance to the tissue planes via a lower abdominal incision and low urinary bladder incision.
2. Transvesical enucleation of all adenomatous tissue within the surgical capsule leaving the remaining vascular, true prostate intact.
3. Accessibility to the vesical neck and proximal prostatic fossa providing direct control and ligation of bleeding vessels near the bladder neck.
4. Accessibility of the bladder for cystolithotomy or diverticulectomy, if indicated.
5. Primary closure of the bladder with urethral and suprapubic catheter drainage.

The exposure of the prostatic fossa is comparable to that in retropubic prostatectomy, without the dissection of the retropubic space and a capsular incision.

Operative Technique

The patient is placed in the supine position with the umbilicus area positioned above the kidney rest. The table is slightly hyperextended with the patient in a mild Trendelenburg's position. The suprapubic area is shaved. The abdomen and genitalia are prepared, from nipple line to mid thigh.

Vasectomy has previously been recommended in all prostatectomies to prevent postoperative epididymitis.

This complication is now less commonly encountered. The procedure is no longer routinely performed but is left to the discretion of the surgeon.

A catheter is introduced into the urinary bladder. The bladder is irrigated and filled with 200 to 250 ml of water or saline. The catheter is then removed. A vertical midline lower abdominal incision is made through the skin and linea alba, with the incision extending from below the umbilicus to the symphysis (Fig. 77–1). The rectus muscles are retracted laterally and the prevesical space is developed, sweeping the peritoneum superiorly. It is not necessary or desirable to expose the retropubic or lateral vesical spaces. For more adequate exposure, a self-retaining retractor is utilized.

Two sutures are placed in the anterior bladder wall below the peritoneal reflection. A vertical cystotomy is made, and the incision is opened down to within 1 cm of the bladder neck (see Fig. 77–1). The bladder is inspected, and the bladder neck and prostate are visualized. A medium-sized Deaver is placed into the open bladder retracting superiorly. A narrow Deaver retractor is then placed over the bladder neck just distal to the trigone. This curved end of the Deaver provides an excellent semilunar line for incising the mucosa around the posterior bladder neck just distal to the trigone (Fig. 77–2). By this method the ureteral orifices are well visualized and are not compromised. Metzenbaum scissors are introduced at the 6-o'clock position, and by gentle dissection the plane between the adenoma and the capsule of the prostate is developed (Fig. 77–3).

The remainder of the procedure is done by digital dissection, freeing the posterior lobes down to the apex of the prostate and circumferentially sweeping anteriorly (Fig. 77–4). The urethra is firmly attached at the apex—it is preferable to use scissors to sharply incise the urethra, keeping close to the prostatic adenoma in order not to cause injury to the sphincter and subsequent incontinence. With large glands, it is often preferable to remove one lobe at a time. In the case of a large intravesical protrusion of the middle lobe, this may be removed separately.

An alternative method for incising the bladder neck and enucleating the prostate is to perform a circumferential incision around the bladder neck with either knife or electrocautery. With the index finger in the prostatic urethra, anterior pressure is exerted, splitting the urethra and the anterior commissure of the prostate. This maneuver delineates a plane between the adenoma and the true prostate or surgical capsule. The adenoma is enucleated by sweeping the finger circumferentially. The urethra at the apex of the prostate may be pinched off; however, sharp excision with Metzenbaum scissors is preferable.

Following removal of the adenoma, the prostatic fossa is inspected and a digital sweep is made to ascertain if there is any remaining nodular adenomatous tissue. Usually, minimal bleeding occurs; however, bleeding frequently occurs in the 5- and 7-o'clock positions. The prostatic arteries enter the capsule and prostate at this level near the bladder neck. Suture ligature of these vessels is done even if there is no active bleeding (Fig. 77–5). Figure-of-eight sutures of 2–0 chromic on a 5/8 circle needle provide good hemostasis. Grasping the bladder neck with Allis forceps aids in the placement of the hemostatic sutures.

A 22 Fr. 30-ml balloon three-way irrigating Foley

Figure 77–1. Suprapubic prostatectomy. Lower abdominal midline incision. A longitudinal bladder incision is made below the peritoneal reflection and extends down near the bladder neck. (From Stutzman, R. E.: Surgery of the prostate. *In* Marshall, F. F. (Ed.): Operative Urology. Philadelphia, W. B. Saunders Co., 1991.)

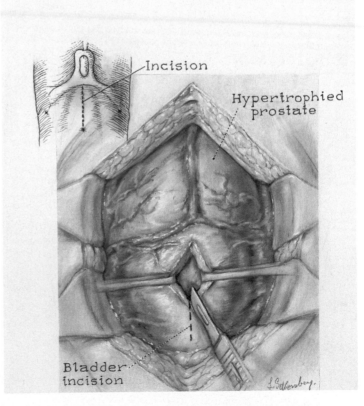

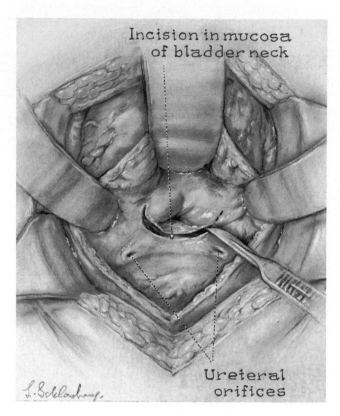

Figure 77–2. Suprapubic prostatectomy. Mucosa sharply incised at the bladder neck. (From Stutzman, R. E.: Surgery of the prostate. *In* Marshall, F. F. (Ed.): Operative Urology. Philadelphia, W. B. Saunders Co., 1991.)

Figure 77–3. Suprapubic prostatectomy. Metzenbaum scissors are used to develop the plane between the adenoma and the prostatic capsule. (From Stutzman, R. E.: Surgery of the prostate. *In* Marshall, F. F. (Ed.): Operative Urology. Philadelphia, W. B. Saunders Co., 1991.)

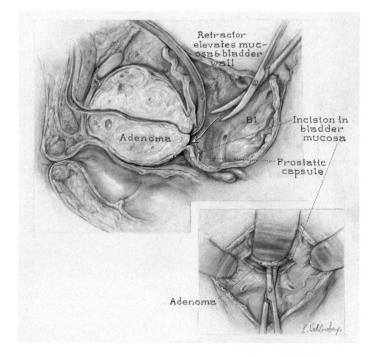

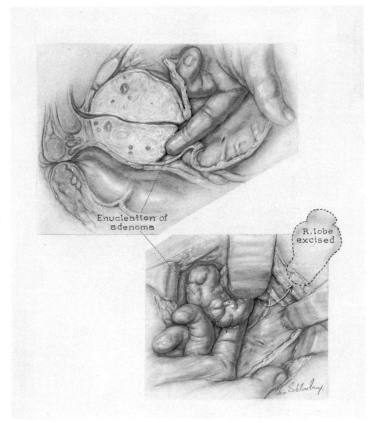

Figure 77–4. Suprapubic prostatectomy. Digital enucleation of the adenoma. (From Stutzman, R. E.: Surgery of the prostate. *In* Marshall, F. F. (Ed.): Operative Urology. Philadelphia, W. B. Saunders Co., 1991.)

catheter is passed per urethra. A 26 or 28 Fr. Malecot suprapubic tube is passed through a separate stab wound in the anterior bladder wall and brought out through a stab wound in the lower abdominal wall (Fig. 77–6). A 4–0 chromic catgut pursestring suture is placed in the bladder wall around the suprapubic tube. This maneuver prevents leakage and secures the suprapubic tube during wound closure.

We prefer a watertight, single layer, interrupted closure of the bladder with either 2–0 chromic catgut or Vicryl, just missing the bladder mucosa but including full thickness of the muscularis and serosa. A multiple layer, running suture closure of the bladder is an alternative method. The balloon of the Foley catheter is inflated to 45 cc. No catheter traction is applied. A Penrose or a closed system drain is placed down to the cystotomy site and brought out through a separate stab wound. The bladder is irrigated clear and checked for significant leakage.

The wound is irrigated and the linea alba is closed

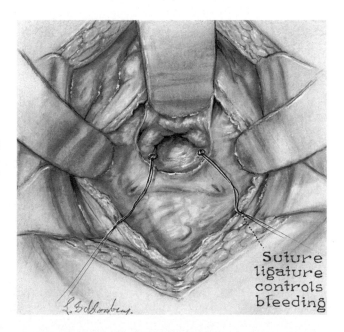

Figure 77–5. Suprapubic prostatectomy. Figure-of-eight sutures are placed at the 4-o'clock and 8-o'clock positions for hemostasis. (From Stutzman, R. E.: Surgery of the prostate. *In* Marshall, F. F. (Ed.): Operative Urology. Philadelphia, W. B. Saunders Co., 1991.)

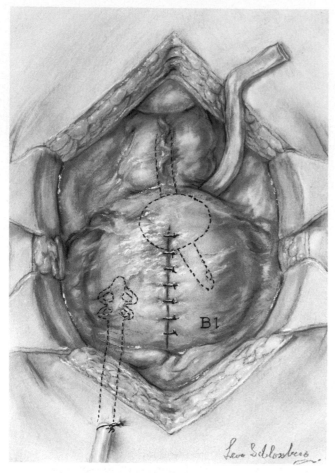

Figure 77–6. Suprapubic prostatectomy. Indwelling urethral Foley catheter, Malecot suprapubic catheter, and Penrose drain are placed with a watertight closure of the bladder incision. (From Stutzman, R. E.: Surgery of the prostate. *In* Marshall, F. F. (Ed.): Operative Urology. Philadelphia, W. B. Saunders Co., 1991.)

with a running No. 2 nylon or No. 1 polydioxanone suture (Poole, 1985). The skin is approximated with skin staples. The drain and suprapubic tube are sutured to the skin with nylon sutures. A dressing is applied.

Complications and Postoperative Management

Excessive blood loss is the most common immediate complication encountered. Approximately 15 per cent of patients require blood transfusions. If excessive bleeding from the prostatic fossa is noted intraoperatively, two techniques are effective in controlling bleeding and should be strongly considered.

Malament (1965) described the placement of a No. 1 or No. 2 nylon pursestring suture around the vesical neck, and the suture was brought out through the skin and tied snugly. This step effectively closes the bladder neck and tamponades the prostatic fossa with control of bleeding. Later, 24 to 48 hours following placement, the suture is cut on one side and removed.

O'Connor (1982) described plication of the posterior capsule using 0 chromic catgut on a 5/8 circle needle.

This plication narrows the fossa and results in effective hemostasis. Point fulguration of bleeders in the fossa may also provide hemostasis.

Surgical mortality for open prostatectomy should be less than 1 per cent. Myocardial infarction, pneumonia, and pulmonary embolus are the most common causes. Early ambulation, leg movement in bed, and breathing exercises decrease morbidity.

The patient is usually limited to intravenous fluids the day of surgery. The following day, he can usually tolerate oral nutrition, often having a full diet. A stool softener or mild laxative is given to decrease straining with bowel movements and fecal impaction. Continuous bladder irrigation via the three-way Foley catheter is maintained for 12 to 24 hours. The Foley catheter is usually removed after 3 days. The suprapubic catheter can be removed first. If the Foley is removed first, the suprapubic tube is clamped at 5 days to give the patient a trial at voiding. It is removed the following day if voiding is satisfactory with little residual. The drain is removed a few hours following removal of the suprapubic tube if there is no drainage.

The skin staples are removed on the 7th postoperative day with Steri-Strip applied. On discharge from the hospital, the patient is encouraged to gradually increase his activity. He should be able to resume full activity 4 to 6 weeks postoperatively, with outpatient visits at 3 and 6 weeks.

Delayed bleeding, as occasionally seen following TURP, is uncommon following suprapubic prostatectomy.

Wound infections occur in less than 5 per cent of patients and are usually limited to the skin and subcutaneous tissue. Urinary fistulas have been reported. Rectal injury is a very rare occurrence. Incontinence of urine is an uncommon complication and usually results from perforation and partial avulsion of the prostatic capsule and/or avulsion of the urethra at the apex of the prostate. With careful enucleation of the adenoma, the capsule should not be perforated; with sharp excision of the urethra at the apex rather than avulsion, incontinence should not occur.

Some patients may experience stress incontinence or urge incontinence, which is often caused by detrusor instability. Urethral stricture and bladder neck contracture are observed most commonly as complications of TURP and are uncommon following suprapubic prostatectomy. Erectile dysfunction following prostatectomy is reported but should not result unless the capsule has been violated. Retrograde ejaculation is common. Postoperative epididymo-orchitis is uncommon and may appear early or late. This complication is most common in patients who have had long-term indwelling catheters or urinary tract infections.

SIMPLE RETROPUBIC PROSTATECTOMY

The retropubic approach offers many advantages over the more blind suprapubic approach. Utilizing the retropubic approach, there is excellent anatomic exposure of the prostate. This enables the surgeon to visualize the interior of the prostatic cavity more easily for detection of residual adenoma and bleeding points. The urethra can be divided more accurately, reducing the risk of incontinence. Accurate control of the venous plexus can reduce intraoperative and postoperative blood loss. However, if the enlargement involves mainly the middle lobe or if one wishes to repair a bladder diverticulum at the time of surgery, the suprapubic approach is preferable. The retropubic approach for simple enucleation is not suitable for the patient with a small fibrous prostate or known prostatic cancer.

Although performed earlier by others, the technique for simple retropubic prostatectomy is credited to Terrence Millin of Ireland, who popularized the procedure and published the monograph *Retropubic Urinary Surgery* in 1947. Following this publication, the technique became widely disseminated throughout the world. It was rapidly adopted for the many virtues it offered over blind suprapubic prostatectomy and the more difficult perineal exposure of the prostate for enucleation or radical surgery.

Operative Technique

Anesthesia, Incision, Vasectomy, and Exposure of the Prostate

Epidural or spinal anesthesia is preferable because of reduced intraoperative blood loss and lower frequency of postoperative pulmonary emboli. Following cystoscopy, the patient is placed in the supine position with the table broken in the midline to extend the distance between the pubis and umbilicus. The table is tilted to 20 degrees in the Trendelenburg position.

The skin is prepared and draped in the usual way. A 22 Fr. catheter is passed into the bladder. The catheter is connected to sterile closed continuous drainage, without inflating the balloon. A right-handed surgeon always stands on the left side of the table.

A midline extraperitoneal lower abdominal incision is made, extending from the pubis to the umbilicus. The rectus muscles are separated in the midline, and the transversalis fascia is opened sharply to expose the space of Retzius. Care is taken to incise the anterior fascia down to the pubis and to incise the posterior fascia above the semicircular line to the umbilicus. Although a transverse incision provides adequate exposure and a better cosmetic result, it is more tedious to perform and may be associated with a higher frequency of subsequent inguinal hernias. The peritoneum is bluntly dissected from the pelvic sidewall, and inspection for indirect and direct hernias is carried out. If a hernia is detected, it can be repaired without difficulty (Schlegel and Walsh, 1987). During this maneuver, the vas deferens is palpated on the edge of the peritoneum, divided, and ligated. Following open simple prostatectomies of all types, the late development of epididymitis is more common because of damage to the ejaculatory ducts with subsequent reflux of infected urine into the vas deferens.

At this point, a self-retaining Balfour retractor is placed. The well-padded malleable blade displaces the bladder, posteriorly and superiorly. In radical retropubic prostatectomy, the balloon on the Foley catheter is positioned beneath the blade to facilitate this maneuver. However, because the catheter is removed early in simple retropubic prostatectomy, the balloon is not inflated and is not positioned beneath the blade. The fibrous, fatty tissue covering the superficial branch of the dorsal vein and puboprostatic ligaments is gently teased away, exposing the anterior surface of the prostate (Fig. 77–7).

Hemostasis

Virtually all investigators have advocated capsular incision and enucleation of the prostate at this point before attempts are made to obtain hemostasis. Recognizing the marked vascularity of the prostate and the excessive bleeding that occurs in many patients during these steps, it is unusual that more surgeons have not attempted to obtain hemostasis *before* enucleation.

Gregoir described a technique in which the prostatic arterial pedicles were ligated prior to enucleation (Walsh and Oesterling, 1990). However, the dorsal vein complex was not completely controlled. Based on our experience with radical retropubic prostatectomy, we have learned the value of ligation of the dorsal vein complex and have applied these principles to simple retropubic prostatectomy. To gain excellent hemostasis, one must also ligate the lateral pedicles. Using this technique it has been possible to perform the enucleation in almost a bloodless field, thus avoiding the need for transfusions (Walsh and Oesterling, 1990).

Small incisions in the endopelvic fascia are made along the pelvic sidewall, and the puboprostatic ligaments are divided. This maneuver is usually much simpler in a patient with marked prostatic enlargement because the prostate protrudes from beneath the pubic symphysis. Next, the lateral wall of the urethra is identified by palpating the indwelling catheter. Employing a right-angle clamp, the surgeon perforates the lateral pelvic fascia and passes the clamp through the avascular plane between the anterior surface of the urethra and the posterior surface of the dorsal vein complex (Fig. 77–8). At this level, the complex with its associated fascia is 1 to 2 cm thick. A 0 chromic catgut ligature is passed around the dorsal vein complex and tied. There is no need to divide the complex. Next, the lateral surface of the prostate at the prostatovesicular junction is exposed for ligation of the lateral pedicles. With 2–0 chromic catgut suture, on a large atraumatic needle, a figure-of-eight ligature is placed rather deep into the soft tissue on the posterolateral surface of the prostate, at the junction of the seminal vesicles. This maneuver should effectively control all venous and most arterial bleeding. The Foley catheter is removed prior to enucleation.

Enucleation

Attention is now turned to the anterior capsule of the prostate. Many investigators advocate the placement of

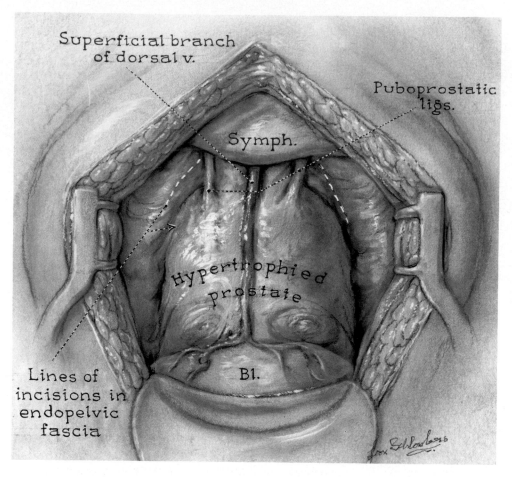

Figure 77–7. Retropubic prostatectomy. Extraperitoneal exposure of the prostate after fibrofatty tissue has been dissected free from the superficial branch of the dorsal vein and puboprostatic ligaments. Incisions in the endopelvic fascia are made on the pelvic sidewall at the site of the dotted lines. (From Walsh, P. C., and Oesterling, J. E.: Improved hemostasis during simple retropubic prostatectomy. J. Urol., 143:1203, 1990. © By Williams & Wilkins, 1990.)

stay sutures in the capsule in an effort to reduce venous bleeding and to aid later in the identification of the capsule. However, if one utilizes maneuvers previously described to control bleeding, it is not necessary to place stay sutures prior to the capsulotomy. At this point, exposure of the anterior capsule is facilitated by using a sponge stick on the bladder neck to displace the bladder posteriorly. The superficial branch of the dorsal vein at the bladder neck should be either coagulated or ligated.

A transverse capsulotomy is made with a No. 15 blade on a long handle. The incision should be made 1.5 to 2 cm distal to the bladder neck (Fig. 77–9). The incision in the capsule should be long enough to allow complete enucleation of the adenoma. Some workers have advocated a longitudinal incision. Although a longitudinal incision may have some advantages, in our opinion it should be avoided because during enucleation the incision can extend through the prostatourethral juncture, leaving the patient incontinent postoperatively. This dire complication does not occur with a transverse incision. The incision is deepened until the adenoma is reached. Next, with sharp scissors the anterior capsule is dissected free from the adenoma (see Fig. 77–7). The surgical plane is then extended with the scissors laterally and inferiorly, until a clear plane has been established around all surfaces of the anterior capsule.

Next, the right index finger is inserted between the adenoma and capsule to separate the adenoma laterally and posteriorly (Fig. 77–10). Once this part has been accomplished, a longitudinal incision is made on the anterior surface of the adenoma dividing the anterior commissure (see Fig. 77–10). At this point, the lateral lobes are separated, the index finger is inserted down to the verumontanum, and the mucosa of the urethra at the apex of the prostate overlying the left lateral lobe is fractured (see Fig. 77–8). Once these procedures have been accomplished, the left lateral lobe is safely enucleated without fear of injury to the external sphincter.

This maneuver is facilitated by grasping the prostatic lobe with a Babcock clamp. Once the left lobe has been removed, the mucosa at the apex of the right lateral lobe is fractured and removed (Fig. 77–11).

The middle lobe is isolated, the mucosa at the bladder neck is divided, and the middle lobe is dissected free. The prostatic fossa is carefully inspected for residual adenoma and bleeders (Fig. 77–12). If arterial bleeding is noted coming from the area of the bladder neck, figure-of-eight sutures of 2–0 chromic catgut should be placed at the 5- and 7-o'clock positions. Care must be taken when placing these sutures to avoid the ureteral orifices. If the ureteral orifices are difficult to visualize, especially if they were not seen during preoperative

Text continued on page 2863

Figure 77–8. Retropubic prostatectomy. After the puboprostatic ligaments have been transected, a right-angle clamp is passed immediately anterior to the urethra and the dorsal vein complex is ligated without division. Using 2–0 chromic catgut on a large atraumatic needle, figure-of-eight suture ligatures are placed rather deep into the soft tissue on the posterolateral surface of the prostate at the junction of the seminal vesicles. Note the location of the neurovascular bundle that is displaced posterior to the urethra at the apex and at the tip of the seminal vesicle at the base, thus avoiding injury during these maneuvers. (From Walsh, P. C., and Oesterling, J. E.: Improved hemostasis during simple retropubic prostatectomy. J. Urol., 143:1203, 1990. © By Williams & Wilkins, 1990.)

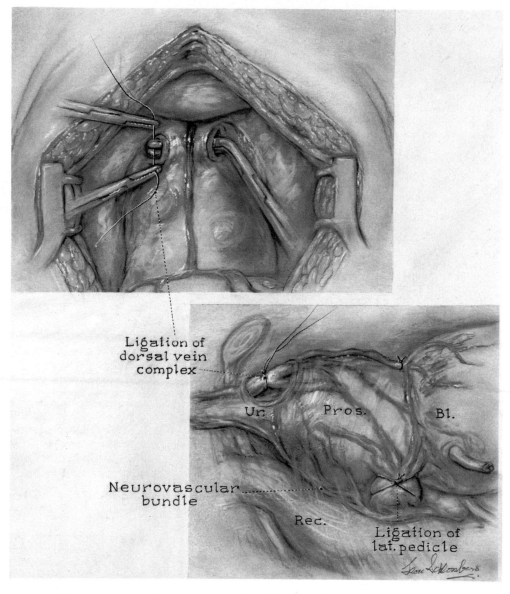

Ligation of dorsal vein complex

Neurovascular bundle

Ur.   Pros.   Bl.

Rec.

Ligation of lat. pedicle

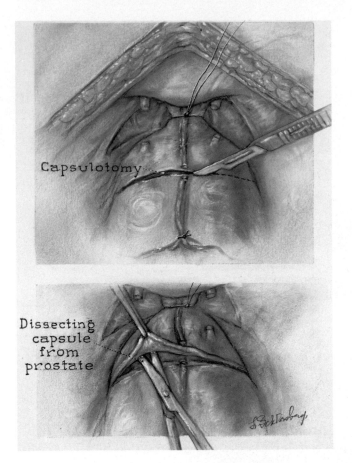

Figure 77–9. Retropubic prostatectomy. Transverse capsulotomy and separation of the anterior capsule from the adenoma. (From Walsh, P. C.: Retropubic prostatectomy for benign and malignant diseases. *In* Marshall, F. F. (Ed.): Operative Urology. Philadelphia, W. B. Saunders Co., 1991.)

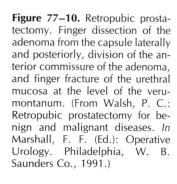

Figure 77–10. Retropubic prostatectomy. Finger dissection of the adenoma from the capsule laterally and posteriorly, division of the anterior commissure of the adenoma, and finger fracture of the urethral mucosa at the level of the verumontanum. (From Walsh, P. C.: Retropubic prostatectomy for benign and malignant diseases. *In* Marshall, F. F. (Ed.): Operative Urology. Philadelphia, W. B. Saunders Co., 1991.)

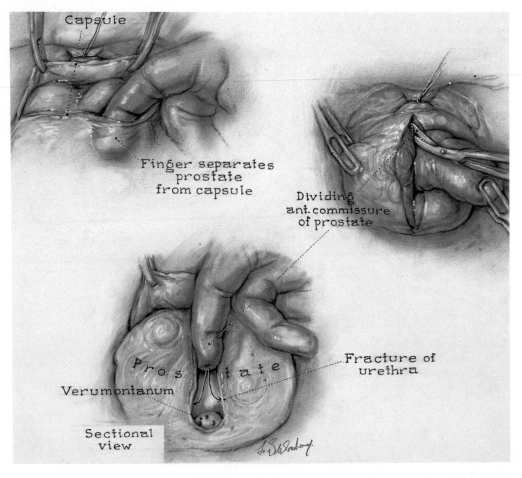

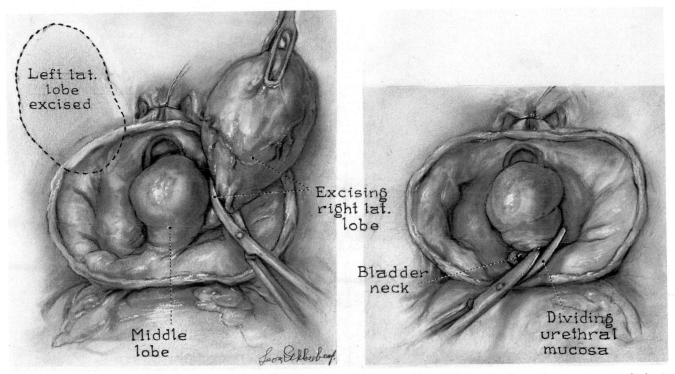

Figure 77–11. Retropubic prostatectomy. Excision of right lateral lobe and middle lobe. (From Walsh, P. C.: Retropubic prostatectomy for benign and malignant diseases. *In* Marshall, F. F. (Ed.): Operative Urology. Philadelphia, W. B. Saunders Co., 1991.)

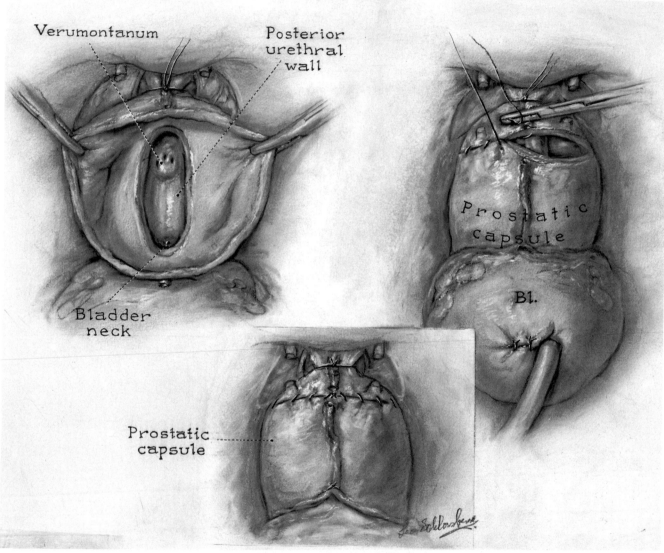

Figure 77–12. Retropubic prostatectomy. Appearance of prostatic fossa following enucleation and closure of prostatic capsule with two running, 2–0 chromic catgut sutures after insertion of the suprapubic tube and the Foley catheter. (From Walsh, P. C.: Retropubic prostatectomy for benign and malignant diseases. *In* Marshall, F. F. (Ed.): Operative Urology. Philadelphia, W. B. Saunders Co., 1991.)

cystoscopy, indigo carmine dye should be injected intravenously to aid in their identification.

Next, the bladder neck should be spread and the interior of the bladder inspected. Some surgeons advise excising a posterior wedge of the bladder neck and advancing the bladder mucosa into the prostatic fossa to avoid the development of a bladder neck contracture.

A No. 22 Foley catheter with a 30-cc balloon is passed into the prostatic fossa and directed through the bladder neck under direct vision. Prior to insertion of the catheter, a No. 24 Malecot suprapubic tube is also placed. The Malecot catheter is secured in place with a purse-string suture of 4-0 chromic catgut. The prostatic capsule is closed with two running 2-0 chromic catgut sutures on 5/8 circle tapered needles.

The first suture begins at the lateral edge of the capsulotomy and is run to the midline. The second suture begins in a similar fashion on the contralateral side. The two sutures are then tied separately in the midline and are then tied together (see Fig. 77–10). The balloon on the Foley catheter is filled with 50 ml of saline, and the catheters are irrigated. Small, closed-suction drains are placed with the ends positioned on the lateral surface of the bladder to avoid direct suction on the capsulotomy closure. The operative site is irrigated vigorously with saline, and the rectus fascia is closed with a running No. 2 nylon monofilament suture. Skin clips are used to close the skin. The catheters are carefully taped to the thigh and abdomen and irrigated.

Postoperative Care

The patient is monitored in the recovery room to make certain that hemostasis is adequate. If excessive bleeding is noted, the Foley catheter should be placed on traction and continuous bladder irrigation initiated with influx through the Foley catheter and efflux out the suprapubic cystostomy. If this step fails to control the bleeding, cystoscopy should be performed and attempts at endoscopic control should be made, before the patient is re-explored.

The patient is fed and ambulated on the 1st postoperative day. If a suprapubic tube is placed, the Foley catheter is removed when the urine is relatively clear. Once the urine is completely clear, the suprapubic tube is clamped. If the patient voids well, it is removed. When no drainage from the suction drains is observed, they can be removed the following day. The patient is discharged from the hospital between the 5th and 7th postoperative day.

Complications

The most troublesome complication of this operation is postoperative bleeding, which can arise from either the prostatic fossa or Santorini's plexus extravesically. However, if one employs the technique described in this chapter excessive bleeding should occur infrequently.

When bleeding does occur in the postoperative period, traction on the Foley catheter controls it in most cases. If this maneuver fails, an attempt at transurethral fulguration should be carried out. In rare circumstances, e.g., an unrecognized bleeding disorder, this may not suffice. One must then consider open packing of the prostatic fossa or selective angiographic embolization of the hypogastric arteries. This embolization technique can be most useful in cases in which all other measures have failed. If care is not taken in closing the prostatic capsule, prolonged urinary drainage may occur. With time and patience and persistent Foley catheter drainage this problem usually resolves without further intervention.

The other complications that may be noted early in the postoperative period are pulmonary emboli, myocardial infarction, and cerebral vascular accident, all of which are not uncommon following any operation on patients in the general age group described. Fortunately, mortality from this operation is less than 1 per cent.

Following discharge from the hospital, patients may return with a late episode of epididymitis. This complication is more common following open prostatectomy because of damage to the ejaculatory ducts with subsequent reflux of infected urine into the vas deferens. Epididymitis can largely be avoided by prophylactic vasectomy at the time of surgery.

Urgency incontinence is common immediately after the catheter has been removed and improves markedly in the first few weeks postoperatively. Severe stress incontinence is extremely uncommon if one is careful in fracturing the urethral mucosa at the verumontanum and removes the prostatic lobes individually. Preservation of the bladder neck may also reduce this possibility.

Bladder neck contractures occur late in approximately 2 per cent of patients. Although many advise wedge resection of the bladder neck with advancement of the bladder mucosa into the prostatic fossa, this maneuver does not completely eliminate the problem. The bladder neck contractures that do develop can usually be treated with cold knife incision.

Retrograde ejaculation occurs in most but not all patients postoperatively, and they should be informed of this possibility prior to surgery. Patients should also be informed of the possibility of impotence, which may affect 15 to 20 per cent. This complication is more common in older than younger men who are undergoing simple retropubic prostatectomy. With improved understanding of the etiology of impotence following radical prostatectomy, it is hoped that impotence may result less commonly.

SUMMARY

Open enucleation of the prostatic adenoma is an excellent procedure applicable in approximately 5 per cent of patients who present with significant bladder outlet obstruction. The operative mortality and morbidity are minimal.

REFERENCES

Freyer, P. J.: A new method of performing prostatectomy. Lancet, 1:774, 1900.

Freyer, P. J.: One thousand cases of total enucleation of the prostate for radical cure of enlargement of that organ. Br. Med. J., 2:868, 1912.

Fuller, E.: Six successful and successive cases of prostatectomy. J. Cutan. Genitourin. Dis., 13:229, 1895.

Fuller, E.: The question of priority in the adoption of the method of total enucleation, suprapubically, of the hypertrophied prostate. Ann. Surg., 41:520, 1905.

Harvard, B. M.: Low transvesical suprapubic prostatectomy with primary closure. *In* Campbell, M. F. (Ed.): Urology. Philadelphia, W. B. Saunders Co., 1954.

Malament, M.: Maximal hemostasis in suprapubic prostatectomy. Surg. Gynecol. Obstet., 120:1307, 1965.

Millin, T.: Retropubic Urinary Surgery. Livingstone, London, 1947.

Nanninga, J. E., and O'Connor, V. J., Jr.: Suprapubic and retropubic prostatectomy. *In* Walsh, P. C., Giltes, R. F., Perlmutter, A. D., and Stamey, T. A. (Eds.). Campbell's Urology, 5th ed. Philadelphia, W. B. Saunders Co., 1986, p. 2739.

O'Connor, V. J., Jr.: An aid for hemostasis in open prostatectomy: Capsular plication. J. Urol., 127:448, 1982.

Poole, G. V., Jr.: Mechanical factors in abdominal wound closure: The prevention of fascial dehiscence. Surgery, 97:631, 1985.

Schlegel, P. N., and Walsh, P. C.: Simultaneous preperitoneal hernia repair during radical pelvic surgery. J. Urol., 137:1180, 1987.

Walsh, P. C., and Oesterling, J. E.: Improved hemostasis during simple retropubic prostatectomy. J. Urol., 143:1203, 1990.

78
RADICAL RETROPUBIC PROSTATECTOMY

Patrick C. Walsh, M.D.

Radical prostatectomy has been employed in the cure of localized prostatic cancer for almost 100 years. Although this procedure was originally performed perineally, in 1947 Millin pioneered the retropubic approach. This technique was rapidly adopted by others and modified (Ansell, 1959; Campbell, 1959; Chute, 1954; Lich et al., 1949; Memmelaar, 1949). This offered an approach to radical prostatectomy that has proved over the years to have many advantages. The retropubic anatomy is less complicated than that in the perineal approach and is more familiar to the surgeon experienced in radical pelvic surgery. In addition, the retropubic approach leads to fewer rectal injuries. Because the urogenital diaphragm is left intact, total urinary incontinence is a rare complication.

Over the past 10 years, further insights into the periprostatic anatomy have evolved. These have led to an anatomic approach to radical prostatectomy, with reduced complications. Initially, a technique for precise control of bleeding from the dorsal vein complex was developed that enabled the surgeon to perform a more precise anatomic dissection, especially at the apex of the prostate (Reiner and Walsh, 1979). Subsequently, the anatomy of the pelvic plexus and the branches that innervate the corpora cavernosa were identified, and modifications in surgical technique were developed that enabled the surgeon to preserve or widely excise the neurovascular bundles (Walsh and Donker, 1982). With the development of techniques for the preservation of the cavernous nerves, it was possible to preserve sexual function in the majority of patients. With a better understanding of the pelvic floor musculature, the technique for apical dissection and vesicourethral anastomosis has been refined.

This chapter describes the anatomic approach to radical prostatectomy that has evolved and emphasizes techniques for vascular control that provide a bloodless field with excellent exposure, precise apical dissection to avoid injury to the pelvic floor musculature, preservation or wide excision of the neurovascular bundles where indicated, and an accurate sutured vesicourethral anastomosis with coaptation of the mucosal surfaces.

SURGICAL ANATOMY

Advances in the knowledge of the anatomy of the prostate and its adjacent structures have minimized the morbidity of retropubic exposure (Lepor et al., 1985; Lue et al., 1984; Reiner and Walsh, 1979; Schlegel and Walsh, 1987; Walsh et al., 1983; Walsh and Donker, 1982). The prostate is confined to a small recess in the pelvis where it is surrounded by the levator ani musculature and pubis and by more vulnerable structures, such as the rectum, the urogenital diaphragm with the striated sphincter, the Santorini plexus, and the autonomic branches of the pelvic plexus to the corpora cavernosa.

Arterial and Venous Anatomy

The prostate receives its arterial blood supply from the inferior vesical artery. According to Flocks (1937), after the inferior vesical artery provides small branches to the inferior, posterior extent of the seminal vesicle and the base of the bladder and prostate, the artery terminates in two large groups of prostatic vessels: the urethral and capsular groups (Fig. 78–1). The urethral vessels enter the prostate at the posterolateral vesicoprostatic junction, providing arterial supply to the vesical neck and the periurethral portion of the gland. The capsular branches run along the pelvic sidewall in the lateral pelvic fascia, traveling posterolateral to the prostate and providing branches that course ventrally and dorsally to supply the outer portion of the prostate. The capsular vessels terminate as a small cluster that supplies the pelvic floor. Histologically, the capsular group of vessels is surrounded by an extensive network of nerves (Lepor et al., 1985; Lue et al., 1984; Walsh and Donker, 1982; Walsh et al., 1983). The capsular vessels, both

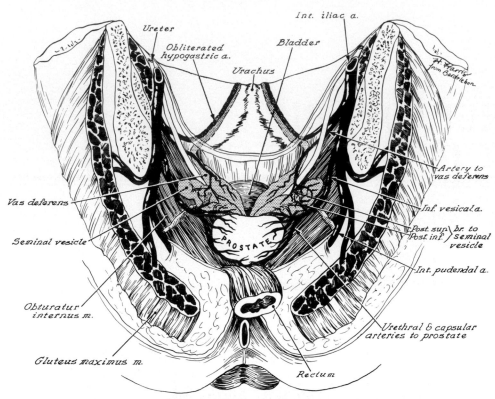

ARTERIAL SUPPLY OF PROSTATE.

Figure 78–1. Posterior view of the arterial supply to the prostate. The rectum has been removed to expose the posterior surface of the prostate and pelvis. (From Weyrauch, H. M.: Surgery of the Prostate. Philadelphia, W. B. Saunders Co., 1959.)

arteries and veins, provide the macroscopic landmark that aids in the identification of the microscopic branches of the pelvic plexus that innervate the corpora cavernosa.

The venous drainage of the prostate is into the Santorini plexus. A complete understanding of these veins is necessary, in order to avoid excessive bleeding and to ensure a bloodless field when exposing the membranous urethra and apex of the prostate. The deep dorsal vein leaves the penis under Buck's fascia between the corpora cavernosa and penetrates the urogenital diaphragm,

dividing into three major branches: the superficial branch and the right and left lateral venous plexuses (Fig. 78–2) (Reiner and Walsh, 1979). The superficial branch, which travels between the puboprostatic ligaments, is the centrally located vein overlying the bladder neck and prostate. This vein is visualized early in retropubic operations and has communicating branches over the bladder itself and into the endopelvic fascia. The superficial branch lies outside the pelvic fascia. The common trunk and lateral venous plexuses are covered and concealed by this fascia.

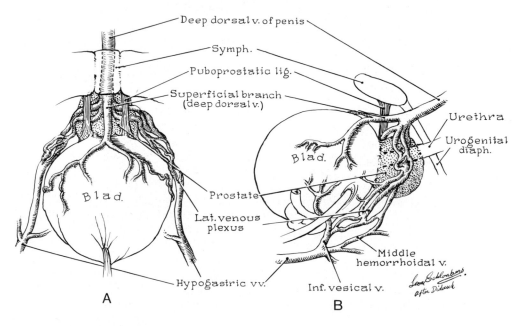

Figure 78–2. Santorini's venous plexus. *A,* View of trifurcation of the dorsal vein of the penis with the patient in the supine position. Relationship of venous branches to puboprostatic ligaments is depicted. *B,* Lateral view shows anatomic relationships at trifurcation. In this schematic illustration, the lateral pelvic fascia has been removed. In reality, these structures are never visualized in this skeletonized manner because they are encased by the lateral pelvic fascia. (From Reiner, W. G., and Walsh, P. C.: J. Urol., 121:198, 1979. © By Williams & Wilkins, 1979.)

The lateral venous plexuses traverse posterolaterally (see Fig. 78–2) and communicate freely with the pudendal, obturator, and vesical plexuses. Frequently, small branches lateral to the puboprostatic ligaments penetrate the pelvic sidewall musculature. These plexuses interconnect with other venous systems to form the inferior vesical vein, which empties into the internal iliac vein. With the complex of veins and plexuses anastomosing freely, any laceration of these rather friable structures can lead to considerable blood loss.

The major arterial supply to the corpora cavernosa is derived from the internal pudendal artery. However, accessory branches to the internal pudendal can arise from the obturator, inferior vesical and superior vesical arteries. Because these aberrant branches travel along the lower part of the bladder and anterolateral surface of the prostate, they are divided during radical prostatectomy. This maneuver may compromise arterial supply to the penis, especially in older patients with borderline penile blood flow (Breza et al., 1989).

Pelvic Plexus

The autonomic innervation of the pelvic organs and external genitalia arises from the pelvic plexus, which is formed by parasympathetic visceral efferent preganglionic fibers that arise from the sacral center (S_2 to S_4) and sympathetic fibers from the thoracolumbar center (T11 to L2) (Lepor et al., 1985; Lue et al., 1984; Schlegel and Walsh, 1987; Walsh and Donker, 1982) (Fig. 78–3). In humans, the pelvic plexus is located retroperitoneally beside the rectum, 5 to 11 cm from the anal verge. This plexus forms a fenestrated rectangular plate that is situated in the sagittal plane, with its midpoint located at the level of the tip of the seminal vesicle.

The branches of the inferior vesical artery and vein that supply the bladder and prostate perforate the pelvic plexus. For this reason, ligation of the so-called lateral pedicle in its midportion not only interrupts the vessels but also transects the nerve supply to the prostate, urethra, and corpora cavernosa. The pelvic plexus pro-

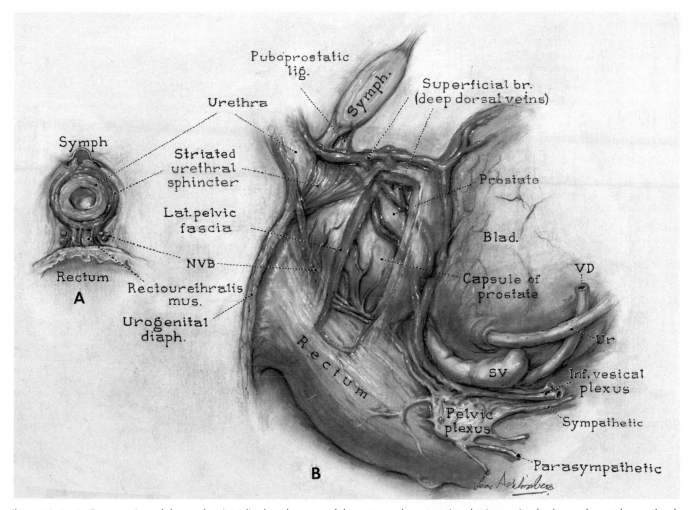

Figure 78–3. *A*, Cross-section of the urethra just distal to the apex of the prostate demonstrating the inner circular layer of smooth muscle, the outer striated urethral sphincter, and the filmy layer of rectourethralis. *B*, Anatomic relationship of the prostate to the pelvic fascia (window of fascia removed to illustrate prostatic capsule), pelvic plexus, and neurovascular bundle. Note the attachment of the striated urethral sphincter to the apex of the prostate.

vides visceral branches that innervate the bladder, ureter, seminal vesicles, prostate, rectum, membranous urethra, and corpora cavernosa. In addition, branches that contain somatic motor axons travel through the pelvic plexus to supply the levator ani, coccygeus, and striated urethral musculature. The nerves innervating the prostate travel outside the capsule of the prostate and Denonvilliers' fascia, until they perforate the capsule where they enter the prostate.

The branches to the membranous urethra and corpora cavernosa also travel outside the prostatic capsule dorsolaterally in the lateral pelvic fascia between the prostate and rectum (see Fig. 78–3). After piercing the urogenital diaphragm, they pass behind the dorsal penile artery and dorsal penile nerve before entering the corpora cavernosa. Although these nerves are microscopic in size, their anatomic location can be estimated intraoperatively by using the capsular vessels as a landmark. For this reason, throughout the remainder of the chapter, I refer to this structure as the neurovascular bundle (see Fig. 78–3).

Pelvic Fascia

The prostate is covered with two distinct and separate fascial layers: Denonvilliers' fascia and lateral pelvic fascia, also called prostatic fascia (Figs. 78–3 and 78–4). Denonvilliers' fascia is a filmy, delicate layer of connective tissue that is located between the anterior wall of the rectum and prostate. This fascial layer extends cranially to cover the posterior surface of the seminal vesicles and lies snugly against the posterior prostatic capsule. This fascia is most prominent and dense near the base of the prostate and seminal vesicles

and thins dramatically as it extends caudally to its termination at the striated urethral sphincter. Microscopically, it is impossible to discern a "posterior" and an "anterior" layer to this fascia (Jewett et al., 1972). For this reason, to obtain an adequate surgical margin, one must excise this fascia completely.

In addition to Denonvilliers' fascia, the prostate is also invested with a second important layer of fascia, the lateral pelvic fascia, which covers the pelvic musculature. This fascia has also been called the prostatic fascia. Anteriorly and anterolaterally this fascia is in direct continuity with the true capsule of the prostate. The major tributaries of the dorsal vein of the penis and the Santorini plexus travel within this fascia (see Figs. 78–3 and 78–4). Posterolaterally, the lateral pelvic fascia separates from the prostate to travel immediately adjacent to the pelvic musculature surrounding the rectum. The prostate receives its blood supply and autonomic innervation through the leaves of this fascia.

In an effort to avoid injury to the dorsal vein of the penis and the Santorini plexus during radical perineal prostatectomy, the lateral pelvic fascia is reflected off the prostate. This maneuver accounts for the reduced blood loss associated with radical perineal prostatectomy. In performing radical retropubic prostatectomy, the prostate is approached from outside the lateral fascia. For this reason, the dorsal vein complex must be ligated and the lateral pelvic fascia must be divided.

Striated Urethral Sphincter

The external sphincter, at the level of the membranous urethra, is often thought of as a series of muscles in the horizontal plane. However, Oelrich (1980) has

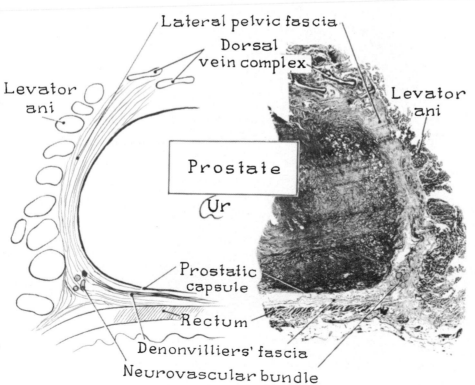

Figure 78–4. Cross-section through an adult prostate demonstrating the anatomic relationships of the lateral pelvic fascia, Denonvilliers' fascia, and neurovascular bundle. (From Walsh, P. C., Lepor, H., and Eggleston, J. C.: Radical prostatectomy with preservation of sexual function: Anatomical and pathological considerations. Prostate, 4:473, 1983.)

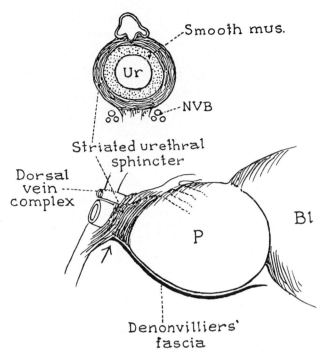

Figure 78–5. Schematic illustration of the striated urethral sphincter and its relation to the dorsal vein complex, smooth musculature of the urethra, and neurovascular bundles (NVB). Arrow points to the site where the striated urethral sphincter is sharply divided posteriorly. Note that this area is anterior to the neurovascular bundles and that it is the distal site of attachment of Denonvilliers' fascia. Sharp division at this point enables the surgeon to identify the correct plane on the anterior surface of the rectum, maintaining all layers of Denonvilliers' fascia on the prostate. (From Walsh, P. C., Quinlan, D. M., Morton, R. A., and Steiner, M. S.: Radical retropubic prostatectomy. Improved anastomosis and urinary continence. Urol. Clin. North Am., 17:679–684, 1990.)

demonstrated clearly that the striated urethral sphincter with its surrounding fascia is a vertically oriented tubular sheath and not a pair of transverse planes. In utero, this sphincter extends without interruption from the bladder to the perineal membrane. As the prostate develops from the urethra, it invades the sphincter muscle thinning the overlying parts and causing a reduction or atrophy of some of the muscle.

In the adult, at the apex of the prostate, the fibers are circular and form a tubular striated sphincter surrounding the membranous urethra. Thus, as Myers and colleagues (1987) have shown, the prostate does not rest atop a flat transverse urogenital diagram like an apple on a shelf, with no striated muscle proximal to the apex. Rather, the external striated sphincter is more tubular and has broad attachments over the fascia of the prostate near the apex (Figs. 78–3 and 78–5). This anatomy has important implications in apical dissection and reconstruction of the urethra for preservation of urinary control postoperatively (Walsh et al., 1990).

SURGICAL TECHNIQUE

Preoperative Preparation

Surgery is deferred for 6 to 8 weeks following needle biopsy of the prostate and 12 weeks following transure-

thral resection of the prostate. These delays enable inflammatory adhesions or hematomas to resolve so that the anatomic relationships between the prostate and surrounding structures are returned to a more normal state prior to surgery. This is especially important if one hopes to preserve the neurovascular bundles intraoperatively and to avoid rectal injury.

Because transfusions are frequently required in the perioperative period, patients are offered the opportunity to donate 3 units of blood for autotransfusion during the 6-to-8-week delay. Patients are advised to avoid taking aspirin or other nonsteroidal anti-inflammatory agents that interfere with platelet function while donating the blood and immediately prior to the surgery. The patients are admitted to the hospital the day before surgery and undergo standard preoperative evaluation. The night before surgery, they are given a Fleets enema and are hydrated intravenously.

Special Instruments

Unlike radical perineal prostatectomy, radical retropubic prostatectomy requires few special instruments. A fiberoptic headlamp is most useful because much of the procedure is performed beneath the pubis in an area where visualization can be difficult. A standard Balfour retractor with a malleable center blade is helpful during the lymph node dissection and is necessary during the radical prostatectomy to provide cranial and posterior retraction on the peritoneum and bladder, respectively. Coagulating forceps, vessel loops, and bulldog clamps are the only other specialized instruments that should be available.

Anesthesia, Incision, and Lymphadenectomy

A spinal or epidural anesthetic is preferable for this procedure. Conduction anesthesia is safer and seems to be associated with less blood loss and a lower frequency of pulmonary emboli (Peters and Walsh, 1985). The patient is placed in the supine position with the table broken in the midline to extend the distance between the pubis and umbilicus. The table is then tilted to effect the Trendelenburg position until the patient's legs are parallel to the floor.

The skin is prepared and draped in the usual way. A No. 22 Foley catheter is passed into the bladder, inflated with 50 ml of saline, and connected to sterile closed-continuous drainage. A right-handed surgeon always stands on the left side of the patient.

A midline extraperitoneal lower abdominal incision is made, extending from the pubis to the umbilicus. The rectus muscles are separated in the midline, and the transversalis fascia is opened sharply to expose the space of Retzius. Care is taken to incise the anterior fascia down to the pubis and to incise the posterior fascia above the semicircular line to the umbilicus. Laterally, the peritoneum is mobilized off the external iliac vessels to the bifurcation of the common iliac artery. This

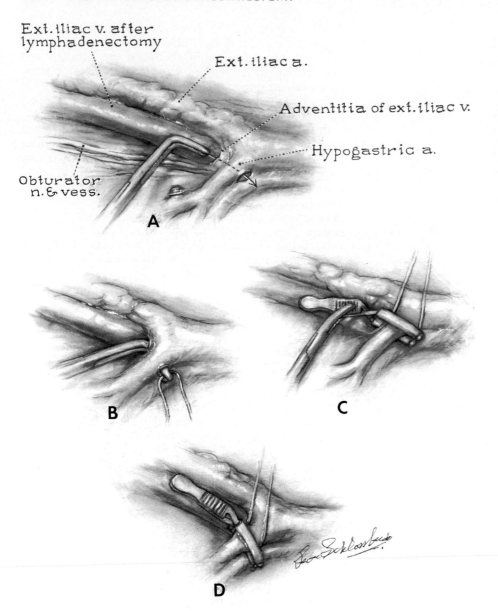

Ext. iliac v. after
lymphadenectomy

Ext. iliac a.

Adventitia of ext. iliac v.

Hypogastric a.

Obturator
n. & vess.

A

B

C

D

Figure 78–6. *A,* View of the right pelvis following completion of the staging lymph node dissection. Note that the fibrofatty tissue overlying the external iliac artery has not been disturbed. In preparation for placement of the bulldog clamp on the hypogastric artery, the adventitia over the external iliac vein has been elevated. *B,* The right-angle clamp is easily passed immediately anterior to the external iliac vein beneath the hypogastric artery. This maneuver provides a bloodless plane through which a vessel loop is passed. *C* and *D,* Placement of the bulldog clamp on the hypogastric artery.

maneuver is accomplished without dividing the vas deferens. Next, a self-retaining Balfour retractor is placed and the staging pelvic lymphadenectomy on the right side is commenced. Exposure is facilitated by utilizing the malleable blade attached to the Balfour retractor to retract the peritoneum superiorly.

Previously, when the vas deferens was routinely divided, some men later complained of persistent testicular pain that I attributed to excessive traction on the spermatic cord during this maneuver. However, if the vas deferens is not divided, the traction on the spermatic cord is absorbed by the vas deferens and persistent testalgia is rare.

The lymphadenectomy is considered a staging and not a therapeutic procedure. Its value is to identify those patients with occult metastases to pelvic lymph nodes in whom radical prostatectomies would be of little benefit. The dissection is initiated along the external iliac vein on the same side as the most prominent clinical induration in the prostate (Fig. 78–6). The lymphatics overlying the external iliac artery are preserved. The dissec-

tion proceeds inferiorly to the femoral canal where care is taken to ligate the lymphatic channels at the node of Cloquet. Next, the obturator lymph nodes are removed with care to avoid injury to the obturator nerve. The obturator artery and vein usually remain undisturbed and are not ligated, unless excessive bleeding occurs.

The dissection proceeds superiorly to the bifurcation of the common iliac artery, where the lymph nodes in the angle between the external iliac and hypogastric arteries are removed. At the completion of the dissection, the vasculature in the hypogastric and obturator fossa should be neatly skeletonized (see Fig. 78–6). These lymph nodes are sent for frozen-section analysis, and a similar procedure is carried out on the contralateral side. The pathologist is requested to section all lymph nodes and to perform frozen-section analysis only on those that look suspicious. To reduce blood loss during the remainder of the procedure, the hypogastric arteries are encircled with vessel loops and bulldog clamps are placed proximal to the origin of the obliterated umbilical artery.

Incision in Endopelvic Fascia

At this point, the malleable blade is repositioned to retract the bladder. If the balloon on the Foley catheter is positioned in the dome of the bladder beneath the well-padded malleable blade, maximal cranial and posterior displacement of the bladder will be achieved, providing excellent exposure of the anterior surface of the prostate. The fibroadipose tissue covering the prostate is carefully dissected away exposing the pelvic fascia, puboprostatic ligaments, and superficial branch of the dorsal vein. The endopelvic fascia is entered where it reflects over the pelvic sidewall, well away from its attachments to the bladder and prostate (Fig. 78–7). This is the site where the visceral pelvic fascia, which covers the anterior surface of the prostate and encases the main trunk of the dorsal vein complex, attaches to the parietal pelvic fascia, which covers the pelvic musculature.

At the point where the fascia is incised, it is often transparent and reveals underlying levator ani musculature. After the fascia has been opened, one can usually visualize the bulging lateral venous plexus, which is located medially. The lateral venous plexuses traverse adjacent to the prostate and the lower portion of the bladder. Therefore, an incision in the endopelvic fascia too close to the bladder or the prostate risks laceration of these important structures with potential severe blood loss. Beneath this venous complex lie the prostatovesicular artery and the branches of the pelvic plexus that course toward the prostate, urethra, and corpora cavernosa.

The incision in the endopelvic fascia is carefully extended in an anteromedial direction toward the puboprostatic ligaments, enabling the surgeon to palpate the lateral surface of the prostate. At this point, often small arterial and venous branches travel from the lateral plexus and perforate the pelvic musculature.

Division of Puboprostatic Ligaments

The fibrofatty tissue covering the superficial branch of the dorsal vein and puboprostatic ligaments is gently teased away to prepare for division of the ligaments without inadvertent injury to the superficial branch of the dorsal vein. Care must be taken to dissect the superficial branch of the dorsal vein away from the medial edge of the ligaments before they are divided (Fig. 78–8). After one teases away all fibrofatty tissue on the medial surface between the superficial branch of the dorsal vein and the ligament, the scissors should be carefully passed immediately behind the ligament, pushing away the anterior prostatic fascia with the enclosed dorsal vein complex that rests on the posterior surface. The ligaments should then be divided along the avascular plane that was created by this maneuver (see Fig. 78–8). Once the major portion of the ligament is divided sharply, the residual fragments can be fractured by careful finger compression.

Alternately, the ligaments can be divided, beginning on their lateral surface and using finger fracture to separate the residual fragments. With the puboprostatic ligaments transected, the superficial branch of the dorsal vein is readily apparent over the bladder neck in the midline. This vein should be dissected carefully from the undersurface of the pubis, thereby exposing the trifurcation of the dorsal vein over the region of the prostatourethral junction.

Figure 78–7. The incision in the endopelvic fascia is made at the junction with the pelvic side wall, well away from the prostate and bladder.

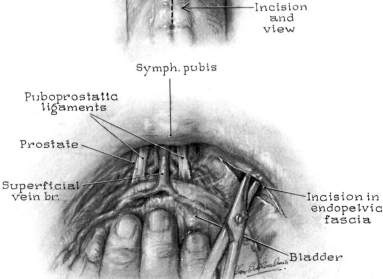

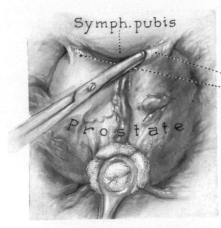

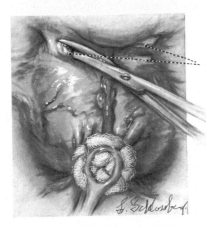

Figure 78–8. Division of the puboprostatic ligaments. A sponge stick is placed on the prostate to displace it posteriorly, exposing the puboprostatic ligaments and placing them on tension. The medial surface of the puboprostatic ligament is dissected free from the superficial branch of the dorsal vein, and the scissors are passed immediately behind the ligament pushing away the anterior prostatic fascia with the enclosed dorsal vein complex. Ligaments are divided along the avascular plane created by this maneuver.

Division of Dorsal Vein Complex

The lateral wall of the urethra is identified by palpating the indwelling catheter. Anterior to the catheter is a thick complex composed of the main trunk of the dorsal vein, the striated urethral sphincter, and the surrounding pelvic fascia (Fig. 78–9). Recognizing that the striated urethral sphincter is a tubular structure that surrounds the urethra and is part of the dorsal vein complex, I attempt to preserve as much of this complex as possible on the anterior surface of the urethra. The complex is identified by palpating its distinct, sharp, shelf-like edge just anterior to the urethra. Utilizing a right-angle clamp, the lateral pelvic fascia is perforated and the clamp is passed through the avascular plane between the anterior surface of the urethra and the posterior surface of the dorsal vein complex. At this level, the complex with its associated fascia and striated urethral sphincter is 1 to 2 cm thick. Care must be taken to avoid fracturing the apex of the prostate or entering the anterior surface of the prostate—the correct plane is between the dorsal vein complex and the urethra.

Next, a large right-angle clamp is gently applied to widen the opening between the dorsal vein complex and the urethra slightly. This maneuver facilitates the subsequent isolation of the urethra. Care should be taken, however, to avoid excessive mobilization of the complex from the anterior surface of the urethra. Because the neurovascular bundles are posterior to the urethra, they cannot be damaged during this maneuver. The dorsal

vein complex is transected. More recently, I have not ligated the dorsal vein complex before dividing it. If the right-angle clamp is under the entire complex, it is possible to divide the complex completely without much blood loss. The technique permits more tissue to be removed from the anterior surface of the prostate and avoids distortion of the striated sphincter from the ligature. Absolute control of venous bleeding from the dorsal vein complex is mandatory so that the remainder of the operation can be performed in a bloodless field. If a silk suture is used to ligate the complex, it should be removed. If a ligature is not used or if an absorbable suture has fallen off, a 2–0 chromic catgut suture is selected to oversew the fascial edges of the ligated dorsal vein so that hemostasis can be perfected (Fig. 78–10).

The striated urethral sphincter is an important component in this complex, and if it is oversewn in a horizontal fashion it provides an excellent hood for the later anastomosis. Generally, there is little or no backflow from the untied lateral plexus because of the valves in the venous system. If back bleeding is a problem, the venous channels over the anterior surface of the prostate can be oversewn with a 2–0 chromic catgut suture.

Division of Urethra

At this point, it is essential to employ a sponge stick for downward displacement of the prostate so that the prostatourethral junction can be visualized. Utilizing

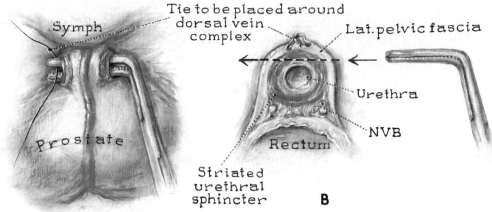

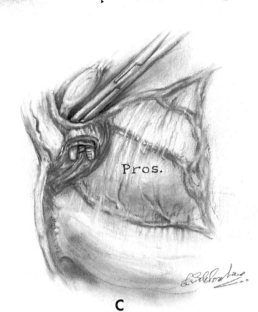

Figure 78–9. Division of the dorsal vein complex. *A,* A right-angle clamp is passed beneath the dorsal vein complex. *B* and *C,* Note that the clamp passes through the anterior fibers of the striated urethral sphincter.

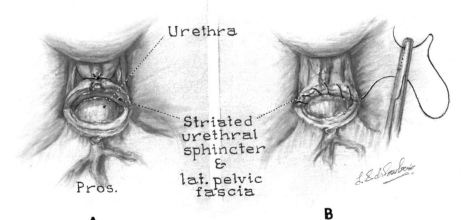

Figure 78–10. If a silk ligature was used it should be removed, or if the absorbable suture has fallen off the dorsal vein complex with the anterior fibers of the striated urethral sphincter can be oversewn horizontally using 2 0 chromic catgut. Large venous channels in the posterolateral edges of the complex can be easily oversewn. This maneuver forms an anterior hood of tissue that will be helpful in the final anastomosis.

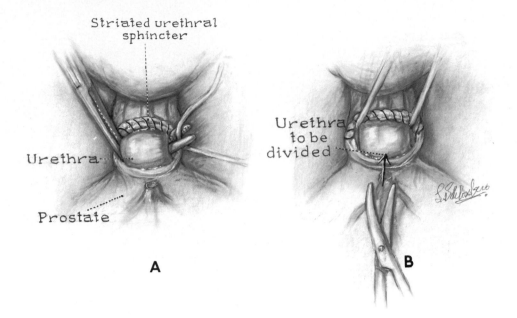

Figure 78–11. Exposure of the prostatourethral junction prior to transection of the urethra. Note that intact bands of fascia and striated urethral sphincter are present on either side of the urethra.

posterior displacement of the prostate with a sponge stick, the prostatourethral junction should be well visualized. Intact bands of fascia and striated urethral sphincter are present on either side of the urethra (Fig. 78–11). The plane between the smooth musculature of the urethra and the striated sphincter is next developed, utilizing sharp dissection. Umbilical tape is passed around the urethra. Care must be taken to avoid excessive traction on the urethra, which might disrupt the attachment of its smooth musculature to the striated sphincter, which can delay the return of urinary control. The anterior wall of the urethra is incised at its junction with the apex of the prostate. This maneuver permits the Foley catheter to be brought through this incision,

clamped, and divided. Next, the posterior wall of the urethra is divided.

Division of Striated Urethral Sphincter

With traction on the catheter, one can visualize a complex of skeletal muscle and fibrous tissue (the residual lateral and posterior components of the striated urethral sphincter) that tethers the apex of the prostate to the pelvic floor musculature (Fig. 78–12). When viewed laterally, this complex attaches to the apex of the prostate and Denonvilliers' fascia anterior to the neurovascular bundles (see Figs. 78–3, 78–5, and 78–

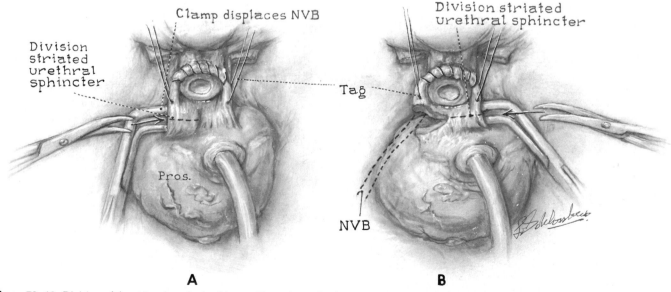

Figure 78–12. Division of the striated urethral sphincter. The right-angle clamp is easily passed immediately beneath the striated urethral sphincter but anterior to the neurovascular bundle. The clamp is individually passed first from the left and then from the right. Tags are placed distally on either side for later identification of the striated urethral sphincter during the anastomosis.

9). I once thought that this complex was composed of muscular bands (the pillars of the prostate) and a medial component, which I incorrectly called the rectourethralis muscle. However, after more observation, I now realize that this entire complex is part of the extensive skeletal muscle sleeve of the external sphincter that attaches to the apex of the prostate.

Identification and precise division of this complex are most important in (1) obtaining adequate margins of resection for apical lesions; (2) identifying the correct plane on the anterior wall of the rectum to ensure that all layers of Denonvilliers' fascia are excised; (3) avoiding blunt trauma to the neurovascular bundles that are located immediately posteriorly; and (4) preserving urinary continence (see subsequent discussion).

Initially, a right-angle clamp is passed immediately beneath the left edge of the complex. The left border is divided with the scissors with care to avoid injury to the neurovascular bundle beneath it. At this point, a stay suture is placed in the distal cut edge. During the urethral anastomoses this suture will be used to identify this component of the external sphincter so that it can be incorporated into the anastomosis. The right-angle clamp is then passed beneath the right edge, and a similar procedure is carried out.

Finally, the central component of the complex, which includes the flimsy bands of the rectourethralis musculature, is divided immediately anterior to the rectum. This sequence of division avoids inadvertent injury to the neurovascular bundles or the rectum.

Identification and Preservation of Neurovascular Bundle

Next, the plane between the anterior wall of the rectum and the prostate with its investment of Denonvilliers' fascia is developed. After this plane has been established, a right-angle clamp separates the superficial lateral pelvic fascia from the lateral surface of the prostate, exposing the neurovascular bundle in a groove at the posterolateral edge of the prostate (Fig. 78–13A). If this superficial fascia is incised from the apex to the bladder neck, the prostate is released, making it more mobile.

The neurovascular bundles are located dorsolateral to

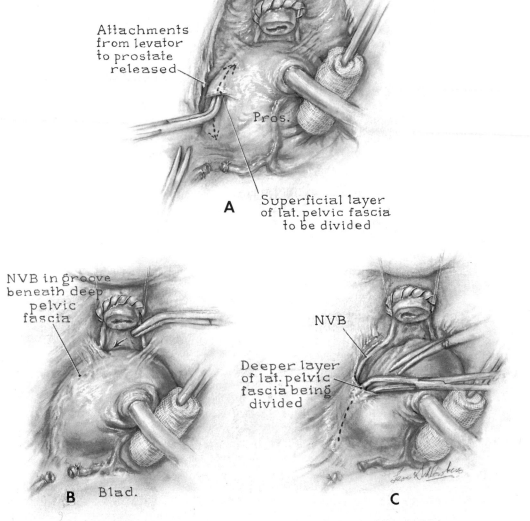

Figure 78–13. The striated urethral sphincter has been divided, and the posterior plane between the anterior rectal wall and prostate has been developed. *A,* Superficial layers of the lateral pelvic fascia are released from the lateral surface of the prostate exposing the location of the neurovascular bundle in a groove at the posterolateral edge of the prostate. *B,* By extending the incision in the superficial fascia from the apex to the bladder neck, the prostate becomes more mobile. The neurovascular bundle is identified at the apex, and the deep layers of the lateral pelvic fascia are gently released from the prostate at a point sufficiently anterior to preserve the neurovascular bundle. *C,* Posterior release of the neurovascular bundle.

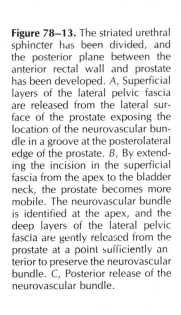

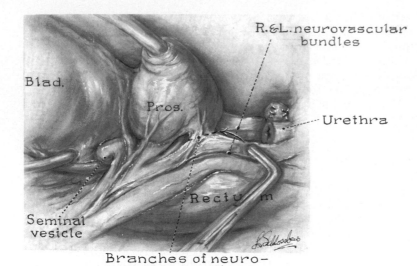

R.&L.neurovascular bundles

Blad.

Pros.

Urethra

Rectum

Seminal vesicle

Branches of neuro-vascular bundle to prostate to be divided

Figure 78–14. The lateral pelvic fascia has been divided bilaterally, releasing the apex of the prostate. The neurovascular bundles are intact. At the apex and midpoint of the prostate, small arterial and venous branches are usually first visualized. These branches are ligated individually, using fine sutures or clips and avoiding mass ligatures, which could produce inadvertent tenting of the bundle into the ligature and subsequent injury.

the prostate. In the past, the incision in the lateral fascia was made at random with blunt dissection. Although the neurovascular bundles were usually not removed with the specimen, they were often injured during the dissection (Walsh, 1987). With the technique described herein, the incision in the lateral fascia is made with precision and with knowledge of the location of the neurovascular bundle. If the induration on the side of the nodule appears to extend into the lateral pelvic fascia or neurovascular bundles, the fascia is divided wherever necessary to excise all evident tumor (see subsequent discussion). The primary objective of the surgical procedure is the removal of all tumor. In this clinical setting, preservation of potency is only of secondary concern. Indeed, it is only necessary to preserve the neurovascular bundles on one side to preserve potency in most patients (see further discussion).

Once the superficial layers of the lateral pelvic fascia have been divided, the neurovascular bundles can be seen in a groove at the posterolateral edge of the prostate (Fig. 78–13B). The lateral pelvic fascia is made up of multiple leaves. As stated earlier, the neurovascular bundle is imbedded in the leaves of this fascia. Up to this point, only the superficial leaves of the lateral pelvic fascia have been divided, i.e., those of the fascia adjacent to the pelvic musculature.

The neurovascular bundles are imbedded in deeper leaves of the fascia and are attached to the prostate by the vessels that supply it. Beginning at the apex, the lateral pelvic fascia is gently released from the prostate (Fig. 78–13B). By identifying the neurovascular bundle distally over the rectum and proximally in the groove, one can determine the exact site at the apex to release the remaining fibers of striated sphincter that cover the neurovascular bundle at this location. Once initiated, the bundle can be released with a right-angle clamp spread posteriorly beneath the bundle. This maneuver assures that Denonvilliers' fascia is not separated from the prostate.

Because the neurovascular bundles supply few vascular branches to the distal third of the prostate, the

bundles can usually be teased away from the prostate at this point. However, at the apex and at the midpoint of the prostate, small arterial and venous branches are usually first visualized. These branches should be ligated individually, employing fine sutures or clips and avoiding mass ligatures that could produce inadvertent tenting of the bundle into the ligature with subsequent injury (Fig. 78–14). As one approaches the base of the prostate, the bundles travel farther posteriorly and are less of a problem.

At this point, the attachment between the rectum and Denonvilliers' fascia should be divided in the midline posteriorly, exposing this fascia covering the posterior surface of the seminal vesicles. The plane between the lateral edges of the seminal vesicles and the overlying lateral pelvic fascia should be developed (Fig. 78–15). Often, prominent arterial branches from the neurovascular bundle supply the posterior surface of the prostate over the seminal vesicles. These posterior vessels should be ligated and divided. After doing so, the lateral pedicles are displaced posteriorly from the prostate facilitating their division without injury to the nerves, as they traverse posteriorly in this tissue (Fig. 78–16).

I have found that it is possible to divide the lateral pedicles on the lateral surface of the seminal vesicles without ligating them. Surprisingly, there is little venous bleeding. The obvious arterial bleeders can be simply controlled with a few hemoclips or sutures. This approach seems to leave more soft tissue on the prostate and may protect the neurovascular bundles from injury.

Excision of Lateral Pelvic Fascia and Neurovascular Bundle

Under certain circumstances, it may be necessary to excise the lateral pelvic fascia and neurovascular bundles completely on one or both sides. This decision can be made either preoperatively or intraoperatively based on a variety of clinical findings.

Figure 78–15. The attachment between the rectum and Denonvilliers' fascia has been divided in the midline posteriorly exposing the posterior surface of the seminal vesicles. Branches from the neurovascular bundle to the posterior surface of the prostate and seminal vesicles are identified and ligated. This maneuver facilitates posterior displacement of the neurovascular bundles and identification of the lateral surface of the seminal vesicles for transection of the lateral pedicles. Illustrated as viewed from the symphysis pubis.

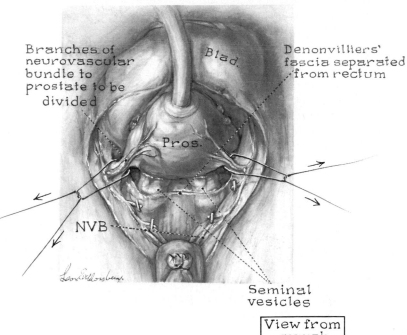

Branches of neurovascular bundle to prostate to be divided

Blad.

Denonvilliers' fascia separated from rectum

Pros.

NVB

Seminal vesicles

View from symph.

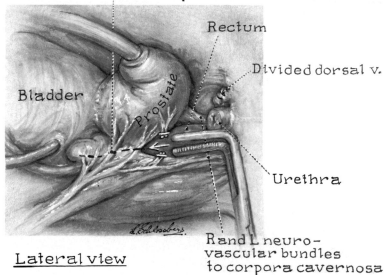

Division of lateral pedicle

Rectum

Divided dorsal v.

Bladder

Prostate

Urethra

R and L neuro-vascular bundles to corpora cavernosa

Lateral view

Figure 78–16. Division of the lateral pedicle. Once the plane between the lateral pedicle and seminal vesicle has been developed the right-angle clamp is placed and spread. The lateral pedicle is divided without ligation. Obvious arterial bleeders are controlled with hemoclips.

1. Surgery on an impotent patient.

2. Induration involving the lateral sulcus found on preoperative physical examination. It has always been obvious to me that the neurovascular bundle was closer to the apex of the prostate than the base (Lepor et al., 1985; Schlegel and Walsh, 1987; Walsh and Donker, 1982). For this reason, the ipsilateral neurovascular bundle is more often excised in patients with apical lesions than in patients with lesions at the base.

3. Induration in the lateral pelvic fascia found intraoperatively after the endopelvic fascia has been opened.

4. Fixation of the neurovascular bundle to the capsule of the prostate detected once the lateral pelvic fascia has been divided. The major determinant is clinical stage (Table 78–1). In 492 clinical stage A and B patients who were potent preoperatively, both neurovascular bundles were preserved in only 58 per cent of the men. In patients with the most favorable pathology (stage A1 and B1N), both neurovascular bundles were preserved in only 83 to 85 per cent. In patients with stage B2 disease, both neurovascular bundles were preserved only 27 per cent of the time.

When excising the neurovascular bundle, the contralateral bundle to be preserved is initially freed from the prostate at the apex. This maneuver is performed first to avoid traction injury during subsequent maneuvers. Next, the neurovascular bundle to be excised is identified at the apex, and a right-angle clamp is passed from medial to lateral immediately on the anterior surface of the rectum. The bundle is divided without ligation in an effort to excise as much soft tissue as possible (Fig. 78–17). Later, if bleeding is troublesome, the distal end can be clipped. Next, the lateral pelvic fascia is divided posterior to the neurovascular bundle on the posterolateral surface of the rectum. This procedure is performed under direct vision, with the dissection terminating at the tip of the seminal vesicle where the neurovascular bundle is ligated and divided. In this way, the neurovascular bundle and the lateral pelvic fascia are excised under direct vision in a more complete way than previously possible. Once this excision has been accomplished, the rectum is dissected free from the posterior surface of the prostate over to the lateral pelvic fascia on the contralateral side. In doing so, the contralateral neurovascular bundle is clearly delineated and skeletonized, enabling it to be preserved in its entirety. Indeed,

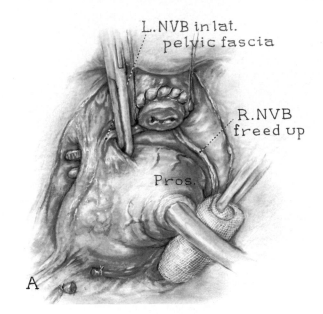

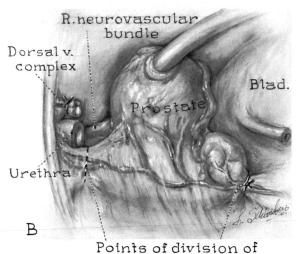

Figure 78–17. Steps in wide excision of the lateral pelvic fascia and neurovascular bundle. *A,* A right-angle clamp is passed from medial to lateral on the anterior surface of the rectum beneath the neurovascular bundle. *B,* The neurovascular bundle is transected at the level of the urethra, the lateral pelvic fascia is divided posterior to the neurovascular bundle on the lateral surface of the rectum, and the pedicle is ligated at the tip of the seminal vesicle.

it is necessary to preserve only one neurovascular bundle to preserve potency (see following discussion).

Following a dissection such as this, the excised specimen demonstrates abundant soft tissue covering the lesion, wide excision of all soft tissue on the ipsilateral side of the rectum, and preservation of the contralateral neurovascular bundle (Fig. 78–18).

Division of Bladder Neck and Excision of Seminal Vesicles

At this point in the procedure, the prostate has been mobilized almost completely. The anesthesiologist is requested to give the patient an ampule of indigo carmine dye to aid later in identification of the ureteral

Table 78–1. CLINICAL STAGE AND OPERATIVE TECHNIQUE IN 492 STAGE A AND B PATIENTS POTENT PREOPERATIVELY

Clinical Stage	Status of Neurovascular Bundles			
	+ +	+ ±	+0	00
A1	83%	13%	4%	—
B1N	85%	12%	3%	—
B1	58%	23%	18%	1%
A2	66%	23%	9%	2%
B2	27%	17%	52%	4%
Total	58%	19%	22%	1%

+ + = preservation of neurovascular bundles bilaterally
+ ± = partial excision of one neurovascular bundle
+0 = wide excision of one neurovascular bundle
00 = wide excision of both neurovascular bundles

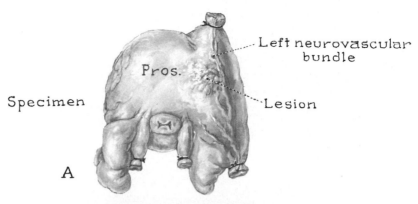

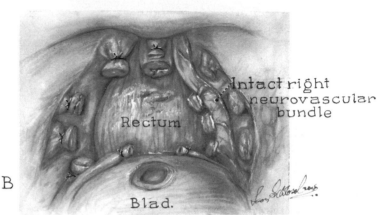

Figure 78–18. Appearance of radical prostatectomy specimen *(A)* and operative field *(B)* following unilateral, complete excision of the lateral pelvic fascia and neurovascular bundle.

orifices. The bladder neck is incised anteriorly at the prostatovesicular junction. The anterior fibromuscular stroma of the prostate contains little or no glandular tissue. For this reason, there should be little fear that tumor is present at this site.

The incision is carried down to the mucosa, the mucosa is incised, the Foley balloon is deflated, and the two ends of the catheter are clamped together to provide traction (Fig. 78–19). Care must be taken to avoid inadvertent dissection within the layers of the trigone resulting in ureteral injury. The correct plane of dissection is identified laterally, between the bladder and seminal vesicles at the level of the prostatovesicular junction. To identify this plane, the lateral pedicles must be divided completely. Having identified the lateral edge of the bladder neck, the posterior bladder wall can be divided distal to the ureteral orifices. Once this maneuver has been accomplished, the bladder neck is retracted with an Allis clamp and the vasa deferentia are divided in the midline. The seminal vesicles are dissected free from surrounding structures.

Residual vascular pedicles along the lateral surface of the seminal vesicles are divided and ligated, facilitating exposure of the tips of the seminal vesicles. Earlier in the operation, the lateral pedicles to the prostate were divided on the lateral surface of the seminal vesicles near their junction with the prostate. Thus, during the process of dissecting out the seminal vesicles, they will be located in a pocket formed by the posterior wall of the bladder and the lateral pelvic fascia with the neurovascular bundle. Care should be exercised not to damage the neurovascular bundles during this step in the operation.

As the tips of the seminal vesicles are dissected free, the small arterial branch at the tip of each seminal vesicle should be identified, divided, and ligated. Any residual attachments of Denonvilliers' fascia are divided, and the specimen is removed. The specimen is inspected carefully to identify any area where the margin of resection is uncertain. If a suspicious area is found, biopsy of the adjacent area or a wider resection is indicated.

The bulldog clamps are removed, and the operative site is inspected carefully for bleeding. Small bleeding vessels on the neurovascular bundle should not be cauterized to avoid coagulating the fine nerve bundles. Bleeding from these small vessels usually ceases spontaneously or can be controlled with small hemoclips.

Bladder Neck Closure and Anastomosis

The bladder neck is reconstructed employing interrupted sutures of 2–0 chromic catgut to approximate full-thickness muscularis and mucosa using a "tennis-racket" closure (Fig. 78–20). The efflux of indigo carmine from the ureteral orifices is noted while placing the sutures—ureteral catheters are not usually necessary. The closure is initiated in the midline and proceeds anteriorly until the bladder neck is narrowed to approximately the diameter of the index finger. Next, interrupted 4–0 chromic catgut sutures advance the mucosa over the raw muscular edges of the bladder neck. In this way, a rosette of mucosa covers the bladder neck facilitating a mucosa-to-mucosa urethrovesical anastomosis (Fig. 78–21). Finally, one or two more 2–0

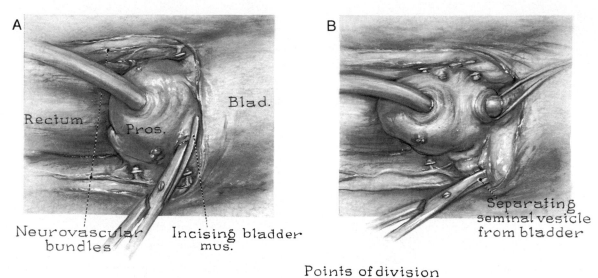

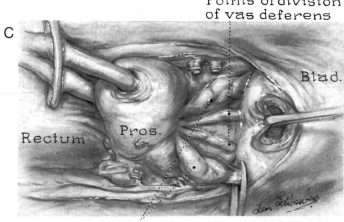

Figure 78–19. Technique for division of the bladder neck. *A,* The bladder neck is incised anteriorly. *B,* The lateral fascia and pedicles overlying the seminal vesicles have been fully divided. This maneuver facilitates identification of the plane between the bladder and the seminal vesicles at the level of the prostatovesicular junction and avoids inadvertent dissection within the layers of the trigone. *C,* An Allis clamp is utilized to elevate the posterior bladder neck during dissection of the plane between the posterior bladder wall and the seminal vesicles, exposing the vasa deferentia and seminal vesicles.

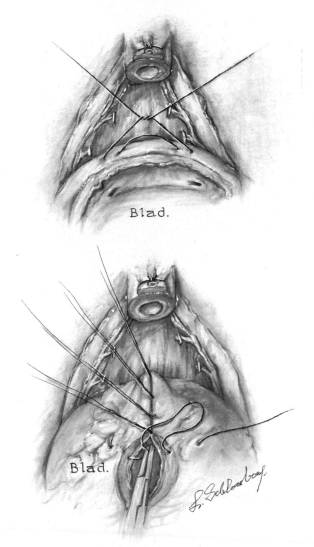

Figure 78–20. "Tennis-racket" technique for bladder neck closure. The closure is initiated in the midline with interrupted 2–0 chromic catgut sutures approximating full thickness of the detrusor musculature and the mucosa. Care should be taken to make this closure both watertight and hemostatic and to avoid injury to the ureteral orifices.

chromic catgut sutures are placed in the bladder neck narrowing it to the caliber of the Foley catheter.

A new Foley catheter (20 Fr., 5-cc balloon) is placed through the urethra, with the tip position just inside the pelvis. The edges of the urethra can be visualized more easily if a silk ligature is placed through the holes in the

catheter and the catheter is pulled back and forth through the distal end of the urethra. This practice facilitates identification of the urethral mucosa for more accurate placement of sutures. In addition, a sponge stick is utilized to displace the rectum posteriorly. With a 2–0 polyglycolic acid suture on a small 5/8 circle tapered needle, the bladder neck is reapproximated to the urethra with four sutures, at 12, 3, 6, and 9 o'clock (Fig. 78–22).

Initially, the posterior suture is placed. The stay sutures in the striated urethral sphincter are grasped and elevated, lifting this complex away from the neurovascular bundles. The 6-o'clock suture is passed through this musculature and into the urethral lumen posteriorly. A Stratte needle holder is useful in placing this stitch. The end of the suture is temporarily held in a clamp. Next, the 3- and 9-o'clock sutures are placed from inside the urethral lumen out, making certain to incorporate the urethral mucosa, the smooth muscle of the urethra, and the striated urethral musculature.

Finally, the 12-o'clock suture is placed from inside the urethral lumen alongside the catheter to the outside catching the dorsal vein complex and anterior fibers of the striated urethral sphincter. Once all the sutures have been placed in the distal urethra, the sutures are placed in their corresponding positions in the bladder neck.

After these four sutures are placed, the balloon and the valve on the catheter are tested, the catheter is positioned in the bladder, and the sutures are tied. The anterior suture is tied initially. The right lateral, posterior, and left lateral sutures are then tied. The balloon is inflated with 15 ml of saline, and the catheter is irrigated. Small suction drains are placed, the operative site is irrigated vigorously with saline, and the incision is closed with a running No. 2 nylon suture and skin clips. The catheter is carefully taped to the thigh.

POSTOPERATIVE MANAGEMENT

The postoperative recovery of men who undergo radical retropubic prostatectomy is usually quite smooth, and the patients ambulate immediately. Intravenous fluids are administered until the patients can tolerate fluid intake by mouth—usually on the 2nd or 3rd postoperative day. The closed suction drains are left in place until they cease to function, usually on the 4th or 5th postoperative day. Occasional patients will have mod-

Figure 78–21. The bladder mucosa is advanced over the raw bladder neck edges with interrupted 4–0 chromic catgut suture material. After this step has been completed, one or two more 2–0 chromic catgut sutures are placed in the bladder neck narrowing it to the caliber of the Foley catheter.

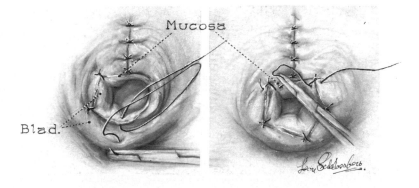

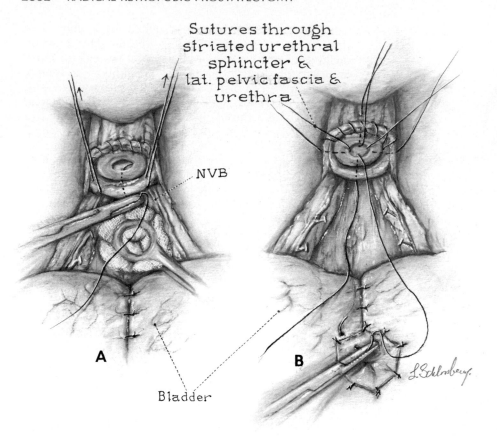

Sutures through striated urethral sphincter & lat. pelvic fascia & urethra

NVB

A

Bladder

B

L. Schlossberg.

Figure 78–22. *A,* The stay sutures in the striated urethral sphincter are grasped with clamps and elevated, lifting this complex away from the neurovascular bundles so that they will not be injured during anastomosis. The 6-o'clock suture of 2–0 polyglycolic acid on a small 5/8 circle tapered needle is passed through this musculature and into the urethral lumen posteriorly. *B,* A Foley catheter with a silk suture through the eye is employed to evert the urethral mucosa. Similar sutures are placed at 3 and 9 o'clock. Finally, a 12-o'clock suture is passed through the urethral lumen, including the dorsal vein complex and anterior fibers of the striated urethral sphincter. Sutures are then placed in their corresponding positions in the bladder neck.

erate amounts of urinary leakage for 7 to 10 days, which is usually of no consequence. Patients are discharged from the hospital with a Foley catheter in place usually within 8 days. They return 3 weeks after the procedure for removal of the catheter.

COMPLICATIONS

Radical retropubic prostatectomy is a procedure that is well tolerated with minimal morbidity and low mortality (0 to 1.7 per cent). In 1000 consecutive patients there were two deaths (0.2 per cent). One patient died 3 weeks postoperatively, while at home, from a pulmonary embolus. A second patient suffered cardiac arrest with the induction of anesthesia before the radical prostatectomy was initiated. Other complications discussed can be divided into those occurring intraoperatively and postoperatively.

Intraoperative Complications

The most common intraoperative problem during radical retropubic prostatectomy is hemorrhage, usually arising from venous structures. Hemorrhage may occur during the pelvic lymphadenectomy if one of the branches of the hypogastric vein is torn inadvertently. Venous injury like this should be repaired with cardiovascular silk sutures. Hemorrhage can also occur (1) during the incision in the endopelvic fascia if the incision is made too close to the prostate; (2) during division of

the puboprostatic ligaments if the ligaments are not dissected free from the superficial branch of the dorsal vein or anterior prostatic fascia; and (3) during exposure of the apex of the prostate with transection of the dorsal vein complex. However, if one understands fully the anatomy of the dorsal vein complex, this bleeding is usually satisfactorily controlled once the dorsal vein has been divided and ligated. Consequently, if there is troublesome bleeding from the complex at any point, the surgeon should aggressively proceed and divide the dorsal vein complex over the urethra and oversew the end. This is the best means to resolve the problem. Any maneuver short of this may only worsen the bleeding. To gain exposure for the prostatectomy, one must put traction on the prostate. If the dorsal vein is not completely divided, this usually worsens the bleeding. It is imperative to obtain excellent hemostasis before the apex of the prostate is approached so that the anatomy can be viewed in a bloodless field.

Most often, blood loss during the procedure occurs gradually from venous back bleeding resulting in an average accumulated loss of 1000 ml (Rainwater and Segura, 1990). We have always applied bulldog clamps to the hypogastric arteries in an attempt to reduce perfusion of the prostate during the procedure. To evaluate whether this practice is helpful, we omitted the bulldog clamps in 50 consecutive patients. Although no patient required transfusions, the average blood loss in this group of patients was 225 ml greater and the operative field was less clear. For these reasons and because it is so easy to place the bulldog clamps, we have continued to do so.

Less common complications include obturator nerve injury during the pelvic lymph node dissection, rectal injury, and ureteral injury. If the obturator nerve is inadvertently severed, an attempt should be made at reanastomosis using very fine nonabsorbable sutures. Rectal injury is an infrequent but serious complication. In 900 consecutive cases, we experienced ten (1 per cent) injuries to the rectum (Borland and Walsh, in press). They occur during apical dissection, when attempting to develop the plane between the rectum and Denonvilliers' fascia.

If a rectal injury occurs, the prostatectomy should be completed, the bladder neck should be reconstructed, and the sutures should be placed in the urethra. Before placing the sutures through the bladder neck, the rectum should be closed in two layers after the edges of the incision have been freshened and the anal sphincter has been dilated widely by an assistant. It is wise to interpose omentum between the rectal closure and the vesico-urethral anastomosis to reduce the possibility of a vesicourethral fistula. This maneuver can be accomplished simply by making a small opening in the peritoneum, dividing the peritoneum in the rectovesical cul-de-sac, and feeding the end of an omental pedicle through this opening.

The wound should be copiously irrigated with antibiotic solution, and the patient should be maintained on broad-spectrum antibiotics for both aerobic and anaerobic bacteria. When this technique without a colostomy was utilized, all patients recovered without developing a wound infection, pelvic abscess, or rectourethral fistula. However, if a patient has received prior radiotherapy, it would be prudent to perform a diverting colostomy. Ureteral injury occurs secondary to inadvertent dissection within the layers of the trigone, while attempting to identify the proper cleavage plane between the bladder and seminal vesicles. If this injury occurs, ureteral reimplantation should be undertaken.

Postoperative Complications

Thromboembolism

Thrombophlebitis and pulmonary embolism are two of the most common and potentially serious complications of the procedure. Thrombophlebitis has been reported to occur in 3 to 12 per cent of patients and pulmonary emboli in 2 to 5 per cent. Some investigators have advocated postoperative anticoagulation with either warfarin sodium or minidose heparin or intermittent compression devices on the lower extremities. If the patient has a history of thrombophlebitis or pulmonary emboli, the morning after surgery the patient is fully anticoagulated with intravenous heparin for the duration of his hospital stay. No patient managed in this way has developed a pulmonary embolus.

In a patient without such a history, my approach to the prevention of thrombophlebitis has been careful attention both intraoperatively and postoperatively to avoid venous stasis. Intraoperatively, patients are placed in the Trendelenburg position to provide adequate venous drainage of the lower extremities. Epidural anesthesia also reduces the incidence of thrombophlebitis, possibly by increasing the circulation to the lower extremities during surgery. Patients are ambulated on the 1st postoperative day; they are encouraged to perform dorsiflexion exercises 100 times every hour, while awake; and they are not permitted to sit with their legs in the dependent position for 3 to 4 weeks postoperatively. In my series of 900 consecutive patients, ten (1 per cent) developed thrombophlebitis or pulmonary emboli.

Disruption of Anastomosis

Disruption of the urethrovesical anastomosis can be a disastrous complication, which may lead to permanent incontinence. This complication occurs most frequently when the Foley catheter is inadvertently removed in the early postoperative period. To avoid this complication, the balloon and valve on the catheter should be tested immediately before the catheter is placed in the bladder. Some workers have advocated making a small cystotomy incision, passing a nylon suture through the eye of the catheter, and tying the suture over a button on the anterior abdominal wall. The catheter should be taped carefully to the thigh. The anchorage of the catheter should be examined each postoperative day. If the catheter falls out prematurely, we usually make one attempt to pass a smaller caliber catheter into the bladder. If this is not successful on the first attempt, the patient undergoes cystoscopy and the catheter is placed under direct vision.

Bladder Neck Contracture

Contracture of the bladder neck has been reported to occur in 3 to 12 per cent of cases. It is usually caused by poor mucosa-to-mucosa apposition of the bladder to the urethra at the time of the anastomosis, but it can also be caused by overzealous reconstruction of the bladder neck. A patient with bladder neck contracture usually complains of a dribbling stream, but at times it may be difficult to make the diagnosis if the patient's only complaint is overflow incontinence.

In any patient who complains of incontinence, a catheter should always be passed to make certain that there is no obstruction or significant residual urine. Bladder neck contractures usually respond to one or two dilations. If this treatment fails, cold knife incision of the bladder neck at 12 o'clock usually resolves the problem (Surya et al., 1990). The mucosal advancement procedure in reconstruction of the bladder neck has markedly reduced this complication.

Incontinence

The most disabling and feared complication following radical prostatectomy is total urinary incontinence. Fortunately, it occurs infrequently in the hands of the experienced surgeon. To achieve continence after radical retropubic prostatectomy, it is mandatory to avoid injury to the pelvic floor mechanism, to reconstruct the vesical neck so that it will provide a passive mechanism of continence, and to avoid stricture formation by coapting the bladder neck to the urethra accurately. To ensure accurate coaptation of the bladder mucosa to the urethra, thereby avoiding a vesical neck contracture, we have modified our technique by exteriorizing the bladder mucosa over the raw edges of the detrusor musculature.

The role of the external sphincter mechanism has come under greater scrutiny. Following a radical prostatectomy, passive urinary control is maintained by the striated urethral sphincter. The striated urethral sphincter is distinct from the levator ani musculature in several important ways. The musculature of the striated sphincter is composed of slow-twitch fibers that are functionally capable of maintaining tone over prolonged time periods without fatigue. Conversely, the periurethral levator ani musculature is composed of fast-twitch fibers that are associated with rapid forceful muscle contraction. These fibers act to increase the force and speed of contraction of the levator ani during events that raise intra-abdominal pressure (Gosling et al., 1981).

Initially, one of the most striking benefits associated with the anatomic approach to radical prostatectomy was a marked reduction in the frequency of total incontinence. Initially, this benefit was attributed to preservation of the autonomic innervation to the pelvic floor musculature. Preservation of the neurovascular bundles may maintain autonomic innervation to the smooth muscle in the distal urethra and somatic motor supply to the striated sphincter. We evaluated 593 consecutive patients who underwent this procedure (Steiner et al., 1991). Complete urinary control was achieved in 92 per cent of the patients. Stress incontinence was present in 8 per cent. Of these, 6 per cent of men wore one or fewer pads per day, and stress incontinence was sufficient to require placement of an artificial sphincter in only two men (0.3 per cent). No patient was totally incontinent.

Age, weight of the prostate, prior transurethral resection of the prostate, pathologic stage, and preservation or wide excision of the neurovascular bundles had no significant influence on urinary continence. These data suggest that anatomic factors rather than preservation of the autonomic innervation are largely responsible for the improved urinary control associated with an anatomic approach to radical prostatectomy.

In the past, the surgeon often retracted the prostate with one hand and divided the dorsal vein complex close to the pelvic floor, where it often retracted. Retraction of the dorsal vein complex made attempts at hemostasis almost impossible and, in retrospect, interfered with reconstruction of the anterior component of the striated urethral sphincter. With the development of an anatomic approach to radical prostatectomy, urinary continence improved because the anterior component of the striated urethral sphincter/dorsal vein complex was preserved.

In this chapter, I have emphasized the importance of making an even greater effort to preserve the striated urethral sphincter and to incorporate it into the anastomosis. Employing this approach, I have noted a more rapid recovery of urinary continence by patients (Walsh et al., 1990).

Impotence

For many years it was assumed that most, if not all, patients, who underwent radical prostatectomy would be impotent postoperatively. However, today it is possible to preserve sexual function in many men. We have completed an analysis of 600 men, ages 34 to 72 years, who underwent radical prostatectomy between 1982 and 1988 (Quinlan et al., 1991). Of the 503 patients who were potent preoperatively, 68 per cent are potent postoperatively. Three factors were identified that correlated with the return of sexual function: age, clinical

Table 78–2. INFLUENCE OF PATHOLOGIC STAGE AND OPERATIVE TECHNIQUE ON RETURN OF SEXUAL FUNCTION IN 503 PATIENTS POTENT POSTOPERATIVELY

Age (Years)	Neurovascular Bundle	% Potent			
		Pathologic Stage			
		− CAP	+ CAP	+ SV	+ LN
<50	+ +	91	100	0	100
	+ ±	100	100	—	—
	+ 0	100	67	100	100
50–59	+ +	79	59	100	100
	+ ±	71	90	100	100
	+ 0	71	47	50	64
60–69	+ +	71	72	44	50
	+ ±	38	45	43	67
	+ 0	62	50	17	43
>70	+ +	17	0	100	—
	+ ±	100	0	0	—
	+ 0	0	0	0	—
All ages	+ +	70	66	50	67
	+ ±	66	80	75	64
	+ 0	70	49	39	59

+ +   = preservation of both neurovascular bundles
+ 0   = wide excision of one bundle
+ ±   = partial excision of one bundle
− CAP = no capsular penetration, seminal vesicle invasion, or lymph node involvement
+ CAP = penetration through the prostatic capsule, negative seminal vesicles, and lymph nodes
+ SV = seminal vesicle invasion, negative lymph nodes
+ LN = positive lymph nodes

and pathologic stage, and surgical technique (i.e., preservation or excision of the neurovascular bundle).

In men younger than age 50 years, potency was similar in those who had both neurovascular bundles preserved (90 per cent) and those who had one neurovascular bundle widely excised (91 per cent). In those older than 50 years, sexual function was better in patients in whom both neurovascular bundles were preserved than in patients in whom one neurovascular bundle was excised. When the relative risk of postoperative impotence was adjusted for age, the risk of postoperative impotence was twofold greater if there was capsular penetration or seminal vesicle invasion or if one neurovascular bundle was excised (Table 78–2).

In addition to neurogenic factors, there are aspects of the return of sexual function that are not completely explained by excision or preservation of the neurovascular bundles. Although the corpora cavernosa receive their primary blood supply from the internal pudendal artery, Breza and co-workers (1989) demonstrated that accessory branches to the internal pudendal artery can arise from the obturator, inferior vesical, and superior vesical arteries. These aberrant branches are divided during radical prostatectomy, and this maneuver may compromise the arterial supply to the corpora cavernosa, particularly in older individuals. Because the intracorporeal injection of papaverine in a patient after nerve-sparing radical prostatectomy produces less of an erection than that in the preoperative state, it has been suggested that erectile dysfunction is predominantly vascular in origin (Bahnson and Catalona, 1988). A number of factors may be responsible for postoperative impotence other than injury to the cavernous nerves.

Potency is defined as an erection that is sufficient for vaginal penetration and orgasm. Although many men who are potent after surgery do not have erections as firm as those preoperatively, there is no good evidence that sexual function is any better following other forms of treatment for prostatic cancer. Following radiotherapy, sexual dysfunction occurs in up to 79 per cent of men (Goldstein et al., 1984). Furthermore, only 63 per cent of men who undergo placement of a penile prosthesis for the treatment of impotence following radical surgery believe that their expectations are met (Fallon and Ghanem, 1989). Thus, regardless of the way men with prostate cancer are treated, it may be difficult to maintain or restore sexual function to normal levels.

CANCER CONTROL

The anatomic approach to radical prostatectomy emphasizes the principle of direct intraoperative visualization and of identification of the extent of disease with wide excision where necessary. This procedure was developed based on sound anatomic and pathologic principles.

1. The autonomic branches of the pelvic plexus to the corpora cavernosa are located outside the capsule of the prostate and Denonvilliers' fascia.

2. During standard radical perineal and retropubic prostatectomy, the cavernous nerves were not purposely or completely excised with the specimen (Walsh, 1987).

3. The delineation of the neurovascular bundles and prostatic fascia has made it possible to obtain a wider margin of excision than previously possible by blunt dissection. Evaluation of the surgical margins of excision obtained with this approach has confirmed the value of this procedure.

In the analysis of the first 100 patients at our institution, the surgical pathologists saw no indication that the nerve-sparing modification compromised the adequacy of the removal of cancer, which was determined primarily by the extent of tumor rather than the operative technique (Eggleston and Walsh, 1985). In a later analysis of 414 consecutive patients who had radical prostatectomies performed for clinical stages A and B cancer, the overall frequency of positive surgical margins was 10 per cent (Walsh, 1988). In this analysis, the frequency of positive surgical margins was always equal to or less than the per cent of patients with involvement of the seminal vesicles and similar to the frequency of patients with positive pelvic lymph nodes. This finding confirms our initial impression that patients with positive surgical margins have extensive disease and are in a high risk category for the development of distant dissemination.

At some institutions, when this approach to radical prostatectomy was compared with the older standard technique, the frequency of positive surgical margins was similar (Catalona and Bigg, 1990; Jones, 1990; Wahle et al., 1990). Although some have expressed difficulty with this technique, they have not excised the neurovascular bundles in the consistent way described herein. The efficacy of this technique, however, will be established only when long-term follow-up evaluation has been performed to determine whether the results of control of local disease and distant metastases are similar to those achieved with standard radical prostatectomy.

We evaluated cancer control following anatomic radical prostatectomy in 586 men with clinical stages A and B disease who had been followed 1.5 to 8 years (median follow-up 4 years; 166 followed 5 years or longer) (Morton et al., 1991). The 5-year actuarial rate for local recurrence was 4 per cent, distant metastases alone 5 per cent, distant metastases in association with local recurrence 2 per cent, death from/with disease 3 per cent, and elevated levels of prostate-specific antigen (PSA) without local recurrence or distant metastases 10 per cent. When the actuarial status at 5 years was evaluated by clinical stage, local recurrence alone occurred in 0 per cent of men with clinical stage A1 or B1 nodule, 4 per cent with stage B1, 7 per cent with stage A2, and 8 per cent with stage B2. When evaluated by pathologic stage at 5 years, local recurrence alone occurred in 2 per cent of men with organ-confined disease, 8 per cent with specimen-confined disease, and 8 per cent of men with disease that involved the surgical margins, seminal vesicles, or pelvic lymph nodes.

From a review of the literature (Morton et al., 1991), the local recurrence rate at 5 years in patients with clinical stage B1 disease is 6 to 7 per cent. This finding compares favorably with the local recurrence rate of 0 per cent in B1 nodules and 4 per cent in stage B1 disease in this series. Based on pathologic examination of the specimens, in the literature at 5 years 8 to 26 per cent of patients with organ-confined cancer will have local recurrence, and local recurrence will occur in 10 to 41 per cent of patients with penetration through the prostatic capsule. In this series, only 2 per cent of patients with organ-confined cancer had local recurrence and local recurrence occurred in only 8 per cent of patients with penetration through the prostatic capsule. Recognizing that two thirds to three quarters of all local recurrences are within the 1st 5 years, these data suggest that the anatomic approach to radical prostatectomy is associated with local control rates that are equal to or greater than those of other series reported in the literature.

SUMMARY

Applying the anatomic approach to radical prostatectomy outlined in this chapter, one should be able to avoid unnecessary injury to the striated urethral sphincter during apical dissection and to make an informed decision about the extent of resection of the lateral pelvic fascia and neurovascular bundles. In performing all procedures, the primary goal of surgery is to remove all tumor. Potency is of secondary concern. Indeed, using the principles outlined in this chapter, one can now obtain wider margins of resection than were achieved with older techniques. The primary goal of surgery should be a reduction in the morbidity of radical prostatectomy without reduction in efficacy. With this goal in mind, radical prostatectomy should be the most effective form of treatment for localized prostatic cancer.

REFERENCES

Ansell, J. S.: Radical transvesical prostatectomy: Preliminary report on an approach to surgical excision of localized prostate malignancy. J. Urol., 2:373, 1959.

Bahnson, R. R., and Catalona, W. J.: Papaverine testing of impotent patients following nerve-sparing radical prostatectomy. J. Urol., 139:773, 1988.

Borland, R. N., and Walsh, P. C.: The management of rectal injury during radical retropubic prostatectomy. J. Urol. (In press).

Breza, J., Abuseif, S. R., Orvis, B. R., Lue, T. F., and Tanagho, E. A.: Detailed anatomy of penile neurovascular structures: surgical significance. J. Urol., 41:437–443, 1989.

Campbell, E. W.: Total prostatectomy with preliminary ligation of the vascular pedicle. J. Urol., 81:464, 1959.

Catalona, W. J., and Bigg, S. W.: Nerve-sparing radical prostatectomy: evaluation of results after 250 patients. J. Urol., 143:538, 1990.

Chute, R.: Radical retropubic prostatectomy for cancer. J. Urol., 71:347, 1954.

Eggleston, J. C., and Walsh, P. C.: Radical prostatectomy with preservation of sexual function: pathologic findings in the first 100 cases. J. Urol., 4:16, 1985.

Fallon, B., and Ghanem, H.: Sexual performance and satisfaction with penile prostheses in impotence of various etiologies. J. Urol., 141:219A, 1989.

Flocks, R. H.: Arterial distribution within prostate gland: its role in transurethral prostatic resection. J. Urol., 37:524–548, 1937.

Goldstein, I., Feldman, M. I., Deckers, P. J., Babayan, R. K., and Krane, R. J.: Radiation induced impotence. JAMA, 251:903, 1984.

Gosling, J. A., Dixon, J. S., Critchley, H. O. D., and Thompson, S. A.: A comparative study of the human external sphincter and periurethral levator ani muscles. Br. J. Urol., 53:35, 1981.

Jewett, H. J., Eggleston, J. C., and Yawn, D. H.: Radical prostatectomy in the management of carcinoma of the prostate. Probable causes of some therapeutic failures. J. Urol., 107:1034, 1972.

Jones, E. C.: Resection margin status in radical retropubic prostatectomy specimens: relationship to type of operation, tumor size, tumor grade, and local tumor extension. J. Urol., 144:89, 1990.

Lepor, H., Gregerman, M., Crosby, R., Mostofi, F. K., and Walsh, P. C.: Precise localization of the autonomic nerves from the pelvic plexus to the corpora cavernosa: a detailed anatomical study of the adult male pelvis. J. Urol., 133:207–212, 1985.

Lich, R., Grant, O., Maurer, J. E.: Extravesical prostatectomy: A comparison of retropubic and perineal prostatectomy. J. Urol., 61:930, 1949.

Lue, T. F., Zeineh, S. J., Schmidt, R. A., Tanagho, E. A.: Neuroanatomy of penile erection: its relevance to iatrogenic impotence. J. Urol., 131:273–280, 1984.

Memmelaar, J.: Total prostatovesiculectomy—retropubic approach. J. Urol., 62:349, 1949.

Millin, T.: Retropubic urinary surgery. Livingstone, London, 1947.

Morton, R. A., Steiner, M. S., Walsh, P. C.: Cancer control following anatomical radical prostatectomy: an interim report. J. Urol., 145:1197–1200, 1991.

Myers, R. P.: Prostate shape, external striated urethral sphincter, and radical prostatectomy: the apical dissection. J. Urol., 138:543–550, 1987.

Oelrich, T. M.: The urethral sphincter muscle in the male. Am. J. Anat., 158:229–296, 1980.

Peters, C., and Walsh, P. C.: Blood transfusion and anesthetic practices in radical retropubic prostatectomy. J. Urol., 134:81–83, 1985.

Quinlan, D. M., Epstein, J. I., Carter, B. S., and Walsh, P. C.: Sexual function following radical prostatectomy: influence of preservation of neurovascular bundles. J. Urol., 145:998–1002, 1991.

Rainwater, L. M., and Segura, J. W.: Technical consideration in radical retropubic prostatectomy: blood loss after ligation of dorsal venous complex. J. Urol., 143:1163, 1990.

Reiner, W. G., and Walsh, P. C.: An anatomical approach to the surgical management of the dorsal vein and Santorini's plexus during radical retropubic surgery. J. Urol., 121:198–200, 1979.

Schlegel, P., and Walsh, P. C.: Neuroanatomical approach to radical cystoprostatectomy with preservation of sexual function. J. Urol., 138:1402–1406, 1987.

Steiner, M. S., Morton, R. A., and Walsh, P. C.: Impact of radical prostatectomy on urinary continence. J. Urol., 145:512–515, 1991.

Surya, B. V., Provet, J., Johanson, K-E., and Brown, J.: Anastomotic strictures following radical prostatectomy: Risk factors and management. J. Urol., 43:755, 1990.

Wahle, S., Reznicek, M., Fallon, B., Platz, C., and Williams, R.: Incidence of surgical margin involvement in various forms of radical prostatectomy. Urology, 36:23, 1990.

Walsh, P. C.: Radical prostatectomy, preservation of sexual function, cancer control: The controversy. Urol. Clin. North Am., 14:663, 1987.

Walsh, P. C.: Radical retropubic prostatectomy with reduced morbidity: An anatomic approach. NCI Monogr., 7:133–137, 1988.

Walsh, P. C., and Donker, P. J.: Impotence following radical prostatectomy: insight into etiology and prevention. J. Urol., 128:492–497, 1982.

Walsh, P. C., Lepor, H., and Eggleston, J. C.: Radical prostatectomy with preservation of sexual function: anatomical and pathological considerations. Prostate, 4:473–485, 1983.

Walsh, P. C., Quinlan, D. M., Morton, R. A., and Steiner, M. S.: Radical retropubic prostatectomy. Improved anastomosis and urinary continence. Urol. Clin. North Am., 17:679–684, 1990.

79
PERINEAL PROSTATECTOMY

David F. Paulson, M.D.

Perineal prostatectomy, both simple and radical, at one time was a popular method to achieve surgical control of prostatic diseases. However, today, the term perineal prostatectomy should be reserved only for radical prostatic surgery. With current transrectal ultrasound enabling the identification and biopsy of nonpalpable lesions within the prostate and with current instrumentation for transurethral resection obviating the need for the open surgical treatment of benign prostatic growth, the perineal approach to the prostate has been discarded by many. Therefore, the comments that follow are directed only to the perineal surgery performed for prostatic malignancy. The perineal approach to the prostate can be used for corrections of rectoprostatic, rectovesical, and rectourethral fistulas, and knowledge of the surgical anatomy of the perineum is of value.

HISTORY

The perineum has been chosen for the approach to the bladder and prostate for over 2000 years. Surgeons first devised and employed a median perineal incision for removal of bladder calculi. In the first century A.D., a semielliptic incision in the perineum was utilized for partial removal of the prostate gland. Thereafter, until approximately 1600, there was little known use of the perineal approach to the prostate. Sporadic accounts of perineal removal of bladder stone or parts of the prostate were noted in the 17th, 18th, and early 19th centuries.

In 1867, the recognition of prostatic carcinoma and the availability of anesthesia prompted the first perineal operation for adenocarcinoma of the prostate. A deliberate but blind enucleation for benign prostatic hyperplasia was described in 1873. Surgical records from the years 1882 and 1891 describe the earliest excisions with urethral reconstruction and the first standardized perineal incisions for benign prostatic enlargement. Later, advances in technique were made by different surgeons. Modifications in the anatomic approach and in the instrumentation assisted in the development of the perineal prostatectomy. This perineal prostatectomy changed from a crude blunt dissection to a precise surgical exercise performed under direct vision with the ability to establish hemostasis, identify local anatomic structures, and appropriately reconstruct the urinary tract. The evolution of this form of surgery was well documented by Weyrauch (1959) (Table 79–1).

INDICATIONS

Multiple modalities may be employed for the treatment of prostatic malignancy. Treatment selection has been standardly based on the stage of the disease and both the patients' and the physicians' bias. The treatment philosophy promoting radical surgery has been based on the observation that many malignancies confined to a single anatomic site are best managed by surgical removal of the primary malignancy. The location of the prostate presents certain technical problems in the removal of this organ without damage to adjacent organ structures.

The two most popular approaches to the prostate are the radical retropubic prostatoseminal vesiculectomy and the perineal prostatoseminal vesiculectomy. Perineal prostatoseminal vesiculectomy has the advantage of providing a relatively avascular field, good exposure for reconstruction of the vesicourethral anastomosis, and dependent postoperative drainage (Belt, 1942; Dees, 1970; Jewett, 1970; Ray, 1975; Weyrauch, 1959). Further, the elderly patient tolerates well the perineal approach, whereas an intra-abdominal approach might very well compromise this patient's postoperative pulmonary function. The principal disadvantage of the perineal approach to the prostate is that it does not afford simultaneous exposure of the pelvic lymphatic drainage, which must be assessed prior to radical prostatectomy. Thus, two incisions are necessary if the patient undergoing perineal prostatectomy is to have a staging lymphadenectomy. Further, preservation of the anatomic innervation of the corporal vasculature may be more difficult through the perineum than through the retropubic approach.

Ankylosis of the hips and previous open prostatic

Table 79–1. LANDMARKS IN DEVELOPMENT OF PERINEAL PROSTATECTOMY

Contribution	Surgeon	Year
Primitive "Blind" Techniques		
First perineal lithotomy: initial step in perineal approach to prostate	Ammonius Lithotomus	460–357 B.C.
Curved incision for perineal lithotomy	Celsus	25 A.D.
Accidental removal of prostatic lobe during perineal lithotomy	Covillard	1639
First perineal prostatectomy: median incision	Guthrie	1834
First perineal prostatectomy for carcinoma: median incision	Billroth	1867
Blind finger enucleation via median perineal urethrotomy	Gouley	1873
Curved incision of Celsus for excision of prostatic carcinoma: reconstruction of urethra	Leisrink	1882
Standardization of technique described by Gouley	Goodfellow	1891
Balloon to pull prostate toward perineum: inflated in bladder	Syms	1900
Operation Performed Under Vision		
Median perineal prostatectomy under vision: a "perineal" table, prostatic tractor, and lobe enucleator	Proust	1901
Conservative perineal prostatectomy: curved skin incision, inverted Y incision for enucleation, preservation of verumontanum and ejaculatory ducts; perineal retractors, prostatic tractor, and lobe forceps	Young	1903
Radical perineal prostatectomy for carcinoma; removal of prostate, seminal vesicles, ampullae of the vasa, and surrounding fascia	Young	1905
Preservation of structures surrounding external sphincter; suture of vesical neck to stump of urethra	Hans Wildbolz	1906
Hemostatic bag for perineal prostatectomy: large drainage tube passing through center of bag	Edwin Davis	1924
Plastic closure: bleeding controlled by suture, obliteration of prostatic fossa	Gibson	1928
Approach Within Anal Sphincter		
Exposure via cleavage plane between external anal sphincter and longitudinal fibers of rectum	Haim	1936
Standardization of approach beneath anal sphincter	Belt	1939

From Weyrauch, H. M.: Surgery of the Prostate. Philadelphia, W. B. Saunders Co., 1959.

surgery, which fixes the bladder and prostate in the pelvis making reconstruction of the vesicourethral junction difficult, are contraindications to the procedure. The patient who is massively obese may have sufficient limitation of diaphragmatic movement when placed in exaggerated lithotomy position that adequate ventilation cannot be achieved. The obese patient with a large panniculous is not at risk; however, the patient with a "large-barrel abdomen" and a large amount of intra-abdominal fat often cannot be adequately positioned.

The patient undergoing perineal prostatectomy is best managed with general anesthesia in order that adequate control of the pulmonary airway can be maintained.

Preoperative Preparation

The patient should be assessed preoperatively to determine whether or not it is believed that the disease is confined to the prostatic primary. This assessment is accomplished by careful digital examination to ensure that there is no evidence of disease extension into the seminal vesicles and that the lateral sulci of the prostate are distinct and not obliterated. Transrectal ultrasound to determine the extent of disease has not yet proved to be of greater advantage than careful digital examination. Patients who have obvious extensions of disease are not candidates for radical perineal prostatectomies. This operation should not be undertaken in patients in whom it is known preoperatively that the disease extends beyond the anatomic borders of the prostate.

Preoperative cystoscopy is not warranted unless the patient has previously undergone a transurethral resection. In this instance, preoperative cystoscopy is appropriate in order that the surgeon can determine that the prostatic fossa is well epithelialized and that no bullous edema from the previous transurethral surgery is evident at the bladder neck. The surgeon also has the opportunity to note the distance between ureteral orifices and the line of the transurethral resection, in order to determine that the ureteral orifices will not be compromised at the time of prostatectomy.

Bowel preparation consists only of repeated enemas until return is clear. A neomycin-containing enema is given several hours prior to the patient's entry to the operating room. Oral laxatives and sterilization of the bowel with antibiotics are unnecessary.

Positioning

The patient is placed in the exaggerated lithotomy position. To achieve this position, the sacrum is brought to the edge of the table, with the buttocks extending several inches over the end of the table. A classic Young table or an operating-room table with appropriately designed leg braces can be used (Fig. 79–1). Padded shoulder braces may be placed against the acromial processes to prevent stress or pressure injury to the brachial plexus. However, with the patient properly positioned, shoulder braces are not necessary. The patient is held in place by the positioning of the lower extremities. When this position can be accomplished, the arms may be taped to the patient's legs rather than being outstretched at the sides. With the arms taped to the patient's legs and in a vertical position, stretch injury to the brachial plexus is extraordinarily uncommon.

The sacrum should be raised on sandbags or folded towels to assist in positioning. This step will help elevate the perineum. The legs are always well padded to prevent damage to vessels and nerves. After correct positioning, the perineum is parallel to the floor and optimum exposure may be accomplished following surgical incision.

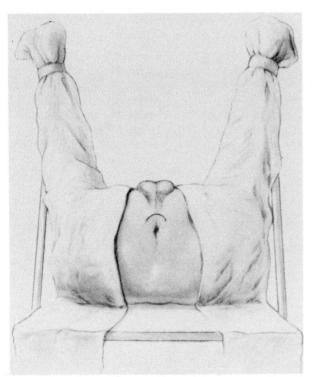

Figure 79–1. Exaggerated lithotomy position for radical perineal prostatectomy with line of incision indicated. (From Skinner, D. G. (Ed.): Diagnosis and Management of Genitourinary Cancer. Philadelphia, W. B. Saunders Co., 1988.)

Exposure of the Prostate

After the patient has been placed in the exaggerated lithotomy position, a Lowsley retractor may be passed retrograde through the urethra into the bladder and the blades extended (Fig. 79–2). If a Lowsley retractor cannot be passed into the bladder because of anatomic abnormalities, either a sound or a Foley catheter may be employed. A ureteral catheter may be of assistance in the bypass of false passages or strictures and is secured to the end of the Lowsley retractor with either waterproof surgical tape or silk sutures. The ureteral catheter will guide the Lowsley retractor into the bladder.

Following placement of the retractor, attention is directed to the line of incision. The skin incision is made approximately 1 cm anterior to the anal verge and curved posterolaterally on either side within the medial borders of the ischial tuberosities. The skin incision should be extended level to a line extending transversely behind the posterior anal margin. The superficial perineal fascia is incised utilizing cutting cautery, and a surgical space in the ischial rectal fossa is developed (Fig. 79–3).

The superficial central muscles of the perineum are divided with the cautery at the most anterior margin of the incision. Following division of the central tendon, the rectal sphincter is visualized as an arch overlying the rectum (Figs. 79–4 and 79–5). An anterior retractor stretches the rectal sphincter superiorly. With this maneuver accomplished, the glistening fibers of the anterior rectal fascia can be identified. Using these anterior

fascial fibers as a guide, with either sharp or blunt dissection, the rectum can be mobilized on either side of the rectourethralis to gain entry to the prostate. The surgeon should recognize that the rectum is pulled forward in the midline by the rectourethralis. Therefore, division of the rectourethralis should be accomplished closer to the bulb of the penis than to the anterior surface of the rectum. Division of the rectourethralis is accomplished with the surgeon's finger in the rectum to define the course of the rectum (Figs. 79–6 and 79–7).

CLASSIC RADICAL PERINEAL PROSTATECTOMY

The rectum is separated from the posterior surface of the prostate by blunt dissection between Denonvilliers' fascia anteriorly and rectal fascia posteriorly. Following posterior displacement, the rectum is protected by folded moist gauze with inferior retraction of the rectum maintained with a weighted posterior speculum. Blunt dissection now permits exposure of the lateral and posterior margins of the prostate (Fig. 79–8). A white and glistening fascia overlies the prostate. This fascia is multilayered and may be incised to identify a plane between it and prostatic substance; however, the fascia is usually carried with the specimen, employing the anterior rectal fascia to protect the rectum (Figs. 79–9 and 79–10).

With blunt dissection, the prostate is mobilized lat-

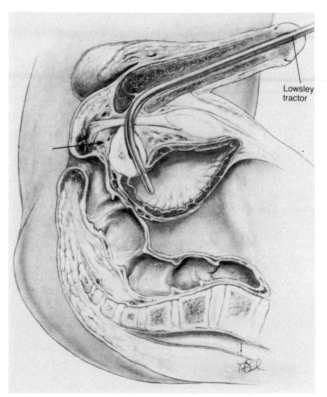

Figure 79–2. Positioning of the Lowsley retractor for traction. The approach to the prostate is indicated by the arrow. (From Skinner, D. G. (Ed.): Diagnosis and Management of Genitourinary Cancer. Philadelphia, W. B. Saunders Co., 1988.)

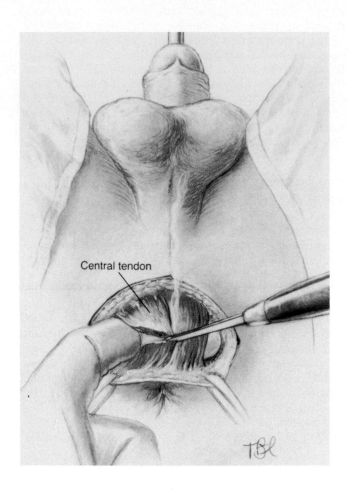

Figure 79–3. The central tendon is the muscular sheet that extends anterior to the rectum and is superficial to the external anal sphincter. Incision of the central tendon alone with division of the projection of the external sphincter to the perineal body will permit the dissection to be carried out beneath the triangle formed by the superficial external anal sphincter. (From Skinner, D. G. (Ed.): Diagnosis and Management of Genitourinary Cancer. Philadelphia, W. B. Saunders Co., 1988.)

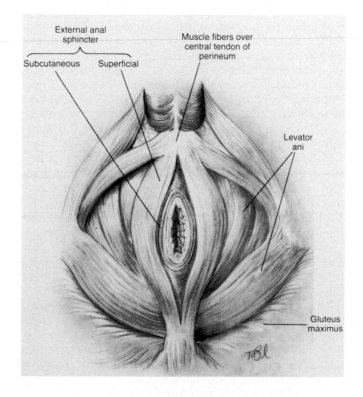

Figure 79–4. The fibers of the external anal sphincter can be visualized following division of the central tendon. A retractor can be placed in the triangle formed by the superficial external anal sphincter and those muscle fibers elevated to provide visualization of the rectal wall. (From Skinner, D. G. (Ed.): Diagnosis and Management of Genitourinary Cancer. Philadelphia, W. B. Saunders Co., 1988.)

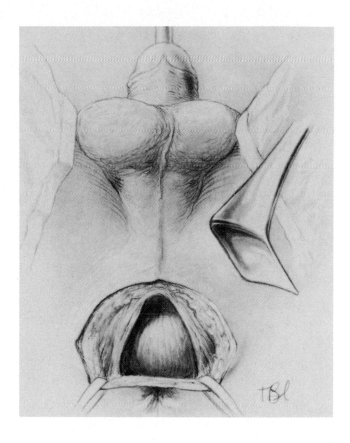

Figure 79–5. The anterior retractor has been removed for this diagrammatic representation of the subsphincteric approach. The anterior rectal fascia can be followed to the level of the rectourethralis. (From Skinner, D. G. (Ed.): Diagnosis and Management of Genitourinary Cancer. Philadelphia, W. B. Saunders Co., 1988.)

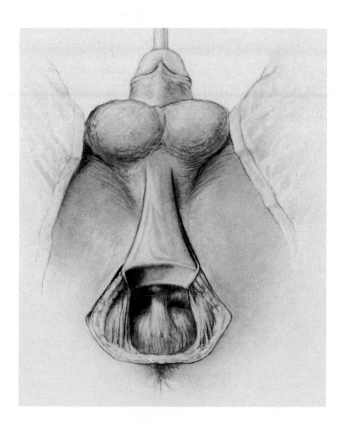

Figure 79–6. With the sphincter retracted superiorly (lateral retractor can be placed beneath the muscle to produce additional exposure), the rectourethralis can be visualized. The extent of development of this muscle is variable. (From Skinner, D. G. (Ed.): Diagnosis and Management of Genitourinary Cancer. Philadelphia, W. B. Saunders Co., 1988.)

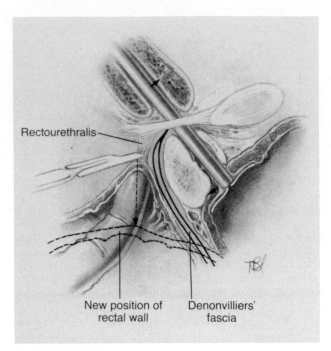

Figure 79–7. Lateral view of the rectourethralis. The surgeon's finger has been placed in the rectum to assist in identification of the rectal wall. (From Skinner, D. G. (Ed.): Diagnosis and Management of Genitourinary Cancer. Philadelphia, W. B. Saunders Co., 1988.)

erally. This mobilization is carried to the level of the bladder, at which point a line of demarcation can be identified between the bladder and the prostate itself. The dissection is carried anteriorly until a line of cleavage can be developed on either side of the membranous urethra just distal to the prostatic apex. At this point, a right-angle clamp is placed around the membranous urethra distal to the prostatic apex, the Lowsley retractor removed, and the urethra sharply divided.

The urethra is divided in two stages. After the urethra is partially cut, the urethra on the patient's side is tagged with 2–0 chromic catgut suture in order that it can be exposed at the time of reconstruction (Fig. 79–11). The urethra is always divided distal to the apex of the prostate. Following division of the urethra, a Young prostatic tractor or a Foley catheter can be passed through the prostatic urethra into the bladder and the blades extended or the balloon inflated. With posterior pressure on the retractor to displace the prostate, and with either sharp or blunt dissection, a plane can be developed beneath the venous plexus to the level of the detrusor musculature. At this point, the bladder may be entered and the prostate sharply cut away. Alternatively, a plane is developed bluntly between the detrusor musculature and the prostatic substance (Fig. 79–12). As the prostate is dissected from the bladder neck anteriorly, a "horse collar" of fibers at the bladder neck can be identified. The dissection may be carried around

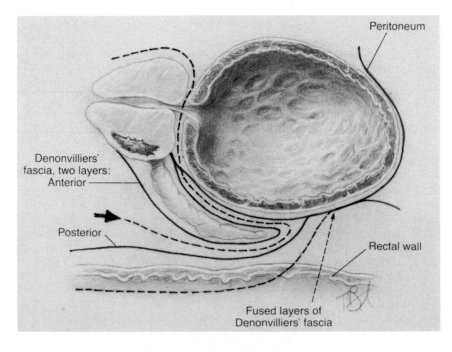

Figure 79–8. Limits of dissection for the radical prostatectomy. Solid area with dashed line indicates surgical route. (From Skinner, D. G. (Ed.): Diagnosis and Management of Genitourinary Cancer. Philadelphia, W. B. Saunders Co., 1988.)

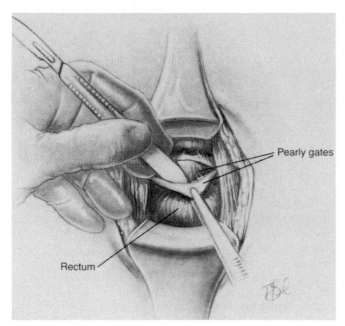

Figure 79–9. Incision of the overlying fascia ("the pearly gates") to expose the true capsule of the prostate. (From Skinner, D. G. (Ed.): Diagnosis and Management of Genitourinary Cancer. Philadelphia, W. B. Saunders Co., 1988.)

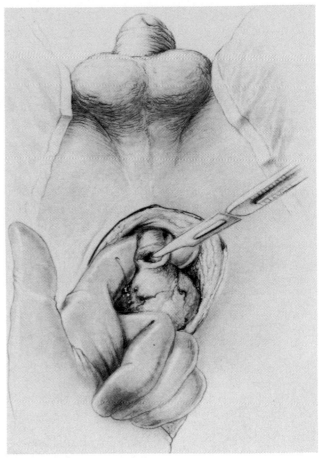

Figure 79–11. The apex of the prostate is identified and the membranous urethra sharply divided. (From Skinner, D. G. (Ed.): Diagnosis and Management of Genitourinary Cancer. Philadelphia, W. B. Saunders Co., 1988.)

the entry of the urethra in the prostatic substance on both sides, and the extension of the prostatic urethra into the bladder is divided at this point at 12 o'clock. This maneuver preserves the continuity of the bladder neck fibers. At this point, the Young retractor is withdrawn and a Foley catheter or Penrose drain passed

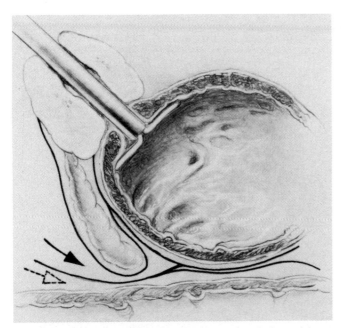

Figure 79–10. The solid arrow identifies the preferred plane of dissection above the anterior rectal fascia (posterior Denonvilliers' fascia) and the fascia of the rectovesical septum (anterior layers of Denonvilliers' fascia). The broken arrow indicates a line of dissection beneath the rectal fascia, which carries the hazard of rectal perforation. (From Skinner, D. G. (Ed.): Diagnosis and Management of Genitourinary Cancer. Philadelphia, W. B. Saunders Co., 1988.)

through the prostatic urethra and brought out superiorly through the line of incision between the prostate and the bladder neck. Traction on the catheter permits the surgeon to displace the prostate posteriorly or laterally as necessary for completion of the dissection (Fig. 79–13).

As the prostate is pulled toward the surgeon, a line of cleavage may be identified between the bladder neck fibers. Often, a right-angle clamp can be passed beneath the extension of the trigonal fibers into the prostate and the fibers sharply divided. When visualization of this structure is difficult because of previous transurethral surgery, digital examination often allows the surgeon to identify the posterior bladder neck as a transverse ridge.

As previously mentioned, the trigonal fibers should be divided just distal to the detrusor muscles of the bladder neck because these fibers course down into the prostatic urethra. With a transverse incision made at this point and carried across the posterior aspect of the specimen, the detrusor fibers are separated from the prostate and the posterior bladder neck rides up into the pelvis. It is advisable to place a traction suture of 0 chromic catgut into the bladder neck fibers in order that the bladder neck can be identified at the completion of the procedure. If this step is not accomplished, as the detrusor muscles contract identification of the bladder neck may become difficult.

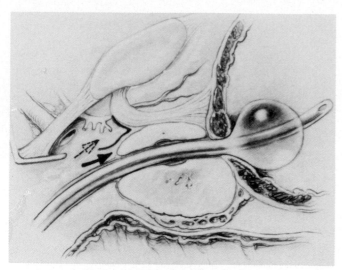

Figure 79–12. The solid arrow indicates the proper plane of dissection beneath the anterolateral fascia and beneath the venous plexus. Dissection above this fascia (dotted arrow) carries the hazard of disruption of the venous sinus and troublesome bleeding. (From Skinner, D. G. (Ed.): Diagnosis and Management of Genitourinary Cancer. Philadelphia, W. B. Saunders Co., 1988.)

If an appropriate line of division has been established, the glistening seminal vesicles are evident coursing beneath the detrusor musculature of the posterior bladder neck. Blunt dissection allows the surgeon to mobilize the bladder superiorly and expose the ampullae of the vas deferens. These can be isolated with a right-angle clamp, controlled on the patient's side with large surgical clips, and divided. At this point, the prostate is attached by some of its fascial attachments at 5 and 7 o'clock, by the posterior extension of Denonvilliers' fascia behind

the seminal vesicles, and by the seminal vesicles themselves. In addition, the prostate is secured posterolaterally by the vascular pedicles (see Fig. 78–13). The vascular pedicles to the prostate cannot be isolated and controlled until the fibrofascial extension of the periprostatic fascia is divided at 5 and 7 o'clock. The vasculature within this fibrovascular fascia may be controlled with surgical clips. Following division of this tissue, the pedicles can be isolated at their point of egress from the specimen at both 5 and 7 o'clock and controlled prior to division either with surgical metal clips or with absorbable sutures.

Following division of the vascular pedicles bilaterally, the specimen is retained only by the seminal vesicles. If the vas deferens have not been previously divided, they are now exposed for a distance of 2 to 3 cm, cross-clamped, and then divided. The seminal vesicles may be removed with the specimen utilizing alternating sharp and blunt dissection. The fibrofilamentous tissue overlying the seminal vesicles may contain small bleeding vessels, which should be controlled with cautery. If the seminal vesicles do not dissect freely, this does not mean that there is perivesicular tumor involvement. This finding may reflect only chronic inflammation. The vesicles themselves may be divided and oversewn with interlocking chromic catgut suture or divided with the patient's side controlled with surgical clips (Fig. 79–14).

After ascertaining that hemostasis has been established, attention should be directed to reconstruction of the bladder neck and to establishing continuity between the bladder neck and the membranous urethra. These are best accomplished by direct anastomosis between

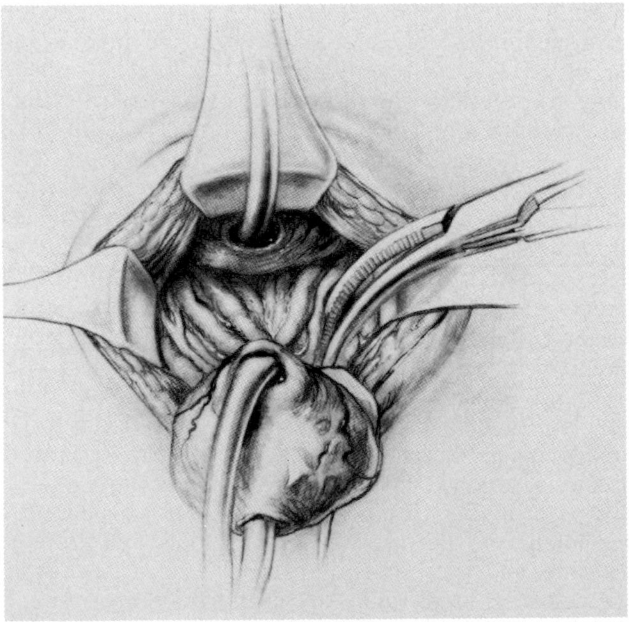

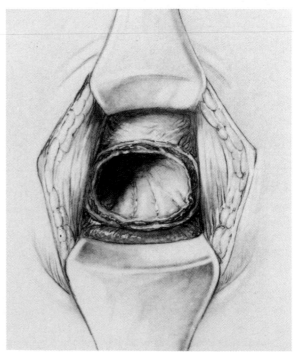

Figure 79–13. The posterior bladder neck has been cut away and the bladder allowed to retract separately. A plane is then developed between the bladder anteriorly and the prostate and seminal vesicles posteriorly. (From Skinner, D. G. (Ed.): Diagnosis and Management of Genitourinary Cancer. Philadelphia, W. B. Saunders Co., 1988.)

Figure 79–14. View of the bladder after removal of the specimen. The bladder neck fibers are preserved anteriorly but may be sacrificed posteriorly and laterally as necessary for removal of the tumor. (From Skinner, D. G. (Ed.): Diagnosis and Management of Genitourinary Cancer. Philadelphia, W. B. Saunders Co., 1988.)

the bladder neck and the urethra, with the direct anastomosis supported by a modification of the vest traction sutures. These steps provide maximum alignment between the reconstructed bladder neck and the membranous urethra and reduce the tension on the direct anastomosis.

The bladder neck is closed from 6 to 12 o'clock with interrupted 0 chromic catgut suture (Fig. 79–15). This maneuver permits the vesicourethral anastomosis to be done superiorly at 12 o'clock, at a maximum distance from ureteral orifices and a minimum distance from the urethra itself. The closure can be conducted by inverting the suture, closing the bladder neck from 12 to 6 o'clock, and making the vesicourethral anastomosis at the 6 o'clock position. This procedure, however, rolls the bladder neck and trigone into a tube and may occlude the ureteral orifices by incorporating them into the bladder closure itself.

Bladder neck reconstruction is begun by placing two mattress sutures of 0 chromic catgut at 1 and 11 o'clock, outside-in, inside-out, approximately 5 mm from the cut margin of the anterior bladder neck. These are tied securely and left long for subsequent placement beneath the perineal skin. At this point, an 18 Fr. Foley catheter is passed through the urethra. Four sutures of 00 chromic catgut now are placed in the membranous urethra at 2, 4, 8, and 10 o'clock. The 00 chromic catgut sutures placed at 4 and 8 o'clock are carried down and placed into the bladder neck at 10 and 2 o'clock. These are the anterior direct anastomotic sutures. The 18 Fr. Foley catheter now is passed into the bladder itself and the balloon inflated (Fig. 79–16). Closure of the bladder neck now begins at 6 o'clock and is carried, with

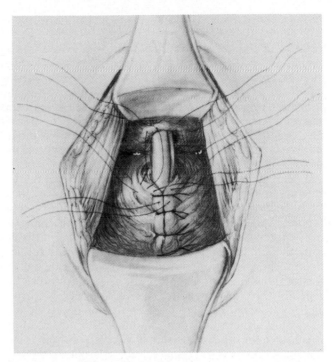

Figure 79–16. The vest sutures at 2, 4, 8, and 10 o'clock of 0 chromic catgut, with placement used for direct anastomosis. (From Skinner, D. G. (Ed.): Diagnosis and Management of Genitourinary Cancer. Philadelphia, W. B. Saunders Co., 1988.)

interrupted 0 chromic catgut sutures, in a racket-handle fashion until the bladder neck is tightly closed around the 18 Fr. Foley catheter. At this point, the two remaining sutures of 00 chromic catgut that were placed in the membranous urethra at 1 and 11 o'clock are placed in the reconstructed bladder neck at 4 and 8 o'clock. The four 00 chromic catgut sutures are secured, first anteriorly and then posteriorly. As these sutures are tightened, the reconstructed bladder neck is approximated to the membranous urethra. The two 0 chromic catgut sutures, previously placed at 11 and 1 o'clock in the bladder neck are drawn through on each side of the perineal body and tied subcutaneously. The last two 0 chromic sutures used to create the racket-handle closure of the bladder neck are also brought through on either side of the perineal body and tied subcutaneously.

These four modified vest sutures of double 0 chromic catgut support the direct anastomosis between the bladder neck and the urethra. The wound now is closed. Drainage is established with a Penrose drain, which may be brought out either through a stab wound or through the lateral aspect of the incision. During closure of the perineum, the levator ani musculature is approximated in the midline with absorbable suture material. Reconstruction of this area supports the new bladder neck and reduces the likelihood of both bladder and rectal incontinence.

POTENCY-SPARING RADICAL PERINEAL PROSTATECTOMY

In the classic perineal prostatectomy, the investing periprostatic fascia, or the posterior layer of Denonvil-

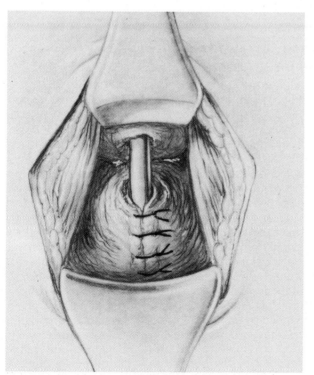

Figure 79–15. Closure of the bladder neck from 6 o'clock. (From Skinner, D. G. (Ed.): Diagnosis and Management of Genitourinary Cancer. Philadelphia, W. B. Saunders Co., 1988.)

liers' fascia, is incised in a left-to-right fashion, usually just below the apex of the prostate. Review of the location of the corporal nerves would indicate that the likelihood of division of the nerves is extremely high when the incision is so placed. Further, as the "posterior layer" of Denonvilliers' fascia is dissected from the prostatic surface and retractors are placed beneath this posterior layer, stretch injury or tearing of the nerves may occur. Slight modification of the operative procedure permits the surgeon to preserve the neurovascular plexus (Fig. 79–17).

If the incision into the fascial layer overlying the prostate is made in the midline from 6 to 12 o'clock, the dissection may be carried beneath the neurovascular bundle, which lies in the periprostatic fascia (Fig. 79–18). Employing both alternating sharp and blunt dissection, the prostate may be exposed within this surgical plane. The dissection develops on either side of the membranous urethra just distal to the prostatic apex but beneath the puboprostatic venous plexus. A curved clamp can then be placed beneath the neurovascular plexus but around the membranous urethra distal to the prostatic apex and the urethra divided as previously described. After the Young retractor is placed through the prostatic urethra and into the bladder, the prostate may be dissected from the bladder neck itself in the midline and from beneath the neurovascular plexus in such a manner as to "deliver" the prostate without damage to the neurovascular plexus. However, if the surgeon suspects that disease may involve the periprostatic fascia and is concerned that a cancer-negative surgical margin may not be obtained should the periprostatic fascia remain, he or she may modify the

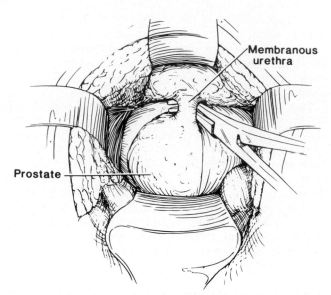

Figure 79–18. The periprostatic fascia has been removed from the right lobe of the prostate but preserved on the left lobe. A dissection plane has been developed between the periprostatic fascia and the prostatic substance on the left side. A right-angle clamp is then passed around the membranous urethra, beneath the lateral pelvic fascia. The membranous urethra is sharply incised.

procedure as described subsequently—to conduct a "wide-field" radical perineal prostatectomy. Alternatively, one may resect the periprostatic fascia on one side and submit it either with the specimen or as a separate specimen (Fig. 79–19). It is difficult to determine with accuracy whether or not periprostatic fascia will be tumor-positive or tumor-negative on the basis of palpation or the characteristics with which it dissects from the prostate.

WIDE-FIELD RADICAL PERINEAL PROSTATECTOMY

When performing a radical perineal prostatectomy, the surgeon should adhere to the principle of establishing margins as far from the malignancy as possible without sacrificing normal tissue. The surgical margins of the perineal prostatectomy may be extended to encompass the fibrovascular fascia surrounding the prostate, the periprostatic fascia or the lateral pelvic fascia, as named by Walsh, which is usually not removed with the specimen in the classic perineal prostatectomy.

The wide-field radical perineal prostatoseminal vesiculectomy always results in sacrifice of the periprostatic neurovascular corporal nerves, because the margin of dissection always includes the periprostatic fascia. The prostate is exposed as described. However, after the rectum has been placed posteriorly, a surgical plane is developed between the posterior layers of Denonvilliers' fascia—the anterior rectal surface posteriorly and the levator musculature anteriorly. The prostate remains surrounded by the periprostatic lateral pelvic fascia.

A right-angle clamp is placed outside the fibrovascular fascia and around the apex of the prostate. The urethra

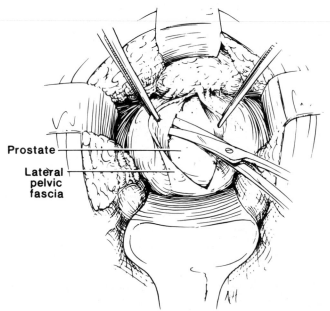

Figure 79–17. Following exposure of the prostate, which is enclosed in the periprostatic fascia here labeled the lateral pelvic fascia in accordance with Walsh's terminology, should the surgeon desire to spare the corporal nerves, the periprostatic fascia is split in the midline. A plane is then developed between the periprostatic fascia and the capsule of the prostate itself. This maneuver can be done by alternating sharp and blunt dissection.

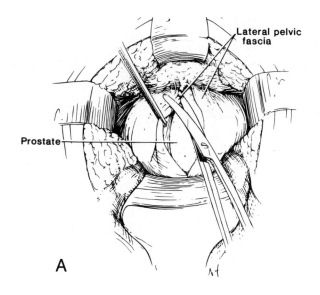

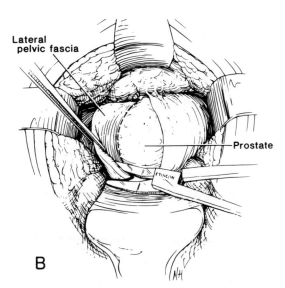

Figure 79–19. *A,* The surgeon may be uncertain as to whether disease has invaded into the lateral pelvic fascia. When this uncertainty arises, the surgeon may separately take the periprostatic fascia (lateral pelvic fascia). The vasculature that flows in the periprostatic fascia may be controlled with surgical clips both at the apex of the prostate and at the base. The fascia is elevated from prostatic substance.

B, The periprostatic fascia has been controlled superiorly and is now being controlled at the base. The clips of the base may be placed back behind the exit of the seminal vesicles, ensuring that all of this tissue can be removed. The lateral pelvic fascia may be sharply incised at the point of its reflection onto the bladder and the bleeding controlled after removal of the prostate. Alternatively, the bleeding points may be controlled with surgical clips because the periprostatic fascia has been removed.

is divided at this level. The prostate is sharply mobilized anteriorly. Bleeding from the venous plexus frequently occurs but can be controlled by pressure from a narrow Deaver retractor. The periprostatic fascia is sharply cut away at the point of its reflection onto the bladder, with bleeding points to be controlled either with surgical clips prior to being cut away from the bladder or with electrocautery. Although venous bleeding may occur, it

stops once the prostate has been removed and tension on the bladder neck fibers is released. Further, after the bladder is brought into the pelvis for reconstruction of the bladder neck and anastomosis to the urethra, previous troublesome bleeding points become occluded.

At the base of the prostate, posterior layers of Denonvilliers' fascia that overlie the seminal vesicles are sharply incised in order to expose the vesicles. This layer of fascia is multilaminated. Surgeons should recognize that they may have to go through several layers of fascia before identifying the seminal vesicle. The fibrovascular pedicles are taken as far distant to the prostatic base as possible, thus ensuring sacrifice of the neurovascular complex at this level also. Following exposure of the seminal vesicles, they are controlled as previously described. The specimen is removed. After removal of the specimen, reconstruction of the bladder neck may be accomplished as previously described.

COMPLICATIONS AND THEIR MANAGEMENT

Loss of Anatomic Landmarks

Following completion of the skin incision, the surgeon must be certain that the central tendon is mobilized and completely divided. The rectum can be palpated beneath the central tendon. With blunt dissection, a tunnel approximately 2 cm anterior to the anal verge is created beneath the central tendon and anterior to the rectum. The central tendon is then divided, employing the cutting cautery. Following division of the central tendon, the surgeon usually identifies the anal sphincter and the anterior rectal fascia. Every attempt must be made to identify the anterior rectal fascia because this provides a path to the prostatic apex and prostate. Failure to identify this anatomic landmark may cause the surgeon to carry the dissection anteriorly into the perineum, injuring either the bulbocavernosus or the membranous urethra.

When the anterior rectal surface cannot be identified with certainty, the surgeon should place a finger into the rectum and, with sharp dissection being conducted toward the rectal surface, the perineal musculature sharply cut away until the anterior rectal surface is identified. Once this maneuver is accomplished, the dissection can be carried to the prostatic apex without difficulty.

The rectourethralis is variously developed and may consist of a few rudimentary fibers between the apex of the prostate and the rectum or it may consist of a vertical band of fibromuscular tissue several centimeters in length. In order to permit proper identification of the rectourethralis, the dissection along the anterior rectal surface should be carried just to the left and right of the midline. This procedure can be accomplished with blunt dissection and even conducted to such an extent that the rectum may be bluntly separated from the prostate and its investing fascia prior to division of the rectourethralis.

Control of Bleeding from the Periprostatic Venous Plexus

Vigorous venous bleeding may be encountered during dissection at the apex of the prostate or after division of the membranous urethra when the prostate is being separated from the bladder anteriorly and anterolaterally. Although one is tempted to stop the dissection and control the venous bleeding, it is best to provide temporary control of the bleeding by pressure behind a curved narrow Deaver retractor, until the prostate is separated from the bladder neck anteriorly and antero-laterally. Once the prostate is so separated, most of the venous bleeding spontaneously ceases. Any troublesome persistent bleeding may be controlled by use of a 4 × 8 sponge wrapped around a curved narrow Deaver retractor at the level of the anterior bladder neck.

The line of incision at the posterior bladder neck must be carried in a transverse manner between 5 and 7 o'clock in order to separate the prostate from the bladder. This line of incision should be carried posteriorly until the fascia that overlies the seminal vesicles is identified. Failure to carry the incision directly posterior will result in thinning of the posterior bladder neck fibers, compromising subsequent reconstruction. Further, if the dissection is not carried posteriorly until the fascia that surrounds the seminal vesicles is identified, subsequent blunt dissection in the purported plane between the seminal vesicles and bladder neck may result in fragmentation of the detrusor musculature, also compromising subsequent reconstruction.

A large median lobe may complicate the separation of the prostate from the posterior bladder neck. If the median lobe is pedunculated and can be delivered through the bladder neck into the operative field, the incision should be proximal to the lobe in such a manner that the bladder neck fibers are sharply cut away and the prostatic tissue is delivered into the operative field. As previously discussed, the dissection should be carried sharply and posteriorly until the fascia surrounding the seminal vesicles is identified. If the median lobe cannot be delivered through the bladder neck into the operative field, it may be sharply amputated, to be removed following completion of the radical prostatectomy. This can be accomplished with little chance of seeding tumor, because the incidence of involvement of median lobe tissue by malignancy is minimal.

Problems in Reconstruction

Problems in reconstruction of the bladder neck usually occur when the posterior margin of the incision has been carried so close to the ureteral orifices that their drainage is compromised. When concern exists regarding bladder neck closure and occlusion of the ureteral orifices, two maneuvers may prevent difficulties. Frequently, as the bladder neck is closed from 6 to 12 o'clock, the posterior portion of the closure can be accomplished by placing the sutures in the detrusor musculature only, not incorporating the bladder mucosa. This step provides the opportunity to bring the detrusor musculature together while keeping the suture line at a distance from the ureteral orifice. Should such a maneuver cause discomfort, the orifices may be catheterized. The ureteral catheters are brought out through the perineum; one is removed on the 5th, and the other on the 7th postoperative day.

Problems in Voiding

Retention is usually a transient phenomenon, most commonly reflecting edema at the site of the urethrovesicle anastomosis. When this problem occurs, we attempt to pass a catheter retrograde through the urethra and across the anastomosis into the bladder. If this passage cannot be accomplished, a trocar-introduced suprapubic cystotomy is placed. The patient remains on cystostomy drainage for several additional days. The cystostomy catheter is then clamped, and the patient is encouraged to void per urethra. In no instance have we found the patient unable to do so. Aggressive attempts to pass a catheter retrograde through the urethra across the fresh anastomosis may disrupt the anastomosis and produce postoperative incontinence.

Urine Leakage from the Incision

Urinary leakage always stops. If the patient experiences this problem only when voiding, the leak is distal to the reconstructed bladder neck. In these instances, the Foley catheter is not replaced and the patient is allowed to go home but is instructed to void only when seated or in the shower. With time, the leak will close and the patient will maintain perfect continence. If the patient drains continually through the perineal incision, the catheter is replaced and the patient remains on catheter drainage. In all instances, this practice has provided cessation of the urinary leakage. It is important that the Foley catheter be in the most dependent portion of the bladder. Failure to place the Foley catheter properly puts the drainage holes high in the bladder. Leakage continues through the defect; if leakage continues with the Foley catheter in place, a gentle cystogram should be performed to determine placement. If it can be determined that the Foley catheter is not seated deep in the reconstructed bladder neck, it should be so placed. With appropriate positioning of the Foley, the leakage will cease.

Three forms of obstruction may occur at the urethrovesical junction. These may be classified as early, intermediate, and late. Early obstruction occurs at the time the Foley catheter is removed, and this problem has been addressed previously. Intermediate obstruction at the urethrovesical anastomosis usually appears within several months after the radical prostatectomy. Although the onset of the obstruction may be gradual, the patient usually presents and complains of a progressive decrease in the size and force of the stream and the necessity to strain to void, often to the point of dribbling. This complication usually reflects postoperative cicatricial stricture and is best handled by gentle dilatation, usually with a filiform and follower catheter to ensure that the sound is not misdirected. The dilatation preferably is not carried above 18 to 20 Fr. Repetitive dilatation may be necessary. However, we have found it seldom necessary to dilate more than twice. On occasion, when the stricture has not responded well to gentle dilatation, direct-vision internal urethrotomy, cutting only in one position, may provide the ability to void without difficulty.

Late stricture, appearing several years after the operative procedure, usually heralds local recurrence. Similarly, local recurrence should be suspected when dilatation is accomplished and the patient is unable to void immediately afterward. When local recurrence is suspected, every effort should be made to confirm or deny this diagnosis. If local recurrence is identified, the stricture is managed in a very conservative manner. The most gentle dilatation is accomplished to permit reasonable voiding, until such time as the local recurrence has been managed by either radiation therapy or androgen deprivation. Any one of these treatments may have an impact on the local recurrence. Ablating the cause of the obstruction by aggressive incision or dilatation may result in incontinence following the definitive treatment of recurrence.

Urinary incontinence may be divided into early and late incontinence. Although the incidence of postoperative incontinence is reported to be between 10 and 18 per cent, this incidence most probably reflects the lack of experience of many surgeons in the reported series. In the hands of surgeons who are skilled in radical prostatectomy, the actual incidence of incontinence is probably less than 2 per cent. The comments that follow reflect my experience in treating referred patients.

Early urinary incontinence may be either functional or mechanical. Functional incontinence is characterized by urgency and frequency with a stream of adequate caliber. When seen in the early postoperative period, the patient is managed with an antispasmotic, usually oxybutynin (Ditropan) at a dosage of 5 mg, two to three times daily. This form of functional incontinence is believed caused by residual inflammation from the surgery. It may persist for several months but gradually the patient will recognize that the antispasmotic is no longer necessary and will stop the drug.

Mechanical incontinence occurs as a result of damage to the distal sphincteric mechanism or failure to reconstruct adequately the bladder neck. The patients may be persistently wet in the early postoperative period. However, as time passes, they will demonstrate a pattern of incontinence early in the day with some leakage, usually exacerbated by stress, beginning in the early or late afternoon as they fatigue. Although phenylpropanolamine-chlorpheniramine maleate (Ornade) Spansules, once or twice daily, may provide some benefit, this is not a reasonable long-term therapeutic modality. The patients are best treated with encouragement and time. Those who demonstrate the aforementioned pattern usually become continent with time.

The patient who presents with persistent incontinence usually has mechanical damage that was done at the time of surgery. This damage is most difficult to manage, and these patients usually have to undergo some form of artificial sphincter placement to establish continence. The scarring produced by the previous surgery usually requires that the artificial sphincter be placed around the bulb of the urethra. Although previous prostatic surgery may have partially compromised blood supply in this area, using delayed activation of the sphincter, we have not found erosion to be a major problem.

Loss of Potency

Despite the most careful attempts to preserve erectile function, a patient may experience lack of potency in the postoperative period. Restoration of erectile potency should be in response to patient demand. Our current belief is that placement of a prosthetic device at the time of primary prostatic surgery is not appropriate. When voluntary erectile function is lost as a result of the operative procedure, the patient and his partner should participate in the decision to restore erectile function. A considerable number of patients will not seek restoration of sexual function either because they have found alternative means for sexual gratification or because intercourse is no longer important to them or their partner in the maintenance of their relationship. Furthermore, as erectile function may be restored by vacuum devices, prosthetics, or pharmaceutic means, the patient and his partner are provided considerable flexibility in choosing the mechanism by which potency is to be restored.

Careful attention to the principles inherent in the conduct of any surgery reduces the incidence of complications directly related to the procedure itself. Those problems that are attendant to the specific nature of the surgery can be thoughtfully managed without risk to the patient and with every likelihood of a successful outcome (Carlton, 1972; Golimbu, 1979; Paulson, 1982, 1984, and 1987; Walsh, 1983).

REFERENCES

Belt, E.: Radical perineal prostatectomy in early carcinoma of the prostate. J. Urol., 78:287–299, 1942.

Carlton, C. E., et al.: Irradiation treatment of carcinoma of the prostate. J. Urol., 108:924, 1972.

Dees, J. E.: Radical perineal prostatectomy for carcinoma. J. Urol., 104:180, 1970.

Golimbu, M., et al.: Extended pelvic lymphadenectomy for prostatic cancer. J. Urol., 121:617, 1979.

Jewett, J. H.: The case for radical perineal prostatectomy. J. Urol., 103:195, 1970.

Paulson, D. F., et al.: Radical surgery vs. radiotherapy for adenocarcinoma of the prostate. J. Urol., 118:502, 1982.

Paulson, D. F.: Technique of radical perineal prostatectomy. In Skinner, D. G. and Lieskovsky, G. (Eds.): Diagnosis and Management of Genitourinary Cancer. Philadelphia, W. B. Saunders Co, 1988, p. 721.

Paulson, D. F.: The prostate. In Genitourinary Surgery. Paulson, D. F. (Ed.): New York, Churchill Livingstone, 1984.

Paulson, D. F.: Management of prostatic malignancy. In deKernion, J. B. and Paulson, D. F. (Eds.). Genitourinary Cancer Management. Philadelphia, Lea & Febiger, 1987.

Ray, G. R., Cassady, J. R., and Bagshaw, M. A.: External beam megavoltage radiation therapy in treatment of prostatectomy residual or recurrent tumor: Preliminary results. J. Urol., 114:98–101, 1975.

Walsh, P. C., Lepor, H., and Eggleston, J. C.: Radical prostatectomy with preservation of sexual function: Anatomical and pathological considerations. Prostate, 4:473, 1983.

Weyrauch, H. M. (Ed.): Surgery of the Prostate. Philadelphia, W. B. Saunders Co., 1959.

80
TRANSURETHRAL SURGERY

Winston K. Mebust, M.D.

Transurethral resection of the prostate (TURP) is one of the most common operations performed. In 1985, 350,000 were performed. It was the second, after cataract extraction, most costly operation under Medicare, accounting for 1.4 per cent of total allowable charges. In 1987, a survey of urologists revealed that TURP accounted for 38 per cent of their major operations. With an aging population, therefore, one would expect a further increase in the number of these operations performed, with a corresponding impact on money spent for medical care (Holtgrewe et al., 1989). Although TURP has been associated with a low surgical mortality rate and a good outcome, the need to control rising medical costs has caused the federal government and the medical profession to re-evaluate prostatectomy with regard to the indications for therapeutic intervention and the long-term, as well as short-term, results.

What diagnostic tests, if any, can be used to predict which patients will benefit the most from therapeutic intervention? Alternative forms of medical and surgical intervention in patients with bladder outlet obstructions, secondary to benign prostatic hypertrophy (BPH), are being developed. Some of the newer surgical procedures are commented on briefly in this chapter. Indications for intervention, diagnostic procedures, and surgical outcomes are reviewed as well.

HISTORICAL REVIEW

The development of transurethral surgery for BPH occurred primarily in the United States. However, Ambrose Pare, in the 16th century, is given credit for doing the first transurethral surgery to relieve bladder outlet obstruction (Mebust and Valk, 1983). He recognized obstruction from urethral strictures, which he called carnosities. He used a curet and a sharpened, hollow sound to shear off these carnosities to relieve obstruction. In 1830, the French surgeons, Mercier, Civiale, and D'Etoilles, modified the lithotrite so that the narrow blade was sharp. The instrument was inserted, per urethra, and the bladder neck incised blindly. This surgical approach was associated with significant hemorrhage, infection, incontinence, and operative mortality. Thus, the technique was never widely accepted.

In reviewing the development of transurethral prostatectomy, Nesbit (1975) cited three factors that are important in today's modern surgical procedure. First was the development of the incandescent lamp, by Edison, in 1879. In 1887, Nitze and Leiter independently developed cystoscopes illuminated by the incandescent lamp. The second factor was the development of a high frequency, electrical current that could be utilized to cut tissue. The high frequency current was discovered by Hertz in 1888. In 1908, DeForest's invention of the vacuum tube permitted the production of a continuous high frequency current. DeForest suggested this current could be used to cut tissue in surgery. In 1924, Reinholdt Wappler, along with George Wyeth, introduced the first practical cutting current. Spark gap generators were also being improved at this time. Bovie, of Harvard, built a generator with a heavily dampened current for coagulation hemostasis. The two types of currents were placed together in one unit, by Frederick Wappler in 1931, and marketed as the "complex oscillator" by the American Cystoscope Manufacturers, Incorporated. The third important factor, noted by Nesbit, was the concept of a fenestrated tube, introduced by Hugh Young in 1909. He engaged tissue in the fenestration of the tube and blindly sheared off the obstructing tissue with a tubular knife.

In 1926, Bumpus combined the cystoscope with a tubular punch concept and cauterization for prostate surgery. In 1926, Stern introduced a tungsten wire loop, which could be utilized with a high frequency current to resect tissue. All of these developments were brought together by McCarthy in 1932, when he introduced the direct vision resectoscope with a Foroblique lens, the wire loop for resection, and the cautery of obstructing prostatic tissue.

Originally, distilled water was the most common irrigating fluid. Creevy and Webb (1947) pointed out the danger of water in causing intravascular hemolysis, resulting in higher morbidity and death rates. Emmett and co-workers (1969), in reviewing two large series from the Mayo Clinic in which water or a nonhemolytic

2900

solution was chosen, found a distinct advantage in a nonhemolytic solution, reducing the mortality rate associated with TURP. Later, studies by Madsen and Nader (1973) and Oester and Madsen (1969) pointed out the relationship of fluid absorption to pressure in the prostatic fossa and the intravascular absorption occurring toward the end of the resection, as venous sinuses are exposed.

Since Fleming's discovery of penicillin in the 1940s, a great variety of antibiotics have become available. Preexisting infections are treated properly, prior to surgery. Although prophylactic antibiotic therapy is somewhat controversial, one cannot help but be impressed to observe a reduction in infections following TURP when it is used (Mebust et al., 1979).

In the 1970s the development of a fiberoptic lighting system, together with the Hopkins (1976) rod lens wide-angle system, significantly improved visualization for endoscopic surgery. Previously, the optical system was a series of small lenses placed in a rigid tube. In the Hopkins rod lens wide-angle system, the air spaces were replaced by solid glass rods. The spacer tubes were shorter and thinner, resulting in minimal obstruction and increased admission of light.

The fiberoptic light system is basically a glass core surrounded by a material of lower refractive index. Light is then transmitted, from a source through the glass fibers, and is trapped and reflected at the inner surface between the primary core and a layer of less refractive index through the flexible cord to the scope, where it is transmitted into the field.

In 1985, 95 per cent of prostatectomies performed in Medicare patients were transurethral (Roos et al., 1989). However, new modalities of therapeutic intervention are being evaluated. Drugs (e.g., alpha-adrenergic blockers and 5 alpha-reductase inhibitors) are being considered as medical alternatives to surgery. Less invasive surgical procedures, such as dilating the prostatic fossa with a balloon, are being evaluated. The thermal effects of transrectal and transurethral microwave hyperthermia on the prostate, to relieve obstruction, are also being studied. Some of these newer medical and surgical techniques will find a place in managing the patient with an obstructing prostate. However, today, the gold standard, in treating a patient with bladder outlet obstruction, remains the transurethral prostatectomy.

INDICATIONS FOR PROSTATECTOMY

Lytton and colleagues (1968) estimated that the chance of a 40-year-old man having a prostatectomy in his lifetime was approximately 10 per cent. However, Glynn and co-workers (1985) raised the estimate to 29 per cent. McPherson and associates (1982) noted that the incidence of prostatectomy, per 100,000 population, was 264 in New England (United States), compared with 122 in England (United Kingdom). Wennberg and Gittelsohn (1982) observed marked variation in incidence of TURP within the United States. These studies raised the question as to whether or not different criteria were chosen to select patients for surgery, not only internationally, but also nationally (within the United States). However, Holtgrewe and co-workers (1989) divided the United States into four geographic regions (northeast, midwest, south, and west). They found that the percentage of the total number of TURP procedures done in 1985 was almost identical to the percentage of the national population over the age of 65 within that geographic region.

Very few studies have been done on the natural history of patients who are seen initially because of modest symptoms of prostatism without absolute indications for intervention (e.g., acute urinary retention). Ball and co-workers (1981), in following 97 patients over 5 years, found that the symptoms were essentially the same in 52 per cent and worse in only 16.5 per cent. Their urodynamic studies revealed little change in that particular group and only 1.6 per cent developed retention. Conversely, Birkhoff and colleagues (1976), in following 26 patients for 3 years, found a 50 to 70 per cent deterioration in the patient's subjective symptoms and 71 per cent deterioration in objective criteria. Further, acute retention was unpredictable.

However, certain indications have been accepted as standards over the years by urologists (e.g., acute retention, significant residual urine, hematuria, recurrent infections, and azotemia). In the AUA Cooperative Study (Mebust et al., 1989), 27 per cent of the patients had the primary indication for surgery of acute urinary retention (Table 80–1). It is impossible to predict which patient will have modest symptoms of prostatism (those of bladder outlet obstruction and bladder hyperreflexia) and will subsequently develop acute urinary retention. However, Breum and associates (1982) found that 90 per cent of patients, presenting with acute retention, required surgery in 1 year. Craigen and co-workers (1969) found that 58 per cent required surgery within 3 months. The unpredictability of acute retention implies another mechanism, rather than just the accumulative effect of natural progression of BPH. Prostatic infarction has been noted in 85 per cent of patients operated on for acute retention but in only 3 per cent of patients

Table 80–1. INDICATIONS FOR PROSTATECTOMY AND COMBINATION OF OPERATIVE INDICATIONS

Indications for Prostatectomy	Number	(%)
Symptoms of prostatism	3522	(90.7)
Significant residual urine	1336	(34.4)
Acute urinary retention	1053	(27.1)
Recurrent urinary infection	479	(12.3)
Hematuria	465	(12.0)
Altered urodynamic function	385	(9.9)
Renal insufficiency	176	(4.5)
Bladder stones	116	(3.0)
Combination of Operative Indications		
Symptoms of prostatism only	1145	(29.5)
Prostatism, residual urine	577	(14.9)
Prostatism, acute retention	372	(9.6)
Prostatism, acute retention and residual urine	217	(5.6)

From Mebust, W. K., Holtgrewe, H. L., Cochett, A. T. K., Peters, P. C., and the Writing Committee: J. Urol., 141:243–247, 1989. AUA Cooperative Retrospective Study of 3885 Patients.

with BPH, without retention (Spiro et al., 1974). However, infarction may be a secondary event to another specific cause.

Residual urine and chronic retention have been considered to be signs of bladder decompensation in patients with obstructing BPH. However, failure to find residual urine does not mean that the patient does not require surgery. Hinman (1983), in following a series of patients over several years, noted a possible gradual increase in residual urine. He suggested that 60 ml might be the indication for intervention. However, a progressive increase in residual urine or chronic urinary retention did not necessarily mean the patient would ultimately experience acute retention.

Bruskewitz and associates (1982), in comparison, have noted individual variations and they question the value of residual urine in selecting those patients requiring surgery. The amount of residual urine, at which point surgical intervention would be recommended, is controversial. Bruskewitz's group found no positive correlation between preoperative residual urine volume and postoperative outcome. However, Drach and colleagues (1982), in looking at flow rates and residual urines, noted that when patients had residual urine greater than 150 ml, they seem to do worse than when patients had 70 ml or less. In the AUA Cooperative Study (Mebust et al., 1989), the amount of residual urine, considered to be significant, was left to the individual investigators. Of the patients studied, 35 per cent had significant residual urine, which was used as one of the indications for surgical intervention.

Recurrent gross hematuria has also been considered as an indication for intervention. This finding occurred in 12 per cent of the patients in the AUA Cooperative Study. The exact pathophysiology of hematuria, secondary to BPH, is unclear but can lead to significant complications for the patient (e.g., clot urinary retention). My clinical experience has been that hematuria usually is associated with larger glands.

Recurrent preoperative infection has also been considered as an absolute indication for intervention. Preoperative infection was found in 12 per cent of patients in the AUA Cooperative Study. However, the incidence (21 per cent) was significantly higher in the black population. In contrast, Melchior and co-workers (1974) found an incidence of 25 per cent, in a study of over 2000 consecutive cases in which preoperative urinary cultures were done routinely. Conversely, Hasner (1962) found an incidence of 8.6 per cent in a smaller series of patients. The source of infection presumably involves the prostate and is related to the presence or absence of residual urine. Unfortunately, the recurrence of infection is not necessarily related to the amount of residual urine. Therefore, infection related to bladder outlet obstruction will probably recur, unless the obstructing prostate is surgically corrected.

The most common reasons for TURP are bladder outlet obstruction symptoms (e.g., decrease in force and caliber of the urinary stream, hesitancy, straining to void, and so forth) and bladder hyperreflexia symptoms (e.g., urinary urgency, frequency, and nocturia). Of the patients in the AUA Cooperative Study, 90 per cent had significant symptoms of prostatism. However, 70 per cent had another indication other than symptoms. Attempts have been made to quantitate patient symptoms. The Madsen/Iversen scoring sheet is noted in Table 80–2, but the initial recommendations were published by Boyarsky and associates (1977). Quantitating symptoms is difficult and making comparisons of symptoms, before and after treatment, even more difficult.

Symptoms vary over time in a patient who has an obstructing prostate. Ball and Smith (1981) noted, in their series of patients who were followed conservatively over a 5-year period of time, that 31 per cent had improvement in symptoms. Further, it has been noted by Abrams (1977), in studying the effect of candicidin on patients awaiting prostatectomy, that 45 per cent of the placebo group were much improved. Therefore, any intervention has a tremendous placebo effect on patients, as far as symptoms are concerned. One of the problems in trying to quantitate symptoms is that it really does not reflect the symptom that was most significant for the patient seeking medical attention (e.g., one patient may not be bothered by nocturia X2, but another patient is significantly concerned to the point that he will demand something be done).

Following TURP, well over 80 per cent of patients experience improvement in urinary flow rates. Abrams (1985) cited the incidence of detrusor instability, in patients with outlet obstruction, secondary to prosta-

Table 80–2. SYMPTOM SCORE SHEET

Symptom	0	1	2	3	4
Stream	Normal	Variable		Weak	Dribbling
Voiding	No strain		Abdominal strain or Credé method		
Hesitancy	None			Yes	
Intermittency	None			Yes	
Bladder emptying	Don't know or complete	Variable	Incomplete	Single retention	Repeated retention
Incontinence			Yes (including terminal dribbling)		
Urge	None	Mild	Moderate	Severe (incontinence)	
Nocturia	0–1	2	3–4	>4	
Diuria	q > 3 hours	q 2–3 hours	q 1–2 hours	q <1 hour	
TOTAL SCORE					

From Madsen, P. O., and Iversen, P.: A point system for selecting operative candidates. *In* Hinman, F., Jr.: Benign Prostatic Hypertrophy. New York, Springer-Verlag, 1983, pp. 762–765.

tism, as ranging from 53 to 80 per cent. The high reversal rate of the phenomena, following prostatectomy (45 to 100 per cent), is cited by Abrams as supporting this association. Well over 80 per cent of patients will have improvement in symptoms following a TURP.

Urodynamic studies have been employed to evaluate the pathophysiology of bladder outlet obstruction, secondary to BPH. It had been hoped that these studies would clearly identify which patients would benefit the most from intervention. Perhaps the simplest and most noninvasive observation is urinary flow rate. However, flow rate is dependent on not only the degree of obstruction caused by the prostate but the contractility of the bladder. Nevertheless, most men with bladder outlet obstructions from BPH have altered flow patterns compared with the normal.

Siroky and co-workers (1979) developed a nomogram for average and peak flow rates, adjusted for initial bladder volume. It was suggested that a patient whose flow rate was greater than a -2 standard deviation from the mean was definitely experiencing obstruction (Fig. 80–1). Drach and co-workers (1982) developed a nomogram adjusted for peak flow rates, taking into consideration the volume voided and the age of the patient (Fig. 80–2). Using this nomogram, an adjusted peak flow rate of less than 16 ml per second, or greater than 1.3 standard deviation below the mean, was considered as suspicious for bladder outlet obstruction. Abrams (1977) found that those who had peak flow rates of less than 10 ml per second seemed to do better after surgery than those who had higher flow rates. However, it is important to know what the pressure is in the bladder when evaluating a flow rate.

Iversen and associates (1983) noted in a group of patients with a 15 ml per second peak flow rate that there was definite obstruction because they had increased intravesical pressure.

Pressure flow rates are certainly the most appropriate way of evaluating a given patient's urinary flow, as to whether it is normal or abnormal. Unfortunately, pressure flow studies are not readily available to most urologists. Other problems with flow rates involve patients who do not void with an adequate volume or void with an interrupted stream. They also void in an artificial situation, when being evaluated, and pattern may not reflect the usual one. Nevertheless, of all the urodynamic studies, urinary flow rates adjusted for volume voided and age seem to be the most helpful.

The cystometrogram (CMG) was noted to be of assistance by Abrams (1985) in determining uninhibited contractions. Andersen (1982) correlated CMG changes with hyperreflexic symptoms. However, Frimodt-Moller and co-workers (1984) could find no correlation with CMG-determined uninhibited contractions and symptoms. Conversely, a CMG may indicate that the patient has significant bladder decompensation. However, it is impossible to predict whether removing the obstructing prostate, in a given patient with a decompensated bladder, will permit him to void adequately with a minimal amount of residual urine.

Azotemia, secondary to obstruction, is also an indication for intervention. I have defined azotemia as a creatinine level greater than 1.5 mg. The incidence was noted by Holtgrewe and Valk (1962) (7 per cent); Melchior and co-workers (1974) (18 per cent); and the AUA National Cooperative Study (1989) (9 per cent). In the AUA Cooperative Study, the indication for TURP was azotemia (4.5 per cent). In following a group of patients with symptoms of prostatism, it is impossible to predict who will develop azotemia, unless they

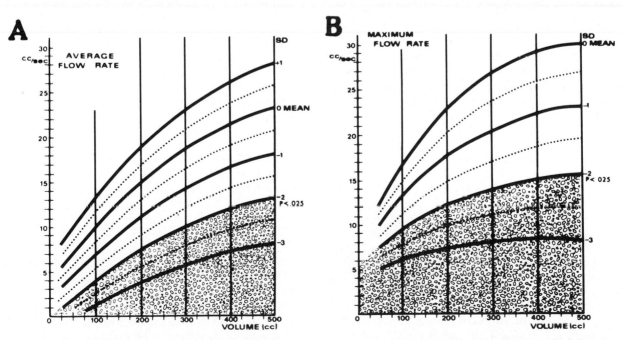

Figure 80–1. *A* and *B*, Siroky nomogram relating peak urinary flow and initial bladder volume of urine voided. The 2 standard deviations below the mean were believed to be obstruction secondary to benign prostatic hypertrophy. (From Siroky, M. B., Olsson, C. A., and Krane, R. J.: The flow rate nomogram. I. Development. J. Urol., 122:665, © by Williams & Wilkins, 1979.)

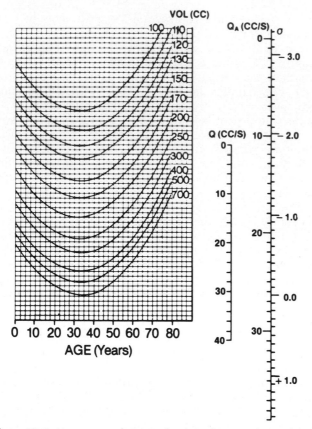

Figure 80–2. Nomogram relating peak urinary flow to volume of urine voided corrected for age. (From Drach, G. W., Laylon, T., and Bottaccini, M. R.: A method of adjustment of male peak flow rate for varying age and volume voided. J. Urol., 128:960, © Williams & Wilkins, 1982.)

undergo therapeutic intervention. The patients usually present with significant symptoms or retention and are found to be azotemic. Many patients presenting with azotemia are improved with relief of bladder outlet obstruction.

The following are my thoughts on the indications for prostatectomy, based on my clinical experience and a careful review of the literature of urodynamic studies and quantitation of symptoms in patients with bladder outlet obstruction, secondary to BPH. The most significant indications are usually the symptoms of bladder outlet obstruction and bladder irritability, when they are persistent and progressive and, particularly, troublesome to the patient. In this instance, the patient must participate in the decision to intervene. Certain absolute indications for intervention are recurrent urinary tract infection, recurrent bleeding, acute urinary retention, azotemia, and upper urinary tract changes. Further, as I review the controversy over urodynamics and chronic urinary retention or persistent residual urine, I believe that urinary flow rate is the simplest and most noninvasive method of documenting bladder outlet obstruction. Siroky and Drach nomograms are helpful. As a general rule, given an adequate volume, a peak flow rate of less than 13 ml per second is considered to be an indication for intervention.

The significance of residual urine is, however, most difficult to determine. It would seem logical that the greater the amount of residual urine the greater the bladder decompensation. Although a poorly functioning bladder can be secondary to a problem other than obstructing BPH, in usual clinical circumstances, it is probably secondary to BPH. Therefore, arbitrarily, I have selected 60 ml of residual urine as an indication to consider intervention. Admittedly, this value is not based on scientific data. In the AUA Cooperative Study, it should be remembered, 70 per cent of the patients had more than one indication for intervention.

PREOPERATIVE EVALUATION

At the present time, patients are usually admitted to the hospital on the day of surgery. Therefore, the general evaluation must be completed on an outpatient basis. In the AUA Cooperative Study only 23 per cent of the patients did not have significant prior medical problems. The most common problems were pulmonary (14.5 per cent), gastrointestinal (13.2 per cent), myocardial infarction (12.5 per cent), cardiac arrhythmia (12.4 per cent), and renal insufficiency (9.8 per cent).

In the AUA Cooperative Study, the most common cause of death following TURP was sepsis. The deaths occurred in debilitated patients with multisystem diseases. The operation may not have been a significant factor in their deaths. However, prior to the study, the most common cause of death following TURP was cardiovascular complication. The patient with renal insufficiency was also noted to be at higher risk. Therefore, we still believe it is critically important to evaluate the cardiac, pulmonary, and renal status of patients prior to surgery. Hematogram, chemistry profile, chest radiograph, and electrocardiogram are usually done.

The indications for visualization of the upper urinary tract are usually histories of hematuria, infections, or stones. However, over 60 per cent of the patients in the AUA Study had the upper tracts evaluated. This suggests the urologist's concern to completely evaluate patients, even those not having the indications previously noted. Pre-existing medical problems did not predispose the patient to postoperative exacerbation of those problems.

The evening prior to surgery, we suggest a diet of clear liquids and a cleansing enema. The hope is that the patient will not strain during a bowel movement in the immediate postoperative period, which may exacerbate bleeding.

ANESTHESIA

Sinha and colleagues (1986) have reported doing TURP with local anesthesia. However, most patients are given a general anesthetic or an epidural or a subdural spinal block. Nielsen and co-workers (1987) noted no difference in blood loss between an epidural or a general anesthesia. McGowan and Smith (1980) evaluated spinal anesthetic versus general anesthetic and found no difference in blood loss, postoperative morbidity, or mortality. However, there was a higher incidence of cardiac arrhythmias with general anesthesia.

Our conclusion is that surgery can be done with either form of anesthesia and should be tailored to the particular patient. During the procedure, the anesthetist should monitor the patient's tissue oxygen saturation, electrocardiogram, and, if warranted, the serum sodium level, in addition to the usual parameters.

PERIOPERATIVE ANTIBIOTICS

Preoperative infection should be treated with appropriate antibiotics prior to surgery. However, the role of prophylactic antibiotics remains controversial. Gibbons and associates (1978) and Hall and Rous (1982) found that prophylactic therapy did not reduce postoperative infection, but Nielsen (1981) and others (Goldwasser et al., 1983; Grabe et al., 1984; Grabe and Hellsten, 1985; Prokocimer et al., 1986) found it to be beneficial.

The appropriate length of time during which prophylactic antibiotics should be administered in the perioperative period is not clear. In the AUA Cooperative Study, 61 per cent of the patients were given prophylactic antibiotics and 49 per cent beyond 8 days. We believe that the patient should begin a systemic prophylactic antibiotic (e.g., a first generation cephalosporin) just before surgery. Patients should then change to an oral antibiotic (e.g., nitrofurantoin) when intravenous fluids are discontinued. The antibiotics should be continued for 2 to 3 days after the catheter is removed.

SURGICAL TECHNIQUES

General Comments

The patient is placed in the lithotomy position, with the buttocks just off the end of the table. We prefer the Alcock holders over knee crutches for leg support. The perineum is not shaved but is scrubbed for 5 minutes with a germicidal soap. An O'Connor rectal shield is inserted for manipulation of the gland during the surgical procedure.

At the time of surgery, the urethra is calibrated with bougie à boule (Fig. 80–3). The majority calibrate at 28 Fr. or greater, but a significant number are less, as pointed out by Emmett and co-workers (1963). If the distal urethra is inadequate to accommodate the more commonly selected 28 Fr. resectoscope, a smaller size should be selected. For several years, we have successfully utilized a 24 Fr. resectoscope sheath, even in cases of very large glands. However, if the distal urethra is

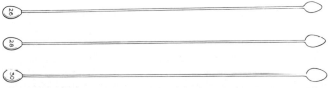

Figure 80–3. Bougie à boule or Otis bulb is to calibrate the urethra.

inadequate to accommodate a resectoscope sheath, a perineal urethrostomy may be performed. By inserting the resectoscope, through the more commodious bulbous urethra, the incidence of postoperative stricture is reduced (Melchior et al., 1974).

The technique of perineal urethrostomy has been described elsewhere (Mebust et al., 1972). Basically, a 24 Fr., grooved, van Buren sound is inserted into the urethra and the perineum is tented upward. The sound is stabilized with a Conger clamp and a 2-cm long, midline incision is made in the bulbous urethra. The cut edges of the urethra are stabilized with stay sutures of 0 chromic to facilitate insertion of the resectoscope sheath and, subsequently, the catheter (Fig. 80–4). Alternatively, an internal urethrotomy can be done, as advocated by Emmett and co-workers (1963) and by Bailey and Shearer (1979). A common area of narrowing is at the meatal postnavicular region. In this instance, we would either perform a dorsal internal urethrotomy with the Otis urethrotome (Fig. 80–5) or a curved blade (Fig. 80–6). A generous ventral meatotomy often leads to either a splattering or an errant direction of the urinary stream.

PRELIMINARY CYSTOSCOPIC EXAMINATION

The bladder is examined and any abnormality or pathology noted. Particular attention is paid to the presence of vesical diverticula, which should be entered, if possible, and examined. The diverticula may also retain prostatic chips and, therefore, should be inspected at the end of the procedure. Small bladder tumors may be encountered and can be resected at the same time. More extensive, possibly invasive, tumors should be liberally biopsied. Prostate surgery is deferred, because the patient may be a candidate for radical cystoprostatectomy.

The prostate should now be estimated as to size, to judge whether it can be resected transurethrally. With experience, one can determine the approximate size of the prostate by palpating the prostate with the finger in the O'Connor shield and estimating the length. Although we routinely resect prostates up to 100 g, the incidence of complications increases when the gland is more than 75 g. At that point, the patient should be considered for open prostatectomy.

Surgical Technique

A variety of surgical techniques have been espoused by urologists for removing prostate adenomas transurethrally. The procedures all employ the basic principle that the resection should be done in a routine step-by-step manner. The resection technique may vary according to the size or configuration of the adenoma but should be based on an orderly plan. Further, all techniques employ the principle of resecting ventrally first so that the adenomatous tissue drops down, allowing the surgeon to resect from the top downward rather

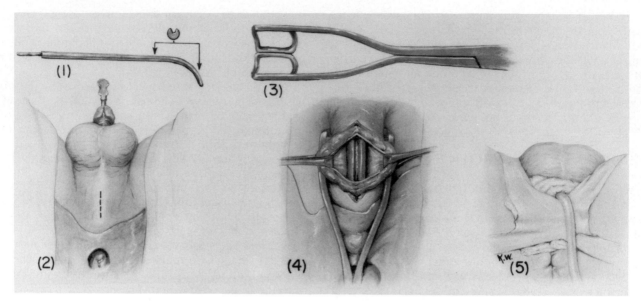

Figure 80–4. Technique of perineal urethrostomy. The incision in the perineum is made over a grooved van Buren sound (1 and 2). A Conger clamp is used to stabilize the sound (3). The cut edges of the urethra are stabilized with Stay sutures or Allis clamps to facilitate insertion of the resectoscope (4). The urethral catheter may be brought out through the urethrostomy or through the full length of the urethra with closure of the urethrostomy (5).

than from the floor upward. However, some surgeons have suggested resecting the floor and the median lobe tissue, initially, to improve water flow. They then proceed with the ventral resection of the prostate.

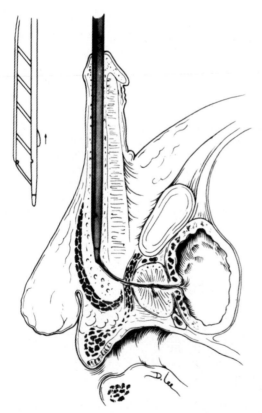

Figure 80–5. The Otis urethrotome is inserted into the urethra and expanded to allow a dorsal incision with the blade. This may be used to enlarge the entire anterior urethra or just the postnavicular area.

As a teaching technique, we often resect one lobe of the prostate, allowing the resident to resect the other. Our standard technique is that described by Nesbit in 1943. The Nesbit surgical technique is divided into three stages. In the first stage, the surgeon resects the fibers at the bladder neck and the immediately adjacent prostatic adenoma. The second stage is the mid-fossa—starting at the 12-o'clock position and resecting the lateral lobes so that they drop down to the floor. The final stage is resecting the apex.

STAGE I (Fig. 80–7). Following the preliminary endoscopy and urethral calibration, the bladder is filled with approximately 150 ml of a nonhemolytic irrigation solution (e.g., 1.5 per cent glycine). The resection begins at the bladder neck, starting at the 12-o'clock position and carried down to the 9-o'clock position, in a stepwise fashion. The adenoma is resected down to the level where the apparent circular fibers of the bladder neck become visible. Over-resection of the entire neck, or excessive cauterization, may lead to vesical neck contracture. The anterior quadrant, from 12 to 3 o'clock, is now resected. The posterior quadrants are then individually resected, down to the 6-o'clock position. If, at the completion of the entire resection, the bladder neck appears to be partially obstructing, which is particularly true of glands weighing less than 20 g, we advise incising the bladder neck with a Collings knife at the 6-o'clock position. This step is recommended by Kulb and associates (1987) to reduce the incidence of postoperative vesical neck contracture.

STAGE II (Figs. 80–8 to 80–10). The adenoma is resected in quadrants. The resectoscope is placed in front of the verumontanum. The resection begins at 12 o'clock, so that the lateral lobe tissue falls into the mid-fossa. The resection is carried down to the prostatic capsule, which is recognized as a rather fibrous structure

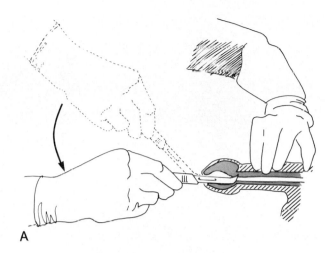

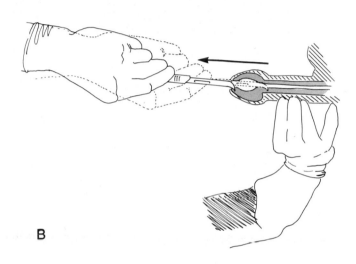

Figure 80–6. The curved blade is inserted into the urethra *(A)* and then retracted *(B)* through the dorsal portion of the urethra, in those patients with inadequate postnavicular areas to allow insertion of the resectoscope. (From Mebust, W. K.: A Review of TURP Complications and the AVA National Cooperative Study, Lesson 24, Volume VIII, 1989, pp. 189–190.)

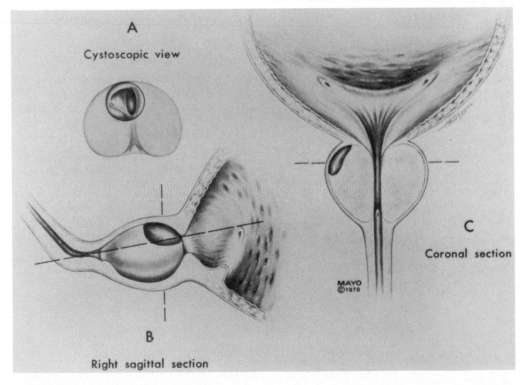

Figure 80–7. First stage of resection of the prostate. The resection is begun at 12 o'clock and the tissue at the bladder neck and adjacent adenoma resected in quadrants.

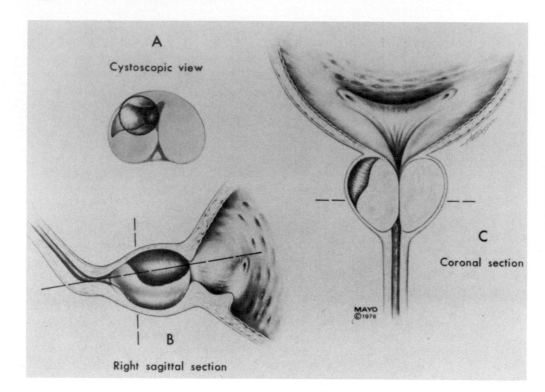

A
Cystoscopic view

C
Coronal section

B
Right sagittal section

Figure 80–8. The midportion of the gland is resected starting at 12 o'clock, carrying it down to the 9-o'clock position (A). The sagittal and coronal section views are noted (B and C).

compared with the granular appearance of the prostatic adenoma. The right lateral lobe and then the left lateral lobe are resected so that the tissue now falls to the floor. With the right lateral lobe on the floor of the prostatic fossa, resection of this fallen lobe is started at the 9-o'clock position, approximately. The posterior portion, on the floor of the prostatic fossa, is resected. Care must be taken not to resect too deeply in the region of the posterior aspect of the vesical neck to prevent under-

mining of the trigone. The resection is carried to the right side of the verumontanum. A similar procedure is started at approximately 3 o'clock. The posterior portion of the lobe is resected to the left side of the verumontanum. The apical portion of the lobe remains. At this stage, therefore, the posterior portions of the lateral lobe, including the floor tissue, have been resected to the verumontanum. As one resects the lower two quadrants in the floor of the prostate, the capsule fibers

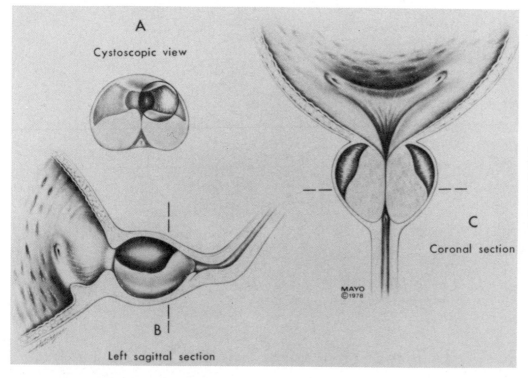

A
Cystoscopic view

C
Coronal section

B
Left sagittal section

Figure 80–9. The resection is now begun at 12 o'clock and the left side of the patient's gland in the mid-fossa is resected down to the 3-o'clock position as noted in (A). Sagittal and coronal sections are noted (B and C).

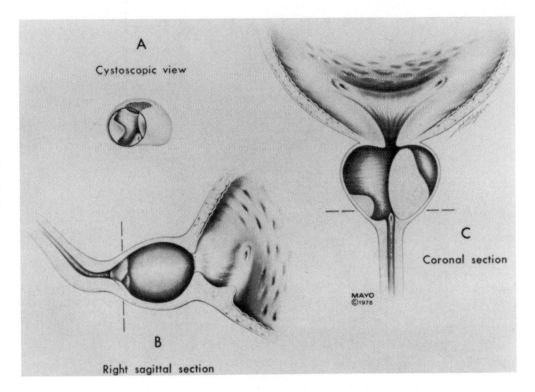

Figure 80–10. The midportion of the gland is resected further from the 9-o'clock to 6-o'clock positions as noted in *(A)* with sagittal views in *(B and C).*

become less distinct. The resection is done with an O'Connor rectal shield in place. We employ the Iglesias modification of the Nesbit scope so that one hand is free to palpate the depth of resection as the floor tissue is removed.

STAGE III (Figs. 80–11 to 80–13). The adenoma is removed immediately proximal to the external sphincter mechanism, preserving the verumontanum. The prostatic apex is concave. A sweeping motion is used so that the loop is moved from a lateral-to-medial direction, as it approaches the sphincter mechanism. However, Shah and co-workers (1979) observed that 10 to 20 per cent of the prostate projects below the verumontanum. Therefore, it may be necessary to leave a small rim of adenoma to avoid sphincter injury.

Turner-Warwick (1983) has divided the sphincter mechanism into three areas: first, immediately adjacent to the verumontanum; second, from the verumontanum

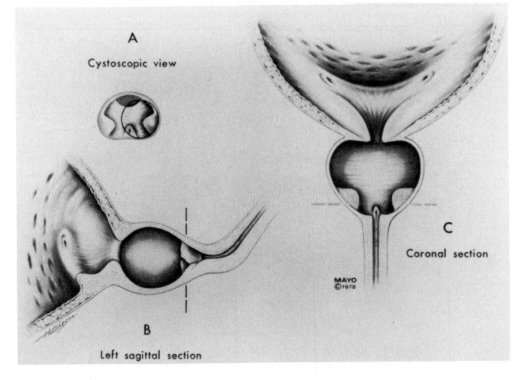

Figure 80–11. The tissue remaining at the apex is now resected. Begin by initiating the resection next to the verumontanum and carrying it toward the 12-o'clock position. Small amounts of residual tissue at the apex are noted *(A, B, and C).*

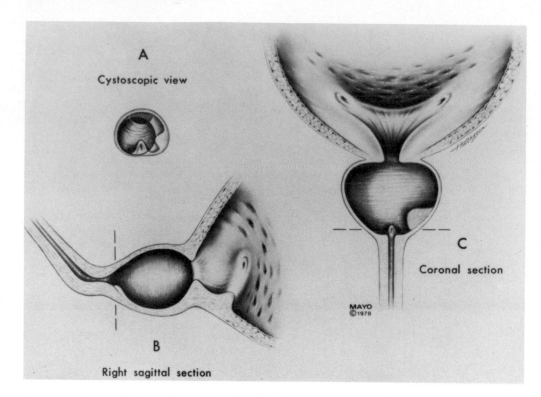

Figure 80–12. Residual tissue is carefully cleared on the patient's right side.

to the capsule; and third, beyond the capsule of the prostate. Injury to the second or third portion of the sphincter mechanism can result in significant urinary incontinence. Therefore, we begin our resection by placing the resectoscope next to the verumontanum. We continue the resection up to the 12-o'clock position, rather than starting at the 12-o'clock position as in the prior two steps.

With the patient in the lithotomy position, the distal portion of the prostate is not always parallel to the surgical table but is tilting slightly toward the cephalad end. The most common area of damage to the external sphincter is at the 12-o'clock position. Thus, care must be taken as one approaches the 12-o'clock position.

When the resection is completed, the surgeon should pull the resectoscope into the urethra, just distal to the verumontanum, and note that there is no falling and obstructing tissue. Some small wings of adenoma may

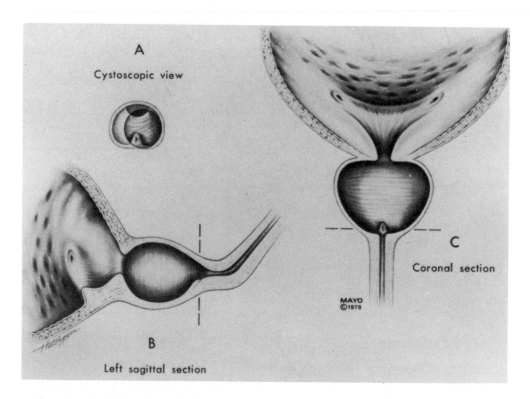

Figure 80–13. The remaining residual tissue is cleared from the patient's left side, leaving an unobstructed view from the verumontanum through the bladder neck into the bladder.

be attached to the sphincter area. These can be judiciously trimmed. Care must be taken not to cut too deeply and thus damage the sphincter mechanism. Occasionally, there is tissue that is nothing more than mucosal tags, which are unimportant. They will slough and will not cause obstruction. When significant tissue drops into the prostatic fossa, with the scope in the distal urethra, it is usually the tissue that remains at the roof of the mid-fossa area. The surgeon should replace the scope in the mid-fossa and resect the adenoma down to the fibrous capsule.

Hemostasis

The extent of bleeding depends on the size of the gland and the extent of the surgeon's skill. Arterial bleeding is controlled by electrocoagulation. It is a cardinal rule to control all arterial bleeding, in one stage, before moving to the next stage of the resection. After the catheter is inserted, at the end of the surgical procedure, the irrigation fluid should be light pink. However, if the irrigation fluid has a continued red color, one should suspect arterial bleeding. The surgeon should then reinsert the resectoscope and coagulate the arterial bleeding. Venous bleeding is apparent at the end of the procedure when upon irrigating the catheter, the return is initially clear but dark blood later oozes from the catheter. Venous bleeding can be controlled by filling the bladder with 100 ml of irrigating fluid and placing the catheter on traction for 7 minutes at the operating table. The balloon of the catheter is overinflated to 50 ml of fluid.

Evacuation of Prostatic Chips

At the end of the surgical procedure, all prostatic chips must be evacuated from the bladder. An Ellik evacuator is a piece of blown glass that permits the injection of irrigating fluid into the bladder and removal of fragments by suction (Fig. 80–14). The distal end of the resectoscope sheath is directed toward the base of the bladder and the bulb of the Ellik compressed. The

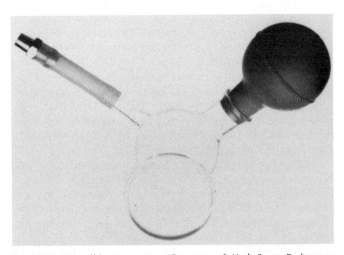

Figure 80–14. Ellik evacuator. (Courtesy of Karl Storz–Endoscopy America, Inc.)

fragments that are drawn into the upper chamber are allowed to settle into the lower bulbous chamber. When all the prostatic chips are removed by the Ellik evacuator, the bladder is reinspected to be sure that there are no chips in the bladder diverticulum or within the prostatic fossa.

POSTOPERATIVE CARE

Currently, we use a 22- or 24-Fr., three-way catheter with a 30-cc balloon. When comparing this catheter with our standard two-way catheter, we found less of a problem in forming clots, less nursing time in evacuating clots, and improved patient comfort. The constant irrigation is approximately 500 ml per hour or that sufficient to keep the drainage light pink. The drainage system employed should be closed to reduce the incidence of urinary tract infection. If there is still concern about venous bleeding, the catheter may be placed on light traction. Although most surgeons consider that the balloon is just next to the bladder neck, Greene (1986) has shown that it is actually in the prostatic fossa when on traction, helping in hemostasis. The catheter should be removed as soon as the urine is sufficiently clear of blood, which is within 24 to 48 hours following surgery. The patient is given a light supper the evening of surgery. He is ambulated that night or, certainly, early the following morning. As noted, we prefer to give prophylactic antibiotics for approximately 2 to 3 days after the catheter has been removed.

RESULTS OF TRANSURETHRAL PROSTATECTOMY

Over the past 60 years, a gradual reduction has been reported in the mortality rate associated with TURP. Perrin and associates (1976) found an incidence of 5 per cent in the 1930s. Holtgrewe and Valk reported 2.5 per cent in 1962; Melchior and colleagues, 1.3 per cent in 1974; and the AUA Cooperative Study, 0.2 per cent in 1989. Prior to the AUA Cooperative Study, the most common cause of death reported was cardiovascular complication. In the study, the most common cause of death was sepsis, occurring in patients who were debilitated and had other systemic disease processes. However, the incidence of sepsis, in this study, was less than that reported in prior studies, as was the incidence of deaths secondary to sepsis. The morbidity rate, however, was 18 per cent. This was similar to that reported by Holtgrewe and Valk (1962) and Melchior and associates (1974).

Intraoperative and postoperative complications were defined as any untoward event that deviated from the expected result, irrespective of the effect of the event. Although the morbidity rate was similar to that in previous studies, the hospital stay was much less, suggesting that these events were either less significant or better managed than previously.

Intraoperative bleeding was defined as that requiring a transfusion, which was found to occur in 2.5 per cent.

Postoperative bleeding occurred in 3.7 per cent. However, 85 per cent required 2 or less units of blood. The average blood loss, per TURP, has been noted to be 250 to 400 ml. Intraoperative bleeding is related to the size of the prostate and length of surgery. The AUA Cooperative Study found that if the surgery was greater than 90 minutes, the incidence of bleeding was 7.3 per cent compared with 0.9 per cent, if less than 90 minutes. If the gland was over 45 g, bleeding incidence was 10 per cent compared with 1.7 per cent if less than 45 g.

TRANSURETHRAL RESECTION (TUR) SYNDROME

In the AUA Cooperative Study, the transurethral resection (TUR) syndrome occurred in 2 per cent of patients. Since Creevy and Webb (1947) pointed out the danger of hemolysis caused by water, the emphasis has been on a nonhemolytic fluid. Although water is of course less expensive and surgery can be done safely with it, probably 80 per cent of surgeons employ a nonhemolytic solution because of the risk of intravascular hemolysis with water. A variety of fluids are used today—1.5 per cent glycine and Cytol (a combination of sorbitol and mannitol). These are not isotonic fluids but rather nonhemolytic fluids—1.5 per cent glycine has an osmolarity of approximately 200 compared with a normal serum osmolarity of approximately 290. Although these fluids do not cause hemolysis, they can be associated with the TUR syndrome.

The TUR syndrome is characterized by mental confusion, nausea, vomiting, hypertension, bradycardia, and visual disturbances. In the 1950s, several studies were undertaken to determine the amount of fluid absorbed during a TURP. Hagstrom (1955) weighed patients preoperatively and postoperatively and calculated that about approximately 20 ml/minute of fluid was absorbed by the patient. However, there appeared to be a wide variation among patients. Oester and Madsen (1969), utilizing a double-isotope technique, demonstrated that the average was approximately 1000 ml. Furthermore, one third of the fluid was absorbed, intravenously, when the venous sinuses were opened, meaning that most of the fluid was in the periprostatic area.

Madsen and Naber (1973) demonstrated that the pressure in the prostatic fossa and the amount of fluid absorbed was dependent on the height of the fluid above the patient. They noted that when the height of the fluid was changed from 60 to 70 cm, fluid absorption was greater than twofold. They also reported that approximately 300 ml of fluid per minute was needed for a good visual field. This could not be achieved when the fluid was below 60 cm.

Harrison and colleagues (1956) observed that the TUR syndrome appeared to be related to dilutional hyponatremia. Glycine is metabolized to glycolic acid and ammonium. Ammonia intoxication has also been suggested as a possible cause of the TUR syndrome or, perhaps, a direct toxic effect of glycine (Hoekstra et al., 1983; Roesch et al., 1983). Glycine is a neurotransmit-

ter, and the visual disturbances in TUR syndrome are not the same as those one would expect in cortical edema. Light perception is usually lost in cortical edema but not usually in TUR syndrome (Ovassapian et al., 1982). Measurement of intraocular pressure has also been noted to remain unchanged in TUR syndrome (Peters et al., 1981). O'Donnell (1983) has suggested the cause of the TUR syndrome could be absorption of substances from the prostate occurring during the resection. However, the correction of the TUR syndrome is quickly achieved with hypertonic saline and/or diuretics. Therefore, the TUR syndrome is probably dilutional hyponatremia.

Patients usually do not become symptomatic until the serum sodium concentration reaches 125 mEq/L. As noted in the AUA Cooperative Study, the risk is higher if the gland is greater than 45 g and the resection time is over 90 minutes. The incidence of the TUR syndrome was 2 per cent, and 66 per cent of cases were corrected simply with diuretics and observation. The relative sodium deficit can be calculated by assuming that 20 per cent of the body weight is extracellular fluid. One then calculates the difference between the preoperative and postoperative serum sodium values, thus determining the relative sodium deficit. However, this is not a true sodium deficit, as the patient is merely water overloaded. In general, the average case of TUR syndrome can be corrected with 200 ml of 3 per cent saline. This must be given slowly, preferably, in divided doses, with monitoring of the serum sodium level in between. This treatment should be accompanied by diuretics, to avoid pulmonary edema.

EXTRAVASATION

Extravasation, or perforation of the prostatic capsule, occurs in 2 per cent of patients. The symptoms of extravasation are restlessness; nausea; vomiting; and abdominal pain, despite spinal anesthesia. The pain is usually localized to the lower abdomen or to the back. If extravasation is suspected, the operation should be terminated as rapidly as possible, but hemostasis must be secured. Bleeding must be controlled, even if the extravasation is increased, because simultaneous management of extravasation and hemorrhage is difficult. Cystography may be performed to establish the diagnosis and to provide some measurement of the extent of the extravasation.

In the AUA Cooperative Study, 92 per cent of patients were simply managed by urethral catheter drainage and cessation of the operative procedure. If there is extensive extravasation and concern about infecting the perivesical tissue, suprapubic drainage should be instituted.

During the surgical procedure, a penile erection may occur, which may obviate the surgery, unless a perineal urethrostomy is performed. We have found success with ketamine (0.5 to 0.7 mg/kg) in reducing penile erection. However, others have not found it to be successful. Currently, we are injecting dilute epinephrine or ephedrine directly into the corpora cavernosa (0.1 ml 1:1000 epinephrine).

IMMEDIATE POSTOPERATIVE COMPLICATIONS

In the postoperative period, the most common problem, according to the AUA Cooperative Study, was failure to void. This occurred in 6.5 per cent of patients. Half of these patients had hypotonic bladders. Postoperatively, bleeding was a factor in 3.9 per cent. A bleeding complication was defined as that requiring transfusion, but 74 per cent of patients required 2 or less units of blood. The incidence was higher in those patients who had glands greater than 45 (7.5 per cent versus 1.5 per cent) or resection time greater than 90 minutes (7.3 per cent versus 0.2 per cent). Clot retention was noted in 3.3 per cent and infection in 2.3 per cent. In this series, preoperative infection was observed in 11 per cent. An additional 60 per cent of patients received postoperative antibiotics. The incidence of preoperative infection was certainly less than that reported by Chilton and colleagues (1978) (20 per cent), Murphy and colleagues (1984) (30 per cent), and Melchior and colleagues (1974) (23 per cent). In the last study, all patients had cultures done preoperatively, which was not necessarily the case in the AUA Cooperative Study. Therefore, the incidence of infection, preoperatively, could have been higher. Nevertheless, the postoperative infection rate, documented by culture-based data, was 2.3 per cent, comparable to the 5 per cent reported by Symes and co-workers (1972).

In managing immediate postoperative complications, patients who failed to void after a second trial, should undergo reinstrumentation. The prostate is then inspected to be sure that there is no residual adenoma. Furthermore, if not already done, a cystometrogram should be performed to determine if the patient has hypotonic bladder. In those patients with severely hypotonic bladders, occasionally, it has been necessary to discharge them from the hospital while on a catheter for a week or two. During this time, the bladder tone seems to return and they can void satisfactorily. Cholinergic drugs (e.g., bethanecol chloride, 25 to 50 mg, four times a day) may also be tried.

Postoperative bleeding can be secondary to inadequate control of bleeding during the intraoperative period. It can also occur with increased activity of the patient (e.g., straining with a bowel movement). Therefore, we recommend a stool softener to reduce straining. Should the patient continue to bleed, we recommend returning him to the operating room where clots can be washed from the bladder. With the removal of the clots, usually the site of bleeding is not apparent. The patient usually does well with complete evacuation of the clots in the bladder and prostate fossa. Occasionally, a patient will have persistent bleeding, even though cystoscopy was done, no bleeding point was found, and no blood dyscrasia was identified. Empirically, we have occasionally given aminocaproic acid (Amicar) to control the bleeding. This therapy is associated with the formation of tenacious clots that can be difficult to remove from the bladder, however.

RISK FACTORS

In the AUA Cooperative Study, certain risk factors were noted. In those patients over the age of 80, the postoperative morbidity was 22.6 per cent. The most common problems were failure to void and infection. Acute retention (27 per cent) was associated with an increase in postoperative complications—infection (4.3 per cent versus 1.5 per cent), failure to void (11 per cent versus 3.6 per cent), and hypotonic bladder (8.4 per cent versus 1.7 per cent). Black patients were also found to present more commonly with acute retention—44.7 per cent versus white patients, 24.7 per cent; they also had a higher incidence of preoperative infection (21 per cent versus 10 per cent), and a higher incidence of pre-existing disease (stroke).

LATE RESULTS OF TRANSURETHRAL RESECTION OF THE PROSTATE

In the AUA Cooperative Study, 92 per cent of the patients were seen at least once postoperatively and 85 per cent at least twice. The average follow-up time for the first visit was 2.5 weeks and the second visit 2 months. At the second visit, 97 per cent of the patients stated that they were voiding with a good stream; however, vesical neck contracture (2.7 per cent), urethral stricture (2.5 per cent), mild stress incontinence (1.2 per cent), and significant incontinence (0.5 per cent) were found.

Vesical neck contracture usually occurs within the first 4 to 6 weeks following surgery. Classically, the patient has had a good urinary stream and then a marked reduction. Contracture is diagnosed endoscopically and can be treated by incising the neck with the Collings knife or cold knife urethrotome. We have injected triamcinolone at the time of incision, to soften recurrent scar formation (Damico et al., 1973).

The incidence (2.5 per cent) of urethral stricture noted here is significantly less than that (6 to 7 per cent) reported by others (Lentz et al., 1977). New strictures are undoubtedly related to urethritis, which can be caused by an indwelling catheter. This is particularly true if the catheter has been indwelling for some time and is of a larger caliber. However, the most common cause of urethral stricture, after TURP, is probably the trauma from the resectoscope. Its prevention is by adequately calibrating the urethra, preoperatively, and by determining the appropriate size resectoscope sheath. If the urethra is inadequate, we would recommend either a perineal urethrostomy or an internal urethrotomy. Urethral stricture is related to the size of the gland and length of resection time. We found a significant increase (30 per cent versus 1 per cent) when the gland was over 45 g and a perineal urethrostomy was not done.

Although the incidence of urinary incontinence is relatively low, it is a risk of surgery and the source of many malpractice suits. The internal sphincter mechanism at the bladder neck is destroyed with the TURP.

The patient is dependent on the external sphincter mechanism. The external sphincter mechanism is composed of striated muscles, some of which are the slow-twitch type, which give constant tone, and the fast-twitch type, which give voluntary control. The mechanism is also composed of smooth muscle and elastic fibers, which contribute to sphincteric tone. The external sphincter is not a simple circular muscle located in the pelvis but is rather more complex. This external sphincter mechanism has been described by Turner-Warwick (1983).

In reviewing 68 patients, with postprostatectomy incontinence, Fitzpatrick and associates (1979) noted that sphincteric damage was the cause of incontinence in 47 patients and was responsible alone in 18, with detrusor instability in 28, and with residual obstruction in three. Detrusor instability, however, was present in 45 of the 68 patients and was associated with sphincteric damage in 28. Instability alone was present in 11 patients and associated with residual obstruction in six patients. Therefore, three factors are important in postoperative incontinence: sphincteric injury, bladder hyperreflexia, and residual obstruction that impairs the external sphincter mechanism. Obviously, little data concerning the actual mechanism causing sphincteric injuries are available. The surgical technique is important and the limit of resection should be at the verumontanum, even if a small rim of adenoma is left behind. Bleeding should be well controlled so that the visual field is not obstructed. Electrocoagulation of vessels around the sphincter should be done carefully so that the muscle is not injured with cautery. The patient should be carefully positioned and further caution taken when resection approaches 12 o'clock.

Although temporary urgency and stress incontinence are common immediately after the catheter is removed, persistent stress incontinence and total incontinence, although rare, should be investigated. If a patient complains of incontinence a few weeks after surgery, we do a cystometrogram to determine if bladder hyperreflexia is a contributing factor. We will also perform cystoscopy to be sure that there is no obstructing adenoma at the apex. Patients are placed on Kegel exercises to strengthen the sphincter and anticholinergic drugs, if necessary. The urinary leakage is managed with a diaper-type padding or an external catheter. Fortunately, many of the patients improve with time. We generally do not recommend an artificial sphincter until 1 year after surgery.

Impotency has been reported from 4 to 40 per cent (Hargreave and Stephenson, 1977; Holtgrewe and Valk, 1964). The incidence of impotence, in the AUA Cooperative Study, was 4 per cent, but in only 1000 patients were there adequate data. In this subset of patients, the incidence was 13 per cent. In my opinion, the incidence of impotence is closer to 4 per cent than 40 per cent. However, it is extremely difficult to obtain valid data on the true incidence of impotence. It is very dependent on the presence or absence of a sexual partner and the patient's perception of his sexual ability, before and after surgery. So and colleagues (1982) found little correlation between nocturnal penile tumescence and the patient's perception of his sexual ability when these studies were done before and after surgery.

About 50 per cent of those with TURP will have retrograde ejaculation, which the patients may confuse with impotence. Therefore, we advise the patient of the higher risk of retrograde ejaculation as well as the smaller risk of erectile impotence. Patients who are sexually active will probably continue to be so. Patients who were already having sexual difficulty may worsen or date the onset of the problem to the operation.

The cause of impotence following a TURP is unknown. It is possible that excessive coagulation on the lateral floor of the prostate may injure the nerves important in potency. Many patients may already have compromised arterial supply to the penis because of age. In any event, we know of no technical procedure or variation that can reduce the incidence of impotence. It remains a risk of surgery.

LONG-TERM FOLLOW-UP

Interestingly, very little data exist on patients followed for several years after TURP. Bruskewitz and co-workers (1986), in following a series of patients over 3 years, noted, at 1 year, the symptoms were improved in 84 per cent and 10 per cent were approximately the same. At 3 years, 75 per cent remained improved, with 13 per cent the same. The change in symptomatology was the development of urge incontinence, occurring in these patients several years after surgery. Only one patient, in the 84 patients studied, required a repeat resection for an incidence of 2 per cent. However, 10 per cent of the patients developed vesical neck contracture and all of these had small prostates preoperatively. Three deaths (3.5 per cent) from cancer were recorded later.

Malone and associates (1988) reviewed 500 consecutive prostatectomies. Patients were followed between 5 and 8 years. These investigators noted a significant difference in the 3-year mortality rate between those who presented with acute or chronic retention. The survival rate, at 3 years for those with acute retention, was 80 per cent, whereas, those with chronic retention, 65 per cent. Of these patients, 80 per cent were asymptomatic. However, those with chronic retention (36 per cent) still had residual symptoms—a poor stream and nocturia and a flow rate compatible with failed detrusor.

Chilton and associates (1978), in studying a large series of patients for 5 years, noted that 4 per cent required a second resection for benign disease during that time. A delayed mortality rate of 0.8 per cent was seen in a group of patients who died from cancer that was unrelated to surgery.

Meyhoff and Nordling (1972) noted that 90 per cent of their patients were considered to have satisfactory results at 5 years after TURP. Flow rates were improved from preoperative values, although there had been a slight decline in flow rates over the 5-year period. These workers, however, noted an 8 per cent "re-resection" rate, but all were in patients with essentially small glands, suggesting that these might have been postoperative vesical neck contractures.

Bergman and associates (1955) noted a re-resection rate of 2.8 per cent at 5.5 years. Ball and Smith (1982), in following a series of patients, noted that flow rates remained improved, postoperatively, but a slight decrease occurred over the 5 years of follow-up. Assuming a linear progression, it would take approximately 24 to 30 years to return to preoperative flow rates.

However, Roos and Ramsey (1987) found a significant difference in the re-resection rate and late mortality following TURP. Using insurance claims data in Manitoba, Canada, they noted a re-resection rate of 2 per cent per year or 16 per cent at 8 years. Information as to the initial size of gland requiring repeat resection was not available nor was the amount of tissue removed at the time of the second resection known. These investigators also noted a mortality rate of 2.5 per cent at 90 days following surgery.

Roos and colleagues (1989), in a subsequent publication using insurance claims data information from England, Denmark, and Manitoba, noted that the reoperation rate for TURP ranged from 2.7 to 6.7 times that for a TURP compared with the open operation. Death rate at 90 days was higher than that previously recognized. It was definitely higher in those who had TURP compared with those who had open prostatectomy. One might assume that the difference in mortality rate was based on patient selection. However, Malenka and co-workers (1990) did a careful chart review of the patients in Manitoba, comparing those having transurethral prostatectomy with those having open prostatectomy. The mortality rate seemed to be higher with transurethral prostatectomy. The cause of death most commonly was myocardial infarction in the TURP group. There did not seem to be any differences in the comorbidity factors between the two groups.

This information, based on insurance claims data, is clearly different with respect to mortality and reoperation rate, when compared with previous studies that were based on chart review, retrospective analysis. The re-resection rate could be related to the skill of the surgeon or perhaps to a higher incidence of vesical neck contracture than had been noted in the other studies. The mortality rate could also be influenced by many factors, such as the type of hospital where the surgery was performed, the skill of the surgeon, the size of the gland, the length of operating time, and the predisposing cardiovascular problems.

Because of the uncertainties and the significance pointed out by these review studies based on insurance claims data, a national cooperative prospective study is being undertaken by the AUA and Dr. John Wennberg and his associates at Dartmouth Medical School.

OTHER SURGICAL TECHNIQUES FOR TRANSURETHRAL PROSTATECTOMY

Constant Flow Resectoscope

In 1975, Iglesias introduced the constant flow resectoscope, suggesting that it would allow a continuous resection, clearer visual field, and lower intraprostatic

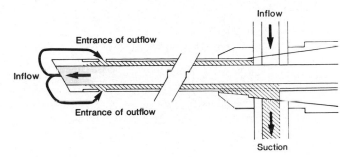

Figure 80–15. Constant flow resectoscope in which fluid is introduced through the center core and removed through the outer core, using suction.

fossa pressure with decreased fluid absorption (Fig. 80–15). The time for surgery should also be reduced. However, Stephenson and co-workers (1980) compared constant flow with standard interrupted flow and could find no difference in speed of resection, blood loss, or glycine absorption. Similarly, Flechner and Williams (1982) found no difference between the two techniques. However, Gellman (1980) cautioned that it was important to resect the floor tissue first to improve flow characteristics. At this time, the problem seems to be maintaining a constant inflow and outflow, while keeping the pressure low within the prostatic fossa and maintaining good visibility. Therefore, there does not appear to be a clear-cut advantage of constant flow irrigation, as opposed to the more standard intermittent irrigation, during transurethral prostatectomy.

Suprapubic Drainage During TURP

In the early 1970s, Bergman (1971) and Reuter and Jones (1974) suggested that a temporary suprapubic cannula could facilitate TURP by allowing a continuous flow system with a reduced absorption of fluids. In 1984, Madsen and Frimodt-Moller (1984) reported 577 cases with no problems of fluid absorption but noted a slightly higher blood loss compared with conventional TURP. The pressure of the irrigating fluid in the bladder was 8 cm H_2O and, thus, significantly less than the 10 to 15 cm H_2O of pelvic venous pressure. Comparing the suprapubic drainage technique to the Iglesias suction constant flow, Holmquist and associates (1979) found a shorter operating time for the suprapubic technique. The intravesical pressure was lower than that with the Iglesias procedure.

Transurethral Incision of the Prostate

Transurethral incision of the prostate (TUIP) is not a new procedure. Edwards (1985) credits Bottini in 1887 with describing the technique, but Hedlund and Ek (1985) credit Guthrie in 1834. In 1973, Orandi (1973) published the first significant series on TUIP. The procedure seemed to be most useful in those who had small prostates, which have been called primary vesical neck contractures, median bars, and sclerosed du Col, and

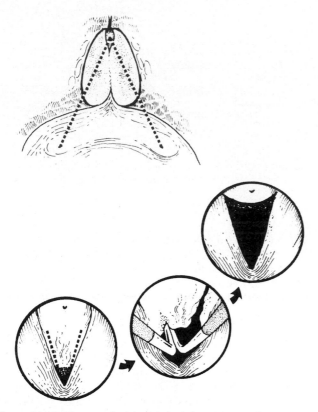

Figure 80–16. Transurethral incision of the prostate. The incision is started at the ureteral orifice and carried through the bladder neck up to the verumontanum. This procedure is done bilaterally. (From Mebust, W. K.: A Review of TURP Complications and the National Cooperative Study, Lesson 24, Volume VIII, 1989, pp. 189–190.)

who had obstructive bladder outlet symptoms. Classically, the patient was a younger man, compared with those undergoing TURP. The advantages of TUIP were that it was quicker and technically simpler and associated with less morbidity. A decrease in retrograde ejaculation was also noted, as compared with TURP. Retrograde ejaculation, following TURP, is from 50 to 95 per cent. Following a transurethral incision of the bladder neck, it has been reported as from 0 to 37 per cent (Edwards et al., 1985). Turner-Warwick (1979) noted that with one incision, the incidence of retrograde ejaculation was less than 5 per cent; but with two incisions, it was 15 per cent. Hedlund and Ek (1985) reported no difference between one and two incisions.

Few comparative studies have been done to determine the differences between TURP and TUIP. However, Nielsen (1988) noted similar results in a group of patients who had small glands and were randomized to either TURP or TUIP. He noted a better flow rate after TURP (12 ml) than TUIP (9 ml). Helstrom and colleagues (1986) noticed a better reduction in the maximum bladder pressure flow at maximum voiding, although a difference was noticed in flow rate favoring TURP. The investigators did not believe this was statistically significant.

The surgical technique is relatively simple. Using a Collings knife, the incision is performed at the 5-o'clock and 7-o'clock position, starting at the ureteral orifice and carrying it to the verumontanum (Fig. 80–16). The

incision should be carried so that the deeper portion of the prostatic incision has the fine filaments of the external capsule, with the occasional protrusion of fat. Care must be taken not to cause undue extravasation and not to enter into the rectum. With completion of the incisions and with the scope in the more distal urethra, there should be no visual obstruction to the bladder. Additionally, a biopsy of the prostate should be performed to ensure that carcinoma is not overlooked.

Balloon Dilatation

Mercier is given credit for the first dilatation of the prostate in 1844 (Castaneda et al., 1987). However, it was Deisting (1956) who, using an instrument in which the blades could be distracted, first stretched the prostate in the anteroposterior diameter 6 to 8 cm and caused a rent in the anterior commissure. He reported good results in 95 per cent of cases (Fig. 80–17). Backman (1963), in 130 patients followed 1 to 2 years, noted an 11.3 per cent reoperation rate and a 3.8 per cent redilatation rate. Aalkjer (1965) followed 186 patients for 7 years after dilatation, employing the Deisting technique. These patients were compared with 110 patients who had TURP. In those who were dilated, 38 per cent required a reoperation within that period of time. A progressive rate of increase of reoperation was reported, according to the increasing size of the gland. The larger glands did not do well with dilatation. The reoperation rate, during that period of time for the TURP patients, was 8 per cent.

However, interest in balloon dilatation of the prostate again became apparent in the 1980s, because of experience with balloon dilatation of the vascular system. Castaneda and colleagues (1987) reported good short-term results in a small series of patients. Moreover, Reddy (1990), using a 90 Fr. balloon, reported improve-

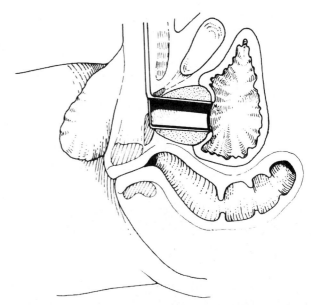

Figure 80–17. Dilatation of the prostatic fossa by distraction of the blades in the anteroposterior diameter, as described by Deisting.

ment at 6 months of 70 per cent and at 1 year of 58 per cent. Dowd and Smith (1990) reported, in 31 patients followed for 3 to 48 months, acceptable results in 58 per cent. Conversely, McLoughlin and associates (1990) found only 10 per cent of patients remained unobstructed at 8 months, utilizing urodynamic criteria. Patients have improvement in symptoms to a greater degree and lasting longer than they have in objective responses, as measured by urodynamic criteria.

At this time, the candidates are patients who are at high risk for surgical procedures, with perhaps limited life expectancy, who need relief of small obstructing prostates. The contraindications would be cases of median lobes and possibly carcinomas. Some concern exists that the increase in pressure within the prostatic fossa could disseminate the cancer. The advantage of the procedure is that it is done in a short period of time, under a periprostatic block with sedation. Also, a minimal hospital stay is required. The greatest risk is external sphincteric injury.

Surgical Technique

At this time, most surgeons select a 90 Fr. balloon, which is distended to 4 atm of pressure within the prostatic fossa and left in place for 10 minutes. The critical part of the procedure is the proper positioning of the balloon, so that it does not injure the external urethral sphincter. The balloon must be maintained within the prostatic fossa, because of a tendency for it to migrate into the bladder with distention. The actual technique of positioning the balloon is dependent on how the balloon is constructed. Several manufacturers are making these balloons at this time.

The technique described by Reddy (1990) employs radiographic control to position the balloon. A retrograde urethrogram is done to define the external sphincter. The area of the external sphincter is marked on the patient's drapes with a metallic object. A .038-cm guide wire is passed through the Councill catheter and the balloon positioned in the fossa, confirming its position in relationship to the metallic marker. The positioning balloon is inflated in the bulbous urethra, and its position is confirmed by palpating it through the rectum. The dilating balloon is then inflated.

The Dowd balloon is similarly inserted into the bladder, over a guide wire, but it has a firm positioning button that can be palpated transrectally (Fig. 80–18). This button is positioned directly at the apex of the prostate and the balloon inflated. Gentle traction is applied to the catheter to prevent its migration into the bladder. A LeVeen inflator with a pressure gauge is used in the final inflation of the dilating balloon and is used in monitoring the pressure within the balloon. With distention of the prostate, additional fluid may be required to keep the pressure constantly at 4 atm, during the 10-minute period of dilatation time.

Klein and co-workers (1990) have described another technique of positioning the balloon. The length of the prostate is measured with a graduated urethral catheter inserted cystoscopically. The catheter is secured to the bladder neck with a balloon and inflated within the

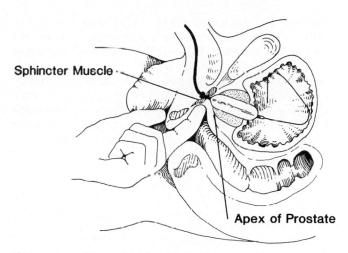

Figure 80–18. Positioning of the Dowd balloon within the prostatic fossa. The positioning button is palpated transrectally just outside the apex of the prostate.

bladder. As the cystoscope is withdrawn, the distance from the bladder neck to the external sphincter is measured. A dilating balloon of proper length is then inserted through the cystoscope. The catheter has an anchoring balloon that is inflated in the bladder and holds the dilating balloon in place. A localization ring is imprinted on the catheter 0.5 cm distal to the dilating balloon. This is observed through the cystoscope to be in the bulbous urethra, just distal to the external sphincter, when the balloon is properly positioned. The balloon is then inflated to 75 Fr., with 3 atm of pressure for 10 minutes.

The common factor in all these positioning techniques is to be sure that when the dilating balloon is inflated, the external sphincter is not injured.

In summary, this is an old technique, revisited. It would appear that it is of help in a select group of patients. It would appear that the objective, long-term results will be measured in months rather than years.

MANAGING BENIGN PROSTATIC HYPERTROPY (BPH) WITH INTRAPROSTATIC THERMAL CHANGES

Heating or freezing the prostate to relieve obstructing tissue was utilized 20 to 30 years ago. Gonder and colleagues (1966) employed transurethral cryoprostatectomy in the early 1960s. However, the procedure was abandoned because of post-treatment sloughing of large fragments of prostatic tissue, causing acute obstruction and infection. Ablin and co-workers (1977) suggested that freezing the prostate might evoke an autoimmune response that could have clinical applications in treating carcinoma of the prostate. Whether or not an autoimmune response was evoked became immaterial, because no obvious clinical beneficial response was seen in patients with prostate cancer treated with cryoprostatectomy.

Mebust and associates (1972, 1977) used a transurethral probe, with direct vision capabilities, to heat and desiccate the prostate. The energy source was the cutting current of the electrosurgical unit. The procedure was chosen for high-risk patients, as it could be quickly performed without blood loss. Sloughing of tissue after the procedure was not a problem. Improved flow rates were obtained. Some patients, however, did experience prolonged pyuria with prostatitis-like symptoms.

In the mid 1980s, Harado and associates (1985) and Lindner and associates (1987) introduced the concept of heating the prostate with microwaves. A probe was placed in the rectum, and the prostate was heated to 42 ± 1.5° C, with microwaves at 950 MHz. Treatment sessions lasted 30 to 60 minutes and were repeated several times. Lindner and colleagues (1990a) reported a 50 per cent success rate and an overall complication rate of 6.6 per cent in 435 patients. Complications were urinary tract infections, hematuria, and epididymitis. However, the mechanism of action is unclear. Lindner and colleagues (1990b) reported no change in the postoperative prostate-specific antigen value compared with the preoperative value. This finding suggests that tissue destruction is not the mode of action. Pre-treatment and post-treatment ultrasound evaluations of prostate size showed no change in 25 of 28 patients and only three patients had improvement in voiding, as reported by Strohmaier and co-workers (1990).

Conversely, Watson (1990) reported only 25 per cent of 30 patients had improvement in flow rate, but the majority, following transrectal hyperthermia, had improvement in symptomatology. At least 40 per cent of patients improve symptomatically with placebo. However, Zerbib and associates (1990) incorporated a placebo in a prospective, randomized study of transrectal microwave hyperthermia and found that those who received active treatment did better. Lindner and colleagues (1990a) list the contraindications as cases of rectal pathology, urethral stricture, and intravesical pathology, and prostates more than 55 mm in the anteroposterior diameter.

At this time, it is too early to determine what the role of transrectal hyperthermia will be. We don't know if all patients will benefit from the procedure. It is also unknown whether the benefit will be improvement in objective urodynamic data, as well as symptoms. The long-term results are also unclear. Sapozink and coworkers (1990) reported their experience in 21 patients with transurethral microwave hyperthermia at 630 or 950 MHz (Fig. 80–19). The procedure was done using local anesthesia, on an outpatient basis. The treatments were for 1 hour, and there were ten treatment sessions. The investigators believed that 71 to 81 per cent had good subjective and objective responses at a median follow-up of 12 months. However, this report is preliminary, from one institution. Wider usage, with longer follow-up of patients, will be necessary for determining the role of transrectal hyperthermia in managing BPH.

VESICAL LITHOLAPAXY AND LITHOTRIPSY

The etiology of bladder stones is primarily bladder outlet obstruction and urinary infection. Diet may play a role. Patients who have a very minimal animal protein diet and a more alkaline urine may be more prone to bladder stones. Bladder stones have always plagued humanity. Classically, they were removed transvesically. However, Bigelow introduced the transurethral lithotrite, which mechanically crushed the stone. This instrument was introduced transurethrally. The stone was engaged in the forceps blindly and crushed. The patient then voided the fragments transurethrally.

Mechanical Litholapaxy

The Hendrickson lithotrite allowed the crushing of stones mechanically under direct vision. The contraindications to the procedure were cases of small capacity bladders; multiple stones; large stones, which could not be engaged; and inadequate urethras.

The procedure was somewhat difficult to perform because of poor water flow, resulting in poor visualization within the bladder. The risk of bladder injury was always there. The technique is to fill the bladder with 150 ml of fluid, grasp the stone, rotate the lithotrite with the stone engaged so that it is away from the mucosa, and crush the stone manually (Fig. 80–20). This procedure is repeated several times to reduce the stone to small fragments. By rotating the jaws of the lithotrite with the stone in it, it is hoped that the mucosa would not become engaged and the bladder injured. Stone fragments are then removed with small, alligator jaw forceps or triradial forceps. The stone fragments can

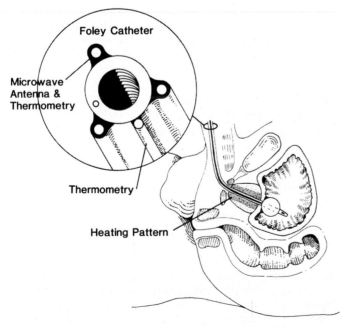

Figure 80–19. Transurethral microwave hyperthermia of the prostate. (Modified from Saponzink, M. D., Boyd, S., Astrahan, M., Joseph, G., and Petrovich, Z.: Transurethral hyperthermia for benign prostate hyperplasia with preliminary clinical results. J. Urol., 143:944–950, 1990.)

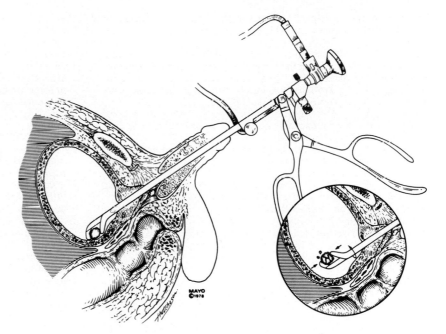

Figure 80–20. Mechanical litholapaxy using the visual Hendrickson lithotrite.

also be washed out with the Ellik evacuator. A resectoscope, with a modification of the loop so that it is a scoop, can also remove stone fragments. Not uncommonly, we will perform a TURP, assuming that the basic pathology is an obstructing prostate.

Electrohydraulic Lithotripsy

Bergman and associates (1982) credit Yutkin for the discovery of the principle of electrohydraulic lithotripsy (EHL). The URAT I was developed by Goligowsky of the Soviet Union in the 1960s. Now, EHL is used in the kidney and ureter as well as the bladder.

Numerous companies manufacture EHL units. The technique involving the EHL is somewhat dependent on the manufacturers' recommendations. The generator usually permits variations in power settings and whether or not the shock impulse is to be single or repetitive. Physiologic saline (l/6 normal) has been recommended as the best solution for bladder irrigation. However, we have used sterile water with reasonable results. The electrode is usually 9 Fr., although smaller electrodes may be chosen for smaller stones. The tip of the electrode is placed 1 to 2 mm in proximity to the stone, and the tip must also be 1 cm away from the lens system. The tip should also be 1 cm away from the bladder wall to avoid injury. We prefer a short burst of energy to conserve the electrode, and we try to concentrate the shock wave at one location on the stone, to facilitate breaking.

Following the breaking up of the stone, the fragments are removed with the Ellik evacuator. The remaining fragments can be removed, transurethrally, with grasping forceps. A modified resectoscope loop, that looks like a scoop, is also helpful in removing stones.

The contraindications to EHL would appear to be the presence of large stones (over 5 cm), the presence of other pathology in the bladder that needs surgical correction (e.g., diverticulum), and the necessity of doing an open prostatectomy.

Bulow and Frohmuller (1981) completed a TURP in 70 per cent of their cases, at the time of the EHL. They reported an overall success rate of EHL of 92 per cent. Bergman and co-workers (1982) reported a 95 per cent success rate. Short and co-workers (1984), in comparing the rates of recurrence of calculi in the bladder in patients with an indwelling Foley following vesicolithotomy, litholapaxy, and EHL, found the respective recurrence rates of 7.4 per cent, 44.1 per cent, and 50 per cent. Obviously, those patients who are at high risk for recurrent calculi should have cystoscopy sometime after the procedure to be sure that all the stone fragments have been satisfactorily removed from the bladder.

Except in a patient with an indwelling catheter, most bladder stones are considered to be secondary to bladder outlet obstruction and infection. We would, therefore, recommend, in addition to the removal of the stone, that the bladder outlet obstruction be corrected. Patients who have prostate glands amenable to TURP can have this correction done at the time of transurethral litholapaxy. Patients with larger glands, requiring open surgery, can also have bladder outlet obstruction correction done at the time the stone is removed, transvesically.

REFERENCES

Aalkjer, V.: Transurethral resection/prostatectomy versus dilatation treatment in hypertrophy of the prostate. II. A comparison of late results. Urol. Int., 20:17–22, 1965.

Ablin, R. J., Bruns, G. R., Guinan, P. D., Sadoughi, N., Sheik, H. A., and Bush, I. M.: Alterations in host responsiveness in patients with prostatic cancer following cryosurgery or transurethral resection. Am. Surg., 43:144–150, 1977.

Abrams, P. H.: Detrusor instability and bladder outlet obstruction. Neurol. Urodynsm., 4:317, 1985.

Abrams, P. H.: A double-blind trial of the effects of candicidin on patients with benign prostatic hypertrophy. Br. J. Urol., 49:67–71, 1977.

Abrams, P. H.: Prostatism and prostatectomy: The value of urine flow rate measurement in the preoperative assessment for operation. J. Urol., 117:70–71, 1977.

Andersen, J. T.: Prostatism: Clinical, radiologic and urodynamic aspects. Neuro. Urodynam., 1:241, 1982.

Backman, K. A.: Dilatation of the prostate according to Deisting: Results of follow up one and two years after operation. Acta Chir. Scand., 126:266–274, 1963.

Bailey, M. J., and Shearer, R. J.: The role of internal urethrotomy in the prevention of urethral stricture following transurethral resection of prostate. Br. J. Urol., 51:28–31, 1979.

Ball A. J., Feneley, R. C. L., and Abrams, P. H.: The natural history of untreated prostatism. Br. J. Urol., 53:613, 1981.

Ball, A. J., and Smith, P. J. B.: The long-term effects of prostatectomy: A uroflowmetric analysis. J. Urol., 128:538–540, 1982.

Bergman, B., Nygaard, E., Osterman, G., and Tomic, R.: Vesical calculi: Experience of electrohydraulic lithotripsy with URAT I. Scand. J. Urol. Nephrol., 16:217–220, 1982.

Bergman, M.: Suprapubic drainage in transurethral electroresection. Urologe, 10:110–111, 1971.

Bergman, R. T., Turner, R., Barnes, R. W., and Hadley, H. L.: Comparative analysis of one thousand consecutive cases of transurethral prostatectomy. J. Urol., 74:533–545, 1955.

Birkhoff, J. D., Wiederhorn, A. R., Hamilton, M. L., and Zinsser H. H.: Natural history of benign prostatic hypertrophy and acute urinary retention. Urology, 7:48–52, 1976.

Boyarsky, S., Jones, G., Paulson, D. F., and Prout, G. R., Jr.: A new look at bladder neck obstruction by the Food and Drug Administration: Guidelines for investigation of benign prostatic hypertrophy. Trans. Am. Assoc. Genitourin. Surg., 68:29–32, 1977.

Breum, L., Klarskov, P., Munck, L. K., Nielsen, T. H., and Nordeslgaard, A. G.: Significance of acute urinary retention due to infravesical obstruction. Scand. J. Urol. Nephrol., 16:21, 1982.

Bruskewitz, R. C., Iversen, P., and Madsen, P. O.: Value of post void residual urine determination in evaluation of prostatism. Urology, 20:602, 1982.

Bruskewitz, R. C., Larsen, E. H., Madsen, P. O., and Dorflinger, T.: Three-year followup of urinary symptoms after transurethral resection of the prostate. J. Urol., 136:613–615, 1986.

Bulow, H., and Frohmuller, H. G.: Electrohydraulic lithotripsy with aspiration of the fragments under vision—304 consecutive cases. J. Urol., 126:454–456, 1981.

Castaneda, F., Reddy, P., Wasserman, N., Hulbert, J., Lund, G., Letourneau, J. G., Hunter, D. W., Castaneda-Zuniga, W. R., and Amplatz, K.: Benign prostatic hypertrophy: Retrograde transurethral dilation of the prostatic urethra in humans. Radiology, 163:649–653, 1987.

Chilton, C. P., Morgan, R. J., England, H. R., Paris, A. M. I., and Blandy, J. P.: A critical evaluation of the results of transurethral resection of the prostate. Br. J. Urol., 50:542–546, 1978.

Craigen, A. A., Hickling, J. B., Saunders, C. R. G., and Carpenter, R. G.: Natural history of prostatic obstruction. J. Roy. Coll. Gen. Prac., 18:226–232, 1969.

Creevy, C. D., and Webb, E. A.: A fatal hemolytic reaction following transurethral resection of the prostate gland: A discussion of its prevention and treatment. Surgery, 21:56–66, 1947.

Damico, C. F., Mebust, W. K., Valk, W. L., and Foret, J. D.: Triamcinolone: Adjuvant therapy for vesical neck contracture. J. Urol., 110:203–204, 1973.

Deisting, W.: Transurethral dilatation of the prostate: A new method in the treatment of prostatic hypertrophy. Urol. Intervent., 2:158–171, 1956.

Dowd, J. B., and Smith, J. J., III: Balloon dilatation of the prostate without imaging: Comparison with transurethral resection of the prostate. Presented at the Meeting of the American Urological Association, New Orleans, May, 1990.

Drach, G. W., Laylon, T., and Bottaccini, M. R.: A method of adjustment of male peak urinary flow rate for varying age and volume voided. J. Urol., 128:960, 1982.

Edwards, L. E., Bucknall, T. E., Pittam, M. R., Richardson, D. R., and Stanek, J.: Transurethral resection of the prostate and bladder neck incision: A review of 700 cases. Br. J. Urol., 57:168–171, 1985.

Emmett, J. L., Gilbaugh, J. H., Jr., and McLean, P.: Fluid absorption during transurethral resection: Comparison of mortality and morbidity after irrigation with water and nonhemolytic solutions. J. Urol., 101:884–889, 1969.

Emmett, J. L., Rous, S. N., Greene, L. F., DeWeerd, J. H., and Utz, D. C.: Preliminary internal urethrotomy in 1036 cases to prevent urethral stricture following transurethral resection; caliber of normal adult male urethra. J. Urol., 89:829, 1963.

Fitzpatrick, J. M., Gardiner, R. A., and Worth, P. H. L.: The evaluation of 68 patients with post-prostatectomy incontinence. Br. J. Urol., 51:552–555, 1979.

Flechner, S. M., and Williams, R. D.: Continuous flow and conventional resectoscope methods in transurethral prostatectomy: comparative study. J. Urol., 127:257–259, 1982.

Frimodt-Moller, P. G., Jensen, K. M. E., Iversen, P., Madsen, P. O., and Bruskewitz, R. C.: Analysis of presenting symptoms in prostatism. J. Urol., 132:272, 1984.

Gellman, A. C.: Endoscopic prostatectomy with the continuous flow resection technique. Int. Surg., 65:433–436, 1980.

Gibbons, R. P., Stark, R. A., Correa, R. J., Jr., Cummings, K. B., and Mason, J. T.: The prophylactic use—or misuse—of antibiotics in transurethral prostatectomy. J. Urol., 119:381, 1978.

Glynn, R. J., Campion, E. W., Bouchard, G. R., and Silbert, J. E.: The development of benign prostatic hyperplasia among volunteers in the normative aging study. Am. J. Epidemiol., 121:78, 1985.

Goldwasser, B., Bobokowsky, B., Nativ, O., Sidi, A. A., Jonas, P., and Many, M.: Prophylactic antimicrobial treatment in transurethral prostatectomy. How long should it be instituted? Urology, 22:136–138, 1983.

Gonder, M. J., Soanes, W. A., and Shulman, S.: Cryosurgical treatment of the prostate. Invest. Urol., 3:372–378, 1966.

Grabe, M., Forsgren, A., and Hellsten, S.: The effect of a short antibiotic course in transurethral prostatic resection. Scand. J. Urol. Nephrol., 18:37–42, 1984.

Grabe, M., and Hellsten, S.: Long-term follow-up after transurethral prostatic resection with or without a short perioperative antibiotic course. Br. J. Urol., 57:444–449, 1985.

Greene, L. F.: Transurethral surgery. In Walsh, P. C., Gittes, R. F., Perlmutter, A. D., and Stamey, T. A. (Eds.). Campbell's Urology, 5th ed. W. B. Saunders Co., Philadelphia, 1986, pp. 2815–2843.

Hagstrom, R. S.: Studies on fluid absorption during transurethral prostatic resection. J. Urol., 73:852–859, 1955.

Harado, T., Etori, K., Kumazaki, T., Nishizawa, O., Noto, H., and Tsuchida, S.: Microwave surgical treatment of diseases of prostate. Urology, 26:572, 1985.

Hargreave, T. B., and Stephenson, T. P.: Potency and prostatectomy. Br. J. Urol., 49:683–688, 1977.

Harrison, R. H., III, Boren, J. S., and Robison, J. R.: Dilutional hyponatremic shock: Another concept of the transurethral prostatic resection reaction. J. Urol., 75:95–110, 1956.

Hasner, E.: Prostatic urinary infection. Acta Chir. Scand., (Suppl) 285:1–40, 1962.

Hedlund, H., and Ek, A.: Ejaculation and sexual function after endoscopic bladder neck incision. Br. J. Urol., 57:164–167, 1985.

Helstrom, P., Lukkarinen, O., and Kontturi, M.: Bladder neck incision or transurethral electroresection for the treatment of urinary obstruction caused by a small benign prostate. A randomized urodynamic study. Scand. J. Urol. Nephrol., 20:187–192, 1986.

Hinman, F., Jr.: Residual urine. Measurement and influence in management of obstruction. In Hinman, F. Jr. (Ed.). Benign Prostatic Hypertrophy. New York, Springer-Verlag, 1983, pp. 589–596.

Hoekstra, P. T., Kahnoski, R., McCamish, M. A., Bergen, W., and Heetderks, D. R.: Transurethral prostatic resection syndrome—A new perspective: Encephalopathy with associated hyperammonemia. J. Urol., 130:704–707, 1983.

Holl, W. H., and Rous, S. N.: Is antibiotic prophylaxis worthwhile in patients with transurethral resection of the prostate? J. Urol., 19:43, 1982.

Holmquist, B. G., Holm, B., and Ohlin, P.: Comparative study of the Iglesias technique and the suprapubic drainage technique for transurethral resection. Br. J. Urol., 51:378–381, 1979.

Holtgrewe, H. L., Mebust, W. K., Dowd, J. B., Cockett, A. T. K., Peters, P. C., and Proctor, C.: Transurethral prostatectomy: Practice aspects of the dominant operation in American urology. J. Urol., 141:248–253, 1989.

Holtgrewe, H. L., and Valk, W. L.: Factors influencing the mortality and morbidity of transurethral prostatectomy: A study of 2,015 cases. J. Urol., 87:450–459, 1962.

Holtgrewe, H. L., and Valk, W. L.: Late results of transurethral prostatectomy. J. Urol., 92:51–55, 1964.

Hopkins, H. H.: Optical principles of the endoscope. In Berci, G. (Ed.). Endoscopy. New York, Appleton-Century-Crofts, 1976, pp. 3–26.

Iglesias, J. J., Sporer, A., Gellman, A. C., and Seebode, J. J.: New Iglesias resectoscope with continuous irrigation, simultaneous suction and low intravesical pressure. J. Urol., 114:929–933, 1975.

Iversen, P., Bruskewitz, R. C., Jensen, K. M. E., and Madsen, P. O.: Transurethral prostatic resection in the treatment of prostatism with high urinary flow. J. Urol., 129:995, 1983.

Klein, L., Perez-Marrero, R., Bowers, G. W., Ludwig, J. J., and Herwig K.: Transurethral cystoscopic balloon dilatation of the prostate. J. Endourol. 4:183–191, 1990.

Kulb, T. P., Kamer, M., Lingeman, J. E., and Foster, R. S.: Prevention of post-prostatectomy vesical neck contracture by prophylactic vesical neck incision. J. Urol., 137:230–231, 1987.

Lentz, H. C., Jr, Mebust, W. K., Foret, J. D., and Melchior, J.: Urethral strictures following transurethral prostatectomy: Review of 2,223 resections. J. Urol., 117:194–196, 1977.

Lindner, A., Colomb, J., Siegel, Y. I., and Lev, A.: Local hyperthermia of the prostate gland for the treatment of benign prostatic hypertrophy and urinary retention. Br. J. Urol., 60:567–571, 1987.

Lindner, A., Siegel, Y. I., and Korczak, D.: Serum prostate specific antigen levels during hyperthermia treatment of benign prostatic hyperplasia. J. Urol., 144:1388, 1990a.

Lindner, A., Siegel, Y. I., Saranga, R., Korzcak, D., Matzkin, H., and Braf, Z.: Complications in hyperthermia treatment of benign prostatic hyperplasia. J. Urol., 144:1388, 1990b.

Lytton, B., Emery, J. M., and Harvard, B. M.: The incidence of benign prostatic obstruction. J. Urol., 99:639, 1968.

Madsen, P. O., and Frimodt-Moller, P. C.: Transurethral prostatic resection with suprapubic trocar technique. J. Urol., 132:277–279, 1984.

Madsen, P. O., and Naber, K. G.: The importance of the pressure in the prostatic fossa and absorption of irrigating fluid during transurethral resection of the prostate. J. Urol., 109:446–452, 1973.

Malenka, D. J., Roos, N., Fisher, E. S., McLerran, D., Whaley, F. S., Barry, M. J., Bruskewitz, R., and Wennberg, J. E.: Further study of the increased mortality following transurethral prostatectomy: A chart-based analysis. J. Urol., 144:224–228, 1990.

Malone, P. R., Cook, A., Edmonson, R., Gill, M. W., and Shearer, R. J.: Prostatectomy: Patients' perception and long-term follow-up. Br. J. Urol., 61:234–238, 1988.

McGowan, S. W., and Smith, G. F. N.: Anaesthesia for transurethral prostatectomy: A comparison of spinal intradural analgesia with two methods of general anaesthesia. Anaesthesia, 35:847–853, 1980.

McLoughlin, J., Keane, P., Jager, R., Abel, P., and Williams, G.: The objective assessment of 35 mm balloons in the treatment of bladder outflow obstruction. Presented at the Meeting of the American Urological Association, New Orleans, May, 1990.

McPherson, K., Wennberg, J. E., Hovind, O. B., and Clifford, P.: Small-area variations in the use of common surgical procedures: An international comparison of New England, England, and Norway. N. Engl. J. Med., 307:1310–1314, 1982.

Mebust, W. K., and Damico, C.: Prostatic desiccation: A preliminary report of laboratory and clinical experience. J. Urol., 108:601–603, 1972.

Mebust, W. K., Foret, J. D., and Valk, W. L.: Transurethral surgery. In Harrison, J. H., Gittes, R. F., Perlmutter, A. D., Stamey, T. A., and Walsh, P. C. (Eds.). Campbell's Urology, 4th ed. Philadelphia, W. B. Saunders Co., 1979, pp. 2361–2381.

Mebust, W. K., Holtgrewe, H. L., Cockett, A. T. K., Peters, P. C., and the Writing Committee: Transurethral prostatectomy: Immediate and postoperative complications. A cooperative study of thirteen participating institutions evaluating 3,885 patients. J. Urol., 141:243–247, 1989.

Mebust, W. K., and Valk, W. L.: Transurethral prostatectomy. In Hinman, F., Jr. (Ed.). Benign Prostatic Hypertrophy. New York, Springer-Verlag, pp. 829–846, 1983.

Mebust, W. K., and White, T. G.: Immune reactions following desiccation surgery of the canine prostate. Invest. Urol., 14:427–430, 1977.

Melchior, J., Valk, W. L., Foret, J. D., and Mebust, W. K.: Transurethral prostatectomy: Computerized analysis of 2,223 consecutive cases. J. Urol., 112:634–642, 1974.

Melchior, J., Valk, W. L., Foret, J. D., and Mebust, W. K.: Transurethral resection of the prostate via perineal urethrostomy: Complete analysis of 7 years of experience. J. Urol., 111:640–643, 1974.

Meyhoff, H. H., and Nordling, J.: Long-term results of transurethral and transvesical prostatectomy: A randomized study. Scand. J. Urol. Nephrol., 20:27–33, 1986.

Murphy, D. M., Stassen, L., Carr, M. E., Gillespie, W. A., Cafferkey, M. T., and Falkiner, F. R.: Bacteremia during prostatectomy and other transurethral operations: Influence of timing of antibiotic administration. J. Clin. Pathol., 37:673–676, 1984.

Nesbit, R. M.: A history of transurethral prostatectomy. Rev. Mex. Urol., 35:349–362, 1975.

Nesbit, R. M.: Transurethral prostatectomy. Springfield, IL, Charles C. Thomas, 1943.

Nielsen, H. O.: Transurethral prostatotomy versus transurethral prostatectomy in benign prostatic hypertrophy: A prospective randomized study. Br. J. Urol., 61:435–438, 1988.

Nielsen, K. K., Andersen, K., Asbjorn, J., Vork, F., and Ohrt-Nissen, A.: Blood loss in transurethral prostatectomy: Epidural versus general anaesthesia. Int. Urol. Nephrol., 19:287–292, 1987.

Nielsen, O. S., Maigaard, S., Frimodt-Moller, N., and Madsen, P. O.: Prophylactic antibiotics in transurethral prostatectomy. J. Urol., 126:60–62, 1981.

O'Donnell, P. D.: Serum acid phosphatase elevation associated with transurethral resection syndromes. Urology, 22:388–390, 1983.

Oester, A., and Madsen, P. O.: Determination of absorption of irrigating fluid during transurethral resection of the prostate by means of radioisotopes. J. Urol., 102:714–719, 1969.

Orandi, A.: Transurethral incision of the prostate. J. Urol., 110:229–231, 1973.

Ovassapian, A., Joshi, C. W., and Brunner, E. A.: Visual disturbances: An unusual symptom of transurethral prostatic resection reaction. Anesthesiology, 57:332–334, 1982.

Perrin, P., Barnes, R., Hadley, H., and Bergman, R. T.: Forty years of transurethral prostatic resections. J. Urol., 116:757–758, 1976.

Peters, K. R., Muir, J., and Wingard, D. W.: Intraocular pressure after transurethral prostatic surgery. Anesthesiology, 55:327–329, 1981.

Prokocimer, P., Quazza, M., Gibert, C., Lemoine, J. E., Joly, M. L., Dureuil, B., Moulonguet, A., Manuel, C., and Desmonts, J. M.: Short-term prophylactic antibiotics in patients undergoing prostatectomy: Report of a double-blind randomized trial with 2 intravenous doses of cefotaxime. J. Urol., 135:60–64, 1986.

Reddy, P. K.: Role of balloon dilation in the treatment of benign prostatic hyperplasia. The Prostate Supplement, 3:39–48, 1990.

Reuter, H. J., and Jones, L. W.: Physiologic low pressure irrigation for transurethral resection: Suprapubic trochar drainage. J. Urol., 111:210–212, 1974.

Roesch, R. P., Stoelting, R. K., Lingeman, J. E., Kahnoski, R. J., Backes, D. G., and Gephardt, S. A.: Ammonia toxicity resulting from glycine absorption during a transurethral resection of the prostate. Anesthesiology, 58:577–579, 1983.

Roos, N. P., and Ramsey, E. W.: A population-based study of prostatectomy: Outcomes associated with differing surgical approaches. J. Urol., 137:1184–1188, 1987.

Roos, N. P., Wennberg, J. E., Malenka, D. J., Fisher, E. S., McPherson, K., Andersen, T. F., Cohen, M. M., and Ramsey, E.: Mortality and reoperation after open and transurethral resection of the prostate for benign prostatic hyperplasia. Special Article. N. Engl. J. Med., 320:1120–1123, 1989.

Sapozink, M. D., Boyd, S., Astrahan, M., Joseph, G., and Petrovich, Z.: Transurethral hyperthermia for benign prostatic hyperplasia with preliminary clinical results. J. Urol., 143:944–950, 1990.

Shah, P. J. R., Abrams, P. H., Feneley, R. C. L., and Green, N. A.: The influence of prostatic anatomy on the differing results of prostatectomy according to the surgical approach. Br. J. Urol., 51:549–551, 1979.

Short, K. L., Amin, M., Harty, J. I., and O'Connor, C. A.: Comparison of recurrence rates of calculi of the bladder in patients with indwelling catheters following vesicolithotomy, litholapaxy and electrohydraulic lithotripsy. Surg. Gynecol. Obstet., 159:247–248, 1984.

Sinha, B., Haikel, G., Lange, P. H., Moon, T. D., and Narayan, P.: Transurethral resection of the prostate with local anesthesia in 100 patients. J. Urol., 135:719–721, 1986.

Siroky, M. B., Olsson, C. A., and Krane, R. J.: The flow rate nomogram. I. Development. J. Urol., 122:665, 1979.

So, E. P., Ho, P. C., Bodenstab, W., and Parsons, C. L.: Erectile impotence associated with transurethral prostatectomy. Urology, 19:259–262, 1982.

Spiro, L. H., Labay, G., and Orkin, L. A.: Prostatic infarction: Role in acute urinary retention. Urology, 3:345, 1974.

Stephenson, T. P., Latto, P., Bradley, D., Hayward, M., and Jones, A.: Comparison between continuous flow and intermittent flow transurethral resection in 40 patients presenting with acute retention. Br. J. Urol., 52:523–525, 1980.

Strohmaier, W. L., Bichler, K. H., Fluechter, S. H., and Wilbert, D. M.: Local microwave hyperthermia in benign prostatic hyperplasia (BPH). Presented at the Meeting of the American Urological Association, New Orleans, May, 1990.

Symes, J. M., Hardy, D. G., Sutherns, K., and Blandy, J. P.: Factors reducing the rate of infection after trans-urethral surgery. Br. J. Urol., 44:582–586, 1972.

Turner-Warwick, R.: The sphincter mechanism: Their relation to prostatic enlargement and its treatment. *In* Hinman, F., Jr. (Ed.). Benign Prostatic Hypertrophy. New York, Springer-Verlag, 1983, pp. 809–828.

Turner-Warwick, R.: A urodynamic review of bladder outlet obstruction in the male and its clinical implications. Urol. Clin. North Am., 6:171–192, 1979.

Watson, G. M.: Experience with a transrectal microwave device for hyperthermia treatment of prostatic disease. Presented at the Meeting of the American Urological Association, New Orleans, May, 1990.

Wennberg, J. E., and Gittelsohn, A. M.: Variations in medical care among small areas. Sci. Am., 246:120–134, 1982.

Zerbib, M., Steg, A., Conquy, S., and Debre, B.: A prospective randomized study of localized hyperthermia vs. placebo in obstructive benign hypertrophy of the prostate. Presented at the Meeting of the American Urological Association, New Orleans, May, 1990.

81
UROLOGIC LASER SURGERY

Joseph A. Smith, Jr., M.D.

A laser generates a collimated, monochromatic beam of light with all of the photons in phase with one another. With certain wavelengths, the beam can be propagated along a flexible fiber with little energy loss, facilitating delivery of the light to tissue. Nontoxic fibers for clinical use have not yet been developed for some longer wavelengths, such as carbon dioxide. Regardless of the method of delivery, the therapeutic effects depend on interaction of the laser beam and tissue. Generally, the tissue effects of a laser beam may be characterized as thermal, mechanical, or photochemical.

TISSUE EFFECTS

Thermal

Most therapeutic laser effects depend on thermal transformation of light energy. Up to 60° C, only tissue warming occurs without irreversible cellular damage. Between 60 and 100° C, protein coagulation is observed, resulting in cell death but no loss of structural or architectural integrity of the tissue (Hofstetter et al., 1989). This quality may be of particular importance in hollow organs, such as the bladder. Above 100° C, carbonization and vaporization occur.

Mechanical

A low-energy laser with a short-pulse duration creates an optico-acoustic effect. This can result in mechanical stone fragmentation (Watson et al., 1983). The effects are nonthermal and depend on absorption of the laser energy by the stone. Expansion of a plasma that is formed results in disruption of the stone.

Photochemical

Photosensitizers that are activated by light of a specific wavelength can result in cellular death from a photochemical effect. The photosensitizer most frequently used in clinical studies is hematoporphyrin derivative. After systemic administration, retention of the drug in dysplastic and malignant cells occurs (Benson et al., 1983). Usually, 630 nanometer light from an argon dye laser is applied. The exact mechanism of cellular death is uncertain. It has been theorized that production of singlet oxygen is toxic to the mitochondria. At any rate, low-power laser energy is utilized and the tissue effects are nonthermal.

PARAMETERS AFFECTING TISSUE INJURY

A number of factors influence the tissue effects of a given laser. Some of these are under the precise control of the operating surgeon and others are not. The type and depth of tissue injury may vary, and the surgeon using the laser must choose those parameters that most optimally produce the desired therapeutic effect.

Energy

The power output of a laser can usually be selected precisely and varied as necessary. Power is measured in watts. The power may be emitted continuously, as long as the laser is activated, or in pulses. Continuous-wave lasers are employed for most applications in urologic surgery. However, pulsed lasers allow rapid escalation and may produce tissue effects at lower temperature.

The duration the beam remains in contact with the tissue is another important parameter. This may be controlled by defining the duration of the laser pulse. Alternatively, the laser may be activated continuously and the duration of contact between the beam and the tissue controlled by the speed with which the laser beam is moved across the tissue surface. Often, uniform energy distribution is achieved more readily through a dynamic process of "painting" the tissue with slow movement of the laser beam rather than through a series of adjacent static impulses (Smith, 1989).

The power of the laser (measured in watts) times the duration (measured in seconds) determines the total energy (joules). The ultimate measure of energy delivery is the energy density. This is measured as joules/cm². The size of the area being treated (spot size) depends on the diameter of the fiber as well as the distance between the fiber tip and the tissue surface. Most surgical laser fibers do not emit a true coherent beam—a small angle of divergence is produced.

Wavelength

The active medium of a laser determines the wavelength of the emitted light (Stein, 1989). The active medium may be a solid, liquid, or gas. Wavelength is a critical factor in determining tissue effect and depends primarily on the absorption spectrum for a given wavelength. Water absorption is the most important factor. Absorption by body pigments, such as hemoglobin and melanin, also determines the depth of injury. Wavelengths that are absorbed rapidly usually result in intense heating and carbonization but with superficial tissue effect. Poorly absorbed wavelengths penetrate more deeply with a coagulative necrosis (Smith, 1986).

Carbon Dioxide

The 10,600 nanometer wavelength of a CO_2 laser is rapidly absorbed by water. It produces intense heat with carbonization and vaporization but minimal tissue penetration. Nontoxic fibers for conduction of CO_2 laser energy are not available clinically. The CO_2 laser has been employed most often in urologic surgery for treatment of various lesions of the external genitalia.

Argon Laser

An argon laser has a spectral emission between 488 and 514 nanometers. It is poorly absorbed by water but somewhat selectively absorbed by hemoglobin and melanin. The energy is readily transmitted by a flexible quartz fiber with minimal energy loss. Tissue penetration is about 1.0 mm.

Neodymium: Yttrium-Aluminum-Garnet (YAG) Laser

Over the last decade, the neodymium:YAG laser has been the most versatile and widely utilized laser in urologic surgery. It emits a wavelength of 1060 nanometers, which is poorly absorbed by both water and hemoglobin. A neodymium:YAG laser produces tissue coagulation through protein denaturation, up to a depth of 5 mm. Minimal carbonization and vaporization occur. The energy is readily transmitted by fiber.

KTP-532 Laser

A KTP laser has a potassium titanyl phosphate crystal to double the frequency of a neodymium:YAG laser. The 532 nanometer wavelength produces tissue effects similar to those of an argon laser but with a higher power output. More vaporization but less coagulation occurs with a KTP laser than a neodymium:YAG laser.

Pulsed-Dye Laser

The term pulsed-dye laser usually refers to a laser lithotriptor that employs pulsed output and an active medium of coumarin green. The fiber tip is placed in contact with a stone. Absorption of the laser energy by the stone forms a plasma that rapidly expands. The mechanical effect of plasma expansion results in stone disruption with minimal thermal effect.

Alexandrite Laser

An Alexandrite laser produces a wavelength of 750 nanometers. Short laser pulses can result in stone disruption. Lithotripsy is usually fairly efficient, but some thermal effect is observed.

Argon-Dye Laser

The term argon-dye laser usually refers to an argon-pumped laser, which uses rhodamine B dye as the active medium. A red color of 630 nanometers is produced. The power output is relatively low (~ 2 watts). The laser has little direct effect on tissue when applied alone.

CLINICAL APPLICATIONS

External Genitalia

Condyloma Acuminatum

Lasers have proved to be effective for treatment of condyloma acuminatum of the external genitalia. Cosmetic and therapeutic results are often superior to alternative treatment (Malloy et al., 1989).

Human papillomavirus (HPV) genital infection appears to be increasing in incidence in this country. Previously thought to be primarily a cosmetic problem, an association with certain subtypes of HPV infection with carcinoma of the cervix and, perhaps, carcinoma of the penis has increased the significance of this lesion and drawn greater attention to treatment.

Although multiple subtypes of the virus exist and can be identified by DNA probe technology, most lesions in the male can be divided into two general categories. HPV types 6 and 11 usually are grossly visible in men and are the subtypes with the greatest apparent oncogenic potential. Types 16, 18, and 31 frequently are isolated from microscopic lesions.

For the typical, grossly identifiable condyloma acuminatum, excellent results have been achieved with a CO_2, KTP-532, and neodymium:YAG laser (Fig. 81–1). Gross recurrences are relatively unusual. However, magnified penile surface scanning and biopsy identify residual viral particles in a significant number of patients. When a CO_2 laser is used, vaporization of the lesion occurs. A power output of 3 to 5 watts generally is sufficient. The laser beam is defocused when the base

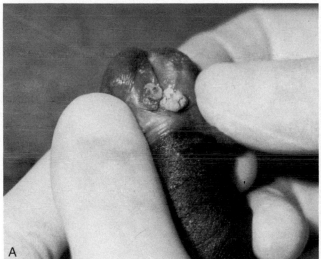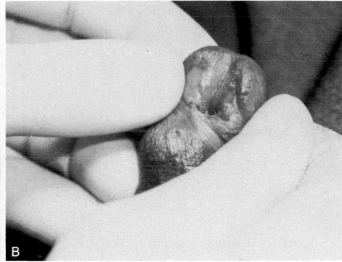

Figure 81–1. *A*, Condyloma acuminatum of the urethral meatus. *B*, After Nd:YAG laser treatment, the lesions are no longer visible. No evidence exists of residual scarring or cosmetic deformity.

of the lesion is treated to avoid excessive penetration and full-thickness injury to the dermis. Studies have shown that there may be viable DNA particles in the laser smoke plume. High-power vacuum smoke evacuators should be utilized as well as special laser masks, with a weave designed to block small particles.

With a neodymium:YAG laser, a focusing hand piece is often used to facilitate energy delivery to the tissue. Unless the lesions are extremely large, a power output of 15 to 20 watts is sufficient. The lesion is treated until it undergoes a characteristic white discoloration. Caution should be taken to avoid excessive energy delivery to the underlying skin. The epithelium surrounding the lesion should be treated, because the HPV virus can extend up to 6 mm into the surrounding normal-appearing skin at the base of the lesion. Laser application to the skin is painful. Anesthesia, usually by local infiltration, is required. For large lesions, treatment can be performed by coagulating the superficial portion of the condyloma and then removing the coagulated necrotic tissue with a saline-soaked sponge. This sequential therapy rapidly debulks the lesion until the base is visible and can be treated.

The KTP-532 laser is also helpful for external genital lesions. A power output of 7 to 9 watts generally is used. This laser may be preferred, because of its affinity for melanin, especially in black patients.

Muschter and Dann (1990) treated 161 patients with urogenital condyloma acuminatum utilizing a neodymium:YAG laser. In total, 80 patients had primary lesions and 81 had recurrent condylomata after previous alternative treatments. With a mean follow-up time of 16 months, 80 per cent of treated patients were free of recurrence.

Carpiniello and associates (1987) reported results in 127 men with biopsy-proven subclinical HPV infections detected by magnified penile surface scanning and treated with CO_2 laser. With a mean follow-up period of 4 months, a 6 per cent recurrence rate of microscopic

condylomata was observed. Thus, with microscopic subclinical lesions, the recurrence rate is high even after adequate destruction of detected lesions. In a follow-up study, Carpiniello and associates (1988) applied adjuvant 5-fluorouracil cream after laser therapy. Despite this treatment, a recurrence rate of 71 per cent was observed. Currently, laser therapy of aceto-white microscopic condyloma acuminatum has not been found to decrease recurrence rates. Effective therapy for this disease has not yet been described.

Carcinoma of the Penis

A laser is capable of providing effective local control for selected penile cancers. Cosmetic and therapeutic results are usually excellent. Patients chosen for primary laser therapy should have only superficially invasive tumors (Fig. 81–2).

Malloy and co-workers (1988) reported 16 patients with carcinoma of the penis treated primarily with a neodymium:YAG laser. Five patients had Tis, nine had T1 tumors, and two had T2 carcinoma. All five patients with Tis were free of tumor. Of the nine patients with T1 lesions, 6 were tumor free. After therapy, the two men with stage T2 carcinomas had reduction of the tumor mass but were not cured.

Boon (1988) reported his experience with 16 patients with penile carcinoma. Follow-up lasted 4 to 36 months (mean 17 months). Eight patients were treated with a contact-tip neodymium:YAG laser, and eight others were treated with surgical excision of the exophytic lesion and neodymium:YAG laser photoirradiation of the tumor base. Of the 16 patients, 13 were free of disease at the time of follow-up.

For tumor ablation, a neodymium:YAG laser is preferable (Smith and Dixon, 1984). However, CO_2 laser excision of penile cancer has been reported. Bandiearmonte and associates (1987) reported a series of 15 patients treated with resection of the surface of the glans

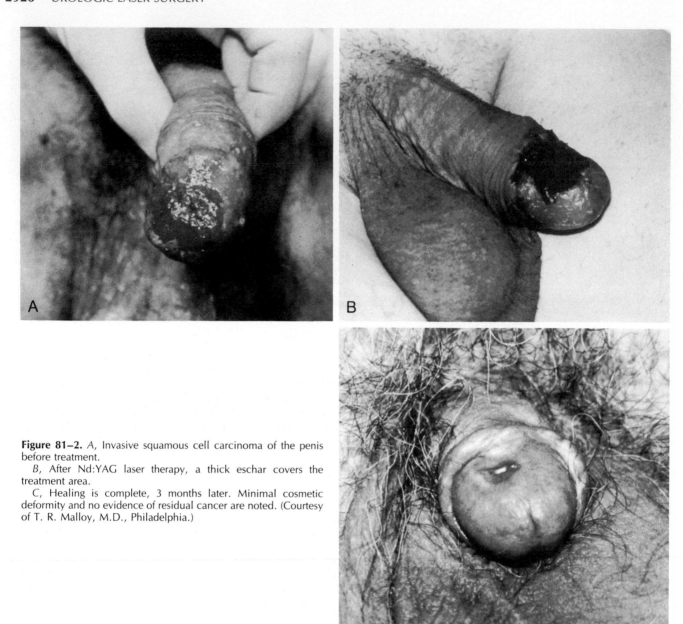

Figure 81–2. A, Invasive squamous cell carcinoma of the penis before treatment.

B, After Nd:YAG laser therapy, a thick eschar covers the treatment area.

C, Healing is complete, 3 months later. Minimal cosmetic deformity and no evidence of residual cancer are noted. (Courtesy of T. R. Malloy, M.D., Philadelphia.)

penis using a CO_2 laser. Cosmetic and functional results were excellent, with satisfactory sexual activity reported in 14 of 15 patients. Only one patient had persistent or recurrent tumor during a follow-up of 2 to 48 months. After a second laser treatment, this patient was free of disease. This technique is similar to Moh's surgery in that it provides excision of tumor with a minimum surgical margin.

Urethra

Although endoscopic access to the urethra is not difficult, treatment of some urethral lesions with conventional methods, such as electrocautery, often is unsatisfactory. With urethral strictures, rapid recurrence of the scar tissue is often observed. In other circum-

stances, such as treatment of urethral condyloma acuminatum, concerns arise that treatment will cause scar tissue and induce strictures. It is the limitations of traditional treatment that have led to the use of lasers within the urethra.

Urethral Condyloma Acuminatum

Condyloma acuminatum of the urethra is being recognized with increased frequency. The disease therapy has two parts: elimination of the existing lesions and prevention of recurrence. Topical therapy using drugs, such as 5-Fluorouracil, is of some value but is often unsuccessful in eliminating gross lesions. Electrocautery carries with it the hazard of inducing scar tissue and urethral stricture. Systemic drugs, such as interferon, are being evaluated but are of unproven value in the treatment or prevention of urethral condyloma acuminatum.

The amount of fibrous tissue and collagen induced by a laser is less than that of a comparable electrocautery injury. Although it is possible for a urethral stricture to develop after laser treatment, the risk seems to be less than after electrocautery. Furthermore, laser coagulation may extend several millimeters into the periurethral tissue, effectively eliminating the adjacent viral particles, which may contribute to local recurrence. These factors combine to enhance the attractiveness of laser treatment of condyloma acuminatum of the urethra.

TECHNIQUE

The choice of wavelength does not seem to be a critical factor in the results achieved with laser treatment of condyloma acuminatum. Lesions at the urethral meatus, which may be visualized by simple eversion of the urethra, are amenable to treatment with CO_2, neodymium:YAG, argon, and KTP 532 lasers. Although some proponents advocate the superiority of an individual wavelength, all wavelengths accomplish the primary task of destruction of the gross lesion with minimal bleeding or scar tissue. No evidence exists that local recurrence due to inadequate treatment of the primary lesion is lower with one wavelength laser than another.

Urethral condyloma acuminatum frequently occurs at the meatus and fossa navicularis. Often, the proximal extent of the lesion is in a critical area several centimeters inside the meatus, which is difficult to visualize by either external inspection or endoscopy. Meatotomy and cystoscopy with pediatric instruments may be helpful.

Nontoxic fibers for conduction of CO_2 laser energy are not available for clinical use. Therefore, for treatment of lesions that require endoscopy for visualization, a neodymium:YAG, argon, or KTP laser must be employed. The fiber tip is positioned several millimeters from the surface of the lesion and energy applied until complete coagulation or vaporization is achieved (Fig. 81–3). Depending on location, contact between the fiber tip and the lesion may be required. Tips constructed of sapphire and other materials have been developed for contact with a neodymium:YAG laser (Fig. 81–4). Condyloma acuminatum can be successfully treated with contact tip lasers, but the tissue effects are not unlike those obtained with a Bugbee electrode.

Fuselier and associates (1980) and Rosemberg and associates (1982) reported on small groups of patients with short follow-up periods, who underwent laser treatment of urethral condylomata. Basically, these studies demonstrated the feasibility of the technique. Krogh and colleagues (1990) reported results in 74 men with condyloma acuminatum of the urethral meatus, who were observed for a mean of 18 months after therapy. Of these patients, 78 per cent had no recurrences if there was an isolated urethral lesion. The recurrence rate was higher if the patient had coexisting lesions on the external skin. One case of urethral stricture and six cases of meatal stenoses were observed more than 3 months after treatment.

Urethral Stricture

Dilation or direct vision urethrotomy increases urethral caliber and provides effective symptomatic improvement in patients with urethral strictures. Recurrence is high, however, and the need for repeated procedures sometimes leads to open surgical repair with variable results. Partly because of the unsatisfactory results achieved with alternative therapy, lasers have been investigated in the treatment of benign strictures of the urethra.

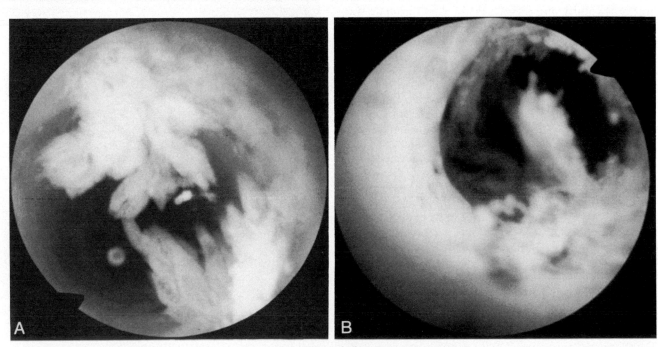

Figure 81–3. A, Condyloma acuminatum of the bulbous urethra before treatment.
B, After Nd:YAG laser therapy (35 watts × 3 seconds) the lesions are thoroughly coagulated without any evident bleeding.

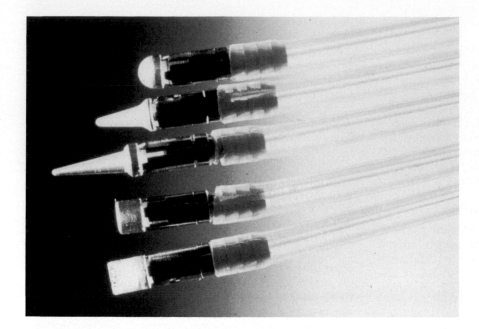

Figure 81–4. Sapphire contact tips for Nd:YAG laser fibers are available in various configurations. They increase the cutting effect of the Nd:YAG laser by concentrating the energy density.

Based on tissue effects, a CO_2 laser seems most appealing for treatment of urethral strictures. Tissue vaporization occurs with minimal forward scatter of the laser energy. Therefore, elimination of the scar tissue with little underlying thermal injury seems feasible. Practical considerations, however, preclude the CO_2 laser within the urethra. The lack of a fiber delivery system limits its feasibility with endoscopy. Furthermore, CO_2 laser energy is rapidly extinguished by water. Gaseous distention of the urethra carries the hazard of air embolus, even with suprapubic venting.

Partly because of availability, the greatest experience with laser treatment of urethral stricture has been with the neodymium:YAG laser. The initially reported technique involved circumferential treatment of the stricture (Fig. 81–5) (Smith and Dixon, 1984). The rationale was based on studies showing less collagen deposition and more elastic fibers after laser treatment compared with electrocautery. It was hoped that sloughing of the laser-treated area would occur with nonstrictured healing. Because minimal tissue vaporization occurs with a neodymium:YAG laser, dilation of the stricture is necessary to provide immediate symptomatic relief until tissue slough occurs. A total of 24 patients were treated by this method (Smith and Dixon, 1984). Although good early results were achieved without complications, recurrence was observed in 13 patients after 6 months. It was concluded that this technique offered no advantage over internal urethrotomy.

Subsequently, several small series have been reported of a technique that involves laser urethrotomy. The rationale for why a urethrotomy with a laser is therapeutically superior to an incision with a cold knife has not been established. However, even though a neodymium:YAG laser is not a "cutting" laser, increasing the energy density by placing the fiber tip in contact with the tissue allows some vaporization and tissue separation to occur. Urethrotomy, then, is technically feasible.

Shanberg and associates (1984) reported their results after performing multiple urethrotomies with a bare neodymium:YAG laser fiber. The overall recurrence rate was greater than 50 per cent. However, because most of the patients had recurrent strictures after previous therapy, these investigators concluded that this technique was effective for treatment of strictures.

Merkle (1990) performed multiple urethrotomies utilizing a neodymium:YAG laser in 26 patients with recurrent urethral strictures. Four patients underwent a second treatment after 6 months, which was not considered a recurrence but a failure to adequately open the

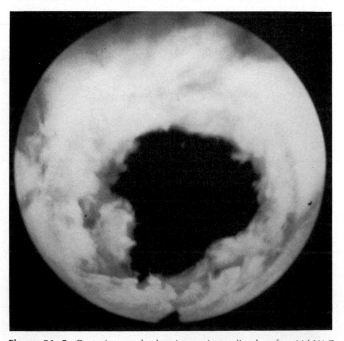

Figure 81–5. Posterior urethral stricture immediately after Nd:YAG laser therapy. Treatment has been applied circumferentially, and the interface between the coagulated tissue and the normal appearing urethra is evident.

stricture with the initial therapy. Otherwise, no recurrence was reported. In addition, for reasons that were unexplained, Merkle reported that ultrasonography after laser therapy showed that scarring, which had been present before treatment, was no longer visible.

The most efficient way to increase the energy density of a neodymium:YAG laser and, thereby, improve the cutting effect, is through contact tips. These tips allow direct contact between the fiber and the tissue, concentrating the energy in a small area. A prospective study utilizing contact tips in patients with recurrent urethral strictures was reported (Smith, 1989). A total of 24 patients were treated but, in 42 per cent, therapy was considered inadequate. The contact tips allow cutting only in an antegrade manner, which creates some boring into the tissue. In addition, tissue vaporization and separation are suboptimal. Over half the patients had recurrences within 6 months of follow-up. It was concluded that laser therapy offered no advantages over cold knife urethrotomy for treatment of most urethral strictures.

A KTP laser has a wavelength of 532 nanometers, similar to that of an argon laser. Some tissue vaporization occurs under water, seemingly making it preferable to a neodymium:YAG laser for performing urethrotomy. Turec and co-workers (in press) reported results in 31 patients treated with KTP laser. The patients underwent circumferential ablation followed by Foley catheter drainage. The follow-up period was variable, but 59 per cent of patients had no further symptoms after treatment.

Undoubtedly, urethrotomy is feasible with a laser. The technique can sometimes be performed without providing anesthesia, and minimal bleeding occurs. However, reported results are difficult to interpret and have not been uniformly favorable. Even more elusive is a convincing rationale for why laser urethrotomy would be therapeutically superior to cold knife urethrotomy. Even though there is less scar tissue after laser therapy than after electrocautery, the least scarring occurs after incision with a cold knife. In addition, no laser has been shown to cut tissue more effectively than a knife.

Bladder Neck Contractures

Incisions in the bladder neck can also be performed with a laser. The technique is similar to that described for urethral strictures and usually involves direct contact between the laser fiber and the strictured tissue of the bladder neck. Little bleeding occurs. Placement of a Foley catheter afterward is optional.

The type of laser used to incise the bladder neck seems relatively unimportant. However, bladder neck contractures often involve dense fibrous tissue; therefore, the optimal cutting effect of a laser is required. This is best achieved with contact between a neodymium:YAG laser fiber and the tissue or by a KTP or an argon laser.

Turec and associates (in press) reported only one recurrence in five patients treated with a neodym-

ium:YAG laser. Shanberg and co-workers (1984) also reported good results using a neodymium:YAG laser to perform incision of bladder neck contractures. Salant and associates (1990) treated 50 bladder neck contractures utilizing a technique involving circumferential application of the laser energy. Recurrences were reported in eight patients (16 per cent).

Prostate

Benign Prostatic Hyperplasia

Surgical intervention in patients with symptoms of bladder outlet obstruction from benign prostatic hyperplasia is intended to decrease outlet resistance by either bulk tissue removal or incision through the prostate and capsule. Lasers have been employed for both purposes.

Sometimes, these efforts to use lasers in surgery have caught the attention of the public. It is important to maintain the distinction between a procedure that has been demonstrated to be feasible and one that has proven therapeutic benefit and clinical value.

The laser wavelengths that can be utilized endoscopically are ineffective for bulk tissue removal. A neodymium:YAG laser exerts its primary tissue effects through coagulation. Kandell and associates (1986) were able to achieve some vaporization in prostates in dogs using a high energy density. However, there seems to be little promise for a noncontact neodymium:YAG laser in the treatment of benign prostate hypertrophy.

Prostatotomy is feasible with a laser. The results could be considered comparable to those achieved with transurethral incision of the prostate (TUIP). Shanberg and co-workers (1984) reported results in 21 men and found improvement in symptoms and greater urine flow in 15. These investigators recommended the procedure as an alternative to transurethral prostatectomy in men with prostates less than 30 g. Clearly, incision of the prostate and prostatic capsule is feasible with a laser. More doubtful, however, is whether there is any less bleeding or some other benefit. In addition, the cutting effect of all available lasers, whether in direct contact with the tissue or not, is less than that achieved with electrocautery.

A transurethral laser-induced prostatectomy (TULIP) has been described. The device utilizes ultrasound localization of a balloon within the prostatic urethra. The prostatic tissue is compressed by inflation of the balloon. Neodymium:YAG laser energy is applied to the compressed tissue. Squeezing the blood out of the tissue and compressing it allows greater penetration of the laser energy into the prostate. Results in dogs show good tissue removal within the prostatic capsule (Roth et al., 1990). Preliminary clinical results have also been favorable, but more data are required before conclusions can be reached regarding the potential clinical role of this device.

Carcinoma

Laser treatment of prostate cancer would require effective ablation of all tumor-bearing tissue. Because of the multifocal nature of prostate cancer and the diffuse location of the tumor within the prostate, ablation of the entire prostate is required.

A neodymium:YAG laser penetrates tissue 5 to 7 mm. Therefore, clinical studies of laser treatment of prostate cancer have involved a preliminary transurethral resection of the prostate for debulking. Prostatic cancer typically arises in the peripheral zone in the posterior portion of the prostate. Direct access to this area with a neodymium:YAG laser fiber is difficult by the transurethral route. Sander and Beisland (1984) have described a method for treatment of prostatic cancer that involves suprapubic puncture and transvesical visualization of the posterior prostate. A neodymium:YAG laser is then employed to coagulate the entire posterior capsule of the prostate. A thermistor was placed in the rectum to ensure that the temperature did not rise over 60° C, the point at which protein denaturation and irreversible tissue damage occur. Preliminary results have shown this to be a low morbidity approach. No prostatorectal fistulas have occurred. Follow-up information is insufficient to draw any conclusions, but postoperative biopsy results have been negative in most patients.

Although the procedure has gained in popularity, especially in Scandinavia, it seemingly is a relatively imprecise method. In question is whether the entire prostate can effectively be ablated by this method. Postoperative prostate-specific antigen levels have decreased in most patients but have not reached zero or undetectable. Until further follow-up and clinical results are available, this must be considered an unproven method for treatment of prostate cancer.

McPhee and associates (1989) have been investigating a method of photosensitization of prostate cancer employing hematoporphyrin derivative. Interstitial implantation of laser fibers emitting red light at 630 nanometers is performed. Red light penetrates tissue 0.5 cm; therefore, multiple fibers must be placed. Clinical studies of photodynamic therapy of prostate cancer have not been conducted.

Littrup and associates (1989) reported a method for percutaneous placement of needles into the prostate by insertion of a neodymium:YAG laser fiber. A study in dogs demonstrated focal areas of necrosis and coagulation extending up to 14 mm. Although the investigators considered this method promising as a treatment for localized prostate cancer, it has major limitations. The needles can be placed accurately with ultrasound, but the laser treatment is imprecise and the penetration depth is variable.

Benign Bladder Disease

Bladder Hemangioma

Hemangioma of the bladder is a rare benign tumor that may occur as an isolated lesion or in association with cutaneous or visceral vascular malformations. Transurethral resection is inadvisable because of the possibility of excessive bleeding. The location of the

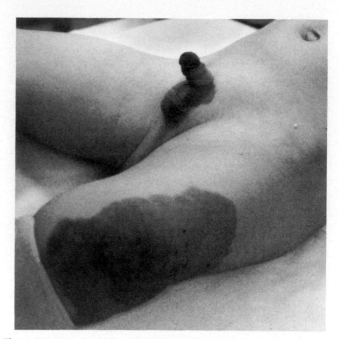

Figure 81–6. 2-year-old boy with Klippel-Trenaunay-Weber syndrome. Extensive hemangiomatous involvement of the left thigh is evident. In addition, involvement of the external genitalia is observed.

lesion or diffuse bladder involvement may preclude segmental cystectomy. The poor tissue absorption of the neodymium:YAG laser wavelength produces an effective thermal coagulation and a characteristic lack of bleeding.

Often, bladder hemangiomas occur as part of congenital vascular malformations (Fig. 81–6). Smith (1990) reported 13 patients with benign hemangiomas of the bladder treated with a neodymium:YAG laser for recurrent bleeding. Treatment was performed with the laser fiber positioned several millimeters from the bladder surface. A power output of 20 to 35 watts was applied, with lower power chosen for young children. The total energy delivery ranged from 2600 to 27,000 joules. No complications were observed, and excellent results were obtained (Fig. 81–7). Based on this experience, neodymium:YAG laser coagulation appears to be an effective method for treatment of bleeding from bladder hemangioma.

Interstitial Cystitis

Lasers have been reported to be effective for the treatment of interstitial cystitis. The mechanism for this remains uncertain but may be related to ablation of sensitive nerve endings in the bladder wall and those surrounding the inflammatory lesions of interstitial cystitis. The lesions of interstitial cystitis often are located on the bladder dome in women. Bowel perforation has been reported in a disproportionate number of patients treated with lasers for interstitial cystitis, probably because of the location and the relatively thin bladder wall.

Shanberg and Malloy (1987) reported their experience in 39 patients (33 females and 6 males) with interstitial

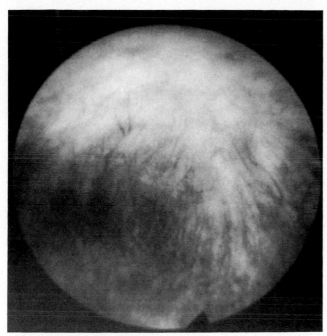

Figure 81–7. Extensive bladder hemangioma 3 months after Nd:YAG laser treatment. The treated area *(bottom)* is contrasted with the untreated area *(top)*.

cystitis treated with a neodymium:YAG laser. A total of 19 patients had obvious Hunner's ulcers and 17 of these had rapid relief of pain with a demonstrated increase in functional bladder capacity (Fig. 81–8). Recurrent symptoms were noted in 12 of the 17 patients between 6 and 18 months post-treatment. Of the 20 patients without Hunner's ulcers, 13 had symptomatic improvement. Two patients in the series developed small

bowel perforation, and these workers thus recommend restricting the total energy to less than 25,000 joules.

Bladder Cancer

The majority of bladder cancers arise from the transitional epithelium of the bladder. Therefore, they are visible endoscopically and accessible for delivery of laser energy through cystoscopes. The safety and efficacy of laser treatment of bladder cancer have been established through the combined experience of medical centers in Europe (Hofstetter et al., 1981), the United States (Smith, 1985), and Japan (Okada et al., 1982). However, a relatively safe and efficient form of treatment for superficial bladder cancer has existed for a number of years. Questions have arisen regarding the advantages of laser therapy over electrocautery transurethral resection of bladder tumors. Patient selection, treatment techniques, and anticipated results are dependent on the stage of the primary tumor.

Superficial Bladder Cancer

Bladder tumors of clinical stages 0 or A by the Jewett classification or Ta, Tis, or T1 by the tumors, nodes, and metastases (TNM) system are included under this discussion as superficial bladder tumors. Such superficial lesions make up some 80 per cent of bladder tumors. Although only a minority of these lesions progress to invasive cancer, they represent a distinct clinical problem because of the high rate of recurrence.

Somewhat over half of new patients with superficial transitional cell carcinoma of the bladder are destined to develop recurrences after electrocautery resection

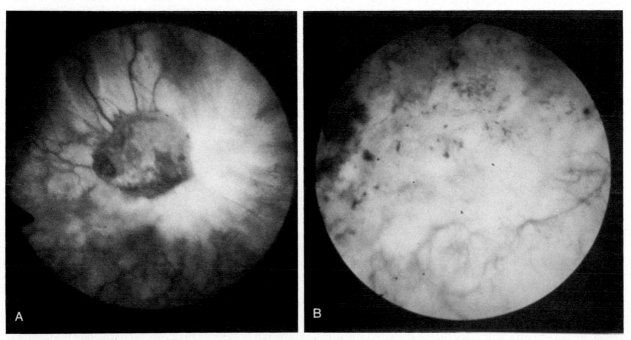

Figure 81–8. *A,* Typical Hunner's ulcer in a patient with interstitial cystitis.
B, After Nd:YAG laser ablation, the coagulated bladder wall is evident. (Courtesy of Alan Shanberg, M.D., Long Beach, California.)

alone. The reason for this relatively high rate is multifactorial. Experimental evidence and clinical observation support the concept that some recurrences are due to implantation of viable tumor cells that may be dislodged at the time of electrocautery resection (Soloway and Masters, 1979). Because laser destruction of superficial bladder tumors occurs in a noncontact manner, it has been theorized that the recurrence rate of superficial bladder cancer is less after a laser treatment than after a comparable electrocautery resection (Malloy et al., 1984). Whether or not this finding translates into a clinically detectable decrease in recurrence rate is, however, uncertain. Uncontrolled, nonrandomized studies of superficial bladder cancers are notoriously inaccurate. Randomized studies comparing laser treatment to electrocautery resection are usually incomplete.

STAGING

An issue of paramount importance in treating cancer is tumor staging. An adequate definition of tumor stage not only influences treatment of the existing tumor but also has implications regarding future tumor behavior. The optimal method of staging bladder cancer treated by neodymium:YAG laser has generated a great deal of discussion.

A number of potential solutions to the problems of tumor staging have been offered. Pretreatment cold-cup biopsy specimens from the tumor base can be obtained. Although these should provide adequate histologic confirmation of the presence of cancer and assist in determining tumor grade, the portion of the lesion most useful for staging, i.e., the tumor base, may be incompletely sampled. A preliminary electrocautery resection would appear to obviate the theoretical advantages of laser treatment, regarding the dissemination of viable tumor cells, and would eliminate many of the practical advantages of laser treatment. Examination of the necrotic tumor after laser therapy is feasible because the lesion maintains some of its architectural integrity. However, detail is not sufficient for optimal tumor staging.

In cases in which adequate histologic material is important, a definitive transurethral resection with electrocautery should be performed. Alternatively, a large number of cases exist in which pathologic material is neither necessary nor useful. Laser therapy can be performed without submitting material for histologic examination. Primarily, the patients are selected for laser therapy if they have previous histories of superficial, papillary transitional cell carcinomas of the bladder; normal or low-grade malignant cells on voided cytology examinations; and tumors that appear to be low grade on cystoscopic examination. If a cold-cup biopsy finding establishes the diagnosis of transitional cell carcinoma, a previous history of bladder cancer is not mandatory for confirmation. Partially because of staging considerations but also because of practical problems with large tumors, lesions to be treated should be limited to less than 2.5 cm. Using these criteria, the risk of significantly understaging cancer during laser therapy appears to be extremely low.

TECHNIQUE

Specialized laser bridges have been developed for rigid cystoscopes, and laser energy can be delivered satisfactorily to most areas of the bladder with one of these devices. However, tumors of the anterior bladder neck and trigone can be relatively inaccessible with a rigid cystoscope. Flexible instruments may facilitate delivery of laser energy to these regions.

Often, when treating superficial tumors, general or regional anesthesia is unnecessary. Topical urethral anesthetics, such as lidocaine (Xylocaine) may lessen the discomfort of cystoscopy. Patients are able to perceive the laser energy when it is applied to the bladder and may describe it as a "burning sensation." However, patients are able to tolerate treatment well without adjuvant anesthesia unless the tumors are large or cover extensive areas of the bladder surface.

The tip of the laser fiber is positioned approximately 2 or 3 mm from the surface of the tumor. In general, a power output of 35 to 40 watts is chosen and laser energy is applied to the base of the tumor and the surrounding mucosa in continuous fashion (Fig. 81–9). Initial application of laser energy to the surrounding mucosa or periphery of the tumor does not seem necessary. Early suggestions that sealing of lymphatic vessels occurs with neodymium:YAG energy have not been fully substantiated. Furthermore, bleeding does not occur during treatment whether the energy is applied initially to the tumor or to the surrounding mucosa.

Treatment is maintained in a given area until a characteristic white discoloration indicative of adequate thermal necrosis is evident. Usually this requires 2 to 3 seconds of energy application in a given area. The duration of the pulse can be controlled from the instrument panel, although it is usually simpler to select a continuous output from the laser and control the pulse duration with the foot pedal. Laser treatment should be a dynamic process rather than a series of static impulses. The beam is slowly moved across the surface of the tumor in a painting fashion.

Employing these specifications, thermal necrosis should extend to the deep lamina propria or superficial detrusor muscle. Excessive forward scatter of laser energy to adjacent organs is unlikely. However, several unpublished reports have been made of small bowel perforation after laser treatment of superficial bladder cancer. With the specifications described, this complication should be unusual. Nevertheless, caution should be maintained, especially when treating tumors on the intraperitoneal portion of the bladder and when previous pelvic surgery or radiation has caused adhesions between small bowel and the bladder dome.

No bleeding is usually encountered during treatment, and a Foley catheter is not necessary postoperatively. Obturator nerve spasm does not occur. Treatment of tumors overlying the ureteral orifice has not resulted in ureteral stricture (Fig. 81–10). The coagulated tumor mass sloughs within 1 week of treatment and is passed in the urine, usually as imperceptible particles. In general, the patients may return immediately to previous

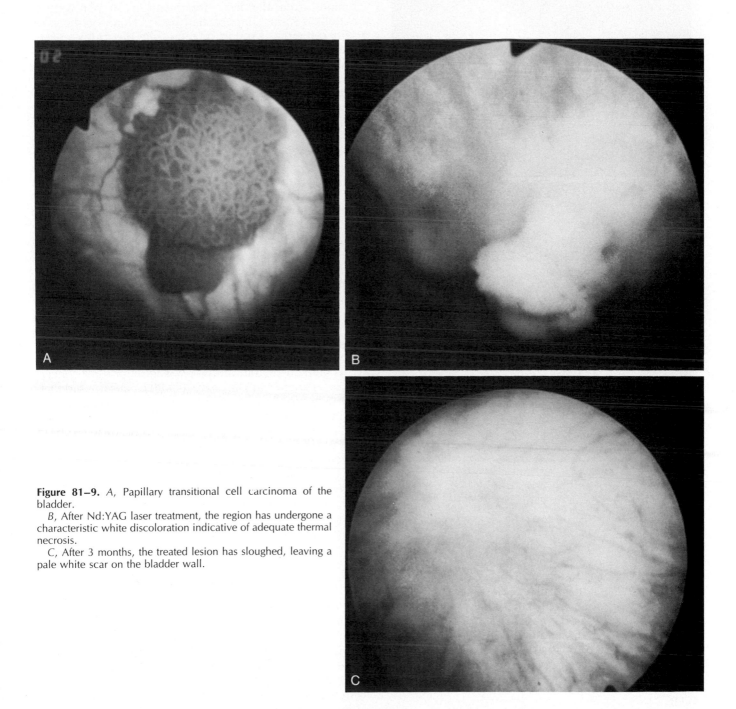

Figure 81–9. *A*, Papillary transitional cell carcinoma of the bladder.

B, After Nd:YAG laser treatment, the region has undergone a characteristic white discoloration indicative of adequate thermal necrosis.

C, After 3 months, the treated lesion has sloughed, leaving a pale white scar on the bladder wall.

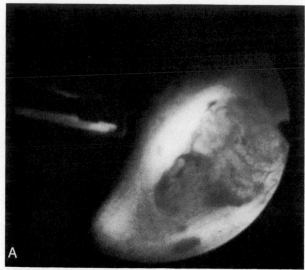

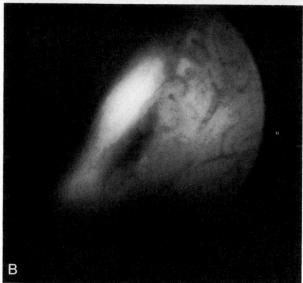

Figure 81–10. *A,* Papillary tumor of the left ureteral orifice. The Nd:YAG laser fiber is evident at the left side of the photograph.
B, At 3 months after laser treatment, no residual tumor and no stricture of the ureteral orifice are noted.

activities. They usually have minimal bladder spasm and discomfort after laser treatment.

Follow-up management should be the same as that after electrocautery resection. The indications for adjuvant intravesical chemotherapy or immunotherapy are also the same. After three months, the laser scar at the area of previous treatment usually is evident as a pale white discoloration of the bladder mucosa.

RESULTS

If superficial bladder tumors are thoroughly coagulated, the local recurrence rate compares favorably with that for electrocautery resection. A more pertinent issue is the impact of laser treatment on overall recurrence in remote areas of the bladder. Malloy and co-workers (1984) initially reported an 18 per cent recurrence rate at 1 year but this increased to 35 per cent with longer follow-up. Beer and associates (1990) found an overall

recurrence rate of 33 per cent for primary tumors and 54 per cent for recurrent T1 tumors treated with a neodymium:YAG laser; local recurrence was only 7 per cent. At the University of Utah, 157 patients have undergone laser treatment of superficial bladder tumors. Recurrence has been detected in areas of the bladder remote from the laser treatment in 36 per cent of patients (Smith, unpublished data). None of these results can either support or refute the theory that recurrence rate is less after laser treatment than after electrocautery resection. Randomized prospective trials are necessary.

Lasers generally appear to offer substantial practical advantages over electrocautery resection. Patient morbidity is diminished, and the procedure can be accomplished simply in an outpatient ambulatory setting. Postoperative discomfort, and Foley catheterization of the bladder are avoided. Comparative cost analysis for those who undergo outpatient laser treatment and those who are hospitalized for electrocautery resection with anesthesia demonstrates an obvious and a substantial savings on an individual basis. Further experience is necessary to confirm the practical advantages, and randomized studies are needed to address the issue of tumor recurrence. However, the simplicity of the procedure and its demonstrated safety indicate a lasting role for lasers in the treatment of superficial bladder tumors.

Invasive Bladder Cancer

Treatment-related morbidity is an important concern in any patient with invasive bladder cancer. Although mortality rates are low and methods of continent urinary reconstruction have lessened the impact of surgery, radical cystectomy remains a major procedure and bladder preservation a worthwhile goal. Laser therapy is a potential means for definitive endoscopic management of some muscle invasive bladder cancers. Obviously, cure rates with laser surgery will not exceed those obtained with radical surgery. The intent, then, is to select the patient in whom endoscopic management with laser therapy can provide survival statistics that equal or approach radical surgery while decreasing morbidity.

Rationale for Laser Therapy

Not all muscle invasive bladder cancers require radical cystectomy for total tumor extirpation. Logically, transurethral resection can totally excise some tumors, especially T2 lesions and some T3a. Furthermore, some cases are downstaged to T0 after TUR alone.

A neodymium:YAG laser produces its tissue effects through thermal transformation of the light energy. The 1060 nanometer wavelength is poorly absorbed by water and body tissues, resulting in deep coagulation necrosis. The thermal injury may extend 5 to 7 mm into the tissue. The laser energy does not result in bleeding, providing superb hemostasis. Moreover, the bladder wall maintains its structural and architectural integrity, even after a transmural laser coagulation.

Viewed simplistically, a laser is capable of extending the margin of resection some 5 to 7 mm after a TUR of an invasive bladder cancer. It is logical, therefore, to conclude that laser therapy would be ineffective for tumors that extend beyond this depth but may be curative for tumors incompletely excised by TUR but otherwise limited to the bladder wall.

TECHNIQUE

Laser treatment of superficial bladder cancer can be performed without providing anesthesia. However, the deep tissue penetration and high total energy in treatment of invasive cancer usually requires that the patient undergo general or regional anesthesia. Although flexible cystoscopes can be used, better visualization is provided by rigid cystoscopes. A 600 μ neodymium:YAG laser fiber is inserted through the working channel of a modified Albarran apparatus. Deep transurethral resection of the tumor precedes laser therapy, serving two purposes. First, it is the TUR that provides the pathologic material upon which staging is based. Second, TUR debulks the tumor. Ideally, a minimum of several days should elapse between TUR and laser treatment so that bleeding has stopped and any overlying clot has dissolved.

The tip of the laser fiber is positioned 2 to 3 mm from the surface of the resected area (Smith, 1989). A power output of 40 to 45 watts is used on a continuous pulse duration. Treatment is maintained in a given area for about 3 seconds. The beam is slowly and systematically moved across the entire tumor crater and at least a 1-cm margin of the normal-appearing peripheral bladder mucosa (Fig. 81–11). Unlike the treatment of superficial bladder tumors, visible changes are unreliable in determining treatment adequacy; therefore, a systematic, thorough application is required. Foley catheter drainage is not needed postoperatively and treatment often can be performed on an outpatient basis. Follow-up

cystoscopy is done after 2 months. Although bladder re-epithelialization may occur over viable tumor deep in the bladder wall, this is a rare event. Usually, complete bladder healing indicates that the tumor has been eliminated (Fig. 81–12). Residual tumor is usually evident cystoscopically.

RESULTS

Various measures can be employed to assess the results of laser treatment of invasive bladder cancer. Undoubtedly, survival is the most meaningful parameter. However, laser treatment of invasive bladder cancer has often been performed in elderly patients or in those with poor overall health, making survival a difficult parameter to follow.

Most often, local ablation of the tumor has been utilized as a parameter by which to assess treatment efficacy. Because laser treatment is by design a means for local control, this approach has seemed reasonable. At the University of Utah, 34 patients with invasive bladder cancer have been treated with a neodymium:YAG laser (Smith, 1986). With a minimum of 6 months of follow-up data, 84 per cent of patients with stage T2 tumors have remained without clinical or biopsy evidence of recurrent cancer at the site of laser therapy. In patients with stage T3a lesions, successful results have been obtained in 54 per cent of patients. Persistent disease at the site of laser therapy has been observed in 68 per cent of patients with clinical stage T3b disease.

McPhee and associates (1987) reported similar results. No local recurrence was observed in 12 patients with stage T2 lesions. In four of seven patients, T3a lesions occurred locally. Local recurrence was observed in six of seven patients with T3b cancers. Beisland and Sanders (1990) have followed 15 patients with solitary T2 bladder tumors treated with neodymium:YAG laser for 56 to 78

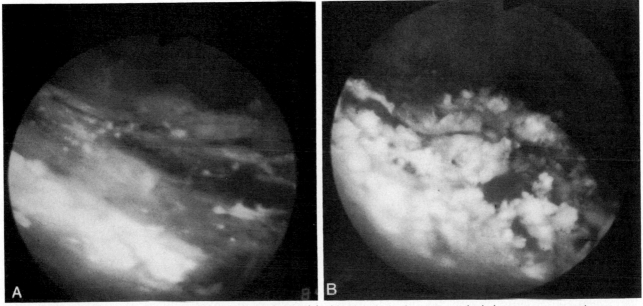

Figure 81–11. *A,* Stage T3a transitional cell carcinoma of the bladder after a deep transurethral electrocautery resection. *B,* After Nd:YAG laser energy has been applied, the entire area shows thermal coagulation.

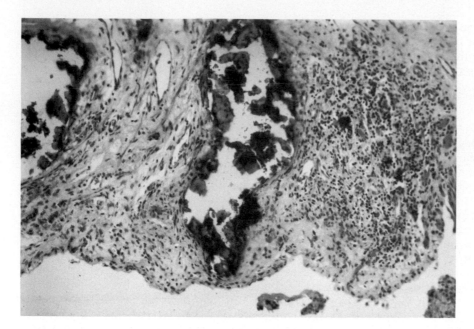

Figure 81–12. Bladder biopsy specimen 3 months after laser treatment for invasive bladder cancer. Some calcium is present in the tissue, but no evidence of residual cancer is present.

months. Ten patients were alive and apparently free of disease, and one died of other causes without cancer. In the remaining four patients, the treatment failed.

LIMITATIONS OF LASER TREATMENT

Although there seems to be a logical rationale for the use of laser therapy in some patients with invasive bladder cancers, major limitations exist. Clinical staging of invasive bladder cancer is notoriously inaccurate. In up to one third of patients, significant understaging occurs (Smith, 1982). Because appropriate patient selection depends directly on accurate clinical staging, this difficulty is a major obstacle.

An additional problem is that the depth of tissue penetration achieved with the Nd:YAG laser is neither predictable nor reproducible. Studies have shown penetration depths between 3 and 7 mm, using the parameters previously described for laser treatment of invasive bladder cancer (Smith and Landau, 1989). Several factors responsible for the depth of penetration are under the precise control of the operating surgeon, including power output, duration, and wavelength. However, the primary determination of tissue effect is energy density, i.e., the amount of energy applied to a given area. The denominator in this equation, the area, is difficult to control in a clinical setting involving endoscopy. Distance between the fiber tip and the bladder wall, angulation at the point of impact, or irregularities in the tissue surface all influence the spot size, and, thereby, the penetration.

A problem common to any focal treatment for invasive bladder cancer is the high incidence of disease recurrence elsewhere in the bladder. Even if laser treatment is successful in eradicating the known tumor, patients with high-grade and invasive disease are at risk for the development of new tumors at remote sites in the bladder. Over the long-term, failure to remove the bladder could compromise survival, because of the development of these new muscle-invasive tumors.

Currently, laser therapy has a role in the treatment of invasive bladder cancer, although a somewhat limited one. Neodymium:YAG laser treatment should not be considered a reasonable alternative to radical cystectomy for most patients. However, for selected patients who have stage T2 tumors or those who are not candidates for radical surgery, laser treatment represents a reasonable alternative, which should be considered.

Carcinoma of the Ureter and Renal Pelvis

Endoscopic access to the ureter or upper urinary collecting system can be achieved with either the ureteroscope or the percutaneous approaches to the kidney. Potentially, transitional cell carcinoma of the ureter or renal pelvis is amenable to treatment with neodymium:YAG laser energy. However, several problems arise. Tumor staging can be difficult, and the prognosis for invasive tumors of the upper urinary system is extremely poor even with radical surgery. Optimal visualization can also be difficult, but the ability to perform the treatment without bleeding offers advantages over resection of the tumor. Although potential exists for ureteral perforation, postoperative indwelling ureteral stents should lessen this problem. When a percutaneous approach is chosen, there is concern that extravasation of fluid into the perinephric space could allow implantation of tumor cells in the extrarenal region.

Favorable results after treatment of lesions of the intramural ureter have been reported from a number of medical centers. Experience is limited in tumors of the mid-ureter or upper urinary tract. Hofstetter (1984) has treated 14 patients with mid-ureteral tumors without ureteral perforation or stricture. Follow-up data are relatively limited, but early results are impressive. Smith (1989) used a neodymium:YAG laser to treat the base of renal pelvis tumors resected by percutaneous access.

Of eight patients treated, five were free of recurrence at the time of follow-up.

The overall indications for laser treatment of the ureter are limited, and appropriate patient selection and treatment make caution mandatory. For superficial transitional cell tumors of the ureter, however, the lack of bleeding and the less intense fibrotic reaction compared with electrical energy make the neodymium:YAG laser a potentially attractive treatment modality.

Kidney

Overall, the application of lasers for partial nephrectomy has been unimpressive. The rapid absorption and tissue vaporizing characteristics of a CO_2 laser allow its use as a "surgical knife" to incise renal parenchyma, but bleeding is usually brisk and beyond the hemostatic capabilities of this laser. In comparison, the tissue coagulation effects of a neodymium:YAG laser make it a poor cutting device. Excessive thermal injury to the renal parenchyma may result when this laser is utilized to produce hemostasis after a guillotine-type partial nephrectomy. Skeletonization of blood vessels employing an ultrasonic surgical aspirator may facilitate utilization of a neodymium:YAG laser for partial nephrectomy, but two expensive and somewhat cumbersome instruments are required (Melzer et al., 1985). The advantages of this technique over standard methods of partial nephrectomy are debatable (Fig. 81–13).

A neodymium:YAG laser has been employed to facilitate local excision of renal cell carcinomas (Malloy et al., 1986). Radical nephrectomy or, perhaps, partial nephrectomy with excision of a generous margin of normal parenchyma is the preferred method of treatment for renal cell carcinoma. In patients with a solitary kidney or compromised renal function, such treatment may not be feasible and enucleation of hypernephromas is sometimes necessary. In these circumstances, tumor margins are precarious. A neodymium:YAG laser has

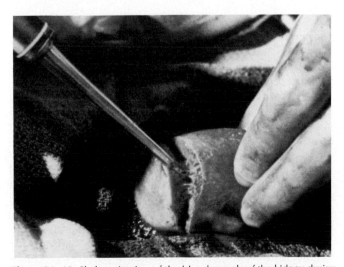

Figure 81–13. Skeletonization of the blood vessels of the kidney during partial nephrectomy using an ultrasonic surgical aspirator. After the vessels are exposed, effective coagulation can be achieved with the Nd:YAG laser.

been employed to coagulate thoroughly the pseudocapsule formed by hypernephroma after enucleation of the primary renal mass. Such treatment should extend the surgical margin some 5 mm and provide good hemostasis. Only anecdotal reports exist, but this theoretically is a promising application of laser energy for treatment of selected renal cell carcinomas.

PHOTODYNAMIC THERAPY

Photodynamic therapy (PDT) defines a methodology that involves photosensitization of cells with subsequent destruction by application of light of a specific wavelength. Preferential destruction of malignant cells occurs by the selective retention of the photosensitizer within the target cells or by the specific direction of the light to the affected areas. Currently, a laser is required to deliver a sufficient amount of the appropriate wavelength.

Several photosensitizers are known to exist but hematoporphyrin derivative has been used most often clinically. The drug is a synthetic derivative of hemoglobin that is retained within malignant or dysplastic cells. HPD is a mixture of porphyrins, which has been further purified to a combination of ethers and esters of dihematoporphyrin (DHE).

HPD is cleared from most tissues within a few hours after systemic administration. However, the drug is retained in liver, spleen, kidneys, and skin as well as in malignant and dysplastic cells. Retention within malignant cells is measurable for several days (Benson, 1989).

The cytotoxic effects of PDT are not fully explained. However, oxygen must be present. Tumors with areas of hypoxia due to poor blood flow respond less favorably. It has been postulated that singlet oxygen production caused by irradiation of DHE is responsible for the toxic effects of PDT on cells (Dougherty et al., 1985).

The optimal light for PDT is one that produces excitation of the photosensitizer coupled with sufficient tissue penetration. However, other molecules within the tissue, such as melanin and hemoglobin, may also absorb light, thereby decreasing the amount available for destruction of tumor cells or producing unwanted thermal effects. The absorption maximum of DHE in aqueous solution occurs at 365 nanometers (in the ultraviolet blue light range). However, light at this wavelength has minimal tissue penetration. Red light (630 nm) penetrates tissue up to 1 cm and has been preferred for clinical PDT.

Cells containing the photosensitizer emit a fluorescence caused by light emission from an excited molecule returning to the ground state. A characteristic salmon-pink color is seen. This fluorescence emission can be used for tumor localization, especially for carcinoma in situ (Benson et al., 1982; Tsuchiya et al., 1983). In the bladder, although malignant cells retain HPD in the greatest proportion, HPD is also observed in dysplastic and inflamed cells, thereby decreasing the specificity of the fluorescence emission.

Light delivery can be focal or nonfocal. A flat cut fiber is employed for focal therapy with emission of light with a small angle of divergence. More useful has been whole bladder therapy (Benson, 1985). A bulb-type diffuser tip illuminates the entire inner surface of the bladder. Depending on the type of fiber chosen, a fairly uniform light distribution can be achieved. Difficulty exists in maintaining the fiber tip in the center of the bladder. Visual placement is relatively inexact in the anteroposterior plane. Ultrasound guidance and monitoring of the fiber tip's placement may facilitate PDT. Alternatively, a lipid-diffusing medium may be utilized.

If applied for an extended period of time, an ordinary light bulb with a red filter can provide sufficient light to produce the cytotoxic effects of PDT. However, the monochromatic intense light produced by a laser is vastly preferable and is preferred in clinical treatment. Most often, an argon pumped-dye laser is chosen. The argon laser serves as an energy source to excite the rhodamine B dye, which serves as the active medium. Pulsed, gold, vapor lasers emit a wavelength of 628 nanometers and may also be utilized for PDT.

Technique

Although the optimal time for delivery of laser energy after drug administration has not been determined, most studies have reported 48 to 72 hours. Most clinical studies for PDT of bladder cancer use a dose of 2 to 2.5 mg/kg of DHE. For whole bladder therapy, an energy density of 15 to 25 joules/cm^2 is desirable. Depending on the bladder volume and laser power output, it may take 45 minutes to an hour to deliver this amount of light. Therefore, the treatment is best performed with the patient under anesthesia to ensure immobility.

The laser fiber is introduced into the bladder through a cystoscope. Optimal positioning is determined by visual inspection as well as by ultrasound guidance. A bulb-type diffusing tip is used with irradiance of the entire bladder wall.

Postoperatively, patients typically experience irritative voiding symptoms manifested by dysuria and frequency for several weeks. Usually, symptoms resolve as some bladder healing occurs. It is imperative that the patient be cautioned to stay out of direct sunlight for a minimum of 6 weeks. Retention of the drug within the skin places the patient at risk for severe sunburn even with limited exposure.

During the first few weeks after PDT, the bladder has an edematous hyperemic appearance. The urine cytology is difficult to interpret at this time. Eventually, complete bladder healing should occur and cytologic examination of the urine should be more reliable.

A temporary functional impairment occurs in the bladder capacity observed in most patients after PDT. Eventually, however, the bladder resumes its pretreatment capacity. However, severe bladder contracture after PDT has been reported, especially at higher energy densities.

Results

PDT remains an investigational procedure with limited clinical data available. Nevertheless, several reports have been made of the results of PDT for superficial bladder cancer. Hisazumi and associates (1984) treated nine patients with Ta and T1 bladder tumors, giving a dose of 2.0 to 3.2 mg/kg of HPD. In tumors less than 1 cm, five of six patients had complete eradication of the lesion. Nseyo and co-workers (1987) reported the results of 23 patients with resistant transitional cell carcinoma of the bladder treated by PDT. All patients had either Ta or T1 tumors. An 83 per cent response rate was reported (seven complete and ten partial).

Song and co-workers (1985) published results of 12 patients with superficial bladder cancer and reported a complete response in ten and partial response in two. Prout and co-workers (1987) reported the results of 19 patients treated with PDT for superficial bladder cancer (Ta to T1). Complete tumor ablation was observed in nine patients (47 per cent), whereas another nine were thought to have evidence of a partial response (i.e., reduction in size of at least 50 per cent). These combined results clearly show an effect of PDT on superficial bladder cancer. However, its role is limited by competing and probably less morbid therapy with resection and intravesical cytotoxic chemotherapy or immunotherapy with bacille Calmette-Guérin.

Potentially more clinically useful is PDT for diffuse carcinoma in situ of the bladder. Cases of diffuse Tis that have failed to be cured with other treatment modalities often require cystectomy as the only available option. Benson (1989) reported complete response in 14 of 16 patients treated by PDT for Tis alone, although six of the patients developed recurrence with longer follow-up.

Photodynamic therapy remains a potentially exciting treatment for bladder cancer. The ability to direct specific therapy at malignant lesions with relatively low morbidity enhances the appeal of this methodology. Nevertheless, many questions of a clinical origin remain. The optimal drug, laser wavelength, time between drug administration and therapy, and amount of light have yet to be defined. Further investigation is necessary before PDT becomes an accepted clinical treatment modality for superficial bladder cancer or carcinoma in situ.

LASER LITHOTRIPSY

In 1968, Mulvaney and Beck successfully fragmented calculi utilizing a ruby laser. However, the accompanying thermal effect produced excessive tissue damage. Likewise, a continuous wave neodymium:YAG laser requires very high energy levels for stone fragmentation, producing extreme heat. Fragmentation of calculi without tissue injury was first achieved with a laser with a short pulse duration and a high peak energy. The ideal wavelength would be absorbed by the calculus but not by the ureter. Initial attemps with a neodymium:YAG laser were unsuccessful because of fiber damage and poor absorption of the wavelength by the stone.

Watson and associates (1987) directed their efforts toward a new class of lasers: tunable pulsed-dye lasers. The energy could be somewhat selectively absorbed by the stone and readily passed down a small, flexible quartz fiber. Minimal tissue damage occurred.

Instrumentation and Mechanisms for Stone Disruption

Pulsed-Dye Laser

The term pulsed-dye laser generally refers to lasers that utilize a coumarin green dye. When excited, this dye generates a wavelength of 504 nm. This wavelength is well absorbed by the yellow color of most calculi but poorly absorbed by body tissues.

Initial studies showed that the most effective laser light was at an energy level of 60 millijoules per pulse for a duration of 1 microsecond. A silica-coated quartz fiber, with a diameter of 250 μ, was utilized. Repetition of the laser pulse at 5 to 10 Hz produces fragmentation of most calculi. Cystine and pure calcium oxalate monohydrate stones are more resistant to fragmentation (Watson, 1989).

TECHNIQUE

The laser fiber may be employed with a rigid or flexible ureteroscope. It may be passed through the scope bare, within a ureteral catheter, or within a specially designed, curved-tip catheter or steerable guide wire. When the calculus is visualized, the laser fiber is placed in direct contact with the stone (Dretler, 1987). A right angle of contact provides the most efficient fragmentation. The laser beam is fired at a discharge rate of 5 Hz. Higher frequencies may impair the surgeon's visual field because of the light flash. Stone fragmentation occurs because of absorption of the laser energy by the stone. A "plasma" bubble is formed on the surface of the stone resulting in an expansion bubble of a column of electrons. This expansion bubble mechanically disrupts the stone along stress lines. Blood clots or fragments of mucosa interposed between the laser and the stone absorb the light and prevent efficient fragmentation (Coptcoat et al., 1988).

Fragments are rarely displaced retrograde during lithotripsy because there is not a great deal of power generated with the laser. Retrograde migration is usually from the irrigant rather than from the laser power. The stone is fragmented into 2- to 3-mm pieces. The fragments may be removed with grasping forceps or allowed to pass spontaneously.

RESULTS

The pulsed-dye laser has proved to be effective in the treatment of ureteral calculi. Even if the probe is inadvertently fired on the ureteral mucosa, no discernible damage is done. The greatest risk of ureteral injury comes from the ureteroscopy itself.

The most easily fragmented calculi are those of struvite and calcium oxalate dihydrate. Power from 20 to 30 millijoules is usually sufficient for these stones. For uric acid calculi and calcium phosphate stones, up to 60 millijoules may be required. Calcium oxalate monohydrate stones are more difficult to fragment, and one may need an energy level of 80 to 120 millijoules. Cystine stones also require high energy but can be fragmented at levels over 90 millijoules.

Dretler (1989) has reported an experience of 127 consecutive ureteral calculi treated with the laser. Complete or partial stone fragmentation was achieved in 87 per cent of the patients. Most of the stones that were not fragmented were composed of calcium oxalate monohydrate. They were described as jet black, smooth, and easy to recognize.

Grasso and Bagley (1990) reported their experience with a pulsed-dye lithotriptor, which was capable of generating power up to 120 millijoules. In 24 patients, this lithotriptor was able to fragment all stones, including those of calcium oxalate monohydrate.

A similar experience has been reported from other medical centers employing a pulsed-dye lithotriptor. Scarpa and associates (1990) successfully fragmented 98 per cent of the stones encountered in 68 patients. No ureteral injuries were reported except those related to the ureteroscopy. Blute and associates (1990) treated 101 consecutive patients and had successful fragmentation in 84 (83 per cent). Seven (7 per cent) cases were considered failures because of difficulty with access. The laser fragmentation was inefficient in ten patients—all with calcium oxalate monohydrate or cystine stones.

The higher energy pulsed-dye laser has obviated some of the problems with stones of hard composition. Moreover, changing the fiber size results in a different energy density. For example, at the same energy output, a 200-micron fiber provides 76 millijoules at the point of impact; a 320-micron fiber, 117 millijoules, and a 400 micron fiber, 123 millijoules. Bhatta and Dretler (1990) utilized a large fiber (320 microns) and a high energy (140 millijoules) pulsed-dye laser and found effective fragmentation of both hard and fragile ureteral calculi without any evident ureteral damage.

Q-Switched Neodymium:YAG Laser

Q-switched neodymium:YAG lasers produce stone disruption by inducing a breakdown in the fluid surrounding the stone. Stone color and composition may be of less importance than with pulsed-dye lasers. The liquid around the calculus acts as an energy converter, propagating the laser-induced shock wave to the stone.

A 20-nanosecond pulse duration and a single pulse energy of up to 80 millijoules produce directional shock waves, with a rise time to peak energy of 3 nanoseconds and a peak pressure of up to 1000 bar. Quartz fibers are utilized for propagation of the energy. However, the high energy pulse durations may result in breakage at the tip of the fiber.

Hoffmann and associates (1990) have reported the largest clinical experience with Q-switched neodymium:YAG laser lithotripsy. Complete stone fragmentation has been achieved in 91 of 120 ureteral stones. Reduction in size was observed in 15 stones. The treatment was considered unsuccessful in only six calculi. Time required for complete stone disruption ranged from 20 seconds to 25 minutes (Hofmann et al., 1990).

Vasovasostomy

A milliwatt CO_2 laser has been utilized for vasovasostomy. The theoretical advantages that have been

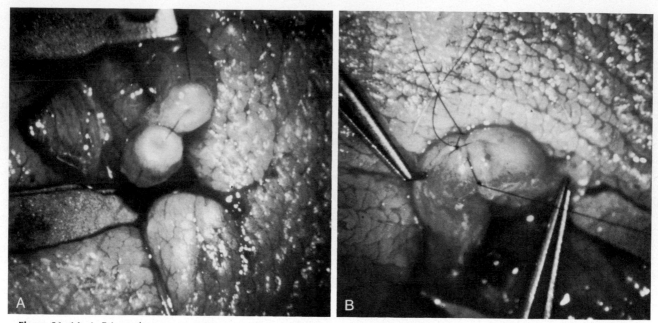

Figure 81–14. *A,* Prior to laser vasovasostomy, sutures are placed to provide alignment.
B, Using a milliwatt CO_2 laser, a weld is created between the sutures. (Courtesy of Alan Shanberg, M.D., Long Beach, California.)

discussed are increased patency, and decreased sperm granuloma, and the ability to perform the laser weld rapidly. Laser-assisted vascular anastomosis has been promising, and many of its principles are applicable to vasovasostomy (Schlossberg and Poppas, 1989).

Seidman and associates (1990) performed vasovasostomy in dogs with a CO_2 milliwatt laser. The vasovasostomy specimens were studied with electron microscopy and histologic evaluation. No evidence was noted of sperm leakage or sperm granuloma in the gross specimens, and minimal local tissue reaction was noted. Histologically, the mucosa at the site of the anastomosis was normal. The electron microscopic data confirmed only minimal scarring at the site of the anastomosis (Seidman et al., 1990). Shanberg and colleagues (1990) have reported results in 32 patients who were undergoing laser-assisted vasectomy reversal. In the 20 patients who had undergone vasectomy less than 10 years prior to reversal, sperm returned to the ejaculate in 19 and a 35 per cent pregnancy rate was observed. In patients whose vasectomies were performed more than 10 years before reversal, sperm returned to the ejaculate in only 36 per cent and the pregnancy rate was only 9 per cent (Fig. 81–14) (Shanberg et al., 1990).

REFERENCES

Bandiearamonte, A., Monte, G., Lepera, P., Marchesini, R., Andreola, S., and Pizzocarara, G.: Laser microsurgery for superficial lesions of the penis. J. Urol., 138:315–319, 1987.

Beer, M., Jocham, D., Beer, A., and Staehler, G.: Adjuvant laser treatment of bladder cancer: 8 years experience with the Nd:YAG laser 1064 nm. Br. J. Urol., 63:476–480, 1990.

Beisland, H. O., and Sander, S.: Nd:YAG laser irradiation of stage T2 muscle invasive bladder cancer: Long-term results. Br. J. Urol., 65:2426, 1990.

Bhatta, K. M., and Dretler, S. P.: Comparison of pulsed-laser lithotripsy using 320 μ and 200 μ quartz fiber on fragmentation and tissue safety: Laboratory studies. J. Endourol., 4:586, 1990.

Benson, R. C.: Hematoporphyrin derivative photodynamic therapy. *In* Smith, J. A., Jr. (Ed.). Lasers in Urologic Surgery. Chicago, Year Book Medical Publishers, 1989, p. 147–165.

Benson, R. C., Jr.: Treatment of diffuse transitional cell carcinoma in situ by whole bladder hematoporphyrin derivative photodynamic therapy. J. Urol., 134:675–678, 1985.

Benson, R. C., Jr., Farrow, G. M., Kinsey, J. H., et al.: Detection and localization of in situ carcinoma of the bladder with hematoporphyrin derivative. Mayo Clin. Proc., 57:548–555, 1982.

Benson, R. C., Jr., Kinsey, J., and Cortese, D.: Treatment of transitional cell carcinoma of the bladder with hematoporphyrin derivative phototherapy. J. Urol., 130:1090–1095, 1983.

Blute, M. L., Patterson, D. E., and Segura, J. Q.: Mayo experience with pulsed-dye laser lithotripsy of ureteral calculi. J. Endourol., 5131, 1990.

Boon, T. A.: Sapphire probe laser surgery for localized carcinoma of the penis. Eur. J. Surg. Onc. 14:193–195, 1988.

Carpiniello, V. L., Malloy, T. R., Sedlacek, T. V., and Zderic, S. A.: Results of carbon dioxide laser therapy and topical 5-fluorouracil treatment for subclinical condyloma found by magnified penile surface scanning. J. Urol., 140:53–54, 1988.

Carpiniello, V. L., Zderie, S. A., Malloy, T. R., and Sedelacek, T. V.: Carbon dioxide laser therapy of subclinical condyloma found by magnified penile surface scanning. Urology, 24:608–610, 1987.

Coptcoat, M. J., Ison, K. T., Watson, G., and Wickham, J. E. A.: Lessons learned. Br. J. Urol., 61:487, 1988.

Dougherty, T. J., Weishaupt, K. R., and Boyle, D. G.: Photodynamic therapy and cancer. *In* De Vita, V. J., Hellman, S., and Rosenberg, S. A. (Eds.). Principles and Practices of Oncology, 2nd ed. Philadelphia, J. B. Lippincott Co., 1985.

Dretler, S. P.: Laser photo-fragmentation of ureteral calculi. Analysis of 75 cases. J. Endourol., 1:9, 1987.

Dretler, S. P.: Urinary stone fragmentation: Clinical application. *In* Smith, J. A., Jr. (Ed.). Lasers in Urologic Surgery. Chicago, Year Book Medical Publishers, 1989, pp. 126–137.

Fuselier, H. Jr., McBurney, E. I., and Brannen, W.: Treatment of condylomata with carbon dioxide laser. Urology, 15:265, 1980.

Grasso, M., and Bagley, D. H.: Flexible ureteroscopic lithotripsy using pulsed-dye laser. J. Endourol., 4:155–160, 1990.

Hisazumi, H., Miyoshi, N., and Misaki, T.: Whole bladder wall photoradiation therapy for carcinoma in situ of the bladder. J. Urol., 131:884–887, 1984.

Hofmann, R., Hartung, R., Schmidt-Kloiber, H., and Reichel, E.: Laser-induced shock wave ureteral lithotripsy using Q-switched Nd:YAG laser. J. Endourol., 4:169–174, 1990.

Hofstetter, A.: Laser application for destroying ureteral tumors. Lasers Surg. Med., 3:152, 1984.

Hofstetter, A., Frank, F., and Keiditsch, E.: Laser treatment of the bladder. Experimental and clinical results. *In* Smith, J. A., Jr. (Ed.). Lasers in Urologic Surgery. Chicago, Year Book Medical Publishers, 1989.

Hofstetter, A., Frank, R., Keiditsch, E., et al.: Endoscopic Nd:YAG laser application for destroying bladder tumors. Eur. Urol., 7:278, 1981.

Kandell, L. B., Harrison, L. H., McCullough, D. L., Boyce, W. H., Woodruff, R. P., and Dyer, R. B.: Transurethral laser prostatectomy: Creation of a technique for using the Nd:YAG laser in the canine model. J. Urol., 135:110A, 1986.

Krogh, J., Beuke, H. P., Miskowiak, J., Honnens De Lichtenberg, M., and Nielsen, O.: Long-term results of carbon dioxide laser treatment of meatal condylomata acuminata. Br. J. Urol., 65:621–623, 1990.

Littrup, P. J., Lee, F., Borlaza, G. S., Sacknoff, E. J., Torp-Pedersen, S., and Gray, J. M.: Percutaneous ablation of canine prostate using transrectal ultrasound guidance, absolute ethanol and Nd:YAG laser. Invest. Radiol., 23:734–741, 1988.

Malloy, T. R., Schultz, R. E., Wein, A. J., et al.: Renal preservation utilizing Nd:YAG laser. Urology, 27:99–103, 1986.

Malloy, T. R., Wein, A. J., and Carpiniello, V. L.: Carcinoma of the penis treated with a Nd:YAG laser. Urology, 31:26–29, 1988.

Malloy, T. R., Wein, O., and Shanberg, A.: Superficial transitional cell carcinoma of the bladder treated with a Nd:YAG laser: A study of recurrence rates within the first year. J. Urol., 131:251, 1984.

Malloy, T. R., Zderic, S. A., and Carpiniello, V. L.: External genital lesions. *In* Smith, J. A., Jr. (Ed.). Lasers in Urologic Surgery. Chicago, Year Book Medical Publishers, 1989, p. 23–35.

McPhee, M. S.: Prostate. *In* Smith, J. A., Jr. (Ed.). Lasers in Urologic Surgery. Chicago, Year Book Medical Publishers, 1989, pp. 41–49.

McPhee, M. S., Arnfield, M. R., Tulip, J., and Lakey, W. H.: Nd:YAG laser "resection" for infiltrating bladder cancer. Presented at the Canadian Urological Association Annual Meeting, Banff, June, 1987.

Merkle, W.: Laser urethrotomy. Urology Times, 18:24, 1990.

Melzer, R. B., Wood, T. W., Landau, S. T., et al.: Combination of CUSA and Nd:YAG laser for partial nephrectomy. J. Urol., 134:620–622, 1985.

Mulvaney, W. P., and Beck, C. W.: The laser beam in urology. J. Urol., 99:112–115, 1968.

Muschter, R., and Dann, T. F.: Laser coagulation of urogenital condylomata acuminata. J. Endourol., 4:549, 1990.

Nseyo, U. O., Dougherty, T. J., and Sullivan, L.: Photodynamic therapy in the management of resistant lower urinary tract carcinoma. Cancer, 12:3113–3119, 1987.

Okada, K., Asoaka, H., Amagai, T., et al.: Transurethral Nd:YAG laser surgery for bladder tumors. Urology, 20:404, 1982.

Prout, G. R., Lin, C., Benson, R. C., Jr., Nseyo, U. O., Daly, J. J., Griffin, P. P., Kinsey, J., Tian, M., Lao, Y., Mian, Y., Chen, X., Ren, F. I., and Qiao, S.: Photodynamic therapy with hematoporphyrin derivative in the management of superficial papillary transitional cell carcinoma of the bladder. N. Engl. J. Med., 317:1251–1255, 1987.

Rosemberg, S. K., Jacobs, H., and Fuller, T. A.: Some guidelines in the treatment of urethral condylomata with carbon dioxide laser. J. Urol., 127:906, 1982.

Roth, R. A., Aretz, T. H. and Lage, A. L.: "Tulip": Transurethral laser induced prostatotomy under ultrasound guidance. J. Urol., 143:285A, 1990.

Salant, R. S., Cohen, M. S., and Warner, R. S.: Neodymium:YAG laser treatment of postoperative bladder neck contractures. Urology, 35:385–387, 1990.

Sander, S., and Beisland, H. O.: Laser in the treatment of localized prostate cancer. J. Urol., 132:280–281, 1984.

Scarpa, R. M., Migliara, R., DeLisa, A., Campus, G., Usai, M., and Usai, E.: Ureteroscopic laser lithotripsy with pulsed-dye laser. J. Endourol., 4:583, 1990.

Schlossberg, S. M., and Poppas, D. P.: CO_2 laser microsurgery and welding. *In* Smith, J. A., Jr. (Ed.). Lasers in Urologic Surgery. Chicago, Year Book Medical Publishers, 1989, pp. 109–118.

Seidman, E. J., Krisch, E. B., Baer, H. M., Phillips, S. J., Tang, C. K., and Shea, F. J.: Vasovasostomy in dogs using the CO_2 milliwatt laser: Part II. Laser Surg. Med., 10:433–437, 1990.

Shanberg, A. M., Chalfin, S. A., and Tansey, L. A.: Neodymium:YAG laser: New treatment for urethral stricture disease. Urology, 24:15, 1984.

Shanberg, A. M., and Malloy, T. R.: Treatment of interstitial cystitis with a Nd:YAG laser. Urology, 24:31–33, 1987.

Shanberg, A., Tansey, L., Baghdassarian, R., Sawyer, D., and Lynn, C.: Laser-assisted vasectomy reversal: Experience in 32 patients. J. Urol., 143:528–530, 1990.

Smith, A. D.: Percutaneous laser use in the upper tract. *In* Smith, J. A., Jr. (Ed.). Lasers in Urologic Surgery. Chicago, Year Book Medical Publishers, 1989.

Smith, J. A., Jr.: Bladder cancer. *In* Lasers in Urologic Surgery. Chicago, Year Book Medical Publishers, 1985, pp. 52–62.

Smith, J. A., Jr.: Endoscopic applications of laser energy. Urol. Clin. North Am., 13:405–419, 1986.

Smith, J. A., Jr.: Laser treatment of invasive bladder cancer. J. Urol., 135:55–57, 1986.

Smith, J. A., Jr.: Treatment of benign urethral strictures using a sapphire-tipped Nd:YAG laser. J. Urol., 142:1221–1222, 1989.

Smith, J. A., Jr.: Invasive bladder cancer. *In* Smith, J. A., Jr. (Ed.). Lasers in Urologic Surgery. Chicago, Year Book Medical Publishers, 1989, pp. 73–80.

Smith, J. A., Jr.: Laser treatment of bladder hemangioma. J. Urol., 143:282–284, 1990.

Smith, J. A., Jr., Batata, M., Grabstald, H., and Whitmore, W. F., Jr.: Preoperative irradiation and cystectomy for bladder cancer. Cancer, 49:869, 1982.

Smith, J. A., Jr., and Dixon, J. A.: Laser photoradiation in urologic surgery. J. Urol., 131:655, 1984.

Smith, J. A., Jr., and Dixon, J. A.: Neodymium:YAG laser treatment of benign urethral strictures. J. Urol., 131:1080–1082, 1984.

Smith, J. A., Jr., and Landau, S. T.: Nd:YAG laser specifications for safe intravesical therapy. J. Urol., 141:1238–1240, 1989.

Soloway, M. S., and Masters, S.: Implantation of transitional tumor cells on the cauterized murine urothelial surface. Proc. Am. Assoc. Cancer Res., 20:256, 1979.

Song, S., Li, J., Zou, J., Shu, M., Zhao, F., Jin, M., and Guo, Z.: Hematoporphyrin derivative and laser photodynamical reaction to the diagnosis and treatment of malignant tumors. Lasers Surg. Med., 51:61–66, 1985.

Stein, B. S.: Laser physics and tissue interaction. *In* Smith, J. A., Jr. (Ed.). Lasers in Urologic Surgery. Chicago, Year Book Medical Publishers, 1989, pp. 1–20.

Tsuchiya, A., Obara, N., Miwa, M., et al.: Hematoporphyrin derivative and photoradiation therapy in the diagnosis and treatment of bladder cancer. J. Urol., 130:79–82, 1983.

Turec, P. J., Malloy, T. R., Cendron, M., Carpiniello, V. L., and Wein, A. J.: KTP-532 laser ablation of urethral strictures. Urology, (In press).

Watson, G. M.: Laser lithotripsy: A theoretical basis. *In* Smith, J. A., Jr. (Ed.). Lasers in Urologic Surgery. Chicago, Year Book Medical Publishers, 1989, pp. 119–125.

Watson, G. M., Murray, S., Dretler, S. P., and Parrish, J. A.: The pulsed-dye laser for fragmenting urinary calculi. J. Urol., 138:195–198, 1987.

Watson, G. M., Wickham, J. E. A., and Mills, T. N.: Laser fragmentation of renal calculi. Br. J. Urol., 55:613–616, 1983.

82
SURGERY OF THE SEMINAL VESICLES

Richard D. Williams, M.D.

The seminal vesicles, paired male organs first described by Fallopius in 1561 (Brewster, 1985), play an important role in reproduction. Primary pathology within the seminal vesicles is rare, but secondary lesions, such as seminal vesiculitis due to prostatitis, or extension of adenocarcinoma of the prostate into the seminal vesicles is more common. In the past, insufficient imaging methods led to infrequent definition of both primary and secondary seminal vesicle pathology. Ultrasonography, computed tomography, and magnetic resonance imaging have improved diagnostic visibility and facilitated selected biopsy of the seminal vesicles. The necessity for surgical intervention is rare but includes congenital cyst with infection and/or obstruction; ureteral ectopy into a seminal vesicle, with resultant obstruction or dysplasia of the ipsilateral kidney; and primary tumor, either benign or malignant. Access to the seminal vesicles is mostly via routes familiar to the urologic surgeon, but a procedure on the seminal vesicles alone without adjacent organ removal is a unique challenge.

EMBRYOLOGY

The seminal vesicle is a strictly male organ, i.e., no female homologue, developing as a dorsolateral bulbous swelling of the distal mesonephric duct at approximately 13 fetal weeks (Arey, 1965; Brewster, 1985). Initially, the cloaca is subdivided by downward growth of the urorectal septum into the posterior anal canal and the anterior urogenital sinus (Fig. 82–1A). The division is completed around the 7th week. The mesonephric duct or wolffian duct is thus included in an area termed the vesicourethral canal within the urogenital sinus. The ureter is a bud initiating from the mesonephric duct at 4 weeks, which eventually attains a separate opening into the bladder by absorption and cranial migration (Fig. 82–1B). The mesonephric duct becomes the vas deferens, which normally drains into the urethra at the ejaculatory duct where it is surrounded by the prostatic glands. Separate symmetric buds extend from the distal mesonephric duct just proximal to the ejaculatory duct at approximately 13 weeks and form the seminal vesicles (Fig. 82–1C).

Developmental anomalies form by alteration of this orderly process. If the ureter does not absorb properly into the bladder, it can enter ectopically anywhere along the vas deferens or posterior urethra. Gordon and Kessler (1972) have shown that 50 per cent of ectopic ureters in males join the posterior urethra, whereas 30 per cent join the seminal vesicle. The remainder enter the vas deferens or the ejaculatory ducts. The seminal vesicles may be congenitally absent. Lack of a vas deferens does not necessarily imply an absent seminal vesicle, unless the ipsilateral ureter is also not present (Goldstein and Schlossberg, 1988). Male patients with cystic fibrosis commonly do not have vas deferens or seminal vesicles (Kaplan et al., 1968).

ANATOMY AND PHYSIOLOGY

The normal adult seminal vesicle is 5 to 10 cm in length and 3 to 5 cm in diameter. The volume capacity of the seminal vesicle averages 13 ml. The right gland is slightly larger than the left in one third of men, but the size of both decreases with age (Redman, 1987). There are three major anatomic types, but the most common contains one central canal with minimal tortuosity and only a few side branches (Aboul-Azm, 1979). The major canal of the seminal vesicle empties into the ejaculatory duct (2.2 cm average length) at the terminal portion of the vas deferens within the prostate.

The blood supply to the seminal vesicle is from the vesiculo-deferential artery, a branch of the umbilical artery (Braithwaite, 1952). Occasionally, the inferior vesical artery provides a communicating vessel. Venous drainage is from the vesiculo-deferential veins and the inferior vesical plexus. The seminal vesicles are inner-

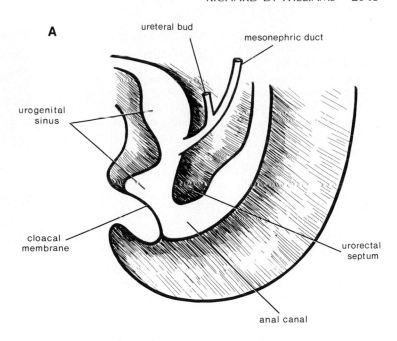

A

ureteral bud

mesonephric duct

urogenital
sinus

cloacal
membrane

urorectal
septum

anal canal

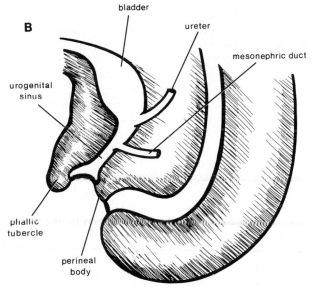

B

bladder

ureter

mesonephric duct

urogenital
sinus

phallic
tubercle

perineal
body

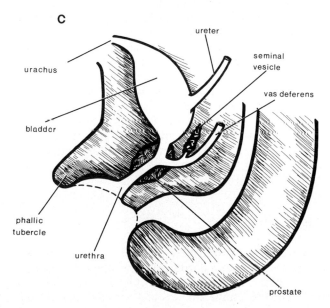

C

ureter

seminal
vesicle

vas deferens

urachus

bladder

phallic
tubercle

urethra

prostate

Figure 82–1. Intrauterine (fetal) development of the seminal vesicles. *A*, Fifth week. *B*, Eighth week. *C*, Thirteenth week. (Redrawn from Langman, J.: Medical Embryology, 4th ed. Baltimore, Williams & Wilkins, 1981, pp. 242–243.)

vated by adrenergic fibers from the hypogastric nerve (Mawhinney, 1983). Lymphatic drainage is via the internal iliac nodes.

The physiologic role of the seminal vesicle is not entirely known; however, the ejaculate contains approximately 2.5 ml of sperm-free semen, which is added by the seminal vesicle. Seminal vesicle secretions contain primarily carbohydrates, such as fructose and prostaglandins E, A, B, and F, as well as a coagulation factor (Tauber et al., 1975 and 1976).

DIAGNOSTIC METHODS

At one time, physical diagnosis and vasography were the only tools available for studying the seminal vesicle. The advent of transrectal ultrasound (TRUS), computed tomography (CT), and magnetic resonance imaging (MRI) have each added substantially to the examination and diagnosis of pathologic conditions of the seminal vesicle.

The normal seminal vesicle and adjacent ducts are not palpable in the normal male. On rectal examination, the area directly craniad to the base of the prostate where the seminal vesicles reside is soft and nondescript. The seminal vesicles lie anterior to the surrounding relatively thick and inelastic two layers of Denonvilliers' fascia, but no anatomic detail of the vesicles or ducts is usually appreciated by palpation, even if the glands are asymmetric. The area immediately above the prostate on rectal examination may be enlarged and relatively compressible in the presence of a seminal vesicle cyst, or it may be solid and firm if there is a seminal vesicle tumor. These lesions may compress the bladder base anteriorly instead and, thus, not be readily palpable. Secondary involvement of the seminal vesicle from the prostate or bladder is palpated as hard areas above the prostate, but these may not be absolutely definable on physical examination.

Laboratory examination of seminal vesicle fluid requires obtaining a semen sample and testing directly for exclusively seminal vesicle excretions, such as fructose. Indirect examination is by measuring the volume and observing the liquefaction of the semen sample. A low semen volume and lack of both fructose and liquefaction imply either absent seminal vesicles or ejaculatory duct obstruction. Although the terminal portion of the ejaculate originates from the seminal vesicles, split ejaculate bacterial cultures are more likely contaminated by the other multiple sites along the lower urinary tract and, thus, are not useful for localizing the site of infection (Stamey, 1980). TRUS–guided perineal aspiration cultures and abscess drainage have been successful, however (Lee et al., 1986).

Vasography

Vasography accomplished by transurethral contrast injection at the seminal colliculus or surgical exposure of the scrotal vas and contrast injection was the preferred means to image the seminal vesicles (Fig. 82–2).

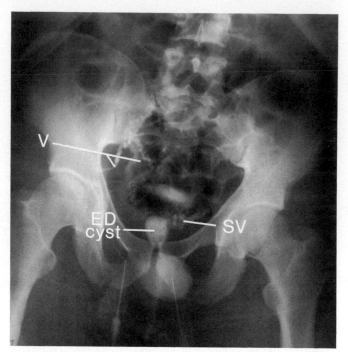

Figure 82–2. Bilateral vasograms in a patient with right ejaculatory duct obstruction (V, vas deferens; SV, seminal vesicle; ED cyst, ejaculatory duct cyst).

Transurethral routes of injection were often unsuccessful owing to the time, special equipment, and expertise required. Antegrade injection through the surgically exposed vas is highly successful, particularly in evaluating duct obstruction in individuals with azoospermia or prior surgical trauma (Al-Omari et al., 1985). Vasography does not, however, provide accurate demonstration of the pathology of the seminal vesicles in patients with vesiculitis, cysts, or tumors (Dunnick et al., 1982; King et al., 1989). Direct transrectal needle seminal vesiculography has also been reported as a method for diagnosis or drug delivery but is not recommended for routine cases (Fuse et al., 1988; Meyer et al., 1979).

Ultrasound

Ultrasound, by either the transabdominal or the transrectal and preferred route, has become one of the most accurate methods of evaluating the seminal vesicle. The advent of probes with high resolution at short focal lengths has allowed rapid, noninvasive, inexpensive, and accurate seminal vesical examination in an outpatient setting.

The normal seminal vesicle on TRUS is an elongated, flat, paired structure between the rectum and bladder just superior to the prostate (Fig. 82–3). The seminal vesicle appears predominately symmetric and is smooth with apparent saccularity. The center of the seminal vesicle is echopenic, with occasional areas of increased echogenicity relating to luminal folds within the vesicle itself (Carter et al., 1989). The ampulla of the vas can usually be seen, particularly near the prostate, as a tortuous tube on sagittal scans. The ejaculatory duct

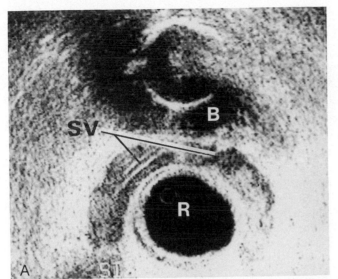

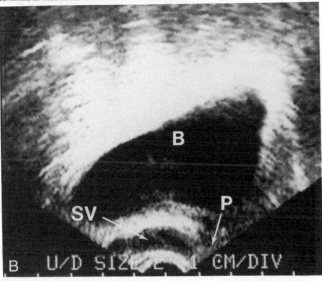

Figure 82–3. Transrectal ultrasound of normal seminal vesicles (B, bladder; SV, seminal vesicles; R, rectum; P, prostate). *A,* Transaxial view showing bilaterally symmetric seminal vesicles. *B,* Sagittal view of normal right seminal vesicle.

may also be visible within the substance of the prostate, but the lumen is not usually visible. The verumontanum is characteristically seen as a more densely echoic structure in the midline at the termination of the ejaculatory ducts. Although sagittal images are best for examining the length of seminal vesicles and adjacent ductal anatomy (Fig. 82–3*A*), transaxial images are best for detecting symmetry and volume (Fig. 82–3*B*). TRUS of the seminal vesicle does not require any special preparation, although a half-full bladder allows better differentiation of the vesicles and adjacent structures.

Abnormal findings on TRUS include seminal vesicle aplasia, atrophy, or cyst formation. Aplasia and atrophy are commonly associated with infertility in up to 2.5 per cent of infertile men (Carter et al., 1989). Cysts, although quite rare, may be congenital and associated with an ipsilateral ectopic ureter and/or an agenetic kidney. Cysts may be acquired as a result of obstruction

following transurethral prostatectomy. The majority of patients with seminal vesicle cysts are asymptomatic. However, they may present with urinary tract symptoms, including dysuria, painful ejaculation, hemospermia, or recurrent epididymitis.

Ultrasound reveals these cystic lesions to be anechoic masses within the substance of the seminal vesicle or larger anechoic saccular lesions, which might rise out of the pelvis and displace the bladder and other pelvic structures (Steers and Corriere, 1986). TRUS can be employed to guide needle placement for drainage or contrast studies to more fully delineate the lesion (Shabsigh et al., 1989). Ultrasound has also been used in the attempt to differentiate inflammatory conditions of the seminal vesicle. However, other than calcifications with chronic bilharziasis, the TRUS findings in patients with chronic prostatourethritis and prostatodynia, for example, are relatively nonspecific (Littrup et al., 1988).

Sonographic findings of a tumor within the seminal vesicle depend on whether the tumor is primary or secondary. Primary tumors are usually unilateral. Secondary tumors more likely involve both seminal vesicles and may be difficult to distinguish as to their origin (i.e., from the rectum, bladder, or prostate). The TRUS image of solid tumors is isoechoic to prostate, but relatively hyperechoic to normal seminal vesicles. No image characteristics are indicative of benign versus malignant or primary versus secondary tumors. However, primary tumors are commonly unilateral and tend not be contiguous with the prostate. Prostate cancer invading the seminal vesicle may be at the base of both seminal vesicles and contiguous with the prostate tumor. Ultrasound-guided transrectal or perineal aspiration cytology or core biopsy findings can be useful to the pathologic diagnosis of seminal vesicle neoplasms.

Computed Tomography

Computed tomography (CT) is a considerable improvement over conventional radiography for evaluation of the pelvis. Evaluation of seminal vesicle pathology by CT, however, has not been systematically studied. Silverman and colleagues (1985) reviewed a group of 50 patients with normal seminal vesicles by CT and determined that the mean length was 3.1 cm, width 1.5 cm, and overall area 3.6 cm. The volume tended to decrease with age. The shape varied from ovoid (70 per cent) to tubular (20 per cent) to round (10 per cent). The seminal vesicles were symmetric in 67 per cent of those studied. The seminal vesicles themselves are medium contrast structures, similar to muscle, routinely seen directly below the bladder (Fig. 82–4). The surrounding Denonvilliers' fascia is not discernible on CT. Goldstein and Schlossberg (1988) studied CT in patients who had absent vas deferens and found that not all had absent seminal vesicles. These workers concluded that CT was accurate for detection of the presence of seminal vesicles. CT has been utilized to detect congenital anomalies. Perhaps, this may be its best use in seminal vesicle diagnosis (Fig. 82–5). Cystic structures have CT attenuation numbers from 0 to 10 Hounsfield units like most

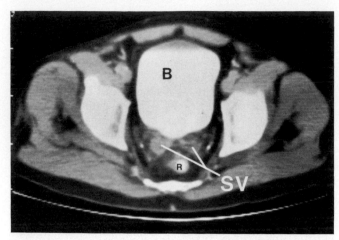

Figure 82–4. Computed tomogram of a normal seminal vesicle (B, bladder; SV, seminal vesicles; R, rectum).

8). This finding is thought to be secondary to the secretions present in the lumen of the seminal vesicle. The surrounding Denonvilliers' fascia is of low intensity on both T1 and T2. Seminal vesicle cysts are similar to cysts in other locations (Fig. 82–9), in that the T1-weighted image is low intensity, and the T2-weighted image is of a unilocular smooth wall with a uniform high intensity and a well-defined margin (Gevenois et al., 1990). Hemorrhagic cysts have high intensity signals on both T1- and T2-weighted images (Sue et al., 1989). Seminal vesiculitis shows a decreased signal intensity on T1. T2 intensity is higher than both that of fat and the normal seminal vesicle.

MRI of seminal vesicle tumors shows a heterogenous mass with a medium intensity on T1 and a heterogenous intensity on T2. No systematic MRI study has been made of seminal vesicle tumors, and MRI cannot distin-

clear fluid-filled structures, although the density may be higher secondary to debris, pus, or hemorrhage.

A primary tumor within the seminal vesicle is readily seen on CT as an enlarged vesicle with a higher attenuation number in the area of the tumor than that in a normal seminal vesicle, with a normal bladder and prostate (Fig. 82–6). The lesion may be cystic, however, as a result of tumor necrosis (King et al., 1989). CT cannot distinguish between benign and malignant tumors and cannot routinely distinguish between primary and secondary tumors, although tissue planes are usually obliterated by secondary tumors that invade from prostate or rectum (Sussman et al., 1986). Inflammatory masses in the seminal vesicles, such as those from tuberculosis or old bacterial abscesses, can be calcified (Birnbaum et al., 1990; Patel and Wilbur, 1987; Schwartz et al., 1988) and thus distinguished from tumors, although a history of infection and related symptoms can usually be elicited. A long-term history of diabetes mellitus has also been associated with seminal vesicle calcification (King et al., 1989).

Magnetic Resonance Imaging

Magnetic resonance imaging (MRI) of the pelvis has become helpful to the management of some urologic diseases. Although MRI is not, in general, more sensitive than CT or US for diagnosis, the anatomic relationships are more clearly seen. In addition, the multiplanar imaging is readily available, and the minimal amount of fat in the pelvis and the characteristics of the MR phenomenon (T1- and T2-weighted images) allow for a more definitive diagnosis of cystic lesions and a more accurate staging of solid neoplasms in the pelvis. Although MRI of the pelvis has been studied extensively, no specific study has compared normal with pathologic seminal vesicles. In the normal situation, the anatomic relationships of the seminal vesicles are similar to those shown on CT, except that on T1-weighted images seminal vesicles are of low signal intensity that increases substantially on T2-weighted images (Figs. 82–7 and 82–

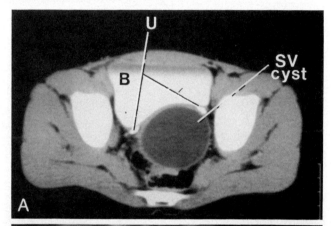

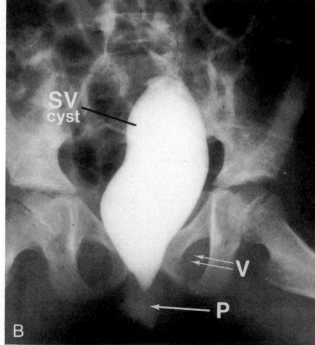

Figure 82–5. Radiologic studies of an 8-year-old boy with a seminal vesicle cyst. *A,* Computed tomogram of a seminal vesicle cyst (SV cyst) (U, ureters; B, bladder). *B,* Retrograde seminal vesiculogram showing a cyst (V, vas deferens; P, prostate).

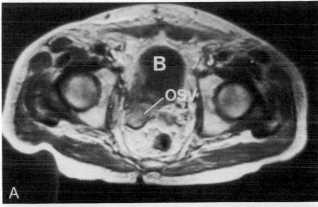

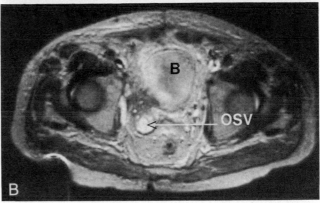

Figure 82–6. Computed tomogram of seminal vesicle lymphoma (SVL) (R, rectum; B, bladder).

guish between benign and malignant solid masses within the seminal vesicle.

Patients with suspected seminal vesicle abnormalities or masses felt on rectal examination should first undergo TRUS. If the mass is solid and noncystic, a transperineal or TRUS–guided biopsy is a reasonable next step. If tumor is confirmed, a CT scan should be done next for

Figure 82–8. Magnetic resonance image (MRI) of an obstructed right seminal vesicle (OSV) as a result of invasive bladder cancer (B, bladder). A, Transaxial T1-weighted MRI. B, Transaxial T2-weighted MRI.

staging purposes. MRI is only necessary to confirm the hemorrhagic nature of the mass or to stage the extent of the mass within the pelvis. Definitive treatment for most seminal vesicle lesions, however, can be appropriately determined without MRI.

PATHOLOGY AND TREATMENT

Congenital Lesions

The previous discussion of embyology identified several congenital abnormalities including cysts, with or without ureteral ectopy and ipsilateral renal agenesis or dysplasia, and seminal vesicle aplasia. Unless these lesions are symptomatic, treatment is not usually necessary (Surya et al., 1988). If the lesion causes symptoms, percutaneous transperineal drainage of the cysts with TRUS guidance can be successful. If not, surgical excision may be necessary. When an ectopic ureter is present, a nephroureterectomy, including removal of the seminal vesicle, should be curative. Seminal vesicle agenesis requires no treatment.

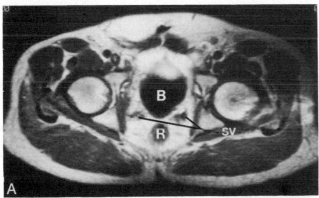

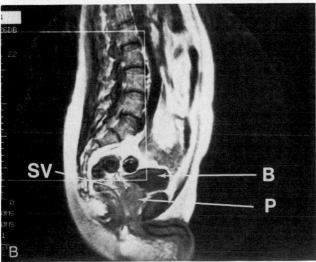

Figure 82–7. Magnetic resonance image (MRI) of normal seminal vesicles (SV) (B, bladder; R, rectum; P, prostate). A, Transaxial T1-weighted MRI. B, Sagittal T1-weighted MRI.

Acquired Benign Lesions

In the United States, infection of the seminal vesicles is an uncommon problem. In less developed countries,

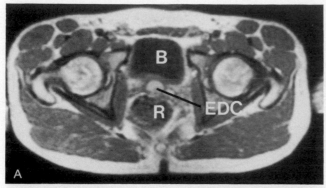

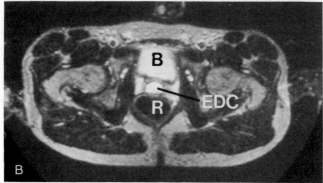

Figure 82–9. Magnetic resonance image (MRI) of a right ejaculatory duct cyst (EDC) of the same patient as in Figure 82–2 (B, bladder; R, rectum). *A,* Transaxial T1-weighted MRI. *B,* Transaxial T2-weighted MRI.

tuberculosis and schistosomiasis remain common causes of seminal vesicle masses, abscesses, and calcifications. Chronic bacterial vesiculitis is rare and difficult to diagnose. However, transrectal/perineal needle aspiration for diagnosis or treatment of abscesses has been successful. Bacterial infections are commonly caused by colon flora and are thought to be secondary to bacterial prostatitis. In the distant past, bilateral seminal vesiculectomy was a treatment for infections of the seminal vesicle. Today, selected systemic antibiotics are usually curative, obviating surgery. Occasionally, chronic bacterial seminal vesiculitis may require surgical removal to eliminate symptoms and prevent recurrent septicemia. Any of the surgical approaches to be described subsequently would be appropriate.

Neoplasms

Tumors of the seminal vesicles are extremely rare. Benign primary tumors are the most common, including papillary adenoma, cystadenoma, fibroma, and leiomyoma (Bullock, 1988; Lundhus et al., 1984; Mazur et al., 1987; Mostofi and Price, 1973; Narayana, 1985). Primary malignant tumors include papillary adenocarcinoma, and less commonly, leiomyosarcoma or hemangiosarcoma (Benson et al., 1984; Chiou et al., 1985; Davis et al., 1988; Kawahara et al., 1988; Schned et al., 1986; Tanaka et al., 1987). One difficulty encountered with seminal vesicle neoplasms is determining whether they are, in fact, primary within the seminal vesicles. Indeed,

it is more common for carcinoma in situ of the bladder, adenocarcinoma of the prostate, lymphoma, or rectal carcinoma to secondarily involve the seminal vesicle (Jakse et al., 1987; Mostofi and Price, 1973; Ro et al., 1987).

To date, very few primary tumors of the seminal vesicles have been reported. This is due in part to the paucity of symptoms, the lack of detection on physical examination for the most common small benign tumors, and the previous lack of diagnostic imaging capable of accurately depicting the seminal vesicles. Less than 100 primary cancers of the seminal vesicles have been reported. Using strict criteria, only approximately 50 are truly primary in the seminal vesicle. It is surprising that a tumor arising from anlage similar to that of the prostate and responding to similar hormonal influences has so few recognized pathologic conditions. Perhaps the extremely low proliferative activity of seminal vesicle epithelium accounts for this characteristic in part (Meyer et al., 1982).

Characteristics of a primary seminal vesicle adenocarcinoma include the following:

1. The tumor commonly occurs in patients over the age of 50.

2. When discovered, the tumor usually extends locally into prostate and bladder and/or rectum.

3. Prostatic and/or ureteral obstruction is common.

4. The pathology reveals a mucin-producing papillary or anaplastic carcinoma that may contain lipofuscin in a patient with no other pelvic primary tumor.

5. The serum markers for prostate cancer, such as prostate-specific antigen (PSA) and prostatic acid phosphatase (PAP) are normal.

6. Serum carcinoembryonic antigen levels may be elevated (Benson et al., 1984; Mostofi and Price, 1973; Tanaka et al., 1987).

The diagnosis of seminal vesical neoplasms can be difficult because they often do not cause symptoms until late in the course. General symptoms that may occur include urinary retention, dysuria, hematuria, and hemospermia. A mass is often palpable above the prostate and is usually not tender. TRUS is usually the next step in diagnosis and may be accompanied by needle aspiration or biopsy. CT would then be appropriate to stage the cancer. Because prostate cancer may be mistaken for primary seminal vesicle cancer, serum PSA and PAP as well as tissue immunohistochemical stains for both enzymes should be helpful. If positive, the prostate is defined as the site of primary malignancy.

When a solid lesion identified in the seminal vesicle shows no evidence of local spread and is benign on biopsy, treatment depends on symptoms. If the patient is asymptomatic, close follow-up consisting of repeat rectal examination and TRUS to determine subsequent growth of the tumor is reasonable, although it may be difficult to be certain the tumor is not malignant. If the mass enlarges or the patient has symptoms referrable to the mass, simple seminal vesiculectomy is advisable. This may be accomplished through one of several routes subsequently described.

If the mass is quite large and solid and has questionable margins or has malignant columnar or poorly differentiated carcinoma cells on biopsy, the treatment of choice is quite different. Because less than 50 accepted cases of seminal vesicle cancer have been described in the literature and less than ten treated at any one institution, it is difficult to define optimum treatment with any degree of certainty. Radical excision, which usually includes a cystoprostatectomy with pelvic lymphadenectomy, is the treatment of choice unless the tumor is extremely small. This recommendation is based on the extensive nature of the majority of the cancers when detected. The excision may include the rectum (i.e., total pelvic exenteration), if it is thought to be invaded. Adjuvant therapy has no proven efficacy, although the only long-term survivors, reported in the literature, had radical surgery with subsequent pelvic radiation therapy or androgen deprivation therapy. No chemotherapeutic regimen is known to be efficacious.

Sarcomas of the seminal vesicles are extremely rare and are also diagnosed late in the course of the disease. Except for the biopsy findings, there are no distinguishing features. Treatment is similar to that for carcinoma.

SEMINAL VESICLE SURGERY

The surgical approaches to the prostate have varied considerably since the first seminal vesicle was removed by Ullmann in 1889 (De Assis, 1952). Descriptions of large series, up to 700 by one surgeon, of seminal vesiculectomies have been described—most for tuberculosis or suspected inflammation. Today, a seminal vesiculectomy is rarely necessary. The most useful open surgical methods include transperineal, similar to that for a radical perineal prostatectomy; transvesical, incising through the posterior bladder wall; paravesical; retrovesical, and transcoccygeal. The choice of surgical approach depends partly on the characteristics of the lesion to be treated but probably more on the experience and expertise of the surgeon. For the most part, congenital lesions require an abdominal approach so that the ipsilateral kidney can be dealt with concomitantly, if necessary. Benign or very small malignancies could be approached perineally. However, the risk of impotence is high even if a nerve-sparing approach is attempted. Larger benign tumors or cysts are best handled by an anterior abdominal approach, although a transcoccygeal method may be as helpful. Patients with malignancy require radical extirpation, which commonly includes a cystoprostatoseminal vesiculectomy and a pelvic lymphadenectomy. This operation is no different than a routine procedure for bladder cancer and, thus, is not described here. The remainder of this chapter describes procedures for excision of the seminal vesicles alone.

Indications

The majority of procedures on seminal vesicles currently are performed in conjunction with the radical surgical treatment of pelvic neoplasms, such as bladder, prostate, or uretheral cancer, and occasionally rectal cancer. The indications and surgical principles for the treatment of these conditions are detailed in other chapters.

Treatment of conditions of the seminal vesicle alone is limited to (1) transperineal/transvesicle aspiration of seminal vesicle cysts or abscesses, (2) transurethral unroofing of seminal vesicle cysts or abscesses, and (3) open resection for chronic infection localized to the seminal vesicle, and (4) open resection for an ectopic ureter emptying into a seminal vesicle, with symptomatic obstruction or a small primary neoplasm in the seminal vesicle.

Patients with small seminal vesicle cysts obstructing ejaculatory ducts or causing local symptoms should undergo an initial attempt at a transperineal or TRUS–guided aspiration. If this attempt is not successful because the cyst reaccumulates, consideration could be given to reaspiration with injection of a sclerosing solution, such as tetracycline. Similarly, an abscess in the seminal vesicle could be aspirated for culture and drained, perhaps even with a short-term indwelling catheter via a transperineal or transvesicle percutaneous route utilizing TRUS or CT guidance (Frye and Loughlin, 1988; Shabsigh et al., 1989). Direct irrigation of the cavity and subsequent antibiotic injection may be curative (Fuse et al., 1988; Fox et al., 1988).

Should these approaches be unsuccessful, and if the cyst or abcess is adjacent to the prostate and not in the mid or distal end of the seminal vesicle, it may be possible to unroof the cavity with a deep transuretheral resection into the prostatic substance just distal to the bladder neck at the 5- or 7-o'clock position (Frye et al., 1988; Honnens de Lichtenberg and Hvidt, 1989). If the aforementioned procedures fail, open surgery will be necessary. If the cyst or abscess is small, a transperineal approach for removal of the cyst or drainage of the abscess will be sufficient. Much larger lesions may require an anterior paravesical approach.

Patients with chronic seminal vesiculitis or small benign tumors of the seminal vesicles can undergo seminal vesiculectomy via the perineal route similar to radical perineal prostatectomy. Large benign tumors or cysts require removal through either an anterior incision or a transcoccygeal approach, because the perineal route limits the ability to reach more than a few centimeters craniad to the bladder neck or to physically remove large masses through the relatively small opening.

A patient with an ectopic ureter into a seminal vesicle cyst requires an anterior approach so that the kidney, ureter, and seminal vesicle can be removed in toto. I prefer a midline incision so that the kidney and ureter can be approached transperitoneally, after mobilizing the colon. The ureter can then be followed and dissected from the bladder in a paravesical approach similar to that in a nephroureterectomy for urothelial cancer.

Preoperative Preparation

Preoperative preparation for open seminal vesicle surgery depends on the extent of the pathology and the planned incision. The transperineal, transcoccygeal, and transvesicle approaches should be prefaced by a complete bowel preparation. I order a mechanical preparation, with Go-LYTELY orally the evening prior to surgery, followed by a standard antibiotic regimen, including oral neomycin/erythromycin. This practice is in anticipation of the uncommon, but not unlikely, possibility of a rectal laceration. A prophylactic systemic antibiotic of choice is administered immediately before surgery.

Routine minidose heparin is not recommended, unless the patient has venous stasis or varices or a history of thromboembolic disease. Little evidence exists in the urologic literature that such treatment is beneficial in routine pelvic surgery. Some method of attempted prevention of phlebothrombosis in the legs, such as intermittent compression stockings during and immediately after surgery, is advisable. Early and frequent ambulation initiated the night of surgery is also stressed. The blood loss expected from seminal vesicle surgery depends on the surgical approach. One to 2 units should be prepared for those involving perineal and transcoccygeal approaches and 2 to 3 units for anterior approaches. Autologous blood should be obtained because these operations are rarely emergencies.

Methods

Transperineal Approach

The transperineal approach follows the standard positioning and incision described in Chapter 79 for a radical perineal prostatectomy. In order to find the seminal vesicles above the prostate, the rectal wall needs to be dissected free and released higher on the base of the prostate and seminal vesicles than is usually necessary for initiation of the radical prostatectomy.

The incision in Denonvilliers' fascia is then made either transversely, just above the level of the base of the seminal vesicles on the prostate (Fig. 82–10), or vertically, if attempting to save the neurovascular bundles responsible for potency (Weldon and Tavel, 1988). In this case, Denonvilliers' fascia is carefully dissected laterally away from the underlying seminal vesicle and ampulla of the vas so as not to tear the longitudinal tissue carrying the neurovascular bundle. The dissection at the base of the seminal vesicle may be enhanced by posterior traction on a Lowsley tractor placed through the urethra into the bladder, thus elevating the prostate and putting tension on Denonvilliers' fascia. The two ampullae of the vas deferens should be dissected directly above the prostate and just under Denonvilliers' fascia. They are somewhat friable but can be clipped with metal clips not placed too tightly, if necessary.

In the case of a simple seminal vesicle cyst or small adenoma, the vas can be spared. The dissection then proceeds to the vesicle of concern. If the reason for surgery is cancer or recurrent infection, a wider resection including the ampulla of the vas may be advisable. If the diagnosis is a benign lesion, the dissection can begin directly on the seminal vesicle. Usually, a simply dis-

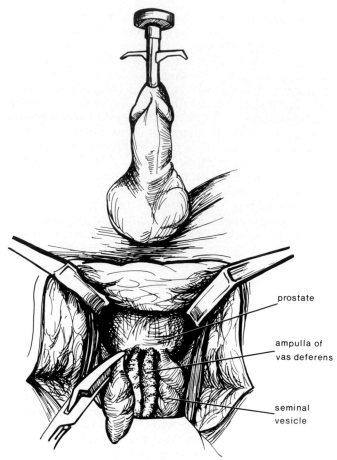

Figure 82–10. Transperineal approach to seminal vesiculectomy. (Redrawn from Hinman, F., Jr.: Atlas of Urologic Surgery. Philadelphia, W. B. Saunders Co., 1989, p. 381.)

sected plane can be found between the seminal vesicle, surrounding retroperitoneal tissue and Denonvilliers' fascia. After dissecting around the seminal vesicle at the base of the prostate, it will usually be possible to pass a right-angle clamp around the seminal vesicle and to use an absorbable 2–0 suture to ligate the stump of the seminal vesicle directly on the prostate. A second tie or clip on the distal seminal vesicle will keep the secretions from obscuring the field after the vesicle is cut across, which is the next step.

Although some surgeons may prefer to attempt to dissect out the seminal vesicle completely before ligating its entry into the prostate, this step makes the operation more difficult and lengthy, as well as serving no purpose when the seminal vesicle is being removed for a benign condition. Once the seminal vesicle has been ligated and cut across at the base, an Allis clamp can be placed on the cut edge. This puts countertraction on the seminal vesicle so that the spreading dissection with Metzenbaum scissors can free the seminal vesicle from the surrounding tissue. The vascular pedicle is usually encountered within 1 cm of the distal tip. After it is ligated with metal clips and cut across, the organ can be removed. The wound is closed in layers, exactly as outlined for a radical perineal prostatectomy. A Penrose drain is left in the bed of the seminal vesicle and removed within 24 hours, if no drainage is noted.

The perineal approach is extremely well tolerated by patients, affording them minimal blood loss, early ambulation, and minimal postoperative pain. Because there is no urethral anastomosis, patients may be ready for discharge from the hospital within 48 to 72 hours. Intraoperative complications primarily entail inadvertent rectal wall laceration, although it is possible to lacerate the trigone area of the bladder or the ipsilateral ureter during deep dissection of the distal tip of the seminal vesicle. If an adequate bowel preparation has been given preoperatively and no gross fecal contamination is seen, a two-layer closure of the rectum with a running mucosal layer of 3–0 absorbable suture and a submucosal layer of interrupted 4–0 silk is usually sufficient. Anal dilatation before awakening the patient may be of assistance. A large laceration and/or fecal contamination should cause consideration of a temporary colostomy, although such a measure has not been necessary in my experience.

If a bladder injury is noted, it should be closed in two layers with absorbable suture as in any other bladder incision. A uretheral catheter is left indwelling for 7 to 10 days postoperatively. If a ureteral injury occurs, an attempt to place a self-retaining (double-J) catheter should be made, and the ureter repaired with absorbable suture. If the ureter cannot be catheterized, flexible cystoscopy and retrograde placement of a ureteral stent should be performed while the patient is still on the table with the stent left in place for 10 to 14 days postoperatively.

Transvesical Approach

The transvesical approach to the seminal vesicle has been described by numerous workers (Politano et al., 1975; Walker and Bowles, 1968). A midline extraperitoneal suprapubic incision is made up to the umbilicus, and the rectus muscles are separated on the midline. The space of Retzius is opened by downward displacement of the transversalis fascia on the pubis, and a Balfour retracter is placed to expose the anterior bladder wall. Care is taken during this dissection not to injure the epigastric vessels on either side of the pubis. The bladder is opened longitudinally, approximately 7 to 10 cm, ending 2 to 3 cm away from the bladder neck. A 1–0 stay suture is placed full thickness on each side of the bladder wall to use as a traction suture. Several moist 4×8 sponges are placed in the dome of the bladder. A Deaver retractor is placed inside the dome to place the open bladder on stretch.

Although it is not absolutely necessary, it is preferable to place long No. 8 feeding tubes in the ureters at this point for definition of the orifices and to help with identification of the subtrigonal ureters in order to prevent their injury later during the dissection. With a Bovie cutting stylet, a vertical incision is made through the trigone on the posterior midline approximately 5 cm in length (Fig. 82–11B). Alternatively, a transverse incision just above the bladder neck could be employed but is not preferred (Fig. 82–11A). The incision is deepened through the bladder muscle, and directly beneath the bladder neck the ampullae of the vas should

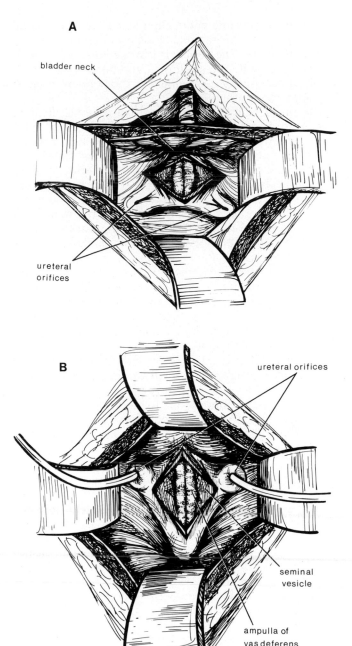

Figure 82–11. Transvesical approach to seminal vesiculectomy. A, Transverse incision 2 cm superior to the bladder neck below the ureteral orifices. B, Vertical incision between the ureteral orifices. (Redrawn from Hinman, F., Jr.: Atlas of Urologic Surgery. Philadelphia, W. B. Saunders Co., 1989, p. 382.)

be recognized. They can be dissected by scissors down to their entrance into the prostate and ligated and divided or left intact, depending on the pathology, as described in the perineal approach.

Just lateral to the ampullae on the prostate base, the seminal vesicles should be identified. The plane surrounding them is entered without difficulty, unless there has been prior inflammatory disease. The seminal vesicles should be encircled and dissected completely free. Metal clips should be placed on the vascular pedicle along with a 2–0 chromic tie on the proximal seminal vesicle at the prostate and a clip placed across the distal end to prevent the seminal vesicle contents from obscuring the field. The vesicle is transected and removed. If there is a moderate-sized cyst, the dissection is more involved but usually is simplified as the perivesicle plane is usually more pronounced.

The plane may be very difficult to establish if there was prior vesiculitis. In this instance, the ureteral catheters are a welcome safeguard—care must be taken not to dissect completely through Denonvilliers' fascia posteriorly and into the rectum. The posterior bladder incision is closed with a running 2–0 absorbable suture in the muscle layer followed by a running 4–0 absorbable suture in the mucosal layer. The ureteral stents and 4×8 sponges are removed, a 20 Fr. urethral catheter is placed, and the anterior bladder wall is closed as was the posterior wall.

Suprapubic tube placement is an option but is not necessary. A suction drain is placed through a separate stab incision and positioned in the prevesical space away from the suture line. The drain is left for 2 to 3 days. It is removed when the drainage has proven not to be urine and is less than 50 ml/day. The urethral catheter is removed in 7 to 10 days. Early ambulation is the rule. The patient is usually discharged within 5 to 6 days after surgery.

This approach is more prone to blood loss and ureteral injury than the perineal approach, but a rectal laceration is much less likely. These complications are handled as described previously.

Paravesical Approach

The paravesical incision is commonly used in children. This approach is also chosen when a large unilateral cyst lies lateral to and above the bladder and when nephroureterectomy is required. A midline or Pfannenstiel extraperitoneal suprapubic incision is made. The bladder is finger dissected away from the lateral pelvic sidewall on the affected side. The vas deferens is identified, placed on tension, and dissected down toward the base of the bladder.

If the seminal vesicle mass is distended, it should be visible rather quickly as the vas comes close to the bladder posteriorly. Placing a catheter in the bladder and emptying it usually allows the plane between the bladder and the cyst to be readily identified. The plane is incised with scissors and the seminal vesicle cyst carefully dissected away sharply. When the tip of the cyst is clearly identified, a 1–0 chromic suture is placed into it to provide traction making further dissection less difficult. As the dissection proceeds, it must be remembered that the ureter crosses the vas and therefore must be identified to prevent its injury. In addition, the superior vesical artery and perhaps the inferior vesical artery may be sacrificed to gain access to the base of the seminal vesicle. This sacrifice will cause no harm and should be done without major concern.

As the dissection proceeds, the bladder is progressively rolled over medially, and the mass dissected away from the bladder laterally. The plane is maintained with sharp dissection. Any vessels feeding the seminal vesicles should be suture ligated or metal clipped. As the

prostate is approached, caution must be taken to stay directly on the mass so as not to injure the neurovascular bundle lying just lateral to the seminal vesicle.

At the prostate base, the neck of the seminal vesicle is encircled and ligated with a 2–0 absorbable suture. A clamp is placed across just distal to the tie, and the seminal vesicle is severed. There may be no need to clip the vas. A suction drain is placed in the bed of the seminal vesicle and brought out through a separate stab incision. The wound is then closed in layers.

Postoperative care is as previously described, except with this approach, the drain can be removed within 24 hours if there is no drainage. The urethral catheter can be removed within 1 to 2 days. The patient may be discharged within 3 to 5 days. Complications can include a ureteral injury and excessive blood loss. If the principles outlined are followed, these are unlikely events.

Retrovesical Approach

The retrovesical approach should be considered in patients requiring bilateral excision of small seminal vesicle cysts or benign masses (De Assis, 1952). A midline suprapubic incision is made into the peritoneal space. A catheter is placed, and the urine is evacuated. The reflection of the peritoneum over the rectum at the posterior bladder wall is incised transversely, being careful not to incise into the rectum (Fig. 82–12A). The bladder is peeled back from the rectum progressively with sharp dissection, until the ampullae of the vasa and tips of the seminal vesicles come into view (Fig. 82–12B). The seminal vesicles are dissected down to the base of the prostate, much as described in the transvesical approach. The neck of the seminal vesicle is ligated and divided bilaterally. The ampullae are usually not taken unless necessary.

A suction drain is left in the area posterior to the bladder and brought out as before. Postoperative care is the same as that for a paravesical resection. Complications include rectal injury, bladder laceration, and hemorrhage. In this situation, a rectal injury would be within the peritoneum well above the levator ani muscles. Following a two-layer closure as before, strong consideration should be given to placement of omentum over the closure between the bladder base and the rectum as well as a temporary colostomy.

Transcoccygeal Approach

The transcoccygeal approach may not be familiar to most urologic surgeons and is unlikely to be a common choice because of the fear of rectal injury and impotence. In individuals in whom the perineal or supine position may be difficult to maintain or in whom multiple suprapubic or perineal surgeries have been done, the transcoccygeal approach may be very useful.

The patient is placed on the table ventral side down (prone) and in a relative jackknife position (Kreager and Jordan, 1965). The incision is made in an L shape, from midway on the sacrum, 10 cm from the tip of the coccyx, and angled at the tip of the coccyx down the gluteal cleft within 3 cm of the anus (Fig. 82–13A). The incision is carried down to the lateral side of the coccyx,

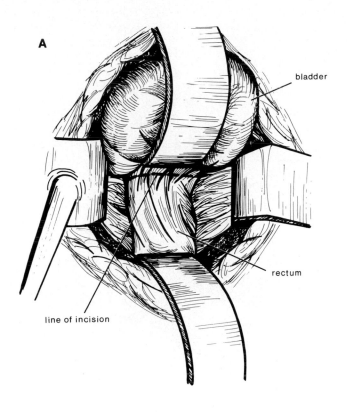

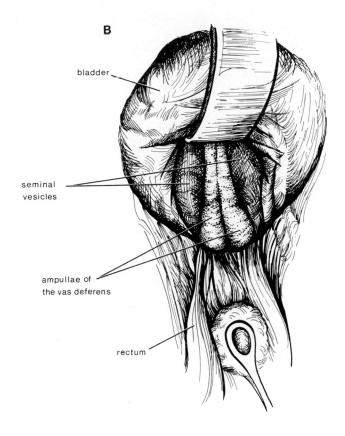

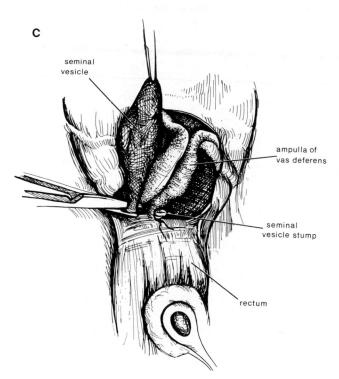

Figure 82–12. Retrovesical approach to seminal vesiculectomy. *A,* Incision line between base of bladder and peritoneal reflection over the rectum. *B,* Caudal dissection reveals the ampullae of the vas deferens on the midline and seminal vesicles immediately lateral to them. *C,* The duct of the seminal vesicle is ligated and transected. (Redrawn from Hinman, F., Jr.: Atlas of Urologic Surgery. Philadelphia, W. B. Saunders Co., 1989, pp. 379–380.)

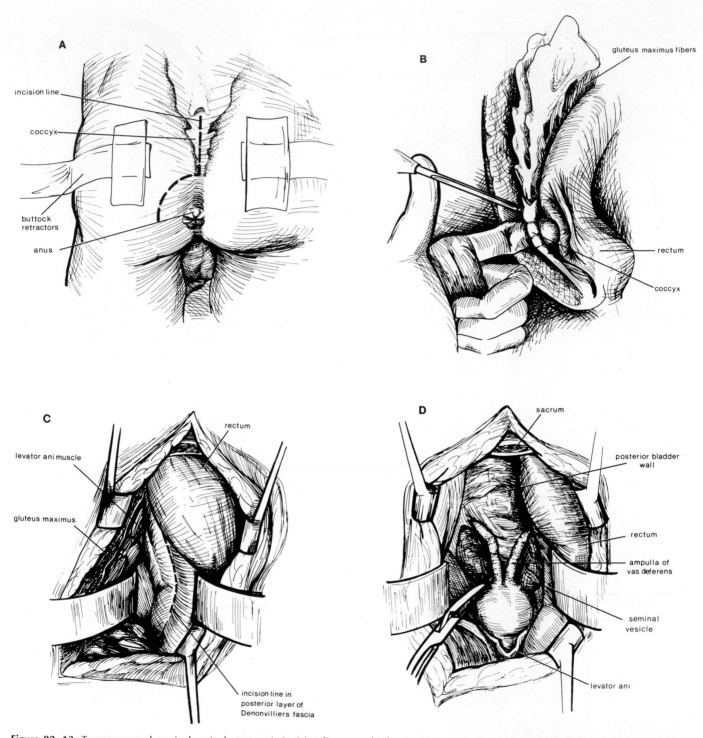

Figure 82–13. Transcoccygeal seminal vesiculectomy. *A,* Incision line over the lower sacrum on coccyx surrounding the anus. *B,* Dissection of the coccyx. *C,* Incising Denonvilliers' fascia after the rectum has been displaced. *D,* Exposure of the prostate and seminal vesicles. (Redrawn from Hinman, F., Jr.: Atlas of Urologic Surgery. Philadelphia, W. B. Saunders Co., 1989, pp. 385–388.)

which is dissected free from the underlying rectum and eventually totally removed (Fig. 82–13*B*). The gluteus maximus muscle layers are moved aside and the rectosigmoid encountered and dissected carefully from the underside of the sacrum.

With careful dissection, the lateral wall of the rectum on the side of the lesion is dissected medially from the levator ani muscle and surrounding tissue until the prostate is encountered (Fig. 82–13*C*). It is possible that the neurovascular bundle will be recognized from this approach. If the dissection is unilateral, injury may be of little consequence. Once the prostate is palpated, dissection of the tissue directly superior to the base on the midline should reveal the ampulla of the vas and, lateral to it, the seminal vesicle (Fig. 82–13*D*).

If difficulty dissecting the rectum away from the prostate is encountered, a finger in the anus via an O'Connor sheath allows the correct plane to be determined. Dissection and removal of the seminal vesicles should follow the principles outlined previously. A Penrose drain should be left in the area, exiting through a separate stab incision at closure. The rectum should be carefully scrutinized for injury and, if found, closed in two layers as previously described. The wound is closed in layers as well. Postoperative care is not very different from that previously described. Similar to the perineal approach, the patient should have a rapid and uneventful recovery. The drain should be removed within 2 to 3 days, if there is no drainage.

CONCLUSION

The seminal vesicles are difficult organs to access, but they fortunately have a small number of primary pathologic conditions. Today, there are very few reasons to operate solely on the seminal vesicles. When the indications are appropriate, the approach and surgical principles are not particularly different from those of other pelvic conditions more frequently encountered by the urologic surgeon.

REFERENCES

Aboul-Azm, T. E.: Anatomy of the human seminal vesicles and ejaculatory ducts. Arch. Androl., 3:287, 1979.

Al-Omari, H., Girgis, S. M., and Hanna, A. Z.: Diagnostic value of vaso-seminal-vesiculography. Arch. Androl., 15:187, 1985.

Arey, L. B.: The urinary system. *In* Developmental Anatomy. Philadelphia, W. B. Saunders Co., 1965, p. 313.

Benson, R. C., Jr., Clark, W. R., and Farrow, G. M.: Carcinoma of the seminal vesicle. J. Urol., 132:483, 1984.

Birnbaum, B. A., Friedman, J. P., Lubat, E., Megibow, A. J., and Bosniak, M. A.: Extrarenal genitourinary tuberculosis: CT appearance of calcified pipe-stem ureter and seminal vesicle abscess. J. Comput. Assist. Tomogr., 14:653, 1990.

Braithwaite, J. L.: The arterial supply of the male urinary bladder. Br. J. Urol., 24:64, 1952.

Brewster, S. F.: The development and differentiation of human seminal vesicles. J. Anat., 143:45, 1985.

Bullock, K. N.: Cystadenoma of the seminal vesicle. J. R. Soc. Med., 81:294, 1988.

Carter, Simon St. C., Shinohara, K., and Lipshultz, L. I.: Transrectal ultrasonography in disorders of the seminal vesicles and ejaculatory ducts. Urol. Clin. North Am., 16:773, 1989.

Chiou, R. K., Limas, C., and Lange, P. H.: Hemangiosarcoma of the seminal vesicle: case report and literature review. J. Urol., 134:371, 1985.

Davis, N. S., Merguerian, P. A., DiMarco, P. L., Dvoretsky, P. M., and Rashid, H.: Primary adenocarcinoma of seminal vesicle presenting as bladder tumor. Urology, 32:466, 1988.

De Assis, J. S.: Seminal vesiculectomy. J. Urol., 68:747, 1952.

Dunnick, N. R., Ford, K., Osborne, D., Carson, C. C., and Paulson, D. F.: Seminal vesiculography: Limited value in vesiculitis. Urology, 20:454, 1982.

Fox, C. W., Jr., Vaccaro, J. A., Kiesling, V. J., Jr., and Belville, W. D.: Seminal vesicle abscess: the use of computerized coaxial tomography for diagnosis and therapy. J. Urol., 139:384, 1988.

Frye, K., and Loughlin, K.: Successful transurethral drainage of bilateral seminal vesicle abscesses. J. Urol., 139:1323, 1988.

Fuse, H., Sumiya, H., Ishii, H., and Shimazaki, J.: Treatment of hemospermia caused by dilated seminal vesicles by direct drug injection guided by ultrasonography. J. Urol., 140:991, 1988.

Gevenois, P. A., Van Sinoy, M. L., Sintzoff, S. A., Jr., et al.: Cysts of the prostate and seminal vesicles: MR imaging findings in 11 cases. AJR, 155:1021, 1990.

Goldstein, M., and Schlossberg, S.: Men with congenital absence of the vas deferens often have seminal vesicles. J. Urol., 140:85, 1988.

Gordon, H. L., and Kessler, R.: Ectopic ureter entering the seminal vesicle associated with renal dysplasia. J. Urol., 108:389, 1972.

Hinman, F., Jr.: Seminal vesiculectomy. *In* Hinman, F., Jr.: Atlas of Urologic Surgery. Philadelphia, W. B. Saunders Co., 1989, p. 379.

Honnens de Lichtenberg, M., and Hvidt, V.: Transurethral, transprostatic incision of a seminal vesicle cyst. Scand. J. Urol. Nephrol., 23:303, 1989.

Jakse, G., Putz, A., and Hofstadter, F.: Carcinoma in situ of the bladder extending into the seminal vesicles. J. Urol., 137:44, 1987.

Kaplan, E., Shawachman, H., Perlmutter, A. D., et al.: Reproductive failure in men with cystic fibrosis. N. Engl. J. Med., 279:65, 1968.

Kawahara, M., Matsuhashi, M., Tajima, M., et al.: Primary carcinoma of seminal vesicle. Urology, 32:269, 1988.

King, B. F., Hattery, R. R., Lieber, M. M., Williamson, B., Hartman, G. W., and Berquist, T. H.: Seminal vesicle imaging. Radiographics, 9:653, 1989.

Kreager, J. A., and Jordan, W. P.: Transcoccygeal approach to the seminal vesicles. Am. Surg., 31:126, 1965.

Langman, J.: Medical Embryology, 4th edition. Baltimore, Williams & Wilkins, 1981, p. 242.

Lee, S. B., Lee, F., Solomon, M. H., Kumasaka, G. H., Straub, W. H., and McLeary, R. D.: Seminal vesicle abscess: diagnosis by transrectal ultrasound. J. Clin. Ultrasound, 14:546, 1986.

Littrup, P. J., Lee, F., McLeary, R. D., Wu, D., Lee, A., and Kumasaka, G. H.: Transrectal US of the seminal vesicles and ejaculatory ducts: clinical correlation. Radiology, 168:625, 1988.

Lundhus, E., Bundgaard, N., and Sorensen, F. B.: Cystadenoma of the seminal vesicle. Scand. J. Urol. Nephrol., 18:341, 1984.

Mawhinney, M. G.: Male accessory sex organs and androgen action. *In* Lipschultz, L. I., and Howards, S. S. (Eds.): Infertility of the Male. New York, Churchill Livingstone, 1983, p. 135.

Mazur, M. T., Myers, J. L., and Maddox, W. A.: Cystic epithelial-stromal tumor of the seminal vesicle. Am. J. Surg. Pathol., 11:210, 1987.

Meyer, J. J., Hartig, P. R., Koos, G. W., and McKinley, C. R.: Transrectal seminal vesiculography. J. Urol., 121:129, 1979.

Meyer, J. S., Sufrin, G., and Martin, S. A.: Proliferative activity of benign human prostate, prostatic adenocarcinoma and seminal vesicle evaluated by thymidine labeling. J. Urol., 128:1353, 1982.

Mostofi, F. K., and Price, E. B.: Tumors of the seminal vesicle. *In* Mostofi, F. K., and Price, E. B. (Eds.). Tumors of the Male Genital System. Washington, D.C., Armed Forces Institute of Pathology, 1973, p. 259.

Narayana, A.: Tumors of the epididymis, seminal vesicles, and vas deferens (spermatic cord). *In* Culp, D. A., and Loening, S. A. (Eds.): Genitourinary Oncology. Philadelphia, Lee & Febiger, 1985, p. 385.

Patel, P. S., and Wilbur, A. C.: Cystic seminal vesiculitis: CT demonstration. J. Comput. Assist. Tomogr., 11:1103, 1987.

Politano, V. A., Lankford, R. W., and Susaeta, R.: A transvesical approach to total seminal vesiculectomy: a case report. J. Urol., 113:385, 1975.

Redman, J. F.: Anatomy of the genitourinary system. *In* Gillenwater,

J. Y., Grayhack, J. T., Howards, S. S., and Duckett, J. W. (Eds.): Adult and Pediatric Urology, Chicago, Year Book Medical Publishers, 1987, p. 45.

Ro, J. Y., Ayala, A. G., el-Naggar, A., and Wishnow, K. I.: Seminal vesicle involvement by in situ and invasive transitional cell carcinoma of the bladder. Am. J. Surg. Pathol., 11:951, 1987.

Schned, A. R., Ledbetter, J. S., and Selikowitz, S. M.: Primary leiomyosarcoma of the seminal vesicle. Cancer, 57:2202, 1986.

Schwartz, M. L., Kenney, P. J., and Bueschen, A. J.: Computed tomographic diagnosis of ectopic ureter with seminal vesicle cyst. Urology, 31:55, 1988.

Shabsigh, R., Lerner, S., Fishman, I. J., and Kadmon, D.: The role of transrectal ultrasonography in the diagnosis and management of prostatic and seminal vesicle cysts. J. Urol., 141:1206, 1989.

Silverman, P. M., Dunnick, N. R., and Ford, K. K.: Computed tomography of the normal seminal vesicles. Comput. Radiol., 9:379, 1985.

Stamey, T. A.: Urinary infections in males. *In* Stamey, T. A. (Ed.): Pathogenesis and Treatment of Urinary Tract Infections. Baltimore, Williams & Wilkins, 1980, p. 417.

Steers, W. D., and Corriere, Joseph N., Jr.: Case profile: seminal vesicle cyst. Urology, 27:177, 1986.

Sue, D. E., Chicola, C., Brant-Zawadzki, M. N., Scidmore, G. F.,

Hart, J. B., and Hanna, J. E.: MR imaging in seminal vesiculitis. J. Comput. Assist. Tomog., 13:662, 1989.

Surya, B. V., Washecka, R., Glasser, J., and Johanson, K. E.: Cysts of the seminal vesicles: diagnosis and management. Br. J. Urol., 62:491, 1988.

Sussman, S. K., Dunnick, N. R., Silverman, P. M., and Cohan, R. H.: Case report: carcinoma of the seminal vesicle: CT appearance. J. Comput. Assist. Tomogr., 10:519, 1986.

Tanaka, T., Takeuchi, T., Oguchi, K., Niwa, K., and Mori, H.: Primary adenocarcinoma of the seminal vesicle. Hum. Pathol., 18:200, 1987.

Tauber, P. F., Zaneveld, L. J. D., Propping, D., et al.: Components of human split ejaculate. J. Reprod. Fertil., 43:249, 1975.

Tauber, P. F., Zaneveld, L. J. D., Propping, D., et al.: Components of human split ejaculate II. Enzymes and proteinase inhibitors. J. Reprod. Fertil., 46:165, 1976.

Walker, W. C., and Bowles, W. T.: Transvesical seminal vesiculostomy in treatment of congenital obstruction of seminal vesicles: case report. J. Urol., 90:324, 1968.

Weldon, V. E., and Tavel, F. R.: Potency-sparing radical perineal prostatectomy: anatomy, surgical technique and initial results. J. Urol., 140:559, 1988.

83
SURGERY OF THE PENIS AND URETHRA

Charles J. Devine, Jr., M.D.
Gerald H. Jordan, M.D.
Steven M. Schlossberg, M.D.

Development of the surgical techniques for transfer of tissue has expanded the ability of urologists to reconstruct congenital and acquired genitourinary abnormalities. Improvements in microvascular and microneurosurgical techniques have made it possible to create a phallus with which a patient may stand to void and enjoy erotic sensibility. We discuss some of the general aspects of this type of surgery before the details.

A graft is tissue transferred from a donor site to a recipient site, where it must pick up its new blood supply. Graft "take" occurs in two phases. The initial phase, imbibition, lasts for 48 hours, during which time the graft survives by absorbing nutrients from the host bed. During the second phase, inosculation, circulation to the graft is re-established by anastomosis of the exposed vessels of the host bed with the vessels of the graft. Growth factors produced in response to hypoxic metabolism within the graft induce capillary sprouting and penetration necessary for the arteries and veins of the host bed to anastomose with the vessels of the graft. As blood flow is established, aerobic metabolism resumes in the graft. This process is complete by 96 hours, by which time connections have also been completed between lymphatics in the graft and the host bed, and the imbibed fluid has been carried off.

Four conditions are necessary to ensure a successful graft take: (1) a well-vascularized host bed, (2) a rapid onset of imbibition, (3) a good apposition and immobilization of the graft at the host site, and (4) a rapid onset of inosculation. Because of its poor vascularity, scar tissue is never a good host bed. A hematoma, a seroma, or a purulent collection established between the graft and even the best host bed will result in the failure of the graft. Grafts must be fixed securely in place and be well bolstered. Also, we recommend prophylactic broad-spectrum antibiotics. After harvesting, grafts must be kept wrapped in a saline-soaked sponge because the surface changes caused by dehydration inhibit imbibition and release of the vascular growth factors produced within the graft, limiting effective revascularization.

Full-thickness skin grafts (FTSGs) contain all of the layers of the skin (Fig. 83–1). Inclusion of the reticular dermis limits the potential for contraction. Removing the fat and subcutaneous tissue from the graft exposes the vessels of the subdermal plexus on its undersurface. Because of the sparsity of these vessels and the thickness of the graft, FTSGs revascularize slowly and require the most favorable conditions for take. Split-thickness skin grafts (STSGs) contain the epidermis and a portion of the dermis. STSGs are harvested at various thicknesses: a medium thickness graft is 0.016 to 0.018 inch, and a thick graft is greater than 0.022 inch. The plentiful, smaller vessels of the interdermal plexus are exposed on the undersurface of the STSGs and inosculation is rapid. Little of the reticular dermis is included; therefore, the grafts tend to be brittle and to have a marked tendency to contract in unsupported tissue. With rapid inosculation and diminished lymph accumulation, STSGs are useful for acute trauma and for coverage after excision of lymphedematous tissue.

A meshed graft is a special application of an STSG. Multiple thin slits are cut into the graft with a meshing dermatome, using a template designed to create an expansion ratio of 1.5:1 or 2:1. Meshed grafts have advantages when the host bed is not optimal or when a potential exists for development of a hematoma or an infection in the host bed. Generally, a meshed graft in genitourinary reconstructive surgery is not expanded, as it would be in extensive burn or large tissue defect treatment.

A dermal graft consists almost entirely of the reticular dermis with a small portion of the adventitial dermis. The epidermis and superficial papillary dermis are re-

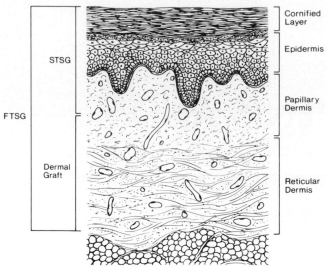

Figure 83–1. Diagram illustrating the portions of the skin included in various grafts. Note the multiple small vessels in the papillary dermis. Skin appendages are not depicted. (From AUA Update Series, Vol. 7, 1988.)

though their survival is subject to the restriction of a length-to-width ratio, no ideal value fits all flaps because of variations in the vascularity of the areas where they might be elevated.

An axial flap has an identifiable artery and vein entering the base of the flap (Fig. 83–2B). The cutaneous vascular territory of an axial flap includes the tissue directly supplied by the artery in the pedicle and the peripheral tissue supplied by the continuation of the dermal and subdermal plexuses.

In a fasciocutaneous flap, the identifiable axial vessels are deep to the fascia (Fig. 83–3A). Perforator vessels penetrate the fascial septa and fan out to form subfascial and suprafascial plexuses, which connect to the subcuticular tissue and overlying skin that are to be transferred with the flap. The dartos fascia with its overlying penile skin and all of the other local flaps that have revolutionized genital reconstruction are essentially fasciocutaneous flaps.

A musculocutaneous flap is an axial flap composed of muscle, subcutaneous fat, and an overlying skin paddle, elevated as a unit based on the vascular supply in the

moved prior to harvesting the graft, and the underlying fat and subcutaneous tissue are removed as the graft is mobilized.

The collagen and elastic network in the reticular dermis resists contraction, and upon maturation the graft will have good extensibility. Multiple vessels are exposed on both sides of the graft so it takes reliably, probably with inosculation occurring on both surfaces of the buried graft. The epidermis and the skin appendages— hair follicles, sweat glands, and so forth—do not regenerate when a dermal graft is buried. However, regeneration will occur if the graft is placed on the surface. Good sized dermal grafts can be harvested freehand by removing the epidermis with a No. 10 or No. 20 scalpel blade or by using a dermatome set to remove a thin STSG at 0.010 or 0.012 inch. The graft should be removed from an area that will allow the donor defect to be closed edge to edge, leaving a linear scar. Choosing the removed epidermis to cover the donor site produces an ugly scar.

A flap is tissue that is transferred from its donor site with its blood supply intact or re-established by a microvascular anastomosis to new vessels at the recipient site. Grafts take; flaps survive. Survival of a flap depends as much on preservation of its venous "runoff" as it does on its arterial supply. The term flap is not limited to a skin flap. A flap can also consist of muscle, fascia, omentum, or intestinal tissue. The British call flaps "pedicle grafts," a locution that sometimes leads to awkward terminology (e.g., a graft as we know it must always be called a "free graft," and a free flap would be called a "free pedicle graft").

The classification of flaps varies with the vascularity and the elevation technique. A random flap lacks an identifiable artery or vein at its base and depends on a random vascularity consisting of the vessels of the dermal and interdermal plexuses (Fig. 83–2A). As these flaps are mobilized, care must be taken to preserve the continuity of the dermal and subdermal vessels. Al-

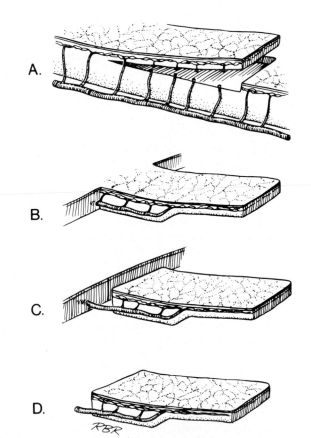

Figure 83–2. *A,* Random flap. The arterial connections have been interrupted and flap survival depends on the dermal and subdermal plexuses.

B, Axial flap. Large vessels enter the base of the flap. Survival depends on them and on the random distal vascularity.

C, Island flap. The vascular pedicle is intact; the skin has been divided. These axial vessels are unsupported. In practice, such a cutaneous paddle would be based on a fascial or muscle flap.

D, Free flap. The skin and vascular connections are interrupted at the base of the flap. Vascular continuity is reconstituted in the recipient area by a microsurgical anastomosis. (From AUA Update Series, Vol. 7, 1988.)

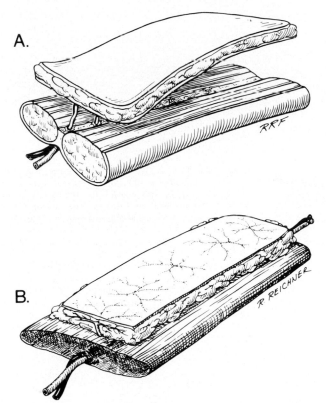

Figure 83–3. *A,* Fasciocutaneous flap. Perforating blood vessels form rich plexuses on the superficial and deep aspects of the fascia connecting to fasciocutaneous vessels that communicate with the vessels of the skin. In genital reconstruction, these are useful as flaps based on the dartos fascia of the penis or as free flaps from the forearm.

B, Musculocutaneous flap. Perforators from an axial artery vascularize a muscle and the skin and subcutaneous fat overlying it. They may be transferred as free flaps but are usually left attached to the vascular pedicle. (From AUA Update Series, Vol 7, 1988.)

pedicle of the muscle (Fig. 83–3*B*). The blood supply to the skin involves perforating vessels that penetrate the fascia and subcutaneous tissue to connect with the dermal plexus of the skin. This composite flap is usually bulky, allowing transfer of a large amount of vascularized tissue to the recipient area. If only vascularized tissue is desired, the muscle can be mobilized as a muscular flap leaving the skin to survive on the random vascularity of the tissues peripheral to the incision. With development of these flaps, the techniques of sequential advancement of tubed flaps and other methods of delayed transfer of tissue have all but been eliminated.

A peninsula flap is elevated with the skin and subcutaneous tissue in continuity at its base (see Fig. 83–2*B*). Because of this restriction, its mobility is limited. It can be advanced, as in a YV-flap. Alternatively, rotation of each of two congruent peninsula flaps into the donor area of the other produces a Z-plasty, used to break up or prevent contraction in a straight line closure.

In an island flap, the vascular pedicle is preserved and the skin and subcutaneous tissue at the base of the flap are divided (Fig. 83–2*C*). Island flaps with unprotected pedicles are insecure. Most island flaps are fascial or muscle flaps carrying an island or a paddle of skin (see Fig. 83–3*A* and *B*). These islands can be moved any-

where within the axis of rotation of the supporting flap (Fig. 83–4).

In a free flap (Fig. 83–2*D*), the artery and vein are interrupted and reconnected to a recipient artery and vein, re-establishing the vascularity of the flap at the recipient site. Any axial flap can be transferred as a free flap. Most fasciocutaneous or myocutaneous flaps also have one or more sensory nerves providing sensibility to the flap. When connected by microsurgical techniques to nerves in the recipient area, the free flap will develop sensation. This is called a sensate flap.

Examples of the usefulness of these various techniques are illustrated further in the chapter. Because an understanding of the anatomy of the area is extremely important in a discussion of the reconstructive surgery of the region, we begin with a discussion of the anatomic relationships of the male genitourinary structures in the penis and male perineum.

ANATOMY OF THE PENIS AND MALE PERINEUM

The penile shaft is made up of three erectile bodies, the two corpora cavernosa and the corpus spongiosum containing the urethra with their enveloping fascial layers, nerves, and vessels, all covered by skin (Fig. 83–5). All of these structures continue into the perineum. The corpora cavernosa make up the bulk of the penis. They contain erectile tissue within a dense elastic sheath of connective tissue called the tunica albuginea. The corpora cavernosa are not separate structures but constitute a single space with free communication through a midline septum, composed of multiple strands of elastic tissue similar to that making up the tunica albuginea. The septum becomes more complete toward the base of the penis, but the corpora truly become independent only as they split to form the crus attached to the inferior ramus of the pubis and ischium.

The erectile tissue containing arteries, nerves, muscle fibers, and venous sinuses lined with flat endothelial cells fills the space of the corpora, making its cut surface look like the cut surface of a sponge. This tissue is separated from the tunica albuginea by a thin layer of areolar connective tissue, which was described by Smith (1966). The paired cavernosal arteries run near the center of the corpora. Blood inflow through these arteries returns through the erectile space of the corpus and numerous anastomotic channels. An artificial erection produced by placing a tourniquet on the base of the penis and injecting a saline solution into one side of the corpora cavernosa fills both sides, the corpus spongiosum, the glans penis, and the superficial and deep veins of the penis. However, with normally functioning erectile vasculature, contrast material injected into one corpus cavernosum, after having established a pharmacologically evoked erection, fills only the two corpora. The other anastomotic channels have been occluded by the neuroendocrine processes of erection.

The third erectile body, the corpus spongiosum, lies in the ventral groove between the two corpora cavernosa. The tunica albuginea of the corpus spongiosum is

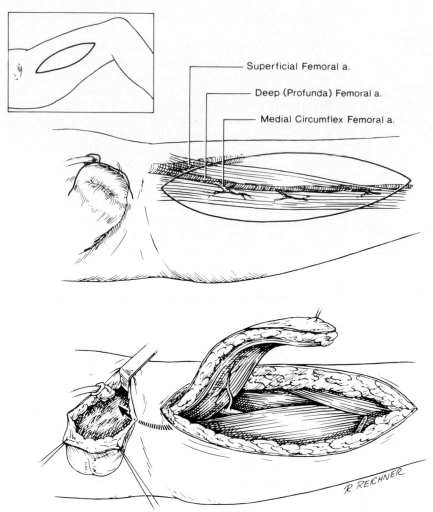

Superficial Femoral a.

Deep (Profunda) Femoral a.

Medial Circumflex Femoral a.

R. REICHNER

Figure 83–4. Gracilis musculocutaneous flap. The muscle originating at the pubic symphysis inserts into the medial tibial condyle and is located by having the patient abduct the thigh prior to being anesthetized. The outline of the muscle and its cutaneous paddle is drawn on the skin of the thigh. As it is mobilized, the skin is sewn to the muscle to prevent trauma to the vessels that penetrate the muscle and join the subdermal plexus. While incising the insertion of the muscle, dissection is continued beneath it, dividing the smaller pedicles distal to its major pedicle. The mobilized muscle flap can be rotated clockwise and passed beneath a skin bridge, effectively transposing skin and vascularized tissue to the genital area. (From AUA Update Series, Vol. 7, 1988.)

thinner than the tunica of the corpora cavernosa, and there is less erectile tissue. Another thin layer of tunica encloses the urethra, which traverses the length of the penis within the corpus spongiosum. At its distal end, the corpus spongiosum expands to form the glans penis, a broad cap of erectile tissue covering the tips of the corpora cavernosa. The urethral meatus is slit-like, lying slightly on the ventral aspect of the tip of the glans with

Superficial Dorsal Vein
Deep Dorsal Vein
Dorsal Artery
Dorsal Nerves
Profunda Artery
Septum
Urethra

Tunica Albuginea
Buck's Fascia
Dartos Fascia

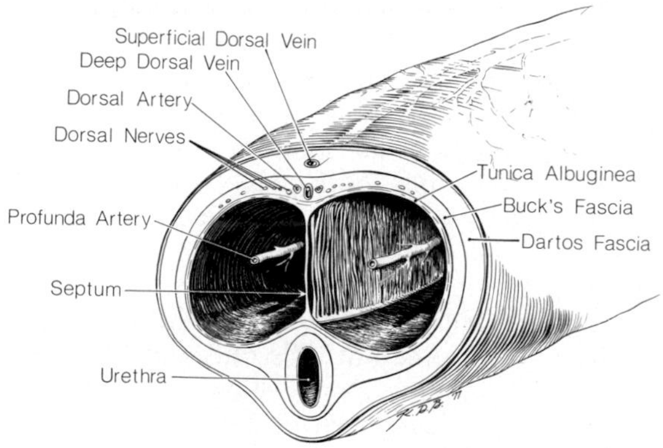

Figure 83–5. Transverse section of the penis at the junction of its middle and distal thirds. Note that the septum is not a solid sheet but is made up of multiple strands that attach to the tunica in the ventral and dorsal midlines.

its long axis oriented vertically. The edge of the glans overhangs the penile shaft, forming a rim called the corona with the sulcus just proximal. A fold of skin, the frenulum, is attached at the most ventral point just proximal to the meatus, where the corona forms a distally pointing V.

At its base, the penis is supported by two ligaments composed primarily of elastic fibers that are continuous with the fascia of the penis. Posterior to this attachment, the right and left corpora cavernosa diverge and the corpus spongiosum broadens between the two crura to form the bulbospongiosum (bulb).

Figure 83–6 illustrates the relationship of the erectile bodies and the urethra to the structures in the perineum. The portions of the urethra are numbered in Figure 83–6. The urethra in the glans *(1)* is lined with stratified squamous epithelium. The pendulous urethra *(2)*, extending to the level of the suspensory ligament, is lined with simple squamous epithelium and maintains a constant lumen size roughly centered in the corpus spongiosum. The urethra in the bulb *(3)* becomes larger and lies closer to the dorsal aspect of the spongy tissue, exiting from its dorsal surface prior to the posterior attachment of the bulbospongiosum to the perineal body. It is lined distally with squamous epithelium, changing gradually to a delicate transitional epithelium

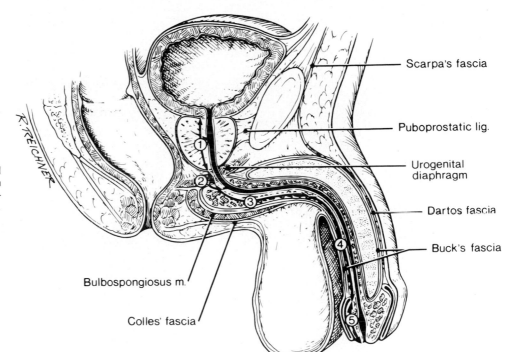

Figure 83–6. Diagram of the sagittal section of the penis and perineum illustrating the fascial layers. The divisions of the urethra are enumerated.

Scarpa's fascia

Puboprostatic lig.

Urogenital diaphragm

Dartos fascia

Buck's fascia

Bulbospongiosus m.

Colles' fascia

and narrowing again as it swings upward to become the membranous urethra *(4)* (Devine, P. C., 1977). Above the triangular ligament (urogenital diaphragm), the urethra enters the prostate *(5)*. Its epithelium is continuous with that of the trigone and bladder.

A submucosal layer is noted throughout the length of the urethra, with an outer sphincter active muscular layer in the prostatic and membranous portions. Numerous glands of Littre open into the urethra along its dorsal surface. At times, these form small diverticula called lacuna of Morgani. Often there is a larger lacuna magna in the dorsal wall of the fossa navicularis. The ducts of Cowper's glands open into the urethra in the bulb and travel to the glands located in the urogenital diaphragm adjacent to the membranous urethra.

In the penis, the erectile bodies are surrounded by Buck's fascia, dartos fascia, and skin. Buck's fascia is the tough, elastic layer immediately adjacent to the tunica albuginea. On the superior aspect of the corpora cavernosa the deep dorsal vein, paired dorsal arteries, and multiple branches of the dorsal nerves, lying on the tunica albuginea, are attached to the inner surface of the fascia. In the midline groove on the underside of the corpora cavernosa, Buck's fascia splits to surround the corpus spongiosum. Consolidations of the fascia lateral to the corpus spongiosum attach it to the tunica albuginea of the corpora cavernosa. Attached distally to the undersurface of the glans penis at the corona, Buck's fascia extends into the perineum enclosing each crus of the corpora cavernosa and the bulb of the corpus spongiosum, firmly fixing these structures to the pubis and ischium and the inferior fascia of the urogenital diaphragm (the perineal membrane).

Distally, the skin of the penis is confluent with the glabrous skin covering the glans. At the corona it is folded on itself to form the foreskin (prepuce), which

overlies the glans. The dartos fascia, a layer of areolar tissue remarkable for its lack of fat, separates these two layers of skin and continues into the perineum where it fuses with the layers of the superficial perineal (Colles') fascia. In the penis, the dartos fascia is loosely attached to the skin and to the deeper layer of Buck's fascia and contains the superficial arteries, veins, and nerves of the penis.

Blood is supplied to the skin of the penis by the left and right superficial external pudendal vessels, which arise from the first portion of the femoral artery; cross the upper medial portion of the femoral triangle; and divide into two main branches, running dorsolaterally and ventrolaterally in the shaft of the penis with a collateralization across the midline. At intervals they give off fine branches to the skin, forming a rich subdermal vascular plexus that can sustain the skin after its underlying dartos fascia has been mobilized. The arteries are accompanied by venous tributaries, which are more prominent than the arteries and can more easily be seen through the skin. Because of its remarkable thinness and mobility and the character of its vascular supply, the skin covering the penis is an ideal substitute in urethral reconstruction. A flap of skin may be elevated, and the fascia containing its blood supply can be mobilized to create a subcutaneous pedicle allowing distal islands of preputial or penile skin to be transferred to virtually any part of the urethra.

Venous Drainage

The penis is drained by three venous systems: the superficial, intermediate, and deep (Fig. 83–7) (Aboseif et al., 1989). The superficial veins contained in the

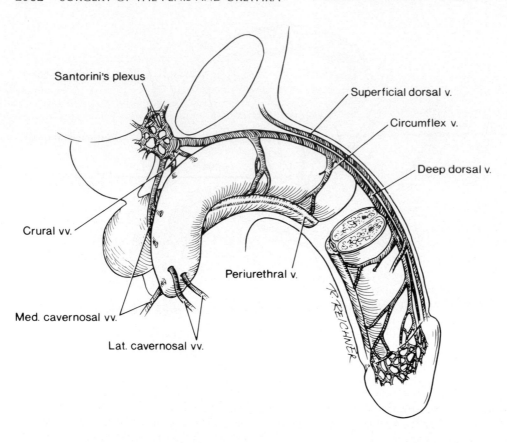

Figure 83–7. Diagram illustrating the venous drainage of the penis.

dartos fascia on the dorsolateral aspects of the penis unite at its base to form a single superficial dorsal vein, usually draining into the left saphenous vein, rarely into the right, and occasionally forming two trunks that drain into both. Veins from more superficial tissue may drain into the external superficial pudendal veins.

The intermediate system contains the deep dorsal and circumflex veins, lying within and beneath Buck's fascia. Emissary veins begin within the erectile space of the penis and, following a perpendicular or oblique course through the tunica albuginea, emerge from the lateral and dorsal surfaces of the corpora cavernosa to empty into the circumflex veins or the deep dorsal vein. The circumflex veins are channels present in the distal two thirds of the penile shaft. They arise from the corpus spongiosum and receive emissary veins, as they travel around the lateral aspect of the corpora passing beneath the dorsal arteries and nerves to empty into the deep dorsal vein. They communicate with one another and those of the opposite side to form three to 12 common venous channels, usually accompanied by branches of the dorsal nerve and artery. The circumflex veins also become confluent ventrally, forming periurethral veins on each side. These become important in the treatment of impotence caused by veno-occlusive incompetence. Additionally, venae comitantes travel with the dorsal arteries and their branches.

The deep dorsal vein is formed by five to eight small veins emerging from the glans penis to form the retrocoronal plexus, which drains into the deep dorsal vein lying in the midline groove between the corporal bodies. In a number of patients, we have found a connection between the superficial and deep dorsal veins. In the shaft of the penis, the deep dorsal vein often consists of

two and sometimes three tributaries that anastomose with each other. The vein gathers blood from the emissary and circumflex veins, and passing beneath the pubis at the level of the suspensory ligament, it leaves the shaft of the penis at the crus and drains into the periprostatic plexus.

The deep drainage system consists of the crural and cavernosal veins. The crural veins arise in the midline in the space between the crura. Normally, they are small and almost undiscernible, joining the deep dorsal vein or the periprostatic plexus. If the deep dorsal vein has been ligated or obliterated following trauma, striking development of these veins can be noted as the intracrural space is entered during the perineal dissection for urethral repair. Emissary veins in the proximal third of the crura near their attachment to the ischial tuberosities join to form several thin-walled trunks on the dorsomedial surface of each corpus cavernosum. Some pass medially, joining the dorsal or crural veins, or extend proximally, entering the periprostatic plexus. Mostly, they consolidate into one or two cavernosal veins on each side. Running in the penile hilum deep and medial to the cavernosal arteries and nerves, they join to form a large venous channel that drains into the internal pudendal vein. Three or four small cavernosal veins emerge from the dorsolateral surface of each crus and course laterally between the bulbospongiosum and the crus of the penis for 2 to 3 cm, before draining into the internal pudendal veins. These usually insignificant vessels become larger and can be noted more readily in patients with veno-occlusive erectile dysfunction. The internal pudendal veins (usually two) run together with the internal pudendal artery and nerve in Alcock's canal to empty into the internal iliac vein.

Arterial System

The blood supply to the deep structures of the penis is derived from the common penile artery, which is the continuation of the internal pudendal artery after it gives off its perineal branch (Fig. 83–8). The common penile artery travels along the medial margin of the inferior pubic ramus, and as it nears the urethral bulb the artery divides into its three terminal branches (Fig. 83–9). These branches are as follows:

1. The bulbourethral artery, a short artery of large caliber, pierces Buck's fascia to enter the bulbospongiosum.

2. The dorsal artery, generally arises as the terminal branch of the internal pudendal artery, travels along the dorsum of the penis between the deep dorsal vein medially and the dorsal nerves laterally, having a coiled rather than a straight configuration. As the penis elongates with erection, the artery uncoils allowing flow to be maintained. Along its course it gives off three to ten circumflex branches that accompany the circumflex veins around the lateral surface of the corpora. Its terminal branches supply the glans penis. Occasionally, a branch will penetrate the tunica to help supply the erectile tissue. Proximally, the circumflex arteries are also a part of the blood supply of the urethra.

3. The cavernosal artery, usually a single artery, arises on each side as the ultimate branch of the penile artery. They enter the corpus cavernosum at the hilum and run the length of the penile shaft giving off the many helicine arteries that constitute the arterial portion of the erectile apparatus. Frequently, the arteries branch prior to entering the corporal body. Sometimes, a branch will enter the opposite corpus. Occasionally, a single artery will branch in the penile shaft to supply both sides. We have seen some of these variations during the course of duplex ultrasound evaluation of the penis following a pharmacologically induced erection.

Lymphatics

Lymph drainage from the glans penis collects in large trunks in the area of the frenulum. The lymph vessels circle to the dorsal aspect of the corona, where they unite with those from the other side. The vessels traverse the penis beneath Buck's fascia, terminating mostly in the deep inguinal lymph nodes of the femoral triangle. Some drainage is to the presymphyseal lymph nodes and by way of these to the lateral lymph nodes of the external iliac group.

Nerve Supply

The nerves of the penis are derived from the pudendal and cavernosal nerves. The pudendal nerves supply somatic motor and sensory innervation to the penis. The cavernosal nerves and a combination of the parasympathetic and visceral afferent fibers constitute the auto-

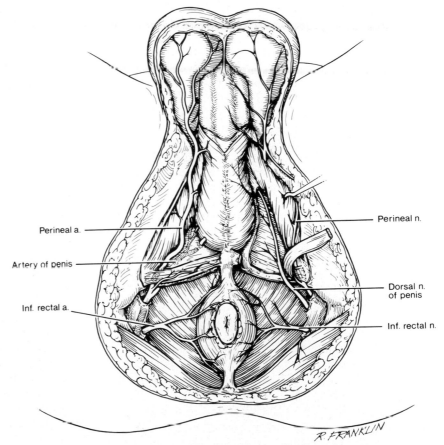

Figure 83–8. Diagram of the perineum illustrating on the left the arterial branches derived from the pudendal artery, and on the right the nerves that accompany the vessels, as they emerge from Alcock's canal.

Perineal a.

Artery of penis

Inf. rectal a.

Perineal n.

Dorsal n. of penis

Inf. rectal n.

R. FRANKLIN

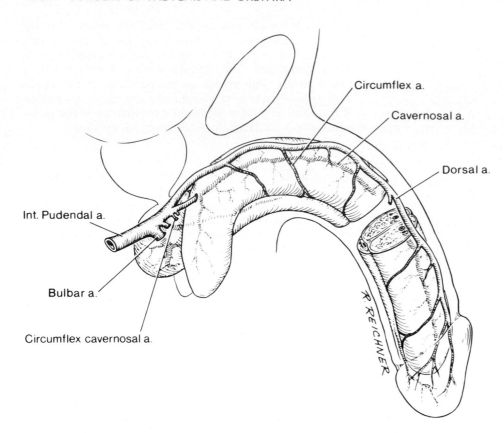

Circumflex a.

Cavernosal a.

Dorsal a.

Int. Pudendal a.

Bulbar a.

Circumflex cavernosal a.

Figure 83–9. Diagram illustrating the arterial supply to the penis. (From Horton, C. E., Stecker, J. F., and Jordan, G. H.: Management of erectile dysfunction, genital reconstruction following trauma, and transsexualism. *In* McCarthy, J. G., May, J. W., Jr., and Littler, J. W. (Eds.): Plastic Surgery, Vol. 6, Philadelphia: W. B. Saunders Co., 1990, p. 88.)

nomic nerves of the penis. These are the nerve supply to the erectile apparatus.

The pudendal nerves enter the perineum with the internal pudendal vessels through the lesser sciatic notch at the posterior border of the ischiorectal fossa. They run in the fibrofascial pudendal canal of Alcock to the edge of the urogenital diaphragm (see Fig. 83–8). Each dorsal nerve of the penis arises in Alcock's canal as the first branch of the pudendal nerve. Traveling ventral to the main pudendal trunk above the internal obturator and under the levator ani, the dorsal nerves perforate the transverse perinei muscles to attain the dorsum of the penis. They continue distally along the respective dorsolateral penile surface lateral to the dorsal artery. On the shaft, their fascicles fan out to supply proprioceptive and sensory nerve terminals in the tunica of the corpora cavernosa and sensory terminals in the skin. These nerves terminate in the glans penis.

The autonomic innervation of the pelvic organs and external genitalia arises from the pelvic plexus. The plexus is formed by preganglionic parasympathetic visceral efferent and afferent fibers arising from the sacral center (S2-S4) and sympathetic preganglionic afferent and visceral afferent fibers from the thoracolumbar center (T11-L2). Beyond the prostate the parasympathetic nerves, the cavernosal nerves, run adjacent to and through the wall of the membranous urethra. As they pierce the urogenital diaphragm, these nerves pass close to and supply Cowper's glands before entering the corpora cavernosa—where they are readily identified in the hilum of the penis dorsomedial to the cavernosal arteries.

Perineum

The perineum is the diamond-shaped pelvic outlet bounded anteriorly, by the pubic arch and the arcuate ligaments of the pubis; posteriorly, by the tip of the coccyx; and laterally, by the inferior rami of the pubis and ischium. A transverse line between the ischial tuberosities divides the perineum into an anterior triangle containing the external urogenital organs and a posterior anal triangle.

Colles' Fascia

In the anterior triangle, Colles' fascia (see Fig. 83–6) attaches at its posterior margin to the perineal body at the posteroinferior margin of the urogenital diaphragm. The fascia curves below the superficial transverse perinei muscles and projects forward as two layers attached laterally to the ischium and the inferior ramus of the pelvis. The loose superficial layer contains much fat and is continuous with the more substantial dartos fascia of the scrotum. In the scrotum the dartos fascia layer contains muscle fibers that cause the rugous appearance of the scrotum. The fascia also projects, but without muscle fibers, into the midline to form the septum between the two halves of the scrotum. The median raphe in the skin delineates the separation of the two halves of the scrotum and is continued anteriorly as a darkly colored streak in the ventral midline of the penis and posteriorly as the median raphe of the perineum, terminating at the anus.

The deep membranous layer of Colles' fascia is a more substantial layer and forms a roof over the scrotal cavity, separating it from the superficial perineal pouch. At the anterior aspect of the scrotum, Colles' fascia joins with the dartos fascia of the scrotum and a fold of this fascia projects backward beneath the fibers of the bulbospongiosus muscle. At the base of the penis, it is continuous with the dartos fascia of the penis. Thickenings of the fascia at this level form the two suspensory ligaments of the penis. First, the outer fundiform ligament, which is continuous with the lower end of the linea alba, splits into laminae that surround the body of the penis and unite beneath it. Second, the inner, triangular-shaped suspensory ligament is attached to the anterior aspect of the symphysis pubis and blends with the dartos fascia of the penis below it.

Anteriorly, Colles' fascia fuses and becomes continuous with the membranous layer of the subcutaneous connective tissue of the anterior abdominal wall (Scarpa's fascia). Laterally, Colles' fascia fuses to the pubic arch and with the fascia lata. Posteriorly, Colles' fascia sweeps beneath the transverse perinei muscles fusing with the posterior aspect of the perineal membrane. The space beneath the continuous plane formed by these fascial attachments is the superficial perineal pouch into which infections or extravasations of urine and collections of blood following trauma to the urethra may be confined.

Superficial Perineal Space

In males, the superficial perineal space contains the continuation of the corpora cavernosa, the proximal part of the corpus spongiosum and urethra, the muscles associated with them, and the branches of the internal pudendal vessels and pudendal nerves.

The ischiocavernosus muscles cover the crura of the corpora cavernosa. They attach to the inner surfaces of the ischium and ischial tuberosities on each side and insert in the midline into Buck's fascia surrounding the crura at their junction below the arcuate ligament of the penis. The bulbospongiosus muscles are located in the midline of the perineum. They are attached posteriorly to the perineal body and to each other in the midline, as they encompass the bulbospongiosum and crura of the corpora cavernosa at the base of the penis. These muscles are confluent with the ischiocavernosus muscles laterally and at their insertion into Buck's fascia, covering the dorsal vessels and nerves at the base of the penis.

Central Perineal Tendon (Perineal Body)

Lying just anterior to the anus, as a part of the plane separating the anterior and posterior perineal triangles, the perineal body is formed by the interconnection of eight muscles of the perineum. The perineal body receives fibers from the anterior portion of the anal sphincter and is the central point of insertion of the superficial transverse perinei muscles, which arise at the ischial tuberosities. The bulbospongiosus muscle is fixed to the perineal body by its most posterior fibers. The deep transverse perinei muscles and fibers from the anterior portions of the levator ani muscles attach to the deep aspect of the perineal body.

Deep Perineal Space

The urogenital diaphragm constitutes the deep perineal space. It is contained within two layers of fascia, and incompletely covers the outlet of the pelvis anterior to the deep layer of the perineal body. The deep layer of fascia is an indistinct structure—the continuation of the endopelvic obturator fascia. The superficial fascia attaches laterally to the ischial rami and the inferior ramus of the pubis. This fascia blends with the deep layer behind the perineal body and anteriorly, where it terminates with a thickened edge—the transverse perineal ligament. A space between this ligament and the arcuate ligament of the pubis accomodates the deep dorsal vein of the penis.

The deep perineal pouch contains the deep transversus perinei muscles, the external sphincter of the urethra, the bulbourethral (Cowper's) glands, and the blood vessels and nerves associated with the structures within it. The sphincter urethrae muscle fibers arise from the medial surface of the inferior pubic rami and pass medially toward the urethra, where they meet the fibers from the opposite side. In males, the muscle encircles the membranous urethra to function as the somatic sphincter of the urethra.

SURGERY FOR PENILE AND URETHRAL LESIONS

Lesions of the penis and urethra may be defined as congenital and acquired. The latter may be considered as either acute or chronic. Congenital lesions are discussed only briefly in this chapter and at length elsewhere in this book.

BALANITIS XEROTICA OBLITERANS

Balanitis xerotica obliterans (BXO) is the most common disease to cause meatal stenosis. It may affect the glans penis, the prepuce, the urethral meatus, and at times the fossa navicularis. Clinically, it appears as a white plaque that histologically shows a think epidermis and an underling dermis filled with collagen and inflammatory cells. In uncircumcised men, the prepuce becomes edematous and thickened and often may be adherent to the glans (Bainbridge et al., 1971). The diagnosis of BXO is made through biopsy, to exclude other inflammatory conditions.

If only the foreskin is involved, circumcision is performed. With glanular and meatal involvement, topical steroids and antibiotics may help to stabilize the inflammatory component, making subsequent surgery simpler and more reliable. Urethral dilation and internal ure-throtomy are seldom curative of the urethral strictures associated with BXO.

Some patients can be managed with an initial internal urethrotomy and a course of long-term self-catheterization. Lubrication of the catheter with 0.1 per cent triamcinolone may soften the scar and allow the patient to increase the time between self-catheterizations. In general, patients so managed are fortunate when this time interval can be prolonged to a week.

Although dilation and meatotomy seldom produce long-term results in isolated meatal stenosis caused by BXO, patients respond very effectively to reconstruction of the meatus and fossa navicularis. Initial reconstruction of the meatus can avert extensive urethral stricture disease, but the reason is unclear. Possibly avoidance of urethral instrumentation limits trauma to the urethra, and reduction of pressure against the stenotic meatus limits scarring secondary to extravasation of urine into the glans of Littre.

We have performed two different procedures for this problem. The first has been to resurface the fossa navicularis with an FTSG (see subsequent discussion) (Devine, 1986). A second procedure employs a ventral transverse preputial island flap (Jordan et al., 1988). An incision is made through the ventral aspect of the strictured fossa and is continued proximally, into the normal urethra. Wings of the glans are mobilized, and a ventral transverse island flap is developed. The flap is transposed and inverted into the defect and the lateral glans wings are closed over the repair (see subsequent discussion). Although we have had success with both approaches, we currently favor the flap over the graft for patients with BXO.

REITER'S SYNDROME

Reiter's syndrome is characterized by inflammatory involvement of three unconnected membranes, producing urethritis, conjunctivitis, and arthritis. In most cases, the systemic effects of the disease far outweigh the local effects on the urethra. However, the urethritis may progress to severe inflammation with necrosis of the mucosa, producing severe stricture disease sometimes involving the full length of the urethra back to the prostate. Multiple attempts at reconstruction only lead to further disease.

In our hands, excising the urethra and replacing it with a tubed skin graft has been unsuccessful. At present, we create a perineal urethrostomy and excise the entire distal urethra. This approach may decrease the rheumatic manifestations (Rubin et al., 1990).

MULTIPLE HEMANGIOMA

These lesions are exceedingly rare but offer challenge to the surgeon. All reported cases have been benign but have demonstrated a persistent nature if not completely excised. Patients with hemangiomas present with hematuria or a bloody urethral discharge. The dilated blood vessels can be seen on cystoscopy. The urethral meatus is a common site, and the lesion usually protrudes. Electrofulguration will not resolve the lesions and should be used only to control an acute episode of bleeding. The lesion consists of vascular spaces lined by endothelial cells. The walls are thin and fragile. Excision of the lesion with adequate margins will help prevent recurrence (Fig. 83–10). They should be managed ag-

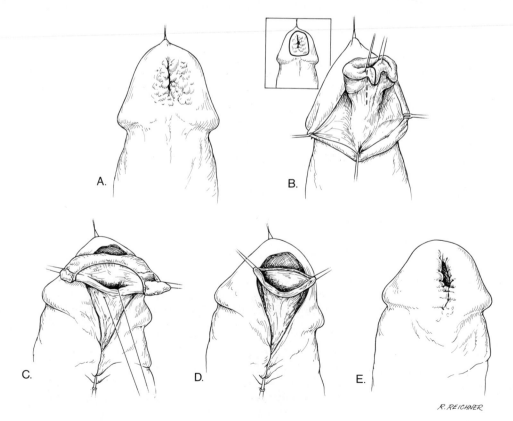

A. B. C. D. E.

Figure 83–10. Excision of a meatal urethral hemangioma. *A,* The hemangioma evident at the meatus involves the distal 1 1/2 cm of the urethra.

B, A skin incision is planned to encompass the entire lesion. Dissection with strabismus scissors is carried out until normal urethra is encountered proximal to the lesion.

C, The urethra is opened, and the extent of the hemangioma marked.

D, The hemangioma is resected.

E, The urethra is reapproximated to the epithelium of the glans.

R. REICHNER

gressively to spare the patient prolonged morbidity. In addition, laser treatment has been attempted with both the argon and KTP-532 laser (Malloy et al., 1989).

CONDYLOMA ACUMINATUM

Condyloma acuminatum or venereal wart is a villous lesion of the genitalia caused by human papilloma virus. Subclinical lesions may also be present. In men, they are common in the warm moist areas under the prepuce or behind the corona of the glans. Lesions can be found in the urethra where they tend to be located in the fossa navicularis. A biopsy must be taken to confirm the diagnosis, especially for large lesions on the glans or lesions within the urethra. Large lesions are best treated with the neodymium:YAG laser, although subclinical lesions can be made more prominent by lavage with acetic acid after which they are fulgurated with a CO_2 laser under microscopic control. This therapy is discussed elsewhere in this book.

SKIN LESIONS

Other skin lesions are frequently seen on the penis. Birthmarks and cysts are common. Hemangiomas may be present at birth and have to be removed because chronic irritation from urine causes ulceration and bleeding. Simple cysts of the penis are likely to be epidermal inclusion cysts. They may grow and become painful. With symptoms, the cysts should be excised. It is not necessary to excise pigmented nevi, but any deeply pigmented nevus of the genital area should be excised when other surgical procedures are being carried out, because of the possibility of its developing into a melanoma.

HYPOSPADIAS

Refinements of tissue transfer techniques (Jordan, 1988) have produced a revolution in the management of hypospadias. Hypospadias is a condition manifested by incomplete development of the phallus caused by a deficiency of the effects of androgen on the development of cells of the external genitalia (see subsequent discussion). The phallus has a hooded prepuce with a urethral meatus located ventral and proximal to its normal location. In addition, the mesenchyme that would normally have formed the corpus spongiosum becomes dysgenetic and develops into a fibrous band, which produces a ventral bend of the penis known as chordee (see Fig. 83–56). More severe cases may be associated with anterior scrotal transposition to a varying degree.

Repair of hypospadias requires a systematic approach to correct these deformities. The approach taken depends on the degree of the curvature, location of the meatus after release of any curvature, quality of the available skin, and preference of the surgeon (Winslow and Horton, 1987). The surgeon needs to address each case with an open mind—ready to use any of the various techniques to accomplish the repair.

ARTIFICIAL ERECTION

In order to assess the amount of chordee, it is necessary to perform an artificial erection to be sure the phallus is straight prior to constructing a neourethra (Gittes and McLaughlin, 1974). To accomplish this assessment, digital pressure can be utilized to compress the corpora behind the scrotum. Alternatively, a red rubber catheter can be secured with a hemostat at the base of the penis. A butterfly needle is introduced into the glans or one corpus cavernosum, being careful to avoid any obvious blood vessels. The penis is filled with injectable normal saline. In a child, only 10 ml or so is required, but in an adult 100 ml or more may be required. When, in adults, we need to produce artificial erections several times during the course of an operation (e.g., in Peyronie's disease and congenital ventral penile curvature), we place the needle in the glans and use the infusion pump from the dynamic cavernosometry setup to introduce the saline solution (Fig. 83–11).

At times, it is not possible for a patient to bring in needed photographs. Discussion of his condition depends on an evaluation of his erect penis. Some patients can accomplish this with minimal self-stimulation, but most cannot and require help. The turgor of an artificial erection depends on continuous inflow of saline. This maneuver can be accomplished, but a pharmacologically evoked erection would allow a much more informative evaluation. We instill 10 to 20 μg of prostaglandin E (PGE) through a 26-gauge needle. Occasionally, if this procedure is not successful, we use a combination of PGE, 12.5 μg with 18 mg of papaverine and 1 mg of phentolamine (Regitine). If the erection lasts longer

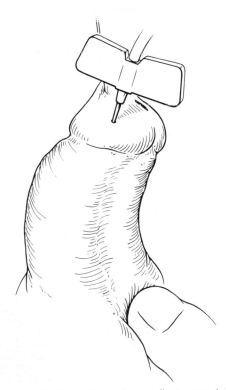

Figure 83–11. Artificial erection. The needle is passed through the glans penis into the tip of one corporal body. Instillation of saline fills all of the vascular structures of the penis.

than 45 minutes or if there is pain, detumescence is accomplished by irrigation of the erectile body with 300 to 500 μg of phenylephrine (Neo-Synephrine).

FAILED HYPOSPADIAS REPAIR

A hypospadias repair may fail owing to an inadequate correction of chordee and/or an inadequate urethra, with a stricture, fistula, or diverticulum (Fig. 83–12) (Winslow et al., 1986). In addition, some patients may have clinical findings, not related to hypospadias, that should have been recognized previously, especially when hypospadias is an aspect of intersex. When treating a patient in whom hypospadias repair has failed, it is important to obtain all available records to help determine what may have contributed to the complication. Generally, problems associated with previous failures may have been caused by errors in design, technique, or postoperative care (Devine et al., 1978).

Evaluation includes retrograde urethrogram, voiding cystourethrogram, and cystoscopy. In an older patient, a reliable preoperative assessment of residual chordee can be made based on history and photographs taken at home. In younger patients, complete evaluation of more complex situations may need to be carried out using anesthesia.

We believe that surgical correction of complex cases requires an aggressive attitude in the surgeon. All residual dysgenetic and scarred tissue causing chordee must be excised and the penis straightened, employing whatever technique is necessary. All of the fibrotic tissue around the neourethra must be excised. If the urethra is inadequate, it must be excised. The most difficult cases clearly present a challenge to the reconstructive surgeon. The techniques for release of chordee and repair of urethral strictures are discussed further on in this chapter.

URETHRAL MEATAL STENOSIS

A small urethral meatus in the newborn will probably not be called to a urologist's attention, unless the

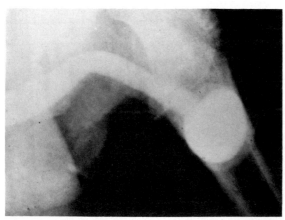

Figure 83–12. Voiding urethrogram demonstrates a diverticulum of the terminal urethra associated with a urethral meatal stricture following hypospadias repair.

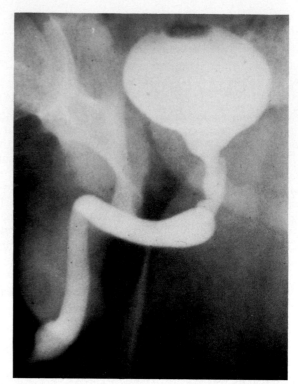

Figure 83–13. Voiding urethrogram of a child with congenital meatal stenosis. The entire urethra is dilated, and the tiny stream distal to the bulging meatus can be seen.

stenosis is associated with other congenital deformities (e.g., hypospadias) or causes voiding difficulties or urinary tract infection (Allen and Summers, 1974).

If the urethral meatus of a boy appears very narrow and if there are associated symptoms, a meatotomy should be considered. To make this decision, voiding should be observed to note that the meatus opens as a full, forceful stream is passed. If the stream is narrow and excessively forceful, stenosis is probably present. The occluding skin is generally a thin layer that can be seen to pouch out with the meatus opening in its center as the child voids (Fig. 83–13).

A urethral meatotomy can be done using local anesthesia (Fig. 83–14). It is important to insert the needle into the skin fold from the underside, so that the tip of the needle can be observed and controlled. If insertion is done from the outside, the needle will pass through both layers of the fold and a wheal cannot be raised because of leakage of the anesthetic solution. After the meatotomy, the edges of the cut will seal together unless they are kept open. The tip of an antibiotic ophthalmic ointment tube is the best instrument for this. The child's parents are instructed to separate the edges gently with the tip of the tube three times a day for 7 to 10 days. One should watch the parents carry out the procedure as they use the ointment for lubrication and the wedge-shape tip for gentle dilation.

In adolescents and adults, it is often necessary to place sutures to approximate the urethral mucosal edge to control bleeding (Fig. 83–15). This step usually requires three sutures: one at the apex and one on either side. We find a dilator made by Cook (Cook Urological, P.O. Box 227, Spencer, IN 47460, Cat. No. 073406) helpful

Meatotomy

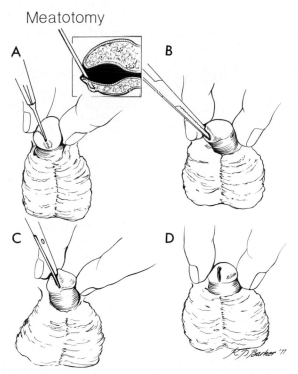

Figure 83–14. Meatotomy. *A,* Introducing the needle into the obstructing leaf of tissue from the inside allows for better control, because about 0.5 ml of anesthetic solution is used to form the wheal.

B, The obstructing tissue is crushed with a mosquito clamp.

C, The crushed tissue is incised.

D, There is no bleeding. The child's parent is instructed in how to keep the meatus open until it heals.

in keeping the meatus open. Meatal stenosis occurs in adults following inflammation, specific or nonspecific urethral infection, and trauma especially in association with indwelling catheters or urethral instrumentation. In these patients so affected, or when meatal stenosis is an aspect of the failure of a previous hypospadias repair, a dorsal instead of a ventral meatotomy may be neces-

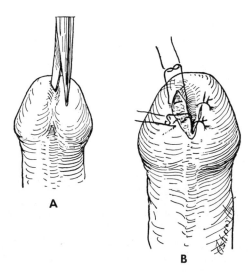

Figure 83–15. Meatotomy in a normally developed penis. *A,* Incision in the ventral aspect of the glans. *B,* Closure of the wound. (From Hand, J. R.: *In* Campbell, M. F., and Harrison, J. H. (Eds.): Urology Vol. 3, 3rd ed. Philadelphia, W. B. Saunders Co., 1970.)

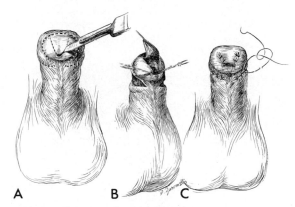

Figure 83–16. The procedure for dorsal Y-V meatotomy. *A,* Skin incisions are outlined by the dotted line. The V-shaped flap of glans is incised and elevated.

B, An incision is made on the dorsal surface of the urethra.

C, The flap of glans has been advanced into the urethra. (From Horton, C. E., and Devine, C. J., Jr.: Hypospadias. *In* Converse, J. M. (Ed.): Reconstructive Plastic Surgery. Philadelphia, W. B. Saunders Co., 1977.)

sary. This can be accomplished as a YV-plasty, after excising any scarred ridge of neourethra (Fig. 83–16).

URETHRAL FISTULA

A fistula is a tract lined with epithelium leading from the urethra to the skin. A urethral fistula may result as a complication of urethral surgery. The fistula may develop secondary to periurethral infection associated with inflammatory strictures or secondary to treatment of a urethral growth (condyloma or papillary tumor). The size of the fistula may vary from a pinpoint to one that is quite large. The treatment must be directed toward the defect but also the underlying process that led to the fistula.

After urethral surgery, a fistula may develop as an immediate or a delayed complication. An early fistula results from poor local healing secondary to hematoma or infection or tension on the tissues. In addition, breakdown of the urethral and skin closure might occur. Occasionally, with aggressive local care and continued urinary diversion, the fistula will close spontaneously. If a fistula is seen after removal of a urethral stent for a voiding trial, urinary diversion is reinstituted. Cystoscopy to determine if meatal stenosis or other factors are present may be helpful prior to reinsertion of a urethral stent in managing such an acute fistula. If these measures fail, repair of the fistula should be delayed for 6 months to allow for all the inflammation to resolve.

We close fistulas in several ways. Endoscopic and radiographic evaluation of the urethra should be performed prior to the repair. If the fistula is small and closure of the hole will not decrease the lumen of the urethra, a button of skin is removed from around the fistula and its edges are cut even with the urethra (Fig. 83–17). The urethra is closed with 7–0 polydioxanone suture (PDS), inverting the mucosal edge. We test the repair to be sure it is watertight. A second layer of tissue is closed over the sutures. A flap of widely

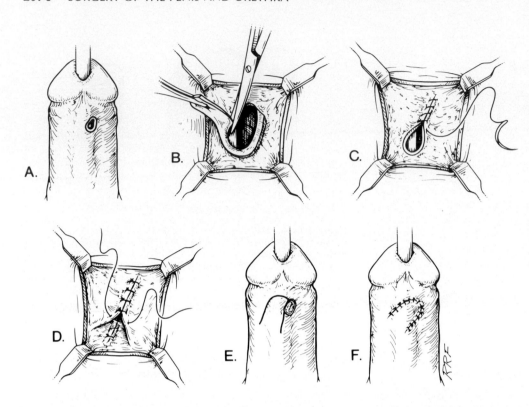

Figure 83–17. *A,* An incision is marked surrounding a fistula—the closure of which will not compromise the lumen of the urethra.

B, The skin is dissected peripherally, and the fistula tract excised.

C, A running extraepithelial 6–0 polydioxanone suture secures a watertight closure.

D, A second layer of sutures buries the urethral closure.

E, A skin flap is designed to cover the repair without overlapping suture lines.

F, The closure is complete—a Bioclusive dressing will be applied. The patient will void through a silicone stent for 2 weeks.

mobilized skin is placed over the repair so that the suture lines are not apposed. A small silicone stent tube is left in the urethra to reduce pressure in the urethra during voiding for 10 to 14 days.

If the fistula is so large that simple closure will compromise the lumen of the urethra, a trap-door flap of penile skin is left attached to one edge of the fistula, and the other edges are incised even with the urethral mucosa (Fig. 83–18). The flap is trimmed to fit exactly and is sewn in place with interrupted 7–0 PDS to invert the mucosa. A urethral stent is left for 10 to 14 days. Occasionally, the urine may be diverted for several days with a feeding tube passed through the stent.

Fistulas associated with inflammatory strictures occur as periurethral tracts and develop secondary to high pressure voiding of infected urine. As multiple tracts develop, this problem becomes what is known as a watering-pot perineum. Repair requires suprapubic drainage and treatment of the infection requires incision and drainage of any abscess. We widely excise the fistula

tracts and the associated inflammatory tissue and wait 4 to 6 months before repairing the underlying stricture. If the tissue is available, a flap urethroplasty would be our first choice; however, in such a situation a meshed graft repair (see further discussion) may be ideal.

Treatment of a fistula occurring after electrocautery or laser destruction of a urethral lesion would follow the same general principles as outlined, but if the original lesion was a papillary tumor or condyloma, it would be imperative to determine if there has been any seeding of the tract that must be excised at the time of repair.

URETHRAL DIVERTICULUM

A diverticulum is an epithelium-lined pouch, which is either a distention of a segment of the urethra or an attachment to the urethra by a narrow neck. In males, a congenital urethral diverticulum may result from in-

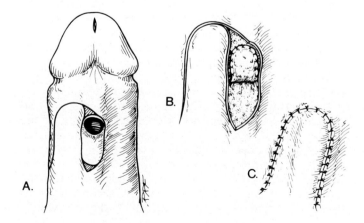

Figure 83–18. *A,* A trap door flap is outlined to fill the defect when simple closure would compromise the urethral lumen.

B, The flap has been mobilized and sewn into the fistula tract with chromic sutures in the epithelium and interrupted polydioxanone sutures placed to make the closure watertight.

C, A skin flap is mobilized to cover the repair without overlapping suture lines. A Bioclusive dressing will be applied. The patient will void through a stent for 2 to 3 weeks.

complete development of the urethra, with a defect in only the ventral wall and subsequent distention of this segment by the hydraulic force of the voiding stream. The downstream lip of the defect may serve as a valvular obstruction, increasing the pressure in the lumen and the rate at which the diverticulum enlarges. Injuries of the urethra may cause defects, such as a diverticulum or a fistula, which are often associated with urethral strictures.

A congenital diverticulum in the prostatic urethra may be a large remnant of the müllerian duct associated with intersex. However, it often occurs in proximal hypospadias and represents an enlarged utricle (Fig. 83–19A) (Devine, 1980). These diverticula may not be demonstrated with voiding urethrography but are demonstrated with cystoscopy or retrograde urethrography. The tip of a urethral catheter tends to catch in this opening, necessitating the use of a catheter guide. Aside from this, however, they usually cause no problems and require no treatment.

Occasionally, a large diverticulum will hold urine post-voiding and will lead to dribbling or recurrent infection (Fig. 83–19B). A surgical approach to small lesions can be through a suprapubic incision, possibly opening the bladder to go through the center of the trigone. How-

ever, large diverticula should be approached transsacrally, using the Peña approach (Peña and Devries, 1982). This is a complex procedure, but it carries much less morbidity than does an abdominal or a perineal approach. Diverticula farther down the urethra will cause obstruction and dribbling, because of delayed passage of contained urine. They are often associated with infection or obstruction. We excise the diverticulum after exposing and dissecting its communication with the urethra. We then close this urethral opening after ensuring that there is no distal obstruction to interfere with healing.

Diverticula of the female urethra may result from dilatation of the periurethral glands or may follow maternal birth trauma. They can cause severe pain when they become infected and distended with pus. Urethral dribbling after voiding may be an early finding. The diagnosis is made by palpation of a mass and expression of urine or infected material from the urethra. Most cases require radiographic confirmation prior to surgery. Sometimes, a diverticulum fills on a voiding urethrogram. However, its delineation may require a special catheter that occludes the bladder neck and external meatus with balloons, while an opening between them allows the urethra to fill with contrast material. Ultra-

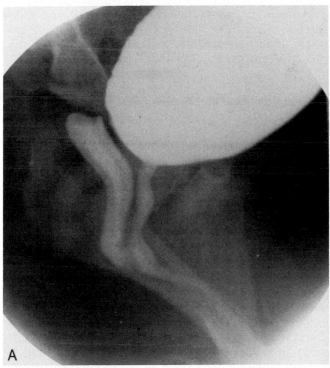

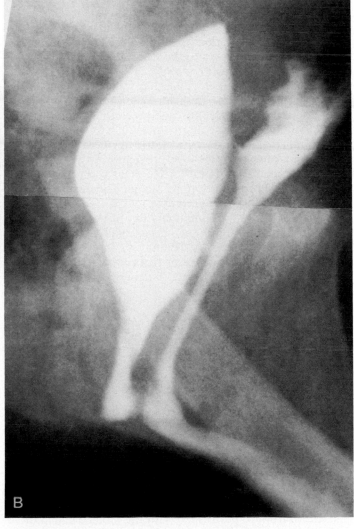

Figure 83–19. *A,* Radiograph showing a posterior urethral diverticulum in a pseudohermaphrodite with hypospadias. The impression of a cervix can be seen in the tip of this structure. A dysgenetic gonad, tube, and upper portion of this diverticulum were removed transabdominally.

B, Composite fluroscopic radiograph of a large utricular diverticulum and partially filled bladder in a patient with hypospadias who is XY. Over time, it dilated to hold over 100 ml of urine, causing dribbling and recurrent urinary tract infection. It was removed via the Peña exposure.

sound can document the presence of a fluid-filled structure and can aid in defining the extent of the diverticulum, especially if it extends anteriorly around the urethra. Cancer may reside in a diverticulum but is extremely rare.

Repair of a urethral diverticulum can be accomplished by excising the diverticulum and closing its neck through a vertical or U-shaped vaginal incision or by simply opening the sac to allow drainage. A catheter in the urethra and, if possible, a Fogarty balloon placed in the sac, aid in the dissection. The urethra may be opened back to the neck of the diverticulum and a urethroplasty done after excision of the diverticulum. Spence and Duckett (1970) and O'Connor and Kropp (1969) have shown that it is possible to marsupialize a distal urethral diverticulum by incising the urethra and the wall of the diverticulum, allowing the tract to granulate. Our experience with this procedure has not been good. We would select it for only very small and distal lesions. Patients have noted considerable tenderness in these opened urethras.

PARAPHIMOSIS, BALANITIS, AND PHIMOSIS

Paraphimosis may occur if the foreskin has been retracted for a prolonged period of time. There may be swelling enough to prevent its subsequent replacement over the glans. To reduce paraphimosis, gentle steady pressure must be applied to the foreskin to decrease the swelling. Especially with a child, it is best done in a quiet room by a parent squeezing it in the hand. At times, an elastic wrap may help. When the swelling has been reduced, the surgeon can push against the glans with the thumbs, pulling on the foreskin with the fingers. Paraphimosis tends to recur. A circumcision should be carried out later as an elective procedure.

Balanitis or inflammation of the glans can occur with poor hygiene from failure to retract and clean under the foreskin. The subsequent swelling makes cleaning more difficult but usually the inflammation responds to local care and antibiotic ointment. Occasionally, an oral antibiotic may be necessary. Phimosis, the inability to retract the foreskin, can result from repeated episodes of balanitis. In older patients, balanitis may be a presenting sign of diabetes.

CIRCUMCISION

Controversy continues to exist as to whether neonatal circumcision should or should not be performed (Poland, 1990; Schoen, 1990). Much attention has been focused on this issue but, despite this, most little boys in the United States are circumcised. Ritual circumcision will continue to be done. However, it is important not to circumcise any boy with a penile abnormality (e.g., hypospadias) that may require the foreskin for repair. In ritual circumcision, it is not necessary to remove the skin but only to draw blood. Most circumcisions done just after birth are performed with the Gomco clamp or one of the plastic disposable devices made for this purpose. It is important to free the foreskin from the glans completely and to apply appropriate tension when pulling the foreskin into the clamp to prevent a too generous or an inadequate circumcision.

The most common complication is bleeding because control with vascular compression has been inadequate. Application of an epinephrine-soaked sponge may help in controlling a minimal ooze. Infection can also occur and responds to local care. Any resulting skin separation should be repaired after the inflammation resolves. Sometimes, too much skin is removed or the urethra may be included in the clamp resulting in a fistula. If the entire penis is "scalped," it may be covered with a STSG but may be best managed by burying the penis in the scrotum and repairing it at a later date. Electrocautery should *never* be used in a neonatal circumcision as penile loss can occur!

At present, the consensus would be that a newborn who has lost his penis as a result of such a mishap should be converted to a girl (Gearhart and Rock, 1989; Oesterling, 1987). Our experience with construction of a penis now includes a number of children and youths. Some of these older patients had been converted to female gender following circumcision accident, and as they passed through puberty they realized that this sexual assignment was wrong. We believe that with the present level of development of techniques, the matter should receive more thought because most of these boys could undergo reconstruction in such a manner as to preserve reproductive function.

The vessels of older boys are more substantial and not easily sealed by compression, no matter how vigorous. Clamps should never be applied, even though larger sizes are available. We favor a sleeve circumcision in older boys and in men (Fig. 83–20). With the foreskin in its proper position, a marking pen outlines an incision following the outlines of the corona and the V of the frenulum on the ventral side. The foreskin is retracted, and a second incision is marked a centimeter proximal to the corona. This mark should go straight across the base of the frenulum, because the skin will retract as it is cut. We make the skin incision and fulgurate bleeding vessels with the bipolar cautery, as the incision is deepened and the skin edge mobilized. The prepuce is now extended over the glans, and the previously marked proximal incision is made. Four stitches are placed in the distal skin edge, which is retracted inverting the prepuce. The dartos fascia is freed from the skin, using the knife. As the prepuce is unfolded, the previously made incision near the corona of the glans can be recognized by the dark color of the blood beneath.

The dissection is completed and the sleeve of prepuce removed, having been turned inside out by this maneuver. All bleeders are controlled, and the skin edges are reapproximated with 4–0 or 5–0 chromic cat gut sutures, the first being placed at the frenulum. A Bioclusive dressing is applied. In adults, circumcision can be done using local anesthesia, by blocking the dorsal nerves at the base of the penis and infiltrating the frenulum.

In smaller boys, this procedure may be considered tedious and too difficult in which case, after marking the skin, a dorsal slit is made through both layers of the

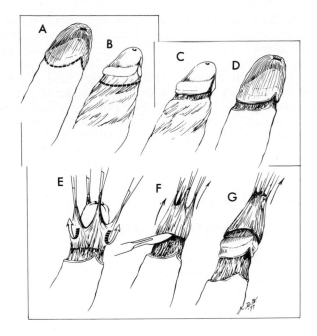

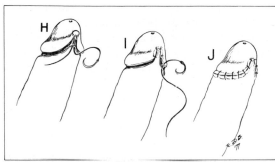

Figure 83–20. Sleeve circumcision. *A* and *B*, The incisions are marked on the skin. Note that the skin incision follows the line of the corona up into the notch of the frenulum, and the mucosal incision goes straight across.

C and *D*, Incisions are made. Note how the "mucosa" retracts into the notch of the frenulum.

E, The sleeve of skin is inverted.

F, At the same time, the dartos fascia is dissected away with the knife, much like skinning a small animal.

G, When the mucosal incision has been completed, the skin is removed.

H, The frenulum stitch is placed, catching the tip of the V of skin and each side of the retracted mucosa.

I, Suturing is completed, giving a good cosmetic effect (*J*).

prepuce back to the level of the corona (Fig. 83–21). Following the marks, the two layers of the prepuce are incised. Bleeders are controlled, and the skin edges are approximated with 5–0 or 6–0 chromic cat gut sutures.

Complications should be uncommon. Most patients develop some hyperesthesia of the glans, which resolves. A hematoma is probably the most common immediate complication. Some patients notice minor cosmetic imperfections that are functionally insignificant. However, one of the most distressing problems we see is a patient who complains that the surgeon has removed too much skin. These men are agonized and litigious. A circumcision should be done precisely and, whatever the procedure to be carried out, the incisions should first be marked with the skin lying undistorted on the shaft.

DORSAL SLIT

In uncircumcised males, phimosis or inability to retract the foreskin may develop secondary to inflammation or poor hygiene. Also, at times it may not be possible to release a paraphimosis. In either of these circumstances, it is necessary to release the constrictive band. This is accomplished by fixing the edge of the prepuce with two clamps at the dorsal midline and making an incision between them to the level of the corona of the glans. Bleeders are fulgurated, and the edges are approximated with interrupted sutures of 4–0 chromic catgut. After the inflammation has resolved, the circumcision may be completed.

RESIDUAL GENITAL ABNORMALITY IN PATIENTS WITH REPAIRED EXSTROPHY

Residual genital defects in adult male patients who have had exstrophy repaired as a child can cause functional, aesthetic, and psychologic problems. These seem to be more severe in men who have undergone urinary diversions and who must wear stomal appliances. Continent boys with epispadias should have a single stage penile reconstruction. We do this at about the second birthday as with hypospadias (Winslow, 1988). When the child is incontinent, the bladder neck should be reconstructed prior to that time. Urogenital reconstruction in exstrophy is usually staged, closing the bladder and reconstructing the abdominal wall 24 to 36 hours after birth. The bladder neck should be closed tightly enough so that increased resistance to outflow of urine will encourage bladder development but not so tightly as to cause obstruction or high pressure vesicoureteral reflux. Small bladders should be closed and, if necessary, subsequently augmented with bowel.

At the time a boy is expected to achieve urinary control, the bladder neck is tightened, usually with bilateral ureteral reimplantation. In some patients, a dysgenetic bladder may remain small, but in most the bladder will have improved in capacity. We reconstruct the external genitalia at that time (Winslow et al., 1988). Except in the most severe forms of bladder exstrophy or cloacal exstrophy when the penis or two halves of the bifid penis are truly inadequate, male-to-female sex reassignment is unusual. Even then, if normal testes are present, the success of newer techniques of phallic construction (see subsequent discussion) should support a decision to raise the child as a boy, preserving his reproductive potential through puberty. Remarkable progress has been made in the treatment of difficult cases (Hendren, 1979; Jeffs, 1979; Johnston, 1975 Snyder, 1990). However, many patients need further genital surgery as they experience the genital growth associated with puberty.

The goals of reconstructive surgery in male patients with exstrophy or epispadias are to produce a dangling penis with erectile bodies of satisfactory length and shape to allow sexual function and a urethra that serves

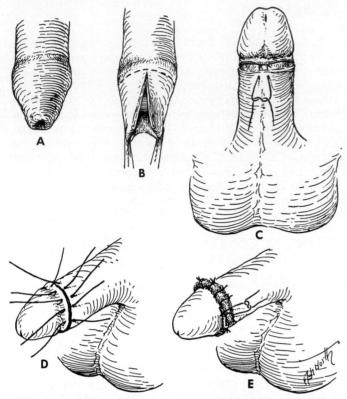

Figure 83–21. Circumcision in a patient with phimosis. *A,* Phimosis to be corrected by circumcision.

B, Incision in the dorsal aspect of the foreskin, which has been drawn over the glans. Broken line indicates point of incision for removal of foreskin.

C, Suture in frenulum.

D, Closure. Note that the sutures have been left long.

E, Sutures are tied around a strip of Xeroform gauze. (From Hand, J. R.: *In* Campbell, M. F., and Harrison, J. H. (Eds.): Urology, Vol. 3, 3rd ed. Philadelphia, W. B. Saunders Co., 1970.)

as a conduit for the passage of urine and ejaculate. Completion of the urethral reconstruction should await complete release and straightening of the penis so that subsequent reconstruction will not be complicated by the need for partial or total reconstruction of a neourethra.

Many patients who have undergone surgery as children do not present for correction of inadequate external genitalia until after they have completed puberty and realize that the situation will not improve. We employ a systematic approach to accomplish the reconstruction necessary to correct the anatomic defects in these patients (Devine et al., 1980; Winslow et al., 1988). Figure 83–22 is an algorithm illustrating the sequence of this process at our medical center and enumerating the individual procedures that may be required to achieve a dangling penis followed by those required to correct the curvature. Surgery is undertaken in a sequential fashion beginning with the simplest procedure, which will achieve the desired functional result.

The W-flap incision allows mobilization of superiorly based random flaps of skin lateral to the base of the penis (Fig. 83–23), affording optimal exposure of the infrapubic region. The penis can then be mobilized by meticulous dissection. When the penis dangles, we proceed using one and then another of several possible

techniques designed to correct intrinsic chordee, until an artificial erection confirms that the penis is straight. We construct a neourethra. In closing the incision, the lower abdominal wall is reconstructed. The bifid escutcheon is brought medially and superiorly into a more normal location by transposing the tips of the W-flap to the midline (Fig. 83–23*C*). Incisions are closed with subcutaneous Vicryl sutures and nylon for the skin. Most patients will also require construction of an umbilicus.

SURGICAL TECHNIQUE

Release and Lengthening of the Penis

The genital dissection is begun by marking a W-shaped skin flap composed of paired superiorly based groin flaps, incorporating the laterally displaced pubic hair on each side of the penis (Fig. 83–23*A*). We excise all of the midline abdominal and penopubic scar tissue and release the attached skin, while preserving the vascularity in the fat layer deep to the skin. The W-flaps have a random vascular distribution.

Care must be taken while mobilizing these flaps in patients who have had inguinal herniorrhaphies—not unusual in exstrophy patients. The presence of herniorrhaphy scars is not a contraindication to use of the W-flap. However, the flap must be more cautiously elevated, preserving all of the remaining blood supply to the tips. A dorsal midline incision in the penile skin may be extended distally to meet a circumcising incision proximal to the corona of the epispadiac glans to expose the shaft of the penis.

A sound placed in the native urethra or neourethra of a patient who has had a previous urethroplasty helps in identifying these structures and avoiding injury to them. Because of the inguinal anomalies associated with exstrophy, the spermatic cord structures may be unusually superficial. On each side they should be identified as the tips of the flaps are elevated. They are mobilized and retracted laterally with Penrose drains (Fig. 83–23*B*). The dorsal penile branches of the pudendal vessels and nerves come onto the dorsal surface laterally at the base of each corporal body and must be preserved in the dissection.

After the flaps are elevated and retracted, we evaluate the corporal bodies. Relative shortening, dorsal chordee, and sometimes torsion of the penis may be caused by one or more of the following factors:

1. Inelastic fibrous bands of scar tissue that attach the penis to the bone or fascia in the anterior part of the ring of the pelvis

2. Shortness of the dorsally placed natural urethra or shortness and possible scarring of a previously constructed neourethra

3. Inelasticity or abnormal attachment of the deeper dartos and Buck's fascial layers

4. Dysgenetic development or inelasticity of the dorsal aspect of the tunica albuginea of the paired corpora cavernosa.

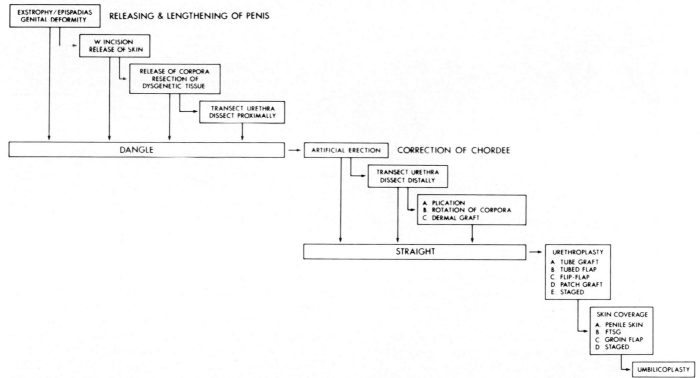

Figure 83–22. Algorithm for repair of the male genital abnormality in exstrophy. This cascade defines the sequence of procedures employed to free the penis so that it dangles, then to straighten the penile shaft and complete the repair. (From Winslow, B. H., et al.: Epispadias and exstrophy of the bladder. *In* Mustarde, J. C., and Jackson, I. T. (Eds.): Plastic Surgery in Infancy and Childhood, 3rd ed. New York, Churchill Livingstone, 1988, p. 526.)

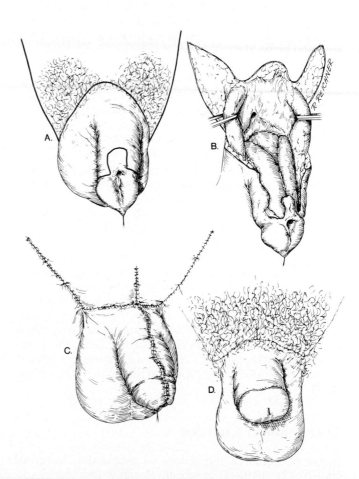

Figure 83–23. Diagram illustrating development of the superiorly based W flap for exposure of the penile shaft and correction of the abnormal distribution of the pubic hair. *A,* The flap is outlined, encompassing the laterally displaced pubic hair.

B, The flap is developed, and the structures of the cord are mobilized and retracted laterally. A midline incision in the skin exposes the penile shaft.

C, At completion of the repair, the penile skin is closed and movement of the limbs of the W flap to the midline has placed the pubic hair above the base of the penis.

D, After healing, the growth of hair hides the scars of the incision.

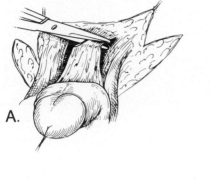

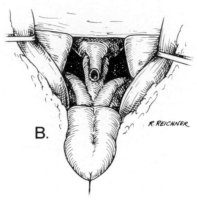

Figure 83–24. Dorsal dissection to get the penis to dangle. *A*, The first step in release of the penis. The fascial band fixing the penis to the rim of the pelvis is being excised.

B, Completion of the dissection. The urethra has been transected, and the corpora have been released from the pubic rami. The corpus spongiosum lies between the divergent corpora cavernosa. (From Winslow, B. H., et al.: Epispadias and exstrophy of the bladder. *In* Mustarde, J. C., and Jackson, I. T. (Eds.): Plastic Surgery in Infancy and Childhood, 3rd ed. New York, Churchill Livingstone, 1988, p. 520.)

We undermine the skin of the penis in order to dissect any restricting tissue from the shaft (Fig. 83–24*A*). If the epispadiac urethra or neourethra prevents release of the penis by this mobilization, we transect the urethra distally and mobilize the proximal portion releasing the very vascular spongy tissue of the corpus spongiosum, which lies deep to the urethra in the midline between the divergent proximal ends of the corporal bodies. Bleeding from the thin-walled venous spaces of the corpus spongiosum may be troublesome, if the structure is injured in the course of the dissection. This bleeding is best controlled by pressure during the dissection and by placement of sutures after the dissection has been completed. The dissection is continued, releasing the proximal portions of the erectile bodies from their attachment to the widespread inferior pubic rami and excising the dysgenetic scar tissue encountered during the dissection (Fig. 83–24*B*). We have not completely detached the corpora, as has been described (Kelley and Eraklis, 1971), for fear of devascularizing the corporal bodies.

When at any point in this dissection the penis has been released so that it dangles, we move to the next stage of the algorithm to straighten the penile shaft. When the penis dangles, there can be some recession at its base, but this will not be of concern after the pubic hair has grown back. The divergent corporal bodies cause the base of the penis to be wide; however, sewing the corporal bodies together to narrow the base of the penis would also shorten the penile shaft. In one patient who had previously undergone an ileal conduit diversion, we were able to gain additional penile length by releasing the retained base of the bladder and advancing it with the proximal end of the urethra, as it was reconstructed as a conduit for the ejaculate. If urethral reconstruction is not undertaken at this time, the proximal urethra should be released and brought between the corporal bodies to open on the underside of the penis.

Correction of Chordee

After release of the penis, we assess the degree of chordee by artificial erection. Because the corpora in

exstrophy/epispadias do not communicate, an artificial erection requires two needles, with injection of sterile physiologic saline into each corporal body (Fig. 83–25*A*). If at artificial erection, the penis is found to be straight, further dissection is not required. This finding seldom is the case—usually, the penis is not straight. We identify the location, direction, and degree of curvature and proceed with its correction. After each step in the sequence of this process, shaft straightness is reassessed with another artificial erection. When the penis is straight, we proceed with urethral construction and penile shaft skin coverage.

The first step in the correction of chordee involves resection of all dysgenetic restrictive bands from the dorsal surface of the corporal bodies, carefully preserv-

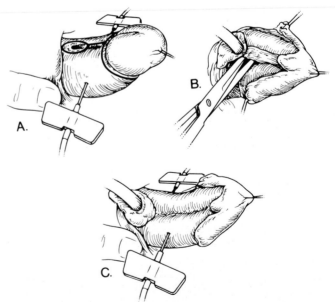

Figure 83–25. Distal dissection to release chordee. *A*, In exstrophy and epispadias, the corpora cavernosa do not communicate and it will be necessary to place a needle in each corpus to achieve an artificial erection. An incision is marked surrounding the urethral meatus and in the skin proximal to the corona of the glans.

B, The urethra is released, and fibrous tissue in the distal midline is being excised. A midline flap is developed in the glans for reconstruction of the urethra.

C, Despite the dissection, ventral chordee persists.

ing the dorsolateral vessels and nerves (Figs. 83–25*B* and 83–25*C*). If chordee persists and the urethra is shown to restrict the dorsum, it is transected and mobilized from the proximal portion of the corporal bodies. Usually, the distal portion of the urethra must also be mobilized, excising all of the dysgenetic tissues remaining on the dorsal aspect of the corporal bodies, sparing the dorsal vessels and nerves (see Fig. 83–25*C*).

If chordee persists following this dissection, the problem will be related to dysgenetic development of the corporal bodies themselves. Three treatment options are possible depending on the extent and location of the chordee.

1. Excision of ellipses of tunica from the convex, in this case *ventral*, aspect of the corporal bodies and approximation of the cut edges can straighten the penis (Fig. 83–26*A*). This technique tends to shorten the length of what is already a short penis but is especially useful for the patient who has a well-functioning urethra that should be preserved (Horton and Devine, 1973; Vorstman and Devine, 1987).

2. Koff (1984) has described inward corporal rotation to correct chordee. After mobilizing the ventral aspects of the corporal bodies, we place several deep midline polydioxanone sutures to rotate the corporal bodies

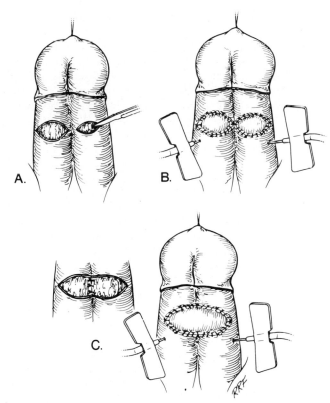

Figure 83–27. Correction of chordee with dermal graft. *A,* Transverse incisions are made in the dorsal aspect of the corporal bodies.

B, A lenticular dermal graft is placed in each of these defects or *(C)* the medial ends of the incision are sewn together with 5–0 polydioxanone sutures, and the conjoined defect is closed with a simple dermal graft.

inward, attaching them in the midline. If the artificial erection now shows the penis to be straight, we incise the tunica of each corporal body and join them by suturing the respective edges together to assure persistence of the rotation (Fig. 83–26*B*).

3. Most commonly, we lengthen the dorsal aspect of the corpora by insertion of a dermal graft. During an artificial erection, we mark the dorsal aspect of each of the corporal bodies at the point of maximum concavity. Incisions at these marks extending from the midline medially to the midline laterally allow the tunica to elongate, leaving erectile tissue exposed (Fig. 83–27*A*). To preserve the increased length, the defects are patched with dermal grafts. We can apply lenticular-shaped grafts, each individually placed in the defects in the corpus (Fig. 83–27*B*). However, in most cases, we approximate the medial aspects of the incisions in the midline and cover the merged defect with a single dermal graft (Fig. 83–27*C*). Because of the contraction that all grafts undergo, this graft should be 30 per cent larger than the size of the defect in the tunica, measured while stretching the corporal body over a finger.

Urethral Construction

At this point, the shaft of the penis should be straight and free to dangle. In each case, the complexity of the procedures required and of those that will be necessary to create a urethra determines whether completion of

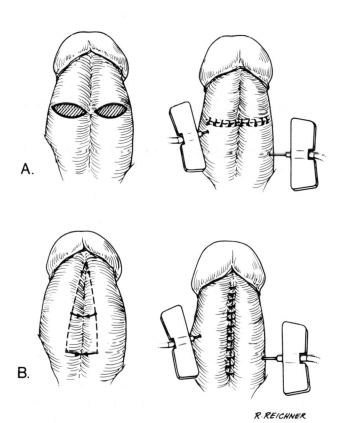

R·REICHNER

Figure 83–26. *A,* Nesbit's type ellipses are excised from the ventral aspect of the two erectile bodies. Closure of these can straighten chordee.

B, Koff's procedure. The corporal bodies are rotated to the midline and tacked in place. If this maneuver corrects the chordee, a longitudinal incision is made in the tunica and the rotation is fixed with polydioxanone sutures. (From Winslow, B. H., et al.: Epispadias and exstrophy of the bladder. *In* Mustarde, J. C., and Jackson, I. T. (Eds.): Plastic Surgery in Infancy and Childhood, 3rd ed. New York, Churchill Livingstone, 1988, p. 527.)

the reconstruction is to be staged or accomplished at the time of this operation. We avoid graft/graft interfaces because a potential exists for interference with take in an area where grafts overly each other. If we have needed a dermal graft to straighten the penis, and it appears that an FTSG will be necessary for the urethroplasty, it might be advisable to proceed with urethral construction at another stage. We would not construct the urethra with a tube graft at this stage unless it could be placed in the ventral groove between the corpora without overlapping the grafts. It is preferable to complete the urethral construction in one stage, and this may be possible utilizing one of two techniques: (1) a tubed graft of full-thickness skin can be brought to the ventral aspect of the penis by passing it between the corporal bodies at its base, keeping it away from the deramal graft, and (2) a flap of ventral penile skin tubed to form a urethra can be brought between the corpora to rest on the dermal graft and can even help furnish a vascular bed for it (Duckett, 1981).

For patients with epispadias and for patients with exstrophy who still have sufficient penile skin, we prefer the skin from the ventrum of the penis for the urethral construction. However, if redundant penile skin is not available, we construct a full-thickness tube graft from the relatively thin and hairless skin taken from the abdominal wall adjacent to the anterior superior iliac spine over the crest of the ilium.

In pediatric patients, we fashion the graft into a tube measuring about 15 Fr., which with graft maturation will become a urethra measuring about 12 Fr. The tube is anastomosed in a widely spatulated fashion to bridge the gap between the native proximal urethra and the tip of the glans penis (Fig. 83–28). After placing the neourethral graft tube, it is splayed by securing it along its length with sutures placed between the dermal surface of the graft and the tunica of the corpora, minimizing the dead space and speeding acquisition of its new blood supply by increasing the surface area of the graft in apposition to its vascularized tissue bed. The intimate graft host bed relationship encourages the ingrowth of new blood vessels. The dorsal glans wings, created by the development of the glans flap, are closed around the neourethra to place the urethral meatus in the tip of the glans. In some patients presenting for secondary exstrophy reconstruction, the midline abdominal skin will not be scarred, and the tumble-tube method of urethroplasty described by Snyder (1990) may be helpful.

If a patient has undergone previous urinary diversion, construction of a urethra may not be necessary and coverage of the penis completes the procedure. However, a sinus must be created in order to allow the escape of prostatic secretion and ejaculate and to avoid the collection of these fluids in a suprapubic cyst. The sinus may be placed in the abdominal wall above the base of the penis or the bladder neck. The posterior urethra may be formed into a tube and brought out between the corpora to open in the skin below the penis. A man with such an arrangement could be fertile. Some men who have undergone urinary diversion wish to ejaculate through the penis. We have constructed a

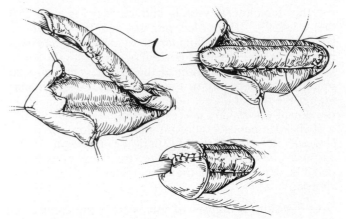

Figure 83–28. Skin graft urethroplasty. A full-thickness skin graft is formed into a tube around a plastic stent. A tongue is left at the base to be spatulated into an incision in the urethra, and a V is left distally into which the midline flap in the glans is inserted. The tube is fixed to the tunica, and the glans wings are brought around to place the meatus at the tip of the penis.

urethra from an FTSG or a tubed flap for this purpose. However, such a defunctionalized reconstructed urethra may tend to stenose.

Escutcheon Repair in Exstrophy

In exstrophy, as part of the midline abnormality, the hair-bearing skin of the escutcheon is located lateral to the penis and scrotum. Usually there is no umbilicus, the cord having entered from the upper edge of the exstrophic bladder. When present, the umbilicus is caudally displaced and prone to form a hernia. The lower abdominal wall exhibits diastasis recti, and this lower midline area may be considerably scarred in patients who have had previous surgery and/or urinary diversion. The escutcheon can be reconstructed rotating the flaps of W-skin to the midline, bringing the hair-bearing skin medially and simultaneously contouring the suprapubic area (see Fig. 83–23C and 83–23D). The large amount of dead space created by the elevation of these flaps needs to be drained. We utilize two small suction drains.

Skin Coverage

If possible, coverage of the penile shaft is accomplished with flaps of local skin. These tissues provide proper sensation and are of appropriate pigmentation. However, in many of these multiply operated patients, skin coverage of the penis is a problem. The remaining genital skin may be scarred and insufficient to cover the length of the straightened penis. If well vascularized, the penile shaft can be covered with a skin graft. If a dermal graft has been employed to correct chordee or a tubed FTSG has been employed to create a neourethra and there is insufficient penile skin, we would not choose an FTSG to cover the penile shaft. Local flaps must be developed to cover the penis—we have used a groin flap (Devine, 1979). Revision of the penile skin coverage can be done in 6 months. Often, the skin of the penis and the graft or flap will have become so elastic that at the time of scar revision we will have been able to excise the redundant tissue and close the wound primarily.

Umbilicoplasty

Not having an umbilicus is a disturbing defect for many younger patients with exstrophy and, for them, reconstruction of the umbilicus is important. One of our patients who was an excellent swimmer had resigned from his swimming team when he realized that his competition bathing suit would make him look different from the other members of his team. An umbilicus is constructed by elevating a small superiorly based semicircular flap in the midline at the level of the iliac crests. After removing the subcutaneous fat and exposing the fascia of the abdominal wall, the flap is sutured to the fascia with 5–0 PDS. The remaining defect at the lower edge of this wound is covered by a graft of full-thickness or split-thickness skin (Fig. 83–29). Taking the graft from the area of the genitalia creates a color contrast further emphasizing the umbilicus.

Urethroplasty as a Second Stage

When it has been necessary to stage the urethral construction, the second stage is carried out 6 to 9 months after healing has occurred. If there is smooth and soft redundant skin on the penis, that skin can be chosen for the urethra. After confirming the straightness of the penis with an artificial erection, we outline and incise a central strip of dorsal skin wide enough to construct the urethra. We elevate the skin lateral to this central strip and secure it into a tube over an appropriately sized catheter, placing the urethral meatus at the tip of the glans. The strip of skin must not be undermined and should be handled meticulously to prevent tissue damage and devascularization, which could lead to stricture or fistula formation. We approximate the edges of the neourethra with interrupted 5–0 chromic catgut sutures, tying the knots in the lumen. We close

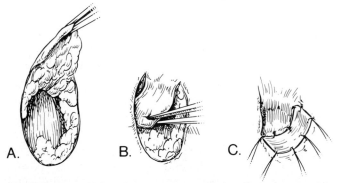

Figure 83–29. Umbilicoplasty. *A,* A cranially based semicircular flap is elevated.
B, The subcutaneous fat is removed, and the flap is secured to the fascia with polydioxanone or Prolene sutures.
C, A split-thickness graft is placed to cover the defect.

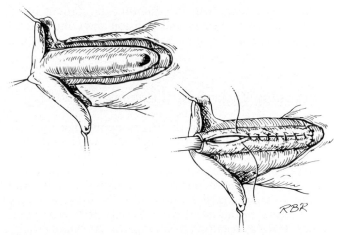

Figure 83–30. Urethroplasty as a second stage. A midline strip of skin is marked and incised but not undermined. The skin of the penis is undermined. The edges of the skin flap are approximated with interrupted sutures and a subcutaneous running polydioxanone suture. The wings of the glans are brought around, and the skin of the penis is closed.

it watertight, with a running 6–0 PDS involving only the dermis of the skin and turning the epithelial edges inside (Fig. 83–30). The dorsal glans wings are approximated to cover the distal urethra. If there is a urethra in the glans, we anastomose the new tube to it over the indwelling catheter. We remove this urethral catheter after insertion of a percutaneous suprapubic catheter and leave a soft silicone stent in the neourethra.

RECONSTRUCTION FOLLOWING TRAUMA

Fracture of the Penis

Acute management of fracture of the penis is covered elsewhere in this book. Fractures occur when the penis is erect. Two factors contribute to the rigidity of the penis: (1) the corporal bodies are distended to near central arterial pressure, stretching the tunica and its internal fibrous framework to the limit of their stretch, and (2) the midline septum is also stretched tightly between the dorsal and ventral tunica albuginea, creating the ultimate vertical rigidity. In young patients with firm erections, vertical rigidity is solid and bends occur in a lateral direction. With lateral buckling, the tunica albuginea tears. Some patients who have sustained a fracture of the penis will have a history of congenital curvature of the penis. One of our patients with Peyronie's disease fractured his penis the weekend prior to his consultation with us. We favor immediate exploration and repair of a fracture of the penis because tears of the tunica managed "conservatively" heal with a scar, which may cause a disabling distortion of the penis.

The goal of reconstruction following fracture of the penis is correction of the curvature. The surgery is not unlike surgery for other cases of curvature of the penis. The curve can be corrected by excising the scar and replacing it with a dermal graft or by excising an ellipse of tunica from the convex aspect of the tunica contralateral to the scar. Not infrequently, the patient has a larger than average penis and excision and contralateral tuck offer the advantage of more rapid healing with a less complex postoperative course.

Penetrating Trauma of the Penis

Penetrating injuries of the penis involve the urethra, the corporal bodies, or both. Our choice when managing an acute injury would be to explore it surgically and to attempt immediate repair, perhaps placing a suprapubic tube. Later reconstruction will be directed at a urethral stricture, which might develop from the urethral injury or curvature of the penis from damage to the corporal bodies. Fistulas resulting from penetrating trauma to the penis are often treated by primary closure and imposition of superficial tissue layers between the urethra and the skin. Large fistulas may require more complex tissue transfer to correct the urethral defect. These principles are discussed elsewhere in this chapter.

Amputation of the Penis

Amputation is the ultimate penile injury. If the patient presents acutely with the amputated distal part of his penis, microvascular replantation is the favored approach. If there is no microvascular surgeon at the center where he presents, the patient should be transferred. The penis should be cleaned, wrapped in a sponge soaked in sterile saline, and placed in a sterile plastic Ziploc bag. This is kept in ice water, and replantation can be accomplished as long as 18 hours following amputation. Often, the amputation is self-inflicted, usually during an acute mental crisis. This should not preclude replantation unless the patient adamantly refuses such treatment. The patient's condition of other circumstances may prevent his transfer for microvascular replantation. If so, replantation by the technique described by McRoberts (1968) should be carried out. His series showed that a high degree of success can be expected following replantation without microvascular reanastomosis.

If the patient presents with the distal part having been disposed of or otherwise unavailable, the wound should be closed. Often the penis will have been stretched out during the amputation, and an excess of skin will have been removed leaving a length of intact but denuded shaft structures proximal to the amputation wound. We close the corporal bodies with 4–0 or 5–0 PDS, spatulate the urethral meatus to the tunica, and immediately cover the penile shaft with an STSG. Others would bury the shaft beneath the skin of the scrotum. In some of these patients, primary grafting of the stump will allow a functional penis. However, most require phallic/penile reconstruction.

A number of sophisticated techniques for reconstruction of the traumatized penis are available. The radial forearm flap has become the mainstay of penile reconstructive procedures (see subsequent discussion). The initial stage of reconstruction of the amputated penis consists of mobilizing the penile and urethral stumps.

Shaft coverage as well as neourethra construction can then be accomplished by microneurovascular transfer of a free flap. We believe that the "cricket-bat" modification of the radial forearm flap offers advantages in the reconstruction of traumatized patients. The portion of the flap designed to repair the urethra can be shortened or lengthened to accommodate the existing urethra, and the portion of the flap designed for shaft coverage can also be tailored in length.

Degloving Injuries of the Penis

Degloving injuries occur when the skin of the penis or scrotum is trapped and stripped from the deeper structures, exposing the uninjured corpora and the testicles. The tear is in the elastic dartos fascia. Bleeding is usually not a problem, because there are not many large vessels in this space. The appearance of the bare testicles and penile shaft, however, is impressive.

After defining the extent of the damage, most degloving injuries can be managed acutely with immediate reconstruction by application of STSGs. The shaft is covered with a sheet graft of split-thickness skin. The testicles are sutured together in the midline, pexed in their anatomically correct position, and covered with a meshed STSG. After take of this graft, the meshing gives the appearance of rugations. With time, the effect of gravity on the testicles causes the reconstructed scrotum to become pendulous and sometimes even redundant. In this repair, STSGs are more successful than FTSGs, because the host bed will be less than optimal following a degloving injury. Although split-thickness grafts cannot be employed for urethroplasty, contraction has not been a problem with such grafts applied to the penile shaft or testicles. Split-thickness skin itself never becomes sensate, but adequate shaft sensation is achieved via the deep structures through the graft.

Some surgeons bury the shaft of the penis in a subcutaneous tunnel on the abdomen and bury the testicles in subcutaneous thigh pouches. McDougal (1983) has described a technique to mobilize the buried testicles with the overlying thigh skin, combining scrotal reconstruction with testicular replacement. In patients so managed, this is a good way of transposing the testicles and overlying tissues to an anatomically correct location. When we have managed patients who have been previously managed acutely with the placement of testicles and penis in subcutaneous tunnels, we have mobilized the testicles and the penile shaft from their tunnels and immediately applied grafts of split-thickness skin, as previously described.

Genital Burns

The ability to reconstruct the damage caused by genital burns often depends on how well the normal structures have been maintained following the acute injury. Careful debridement is the rule in acute management of genital burns. Corporal tissue cannot be replaced with transferred tissue. The physiologic functions of genital tissues cannot be accurately duplicated.

The unique vascularity of genital tissue allows for less aggressive rather than more aggressive debridement.

Devastating urethral injuries occur with many burns. Reconstruction of the urethra is dependent on the nature of the injury. When the urethra has been nearly obliterated, there will not be sufficient uninvolved, nonhirsute local genital tissue that could be transferred for urethral reconstruction. Vascularized tissue must be imported to support reconstruction of the urethra with a graft. In many patients, the penis will have become incarcerated in contracted scar tissue after healing of the acute injury. Successful transposition of a gracilis musculocutaneous flap introduces complaint vascular tissue and skin into the area allowing release of the penile shaft (see Fig. 83–4). Subsequently, the penile shaft can be covered with an STSG. In some patients, the genital scarring is so severe that microvascular transfer of a free flap is necessary to replace the penile shaft.

For many patients, reconstruction will require a number of stages. In several of our patients, the urethra has been obliterated literally from the entry of the membranous urethra into the bulbospongiosus to the tip of the penis. A perineal urethrostomy has been required while transfer of vascular tissues to the area of the perineum and penis was being accomplished. When these tissues are in place, subsequent reconstruction of the urethra can be carried out, with extragenital FTSGs, meshed split-thickness grafts, or bladder epithelial grafts.

Radiation Trauma

Radiation trauma to the penis occurs in two patient subsets: (1) patients in whom radiation has been used therapeutically for a lesion on the penis and (2) those in whom radiation to the pelvis has caused chronic lymphedema. Therapeutic radiation can produce chronic suppurative gangrene. These lesions are not amenable to reconstruction and are best managed by partial penectomy and later by reconstruction. Also, we have treated several patients who developed tissue atrophy and further fibrosis following radiation therapy for Peyronie's disease. Delivered at a near tumoricidal dose, this radiation made dermal graft repair much more difficult. Patients with lymphedema can undergo reconstruction.

Lymphedema of the penis involves the tissues of the dartos fascia and the dermis layer of the skin. In the penis, the lymphedematous tissue can be excised by removing the dartos fascia and skin, dissecting in the layer above Buck's fascia. In the scrotum the external spermatic fascia and skin of the scrotum must be removed. When the lymphedematous tissue has been excised, the testicles will be free and, as in a degloving injury, they must be fixed in the midline in an anatomically correct position. Often scrotal skin peripheral to the edema will be normal and can be advanced to cover the testicles. The shaft of the penis should be covered with an STSG. If the scrotum cannot be closed, a meshed STSG is utilized to cover the testicles. Grafts provide optimal reconstruction in these patients.

Split-thickness skin carries little of the reticular dermis, with minimal lymphatic channels, and does not reaccumulate significant lymphedema. Full-thickness skin, however, contains the lympatic spaces in the dermis. Reaccumulation of lymphedema can occur within the graft. Local skin flaps should be avoided. They seldom give good cosmetic results, and often they will reaccumulate lymph once they have been transposed to the area of the genitalia. As previously noted, grafts do not develop sensation. However, good sensation usually develops, derived from the deep structures. The glans almost never accumulates disabling edema, and the sensation of the glans remains intact because the lymphedematous tissue has been excised in the plane superficial to Buck's fascia, sparing the dorsal nerves of the penis.

We have managed one patient who had organic impotence in addition to chronic lymphedema. He wanted the lymphedematous tissue excised but also desired that a prosthesis be implanted. With lymphedema involving all of the genital tissues, he was not considered to be a good candidate for a hydraulic device. An articulated prosthesis was selected. After excision of the lymphedematous tissue, the articulated device was placed in the penis via subcoronal corporotomies, which were meticulously closed. The subcuticular tissue of the glans was superimposed over the closures of the corporotomy, and an STSG was placed on the shaft of the penis. He had an excellent cosmetic and functional result. We believe that placement of a prosthesis at the same time as the graft carried a diminished possibility of morbidity compared with placement of a prosthesis beneath the graft at a later stage.

Direct radiation to the penis can cause urethral injury. However, it is unusual for the urethra to be injured without damage to adjacent structures. Often, because of the vascularity of the corpus spongiosum, minimal debridement can be accomplished leaving the patient with a fistula that can be reconstructed at a later date. The success of such reconstruction depends on the damage that the radiation has done to the adjacent structures.

DELAYED RECONSTRUCTION OF FEMALE URETHRAL INJURIES

Delayed repair of female urethral injuries may be necessary following pelvic fracture or vaginal surgery. The complexities of subsequent management will depend on the initial injury or surgery. After a pelvic fracture in the female, we would encourage an immediate attempt to restore the continuity of the urethra. Even if not completely successful, a spatulated urethral anastomosis with closure of the vaginal mucosa will facilitate further management. Similarly, if a urethral injury is recognized during vaginal surgery, a repair should be performed, even though some patients who undergo repair primarily will later develop a urethrovaginal fistula and will require subsequent surgery. A delayed urethrovaginal fistula may develop after urethral diverticulectomy or anterior vaginal repair or after treatment of tumors with radiation therapy. Management in these cases is complicated by the relation of the injury to the continence mechanism.

The location and degree of injury also influence the necessity and technique of repair. A distal urethrovaginal fistula may require no therapy or may even remain unrecognized. If symptomatic, because of spraying of the stream within the vagina, division of the urethrovaginal septum with primary closure or with suturing it open is successful. We favor a primary repair. Proximal fistulas are more difficult to repair, especially if the continence mechanism has been affected. In addition, it is important to determine if associated injuries to the bladder and ureters are present prior to planning any repair.

A proximal urethrovaginal fistula can be repaired by excision of the tract and closure of the urethra and vagina. Closure should invert the mucosa into the lumen of the appropriate space to facilitate healing. Interposing a flap of local tissue helps to optimize the healing process and prevents recurrence. The simplest approach would be to use local vaginal tissues. Other options include a labial fat pad, a gracilis muscle, or an omentum as the situation dictates. Of these, the labial fat pad would seem to be the simplest, providing excellent results (Webster et al., 1984). This approach is suitable for small fistulas, regardless of etiology. After surgery or trauma, we wait a minimum of 3, but almost 6 months before attempting a repair. In a patient who has a fistula following radiation therapy, it is better to wait 6 months.

Obliteration of the urethra may occur after pelvic fracture when a complete disruption has occurred and primary alignment has been performed. The importance of preoperative assessment cannot be overemphasized. If the bladder neck appears intact by antegrade cystoscopy through the suprapubic tract and if retrograde urethroscopy reveals a blind-ending urethra, primary repair should be performed. The bladder should be opened and the vesical neck identified. The retropubic space is entered and the proximal end of the urethra identified with the aid of a sound passed through the bladder neck. A similar dissection can identify the severed distal urethra. With as little mobilization as possible, a tension-free, end-to-end, spatulated anastomosis is performed with interrupted sutures. We have used omentum to fill the dead space and to help with healing (Ganesan et al., 1989). A similar technique has been described by Lee and Lee (1988). If the obliteration cannot be repaired, bladder augmentation with creation of a continent catheterizable stoma can be performed.

After reconstruction, some patients experience urinary incontinence. Both urgency and stress incontinence have been reported. A small capacity, poorly compliant bladder may be the result of long-term suprapubic catheterization or may be secondary to the original injury. If medical therapy is unsuccessful, a bladder augmentation will be necessary. A noncompliant urethra can be seen after pelvic fracture with or without disruption of urethral continuity. Our first choice, as that of others (Woodside, 1987), would be to perform a fascial sling procedure. However, in some patients, bladder neck reconstruction using the Young-Dees technique, usually associated with bladder augmentation, may also be necessary.

URETHRAL STRICTURE

Definition

A urethral stricture is a scar resulting from tissue injury or destruction. Contracture of this inelastic scar shortens the circumference of the urethra and reduces the lumen. If a normal urethra measures 30 Fr., its diameter is 10 mm, and the area of its lumen is about $78 mm^2$. If scarring halves the circumference to 15 Fr., its diameter will be 5 mm, reducing the area of the lumen about 25 per cent of normal with significant urodynamic effects.

Anatomy and Etiology

At its proximal end, the urethra is continuous with the epithelium of the bladder neck and trigone. Anatomically we speak of its anterior and posterior divisions. The posterior urethra is the portion proximal to its entry into the bulb, and the anterior urethra lies distal to that point contained within the corpus spongiosum. Division of the urethra into at least five components is more useful in making decisions about surgical therapy of lesions of the urethra (see Fig. 83–6), which are defined as follows:

1. The prostatic urethra proximal to the verumontanum is surrounded by the prostatic glandular tissue.
2. The membranous urethra traverses the deep perineal pouch, where it is surrounded by the external urethral sphincter. This segment of the posterior urethra is essentially unattached to fixed structures, and anterior urethral strictures will often extend into this portion of the urethra.
3. The bulbous urethra is invested by the bulbospongiosum and covered by the midline fusion of the bulbospongiosus muscles.
4. The penile or pendulous urethra, still invested in the corpus spongiosum, lies distal to the suspensory ligaments of the penis.
5. The fossa navicularis is the portion of the urethra within the erectile tissue of the glans penis terminating at the junction of the urethral epithelium with the skin of the glans.

Diagnosis and Evaluation

The scar of urethra stricture is the result of trauma or inflammation. External trauma is caused by an injury in which usually the urethra is crushed against the pubis or by a more severe injury causing a fracture of the pelvis and a distraction or a tearing of the membranous urethra. Internal trauma is usually iatrogenic and associated with the passage of instruments, indwelling urethral catheters, or transurethral surgery. Catheters can also cause inflammation, which penetrates into the glands of Littre, sometimes forming subepithelial microabscesses. Gonorrhea is probably still the most common infection causing urethral stricture, although with early treatment it is less likely that a stricture will follow an uncomplicated episode of gonorrhea. Urethritis caused by *Chlamydia* or *Ureaplasma* has not been positively linked to the occurrence of strictures. This possibility must be suspected, however, in patients who present with an inflammatory stricture without a history of gonorrhea. Today, most urethral strictures are caused by external trauma.

The presence of a stricture is suspected from the history of obstructive symptoms with slowing of the urinary stream, frequency, nocturia, sometimes dysuria, and recurrent urinary tract infections. A stricture in the urethra can also be associated with recurrent prostatitis and epididymitis. Some patients are found to have a stricture when an attempt at passing a catheter in the emergency room or prior to some major surgical procedure has been unsuccessful. The inability to pass this catheter confirms the presence of a stricture. When the catheter will not pass, the nature of the obstruction must be determined. The precise anatomy and character of a stricture must be defined before a plan of treatment is devised. Radiographs and urethroscopy can determine the length and location of the stricture. The depth and density of the scar in the spongy tissue may be deduced from the physical examination, the appearance of the urethra on the contrast studies, the amount of elasticity noted at urethroscopy, and the depth and density of the fibrosis evidenced during real time ultrasound evaluation of the urethra, after it has been filled with lubricating jelly (McAninch et al., 1988).

Radiography must include dynamic studies done while retrograde injection of the contrast material is taking place or while the patient is voiding (Fig. 83–31) (McCallum, 1979). More than one projection may be necessary to visualize the stricture (Fig. 83–32). Radiographic studies should be carried out with contrast material suitable for intravenous injection as, even with gentle technique, extravasation may occur (Fig. 83–33). Contrast material thickened with lubricating jelly may be the source of problems.

These studies are best carried out under the supervision of the surgeon who will be treating the patient and who can proceed with cystoscopic examination when the studies are complete. Development of the flexible urethroscope has simplified this examination. With local anesthesia, there will be little discomfort. The scope can be passed to the stricture before dilating it, and beyond the stricture into the bladder after dilation. Other features of the urethrogram must be considered. Evidence is often present of loss of elasticity in the urethra proximal and distal to the stricture, and the full length of the involved urethra must be treated. During voiding, pressure generated by the bladder is transmitted to the urethra proximal to the stenosis. If normal, this segment of the urethra will be dilated during the voiding urethrogram.

Irregularity or "coning down" of the urethra illustrates its involvement in the scar (Fig. 83–31E and F).

It has been kept dilated by the hydraulic pressure, and unless this segment is included in the repair, it will contract after the obstruction is relieved, causing a recurrence of the stricture. During surgery it is important to evaluate the urethra proximal and distal to the stricture with bougienage and cystoscopy to be sure that all of the involved urethra has been included in the repair.

Treatment

The anatomy of strictures varies (Fig. 83–34), and so must treatment. Treatment is considered in two contexts: cure and management. Urethral strictures have long been managed by trying the simplest treatment first, and only if that were unsuccessful would treatment proceed to more complex or more difficult procedures. Strictures would be dilated. An internal urethrotomy or several would be attempted before the consideration of an open surgical procedure. Usually, the "classic" multistaged procedures, although considered "more forgiving," are fraught with complications. Dissatisfaction with these operations has encouraged this sequence of temporizing procedures called the reconstructive ladder.

The development and application of very successful surgical procedures designed to take advantage of modern tissue transfer techniques have outdated this reconstructive ladder. Figure 83–35 is an algorithm matching the anatomy of the stricture with the methods of treatment, with the goal being cure of the stricture. If a patient has a stricture known to respond to a simple procedure, he should be offered that procedure. A more complex stricture should be treated with a more complex procedure dictated by the anatomy of the stricture. Long-term functional and cosmetic results rather than the simplicity of the procedure should govern the choice of therapy.

Urethral dilation and internal urethrotomy have a place in the treatment of strictures. They can be curative for strictures involving epithelium alone or those involving superficial spongiofibrosis. Dilation is usually a management tool only. If dilation is to be effective, it must be carried out without further traumatizing the urethra. It is not a one-time only treatment and should not disrupt the stricture but should gradually stretch it. When the area of fibrosis is torn, bleeding and further fibrosis occur, with increased scar formation and increased length, depth, and density of the stricture.

When we suspect that a patient has a urethral stricture, we fill the urethra with lubricating jelly containing a local anesthetic and attempt to pass a No. 14 Fr. coudé tip catheter (Rusch Coudé-tipped catheters, Catalog No. 221800, Rusch, Inc., 2450 Meadowbrook Pkwy., Duluth, Georgia 30136). If this catheter does not pass easily, we make a urethrogram. Employing filiforms and followers or inserting a guide wire, using a flexible urethroscope, and passing Cook dilators, the urethra is stretched. We would not use van Buren sounds smaller than 16 or 18 Fr. because the tips of these sounds are sharp enough to penetrate the urethra and cause a false passage. Filiforms with a coudé or spiral tip are less difficult to pass than straight ones and are

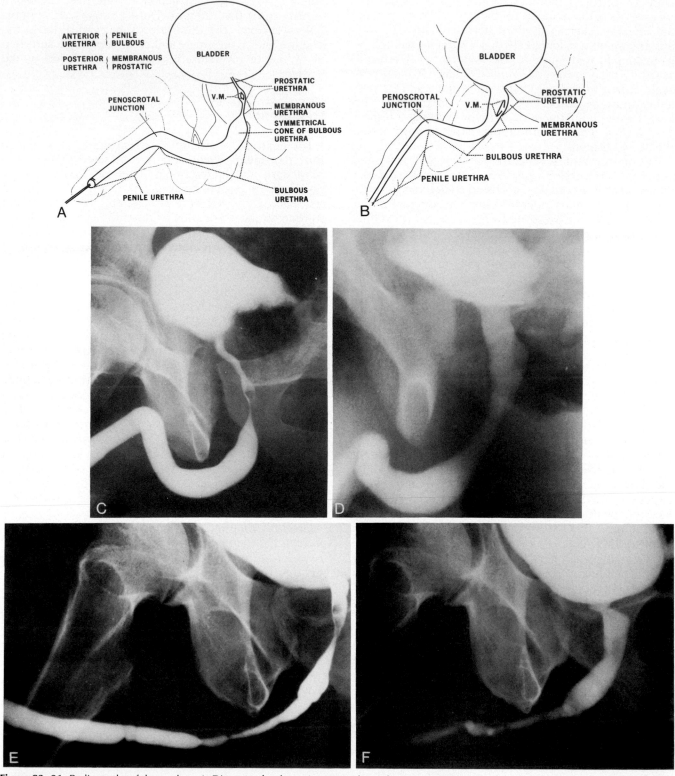

Figure 83–31. Radiographs of the urethra. *A*, Diagram of a dynamic retrograde urethrogram.
B, Diagram of a dynamic voiding urethrogram.
C, Normal retrograde urethrogram.
D, Normal voiding urethrogram. (From McCallum, R. W.: Urol. Clin. North Am., 17:227, 1979.)
E, Retrograde urethrogram—urethral stricture.
F, Voiding urethrogram—urethral stricture. (Note the evidence of urethral involvement proximal and distal to the tight part of the stricture.)

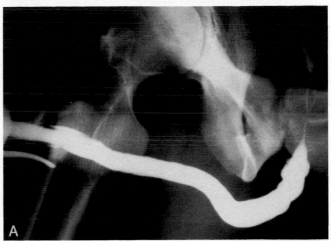

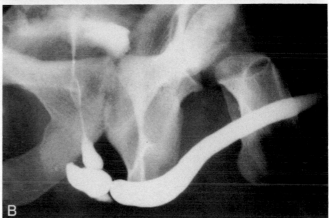

Figure 83–32. *A,* A right posterior oblique dynamic retrograde urethrogram does not define the situation. Contrast material flows past an irregular area in the posterior bulb and through the tonic external sphincter outlining the verumontanum.

B, A left posterior oblique dynamic retrograde urethrogram shows two strictures joined by a diverticulum.

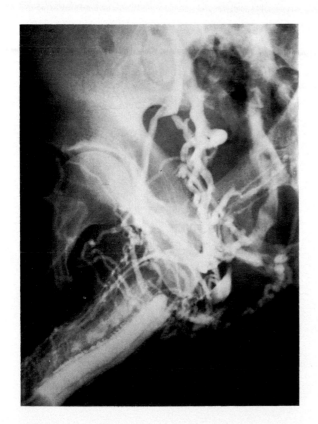

Figure 83–33. Venogram of the penis, pelvis, and inferior vena cava following gentle retrograde urethrogram. (From Horton, C. E., and Devine, P. C.: Strictures of the male urethra. *In* Converse, J. M. (Ed.): Reconstructive Plastic Surgery. Philadelphia, W. B. Saunders Co., 1977.)

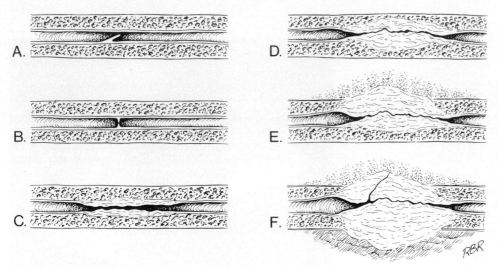

Figure 83–34. The anatomy of strictures. *A*, Mucosal fold.

B, Iris constriction.

C, Full-thickness involvement with minimal inflammation in the spongy tissue.

D, Full-thickness spongiofibrosis.

E, Inflammation and fibrosis involving tissues outside the corpus spongiosum.

F, Complex stricture complicated by a fistula. This can proceed to the formation of an abscess, or the fistula may open to the skin or the rectum. In many strictures, especially those associated with fracture of the pelvis, no continuity will occur between the two ends of the urethra.

followed with woven Phillips catheters, not with LeFort sounds.

After obtaining urine for a culture, we fill the bladder with contrast material and obtain a voiding urethrogram. In the past, if the configuration or the density of the stricture made it difficult to pass larger instruments, we would have left this follower in the urethra and begun a course of dilation by changing to a larger catheter every 2 or 3 days. Today, we insert a suprapubic tube and plan another treatment. Such a stricture will probably call for open surgery.

Dilation

We do not dilate urethral strictures past 24 Fr. and sometimes it takes weeks to attain this caliber. After passing the small catheter, we begin with an 18 Fr. sound and pass larger sounds in sequence until there is resistance—then we stop. The patient will be able to void, and because he has not been hurt he will return for further treatment. (If he has been hurt, he will not return for treatment until he is in trouble again.) We ask him to return at weekly intervals, passing one or two larger sounds at each visit.

When a 24 Fr. sound passes with ease, we double the time between calibrations. Intermittent dilation is a management technique. If dilation were curative, no subsequent treatment should be required. However, dilation can be an acceptable modality if the interval between the need for treatment is between 6 and 12 months.

Recurrent obstructive symptoms requiring shortening

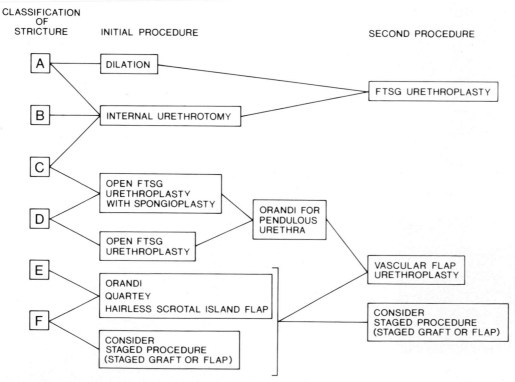

Figure 83–35. Algorithm for selection of the modality of treatment as dictated by the anatomy of the stricture. (From Jordan, G. H.: Management of anterior urethral stricture disease. *In* Webster, G. D. (Ed.): Problems in Urology. Philadelphia, J. B. Lippincott Co., 1987.)

of this interval are evidence of a change in the character of the stricture, which will probably necessitate a change in its treatment. Also, because changes in the character of the stricture can occur without change in the symptoms, the urethra should be examined with the flexible cystoscope from time to time in the course of what seems to be successful therapy. Urethral strictures may soften with the dilations, but it is not unusual for the scar to become worse during the treatment.

Internal Urethrotomy

The next step, in the complex modalities in the treatment of urethral stricture, is to incise the scar and allow the urethra to open, hoping that it will maintain this increase in caliber as healing progresses. This incision can be done blindly with an Otis urethrotome or visually with any of several "cold knife" instruments devised for the procedure (Fig. 83–36). The Otis urethrotome is still useful when the stricture is corrugated, having a number of bands. The urethrotome is passed following a filiform. Its blade is designed to cut the fibrotic tissue while not cutting adjacent compliant urethral epithelium.

When the urethra has been opened, it should be examined with a cystoscope and any "touch up work" that may be needed can be visually done with a urethrotome.

Internal urethrotomy is helpful when the spongiofibrosis associated with the stricture is superficial and the incision extends through the depth of the scar. We prefer to make a single incision at the 12 o'clock position. Other surgeons prefer incisions at 10 and 2 o'clock. In fact, some prefer the 10, 2, and 6, o'clock positions. These multiple cuts must also be full-thickness incisions and not just superficial lacerations.

A ureteral catheter should be passed through the stenotic urethra to guide the blade and prevent protrusion of the urethrotomy into tissues outside the corpus spongiosum. The cut is made by extending the blade and moving the entire operating scope as a unit, not moving the blade to and fro as is done with the loop while doing a transurethral resection (TUR). With a short stricture, one pass with the blade may be enough. With longer strictures with deeper fibrosis, the knife must be advanced through the narrow lumen until the normal urethra proximal to the stricture has been opened. Because he has seen significant extravasation of the irrigation solution into the tissues of the perineum, one of us (CJD) always uses intravenous saline for this procedure, changing to water if electrofulguration of a bleeder becomes necessary.

A soft silicone catheter is left in the urethra after an internal urethrotomy. The length of time the catheter remains depends on the character of the stricture, as this controls the depth of the urethrotomy. The cut is not healed until urethral epithelium has covered the incision. This healing can happen rapidly with a short

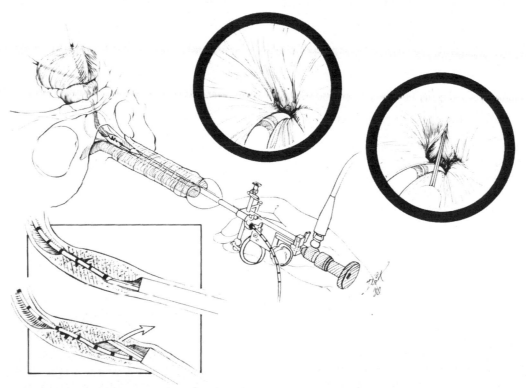

Figure 83–36. Internal urethrotomy under vision with a cold knife. A ureteral catheter is passed through the stricture, and the cold knife is advanced under vision into the stricture guided by this catheter. As the proximal end of the urethrotome is depressed, it cuts upward at 12 o'clock through the stricture. In short strictures, only one cut may be necessary, but in longer ones the ureteral catheter will allow the blade to be advanced farther and the incision to be elongated.

The urethra is incised until a 24 Fr. silicone catheter can be passed with ease in an adult or an appropriately smaller one in a child. (From Devine, C. J., Jr., and Devine, P. C.: Operations for urethral stricture. *In* Stewart, B. H. (Ed.): Operative Urology. Baltimore, Williams & Wilkins, 1982, pp. 243–270.)

relatively superficial stricture, and the catheter need remain only a few days. However, with a deeper urethrotomy, there is far more surface to be epithelialized, and the silicone catheter must be retained for as long as 3 to 6 weeks.

Internal urethrotomy may be a curative modality, but often cure cannot be accomplished with one treatment. If symptoms persist following an internal urethrotomy, the situation must be reassessed. If repeat radiographic studies and flexible cystoscopy show an improvement in the nature of the stricture, another internal urethrotomy is indicated. Two or more attempts should be the limit. If the obstructive symptoms recur rapidly and studies of the stricture show little or no improvement, open surgical treatment should be considered. Currently, unless there are complicating factors, no stricture should be managed by multiple dilations or internal urethrotomies without consideration of urethral reconstruction. Some patients may begin treatment with relatively minimal stricture disease that can be converted to long segment or panurethral strictures by the recurrent trauma of the instrumentation.

The American Medical Systems (11001 Bren Road East, Minnetonka, MN 55343) has embarked on a national protocol to investigate the efficiency of their implantable stainless steel meshed coil urethral stent as an adjunct to dilation and internal urethrotomy. Another stent made of titanium is marketed by Advanced Surgical Intervention (951 Calle Amanecer, San Clemente, CA 92672).

The stainless steel stents have been employed widely in England and Europe. Early results from this experience seem to show that the stents will have a place in the treatment of some but not all strictures. The investigational work is still underway in this country, yet a few observations can be made. The stent does not seem to work well when there is a deep spongiofibrosis or an essentially full-thickness scar. Inflammatory tissue seems to grow right through the stent. This effect seems to stabilize following TUR of the fibrosis, but this is not the best method of treatment for this type of stricture. As an extension of this experience, the stent does not seem to have a place in the treatment of strictures following fracture of the pelvis with posterior urethral distraction. Also, fibrosis may be so deep that there is virtually no corpus spongiosum after laser therapy of strictures, and these strictures produce a similar overgrowth of inflammatory tissue.

It would seem an ideal salvage procedure to place a stent in a patient who has had an unsuccessful urethral reconstruction accomplished by inlaying skin as a graft of flap. Unfortunately, while placement of a stent can maintain the urethral lumen, an aggressive hypertrophic reaction develops in the area of contact between the stent and the imported skin. When the area of skin is large, the hypertrophic reaction increases the surface area of the urethral lining with the result that some patients have almost continuous urinary dribbling. A small layer of urine is trapped after voiding and drains continuously from the hypertrophic "nooks and crannies" in the area of the stent. These patients report this as very troublesome "incontinence."

The European experience suggests that strictures managed by interval dilation and stabilization prior to placement of a stent may respond more favorably than those managed by stent placement at the time of aggressive dilation or an internal urethrotomy. Possibly, the optimal method of employing a urethral stent may begin with dilation or internal urethrotomy followed by a period of soft catheter calibration, which will allow the stricture to stabilize before the urethral stent is placed. At the time of this writing, few other facts concerning the artificial stent can be cited.

PRINCIPLES OF RECONSTRUCTIVE SURGERY

Several general principles need to be addressed when considering reconstructive surgery of the urethra. It is imperative that the vascular supply to the urethral tissues be maintained during urethral surgery. The male urethra has a dual blood supply. Arteries of the bulb and the circumflex arteries of the crura of the corpora cavernosa enter the corpus spongiosum proximally. The dorsal arteries of the penis supply the distal urethra through communicators in the glans penis. Because of this dual vascularity, both ends of the male urethra can survive its being divided at any point (McGowan, 1964). If the artery to the bulb is interrupted, the normal corpus spongiosum serves as a vascular channel between the dorsal arteries of the penis and the proximal portion of the anterior urethra. However, with anterior urethral stricture disease, this channel may be attenuated by attendant fibrosis. The proximal portion of the anterior urethra may not reliably survive once so mobilized. Fibrosis in the proximal portion of the anterior urethra may prevent the circulation provided by the arteries of the bulb from reaching the distal end of the mobilized urethra.

All of the urethral blood supply comes through branches of the pudendal artery (see Fig. 83–9). Pelvic trauma may disrupt one or both of the pudendal arteries or their continuations—the proximal common penile arteries or the dorsal arteries of the penis—and it may not be possible to mobilize the urethra for proximal urethral reconstruction without risking ischemic damage to the mobilized segment. If there are changes in sensation that may be evidence of damage to the pudendal or dorsal nerves of the penis, arteriography is indicated. Such injuries suggest concomitant vascular injury. If the arteriographic studies demonstrate bilateral pudendal or dorsal penile artery damage, it is advisable to employ a method of urethral reconstruction utilizing transfer of a flap instead of excision of the stricture followed by mobilization and reanastomosis.

A number of incisions can afford surgical access to the urethra. The pendulous portion of the penile urethra can be exposed by making a circumcising incision and reflecting the skin of the penis or by making a longitudinal incision in the ventral aspect of the penis. When a fascial flap carrying a skin island is to be utilized to reconstruct a stricture in the distal part of the anterior urethra, placement of the incision will be determined by the location of the skin island and the fascial flap that will support it.

The penile urethra beneath the scrotum can be reached through a ventral incision in the penis or a perineal incision with retraction of the scrotum. Directly, the urethra can be approached by incising the scrotal raphe and scrotal septum and retracting the testicles laterally. In most cases the bulbous, membranous, and apical prostatic portions of the urethra are approached most simply via a perineal incision. This is carried sharply through Colles' fascia anterior to the central tendon of the perineum to expose the bulbospongiosus muscle in the midline. Dissecting distally beneath the scrotum, the univested corpus spongiosum is encountered. The bulbospongiosus muscle can then be elevated from the corpus spongiosum and divided in the midline. Posteriorly, the bulbospongiosus muscles are attached to the central tendon of the perineum at the level of the attachment of the transverse perinei muscles. Deep to that, the bulb of the corpus spongiosum is attached to the perineal body.

In the penis, the urethra is roughly in the center of the corpus spongiosum, but it becomes eccentrically displaced toward the dorsal aspect of the corpus spongiosum in the bulb. The urethra then departs the bulb distal to the attachment of the bulb to the perineal body. Because of this eccentric placement, the incision into the urethra should often be made on the lateral aspect of the bulb, limiting the amount of spongy erectile tissue that must be traversed in exposing the urethra, reducing bleeding and thereby enhancing proximal urethral exposure. However, if there is not much spongiofibrosis, a lateral urethrotomy may preclude mobilization of the spongy tissue necessary to support a tubed FTSG or a patch graft which, in some circumstances, may be the procedure of choice for reconstruction of this portion of the urethra.

Excision and Reanastomosis

Total excision of the fibrotic stricture followed by primary anastomosis of normal urethra to normal urethra is the optimum urethral reconstructive procedure. However, in the anterior urethra this procedure can be considered only for strictures that are discrete and short. Excision with primary anastomosis is limited by the capacity of the penile urethra to be mobilized so that the defect left by excising the stricture can be spanned without producing chordee. Avoiding recurrence is a primary concern in urethral stricture repair. Spatulation of the urethra in primary anastomoses or spatulation of graft or flap inlays limits such recurrences. In the most elastic segment of the urethra in the perineum, the spatulation required for a primary anastomosis following excision of a 2 to 3 cm stricture may approach the limit of such mobilization. The corpus spongiosum must be released from its attachment to the corpora cavernosa from the level of the suspensory ligament to the departure of the urethra from the bulb. After mobilizing the corpus spongiosum, the urethra can be advanced to produce a tension-free anastomosis. The more distal

mobilization of the pendulous portion of the corpus spongiosum in the penis must be approached with caution, lest tension in the repair produce chordee.

The success of primary anastomotic procedures depends on good epithelial apposition, which is best accomplished with a two-layer closure (Fig. 83–37). After excision and spatulation, the dorsal aspect of the corpus spongiosum and its adventitia are reapproximated and secured to the tunica of the corpora and the triangular ligament with PDS, relieving tension on the anastomosis. Good epithelial apposition can be achieved by placing 6–0 chromic catgut sutures, so that they provide optimal epithelial apposition and produce a hairline scar.

Skin Graft Patch

The technique of full-thickness skin graft urethral reconstruction has been considered the most versatile of all open urethral reconstruction procedures (Devine, P. C., et al., 1976), but it clearly has limitations. Best results are obtained with FTSGs in patients who have superficial spongiofibrosis and essentially no scarring in the adjacent tissues. STSGs contract severely and are not useful for this type of urethroplasty. Take of a FTSG in the urethra requires the same conditions as does that of a superficially placed graft. The graft host bed must provide for imbibition and rapid onset of inosculation of an immobilized graft. A FTSG must be well prepared so that its dermal plexus vessels are exposed intimately to the vasculature of the host bed.

A number of areas of hairless or nearly hairless skin can provide suitable tissue for FTSGs. Preputial skin or

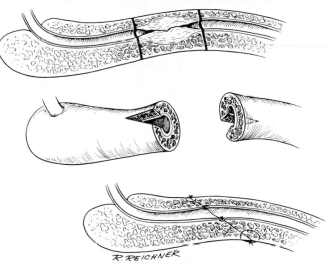

R. REICHNER

Figure 83–37. Urethral stricture primary anastomosis. The stricture involving a short segment of the urethra in the bulb is excised, and the normal ends of the urethra are spatulated and reapproximated. The deep aspect of the tunica of the two ends of the bulb is brought together and sewn to the inferior fascia of the urogenital diaphragm with interrupted 4–0 or 5–0 polydioxanone sutures.

The urethral epithelium is reconstituted with interrupted 5–0 chromic sutures with the knots tied in the lumen and made watertight by a submucosal running polydioxanone suture of 5–0 or 6–0. Closure of the rest of the tunica of the bulb completes the repair. (From Jordan, G. H.: Urethral surgery. *In* Droller, M. (Ed.): Genitourinary Surgery. St. Louis, Mosby-Year Book, Inc., 1992.)

penile shaft skin is best suited for urethral reconstruction. While full thickness, it is thin and takes readily. These grafts undergo minimal contraction, perhaps less than 15 per cent. Extragenital skin grafts contain a thicker dermal layer and contract more than penile skin grafts. An allowance for contraction must be made at the time the graft is tailored.

Bladder epithelium has also been utilized for urethral reconstruction. These grafts are reliable and hairless and, at maturation, tend to maintain good compliance. We have excised a bladder diverticulum resulting from the back pressure produced by a urethral stricture. Tissue from the diverticulum was used as a patch to repair the stricture. Grafted bladder epithelium has been criticized as being prone to diverticular formation. However, if the graft is kept stretched during harvesting, it can be accurately tailored, limiting later redundancy. An incision can be made through the detrusor to the level of the lamina propria. This plane can be developed, allowing the graft to be measured and harvested while the bladder is distended. Others open the bladder and remove the graft from the posterior wall while keeping the tissue stretched. The graft seems to be especially prone to desiccation injury and should be moistened with saline after it is harvested. Bladder epithelium seems to contract in about the same proportion as FTSGs, and a 5 to 15 per cent allowance must be made.

Grafts in the reconstruction of the urethra seem to do better if placed as patches rather than tubes (Fig. 83–38). The stabilizing effect of a dorsal urethral strip, even if narrow, seems to improve results. Also, fixation of the graft to its bed by quilting stitches improves graft

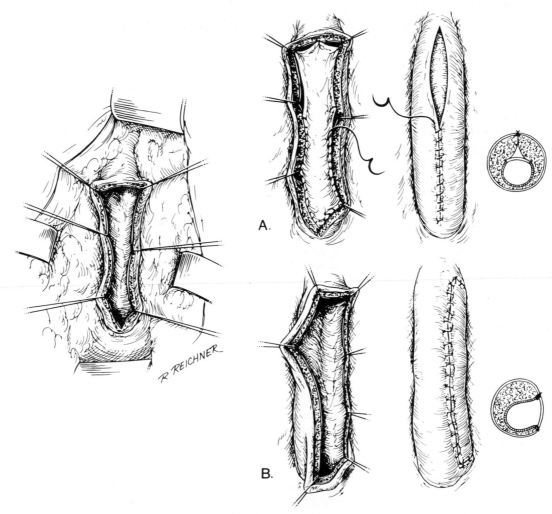

Figure 83–38. Patch graft. With the patient in the exaggerated lithotomy position (see Fig. 83–52), exposure of the urethra in the bulb is achieved as illustrated in Figure 83–55. The spongy tissue of the bulb and the epithelium of the urethral stricture have been opened for placement of a patch of full-thickness skin to repair the stricture. The spongy tissue can be seen between the mucosa of the urethra and the tunica of the bulb, which are approximated by the stay sutures. If there is excessive bleeding a running 5–0 or 6–0 chromic suture will close this gap.

A, The skin graft has been fitted to the urethral mucosa with 5–0 chromic gut tying the knots inside the lumen. A running locked 5–0 polydioxanone suture is placed to approximate the submucosa of the urethra to the dermis of the graft. The erectile tissue is mobilized so that it will cover the graft as the tunica of the bulb is closed with a running 5–0 polydioxanone suture.

B, Because of fibrosis in the spongy tissue, the urethrotomy has been placed laterally. With this amount of spongiofibrosis, we often fill the defect with a flap. In this instance, the graft is anastomosed to both layers—the mucosa and the tunica—with fixing sutures of chromic with the knots tied in the lumen and a running 5–0 polydioxanone suture that turns the epithelial edges into the lumen. The bulbospongiosus muscle serves as the host bed. (From Devine, C. J., and Jordan, G. H.: Surgery of anterior urethral strictures. *In* Marshall, F. F. (Ed.): Operative Urology. Philadelphia, W. B. Saunders Co., 1991, p. 316.)

apposition and hence take. With few exceptions, we employ grafts for reconstruction of the urethra or in the portion of the urethra invested by the bulbospongiosus muscles. When an FTSG tube is employed (Fig. 83–39), the graft must be laid into the widely dissected bulbospongiosus or spread out on the corpora cavernosa to form a flat tube, which is also attached by sutures to the bulbospongiosus muscles as they are brought together to cover the graft ventrally. The application of grafts for fossa reconstruction is discussed subsequently.

FLAP REPAIR OF URETHRAL STRICTURE. Several dartos fascia flaps with a skin island can be applied to the anterior urethra. A ventral longitudinal island of penile skin is well suited to the reconstruction of the pendulous portion of the penile urethra (Fig. 83–40) (Orandi, 1972). Utilization of this flap capitalizes on the marked extensibility of the penile dartos fascia layer, allowing the skin paddle of the flap to be inlayed with minimal mobilization of the pedicle. In designing the flap, the longitudinal incision in the ventral penile skin that will expose the urethra should be placed lateral to the midline. The incision is carried sharply through the dartos fascia to the level of Buck's fascia, allowing the layer of the dartos fascia that contains the vessels to the flap to be elevated reliably, without injury.

After having exposed the urethra, the urethrotomy is made on its lateral aspect, opposite to the original skin incision and ipsilateral to the pedicle of the flap. This placement of the skin incision and urethrotomy allow inversion and inlay of the flap without torsion of the penis or extensive mobilization of the dartos fascial pedicle. If the urethrotomy is located proximal or distal to the island of hairless skin, wider mobilization of the pedicle allows the flap to be recessed beneath the scrotum or advanced into the urethra in the glans.

DORSAL TRANSVERSE ISLAND FLAP. A transverse island of the skin of the prepuce can be mobilized on a dartos fascial pedicle for urethral reconstruction in strictures as well as in hypospadias (Fig. 83–41). Dorsal location of the pedicle, however, limits its use to the proximal portion of the pendulous urethra and, perhaps, to include the very distal subscrotal urethra. A combination of techniques can be employed to repair more

extensive urethral lesions. A dorsal transverse preputial island flap or a longitudinal ventral island flap can be utilized distally in concert with an FTSG or a hairless scrotal skin island (see further on) for the proximal reconstruction.

VENTRAL ISLAND FLAPS. When the stricture involves the fossa navicularis, a transverse flap of penile skin can be advanced on a ventral dartos fascial pedicle for its repair (see subsequent discussion). The vascularity of this pedicle is based on vessels that enter the dartos fascia from the lateral aspects of the scrotum. For proximal strictures, a longitudinal skin flap can be elevated based on the dartos fascia from the ventrum of the penis—its vascular pedicle being elevated on one or the other ventrolateral aspects of the penis, carrying the dissection with ease well beneath the scrotum (Fig. 83–42). The flap can be transposed beneath the scrotum and inverted into the most proximal part of the bulbous urethra and the membranous urethra distal to the sphincter.

As originally described by Quartey (1983), the skin paddle of the flap was developed lateral to the midline with a laterally oriented dartos fascial pedicle. The midline dartos pedicle described here, however, limits the amount of remaining penile skin that must depend on random vascularity. For longer strictures, the flap can be designed much like a "hockey stick," with a midine ventral longitudinal portion and a lateral extension into the distal penile skin. This extended island should still be developed with a midline dartos pedicle. By placing the skin island in the ventral midline, the dartos pedicle can be elevated based on the vessels from both sides of the scrotum, broadening the pedicle and ostensibly improving the reliability of the flap.

Turner-Warwick (1988) has also taken advantage of this vascularity, in what he calls a pedicle island of penile skin (PIPS). He describes two varieties, "UNIPIPS," which is similar to Quartey's flap, and "BIPIPS," which is similar to the flap described here.

HAIRLESS SCROTAL FLAP. A hairless island of scrotal skin raised as a flap on a dartos fascial pedicle can be employed for the repair of proximal urethral strictures (Fig. 83–43). Also, as previously mentioned,

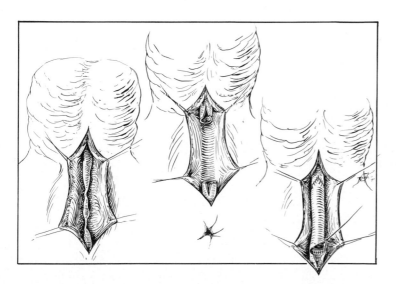

Figure 83–39. Perineal urethral stricture exposed, excised, and replaced with a tubed, full-thickness skin graft. The molding catheter is not shown. If the substance of the bulb is healthy, we open the erectile tissue and excise the strictured epithelial tube. We then insert the graft and close the bulb around it. (From Horton, C. E., and Devine, P. C.: Strictures of the male urethra. *In* Converse, J. M. (Ed.): Reconstructive Plastic Surgery. Philadelphia, W. B. Saunders Co., 1977.)

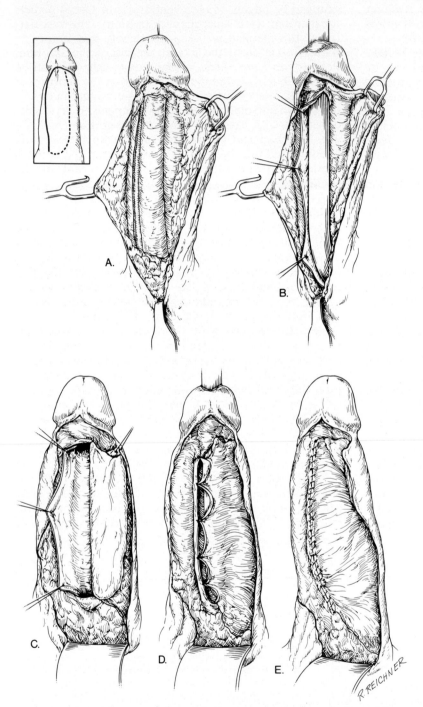

Figure 83–40. Orandi flap. The incisions to be made to mobilize the flap are demonstrated in the box. The heavy line is the primary incision made full thickness through the dartos fascia and Buck's fascia to the level of the tunica of the corporal bodies lateral to the corpus spongiosum. *A,* Dissection beneath Buck's fascia mobilizes the pedicle of the flap well past the corpus spongiosum in the midline.

B, A lateral urethrotomy placed to face the pedicle of the flap has opened the entire length of the stricture. This incision can be continued into the urethra in the glans if that portion of the urethra is involved in the stricture.

C, The skin paddle of the flap has been developed by making the incision outlined by the dotted line in the initial box and undermining the skin lateral to it. The medial edge of the flap has been fixed to the edge of the urethrotomy with sutures of chromic gut and the epithelial edges approximated by a running subepithelial 5–0 polydioxanone suture.

D, The flap is inverted into the defect. Chromic tacking sutures are used to approximate the epithelial edges of the flap and urethra.

E, A watertight subepithelial suture line has been completed with a running 5–0 polydioxanone suture. The skin will be closed with subcutaneous sutures of Vicryl or polydioxanone, using 4–0 chromic for the skin. (From Jordan, G. H.: Management of anterior urethral stricture disease. *In* Webster, G. D. (Ed.): Problems in Urology. Philadelphia, J. B. Lippincott Co., 1987, p. 214.)

Figure 83–41. A dorsal transverse island (Duckett) flap of penile skin applied to a stricture of the urethra. The flap has been elevated upon its vascular pedicle in the dartos fascia, and a lateral incision has been made into the urethra. The flap has been secured in place *(right)*. The edge of the anastomosis that will be covered by the pedicle is sewn first with tacking chromic sutures and a running polydioxanone suture to make a watertight epithelial-to-epithelial anastomosis. With this step completed, the anastomosis of the free edge is carried out. (From Jordan, G. H.: Management of anterior urethral stricture disease. *In* Webster, G. D. (Ed.): Problems in Urology. Philadelphia, J. B. Lippincott Co., 1987, p. 217.)

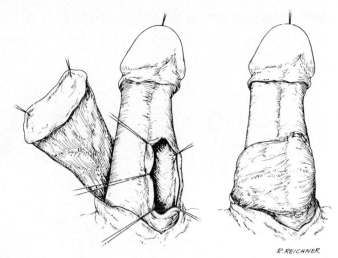

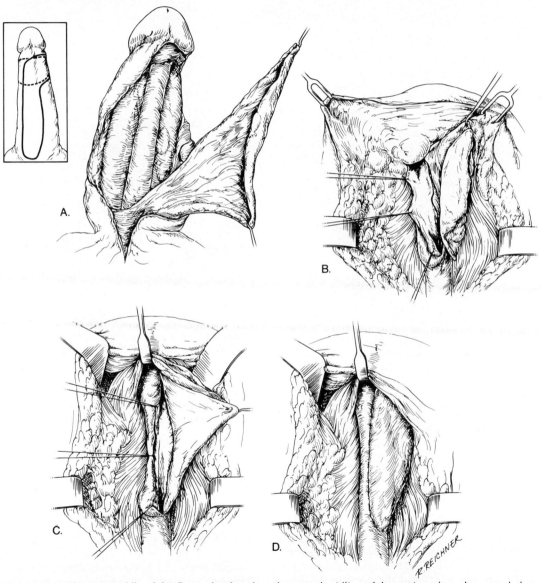

Figure 83–42. Quartey flap. The skin paddle of the flap is developed on the ventral midline of the penis and can be extended around the penile shaft at its distal end. *A,* The paddle of the flap has been incised, and its pedicle elevated. This pedicle includes Buck's and dartos fascia denuding the tunica of the corpus spongiosum and the corpora cavernosa. The pedicle's vascular supply extends into the dartos fascia bilaterally from the perineal vessels and the external pudendal vessels in the scrotum. Development of this pedicle allows the flap to be moved to any area of the urethra.

B, The flap has been passed through a tunnel beneath the scrotum created by dissecting along the corpus spongiosum. A laterally placed urethrotomy has opened the urethral stricture (see Fig. 83–38B).

C, The deep edge of the flap is secured employing the suture techniques previously described.

D, Anastomosis of the flap has been completed. The pedicle can be seen extending beneath the scrotum. (From Jordan, G. H., and McCraw, J. B.: Tissue transfer techniques for genitourinary surgery, Part III. AUA Update Series, Lesson 11, Vol. 7, 1988.)

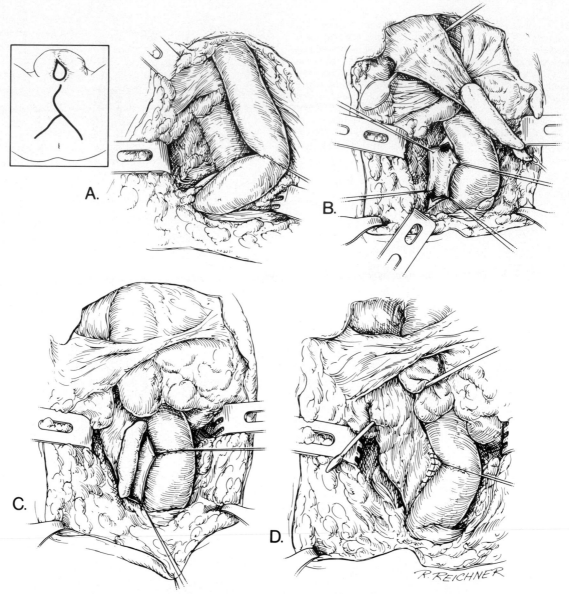

R. REICHNER

Figure 83–43. Hairless scrotal island flap. *A,* In the inset, the incisions are planned so that a hairless area of skin in the midline of the scrotum can be transferred as a flap on a pedicle of the dartos fascia of the scrotum, to repair a stricture in the bulbomembranous portion of the urethra. With the patient in the deep lithotomy position, the inverted Y-incision is made in the perineum. One of the lateral aspects of the bulb is mobilized, isolating the membranous portion of the urethra as it emerges.

B, The skin paddle has been elevated; the bougie lies beneath the pedicle of the flap.

C, The flap has been brought down without tension through a tunnel developed beneath the scrotum. The deep edge of the flap has been anastomosed to the deep edge of the incision in the lateral aspect of the urethra.

D, The superficial edge of the flap has been sewn into place, and the closure is watertight. A probe lies behind the transposed pedicle of the flap. Drains will be placed, and the skin will be closed. A urethral catheter will be left as a stent through the repair, but the urine will be diverted with a suprapubic tube.

the flap can be utilized in concert with a distal flap of penile skin for the repair of extensive urethral stricture disease. The vessels of this flap extend into the scrotum from a posterolateral direction, and the pedicle must be developed with a lateral base. It should not be based on the midline septum as its vascularity is not dependable. The dartos fascia supporting the scrotal skin contains muscle fibers. Scrotal skin flaps, created from skin of remarkable extensibility, do not contract, but are prone to diverticular formation unless properly tailored by stretching the skin to its limit prior to outlining the skin island.

FOSSA NAVICULARIS

Strictures of the fossa navicularis present an additional challenge. As with strictures of other portions of the urethra, careful attention is required to achieve a good functional result, but repair of a stricture in the glans penis must also produce a good cosmetic result. A number of techniques have been described for meatal reconstruction, but some yield good functional results with poor cosmetic results (Blandy and Tresidder, 1967; Brannen, 1976; Cohney, 1963). To reconstruct isolated strictures of the meatus and the urethra in the glans,

Devine (1986) excised the stricture and resurfaced the fossa navicularis with an FTSG, approximating the ventrum of the glans to cover the graft (Fig. 83–44). This procedure has provided good functional and cosmetic results, but it seems more likely for the BXO process to involve grafts rather than flaps used in urethroplasty.

DeSy (1984) has described a skin island based on a dartos fascial pedicle. After mobilizing the fascial pedicle, the skin island is advanced and inverted into the fossa. Jordan (1988) utilizes a ventral transverse preputial skin island based on a broad dartos fascial pedicle (Fig. 83–45). He transposes this flap, inverts it into the urethrotomy defect, and closes the glans. All of these procedures reconstruct the fossa navicularis obtaining cosmetic results that are excellent. Most patients will have virtually no stigmata of stricture or reconstruction.

Staged Repair

A number of staged procedures have been described, most utilizing marsupialization as a first stage. The strictured urethra was incised and deployed onto the ventrum of the penis, scrotum, or perineum, opening the urethra back to the site of a perineal urethrostomy. Revision of the perineal urethrostomy often required two or three operations between the first and last stages of the "two-staged" procedure (Turner-Warwick, 1988). At the ultimate stage, the adjacent tissues are tubed over the marsupialized urethral strip to reconstruct the urethra, in most cases placing hair-bearing skin in the urethra.

UNMESHED SPLIT-THICKNESS GRAFT URE-THROPLASTY. Schreiter and co-workers (1989) have described a staged procedure in which a meshed STSG is placed on the ventrum of the penis and perineum and subsequently tubularized, after the graft has matured. When the graft is placed, the urethra is either totally excised or opened leaving only a dorsal strip (Fig. 83–46). The dartos fascia of the penis and scrotum is mobilized and deployed to cover the defect, providing a good vascularized host bed. An STSG is harvested at about 0.016 inch and meshed on the Padgett mesher, using a 1.5:1 carrier. Without expanding the mesh, the graft is fixed open-faced in the site of the excised urethra, after which it is meticulously bolstered.

A catheter is left in the proximal urethrostomy. In 3 to 6 months, after graft maturation has progressed, the patient is returned to the operating room. In each of our patients, the meshed STSG has been smooth and elastic, assuming a remarkable consistency that can be likened to kid leather. In patients who have undergone reconstruction with this technique, none has demonstrated any tendency of the graft to contract.

The second stage procedure consists of making parallel incisions and tubularizing the isolated strip of the mature graft (Fig. 83–47). The tube is formed by precisely approximating the epithelium with interrupted 5–0 chromic cat gut sutures, tying the knots in the lumen and placing a running extraepithelial PDS, to make the closure watertight. Precise tapering of both ends prevents restenosis at the juncture of this tube with the proximal and distal portions of the native urethra. We leave a suprapubic tube to drain the urine and a 14 Fr.

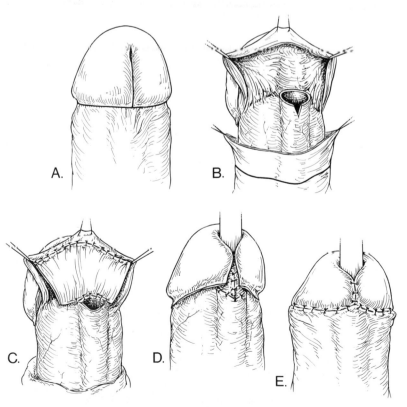

Figure 83–44. Patch graft resurfacing of the fossa navicularis. *A*, When the stricture of the urethra caused by BXO involves only the urethral meatus or the urethra in the glans, a circumcising incision is made just proximal to the corona, and the urethra is incised opening the ventral aspect of the glans penis.

B, The scarred urethra in the glans has been excised, and a spatulating incision has been made in the distal end of the normal urethra. The area from which the graft will be taken is outlined on the mobilized skin of the penis.

C, The skin graft has been sewn to the urethra and the edge of the epithelium of the glans with interrupted 5–0 chromic sutures.

D, The skin graft has been tubed, making a watertight anastomosis with dermal sutures of fine polydioxanone.

E, The glans has been brought around the new urethral tube and the skin edge reapproximated. The penis is covered with Bioclusive dressing, and a short silicone stent is placed, diverting the urine for several days by passing a feeding tube through the stent.

R. REICHNER

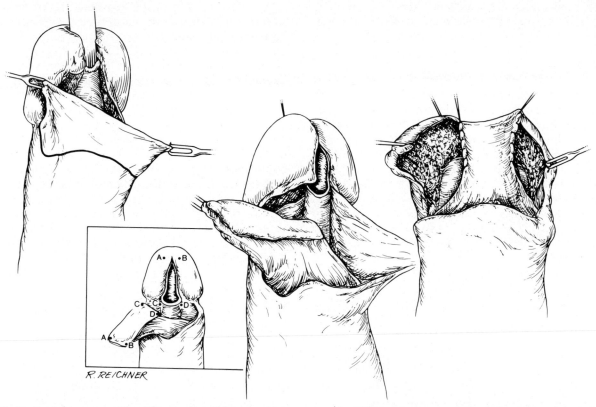

R. REICHNER

Figure 83–45. Ventral transverse island flap (Jordan). When the stricture caused by BXO involves more of the urethra in the glans, repair with a flap is preferred. The urethra in the glans has been opened. The flap has been outlined on the ventral side of the skin of the penis. The wings of the glans are mobilized, leaving the urethra as a strip on the dorsal aspect of the erectile tissue. Note the tips of the corpora cavernosa. The skin proximal to the flap is undermined, leaving the pedicle of the flap in the dartos fascia long enough so that the flap may be rotated to fit the urethral defect.

The diagram in the inset shows the placement of the corners of the flap. When the suture line has been demonstrated to be watertight, the glans is closed replacing the meatus at the tip of the penis. (From Jordan, G. H., and McCraw, J. B.: Tissue transfer techniques for genitourinary surgery, Part III. AUA Update Series, Lesson 11, Vol. 7, 1988.)

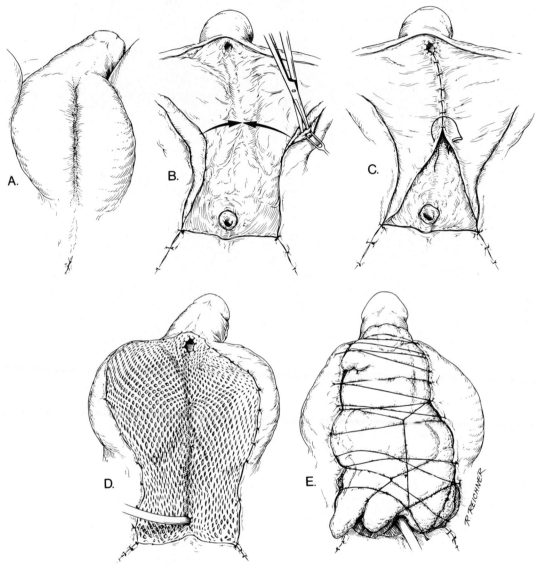

Figure 83–46. Meshed graft urethroplasty, first stage. In patients with lengthy strictures in whom all available tissue has been expended. *A*, The strictured urethra is excised completely or only a dorsal strip of epithelium is left.

B, The dartos fascia is mobilized from the scrotum and *(C)* Brought in to cover the fat and scar in the defect with vascularized tissue.

D, A split-thickness skin graft is harvested from the buttocks or inner surface of the thigh, meshed on the Padgett dermatome with a carrier, using a 1.5:1 ratio, and placed in the site of the excised urethra as an open-faced graft, without expanding the mesh. The epithelium of urethra is sewn to the graft.

E, The graft is covered with Xeroform gauze, and a thick bolster of damp Dacron batting is secured in place with black silk sutures. A Foley catheter is left in the proximal urethra.

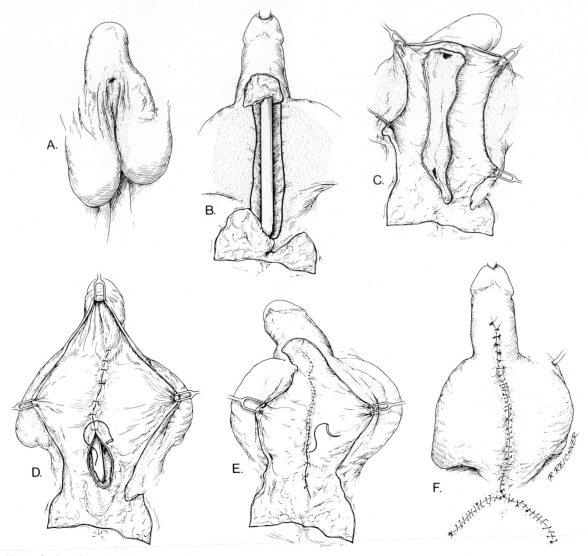

Figure 83–47. Meshed graft urethroplasty, second stage. *A,* In 2 to 3 months, the new epithelial surface is smooth and elastic. The patient is brought back to the operating room. The proximal and distal portions of the urethra are evaluated with bougie à boules and cystoscopy.

B, A catheter is passed through the penile urethra and into the bladder. A 3-cm wide strip is marked to form the new urethra, outlining flaps at each end to tailor the junction of the tube to the existing urethra.

C, The strip is not undermined, but dissection is carried out laterally to mobilize the remaining skin graft and scrotal skin.

D, Interrupted chromic sutures are placed to approximate the epithelial edges, tying the knots in the lumen.

E, A running subepithelial 5–0 polydioxanone suture is placed to roll the edges in and to make the suture line watertight.

F, The skin is closed with chromic sutures leaving suction drains. The urine is diverted with a suprapubic tube. (From Devine, C. J., and Jordan, G. H.: Strictures of the anterior urethra, Part II. AUA Update Series, Lesson 26, Vol. 9, 1990.)

Foley (Rusch) catheter in the urethra for 2 to 3 weeks. If a voiding radiograph at the time the urethral catheter is removed shows a well-formed urethra, the suprapubic tube is clamped for several days and then removed.

POSTERIOR URETHRAL STRICTURES

The urethra from the bladder neck to the striated external sphincter has been shown to have sphincter activity. Posterior urethral strictures located proximal to the junction of the urethra with the bulbospongiosum and distal to the verumontanum involve this sphincter-active portion of the urethra. The sphincter mechanism can be severely affected by the injury that caused the stricture or by the reconstruction attempts. Strictures in

this portion of the urethra generally are the result of distraction injuries accompanying pelvic fracture, but some may be the result of prostatectomy.

Following prostatectomy, the proximal bladder neck sphincter mechanism will have been obliterated by removal of the prostate. This effect must be kept in mind when planning treatment. These strictures initially may respond well to dilation with balloon catheters (American Medical Systems, 11001 Bren Road East, Minnetonka, MN 55343–9058). Many patients require treatment at intervals of greater than 6 months. If these intervals become shorter, the patient is taught self-catheterization, which can be performed at home.

We do not favor internal urethrotomy by either direct vision or Otis urethrotome, because cutting the urethra can injure the remaining active portion of the urethral sphincter leaving the patient incontinent. Should urethral reconstruction be necessary, it must be done with an awareness of the very real risk of external sphincter damage and hence incontinence. Also, future placement of an artificial sphincter around the bulbous urethra may be contraindicated owing to obliteration of the posterior blood supply to the corpus spongiosum. In this patient so affected, incontinence could be managed with an artificial sphincter placed about the bladder neck. However, the technical difficulty of that procedure should not be underestimated. Unanimity concerning the approach to this most difficult patient population is not yet reached. Another alternative for the most difficult case is a continent bladder augmentation, with closure of the bladder neck.

About 10 per cent of pelvic fractures have a concomitant urethral distraction injury, ranging from a mere stretching injury of the bulbomembranous area of the urethra to total distraction with wide displacement of the posterior urethra. Until proved otherwise, all such injuries should be treated as if they had produced

diminished function of the external sphincter mechanism.

In the acute phase, most workers would agree that placement of a suprapubic cystostomy tube helps to manage these patients well. However, our experience has clearly shown that in some patients placement of an aligning catheter without traction simplifies later reconstruction. It fosters the approximation of the two ends of the totally distracted urethra, producing a scar that can be managed in the future with dilation or internal urethrotomy (Fig. 83–48) (Devine, P., 1982).

Fortunately, the more proximal sphincter mechanism is usually not compromised in pelvic fracture patients. Turner-Warwick (1977) has emphasized the frequency with which the bladder neck is incarcerated within the scar and the subsequent fibrosis from the hematoma. This "bound bladder neck" has not been common in our patients but may only represent the different levels of trauma experienced by the two different referral groups. A patient whose bladder neck has become entrapped can become continent following lysis of the

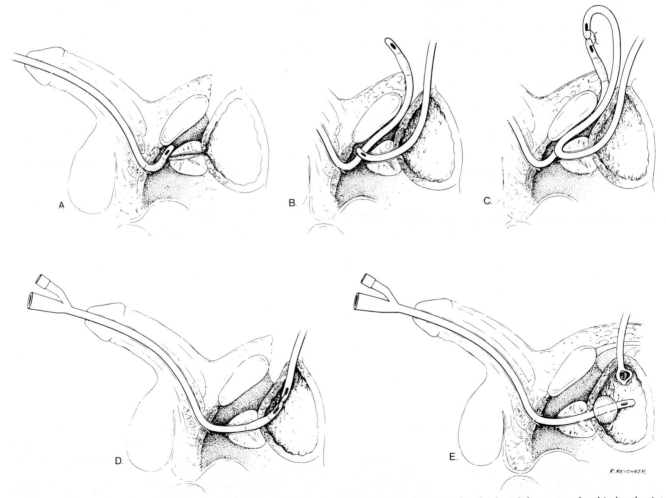

Figure 83–48. In fractured pelvis with ruptured urethra, the prostate may remain attached to the displaced fragment of pubis by the intact puboprostatic ligaments. The prostate will never return to its normal position, and a long defect will have to be made up in a later repair.

When the bladder is exposed to insert a suprapubic tube, the status of the puboprostatic ligaments can be evaluated by putting the finger between the pubis and the prostate. If the ligaments are present, they should be cut, releasing the prostate to return to its normal position. Placing a catheter in the urethra will help to guide the prostate home. An 18 Fr., 5-cc Foley catheter is passed through the urethra and picked up in the wound. A red rubber catheter is passed through the bladder neck and also picked up in the wound. The tips of the catheters are sewn together, and the Foley is pulled into the bladder. The balloon is distended with 10 ml of water and the suture secured to a button on the abdomen. No traction should be applied to this catheter.

scar tissue, reduction of the bladder neck, tapering of the posterior urethra, and creation of a short Young-Dees bladder plication. Ureteroneocystostomy is usually not necessary.

In categorizing posterior urethral strictures, Colapinto and McCallum (1977) noted a higher incidence of incontinence following reconstruction of distraction injuries occurring at the junction of the prostatic urethra with the membranous urethra than those at the bulbomembranous junction. Perhaps more of the intrinsic smooth muscle sphincter is involved in the spatulation required to attach the bulbous urethra to the apical prostatic urethra. Also, the more proximal injury may have been associated with trauma to the bladder neck, even though when studied it may appear relatively normal.

No one ideal approach exists in the management of every posterior urethral distraction injury associated with fracture of the pelvis. Although some can be managed with endoscopic techniques and a few require complete removal of the pubis with re-routing of the corpus spongiosum around a crus of the corpus cavernosum, most can be managed by excision of the stricture, wide mobilization of the urethra, and primary anastomosis. Some patients will have had injury to a portion of the anterior urethra in association with the distraction injury, and it may not be possible to mobilize the urethra for a primary anastomosis. This repair will require one of the tissue transfer techniques to span the gap (see previous discussion). The operation must be selected to fit the circumstances. To manage these potentially very difficult cases, the surgeon must have command of the entire spectrum of reconstructive procedures.

Most of these patients will have been managed acutely with placement of a suprapubic cystostomy and some with placement of a urethral aligning catheter. Reconstruction should be delayed 4 to 6 months to allow fibrosis and scarring to mature. During this time, the hematoma reabsorbs and the posterior structures settle into a fixed position. In most, the bladder neck will be competent. Unless it opens during an attempt to void, the urethra proximal to the stricture will not fill during a cystogram. Hence, radiographic demonstration of the true length of the stricture may be difficult. Yet, if the bladder neck is always open and the posterior urethra is visualized on all of the cystogram films, one must suspect the possibility of a bladder neck injury. With encouragement, most patients with a competent bladder neck can fill the posterior urethra while straining to increase the pressure in the bladder. This will produce a cystogram that, with a simultaneous retrograde urethrogram, will furnish an excellent radiographic demonstration of the stricture defect (Fig. 83–49).

Many patients will not be able to allow the bladder necks to open, therefore, evaluation must include endoscopy. The anterior urethra can be evaluated with a flexible panendoscope to the level of the obliteration to rule out concomitant anterior urethra injury. This instrument can also be introduced through the suprapubic cystostomy tract to visualize the bladder neck and posterior urethra. If the bladder neck appears to be tightly closed, it is probably competent, although this finding

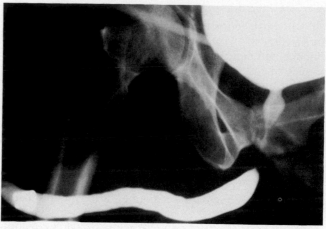

Figure 83–49. Distraction injury. The bladder was filled through the suprapubic tube, and as the pressure rose in the bladder, the bladder neck opened to fill the prostatic urethra. The irregular tapered end of the urethra defines the scarred upper end of the urethra. Retrograde instillation of contrast material demonstrates the other end of the scar and a normal looking distal urethra.

does not correlate 100 per cent with function. With gentle pressure, while reassuring the patient, the scope can be introduced through the bladder neck to visualize the posterior urethra and, in many cases, the external sphincter mechanism with the site of total obliteration just beyond it.

It is safe to say that (1) if the bladder neck is not unreasonably displaced and (2) if the bulbous urethra is an adequate length, with a normal urethra distal to it, the stricture can be repaired. The repair can be accomplished by excising the fibrosis and reanastomosing the spatulated bulbous urethra to the spatulated apical portion of the prostatic urethra.

Transurethral Management of Posterior Urethral Strictures

Although we favor primary reconstruction of these strictures, some can be managed endoscopically. As mentioned, in some patients the ends of the urethra settle back virtually lined up with an extremely short stricture, which may not be totally obstructed. These patients should be managed with dilation and internal urethrotomy. Many are cured with these treatment modalities. A number of procedures can be categorized as "cut for the light." Although some workers have reported success (Barry, 1989; Fishman, 1987), most cut-for-the-light procedures are not done with enough precision to provide for adequate realignment of the urethra. Unfortunately, we have seen disasters that have resulted from them.

Marshall (1989) described his method of using stereotactic techniques for endoscopic realignment of the ends of the urethra. He emphasizes the length of time it takes to obtain precise alignment prior to the endoscopic procedure. He passes a wire through the aligned ends of the urethra, minimally dilating the channel and widening it by transurethral resection. The scar is stabilized by a period of self-catheterization. We do not advocate this as a primary modality. However, patients whose medical condition, age, orthopedic injuries, and so forth prevent their being placed in the exaggerated lithotomy position may be managed with this technique.

In our experience, most posterior urethral strictures can be approached by perineal exposure alone. Only a few patients have required a combined procedure. This statement, however, should not be taken to mean that the dissection is simply done and that the urethral ends will be in broad view "asking" to be reanastomosed. Most of these cases are far from straightforward.

EXAGGERATED LITHOTOMY POSITION. The first step in approaching these strictures via the perineum is to place the patient in the exaggerated lithotomy position (Fig. 83–50). Potentially, this exaggerated position can cause complications by itself. Some patients complain of subsequent discomfort and some demonstrate evidence of neuropraxic injury, usually numbness on the lateral aspect of the foot or, in severe cases, muscle weakness with dorsiflexion. However, we have reviewed a series of 150 of our cases, and the morbidity associated with the position has been mild and has resolved promptly. In only two patients did the neuropraxic symptoms persist beyond 48 hours. In one, the symptoms resolved in 3 to 4 weeks. In the other, they persisted for 6 weeks. Complaints of back pain seem to resolve when the patient is allowed to ambulate.

Placing the patient in the exaggerated lithotomy position by elevation of a buttock plate will reduce this morbidity. A number of tables on the market allow for this elevation. Most of our experience has been with the Stille Scandia table, which is no longer available. Chick Systems has introduced a table with similar capabilities as has Amsco (6480 Dobbin Road, Suite H, Columbia,

MD 21045). The buttock plate on the Chick Systems table is longer than that on the first two tables mentioned.

To support the patient's legs, we have selected the Allen stirrups (Edgewater Medical Systems, Mayfield Heights, OH 44124). They provide optimal management of the feet and legs, but great care must be taken to avoid localized pressure on the extremity while the patient is up in this position. In the exaggerated lithotomy position, the legs of our patients literally hang from their feet secured in the boot pieces of the Allen stirrups without pressure on the legs or thighs. When, as rarely happens, a patient requires a combined approach; the perineal exposure is first achieved. The patient's legs are then very carefully repositioned to allow better access to the abdominal area. In our view the Allen stirrups are virtually a necessity for this intraoperative repositioning.

Prior to the development of the equipment described, we used a wedge-shaped pad, the "candy-cane" stirrups, and the Vac Pac (Olympic Medical Corporation, 4400 7th Street South, Seattle, WA 98108) to achieve the exaggerated perineal position (Fig. 83–51). This technique can still be useful today as the tables described here are not widely available. The Allen stirrups, however, have so many advantages for multiple purposes that they should be in every urology operating room.

PERINEAL APPROACH. After placing the patient in the correct position, all areas of hairless genital skin are marked in case a graft or flap will be necessary. The patient's lower abdomen, genitalia, and perineum are prepared and draped. We make a lambda-shaped incision in the midline of the perineum posterior to the scrotum. This incision provides for wide visualization of the perineal structures (Fig. 83–52). The incision is

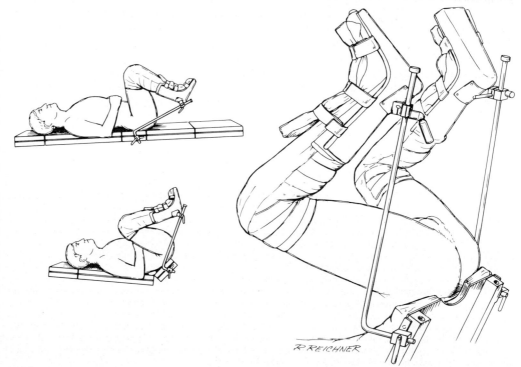

Figure 83–50. Placement of the patient into the exaggerated lithotomy position using the Allen stirrups on the Chick table. The patient is placed on the table flat with the tip of the coccyx at the lower end of the short section of the table. After he is anesthetized, the feet are placed in the Allen stirrups, which are adjusted so that there is no pressure on the calf muscles. After removing the flat sections of the table that supported the legs, his position is adjusted so that the sacrum slightly overlaps the end of the table. A rolled towel is placed to support the lumbar curve of the back. As the short section of the table is elevated, the perineum is brought parallel to the floor. (From Devine, C. J., Jr., and Jordan, G. H.: Surgery of anterior urethral strictures. *In* Marshall, F. F. (Ed.). Operative Urology. Philadelphia, W. B. Saunders Co., 1991, p. 314.)

R REICHNER

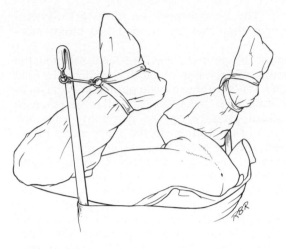

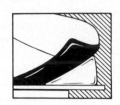

Figure 83–51. Patient in the deep lithotomy position (alternate technique). He has been given a general anesthetic. The inset shows the black Vac Pac, which has been molded to his contour before it is evacuated. This supports him as the pelvis is elevated on a wedge-shaped sandbag supported by a board on the operating table. No shoulder braces are used.

The superior flaps of the Vac Pac are conformed to keep the patient from sliding up on the table. The patient's legs are held flexed by the stirrups, which do not exert pressure on the hip or knee joints. However, the Allen stirrups that will fit this type of table would be advantageous, in that they hold the feet and suspend the legs without compression.

carried sharply through Colles' fascia, and the central tendon of the perineum is attached at the posterior reflection of Colles' fascia. This layer can be vascular, and we generally employ the cutting electrocautery to carry the dissection down to the bulbospongiosus muscles. With careful dissection beneath the scrotum, the corpus spongiosum distal to the muscles is exposed. At this point, a Denis Browne perineal ring retractor is placed. The bulbospongiosus is freed by dissecting between the muscle and the corpus spongiosum and is divided in the midline, dissecting it free from the bulbospongiosum.

The muscles are retracted with gently applied stay sutures. Dissecting beneath the corpus spongiosum, it is detached from the corpora cavernosa to about the mid-scrotal position. The dissection is carried posteriorly to expose the departure of the urethra from the bulbospongiosum. While retracting the transverse perinei muscles to expose the plane of dissection, the posterior aspect of the bulbospongiosum is detached from the perineal body.

Hemostasis is achieved utilizing bipolar electrocautery forceps. The tip of the bulb having been freed, dissection is carried forward to where the arteries to the bulb are encountered. They are divided, being controlled with the bipolar cautery. In some patients, one or more of these arteries will already have been obliterated by the trauma. The circumferential arteries of the corpora

cavernosa come in laterally. These arteries are virtually never obliterated by the trauma process but are controlled with the bipolar cautery.

Eventually, the corpus spongiosum remains attached by only scar fibrosis and the urethral remnant. These are divided, and the corpus spongiosum is retracted out of the field and wrapped with a moist sponge. Some oozing from the bed of the bulb of the urethra is always evident; however, hemostasis is seldom a problem.

We divide the triangular ligament and develop the space between the crura of the corpora cavernosa, improving the surgical exposure and shortening the path that the urethra must take to reach the urethra at the apex of the prostate (Fig. 83–53). Great care must be taken to identify precisely all vessels in the space prior to dividing any of them. Occasionally, the cavernosal arteries are encountered in this space prior to their entry into the corpora. Usually, the dorsal vein of the penis will not have been disrupted by the trauma. Visualization and control of the dorsal vein in this space greatly assists further dissection. If the dorsal vein has been obliterated by the trauma, one can expect to encounter a number of dilated crural or cavernosal veins in this space. They also can be controlled with the bipolar cautery.

The dissection is carried down to the periosteum/perichondrium of the symphysis pubis, which is incised and elevated from the cartilage and bone. By

Figure 83–52. Diagram of a perineal repair of membranous urethral stricture. An inverted Y incision extends from the midline of the scrotum to the ischial tuberosities.

A, Colles' fascia has been opened to expose the bulbospongiosus muscles and the tunica of the corpus spongiosum distal to the edge of the muscles.

B, The scissors are introduced to develop the space between the muscle and the bulb of the urethra.

C, An incision is made in the midline with the scissors exposing the length of the bulb.

D, The transverse perinei muscles are retracted to expose the full length of the bulb.

E, The self-retaining retractor is placed to expose the inferior fascia of the genitourinary diaphragm. The bulb of the corpus spongiosum (bulbospongiosum) can now be mobilized to gain access to the strictured area of the urethra.

F, The strictured urethra is incised, freeing the bulb.

G, The urethra is opened, showing an adequate lumen and the proximal overhang of the spongy tissue of the bulb.

H, The Haygrove staff has been passed through the suprapubic cystostomy. Resection of the scar has allowed it to pass into the perineum.

I, The scar tissue has been removed from the anterior aspect of the prostatic urethra and the urethra opened for the anastomosis.

J, Sutures have been placed to approximate the epithelial edges of the proximal and distal segments of the urethra.

K, The catheter has been passed, the anterior sutures have been tied, and the posterior sutures are about to be tied.

L, Anastomosis completed, with the reinforcing sutures between the tunica of the corpus spongiosum and corpora cavernosa in place. The dead space at the anastomotic site is obliterated by a dartos fascia flap.

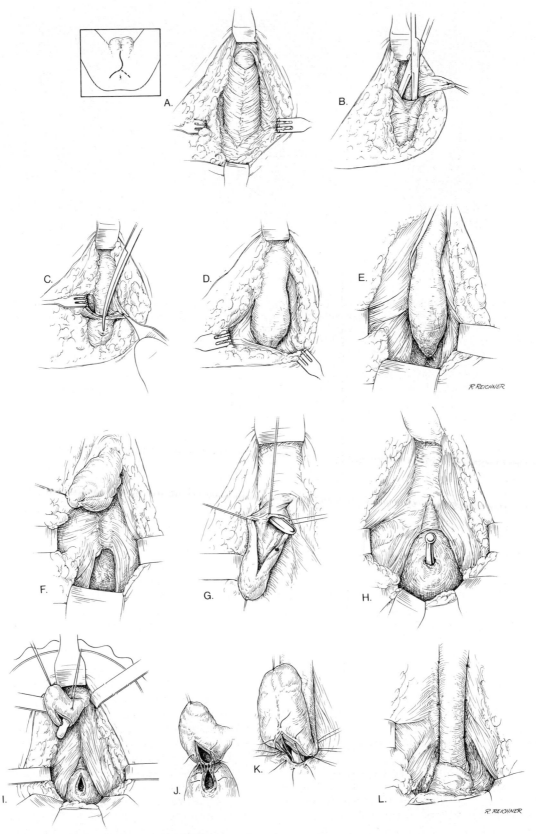

Figure 83–52 *See legend on opposite page*

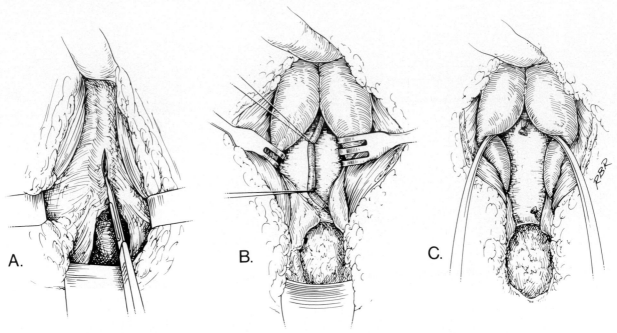

Figure 83–53. Division of the fascia of the genitourinary (GU) diaphragm and dissection of the crura. When the prostatic urethra is displaced and the arc that the urethra must traverse needs to be shortened, the crura of the corpora can be mobilized by (A) incising Buck's fascia that contains them and the inferior fascia of the GU diaphragm to which they are attached.

B, Incision and mobilization of the perichondrium and periosteum of the symphysis pubis allow placement of retractors without trauma to the erectile bodies. Lateral displacement of the crura will expose the dorsal vein of the penis, which after careful identification can be ligated and divided.

C, Completion of this dissection affords additional exposure for resection of the fibrosis that surrounds the prostate and the proximal end of the disrupted urethra. (From Schreiter, F. and Noll, F. (Eds.): Plastic-Reconstructive Surgery in Urology. Stuttgart, Germany. Thieme Publishers, In preparation.)

placing modified Gelpi retractors in the space developed beneath the periosteum/perichondrium, the corporal bodies can be retracted laterally without the danger of damaging the neurovascular bundle on the anterior surface of the corpora.

When adequate exposure has been achieved, the posterior urethra must be identified. We may use the half circle Haygrove staff or pass a flexible cystoscope through the suprapubic sinus into the posterior urethra. After the distal limit of the posterior urethra has been identified, the often laborious process of total excision of the fibrosis is begun. To expose the normal plane of the apical prostatic urethra, all of the scar must be excised and a button of scar at the apex of the prostate must be excised. Although the process may be tedious, one should resect the fibrosis prior to "cutting down" onto the end of the sound rather than cutting down on the sound through the scar tissue. This would allow the posterior urethra to retract so that subsequent excision of the fibrosis would become much more difficult than necessary.

When the tip of the sound is concealed only by the epithelium of the apical prostatic or membranous urethra, the epithelium is opened, and the posterior urethra is controlled by placement of sutures. A silk suture is drawn back through the urethra following the path of the sound.

Endoscopy ensures that the urethrotomy has been made into the distal limit of the posterior urethra. If the disruption of the urethra has occurred distal to the external sphincter, actual prostatic tissue will not be encountered. The widely spatulated anastomosis should be created with the apical portion of the membranous urethra or at the level of the external striated sphincter.

We have treated a number of referred patients in whom the bulbous urethra has been anastomosed to a false passage or to the bladder anterior to the prostate, because the normal structures of the posterior urethra had not been recognized prior to proceeding with the anastomosis. Most of these operations had been done through the transpubic route. We have been able to repair each of them through a perineal approach as previously described.

When the prostatic urethra has been displaced in a cephaloposterior direction, resection of the lower portion of the symphysis pubis further shortens the path the urethra must take and usually allows a primary anastomosis to be accomplished (Fig. 83–54). An infrapubectomy is carried out, accomplished by elevating the soft tissue structures from the undersurface of the pubis and, utilizing Kerrison rongeurs, resecting as much of the pubis as is necessary to provide adequate exposure and a smooth path to the apex of the prostate (see Fig. 83–54). Rarely, partial infrapubectomy does not allow a tension-free anastomosis, and more of the pubis can be resected. In several patients, the entire pubic ramus has been resected through this perineal exposure. Often in these patients, the corpus spongiosum must be rerouted over one crus of the corpus cavernosum (Fig. 83–55). This diminishes the circumference of the arc

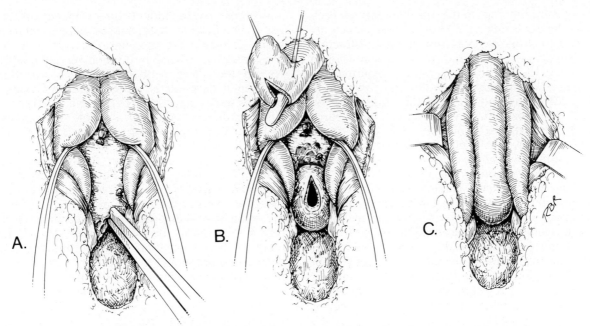

Figure 83–54. Infrapubectomy. If the prostate is elevated behind the symphysis pubis *(A)* the inferior aspect of the symphysis is resected using a Kerrison rongeur. As much of the bone can be removed as necessary *(B)* to afford a simple approximation of the ends of the urethra *(C)*.

that must be traversed so that the corpus spongiosum can be passed directly to the urethra at the apex of the prostate.

The ends of the urethra are adequately spatulated so that they accommodate a 32 Fr. bougie with ease, and the anastomosis can be performed (Fig. 83–52 *J* and *K*).

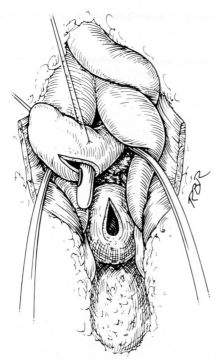

Figure 83–55. Resection of the pubis and re-routing of the urethra over a crus. When the prostate is markedly displaced, it may be necessary to resect the entire depth of the symphysis pubis. Sometimes, despite the crura having been separated to the full extent possible, the two ends of the urethra will not meet when brought directly through the crus. It will be necessary to bring the urethra lateral to one of the crura to make up this length.

Currently, we use alternating 2–0 chromic and 3–0 polydioxanone sutures, placing between eight and 11 sutures in most patients. We mobilize the urethra with the bulbospongiosum intact. The anterior aspect of the bulbous urethra is sewn to the anterior aspect of the prostatic urethra before the sutures placed in the posterior aspect of the repair are tied down. Prior to tying the sutures and seating the anastomosis, a stenting silicone catheter is placed through the repair under direct vision.

The urethra lies in the groove created by splitting the decussation of the corpora cavernosa. To relieve tension, the mobilized urethra is attached to the corpora cavernosa with interrupted sutures of Vicryl or polydioxanone. Because of the careful dissection and the stepwise process in which we proceed, from division of the triangular ligament through development of the intercrural space to infrapubectomy, we have generally created very little dead space that is usually filled very well by the corpus spongosium of the bulb. If this does not fill the dead space, a dartos fascial flap can be mobilized from the scrotum to fill it. When there is marked displacement of the bladder neck, it may be necessary to mobilize a gracilis muscle flap to fill the dead space. With the patient's legs in this position, the gracilis muscle may seem to be markedly displaced in a posterior direction. Care must be taken not to become confused during mobilization of the muscle.

To date, we have not needed a combined procedure for repair of what were only distraction defects. Some patients clearly have an incompetent bladder neck and need a concurrent procedure. These patients require a combined abdominal and perineal exposure. In other medical centers, the combined exposure is utilized for all cases. Their patients are not placed into the exaggerated lithotomy position but rather into a relatively low lithotomy position (Turner-Warwick, 1988). The limited perineal exposure inherent in the low lithotomy position is overcome by dissecting from above. Total pubectomy for the reconstruction of a posterior urethral distraction defect is virtually never required. In patients in whom a combined abdominal perineal exposure is required, the large amount of dead space created by the dissection in the space of Retzius and beneath the pubis must be obliterated. The omentum serves as an excellent source of tissue for transfer to obliterate this dead space (Turner-Warwick, 1989). Failing that, an inferior rectus abdominis muscle flap can be transposed into the retropubic area for obliteration of this dead space.

Fortunately, few patients cannot be managed with primary reanastomosis of the urethra. There are patients, however, who have had a significant amount of damage to the anterior urethra during the same trauma that caused the posterior urethral distraction injury. Vascular occlusion will not allow the corpus spongiosum to be mobilized—one of the tissue transfer techniques must be employed to re-establish the continuity of the urethra. Grafts, even when accompanied by transfer of a muscle flap, are seldom of help in these patients. Penile preputial flaps mobilized on a dartos fascial pedicle have been successful, however. One of us (GHJ) has spanned a 13-cm defect with a tubed penile preputial skin island mobilized on a dartos fascial pedicle. A second defect, measuring 11 cm, has been so reconstructed. Both flaps survived, and both patients are voiding through unencumbered urethras.

Postoperative Management of Posterior Strictures

The urethral stenting catheter that we employ is a 20 Fr. ribbed silicone catheter (Rusch). The urine is diverted by a suprapubic cystostomy with the urethral catheter plugged, serving only as a stent. In most patients, the urethral stenting catheter is left in place for 21 days. At that time, it is removed and a voiding urethrogram is performed. If good healing is documented, the suprapubic cystostomy tube is clamped. The patient is then able to void per urethra, following this office visit.

The suprapubic catheter is removed 5 to 7 days later. Cultures of the urine are obtained during this time so that when he no longer has a catheter, bacterial colonization of the bladder can be managed with organism-specific antibiotics. In patients who require a graft or flap, the catheter may remain a little longer. The operative field and, in particular, the tunnel dissected beneath the scrotum during mobilization of the urethra must be drained. We employ a combination of 10-mm J-Vac drains (Johnson & Johnson, New Brunswick, NJ 08903) and 10 Fr. TLS drains (Porex Medical, Fairburn, GA 30213) left in as long as required. When the drainage becomes serous, the drains can be removed.

Patients generally remain in bed for 5 days postoperatively. In older patients or those with associated orthopedic injuries of the lower extremities, Kendall stockings are worn. We have not routinely ordered prophylactic heparinization. Most patients are ready for discharge from the hospital on the 6th or 7th postoperative day.

Postoperatively, patients are evaluated with urethroscopy. The flexible cystopanendoscope allows for endoscopic evaluation in such an atraumatic fashion that it has virtually replaced postoperative radiographic studies. In the absence of symptoms, this evaluation is performed between 5 and 6 months. Review of our patients shows that strictures that will undergo restenosis will have done so by 1 year. Patients are again evaluated at 1 year with repeat urethroscopy. If, at that time, the repair is widely patent, we believe that the scarring process is mature and further routine follow-up is not done. Flow studies are not valuable in these patients. Repaired strictures can undergo a significant degree of restenosis with no adverse effect on the flow. The reduction of voiding pressure that accompanies the usual recompensation of the hypertrophic bladder, following relief of the obstruction, may be confusing. With this decrease in propelling force, there will be a decrease in flow that is not an indicator of restenosis.

PENILE CURVATURE

Normal elasticity of the tissue layers of the penis is critical for erectile function. As the penis engorges with blood, it expands its girth and extends its length until the tissues of the tunica and the septum of the corpora cavernosa are stretched to the limit of their elasticity. In the normal penis, the tissues are symmetrically elastic, and the erection will be straight. Chordee, a congenital or an acquired bend of the penis, is caused by decreased elasticity in one or more of the fascial layers of the penis, leading to a shortness of one aspect of the erect corporal bodies. The bend may be ventral, dorsal, lateral, or complex.

CONGENITAL CHORDEE

Fetal development of the penis is regulated by the testosterone produced by the fetal testis and is converted to dihydrotestosterone by the enzyme 5-alpha reductase in the target cells of the male external genitalia. The urethra begins as an epithelial groove in the midline on the ventral surface of the developing penis. As the groove extends it deepens; eventually, the edges meet and fuse to form a tube. Fusion begins proximally and progresses distally, until the urethral tube reaches the end of the penis. Proliferating mesenchyme surrounds the tube, separating it from the skin, and differentiates to form the corpus spongiosum, Buck's fascia, and dartos fascia (Fig. 83–56, *left*) (Devine, 1982).

Maturation of these tissues into normal structures depends on the same growth factors that control the formation of the urethra. Even though urethral development has progressed normally, mesenchymal tissue development in the penis may be deficient, resulting in dysgenetic and inelastic fascial layers. Chordee is most frequently associated with hypospadias when the mesenchyme distal to the meatus ceases to differentiate, becoming a fan-shaped band of dysgenetic fascia. The apex of this inelastic tissue surrounds the urethral meatus and inserts into the undersurface of the glans penis, matching the width of the defect in the prepuce (Fig. 83–56, *right*). We believe that in most cases, the anomaly in hypospadias is due to premature cessation of the production of testosterone (Devine and Horton, 1979).

In chordee without hypospadias, development of the urethral epithelial tube has progressed to the tip of the glans. The prepuce is normal in configuration; however, the penis curves ventrally with erection. When present, it is disturbing for affected patients and a challenge for surgeons to repair. If diagnosed in childhood, it should be corrected at that time. However, the patient may not seek treatment until after puberty, because often the curvature worsens or does not become apparent until the growth of the penis that occurs during adolescence. As defined by which fascial layer of the penis is involved, there are five types of chordee without hypospadias (Fig. 83–57) (Devine and Horton, 1973).

In type I, the urethral meatus is at the tip of the glans; however, none of the surrounding layers are normally formed, and the epithelial urethra lies immediately beneath the skin with inelastic fascia deep to it.

In type II, a dysgenetic band of fibrous tissue derived from the mesenchyme that would have produced Buck's fascia and the dartos fascia lies beneath and lateral to the urethra within the normally developed corpus spongiosum.

In type III, the urethra, corpus spongiosum, and Buck's fascia are all normally developed with the inelastic tissue present in the dartos layer. There may be only a short area of involvement with a sharp bend. Abnormal development of the dartos fascia is often associated with torsion of the penis. With extensive involvement, the inelasticity may be sufficient to restrain the penis and conceal the penile shaft within the skin.

In type IV, although the urethra, corpus spongiosum, and fascial layers are normally developed, there is relative shortness or inelasticity of one aspect, usually the ventral, of the tunica albuginea of the corpora cavernosa.

Type V is the so-called congenital short urethra. The term was synonymous with chordee without hypospadias. Discussion of the condition centered on the best location to cut the urethra during the repair. Short urethra occurs so rarely that the urethra should be cut only after the corpora cavernosa have been released and

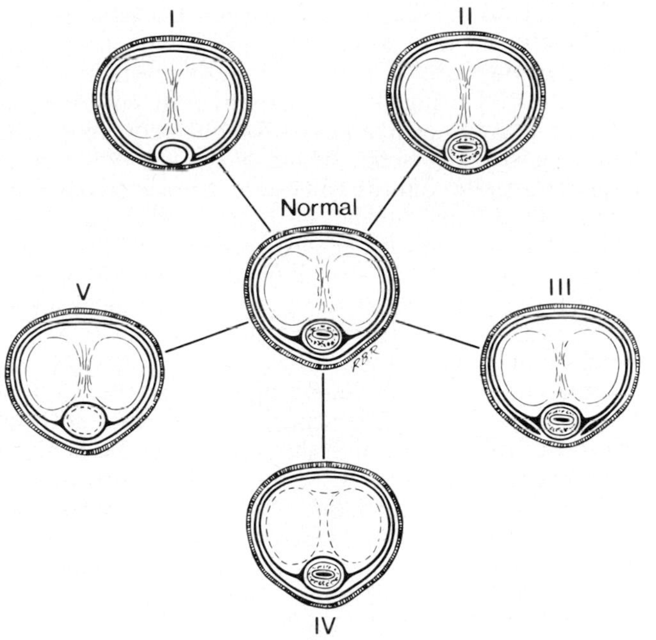

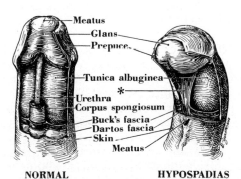

Figure 83–56. Anatomy of the normal penis and one with hypospadias. The fan-shaped band of fibrous tissue marked with an asterisk is the structure that holds the penis in chordee. (From Horton, C. E., and Devine, C. J., Jr.: Hypospadias. *In* Converse, J. M. (Ed.): Reconstructive Plastic Surgery. Philadelphia, W. B. Saunders Co., 1977.)

Figure 83–57. Cross-section of the penis displaying the forms of chordee without hypospadias. The normal penis is in the center.

Class I. Epithelial urethra beneath the skin. Dysgenetic tissue beneath it represents undeveloped corpus spongiosum, Buck's fascia, and dartos fascia.

Class II. Normal urethra and spongiosum but abnormal Buck's and dartos fascia.

Class III. Abnormal dartos fascia only.

Class IV. Normal urethra and fascial layers with abnormal corpocavernosal development.

Class V. "Congenital short urethra" (rare) (From Devine, C. J.: Bent penis. Semin. Urol., 5:252, 1987.)

the corpus spongiosum has been widely mobilized. If, after these maneuvers, the urethra continues to act as a bowstring, it should be divided in its mid-portion. The resultant defect can be repaired with a tube constructed from a flap or a skin graft.

CHORDEE WITHOUT HYPOSPADIAS IN YOUNG MEN

We have seen a number of young adults who have chordee without hypospadias, most commonly type II or IV. In many of these cases, the patients state that erections have always been curved yet their parents remember only straight erections during childhood. These young men tend to have a stretched penile length greater than average (13.1 cm) (Schonfeld and Beebe, 1942), with a gradual curvature throughout the length of the shaft, bending downward 30 to 40 degrees. In some cases, the flaccid penis may seem of average length; however, with tumescence the erect penis is impressively longer than average. Occasionally, there is an element of lateral curvature as well. A dense band of tissue on the ventral side of the penis beneath the corpus spongiosum can be best felt with the penis stretched. The restrictive effect of this tissue can be recognized in that the ventral aspect of the penis will stretch taut while the dorsal side is still loose.

This fibrous band consists of dysgenetic tissue replacing Buck's and the dartos fascial layers on the ventral surface of the corpora cavernosa and inelasticity of the tunica itself. During surgical exploration, we have obtained tissue for evaluation of 5-alpha reductase. The data suggest a deficiency of the enzyme in the ventral dysgenetic tissue, but the values are inconclusive to date (unpublished data, Devine, C. J., Jr., and Pepe, G.).

Corrective surgery is highly successful. In some cases, we have been able to straighten the penis by sharply excising all of the dysgenetic tissue from the ventral side of the penis and by mobilizing the very elastic corpus spongiosum (Fig. 83–58). However, in most patients, the penis will still be curved owing to inelasticity causing shortness of the ventral aspect of the erect corpora cavernosa. In children, this abnormality can be handled by maintaining the erection and by making a longitudinal incision in the ventral midline of the corpora cavernosa, using a new No. 15 knife blade, cutting deliberately and cautiously to dissect between the corporal bodies. As the edges of the tunica move laterally, the penis will straighten (Devine et al., 1988).

When this maneuver is not sufficient, a dorsal ellipse of tunica can be excised. In hypospadias, one must be

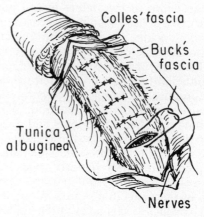

Figure 83–59. Dorsal shortening operation of Nesbit (1964). Silk sutures are being placed in the incised tunica albuginea of the corpora body. (From Hand, J. R.: *In* Campbell, M. F., and Harrison, J. H. (Eds.): Urology, vol. 3, 3rd ed. Philadelphia, W. B. Saunders Co., 1970.)

especially careful when excising a dorsal ellipse of tunica. With incomplete development of the corpus spongiosum, the sole vascularity of the glans is supplied by the dorsal arteries and veins that lie between Buck's fascia and the tunica albuginea. A midline ventral incision is never effective in adults. To equalize the length of the dorsal and ventral aspects of the corporal bodies, it has been necessary to excise one or more ellipses of dorsal tunica albuginea (Fig. 83–59). In one patient, we found a deep longitudinal midline groove on the dorsal aspect of the corpora. We approximated the edges of this groove—in effect rotating the corporal bodies inward—straightening the penile shaft. In 24 of 26 cases, in a two-year period, correction was accomplished in one operation, with two cases needing a second operation to achieve a straight penis (Devine et al., 1991).

We ask each patient to bring a Polaroid photograph of his erect penis documenting the curvature. All patients are screened preoperatively by a sex therapist. Our surgical approach is illustrated in Figure 83–60. Most have been circumcised, and the patterns of venous and lymph drainage of the skin have been established at the time of that procedure. We make an incision through the circumcision scar, which in some cases is nearly half way down the shaft of the penis, and reflect the skin to the base of the penis by dissecting in the dartos fascia layer, immediately superficial to Buck's fascia.

An artificial erection will demonstrate the location and character of the curvature. Ventrally, the dartos and Buck's fascial layers are usually thickened along each side of the urethra. We mobilize this fibrous tissue completely, excising it sharply from the tunica albuginea, and widely mobilize the corpus spongiosum and urethra. After excising all of the obviously dysgenetic tissue, we repeat the artificial erection. In patients with type II chordee without hypospadias, who have normal corporal bodies, the penis will be straightened completely by this dissection. Most patients, however, have a type IV defect with shortness or inelasticity of the ventral aspect of the corporal bodies. Expansion of the circumference of the penile shaft is greatly improved.

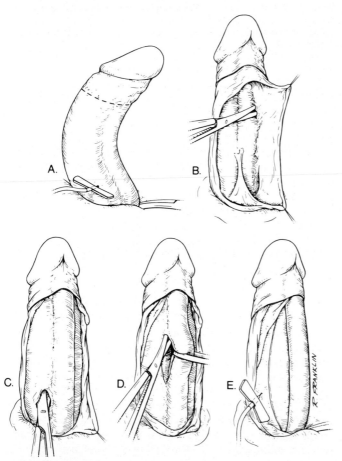

Figure 83–58. Surgery for class II chordee without hypospadias. *A,* Ventral curvature demonstrated with artificial erection.

B, Dysgenetic dartos fascia is elevated and will be excised.

C, The dysgenetic layer of Buck's fascia is undermined by spreading the scissors.

D, The inelastic fascia is excised as the corpus spongiosum and urethra are mobilized.

E, Artificial erection demonstrates correction of the curvature.

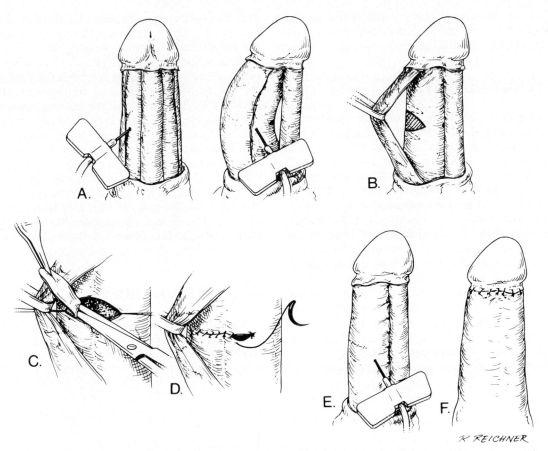

K REICHNER

Figure 83–60. Surgery for class IV chordee without hypospadias. *A,* A circumcising incision has been made and the urethra mobilized by resecting the dartos and Buck's fascia. The needle is in place for an artificial erection. The erection shows continuing chordee. The elastic urethra is not the cause of this curvature. The point of maximum concavity has been marked.

B, An ellipse of tissue is outlined opposite the point of maximum concavity. As an alternative, two smaller ellipses are shown.

C, Excision of the ellipse of tunica. Note the tips of the septal strands in the midline.

D, Closure of the edges of the incision.

E, Artificial erection revealing a straight penis. When the bend is more complex, ellipses must be excised in other locations.

F, The skin is closed. (From Devine, C. J.: Bent penis. Semin. Urol., 5:4, 1987.)

The curvature will be lessened, but significant curvature will persist.

In an adult, when there is still curvature, there are two options for surgical correction: (1) to lengthen the ventral aspect of the penis by making a transverse incision in the ventral tunica with placement of a dermal graft and (2) to shorten the dorsal aspect of the penis by mobilizing the neurovascular bundle, excising an ellipse or several ellipses that cross the midline of the dorsal tunica albuginea and closing the defects in a watertight fashion (the Nesbit procedure) (see Fig. 83–59) (Nesbit, 1965). Because, in this case, the erect penis is usually longer than average, we have chosen the second of these options, since the recovery period is much shorter. However, if the patient has a short penis we will not hesitate to employ a dermal graft (Devine and Horton, 1975).

Having decided to proceed with excision of ellipses of the dorsal tunica, we mobilize the lateral aspects of Buck's fascia and elevate the dorsal neurovascular bundle from the tunica (Fig. 83–60). An artificial erection allows us to mark a narrow ellipse of tunica opposite

the point of maximum concavity. We plicate the edges of this ellipse with several 5-0 Prolene sutures or skin staples and repeat the artificial erection. If the penis is not perfectly straight, we mark and plicate a second and, if necessary, a third ellipse until the penis is straight. With brilliant green marking solution, we mark the edges of the ellipses again before removing the sutures. The ellipses are excised, cutting through the tunica and removing the ellipse of the tunica by dissection in the space of Smith, being careful not to damage the underlying erectile tissue.

The defects are closed with interrupted and running 5–0 PDS. This monofilament is absorbed by hydrolysis over the course of 6 months. By the time the suture is absorbed, healing of the tunica will have progressed with enough strength to withstand the intracorporal pressures associated with intercourse. The resultant scar is usually impalpable. After closure, another artificial erection is performed to confirm the straightening. We close Buck's fascia with interrupted 5–0 PDS and replace the skin sleeve, apposing its edges with interrupted chromic sutures. Two suction drains remain, which are removed in 24 to 36 hours. The patient is discharged from the hospital on the 2nd or 3rd postoperative day, depending on the extent of edema.

LATERAL PENILE CURVATURE

Lateral penile curvature is an uncommon situation in post adolescent males. It is caused by a disparity in the size of the corpora cavernosa, usually the right side being larger than the left with a curvature to the left—we have seen only three to the right. Repair of lateral curvature is similar to that of ventral curvature. In most cases, the lateral bend is uncomplicated, but in others there is an upward or downward component. In simpler cases, after induction of anesthesia, we observe an artificial erection to delineate the deformity. Placing the needle through the glans is associated with fewer problems when an artificial erection is to be done prior to making the skin incisions. We mark the point of maximum concavity on the short side and make a longitudinal incision in the skin opposite that point (Fig. 83–61).

After opening the dartos fascia and Buck's fascia and mobilizing the dorsal neurovascular bundle to expose the tunica albuginea, we place two Prolene sutures, one near the corpus spongiosum and another directly opposite on the dorsal surface of the tunica. While maintaining an artificial erection, with opposing tension on the Prolene sutures, we push on the glans to straighten the penis, thereby generating a fold in the tunica. We mark the edges of this fold and outline the ellipse to be excised. To be sure that the correct amount of tissue will be excised, we place Prolene sutures to plicate these marks together and establish another artificial erection.

We remove the elliptic segment of the tunica that we have marked and sew the edges together with interrupted and running 5–0 PDS. If the bend is more complex, wider exposure is necessary. A circumcising incision is made, and the skin is reflected from the shaft of the penis. While maintaining the artificial erection, we identify the location of multiple incisions, which will be necessary to straighten the penis.

ACQUIRED CHORDEE

Acquired chordee may follow trauma or may be caused by Peyronie's disease. If, during transurethral surgery for a urethral stricture, using a visual cold knife or an Otis urethrotome the incision is extended outside

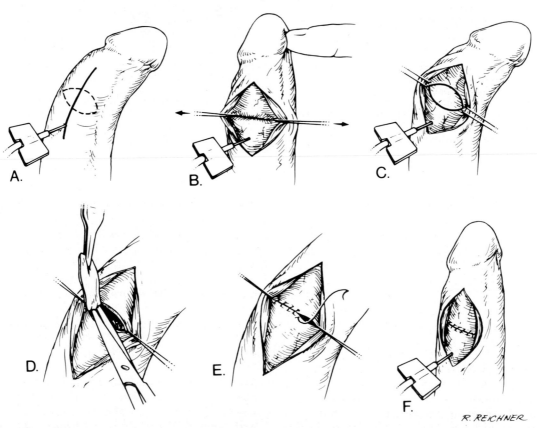

R. REICHNER

Figure 83–61. Lateral curvature. *A,* An artificial erection reveals the curvature. The incision to gain access to the potential ellipse of tissue is marked.

B, The tunica albuginea has been exposed by mobilizing Buck's fascia, and Prolene sutures have been placed at the dorsal and ventral tips of the potential ellipse. While maintaining the artificial erection, tension is established on the two sutures as the penile shaft is straightened. The fold produced in the tunica is marked.

C, When the penis is relaxed, this mark defines the ellipse of tunica to be removed.

D, The tunica is excised.

E, The edges are approximated with interrupted and running 5–0 polydioxanone sutures.

F, The penis is straight. Buck's fascia and the skin will be closed.

the urethra to involve the tunica of the corporal bodies, scarring can cause chordee. Inflammation from a long-standing indwelling catheter can also generate a scar. Correction of this type of curvature involves surgery of the tunica not unlike that described next for Peyronie's disease. Chordee caused by inelasticity of the urethra may follow reconstruction of hypospadias or urethral stricture. In that case, urethral reconstruction will be necessary. With release of the urethral scarring, the penis may be sufficiently straightened making it unnecessary to repair the corpora.

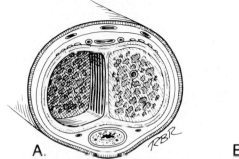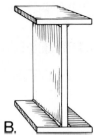

Figure 83–62. *A,* Diagram of the penis as related to the occurrence of Peyronie's disease. The fibers of the septum are attached to the inner surface of the tunica albuginea of the corpora cavernosa along the dorsal and ventral midlines. Plaques of Peyronie's disease occur in the tunica albuginea at the site of attachment of the septal strands.

B, A diagram of an I-beam illustrates the configuration of the septum that is responsible for the ultimate rigidity of the penile erection. This function leads to the occurrence of Peyronie's disease. (From Devine, C. J., Jordan, G. H., and Somers, K. D.: Peyronie's disease: Cause and surgical treatment. AUA Today, Vol. 2, No. 5, September/October, 1989.)

PEYRONIE'S DISEASE

In Peyronie's disease, named for Francois de la Peyronie (Peyronie, 1743) surgeon to Louis XV of France, a scar, called a plaque, in the tunica albuginea of the corpora cavernosa restricts the elasticity of the involved aspect of the penis causing the erection to be bent. The condition is not rare—we have seen it in about 1 per cent of the men in two small groups. None of these men have required surgery, although one had undergone a biopsy prior to consultation. Most patients have been middle-aged, but the youngest was 19. We have also seen it in a number of sexually active men over 70. Only a few patients have been black, none Oriental.

Other physiologically important elastic tissue may be involved by similar processes: palmar fascia by Dupuytren's contracture; plantar fascia by Ledderhose's disease (Magalini, 1990); and ear drum by tympanosclerosis. As many as 25 per cent of our patients have had Dupuytren's contracture. A familial association is noted in patients with these conditions, but no special association with the B7 group of HLA antigens (Leffell, et al., 1982; Nyberg, et al., 1982). No test will identify relatives at risk.

The cause of Peyronie's disease has not been well understood. In 1966, Smith described its pathology and thought that the lesion resulted from perivascular inflammation in the space he described as lying between the tunica albuginea and the erectile tissue. Smith (1969) was never able to define the cause of this inflammation; however, most of the nonsurgical treatment of Peyronie's disease is aimed at controlling it. Inflammation is present in this space, but it is also present in and beneath Buck's fascia where it overlies the lesion. We believe the inflammation to be a result of the underlying process in the tunica. The plaque is a scar not the result of an inflammatory or autoimmune process.

Pathophysiology

Tissue sections from plaques stained using a technique that defines elastic fibers, collagen, and fibrin exhibit characteristically disordered collagen and abnormal deposition of elastic fibers. Extravascular material in these sections has been identified as fibrin through biochemical and immunologic criteria (Devine, 1988). Although there is excessive deposition of collagen in the plaques,

cells derived from plaques do not show excessive collagen production in tissue culture. They do show strongly reduced elastin production (Somers, et al., 1989).

Plaques may extend laterally to involve adjacent aspects of the tunica albuginea, but all plaques that we have seen have been located in the dorsal or ventral midline, where the strands of the septum are attached. The cross-sectional diagram of the penis depicts the structural relationships that we believe cause Peyronie's disease (Fig. 83–62A).

Two layers of elastic fibers are observed in the tunica albuginea, the outer being longitudinal and the inner circular. The fibers of the septal strands fan out and are interwoven with the strands of the inner layer of the tunica (Fig. 83–63A). Normally, the tissues of the corpora are symmetrically elastic and the penis remains relatively straight as it fills with blood and becomes erect. As they stretch, the tissues of the tunica become thinner. Without an inner supporting fibrous structure, the penis would have little rigidity. An intracavernosal fibrous framework contributes to this characteristic (Goldstein and Padma-Nathan, 1990); however, the strands of the septum afford most of the axial rigidity to the erect penis.

When the tunical sheath and the septum have been stretched to the limit of their distensibility, the configuration of the septum forms an inflated "I-beam" (Fig. 83–62B), resisting dorsoventral bending forces. When the penis flexes in this plane, the stress in the system—compression on the concave side and tension on the convex side—is focused at the connection of the septal strands with the tunica, where plaques of Peyronie's disease occur as scars in the tunica albuginea.

Other investigators have associated trauma in a susceptible individual, possibly during sexual intercourse, with the occurrence of Peyronie's disease (DeSanctis, 1967; Godec, 1983; Hinman, 1983; McRoberts, 1969). We agree and think that we can define the process by which it happens. Diminution of the modulus of elasticity of the aging tissues of the tunica is perhaps the first

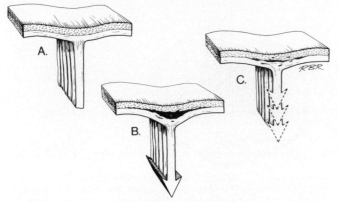

Figure 83–63. *A,* Fibers of the septal strands fan out and are interwoven with the inner circular layer of fibers of the tunica albuginea. The outer layer consists of longitudinal fibers.

B, In the *acute* form of Peyronie's disease, bending the erect penis out of column produces tension on the strands of the septum delaminating the fibers of the tunica albuginea. Bleeding occurs, and the space fills with a clot. The scar generated by the response of the tissue to this process becomes the plaque of Peyronie's disease.

C, In the *chronic* form of Peyronie's disease, less turgid erections allow flexion of the penis during intercourse producing elastic tissue fatigue, further reducing the elasticity of the tissue and leading to multiple smaller ruptures of the fibers of the tunica with smaller collections of blood producing multiple scars. (From Devine, C. J., Jordan, G. H., and Somers, K. D.: Peyronie's disease: Cause and surgical treatment. AUA Today, Vol. 2, No. 5, September/October, 1989.)

step. The rapidity of this loss of elasticity may be genetically determined, accounting for its familial association. Trauma to the penis need not be severe—tension generated at the attachment of the stressed septal strands by an acute bending out of column of the turgid penis can be sufficient to delaminate the fibers of the tunica (Fig. 83–63*B*). This tear disrupts small blood vessels with bleeding and formation of a clot within the tunica.

As the clot resolves, fibrin remains in the injured tissue. Retained fibrin (1) activates fibroblasts causing cellular proliferation, (2) enhances vascular permeability, and (3) generates chemotactic factors for inflammatory cells (histiocytes). This is a normal part of the process of healing, but the tunica is relatively hypovascular. The fibrin is not removed by the remodeling that takes place in the tissue during healing. Because this original stimulus is not cleared or perhaps because of repeated trauma leading to further fibrin deposition, the lesion does not resolve. Inflammation persists, collagen is trapped, and pathologic fibrosis ensues (NIH Grant No. 1546055378A2—Cell Biology and Immunology of Peyronie's Disease—Kenneth D. Somers, Ph.D., Principal Investigator). The other participants in the study are enumerated in the references (e.g., Devine, 1988 and 1989; Schmidt, 1987; Somers, 1982, 1987, and 1989; and VandeBerg, 1981 and 1982). The course of this active process, during which the body is attempting to remodel the scar, generally takes about 1 to 1.5 years.

Peyronie's disease occurs mostly in men of middle-age, less frequently in younger men or older men. Young men accumulate intracorporal pressures sufficient to resist the deforming force and limit flexion during inter-

course. Despite the turgor of the erection or the vigor of the intercourse, should a bend occur the elasticity of the tissue allows the structures to stretch with the stress and spring back. As a man ages, the tissues become less elastic. This rigidity diminishes and, if the vigor of intercourse persists, this same type of force can cause the penis to bend generating a tear as discussed. Many of these patients retain a vivid memory of this acute episode, perhaps a week to a month prior to the onset of the Peyronie's disease. With older men intercourse is often less vigorous and, despite diminished elasticity and rigidity, there is less likelihood of such trauma.

This process can explain the acute onset of Peyronie's disease, but in most patients the onset is insidious. These men will have lost some of the turgor of erection. Tension on the septal strands is decreased during active sexual performance, allowing the attachments to the tunica to work back and forth generating tissue fatigue. This factor further reduces the elasticity of the attachments of the septal strands, leading to multiple small tears with vascular disruption and deposition of fibrin (Fig. 83–63*C*). The result, however, is the same—a scar causing a bend of the penis.

In about half of our patients, the condition has appeared suddenly with little or no further progression. Others may first have noted pain or a lump, followed by minimal curvature that is slowly progressive. These two presentations may represent the two sets of patients noted previously. Although often considered pathognomonic of Peyronie's disease, pain has been present in only two thirds of the patients we have seen (Snow and Devine, 1981). The history and the characteristic physical findings will usually provide the diagnosis. Any association with a previous medication (e.g., beta blockers) or concurrent disease (e.g., diabetes) will be happenstance.

The scar may involve one or several strands of the septum. Although sometimes discussed, the erectile tissue is almost never involved in the scar of Peyronie's disease. The plaque is confined to the tunica albuginea located in the dorsal or ventral midline. In looking for a plaque, physical examination of the penis must be precise. Giving the penis a dorsoventral squeeze will distinguish the lesion but will not define its extent. The examiner must remember that the plaque is on the dorsal or ventral aspect of the corpora confined to the tunica albuginea. While grasping the glans with one hand and stretching the penis to its limit, the edges of the lesion can be palpated between the index finger and thumb of the other hand placed laterally on the shaft. Dorsal plaques can be differentiated from ventral plaques without difficulty.

Most plaques involve the dorsal aspect of the corporal body, causing the penis to bend upward. In contrast, a ventral plaque will cause a downward bend. If involvement of the tunica is not symmetric and there is more overhang of the scar on one side than the other, the curvature will have a lateral component. Combined dorsal and ventral plaques may balance each other, the shaft being straight or curved laterally but shortened with a reduced circumference in the involved area, sometimes causing the penis to be flail at the site of the opposed plaques. In some patients, the part of the penis distal to the plaque will not be as firm as the part proximal to it. The patient may think that the lesion has obstructed the flow of blood into that part of the penis. Doppler studies, however, have shown that the plaque, confined to the tunica, does not obstruct the arteries in the penis. We are not sure of the cause of this disparity in erection, but the plaque does restrict the extension of the elastic fibers of the tunica and the intercavernosal fibrous framework that are attached to it. Until these elastic tissues are stretched to their limit, they have no strength.

Peyronie's disease and erectile dysfunction are often associated (Godec and Van Beek, 1983). Peyronie's disease in and of itself does not cause impotence, and some degree of dysfunction may be a precursor of Peyronie's disease. The distortion and pain can also have a profound psychologic effect. It is unlikely that a patient will not be able to achieve an erection, but he may lose it quickly—especially if pain is present. If some degree of venous occlusive dysfunction (venous leak) is present, he may note that the erect penis is not as firm as it used to be.

Diminution of the elasticity of the aging tissue of the corpora cavernosa, which plays a part in the pathogenesis of Peyronie's disease, also plays a major part in the impotence that may accompany it. Proponents of the implantation of a prosthesis as the first line of therapy for Peyronie's disease have argued that all patients with Peyronie's disease will become impotent. This is not the case, and there is no rationale for putting a device in a man still capable of achieving his own erection.

Course: When the active remodeling process in the scar in the tunica has run its course, the effects of the lesion may remain static or recede, occasionally disappearing completely. Pain that is associated with the inflammation present during the active phase of Peyronie's disease disappears with resolution of the inflammation. For this reason, medical therapy directed at the inflammation may have a beneficial effect early in the course of the disease.

During the year and a half that it takes for the situation to resolve and for the scar to become fixed, most patients have been able to maintain sexual activity. However, they will never be the same as they were prior to the onset of this condition. When the scar has matured, there will be no further change in the configuration of the penis (Gelbard, et al., 1990). If at that time, the patient and his partner are satisfied with their sexual function, no medical therapy will benefit the situation. They should be advised that he should not have surgery. If, however, the distortion does not allow intercourse satisfactory for both, surgery will be required. A plaque can reach maturity without calcification, but calcification is a sign of the end stage of the healing process and may be present in as short a time as 6 months.

Extensive investigation is not required to diagnose the disease, but a simple radiograph to discern calcification aids the prognosis. In a quarter of our patients, radiography of the plaque has revealed calcium. In one of every four of these, there has been ossification. Xeroradiography, which is more complex and costly, can also show the presence of calcification. We have not seen it demonstrate the extent of an uncalcified lesion.

Ultrasound can show the plaque, but this study adds little to the digital examination (Altaffer, 1981). Ultrasound can also demonstrate calcification at which time the sonic shadow of the lesion in the tunica will obscure the spongy tissue beneath it. This irregularity has been interpreted as evidence of involvement of the erectile tissue by Peyronie's disease. The erectile tissue has not been involved in any of the many patients we have operated upon. Simple corpus cavernosography can delineate the extent of a plaque, but rarely will this study furnish information that will change the course of therapy. Expensive tests, such as magnetic resonance imaging, have contributed nothing to our evaluation of the situation in individual patients nor to our understanding of the disease. In younger patients there is a possibility of sarcoma, but a biopsy will be necessary only if the lesion is uncharacteristic.

Treatment: During the acute phase, most medical therapy has been aimed at control of inflammation. This may help to relieve discomfort in the very early stages. Dimethyl sulfoxide (DMSO), ultrasound therapy, iontophoresis of steroids, and other treatment modalities have been tried. No controlled studies have been done to show that the patients receiving these treatments do better than those receiving no treatment at all (Williams and Thomas, 1970). Collagenase injections sound reasonable (Gelbard, 1985), but a double-blind evaluation did not encourage their continuation (Gelbard, 1989). Though often prescribed as a specific agent for the "bent spike," *p*-aminobenzoate (Potaba) requires 24 tablets per day, carries a significant incidence of gastrointestinal distress, and costs $2000 per year. Many patients we have seen have been taking this medication without specific effect, although some believe that it has relieved pain.

We have seen little benefit and have seen tissue atrophy in patients who have had steroids injected. We do not, therefore, inject plaques with steroids. We have also seen tissue atrophy following radiation therapy delivered in the tumoricidal doses sometimes reported in the literature. Radiation will not affect the outcome of the scarring process. Persistence of pain is, to our minds, the only indication for radiation therapy. Pain slowly resolves, persisting in only 1 per cent of our patients (Snow and Devine, 1981). A small dose of radiation delivered by a soft modality (in our hands, 450 rad by the beta beam of a linear accelerator), much as is used to treat a keloid (El-Mahdi, 1990), can allay residual pain. Some patients have told us that terfenadine (Seldane), an antihistamine with no sedative side effects, may help relieve painful erections in the active phases of the disease.

We have found Peyronie's disease to resolve or improve or to become static with continuing function in two thirds of our patients taking vitamin E, 200 mg, with each meal or 400 mg twice a day, and we continue to advise this treatment (Devine, 1974).

EVALUATION. When we first see a patient we insist that his wife or sex partner accompany him so that an explanation of the condition can be given to both. However, because the trauma that led to the scar may have occurred during his involvement with another sex partner, it may be best to question him alone. We also ask each patient to bring two Polaroid photographs of his erect penis. These define the angle of the bend and the quality of the erection. The bend will increase with the turgor of the erection. After the examination, we explain the disease and discuss the situation with him and his sex partner, drawing diagrams and outlining the process by which it has come about. We reassure both that this is not cancer and that it does not mean the end of their sex life. We discuss therapy and the fact that there is no quick cure for the lesion—just slow healing of a scar in the not well-vascularized tunica albuginea. If they are still able to function sexually, we prescribe vitamin E and arrange for follow-up examinations.

Most patients and their wives or sex partners are able to understand this explanation and ask cogent questions. In years past this may have been the first time that the husband will have discussed the problem with his wife, but lately most couples have already discussed it. At the time of our discussion, some women have indicated that intercourse is not the center of their lives and that a decision for surgery is his to make. Others have been quite distraught. Both of these attitudes must be considered in the treatment of the patient, and most couples should have the benefit of consultation with a sex therapist who understands Peyronie's disease (Jones, 1984). Patients with an upward bend of less than 45 degrees can usually continue to have satisfactory intercourse. When the bend is down or to the side, however, the critical angle is 30 degrees. When the bend is worse, attempts at intromission are frequently met with further folding and failure.

In 1978 and 1979, we saw 200 patients, 75 of whom required surgery. In 1981, we were able to contact 105 of those who were sent home with vitamin E and our encouragement (Snow and Devine, 1981). Two thirds of these had continued to function in a satisfactory manner, and some had improved. In four, the lesion had disappeared. In 11 patients, the deformity had increased and they underwent surgery. Originally, four had been impotent; at resurvey, eight were impotent. We subsequently inserted penile prostheses in three of these. The other five declined further treatment. If the plaque has been present for at least a year or is calcified and the distortion precludes intercourse, we offer the patient surgical treatment. This consists of excision of the plaque and replacement of the diseased area of the tunica with a graft from the dermal layer of the skin, as described by Devine and Horton (1974) and Horton and Devine (1973). We have modified the operation over the years (see the following discussion).

Some surgeons have utilized other materials for this patch. Full-thickness skin from the prepuce is unacceptable because buried skin will form a sebaceous cyst. Tunica vaginalis (Das and Maggio, 1979) is thin and, although acceptable for small lesions, does not have the strength for large grafts. Arterial and venous segments and pieces of fascia are flexible but have no elasticity (Horton and Devine, 1973). Gore-Tex and other artificial materials are also not elastic and produce an inflammatory collection of collagen beneath them. We have removed pieces of all of the aforementioned materials from patients who have had prior unsuccessful surgery.

The Nesbit procedure (Nesbit, 1965) has been employed for correction of the bend of the penis in Peyronie's disease (Pryor, 1979). As noted, we use plication to correct other bends in the patient who has a good-sized penis. Despite this practice, we believe plication to be inappropriate for patients who are not functional because of a significant bend caused by Peyronie's disease. We would not want to shorten the penis of a patient who is already distressed by its decreased size. However, the problem is often merely the presence of the bend rather than its severity that incapacitates a man without a sex partner who cannot bring himself to expose his distorted penis to a new sex partner. Minimal distortion can be corrected by a Nesbit tuck or two on the side opposite the bend. We have done this, and we have also employed plication to complete the repair when the penis still has a minimal bend after a dermal graft operation.

Having decided that surgery is necessary, we plan our approach. The Polaroid photographs demonstrate the distortion of the penis, palpation of the penis locates the plaque, and radiography identifies calcification. If, in the past, impotence was a factor, we utilized a duplex ultrasound scan with pulsed Doppler to evaluate a pharmacologically induced erection (Lue et al., 1985). If this study revealed a disorder of vascular function, we proceeded to dynamic infusion corpus cavernosometry (DICC) with corpus cavernosography to evaluate the patient's erectile capacity. Currently, all of our patients who come to surgery undergo this detailed preoperative evaluation (Jordan et al., 1990). Criteria for normalcy have been developed for various phases of DICC (Padma-Nathan, 1989). A man does not have to measure up to these values to have sexual relations that he considers satisfactory. Separate criteria must be considered for patients with Peyronie's disease.

The association of preoperative erectile function with postoperative results is at present the basis of our counseling and recommendations for surgery. Most of our patients who have been able to accumulate 50 mm Hg or more of intercorporal pressure in response to provoked pharmacologic erection (PEP) have been able to have intercourse following straightening of the penis and application of a dermal graft, as have about 60 per cent of the patients who have been able to accumulate 40 to 50 mm Hg of intercorporal pressure. Patients who are unable to have intercourse require placement of a prosthesis. After surgery, a patient who has not been able to accumulate at least 40 mm Hg of intercorporal pressure will have a straight penis that is not turgid enough for intercourse. We advise these men to have prostheses placed at the time of the straightening procedures.

Even in patients who are happy that they can function after surgery, the penis is never "like it used to be." It may be shorter than it was prior to the onset of the Peyronie's disease, and it will have some degree of distortion possibly with patchy areas of hypoesthesia. A patient whose straight penis lacks rigidity may respond to PEP or may require placement of a prosthesis.

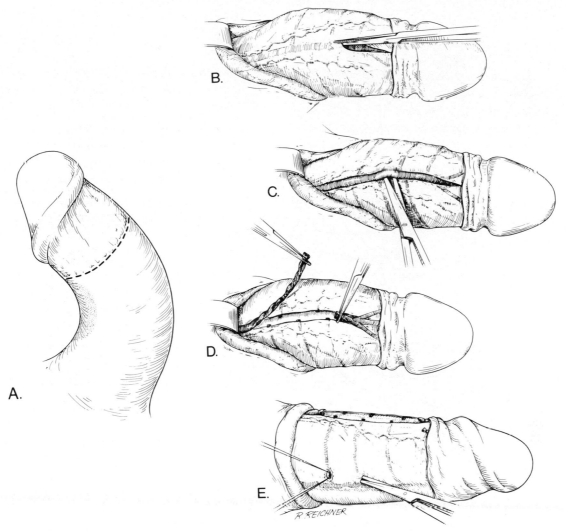

Figure 83–64. *A,* An erection demonstrates the dorsal curvature of the penis caused by the inelastic scar tissue in a dorsal plaque of Peyronie's disease. The incision to be made in the scar of the previous circumcision has been marked.

B, The skin has been reflected to the base of the penis by dissecting in the layer of the dartos fascia. An incision made with scissors in the dorsal midline of Buck's fascia exposes the deep dorsal vein. The coiled dorsal arteries and the circumflex veins are demonstrated.

C, The deep dorsal vein is mobilized by dissecting beneath it with blunt-tipped iris scissors.

D, After dividing the deep dorsal vein, it is dissected proximally, dividing the emissary veins and ligating them with fine black silk sutures. Distally, the vein is mobilized and followed to the point where the veins draining the glans penis combine to form the deep dorsal vein and then dividing and ligating each of these.

E, The circumflex veins are isolated and are oversewn with sutures of 4–0 black silk on each side where they join the vein running lateral to the corpus spongiosum.

Illustration continued on following page

Perhaps 25 per cent of the patients who underwent surgery prior to routine preoperative functional evaluation developed this situation following surgery. Our dermal graft procedure does not preclude later placement of such a device.

Vascular anastomoses become established on both sides of the dermal graft, and we have been concerned that venous "short circuits" not controlled by the normal occlusive mechanism could occur. Therefore, in operations on dorsal plaques (Fig. 83–64), even in patients with normal preoperative vascular function, we remove the penile segment of the deep dorsal vein and expose the lesion by dissecting laterally beneath Buck's fascia through the bed of the vein. This maneuver has improved postoperative function, but to obviate all of these connections it has also been necessary to ligate

the circumflex veins at their junction with the deep veins that run lateral to the corpus spongiosum.

When the plaque is ventrally located and penile vascularity seems normal, similar uncontrolled venous connections can occur between the graft and the corpus spongiosum. We do not excise the deep dorsal vein but ligate the circumflex veins in mobilizing the corpus spongiosum and impose a flap of dartos fascia between the graft and the corpus spongiosum before closing the skin over the urethra (Fig. 83–65).

SURGERY. At surgery, the incision will depend on the location of the lesion. With a ventral plaque, we make a midline incision on the ventral aspect of the penis and mobilize the corpus spongiosum and urethra (Fig. 83–65). Most patients have been circumcised, and for dorsal plaques we make the incision through the scar

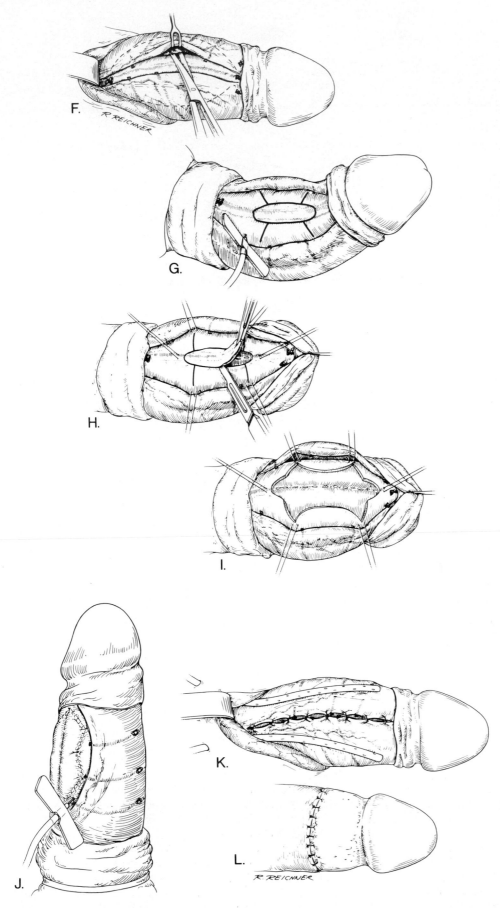

R. REICHNER

Figure 83–64 *Continued F,* Using the blunt-tipped scissors, Buck's fascia is elevated from Peyronie's plaque. The area of dissection is outlined by the dashed line in the diagram, continued far enough proximally, distally, and laterally to allow excision of the plaque without distraction injury to the dorsal arteries and the nerves in Buck's fascia, which are clearly seen and avoided during this dissection.

G, An artificial erection demonstrates the curvature caused by the inelastic plaque, which has been outlined on the tunica. Stellate releasing incisions have also been marked.

H, Prolene sutures have been placed distal and proximal to the plaque and at the tip of each of the releasing incisions. Each suture has been tagged to control the tunica as the surgery progresses. An incision has been made outlining the plaque, and the tip of the plaque is grasped with forceps as it is being excised, using sharp dissection to separate it from the erectile tissue. The strands of the septum have been incised and are seen in the midline of the defect being created.

I, The plaque has been excised, and the lateral incisions have released the shortness of the dorsal aspect of the penis. This defect must now be filled with a dermal graft. To determine the size of the patch we measure the defect in the tunica while stretching it first longitudinally, then laterally.

J, The dermal graft has been obtained (see Fig. 83–69) and applied to the defect (see Fig. 83–70). An artificial erection shows the penis to be straight. If there is a leak in a suture line, it is oversewn with 5–0 polydioxanone sutures.

K, Buck's fascia is loosely reapproximated in the midline with interrupted 5–0 polydioxanone sutures. One or two small suction drains are left in the space above Buck's fascia.

L, The skin closure is completed using several sutures of 5–0 Vicryl in the subcutaneous tissue and 4–0 chromic catgut to approximate the skin. A Bioclusive dressing is applied. A light pressure wrap of Kling dressing is left on for 3 to 4 hours. A 14 Fr. urethral catheter is placed and removed next morning.

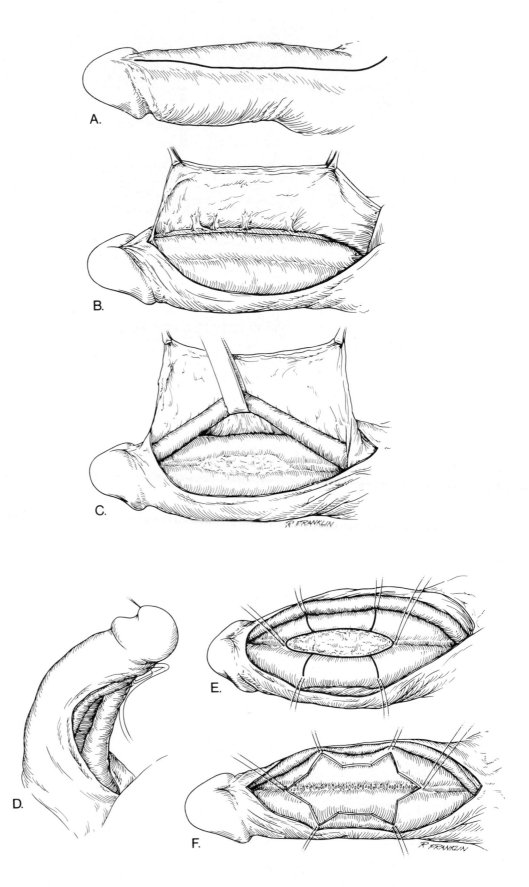

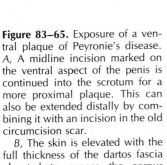

Figure 83–65. Exposure of a ventral plaque of Peyronie's disease.

A, A midline incision marked on the ventral aspect of the penis is continued into the scrotum for a more proximal plaque. This can also be extended distally by combining it with an incision in the old circumcision scar.

B, The skin is elevated with the full thickness of the dartos fascia elevated to expose the corpus spongiosum.

C, The corpus spongiosum is mobilized by incising Buck's fascia on each side. The connections of the circumflex veins with the veins running lateral to the corpus spongiosum are ligated during this dissection. The inelastic plaque of Peyronie's disease is seen on the ventrum of the corporal bodies.

D, An artificial erection demonstrates the extent of the curvature.

E, The incision to excise the plaque and the releasing incisions have been marked. Stay sutures of Prolene are placed at the ends of the plaque and of the releasing incisions.

F, Resection of the plaque is complete. The defect is ready for the dermal graft. Note the ends of the strands of the septum in the midline of this space.

Illustration continued on following page

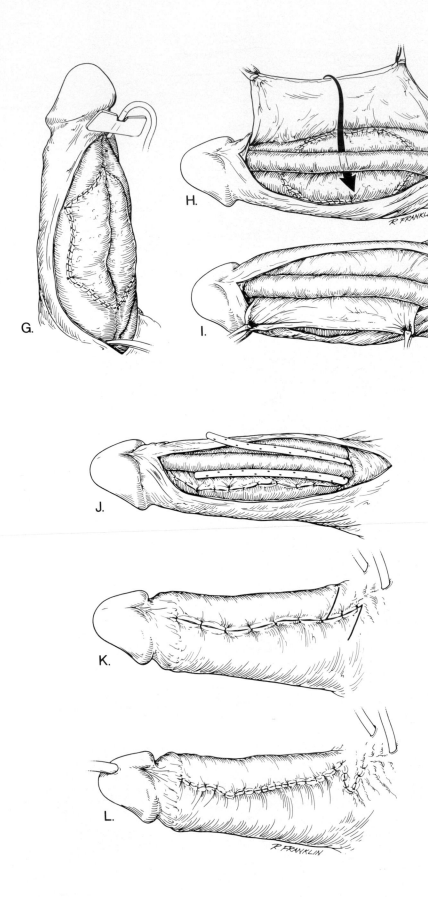

Figure 83–65 *Continued G,* A dermal graft has been obtained (see Fig. 83–69) and placed in the defect (see Fig. 83–70). An artificial erection shows the penis to be straight. Note that the expansion of the graft is restrained by its attachment to the strands of the septum in the midline.

H, A dartos fascial flap has been mobilized from one edge of the penile skin. It will be passed between the graft and the overlying corpus spongiosum. The edges of the layer of Buck's fascia are tacked to the tunica albuginea but are not closed over the graft.

I, The flap has been brought across the graft and will be secured to the dartos fascia on the other side.

J, Closure of the dartos fascia is complete. Two TLS suction drains are in place.

K, The skin is approximated and a Z-plasty has been marked where the incision crosses the penoscrotal junction.

L, Closure is complete. A Bioclusive dressing will be applied, and the 14 Fr. catheter will be removed on the following morning. The patient remains in the hospital for about 3 days.

left by this previous procedure (Fig. 83–64). The skin is mobilized to the base of the penis. This maneuver works well for midshaft lesions with normal venous drainage. For more proximal plaques and for cases in which we plan to excise the most proximal portion of the deep dorsal vein, we make an incision in the scrotum lateral to the base of the penis. Having freed the shaft of the penis, we deliver it into the scrotal incision, laying the penile shaft skin to the side and covering it with a warm sponge (Fig. 83–66). This protects the penile skin from trauma. At the end of the procedure, we replace the penile shaft within the sleeve of skin and close the incision. This technique also works well for uncircumcised patients who do not wish to have the foreskin removed, although there is always more edema in this circumstance.

In the past, we approached a dorsal plaque by reflecting the skin of the penis and made longitudinal incisions in Buck's fascia close to the corpus spongiosum. We extended these incisions on the shaft distal and proximal to the plaque, using blunt-tipped dissecting scissors (Devine-Horton Scissors No. 32–0933–1, Adler Instrument Company, 6191 Atlantic Blvd. Norcross, GA 30071). We then elevated Buck's fascia to mobilize the dorsal nerves and arteries and deep dorsal vein. The inflammation in this tissue plane between the tunica involved by Peyronie's disease and the overlying fascia makes it necessary to dissect sharply to free Buck's fascia and expose the plaque. Where the underlying tunica is normal, Buck's fascia is simply lifted off the tunica by spreading the tips of the scissors between the two tissue layers. We ligated the encircling vessels and emissary veins as we encountered them.

Today, we approach dorsal plaques by dissecting sharply through the bed of the deep dorsal vein, but the same techniques apply. We retract the tunica with hooks and lift Buck's fascia with Beasley forceps to define a sharp angle between the tissue layers, allowing us to cut with the tips of the scissors to open this space. We excise the deep dorsal vein from its origin where the veins draining the coronal sinus come together to the level of the suspensory ligament proximally (Fig. 83–64D). Usually, there is not one single dorsal vein but several veins running in this space anastomosing with one another. It is not unusual to find a venous connection between the deep vein and the superficial drainage system. We ligate the emissary veins and the circumflex veins where they enter the deep dorsal vein. If studies have shown evidence of leakage from the crural veins, we free the penis by cutting the suspensory ligament and follow the deep dorsal veins to the crus, where we ligate the veins as they enter the pampiniform plexus. Crural veins are isolated and ligated as they are identified, being careful not to injure the dorsal or cavernosal arteries or the dorsal or cavernosal nerves, which run close to the venous structures in this area.

We expose the circumflex veins and the longitudinal veins that run lateral to the corpus spongiosum on the ventral side of the penis by making small openings in Buck's fascia with the tips of the dissecting scissors over each vein as we identify it (Fig. 83–64E). Unless the vein is very large, we simply ligate it with a 4-0 silk

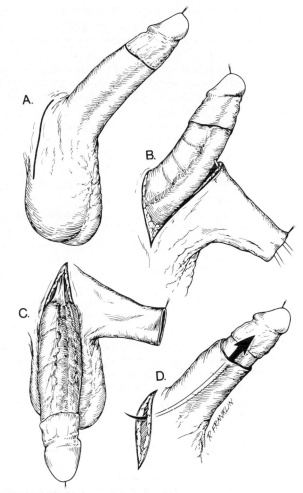

Figure 83–66. *A,* When exposure of the full length of the shaft of the penis is necessary, two incisions are marked: one in the scar of the previous circumcision and the other lateral to the base of the penis and carried down into the scrotum.

B, The two incisions are completed, and the shaft of the penis is freed by dissecting close to Buck's fascia leaving most of the dartos fascia with the skin. The shaft of the penis is delivered into the scrotal incision.

C, Retraction of the penis exposes the full length of the shaft and with minimal dissection the suspensory ligaments can be visualized. With further dissection, complete resection of the dorsal vein can be accomplished.

D, At the conclusion of the surgical procedure, the shaft of the penis is replaced within the relatively untraumatized sleeve of skin.

suture. We coagulate smaller veins with the bipolar cautery and mobilize, cut, and tie larger ones. Having excised or ligated the veins as noted, we expose the tunica in the midline through the bed of the dorsal vein and dissect laterally, elevating Buck's fascia to expose the plaque and the uninvolved tunica peripheral to it (Fig. 83–64F). This dissection affords excellent exposure of dorsal plaques, but care must be taken to protect the prominent dorsal arteries and nerves running on each side close to the deep dorsal vein within Buck's fascia or attached to its deep surface. Mobilization must be continued proximally far enough so that the dorsal nerves are not stretched as the fascia is retracted during resection of the plaque.

For a ventral approach we make a midline incision and after mobilizing the skin by dissecting deep to the dartos fascia, we free up the corpus spongiosum containing the urethra (Fig. 83–65C). As we make this incision in Buck's fascia just lateral to the corpus spongiosum, we ligate the venous connections between the circumflex veins and the veins running lateral to the corpus spongiosum with fine silk or Vicryl sutures. Tiny veins may be coagulated with the bipolar cautery. We dissect beneath the corpus spongiosum with the blunt-tipped dissecting scissors, keeping the tips against the tunica to lessen the chance of opening the corpus spongiosum. Mobilization of this structure is continued well proximal and distal to the lesion.

When the tunica has been exposed, the inelasticity of the plaque will be evident and its extent can be delineated by the rough feel of its surface. An artificial erection defines the curvature (Figs. 83–64G and 83–65D). Incisions can be planned to remove the plaque and correct the curvature (Figs. 83–64G and 83–65E). We place stay sutures of Prolene in the midline proximal and distal to the plaque and beyond the tips of the lateral releasing incisions that will be made. We incise following the marks through the full thickness of the tunica albuginea around the plaque. The tip of the plaque is lifted, and the plaque is resected employing a knife or sharp pointed scissors (Devine Scissors No. 32–0703–1, Adler Instrument Company, 6191 Atlantic Blvd. Norcross, GA 30071) to dissect in the space of Smith (Fig. 83–64H).

The disease process does not extend into the spongy erectile tissue, which must not be injured during excision of the plaque. It will be necessary, however, to cut across the strands of the septum, the ends of which will lie prominently in the midline (Figs. 83–64I and 83–65F). Matching lateral stellate incisions in the tunica will release the tightness of the edges of the defect and increase its area to about 1.5 to 2 times the size of the plaque that has been removed. We apply a dermal graft, which measures 30 per cent larger than the resulting corporotomy defect. Rarely, with a very extensive lesion, we have resected a portion of the plaque and made releasing incisions to straighten the penis covering these defects with dermal grafts (Devine, 1987).

A tourniquet is not necessary to control bleeding during this dissection and actually would be in the way. When the penis is flaccid, the erectile space is primarily a venous one requiring only a little pressure to control bleeding. However, the level of anesthesia must be as deep as that required for an open abdominal operation.

Having excised the plaque and made the lateral incisions, we measure the defect while stretching it first longitudinally, then laterally—allowing a little extra for the roundness of the penis. The dermal graft is outlined on the donor site. We prefer the skin of the abdomen just above the iliac crest lateral to the hairline (Fig. 83–67A). The epidermis is usually removed freehand (Fig. 83–67B) or sometimes with a dermatome. The epidermis is discarded, and the dermal patch is harvested. After making an incision around it, we leave a few millimeters of dermal cuff to aid in closure (Fig. 83–67C). One end of the graft is elevated, and it is removed excising the

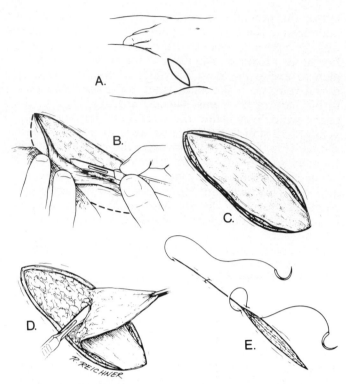

Figure 83–67. Harvesting a dermal graft. We excise a portion of dermis from the skin over the crest of the ilium lateral to the hair line. *A,* The area is marked on the skin.

B, The epidermis is removed freehand with a knife. A dermatome could also be used.

C, An incision is made around the dermal graft leaving a narrow cuff of dermis to aid in closure of the skin.

D, One end of the graft is elevated while the fat is trimmed off the underside.

E, The skin is closed with dermal sutures of Vicryl and a running subcuticular double ended suture of Prolene or nylon. Closure is begun in the middle of the incision placing each needle from the outside in, leaving a loop of suture outside the wound to aid in its removal. Sewing is continued to the two ends, bringing another loop to the surface half way there. The two ends are tied together loosely and a Bioclusive dressing applied.

fat from its underside to expose its subdermal plexus (Fig. 83–67D). The graft is about 1-mm thick. The donor area is closed primarily. We do a full-thickness closure with interrupted Vicryl sutures placed in the dermis and a pull-out subcuticular suture of 3.0 Prolene (Fig. 83–67E). This suture is removed in 3 weeks, leaving a linear scar that widens slightly.

The graft is placed into the corporotomy defect approximating its edges to the edges of the tunica with a watertight running 5–0 PDS, fixing its midline to the strands of the septum. Tacking 4–0 polydioxanone sutures are placed securing the graft at the proximal and distal points of the defect and at the tips of the releasing incisions on one side (Fig. 83–68A). Then, with a cutting needle, a 5–0 running PDS is placed to secure the graft to the tunica, producing an edge-to-edge closure with no overlap. When one side of the graft has been closed, we fold the graft and mark its midline so that we will not lose this relationship, as we place another line of 5–0 polydioxanone sutures to secure the graft to the strands of the septum (Fig. 83–68B). The graft is un-

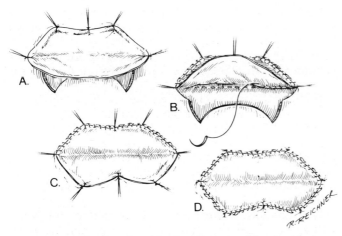

Figure 83–68. The dermal graft is placed into the defect fat side down.
A, Stay sutures of 4–0 polydioxanone are placed, securing the midline of the graft proximally and distally at the ends of the defect and at the tips of each of the releasing incisions, on just one edge of the repair. That edge of the graft will be sewn to the tunica with a running 5–0 polydioxanone suture, locking every second or third throw.

B, The graft is folded, and the midline is marked with a brilliant green solution. This midline of the graft is secured to the tips of the strands of the septum with a running 5–0 polydioxanone suture. This anastomosis will help to ensure continued function of the septum in erections subsequent to the surgery.

C, Stay sutures are applied on the opposite side.

D, The remaining edge of the graft is secured to the tunica with a running 5–0 polydioxanone suture to make a watertight anastomosis. (From Devine, C. J., Jr.: Peyronie's disease. *In* Glenn, J. F. (Ed.): Urologic Surgery, 4th ed. Philadelphia, J. B. Lippincott Co., 1991, p. 873.)

folded and the other edge secured, in the same manner as the first (Fig. 83–68C and D).

When the sutures have been placed, another artificial erection demonstrates that the penis is straight. We check the suture line for leaks (Figs. 83–64J and 83–65G). Leaks are oversewn with another PDS or two. If the penis is straight, we close the superficial tissue layers. If curvature persists, incisions will have to be extended and further grafts applied.

Closure depends on the incision that has been made to access the plaque. On the dorsal side, Buck's fascia is approximated at the midline with interrupted 5–0 PDS, carefully avoiding the dorsal arteries and nerves (Fig. 83–64K). Small suction drains are placed superficial to Buck's fascia but deep to the dartos layer. The skin incisions are closed (Fig. 83–64L).

When a ventral midline incision has been made, we develop a flap of the dartos fascia (Fig. 83–65H) and pass this between the graft and the corpus spongiosum, securing it with interrupted 5–0 Vicryl sutures to the dartos fascia on the other side (Fig. 83–65I). Drains are placed (Fig. 83–65J), and the skin is closed over the urethra (Fig. 83–65K and L).

We use Bioclusive (Johnson & Johnson, New Brunswick, NJ 98903) to dress the penis, applying it loosely and extending from the base of the penis to the level of the mid glans. We leave a 14 Fr. Foley catheter until the patient ambulates, usually the next morning. The suction drains are removed at 24 to 48 hours. Erections are suppressed with diazepam (Valium) and amyl nitrate. Patients are discharged between the 3rd and 5th day.

Dermal grafts go through the same phases of maturation as other grafts. At first they are nourished by imbibition of tissue fluids, while blood vessels from the bed are forming buds that penetrate the graft and anastomose with the arteries and veins in the graft. By the 5th day, this process (inosculation) has been completed. The dermis continues to undergo remodeling for at least 6 months to a year. All grafts contract as they mature. Dermis may contract 30 per cent. In the first 3 months, the graft contracts before it softens and some curvature may recur. However, as remodeling progresses the graft becomes more elastic and the shape of the penis improves.

After the first 2 weeks, we encourage erections but discourage intercourse for another month. During that time it is desirable for the penis to be manipulated so that the skin will not adhere to the deeper layers of the penis. Additionally, erections stretch the graft. We ask that the patient's wife or sex partner carry out this physical therapy—which is also sexual therapy in that it intimately involves her in the patient's rehabilitation. When the suture line can withstand the stress, this activity can lead directly to intercourse. During the follow-up period, patients continue to take vitamin E, 400 mg, twice a day with vitamin B, 150 mg, daily and vitamin C, 500 mg, twice a day.

At least 75 per cent of the patients who have been treated with these grafts have been happy with the results (Wild et al., 1979). This experience compares well with the results of other penile surgery:

1. Penile prosthesis, 50 per cent satisfied and 30 per cent somewhat satisfied (Kaufman, 1981).

2. Nesbit procedure for Peyronie's disease, 44 per cent excellent and 37 per cent moderately satisfied (Frank, 1981).

As we continue to evaluate the results in patients who have had erectile function tests carried out prior to surgery, we may be able to further refine statistics. Most patients with Peyronie's disease will continue to function sexually without surgery despite the distortion caused by the disease. A third will need surgery to function, and the odds are good that they will continue to function after the surgery.

It is extremely important for patients to have reasonable expectations concerning the outcome of any surgery on the penis. In addition to our counseling, all patients are screened by our sex therapist colleague. He may discover problem areas that must be dealt with before surgery. Additionally, he helps ensure that the patient and his sex partner have proper expectations to deal with the surgery and the recovery of function (Jones, 1984). Patients having surgery for congenital chordee will, in general, have a normal penis with function within 2 months of surgery. Rehabilitation of patients with Peyronie's disease is more protracted.

REOPERATION. Not including patients who have required a penile prosthesis because of postoperative impotence, we have re-explored a number of patients who have had previous surgery for Peyronie's disease, a few by us—most by others. Half these patients have functioned sexually after our reoperation. We were able to straighten the penis with a Nesbit tuck in two of our patients who had a significant bend after our dermal graft operation. One regained function. The other had difficulty and has been lost to follow-up. We have seen patients who have had a Nesbit tuck and, because of the rigidity of a large apposing plaque, removal of enough tissue to straighten the shaft resulted in a narrow penis with poor rigidity. In one, placement of a dermal graft restored the penile configuration, but he needed a prosthesis for function.

One patient had had a lesion repaired with a dermal graft that was too small and that had been removed from the middle of the pubic escutcheon area. We excised multiple sebaceous cysts, incised the graft in the midline, and covered this defect with a proper dermal graft. His penis is straight, and he has resumed sexual function. In several patients who have had tunica vaginalis grafts applied, tightness of the unreleased edges of the defects continued to restrict their erections. The tunica vaginalis graft was simply a scar.

We have removed patches of artificial materials. Because of the inflammation associated with these materials, dissection has been more difficult than in patients who have had only their own tissue involved in previous operations. In one patient, a clot of collagen had formed beneath a sheet of Gore-Tex. Contraction of this scar pulled the edges together forming a tent of the material. When we removed the Gore-Tex, the edges of the tunica relaxed. We then applied a dermal graft. Artificial erection showed the penis to be straight, and the patient has regained sexual function.

TOTAL PENILE RECONSTRUCTION/PHALLIC CONSTRUCTION

The major methods for reconstruction of the penis have been developed to repair injuries. In 1936, Bogoraz reported a series of cases and described a technique for phallic construction in war-injured patients. In 1944, Frumkin followed with another series from the Soviet Union. Gilles (1948) who was aware of their work was stationed at a major hospital in the outskirts of London during World War II. In 1948, he reported a series of patients in whom he had reconstructed the penis. In that series there were patients with congenital absence of the penis. However, much of his experience with the procedure was obtained from war injuries.

Initially, all procedures involved the delayed formation and transfer of tubed abdominal flaps. These tubes were produced from random flaps of skin, and because of their size their blood supply was tenuous. They were formed in stages with a "delay" between the stages to allow new vascular patterns to become established. In the "tube-within-a-tube" design, the inner tube allowed for placement of a baculum for intercourse, while the outer tube provided skin coverage. Patients generally voided through a proximal urethrostomy. This was "state-of-the-art" penile reconstruction until Orticochea (1972) described total reconstruction of the penis with a gracilis musculocutaneous flap.

Puckett (1978) reported a series in which he constructed a penis utilizing a tubed groin flap. In the initial cases in this series, he tubed a groin flap and delayed its transfer to the area of the penile stump. In the latter part of his series, the tissue was transferred as a microvascular free flap.

In 1984, Chang popularized the forearm flap based on the radial artery for penile construction (Fig. 83–69). Biemer (1988) reported a modification of the forearm flap (Fig. 83–70). In 1990, Farrow and associates reported their cricket-bat modification of the radial forearm flap (Fig. 83–71). Currently, forearm flaps are the most commonly employed method of total phallic reconstruction.

For patients undergoing reconstruction following trauma or extirpative surgery for carcinoma, we have found the cricket-bat modification to be of most help. Disadvantages of the forearm flap include the obvious donor site deformity. At best, the scar is ugly. Also, there is the possibility that cold intolerance might develop in the hand on the donor side; however, that has not been the case in our patients. In male patients or virilized transsexual patients, the forearm skin is hirsute and this hair may create a problem when it is included in urethral reconstruction. A portion of the radius could be included in the flap to provide rigidity to the new penis. However, inclusion of this bone carries the potential for loss of function in the hand.

Early in our series, we reconstructed the radial artery by interposition of a vein graft. However, we do not now reconstruct the radial artery because our patients have had no limitation of function of the distal forearm due to interruption of the radial artery. Its loss is replaced by blood flow from the ulnar artery. The radial and the ulnar arteries communicate distally through the superficial and deep palmer arches, and neither gives off any large branches in the forearm. The flap is customarily taken from the nondominant forearm. Patients are carefully screened preoperatively for arterial insufficiency with the Allen test. The radial and ulnar arteries are palpated in the wrist, and the patient makes a tight fist to express blood from his hand. The observer compresses both arteries impeding the flow of blood to the hand. After the patient has opened his fist, the fingers will be pale, but they will "pink-up" on release of either artery if circulation is normal. If there is any doubt that the distal vascular arcade is intact, upper extremity angiography is performed.

The radial forearm flap is a fasciocutaneous flap vascularized via the radial artery with paired vena comitans. The radial artery arises as a continuation of the brachial artery. Proximally, the artery lies beneath the belly of the brachioradial muscle, becoming more superficial at the wrist. The radial artery perfuses the skin and the underlying adipose tissue via the fascial plexus. The ulnar artery vascularizes a similar area of skin and underlying adipose tissue. Vascularity of the overlying skin is achieved entirely via the underlying (antebrachial) fascia, which is the superficial fascia investing the musculature of the forearm. The lateral and medial antebrachial cutaneous nerves appear proximally beneath this fascia. The cephalic, basilic, and medial

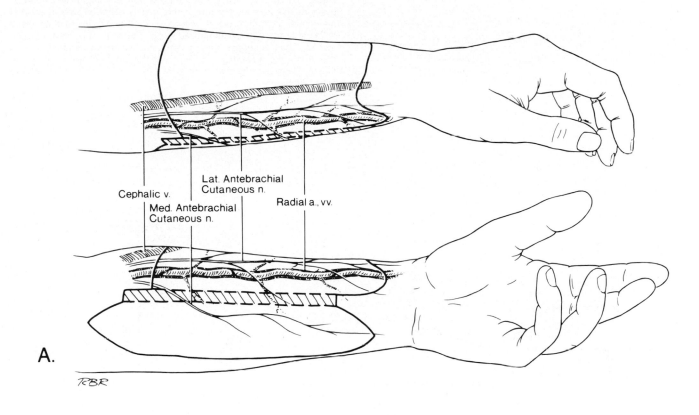

A.

Cephalic v.

Lat. Antebrachial
Cutaneous n.

Med. Antebrachial
Cutaneous n.

Radial a., vv.

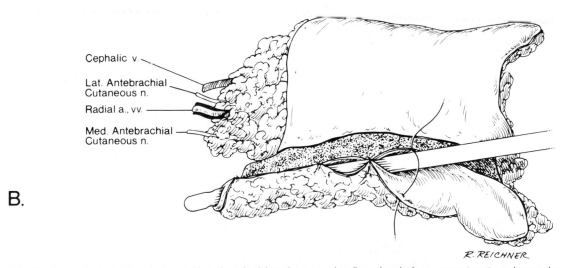

B.

Cephalic v.

Lat. Antebrachial
Cutaneous n.

Radial a., vv.

Med. Antebrachial
Cutaneous n.

Figure 83–69. Radial forearm flap similar to that described by Chang. In this flap, the shaft coverage is oriented over the radial artery. A de-epithelialized strip is created between a second portion of the flap, which will become the urethra. That portion is centered over the ulnar aspect of the forearm. The urethral portion is tubed and that tube is rolled inside the shaft coverage portion of the flap.

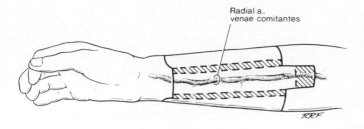

Figure 83–70. Modification of the radial forearm flap as described by Biemer. The urethral portion of this flap is centered over the radial artery with an epithelialized strip on each side. Skin for shaft coverage is lateral to these de-epithelialized strips. The urethral portion is tubed, and the shaft coverage portions are tubed over the neourethra. This flap offers the advantage of centering the urethral portion over the radial artery, making that portion of the cutaneous vascular territory most reliable.

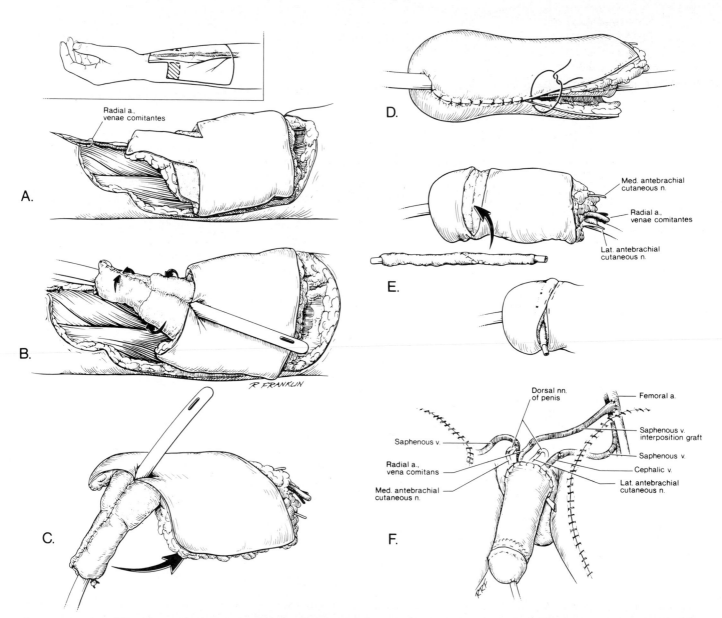

Figure 83–71. Radial forearm flap described by Farrow and Boyd ("cricket-bat" modification). In this modification, the urethra extends distally onto the forearm centered over the radial artery. The shaft portion lies on the more proximal forearm. In this flap, the urethral portion is tubed and inverted onto the shaft coverage, which is tubed over the neourethra. Coronoplasty is achieved by burying a tubed skin graft in a groove created in the flap. The epithelial portion of the flap is closed over the tubed buried graft. In a second stage, the buried graft is opened. The flap is then transposed to the area of the perineum, where the radial artery is anastomosed to a vein interposition graft from the common femoral artery. The dominant venous supply is anastomosed to the saphenous veins bilaterally.

antebrachial veins are included in the flap and constitute its superficial venous drainage. In some patients the deep system (the venae comitantes) will be the dominant drainage system; in others, the veins of the superficial system will be dominant. At the time of transfer of the flap, it is imperative to assess these veins after the arterial anastomosis has been accomplished and to then anastomose the dominant system to the largest of the branches of the saphenous veins.

The lateral antebrachial cutaneous nerve arises at the elbow as the distal continuation of the musculocutaneous nerve. This nerve provides sensation to both the volar and dorsal radial aspects of the forearm. The medial antebrachial cutaneous nerve divides distally into an anterior and an ulnar branch and innervates similar areas on the ulnar aspect of the forearm. The superficial branch of the radial nerve arises from beneath the belly of the brachioradialis muscle and runs close to the radial artery. Care must be taken to avoid inclusion of this nerve in the flap. Division of the nerve creates an area of numbness in the region of the thenar eminence, and a painful neuroma may develop. Should the nerve be injured during flap elevation, primary reconstruction should be accomplished at the time of surgery.

The various modifications of the forearm flap are not modifications in the technique of flap elevation, but rather are modifications in the design of the skin island and the relative position of the urethral strip in relation to the skin that will cover the shaft. Each of these modifications has advantages in various situations. In the radial forearm flap, as described by Chang (see Fig. 83–69), shaft coverage is accomplished with the radial aspect of the flap, leaving a de-epithelialized strip between it and a second skin island that will be tubed to form the urethra. The urethral tube is rolled within the tube of the skin that will cover the shaft.

In the cricket-bat modification described by Farrow and Boyd (see Fig. 83–71), the urethral tube extends distally overlying closely the radial artery. Proximal to that, the broader portion of the flap will cover the shaft. The urethral portion is tubed and transposed by inverting it into the center of the portion of the flap designed for shaft coverage. The advantage of this modification is that the urethral portion of the island is centered over the radial artery. However, in patients with large forearms, this vascular territory in the area of the urethral tube may be tenuous, leading to areas of ischemia in the reconstructed urethra after its transfer.

Beimer's modification (see Fig. 83–70) addresses the potential for ischemia in this area of the flap. He centers the urethral portion over the radial artery, separated from the two parts of the flap that will cover the shaft by two de-epithelialized strips. In designing the flap, the urethral strip is generally planned to be 3 to 3.5 cm wide. The de-epithelialized strips are generally 1.0 to 1.5 cm in width. The width of the flap for shaft coverage must be modified, depending on the thickness of the fat layer in the flap. After the urethra is tubed, shaft coverage is achieved by sewing these two outer skin islands together so that they surround the urethral tube in somewhat of a clamshell-like fashion.

The skin islands of all of these flaps can be modified by omitting the urethral segment, employing only the shaft portion of the flap for patients requiring only coverage with vascularized tissue. For patients who need only vascularized tissue to cover the shaft, the upper lateral arm flap has been a helpful alternative (Fig. 83–72). This is an axial fasciocutaneous flap, with its cutaneous vascular territory centered on the radial collateral artery. It is thin with little subcutaneous adiposity. A line drawn joining the insertion of the deltoid with the lateral epicondyle marks the location of the lateral

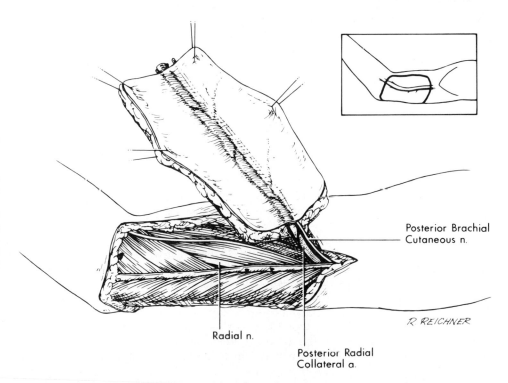

Figure 83–72. Upper lateral arm flap. This fasciocutaneous flap based on the posterior radial collateral artery, one of the first branches of the axillary artery located in the interosseous septum in the upper forearm, is elevated with the superficial fascia of the upper arm. The cutaneous vascular territory is centered roughly on a line between the groove of the deltoid and the lateral epicondyle of the elbow. In elevating the vessels, care must be taken to not injure the radial nerve, which runs proximate to the posterior radial collateral artery.

Posterior Brachial Cutaneous n.

Radial n.

Posterior Radial Collateral a.

R. REICHNER

intramuscular septum and the course of the superior radial collateral artery. Dissection is begun posteriorly, elevating the superficial fascia until the posterolateral portion of the intermuscular septum has been identified. The cutaneous vascular branches are readily identified and the septum is separated from the triceps revealing the vascular pedicle. The fascia of the triceps, which will remain as the deep layer of the flap, is dissected as the flap is elevated.

This flap has a potential disadvantage in that in most patients its venous drainage is totally dependent on a single vena comitans. Superficial veins traverse the flap, but none of them seem to provide significant venous drainage. This is somewhat disquieting, but, in our hands, the flap has evidenced no venous insufficiency. Occasionally, the upper lateral arm flap donor site can be closed primarily, but usually it must be covered with an STSG. The flap donor site is unsightly but does not impair function. This scar on the upper arm may be more readily concealed than the donor site of the forearm flap. In the intermuscular septum one encounters the following: (1) the cutaneous nerve, (2) the radial collateral artery and its accompanying vena comitans, and (3) the radial nerve that passes very close to the radial collateral artery in the intermuscular septum. This nerve must be identified and retracted out of harm's way.

All of the flaps described here allow microneurosurgical coaptation of the cutaneous nerves of the flap to recipient nerves at the site of transposition. With phallic construction, the cutaneous nerves can be attached to either the dorsal nerves of the penis (in transsexual patients the dorsal nerves of the clitoris) or to a pudendal nerve (perhaps through a nerve graft in patients in whom the dorsal nerves have been obliterated). These recipient nerves provide the best restoration of erogenous sensibility.

The cricket-bat modification of the radial forearm flap is a fasciocutaneous flap with the superficial fascia of the forearm (see Fig. 83–71). Customarily, the portion of the flap for male urethral construction is outlined on the distal part of the forearm, centered over the radial artery, trying to avoid hairy areas of the skin. In adults, this strip should be about 3.5 cm wide. Its length is adjusted to fit that of the existing native urethra. The epithelium will be removed from areas of skin, which are outlined adjacent to the portion of the urethra and which will become the "glanular" urethra. As the flap is rolled, these de-epithelialized areas are buried, defining the distal end of the phallus by adding additional bulk to produce a more normal looking "glans." The shaft portion of the flap is outlined, adjusting its length to accommodate the existing penile shaft and the remaining skin coverage. Optimally, the technique can achieve a penile length of approximately 13 cm. The flap will contain all of tissues between the skin and the superficial fascia, and its width must be adjusted to accommodate for that. A person with more fat in his forearm will require a wider flap.

The incisions are carried sharply down to the fascia. The initial incision through the fascia is made at the base of the flap over the radial artery, which runs in a groove beneath the edge of the brachioradialis muscle distally throughout the extent of the forearm. The artery is left intact and dissected from beneath the brachioradialis muscle. The superficial fascia is mobilized, including the lateral and medial antebrachial cutaneous nerves along with the venae comitantes, the deep venous system, and the cephalic vein. The vascular pedicle is dissected as far as the junction of the radial artery with the brachial artery. The recipient area in the perineum and the recipient vessels must be totally prepared prior to transfer of the flap.

After the flap is elevated, the arm tourniquet is released and the flap is left for a period of time as its circulation is confirmed. The flap is conformed into a phallus while still attached to the forearm. With the cricket-bat modification, the urethral strip is rolled into a tube over a plastic stent usually with a two-layer closure (Fig. 83–71B). When this maneuver is complete, the urethra is transposed into the central portion of the flap (Fig. 83–71C). The distal portion of the flap is closed, covering the urethra (Fig. 83–72D). The ventral aspect of the base of the flap is left open on the proximal shaft of the neophallus to accommodate the residual corpora. The formed flap is left attached to the vessels of the forearm with warm soaks applied until preparation of the recipient area is complete.

Currently, the recipient vessels include both saphenous veins and the femoral artery through a saphenous vein graft. On one side, the full length of the saphenous vein is mobilized. The distal end of the vein is brought up and attached end-to-side to the femoral artery. This arteriovenous (AV) fistula remains patent until it is time to re-establish circulation in the flap. Meanwhile, the other saphenous vein and the nerves are prepared. Venous drainage of the transferred flap will be via the saphenous vein on each side. Often, a number of the branches of the saphenous vein can be elevated with it allowing for the connection of multiple veins from the flap. The recipient nerves are generally the remaining dorsal nerves of the penis, which are dissected from the shaft of the penis and elevated pending flap transfer. The skin medial to the inguinal incisions is widely undermined, making a tunnel that will allow the saphenous veins and saphenous vein interposition graft to be passed to the area of the penile stump.

The flap is readied for transfer, first dividing and meticulously marking the nerves. Next the artery is divided and marked. Lastly, the venae comitantes and the superficial veins are divided and marked. Transfer of the flap to the area of the penile stump is begun with a two-layer urethral anastomosis. Epithelial apposition is accomplished with chromic cat gut sutures, with the knots placed in the lumen. The second layer is an extraepithelial PDS. Making the urethral connection first allows for a reliable anastomosis, and the time necessary to complete the anastomosis does not compromise the survival of the flap.

The operating microscope is brought into the field. The loop of the AV fistula is divided in the midline, and the radial artery is anastomosed to the arterial end of the saphenous vein interposition graft with interrupted 10–0 nylon or Prolene sutures. The venae comitantes and superficial veins are inspected. In many patients, distention of the veins will clearly indicate predominance of one venous drainage system over another. Veins are anastomosed to the largest of the branches of the recipient saphenous veins. The saphenous vein not utilized for the graft interposition usually has several branches allowing for multiple venous connections. Optimally, the basilic and cephalic veins and all venae comitantes are anastomosed to recipient vessels. Flap vascularity is assessed with a Doppler probe, and the vascular anastomoses are carefully investigated for patency. Ponten (1981) has shown fasciocutaneous flaps to be very high resistance flaps. High resistance systems present difficult problems in microvascular surgery, but this high pressure and high volume arterial anastomosis, and the multiple venous connections, provide excellent flow through the flap as evidenced by the volume of the venous return.

The flap is wrapped with warm saline sponges and is watched for development of vascular spasm. When good revascularization of the flap has been observed, coaptation of the medial and lateral antebrachiocutaneous nerves to the recipient dorsal penile nerve stump is accomplished with 9–0 or 10–0 nylon or Prolene sutures (Fig. 83–71F).

The remainder of the phallic skin flap is closed around the existing penile shaft, and the glans is defined. An incision is made around the distal end of the phallus forming a groove at the location of the coronal margin (Fig. 83–71E). An STSG is harvested from the genital area and formed into a tube by sewing it over a small catheter. This tube is buried in the groove, and the skin is closed. The second stage of this coronoplasty is accomplished at about 6 weeks following the initial surgery by opening this buried tube of skin. Implantation of this tissue allows for a difference in skin color and texture at the site of the coronal margin, emphasizing the shape of the glans.

The donor site of forearm flaps must always be covered with STSGs, which are obtained from the skin of the thigh. The donor areas of these STSGs are dressed with gauze soaked with Congo red.

The flap is meticulously surveyed with a Doppler probe, marking the site of strong signals so that circulation may be evaluated continuously during the postoperative period. We have also employed a pH monitoring device to assess the status of the tissues of the flap. Development of acidosis in the flap generally implies vascular compromise. Combined with Doppler inspection accomplished at very frequent intervals, this practice has allowed for close monitoring of the flaps. The patient is kept at bedrest in a room between 80° and 85° F, for 5 to 7 days. He remains in the intensive care unit for the first 2 or 3 days. With the exception of a baby aspirin a day, we do not routinely administer anticoagulants.

In all patients, urine is diverted via a suprapubic cystostomy tube. The urethra is stented with a No. 14 silicone ribbed catheter (Rusch). A voiding study is generally performed between the 21st and 28th days following surgery by filling the bladder with contrast material and removing the catheter from the urethra.

Development of a fistula at the site of the urethral anastomosis has been a major problem. This finding does not seem to be dependent on the adequacy of the anastomosis at the time of the procedure. Because of the frequency of a fistula, we now elevate a gracilis muscle flap and transpose it to the area of urethral anastomosis. The addition of this tissue with its increased vascularity has helped alleviate the fistula problem. Because the flap is denervated in the process of its transposition to the area of the perineum, it does not persist with any meaningful bulk beneath the area of scrotal construction. Nonetheless, all patients undergoing this type of reconstruction must be counseled as to the frequent occurrence of fistulas. In most patients the fistulas are small. If not associated with distal urethral stenosis, many close spontaneously or can be readily closed at a second procedure.

RECONSTRUCTION FOLLOWING TRAUMA

We have treated patients who have had devastating injuries of the penis following complicated prosthetic surgery or surgery to correct penile curvature or Peyronie's disease. In many ways, the problems have been more challenging to solve than those of patients who have had the penis amputated. Most of the aforementioned patients have developed gangrene, which in many began with a leakage of blood from an opening into the intercorporal space, forming a hematoma which if not drained became secondarily infected. In some patients, delay in removing the prosthesis has led to massive destruction of the urethra and corporal bodies. Inevitably, the abscess decompresses spontaneously devastating the nerves or vascular bundle, if it opens through the dorsal aspect of the penis, or the urethra and corpus spongiosum, if it drains ventrally.

We always try to save as many of the structures of the penis as possible. Acutely, the urine must be diverted and the necrotic tissue carefully debrided. If acute wound management is successful, the wounds will be uninfected and active granulation will be progressing. Primary reconstruction can begin in 3 to 6 weeks and can continue after 3 to 6 months.

When there has been a significant loss of tissue, new well-vascularized tissue must be moved into the area, using local muscle flaps or free flaps. In some patients, we have employed a radial forearm flap, and in others an upper lateral arm flap (Fig. 83–72) has seemed better, although it is difficult to accomplish a total phallic construction with an upper lateral arm flap. This flap is optimal for providing good vascular coverage to remnants of the corporal bodies and urethra in the penis. Later, the penis can be reconstructed combining this flap tissue with a gracilis muscle flap, reconstructing a urethra from an FTSG.

Initially, the cosmetic appearance is somewhat stubby and bulky, but subsequent atrophy of the gracilis muscle combined with further debulking surgical procedures can provide a very adequate cosmetic result. Importation of well-vascularized tissues into the area of the obliterated penis allows hope that in the future a prosthesis may be implanted for erectile function. Amazingly, considering the bulk of the flap, many of these patients have had enough residual tumescence for penetration and what they considered to be adequate sexual interaction.

FEMALE-TO-MALE TRANSSEXUALISM

Female-to-male transsexual patients are a unique challenge. No person should have gender reassignment surgery without having undergone complex screening and evaluation by a team consisting of mental health professionals as well as the surgeons who will be doing the transgender surgery. The psychologists on our team serve to screen the patients, and it is imperative that an ongoing stable therapeutic relationship with an individual mental health professional be underway at the time of definitive gender reassignment surgery. Once the surgery has been approved we, in association with the gynecologists on the team, proceed with transabdominal hysterectomy and bilateral salpingo-oophorectomy.

In some patients, a vaginectomy can be done at the same operation. In most of our patients, however, we have removed the vagina as a second procedure at the time we lengthen the urethra. To lengthen the female urethra, an anterior vaginal wall flap is flipped onto a ventral strip created from the opened urethra extending it to the glans clitoris to begin a more anterior redirection of the urinary stream. Extending the urethra in this fashion has made the urethral anastomosis at the time of phallic construction technically much more straightforward, reducing the incidence of fistulization. After the vaginectomy and urethral lengthening, the urine is diverted via a suprapubic cystostomy tube with a stenting urethral catheter left in place for a period of 14 to 21 days. When the stenting catheter has been removed and the patient has been able to void, the suprapubic tube is removed.

Approximately 3 to 4 months later, the patient returns for phallic construction. Our approach to transsexual patients is a bit different from our approach to trauma patients or patients who have had extirpative surgery for carcinomas. In men, the penis is suspended from the crest of the pubis, while the clitoris is essentially displaced caudally and posteriorly. Therefore, in transsexual patients, we elevate a bipedicled flap of skin from the area where the phallic structure will be implanted and transpose it to the undersurface of the shaft of the clitoris. This maneuver places more tissue beneath the shaft allowing for more anatomically correct positioning of the phallus and transposes redundant tissue to the ventral side of the phallic shaft for later scrotal construction. Additionally, moving this flap affords skin coverage for the gracilis muscle flap, which we will transpose to the area of the urethral anastomosis.

The postoperative period for transsexual patients is the same as that for patients treated following trauma or carcinoma resection. The urethra is evaluated in 6 months. If it is widely patent, the patient is a candidate for placement of testicular prostheses should that be desired. The testicular prostheses are implanted through an inguinal incision, developing the potential canal of Nuck down into the area of the scrotal construction. If there is any concern about the urethra, prosthetic placement is delayed until this concern has been resolved.

After a period of a year has elapsed, erogenous sensibility can be tested. If the patient is found to have adequate sensation in the phallic flap and has a good urethra, erectile prosthetic placement can be considered. Prosthetic placement in a Gore-Tex sleeve has not been a problem when the distal corpora have been reconstructed in patients following trauma and carcinoma of the penis. In transsexual patients, however, prosthetic placement, although seemingly straightforward relatively, has been a source of difficulty for us. We have used the Duraphase prosthesis and a custom modification of the Uniflate 1000 prosthesis implanted in a Gore-Tex sleeve, hoping that tissue ingrowth into the Gore-Tex will help to stabilize the prosthesis in the flap. With the Uniflate 1000 prosthesis, one of the testicular prostheses is removed, placing the Uniflate pump/reservoir mechanism in this foreign body capsule.

Patients remain in the hospital on broad-spectrum antibiotics for a period of at least 72 hours after prosthetic placement. They are then discharged and are prescribed a cephalosporin for an additional 2 to 3 weeks. Despite these precautions in transsexual patients, erosion and late infection have been a worry and a problem.

VAGINAL CONSTRUCTION

A number of procedures for vaginal construction have been described. In most cases, the type of procedure is dictated by the patient's circumstances. None of the graft techniques has proved to be satisfactory in patients with vaginal agenesis. STSGs have been widely employed for vaginal construction, but they all require constant stenting. Clearly, in a young child with vaginal agenesis, the necessity for stenting is unacceptable. The FTSG technique was thought to offer the possibility of grafts for vaginal construction, without the constant threat of contraction and stenosis. However, over the long-term, these grafts also tend to contract and need either frequent sexual activity or constant stenting to remain open. Again, in young children with absent vaginas, these constraints eliminate graft techniques from reasonable consideration.

Reconstruction after radical pelvic surgery requires the transfer of a large bulk of vascular tissue to the defect in the pelvic floor, in addition to construction of a vaginal vault. Immediate vaginal reconstruction has greatly reduced the postoperative morbidity. Filling the pelvic defect with vascularized tissue improves healing and lessens the possibility of pelvic abscess. A number of techniques have been employed for vaginal construction in these patients. First, bilateral gracilis musculocutaneous flaps (see Fig. 83–4) are elevated and transposed to the area of the perineum. The skin islands are sewn together to form a pouch, which is placed in the vaginal defect. Placing the gracilis muscles into the pelvis moves a bulk of tissue into the defect. Second, inferior rectus abdominis musculocutaneous flaps also allow for transfer of a skin island for vaginal vault construction in addition to transposing a bulk of vascular tissue into the defect in the pelvis. Inferior rectus abdominis muscle flaps with a *vertical* paddle of skin are useful. McCraw (1986) has improved upon that technique using an inferior rectus abdominis muscle flap with a *transverse* skin paddle. These flaps seem to have advantages over flaps with vertical paddles for immediate vaginal construction at the time of radical pelvic surgery. Because of the android shape of the pelvis in transsexual patients, bulky musculocutaneous flaps may leave little space for the actual vaginal vault. McCraw's modification may obviate some of these problems and should find a place in vaginal construction in intersex patients. It can carry as much or as little of the rectus muscle as the surgeon desires. Characteristically, McCraw includes only the portion of rectus abdominis muscle at the periumbilical area.

Bowel segments have been widely chosen for vaginal construction in both intersex and transsexual patients. Reports to date do not indicate any significant increase in complication rates associated with the attendant laparotomy and bowel resection. The better recognition of mesenteric blood supply and the principles of flap transfer added to the advantages of stapled enteric anastomoses allow these procedures to be accomplished with more than acceptable results. Ileum has been utilized for vaginal construction. Although it tends to be fragile and easily traumatized during intercourse, it produces less mucus and this may be an advantage. The transverse colon has more mucus secretion but is a more durable bowel segment. The distal portion of the sigmoid colon seems to offer a good compromise with reduced mucus secretion and with colon durability. The sigmoid colon segment is transferred on the distal branches of the inferior mesenterics or in some cases on the marginal artery of Drummond.

In transsexual patients, vaginal construction is accomplished at the same time as feminizing genitoplasty and bilateral orchidectomy. The patient is treated with female hormones, but we believe strongly that the testicles should not be removed until the patient has been approved for definitive gender reassignment surgery. Bilateral orchiectomy done at the time of feminizing genitoplasty and vaginal construction adds little time and no morbidity. The patient is placed in a low lithotomy position to allow for concurrent laparotomy and perineal incision. In most patients, we make a transverse abdominal incision. The android pelvis does somewhat limit the exposure through such an incision unless it is done in a true Pfannenstiel fashion with the fascial and peritoneal incisions oriented vertically.

Before making the abdominal incision, the feminizing genitoplasty is completed. A number of techniques for accomplishing this have been described. We preserve a section of the glans penis to serve as a glans clitoris, leaving it on the dorsal neurovascular bundle. A circumcising incision is made at the site of the old circumcision scar or a centimeter or so proximal to the corona, if the patient has not been circumcised. An incision is made

in the ventral midline and the skin is reflected off the shaft of the penis by dissecting in the dartos fascia layer. The urethra is detached from the corporal bodies at the midscrotal level and divided. A catheter is passed to the bladder, and the bulbospongiosus and urethra are dissected free to the point where the membranous urethra enters the bulb. It is imperative that the corpus spongiosum be totally freed from its attachment to the corpora cavernosa and the triangular ligament, allowing the residual bulbous urethra to be straightened so that the urinary stream may be directed straight down.

The corpora cavernosa are dissected to the midportion of the crus and divided. The ends of the crura are oversewn with 4–0 PDS. The glans is removed from the tips of the corpora, and the tunica is incised so that a strip of tunica is left to support the dorsal vessels and nerves. This strip is folded behind the pubis, and the segment of glans is secured to the posterior rim of the symphysis. The skin of the penis and scrotum will be distributed to form the labia as the perineal incision is closed.

After making the abdominal incision, the testicles are removed by mobilizing them from the scrotum and passing them into the area of the abdominal wound. The cord is ligated proximal to the internal inguinal ring. We are aware of a single transsexual patient who, at the time of orchiectomy, was found to have an occult focus of carcinoma. This type of orchiectomy done in a "radical" fashion adds little to the time or morbidity of the procedure.

An incision is made in the perineum creating a posteriorly based V-flap just anterior to the anus. Dissection is carried just superficial to the circular fibers of the anal sphincter developing the plane along the anterior rectal vault. The rectourethralis muscle is identified and divided. This is a potential source of complication in that tension on the muscle tends to tent slightly the rectum anteriorly. Dissection is continued beneath the prostate. In transsexual patients who have had estrogen therapy, the prostate is virtually not palpable. Denonvilliers' fascia is usually not visualized. At this point the surgeon working from above will have mobilized the colon. The rectovesical space is developed behind the prostate, and the surgeon at the perineum dissects bluntly toward the surgeon at the abdomen. This dissection is accomplished without difficulty, creating a broad vaginal vault without much blood loss.

The sigmoid segment, having been identified, is resected from its continuity with the bowel and mobilized so that it passes simply into the area of the perineum. The bowel segment is passed into the abdomen, and a low anterior anastomosis of the colon is accomplished using the EEA stapler (U.S. Surgical Corp., 150 Glover Avenue, Norwalk, CT 06856). This stapler produces a technically straightforward anastomosis which is watertight and airtight. We reinforce the stapled anastomosis with silk sutures. After completion of the anastomosis, proctoscopy is performed examining the anastomosis line directly and distending the bowel to check for any leak of gas. When the anastomosis has proved reliable, the bowel segment is passed through the dissected tunnel and is incorporated into the closure of the perineum.

With hemostasis assured, the abdominal incision is closed in the usual fashion.

In patients in whom we have employed FTSGs for vaginal construction, no laparotomy incision has been required. Dissection of the vaginal vault is carried out with the patient in an exaggerated lithotomy position in the fashion of a radical prostatectomy. The full-thickness skin is harvested from nonhirsute areas of the lower part of the abdomen, which extend over the anterior superior iliac crests. In some patients, the graft donor sites are excised by doing a small abdominal panniculectomy. The full-thickness skin is meticulously cleared of the underlying adipose tissue and wrapped about a foam-rubber bolster with the epithelial surface inside.

In some medical centers, perineal dissection is carried out with more of an anterior orientation necessitating division of the transverse perinei muscles. This maneuver does allow for a more anatomically correct anterior placement of the vaginal introitus. However, the bulbospongiosum bulges into the anterior vaginal wall and, cosmetically, is less acceptable than the slight posterior displacement of the vaginal vault when dissection is carried out posterior to the transverse perinei musculature.

STSGs were used in large series in the past, but probably have little place in the current techniques of vaginal construction. Invariably, STSGs are attended by stenosis, frequent acute loss of the graft, and occasional rectovaginal urethral or vesicovaginal fistula due to the necessity of wearing a stent long-term. The take of FTSGs may be more precarious than the take of STSGs, because of the necessity of having a more optimal host bed. However, FTSGs can provide an adequate vaginal vault for patients who will soon engage in sexual activity but, without sexual activity, these patients must also wear a stent. Squamous carcinoma has been reported in vaginas constructed of skin grafts, and careful follow-up examination is a necessity.

Some urology centers favor a penile inversion procedure in transsexual surgery. This procedure provides a shallow vaginal cavity limited by how far the penile skin may stretch from the crest of the pubis into the depth of the vaginal vault. The Frank technique (1938) of intermittent perineal pressure has fallen from common usage even for children with congenital absence of the vagina. In this technique, small vaginal dilators were placed at the site of the vaginal dimple or the foreshortened vagina and with increasing pressure and increasing size of the dilators, a vaginal cavity was formed.

The sigmoid colon segment offers a number of advantages for vaginal construction. It is a reliable flap for transfer. Elevation of the flap requires a laparotomy. However, in large series, this maneuver has not increased surgical morbidity. The vaginal vault does not require stenting; hence, the many complications attendant to long-term stenting are avoided. To our knowledge, there has not been a report of adenocarcinoma developing in a colon segment mobilized for vaginal construction. However, patients should be closely monitored. Mucus discharge can be limited by tailoring the length of the colon and by selecting the distal sigmoid.

If it does become a problem, intermittent douches with 3 per cent saline have been shown to resolve any associated complications.

REFERENCES

Aboseif, S. R., Breza, J., Lue, T. F., and Tanagho, E.: Penile venous drainage in erectile dysfunction: Anatomical, radiological and functional considerations. Br. J. Urol., 64:183–190, 1989.

Allen, J. S., and Summers, J. L.: Meatal stenosis in children. J. Urol., 112:526, 1974.

Altaffer, L. F., III, and Jordan, G.: Sonographic demonstration of Peyronie's plaques. Urology, 17:292, 1981.

Bainbridge, D. R., Whitaker, R. H., and Shepheard, B. G. F.: Balanitis xerotica obliterans and urinary obstruction. Br. J. Urol., 43:487, 1971.

Barry, J. M.: Visual urethrotomy in the management of the obliterated membranous urethra. Urol. Clin. North Am., 16:2, 1989.

Biemer, E.: Penile construction by the radial arm flap. Clin. Plast. Surg., 15:425, 1988.

Blandy, J. P., and Tresidder, G. C.: Meatoplasty. Br. J. Urol., 39:633–634, 1967.

Bogoraz, N. A.: Plastic restoration of the penis. Sovet Khir. No., 8:303–307, 1936.

Brannen, G. E.: Meatal reconstruction. J. Urol., 116:319, 1976.

Chang, T. S., and Hwang, W. Y.: Forearm flap in one-stage reconstruction of the penis. Plast. Reconstr. Surg., 74:251, 1984.

Cohney, B. C.: A penile flap procedure for the relief of meatal strictures. Br. J. Urol., 35:182, 1963.

Colapinto, V., and McCallum, R. W.: Injury to the male posterior urethra in fractured pelvis. J. Urol., 118:575, 1977.

Das, S., and Amar, A. D.: Peyronie's disease: Excision of the plaque and grafting with tunica vaginalis. Urol. Clin. North Am., 9:1, 1982.

Das, S., and Maggio, A. J.: Tunica vaginalis autografting for Peyronie's disease. An experimental study. Invest. Urol., 17:186, 1979.

DeSanctis, P. N., and Furey, G. A.: Steroid injection therapy for Peyronie's disease: A 10-year summary and review of 38 cases. J. Urol., 97:114, 1967.

DeSy, W. A.: Aesthetic repair of meatal stricture. J. Urol., 132:678, 1984.

DeSy, W. A., Oosterlinck, W., and Verbaeys, A.: European experience with one-stage urethroplasty with free full thickness skin graft. J. Urol., 125:502, 1981.

Devine, C. J., Jr.: Embryology of the genitourinary tract. In Urologie in Klinik and Praxie. Hohenfellner, R., and Zingg, E. J. (Ed.). Stuggart, Germany. George Thieme Verlag Publisher, 1982, pp. 830–850.

Devine, C. J., Jr.: Surgery of the urethra. In Walsh, P. C., Gittes, R. F., Perlmutter, A. D., and Stamey, T. A. (Eds.). Campbell's Urology, 5th ed. Philadelphia, W. B. Saunders Co., 1986, pp. 2853–2887.

Devine, C. J., Jr.: Commentary: Urethroplasty for anterior urethral stricture. In Current Operative Urology. Whitehead, E. Douglas, (Ed.). Philadelphia, J. B. Lippincott Co., 1991, pp. 336–346.

Devine, C. J., Jr., Blackley, S. K., Horton, C. E., and Gilbert, D. A.: The surgical treatment of chordee without hypospadias in post adolescent men. J. Urol., 146:325–329, 1991.

Devine, C. J., Jr., Franz, J. P., and Horton, C. E.: Evaluation and treatment of patients with failed hypospadias repair. J. Urol., 119:223–226, 1978.

Devine, C. J., Jr., Gonzales-Serva, L., Stecker, J. F., Jr., and Devine, P. C.: Utrical configuration in hypospadias and intersex. J. Urol., 123:407, 1980.

Devine, C. J., Jr., and Horton, C. E.: Bent penis. Semin. Urol., 5:251–261, 1987.

Devine, C. J., Jr., and Horton, C. E.: Chordee without hypospadias. J. Urol., 110:264–271, 1973.

Devine, C. J., Jr., and Horton, C. E.: The surgical treatment of Peyronie's disease with a dermal graft. J. Urol., 111:44, 1974.

Devine, C. J., Jr., and Horton, C. E.: Use of dermal graft to correct chordee. J. Urol., 113:56, 1975.

Devine, C. J., Jr., and Horton, C. E.: Penile reconstruction of epispadias associated with exstrophy. Norwich Eaton Professional Services (16 mm color and sound, 925), 1979.

Devine, C. J., Jr., Horton, C. E., Gilbert, D. A., and Winslow, B. H.: Hypospadias. *In* Plastic Surgery in Infancy and Childhood, 3rd ed. Mustarde, J. C., and Jackson, I. T. (Ed.). New York, Churchill Livingstone, 1988, pp. 493–509.

Devine, C. J., Horton, C. E., and Scarff, J. E.: Epispadias. Urol Clin. North Am. 7:465–476, 1980.

Devine, C. J., Jr., and Jordan, G. H.: Strictures of the anterior urethra. Parts I and II. AUA Update Series. Lessons 25 and 26, Volume IX, 1990.

Devine, C. J., Jr., Jordan, G. H., and Somers, K. D.: Peyronie's disease: Cause and surgical treatment. AUA Today, 2:1–3, 1989.

Devine, C. J., Jr., and Pepe, G.: Unpublished data.

Devine, C. J., Jr., Somers, K. D., Wright, G. L., Jr., et al.: A working model for the genesis of Peyronie's disease derived from its pathobiology. Abstract 495. J. Urol., 139:286A, 1988.

Devine, P. C., et al.: Use of full thickness skin grafts in repair of urethral stricture. J. Urol., 90:67, 1963.

Devine, P. C., and Devine, C. J., Jr.: Posterior urethral injuries associated with pelvic fractures. Urology, 20:467, 1982.

Devine, P. C., Fallon, B., and Devine, C. J., Jr.: Free full thickness skin graft urethroplasty. J. Urol., 116:444, 1976.

Devine, P. C., and Horton, C. E.: Strictures of the male urethra. *In* Converse, J. M., (Ed.). Reconstructive Plastic Surgery, vol. 7, 2nd ed. Philadelphia, W. B. Saunders Co., 1977, pp. 3883–3895.

Duckett, J. W.: The island flap technique for hypospadias repair. Urol. Clin. North Am., 8:503, 1981.

El-Mahdi, A. M.: Personal communication, 1990.

Farrow, G. A., Boyd, J. B., and Semple, J. L.: Total reconstruction of the penis employing the "cricket bat flap" single stage forearm free graft. AUA Today, 3:7, 1990.

Fishman, I. J., Hirsch, I. H., and Toombs, B. D.: Endourological reconstruction of posterior urethral disruption. J. Urol., 137:283–286, 1987.

Frank, J. D., Mor, S. B., and Pryor, J. P.: The surgical correction of erectile deformities of the penis of 100 men. Br. J. Urol., 53:645, 1981.

Frank, R. T.: The formation of an artificial vagina without operation. Am. J. Obstet. Gynecol., 35:1053, 1938.

Frumkin, A. P.: Reconstruction of male genitalia. Am. Rev. Sov. Med., 2:14–21, 1944.

Ganesan, G. S., Jordan, G. J., Winslow, B. H., and Devine, C. J., Jr.: Traumatic disruption of the female urethra—its pathogenesis, sequelae and management in a study of five patients. Abstract 1570. J. Urol., 141:557A, 1989.

Gearhart, J. P., and Rock, J. A.: Total ablation of the penis after circumcision with electrocautery: A method of management and long-term followup. J. Urol., 42:799, 1989.

Gelbard, M. K.: Personal communication. At, The Peyronie's Disease Conference, Norfolk, October 14, 1989.

Gelbard, M. K., James, K., and Dorey, F.: the natural history of Peyronie's disease. J. Urol., 144:1376–1379, 1990.

Gelbard, M. K., Linder, A., and Kaufman, J. J.: The use of collagenase in the treatment of Peyronie's disease. J. Urol., 134:280, 1985.

Gilbert, D. A.: Radial forearm flap for phallic reconstruction. *In* Strauch, B., Vasconez, L. O., Hall-Findlay, E. J., (Eds.). Grabb's Encyclopedia of Flaps. Boston, Little, Brown & Co., 1990, pp. 1515–1520.

Gilles, H. D., and Harrison R. H.: Congenital absence of the penis. Br. J. Plast. Surg., 1:8–28, 1948.

Gittes, R. F., and McLaughlin, A. P.: Injection technique to induce penile erection. Urology, 4:473, 1974.

Godec, C. J., and Van Beek, A. L.: Peyronie's disease is curable—is it also preventable? Urology, 21:257, 1983.

Goldstein, A. M., and Padma-Nathan, H.: The microarchitecture of the intracavernosal smooth muscle and the cavernosal fibrous skeleton. J. Urol., 144:1144, 1990.

Hinman, F., Jr.: Peyronie's disease: Etiological considerations. Prog. Reprod. Biol. Med., 9:5–12, 1983.

Hendren, W. H.: Penile lengthening after previous repair of epispadias. J. Urol., 121:527, 1979.

Horton, C. E., and Devine, C. J., Jr.: Plication of the tunica albuginea to straighten the curved penis. Plast. Reconstr. Surg., 52:32, 1973.

Horton, C. E., and Devine, C. J., Jr.: Peyronie's disease. Plast. Reconst. Surg., 52:503, 1973.

Horton, C. E., Sadove, R. C., and Devine, C. J., Jr.: Peyronie's disease. Ann. Plast. Surg., 18:121–127, 1987.

Horton, C. E., Sadove, R. C., Devine, C. J., Jr., and Vorstman, B.: Hypospadias, epispadias, and exstrophy of the bladder. *In* Smith, J. W., and Aston, S. J., Grabb and Smith's Plastic Surgery, 4th ed. Boston, Little, Brown & Co., 1991.

Jeffs, R. D.: Exstrophy. *In* Harrison, J. H., Gittes, R. F., Perlmutter, A., et al. (Eds.). Campbell's Urology, 4th ed. Philadelphia, W. B. Saunders Co., 1979.

Johnston, J. H.: The genital aspects of exstrophy. J. Urol., 113:701, 1975.

Jones, W. J., Jr.: The evaluation and treatment of psychosexual dysfunction in men. AUA Update Series. Vol. III, Lesson 33, 1984.

Jones, W. J., Jr., Horton, C. E., Stecer, J. F., Jr. et al.: The treatment of psychogenic impotence after dermal graft repair for Peyronie's disease. J. Urol., 131:286, 1984.

Jordan, G. H.: Reconstruction of the fossa navicularis. J. Urol., 138:102–104, 1987.

Jordan, G. H., and Devine, P. C.: Management of urethral stricture disease. Urol. Clin. North Am., 15:277–289, 1988.

Jordan, G. H., Kodama, R. T., Rowe, D. F., and Devine, C. J., Jr.: Interpretation of penile duplex ultrasound wave forms and measurements in pharmacologically induced erections. Abstract 33. J. Urol., 143:197A, 1990.

Jordan, G. H., Schlossberg, S. M., and McCraw, J. B.: Tissue transfer techniques for genitourinary reconstructive surgery. Parts I-III. AUA Update Series, Vol. VII, Lessons 9-12, 1988.

Kaufman, J. J., Boxer, B., and Quinn, M. C.: Physical and psychological results of penile prostheses: A statistical survey. J. Urol., 126:173, 1981.

Kelley, J. H., and Eraklis, A. J.: A procedure for lengthening the phallus in boys with exstrophy of the bladder. J. Pediatr. Surg., 6:645, 1971.

Koff, S. A., and Eakins, M.: Treatment of penile chordee using corporal rotation. J. Urol., 131:931, 1984.

Lee, Y. T., and Lee, J. M.: Delayed retropubic urethroplast of completely transected female membranous urethra. Urology, 31:499–502, 1988.

Leffell, M. S., Devine, C. J., Jr., Horton, C. E., et al.: Nonassociation of Peyronie's disease with HLA B7 cross-reactive antigens. J. Urol., 127:122, 1982.

Lue, T. F.: Penile venous surgery. Urol. Clin. North Am., 16:607–611, 1989.

Lue, T. F., Hricak, H., Marich, K. W., and Tanagho, E. A.: Vaculogenic impotence evaluated by high-resolution ultrasonography and pulsed Doppler spectrum analysis. Radiology, 155:777, 1985.

Magalini, S. (Ed.): Dictionary of Medical Syndromes, 3rd ed. Philadelphia, J. B. Lippincott Co., 1990, p. 526.

Malloy, T. R., Zderic, S. A., and Carpiniello, V. L.: External genital lesions. *In* Smith, J. A., Jr., Stein, B. S., and Benson, R. C., Jr., (Eds.). Lasers in Urologic Surgery, 2nd ed. Chicago, Year Book Medical Publishers, 1989, pp. 23–34.

Marshall, F.: Endoscopic reconstruction of traumatic urethral transections. Urol. Clin. North Am., 16:313–318, 1989.

Martius, H., McCall, J., and Bolster, K. A. (Eds.). Operative Gynecology. Boston, Little, Brown & Co., 1956.

McAninch, J. W., Laing, F. C., and Jeffrey, R. B., Jr.: Sonourethrography in the evaluation of urethral strictures: a preliminary report. J. Urol., 139:294, 1988.

McCallum, R. W.: The adult male urethra: Normal anatomy, pathology and method of urethrography. Radiol. Clin. North Am., 17:227, 1979.

McCraw, J. B., and Arnold, P. G.: McCraw and Arnold's Atlas of Muscle and Musculocutaneous Flaps. Norfolk, Hampton Press Publishing, 1986, pp. 265–294.

McDougal, W. S.: Scrotal reconstruction using thigh pedicle flaps. J. Urol., 129:757–759, 1983.

McDougal, W. S., and Persky, L.: Traumatic injuries of the genitourinary system. *In* International Perspectives in Urology. vol. 1. Baltimore, Williams & Wilkins, 1981.

McGowan, A. J., and Waterhouse, K.: Mobilization of the anterior urethra. Bull. NY Acad. Med., 40:776, 1964.

McRoberts, J. W.: Peyronie's disease. Surg. Gynecol. Obstet., 12:1291, 1969.

McRoberts, J. W., Chapman, W. H., and Ansell, J. S.: Primary anastomosis of the traumatically amputated penis: Case report and summary of literature. J. Urol., 100:751, 1968.

Nesbit, R. M.: Congenital curvature of the phallus: A report of three cases with description of corrective operation. J. Urol., 93:230, 1965.

Nyberg, L. M., Bias, W. B., Hochberg, M. C., and Walsh, P. C.: Identification of an inherited form of Peyronie's disease with autosomal dominant inheritance and association with Dupuytren's contracture and histocompatibility B7 cross-reacting antigens. J. Urol., 128:48, 1982.

O'Connor, V. J., Jr., and Kropp, K. A.: Surgery of the female urethra. In Glen, J. F., and Boyce, W. H. (Eds.). Urologic Surgery. New York, Harper and Row, 1969, p. 572.

Oesterling, J. E., Gearhart, J. P., and Jeffs, R. D.: A unified approach to early reconstructive surgery of the child with ambiguous genitalia. J. Urol., 138:107, 1987.

Orandi, A.: One-stage urethroplasty. Br. J. Urol., 40:77, 1968.

Orandi, A.: One-stage urethroplasty: Four year follow-up. J. Urol., 107:977, 1972.

Orticochea, M.: Musculo-cutaneous flap method: immediate and heroic substitute for the method of delay. Br. J. Plast. Surg., 25:106, 1972.

Orticochea, M.: New method of total reconstruction of the penis. Br. J. Plast. Surg., 25:347, 1972.

Padma-Nathan, H.: Evaluation of the corporal veno-occlusive mechanism: Dynamic infusion cavernosometry and cavernosography. Semin. Intervent. Radiol. 6:205–211, 1989.

Peña, A., and Devries, P. A.: Posterior sagittal anorectoplasty. Important technical considerations and new applications. J. Pediatr. Surg., 17:796–811, 1982.

Peyronie, F. de la: Sur quelques obstacles qui s'opposent a l'ejaculation naturelle de la semence. Memoires de l'Academie de Chirurgie 1:318, 1743.

Poland, R. L.: The question of routine neonatal circumcision. Sounding Board. N. Engl. J. Med., 322:1312–1315, 1990.

Ponten, B.: The fascio-cutaneous flap: its use in soft tissue defects of the lower leg. Br. J. Plast. Surg., 34:215, 1981.

Pontes, J. E., and Pierce, J. M., Jr.: Anterior urethral injuries: four years of experience at the Detroit General Hospital. J. Urol., 120:563–564, 1978.

Pressman, D., and Greenfield, D.: Reconstruction of the perineal urethra with a free full thickness skin graft from the prepuce. J. Urol., 69:677, 1953.

Pryor, J. P., and Castle, W. M.: Peyronie's disease associated with chronic degenerative arterial disease and not with beta-adrenoceptor blocking agents. Lancet, 4:917, 1982.

Pryor, J. P., and Fitzpatrick, J. M.: A new approach to the correction of the penile deformity in Peyronie's disease. J. Urol., 122:622, 1979.

Puckett, C. L., and Montie, J. E.: Construction of male genitalia in the transsexual using a tubed groin flap for the penis and a hydraulic inflation device. Plast. Reconstr. Surg., 61:523, 1978.

Puckett, C. L., Reinisch, J. F., and Montie, J. E.: Free flap phalloplasty. J. Urol., 128:294, 1982.

Quartey, J. K. M.: One-stage penile/preputial cutaneous island flap urethroplasty for urethral stricture: A preliminary report. J. Urol., 129:284, 1983.

Rubin, R. A., Goldfarb, R. A., Lidsky, M. D., and Abrams, J.: Decreased activity of Reiter's syndrome after urethrectomy. Arthritis Rheum., 33:885–887, 1990.

Schlossberg, S. M., Jordan, G. H., and Devine, C. J., Jr.: Unpublished data.

Schmidt, K. H., Somers, K. D., Devine, C. J., Jr., et al.: Development of an in vivo model of Peyronie's disease in the nude mouse. Abstract 147. J. Urol., 137:140A, 1987.

Schoen, E. J.: The status of circumcision of newborns. Sounding Board. N. Engl. J. Med. 322:1309–1311, 1990.

Schonfeld, W. A., and Beebe G. W.: Normal growth and variation in the male genitalia from birth to maturity. Am. J. Dis. Child., 64:759: 1942.

Schreiter, F., and Noll, F.: Mesh graft urethroplasty using split thickness skin graft or foreskin. J. Urol., 142:1223–1226, 1989.

Singh, M., and Blandy, J. P.: The pathology of urethral stricture. J. Urol., 115:673, 1976.

Smith, B. H.: Peyronie's disease. Am. J. Clin. Pathol., 45:670, 1966.

Smith, B. H.: Subclinical Peyronie's disease. Am. J. Clin. Pathol., 52:385, 1969.

Snow, R., and Devine, C. J., Jr.,: The conservative management of Peyronie's disease. Unpublished data. 1981.

Snyder, H.: The surgery of bladder exstrophy and epispadias. In Frank, J. D., Johnston, J. H. (Eds.). Operative Paediatric Urology. London, Churchill Livingstone, 1990, pp. 153–185.

Somers, K. D., Dawson, D. M., Wright, G. L., Jr., et al.: Cell culture of Peyronie's disease plaque and normal penile tissue. J. Urol., 127:585, 1982.

Somers, K. D., Sismour, E. N., Wright, G. L., Jr., Devine, C. J., Jr., et al.: Isolation and characterization of collagen in Peyronie's disease. J. Urol., 141:629, 1989.

Somers, K. D., Sismour, E. N., Wright, G. L., Jr., Devine, C. J., Jr., et al.: Isolation and characterization of collagen in Peyronie's disease. J. Urol., 141:629, 1989.

Somers, K. D., Winters, B. A., Dawson, D. M., et al.: Chromosome abnormalities in Peyronie's disease. J. Urol., 137:672, 1987.

Song, R., Gao, Y., Song, Y., Yu, Y., and Song, Y.: The forearm flap. Clin. Plast. Surg. 9:21, 1982.

Spence, H. M., and Duckett, J. W., Jr.: Diverticulum of the female urethra: clinical aspects and presentation of a simple operative technique for cure. J. Urol., 104:432, 1970.

Turner-Warwick, R.: A personal view of the management of traumatic posterior urethral stricture. Urol. Clin. North Am., 4:111, 1977.

Turner-Warwick, R.: Urethral stricture surgery. Current Operative Surgery: Urology. London, Bailliere Tindal, 1988.

Turner-Warwick, R.: Prevention of complications resulting from pelvic fracture urethral injuries and from their surgical management. Urol. Clin. North Am., 16:335–358, 1989.

VandeBerg, J. S., Devine, C. J., Jr., Horton, C. E., et al.: Peyronie's disease: an electron microscopic study. J. Urol., 126:33, 1981.

VandeBerg, J. S., Devine, C. J., Jr., Horton, C. E., et al.: Mechanisms of calcification in Peyronie's disease. J. Urol., 127:52, 1982.

Vorstman, B., and Devine, C. J., Jr.: Penile torsion, curvature and Peyronie's disease. In Pryor, J. P., and Lipshultz, L. I. (Eds.). Andrology. London, Butterworths, 1987, pp. 69–91.

Waterhouse, K., Abrahams, H. G., Hackett, R. E., and Peng, B. K.: The transpubic approach to the lower urinary tract. J. Urol., 109:486, 1973.

Webster, G. D., Sihelnik, S. A., and Stone, A. R.: Urethrovaginal fistulas: a review of surgical management. J. Urol., 132:460–462, 1984.

Wild, R. M., Devine, C. J., Jr., and Horton, C. E.: Dermal graft repair of Peyronie's disease. Survey of 50 patients. J. Urol., 121:47–50, 1979.

Williams, J., and Thomas, G.: The natural history of Peyronie's disease. J. Urol., 103:75, 1970.

Winslow, B. H., and Horton, C. E.: Hypospadias. Semin. Urol., 5:236–242, 1987.

Winslow, B. H., Horton, C. E., Gilbert, D. A., and Devine, C. J.: Epispadias and exstrophy of the bladder. In Plastic Surgery in Infancy and Childhood, 3rd ed. Mustarde, J. C., and Jackson, I. T. (Eds.). New York, Churchill Livingstone, 1988, pp. 511–527.

Winslow, B. H., Vorstman, B., and Devine, C. J., Jr.: Complications of hypospadias surgery. In Marshall, F. F. (Ed.). Urologic Complications, Medical and Surgical, Adult and Pediatric. Chicago, Year Book Medical Publishers, 1986, pp. 411–426.

Woodside, J. R.: Pubovaginal sling procedure for the management of urinary incontinence after urethral trauma in women. J. Urol., 138:527–528, 1987.

84

DIAGNOSIS AND THERAPY OF ERECTILE DYSFUNCTION

Irwin Goldstein, M.D.
Robert J. Krane, M.D.

DIAGNOSIS OF ERECTILE DYSFUNCTION

It is the goal of this discussion on the diagnosis of erectile dysfunction to review the rationale for the diagnostic evaluation of the impotent male. The diagnostic evaluation is designed to help the patient understand the probable basis for his sexual problem so that an appropriate treatment plan may be formulated.

The evaluation begins with a sexual, a psychosocial and medical history, a physical examination, and routine laboratory tests (Krane et al., 1989). The initial diagnostic evaluation is designed to gain information in both major pathophysiologic areas—the psychologic and the physical. The impressions discovered on the initial evaluation may be subsequently corroborated by a series of additional diagnostic examinations, such as nocturnal penile tumescence and neurologic, psychologic, hormonal, and vascular testing (Barry and Hodges, 1978; Melman et al., 1984; Padma-Nathan et al., 1986).

The evaluation should be tailored to the individual patient (Table 84–1). No universally agreed upon diagnostic algorithm for the evaluation of all impotent patients is available as yet. Many noninvasive and invasive erectile function tests are available, ranging from nocturnal penile tumescence testing, which has been done for over 4 decades (Ohlmeyer et al., 1944), to newer diagnostic evaluations, such as cavernosal tissue biopsy (Meulerman et al., 1990), dynamic nuclear magnetic resonance (NMR) (Sohn et al., 1990), determination of corporal blood Po_2 (Vardi et al., 1990), visual sexual stimulation (Morales et al., 1990), cavernous electric activity (Stief et al., 1990; Wagner et al., 1989), and gravity cavernosometry (Puech-Leao et al., 1990). Many of the erectile function tests are in evolution, and their standardization and reliability have not been fully determined.

A number of factors need to be considered when selecting diagnostic procedures for the impotent male, including test morbidity, the patient's wish for treatment, the cost, and the patient's age and general health. As the diagnostic evaluation becomes more intricate and sophisticated, primary organic factors influencing erectile performance will be found with increasing frequency. The secondary psychologic reaction to these organic factors should not be ignored. Successful management of the patient with primary organic and sec-

Table 84–1. SUMMARY OF ERECTILE FUNCTION TESTING

Tests	Recommendations
Initial examination	Perform as described in all patients.
Nocturnal penile tumescence (NPT) or visual sexual stimulation (VSS)	May be obtained; results need to be corroborated with other test results.
Neurologic	Biothesiometry may be routinely performed in all patients; neurophysiologic testing may be performed as suggested by the history and physical examination.
Psychologic	Psychologic interview and questionnaires may be obtained as suggested by history.
Hormonal	Hormonal studies may be obtained if libido is diminished.
Vascular	
Arterial—flaccid state	May be obtained as part of initial evaluation in all patients.
Arterial—dynamic state	May be obtained in order of invasiveness based on history, previous arterial testing, NPT, or VSS studies.
Corporal veno-occlusive function	Pharmacocavernosometry by pump or gravity methodology may be obtained based on history, previous arterial testing, NPT, or VSS studies.

ondary psychologic impotence may commonly demand attention to both dysfunctions (Melman et al., 1988).

An estimated 10 million American males (Shabsigh et al., 1988) have impotence. In 1985, over 400,000 outpatient visits to a physician and over 30,000 inpatient hospital admissions for impotence were recorded. This resulted in a total cost for the evaluation and treatment of impotence of 146 million dollars (National Center for Health Statistics data, from Fitzsimmons, 1989).

Initial Examination

The patient's history is the most important element in the evaluation of the impotent male. Even though there are numerous noninvasive and invasive erectile function tests available, the history helps define the actual sexual problem, the presence or absence of potency, the presence of normal erections, the erectile insufficiency or erectile failure as well as the interaction of physical and psychologic factors.

The evaluation should include a detailed sexual history; a psychosocial history; a medical history, involving a review of neurologic, vascular, and genitourinary systems, as well as a surgical history. The physical examination and routine laboratory tests usually follow, enabling the complete evaluation to be performed in usually an hour or less.

The physician should help allay the anxieties about the erectile dysfunction by informing the patient about the incidence and age-dependent nature of the disorder. Impotence is common and age-dependent with an incidence of 1.9 per cent at 40 years of age and 25 per cent at 65 years of age (Kinsey, 1948). Physicians should inform their patients that they are fully aware that the subject material may be difficult to discuss. A previsit questionnaire may help eliminate some of the initial embarrassment. Patients should express in their own words their sexual problems and their expectations from the diagnostic evaluation. Patients must be confident that all information obtained throughout the evaluation and treatment will remain private and confidential. If the patient wishes, his partner should be included in the initial evaluation.

Sexual History

The first issue in the interview should be to establish the nature of the sexual complaint. It is important to determine whether it is a problem of penile erection, ejaculation, libido, or orgasm.

When the primary complaint is an abnormal penile erection, one must establish whether the patient is potent, that is, does he have the ability to achieve successful penetration and maintain penetration until ejaculation. Erectile potency is a functional term and its presence does not imply the existence of a normal erection. Individuals may be functionally potent but still complain of diminished quality of erectile performance, either in terms of rigidity or sustaining capability. Questions, such as when was the last successful intercourse, what is the present frequency of intercourse, and what was the frequency of intercourse years ago, should be asked early in the interview to establish the patient's potency status.

The next step is to identify the quality of the penile erection in terms of maximum rigidity and sustaining capability; the consistency among morning, masturbatory, and coital erections; and the duration and onset of the initial complaint.

Maximum rigidity may be expressed in terms of a comparison of peak rigidity to a known reference rigidity. The reference may be the rigidity of previously normal capabilities or the rigidity of a typical hard object taken as a 100 per cent reference. The percentage of the maximal rigid erections commonly reflects the maximal pressure that can be achieved within the corporal body, because the maximal physiologic pressure at equilibrium is approximately 100 mm Hg. For example, an individual whose maximum rigidity of morning and coital erections is 60 per cent that of previous capabilities may be able to achieve only an intracavernosal pressure of approximately 60 mm Hg, possibly suggesting the existence of a hemodynamic impairment.

Sustaining capability is best expressed in terms of the duration in minutes that functional rigidity is able to be maintained with minimal stimulation. This value may then be compared with previous capabilities. It is important to know if sustaining capability is consistent in morning and coital erections. In many patients, the inability to sustain the various erections suggests the presence of corporal veno-occlusive dysfunction.

The *onset* of the dysfunction is also important. Classic features suggesting primary psychogenic impotence include an acute onset, which may be related to a specific loss, such as a divorce or financial crisis. Such a patient may also provide a history of normal erections upon awakening and with masturbation. In contrast, a slow insidious and progressive loss of erectile capabilities with a consistent change in the rigidity or sustaining capability of the erections for over 1 year, involving morning, coital, or masturbation-related erections, is usually indicative of a primary organic etiology. Such a patient may be considered to have *erectile insufficiency* or *erectile failure*, depending on the degree of the dysfunction. A patient with erectile insufficiency may be "potent" but may still have abnormalities in the erection mechanism—reduced rigidity or reduced sustaining capability (Padma-Nathan et al., 1987).

Other questions concerning the quality of the patient's erection should include the existence of pain or curvature, because such a history may be indicative of Peyronie's disease (Roddy et al., 1991). Questions concerning libido or sexual interest should be posed. Diminished libido may result from endocrine disorders, such as hypogonadism, or psychosocial factors, especially secondary or reactive to the impotence itself. One useful discriminator of a reactive loss of libido versus a primary endocrine dysfunction is the expression by the patient of the desire to immediately increase sexual activity if his erectile performance were to be corrected. If doubt remains as to the explanation of the loss of libido, an endocrine evaluation should be considered.

Psychosocial History

A psychosocial history is directed toward identifying psychologic factors that may adversely affect erectile performance, either in a primary or secondary sense. Such a history may be obvious, especially in patients with a history of affective disorders, psychopathology, psychologic counseling, or utilizing psychotropic medication. In such a patient, additional consultation with the primary mental health professional may be indicated.

The urologist may also wish to explore more subtle psychologic factors such as how the patient has dealt with his dysfunction, especially in terms of behavior, self-confidence, partner relationship (supportive or adversarial), and work and family relationships. Is there any presence of anger, fear, guilt, denial, anxiety, depression, or obsession? Is there a history of drug or alcohol abuse, marital discord, or numerous unexplained physical complaints? Is there evidence of a litigious personality? More detailed psychosocial evaluation in impotent patients is generally helpful in providing "total" and not exclusively "penis" care. Detailed psychologic evaluation is generally performed by a trained mental health professional (Smith, 1988).

Medical History

The medical history should include details concerning the management, treatment, and associated complications of any chronic systemic medical disorders, such as multiple sclerosis, cirrhosis of the liver, chronic alcoholism, chronic renal failure, and diabetes mellitus (Table 84–2). Diabetes mellitus, in particular, represents one of the systemic medical disorders most frequently associated with impotence, with a prevalence of impotence estimated to be 35 to 50 per cent (McCulloch et al., 1980). The vascular and neurologic complications associated with the natural history of diabetes are thought to be the main causes of diabetic impotence (Blanco et al., 1990; Ellenberg, 1971; Kolodny et al., 1974; Lehman et al., 1983; Saenz de Tejada et al., 1989). A history of spinal cord injury (Amelar et al., 1982; Torrens, 1983) or of concomitant symptoms, such as changes in bladder and bowel function, paresthesias, changes in balance, strength, or penile sensation, may suggest an underlying neurologic etiology. A history of previous pelvic surgery, such as radical prostatectomy (Catalona and Dresker, 1985; Eggleston et al., 1985; Lepor et al., 1985; Walsh, 1982), cystoprostatectomy, and proctocolectomy, or of vascular surgery, such as aortoiliac procedures (Dewar et al., 1985) may be relevant.

Alterations in the inflow and outflow of blood to and from the penis are thought to be the most frequent causes of organic impotence. Vascular risk factors that may be associated with the development of either atherosclerotic or traumatic arterial occlusive disease of the hypogastric cavernous arterial bed should be carefully identified in the history. Common risk factors associated with arterial insufficiency include hypertension, hyperlipidemia, cigarette smoking, diabetes mellitus, blunt perineal or pelvic trauma, and pelvic irradiation (Gold-

Table 84–2. MEDICAL HISTORY

Chronic medical disorders	Management, treatment, and associated complications of such disorders as multiple sclerosis, liver cirrhosis, chronic renal failure, chronic alcoholism, and diabetes mellitus
Neurologic disorders	Spinal cord injury, changes in bladder and bowel function, paresthesias, changes in balance and strength or penile sensation
Previous surgery	Radical prostatectomy, cystoprostatectomy, proctocolectomy, or vascular surgery such as aortoiliac surgery, surgery to the penis
Vascular risk factors adversely influencing arterial inflow	Hypertension, hyperlipidemia, cigarette smoking, diabetes mellitus, blunt perineal or pelvic trauma, and pelvic irradiation
Factors adversely influencing fibroelastic integrity of erectile tissue	Diabetes mellitus, aging, vascular risk factors such as hyperlipidemia, Peyronie's disease, injury to the erect penis during coitus or masturbation, surgery to the penis, priapism
Medications	
Central neuroendocrine control	Cimetidine, antipsychotics, antidepressants, central-acting antihypertensives
Antihypertensives	Sympatholytics (e.g., alpha methyldopa, guanethidine, clonidine), alpha-adrenoceptor blocking agents (e.g., prazosin), beta-adrenoceptor blocking agents (e.g., propranolol), vasodilators (e.g., hydralazine), and diuretics (e.g., thiazide)

stein et al., 1984; Levine et al., 1990; Michal, 1982; Rosen et al., 1991; Ruzbarsky et al., 1977; Sharlip, 1981; Virag et al., 1985).

Corporal veno-occlusive dysfunction may occur as a result of a structural alteration in the fibroelastic components of the trabeculae. This effect would result in a loss of corporal tissue compliance and an inability to expand the trabeculae against the tunica albuginea and thus compress the subtunical venules. Diabetes mellitus associated with nonenzymatic glycosylation of collagen; aging; and vascular risk factors, such as hypercholesterolemia associated with altered synthesis of collagen, are factors that may be involved in the development of corporal tissue stiffness (Azadzoi and Goldstein, 1987; Cerami et al., 1987; Fischer et al., 1980; Hayashi et al., 1987). The presence of Peyronie's disease (Gasior et al., 1990), a history of injury to the erect penis during coitus or masturbation (Lurie et al., 1988; Penson et al., 1991), as well as a history of surgery to the penis (Montague, 1988) or priapism (Hinman, 1960) should be sought, because they may be associated with corporal veno-occlusive dysfunction.

A detailed history of the patient's medications should be obtained because various classes of therapeutic drugs can cause the undesired side effect of impotence (Seagraves et al., 1985; Slag et al., 1983; Wein et al., 1988).

In general, drugs that interfere with central neuroendocrine control have a potential for causing impotence. Cimetidine, a histamine (H_2 type) receptor antagonist, has been associated with impotence and, reportedly, has antiandrogenic effects (Penden et al., 1979). Central neurotransmitter pathways, including 5-hydroxytryptaminergic, noradrenergic, and dopaminergic pathways, involved in sexual function (de Groat et al., 1988) may be interfered with by a variety of drugs, such as certain antipsychotics and antidepressants and some central-acting antihypertensive drugs (Shader and Elkin, 1980).

The most common prescribed medications that have the potential for causing impotence are the antihypertensives. Antihypertensive agents that have been reported to cause impotence include sympatholytics (e.g., alpha methyldopa, guanethidine, clonidine), alpha-adrenoceptor blocking agents (e.g., prazosin), beta-adrenoceptor blocking agents (e.g., propranolol), vasodilators (e.g., hydralazine), and diuretics (e.g., thiazide) (Seagraves et al., 1985; Slag et al., 1983; Wein et al., 1988). Sympatholytics, alpha-adrenoceptor blockers, or vasodilators are unlikely to cause impotence by direct interference with the local neurovascular control of penile smooth muscle, because reduction in adrenergic tone or direct smooth muscle relaxation would be expected to facilitate erection. A possible explanation for this drug-associated impotence is that many patients with hypertension also have generalized atherosclerotic occlusive disease. Antihypertensive agents decrease systemic blood pressure which, in those patients with pre-existing occlusive disease of the hypogastric cavernous arterial bed, may result in significant decrease in the perfusion pressure to the lacunar spaces. The hemodynamic consequence to erection would be reduced penile rigidity. One study in animals has suggested that the effect of alpha methyldopa on sexual function is a result of both peripheral and central effects (Melman et al., 1983).

Physical Examination

Physical examination of the impotent male should include evaluation of the endocrine, nervous, and vascular systems as well as the local penile factors. A rectal and prostate examination should be performed in patients over 40 years of age.

The endocrine examination involves observation of a gross index of androgen stimulation, such as the normal development of secondary sex characteristics, including body and facial hair patterns, and normal development of external genitalia. The neck should be examined for thyroid disease. The presence or absence of gynecomastia and the size and consistency of the testis should be noted.

The neurologic examination should refer to the sacral dermatomes and should include sensory testing of the penis and perineum. Evaluation of the bulbocavernosus reflex is done during the rectal examination. On initially entering the examination room, the patient's ability to walk and the gait, leg strength, and balance should be observed.

The vascular examination involves the assessment of the arteries in the eyes, in the neck for carotid bruits, in the abdomen for aneurysms, and in the penis and lower extremities. The femoral, pedal, and posterior tibial pulses are noted. Hair loss and skin changes of the feet and lower extremities should be observed.

The penis should be examined for Peyronie's plaques (Horton et al., 1987) and overall erectile tissue stiffness or scarring (Bondil et al., 1990). This evaluation may be performed by retracting the foreskin, grasping the penis by the corona, and pulling. Typically, the penis will stretch at least several centimeters. Patients with Peyronie's plaques or with overall erectile tissue stiffness (e.g., postpriapism) will have penile shafts that do not stretch easily. Furthermore, with the penis taut, it is simpler to palpate for Peyronie's plaques.

Laboratory Tests

No one laboratory test, or series of laboratory tests, is exclusively diagnostic of impotence. Most physicians order routine laboratory tests for occult systemic medical disorders, for vascular risk factors, and for endocrine disorders.

Systemic medical disorders, such as diabetes mellitus, renal insufficiency, and blood dyscrasias, may be screened with routine complete blood counts, liver enzymes, blood urea nitrogen, creatinine, and serum electrolyte (SMA profile) determinations. Vascular risk factors, such as hyperlipidemia, may be determined by recording fasting cholesterol, low-density lipoprotein, high-density lipoprotein, and triglycerides.

Especially if the libido is diminished, endocrine abnormalities may be screened with a serum testosterone test (see Hormonal Testing).

Nocturnal Penile Tumescense (NPT) Testing

The monitoring of sleep-associated erections for the evaluation of impotence has been in existence for many years. The quality of nocturnal penile erections has been traditionally used to differentiate psychogenic from organic impotence (Fisher et al., 1965; Karacan, 1970; Karacan et al., 1978). In the normal male, periodic physiologic erections (three to five per night), each lasting 25 to 35 minutes, and usually associated with rapid eye movement (REM) sleep, will occur each night. The validity of NPT testing is based on the assumption that psychologic factors do not influence this form of erectile activity. Therefore, patients with psychogenic impotence would be expected to exhibit a normal pattern of nocturnal erections, whereas patients with organic impotence exhibit impaired or absent erectile activity.

However, some organic conditions, such as abnormalities in the sensory afferent dorsal nerve pathway and alteration in the pathways between cortical centers and brain stem, do not impair sleep-related tumescense but may result in dysfunctional sexual erections (Kessler, 1988; Morales et al., 1990; Ware, 1987). In addition, nocturnal erections and erections associated with awake erotic behavior cannot always be equated (Kessler, 1988;

Morales et al., 1990a). Furthermore, age (Schiavi et al., 1990), hormonal status, and some emotional states may influence the quality of the nocturnal penile erection (Ware, 1987). In sexually active men over the age of 70 years, a decrease in the frequency, number, and rigidity of nocturnal erections has been documented. In hypogonadal men, there is a reported decrease in normal sleep-associated erectile events (Kwan et al., 1983). Decreased nocturnal penile erectile activity has been observed in various emotional states, including anxiety, clinical depression, and hypoactive sexual desire (Thase et al., 1988). In addition, some illnesses, certain sleep disorders, and various medications adversely influence nocturnal penile erections (Ware, 1987).

Instrumentation influences the accuracy of the measurement of sleep-associated erections. In formal NPT testing, penile circumference changes are monitored at the base and the tip of the penis with mercury strain gauges during three consecutive nights in a specialized sleep facility. In addition, electroencephalographic, electro-oculographic, and electromyographic activities are simultaneously recorded, because the quality and quantity of sleep affect the erectile activity (Fisher et al., 1965; Karacan, 1970; Karacan et al., 1978). During the study, the patient is awakened in the midst of an erectile episode. The axial rigidity of the erection is determined by assessing the resistance of the penis to buckling when applying a known weight against the glans. Such measurements are necessary because normal penile circumferential changes may occur with inadequate penile rigidity. The high cost and the inconvenience to the patient of sleep laboratory testing have led to a variety of portable devices for home NPT testing. Devices utilizing strain gauges to measure changes in penile circumference to detect the presence of nocturnal erections do not record penile rigidity. The stamp test, Snap-Gauge band, and Rigiscan device (Fig. 84–1A and B) have been designed to measure penile rigidity during home nocturnal monitoring but fail to document sleep quality (Anders et al., 1983; Barry et al., 1980; Bradley et al., 1985; Karacan, 1989; Marshall et al., 1983; Procci and Martin, 1984; Wein et al., 1981).

NPT monitoring is considered an important evaluation in erectile function testing, especially when it is combined with measuring nocturnal penile rigidity. In one study, NPT testing with rigidity monitoring and sleep pattern analysis corroborated with other diagnostic studies predicted organic from psychogenic impotence in 68 per cent of cases (Bock et al., 1990). Numerous false-positive and false-negative results occur with sleep-associated erection recording. Nevertheless, the test is appropriately performed when doubt remains as to whether a patient's primary pathophysiology is psychogenic or organic impotence. NPT testing is neither specific nor sensitive enough to be utilized as a single diagnostic evaluation. Its results should be corroborated with other aspects of the diagnostic evaluation.

Visual Sexual Stimulation

The issues concerning the validity and reliability of NPT, as well as the problems of financial and time

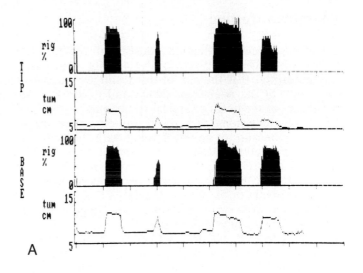

A

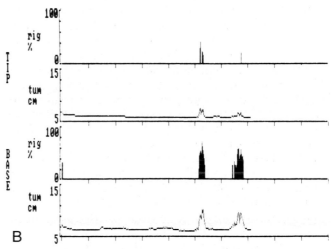

B

Figure 84–1. The Rigiscan device has been designed to measure penile rigidity during home nocturnal monitoring. *A,* A study in a patient with at least two episodes of well-sustained, completely rigid nocturnal erections. *B,* A study with two episodes of poorly sustained, poorly rigid nocturnal erections. Such home studies fail to document sleep quality.

expenditure, have led to the development of an alternative monitoring of nonsleep-associated, erotically stimulated penile erections. Visual sexual stimulation (VSS) utilizes video taped erotic material in a laboratory setting to facilitate penile erection (Morales et al., 1990b; Schouman et al., 1988). During the erotic exposure, there is continuous tumescence and rigidity monitoring of penile responses.

A prospective study was performed to determine the usefulness of VSS (Morales et al., 1990). VSS demonstrated different responses in organic, psychogenic, and mixed diagnostic groups. A high degree of agreement was found between NPT with full polysomnographic recording and VSS penile responses. VSS, which records the responses to erotic and nonsleep-associated erections, may be a cost-effective and reliable alternative to NPT testing in the differentiation of organic from psychogenic impotence. Further corroboration of this observation is needed.

Neurologic Testing

The neurologic evaluation consists of the physical examination (described previously) and the neurophysiologic testing. It is the aim of this testing to document the extent of the neurologic deficit and to identify any possibility of medical or surgical treatment.

Neurologic lesions that result in impotence do so ultimately because of an interference with the ability of the motor efferent autonomic cavernosal nerves to the penis to cause relaxation of penile smooth muscle. These motor efferent autonomic cavernosal nerves may be either indirectly or directly tested.

Indirect testing of cavernosal nerve integrity is performed by recording an impaired NPT activity, in conjunction with evidence of intact hemodynamic integrity, as assessed by the erectile response to the intracavernosal administration of vasoactive agents. The presence of bladder areflexia and concomitant bladder or bowel dysfunction provides further indirect support for the impairment of the motor efferent autonomic cavernosal nerves. Vascular reflexes, such as single breath beat-to-beat variation, provide other indirect measurements of autonomic parasympathetic neuropathy (Nisen et al., 1990). A normal variation of heart rate during shallow breathing is 10 or more beats per minute. Autonomic parasympathetic neuropathy should be considered when a heart rate variation during shallow breathing of less than 10 beats per minute is measured.

Direct testing of the autonomic cavernous innervation may be done by recording the electrical activity of the corporal smooth muscle utilizing either intracavernosal electromyographic needles (Stief et al., 1990; Wagner et al., 1989) or surface electrodes on the penile shaft (Stief et al., 1990). Such direct testing offers the ability to identify neurologic abnormalities at the level of the autonomic neuron-corporal smooth muscle interface. Using single potential analysis of this cavernous electrical activity, waveforms of a defined duration, amplitude, and polyphasity have been recorded in a reproducible pattern from normal subjects (Buvat et al., 1990; Stief et al., 1990). Following VSS, these potentials decrease in amplitude and duration and increase in frequency. Following smooth muscle relaxation induced by intracavernosal vasoactive drug administration, electrical silence of these potentials has been noted.

Suprasacral neurologic lesions may cause impotence even though the reflexogenic sacral erectile mechanism is preserved. In such cases, the erections may be poorly maintained without constant tactile stimulation because of lack of control from higher centers (Dahlof and Larsson, 1976; Herbert, 1973). In patients with upper motor neuron spinal cord lesions (e.g., spinal cord injuries), the single potential analysis of cavernous electrical activity may demonstrate potentials with longer duration and potentials with whips and bursts (Fig. 84–2) (Stief et al., 1990).

In lower motor neuron spinal cord lesions, such as from multiple sclerosis; in peripheral neuropathy, such as secondary to diabetes mellitus and alcoholism; and in pelvic surgery, such as radical prostatectomy, cysto-prostatectomy, and proctocolectomy, the single poten-tial analysis of cavernous electrical activity may reveal potentials that are of short duration and high amplitude or that are of low amplitude (Stief et al., 1990).

With such direct analysis, cavernous electrical activity may be monitored and a specific diagnosis of autonomic cavernous neuropathy may be made. Utilizing indirect recording of cavernous nerve integrity, it has been an uncommon experience to diagnose neurogenic impotence in a patient without a previous history of a known neurologic disorder or without concomitant neurologic symptoms. However, in a group of 112 consecutive impotent patients with a normal neurologic history, the incidence of abnormal single potential analysis of the cavernous electrical activity, indicative of pathology in the autonomic cavernous nerve, was 34 per cent (Stief et al., 1990).

Erectile dysfunction may also result from an alteration of the afferent somatic fibers in the pudendal nerve or their representation in the sacral spinal cord (Herbert, 1973). This effect may be due to an alteration of the tactile perception or interruption of the afferent limb of the reflexogenic erection, with projections to supraspinal centers which may be important in maintaining psychogenic erections.

Testing of these afferent somatic dorsal nerve pathways may be initially performed by penile biothesiometry to measure sensory perception thresholds to vibratory stimulation (Goldstein, 1983; Lavoisier et al., 1990; Newman, 1970; Padma-Nathan et al., 1987a). The biothesiometer is a hand-held electromagnetic device with an amplitude of vibration that is variable but a frequency of vibration that is fixed (Fig. 84–3). The tactor of the device is placed on the pulp of the right and left index fingers and is compared with the right and left sides of the penile shaft as well as the glans penis. The accompanying nomogram has been obtained in our facility from potent controls (Table 84–3). If there is suggestive evidence for sensory loss, neurophysiologic testing determining dorsal nerve conduction velocity or bulbocavernosus reflex latency testing will identify peripheral and sacral spinal pathology (Ertekin et al., 1985). Dorsal nerve somatosensory-evoked response testing is helpful for identifying neuropathology involving the entire peripheral and central afferent conduction pathways (Fig. 84–4).

Psychologic Testing

The principal methods of assessing the psychologic contribution to erectile dysfunction include the interview and sexual, personality, or stress factor questionnaires. The most common causes of psychologic impotence are performance anxiety, relationship conflict, sexual inhibition, sexual preference issues, childhood sexual abuse consequences, and fear of pregnancy or sexually transmitted disease.

Psychogenic stimuli are necessary to initiate and facilitate a sexually induced penile erection. This is achieved by psychogenic input activating the parasympathetic dilator nerves in the sacral cord to the penis as well as by diminishing sympathetic outflow to the penis.

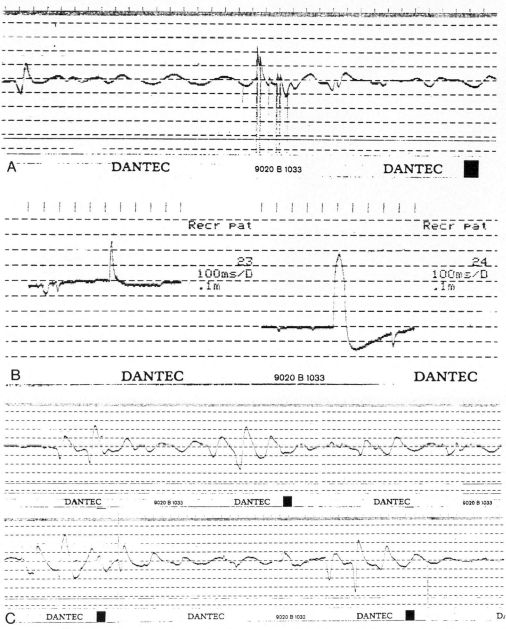

Figure 84–2. Direct testing of the autonomic cavernous innervation may be studied by recording the electrical activity of the corporal smooth muscle utilizing intracavernosal electromyographic needles or even surface electrodes on the penile shaft. Such direct testing offers the ability to identify neurologic abnormalities at the level of the autonomic neuron-corporal smooth muscle interface. Using single potential analysis of this cavernous electrical activity, waveforms of a defined duration, amplitude, and polyphasity have been recorded in a reproducible pattern from normal subjects. In patients with neurologic injuries, the single potential analysis of cavernous electrical activity may demonstrate potentials of longer duration and the presence of whips and bursts potentials. *A,* Bursts. *B,* Whips. *C,* A continuous recording in a patient with a neurologic injury.

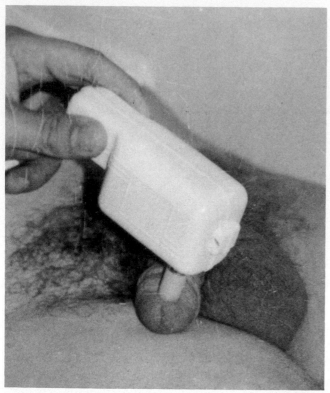

Figure 84–3. Testing of the afferent somatic dorsal nerve pathway may be initially performed by penile biothesiometry to measure sensory perception thresholds to vibratory stimulation. The biothesiometer is a hand-held electromagnetic device with a variable amplitude of vibration but a fixed frequency of vibration. The tactor of the device is placed on the pulp of the right and left index fingers and is compared with the right and left sides of the penile shaft as well as the glans penis. A nomogram has been obtained in our facility using potent controls. If there is suggestive evidence for sensory loss then neurophysiologic testing, determining dorsal nerve conduction velocity or bulbocavernosus reflex latency, will identify peripheral and sacral spinal pathology.

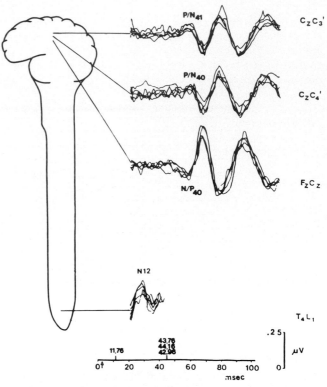

Figure 84–4. If there is suggestive evidence for sensory loss then neurophysiologic testing, such as dorsal nerve somatosensory-evoked response, should be considered. This is useful for identifying neuropathology involving the entire peripheral and central afferent conduction pathways. The study involves the electrical stimulation of the skin of the penis and the recording of the evoked response in the region of the sacral spinal cord as well as over the sensory cortex.

In a similar fashion, cerebral input may inhibit the erectile response (de Groat et al., 1988). It is hypothesized that adverse psychogenic input to the sacral cord, such as in anxiety, may inhibit the sacral cord–mediated reflexogenic erections and, therefore, prevent the activation of the parasympathetic dilator nerves to the penis. Also, excessive sympathetic outflow and elevated blood catecholamine levels may increase penile smooth muscle tone, opposing the smooth muscle relaxation necessary for erection (Benard et al., 1988; Diederichs et al., 1988; Euler, 1964).

The interview is the primary method of psychologic evaluation and should include the patient and partner's subjective experience of the sexual problem and identification of patterns of sexual avoidance. An important goal of the interview is to identify factors that increase performance anxiety (Smith, 1988).

A number of questionnaires have been created to assess sexual attitudes and sexual function as well as personality and stress factor information. The Minnesota Multiphasic Personality Inventory has been one of the most popular questionnaires in sexual dysfunction evaluation and has been successful in detecting gross psychologic aberrations, which suggest the need for more detailed psychologic evaluation. In general, no questionnaires have been useful in the differentiation of psychogenic from organic impotence; however, they have been beneficial in assessing the need and the outcome of sex therapy intervention. The role of the mental health

Table 84–3. PENILE BIOTHESIOMETRY*

Patient Age Range	(N)	Mean age	Right finger	Left finger	Right shaft	Left shaft	Glans	Frequency coitus/ month
17–29	15	23 ± 4	5	5	5	5	6	3 ± 3
30–39	22	34 ± 3	5	5	6	6	7	8 ± 5
40–49	31	44 ± 3	5	5	6	6	7	4 ± 2
50–59	31	54 ± 3	6	6	8	8	9	3 ± 2
60–69	10	64 ± 3	6	6	9	9	10	3 ± 3
70	9	73 ± 3	7	7	14	14	16	2 ± 2

*Average vibration perception threshold to nearest whole number.
Non-neurologic potent controls.

professional in evaluating impotent patients is not confined to diagnosing primary psychogenic impotence. Impotent men with recognized primary organic factors adversely influencing erection may undergo psychologic counseling to reduce anxiety, sexual inhibition, or relationship conflict (LoPiccolo, 1988).

Hormonal Testing

Testosterone influences the growth and development of the male reproductive tract and secondary sexual characteristics as well as sexual libido and sexual behavior (Bancroft et al., 1983; Davidson, 1975; Kwan et al., 1983; Wilson et al., 1981). The effect of testosterone on the erectile mechanism, however, remains unclear. Patients with "castrated" levels of testosterone can achieve erections in response to VSS, which are comparable in quality to erections in men with normal levels of testosterone. In contrast, it has been shown that hypogonadal men have decreased nocturnal penile erectile activity that responds to androgen replacement (Kwan et al., 1983). Furthermore, a wide variation exists in serum testosterone levels in normal men with values ranging from approximately 100 ng/dl to 1300 ng/dl, as related to the episodic secretion of luteinizing hormone. Typically, higher values are noted in the morning (Spratt et al., 1988).

Because of these aforementioned factors, many physicians do not routinely screen for testosterone in all impotent men. If, however, diminished sexual desire is a concomitant part of the patient's complaint, serum testosterone measurement should follow. Because of the variability of testosterone secretion, the diagnosis of a low serum testosterone level should be based only on repeated findings of low levels. In our facility, we study several repeated early morning specimens.

The three main endocrinologic disorders associated with impotence are hypogonadotrophic hypogonadism, hypergonadotrophic hypogonadism, and hyperprolactinemia. Other associated disorders include hyperthyroidism and hypothyroidism.

If hypogonadism is suspected based on several repeated low serum testosterone values, it is recommended to obtain a serum luteinizing hormone (LH) to determine the underlying pathophysiology. Low testosterone levels associated with low serum LH levels, for example, would suggest hypogonadism secondary to a hypothalamic or pituitary defect, such as pituitary tumor or infiltrative disease of the hypothalamus, or a congenital disorder, such as the Kallmann, Prader-Willi, or Lawrence-Moon-Biedl syndrome. A computed tomography scan of the brain as well as an evaluation of other abnormalities of panhypopituitarism is suggested. An elevated serum LH level suggests primary hypogonadism from testicular failure. Causes include Klinefelter's syndrome, chemotherapy, and radiation therapy.

Low serum testosterone values can also be associated with hyperprolactinemia. In a patient so affected, declining libido and impotence may be early symptoms. The low circulating serum testosterone levels appear to be secondary to the inhibition of normal gonadotropin-releasing hormone pulsation by elevated prolactin levels.

In impotent patients with hyperprolactinemia and low testosterone levels, treatment with exogenous testosterone does not restore potency in approximately half of the patients. This is so despite the normalization of serum testosterone levels, thus possibly implying some degree of antagonism by prolactin to the peripheral action of testosterone. Hyperprolactinemia may be observed secondary to pituitary microadenoma, to drug-induced, and chronic renal failure, and to idiopathic causes (Carter et al., 1978; Franks et al., 1978; Pogach et al., 1983; Spark et al., 1980).

Complaints by patients regarding erections may also be associated with both the hyperthyroid and hypothyroid states. Hyperthyroidism is commonly associated with diminished libido and, less often, with impotence (Pogach and Vaitukaitis, 1983; Spark et al., 1980). In hyperthyroidism, elevated testosterone values exceeding 1000 ng/dl may be found. Hyperthyroidism may be associated with a recent weight loss, a change in shirt collar size, a rapid pulse, an arrythmia, and irritability. However, older men may not display these obvious signs and symptoms and may present only with diminished libido. Hypothyroidism may be a cause of impotence secondary to associated low testosterone and elevated prolactin levels (Pogach and Vaitukaitis, 1983).

Vascular Testing

Erectile function is dependent on the hemodynamic interaction of not only arterial inflow and perfusion pressure but also on the development of an adequate venous outflow resistance. Functional impairment of arterial inflow, veno-occlusive function, or both may result in erectile dysfunction. To accurately assess the integrity of the hemodynamic components of erection in an impotent patient, both arterial and veno-occlusive function testing should be performed.

Arterial Testing

FLACCID STATE. Evaluation of the integrity of the penile arteries should ultimately determine the perfusion pressure and arterial inflow of the cavernosal arteries, because both variables have an impact on the rigidity and speed with which erection develops. At present, evaluation may be performed of the penile arteries in the flaccid state and in the dynamic state following intracavernosal vasoactive agent administration.

In the flaccid state, the penile arteries may be evaluated by determining penile artery systolic blood pressure utilizing either a Doppler ultrasound probe or penile plethysmography (Abelson, 1975; Goldstein et al., 1982; Kedia, 1984). The value may then be compared with the brachial artery systolic blood pressure providing a ratio entitled—the penile brachial index. Alternatively, the penile arteries may be evaluated by analyzing the Doppler waveform.

A shortcoming of the previous techniques is the inability to consistently measure blood pressure or flow in the cavernosal artery as opposed to the dorsal or spongiosal arteries. It is the cavernosal artery systolic pressure, exclusively, that represents the highest intracavernosal pressure that can be achieved in a physiologic erection. It is further unclear what penile brachial index ratio value represents an abnormal study. Furthermore, testing in the flaccid state, as opposed to the dynamic state, does not address the ability of the cavernosal artery to dilate and increase blood flow. Flaccid state determination of the arterial system has a low sensitivity and specificity and a poor correlation of the penile brachial index to other evaluations of the arterial system, including penile arteriography (Padma-Nathan et al., 1988; Washecka and Zorgniotti, 1988).

Nevertheless, the flaccid state arterial study is commonly obtained. It is utilized as a noninvasive screening test of the penile arterial blood supply, which can be performed as part of the initial physical examination.

DYNAMIC STATE. A test that is done in the physician's office, in which the erectile response is observed following the intracavernosal injection of vasoactive agents, may aid in the diagnosis of vascular-related impotence (Abber and Lue, 1987). A normal rigid erection should develop within 5 to 10 minutes and last approximately 45 minutes. If such an erection develops in an impotent patient, a normal vascular status is implied and neurologic or psychologic impotence should be considered. A prolonged erectile response may require the intracavernosal administration of phenylephrine (Neo-Synephrine) to induce detumescence.

If only a partial, a short-lived, or an absent erection results, hemodynamic impairment, either arterial insufficiency or corporal veno-occlusive dysfunction, may be present. Purely arterial insufficiency may be suspected if the erection is partially rigid and delayed in onset and, ultimately, requires intracavernosal adrenergic agonist administration to achieve detumescence. Alternatively, corporal veno-occlusive dysfunction may be suspected if the response achieves a partial erection quickly and loses rigidity with time. In such cases, there is virtually no need to utilize intracavernosal adrenergic agonist administration to achieve detumescence.

Failure to produce an erection in this test setting, however, may be due to excessive adrenergic constrictor tone secondary to anxiety about the test conditions. This occurrence represents a common problem in all invasive testing in the dynamic state. The goal of invasive testing is to achieve an erectile response that represents, as closely as possible, the maximal erectile response. Anxiety, however, prevents adequate relaxation of the corporal smooth muscle, a necessary factor in obtaining an erection. In order to reduce adverse psychologic influences and to facilitate maximal smooth muscle relaxation, this test has been performed in conjunction with manual, vibratory, or audio-visual sexual stimulation. Thus, a negative result from a single intracavernosal injection without adjunctive stimulation is inconclusive.

At present, no standardized approach is used regarding the pharmacologic agent, the dose, the method of monitoring the erectile response, and the adjunctive stimulation. Such testing is selected as a screening procedure for abnormal erectile hemodynamics. However, the lack of a rigid erectile response may be noted with arterial insufficiency, corporal veno-occlusive dysfunction, or psychogenic impotence due to increased adrenergic activity. Conversely, a rigid response may be seen with neurogenic and psychogenic impotence and, in cases of arterial insufficiency, with normal corporal veno-occlusion. With proper standardization of the variables mentioned, it is hoped that in the future this evaluation may increase in sensitivity and specificity. In general, this form of testing should precede other more invasive diagnostic techniques, such as pharmacocavernosometry and arteriography.

Duplex ultrasonography utilizes the combination of real-time high-frequency ultrasonography with pulsed Doppler analysis to provide the ability to focus on specific penile structures and, in particular, the cavernosal arteries (Lue et al., 1985). If the cavernosal arteries are studied before and after the intracavernosal administration of vasoactive agents, the study may help determine changes in cavernosal artery diameter and in calculated peak flow velocity. The normal postintracavernosal injection values in potent patients are cavernosal artery diameter of more than 0.08 cm and peak flow velocity of more than 30 cm/second, and strong pulsation of the thin-walled cavernosal arteries. Cavernosal arteries in atherosclerosis show a postinjection diameter of less than 0.07 cm, and a blood flow velocity measurement in the dynamic state below 25 cm/second. Younger patients with proximal traumatic arterial occlusive disease may show a normal postinjection diameter but should show a low postinjection peak flow velocity. In one study, an abnormal flow velocity response had a 58 per cent sensitivity, whereas an abnormal diameter response had an 88 per cent sensitivity in detecting significant occlusive disease at arteriography (Padma-Nathan et al., 1988).

Duplex ultrasonography is an invasive test, utilizing intracavernosal vasoactive agent administration. Therefore, this study has the common problem of all dynamic studies—the overriding effects of anxiety on intracavernosal vasoactive agent–induced smooth muscle relaxation. It may be necessary to study duplex ultrasonography not only after intracavernosal agent administration but also after adjunctive erotic stimulation. The major disadvantages of duplex ultrasonography are the high cost of the equipment and the importance of the operator's efficiency in utilizing the ultrasound probe. The timing of the study following an intracavernosal or a genital stimulated erection is important in duplex ultrasonography. As previously mentioned in the section on erectile physiology, the arterial diameter of the cavernosal artery and the blood flow changes in the cavernosal artery vary during different phases of the erection. It is essential to perform duplex ultrasonography within 5 minutes of the onset of the erection, during the initial filling phase, prior to the development of the tumescence phase (i.e., increasing intracavernosal pressure with diminishing inflow) or the full erection phase during steady-state equilibrium (i.e., intracavernosal pressure approximates systemic mean arterial pressure with minimal arterial inflow at approximately 3 to 5 ml/minute). Duplex ultrasonography does not provide any information on cavernosal artery perfusion pressure—the maximal intracavernosal pressure able to be achieved at equilibrium independent of ischiocavernosal muscle contraction.

The technologic advances utilizing color duplex ultrasonography have the advantages of visualizing multiple arteries and veins at the same time and demonstrating the direction of blood flow in the respective blood vessels. Further work is required to determine the benefits of this new technology (Porst, 1990).

The determination of cavernosal artery perfusion pressure in the dynamic state is obtained by recording the intracavernosal pressure and simultaneously monitoring the pulsatile flow of the cavernosal artery utilizing a continuous wave Doppler ultrasound probe (Fig. 84–5). The intracavernosal pressure is raised by infusion of heparinized saline until the cavernosal artery Doppler signal disappears. When saline infusion is terminated, the intracavernosal pressure will diminish below the cavernosal artery systolic pressure, with the resultant reappearance of cavernosal artery pulsatile flow. The intracavernosal pressure, at which cavernosal artery pulsations return, is defined as the effective cavernosal artery systolic pressure, implying the maximal arterial pressure that can be delivered to the lacunar space during erection. The brachial artery systolic pressure is simultaneously recorded. Normal study findings exist when the two pressures are similar. A gradient between the cavernosal and brachial pressures of less than 35 mm Hg has been defined as normal (Goldstein, 1987 and 1988) in individuals with normal intracavernosal pressure responses to intracavernosal pharmacologic agents as controls.

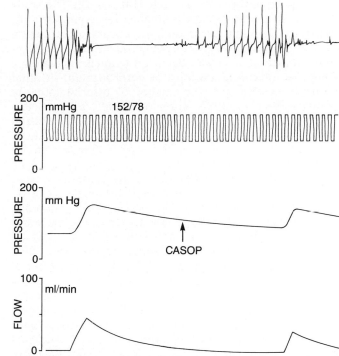

Figure 84–6. This tracing depicts four simultaneous variables obtained during the third phase of dynamic infusion cavernosometry and cavernosography. From top to bottom includes cavernosal artery flow recorded by utilizing a continuous wave Doppler ultrasound probe, systemic brachial systolic and diastolic arterial blood pressure (150/87 mm Hg), intracavernosal pressure, which varied from 70 to 160 mm Hg in this tracing, and intracavernosal heparinized saline inflow. The intracavernosal pressure at which the cavernosal artery pulsations returned, the effective cavernosal artery systolic occlusion pressure (CASOP), was 108 mm Hg. The gradient between the brachial and cavernosal artery systolic occlusion pressures was 150 to 108 or 42 mm Hg, which is abnormal.

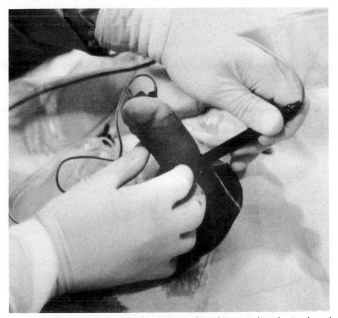

Figure 84–5. The continuous wave Doppler ultrasound probe is placed at the 3-o'clock and 9-o'clock positions along the right and left lateral penile shafts to record the pulsatile flow of the artery within the corporal body. A pulsatile pump is utilized to infuse heparinized saline intracavernosally. The intracavernosal pressure is recorded by a needle via saline-filled tubing to a pressure transducer. The intracavernosal pressure is raised by infusion of heparinized saline until the cavernosal artery Doppler signal disappears. When the infusion is terminated, the intracavernosal pressure will diminish below the cavernosal artery systolic pressure, with the resultant reappearance of cavernosal artery pulsatile flow. The intracavernosal pressure at which cavernosal artery pulsations return is defined as the effective cavernosal artery systolic pressure, implying the maximal arterial pressure that can be delivered to the lacunar space during erection.

In one study, the sensitivity of cavernosal artery systolic occlusion pressure was 77 per cent in predicting arterial occlusive disease as diagnosed by arteriography (Padma-Nathan et al., 1988). Because the test records perfusion pressure, it is the only one that can predict the maximal intracavernosal pressure obtained in a penile erection at equilibrium. Cavernosal artery systolic occlusion pressures can be monitored on a multichannel recorder in which heparinized saline flow, intracavernosal pressure, systemic blood pressure, and continuous wave Doppler ultrasound of this artery can be simultaneously displayed (Fig. 84–6). The study is, however, usually performed during a simultaneous evaluation of corporal veno-occlusive function and, as such, requires indwelling intracavernosal needles. It is, therefore, more invasive than pulsed-Doppler ultrasonography. Because the test records cavernosal artery perfusion pressure, it is less subject to the adverse effects of all dynamic studies, that is, the corporal smooth muscle vasoconstrictive effects of anxiety.

Selective internal pudendal pharmacoarteriography is usually reserved for those patients being considered for arterial reconstructive surgery (Rosen et al., 1990). The study is performed using local anesthesia and intravenous sedation. Intracavernosal and intra-arterial vasoactive agents allow for optimal visualization of the penile arterial tree in the dynamic state (Fig. 84–7). The study is expensive and has the potential for complications, including bleeding, thrombosis or aneurysm formation of the femoral artery, and embolism of the distal peripheral arteries. Because the arteriogram is an anatomic study, its interpretation must be corroborated with that of other erectile function studies of arterial integrity (Bookstein et al., 1987; Zorgniotti et al., 1983). Selective internal pudendal arteriography may also be utilized to diagnose and subsequently treat, via embolization, patients suspected of arterial priapism (Walker et al., 1990; Witt et al., 1990).

New studies of cavernosal artery perfusion have been introduced. Intracavernosal arterial blood flow can be said to "percolate" through the lacunar spaces, in much the same fashion that blood flow traverses the placenta. It is for this reason that arteriographic studies, which require laminar flow for visualization, rarely record flow through the lacunar spaces. NMR, using gadolinium-DTPA as the contrast medium, has the ability to enhance the proton density of such specialized vascular regions. In a study of dynamic NMR with gadolinium-DTPA (Austoni et al., 1990; Sohn et al., 1990), a time-related enhancement of the corpora cavernosa and corpus spongiosum can be achieved. Such studies have the capability of observing blood flow through the erectile tissue. Preliminary work with time enhancement dynamic-NMR in normal penile erections has demonstrated a homogeneous distribution pattern requiring several minutes to fill the entire corporal chamber. In atherosclerotic occlusive disease, a patchy distribution of contrast material is seen, suggesting the possibility of multiple localized regions of arteriolar disease. Dynamic NMR has an obvious potential as a measure of cavernosal artery perfusion to determine the efficacy of vascular reconstructive surgery.

Another new study for arterial perfusion of the erectile tissue measures the intracavernosal blood partial pressure of oxygen (Po$_2$) level following pharmacologic stimulation. In one study (Vardi et al., 1990), the mean cavernosal blood Po$_2$ determinations at 0, 1, 5, 10, and 15 minutes following intracavernosal vasoactive agent administration were 36.2, 88, 92.7, 97.3, and 95.5 mm Hg, respectively, in eight potent control patients. In contrast, in 19 patients with arteriogenic impotence, the mean Po$_2$ values at similar times were 30.5, 72.2, 77.2, 79.8, and 80.5 mm Hg, respectively. Statistical significance ($p < .001$) was obtained at the 1-, 5-, 10-, and 15-minute measurements. The technique of determining cavernous Po$_2$ levels in response to vasoactive medications may again have ultimate use in documenting the functional existence of arteriogenic impotence as well as postoperative changes in cavernosal tissue perfusion following vascular reconstructive procedures.

Corporal Veno-Occlusive Function Testing

PHARMACOCAVERNOSOMETRY AND PHARMACOCAVERNOSOGRAPHY. Alterations in the outflow of blood from the penis are thought to be frequent causes of organic impotence (Krane et al., 1989). The cavernosal artery perfusion pressure and inflow may not be able to compensate for the presence of an abnormal regulation of venous outflow. Thus, functional impairment of veno-occlusive function may result in erectile dysfunction by preventing adequate penile rigidity and adequate sustaining capability.

Hemodynamic testing of the corporal veno-occlusive mechanism is primarily utilized for those impotent patients who wish to consider vascular reconstructive surgery as a treatment option. Testing of the veno-occlusive mechanism may also be performed in those individuals who after noninvasive testing wish a more precise delineation of the hemodynamic status to help them select appropriate therapy. Such an indication is particularly applicable to those impotent patients who experience intracavernosal pharmacotherapy failure and wish to consider treatment alternatives prior to possible penile implantation. Other indications for veno-occlusive testing include Peyronie's disease prior to therapy (Gasior et al., 1990), medico-legal conditions in which the impotence is alleged to have occurred after a specific incident, and follow-up after vascular reconstructive surgery.

To accurately assess the integrity of veno-occlusive function in an impotent patient, testing must be performed in the dynamic state, following intracavernosal vasoactive agent administration. The corporal veno-occlusive mechanism is activated when corporal smooth muscle is relaxed. Subsequent erectile tissue expansion against the tunica albuginea compresses the plexus of subtunical venules, thus reducing lacunar space venous outflow. It is only in the erect state, following smooth muscle relaxation, that resistance to the flow of blood through the corpora is developed. As previously mentioned, the dilemma of any study in the erect state, especially in the diagnostic assessment of corporal veno-occlusive function, is the presence of contracted corporal smooth muscle, secondary to anxiety or inadequate doses of intracavernosal vasoactive agents. In such situations, there are inadequate compression of subtunical venules and inadequate resistance to venous outflow.

An animal study investigating the role of smooth muscle tone in the determination of venous outflow resistance utilized relaxing and contracting infusing solutions (Saenz de Tejada et al., 1991). It was determined that in the presence of complete smooth muscle relaxation, venous outflow resistance was maximal at intracavernosal pressures as low as 30 mm Hg. The flow-to-maintain various intracavernosal pressures was minimal. A linear relationship was found between flow-to-maintain and intracavernosal pressures (i.e., constant venous outflow resistance), through the range of 30 to 150 mm Hg. In the presence of smooth muscle contraction, a nonlinear relationship exists between the flow-to-maintain and the intracavernosal pressures (i.e., variable venous outflow resistance), through the pressure range of 30 to 150 mm Hg (Saenz de Tejada et al., 1991).

Applying these principles to humans we have observed, through the range 30 to 150 mm Hg, a nonlinear relationship between flow-to-maintain and intracavernosal pressures in the absence of vasoactive agents or

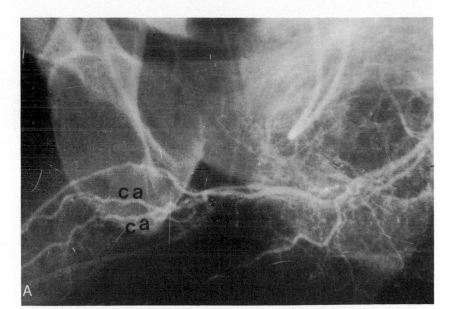

Figure 84–7. Selective internal pudendal pharma-coarteriography is usually reserved for a patient being considered for arterial reconstructive surgery. The study is performed using local anesthesia and intravenous sedation. Intracavernosal and intra-arterial vasoactive agents allow for optimal visualization of the penile arterial tree in the dynamic state. The study is expensive and has potential complications, including bleeding, thrombosis or aneurysm formation of the femoral artery, as well as embolism of the distal peripheral arteries. As the arteriogram is an anatomic study, its interpretation must be corroborated with the results of other erectile function studies of arterial integrity.

A, A normal right selective study in a patient complaining of impotence. The radiograph reveals visualization of the distal internal pudendal, common penile, right and left cavernosal arteries (ca) and dorsal artery.

B, An abnormal right selective study in an impotent patient revealing the visualization of the distal internal pudendal, common penile origin of the right cavernosal artery and dorsal artery. Abrupt occlusion of the proximal cavernosal artery occurs approximately 1 cm from the origination *(arrow)*. Selective internal pudendal arteriography may also be utilized to diagnose and subsequently treat, via embolization, a patient suspected to have arterial priapism.

C, A left selective study in a potent patient with arterial priapism. The radiograph reveals a filling defect in the proximal penile shaft from a lacerated cavernosal artery branch. The remainder of the cavernosal artery (ca) in this potent man with a nonpharmacologically induced erection is normal and is approximately 1.2 mm in diameter—the same diameter as the dorsal artery.

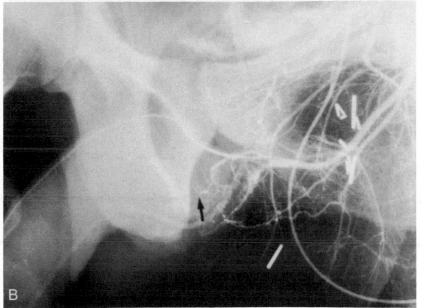

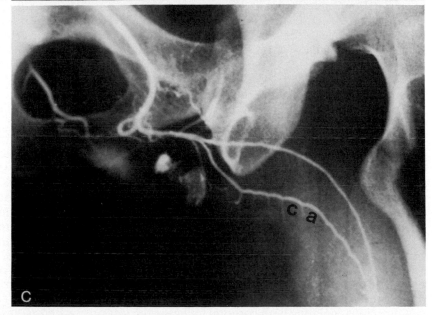

in the presence of minimal doses of vasoactive agents. This finding would suggest a variable venous outflow resistance consistent with the presence of contracted smooth muscle. In the same patients, administering additional intracavernosal vasoactive agents or the same agents at higher doses resulted in a marked reduction in the flow-to-maintain various pressures. In addition, the variable relationship between flow-to-maintain and intracavernosal pressures over the range of 30 to 150 mm Hg converted to a linear one. This finding suggested that smooth muscle relaxation was complete, with a constant venous outflow resistance. When smooth muscle relaxation is presumed complete, the flow-to-maintain various intracavernosal pressures has been found to be 3 ml/minute or less. Under normal physiologic conditions during equilibrium, the pudendal arterial inflow is approximately 3 to 5 ml/minute. Further research needs to be performed to confirm the presence of complete pharmacologic smooth muscle relaxation in humans during dynamic testing. When such information is universal, the standardization of such dynamic testing will be able to be realized.

Corporal veno-occlusive dysfunction may be said to exist if flow rates to maintain various intracavernosal pressures are elevated—greater than 3 ml/minute—under conditions of presumed maximal smooth muscle relaxation. This effect may occur when the collagen/elastin erectile tissue stiffness is high, such as in aging, diabetes mellitus, atherosclerosis, Peyronie's disease, and after trauma (Azadzoi et al., 1987; Ceramiet et al., 1987; Fischer et al., 1980; Gasior et al., 1990; Hayashi et al., 1987; Lurie et al., 1988; Montague, 1988; Penson et al., 1991). Under such conditions, an inadequate subtunical venule compression and a low venous outflow resistance are observed.

Diagnostic testing of the veno-occlusive mechanism may be performed, not only by recording the flow-to-maintain various intracavernosal pressures, but also by recording the intracavernosal pressure decay. This practice is based on the principle that the corpora cavernosa act as a pressure energy storage chamber in the presence of normal subtunical venule compression. Intracavernosal pressure energy is released over time through the subtunical venules. The time constant may be defined as the time associated with decay of an initial intracavernosal pressure to 1/e (36.8 per cent, where e is a fixed number of value 2.718) of the initial intracavernosal pressure. Determination of the time constant of any pressure energy storage chamber is utilized to identify the capacitance or energy storage capability of the chamber. Because capacitance and venous outflow resistance are related by the time constant, as long as complete smooth muscle relaxation is presumed, the method of determining venous outflow resistance, either by flow-to-maintain pressure or intracavernosal pressure decay will be the same (Saenz de Tejada et al., 1991). In our experience, pressure decay may be performed clinically, with an initial intracavernosal pressure of 150 mm Hg, observing the pressure fall over 30 seconds following termination of the saline infusion (Goldstein et al., 1990).

In our facility, we have performed pump cavernosometry by cannulating both corporal bodies in the distal dorsal aspect of the penile shaft with 21-gauge needles, following the initial administration of 5 ml 1 per cent lidocaine to the area (Fig. 84–8A). One needle is connected to a pressure transducer, and the other to an infusion pump with intracavernosal pressure feedback (Life-Tech, Inc. Houston, TX). The initial intracavernosal injection of vasoactive agents has been of papaverine hydrochloride (45 mg) and phentolamine mesylate (2.5 mg). The intracavernosal pressure to these pharmacologic agents is recorded on a strip chart recorder. When a steady-state equilibrium has been reached (usually in 10 minutes) (Fig. 84–8B), provocative tests of corporal veno-occlusive function are subsequently performed. The flow of heparinized saline necessary to maintain various intracavernosal pressures is determined, in increasing intervals of 30 mm Hg to a pressure of 150 mm Hg (Fig. 84–9). At 150 mm Hg, the flow of heparinized saline is terminated and the corporal body pressure drop, over a 30-second period, is determined. The pressure decay is then repeated in the presence of perineal compression to examine if this manuever reduces the maintenance flow rates or if the pressure falls over 30 seconds (Fig. 84–10). If the flow-to-maintain intracavernosal pressure values at 30, 60, 90, 120, and 150 mm Hg are elevated, especially if the values are not linearly related to increasing intracavernosal pressures (Fig. 84–9A), one should consider the possibility that the results are abnormal secondary to incomplete smooth muscle relaxation. The administration of additional papaverine and phentolamine or prostaglandin E_1 should be performed. After waiting for a new steady-state equilibrium (an additional 10 minutes), the flow-to-maintain various intracavernosal pressures as well as pressure decay values should be repeated and compared with the pressures and values obtained previously. A linear response of flow-to-maintain various intracavernosal pressures should be observed, implying that complete smooth muscle relaxation has been achieved (Fig. 84–9B).

Normal values for the provocative testing of the corporal veno-occlusive mechanism have been studied in patients who have responded to the intracavernosal administration of vasoactive agents by achieving an intracavernosal pressure approximating the mean systemic brachial arterial blood pressure (Fig. 84–8B). In such cases, erectile hemodynamic responses have been assumed to be normal. The flow of heparinized saline necessary to maintain various intracavernosal pressures in these patients has been 3 ml/minutes or less, throughout the range of intracavernosal pressures. The fall of corporal body pressure over a 30-second period from a suprasystolic pressure of 150 mm Hg has been less than 45 mm Hg (Fig. 84–10B).

Anatomic visualization of veins draining the corporal bodies during erection by pharmacocavernosography may confirm the findings of cavernosometry, flow-to-maintain pressure, or pressure decay and may provide anatomic information for surgical reconstruction (Payau et al., 1983). When normal corporal veno-occlusive function is present, minimal or absent venous drainage is demonstrated radiographically (Fig. 84–11). In patients with corporal veno-occlusive dysfunction, various patterns of drainage have been noted. In patients with

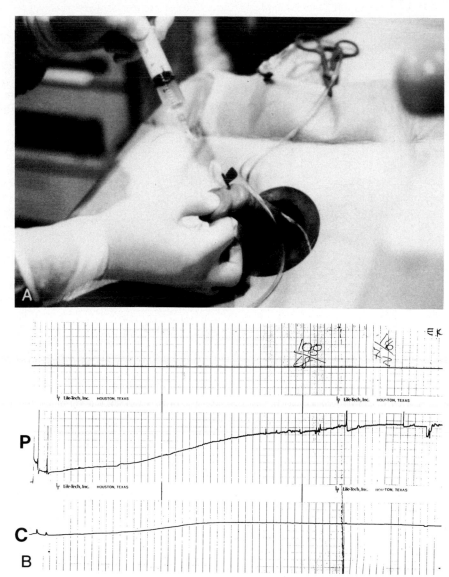

Figure 84–8. In our facility, we have performed pump cavernosometry by cannulating both corporal bodies in the distal dorsal aspect of the penile shaft with 21-gauge needles following the initial administration of 5 ml 1 per cent lidocaine to the area (A). One needle is connected to a pressure transducer while the other, to an infusion pump with intracavernosal pressure feedback. Intracavernosal injection of vasoactive agents follows. The intracavernosal pressure to these pharmacologic agents is recorded on a recorder. A steady-state equilibrium is reached in usually 10 minutes. In a normal study (B), the intracavernosal pressure (P) recorded in the upper tracing at a value of 83 mm Hg approximates the mean systemic arterial blood pressure 108/68 or 82 mm Hg and 116/72 or 87 mm Hg. The lower tracing, the circumferential girth (C) reaches maximum girth change at approximately 60 mm Hg intracavernosal pressure.

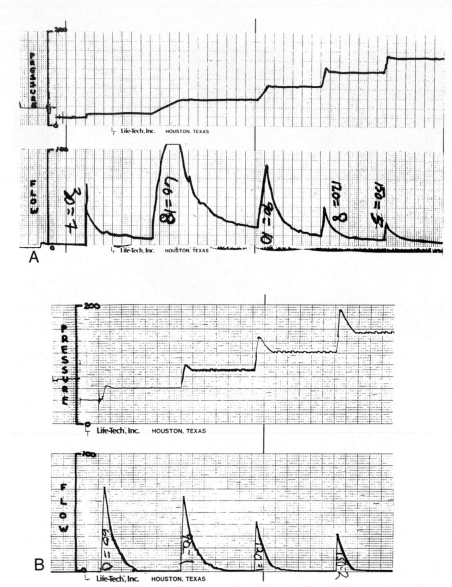

Figure 84–9. After equilibrium intracavernosal pressure is reached following vasoactive agent administration, provocative tests of corporal veno-occlusive function are performed. The flow of heparinized saline necessary to maintain various intracavernosal pressures is determined, in increasing intervals of 30 mm Hg, to a pressure of 150 mm Hg (A). If the flow-to-maintain intracavernosal pressure values at 30, 60, 90, 120, and 150 mm Hg are elevated, i.e., greater than 3 ml/min, especially if the values are not linearly related to increasing intracavernosal pressures (A), then one should consider the possibility that the results are abnormal secondary to incomplete smooth muscle relaxation. The administration of additional papaverine and phentolamine or prostaglandin E_1 should be performed. After waiting for a new steady-state equilibrium for an additional 10 minutes, the flow-to-maintain various intracavernosal pressure values should be repeated and compared with the values obtained previously (B). A linear response of flow-to-maintain various intracavernosal pressure values should be observed, implying that complete smooth muscle relaxation has been achieved.

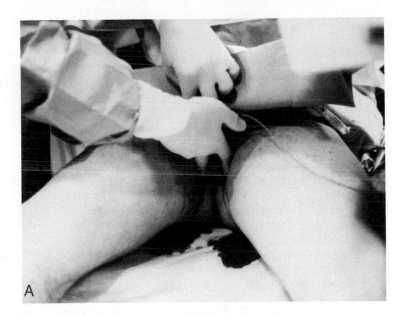

Figure 84–10. At 150 mm Hg intracavernosal pressure, the flow of heparinized saline is terminated and the fall in corporal body pressure over a 30-second period is determined. If the pressure decay is abnormal, i.e., the intracavernosal pressure falls more than 45 mm Hg over 30 seconds, the pressure decay is repeated in the presence of perineal compression *(A)* to examine if this maneuver will reduce the fall in pressure over 30 seconds *(B)*. The normalization of an abnormal pressure decay with perineal compression implies that the location of the abnormal corporal veno-occlusion is proximal and focal in the crura.

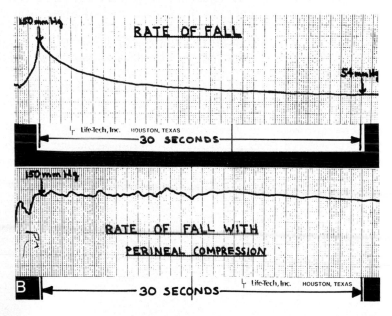

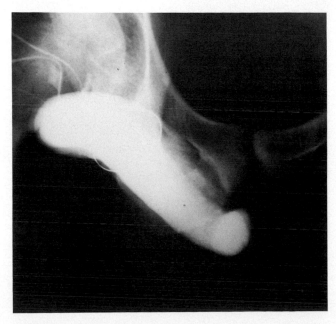

Figure 84–11. Anatomic visualization of veins draining the corporal bodies during erection by pharmacocavernosography is used to confirm the findings of cavernosometry, flow-to-maintain or pressure decay, and may provide anatomic information regarding surgical reconstruction. When normal corporal veno-occlusive function is present, minimal or absent venous drainage is demonstrated radiographically.

generalized atherosclerosis or diabetes mellitus, a diffuse pattern of draining veins is observed including the glans and corpus spongiosum and the dorsal, cavernosal, and crural veins (Fig. 84–12). In patients with Peyronie's disease, a focal pattern (pitchfork sign) demonstrating abrupt visualization of the corpus spongiosum and dorsal vein from the site of the penile curvature has been observed (Fig. 84–13A) (Gasior et al., 1990). In a patient with pelvic fracture or blunt perineal trauma, exclusive visualization of the proximal draining veins and the cavernosal and crural vein has been noted (Fig. 84–13B) (Levine et al., 1990). In a patient with impotence following a penile fracture from coitus, masturbation, or accident during erection, a site-specific leak is noted in the dorsal vein at an abrupt location along the penile shaft (Fig. 84–13C) (Penson et al., 1991).

Currently, the only absolute contraindication to pharmacocavernosometry testing is in the impotent patient who is receiving a monoamine oxidase inhibitor. With such medication there is the potential for a hypertensive crisis if intracavernosal alpha-adrenergic therapy is needed. Otherwise, minor modifications in methodology may be required when specific medical problems exist, such as a history of contrast-medium reactions, significant cardiac disease, mitral or aortic valve disease, or anticoagulant therapy.

GRAVITY PHARMACOCAVERNOSOMETRY TESTING. The same principles that apply to pump-infusion, with pressure feedback, pharmacocavernosometry also apply to gravity-based pharmacocavernosometry (Puech-Leao et al., 1990). After achieving presumed complete smooth muscle relaxation, the corpora are exposed to a volume of heparinized saline placed at a certain height above the level of the penis (Fig. 84–14). In the presence of elevated venous outflow resistance, the volume infused will be minimal. Intracavernosal pressure may also be recorded during the gravity infusion. The closer the intracavernosal pressure is to the pressure equivalent of the heparinized saline source, the better is the status of the veno-occlusive mechanism.

In our own experience studying 50 patients, recording the volume of saline infused by gravity over 20 minutes correlated well with values obtained for either flow-to-maintain pressure or pressure decay in the same patients (Levine et al., 1990a). Normal subjects in the three studies of veno-occlusive testing demonstrated volume infused over 20 minutes of less than 20 ml, flow-to-maintain pressures of 3 ml/minutes or less, and pressure decays from 150 mm Hg to less than 45 mm Hg over 30 seconds.

The advantages of gravity-based cavernosometry include the lack of expensive equipment and the safety to the patient in not needing elevated, unphysiologic intracavernosal pressures typically needed during pump-based cavernosometry.

RADIOISOTOPE MEASUREMENT OF VENOUS OUTFLOW. Nuclear medicine techniques involving ^{133}Xe have been utilized to evaluate impotence. Alternatively, ^{99m}Tc labeled autologous red blood cells have also been employed to record the efficiency of the corporal veno-occlusive mechanism. This radioisotope is the agent of choice for blood pool imaging with high tagging efficiency and virtually no diffusion out of the

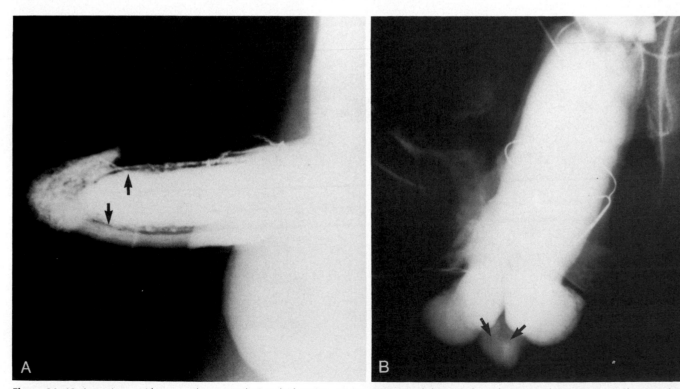

Figure 84–12. In patients with corporal veno-occlusive dysfunction, various patterns of drainage have been noted. In patients with generalized atherosclerosis or diabetes mellitus, a diffuse pattern of draining veins is observed including the glans, corpus spongiosum *(lower arrow)*, dorsal *(upper arrow)*, cavernosal, and crural veins *(A and B)*. Note in the anterior-posterior view the spongiosum *(angled arrows)* is visualized between the separated crura.

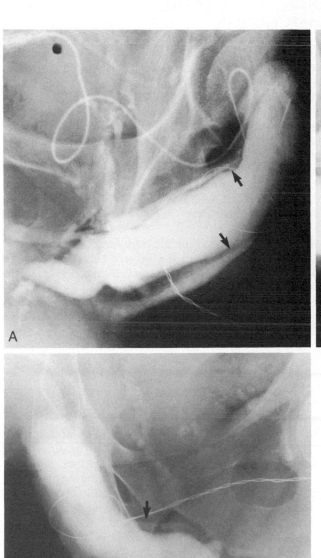

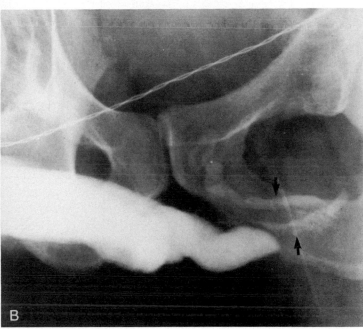

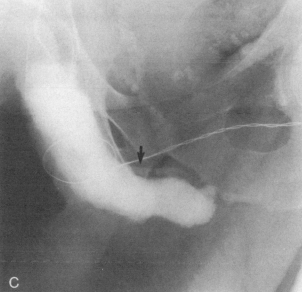

Figure 84–13. *A,* In patients with Peyronie's disease, a focal pattern (pitchfork sign) demonstrating abrupt visualization of the corpus spongiosum *(lower arrow),* and dorsal vein *(upper arrow),* from the site of the penile curvature has been observed.

B, In patients with pelvic fracture or blunt perineal trauma, exclusive visualization of the proximal draining veins, the cavernosal and crural vein *(arrows),* has been noted.

C, In a patient with impotence following a penile fracture from a coital, a masturbation, or an accidental injury during penile erection, a site-specific leak is noted in the dorsal vein at an abrupt location along the penile shaft *(arrow).*

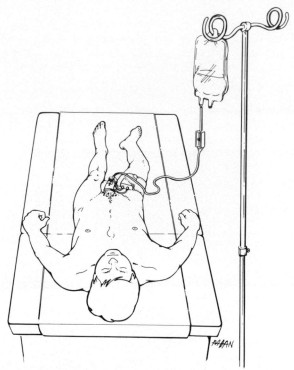

Figure 84–14. After achieving complete smooth muscle relaxation, the corpora are exposed to a volume of heparinized saline placed at a certain height above the level of the penis in gravity cavernosometry. In the presence of elevated venous outflow resistance, the volume infused will be minimal. Intracavernosal pressure may also be recorded during the gravity infusion. The closer the intracavernosal pressure is to the pressure equivalent of the heparinized saline source, the better is the status of the veno-occlusive mechanism.

intravascular space. With the patient in the supine position after pharmacologic stimulation, 0.5 mCi of Tc^{99m} labeled autologous red blood cells is injected intracavernosally. With a digital gamma-counter imaging the pelvis in the anterior view, the region of the penis is defined and a time-activity curve is performed (Groshar et al., 1990). A high disappearance of activity has been correlated with veno-occlusive dysfunction. Sampling of activity in the antecubital veins over time can be utilized to quantify the amount of corporal venous drainage.

CAVERNOUS BIOPSY. Correlations have been found between clinical impotence and structural changes in cavernous tissue (Persson et al., 1989). Histomorphometric studies of human cavernous tissue samples may be a useful tool, therefore, in selecting patients for vascular reconstructive surgery. The presence of excessive scarring or the loss of smooth muscle cells would imply a reduced chance of surgical success.

One study assessed the corporal tissue samples for volume percentage of smooth muscle and volume percentage of fibrous tissue in aging. A slight age-correlated decrease of cavernous smooth muscle tissue was noted, with a large biologic variation among individuals (Meulerman et al., 1990). In the same study, no significant differences occurred between the histomorphologic analysis in the proximal and distal portions of the penile shaft suggesting that the majority of cavernosal abnormalities are diffuse. The Biopty gun has been success-

fully utilized to obtain cavernosal tissue samples for histologic analysis (Wespes et al., 1990).

Further work needs to be done in this area, especially in the ultrastructural analysis of this cavernosal tissue and in the correlation of pathologic findings to the presence of corporal veno-occlusive dysfunction.

THERAPY OF ERECTILE DYSFUNCTION

Therapeutic options available for erectile dysfunction are discussed under two broad categories: noninvasive and invasive. Noninvasive treatments include psychologic therapy, oral and transcutaneous agents as well as vacuum erection devices. Invasive therapies include intracavernosal injections of vasoactive agents, implantation of penile prostheses, and surgical procedures directed toward the amelioration of arterial insufficiency and corporal veno-occlusive dysfunction.

Psychologic Therapy

Traditional psychodynamic approaches for treating psychogenic impotence have largely been replaced by behaviorally oriented sex therapy (Golden, 1982; Smith, 1988). Modern psychosexual therapy aims more at correcting the immediate causes of erectile dysfunction and less at treating remote underlying psychologic causes. The goals of sex therapy are primarily to decrease the performance anxiety that interferes with erectile development and to promote an adequate level of stimulation by increasing the repertoire of sexual activities that do not depend on achieving or maintaining an erection sufficient for vaginal intercourse. When repeated attempts at coitus fail, men become anxious, preoccupied with fears of failure, and apprehensive about their partner's reactions. Whenever possible, psychosexual therapy involves the sexual partners together. This approach is preferable for both evaluation and treatment. One component of this therapy is sensate focus exercises, which are designed to progressively and slowly return potency and to decrease anxiety and guilt by the couple's mutual enjoyment of noncoital activity (Masters and Johnson, 1970). When erectile function returns, the couple continues the exercises until coitus is possible.

Masters and Johnson (1970) initially reported a 70 per cent success rate in patients with impotence. Others have reported success rates of 35 to 80 per cent (LoPiccolo et al., 1986). The major problem with discussing success rates is that most patients were assumed to have psychogenic impotence and were not appropriately evaluated for organic impotence. This factor would be expected to negatively bias published results. Only a few long-term follow-up studies of sex therapy have been performed, and those available suggest a significant recurrence rate of impotence with time after sex therapy (Hengeveld, 1983). This type of therapy is also utilized in the treatment of premature ejaculation. In such a case, relaxation exercises serve to desensitize the patient.

Factors that reduce the likelihood of success using this therapy include long-term erectile dysfunction, older age, diminished libido, and significant mental disorders (Cooper, 1981). The role of the psychotherapist in treating such patients is not confined to psychogenic impotence. Some impotent men, receiving medical or surgical treatment for organic impotence, should also receive psychologic counseling before and after such treatment to reduce anxiety, sexual inhibition, and relationship conflict.

Nonhormonal Medical Therapies

The understanding of the neurologic and vascular mechanisms concerned with creating and maintaining an erection has lead to a greater interest in medical therapies for this disorder. Although much activity has been generated in this area, little in the way of viable treatment options has been forthcoming. The most widely used oral medication has been yohimbine hydrochloride, an alpha$_2$-adrenergic blocking agent. Yohimbine has long been considered an aphrodisiac. Its positive effect on erectile dysfunction was first published by Margolis and co-workers in 1971. In a prospective, double-blind, placebo-controlled study in patients with predominantly organic disease, yohimbine did not show a statistically significant response rate over placebo control. However, 21 per cent of patients did receive a complete response when given yohimbine (Morales et al., 1987). A similarly designed study performed in patients with psychogenic impotence demonstrated that yohimbine provided a statistically significant response rate (31 per cent) over the placebo control rate (5.3 per cent) (Morales et al., 1988).

Attempts at neuropharmacologic therapy of erectile dysfunction have largely involved dopaminergic and serotoninergic agonists (Foreman et al., 1990). The positive erectile effects of dopaminergic agonists was first noted in patients treated with L-dopa (Brown et al., 1978). In addition, subcutaneously administered apomorphine, a dopaminergic agonist, has been shown to enhance erectile responses in men. Laboratory investigations in rats and monkeys have corroborated this observation (Gower et al., 1984). A further study has shown that a dopaminergic compound that mimics the action of apomorphine and lengthens the duration of clinical response (methylenedioxy-N-propylnoraporphrine) was found to induce penile erections when given orally in the rat model (Heaton et al., 1990).

Trazodone, a drug administered clinically for depression, has been reported to be associated with priapism (Scher et al., 1983). Metachlorophenylpiperazine, a serotoninergic agonist and metabolite of trazodone, has been shown to induce erections in rats and monkeys (Szele et al., 1988). A case report showing the beneficial qualities of trazodone in the treatment of organic erectile dysfunction has been published (Lal et al., 1990). A later study in which six potent subjects were treated with oral trazodone, trimiprimine (a tricyclic antidepressant), and placebo demonstrated a statistically significant increase in nocturnal erectile activity with tra-

zodone compared with the other two agents (Saenz de Tejada et al., 1991). In vitro studies suggest that the potential mechanism for prolonging erectile activity is blockade of sympathetic mediated–detumescence (Azadzoi et al., 1990). Further clinical trials in impotent patients are required.

Nitroglycerin, a smooth muscle relaxant, has been employed widely in paste form for transcutaneous delivery in the treatment of angina. It has also been provided in a similar manner for the treatment of impotence (Claes et al., 1989). In a study of 30 patients, 1 cm of nitroglycerin paste or placebo paste was placed on the penis and the patients were then shown VSS. The group receiving nitroglycerin paste developed erections of better quality than those receiving placebo paste (Morales et al., 1988 and 1990). This study is obviously limited and was performed in a clinical laboratory. Further clinical testing does, however, appear warranted.

Hormonal Therapy

Hormonal therapies for impotence should be reserved only for patients with hypogonadal disorders or hyperprolactinemia. In patients with hypogonadal disorders (hypogonadotropic hypogonadism and hypergonadotropic hypogonadism), testosterone replacement is employed to maintain normal serum levels and thereby restore potency and libido. Because of the relatively unpredictable serum levels obtained by oral administration of testosterone preparations, we generally administer testosterone enanthate intramuscularly in doses of 200 to 300 mg, every 2 to 3 weeks (Snyder et al., 1980). The amount and frequency of administration will vary with the individual and can be titrated. One should not treat with testosterone preparations solely on the basis of a single low serum testosterone level. Testosterone may induce a marked increase in libido without a positive effect on erectile capabilities in patients not suffering from hypogonadal disorders. Oral preparations may also have hepatotoxic effects and may produce abnormalities of serum lipid levels (Wilson and Griffin, 1982). Many impotent patients are older men who may have adenocarcinoma of the prostate. Testosterone in these individuals may increase the rate of growth of the prostatic adenocarcinoma. Two patients in whom clinical adenocarcinomas of the prostate developed following normal prostatic rectal examinations prior to testosterone therapy have been reported (Jackson et al., 1989). Before beginning testosterone replacement therapy in men over the age of 50, serum prostate-specific antigen levels and possibly transrectal ultrasound studies should be performed. For all of the aforementioned reasons, it should become apparent that the indiscriminate administration of testosterone in impotent men should be avoided.

The treatment of hyperprolactinemia is cessation of medication causing hyperprolactinemia (e.g., estrogens, alpha methyldopa), administration of bromocriptine, or surgical ablation or extirpation of a pituitary prolactin-secreting tumor (Carter et al., 1978; Franks et al., 1978). Treatment with exogenous testosterone to restore the diminished levels of serum testosterone usually seen with this disorder does not appear to reverse the erectile dysfunction.

Vacuum Constrictor Devices

A variety of external penile appliances have been chosen for the management of impotence for many years (Nadig, 1990). Although many different devices are now manufactured, the majority have three common components: a vacuum chamber, a vacuum pump that creates negative pressure within the chamber, and a constrictor or tension band that is applied to the base of the penis after erection is achieved (Fig. 84–15). The patient while standing places his penis within a preformed suitably sized chamber that is attached to a pump mechanism able to achieve negative pressure within the chamber. Prior to pump activation and creation of a vacuum, a correct airtight fit of the chamber is required. When the vacuum pump is activated, a vacuum or negative pressure is created within the chamber

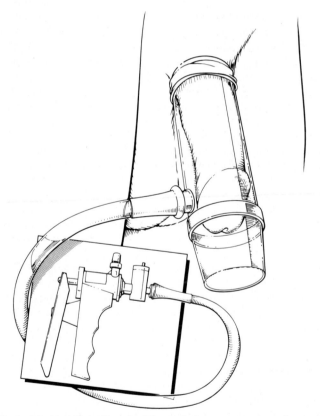

Figure 84–15. Although many different devices are now manufactured, the majority have three common components: a vacuum chamber, a vacuum pump that creates negative pressure within the chamber, and a constrictor or tension band that is applied to the base of the penis after erection is achieved. The patient while standing places his penis within a preformed suitably sized chamber, which is attached to a pump mechanism able to achieve negative pressure within the chamber. Prior to pump activation and creation of a vacuum, a correct airtight fit of the chamber is required. When the vacuum pump is activated, a vacuum or negative pressure is created within the chamber, thereby drawing blood into the penis to produce an erection-like state. At the point of achieving adequate tumescence and rigidity, a constrictor band at the base of the chamber is transferred to the base of the penis, thereby "trapping" blood within the penis.

thereby drawing blood into the penis to produce an erection-like state. This effect usually requires 5 to 7 minutes of pump activation. At the point of achieving adequate tumescence and rigidity, a constrictor band at the base of the chamber is transferred to the base of the penis thereby "trapping" blood within the penis (Witherington, 1990).

A vacuum-induced erection is significantly different from a physiologically induced erection. The second type is achieved by the initial relaxation of the corporal smooth musculature, thus allowing for engorgement of blood into the lacunar spaces. In the case of a vacuum-induced erection, corporal smooth muscle relaxation does not occur initially and blood is simply trapped in both the intra-corporal and extracorporeal compartments of the penis. Distal to the constricting band that is placed at the base of the penis, one sees venous stasis and decreased arterial inflow, which may result in penile distention, edema, and cyanosis if the device is used for too long. In most cases, manufacturers recommend that the vacuum-induced erection be maintained for less than 30 minutes. A physiologically induced erection will cause rigidity along the entire length of the corpora in contradistinction to a vacuum-induced erection, which only causes rigidity distal to the constricting band allowing for the penis to pivot at its base.

In monkeys, increases in cross-sectional corporal area secondary to vacuum-induced erections were found to be only 50 per cent of cross-sectional area changes induced by intracavernosal papaverine (Diederichs et al., 1989). This finding may be secondary to the continued smooth muscle contraction of the corpora limiting corporal expansion. In humans, vacuum constrictive devices may induce a penile diameter equal to or greater than that attained during a physiologically induced erection, presumably secondary to blood trapped in extracorporeal tissues (Nadig et al., 1986). In addition, cavernosography before and after application of a vacuum constrictor device demonstrated the disappearance of blood from the previously opacified glans penis, corpus spongiosum, and dorsal vein. Venous drainage from the corpora proximal to the constrictor device was not altered (Wespes et al., 1990).

Theoretically, the vacuum constrictor devices should create penile rigidity sufficient for vaginal penetration in almost all impotent men who are so treated. Patients with significant intracorporeal scarring, however, such as those with severe Peyronie's disease, postpriapism, or previously infected penile implants, may not be able to develop an adequate rigidity. Men who have penile prostheses explanted may still be successfully treated with a vacuum constrictor device (Moul and McLeod, 1989). Theoretically, a more physiologic erection may result from vacuum constrictor devices when used in conjunction with intracavernosal vasoactive agents capable of relaxing corporal smooth musculature. A patient who does not obtain sufficient penile rigidity from intracavernosal pharmacotherapy alone could be a candidate for a vacuum constrictor device, while continuing self-injection therapy.

To date, the complications from the utilization of these devices have been minor and self-limited (Witherington, 1988, 1989, and 1990). They have included difficulty with ejaculation, penile pain, ecchymoses, hematomas, and petechiae. Patients taking aspirin or coumadin are more likely to develop vascular complications. Many of the devices manufactured have a valve that limits the vacuum pressure (< 250 mm Hg), which might aid in decreasing the complication rate.

Patient acceptance and satisfaction with vacuum constrictive devices have been reported to range from 68 to 83 per cent (Nadig, 1990). The reasons for discontinuing this treatment have included premature loss of penile tumescence and rigidity, penile pain, pain during ejaculation, and inconvenience (Sidi et al., 1990).

Vacuum constrictive devices are a viable therapeutic option for patients with erectile dysfunction by virtue of their lack of significant complications and their high degree of acceptance in patients who elect this therapy.

Intracavernosal Injection of Vasoactive Agents

One of the most important advances in the treatment of impotence over the past decade has been self-administered intracavernosal injection of vasoactive agents. As mentioned elsewhere in this text, the neurophysiologic mechanism required to initiate an erection is neurotransmitter-induced relaxation of the corporal smooth musculature. Vasoactive agents that have been administered by intracavernosal injection either directly relax the corporal smooth musculature or block the adrenergic tone (Jünemann et al., 1986).

The pioneering work in this area involved papaverine hydrochloride, a direct smooth muscle relaxant (Virag, 1982a), or phenoxybenzamine (Brindley, 1986) or phentolamine mesylate (Zorgniotti et al., 1985), both alpha blocking agents. As the use of these agents became more clinically widespread, several issues became apparent. Intracavernosal injection of phentolamine alone was not as effective as papaverine in producing an erection. In addition, papaverine alone was not as effective as the combination of papaverine and phentolamine when injected together. Later, the synthetic prostaglandin E_1, a direct smooth muscle relaxant, has been successful when injected intracavernosally to restore potency (Stackl et al., 1988). A variety of solutions containing these agents are currently being employed in clinical practice as papaverine alone, papaverine and phentolamine, prostaglandin E_1 alone, phentolamine and prostaglandin E_1, or a mixture of all three (Lee et al., 1989). The mechanism of action of papaverine hydrochloride and prostaglandin E_1 is direct smooth muscle relaxation. Therefore, when injected intracavernosally, they will maximize arterial inflow as well as corporal veno-occlusion by relaxation of both arterial and trabecular smooth musculature. Phentolamine, however, blocks adrenergically induced muscle tone and therefore does not alone initiate erections (Azadzoi et al., 1990).

Patients with normal arterial inflow and normal corporal veno-occlusion mechanism will be those in whom intracavernosal injections will work the best. These would include patients with purely neurogenic impotence (Wyndaele et al., 1986) or those with psychogenic impotence (Kiely et al., 1987). Patients with arterial insufficiency may also respond by virtue of the long-acting nature of the smooth muscle relaxation that is being provided (Buvat et al., 1986). Patients with significant corporal veno-occlusive dysfunction, however, would be the least likely to respond to this form of therapy. In general, we offer intracavernosal pharmacotherapy to most of our patients with organic dysfunction. Those with poor manual dexterity, poor visual acuity, or morbid obesity, or those in whom a transient hypotensive episode may have a deleterious effect (e.g., unstable cardiovascular disease and transient ischemic attacks) should be carefully considered prior to being offered this therapeutic option (Padma-Nathan et al., 1987b). We have successfully treated patients with this therapy who are concomitantly taking aspirin or coumadin. Patients with significant psychiatric disease or potential for misuse or abuse of this therapy should be excluded from treatment. Once offered intracavernosal pharmacotherapy, the patient should be informed of its risks and complications (see subsequent discussion). He should also be told that this form of therapy will not affect orgasm or ejaculation and is solely for restoration of erectile capabilities. The usual therapeutic goal is to create a rigid enough erection satisfactory for vaginal penetration that lasts between 30 minutes and 1 hour.

Patients who enter a pharmacologic erection program should be asked first to read and sign a detailed informed consent, which states the known complications of this treatment and discusses the possibility of long-term side effects. Initially, the objective of the dosage determination phase is to define the lowest dose required for achieving an appropriate erectile response. Patients are injected initially with low doses, which are increased incrementally. In patients with purely neurogenic impotence, one would begin with an extremely low dose—as they are most likely to respond. Patients with vascular disease will usually begin the dosage determination phase with a higher dose and subsequently higher increments in dose. An insulin syringe with a 27- to 30-gauge needle is usually employed, which minimizes pain and bleeding. Patients are also taught to compress the site of injection for 3 minutes following therapy. The vasoactive solutions currently recommended at our institution are included in Table 84–4.

After an appropriate dose has been determined, the patient is instructed in the proper injection techniques by reviewing printed material showing him the site and the technique, followed by nurse- or physician-monitored self-injection (Fig. 84–16) (Sidi, 1988; Sidi and Chen, 1987). It is very common that dosages determined in the physician's office will be decreased by the patient at home because he will be in a more sexually stimulating environment. The patient is also instructed in sterile technique. Patients are told not to inject more frequently than once per day.

The follow-up of approximately 4,000 patients treated worldwide with papaverine alone or in combination with phentolamine has been published (Zentgraf et al., 1988). Reported side effects have included hematomas, burning pain after injection, urethral damage, cavernositis or

Table 84–4. VASOACTIVE DRUGS IN INTRACAVERNOSAL INJECTIONS

Vasoactive drugs	Drug mg (μg)/ml	Amount of drug in ampule (ml)	Amount of drug in ampule (mg(μg))	Amount of drug in ampule (mg(μg)/ml)	Amount of drug (0.2 ml mg (μg))
Papaverine	30	10	300	30	6
Papaverine	30	9	270	22.5	4.5
Phentolamine	5	3	15	1.25	0.25
(Normal saline)		3			
Prostaglandin E₁	500	1	500	20	4
(Normal saline)		24			
Papaverine	30	9	270	24.11	4.82
Phentolamine	5	2	10	0.89	0.18
Prostaglandin E₁	500	0.2	100	8.93	1.79

local infections, fibrotic changes of the corpora cavernosa, curvature, and prolonged erections or priapism. Cavernositis or infection due to injections has been an extremely rare event. Burning pain at the time of injection has been seen most commonly with prostaglandin E_1 (Waldhauser and Schramek, 1988) and appears to be less of a problem when prostaglandin E_1 is mixed with other agents. Hematomas were noted in a small percentage of patients undergoing autoinjection therapy and usually resolve within a few days without any permanent sequelae.

The two most important complications are prolonged erections and localized fibrotic changes of the corpora cavernosum. Prolonged erections are usually encountered during the dosage determination phase and have been reported in 2.3 to 15 per cent of patients treated (Zentgraf et al., 1988). Patients must be cautioned to call their physician if an erection persists for 4 hours or longer. The majority of these prolonged erections will detumesce on their own; however, some require an intracavernosal injection of an alpha agonist to produce

detumescence (Padma-Nathan et al., 1986). Alpha agonists that have been utilized for this purpose include epinephrine, phenylephrine, and metaraminol (Trapp, 1987). At present, we administer an initial intracavernosal injection of 200 μg of phenylephrine. This may be repeated as necessary until detumescence. Following the dosage determination phase, the complication of prolonged erection is quite rare and is seen in less than 1 per cent of injections. If treated by the protocol presented here, should not see any permanent sequelae from this side effect.

The most distressing side effect of intracavernosal pharmacologic therapy is the formation of painless fibrotic nodules within the corpora cavernosa, which at times leads to penile curvature. This problem has been reported in 1.5 to 60 per cent of patients treated for 1 year (Levine et al., 1989; Padma-Nathan et al., 1987). In one series, the development of fibrotic nodules was related to the frequency of injection and the duration of treatment (Levine et al., 1989). It appears that fibrosis is not related to the pH of the solution injected. The

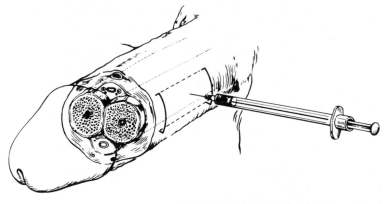

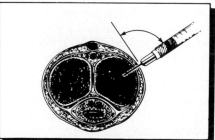

Figure 84–16. The objective of the dosage determination phase of the pharmacologic erection program is to define the lowest dose required for achieving an appropriate erectile response. Patients are injected initially with low doses, which are increased incrementally. An insulin syringe with a 27- to 30-gauge needle is usually employed, which minimizes pain and bleeding. Patients are also taught to compress the site of injection, typically the proximal lateral aspect of the penile shaft, for 3 minutes following therapy. Patients are told not to inject more frequently than once per day.

complications of corporal fibrosis and prolonged erections have been experienced less often when prostaglandin E_1 alone has been utilized (Schramek et al., 1989 and 1990). It is our thinking that to some extent cavernosal fibrotic nodules are secondary to trauma and bleeding within the corpus. To that end, we stress compression over the injection site for 3 minutes and attempt to decrease the amount of fluid injected when possible. We would like most patients to inject less than 0.5 ml of fluid. In patients who are injecting 1 ml or more of the papaverine and phentolamine mixture, we have found that this volume can be decreased by the addition of prostaglandin E_1 (Goldstein et al., 1990). Several cases have been reported of diffuse fibrosis of the corpora following intracorporal injections, almost invariably associated with markedly prolonged erections. A case of diffuse fibrosis, following a test dose of intracavernosal papaverine leading to a prolonged erection of greater than 36 hours, has been reported in which the patient was still able to be successfully treated intracavernosally with a combination of papaverine and phentolamine (Lakin et al., 1988). Therefore, the degree of corporal scarring and fibrosis required to obviate the positive results of intracavernosal pharmacotherapy has not been determined.

We have treated a small group of psychogenically impotent patients with intracavernosal pharmacotherapy in conjunction with sex therapy. This practice has been reported elsewhere with good results (Dhabuwala et al., 1990). The patients must fully understand the undesired side effects of this therapy, especially the potential for the formation of fibrotic nodules within the corpora.

Systemic side effects of this treatment have included vasovagal episodes and syncope, probably related to hypotension. These side effects remain infrequent and are usually seen during the dosage determination phase. It would be expected that patients with significant corporal veno-occlusive dysfunction will exhibit an increase in systemic absorption of intracavernosal agents and therefore be more susceptible to this side effect. As previously mentioned, patients in whom transient hypotensive episodes may be significantly deleterious should be carefully evaluated before this therapy is begun. Intracavernosal pharmacotherapy with papaverine has been associated with hepatotoxicity. During a mean follow-up of 26 months, we have reported only three cases of abnormal liver function test results in the first 201 patients that we treated (1.5 per cent) (Padma-Nathan and Goldstein, 1987b). Others have essentially observed no changes in liver function. However, in one series it has been reported that 40 per cent of patients have at least one chemical abnormality in liver function following this therapy (Levine et al., 1989).

Cavernosal injection of vasoactive agents has clearly been one of the most important contributions to the urologist's armamentarium in treating the patient with erectile dysfunction. The relative lack of side effects and the simplicity of delivery have made this therapy well accepted worldwide. In our institution, a mixture of papaverine, phentolamine, and prostaglandin E_1 is now administered initially in the majority of patients. In the future, two potential alterations in drug delivery deserve investigation. First, a prosthetic implant consisting of a subcutaneous pump/reservoir mechanism connected to a tube going directly into the corpora cavernosa, which could deliver a predetermined dosage without repetitive injections, has been proposed and is undergoing investigation (Turini et al., 1988). Second, the ability to deliver drugs into the corpora without injection by transcutaneous means or by iontophoresis has not been successful heretofore. However, one might envision an iontophoretic system that has the ability to deliver drugs transcutaneously and directly into the corporal tissue (Vaccari et al., 1990).

Penile Prosthesis

In the early 1970s, the urologic subspeciality of erectile dysfunction followed the introduction of an intracorporeal penile prosthesis. Credit must be given to Small and Carrion (1975) as well as to Bradley, Scott, and Timm (1973) for introducing these functional prosthetic devices based on the principle of intracorporeal surgical placement. It was the availability of such devices that made it necessary for urologists to evaluate patients with erectile dysfunction in order to determine etiology (i.e., psychogenic versus organic). Through the 1970s and early 1980s, the development of penile prostheses proceeded along distinct lines: the malleable or rigid prosthesis and the multicomponent inflatable prosthesis (Figs. 84–17 and 84–18A). A mechanical device (Omniphase prosthesis) was later introduced as well as a self-contained inflatable device. Lastly, modifications of the three-piece inflatable device have lead to the introduction of a two-piece inflatable device. The currently available penile prostheses are listed in Table 84–5.

It is not within the scope of this chapter to critique these prostheses. The discussion is of generic prostheses. Where applicable, differences among malleable, mechanical, and inflatable devices are mentioned. Initially, the malleable devices were shown to have relatively low postoperative complication rates accompanied by a relative simplicity of implantation. Component failure and reoperation rate were therefore kept to a minimum. The length and girth of the penis did not change in the

Table 84–5. PENILE PROSTHESES

Malleable devices
  Small-Carrion
  Jonas
  AMS 600
  Mentor Acu-form
  Flexirod
  Duraphase
Mechanical devices
  Omniphase
Inflatable devices
  3-piece—AMS 700 CX, Mentor Alpha-1
  2-piece—Uniflate 1000, Mentor Mark II GFS resipump
Self-contained
  Flexiflate
  Flexiflate 2
  Hydroflex
  Dynaflex

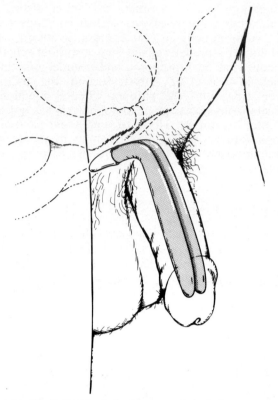

Figure 84–17. Malleable devices have a relatively low postoperative complication rate accompanied by a relative ease of implantation. The length and girth of the penis do not change in the "tumescent" and "detumescent" phases.

combine the relative lack of component failure and simplicity of implantation with a more physiologically appearing detumescent phase. Self-contained inflatable devices, such as the Flexiflate and Hydroflex, were introduced to preserve the aesthetic qualities of an inflatable device and to combine them with simplicity of surgical implantation and potential decrease in component failure. Further simplicity in the implantation of an inflatable device was attained with the introduction of the two-piece inflatable devices, the Uniflate 1000 and Mentor Mark II. Lastly, improvements in semirigid rod prostheses have led to greater malleability, particularly with the introduction of the Duraphase prosthesis (Petrou et al., 1990) and the Mentor Acu-form.

Second- and third-generation prostheses have attempted to improve aesthetic results, at times provide greater girth, decrease likelihood of component failure, and if possible increase simplicity of implantation. As previously mentioned, this discussion is of generic penile prosthesis, focusing on the areas of patient selection, device selection, operative techniques, and complications.

Initially, penile implants were offered to all patients with organic impotence. In addition, patients with psychogenic impotence who failed appropriate psychologic and/or psychiatric therapy were also candidates for prosthetic surgery. Prostheses have also been used in paraplegics and quadriplegics to add bulk to the penis in order to support an external drainage device. With the advent of newer treatments, such as intracavernosal pharmacotherapy, vacuum erection devices, and vascular surgical procedures, implantation of penile prosthesis has become in the opinion of many physicians as well as patients the last treatment option to be considered after attempting therapy with other modalities. In our practice, patients with organic impotence who are not candidates for a vascular procedure are offered self-injection with vasoactive agents and vacuum constrictor devices initially. If they do not choose one of these options or if these options do not result in an appropriate erectile response, they are considered for prosthetic surgery. It is also our belief that patients who are thought to have psychogenic impotence and who have failed appropriate psychologic or behavioral sex therapy and who have no psychologic contraindications should be treated in the same manner. Certainly, the appropriate counseling of patients before the implantation of a prosthesis is essential to the success of this surgery.

"tumescent" and "detumescent" phases, which at times lead to an aesthetically less desirable detumescent phase. In contradistinction to the malleable device, the inflatable devices were based on hydraulic principles, thus allowing the patient to inflate and deflate his device to simulate tumescent and nontumescent phases. This ability provided an improved aesthetic result, especially in the "detumescent" phase but was initially coupled with a relative increase in component failure and reoperation. Again, in contradistinction to the malleable device, activation of the multicomponent inflatable device allowed for an increase in penile girth during the tumescent phase. Subsequent improvements of inflatable devices have markedly reduced the likelihood of reoperation and component failure. Introduction of a mechanical device, the Omniphase prosthesis, sought to

Figure 84–18. Inflatable devices are based on hydraulic principles, thus allowing the patient to inflate and deflate his device to simulate tumescent and nontumescent phases. *A,* The multicomponent inflatable device allows for an increase in penile girth during the "tumescent" phase.

B, At present, our approach for all prostheses is a transverse scrotal incision. This is simply defined using a Scott retractor as shown. The advantages of this incision are that the entire length of the tunica albuginea from the glans to the crus can be exposed, the pump can be placed directly into a dartos pouch in the scrotum, and there is no scar on the penile shaft.

C, The incision is carried down through subcutaneous tissues until the plane between the corpus cavernosum (CC) and the corpus spongiosum (CS) is identified.

D, Following the exposure of the tunica albuginea, stay sutures are placed in both corpora and vertical corporotomies are performed. In this particular example, the central structure in the corporotomy is the cavernosal artery.

E, The corporal spongy tissue is then visualized, and a plane is created and dilated (with Hegar dilators, straight sounds, or a Dilamezinsert) between this tissue and the overlying tunica albuginea along the entire length of each corpus. The Dilamezinsert is shown dilating the proximal crus. Total corporal length is measured, and an appropriately sized device with appropriately sized components is selected.

F, When implanting paired malleable devices, each device is initially placed into the proximal corpus and then inserted distally. In the case of paired inflatable devices, the Dilamezinsert or Furlow passer is required to bring the device to the distal end of each corpus. A Mentor Alpha-1 is being passed into the distal corporal body. Care is taken to have the device avoid touching the surface of the patient's skin during insertion to help prevent infection. During the entire procedure copious amounts of antibiotic irrigation are applied throughout the operative field. After the device is in place and the surgeon has determined that it is neither too long nor too short, the corporotomies are closed with a continuous suture.

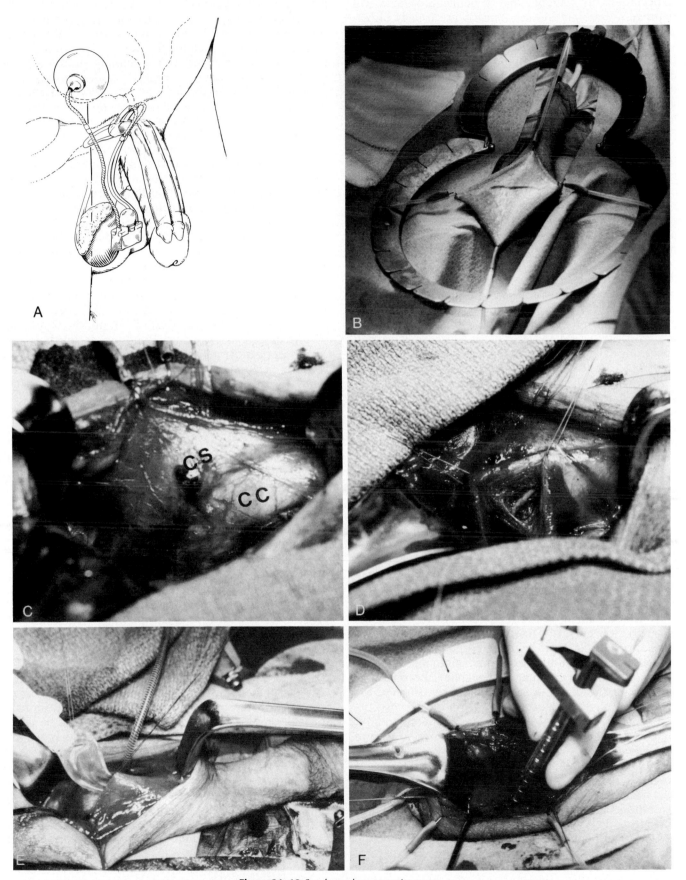

Figure 84–18 *See legend on opposite page*

Expectations by patients that a penile prosthesis will improve a deteriorating relationship are usually unreasonable. The purpose of the prosthesis is only to simulate an erection by providing penile rigidity sufficient for intercourse. The ability to ejaculate and have an orgasm is not altered by the implantation of a prosthesis, but in some cases may be restored. In addition, patients undergoing the surgery should be informed of the potential complications of prosthetic surgery as well as their frequencies and sequelae.

In discussing surgical technique, we divide prostheses into paired devices, simply requiring implantation into both corpora, and multicomponent devices, requiring corporal implantations and implantation of a pump and reservoir. Incisions for this prosthetic surgery have been perineal, penoscrotal, suprapubic, and penile. A perineal approach was the first chosen in the implantation of a noninflatable prosthesis but has essentially been replaced by other incisions (Small and Carrion, 1975). Penile incisions can only be utilized for paired devices, and a distal penile incision is required for the implantation of an Omniphase prosthesis (Krane, 1988). At present, our approach for all prostheses is a transverse scrotal incision (Fig. 84–18B). The incision is carried down through subcutaneous tissues until the urethra is identified (Fig. 84–18C). The soft tissue overlying both corpora is sharply dissected to expose both tunica albuginea. Through a transverse scrotal incision, the entire length of the tunica albuginea from the glans to the crus can be exposed. This is particularly important when one is performing reoperative surgery. Following the exposure of the tunica albuginea, stay sutures are placed in both corpora and vertical corporotomies are performed (Fig. 84–18D). The corporal spongy tissue is visualized, and a plane is created and dilated with Hegar dilators, straight sounds, or a Dilamezinsert between this tissue and the overlying tunica albuginea, along the entire length of each corpus (Fig. 84–18E). Total corporal length is measured, and an appropriately sized device with appropriately sized components is selected. When implanting paired malleable devices, each one is initially placed into the proximal corpus and then inserted distally. In the case of paired inflatable devices, the Dilamezinsert or Furlow passer is required to bring the device to the distal end of each corpus (Fig. 84–18F). During the entire procedure, copious amounts of antibiotic irrigation are applied throughout the operative field. After the device is in place and the surgeon has determined that it is neither too long nor too short, the corporotomies are closed with a continuous suture. Hemostasis is achieved, and a standard wound closure is accomplished.

Implantation of a multicomponent inflatable device proceeds along the same previously described steps. After inflatable cylinders are within each corpus, implantation of other components is carried out. When implanting devices that have a separate reservoir, blunt dissection through the scrotal incision to the external inguinal ring is carried out. At this point, the space of Retzius can usually be entered by pushing through the medial aspect of the external ring. On occasion, blind sharp dissection is required. The bladder must be empty prior to this maneuver. The reservoir can then be implanted manually through this aperture. The pump or pump/reservoir is placed in the scrotum. We prefer creating a dartos pouch for the pump or pump/reservoir and suturing it in place with a running suture. At this point in the procedure, tubing from the various components must be connected and the device tested. Copious amounts of antibiotic solution should be used to irrigate at all stages of the procedure. After hemostasis is achieved, wound closure is carried out. We prefer a Jackson-Pratt drain overnight after inflatable prosthesis implantation and have found that postoperative scrotal swelling and edema have been markedly reduced with this technique. It is not within the scope of this chapter to present in detail the nuances of surgical techniques required for the variety of prostheses that are available to the urologist. Whatever device is placed, attention to hemostasis, lack of unnecessary dissection, and copious antibiotic irrigation are essential.

In complicated prosthetic insertion, such as that following priapism, infection, or previously removed devices, our approach is to expose as much of each corpus as possible. Usually, one will find an inordinate amount of intracavernosal scarring. Exposing as much of the corpus as possible will obviate in most cases inadvertent corporal perforation during dilatation or sharp intracavernosal dissection. In some cases, corporal reconstruction with an overlying Gore-Tex graft is necessary.

Several complications that may occur during the placement of a device include corporal perforation either distally or proximally and inability to seat the device distally, resulting in an SST deformity. Distal corporal perforation occurs into the distal urethra. This problem will usually be obvious during the procedure by seeing either blood at the urethral meatus or the dilator itself protrude out the meatus. In this situation, placement of an ipsilateral cylinder should be aborted and the contralateral cylinder alone should be placed. The patient should then have an indwelling urethral catheter for 7 days. At least 3 months after the procedure, the ipsilateral cylinder can be implanted. One may perforate through the proximal end of the corpus (crus) or into the contralateral corpus. Perforation into the contralateral corpus is usually handled by redirecting the dilator to the appropriate ipsilateral space and proceeding with the surgery. Crural perforation is treated by creating a Gore-Tex sleeve around the proximal part of the ipsilateral cylinder and suturing this sleeve to the tunica albuginea in the area of the corporotomy with nonabsorbable sutures (Mulcahy, 1987). Care should be taken to create the sleeve so that cylinders are of equal length. In our experience, closure of perforations in the area of the crus has usually resulted in reperforation and proximal migration. The SST deformity may be produced when there is improper seating of the distal end of the prosthesis into the distal end of the corpus. This deformity may be secondary to inadequate sizing or inadequate distal corporal dilation or to distal corpora that do not protrude into the glans penis.

The postoperative complications of penile implant surgery are usually relegated to those of component failure, postoperative infection, or device erosion. Probably the most significant complication of prosthetic surgery is infection. The best defense against infection is prophylaxis. As previously mentioned, copious irrigation of antibiotic solutions throughout the procedure is required. In addition, our patients all scrub their genitalia and perineum for 10 minutes each day for 7 days with Hibiclens soap prior to implantation. Patients are treated with perioperative intravenous antibiotics. A 5-minute intraoperative scrub by the surgeon is used, and care is taken to avoid unnecessary traffic within the operating room. The device remains in an antibiotic solution and does not touch other parts of the operative field until the moment of implantation. By paying specific attention to the details described here, we have reduced the infection rate below 2 per cent in the last 80 penile implantations.

The incidence of infection following penile prosthetic surgery has varied between 1 and 9 per cent (Carson, 1989). Following implantation, the time until an infection develops will vary, depending on the organism involved. Infections with more virulent and aggressive bacteria usually occur within the first few postoperative days with fever, pain, and swelling overlying the prosthesis accompanied by purulent wound drainage. A group of patients, however, will complain of prolonged pain overlying the device without any obvious purulent drainage from the wound. Prolonged pain, fixation of the pump or tubing to the overlying scrotal skin, and elevated white blood cell count and sedimentation rate may all contribute to the diagnosis of a possible infection by less virulent organisms. When infection of this type is highly suspected, wound exploration is mandatory. At the time of exploration, if no obvious purulence is demonstrated, Gram's stain of the fluid surrounding the prosthesis should be made. Obviously, if no apparent infection is seen, the wound may be closed without further therapy.

When infection of a prosthesis is diagnosed, it has been our approach to remove the entire prosthesis and reimplant another prosthesis several months later. During this procedure after the prosthesis is removed, the area is copiously irrigated with antibiotic solution and if required drains are placed. Removal of an infected penile prosthesis will usually lead to secondary corporal fibrosis, decreased penile size, and a more difficult operation to place the next prosthesis. Therefore, two attempts at prosthesis salvage have been proposed. The first procedure involves removing the infected prosthesis and leaving the Jackson-Pratt drains in contact with all parts of the wound. The wound is closed, and the drains are irrigated every 8 hours for several days with antibiotic solution. At that time, culture reports from the original procedure are compared with the antibiotic solution used. If organisms are sensitive to antibiotics in the irrigation solution, a new prosthesis is reinserted. If that is not the case, appropriate antibiotics are substituted for another 2 days of irrigation before prosthesis reinsertion (Mulcahy, 1990). The second approach that may be considered is immediate salvage. All parts of the infected prosthesis are removed, the wound is copiously irrigated with antibiotic solution, and insertion of a new prosthesis is accomplished (Fishman et al.,

1987). It is very important with all of these approaches never to leave behind any part of the infected prosthesis. Immediate salvage or rescue has been successful in approximately 85 per cent of those cases published (Fishman et al., 1987). The purposes of salvage procedures are to maintain penile length and obviate the need for a particularly difficult prosthetic reimplantation. Before undergoing a salvage procedure, the patient should understand the possibility that his second implant may have to be removed.

Although erosion of a component of a prosthesis may or may not be associated with infection, it has been our approach to treat this erosion in the same manner as that of an infected prosthesis. Therefore, we remove the entire prosthesis and copiously irrigate all areas of the wound with antibiotic solution prior to closure. Others have reported good results with removal of the eroded component and repositioning of a new component (Furlow et al., 1987). This practice is particularly applicable to an eroded pump or eroded reservoir but not to an eroded cylinder. In our experience, distal erosion of a prosthesis is most usually seen in patients with decreased distal sensation, such as paraplegics, quadriplegics, and diabetics. In addition, we have observed this complication in patients who have received previous pelvic irradiation and patients who are immunosuppressed.

The reoperative rate for penile prosthetic surgery has been reported to be between 14 and 44 per cent (Kessler, 1980), with newer series showing a decreased rate (Furlow et al., 1988). Patient and physician acceptance of penile prostheses has virtually become worldwide, with over 90 per cent of patients reporting satisfaction after surgery (Malloy et al., 1986).

Vascular Surgery

ARTERIAL PROCEDURES. The aim of arterial reconstructive surgery for impotence is to increase blood flow to the penis by the bypassing of arterial obstruction. Revascularization of the penis may be divided into aortoiliac and distal microvascular procedures. In the past, aortoiliac reconstruction or endarterectomy procedures have met with low success rates (Dewar et al., 1985). The failure of these procedures to restore potency was probably due to concomitant distal arterial occlusive disease and to unrecognized corporal veno-occlusive dysfunction.

Microvascular bypass procedures were first introduced for the treatment of erectile dysfunction in the early 1970s (Michal et al., 1973). The initial procedure involved the anastomosis of the inferior epigastric artery directly to the tunica albuginea. This maneuver unfortunately resulted in a modest percentage of priapism as well as an eventual thrombosis of the anastomosis secondary to poor runoff within the corporal tissue (LeVeen, 1978). The importance of this procedure, however, was that it showed for the first time that bringing a new source of blood to the corporal tissue could result in the restoration of potency, albeit for a brief time. Penile revascularization procedures that followed in-

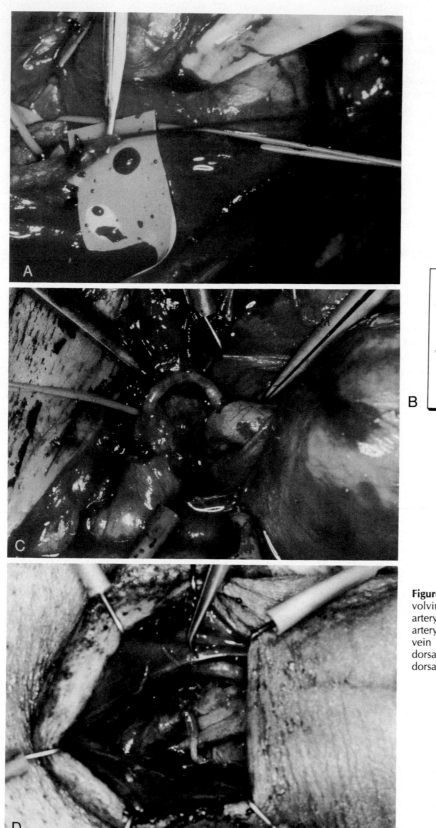

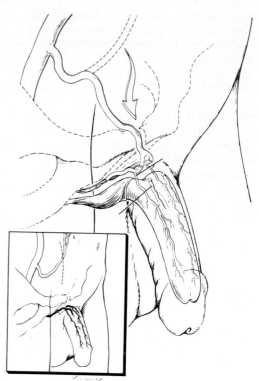

Figure 84–19. Penile revascularization procedures involving the neoarterial inflow source, inferior epigastric artery (A) anastomosed end-to-end to the dorsal penile artery (B, schematic), end-to-side to the deep dorsal penile vein (C) or some combination (D), end-to-side to the dorsal penile vein *(small arrow)*, and end-to-end to the dorsal penile artery *(larger arrow)*.

volved anastomosing a neoarterial inflow source, either the inferior epigastric artery (Fig. 84–19*A*) or an arterialized saphenous vein, to the dorsal penile artery (Fig. 84–19*B*, schematic) (Levine et al., 1990), the cavernosal artery (Konnak et al., 1989), the deep dorsal penile vein (Fig. 84–19*C*) (Virag, 1982b), or some combination of these vessels (Fig. 84–19*D*).

It appears that patient selection for these procedures is most critical and has a strong impact on the results of this surgery. The best candidates appear to be younger men with discrete lesions in the pudendal artery, the common penile artery, or both due to pelvic or perineal trauma rather than older men with more generalized arteriosclerotic occlusive disease involving the hypogastric system. Patients who are considered for these procedures should have undergone some form of sophisticated arterial examination as described in the previous part of this chapter as well as pharmacocavernosometry, pharmacocavernosography, and pudendal arteriography. Many of the younger patients who are, as described, good candidates for these procedures have histories of trauma (Fig. 84–20). Their impotence may begin shortly after the blunt traumatic event or may be delayed for years. One explanation for this delay in impotence is that the perineal injury may cause arterial endothelial disruption, which by itself or in combination with other vascular risk factors eventually causes arteriosclerotic changes and discrete arterial disease leading to penile vascular insufficiency (Levine et al., 1990).

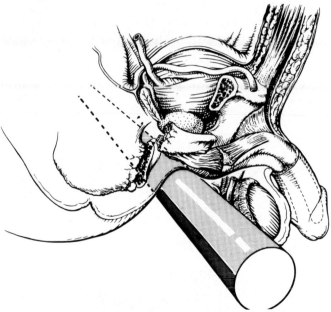

Figure 84–20. The best candidates for penile revascularization appear to be younger men with discrete arterial occlusive lesions in the pudendal artery, the common penile artery, or the cavernosal artery due to pelvic or perineal trauma rather than older men with more generalized arteriosclerotic occlusive disease involving the hypogastric system. Many younger patients will have histories of blunt perineal or pelvic trauma. Their impotence may begin shortly after the traumatic event or may be delayed for years following the blunt traumatic episode. One explanation for this delay in impotence is that the perineal injury may cause arterial endothelial disruption, which by itself or in combination with other vascular risk factors eventually causes arteriosclerotic changes and discrete arterial disease leading to penile vascular insufficiency.

In 1983, Michal introduced an operation involving the end-to-side microvascular anastomosis between the inferior epigastric artery and the dorsal artery of the penis. This procedure has been modified by performing an end-to-end anastomosis between the inferior epigastric artery and the proximal portion of the transected dorsal artery of the penis (Goldstein et al., 1988). The success of this procedure requires the integrity and patency of the bifurcation of the penile artery into the dorsal and corporal arteries. Thus, blood flowing in a retrograde fashion through the proximal dorsal artery of the penis may then enter the corporal artery. The rate of success for this type of procedure varies considerably from 31 to 80 per cent (Fig. 84–21) (Goldstein, 1988; Sharlip, 1988).

We have reported on 29 patients who underwent arterial reconstructive procedures involving the anastomosis of the inferior epigastric artery to the proximal dorsal penile artery at our institution in 1988 and 1989. These patients then returned questionnaires concerning clinical response. Follow-up in this group was from 6 months to 2 years. Of these patients, 72 per cent reported an improved erectile quality, including rigidity and/or sustaining capability. Improved satisfaction of erections and increased spontaneity of erections were reported in 61 per cent each. Intercourse quality was also graded by determining what percentage of coital episodes were satisfying to the patient. Coital episodes were satisfactory in 25 per cent of cases preoperatively, which improved to 78 per cent postoperatively. Some 74 per cent claimed a greater frequency of intercourse. An increase in self-confidence and/or self-image was stated in 69 per cent. Increased partner satisfaction was noted in 63 per cent. When asked if they would undergo the same procedure again if necessary, 93 per cent said they would. Complications were reported in five patients, including two claiming a minor loss of sensation, two some loss of erectile length, and one glans hypervascularization (Levine et al., 1990).

When proximal obstruction to the cavernosal artery is noted and no direct connections between the dorsal artery and the cavernosal artery are apparent, a direct anastomosis between the inferior epigastric artery and the cavernosal artery has been reported in several series. Because of the small luminal diameter (0.3 to 0.5 mm) of the cavernosal artery, this procedure is often technically impossible to perform. Because of the few patients who have been reported who have undergone this operation, it is difficult at this time to assess long-term results. One case of focal corporal veno-occlusive dysfunction has been reported as a result of injury to the erectile tissue during this procedure (Levine et al., 1990).

In cases of bilateral cavernosal artery occlusion, arterialization of a deep dorsal vein segment may be considered. The approach of arterialization of the deep dorsal vein was originally described by Virag and coworkers (1981). The operation is performed by anastomosing the inferior epigastric artery to a segment of the deep dorsal vein after proximal and distal venous ligation (Fig. 84–19*C*). The conceptual basis of this procedure is that arterializing the deep dorsal vein may provide additional blood flow to the corpora cavernosa

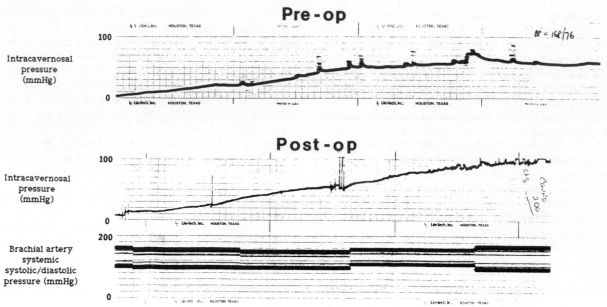

Figure 84–21. The success of the inferior epigastric artery to dorsal penile artery procedure requires the integrity and patency of the bifurcation of the penile artery into the dorsal and corporal arteries. Thus, blood flowing in a retrograde fashion through the proximal dorsal artery of the penis may then enter the corporal artery. The rate of success for this type of procedure varies considerably, ranging from 31 to 80 per cent. This patient's preoperative and postoperative (12 months) intracavernosal pressure response to intracavernosal vasoactive agents demonstrates an improved, virtually normal equilibrium pressure response.

PRE-OPERATIVE

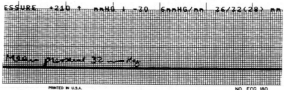

POST-OPERATIVE

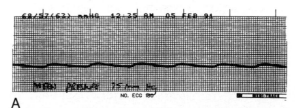

A

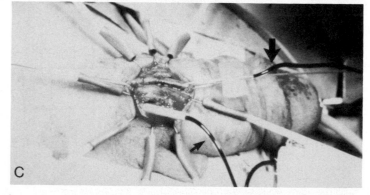

Figure 84–22. In cases of bilateral cavernosal artery occlusion, arterialization of a deep dorsal vein segment may be considered. The operation is performed by anastomosing the inferior epigastric artery to a segment of the deep dorsal vein after proximal and distal venous ligation. The conceptual basis of this procedure is that arterializing the deep dorsal vein may provide additional blood flow to the corpora cavernosa by retrograde flow through the emissary veins. *A,* The ability to arterialize a dorsal vein segment is demonstrated. The preoperative and postoperative P_{O_2} values were 114 mm Hg and 188 mm Hg, whereas the preoperative and postoperative dorsal vein pressures were 32 mm Hg (nonpulsatile) and 75 mm Hg (pulsatile), respectively. Numerous operative issues must be resolved in the dorsal vein arterialization vascular reconstructive procedure, including the need to ablate emissary and dorsal veins valves.

B and *C,* The injection of methylene blue (25-gauge butterfly, *large arrow*) into the isolated dorsal vein segment and the retrograde recovery of methylene blue from the corpus cavernosum (19-gauge butterfly, *small arrow*, initially venous blood which converts to methylene blue) are demonstrated.

by retrograde flow through the emissary veins (Fig. 84–22). To further ensure increased blood flow to the corpora, a side-to-side anastomosis of the deep dorsal vein and the tunica albuginea (corporovenous window) was added to the operation previously described but has largely been abandoned. The rate of success for this operation varies considerably from 20 to 75 per cent (Bennett, 1988; Sharlip et al., 1988). Reports have been published of long-term graft patency (Sohn et al., 1990).

Numerous issues need to be resolved in the dorsal vein arterialization vascular reconstructive procedure, including the optimum length of the dorsal vein segment; the need to ablate emissary and dorsal veins valves; the location of the proximal and distal dorsal vein ligatures; the removal of circumferential veins; the most effective arterial-venous anastomosis (end-to-side or end-to-end); the need for postoperative anticoagulation; the need for additional arterial anastomoses, such as one or both dorsal arteries; and the most effective means of reducing the complication of glans hyperemia. This last complication, a painful, swollen glans penis that can result in glans ischemia and necrosis occurs because of excessive arterial inflow to the glans penis. This is a result of the arterialized blood in the dorsal vein preventing venous

drainage from the glans. Should glans hyperemia occur, re-exploration must be performed to ligate the distal arterialized dorsal vein segment more proximally along the penile shaft.

VENOUS PROCEDURE. Patients demonstrating corporal veno-occlusive dysfunction may undergo vascular reconstructive procedures with the aim of increasing venous outflow resistance. As early as 1908, Lydston performed the first of these procedures for impotence in more than 100 cases. His operation consisted of ligating both the superficial and deep dorsal veins of the penis. Lydston believed that this type of obstruction to venous outflow increased the ability to initiate an erection. In 1936, Lowsley and Bray described a procedure that consisted of plicating the ischiocavernous muscles in addition to ligating the deep dorsal vein of the penis. This was performed in 51 patients with excellent results in 31.

At present, patients who have evidence of corporal veno-occlusive dysfunction, as demonstrated by pharmacocavernosometry and cavernosography, have undergone various procedures in the hope of increasing venous resistance. These procedures have included crural plication (Fig. 84–23A), ligation or excision of the deep

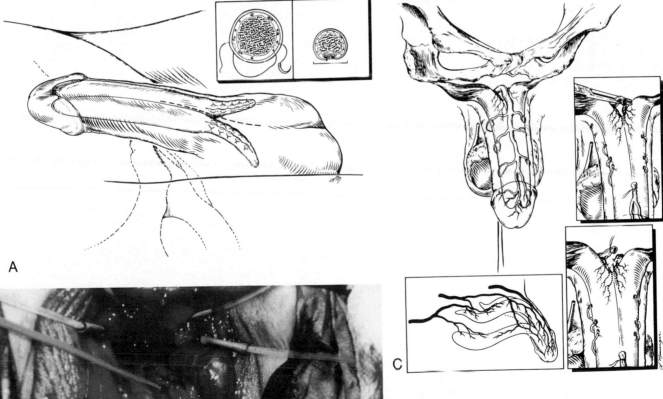

Figure 84–23. At present, patients who have evidence of corporal veno-occlusive dysfunction as demonstrated by pharmacocavernosometry and cavernosography have undergone various procedures in the hope of increasing venous resistance. These procedures have included crural plication (A), ligation or excision of the deep dorsal vein of the penis (B shows the proximal dorsal vein under the pubic symphysis), ligation of cavernosal veins (B and C), spongiolysis, or their combination.

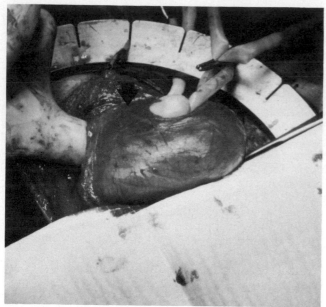

Figure 84–24. Complications reported from the various procedures, especially those involving proximal penile dissection, include diminished penile sensation and shortened penile length. The fundiform ligament *(arrow)* is shown, which is the continuation of Scarpa's fascia onto Buck's fascia. In venous surgery, preservation of the fundiform ligament has reduced the complication of numbness and shortening.

dorsal vein of the penis (Fig. 84–23*B*), ligation of the cavernosal veins (Fig. 84–23*B* and *C*), spongiolysis, or their combination. Success rates of these procedures describing subjective improvement have ranged from 28 to 76 per cent, with an average follow-up of 3 to 26 months (Bar-Moshe et al., 1988; Lewis, 1988). Complications reported from the various procedures, especially those involving proximal penile dissection, include diminished penile sensation and shortened penile length (Levine et al., 1990). The fundiform ligament is the continuation of Scarpa's fascia onto Buck's fascia. In venous surgery, preservation of the fundiform ligament has reduced the complication of numbness and shortening (Fig. 84–24).

The variable success rate with venous procedures may be explained by the underlying pathophysiology of corporal veno-occlusive dysfunction. In some patients, the pathology may be related to a pancavernosal alteration in corporal tissue compliance. In such a case, cavernosography may reveal a more generalized corporal veno-occlusive dysfunction with visualization of the glans, corpus spongiosum, dorsal vein, and cavernosal vein. In particular, patients in our series who are noted to have spongiosal leaks have rarely demonstrated, on follow-up pharmacocavernosometry, restored veno-occlusive function. We believe that there are patients, however, with more localized corporal veno-occlusive dysfunction who may benefit from these procedures. During the performance of pharmacocavernosometry, if abnormal findings can be corrected with perineal compression as originally proposed by Puech-Leao (1987) and if pharmacocavernosograms reveal drainage only through dorsal or crural veins, we have treated patients with crural plication, proximal dorsal vein excision, and cavernosal

vein ligation (Levine et al., 1990). The rationale for this procedure has been that these patients are not suffering from a pancavernosal abnormality but rather from a local abnormality possibly due to pre-existing trauma.

It has been our experience that patients who present with corporal veno-occlusive dysfunction usually have a concomitant arterial insufficiency. Such arterial occlusive disease prevents any arterial compensation for the abnormal venous outflow. Therefore, it is our belief that venous procedures should probably be performed in conjunction with surgery to increase arterial inflow to the corpora.

Obviously, procedures to correct corporal veno-occlusive dysfunction are still in evolution. We must first understand the true nature of this dysfunction. With time, we may be able to define a subset of patients with abnormalities who will be appropriately treated with venous surgery.

SUMMARY

Major advances have been made in the understanding of erectile physiology and pathophysiology. The ability to relax and contract corporal smooth muscle, and thus control the state of penile erection, has led to the development of new and innovative evaluation procedures and therapeutic options. In the future, we look to the performance of prospective studies to investigate the reliability and validity and ultimately the standardization of these procedures. The demand for treatment will continue to foster the development of research in the field.

REFERENCES

Diagnosis and Therapy of Erectile Dysfunction

Abber, J. C., and Lue, T. F.: Evaluation of impotence. *In* deVere White, R. (Ed.). Problems in Urology. Sexual Dysfunction. Philadelphia, J. B. Lippincott Co., pp. 476–486, 1987.

Abelson, D.: Diagnostic value of the penile pulse and blood pressure: A Doppler study of impotence in diabetics. J. Urol., 113:636, 1975.

Amelar, R. D., and Dubin, L.: Sexual function and fertility in paraplegic males. Urology, 20:61, 1982.

Anders, E. K., Bradley, W. E., and Krane, R. J.: Nocturnal penile rigidity measured by the snap-gauge band. J. Urol., 129:964, 1983.

Austoni, E., Cazzaniga, A., Colombo, F., Toia, G., and Pisani, E.: Use of dynamic N.M.R. in the diagnostic evaluation of penile pathology. Int. J. Impotence Res., 2:Supplement 2, 161, 1990.

Azadzoi, K. M., and Goldstein, I.: Atherosclerosis-induced corporal leakage impotence. Surg. Forum, 38:647–648, 1987.

Azadzoi, K. M., Payton, T., Krane, R. J., and Goldstein, I.: Effects of intracavernosal trazodone hydrochloride: Animal and human studies. J. Urol., 144:1277, 1990.

Bancroft, J., and Wu, F. C. W.: Changes in erectile responsiveness during androgen replacement therapy. Arch. Sex. Behav., 12:59, 1983.

Bar-Moshe, O., and Vandendris, M.: Treatment of impotence due to perineal venous leakage by ligation of crura penis. J. Urol., 139:1217, 1988.

Barry, J. M., Blank, B., and Boileau, M.: Nocturnal penile tumescence monitoring with stamps. Urology, 15:171, 1980.

Barry, J. M., and Hodges, C. V.: Impotence: a diagnostic approach. J. Urol., 119:575, 1978.

Benard, F., Stief, C. G., Bosch, R., et al.: Systemic infusion of epinephrine: its effect on erection. *In* Proceedings of the Sixth Biennial International Symposium for Corpus Cavernosum Revascularization and Third Biennial World Meeting on Impotence, Boston, October 6, 1988, p 16.

Bennett, A. H.: Venous arterilization for erectile impotence. Urol. Clin. North Am. 15:111–113, 1988.

Blanco, R., Saenz de Tejada, I., Goldstein, I., Krane, R. J., Wotiz, H. H., and Cohen, R. A.: Dysfunctional penile cholinergic nerves in diabetic impotent men. J. Urol., 144:278, 1990.

Bock, D. B., and Lewis, R. W.: NPT: Is it really the gold standard? Int. J. Impotence Res., 2:Supplement 2, 101, 1990.

Bondil, P., Daures, J. P., Louis, J. F., Costa, P., Lopez, C., and Navratil, H.: Measurement of penile longitudinal extensibility: a new clinical test for impotence. Int. J. Impotence Res., 2:Supplement 2, 181, 1990.

Bookstein, J. J., Valji, K., Parsons, L., and Kessler, W.: Pharmacoarteriography in the evaluation of impotence. J. Urol., 137:333, 1987.

Bradley, W. E., Timm, G. W., Gallagher, J. M., et al.: New method for continuous measurement of nocturnal penile tumescence and rigidity. Urology, 26:4, 1985.

Brindley, G. S.: Pilot experiments on the actions of drugs injected into the human corpus cavernosum penis. Br. J. Pharmacol., 87:495, 1986.

Brown, E., Brown, G. M., Kofman, O., et al.: Sexual function and affect in Parkinson men treated with L-dopa. Am. J. Psychiatry, 135:1552–1555, 1978.

Buvat, J., Buvat-Herbaut, M., Dehaene, J. L., and Lemaire, A.: Is intracavernosus injection of papaverine a reliable screening test for vascular impotence? J. Urol., 135:476, 1986.

Buvat, J., Quittelier, E., Lemaire, A., Buvat-Herbaut, M., and Marcolin, G.: Electromyography of the human penis, including single potential analysis during flaccidity and erection induced by vasoactive agents. Int. J. Impotence Res., 2:Supplement 2, 85, 1990.

Carson, C. C.: Infections in genitourinary prostheses. Urol. Clin. North Am., 16:139, 1989.

Carter, J. N., Tyson, J. E., Tolis, G., et al.: Prolactin-secreting tumors and hypogonadism in 22 men. N. Engl. J. Med., 299:847, 1978.

Catalona, W. J., and Dresner, S. M.: Nerve-sparing radical prostatectomy: extraprostatic tumor extension and preservation of erectile function. J. Urol., 134:1149, 1985.

Cerami, A., Vlassara, H., and Brownlee, M.: Glucose and aging. Sci. Am., 256:90, 1987.

Claes, H., and Baert, L.: Transcutaneous nitroglycerin therapy in the treatment of impotence. Urol. Int., 44:309–312, 1989.

Cooper, A. J.: Short-term treatment in sexual dysfunction: A review. Compr. Psychiatry, 22:206, 1981.

Dahlof, L. G., and Larsson, K.: Interactional effects of pudendal nerve section and social restriction on male rat sexual behavior. Physiol. Behav., 16:757, 1976.

Davidson, J. M.: Hormones and sexual behavior in the male. Hosp. Pract., 18:126, 1975.

de Groat, W. C., and Steers, W. D.: Neuroanatomy and neurophysiology of penile erection. *In* Tanagho, E. A., Lue, T. F., and McClure, R. D. (Eds.). Contemporary Management of Impotence and Infertility. Baltimore, Williams & Wilkens, 1988, p. 3.

Dewar, M. L., Blundell, P. E., Lidstone, D., Herba, M. J., and Chiu, R. C.: Effects of abdominal aneurysmectomy, aortoiliac bypass grafting and angioplasty on male sexual potency: A prospective study. Can. J. Surg., 28:154, 1985.

Dhabuwala, C. B., Kerkar, P., Bhutwala, A., Kumar, A., and Pierce, J. M.: Intracavernous papaverine in the management of psychogenic impotence. Arch. Androl., 24:185–191, 1990.

Diederichs, W., Kaula, N. F., Lue, T. F., and Tanagho, E. A.: The effect of subatmospheric pressure on the simian penis. J. Urol., 142:1087, 1989.

Diederichs, W., Stief, C. G., Lue, T. F., and Tanagho, E. A.: Sympathetic inhibition of papaverine-induced erection. *In* Proceedings of the Sixth Biennial International Symposium for Corpus Cavernosum Revascularization and Third Biennial World Meeting on Impotence, Boston, October 6, 1988, p. 79.

Eggleston, J. C., and Walsh, P. C.: Radical prostatectomy with preservation of sexual function: pathological findings in the first 100 cases. J. Urol., 134:1146, 1985.

Ellenberg, M.: Impotence in diabetes: The neurologic factor. Ann. Intern. Med., 75:213, 1971.

Ertekin, C., Akjurekli, O., Gruses, A. N., et al.: The value of somatosensory-evoked potentials and bulbocavernous reflex in patients with impotence. Arch. Neurol. Scand., 71:48, 1985.

Euler, U. S.: Quantification of stress by catecholamine analysis. Clin. Pharmacol. Ther., 5:398, 1964.

Fischer, G. M., Swain, M. L., and Cherian, K.: Increased vascular collagen and elastin synthesis in experimental atherosclerosis in the rabbit. Atherosclerosis, 35:11, 1980.

Fisher, C., Gross, J., and Zuch, J.: Cycle of penile erections synchronous with dreaming (REM) sleep. Arch. Gen. Psychiatry, 12:29, 1965.

Fishman, I. J., Scott, F. B., and Selim, A. M.: Rescue procedure: an alternative to complete removal for treatment of infected penile prosthesis. (Abstract) J. Urol., 137:202A, 1987.

Foreman, M. M., and Wernicke, J. F.: Approaches for the development of oral drug therapies for erectile dysfunction. Semin. Urol. 8:107–112, 1990.

Franks, S., Jacobs, H. S., Martin, N., and Nabarro, J. D. N.: Hyperprolactinemia and impotence. Clin. Endocrinol., 8:277, 1978.

Furlow, W. L., and Goldwasser, B.: Salvage of the eroded inflatable penile prosthesis: A new concept. J. Urol., 138:312–314, 1987.

Furlow, W. L., Goldwasser, B., and Gundian, J. C.: Implantation of model AMS 700 penile prosthesis: long-term results. J. Urol., 139:741, 1988.

Gasior, B. L., Levine, F. J., Howannesian, A., Krane, R. J., and Goldstein, I.: Plaque-associated corporal veno-occlusive dysfunction in idiopathic Peyronie's disease: A pharmacocavernosometric and pharmacocavernosographic study. World J. Urol., 8:90–96, 1990.

Golden, J. S.: Behavioral approaches to the treatment of sexual problems. *In* Zales, M. (Ed.). Eating, Sleeping and Sexuality; Treatment of Disorders in Basic Life Functions. New York, Brunner-Mazel, 1982, p. 236.

Goldstein, I.: Electromyography: Evoked response evaluations. *In* Controversies in Neuro-Urology. Barrett, D., and Wein, A. J. (Eds.). New York, Churchill Livingston, 1983, pp. 117–129.

Goldstein, I.: Penile revascularization. Urol. Clin. North Am., 14:805–813, 1987.

Goldstein, I.: Overview of types and results of vascular surgical procedures for impotence. Cardiovas. Intervent. Radiol., 11:240–244, 1988.

Goldstein, I., Borges, F. D., Fitch, W. P., Kaufman, J., Moreno, J., Payton, T., Yingst, J., and Krane, R. J.: Rescuing the failed papaverine/phentolamine erection: A proposed synergistic action of papaverine, phentolamine and prostaglandin E_1. Int. J. Impotence Res., 2:Supplement 2, 277, 1990.

Goldstein, I., Feldman, M. I., Deckers, P. J., et al.: Radiation-associated impotence. A clinical study of its mechanism. JAMA, 251:903, 1984.

Goldstein, I., Krane, R. J., Greenfield, A. J., and Padma-Nathan, H.: Vascular diseases of the penis: Impotence and priapism. *In* Pollack, H. M. (Ed.). Clinical Urography. Philadelphia, W. B. Saunders Co., 1990, pp. 2231–2252.

Goldstein, I., Siroky, M. B., Nath, R. L., et al.: Vasculogenic impotence: Role of the pelvic steal test. J. Urol., 128:300, 1982.

Gower, A., Berendsen, H., Princen, M., et al.: The yawning-penile erection syndrome as a model for putative dopamine autoreceptor activity. Eur. J. Pharm., 103:81, 1984.

Groshar, D., Vardi, Y., and Lidgi, S.: Radioisotope measurement of corporal outflow using Tc-99m labelled autologous red blood cells. Int. J. Impotence Res., 2:Supplement 2, 113, 1990.

Hayashi, K., Takamizawa, K., Nakamura, T., Kato, T., and Tsushima, N.: Effects of elastase on the stiffness and elastic properties of arterial walls in cholesterol-fed rabbits. Atherosclerosis, 66:259, 1987.

Heaton, J. P. W., Varrin, S., Ge, S. P., and Morales, A.: Preliminary studies showing erectogenic activity in an oral agent. Int. J. Impotence Res., 2:Supplement 2, 285, 1990.

Hengeveld, M. W.: Erectile dysfunction: A sexological and psychiatric review. World J. Urol., 1:227, 1983.

Herbert, J.: The role of the dorsal nerves of the penis in the sexual behavior of the male rhesus monkey. Physiol. Behav., 10:293, 1973.

Hinman, F.: Priapism: reasons for failure of therapy. J. Urol., 83:420, 1960.

Horton, C. E., Sadove, R. C., and Devine, C. J., Jr.: Peyronie's disease. Ann. Plast. Surg., 18:122, 1987.

Jackson, J. A., Waxman, J., and Spiekerman, A. M.: Prostatic complications of testosterone replacement therapy. Arch. Intern. Med., 149:2365–2366, 1989.

Jünemann, K. P., Lue, T. F., Fournier, G. R., Jr., and Tanagho, E. A.: Hemodynamics of papaverine and phentolamine-induced penile erection. J. Urol., 136:158, 1986.

Karacan, I.: The dilemma of diagnosing erectile dysfunction. In Carlton, C. E., Jr. (Ed.). Controversies in Urology. Chicago, Year Book Medical Publishers, 1989, p. 99.

Karacan, I.: Clinical value of nocturnal erection in the prognosis and diagnosis of impotence. Med. Aspects Hum. Sex., 4:27, 1970.

Karacan, I., Salis, P. J., and Williams, R. L.: The role of the sleep laboratory in the diagnosis and treatment of impotence. In Williams, R. L., and Karacan, I. (Eds.). Sleep Disorder, Diagnosis, Treatment. New York, John Wiley & Sons, 1978, p. 351.

Kedia, K. R.: Vasculogenic impotence: Diagnosis and objective evaluation using quantitative segmental pulse volume recorder. Br. J. Urol., 56:516, 1984.

Kessler, R.: Surgical experience with the inflatable penile prosthesis. J. Urol., 124:611, 1980.

Kessler, W. O.: Nocturnal penile tumescence. Urol. Clin. North Am., 15:81, 1988.

Kiely, E. A., Williams, G., and Goldie, L.: Assessment of the immediate and long-term effects of pharmacologically induced penile erections in the treatment of psychogenic and organic impotence. Br. J. Urol., 59:164, 1987.

Kinsey, A. C., Pomeroy, W., and Martin, C.: Age and sexual outlet. In Kinsey, A. C., Pomeroy, W., and Martin, C. (Eds.). Sexual Behavior in the Human Male. Philadelphia, W. B. Saunders Co., 1948, p. 218.

Kolodny, R. C., Kahn, C. B., Goldstein, A., et al.: Sexual dysfunction in diabetic men. Diabetes, 23:306, 1974.

Konnak, J. W., and Ohl, D. A.: Microsurgical penile venascularization using central corporeal penile artery. J. Urol., 142:305–308, 1989.

Krane, R. J.: Sexual function and dysfunction. In Walsh, P. C., Gittes, R. F., Perlmutter, A. D., and Stamey, T. A. (Eds.). Campbell's Urology, 5th ed. Philadelphia, W. B. Saunders Co., 700, 1986.

Krane, R. J.: Penile prostheses. Urol. Clin. North Am., 15:103, 1988.

Krane, R. J., and Goldstein, I.: Surgery for impotency. Prosthesis implantation and penile revascularization. In Libertino, J. A. (Ed.). Adult and Pediatric Reconstructive Urologic Surgery. Baltimore, Williams & Wilkins, 1987, pp. 598–614.

Krane, R. J., Goldstein, I., and Saenz de Tejada, I.: Medical progress: Impotence. N. Engl. J. Med., 321:1648–1659, 1989.

Kwan, M., Greenleaf, W. J., Mann, J., Crapo, L., Davidson, J. M.: The nature of androgen action on male sexuality: a combined laboratory/self-report study on hypogonadal men. J. Clin. Endocrinol. Metab., 57:557, 1983.

Lakin, M. M., and Montague, D. K.: Intracavernous injection therapy in post-priapism cavernosal fibrosis. J. Urol., 140:828–829, 1988.

Lal, S., Rios, O., and Thavundayil, J. X.: Treatment of impotence with trazodone: A case report. J. Urol., 143:819–820, 1990.

Lavoisier, P., Courtois, F., Galaup, J. P., and Meunier, P.: Normality criteria for penile sensitivity to pressure, touch and vibration. Int. J. Impotence Res., 2:Supplement 2, 89, 1990.

Lee, L. M., Stevenson, R. W. D., and Szasz, G.: Prostaglandin E₁ versus phentolamine/papaverine for the treatment of erectile impotence: a double-blind comparison. J. Urol., 141:549, 1989.

Lehman, T. P., and Jacobs, J. A.: Etiology of diabetic impotence. J. Urol., 29:291, 1983.

Lepor, H., Gregerman, M., Crosby, R., Mostofi, F. K., and Walsh, P. C.: Precise location of the autonomic nerves from the plexus to the corpora cavernosa: a detailed anatomical study of the adult male pelvis. J. Urol., 133:207, 1985.

LeVeen, H. H.: Vein graft for vascular impotence. Med. World News, 3:73, 1978.

Levine, F. J., Payton, T. R., Goldstein, I., and Krane, R. J.: Gravity infusion cavernosometry: An office test utilizing intracavernosal pharmacologic stimulation and real time radial rigidity monitoring to determine veno-occlusive function. J. Urol., 143:62A, 1990a.

Levine, F. J., and Goldstein, I.: Vascular reconstructive surgery in the management of erectile dysfunction. Int. J. Impotence Res., 2:59–78, 1990.

Levine, F. J., Greenfield, A. J., and Goldstein, I.: Arteriographically determined occlusive disease within the hypogastric-cavernous bed in impotent patients following blunt perineal and pelvic trauma. J. Urol., 144:1147, 1990.

Levine, S. B., Althof, S. E., Turner, L. A., Risen, C. B., Bodner, D. R., Kursh, E. D., and Resnick, M. I.: Side effects of self-administration of intracavernous papaverine and phentolamine for the treatment of impotence. J. Urol., 141:54–57, 1989.

Lewis, R. W.: Venous surgery for impotence. Urol. Clin. North Am., 15:115, 1988.

Lewis, R. W., and Pauyau, F. A.: Procedures for decreasing venous drainage. Semin. Urol., 4:263, 1986.

LoPiccolo, J.: Management of psychogenic erectile failure. In Tanagho, E. A., Lue, T. F., and McClure, R. D. (Eds.). Contemporary Management of Impotence and Infertility. Baltimore, Williams & Wilkens, 1988, p. 133.

LoPiccolo, J., and Stock, W. E.: Treatment of sexual dysfunction. J. Consult. Clin. Psychol., 54:158, 1986.

Lowsley, O. S., and Bray, J. L.: The surgical relief of impotence. Further experiences with a new operative procedure. JAMA, 107:2029–2035, 1936.

Lue, T.: Treatment of venogenic impotence. In Tanagho, E. A., Lue, T. F., and McClure, R. D. (Eds.). Contemporary Management of Impotence and Infertility. Baltimore, Williams & Wilkins, 1988, p. 175.

Lue, T. F., Hricak, H., Marich, K. W., et al.: Vasculogenic impotence evaluated by high-resolution ultrasonography and pulsed Doppler spectrum analysis. Radiology, 155:777, 1985.

Lurie, A. L., Bookstein, J. J., and Kessler, W. O.: Angiography of post-traumatic impotence. Cardio. Intervent. Radiol., 11:232, 1988.

Lydston, G. F.: The surgical treatment of impotency. Am. J. Clin. Med., 15:1571–1573, 1908.

Malloy, T. R., Wein, A. J., and Carpiniello, V. L.: Reliability of AMS 700 inflatable penile prosthesis. Urology, 27:385, 1986.

Margolis, R., Prieto, P., Stein, L., et al.: Statistical summary of 10,000 male cases using Aphrodex in the treatment of impotence. Curr. Ther. Res., 13:616, 1971.

Marshall, P. G., Morales, A., Phillips, P., et al.: Nocturnal penile tumescence with stamps: A comparative study under sleep laboratory conditions. J. Urol., 130:80, 1983.

Masters, W. H., and Johnson, V. E.: Human Sexual Inadequacy. Boston, Little, Brown & Co., 1970.

McCulloch, D. K., Campbell, I. W., Wu, F. C., Prescott, R. J., and Clarke, B. F.: The prevalence of diabetic impotence. Diabetologia, 18:279, 1980.

Melman, A., Kaplan, D., and Redfield, J.: Evaluation of the first 70 patients in the Center for Male Sexual Dysfunction of Beth Israel Medical Center. J. Urol., 131:53, 1984.

Melman, A., Libin, M., and Tendler, C.: The effect of chronic alpha-methyldopa upon sexual function in the adult male rat. J. Urol., 129:643, 1983.

Melman, A., Tiefer, L., and Pederson, R.: Evaluation of the first 406 patients in urology department–based center for male sexual dysfunction. Urology, 32:6, 1988.

Meulerman, E. J. H., Naudin ten Cate, L., Bemelmans, B. L. H., de Wilde, P. C. M., Vooys, G. P., and Debruyne, F. M. J.: The role of penile biopsies in the evaluation of erectile dysfunction: A histomorphometric study of the human cavernous body. Int. J. Impotence Res., 2:Supplement 2, 230, 1990.

Michal, V.: Arterial disease as a cause of impotence. Clin. Endocrinol. Metab., 11:725, 1982.

Michal, V., Kramar, R., Pospichal, J., and Hejhal, L.: Direct arterial anastomosis on corpora cavernosa penis in the therapy of erectile impotence. Rozhl. Chir., 52:587–590, 1973.

Montague, D. K.: Penile prostheses. In Montague, D. K. (Ed.). Disorders of Male Sexual Dysfunction. Chicago, Year Book Medical Publishers Inc., 1988, p. 154.

Morales, A., Condra, M., Owen, J. E., Fenemore, J., and Surridge, D. H.: Oral and transcutaneous pharmacologic agents in the treatment of impotence. Urol. Clin. North Am., 15:87–93, 1988.

Morales, A., Condra, M., Owen, J. A., Surridge, D. H., Fenemore, J., and Harris, C.: Is yohimbine effective in the treatment of organic impotence? Results of a controlled trial. J. Urol., 137:1168, 1987.

Morales, A., Condra, M., and Reid, K.: Role of nocturnal penile tumescence monitoring in diagnosis of impotence: review. J. Urol., 143:441, 1990a.

Morales, A., Harris, C., Condra, M., and Heaton, J. P.: Validation of visual sexual stimulation in the etiological diagnosis of impotence. Int. J. Impotence Res., 2:Supplement 2, 109, 1990b.

Morales, A., and Heaton, J. P. W.: The medical treatment of impotence: an update. World J. Urol., 8:80–83, 1990.

Moul, J. W., and McLeod, D. G.: Negative pressure devices in the explanted penile prosthesis population. J. Urol., 142:729, 1989.

Mulcahy, J. J.: A technique of maintaining penile prosthesis position to prevent proximal migration. J. Urol., 137:294–296, 1987.

Mulcahy, J. J.: The management of infected penile implants. World J. Urol., 8:111–113, 1990.

Nadig, P. W.: Vacuum erection devices. A review. World J. Urol., 8:114–117, 1990.

Nadig, P. W., Ware, J. C., and Blumoff, R.: Noninvasive device to produce and maintain an erection-like state. Urology, 27:126, 1986.

National Center for Health Statistics. National ambulatory medical care survey, 1985. Department of Human and Health Services Publication Number 88-1754. Data from Fitzsimmons, S. C., Bethesda, April 24, 1989a and b.

Newman, H. F.: Vibratory sensitivity of the penis. Fertil. Steril., 21:791, 1970.

Nisen, H. O., Alfthan, O. S., Lindstrom, B. L., Ruutu, M. L., and Virtanen, J. M.: Single breath beat-to-beat variation testing in the diagnosis of autonomic neuropathy in impotence. Int. J. Impotence Res., 2:Supplement 2, 136, 1990.

Ohlmeyer, P., et al.: Periodische vorgauge in schlaf. Pflugers Arch., 248:559, 1944.

Padma-Nathan, H., and Goldstein, I.: Neurologic assessment of the impotent male. In Montague, D. K. (Ed.). Disorders of Male Sexual Functions. Chicago, Year Book Publishers, 1987a, pp. 86–94.

Padma-Nathan, H., and Goldstein, I.: Treatment for organic impotence: Alternatives to the penile prosthesis. Part I and Part II, Lesson 11 and Lesson 12, AUA Update Series, 1987b.

Padma-Nathan, H., Goldstein, I., and Krane, R. J.: Evaluation of the impotent patient. Semin. Urol., 4:225, 1986.

Padma-Nathan, H., Goldstein, I., and Krane, R. J.: Treatment of prolonged or priapistic erections following intracavernosal papaverine therapy. Semin. Urol., 4:236, 1986.

Padma-Nathan, H., Goldstein, I., Payton, T. R., and Krane, R. J.: Intracavernosal pharmacotherapy: The pharmacologic erection program. World J. Urol., 5:160–170, 1987.

Padma-Nathan, H., Klavans, S., Goldstein, I., and Krane, R. J.: The screening efficacy of PBI versus duplex ultrasound versus cavernosal artery systolic occlusion pressure. In Proceedings of the Sixth Biennial International Symposium for Corpus Cavernosum Revascularization and Third Biennial World Meeting on Impotence, Boston, October 6, 1988, p. 32.

Payau, F. A., and Lewis, R. W.: Corpus cavernosography. Pressure flow and radiography. Invest. Radiol., 18:517, 1983.

Penden, N. R., Cargill, J. M., and Browning, M. C. K.: Male sexual dysfunction during treatment with cimetidine. Br. Med. J., 1:659, 1979.

Penson, D. F., Seftel, A. D., Krane, R. J., Frohrib, D., and Goldstein, I.: The hemodynamic pathophysiology of impotence following blunt trauma to the erect penis. J. Urol., Accepted, 1992.

Persson, C., Diederichs, W., Lue, T. F., Yen, B., Fishman, I. J., McLin, H., and Tanagho, E. A.: Correlation of altered penile ultrastructure with clinical arterial evaluation. J. Urol., 142:1462, 1989.

Petrou, A. P., and Barrett, D. M.: The use of penile prosthesis in erectile dysfunction. Semin. Urol., 8:138–152, 1990.

Pogach, L. M., and Vaitukaitis, J. L.: Endocrine disorders associated with erectile dysfunction. In Krane, R. J., Siroky, M. B., Goldstein, I. (Eds.). Male Sexual Dysfunction. Boston, Little Brown and Co., 1983, p. 63.

Porst, H.: Hemodynamic evaluation of penile circulation with duplex-sonography and color Doppler: Results in 133 patients. Int. J. Impotence Res., 2:Supplement 2, 212, 1990.

Procci, W. R., and Martin, D. J.: Preliminary observations of the utility of portable NPT. Arch. Sex. Behav., 13:569, 1984.

Puech-Leao, P., Glina, S., Chao, S., and Reichelt, A. C.: Gravity cavernosometry—a simple diagnostic test to cavernosal incompetence. Br. J. Urol., 1990.

Puech-Leao, P., Reis, J. M. S. M., Glina, S., and Reischelt, A. C.:

Leakage through the crural edge of the corpus cavernosum. Diagnosis and treatment. Eur. Urol., 13:163, 1987.

Roddy, T. M., Goldstein, I., and Devine, C., Jr.: Peyronie's Disease Part 1 and Part 2. AUA Update Series, Lesson 1 and Lesson 2, Volume 10, 1–15, 1991.

Rosen, M. P., Greenfield, A. J., Walker, T. G., Grant, P., Dubrow, J., Bettmann, M. A., Fried, L. E., and Goldstein, I.: Cigarette smoking: An independent risk factor for atherosclerosis in the hypogastric-cavernous arterial bed of men with arteriogenic impotence. J. Urol., 145:759–763, 1991.

Rosen, M. P., Greenfield, A. J., Walker, T. G., Grant, P., Guben, J. K., Dubrow, J., Bettmann, M. A., and Goldstein, I.: Arteriogenic impotence: Findings in 195 impotent men examined with selective internal pudendal angiography. Radiology, 174:1043–1048, 1990.

Ruzbarsky, V., and Michal, V.: Morphologic changes in the arterial bed of the penis with aging: relationship to the pathogenesis of impotence. Invest. Urol., 15:194, 1977.

Saenz de Tejada, I., Goldstein, I., Azadzoi, K., Krane, R. J., and Cohen, R. A.: Impaired neurogenic and endothelium-mediated relaxation of penile smooth muscle from diabetic men with impotence. N. Engl. J. Med., 320:1025, 1989.

Saenz de Tejada, I., Moroukian, P., Tessier, J., Kim, J. J., Goldstein, I., and Frohrib, D.: The trabecular smooth muscle modulates the capacitor function of the penis. Studies on a rabbit model. Am. J. Physiol., 260 (Heart Circ. Physiol. 29):H1590–H1595, 1991.

Saenz de Tejada, I., Ware, J. C., Blanco, R., Pittard, J. T., Nadig, P. W., Azadzoi, K., Krane, R. J., and Goldstein, I.: Pathophysiology of prolonged penile erection associated with trazodone use. J. Urol., 145: 1991.

Scher, M., Krieger, J., and Juergens, S.: Trazodone and priapism. Am. J. Psychiatry, 140:1362–1363, 1983.

Schiavi, R. C., Schreiner-Engel, P., Mandeli, J., Schanzer, H., and Cohen, E.: Healthy aging and male sexual function. Am. J. Psychiatry, 147:766, 1990.

Schouman, M. R., and Amer, M. K.: Visual sexual stimulation test as the first screening test for male impotence. The value of thymoxamine in combination or in the place of papaverine. In Proceedings of the Sixth Biennial International Symposium for Corpus Cavernosum Revascularization and Third Biennial World Meeting on Impotence. Boston, October 6, 1988, p. 33.

Schramek, P., Dorninger, R., Waldhauser, M., Konecny, P., and Porpacz, P.: Prostaglandin E₁ in erectile dysfunction. Efficiency and incidence of priapism. Br. J. Urol., 65:68–71, 1990.

Schramek, P., and Waldhauser, M.: Dose-dependent effect and side effect of prostaglandin E₁ in erectile dysfunction. Br. J. Clin. Pharm., 38:567–571, 1989.

Scott, F. B., Bradley, W. E., and Timm, G. W.: Management of erectile impotence: Use of implantable inflatable prosthesis. Urology, 2:80, 1973.

Seagraves, R. T., Madsen, R., and Carter, C. S.: Erectile dysfunction associated with pharmacological agents. In Seagraves, R. T., and Schoenberg, H. W. (Eds.). Diagnosis and Treatment of Erectile Disturbances. New York, Plenum Publishing Corp., 1985, p. 22.

Shabsigh, R., Fishman, I. J., and Scott, F. B.: Evaluation of erectile impotence. Urology, 32:83, 1988.

Shader, R. I., and Elkin, R.: The effects of antianxiety and antipsychotic drugs on sexual behavior. Mod. Prob. Pharmacopsychiatry, 15:19, 1980.

Sharlip, I. D.: Penile arteriography in impotence after pelvic trauma. J. Urol., 126:477, 1981.

Sharlip, I. D.: Treatment of arteriogenic impotence by penile revascularization. In Proceedings of the Sixth Biennial International Symposium for Corpus Cavernosum Revascularization and Third Biennial World Meeting on Impotence. Boston, October 6, 1988, p. 135.

Sharlip, I. D.: The role of vascular surgery in arteriogenic and combined arteriogenic and venogenic impotence. Semin. Urol., 8:129–137, 1990.

Sidi, A. A.: Vasoactive intracavernous pharmacotherapy. Urol. Clin. North Am. 15:95–101, 1988.

Sidi, A. A., Becher, E. F., Zhang, G., and Lewis, J. H.: Patient acceptance of and satisfaction with an external negative pressure device for impotence. J. Urol., 144:1154–1159, 1990.

Sidi, A. A., and Chen, K. K.: Clinical experience with vasoactive intracavernous pharmacotherapy for treatment of impotence. World J. Urol., 5:156, 1987.

Slag, M. F., Morley, J. E., and Elson, M. K.: Impotence in medical clinic outpatients. JAMA, 249:1736, 1983.

Small, M. P., and Carrion, H. H.: A new penile prosthesis for treating impotence. Contemp. Surg., 7:29, 1975.

Smith, A. D.: Psychologic factors in the multidisciplinary evaluation and treatment of erectile dysfunction. Urol. Clin. North Am., 15:41, 1988.

Snyder, P. J., and Lawrence, D. A.: Treatment of male hypogonadism with testosterone enanthate. J. Clin. Endocrinol. Metab., 51:1335, 1980.

Sohn, M., Wein, B., Sikora, R., Bohndorf, K., Dahms, S., and Jakse, G.: The correlation of selective and superselective dynamic pharmaco-angiography of penile vessels to intraoperative finding during penile revascularization. Int. J. Impotence Res., 2:Supplement 2, 354, 1990.

Spark, R. F., White, R. A., and Connolly, P. B.: Impotence is not always psychogenic: newer insights into hypothalamic-pituitary-gonadal dysfunction. JAMA, 243:750, 1980.

Spratt, D. I., O'Dea, L. S. T. L., Schoenfeld, D., Butler, J., Rao, P. N., and Crowley, W. F.: Neuroendocrine-gonadal axis in men: frequent sampling of LH, FSH, and testosterone. Am. J. Physiol. (Endocrinol. Metab. 17), E658, 1988.

Stackl, W., Hasun, R., and Marberger, M.: Intracavernous injection of prostaglandin E_1 in impotent men. J. Urol., 140:66, 1988.

Stief, C. G., Djamilian, M., Schaebsdau, F., Truss, M. C., Schlick, R. W., Abicht, J. H., Allhoff, E. P., and Jonas, U.: Single potential analysis of cavernous electric activity—a possible diagnosis of autonomic impotence? World J. Urol., 8:75, 1990.

Stief, C. G., Thon, W. F., Djamilian, M., Schaebsdam, F., and Jonas, U.: Single potential analysis of cavernous electric activity: a possible diagnosis of autonomic cavernous dysfunction and of cavernous smooth muscle degeneration. Int. J. Impotence Res., 2:Supplement 2, 91, 1990.

Szele, F. G., Murphy, D. L., and Garrick, N. A.: Fenfluramine, m-chlorophenylpiperazine and other serotonin re-uptake agonists and antagonists on penile erections in non-human primates. Life Sci., 43:1297–1303, 1988.

Thase, M. E., et al.: Nocturnal penile tumescence is diminished in depressed men. Biol. Psychiatry, 24:33, 1988.

Torrens, M. J.: Neurologic and neurosurgical disorders associated with impotence. In Krane, R. J., Siroky, M. B., Goldstein, I. (Eds.). Male Sexual Dysfunction. Boston, Little, Brown and Co., 1983, p. 55.

Trapp, J. D.: Pharmacologic erection program for the treatment of male impotence. South. Med. J., 80:426, 1987.

Turini, D., Barbanti, G., Beneforti, P., Canavaro, G., Misuri, D.: Experimental study on an implantable drug delivery system in the treatment of erectile dysfunction. In Proceedings of the Sixth Biennial International Symposium for Corpus Cavernosum Revascularization and Third Biennial World Meeting on Impotence. Boston, October 6, 1988, p. 93.

Vaccari, R., Zucca, R., and Scuzzarella, S.: The cavernoiontophoresis in the therapy of erectile impotence. Int. J. Impotence Res., 2:Supplement 2, 338, 1990.

Vardi, Y., Lidgi, S., and Levin, D. R.: Intracavernous pO_2 response to vasoactive drugs as an indicator of corporal vascular dysfunction. Int. J. Impotence Res., 2:Supplement 2, 242, 1990.

Virag, R.: Intracavernous injection of papaverine for erectile failure. Lancet, 1:938, 1982a.

Virag, R.: Revascularization of the penis. In Bennett, A.H. (Ed.). Management of Male Impotence. Baltimore, Williams & Wilkins, 1982b, pp. 219–233.

Virag, R., Bouilly, P., and Frydaman, D.: Is impotence an arterial disorder? A study of arterial risk factors in 400 impotent men. Lancet, 1:181, 1985.

Virag, R., Zwang, G., Dermange, H., and Legman, M.: Vasculogenic impotence: a review of 92 cases with 54 surgical operations. Vasc. Surg., 15:9, 1981.

Wagner, G., Gerstenberg, T., and Levin, R. J.: Electrical activity of corpus cavernosum during flaccidity and erection of the human penis. J. Urol., 142:723, 1989.

Waldhauser, M., and Schramek, P.: Efficiency and side effects of prostaglandin E_1 in the treatment of erectile dysfunction. J. Urol., 140:525, 1988.

Walker, T. G., Grant, P. W., Goldstein, I., Krane, R. J., and Greenfield, A. J.: High-flow priapism: Treatment with superselective transcatheter embolization. Radiology, 174:1053–1054, 1990.

Walsh, P. C., and Donker, P. J.: Impotence following radical prostatectomy: Insight into etiology and prevention. J. Urol., 128:492, 1982.

Ware, J. C.: Evaluation of impotence. Monitoring periodic penile erections during sleep. Psychiatric Clin. North Am. 10:675, 1987.

Washecka, R., and Zorgniotti, A.: Non-correlation of penile brachial index to angiograms. In Proceedings of the Sixth Biennial International Symposium for Corpus Cavernosum Revascularization and Third Biennial World Meeting on Impotence. Boston, October 6, 1988, p. 31.

Wein, A. J., and van Arsdalen, K.: Drug-induced male sexual dysfunction. Urol. Clin. North Am., 15:23, 1988.

Wein, A. J., Fishkin, R., Carpiniello, V. L., et al.: Expansion without significant rigidity during nocturnal penile tumescence testing: A potential source of misinterpretation. J. Urol., 126:343, 1981.

Wespes, E.: Penile venous surgery for cavernovenous impotence. World J. Urol., 8:97–100, 1990.

Wespes, E., Depierreux, M., and Schulman, C. C.: Use of Biopty gun for cavernous biopsy. Int. J. Impotence Res., 2:Supplement 2, 228, 1990.

Wespes, E., and Schulman, C. C.: Venous leakage: Surgical treatment of a curable cause of impotence. J. Urol., 133:796, 1984.

Wespes, E., and Schulman, C. C.: Hemodynamic study of the effect of vacuum device on human erection. Int. J. Impotence Res., 2:Supplement 2, 337, 1990.

Wilson, J. D., George, F. W., and Griffen, J. E.: The hormonal control of sexual development. Science, 211:1278, 1981.

Wilson, J. D., and Griffin, J. E.: The use and misuse of androgens. Metabolism, 29:1278, 1982.

Witherington, R.: Suction device therapy in the management of erectile impotence. Urol. Clin. North Am., 15:123, 1988.

Witherington, R.: Vacuum constriction device for management of erectile impotence. J. Urol., 141:320, 1989.

Witherington, R.: External penile appliances for management of impotence. Semin. Urol., 8:124–218, 1990.

Witt, M. A., Goldstein, I., Saenz de Tejada, I., Greenfield, A., and Krane, R. J.: Traumatic laceration of intracavernosal arteries: The pathophysiology of nonischemic, high flow, arterial priapism. J. Urol., 143:129, 1990.

Wyndaele, J. J., De Meyer, J. M., de Sy, W. A., and Claessens, H.: Intracavernous injection of vasoactive drugs, an alternative for treating impotence in spinal cord injury patients. Paraplegia, 24:271, 1986.

Zentgraf, M., Baccouche, M., and Jünemann, K. P.: Diagnosis and therapy of erectile dysfunction using papaverine and phentolamine. Urol. Int., 43:65, 1988.

Zorgniotti, A. W., and Lefleur, R. S.: Auto-injection of the corpus cavernosum with a vasoactive drug combination for vasculogenic impotence. J. Urol., 133:39, 1985.

Zorgniotti, A. W., Padula, G., and Shaw, W.: Selective arteriography for vascular impotence. World J. Urol., 1:213, 1983.

Surgical shunting procedures should be considered if the presumptive diagnosis is veno-occlusive priapism and if the medical therapy for veno-occlusive priapism has failed.

Priapism, a prolonged erection not associated with sexual stimulation, may require urgent evaluation if a closed compartment syndrome develops with compression of the cavernosal arteries and resultant corporal ischemia. Veno-occlusive priapism results from persistent obstruction of lacunar space venous outflow. The lack of outflow once the corporal bodies have been fully expanded impedes arterial blood inflow leading to ischemia and pain. Fibrosis of the corpora cavernosa secondary to ischemic necrosis can lead to permanent impotence. Obstruction of lacunar space outflow can be secondary to the extravascular compression of subtunical venules or, more rarely, to intravascular obstruction of the draining veins. Corporal pain and tenderness are characteristic symptoms of veno-occlusive priapism. The status of flow in the cavernosal artery should be established by Doppler ultrasonography or by examination of the corporal blood aspirate in all patients with priapism. Absence of cavernosal artery pulsations or blood gas determinations of the corporal aspirate demonstrating hypoxemia and acidosis are pathognomonic of veno-occlusive priapism.

Medical management of veno-occlusive priapism consists initially of corporal aspiration and corporal irrigation with heparinized saline. If this therapy is unsuccessful in re-establishing arterial inflow, intracavernosal adrenergic agonist administration should be utilized to pharmacologically contract the corporal smooth muscle. If arterial inflow is not re-established, as evidenced by persistent or recurrent dark corporal aspirates, medical management should be considered unsuccessful. Surgical shunting to the glans or corpus spongiosum should then be performed. The aim of all priapism management, medical or surgical, is to re-establish arterial blood inflow to the erectile tissue by augmenting drainage from the corpora cavernosa (Lue et al., 1986 and 1988; Padma-Nathan et al., 1986).

CORPOROGLANULAR SHUNT

Winter (1976) described a procedure in which a percutaneous communication is established between the distal corpus cavernosum and the spongiosum tissue of the glans penis. This fistula provides a path for venous outflow from the corpora, thereby, eliminating the condition for the closed compartment syndrome. In the presence of venous outflow, arterial inflow may subsequently return.

Utilizing local anesthesia with lidocaine, a large-bore needle attached to a syringe is inserted through the glans away from the meatus in the dorsal midline into one corporal body. Corporal aspiration and, if necessary, saline irrigation of the corporal tissue are performed. When the aspirate becomes bright red, the needle is withdrawn and a biopsy needle is reinserted. Multiple core biopsy samples are taken from the distal end of the corporal body in order to create multiple corporoglanular fistulas. The skin puncture wound is closed with an absorbable chromic suture (Winter, 1978).

Alternative corpus glanular shunts have been reported. Ebbehoj (1975) described the insertion of a narrow-blade scalpel knife into the glans to create a fistulous opening of the distal tip of the corpus cavernosum. In this procedure, no core is removed. However, the scalpel blade is rotated 90 degrees to obtain a larger fistulous communication. Ebbehoj later described a similar procedure in which the scalpel was advanced into the corpora at the lower coronal ridge, thus avoiding the glans incision.

Ercole and colleagues in 1981 reported a modification of the previously described shunts that offered the ability to directly visualize and control the size of the fistulous communication between the tips of the corpora cavernosa and the glans. After placing a tourniquet over the base of the penis, a 2-cm transverse incision is fashioned on the dorsal glans, approximately 1 cm distal to the coronal edge. The distal ends of each corpora are dissected from the spongiosum tissue in the glans and are tagged with a heavy stay suture. A 5 × 5–mm segment of the tip of each tunica is excised sharply. It is important, with this procedure, to identify both corporal tips before the first distal tunica incision. Detumescence may result quickly, and the second exposure of the corporal tips may become quite difficult. After corporal irrigation, the fistulous connections are left in place with the skin incision closed with an absorbable suture.

CORPUS SPONGIOSUM SHUNT

In veno-occlusive priapism that has progressed for several days, the distal corpus cavernosum may be the most susceptible to the adverse effects of the persistent ischemia simply because of the long distance the cavernosal artery must travel. Therefore, distally placed shunts may not provide adequate drainage because of tissue edema or fibrosis.

If severe tissue changes are noted distally at the time of the distal shunt, simultaneous creation of a second more proximally located corpus spongiosum shunt should be considered. This procedure was originally described by Quackels in 1964, 12 years before the Winter procedure was first reported. The corpus spongiosum shunt operation requires more surgical dissection than the previously described distal shunts and has the potential for creating a urethrocavernous fistula. As a result, the proximal corpus spongiosum shunt is commonly performed in the surgical management of priapism if the distal shunt fails.

The principle is to utilize the thickest portion of the corpus spongiosum to avoid a urethral fistula and that

3071

implies performing the shunt as proximally as possible. A Foley catheter is utilized to help localize the urethra. The skin incision may be perineal, transverse scrotal, or penoscrotal. Following the skin incision, the corpus spongiosum and the corpus cavernosum are isolated for a distance of at least 3 cm. A 2-cm longitudinal incision is made in the medial side of the tunica albuginea of the corpus cavernosum. This incision can be widened slightly, taking a small ellipse of either side of the tunica for approximately 1 cm. A second 2-cm longitudinal incision is fashioned in the lateral aspect of the tunica of the corpus spongiosum exactly opposite the previous incision, which may also be widened into a 1-cm ellipse. Care is taken not to incise the urethra. This fistula is fashioned with continuous 4-0 nonabsorbable suture on a tapered needle. If one shunt does not result in detumescence, a contralateral one can be performed but at a slightly different level to avoid tension on the suture line.

CORPUS SAPHENOUS SHUNT

Grayhack and co-workers (1964) described a corpus saphenous shunt that established return of lacunar venous blood to the systemic venous circulation via the saphenous vein. The procedure first employs skin incisions on the groin overlying the saphenous vein. Approximately 10 cm of vein is carefully harvested, leaving the attachment to the femoral vein intact. The saphenous vein is brought through a subcutaneous tunnel in the groin to a second incision at the base of the penis. An ellipse of tunica albuginea of the corpus cavernosum approximately 1 1/2 times the size of the lumen of the saphenous vein is created. The saphenous vein is spatulated, and the corpus saphenous anastomosis is created with 5-0 nonabsorbable suture.

SUMMARY

Complications associated with surgical shunting for veno-occlusive priapism are unusual. Compressing cuffs or tight dressings applied after the creation of shunts may produce undesired cavernosal or dorsal artery occlusion leading to further ischemia and possibly to penile gangrene and skin necrosis. Venous drainage may also be impaired, thus possibly contributing to priapism recurrence. Infection of the shunt can result in either glans loss or proximal shaft loss depending on the procedure.

REFERENCES

Surgery of Priapism

Ebbehoj, J.: A new operation for priapism. Scand. J. Plast. Reconst. Surg., 8:241, 1975.

Ercole, C. J. J., Pontes, J. E., and Pierce, J. M.: Changing surgical concepts in the treatment of priapism. J. Urol, 125:210–211, 1981.

Grayhack, J. T., McCullough, W., O'Connor, V. J. Jr., and Trippel, O.: Venous bypass to control priapism. Invest. Urol., 1:509–513, 1964.

Lue, T. F., Hellstrom, W. J. G., McAninch, J. W., and Tanagho, E. A.: Priapism: A refined approach to diagnosis and treatment. J. Urol., 136:104–108, 1986.

Lue, T. F., and McAnnich, J. W.: Priapism. In Tanagho, E. A., Lue, T. F., and McClure, R. D. (Eds.). Contemporary Management of Impotence and Infertility. Baltimore, Williams & Wilkins, 1988.

Padma-Nathan, H., Goldstein, I., and Krane, R. J.: Treatment of prolonged or priapistic erections following intracavernosal papaverine therapy. Semin. Urol. 4:236, 1986.

Quackels, R.: Cure d'un cas de priapisme par anastomose caverno-sospongieuse. Act. Urol. Belg., 32:5, 1964.

Winter, C. C.: Cure for idiopathic priapism. New procedure for creating fistula between glans penis and corpora cavernosa. Urology, 8:389, 1976.

Winter, C. C.: Priapism cured by creation of fistulas between glans penis and corpora cavernosa. J. Urol., 119:227, 1978.

85
SURGERY OF PENILE AND URETHRAL CARCINOMA

Harry W. Herr, M.D.

Carcinoma arising from the prepuce, glans, or shaft of the penis often remains localized for prolonged periods. When metastasis occurs, it follows a stepwise pattern—first to the inguinal (groin) lymph nodes and second to the pelvic lymph nodes. Distant dissemination is usually later. A favorable natural history permits surgical cure of most localized penile cancers and of many with inguinal metastases.

Urethral carcinoma in both males and females, in comparison, tends to invade locally and to metastasize to adjacent soft tissues, regional lymph nodes, and distant sites early in its evolution. Most of these tumors are far advanced locally when diagnosed. This feature accounts for the overall poor prognosis of urethral cancer despite aggressive surgical procedures.

ANATOMIC CONSIDERATIONS

The lymphatic anatomy of the penis and its cutaneous envelopes has been thoroughly studied (Rouviere, 1938). The lymphatics of the prepuce and penile skin converge on the dorsum of the penis and coalesce into several trunks. Coursing together toward the base of the penis, these trunks separate to terminate bilaterally in the superficial inguinal nodes, particularly the superomedial group. The lymphatics decussate at the base of the penis accounting for unilateral and, on occasion, bilateral regional node involvement.

The network of lymphatics arising from the glans penis is more complex. All the lymphatics of the glans initially converge on the frenulum. They then ascend along the corona to pass onto the dorsum of the penis as one to four larger collecting trunks. The termination of these trunks is a matter of some debate. The superomedial group of superficial inguinal lymph nodes on either side can act as the first lymphoid echelon for lymphatics originating in the glans penis (Cabanas, 1977). Alternate pathways that terminate in nodes of the deep inguinal, external iliac, or hypogastric region have been described, but a direct lymphatic route from the penis to the pelvic lymph nodes has not (Riveros et al., 1967; Sen et al., 1967).

The corporal bodies are drained by lymphatic trunks that course beside the dorsal vein of the penis to a presymphyseal plexus. There, they anastomose and may join the previously described pathway to the inguinal region. Direct drainage to the deep inguinal and external iliac regions has also been demonstrated.

The lymphatic anatomy of the male urethra includes a rich mucosal network that extends throughout the length of the urethra and is particularly abundant in the region of the fossa navicularis. This network is continuous posteriorly with that of the prostate and bladder and anteriorly with that of the penis. Collecting ducts arise from the mucosal plexus to join with those from the glans and shaft in the anterior urethra and pass to the superficial inguinal nodes via the presymphyseal plexus. Those collecting ducts of the bulbomembranous urethra course through the urogenital diaphragm to join prostatic and bladder lymphatics and terminate in the obturator and medial external iliac nodes. The scrotum has abundant lymphatic channels that anastomose freely along the medial raphe. Superiorly, trunks arise in the region of the median raphe and course around the base of the penis to terminate in the superomedial group of the superficial inguinal nodes. Inferiorly, the trunks initially pass transversely and upward and then along the genitofemoral sulcus to the inferomedial group of superficial inguinal nodes. The abundance and free intercommunication of the scrotal lymphatics necessitates a very wide local excision of a primary carcinoma involving the scrotum.

In the female, the lymphatics of the proximal urethra course to the external iliac, hypogastric, and obturator nodes with the collecting ducts from the bladder and vagina. Lymphatic channels of the distal urethra and meatus freely communicate with vulvar lymphatics and course toward the mons veneris to terminate in the superomedial group of the superficial inguinal nodes.

Inguinal metastases may be seen, therefore, from distal urethral cancers. With proximal urethral cancers, inguinal metastases are the result of retrograde spread from extensive pelvic lymph node involvement.

HISTOLOGIC CORRELATES

The pattern of progression of a particular malignancy can vary with its histology and can have an impact on specific therapeutic considerations. Squamous carcinoma of the penis slowly enlarges, invades, produces significant local destruction, and embolizes through the local lymphatics to the regional lymph nodes of the groin and pelvis in an orderly fashion. In general, the skin of the penis and prepuce drain primarily into the superficial inguinal nodes and the glans and corpora into the superficial and deep inguinal and iliac nodes. Pathologic evaluation of the resected primary tumor often fails to show permeated lymphatic channels justifying the separate management of the primary tumor and its regional drainage. This unusual circumstance, unlike melanoma, for example, that manifests in transit lymphatic extensions, contributes to surgical cures in patients with regional metastases. This approach is supported by wide clinical experience.

Adenocarcinoma of the female urethra generally arises from the proximal urethra or periurethral glans and tends to be a locally aggressive and highly metastatic lesion. Adenocarcinoma, on occasion, may arise within a urethral diverticulum without adjacent soft tissue or urethral involvement. Location within a diverticulum may allow successful local excision. Squamous carcinoma may involve the entire female urethra or may be localized to the distal third. The distal squamous carcinoma tends to remain localized and amenable to surgical cure by distal urethrectomy.

Secondary transitional cell carcinoma generally involves the urethra as a manifestation of bladder carcinoma. Routine en bloc urethrectomy in the male at the time of cystectomy for transitional cell carcinoma removes current or future sites of tumor formation and may improve local control by obviating tumor cell spillage with transection of the membranous urethra. This maneuver is associated with a slight increase in operative time, morbidity, and blood loss but simplifies postcystectomy follow-up management. Incontinuity urethrectomy is indicated for bladder tumors that involve the bladder neck or prostatic urethra. Total en bloc urethrectomy is routinely included as part of a radical cystectomy in the female.

NONSURGICAL TREATMENT

The therapeutic alternatives in carcinoma of the penis and of the male and female urethra are varied and depend on the extent of the disease. For a given stage of disease, the application of a particular modality depends on factors such as available soft tissue margin, acceptance by the patient, previous therapy, general condition of the patient, and personal bias of the treating physician.

Cancer of the Penis

In situ lesions of the penis may be effectively controlled with topical chemotherapy (Goette, 1976). 5-Fluorouracil (5-FU) cream (Efudex, 5 per cent) applied to superficial lesions twice daily for 2 to 4 weeks is preferred. A biopsy is necessary after 2 months to confirm the response. Excisional biopsy findings may help provide both diagnosis and cure in selected cases. Radiotherapy has also been successfully applied to in situ carcinoma of the penis (Kelley et al., 1974; Mantell and Morgan, 1969). Prophylaxis, however, is not afforded by any of these modalities, and careful follow-up is mandatory.

Radiotherapy for penis cancer has obvious psychologic and cosmetic advantages over surgery, particularly for invasive lesions. Many forms of delivery have been successfully applied, including radium and iridium mould and interstitial and megavoltage external beam techniques. Whereas local control increases with external beam therapy compared with mould techniques, morbidity increases as well (e.g., meatal stenosis, urethral stricture, penile pain, and radionecrosis). Pretreatment circumcision and generous meatotomy are mandatory to minimize acute inflammatory complications, such as phimosis, paraphimosis, and balanitis. Therapy is more morbid if there is associated infection. The high doses of radiation required to cure invasive lesions may result in a "woody," painful organ that is neither cosmetically acceptable nor functional.

Tumor persistence after irradiation is much more common than new tumor formation (Grabstald and Kelley, 1980). Locally recurrent carcinoma ranges from 10 to 50 per cent, depending on lesion size, invasion depth, and radiation technique. Salvage penectomy is often successful therapy for patients who have failed primary irradiation (El-Demiry et al., 1984) or who have debilitating complications (e.g., radionecrosis and pain).

Time to regression of a penile cancer treated by irradiation may be prolonged. Up to 12 months of observation may be required to verify local control (Pointon, 1975). With palpable inguinal adenopathy, a more expedient form of primary therapy, namely surgery, is appropriate.

Cryosurgery has been successfully utilized for verrucous carcinoma of the penis with anatomic and functional preservation of the penis (Carson, 1978; Hughes, 1979).

Cancer of the Male Urethra

Intraurethral instillation of 5-FU, podophyllin, thiotepa, colchicine, and bleomycin has been reported for extensive condyloma acuminatum (Danoff et al., 1981). Thiotepa, 5-FU and bacillus Calmette-Guérin (BCG) have been used with minimum morbidity as adjuncts for low-grade, superficial urethra cancer arising primarily or secondarily after successful bladder cancer management (Bretton and Herr, 1989; Konnak, 1980; Leissner and Johansson, 1980). Concomitant transurethral resection probably plays a primary role, particularly with lesions of the posterior urethra where prostatic tissue may be safely sacrificed.

Radiotherapy for this lesion is palliative. Bulbomembranous tumors are often sizable, regionally metastatic, and incurable at presentation. Some early distal urethral cancers have been controlled with external beam irradiation alone or judiciously combined with intraurethral radium (Billingwood and Million, 1983; Raghavaiah, 1978).

Cancer of the Female Urethra

Radiotherapy is a proven modality in female urethral cancer arising in the distal segment. External beam, intracavitary, and interstitial or combination radiotherapy techniques have been effective (Grabstald et al., 1966; Prempree et al., 1984). Distal urethral tumors are controlled equally satisfactorily by simple excision. Lesions of the entire urethra are difficult to eradicate by either surgery or radiotherapy, prompting a combination radiation-chemotherapy trial (Bracken et al., 1976; Johnson and O'Connell, 1983).

ADJUNCTS TO SURGICAL TREATMENT

Cytotoxic agents with demonstrated activity, alone or in combination, in metastatic penile carcinoma include bleomycin (Ichikawa et al., 1969; Kyalwazi et al., 1974; Yagoda et al., 1972), methotrexate (Garnik et al., 1979; Sclaroff and Yagoda, 1980), and cisplatin (Sklaroff and Yagoda, 1979). 5-FU with cisplatin is being used in clinical trials. Adjuvant chemotherapy in carcinoma of the penis has not yet been initiated but would seem logical for patients with poor prognostic features, such as multiple metastatic lymph nodes.

Preoperative chemotherapy (cisplatin, 5-FU, bleomycin) for locally extensive groin metastasis from penile carcinoma may render some inoperable lesions resectable and may improve soft tissue margins. Similarly, M-VAC (methotrexate, vinblastine, adriamycin, and cisplatin) chemotherapy may improve the surgical therapy of invasive male and female urethral cancers; in some cases, M-VAC may permit less radical surgery (Scher et al., 1988). M-VAC is effective only against transitional cell carcinoma and not against squamous carcinoma or adenocarcinoma. The fact that bulky groin metastases from penile cancers and locally advanced invasive urethral cancers are apt to recur locally, even after aggressive surgical excision, fosters the application of chemotherapy and radiation therapy adjuncts to improve control.

SURGICAL TREATMENT

Penis Cancer

Primary Tumors

TISSUE CONFIRMATION. Histologic verification of penis cancer is the essential first step to staging and the formulation of a treatment plan. Tumors of the penis lend themselves to convenient excisional, incisional, or needle aspiration or to punch biopsy. Adjacent normal tissue should be included to provide a demonstration of the invasion, a critical differential point with regard to planning definitive surgery.

General Considerations

Superficial lesions of the prepuce can be successfully excised primarily by circumcision with adjustment for adequate margins. The patients so affected are prone to local recurrences; therefore, new tumor formation must be followed closely (Hardner et al., 1972; Jensen, 1977; Narayana, 1982). Carefully selected superficial lesions of the skin of the penile shaft can also be simply excised. Excisional biopsy of lesions of the glans penis has not been uniformly successful and may result in a diminished prognosis on recurrence (Ekstrom and Edsmyr, 1958; Hanash et al., 1970).

Superficial or superficially invasive penile cancers may be managed by microsurgical excision using the CO_2 laser (Bandieramonte et al., 1987) or by sharp microexcision (Mohs et al., 1985). The Mohs technique, adopted from the local excision of skin cancers, involves excision of the neoplasm of the penis layer by layer and microscopic examination of the undersurface of each layer by systematic frozen sections. The tumor may be excised using a fresh tissue technique or after a zinc chloride fixative paste has been applied. Multiple (one to seven) daily excisions may be necessary.

Invasive penile cancer not suitable for irradiation, local excision, or micrographic surgery, by virtue of its size, location, depth, or degree of invasion, is best managed by total or partial penectomy. Attainment of a 2-cm gross tumor margin affords excellent local control (Dean, 1952). Local recurrence after a properly performed partial or total penectomy is rare. Penile length sufficient to permit upright and directable micturition may be retained after partial penectomy. At least 3 cm of proximal shaft should be available for consideration of this technique. In selected cases in which the residual stump is of inadequate length (<2 cm from penoscrotal junction), its mobilization from the suspensory ligament and transposition to the perineum can supply additional length to allow directed voiding (deSouza, 1976). Total penectomy is necessary when adequate tumor margin precludes conservative resection.

Penile reconstruction is feasible following partial and total penectomy. However, sexual, urinary, and cosmetic considerations need to be evaluated. Both single and multistage procedures (McDougal and Koch, 1989; Mukherjee, 1980) have been described for reconstruction following total loss of the phallus.

For extensive, proximal invasive lesions or for involvement of the scrotum, perineum, abdominal wall, or pubis, it may be necessary to perform emasculation, incontinuity cystectomy, or resection of the pubic arch (Shuttleworth and Lloyd-Davies, 1969), pubic symphysis (Mackenzie and Whitmore, 1968), or portions of the abdominal wall (Arconte and Goodwin, 1956; Bracken and Grabstald, 1975; Skinner, 1974).

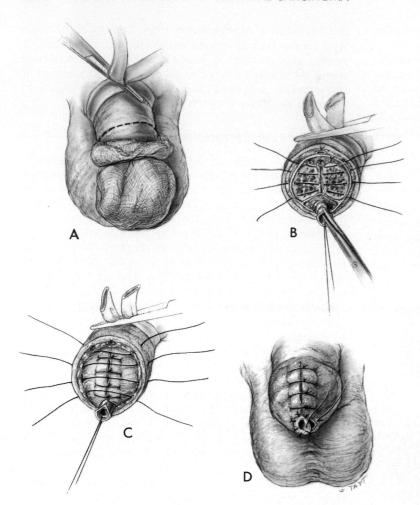

Figure 85–1. Partial penectomy. *A* and *B,* After exclusion of the lesion from the field, the corpora are divided with a 2-cm gross margin.

C, The dorsal vessels are ligated, the cut margins of the tunica albuginea approximated, and the urethra spatulated.

D, Simple skin closure and urethral meatus formation complete the procedure.

SPECIFIC SURGICAL TECHNIQUES

Partial Penectomy

Successful local control by partial penectomy depends on division of the penis 2 cm proximal to the gross tumor extent (Fig. 85–1). After the lesion is excluded by a towel or surgical glove secured along the proposed line of amputation, a tourniquet is applied at the base of the penis. The skin is incised circumferentially, and the cavernous bodies are divided sharply to the urethra. The dorsal vessels are ligated, and the urethra is dissected proximally and distally to attain a 1-cm distal redundancy. The urethra is divided without sacrifice of the tumor margin, and the corpora are secured with interrupted sutures opposing the margins of Buck's fascia. The tourniquet is removed, and additional hemostasis is obtained as necessary. The urethra is spatulated on both its dorsal and ventral surfaces. A skin-urethra anastomosis is performed using 3-0 or 4-0 chromic or Dexon absorbable suture material. The redundant skin is approximated dorsally to complete the closure (Pack and Ariel, 1963). A small urinary catheter is placed and a light dressing applied. Both may be removed the following day.

Modified Partial Penectomy

When the penile stump after partial penectomy is too short for directing the urinary stream, further length can be obtained by releasing the corpora from the suspensory ligament, dividing the ischiocavernosus muscle, and partially separating the crura from the undersurface of the pubic rami. The scrotum is incised along the raphe, and skin flaps are fashioned for penile coverage. The testes are secured in subcutaneous pouches, and the scrotum is reconstructed cephalad to the transposed phallus (deSouza, 1976).

Total Penectomy

The urethra is transposed to the perineum if the size of the primary lesion precludes a partial penectomy (Fig. 85–2). After appropriate draping of the primary lesion, an elliptic incision is made around the base of the penis. Dissection along the corpora is performed with division of the suspensory ligament and dorsal vessels. The urethra is dissected sharply from the corpora to the bulbar region. This dissection is aided by distal division of the urethra and ventral traction. The

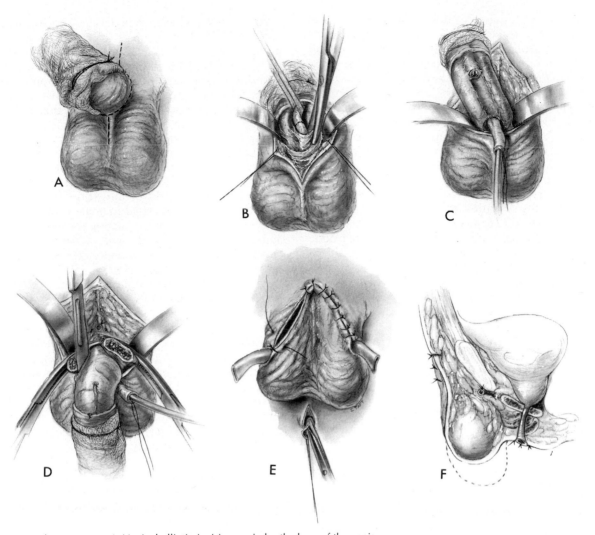

Figure 85–2. Total penectomy. *A*, Vertical elliptic incision encircles the base of the penis.
  B, The urethra is isolated at least 2 cm proximal to the gross lesion.
  C, The suspensory ligament has been divided. The urethra is transected and dissected from the corpora.
  D, The dorsal vessels are ligated, and the crura are transected with the stumps ligated.
  E, A button of perineal skin is excised, and the urethra is transposed and spatulated to form the perineal urethrostomy.
  F, Horizontal closure of the primary incision with drainage serves to elevate the scrotum away from the urinary stream.

corpora are further dissected from their attachments to the inferior pubic rami, divided, and ligated with chromic sutures.

A 1-cm ellipse of skin is removed from the region of the perineal body and a tunnel created bluntly in the perineal subcutaneous tissue. The urethra is grasped and transposed through the perineum without angulation. Spatulation of the urethra and skin-to-urethra anastomosis are performed. The primary incision is closed superiorly, with drainage transversely to elevate the scrotum away from the new meatus. A urethral catheter is placed and the wound dressed.

REGIONAL DISEASE

Anatomic Considerations

The inguinal lymph nodes are divided into superficial and deep groups, which are anatomically separated by the deep fascia of the thigh—the fascia lata. The superficial group of nodes is composed of four to 25 glands (average of eight), which are situated in the deep membranous layer of the superficial fascia of the thigh—Camper's fascia (Daseler et al., 1948). The superficial group drains to the two or three deep inguinal nodes that lie along the femoral vessels within the femoral sheath. The node of Cloquet is the most cephalad of this deep group and is situated within the femoral canal (medial to the femoral vein). The external iliac lymph nodes receive drainage from the deep inguinal, obturator, and hypogastric groups. In turn, drainage progresses to the common iliac and para-aortic nodes.

The blood supply to the skin of the inguinal region derives from branches of the common femoral artery—the superficial external pudendal, the superficial circumflex iliac, and the superficial epigastric arteries. Complete inguinal dissection necessitates ligation of these branches. Viability of the skin flaps raised during the dissection depends on anastomotic vessels in the superficial fatty layer of Camper's fascia that course parallel to the natural skin lines. Because lymphatic drainage of the penis to the groin runs beneath Camper's fascia, this layer can be preserved and left attached to the overlying skin in fashioning the superior and inferior skin flaps. This technique prevents serious skin slough, especially if an oblique incision with a removal of an ellipse of skin overlying adherent nodes is employed. Such incision least disrupts the collateral circulation and best preserves vascular integrity to the reapproximated skin margins. The femoral nerve lies deep to the iliacus fascia and supplies motor function to the pectineus, quadriceps femoris, and sartorius muscles. In addition, this nerve provides cutaneous sensation to the anterior thigh and should be preserved. However, some of the sensory branches are commonly sacrificed in the regional node dissection.

The femoral triangle, the area that contains the pertinent lymphatic groups, is bounded by the inguinal ligaments superiorly, the sartorius laterally, and the adductor longis medially. The floor of the triangle is composed of the pectineus medially and the iliopsoas laterally.

Clinical Correlates

The controversy persists regarding the timing of regional lymphadenectomy in the management of penile carcinoma.

Approximately 30 to 60 per cent of patients with penile carcinomas present with palpable inguinal lymphadenopathy. After treatment of the primary lesion and resolution of the lymphadenitis, half of these patients will have metastatic deposits at node dissection. The likelihood of metastatic disease within palpable adenopathy is increased when the primary lesion is sizable, high grade, or not inflamed; when it shows stromal, vascular, or lymphatic invasion; or when the regional adenopathy is massive (Bassett, 1952; Johnson et al., 1973; Marcial et al., 1962).

Approximately 5 to 20 per cent of patients with initially uninvolved nodes develop metastatic adenopathy or harbor metastases at prophylactic lymphadenectomy (Beggs and Spratt, 1964; Hardner et al., 1972).

At initial diagnosis, if positive nodes are detected ipsilaterally, metastases are present contralaterally in 60 per cent of cases (Ekstrom and Edsmyr, 1958). When delayed dissection is performed for subsequent adenopathy, metastatic deposits are usually found (85 per cent); if the contralateral groin is clinically negative, subsequent metastatic deposits in that location are uncommonly found (<10 per cent) (Ekstrom and Edsmyr, 1958). No overall survival advantage exists for patients having prophylactic dissections compared with those having secondary therapeutic dissection for delayed lymphadenopathy (Beggs and Spratt, 1964; Ekstrom and Edsmyr, 1958; Johnson et al., 1973). Evidence suggests, however, that if occult micrometastases are completely removed, such patients with minimal metastatic deposits may in fact experience a better survival (Fraley et al., 1989; Srinivas et al., 1987).

A sentinel node concept has been proposed by Cabanas (1977). This involves a limited dissection of the primary "landing" site of regional nodes most likely to be first involved by metastatic penile cancer. When the superior medial superficial inguinal lymph node is negative, all other groin nodes are negative at dissection; when only one node is positive, it is the sentinel node; and when multiple nodes are positive, the sentinel node is always involved as well. Patients with a negative sentinel node biopsy finding can avoid a more extensive dissection with a relatively good prognosis. However, patients with a positive sentinel node biopsy finding still need a radical groin dissection. If the sentinel node only is involved, 5-year survival increases overall from 50 to 70 per cent. This concept needs further clinical confirmation, because patients with negative sentinel node biopsy findings have developed extensive regional metastases (Perinetti et al., 1980).

A modified groin lymphadenectomy has been proposed by Catalona (1988). This procedure offers the advantage of a more therapeutic dissection for patients with limited metastases, allows prognostic stratification of nodal status, and reduces morbidity of the procedure.

Stratification of treatment results, based on the anatomic extent of ilioinguinal nodal involvement by metastatic carcinoma of the penis, shows a 90 per cent survival rate with uninvolved nodes that falls to 70 per cent, 50 per cent, and 20 per cent with metastases to a solitary inguinal node, multiple inguinal nodes, and pelvic nodes, respectively (Cabanas, 1977; Srinivas et al., 1987). Patients with common iliac or para-aortic nodal metastases have not been surgically salvaged. A minimal therapeutic dissection should clear the superficial and deep inguinal as well the external iliac and obturator regions to the common iliac bifurcation.

Patients who cannot be followed are best treated by bilateral radical ileoinguinal lymphadenectomy. In other patients with palpably negative groins, a bilateral modified lymphadenectomy or close observation at 2- to 3-month intervals for at least 3 years is a reasonable option.

SURGICAL OPTIONS

General Considerations

Ilioinguinal lymphadenectomy has been associated with a significant incidence of lymph collection, lymphedema, skin slough, and infection (Table 85–1). In view of this morbidity, many clinicians are reluctant to advise routine groin dissection for penile carcinoma (Grabstald, 1981; Johnson and Lo, 1984; Ray and Guinan, 1979). Others (Fegen and Persky, 1969; Fraley et al., 1989; Hardner et al., 1972) advocate routine prophylactic dissection. These workers believe that this approach will eradicate subclinical disease early and thereby improve the survival rate in this patient group with metastases. Some have performed percutaneous aspiration or excisional biopsy of suspected adenopathy (Edwards and Sawyers, 1968; Hanash et al., 1970) or even clinically negative nodes (DeKernion et al., 1973) to obtain his-

Table 85–1. ILIOINGUINAL NODE DISSECTION

Complication	Incidence	Perioperative Countermeasures
Skin flap necrosis	14–65%	Oblique inguinal incision Skin flap thickness Care in tissue handling Transposition of sartorius muscle Excision of ischemic flap margins
Wound infection	10%	Interval resolution of region inflammation Mechanical bowel preparation Prophylactic antibiotics
Seroma/ lymphedema	19–50%	Ligation of transected lymphatics Transposition of sartorius muscle Closed catheter, suction drainage Immobilization of dissected extremity Elastic support stockings

tologic verification before proceeding with regional lymphadenectomy.

When regional disease has been proved by biopsy (N+) surgical dissection of the ilioinguinal lymph nodes should follow. For penile cancer, if metastatic adenopathy is present in either groin at the time of presentation, bilateral regional node dissections should be done in view of the high incidence of bilateral deposits in this setting. Alternatively, if the regional nodes are judged initially free of disease, the delayed appearance of metastatic adenopathy should prompt ipsilateral dissection alone (Ekstrom and Edsymer, 1958).

Adherence of advanced inguinal disease (N3, N4) to the femoral vessels may require en bloc resection with vascular reconstruction. Autologous tissue is preferable in this repair in view of the potential for suppurative complications. Alternatively, bypass prosthetic grafting through the obturator foramen can successfully revascularize the leg (Cockburn et al., 1982; Dardik et al., 1980). Resection of the femoral nerve, if necessitated by tumor or extension, allows for maintenance of a useful extremity (Cockburn et al., 1982; Whitmore, 1970). After extensive groin dissections, a myocutaneous vascular pedicle or other suitable flap may be required to close the defect. If the soft tissue is extensively involved beyond even an extended radical groin dissection, hemipelvectomy may offer a reasonable chance for control of disease; however, muscle and/or contiguous bone invasion seems to denote incurability (Block et al., 1973).

The pelvic and inguinal dissections may be accomplished in a single stage or two stage procedure. When bilateral groin dissections are required, I prefer a bilateral pelvic dissection and an ipsilateral groin dissection, followed 1 to 2 weeks later with groin dissection of the other side.

A palliative groin dissection may be required even with distant metastasis if the regional adenopathy is judged likely to ulcerate and/or erode the femoral vessels. This prophylactic measure can obviate the development of significant pain, sepsis, and hemorrhage from uncontrolled disease. Further, such a procedure may help preserve the patient's self-image and his relationships with family and friends.

Sentinel Node Biopsy

The location of the saphenofemoral junction is estimated to be at a point two fingerbreadths lateral and inferior to the pubic tubercle. A transverse incision through this point exposes the fossa ovalis and the greater saphenous vein with its medial tributaries—the superficial epigastric and the external pudendal veins (Fig. 85–3). Within the space bounded by these branches, the tissue is excised and submitted for microscopic examination. The superomedial area may contain several nodes, and all should be removed to assure complete sampling. With histologic confirmation of metastatic involvement, complete dissection should be undertaken.

The surgeon should anticipate the direction of the preferred incision for groin dissection so that the biopsy incision may be included with the specimen if the results should dictate a complete ilioinguinal lymphadenectomy.

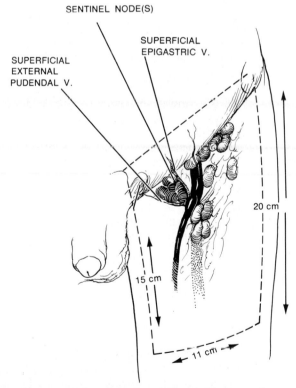

Figure 85–3. Sentinel node biopsy. An incision is centered on a point two fingerbreadths lateral and inferior to the pubic tubercle. The saphenous vein and its medial tributaries are isolated at the fossa ovalis. All fibroadipose node-bearing tissue is removed from this region and submitted for pathologic study. This figure also depicts the topography and dimensions of the quadrangle within which all inguinal nodal tissue is predictably situated. This area can be marked after positioning and draping in order to avoid excessive dissection and excessive compromise of collateral blood supply to the skin flaps. (From Spaulding, J.: In Javadpour, N. (Ed.): Principles and Management of Urologic Cancer. Baltimore, Williams & Wilkins, 1979.)

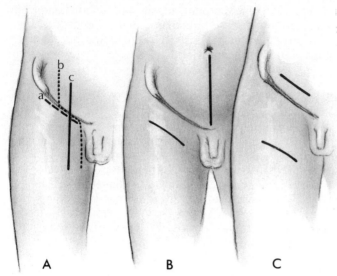

Figure 85–4. *A,* Single incisional approaches include (a) oblique, (b) S-shaped, and (c) vertical techniques.

B, Double incisional techniques may combine a lower midline with an inguinal incision.

C, Alternatively, an oblique abdominal incision may provide unilateral access to the pelvic nodes.

RADICAL ILIOINGUINAL NODE DISSECTION

A 6-week interval following treatment of the penile lesion allows for reduction of any inflammatory component of the regional adenopathy and minimizes the incidence of wound suppuration. Preliminary preparations for regional node dissection include mechanical preparation of the bowel, wearing of elastic support wraps or stockings for the legs, and administration of preoperative antibiotics.

The patient is positioned with the involved thigh slightly abducted and externally rotated. The slightly flexed knee is supported as necessary. A urethral catheter is placed and the scrotum positioned or sutured out of the operative field. A fungating tumor is excluded from the field by suturing a laparotomy sponge to the skin around the lesion prior to the routine skin preparation.

Various incisional approaches to the regional nodes in carcinoma of the penis have been described (Fig. 85–4). For cases that require bilateral dissection, an oblique or elliptic incision below and parallel to the inguinal ligament is commonly used for excision of the superficial and deep inguinal nodes. Addition of a lower midline extraperitoneal incision allows access to the pelvic nodal component and is recommended for bilateral management. Such an approach is preferred because these incisions, coupled with thick skin flaps, virtually eliminate problems of skin necrosis (Whitmore and Vagaiwala, 1984).

A double incisional unilateral approach has been promoted with reported decreased wound morbidity (Fraley and Hutchens, 1972). The inability to conveniently excise a previous biopsy scar or areas of cutaneous involvement is a limitation of the double incision technique. The single oblique incision is recommended for cases that require unilateral dissection.

The inguinofemoral dissection is performed through a separate elliptic incision centered on the saphenofemoral junction at the base of the femoral triangle. The dimensions are determined by the patient's size, and subcutaneous fat distribution and by the features of the inguinal adenopathy. The incision is planned to encompass a liberal soft tissue margin peripheral to metastatic lymph nodes and, simultaneously, to remove the skin at greatest risk of devitalization from dissection.

The elliptic incision extends from the anterosuperior iliac spine toward the pubic tubercle, parallel to the inguinal ligament and usually about 4 to 6 cm. The incision is beveled outward, while it is deepened through the subcutaneous tissue, so that a pyramidal wedge of skin and subcutaneous fat, truncated by the skin surface results. The base of this pyramid rests on the external oblique aponeurosis superiorly, the sartorius muscle laterally, and the adductor muscles medially.

The encompassed fat and areolar tissue are dissected from the external oblique aponeurosis and the spermatic cord to the inferior border of the inguinal ligament. This maneuver usually begins 4 to 5 cm above the level of the inguinal ligament. The inferior angle of the inguinofemoral exposure is at the apex of the femoral triangle, during which dissection the long saphenous vein is identified and divided. Dissection is deepened through the fascia overlying the sartorius muscle laterally and adductor muscle medially. At the apex of the femoral triangle, the femoral artery and vein are identified and dissection continued superiorly along the femoral vessels. The saphenous vein is divided at the saphenofemoral junction and the dissection continued superiorly until continuity with the pelvic dissection is attained at the femoral canal (Fig. 85–5). The anterior and lateral aspects of the femoral vessels are dissected, but the

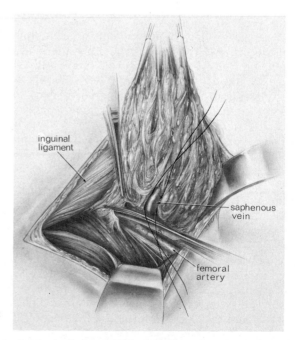

Figure 85–5. The flaps having been dissected, the entire circumference of this area is divided and the ascending lymphatics are ligated. The tissue is mobilized from lateral to medial with exposition and skeletonization of the femoral vessels. Branches and tributaries are sacrificed, including the greater saphenous vein, which is double-ligated at its junction with the common femoral vein.

femoral vessels are not skeletonized nor is the femoral nerve necessarily seen as it will be beneath the iliac fascia.

After dissection of the femoral triangle, the sartorius muscle is mobilized from its origin at the anterior superior spine and either transposed or rolled medially to cover the femoral vessels (Fig. 85–6). Its origin is sutured to the inguinal ligament superiorly, and its margins are sutured to the muscles of the thigh immediately adjacent to the femoral vessels. The femoral canal is closed by suturing the shelving edge of Poupart's ligament to Cooper's ligament, being careful not to compromise the lumen of the external iliac vein or injure the inferior epigastric vessels in the process.

Primary closure of the inguinofemoral dissection, in spite of the skin excision, is usually possible with no or minimal further mobilization of the excision margins. When circumstances demand a particularly large area of inguinal soft tissue sacrifice, primary closure utilizing scrotal skin rotation flaps may suffice. With extensive defects, coverage by a myocutaneous flap is preferred.

The groin dissection is usually drained by a suction catheter placed through a stab wound inferiorly. Light pressure dressings are applied.

Pelvic lymphadenectomy is best accomplished through the lower midline extraperitoneal approach familiar to most urologic surgeons and is not reviewed here. For unilateral dissection, however, there are three basic routes to this region through the recommended single oblique inguinal incision described by Spratt and co-workers (1965). The inguinal ligament can be divided vertically over the vessels or at the anterior superior iliac spine. Another approach is incision of the external oblique fascia and, reflecting the spermatic cord cephalad, division of the inguinal floor from the internal ring to the pubic tubercle, with ligation of the inferior

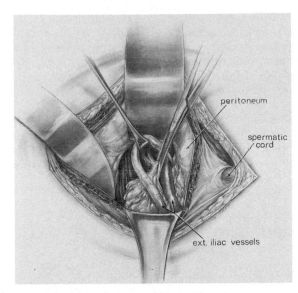

Figure 85–7. When only the ipsilateral pelvic component is to be addressed, access is readily gained to the retroperitoneum through an abdominal incision 4 to 5 cm above and parallel to the inguinal ligament. Nodal tissue is dissected from the iliac vessels, specifically including the external iliac and obturator groups.

epigastric vessels. This maneuver permits wide pelvic and retroperitoneal access. The preferred approach is incision in the anterior abdominal musculature 4 to 5 cm above and parallel to the inguinal ligament with medial mobilization of the peritoneum. This approach widely exposes the iliac region for nodal dissection (Fig. 85–7). The pelvic lymphadenectomy includes the distal common iliac, external iliac, and obturator groups of nodes (Spratt et al., 1965). No further therapeutic benefit is gained from proximal iliac or para-aortic dissection.

The specimen is delivered from the pelvis en bloc through the femoral canal and should be carefully labeled. Alternatively, the inguinal and pelvic components are submitted separately, so that the extent of regional disease can be accurately determined.

Closed-suction catheters are introduced into the area of dissection from a point peripheral to the skin flaps to obliterate dead space and prevent seroma formation. The catheters eliminate the need for compressive dressings over skin flaps. The catheters are removed after 5 to 7 days, when the aspirate volume is negligible and good flap adherence is evident. The skin is closed with fine absorbable sutures without tension. Scrotal flaps may be fashioned to cover some residual groin skin defects. This technique or other rotational or myocutaneous flaps are preferable to primary closure under tension.

Efforts should be made to minimize lymph flow during the initial postoperative period. Thigh length elastic wraps or stockings should be worn. The foot of the bed is elevated slightly. Because the patient should be at bed rest for at least 5 days, postoperative anticoagulation has been recommended (Skinner et al., 1972). The incidence of clinical phlebitis and embolism after this procedure is low. Fortner and associates (1964) noted thrombophlebitis and nonfatal pulmonary embolism in nine and four cases, respectively, among 206 patients with extensive groin dissections. Prophylactic low-dose

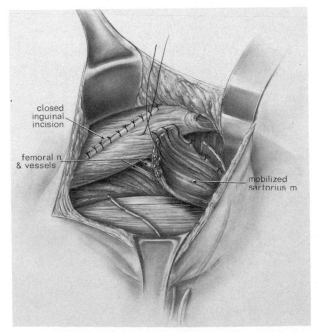

Figure 85–6. Closure of the wound includes repair of the access to the retroperitoneum, transposition of the sartorius muscle, placement of closed suction catheter drainage, and approximation of the skin edges without tension.

heparin therapy has also been recommended (Hindsley et al., 1980; Sogani et al., 1981) but may increase postoperative complications (e.g., prolonged lymphatic drainage, infection, and lymphocele).

A low-residue diet is introduced to minimize fecal contamination. The urinary catheter may be removed on the 1st or 2nd postoperative day. When primary healing appears well established, ambulation can be resumed. Prophylactic application of fitted elastic stockings and limb elevation reduce the incidence and severity of lymphedema following groin dissection (Karakousis et al., 1983).

MODIFIED GROIN LYMPHADENECTOMY

For patients with clinically negative nodes or with equivocally or minimally enlarged nodes, a modified (limited) therapeutic lymphadenectomy has been proposed (Catalona, 1988). This procedure is a compromise between the sentinel lymph node biopsy, which may not be therapeutic for patients with more than one positive node, and the standard extended inguinal lymphadenectomy, which may not be absolutely necessary in patients with minimal regional metastases. The second is also associated with morbidity.

The modified groin dissection (Fig. 85–8) differs from the standard dissection in that (1) the skin incision is shorter; (2) the node dissection is limited, excluding regions lateral to the femoral artery and caudal to the fossa ovalis; (3) the saphenous veins are preserved, and (4) the transposition of the sartorius muscles is eliminated. The dissection is designed to completely remove the superficial inguinal lymph nodes, situated at the anterior and medial aspects of the saphenofemoral junction and the deep inguinal nodes, which are clustered around the femoral vessels situated deep to the fascia lata.

The patient is positioned in a manner similar to that for radical ilioinguinal lymphadenectomy. The skin is opened with a 10-cm incision placed 1.5 cm below the groin crease, deepened to the level of Scarpa's fascia. The superior flap is developed deep to Scarpa's fascia for a distance of about 8 cm. A funiculus of adipose and lymphatic tissue, coursing from the base of the penis to the superficial inguinal lymph nodes, is divided. The spermatic cord is identified and reflected medially. All fibrofatty tissue below this structure is reflected caudally as a "package," which contains the superficial inguinal nodes.

The inferior flap is now developed for a distance of 6 cm below the incision. The saphenous vein is seen in the center of the field, emerging from the package of lymph node–bearing tissue. This tissue is dissected off the fascia lata and the fossa ovalis in the lateral-to-medial fashion. The saphenous vein is carefully preserved. The superficial inguinal lymph nodes are then dissected laterally and off the saphenofemoral junction and surrounding surfaces (Fig. 85–9). As the dissection proceeds, the numerous lymphatic channels encountered are isolated and ligated.

The deep inguinal nodes, clustered around the femoral vessels are dissected superiorly to the level of the inguinal ligament and excised (Fig. 85–10). At the end of the procedure, the saphenofemoral junction is intact. The medial margin of the dissection is the adductor longis muscle; the lateral margin is the femoral artery;

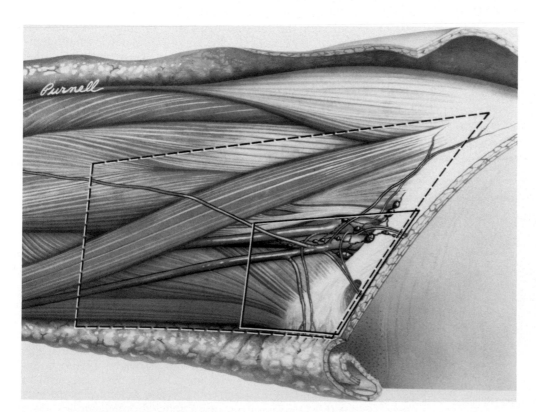

Figure 85–8. Boundaries of the standard ilioinguinal lymph node dissection and the modified (limited) groin dissection.

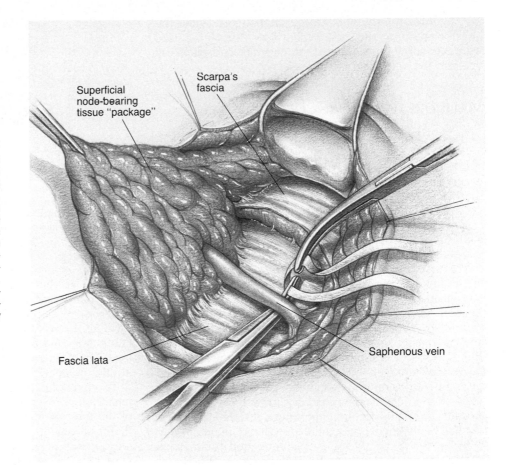

Figure 85–9. Development of the inferior flap has been extended deep to Scarpa's fascia for a distance of approximately 6 cm below the incision. The saphenous vein is seen in the center of the field, emerging from the "package" of lymph node–bearing tissue. This tissue will be dissected off the fascia lata and the fossa ovalis in a lateral-to-medial fashion. (From Catalona, W. J.: Urologic Surgery: Modified Groin Lymphadenopathy for Carcinoma of the Penis. Conferee: Jean B. deKernion. Drawings by William B. Westwood. Courtesy of LTI Medica and Bristol-Myers Company. Copyright 1988 by Learning Technology Incorporated.)

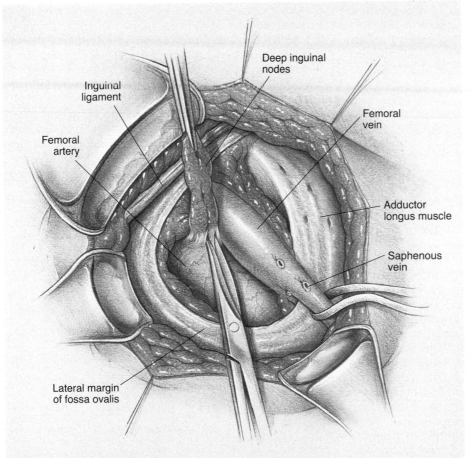

Figure 85–10. The deep inguinal nodes, clustered around the femoral vessels, are dissected out superiorly to the level of the inguinal ligament. (From Catalona, W. J.: Urologic Surgery: Modified Groin Lymphadenopathy for Carcinoma of the Penis. Conferee: Jean B. deKernion. Drawings by William B. Westwood. Courtesy of LTI Medica and Bristol-Myers Company. Copyright 1988 by Learning Technology Incorporated.)

the superior margin is the spermatic cord; and the inferior margin is the fossa ovalis. The incision is closed with skin staples. Suction catheters are placed inferiorly to drain the skin flaps.

MALE URETHRAL CANCER

Primary Tumor

GENERAL CONSIDERATIONS. Urethral tumors occurring at the meatus are simply excised. The entire urethra should be assessed. Urethral tumors not at the meatus can be sampled by transurethral resection or biopsy. Urethral washings may provide the cytologic confirmation of malignancy. A periurethral mass can be sampled by needle or incisional biopsy.

Transurethral resection can be effective therapy for low-grade and superficial lesions of the penile or prostatic urethra (Konnak, 1980; Mullen et al., 1974). For isolated lesions of similar low grade and stage, a segmental urethrectomy with reanastomosis has occasionally been successful (Grabstald, 1973; Kaplan et al., 1967). Invasive lesions of the distal penile urethra are surgically managed by partial penectomy. In selected cases, the corporal bodies may be spared if the invasion seems superficial and limited within the corpus spongiosum. Proximal bulbomembranous lesions are prone to local recurrence, and extended excision, including the pubic arch or symphysis, is recommended to improve primary control (Bracken, 1982; Klein et al., 1983).

Invasive transitional cell carcinoma of the prostatic urethra is an uncommon but aggressive tumor. Management currently consists of radical cystourethrectomy with or without chemotherapy and/or radiotherapy (Grabstald, 1973; Levine, 1980; Scher et al., 1988).

Extended Excision

With proximal urethral lesions or large genital tumors extensively involving the perineum, additional soft tissue clearance is recommended to maximize local control. In addition to en bloc cystectomy, excision of the pubic arch or its subsymphyseal segment has been utilized as a surgical adjunct in these circumstances (Bracken, 1982; Klein et al., 1983; MacKenzie and Whitmore, 1968; Shuttleworth and Lloyd-Davies, 1969).

With the patient in a low lithotomy position to allow perineal access, the standard abdominal mobilization of the bladder is completed, except for preservation of the endopelvic fascia and the anterior pubic attachments. In the male, an inverted U-shaped perineal incision is initiated, based just medial to the ischial tuberosities, with the apex in the mid perineum. The ischiorectal fossae are developed as in perineal prostatectomy and a tunnel is bluntly dissected just anterior to the rectum, extending from one fossa to the other. The inferior skin flap is mobilized by sharply dividing the intervening subcutaneous tissue and rectourethralis muscle.

The superior flap is mobilized by sharply incising the subcutaneous tissue to the superficial Colles fascia. The

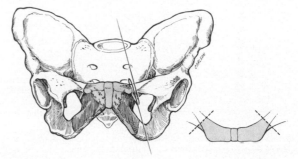

Figure 85–11. The shaded area is excised; beveling as shown facilitates removal of the bony segment. Total symphyseal excision should be considered for all bulky penile and proximal urethral (male and female) lesions. (From Bracken, R. B.: *In* Johnson, D., and Boileau, M. (Eds.): Genitourinary Tumors: Fundamental Principles, New York, Grune & Stratton, 1982.)

dissection is continued bilaterally to the adductor musculature at the inferior pubic rami. Anteriorly, the dissection is carried along the phallus to the penoscrotal junction. Wider exposure, if necessary, results from dividing the scrotum in the midline. Bulky tumors may necessitate sacrifice of portions of the scrotum or perineal skin. The testicles may still be preserved and placed in thigh pouches.

To complete the pubic arch resection, the adductor musculature is sharply divided bilaterally from the length of the inferior pubic ramus along the medial margin of the obturator foramen. A Gigli saw is passed along the inferior ramus just posterior to the origins of the transverse perineal muscles. An inferiorly beveled transection is made bilaterally. The bevel is important to simplify perineal delivery of the specimen. The entire symphysis is resected for bulky urethral lesions involving the presymphyseal tissues and is accomplished by division of the superior rami at their junction with the symphysis. The Gigli saw is introduced and laterally beveled ostomies are completed (Fig. 85–11).

For smaller lesions, the bulk of the symphysis can be preserved with resection of the subsymphyseal arch. This procedure is preferred, where possible, to preserve stability of the pelvic girdle. The Gigli saw is passed through the obturator foramina to incise the symphysis

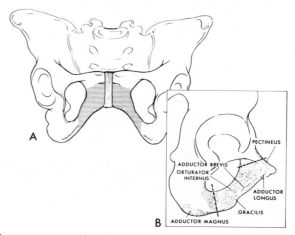

Figure 85–12. *A,* The shaded area is resected. *B,* The muscle groups encountered in resection of the pubis. (From Klein, F. A., et al.: Cancer, 51:1241, 1983.)

transversely, joining the foramina with an upward beveled osteotomy (Fig. 85–12). The specimen is delivered en bloc. After hemostasis is secure, the omentum is mobilized to cover the bowel. Myocutaneous flaps can be fashioned to close large perineal defects (Larson and Bracken, 1982).

REGIONAL DISEASE

Clinical Correlates

The incidence of metastatic inguinal adenopathy from distal male urethral cancers is 50 to 60 per cent (Ray et al., 1977; Riches and Cullen, 1951). In contradistinction to penile primary lesions, there is little inflammation associated with these lesions. Clinical adenopathy in this setting is a highly reliable sign of metastasis. Therapeutic dissection has been successful, but there is no documented advantage to prophylactic surgery (Ray et al., 1977).

Tumors arising from the bulbomembranous and prostatic urethra drain primarily to the external iliac, obturator, and hypogastric nodes. Involvement of the inguinal nodes may result indirectly from retrograde filling from extensive adenopathy or directly from invasion from the perineum or genitals. Although the incidence of metastatic pelvic or inguinal adenopathy is undefined, it carries an ominous prognosis. Only an occasional survivor has been reported following lymphadenectomy (Marshall, 1957).

Although the treatment of inguinal and pelvic metastases from urethral male cancer is primarily surgical, the overall results are poor. For this reason, consideration should be given to pretreatment with combination chemotherapy. In the event of a response, a surgical procedure can be considered that is designed to excise the primary tumor and all regional lymph nodes (Scher et al., 1988). It remains to be seen whether a combination approach will better control the primary tumor and/or offer survival advantages over surgery alone.

The surgical procedure required is the standard ilioinguinal lymphadenectomy as described for invasive penile cancers.

Radiotherapy has been provided as a palliative measure, as an adjunct to surgical excision, and as a primary therapy. Radiotherapy effect in regional disease is unproved, primarily owing to lack of histologic documentation. The induration that may follow radiotherapy to the groin makes clinical examination for recurrent disease more difficult. Induration also increases the local morbidity should surgery subsequently become necessary for uncontrolled regional disease.

MANAGEMENT OF THE RETAINED URETHRA AFTER CYSTECTOMY

General Considerations

The potentially multifocal nature of transitional cell carcinoma places the entire urothelium at risk in the patient with bladder cancer. The prostatic and penile urethra is uncommonly involved, at least clinically recognized, at the time of cystectomy. Therefore, the entire urethra from the membranous portion to the meatus is generally not removed with the specimen. Because this urothelium remains at risk, close follow-up with urethral washings for cytology, flow cytometry (if available), and biopsy (if necessary) is required at 3- to 4-month intervals for at least 5 years. It is important to maintain a high index of suspicion if incontinuity urethrectomy is not performed at the time of cystectomy. The incidence of subsequent severe epithelial atypia or frank in situ urethral carcinoma is estimated at 12.5 per cent in male patients in whom urethrectomy was not performed prophylactically during total cystectomy for bladder cancer (Schellhammer and Whitmore, 1976).

Urethrectomy is indicated as an isolated procedure after cystectomy if the findings determined from urethral washings become positive for malignant cells or if a bloody urethral discharge develops. Secondary urethrectomy may be a less adequate operation than primary urethrectomy, because the perineal scarring and proximity of the small bowel to the urogenital diaphragm after radical cystectomy render complete excision of the membranous portion of the urethra more difficult and less certain.

Operative Technique

A modified lithotomy position is employed for urethrectomy, with hips and knees gently flexed and the lower limbs adducted in foot stirrups.

A 5-cm midline or an inverted U–shaped perineal incision may be used (Fig. 85–13). The perineal incision

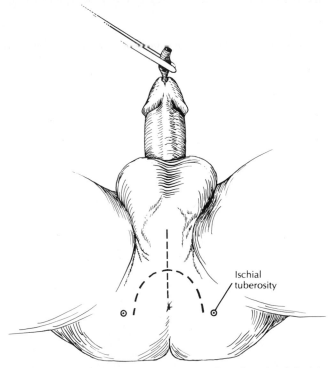

Figure 85–13. A midline or inverted U–shaped perineal incision between the ischial tuberosities or a combination thereof is used to expose the urethral bulb. (From Herr, H. W.: Urethrectomy. *In* Glenn, J. F. (Ed.) Urologic Surgery, 3rd ed. Philadelphia, J. B. Lippincott Co., 1983.)

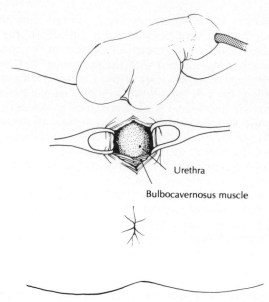

Figure 85–14. The bulbocavernosus muscle is retracted, demonstrating the underlying urethral bulb. (© Royal Victoria Hospital.) (From Herr, H. W.: Urethrectomy, In Glenn, J. F. (Ed.). Urologic Surgery, 3rd ed. Philadelphia, J. B. Lippincott Co., 1983.)

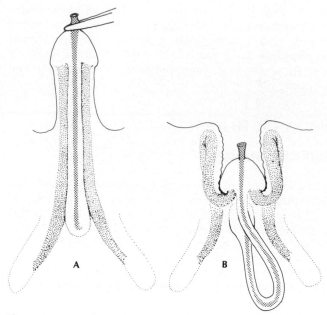

Figure 85–16. Schematic representation of catheterized pendulous urethra (A) prior to dissection and (B) with penis inverted at completion of distal dissection to glans penis. (© Royal Victoria Hospital.) (From Herr, H. W.: Urethrectomy. In Glenn, J. F. (Ed.). Urologic Surgery, 3rd ed. Philadelphia, J. B. Lippincott Co., 1983.)

affords simpler access to the urethral arteries and greater exposure of the urethral bulb and urogenital diaphragm. The subcutaneous tissues and bipenniform bulbocavernosus muscle are divided in the midline and retracted to expose the corpus spongiosum (Fig. 85–14), which is isolated. A small tape is passed around the urethra, and traction is applied to facilitate sharp dissection of the urethra distally, thus separating the corpus spongiosum from the adjacent corpora cavernosa (Fig. 85–15).

As dissection proceeds, the penis becomes inverted as the corpora cavernosa become bowed and the glans recedes into the phallus as it follows the line of traction on the urethra (Fig. 85–16). In this manner, the penis

is turned inside out onto the perineum and dissection is completed to the base of the glans (Fig. 85–17). To excise the meatus and glandular urethra, the penis is replaced in its anatomic position and an incision is made around the meatus and extended on either side down the ventral aspect of the glans (Fig. 85–18). The distal urethra is then freed from its investments within the glans penis employing sharp dissection. The isolated pendulous urethra may now be delivered onto the perineum, and the filleted glans penis is reapproximated to minimize blood loss.

Proximal sharp dissection of the urethral bulb is completed to the level of the perineal membrane and

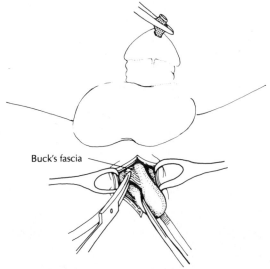

Figure 85–15. Sharp dissection of Buck's fascia with traction on the urethra separates the corpus spongiosum from the corpora cavernosa. (© Royal Victoria Hospital.) (From Herr, H. W.: Urethrectomy, In Glenn, J. F. (Ed.). Urologic Surgery, 3rd ed. Philadelphia, J. B. Lippincott Co., 1983.)

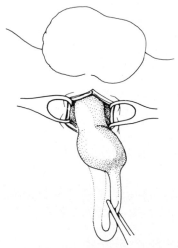

Figure 85–17. Completion of distal dissection to the undersurface of the glans penis. (© Royal Victoria Hospital.) (From Herr, H. W.: Urethrectomy. In Glenn, J. F. (Ed.). Urologic Surgery, 3rd ed. Philadelphia, J. B. Lippincott Co., 1983.)

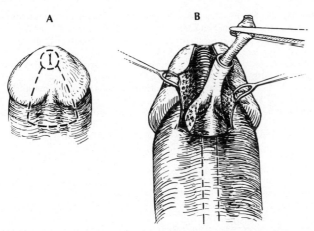

Figure 85–18. *A* Incision used for *B* dissection of the urethral meatus and the glandular urethra. Note that the penis has been placed in its normal anatomic position. (From Herr, H. W.: Urethrectomy. *In* Glenn, J. F. (Ed.). Urologic Surgery, 3rd ed. Philadelphia, J. B. Lippincott Co., 1983.)

inferior fascia of the urogenital diaphragm. Further sharp and blunt dissection is used to enlarge the urethral hiatus and to free the urethra above the level of the urogenital diaphragm, all or a portion of which may be included with the specimen. Vigorous traction on the urethra during this phase of the operation should be avoided to prevent tearing or avulsing the urethra at the prostatomembranous junction.

The urethral branches of the internal pudendal arteries are isolated, ligated, and divided as they enter the bulb at 4 and 8 o'clock, just inferior to the perineal membrane (Fig. 85–19). Care must be exercised in completing the proximal dissection in view of the possible postcystectomy adherence of intestine to the superior surface of the urogenital diaphragm. All that remains of the membranous urethra proximally is an ill-defined fibrotic band. Frozen-section analysis of this region adds some assurance that a negative proximal margin has been attained.

Closure of the bulbocavernosus muscle, subcutaneous tissue, and skin with interrupted absorbable sutures completes the procedure. A light pressure dressing is applied. A small Penrose drain exiting near the frenulum is used to drain the urethral bed. Defects created in the corpora cavernosa during sharp dissection of the urethra

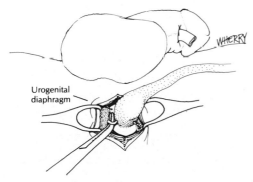

Figure 85–19. Isolation and division of the artery to the urethral bulb, with a drain in the bed of the corpus spongiosum. (© Royal Victoria Hospital.) (From Herr, H. W.: Urethrectomy. *In* Glenn, J. F. (Ed.). Urologic Surgery, 3rd ed. Philadelphia, J. B. Lippincott Co., 1983.).

require suture ligature to control bleeding prior to closure. The patient is ambulated on the 1st postoperative day, and the Penrose drain is removed.

The urethrectomy is completed in approximately 30 to 45 minutes. Superficial hematoma, edema along the penile shaft, and infection are uncommon complications.

FEMALE URETHRAL CANCER

General Considerations

Radiotherapy and/or chemotherapy followed by radical excision with anterior transvaginal pelvic exenteration is recommended for cancer involving the proximal or entire female urethra. Pubic arch or symphyseal resection has been suggested as a surgical adjunct to improve soft tissue margin and local control (Klein, 1983).

Therapy is based primarily on tumor extent and to a lesser degree on histologic type. Anterior or distal lesions are predominately squamous cell type and, if of limited size, can be effectively controlled by partial urethrectomy alone. Urinary continence is maintained after such procedure. Urethral tumors arising in association with urethral diverticula, particularly adenocarcinomas, can also be successfully managed by local excision (Cea et al., 1977; Evans et al., 1981). Restriction to superficial lesions, pathologic assessment of surgical margins, excision without violation and spillage, and careful follow-up are features essential to the successful application of conservative surgery.

The diagnosis of a urethral carcinoma requires biopsy and histopathologic confirmation. Lesions arising at or near the meatus are best diagnosed by excisional biopsy, depending on size. These include suspicious-looking caruncles. Biopsies of lesions occurring in the mid or proximal urethra are usually more satisfactorily obtained utilizing transurethral techniques (cold-cup biopsy forceps, electroresection). Palpable induration requires transurethral biopsy, transvaginal needle biopsy, and rarely open biopsy to substantiate origin and invasion of malignancy.

Specific Surgical Techniques

Local Excision

Circumferential local excision of the distal urethra and adjacent portions of the anterior vaginal wall can be accomplished for small, exophytic, and well-differentiated lesions of the external meatus or distal third of the urethra. Spatulation of the urethra and approximation to the subjacent vagina and labia provide a patent meatus and preserve urinary continence.

For entire or proximal urethral invasive lesions, cystourethrectomy (anterior exenteration), including a wide margin of vagina and in some cases the entire vagina, is required. For bulky female urethral lesions, and/or local recurrences, an extended excision may be necessary. The perineal incision is similar to but wider than that for standard transvaginal anterior pelvic exenterations.

The labia majora are retracted, and the introital incision is initiated anterior to the clitoris. The incision continues inferiorly to include the labia minora to the lower mid-vagina where it joins the vaginotomies initiated from the pelvis. Dissecting anteriorly, the symphysis is cleared, while lateral dissection exposes the fascia overlying the origins of the adductors along the inferior pubic rami. If resection of the pubic arch or its subsymphyseal portion is required, this is accomplished in a manner similar to that described for the male.

Regional Metastasis

The significant morbidity associated with groin dissections and the observation that cancer of the female urethra often metastasizes systemically without regional node involvement caution against the indiscriminate, routine, or prophylactic employment of lymphadenectomy in a patient with no clinically suspected regional lymphatic spread. Groin dissection is reserved for the patient who presents initially with histologically confirmed regional lymph nodes without distant metastases or one who subsequently demonstrates lymph node involvement. Groin dissections in the female are performed in a fashion identical to that in the male for penile cancer. For transitional carcinomas metastatic to the inguinal or pelvic lymph nodes, chemotherapy is expected to play a greater role in combination with surgery.

REFERENCES

Ahmed, T., et al.: Sequential trials of methotrexate, cisplatin, and bleomycin for penile cancer. J. Urol., 132:465, 1984.

Airhart, R. A., DeKernion, J. B., and Guillermo, E. O.: Tensor fascia lata myocutaneous flap for coverage of skin defect after radical groin dissection for metastatic penile carcinoma. J. Urol., 128:599, 1982.

Arconti, J. S., and Goodwin, W. E.: Use of scrotal skin to cover wound defects in the groin and pubic area. J. Urol., 75:292, 1956.

Bandieramonte, G., Lepera, P., Marchesiviv, R., et al.: Laser microsurgery for superficial lesions of the penis. J. Urol., 138:315–319, 1987.

Bassett, J. W.: Carcinoma of the penis. Cancer, 5:530, 1952.

Beggs, J. J., and Spratt, J. S.: Epidermoid carcinoma of the penis. J. Urol., 91:166, 1964.

Block, N. L., et al.: Hemipelvectomy for advanced penile cancer. J. Urol., 110:73, 1973.

Bracken, R. B.: Exenterative surgery for posterior urethral cancer. Urology, 19:248, 1982.

Bracken, R. B., and Grabstald, H.: Bladder carcinoma involving the lower abdominal wall. J. Urol., 114:715, 1975.

Bracken, R. B., et al.: Primary carcinoma of the urethra. J. Urol., 116:188, 1976.

Bretton, P. R., and Herr, H. W.: Intravesical BCG therapy for in situ transitional cell carcinoma involving the prostatic urethra. J. Urol., 141:853–856, 1989.

Cabanas, R. M.: An approach for the treatment of penile carcinoma. Cancer, 39:456, 1977.

Carson, T. E.: Verrucous carcinoma of the penis. Arch. Dermatol., 114:1546, 1978.

Catalona, W. J.: Modified inguinal lymphadenectomy for carcinoma of the penis with preservation of saphenous vein: Technique and preliminary results. J. Urol., 140:306–310, 1988.

Cea, P. C., et al.: Mesonephric adenocarcinomas in urethral diverticula. Urology, 10:58, 1977.

Cockburn, A. G., et al.: Bypass graft for femoral artery involvement by metastatic carcinoma of the penis. J. Urol., 127:1191, 1982.

Danoff, D. S., et al.: New treatment for extensive condylomata acuminata: External radiation therapy. Urology, 18:47, 1981.

Dardik, H., et al.: Remote profunda femoral bypass for limb salvage. Surg. Gynecol. Obstet., 151:625, 1980.

Daseler, E. H., et al.: Radical excision of the inguinal and iliac lymph glands. Surg. Gynecol. Obstet., 87:679, 1948.

Dean, A. L.: Conservative amputation of the penis for carcinoma. J. Urol., 68:374, 1952.

DeKernion, J. B., et al.: Carcinoma of the penis. Cancer, 32:1256, 1973.

deSouza, L. J.: Subtotal amputation for carcinoma of the penis with reconstruction. Ann. R. Coll. Surg., 58:398, 1976.

Duncan, W., and Jackson, W. M.: The treatment of early cancer of the penis with megavoltage X-rays. Clin. Radiol., 23:246, 1972.

Edwards, R. H., and Sawyers, J. L.: The management of carcinoma of the penis. South. Med. J., 61:843, 1968.

Ekstrom, T., and Edsmyr, F.: Cancer of the penis. Acta Chir. Scand., 115:25, 1958.

El-Demiry, M. I. M., et al.: Reappraisal of the role of radiotherapy and surgery in the management of carcinoma of the penis. Br. J. Urol., 56:724, 1984.

Ellingwood, K. E., and Million, R. R.: Carcinoma of the male urethra. Personal communication, 1983.

Evans, K. L., et al.: Adenocarcinoma of a female urethral diverticulum: A case report and review of the literature. J. Urol., 126:124, 1981.

Fegen, P., and Persky, L.: Squamous cell carcinoma of the penis. Arch. Surg., 99:117, 1969.

Fortner, J. G., et al.: Results of groin dissection for malignant melanoma in 220 patients. Surgery, 55:485, 1964.

Fraley, E. E., and Hutchens, H. C.: Radical ilioinguinal node dissection—skin bridge technique. J. Urol., 108:279, 1972.

Fraley, E. E., Zhoug, G., Manivel, C., et al.: The role of ilioinguinal lymphadenectomy and significance of histological differentiation in treatment of carcinoma of the penis. J. Urol., 142:1478–1482, 1989.

Garnick, M. B., Skarin, A. T., and Steele, G. D.: Metastatic carcinoma of the penis: Complete remission after high dose methotrexate chemotherapy. J. Urol., 122:265, 1979.

Goette, D. K.: Review of erythroplasia of Queyrat and its treatment. Urology, 8:311, 1976.

Grabstald, H: Tumors of the urethra in men and women. Cancer, 32:1236, 1973.

Grabstald, H.: Controversies concerning lymph node dissection for cancer of the penis. Urol. Clin. North Am., 7:793, 1981.

Grabstald, H., and Kelley, C. D.: Radiation therapy of penile cancer. Urology, 15:575, 1980.

Grabstald, H., et al.: Cancer of the female urethra. JAMA, 197:835, 1966.

Hanash, J. A., et al.: Carcinoma of the penis: A clinicopathologic study. J. Urol., 104:291, 1970.

Hardner, G. J., et al.: Carcinoma of the penis: Analysis of therapy in 100 consecutive cases. J. Urol., 108:428, 1972.

Hindlsey, J. P., et al.: Mini-dose heparin therapy in pelvic lymphadenectomy and I-125 implantation of localized prostatic cancer. Urology, 15:272, 1980.

Hughes, P. S. H.: Cryosurgery of verrucous carcinoma of the penis. Cutis, 24:43, 1979.

Ichikawa, T.: Chemotherapy of penis carcinoma. Recent results. Cancer Res., 60:140, 1977.

Jensen, M. S.: Cancer of the penis in Denmark, 1942-1962. Dan. Med. Bull., 24:66, 1977.

Johnson, D. E., and Lo, R. K.: Complications of groin dissection in penile cancer. Urology, 24:312, 1984.

Johnson, D. E., and O'Connell, J. R.: Primary carcinoma of female urethra. Urology, 21:42, 1983.

Johnson, D. E., et al.: Carcinoma of the penis. Urology, 1:404, 1973.

Johnson, D. E., et al.: Rotational skin flaps to cover defect in groin. Urology, 6:461, 1975.

Kaplan, G. W., et al.: Carcinoma of the male urethra. J. Urol., 98:365, 1967.

Karakousis, C. P., et al.: Lymphedema after groin dissection. Am. J. Surg., 145:205, 1983.

Kelley, C. D., et al.: Radiation therapy of penile cancer. Urology, 4:571, 1974.

Klein, F. A., et al.: Inferior pubic rami resection with en bloc radical excision for invasive proximal urethral carcinoma. Cancer, 51:1238, 1983.

Konnak, J. W.: Conservative management of low-grade neoplasms of the male urethra: A preliminary report. J. Urol., 123:175, 1980.

Kyalwazi, S. K., Bhana, D., and Harrison, N. W.: Carcinoma of the penis and bleomycin chemotherapy in Uganda. Br. J. Urol., 46:689, 1974.

Larson, D. L., and Bracken, R. B.: Use of gracilis musculocutaneous flap in urologic cancer surgery. Urology, 14:148, 1982.

Leissner, K. H., and Johansson, S.: Topical application of 5-fluorouracil cream: A therapeutic alternative in the treatment of urothelial tumors of the distal urethra. Scand. J. Urol. Nephrol., 14:115, 1980.

Levine, R. L.: Urethral cancer. Cancer, 45:1965, 1980.

Macdonald, I., et al.: Exposure and suction drainage in the management of major dissective wounds. Surg. Gynecol. Obstet., 107:532, 1958.

Mackenzie, A. R., and Whitmore, W. F.: Resection of pubic rami for urologic cancer. J. Urol., 100:546, 1968.

Mantell, B. S., and Morgan, W. Y.: Queyrat's erythroplasia of the penis treated by beta particle irradiation. Br. J. Radiol., 12:855, 1969.

Marcial, V. A., et al.: Carcinoma of the penis. Radiology, 79:209, 1962.

Marshall, V. F.: Radical excision of locally extensive carcinoma of the deep male urethra. J. Urol., 78:252, 1957.

McDougal, W. S., Koch, M. O.: Phallic reconstruction during exenterative surgery for invasive urethral carcinoma. J. Urol., 141:1201–1203, 1989.

Mohs, T. E., Snow, S. N., Messing, E. M., et al.: Microscopically controlled surgery in the treatment of carcinoma of the penis. J. Urol., 133:961–966, 1985.

Mukherjee, G. D.: Reconstruction of penis with urethra from groin and midthigh flap. J. Indian Med. Associ., 75:124, 1980.

Mullen, E. M., Anderson, E. E., and Paulson, D. F.: Carcinoma of the male urethra. J. Urol., 112:610, 1974.

Murrell, D. S., and Williams, J. L.: Radiotherapy in the treatment of carcinoma of the penis. Br. J. Urol., 37:211, 1965.

Narayana, A. S., et al.: Carcinoma of the penis. Cancer, 49:2185, 1982.

Pack, G. T., and Ariel, I. M. (Eds.): Treatment of tumors of the penis. In Treatment of Cancer and Allied Diseases: Tumors of the Male Genitalia and the Urinary System, 2nd ed. New York, Harper & Row, 1963, p. 15.

Perinetti, E., et al.: Unreliability of sentinel lymph node biopsy for staging penile carcinoma. J. Urol., 124:734, 1980.

Pointon, R. C.: Carcinoma of the penis: External beam therapy. Proc. R. Soc. Med., 68:779, 1975.

Prempree, T., et al.: Radiation therapy in primary carcinoma of the female urethra. Cancer, 54:729, 1984.

Raghavaiah, N. V.: Radiotherapy in the treatment of carcinoma of the male urethra. Cancer, 41:1313, 1978.

Ray, B., and Guinan, P. D.: Primary carcinoma of the urethra. In Javadpour, N. (Ed.). Principles and Management of Urologic Cancer. Baltimore, Williams & Wilkins, 1979, pp. 445–473.

Ray, B., et al.: Experience with primary carcinoma of the male urethra. J. Urol., 117:591, 1977.

Riches, E. W., and Cullen, T. H.: Carcinoma of the urethra. Br. J. Urol., 23:209, 1951.

Riveros, M., et al.: Lymphadenography of the dorsal lymphatics of the penis. Cancer, 20:2026, 1967.

Rouviere, H.: Anatomy of the Human Lymphatic System. Tobias, M. J. (transl.), Ann Arbor, Edwards Brothers, Inc., 1938.

Sen, A., et al.: Study of the lymphatic drainage from the growth in the penis by radioactive colloidal gold. Indian J. Cancer, 4:295, 1967.

Schellhammer, P. F., and Whitmore, W. F., Jr.: Transitional cell carcinoma of the urethra in men having cystectomy for bladder cancer. J. Urol. 115:56, 1976.

Scher, H. I., Herr, H. W., Yagoda, A., et al.: Neoadjuvant M-VAC (methotrexate, vinblastine, doxorubicin and cisplatin) for extravesical urinary tract tumors. J. Urol., 139:475–477, 1988.

Shuttleworth, K. E. D., and Lloyd-Davies, R. W.: Radical resection for tumors involving the posterior urethra. Br. J. Urol., 41:739, 1969.

Skinner, D. G.: Management of extensive localized neoplasms of the lower abdominal wall. Urology, 3:34, 1974.

Skinner, D. G., et al.: The surgical management of squamous cell carcinoma of the penis. J. Urol., 107:273, 1972.

Sklaroff, R. B., and Yagoda, A.: Cis-diaminedichloride platinum II (DDP) in the treatment of penile carcinoma. Cancer, 44:1563, 1979.

Sklaroff, R. B., and Yagoda, A.: Methotrexate in the treatment of penile carcinoma. Cancer, 45:214, 1980.

Sogani, P. C., et al.: Lymphocele after pelvic lymphadenectomy for urologic cancer. Urology, 17:39, 1981.

Spratt, J. S. et al.: Anatomy and Surgical Technique of Groin Dissection. St. Louis, C. V. Mosby, 1965.

Srinivas, V., Morse, M. J., Herr, H. W., et al.: Penile cancer—relation of extent of nodal metastasis to survival. J. Urol., 137:880–882, 1987.

Whitmore, W. F., Jr.: Tumors of the penis, urethra, scrotum and testis. In Campbell, M. F., and Harrison, J. H. (Eds.): Urology, Philadelphia, W. B. Saunders Co., 1970, p. 1201.

Whitmore, W. F., Jr., and Vagaiwala, M. R.: A technique of ilioinguinal lymph node dissection for carcinoma of the penis. Surg. Gynecol. Obstet., 159:573, 1984.

Yagoda, A., et al.: Bleomycin, an antitumor antibiotic: clinical experience in 274 patients. Ann. Intern. Med., 77:861, 1972.

86
SURGERY OF TESTICULAR NEOPLASMS

Eila C. Skinner, M.D.
Donald G. Skinner, M.D.

The treatment of testicular cancer has changed considerably in the past 40 years. Prior to 1960, surgery and radiation were the mainstays of treatment, with only 50 per cent overall survival (Whitmore, 1983). Since the advent of cisplatin-based chemotherapy, we have seen cure rates of over 95 per cent for early stage disease and over 70 per cent for advanced stage disease (Skinner, 1984a). During this time, the role of surgery has been re-examined and continues to be the subject of some controversy. In spite of the effectiveness of current chemotherapy regimens, however, there is no doubt that surgery remains a key element in the treatment and eventual cure of many patients.

PRIMARY TESTIS CANCER

Diagnosis

The majority of patients with testicular cancer present with a painless lump in the scrotum. However, the presentation can be quite diverse. Many of the symptoms are caused by metastatic disease, and 10 per cent of patients have chief complaints referable to areas other than the testes. Of special note is that up to 25 per cent of patients present with sudden testicular pain and swelling, with physical signs that may be indistinguishable from acute epididymitis (Richie, 1988). In addition, patients often will ascribe an enlarged testis to a recent acute trauma to the scrotum. In both of these cases, scrotal ultrasound and careful follow-up evaluations are important to arrive at the correct diagnosis.

Scrotal ultrasound is over 90 per cent sensitive and specific for the diagnosis of a solid testis mass and is an inexpensive, noninvasive study (Benson, 1988). However, when ultrasound is inconclusive, inguinal exploration and biopsy are indicated. Ultrasound is an unnecessary expense for the patient with unequivocal examination findings, however.

Blood for serum human chorionic gonadotropin–beta subunit (hCG–β subunit), alpha$_1$-fetoprotein (AFP), and lactate dehydrogenase (LDH) determinations, which are discussed in detail in Chapter 30, should be drawn prior to orchiectomy when a testis tumor is suspected. These cannot be used as screening tests—90 per cent of seminomas and 33 per cent of nonseminomas have normal serum marker levels on presentation (Catalona, 1979). However, serum marker levels are critical in staging and in planning eventual therapy and follow-up.

Radical Orchiectomy

Little controversy exists about the role of radical inguinal orchiectomy in the treatment of primary testicular cancer. The inguinal approach avoids interruption of the scrotal lymphatics, which could potentially change the metastatic pathway of the tumor, and allows complete removal of the spermatic cord up to the internal ring.

The technique is straightforward. A transverse or oblique inguinal incision is made approximately 4 cm in length, beginning 2 cm lateral and superior to the pubic tubercle. Scarpa's fascia is divided in line with the incision, and the external oblique fascia exposed. The external inguinal ring is identified, and the external oblique fascia is divided in line with its fibers down to the external ring (Fig. 86–1). The ilioinguinal nerve is identified and retracted to one side, and the cord is gently mobilized at the internal ring. We place a noncrushing clamp across the cord at this point to avoid any potential tumor spread via veins or lymphatics during the subsequent mobilization of the testis. When the cord has been controlled proximally, it is further freed along its course in the inguinal canal.

The testis is then mobilized from the scrotum into the wound, using blunt dissection (Fig. 86–2). In an occa-

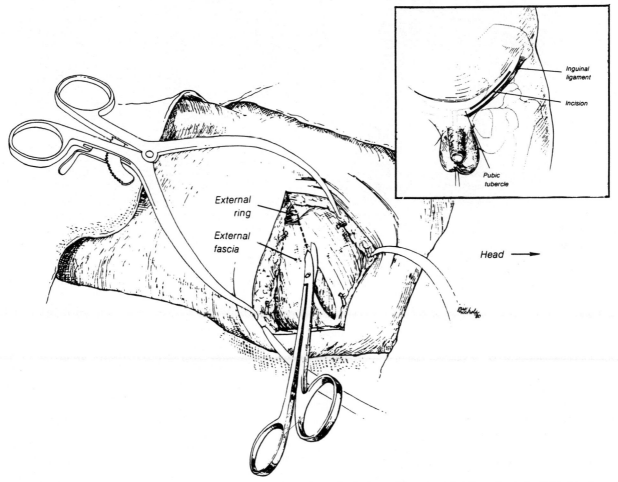

Head ⟶

Figure 86–1. Approach for radical inguinal orchiectomy. The incision is shown in the inset. The external oblique fascia is divided in line with its fibers down to the external inguinal ring. (From Gottesman, J. E.: *In* Crawford, E. D. (Ed.): Current Genitourinary Cancer Surgery. Philadelphia, Lea & Febiger, 1990, p. 319.)

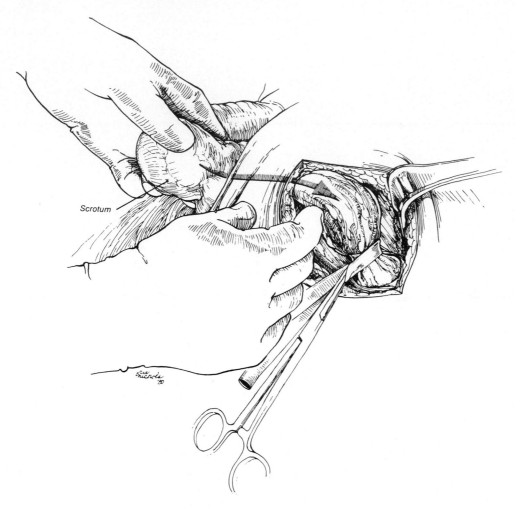

Figure 86–2. After the cord has been controlled with a tightened Penrose drain or rubber-shod clamp, the testicle is mobilized out of the scrotum using blunt dissection. (From Gottesman, J. E.: *In* Crawford, E. D. (Ed.): Current Genitourinary Cancer Surgery. Philadelphia, Lea & Febiger, 1990, p. 319.)

sional patient with a very large testicular mass, it may be necessary to extend the incision. If the diagnosis is in doubt, the testis may undergo biopsy at this point for frozen-section analysis. To do this, we carefully drape off the wound with sterile towels prior to opening the tunica vaginalis. After the wedge biopsy sample has been taken, the spermatic cord is kept clamped until negative results have been verified by pathology.

To complete the orchiectomy, the spermatic cord is mobilized to at least 1 or 2 cm inside the internal inguinal ring. There, it is carefully ligated with a large permanent suture to allow the identification of the stump should subsequent retroperitoneal lymph node dissection be required. The vas should be ligated separately with 3–0 silk or controlled with a hemoclip.

The wound and scrotum are irrigated, applying an antibiotic solution if a testis prosthesis is to be placed. The internal inguinal ring is obliterated with a No. 1 polyglycolic acid (PGA) suture, and the external oblique fascia is closed with a running 3–0 PGA suture. The skin is approximated with clips or a subcuticular closure.

This procedure can usually be done as outpatient surgery, and complications are very rare. The most serious is bleeding from the spermatic cord stump, which can be profuse. Therefore, the ligated cord should be carefully inspected prior to allowing it to retract into the retroperitoneum. Other complications, such as wound infection and subcutaneous seroma formation, are seen only occasionally (Moul, 1989).

Management of Scrotal Orchiectomy

The urologist must occasionally treat patients who have undergone transscrotal biopsies or orchiectomies for testicular cancer. These made up 14 per cent of all patients referred for definitive treatment to one major medical center (Boileau and Steers, 1984). It has long been believed that prior scrotal surgery markedly increases the incidence of local recurrence and inguinal nodal metastasis (Markland et al., 1973). However, further evidence suggests that the risk has been overestimated. With the availability of more effective chemotherapy, the probability of this problem becoming life-threatening has been greatly decreased (Giguere et al., 1988; Boileau and Steers, 1984). Most workers agree that a full hemiscrotectomy or prophylactic inguinal node dissection is no longer necessary in this situation. However, the following management is recommended (see also Staging):

1. In stage A seminoma, prophylactic retroperitoneal radiation should be extended to include the hemiscrotum and ipsilateral inguinal nodes.

2. In stage A nonseminoma, the previous scrotal incision should be excised at the time of retroperitoneal lymph node dissection. The remaining stump of spermatic cord must also be completely removed, either from above or through an inguinal incision.

3. If an observation protocol for stage A nonseminoma is considered, the cord and scrotal incision should be excised as a separate procedure. Inguinal nodes must be monitored carefully for metastases.

4. In advanced disease treated with full-dose platinum chemotherapy, no further treatment of the scrotum is probably necessary. The inguinal nodes and scrotum should be carefully examined at each follow-up visit.

Role of Delayed Orchiectomy in Advanced Disease

A patient with advanced testicular cancer, usually with a testicular mass, elevated serum marker levels, and obvious metastatic disease, occasionally presents with severe or even life-threatening complications. Others may have the tissue diagnosis already established from the biopsy of a metastatic focus. In these cases, it may be in the best interest of the patient to proceed directly to immediate chemotherapy without orchiectomy.

It is important in these patients that eventual inguinal orchiectomy be carried out, even if a complete response from chemotherapy is achieved. Fowler and Whitmore (1981) reported two patients with residual tumor in the testis after extended chemotherapy with vinblastine and bleomycin. In 1983, Calvo and associates reported that three of five patients had persistent viable tumor in the testis following platinum-based chemotherapy, including one in whom the testicular tumor progressed while the metastasis regressed. Thus, the testis may act as a "privileged site" protected from the effects of chemotherapy.

Our general approach is to perform an orchiectomy at the time of retroperitoneal node dissection. This procedure can be done through the abdominal incision by pulling the spermatic cord and testis up through the inguinal canal from above. The gubernacular scrotal attachments must be carefully coagulated as they are divided to prevent postoperative scrotal hematoma. In a patient who does not require node dissection, orchiectomy should be performed shortly after completing chemotherapy. In a patient with normal testes by both palpation and ultrasound throughout the course of treatment, who is believed to have extragonadal germ cell malignancy, the testes may be left in place and monitored carefully at follow-up visits. If the retroperitoneal disease localizes to one side, however, it has been our recommendation that the ipsilateral testis be removed at the time of lymphadenectomy. In several of these patients so affected, we have found a scar or small focus of germ cell tumor within the palpably normal testis.

Pathology

Approximately 40 to 50 per cent of testicular tumors are pure seminomas on histologic sectioning, with the remainder including both pure and mixed nonseminomatous tumors (Smith, 1987). A detailed discussion of testis cancer pathology is presented elsewhere (see Chapter 30). Only a few comments relevant to the surgical plan are discussed here.

Seminoma

It is of central importance that the diagnosis of pure seminoma be made only after step sectioning of the testis. The differentiation between various types of seminoma is thought not to be of prognostic significance, including the ominous sounding anaplastic seminoma (Wetlaufer, 1984).

The significance of the finding of elevated serum marker levels in the presence of pure seminoma has been an area of some controversy. Most investigators agree that any elevation of AFP, which is normally produced by embryonal tumor cells, should be considered a hallmark of occult nonseminomatous disease. The patient should be treated for this disease.

Elevation of hCG–β subunit has been reported in 8 to 40 per cent of pure seminomas (Fossa, 1989a; Javadpour, 1978). Kurman and associates (1977) localized the hCG–β subunit to syncytiotrophoblastic giant cells identified within the primary tumor. The natural history of this cell type in pure seminoma is unknown. Reports have suggested a worse prognoses for patients with elevated hCG–β subunit levels (Maier and Sulak, 1972), but others have failed to confirm this relationship (Lange et al., 1980; Schwartz et al., 1984).

Very high levels of hCG–β subunit (>200 mIU/ml) almost certainly reflect occult metastatic nonseminomatous elements, but lower levels do not exclude them. We have seen one patient with a mild elevation (47 mIU/ml), who was found at retroperitoneal lymph node dissection to have a 4-cm metastasis consisting entirely of embryonal cell carcinoma (Pritchett, 1985).

We recommend that a patient with a primary pure seminoma and an hCG–β subunit >20 mIU/ml, or a patient with a lower hCG–β subunit level but no identifiable syncitiotrophoblastic giant cells in the testis, be treated as having nonseminoma.

Nonseminoma

Interest has been renewed in the pathologic extent of the primary testicular tumor in low-stage nonseminomatous disease because of the development of surveillance protocols (see subsequent discussion). Whitmore (1983) documented that tumors that extend outside the testis parenchyma to invade the tunica albuginea, rete testis, epididymis, or spermatic cord (stage T2 to T4) are associated with a higher risk of metastatic disease and relapse following negative findings on lymphadenectomy. This finding has been confirmed in patients undergoing node dissections (Fung, 1988; Rodriguez, 1986) and in patients in surveillance protocols that did not exclude higher stage primary tumors (Freedman, 1987).

Additional histologic features that appear to correlate with a higher risk of metastatic disease include predominant embryonal cell type or undifferentiated tumor and the presence of vascular or lymphatic invasion (Freedman et al., 1987; Hoskins et al., 1986; Wishnow et al., 1989b). The presence of yolk sac elements had a protective effect in one study, but this was not confirmed in others (Fossa, 1989b; Freedman, 1987). These data have also been reviewed in terms of the need for adjuvant chemotherapy for stage I or IIA patients following retroperitoneal node dissection. Some workers believe that the high relapse rate for T2–T4 tumors warrants adjuvant chemotherapy (Rodriguez, 1986; Sandeman, 1988). Others believe that patients experiencing relapses can be salvaged with full-dose chemotherapy, sparing the 40 to 50 per cent of patients who did not experience relapse the need to undergo any further therapy (Dunphy et al., 1988). This issue has not been addressed to date in a randomized prospective trial.

Nongerm Cell Tumors

Nongerm cell malignancies make up less than 10 per cent of all testicular tumors and are discussed in detail in Chapter 30. The initial approach to all of these tumors is inguinal orchiectomy, which establishes the pathologic diagnosis. Nongerm cell tumors include gonadal stroma tumors (Leydig's and Sertoli's cell tumors), gonadoblastomas, and sarcomas of the cord or testis. Retroperitoneal lymph node dissection is generally recommended for these tumors, although there are a few exceptions. The techniques are the same as those for germ cell tumors.

Lymphomas also occur in the testis and account for the majority of testicular tumors in men over 50. The diagnosis is usually arrived at through radical orchiectomy, although scrotal ultrasound may provide the diagnosis in patients with other sites of documented lymphomas (Benson, 1988). Testicular lymphoma may be the presenting manifestation of occult disseminated disease, but over half of 33 patients in one study had apparently localized disease (Turner, 1981). Seven of these patients subsequently experienced relapses systemically. Retroperitoneal lymphadenectomy is not therapeutic in this disease. Chemotherapy is generally recommended and is best directed by hematology and oncology specialists who are versed in the treatment of other types of lymphoma.

STAGING

The spread of testicular tumors occurs along predictable routes in the majority of patients. Most staging systems group cases by three levels of tumor involvement: confined to the testis (stage A or I), spread to the retroperitoneal nodes (B or II), and spread beyond the retroperitoneal lymphatics (C or III). The most commonly used staging systems are summarized in Table 86–1. Stage III or C includes subcategories of patients with widely varied prognoses—minimal pulmonary disease versus extensive pulmonary disease and visceral, bony, or central nervous system involvement. None of these staging systems differentiates patients further along these lines, stimulating several medical centers to develop more extensive staging systems for advanced disease (Montie, 1984; Williams et al., 1984).

The basic staging work-up currently includes serum tumor markers (AFP, hCG–β subunit, and LDH) before and after orchiectomy, chest radiography, and abdominal and pelvic computed tomography (CT) scans. Although whole lung tomograpy and chest CT scan have been helpful as baseline studies for a patient with advanced disease, they have not been shown to alter initial therapy (Jochelson et al., 1984; Richie, 1988).

Considerable controversy still exists over the role of bipedal lymphangiogram (LAG) in staging testicular cancer. Overall accuracy of the test in detecting retroperitoneal metastases has ranged from 62 to 90 per cent, which is similar to CT scan alone (Ehrlichman et al., 1981; Richie, 1982). Although Pizzocaro and Musumeci (1985c) found that combining CT and LAG reduced the false-negative rate from 27 to 10 per cent, others have not confirmed this finding (Ehrlichman; 1981; Wishnow, 1989a). False-positive results are also common and seen in up to 41 per cent of studies (Storm et al., 1977). LAGs are difficult to perform and interpret accurately, and they are uncomfortable for the patient. In addition, the contrast material can cause significant inflammatory response in the retroperitoneum, which may make subsequent node dissection more difficult. Therefore, we believe that in the case of a planned node dissection little information is to be gained over that available from CT scan. Whether a LAG should be required prior to entrance to a surveillance protocol is controversial (Thompson, 1988; Wishnow, 1989). Perhaps the primary

Table 86–1. COMPARISON OF PATHOLOGIC STAGING SYSTEMS FOR TESTICULAR CANCER

ABC System	Modified Walter Reed	TMN System	Description
A	I	N0	Tumor confined to testis
B1	IIA	N1, N2	Minimal retroperitoneal disease (< six positive nodes, no node >2 cm diameter at node dissection, or elevated serum marker levels with normal preoperative CT scan)
B2	IIB	N2	Moderate retroperitoneal disease (> six positive nodes or node >2 cm at node dissection, or mass <5 cm on preoperative CT scan)
B3	IIC	N3	Palpable abdominal mass or mass >5 cm on CT scan, without spread above diaphragm or to visceral organs
C	III	M+	Lymphadenopathy above diaphragm, pulmonary, visceral, central nervous system, or bony disease.

Adapted from Lieskovsky, G., Weinberg, A. C., and Skinner, D. G.: Semin. Urol., 2:208, 1984.

role of LAG today is in the management of seminoma. Many oncologists employ the LAG to plan radiation fields for low-stage disease.

The accuracy of magnetic resonance imaging (MRI) in detecting retroperitoneal adenopathy appears to be no better than CT scanning (Dooms, 1984), although the technology is changing rapidly. Data are insufficient to recommend its routine use in staging testicular cancer at this time.

All of the currently available staging studies, including CT scanning, tumor serum marker levels, LAG, and MRI, are quite accurate in detecting more advanced retroperitoneal disease with nodes more than 2 cm in diameter (Rowland et al., 1982). The challenge lies in the detection of microscopic or small volume metastases, which is still best accomplished by the retroperitoneal lymph node dissection.

SURGERY FOR LOW-STAGE NONSEMINOMATOUS GERM CELL TUMORS

Surgery versus Observation for Clinical Stage I Disease

Recognition of the marked efficacy of cisplatin-based chemotherapy regimens, plus the high incidence of anejaculation following lymphadenectomy, intensified the search in the 1970s for means to limit the need for this surgery in cases of low-stage nonseminoma. Protocols were designed at several major medical centers using careful follow-up alone for patients with clinical stage I, with full-dose chemotherapy either with or without surgery for patients who develop metastatic disease. Employing this approach, it was expected that 75 to 80 per cent of patients with stage I disease would be able to avoid both retroperitoneal node dissection and chemotherapy and that survival would not be compromised

for the remainder (Peckham et al., 1982; Sogani et al., 1984).

Results are now available from surveillance protocols, including those from several large patient cohorts (Dunphy et al., 1988; Freedman, 1987; Fossa, 1989b; Gelderman, 1987; Raghavan, 1988). Consistently, 25 to 35 per cent of patients eventually develop metastatic disease and, importantly, a few experience recurrences 2 to 4 years after diagnosis. Approximately 50 to 75 per cent of the patients with recurrences have disease in the retroperitoneum and the remainder in the lungs or elsewhere. The results in terms of survival and the treatment required compared with those in a group whose treatment was initial node dissection are summarized in Table 86–2.

Several investigators have identified factors in the histology of the primary testicular tumor that are correlated with a higher risk of recurrence in surveillance protocols. As previously discussed, most workers agree that T2 or higher lesions, involving the tunica vaginalis, rete testis, epididymis, or cord structures, should be eliminated from observation protocols because of the recognized high risk of recurrence of this lesion. However, within T1 lesions the presence of vascular or lymphatic invasion and the presence of embryonal cell histology have been shown to be poor prognostic factors in several studies (Fossa, 1989b; Freedman, 1987; Wishnow, 1989b). Wishnow and co-workers identified a low-risk group of patients with T1 cancer who have no vascular or lymphatic invasion, less than 80 per cent embryonal cell carcinoma, and preorchiectomy serum AFP level of less than 80 ng/dL. They saw no recurrences in 30 patients with all three of these factors, compared with 24/52 recurrences (46 per cent) among patients in the high risk group (Wishnow, 1989b). Freiha and Torti (1989) followed 23 selected patients who had T1 tumors without lymphatic or vascular invasion and compared the findings to 17 patients who had pathologic stage I disease treated with node dissection. With a minimum of 24 months follow-up, they observed re-

Table 86–2. RESULTS OF SURVEILLANCE PROTOCOLS FOR CLINICAL STAGE I NONSEMINOMATOUS TESTIS CANCER

Reference	Number of Patients	Follow-up (mean in months)	Recurrences Number	Recurrences %	Time to Recurrence (months)	Retroperitoneal Metastases (%)	Deaths	Survival (%)
Sogani et al., 1984	45	(19.5)	9	(20)		77	2	95.5
Pizzocaro et al., 1985	71	12–46 (27)	21	(29.5)	2–36	52	2	97.2
Freedman et al., 1987	259	10–63 (30)	70	(26)	1–48	54	3	98.8
Gelderman et al., 1987	54	12–48 (29)	11	(20)	2–8	82	NA	NA
Raghavan et al., 1988	46	6–88 (40+)	13	(28)	1–36	39	2	95.7
Dunphy et al., 1988	93	12–61 (34)	28	(30)	2.5–25	52	NA	NA
Thompson et al., 1988	36	14–92 (36)	12	(33)	2–28	33	2	94.4
Freiha and Torti, 1989	23	24–66 (44)	3	(13)	3–8	66	0	100
TOTAL	627		167	(26.6)			11	98

lapses in three patients in each group. This finding suggests that surveillance may be able to achieve much lower relapse rates if only offered to a highly selected group of patients.

Both surveillance and primary node dissection are highly effective in terms of survival. However, several other important points must be considered. First, Lange and colleagues (1984) analyzed in detail the expected gain in fertility from surveillance instead of primary node dissection. Using conservative estimates of primary sterility among these patients, the effects of chemotherapy, and the recovery of ejaculation after modified versus postchemotherapy node dissection, these investigators estimated 69 per cent ultimate fertility with surveillance compared with 52 per cent with primary node dissection. In addition, sympathomimetics and electroejaculation allow some of the anejaculatory men in the node dissection group to father children (Bennett et al., 1987). This finding adds an important perspective to the discussion, because it was concern over fertility that initially stimulated the development of surveillance protocols.

Second, achieving a high cure rate for the patients who experience relapse under surveillance protocols requires absolute compliance with the follow-up plan. Because of the extremely short doubling time of germ cell tumors, patients who miss one or two follow-up appointments are at risk of massive disease, which may be refractory to chemotherapy. Thus, any surveillance protocol must be carried out in a medical center with well-established mechanisms for identifying and locating patients who drop out of the system.

Third, 50 to 75 per cent of recurrences in patients in surveillance protocols occur in the retroperitoneum, compared with less than 1 per cent in patients following lymph node dissection. Retroperitoneal recurrence may be difficult to detect despite frequent CT scans and more difficult to eradicate with chemotherapy than pulmonary disease. In addition, the 25 to 35 per cent of patients who experience relapse in the surveillance protocols require full-dose cisplatin-based combination chemotherapy, with all of its known toxicity (Einhorn, 1989; Moul, 1989; Roth, 1988). By comparison, the adjuvant chemotherapy regimens for pathologic stage II cancers are shorter and less toxic, and the risk of retroperitoneal recurrence is essentially eliminated.

Finally, there are significant psychologic aspects in both programs that are very difficult to quantitate. A program with initial node dissection with or without adjuvant chemotherapy is completed within 3 months. At that point, the patient knows he has less than a 10 per cent risk of recurrence and can go on with his life with less frequent follow-up visits and without the need for additional CT scans. By comparison, patients in a surveillance protocol require frequent CT scans and follow-up visits, which may cause considerable anxiety. They must contend with the fact that at least a third of them will need chemotherapy and perhaps a delayed node dissection sometimes months to years later, making it difficult to make plans for work, school, marriage, and other activities.

Clearly, the winners in the surveillance protocol are the patients who remain free of disease with no further treatment beyond orchiectomy. Many patients may be willing to take that gamble, which we believe should only be offered by a major medical center with a well-defined protocol for patient follow-up. It may make the most sense to offer this option only to patients who fall in the lowest risk pathologic categories, as previously discussed. For most patients, however, we believe that an initial limited node dissection followed by adjuvant chemotherapy for node-positive disease is the best option.

Rationale for a Limited Retroperitoneal Lymph Node Dissection

As the cure rate for low-stage nonseminoma surpassed 90 per cent, concern became focused appropriately on the morbidity of the treatments. Anejaculation with resultant infertility is not a trivial problem for young men in their twenties and thirties. As interest rose in the surveillance of patients with low-stage nonseminoma, surgeons focused on developing a limited node dissection that could preserve ejaculation.

Lange and co-workers (1984) and others developed such an approach, based on studies by Ray and co-workers (1974), and later by Donohue and co-workers (1989), mapping the location of positive nodes in stage IIA and IIB disease (Fig. 86–3). This approach was also based on a better understanding of the anatomy of the lumbar sympathetics and their role in ejaculation. Most investigators agree that the most important area to preserve is the hypogastric plexus overlying the aorta and sacrum below the origin of the inferior mesenteric artery. Beyond that, however, there are important differences in the limits of dissection defined by various investigators. Fossa and colleagues (1985) and Pizzocaro and colleagues (1985a) both suggest a true unilateral dissection, which preserves the interaortocaval area on left-sided cases. Although this approach preserves ejaculation in up to 86 per cent of cases, reference to Donohue's mapping studies indicates that this dissection may miss positive nodes in up to 25 per cent of stage IIA cases.

Some workers have advocated dissecting out the postganglionic nerve fibers of the lumbar sympathetic chain, which course anteriorly over the aorta and fuse into multiple common trunks (Donohue et al., 1989; Jewett et al., 1988). This approach reportedly achieves preservation of ejaculation in up to 100 per cent of cases. We are concerned about the completeness of the dissection with such an approach, which requires teasing out the nodal tissue between the nerve fibers. It remains to be seen whether the incidence of retroperitoneal recurrences will be increased with this surgical technique.

We have adopted the "template" method of dissection, with the limits described by Wise and Scardino (1988) and Lange and co-workers (1984) (Fig. 86–4). This dissection reliably includes 90 to 95 per cent of the nodes that are at risk of harboring metastases in stage IIb disease. We have employed this approach in 45 patients since 1983 and ejaculation has been preserved

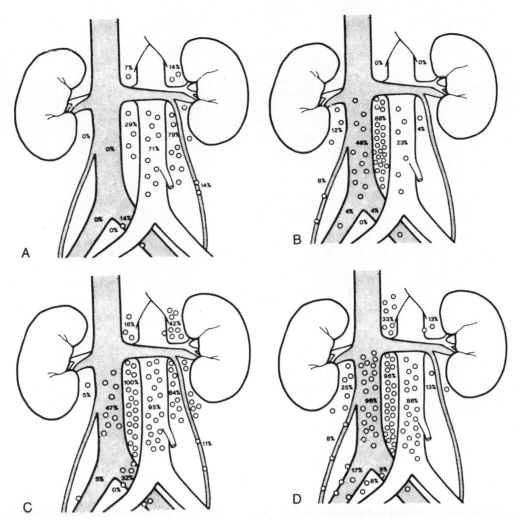

Figure 86–3. Distribution of positive nodes in patients with various pathologic stages of disease. *A,* Left-sided stage IIA. *B,* Right-sided stage IIA. *C,* Left-sided stage IIB. *D,* Right-sided stage IIB. (From Donohue, J. P., et al.: J. Urol., 128:315, 1982. © By Williams & Wilkins, 1982.)

in 88 per cent of those with right-sided and 62 per cent of those with left-sided dissections. Of these, 31 cases were pathologic stage I, 12 stage IIA, and two stage IIB. To date, there have been no retroperitoneal recurrences, with a mean follow-up of 24 months. In this approach it is important to preserve the ipsilateral sympathetic ganglia and postganglionic nerves running parallel to the psoas muscles adjacent to the vertebral bodies, as well as the tissue overlying the aorta below the inferior mesenteric artery.

Management of Stage II Disease

Extension to Full Bilateral Dissection

Approximately 10 per cent of patients thought to suffer clinical stage A disease will be found to have grossly positive nodes at surgery (Fung et al., 1988). Because the limited dissection has been shown in many studies to be adequate for stage IIA disease, we do not routinely perform frozen-section analysis on normal-appearing nodes at the time of surgery. When enlarged or indurated nodes are discovered at surgery, the decision must be made whether or not to extend the limits of dissection. We are influenced by the location of the positive nodes, which can be confirmed by frozen-section analysis in questionable cases. If positive nodes are discovered near the origin of the inferior mesenteric artery, it is necessary to extend the dissection over the lower aorta and down the contralateral common iliac artery. Retrograde lymphatic spread of tumor can occur when these nodes are blocked. However, when positive nodes are located only superiorly, we still attempt to preserve the lower aorta. In probable stage IIB disease, however, the dissection should be extended to the contralateral side with full mobilization of the aorta and vena cava. The sympathetic ganglia usually can be preserved in these cases unless the disease is adherent to the psoas adjacent to the vertebral bodies.

Primary Surgery versus Chemotherapy for Clinical Stage IIA or IIB

Patients are classified as having clinical stage IIA or IIB disease when they have persistent elevation of hCG–β subunit or AFP levels following orchiectomy or a moderate amount of retroperitoneal adenopathy evident on CT scan. Currently, two approaches are taken to the

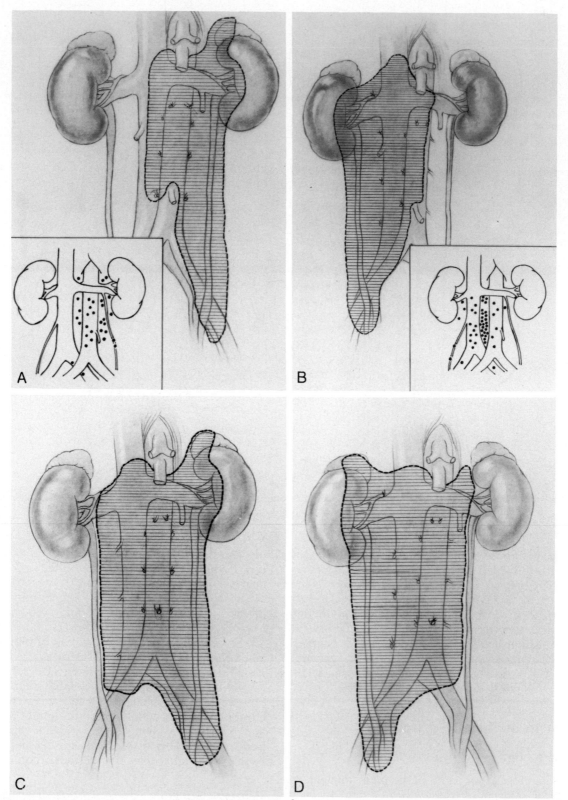

Figure 86–4. Our adopted limits of dissection for retroperitoneal lymphadenectomy. Insets in *A* and *B* show distribution of positive nodes in patients with microscopic disease, stage IIA. *A*, Limited left-sided dissection.

B, Limited right-sided dissection.

C, Full bilateral left-sided dissection.

D, Full bilateral right-sided dissection. (From Wise, P. G., and Scardino, P. T.: *In* Skinner, D. G., and Lieskovsky, G. (Eds.): Diagnosis and Management of Genitourinary Cancer. Philadelphia, W. B. Saunders Co., 1988, p. 779.)

treatment of these patients: (1) primary chemotherapy followed by node dissection for residual disease and (2) primary lymph node dissection with or without adjuvant chemotherapy (Logothetis et al., 1985; Socinski, 1988; Vugrin and Whitmore, 1985). The results in terms of survival are comparable, but there are various advantages and disadvantages with each approach.

Patients treated with primary surgery generally require less chemotherapy, with associated lower morbidity. The staging is more accurate. Occasional patients with apparent lymphadenopathy on CT scan will have been overstaged and will require no chemotherapy at all. With small volume disease, the surgery may be less difficult with lower morbidity prior to exposure to chemotherapy.

Alternatively, up to 75 per cent of patients with stage II disease, primarily those with pure embryonal cell type, achieve complete remission with primary chemotherapy and do not require node dissection (Logothetis et al., 1985; Socinski et al., 1988). In our experience, the CT scan more often underestimates the extent of adenopathy than overestimates it. Clearly, the surgeon must avoid the situation of an incomplete resection or a surgical injury due to more extensive disease than expected. With larger volume disease, the lymph node dissection may be safer following chemotherapy because of the fibrous capsule that forms around the tumor, decreasing the probability of spill. The ability to preserve ejaculation following surgery may be enhanced by the significant reduction in tumor bulk that usually results from chemotherapy.

The decision to approach a particular patient with primary surgery or chemotherapy will ultimately depend on the relative weight of these advantages and disadvantages as well as the skill and experience of the surgeon. We currently recommend an initial node dissection for most patients with questionable disease or a mass less than 3 cm. We are also more likely to do primary dissections on patients with teratomas in the primary testes tumors. We believe that all of these patients require node dissections, regardless of the results of chemotherapy. For those with disease or a mass more than 5 cm diameter on CT scan, we recommend primary chemotherapy with subsequent node dissection for residual disease. Intermediate-sized tumors are approached on a case-by-case basis.

Adjuvant Chemotherapy for Pathologic Stage IIA and IIB after Node Dissection

The risk of tumor recurrence following node dissection alone is 37 to 49 per cent for pathologic stage IIA and IIB disease combined (Scardino, 1980; Williams et al., 1987). This risk can be decreased to 0 to 15 per cent with adjuvant chemotherapy regimens, using actinomycin D alone, "mini" vinblastine, actinomycin D, and bleomycin (VAB), two cycles of platinol (cisplatin), vinblastine, and bleomycin (PVB), or vinblastine and bleomycin alone (Scardino, 1980; Skinner, 1976; Williams et al., 1987). However, this requires the treatment of all patients. The results must be compared with the

results obtained in delayed chemotherapy upon evidence of recurrence.

A multicenter trial was completed in 1984, with 195 patients randomized to observation or chemotherapy (with two courses of VAB or PVB) following bilateral node dissection. Three deaths due to cancer occurred in the observation group and one in the chemotherapy group. The latter patient had undergone a unilateral node dissection. The difference in survival in the two groups was not statistically significant (Williams et al., 1987).

This study did not show a wide variation in the relapse rate of patients with minimal versus moderate retroperitoneal disease (40 to 60 per cent). Others have suggested that patients with microscopic nodal involvement (stage IIA) in fact have a much lower risk of recurrence, as low as 6 to 8 per cent, and do not warrant adjuvant chemotherapy (Richie, 1990; Socinski et al., 1988). Patients with stage IIB disease, however, have reported relapse rates as high as 66 per cent without adjuvant chemotherapy (Skinner, 1976).

Other issues must be discussed in relation to this question. In many ways, they parallel those discussed in the observation protocols for patients with stage I disease.

First, follow-up in patients who are 15- to 35-year-old males is notoriously poor. In the randomized trial previously cited, the mean number of visits per year was nine (of 12 planned), with 25 per cent of patients making six or fewer visits (Williams et al., 1987). Thus, the risk of a patient being lost to follow-up and presenting again with extensive disease is real and may result in an unsalvageable case.

Second, the toxicity of the full platinum-based chemotherapy regimen is significant, with serious acute side effects including an incidence of sepsis up to 10 per cent and occasional treatment-related deaths (Moul, 1989). Long-term side effects include peripheral neuropathy, Raynaud's phenomenon, and azospermia (in up to 50 per cent), and possibly an increased risk of cardiac ischemic events (Doll et al., 1986; Roth et al., 1988; Vogelzang et al., 1981). Adjuvant treatment protocols without cisplatin are less toxic, but they also may be less effective in avoiding recurrence (Skinner, 1976). To date, there has been no direct comparison of the toxicity of two cycles of a platinum-based combination with that of three or four cycles. The philosophic question is whether it is better to expose all patients to a lower level of toxicity in order to avoid the greater toxicity for 50 to 60 per cent.

Third, the issues of the anxiety and the disturbance of normal lifestyles caused by the two approaches are impossible to quantitate. Patients treated with adjuvant chemotherapy have completed treatment in less than 3 months, with a very low risk of recurrence thereafter. By comparison, the patients who are observed are aware of a great chance that they will need full-dose chemotherapy sometime in the next 2 years.

We continue to recommend adjuvant chemotherapy for all patients with stage IIB disease, using 4 weekly cycles of bleomycin, Oncovin (vincristine), platinum, and VP16 (BOP-VP16) or 2 monthly cycles of platinum, etoposide, bleomycin (PEB). Patients with stage IIA disease are offered the alternatives of 1 week of a vinblastine and bleomycin combination and observation alone.

SURGICAL TECHNIQUE OF RETROPERITONEAL NODE DISSECTION

Choice of Surgical Approach

Multiple surgical approaches to the retroperitoneum have been described. The two most popular currently are the thoracoabdominal and transabdominal incisions. Each type of incision has specific advantages. The thoracoabdominal incision provides superb exposure to the upper retroperitoneum, with the renal hilum essentially in the middle of the field. This approach is crucial in the patient with advanced disease who may have a large retroperitoneal mass and who may require a thorough suprahilar dissection. In most patients, the node dissection can be performed entirely outside the peritoneal cavity, reducing postoperative ileus and eliminating the risk of late bowel obstruction, which is approximately 3 per cent in transabdominal surgery.

The transabdominal approach, however, offers a faster opening and closure of the incision and is a more familiar procedure to most surgeons. Exposure to the suprahilar area can be achieved but requires mobilization of the pancreas and spleen. No need exists to enter the chest cavity, decreasing the potential complications related to atelectasis and accumulation of pleural fluid.

The overall incidence of major morbidity in low-stage disease, in our experience and that of others, is 3 to 4 per cent with each type of incision, although specific complications vary (Donohue, 1981 and 1986; Skinner, 1982). However, others report early complication rates up to 27 per cent (Moul, 1989). In low-stage disease, the choice between the two approaches primarily reflects the training of the surgeon.

Preoperative Preparation and Position

After a routine preoperative work-up, the patient undergoes hydration overnight with Ringer's lactate. We administer a combined continuous epidural and general anesthesia for most cases. The epidural is also used postoperatively for analgesia. We generally provide perioperative antibiotics, although they are optional. No bowel preparation is used routinely in low-stage disease.

Technique of Thoracoabdominal Node Dissection

The technique of a full bilateral dissection on the left side is described in detail, with specific comments about the right-sided dissection. A demonstration of the technique is also available on film (Skinner and Lieskovsky,

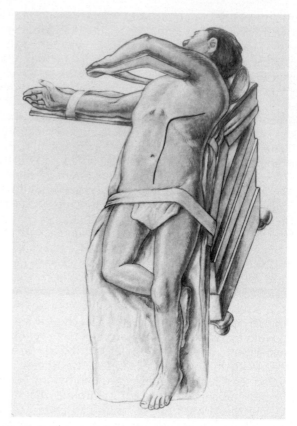

Figure 86–5. Thoracoabdominal position. Patient is positioned at the very edge of the table, with the break just above the iliac crest. The contralateral leg is flexed 30 degrees at the hip and 90 degrees at the knee, and the ipsilateral leg lies over the top with a pillow in between. The ipsilateral arm is supported on an "airplane," and the table is fully flexed. The incision is made over the 9th rib and carried down to the symphysis pubis as a paramedian incision. (From Skinner, D. G., and Lieskovsky, G. (Eds.): Diagnosis and Management of Genitourinary Cancer. Philadelphia, W. B. Saunders Co., 1988, p. 779.)

1984b). Modifications of the technique for a limited dissection for stage I disease are noted in the text.

The patient is positioned as in Figure 86–5. He is placed supine near the edge of the table, with the break in the table located just above the iliac crest. The ipsilateral arm is rotated over the head onto an adjustable arm rest. The lower leg is flexed 30 degrees at the hip and 90 degrees at the knee, and the upper leg is placed straight on a pillow. Sheet rolls are placed longitudinally under the back and abdomen. All potential pressure points are carefully padded, and the table is fully hyperextended. The patient is secured in place with wide adhesive tape.

An incision is made over the bed of the 8th or 9th rib from the midaxillary line to the midepigastrium. It is then carried down as a paramedian incision. The anterior rib is resected subperiosteally (Fig. 86–6), and the anterior rectus fascia is divided. The body of the ipsilateral rectus is mobilized and retracted laterally to avoid damaging the nerves to the muscle, which enter laterally. The proximal rectus is divided with electrocautery.

The pleural cavity is entered through the posterior periosteum of the rib. Blunt Mayo scissors are passed behind the costochondral junction anterior to the peritoneum, and the cartilage divided (Fig. 86–7). This maneuver allows the surgeon to develop the plane between the abdominal wall muscles and fascia and the peritoneal cavity utilizing blunt and sharp dissection. This dissection begins laterally and continues medially, where the peritoneum may be quite adherent along the lateral rectus sheath. A small peritoneotomy is not uncommon, but an attempt should be made to complete the extraperitoneal dissection. The posterior rectus fascia is freed from the peritoneum to its terminus at the arcuate line and is divided longitudinally.

Using the left hand with gentle downward traction on the spleen (or liver on the right), the attachments between the peritoneum and the underside of the diaphragm are separated back to the area of the central tendon of the diaphragm (Fig. 86–8A). This maneuver is best achieved by gently pushing off the muscular fibers of the diaphragm as they attach to the peritoneum. This move is important to subsequently allow the peritoneal envelope to be fully mobilized medially. The diaphragm is then divided for a few centimeters from the costochondral junction posteriorly in the direction of its fibers. A Finochietto retractor is placed with the protruding costal cartilage fixed in the holes in the retractor blades. Palpation of the ipsilateral lung is carried out to detect any unexpected nodules. If found, these nodules are wedge resected at the end of the procedure.

The next step is the mobilization of the posterior peritoneum off the anterior surface of Gerota's fascia. This step is the key to performing a completely extraperitoneal dissection. It is initiated superiorly where one can usually identify the plane between the cephalad extension of Gerota's fascia and the peritoneum. The fibers of the transversalis fascia must be incised sharply to enter the loose fibroareolar tissue in the avascular plane (Fig. 86–8B), which can then be developed bluntly

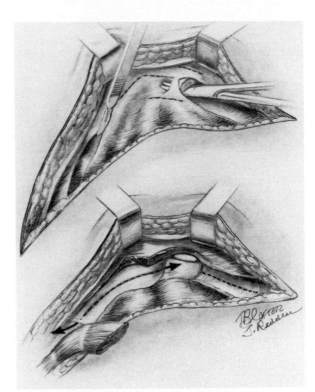

Figure 86–7. A subperiosteal rib resection has been completed. The anterior rectus fascia is divided in the abdominal portion of the wound. Scissors are passed behind the costochondral junction anterior to the peritoneum, allowing the surgeon to bluntly develop the plane between the peritoneum and the transversalis fascia. (From Wise, P. G., and Scardino, P. T.: In Skinner, D. G., and Lieskovsky, G. (Eds.): Diagnosis and Management of Genitourinary Cancer. Philadelphia, W. B. Saunders Co., 1988, p. 779.)

over the top of Gerota's fascia to the anterior aorta and vena cava. Only three structures penetrate through the anterior Gerota's fascia: the celiac artery, superior mesenteric artery (SMA), and inferior mesenteric artery (IMA). In advanced disease (stage IIA or IIB), we routinely divide the IMA as it is encountered entering the peritoneal envelope, which allows full mobilization of the peritoneum to the opposite side. This step is avoided in elderly individuals who may have compromise of the collateral blood supply to the colon. In a limited dissection, the IMA is preserved and represents the distal limit of dissection on the aorta.

The next step is the identification of the root of the SMA, which is a key landmark in the retroperitoneum. The inferior mesenteric vein is traced superiorly to its junction with the splenic vein, and the SMA is located immediately medially, arising from the aorta just superior to the crossing of the left renal vein. The origin of the SMA is skeletonized, carefully clipping the lacteals running alongside it with small hemoclips. The left crus of the diaphragm is identified, and the tissue overlying it, including the celiac plexus, is clipped and divided (Fig. 86–9).

Gerota's fascia is dissected from its cephalad attachments to the diaphragm, clipping and dividing the small arterial branches from the phrenic vessels to the adrenal. In a limited dissection on the right the adrenal gland can be preserved, coming instead across Gerota's fascia between the adrenal and kidney. On the left, the adrenal

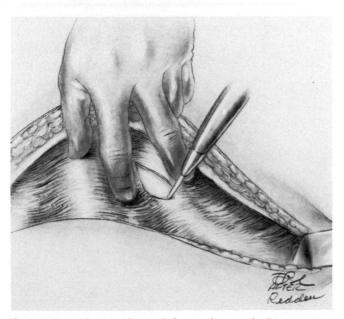

Figure 86–6. The muscles and fascia along with the periosteum overlying the 9th rib are divided using electrocautery. (From Wise, P. G., and Scardino, P. T.: In Skinner, D. G., and Lieskovsky, G. (Eds.): Diagnosis and Management of Genitourinary Cancer. Philadelphia, W. B. Saunders Co., 1988, p. 779.)

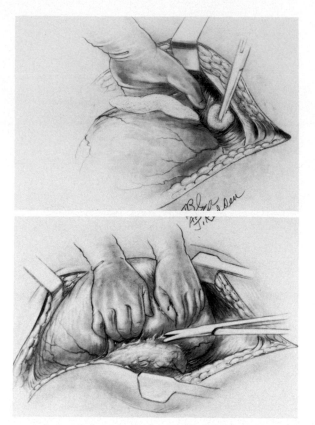

Figure 86–8. The attachments between the diaphragm and peritoneal envelope are divided back to the central tendon of the diaphragm. The peritoneum and Gerota's fascia together are mobilized off the posterior abdominal wall muscles. The avascular plane between the posterior peritoneum and the anterior leaf of Gerota's fascia is then identified and developed across the midline to the vena cava. The inferior mesenteric artery can be divided, if necessary. (From Wise, P. G., and Scardino, P. T.: *In* Skinner, D. G., and Lieskovsky, G. (Eds.): Diagnosis and Management of Genitourinary Cancer. Philadelphia, W. B. Saunders Co., 1988, p. 779.)

becomes devascularized during the remainder of the dissection, so it is not generally preserved.

Gerota's fascia is next split over the left renal vein. The left gonadal and ascending lumbar veins are ligated and divided. The renal vein is skeletonized, allowing it to be retracted inferiorly. The fibroareolar tissue overlying the aorta below the SMA is split and dissected laterally to identify the renal arteries on each side. The left renal artery is skeletonized toward the hilum as far as possible. Prior to this dissection the patient is given 12.5 g of intravenous mannitol to help maintain renal perfusion and decrease arterial spasm. Gerota's fascia is then split laterally over the the kidney, allowing half to be passed anterior and half posterior to the renal pedicle. The ureter is dissected out, mobilized down to the level of the common iliac artery, and retracted out of harm's way. The fibroareolar tissue is then further dissected off until it is free from its renal attachments.

Attention is then turned to the anterior aorta. The fibroareolar tissue is further split from the left renal vein down to the origin of the IMA. In a limited dissection we stop here, taking care not to disturb the aorta below the IMA. In a full dissection, the IMA is again ligated at its origin. It had been previously ligated more distally

with mobilization of the peritoneum. The tissue over the aorta is split down to the bifurcation. The aorta is then further skeletonized. All lumbar arteries are ligated in situ and divided (Fig. 86–10). We believe ligation of the lumbar arteries is necessary in both the limited and full dissections to allow adequate access to the nodal tissue behind the aorta and between the aorta and vena cava. The lumbar arteries arise as three evenly spaced pairs posteriorly. The ligatures should be carefully placed, as a dislodged tie will result in troublesome bleeding and probable damage to the sympathetic chain during attempts to control it.

Dissection continues over the left renal vein to the top of the inferior vena cava and is carried down the contralateral side. In a full bilateral dissection, we extend this over to the medial side of the right ureter. This tissue represents the lateral limit of dissection and should be clipped with hemoclips. The dissection continues down to the origin of the right gonadal vein. In a full dissection we ligate and divide this vein, taking the proximal few centimeters of it within the contralateral nodal "package." We then continue inferiorly to the crossing of the right common iliac artery. The fibroareolar tissue is dissected off the vena cava, and all lumbar veins are ligated and divided (Fig. 86–11).

In a limited dissection, we divide the tissue medial to the origin of the right gonadal, continuing inferiorly to 1 to 2 cm distal to the level of the IMA. The medial side of the cava is dissected free, only ligating the left lumbar veins.

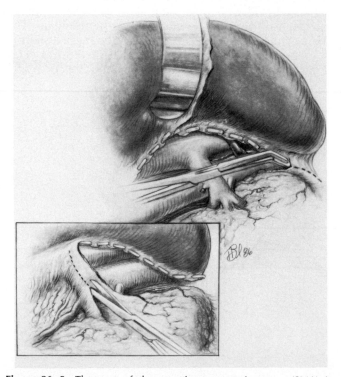

Figure 86–9. The root of the superior mesenteric artery (SMA) is identified just medial to the junction of the inferior mesenteric vein and splenic vein. The lacteals running parallel to the SMA are clipped distally, and the root of the SMA is cleaned off. The tissue over the left renal vein is divided anteriorly, and the left renal artery is identified. (From Wise, P. G., and Scardino, P. T.: *In* Skinner, D. G., and Lieskovsky, G. (Eds.): Diagnosis and Management of Genitourinary Cancer. Philadelphia, W. B. Saunders Co., 1988, p. 779.)

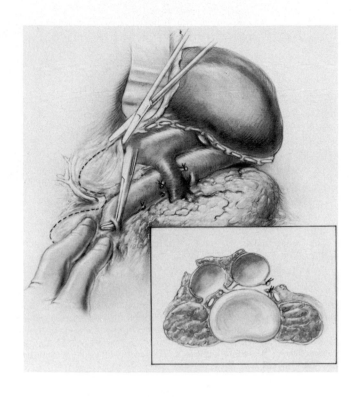

Figure 86–10. The tissue overlying the aorta is split down to the origin of the inferior mesenteric artery (IMA), and the ipsilateral lumbar arteries are ligated and divided. Care must be taken to identify and protect any accessory renal arteries that may be present. The tissue over the inferior vena cava is then split in the midline, clipping the lateral limits of the dissection. Inset shows the great vessels in cross-section, demonstrating the "split-and-roll" technique. (From Wise, P. G., and Scardino, P. T.: *In* Skinner, D. G., and Lieskovsky, G. (Eds.): Diagnosis and Management of Genitourinary Cancer. Philadelphia, W. B. Saunders Co., 1988, p. 779.)

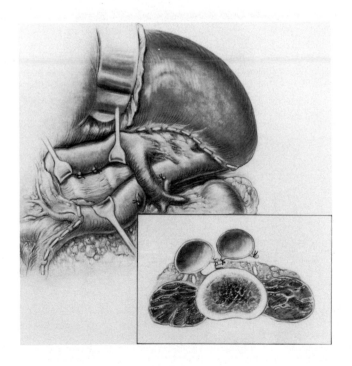

Figure 86–11. The opposite renal artery has been identified, and the tissue overlying the right crus of the diaphragm has been swept inferiorly. Gerota's fascia surrounding the left kidney has been split along the back of the kidney and swept inferiorly with the specimen. (From Wise, P. G., and Scardino, P. T.: *In* Skinner, D. G., and Lieskovsky, G. (Eds.): Diagnosis and Management of Genitourinary Cancer. Philadelphia, W. B. Saunders Co., 1988, p. 779.)

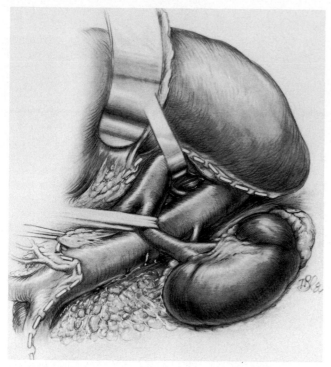

Figure 86–12. The right lumbar arteries and left lumbar veins have been ligated, completely freeing the aorta off the posterior abdominal wall. The interaortocaval tissue is then swept under the aorta to the left side. (From Wise, P. G., and Scardino, P. T.: *In* Skinner, D. G., and Lieskovsky, G. (Eds.): Diagnosis and Management of Genitourinary Cancer. Philadelphia, W. B. Saunders Co., 1988, p. 779.)

Superiorly, the right renal artery is dissected out to the point where it crosses the right crus of the diaphragm, behind the vena cava. The lymphatic tissue around the right renal artery is swept inferiorly, and the superior limit of dissection is clipped and divided (Fig. 86–12). Special care must be taken to clip the tissue behind the right renal artery, where the origin of the cisterna chyli is located. The dissection is continued inferiorly behind the vena cava, sweeping the tissue medially and inferiorly. Care is taken not to injure the contralateral sympathetic chain in this maneuver. Tiny vessels coursing from the lymphatic tissue to the sympathetic ganglia should be clipped rather than avulsed to minimize the risk of bleeding in this area. The contralateral ureter must also be protected from being inadvertently pulled under the vena cava with the nodal package.

The aorta is elevated with a vein retractor, and all the interaortocaval lymphatic tissue is swept to the left side of the aorta. As the intervertebral ligaments are exposed, the previously ligated stumps of the right lumbar arteries are seen coursing medial to the sympathetic chain. These must be carefully clipped and divided again, taking care not to place clips into the groove along the right side of the vertebral bodies where the sympathetic chain runs (Fig. 86–13).

At this point, the stump of the ipsilateral spermatic cord is dissected out of the internal inguinal ring, taking care not to injure the ureter or the peritoneum. The distal limit of dissection is then defined. In a full bilateral dissection, this maneuver will include all of the fibroare-

olar tissue between the common iliac arteries and will require cleaning off the left common iliac vein and sacral promontory. In a limited dissection, the tissue is split over the left lateral aorta from the IMA down the left common iliac artery, as shown in the template, leaving the distal anterior aorta and bifurcation area intact.

The ipsilateral sympathetic chain is identified at the pelvic brim, between the psoas muscle and sacrum behind the right common iliac artery. From there it can be traced superiorly as the nodal package is dissected off the psoas fascia. Each left lumbar artery and vein should be again clipped individually as it dives adjacent to the sympathetic ganglia. This step completes the dissection, and the specimen can be removed en bloc.

Closure

Careful inspection is undertaken to detect any bleeding. The origin of each lumbar artery should be reinforced with a hemoclip for added security. A chest tube is inserted routinely. The diaphragm is closed with two running layers of No. 0 polyglycolic acid (PGA) suture. The abdomen and chest are both closed with

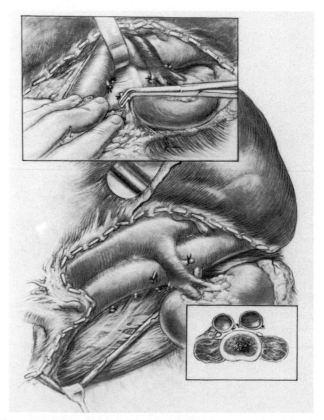

Figure 86–13. The ureter is skeletonized and the stump of the spermatic cord is removed from the internal inguinal ring. As the specimen is dissected off the anterior spinous ligaments, the lumbar vessels are again clipped with hemoclips as they dive into the foramena. The sympathetic chain, not shown here, can usually be clearly identified in the groove between the vertebral body and the psoas muscle and should be protected. Note that the dissection does not disturb any tissue anterior to the aorta below the origin of the inferior mesenteric artery. (From Wise, P. G., and Scardino, P. T.: *In* Skinner, D. G., and Lieskovsky, G. (Eds.): Diagnosis and Management of Genitourinary Cancer. Philadelphia, W. B. Saunders Co., 1988, p. 779.)

inverted, interrupted figure-of-eight sutures of No. 1 nylon in a single layer. In the medial portion of the chest incision, the diaphragm should be included in this suture layer to avoid a leak at this point. This is made less difficult by placing all of the sutures prior to tying them.

Right-Sided Dissection

The initial exposure to the right side is identical to the left, with the exception that the IMA is not generally sacrificed in low-stage disease. The dissection begins with skeletonization of the root of the SMA. In a limited dissection the aorta is cleaned off from the midpoint over, taking only the right lumbar arteries. The vena cava is completely skeletonized, ligating all lumbar veins bilaterally. These are much less predictable in their location than the lumbar arteries. The left sympathetic chain is generally not visualized in a limited dissection, and the right is preserved as previously described. All tissue overlying the aorta distal to the IMA is left intact, as is the area between the common iliac arteries.

Complications

The most common intraoperative complications result from damage to one of the major vascular structures. Aortic injuries can usually be repaired with sutures, but large defects may require patch graft. Vena cava injuries can almost always be oversewn. Damage to the main renal artery can also occur and should be repaired if possible. Primary repair may risk subsequent stenosis and loss of the renal unit, and a patch graft may be necessary. If a small polar vessel is ligated or injured it is best left alone. Hypertension appears to be extremely rare in such instances, probably because the kidney has been stripped of any potential collateral arterial supply through Gerota's fascia (Skinner et al., 1982). Bleeding from an avulsed lumbar vessel should be controlled with an Allis clamp until the area is fully dissected and carefully clipped or oversewn, taking care to avoid damage to the sympathetic chain if possible.

Ureteral injury during dissection is best repaired by ureteroneocystostomy when possible. A mid- or proximal ureteral injury is problematic because of the extensive mobilization of the ureter during the node dissection. Ureteroureterostomy can be attempted but may result in a leak or stenosis due to compromised vascular supply. Such a primary repair should be stented. Other alternatives include placement of a nephrostomy tube with a planned second stage ileal ureteral replacement or autotransplantation of the kidney into the pelvis. Nephrectomy may also be considered in the presence of a normal opposite kidney.

Concern about compromise of the vascular supply to the spinal cord resulting from ligation of the lumbar arteries is unwarranted. The anterior spinal artery syndrome, which has been reported rarely in patients undergoing abdominal aortic aneurysm repair, has not been seen in our experience or that of others in large medical centers (Donohue, 1986; Skinner et al., 1982). Other complications, such as wound infection, are rare. The most common long-term complication is anejaculation, which is discussed in detail previously in this chapter.

Postoperative Care

Generally, the chest tube can be removed on the 1st postoperative day. Occasional high serous output from the chest tube reflects a leak in the retroperitoneal lymphatics and resolves with time. Postoperative pain control can be improved with epidural morphine or intercostal block, which improves respiratory effort and minimizes atelectasis. Postoperative ileus is minimized by the extraperitoneal approach, and most patients are discharged in 4 to 7 days.

Technique of Transabdominal Node Dissection

This procedure has been described in detail (Donohue, 1977 and 1988). The advantages of the transabdominal approach are discussed earlier in this chapter. The details of the incision and the exposure of the retroperitoneum are described here, with comments about the differences from the thoracoabdominal approach.

The incision is made in the midline from the xiphoid to the symphysis pubis. It is carried down through the subcutaneous tissues and the linea alba, and the peri-

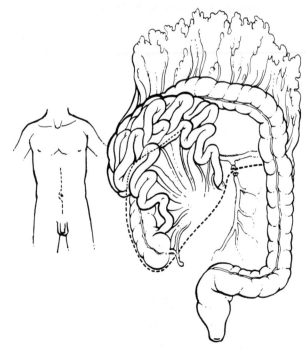

Figure 86–14. Incisions in the posterior peritoneum that provide exposure to the retroperitoneum. In a limited dissection, the incision extends only down to the area of the cecum. In a full dissection, the right colon is completely mobilized and the small bowel and ascending colon are placed in a plastic bag on the chest. (From Donohue, J. P.: Urol. Clin. North Am., 4:509, 1977.)

toneal cavity is entered. The abdomen is explored carefully for any unexpected pathology. A self-retaining ring retractor is placed.

The posterior peritoneum is divided along the root of the small bowel mesentery from the ligament of Treitz to the cecum. Superiorly, the inferior mesenteric vein is divided between ligatures to facilitate mobilization of the mesentery of the left colon. For a limited dissection the right colon is not mobilized. Deaver retractors over laparotomy pads are used to expose the retroperitoneum (Fig. 86–14).

For a bilateral dissection, the incision in the posterior peritoneum is carried around the cecum and up the right side of the colon to the foramen of Winslow, and the right colon is mobilized off Gerota's fascia. The entire small bowel and right colon are placed in a Lahey bag on the chest. The IMA can also be divided at its origin to allow full lateral mobilization of the sigmoid mesentery.

Suprahilar Dissection

In stage IIB disease, the suprahilar areas must be dissected bilaterally. To accomplish this, the head and body of the pancreas are elevated and retracted under two deep Harrington retractors protected by laparotomy pads. The origin of the SMA is identified and skeletonized, clipping the lymphatics that surround it. It is usually necessary to ligate and divide the inferior mesenteric vein near its junction with the splenic vein to complete the suprahilar dissection on the left. The fibroareolar tissue overlying either crus of the diaphragm is clipped as high as possible, including the celiac ganglia bilaterally, and mobilized inferiorly.

On the right, the cisterna chyli is identified and clipped. The dissection continues over the inferior vena cava just distal to the first hepatic vein. The right adrenal vein is ligated and divided. The tissue is dissected off the medial adrenal gland and posterior body wall down to the renal vessels, which are skeletonized out to the renal hilum. The tissue can be either removed separately or passed behind the renal vessels and removed en bloc with the rest of the specimen (Fig. 86–15*A*).

On the left, the adrenal vein and small arterial branches from the aorta to the adrenal gland are divided between clips or ligatures. The attachments to the medial border of the adrenal are clipped, and the tissue is mobilized off the posterior muscles. The renal vessels are mobilized, ligating the ascending lumbar and left gonadal veins as they enter the left renal vein. The tissue is removed separately or en bloc with the infrahilar dissection (Fig. 86–15*B*).

Infrahilar Dissection

The infrahilar dissection is essentially identical to that described previously in the thoracoabdominal approach. The limits of the dissection are those outlined in Figure 86–4. The dissection begins with splitting the fibroareolar tissue overlying the aorta and vena cava anteriorly (Fig. 86–16). Although some workers state that ligation of the lumbar vessels is not necessary in a limited dissection (Donohue, 1988), we believe that it is safer to do so and allows more complete dissection of the posterior package of nodes that lies behind the great vessels. A "split-and-roll" technique is employed to dissect the nodal package off the great vessels and posterior abdominal wall muscles (Fig. 86–17). For a

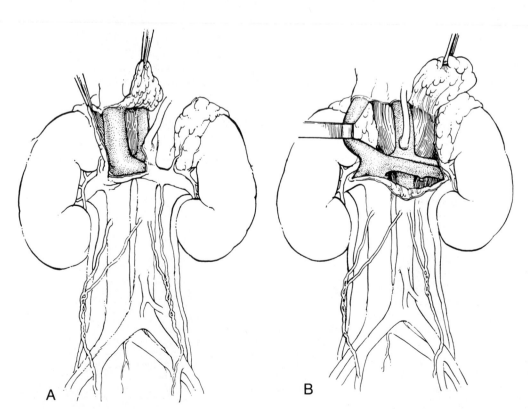

Figure 86–15. Right (*A*) and left (*B*) suprahilar dissections extending 4 to 6 cm above the renal arteries, exposing the crura of the diaphragm. (From Donohue, J. P.: Urol. Clin. North Am., 4:509, 1977.)

A   B

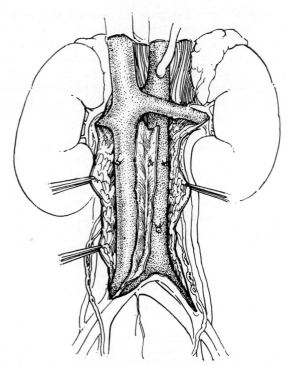

Figure 86–16. Infrahilar transabdominal dissection. When the lumbar arteries and veins have been divided, the great vessels are elevated and the nodal package swept off the anterior vertebral ligaments and posterior abdominal wall muscles. In a limited dissection, the division of the tissue overlying the aorta would extend only down to the origin of the inferior mesenteric artery. (From Donohue, J. P.: Urol. Clin. North Am., 4:509, 1977.)

limited dissection, both sympathetic chains are carefully preserved, as is all tissue overlying the aorta below the IMA.

Postoperative Care and Complications

Management of intraoperative complications is identical to that outlined under the thoracoabdominal technique. Postoperatively, patients require nasogastric suction drainage for several days until the ileus resolves. Otherwise, routine postoperative care techniques apply.

Technique of Prospective Nerve-Sparing Node Dissection

Interest has been evolving in attempting to improve on the 50 to 75 per cent preservation of ejaculation, which is attainable with template-type limited dissections, such as those previously described. Based on autopsy studies of the sympathetic nerve supply to the pelvis, Jewett and associates (1988) and Donohue and associates, (1990) and others developed the so-called prospective nerve-sparing node dissection. This technique involves the early identification of the postganglionic fibers emanating from the lumbar ganglia at L1 to L4, which course anteriorly over the aorta and coalesce into multiple trunks, forming the hypogastric plexus overlying the inferior aorta and sacral promontory (Fig. 86–18). When these roots have been identified and marked with fine vessel loops, the nodes over and around the aorta are dissected out and removed in multiple small packages. No attempt is made to ligate the lumbar arteries.

This technique adds at least 1 hour to the operative time in the hands of those who do it routinely (Jewett et al., 1988), but it reliably results in close to 100 per cent preservation of ejaculation.

The primary issue concerns the adequacy of the dissection in preventing subsequent tumor relapse in the retroperitoneum. Donohue and colleagues (1990) reported that none of 61 patients with pathologically negative nodes experienced recurrence in the retroperitoneum with a minimum follow-up period of 24 months. However, one definite and possibly two retroperitoneal recurrences were noted among 14 patients with stage IIA and IIB disease, all of whom were salvaged with chemotherapy. Longer follow-up of these patients and confirmation of the results by other workers in other

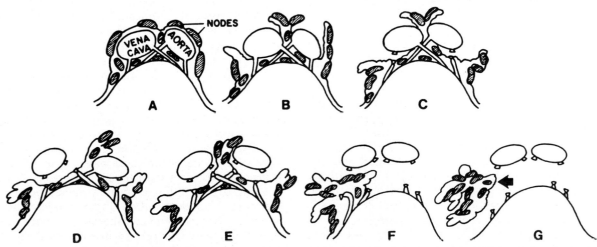

Figure 86–17. A to G, This diagram illustrates the "split-and-roll" technique allowing en bloc removal of the nodal package. The lumbar vessels must be divided twice, first at the wall of the great vessels, and again as they enter the foramina alongside the vertebral bodies. The sympathetic ganglia run in the lateral grooves between the great vessels and psoas muscles, just lateral to the lumbar vessels as they enter the foramina. (From Donohue, J. P.: Urol. Clin. North Am., 4:509, 1977.)

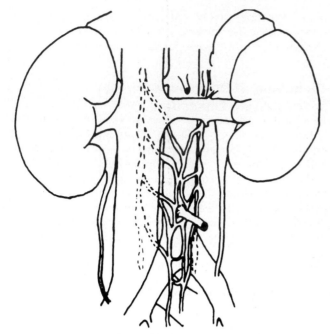

Figure 86–18. Postganglionic fibers course anteriorly off the lumbar sympathetic ganglia to coalesce into trunks passing anterior to the aorta. (From Jewett, M. A. S., et al.: J. Urol., 139:1220, 1988. © Williams & Wilkins.)

medical centers will be required before this approach can be endorsed without reservation. If retroperitoneal recurrence becomes a problem and routine CT scans are required in follow-up, the prospective surgical approach may not really offer any advantage over surveillance for stage I disease. In the meantime, the template modified dissection previously described provides an alternate approach that is surgically straightforward and has a very low retroperitoneal recurrence rate.

SURGERY FOR ADVANCED STAGE DISEASE

Timing of Retroperitoneal Dissection in Stage III

All workers currently agree that any patient with advanced testicular cancer, stage IIC (retroperitoneal disease >10 cm or palpable), or stage III (disease beyond the retroperitoneal lymphatics) should be treated primarily with full-dose platinum-based chemotherapy. The specifics of the chemotherapy are beyond the scope of this chapter. We are currently utilizing a weekly combination of platinum, vincristine, bleomycin, and VP16, which seems to be better tolerated than the standard Einhorn regimen of monthly PEB. The patients are treated for at least 6 weeks, or 2 weeks beyond the time when serum marker levels normalize. Repeat CT scan of the abdomen and chest is then performed.

If the patient has any evidence of residual retroperitoneal disease on CT scan, or if the primary tumor contained teratomatous elements, he is scheduled for a node dissection 4 to 6 weeks following the last treatment.

Patients who have evidence of residual disease in the lungs, or who had supraclavicular adenopathy on presentation, undergo surgical exploration and dissection of those areas prior to retroperitoneal dissection, under separate anesthesia. The rationale for this practice is that if these areas cannot be cleared of all viable tumor there is little reason to subject the patient to the more extensive retroperitoneal dissection and its potential morbidity.

Patients with significant retroperitoneal masses (>10 cm) rarely in our experience have completely normal CT scans after chemotherapy alone (Carter et al., 1987). These men all undergo node dissection. However, the patient with minimal-to-moderate retroperitoneal disease and lung metastases (i.e., stage IIB-III) may have normal serum marker levels and CT scan following chemotherapy in up to 86 per cent of cases (Dexeus et al., 1989). We are willing to follow these patients without a node dissection providing the primary tumor contains no teratomatous elements. Mature teratoma in the retroperitoneum generally is not eradicated by chemotherapy and has a tendency for persistent growth over many years (Logothetis et al., 1982). Although the metastatic potential of such growth is controversial, there is no doubt that it can cause significant and potentially life-threatening problems for the patient, with renal obstruction, mediastinal compression, and possible malignant degeneration. Therefore, we believe that all patients with teratomatous elements in the primary tumor should undergo lymphadenectomy at the time of least disease, shortly after finishing chemotherapy.

Patients who do not achieve normalization of elevated hCG–β subunit or AFP levels with chemotherapy are rarely cured with surgery. Their ultimate cure depends on the response to alternative chemotherapy programs. Therefore, except in rare circumstances, these patients should undergo salvage chemotherapy prior to resection of any residual disease.

The histology of the residual mass in postchemotherapy dissections is scar tissue in 27 to 58 per cent, mature teratoma in 22 to 38 per cent, and viable carcinoma in 12 to 35 per cent (Carter et al., 1987; Donohue, 1984; Loehrer, 1986; Stoter et al., 1984; Vugrin et al., 1981). We recommend additional chemotherapy for any patient with residual viable carcinoma, because more than 50 per cent will relapse following surgery alone (Skinner, 1976). The patients with mature teratoma histology may be at higher risk of tumor recurrence in the future than the patients with scar tissue (Loehrer et al., 1986). These recurrences may be in the form of mature or immature teratoma or frank carcinoma and may occur late (>24 months) after the initial treatment. To date, most of the late recurrences have occurred outside or adjacent to the retroperitoneal dissection. We believe this risk can be minimized by a meticulous dissection. We have elected to follow these patients rather than provide any further chemotherapy. Clearly, continued careful follow-up management is essential for at least 3 years, and, preferably, 5 years.

Occasionally, the histology of the residual mass demonstrates sarcomatous elements, such as embryonal rhabdomyosarcoma or angiosarcoma. This finding occurred in 11 of 269 patients at Indiana University over 6 years. Often the nongerm cell elements were present in the primary testis tumor and, perhaps, were "unmasked" by the disappearance of the metastatic germ cell elements with chemotherapy. Regardless of etiology, the presence of these sarcomatous elements carries a poor prognosis, and the optimum therapy is unknown (Loehrer et al., 1986).

Management of a Residual Mass in Advanced Seminoma

Like nonseminomatous disease, advanced seminoma is now primarily treated with platinum-based chemotherapy, with equally good results (Loehrer et al., 1987; Peckham et al., 1985). However, the management of residual bulk tumor following chemotherapy remains controversial. Viable tumor cells are discovered in the residual mass in 0 to 42 per cent of patients, depending in part on the size of the residual mass (Motzer, 1988; Schultz, 1989). Completing a thorough retroperitoneal lymph node dissection in these cases is often very difficult or impossible, owing to a thick sheet of fibrous reactive tissue that encases the great vessels. Many workers recommend an excision of the mass alone, rather than a full node dissection (Motzer et al., 1988).

All series have relatively small numbers, and it has not been proven that resection of residual masses translates to a survival advantage in these cases. However, the presence of viable tumor does identify those patients who should receive further treatment in the form of either salvage chemotherapy or radiation therapy. Routine "consolidation" radiation therapy of residual masses does not appear to prevent relapse and can limit the tolerance of further chemotherapy (Peckham et al., 1985).

Our current policy is to surgically resect any residual retroperitoneal mass greater than 3.0 cm following chemotherapy. Masses less than 3.0 cm are observed with CT scan every 3 months the first year, and every 6 months the 2nd and 3rd years.

Technique of Retroperitoneal Node Dissection for Advanced Disease

Preoperative Preparation

Patients who have been exposed to chemotherapy require special attention to prepare them for such extensive surgery. The white blood cell and platelet counts must be at normal levels prior to surgery. Patients exposed to bleomycin should have a pulmonary function evaluation. The anesthesiologist must be advised about the need to maintain low inspired oxygen and low crystalloid replacement intraoperatively and postoperatively. In addition, patients may have other problems, such as renal insufficiency or anemia, which should be addressed. We do a routine mechanical bowel preparation on these patients. A full antibiotic preparation is done in cases with suspected large or small bowel invasion by the tumor.

Incision

Patients requiring a postchemotherapy node dissection, especially those with a significant retroperitoneal mass, are best approached by a thoracoabdominal incision. Suprahilar dissections, often extending into the retrocrural space are necessary, and the exposure to this area is clearly superior through a high (6th to 8th rib) thoracoabdominal incision. In patients with minimal residual disease, the dissection may be completed entirely retroperitoneally, as previously described. With a significant mass, however, we open the peritoneal cavity routinely, as subsequently described.

The patient positioning and initial steps of the exposure are identical to those described in a low-stage dissection. It is helpful to separate the peritoneal envelope from the diaphragm even when a transperitoneal approach is planned, because this facilitates mobilization of the liver or spleen and pancreas. The peritoneum is opened, and the right colon and root of the small bowel mesentery are mobilized off the retroperitoneum (Fig. 86–19). The bowel is placed in a Lahey bag on the chest. It is not uncommon to find invasion of the duodenum by the mass, which may require duodenal resection. The posterior peritoneum is divided lateral to the left colon. The sigmoid mesentery is similarly mobilized off Gerota's fascia. This mesentery is often

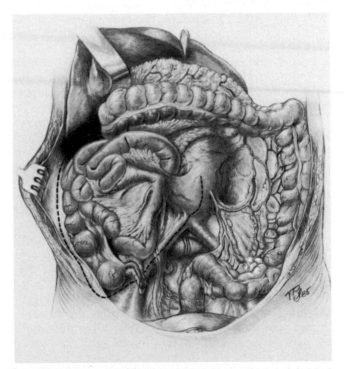

Figure 86–19. Exposure of the retroperitoneum via a thoracoabdominal, transperitoneal approach for advanced disease following chemotherapy. The posterior peritoneum is incised from the ligament of Treitz down along the root of the small bowel mesentery, around the cecum and up the right colic gutter. This maneuver allows all of the small bowel and ascending colon to be placed into a plastic bag on the chest.

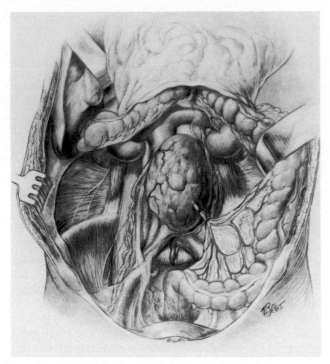

Figure 86–20. The inferior mesenteric artery, which often is encased in the mass, is divided. The left colon is mobilized off Gerota's fascia. The sigmoid mesentery may be adherent to the mass and can be resected, provided the marginal artery remains intact.

involved with the tumor mass and can be divided, providing the marginal artery is carefully protected. The IMA may also be encased in the tumor mass and must be carefully identified and ligated (Fig. 86–20).

The SMA must be identified early. If the area of the left renal vein is involved with tumor, normal areas of the inferior vena cava above and below the tumor should be identified and controlled with Rumel tourniquets prior to dissecting out the left renal vein.

The tumor mass is divided over the inferior vena cava, developing the subadventitial plane under the fibrous capsule formed by the tumor after chemotherapy. The basic technique of "split and roll" is followed throughout the dissection. The lumbar veins are ligated and divided until the entire cava is mobilized. Care must be taken to watch for accessory right renal arteries coursing over the top of the vena cava.

The contralateral ureter is identified and protected during the dissection. The ipsilateral ureter is often encased in the tumor mass. This ureter should be dissected out early, to allow the surgeon to decide if it can be salvaged. If the ureter is damaged during the dissection or cannot be separated from the tumor, a nephrectomy should be performed with the dissection.

Once the vena cava is fully mobilized, the aorta is identified inferiorly. The tumor should be split in its thinnest area over the aorta. Dissection under the adventitia of the aorta should be avoided as much as possible. If this injury occurs it should be repaired, with graft material if necessary, as it may result in a late aortic rupture. The renal arteries are identified, and the right and left lumbar arteries are ligated and divided. This maneuver is difficult, especially in cases of significant retroaortic disease.

Specialized vascular techniques may be required during the dissection, including suture repair, patch graft or segmental replacement of the aorta, and repair or resection of the vena cava. The vena cava can safely be resected below the renal veins if the tumor extends into it as a thrombus or is obliterated by the tumor. The patient may develop significant lower extremity edema if the cava has not been previously obstructed, but this will gradually resolve (Ahlering and Skinner, 1989).

When the great vessels are fully mobilized, the tumor is dissected off the posterior body wall. The lumbar vessels are again clipped as they dive into the foramina. Tongues of tumor may be growing alongside the lumbar vessels, which should be teased out of the foramina if possible. If necessary, the anterior psoas fascia can be removed with the tumor. Generally, no attempt is made to preserve the sympathetic chain during this dissection.

Superiorly, the tissue overlying the crura of the diaphragm is clipped and swept inferiorly with the nodal package. If there is any question of retrocrural disease, the crura can be divided with cautery alongside the vertebral body. When the retrocrural tissue has been dissected out as far superiorly as possible, the crura should be repaired. Special care must be taken on the right to adequately clip the thoracic duct and the azygous vein complex during this dissection.

When the tumor has been removed the aorta should be carefully inspected for hemostasis, and all ligated branches reinforced with hemoclips. We do not routinely leave any drains except for a chest tube.

Complications

Major intraoperative and postoperative complications are more common in patients with large volume retroperitoneal disease (Donohue, 1981 and 1986; Moul, 1989; Skinner et al., 1982). Vascular complications, discussed in detail previously, are common but should not pose a problem if the surgeon is prepared. Injuries to the renal vessels or ureter also occur, resulting in occasional nephrectomy.

Major postoperative complications occurred in nine of 52 (17 per cent) patients with stage IIC or III disease in our series (Skinner et al., 1982), and in six of 45 (13 per cent) in the Indiana series (Donohue, 1986). The most devastating potential complication is fatal adult respiratory distress syndrome associated with bleomycin toxicity. Goldfinger and Schweizer (1979) associated this risk with increased inspired oxygen and overhydration. This risk must be kept in mind constantly and requires the cooperation of the anesthesiologist and surgeon to avoid problems. We generally ventilate the patient with room air during surgery, never raising inspired FiO_2 to exceed 25 to 30 per cent. We also use a colloid:crystalloid ratio of 2:1 during the perioperative period and carefully avoid overhydration.

Other major postoperative complications that have occurred include thrombophlebitis, small bowel obstruction, wound dehiscence, and appendiceal abscess. We no longer perform routine appendectomy because of this last complication.

In spite of the magnitude of the surgery, patients tolerate this procedure remarkably well, and there are few long-term complications other than anejaculation.

The efficacy of the procedure is attested to by the fact that we reported only one retroperitoneal recurrence in 147 patients undergoing retroperitoneal node dissection, including 52 patients with advanced disease (Skinner et al., 1982).

REFERENCES

Ahlering, T. A., and Skinner, D. G.: Vena caval resection in bulky metastatic germ cell tumors. J. Urol., 142:1497, 1989.

Bennett, C. J., Seager, S. W. J., and McGuire, E.: Electroejaculation for recovery of semen after retroperitoneal lymph node dissection: case report. J. Urol., 137:513, 1987.

Benson, C. J.: The role of ultrasound in diagnosis and staging of testicular cancer. Semin. Urol., 6:189, 1988.

Boileau, M. A., and Steers, W. D.: Testis tumors: the clinical significance of the tumor-contaminated scrotum. J. Urol., 132:51, 1984.

Calvo, F., Hodson, N., Barrett, A., and Peckham, M. J.: Chemotherapy of primary (in situ) testicular tumours: response in advanced metastatic disease. Br. J. Urol., 55:560, 1983.

Carter, G. E., Lieskovsky, G., Skinner, D. G., and Daniels, J. R.: Reassessment of the role of adjunctive surgical therapy in the treatment of advanced germ cell tumors. J. Urol., 138:1397, 1987.

Catalona, W. J.: Tumor markers in testicular cancer. Urol. Clin. North Am., 6:613, 1979.

Dexeus, F. H., Shirkhoda, A., Logothetis, C. J., Chong, C., Sella, A., Ogden, S., and Swanson, D.: Clinical and radiological correlation of retroperitoneal metastasis from nonseminomatous testicular cancer treated with chemotherapy. Eur. J. Can. Clin. Oncol., 23:35, 1989.

Doll, D. C., List, A. F., Greco, A., Hainsworth, J. D., Hande, K. R., and Johnson, D. H.: Acute vascular ischemic events after cisplatin-based combination chemotherapy for germ-cell tumors of the testis. Ann. Int. Med., 105:48, 1986.

Donohue, J. P.: Retroperitoneal lymphadenectomy: the anterior approach including bilateral suprarenal-hilar dissection. Urol. Clin. North. Am., 4:509, 1977.

Donohue, J. P.: Complications of lymph node dissection. In Marshall, F. F. (Ed.): Urologic Complications: Medical and Surgical, Adult and Pediatric. Chicago, Year Book Medical Publishers, 1986, p. 281.

Donohue, J. P., Einhorn, L. H., and Williams, S. D.: Is adjuvant chemotherapy following retroperitoneal lymph node dissection for nonseminomatous testis cancer necessary? Urol. Clin. North Am., 7:747, 1980.

Donohue, J. P., Foster, R. S., Rowland, R. G., Bihrle, R., Jones, J., and Geier, G.: Nerve-sparing retroperitoneal lymphadenectomy with preservation of ejaculation. J. Urol., 144:287, 1990.

Donohue, J. P., and Rowland, R. G.: Complications of retroperitoneal lymph node dissection. J. Urol., 125:338, 1981.

Donohue, J. P., and Rowland, R. G.: The role of surgery in advanced testicular cancer. Cancer, 54:2716, 1984.

Donohue, J. P., Rowland, R. G., and Bihrle, R.: Transabdominal retroperitoneal lymph node dissection. In Skinner, D. G., and Lieskovsky, G. (Eds.). Diagnosis and Management of Genitourinary Cancer. Philadelphia, W. B. Saunders Co., 1988, p. 802.

Donohue, J. P., Zachary, J. M., and Maynard, B. R.: Distribution of nodal metastases in nonseminomatous testis cancer. J. Urol., 128:315, 1982.

Dooms, G. C., Hricak, H., Crooks, L. E., and Higgins, C. B.: Magnetic resonance imaging of the lymph nodes: comparison with CT. Radiology, 153:719, 1984.

Dunphy, C. H., Ayala, A. G., Swanson, D. A., Ro, J. Y., and Logothetis, C.: Clinical stage I nonseminomatous and mixed germ cell tumors of the testis: a clinicopathologic study of 93 patients on a surveillance protocol after orchiectomy alone. Cancer, 62:1202, 1988.

Ehrlichman, R. J., Kaugman, S. L., Siegelman, S. S., Trump, D. L., and Walsh, P. C.: Computerized tomography and lymphangiography in staging testis tumors. J. Urol., 126:179, 1981.

Fossa, A., and Fossa, S. D.: Serum lactate dehydrogenase and human choriogonadotrophin in seminoma. Br. J. Urol., 63:408, 1989a.

Fossa, S. D., Ous, S., and Abyholm, T.: Post treatment fertility in patients with testicular cancer. I. Influence of retroperitoneal lymph node dissection on ejaculatory potential. Br. J. Urol., 57:204, 1985.

Fossa, S. D., Stenwig, A. E., Lien, H. H., Ous, S., and Kaalhus, O.: Non-seminomatous testicular cancer clinical stage I: prediction of outcome by histopathological parameters. A multivariate analysis. Oncology, 46:297, 1989b.

Fowler, J. E., and Whitmore, W. F., Jr.: Intratesticular germ cell tumors: observations on the effect of chemotherapy. J. Urol., 126:412, 1981.

Freedman, L. S., Jones, W. G., Peckham, M. J., Newlands, E. S., Parkinson, M. C., Oliver, R. T. D., Read, G., and Williams, C. J.: Histopathology in the prediction of relapse of patients with stage I testicular teratoma treated by orchidectomy alone. Lancet, 2:295, 1987.

Freiha, F., and Torti, F.: Orchiectomy only for clinical stage I nonseminomatous germ cell testis tumors. Comparison with pathologic stage I disease. Urology, 34:347, 1989.

Fung, C. Y., Kalish, L. A., Brodsky, G. L., Richie, J. P., and Garnick M. B.: Stage I nonseminomatous germ cell testicular tumor: prediction of metastatic potential by primary histopathology. J. Clin. Oncol., 6:1467, 1988.

Gelderman, W. A. H., Koops, H. S., Sleijfer, D. T., Oosterhuis, J. W., Marrink, J., de Bruijn, H. W. A., and Oldhoff, J.: Orchidectomy alone in stage I nonseminomatous testicular germ cell tumors. Cancer, 59:578, 1987.

Giguere, J. K., Stablein, D. M., Spaulding, J. T., McLeod, D. G., Paulson, D. F., and Weiss, R. B.: The clinical significance of unconventional orchiectomy approaches in testicular cancer: a report from the testicular cancer intergroup study. J. Urol., 139:1225, 1988.

Goldfinger, P. L., and Schweizer, O.: The hazards of anesthesia and surgery in bleomycin treated patients. Semin. Oncol., 6:121, 1979.

Hoskins, P., Dilly, S., Easton, D., Horwich, A., Hendry, W., and Peckham, M. J.: Prognostic factors in stage I nonseminomatous germ-cell testicular tumors managed by orchiectomy and surveillance: implications for adjuvant chemotherapy. J. Clin. Oncol., 4:1031, 1986.

Javadpour, N.: Biological tumor markers in the management of testicular and bladder cancer. Urology, 12:177, 1978.

Jewett, M. A. S., Kong, Y.-S. P., Goldberg, S. D., Sturgeon, J. F. G., Thomas, G. M., Alison, R. E., and Gospodarowicz, M. K.: Retroperitoneal lymphadenectomy for testis tumor with nerve sparing for ejaculation. J. Urol., 139:1220, 1988.

Jochelson, M. S., Garnick, M. B., Balikian, J. P., and Richie, J. P.: The efficacy of routine whole lung tomography in germ cell tumors. Cancer, 54:1007, 1984.

Kurman, R. J., Scardino, P. T., MacIntire, K. R, Waldmann, T. A., and Javadpour, N.: Cellular localization of alpha fetoprotein and human chorionic gonadotropin in germ cell tumors of the testis using indirect immunoperoxidation techniques: a new approach to classification utilizing tumor markers. Cancer, 40:2136, 1977.

Lange, P. H., Narayan, P., and Fraley, E. E.: Fertility issues following therapy for testicular cancer. Semin. Urol., 2:264, 1984.

Lange, P. H., Nochomovitz, L. E., Rosai, J., Fraley, E. E., Kennedy, B. J., Gosl, G., Brisbane, J., Catalona, W. J., Cochran, J. S., Comisarow, R. H., Cummings, K. B., deKernion, J. B., Einhorn, L. H., Hakala, T. R., Jewett, M., Moore, M. R., Scardino, P. T., and Streitz, J. M.: Serum alpha-fetoprotein and human chorionic gonadotropin in patients with seminoma. J. Urol., 124:472, 1980.

Lieskovsky, G., Weinberg, A. C., and Skinner, D. G.: Surgical management of early-stage nonseminomatous germ cell tumors of the testis. Semin. Urol., 2:208, 1984.

Loehrer, P. J., Sr., Birch, R., Williams, S. D., Greco, A., and Einhorn, L. H.: Chemotherapy of metastatic seminoma: the Southeastern Cancer Study Group experience. J. Clin. Oncol., 5:1212, 1987.

Loehrer, P. J., Sr., Hui, S., Clark, S., Seal, M., Einhorn, L. H., Williams, S. D., Ulbright, T., Mandelbaum, I., Rowland, R., and Donohue, J. P.: Teratoma following cisplatin-based combination chemotherapy for nonseminomatous germ cell tumors: a clinicopathological correlation. J. Urol., 135:1183, 1986.

Logothetis, C. J., Samuels, M. L., Selig, D. E., Johnson, D. E.,

Swanson, D. A., and von Eschenbach, A. C.: Primary chemotherapy followed by selective retroperitoneal lymphadenectomy in the management of clinical stage II testicular carcinoma: a preliminary report. J. Urol., 134:1127, 1985.

Logothetis, C. J., Samuels, M. L., Trindade, A., and Johnson, D. E.: The growing teratoma syndrome. Cancer, 50:1629, 1982.

Maier, J. G., and Sulak, N. H.: Radiation therapy in malignant testis tumors: carcinoma. Cancer, 32:1217, 1972.

Markland, C., Kedia, K., and Fraley, E. E.: Inadequate orchiectomy for patients with testicular tumors. JAMA, 224:1025, 1973.

Montie, J. E.: Testicular cancer: diagnosis and staging. Semin. Urol., 2:194, 1984.

Mostofi, F. K., Sesterhenn, A., and Davis, C. J., Jr.: Developments in histopathology of testicular germ cell tumors. Semin. Urol., 6:171, 1988.

Motzer, R. J., Bosl, G. J., Geller, N. J., Penenberg, D., Yagoda, A., Golbey, R., Whitmore, W. F., Jr., Fair, W. R., Sogani, P., Herr, H., Morse, M., Carey, R., and Vogelzang, N.: Advanced seminoma: the role of chemotherapy and adjunctive surgery. Ann. Int. Med., 108:513, 1988.

Moul, J. W., Robertson, J. E., George, S. L., Paulson, D. F., and Walther, P. J.: Complications of therapy for testicular cancer. J. Urol., 142:1491, 1989.

Oliver, R. T. D., Freedman, L. S., Parkinson, M. C., and Peckham, M. J.: Medical options in the management of stage 1 and 2 (N0-N3, M0) testicular germ cell tumors. Urol. Clin. North Am., 14:721, 1987.

Peckham, M. J., Barrett, A., Husband, J. E., and Hendry, W. F.: Orchidectomy alone in testicular stage I non-seminomatous germ cell tumours. Lancet, 2:678, 1982.

Peckham, M. J., Horwich, A., and Hendry, W. F.: Advanced seminoma: treatment with cis-platinum–based combination chemotherapy or carboplatin (JM8). Br. J. Cancer, 52:7, 1985.

Pizzocaro, G., and Musumeci, R.: The relative value of lymphangiography (LAG) and computed tomography (CT) in diagnosis small retroperitoneal metastases. In Khoury, S. (Ed.). Testicular Cancer. New York, A. R. Liss, 1985c, p. 261.

Pizzocaro, G., Salvioni, R., and Zanoni, F.: Unilateral lymphadenectomy in intraoperative stage I nonseminomatous germinal testis cancer. J. Urol., 134:485, 1985a.

Pizzocaro, G., Zanoni, F., Salvioni, R., Milani, A., and Piva, L.: Surveillance or lymph node dissection in clinical stage I nonseminomatous germinal testis cancer? Br. J. Urol., 57:759, 1985b.

Pritchett, T. R., Skinner, D. G., Selser, S. F., and Kern, W. H.: Seminoma with elevated human chorionic gonadotrophin: the case for retroperitoneal lymph node dissection. Urology, 25:244, 1985.

Raghavan, D., Colls, B., Levi, J., Fitzharris, B., Tattersall, M. H. N., Atkinson, C., Woods, R., Coorey, G., Farrell, C., and Wines, R.: Surveillance for stage I nonseminomatous germ cell tumours of the testis: the optimal protocol has not yet been defined. Br. J. Urol., 61:522, 1988.

Ray, B., Hajdu, S. I., and Whitmore, W. F., Jr.: Distribution of retroperitoneal lymph node metastases in testicular germinal tumors. Cancer, 33:341, 1974.

Richie, J. P.: The surgical management of advanced abdominal disease. Semin. Urol., 2:238, 1984.

Richie, J. P.: Diagnosis and staging of testicular tumors. In Skinner, D. G., and Lieskovsky, G. (Eds.). Diagnosis and management of genitourinary cancer. W. B. Saunders Co., Philadelphia, 1988, p. 498.

Richie, J. P.: Is adjuvant chemotherapy necessary for patients with stage B1 testicular cancer? Abstract, J. Urol., 143:395a, 1990.

Richie, J. P., Garnick, M. B., and Finberg, H.: Computerized tomography: how accurate for abdominal staging of testis tumors? J. Urol., 127:715, 1982.

Rodriguez, P. N., Hafez, G. R., and Messing, E. M.: Nonseminomatous germ cell tumor of the testicle: does extensive staging of the primary tumor predict the likelihood of metastatic disease? J. Urol., 136:604, 1986.

Roth, B. J., Greist, A., Kubilis, P. S., Williams, S. D., and Einhorn, L. H.: Cisplatin-based combination chemotherapy for disseminated germ cell tumors: long-term follow-up. J. Clin. Oncol., 6:1239, 1988.

Rowland, R. G., Weisman, D., Williams, S. D., Einhorn, L. H., Klatte, E. C., and Donohue, J. P.: Accuracy of preoperative staging in stage A and B nonseminomatous germ cell testis tumors. J. Urol., 127:718, 1982.

Sandeman, T. F., and Yang, C.: Results of adjuvant chemotherapy for low-stage testicular cancer. Cancer, 62:1471, 1988.

Scardino, P. T.: Adjuvant chemotherapy is of value following retroperitoneal lymph node dissection for nonseminomatous testicular tumors. Urol. Clin. North Am., 7:735, 1980.

Schultz, S. M., Einhorn, L. H., Conces, D. J., Jr., Williams, S. D., and Loehrer, P. J.: Management of postchemotherapy residual mass in patients with advanced seminoma: Indiana University experience. J. Clin. Oncol., 7:1497, 1989.

Schwartz, D. A., Johnson, D. E., and Hussey, D. H.: Should an elevated human chorionic gonadotropin titer alter therapy for seminoma? J. Urol., 131:63, 1984.

Skinner, D. G.: Non-seminomatous testis tumors: a plan of management based on 96 patients to improve survival in all stages by combined therapeutic modalities. J. Urol., 115:65, 1976.

Skinner, D. G.: The management of germ cell tumors of the testis: an overview. Semin. Urol., 2:189. 1984a.

Skinner, D. G., and Lieskovsky, G.: The thoracoabdominal approach for management of nonseminomatous germ cell tumors of the testis. (Movie) 1984b. Available from Norwich Eaton, Inc., by request.

Skinner, D. G., Melamud, A., and Lieskovsky, G.: Complications of thoracoabdominal retroperitoneal lymph node dissection. J. Urol., 127:1107, 1982.

Smith, R. B.: Diagnosis and staging of testicular tumors. In Skinner, D. G., and deKernion, J. B. (Eds.). Genitourinary Cancer. W. B. Saunders Co., Philadelphia, 1987, p. 448.

Socinski, M. A., Garnick, M. B., Stomper, P. C., Fung, C. Y., and Richie, J. P.: Stage II nonseminomatous germ cell tumors of the testis: an analysis of treatment options in patients with low volume retroperitoneal disease. J. Urol., 140:1437, 1988.

Sogani, P. C., Whitmore, W. F., Jr., Herr, H. W., Bosl, G. J., Golbey, R. B., Watson, R. C., and DeCosse, J. J.: Orchiectomy alone in the treatment of clinical stage I nonseminomatous germ cell tumor of the testis. J. Clin. Oncol., 2:267, 1984.

Storm, P. B., Kern, A., Loening, S. A., Brown, R. C., and Culp, D. A.: Evaluation of pedal lymphangiography in staging nonseminomatous testicular cancer. J. Urol., 118:1000, 1977.

Stoter, G., Vendrick, C. P., Struyvenberg, A., Sleyfer, D. T., Vriesendorp, R., Schrafford Koops, H., van Oosterom, A. T., ten Bokkel Huinink, W. W., and Pinedo, H. M.: Five-year survival of patients with disseminated nonseminomatous testicular cancer treated with cisplatin, vinblastine, and bleomycin. Cancer, 54:1521, 1984.

Thompson, P. I., Nixon, J., and Harvey, V. J.: Disease relapse in patients with stage I nonseminomatous germ cell tumor of the testis on active surveillance. J. Clin. Oncol., 6:1597, 1988.

Turner, R. R., Colby, T. V., and MacKintosh, F. R.: Testicular lymphomas: a clinicopathologic study of 35 cases. Cancer, 48:2095, 1981.

Vogelzang, N. J., Bosl, G. J., Johnson, K, and Kennedy, B. J.: Raynaud's phenomenon: a common toxicity after combination chemotherapy for testis cancer. Ann. Int. Med., 95:288, 1981.

Vugrin, D., and Whitmore, W. F., Jr.: The role of chemotherapy and surgery in the treatment of retroperitoneal metastases in advanced nonseminomatous testis cancer. Cancer, 55:1874, 1985.

Vugrin, D., Whitmore, W. F., Jr., Nisselbaum, J., and Watson, R. C.: Correlation of serum tumor markers and lymphangiography with degrees of nodal involvement in surgical stage II testis cancer. J. Urol., 127:683, 1982.

Vugrin, D., Whitmore, W. F., Jr., Sogani, P. C., Bains, M., Herr, H. W., and Golbey, R. B.: Combined chemotherapy and surgery in treatment of advanced germ-cell tumors. Cancer, 47:2228, 1981.

Wetlaufer, J. N.: The management of advanced seminoma. Semin. Urol., 2:257, 1984.

Whitmore, E. F., Jr.: Germinal testis tumors: guest overview. In Skinner, D. G. (Ed.). Urological Cancer. New York, Grune & Stratton, 1983, p. 335.

Williams, S. D., Loehrer, P. J., Sr., and Einhorn, L. H.: Chemotherapy of advanced testicular cancer. Semin. Urol., 2:230, 1984.

Williams, S. D., Stablein, D. M., Einhorn, L. H., Muggia, F. M., Weiss, R. B., Donohue, J. P., Paulson, D. F., Brunner, K. W., Jacobs, E. M., Spaulding, J. T., DeWys, W. D., and Crawford, E. D.: Immediate adjuvant chemotherapy versus observation with treatment at relapse in pathological stage II testicular cancer. New Engl. J. Med., 317:1433, 1987.

Wise, P. G., and Scardino, P. T.: Thoracoabdominal retroperitoneal lymphadenectomy for testicular cancer. *In* Skinner, D. G., and Lieskovsky, G. (Eds.). Diagnosis and Management of Genitourinary Cancer. Philadelphia, W. B. Saunders Co., 1988, p. 779.

Wishnow, K. I., Johnson, D. E., and Tenney, D. M.: Are lymphan-giograms necessary before placing patients with nonseminomatous testicular tumors on surveillance? J. Urol., 141:1133, 1989a.

Wishnow, K. I., Johnson, D. E., Tenney, D. M., Swanson, D. A., Babaian, R. J., Dunphy, C. H., Ayala, A. G., Ro, J. Y., and von Eschenbach, A. C.: Identifying patients with low-risk clinical stage I nonseminomatous testicular tumors who should be treated by surveillance. Urology, 34:229, 1989b.

87
SURGERY OF MALE INFERTILITY AND OTHER SCROTAL DISORDERS

Marc Goldstein, M.D.

A dramatic increase has taken place in the importance of male infertility surgery as a part of the urologist's practice. Whereas surgery for stones, heretofore, a large part of the urologist's surgical practice, yields to extracorporeal shock wave lithotripsy, and benign prostatic hyperplasia increasingly yields to balloon dilation or medical treatment, the surgery of male infertility has expanded in scope and risen in demand. Part of the reason for the greater demand is caused by the delay in starting families until much later in life. In addition, the epidemic levels of sexually transmitted diseases take their toll, resulting in an apparent rise in the incidence of excurrent ductal obstruction.

Vasectomy has become a more popular form of safe, effective, permanent contraception, but with divorce rates still hovering around 50 per cent, demand for reversal of vasectomy has grown proportionately. Newer, less traumatic, even percutaneous methods of vasectomy described in this chapter promise to further increase the popularity of vasectomy, making both vasectomy and, consequently, reversal an even more important part of the urologist's practice.

Varicocele, long known to be associated with male infertility, has now been shown to result in progressive, duration-dependent testicular injury (Gorelick and Goldstein, 1989; Hadziselimovic et al., 1989; Harrison et al., 1986; Kass et al., 1987; Lipshultz and Corriere, 1977; Nagler et al., 1985; Russell, 1957). Whereas surgical repair of varicocele has previously been reserved for the already infertile male, early repair of varicocele, employing safer and more effective surgical techniques, promises to transform the urologist's role from that of salvaging remaining testicular function to that of preventing future infertility.

New surgical and reproductive technologies have expanded the horizon of male infertility surgery beyond anything previously imaginable. Microsurgical techniques have resulted in marked improvements in the repair of obstructions of the vas deferens and epididymis. The ability to definitively identify the very small structures of the spermatic cord allows the urologic microsurgeon to repair varicoceles with a resultant lower morbidity.

The techniques of in vitro fertilization (IVF), initially thought of by urologists as a possible replacement for male infertility treatment, have instead advanced male reproductive surgery. Pregnancies have been achieved using sperm retrieved from men with previously untreatable disorders, such as congenital absence of the vas deferens. When the urologist collaborates with an IVF team, sperm can be aspirated directly from epididymal tubules and even from efferent ductules with unreconstructable obstructions (Pryor et al., 1984; Silber et al., 1987; Temple-Smith et al., 1985). Micromanipulation techniques perfected by embryologists have allowed fertilization of eggs with sperm too few in number or too feeble in motility to penetrate oocytes on their own (Cohen et al., 1989; Gordon et al., 1988). The ability to achieve fertilization with fewer and less motile sperm now offers hope to men with severe impairment of spermatogenesis. Improvement of in vitro technology obligates the urologist to improve the patient's sperm quality as much as possible before couples undergo these complex and expensive procedures.

SURGICAL ANATOMY

The scrotal contents are unique in their accessibility for physical examination, imaging modalities, and surgical intervention. The success of surgery for male infertility and scrotal disorders is predicated on the selection of the correct operation and the most appropriate approach. The details of the history and careful physical examination, followed by confirmatory, judiciously selected laboratory and imaging procedures, are presented in Chapter 15. When surgical intervention for diagnostic or therapeutic purposes is indicated, a thorough understanding of the anatomy and physiology of the male reproductive system (see Chapter 6) is requisite for planning and carrying out the procedure with the highest probability of success and lowest morbidity.

When surgery for male infertility and scrotal disorders is undertaken, only rarely is the life of the patient at stake. What is at stake when the surgery described in this chapter is undertaken, is new life, with the potential for altering not only the quality of a couple's life but the future of the species. The responsibilities assumed by the surgeon in these circumstances demand the utmost in judgment and skill. Many of the procedures described here are among the most technically demanding in all of urology. Acquisition of the skills required to perform them demands intensive laboratory training in microsurgery and a thorough knowledge of the anatomy and physiology of the male reproductive system. Attempting such surgery only occasionally and without proper training is a terrible disservice to the patient and the couple, and the future of humanity.

TESTIS BIOPSY

Indications

The indications for testis biopsy are detailed in Chapter 15. Briefly, it is indicated in azoospermic men with testes of normal size and consistency, palpable vasa deferentia, and normal serum follicle stimulating hormone (FSH) levels. Under these circumstances, biopsy will distinguish obstructive azoospermia from primary seminiferous tubular failure. In men with absent vasa, IVF with aspirated epididymal sperm offers a chance for pregnancy. Although biopsy findings of such men usually reveal virtually normal spermatogenesis (Goldstein and Schlossberg, 1988), those with slightly elevated serum FSH levels or small soft testes should undergo biopsy prior to sperm aspiration and in vitro procedures. Biopsy should usually be performed bilaterally. Good spermatogenesis is sometimes found in small firm testis. Large healthy testis may reveal maturation arrest.

Open Testis Biopsy

Open testis biopsy can be performed using local, general, or spinal anesthetic. In rats, the incidence of accidental damage to the testicular artery during blind cord block is 5 per cent (Goldstein et al., 1983). Biopsy with only local anesthesia of the skin and tunics, without a cord block, is sometimes painful.

When performing testis biopsy, the surgeon must provide an adequate tissue sample and employ a technique that avoids trauma to the specimen as well as the epididymis and testicular blood supply. Open biopsy under direct vision satisfies these requirements.

An assistant stretches the scrotal skin tightly over the anterior surface of the testis and ensures that the epididymis is posterior. Bilateral, 1-cm transverse incisions

provide good exposure with a minimum of scrotal skin bleeding. Alternatively, a single vertical incision in the median raphe may be made. The incision is carried through the skin and dartos muscle, and the tunica vaginalis is opened. The edges of the tunica vaginalis are held open with hemostats and bleeders cauterized. The area chosen for biopsy should be on the medial or lateral aspects of the upper pole in a site relatively free of visible surface vessels. These locations are the least likely to contain major branches of the testicular artery running superficially under the tunica albuginea (Jarow, 1990). The tunica albuginea of the testis is transfixed with a 4-0 catgut suture armed with a small tapered needle, because cutting needles cause bleeding. The wound should be dry prior to incising the tunica to prevent saturation of the biopsy with blood. A 3- to 4-mm incision is made with the point of the scalpel into the tunica. A pea-sized sample of seminiferous tubules is excised with razor-sharp iris scissors (Fig. 87–1) and deposited directly into Bouin's, Zenker's, or collidine buffered glutaraldehyde solution. Formalin distorts testicular histology and should not be used for testis biopsy. A second specimen may be cut for a wet preparation and placed on a slide. A drop of saline is added and the specimen crushed under a coverslip. Immediate analysis by an experienced pathologist, with phase contrast microscopy, can confirm the presence or absence of spermatozoa, but this method is not reliable for quantitative evaluation.

Testis biopsy material for permanent fixation should not be handled or traumatized in any way, because this may distort the testicular architecture. The specimen should be dropped directly from the scissors into the fixative solution. Using the previously placed transfixing

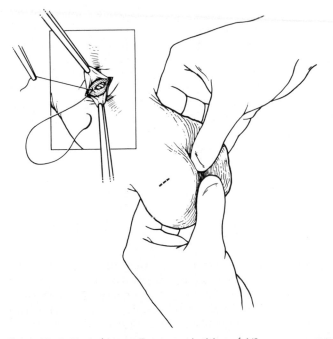

Figure 87–1. Testis biopsy. Transverse incision of 1/2 cm over upper lateral or medial aspect of testis. Transfixing suture in tunica albuginea maintains control and is used for closure. Hemostats hold open edges of tunica vaginalis.

suture, the tunica albuginea is closed with continuous sutures. The tunica vaginalis is closed with a running absorbable suture for hemostasis. The small skin incisions are left open to minimize the risk of hematoma. The wounds are covered with bacitracin ointment, and a fluff-type dressing is held in place with snug scrotal supporter. Antibiotics are unnecessary.

Percutaneous Testis Biopsy

Percutaneous testicular biopsy utilizing a device similar to that for prostatic biopsy is a blind procedure and could result in unintentional injury to either the epididymis or testicular artery coursing on the surface of the tunica albuginea. In addition, specimens obtained in this way often contain few tubules with poorly preserved architecture. When performed using local anesthesia, the procedure can be painful.

Testicular Aspiration Cytology and Flow Cytometry

Testicular aspiration performed with a very fine gauge needle is less risky and painful than percutaneous biopsy. Flow cytometric evaluation of this aspirated material can distinguish haploid from diploid cells and therefore may predict the absence of late stages of spermatogenesis (Chan et al., 1984). Until standards for the cytologic evaluation of testis aspirates are established, open testis biopsy is the diagnostic procedure of choice.

Complications of Testis Biopsy

Carefully performed, testis biopsy is associated with few complications. The most serious mistake associated with biopsy of the testis is inadvertent biopsy of the epididymis. If histologic evaluation of the biopsy material reveals epididymis with sperm within its tubule, obstruction of the epididymis at the site of the biopsy is certain. If, however, there are no sperm within the epididymal tubules, the obstruction is above the level of the biopsy or primary seminiferous tubular failure is present, and no harm has been done.

Hematoma is the most common complication of testis biopsy. Hematomas can grow to a large size and can require drainage. Placement of a transfixing suture in the tunica albuginea prior to incision, to avoid inadvertent loss of the biopsy site, helps prevent this complication. If the biopsy site is lost before closure, the incision should be enlarged and the testis delivered. The tunica vaginalis also has an impressive blood supply and its edges should be carefully oversewn or approximated.

Because of the rich blood supply of the scrotum and its contents, wound infection is rare in the absence of hematoma. Antibiotics are unnecessary.

If the biopsy material is placed in the incorrect fixative, such as formalin, or if sampling of the testicular tissue is inadequate, the biopsy must be repeated.

VASOGRAPHY

Vasography with contrast material and intraoperative radiography is rarely indicated. No need exists to perform vasography at the time of testis biopsy unless a wet preparation biopsy evaluation and an immediate reconstruction are undertaken. If performed carelessly, vasography can cause stricture or even obstruction at the vasography site that can complicate subsequent reconstruction. In addition, because the majority of nonvasectomy-related obstructions are epididymal, vasography is of no diagnostic value.

If testis biopsy reveals normal spermatogenesis and the vasa are palpable, vasography, if necessary, should be performed at the time of scrotal exploration and definitive repair of obstruction.

General anesthesia provides the most flexibility for scrotal exploration, vasography, and obstruction repair. Although local anesthesia can provide adequate analgesia, patients are often unable to remain still through several hours of microsurgery. Long-acting hypobaric spinal or continuous epidural anesthesia can be satisfactory.

Technique of Vasography

A high vertical scrotal incision overlying the testis is made large enough to deliver the testis. This incision allows extension into the inguinal region if necessary.

In a man with probable inguinal obstruction of the vas deferens, most often from previous hernia repair, incision should be made through the previous hernia scar. In this case, the obstructed ends of the vasa are most often found at the site of previous surgery and formal vasography is not necessary. This occurrence eliminates the need to make a separate scrotal vasotomy for vasography and then, later in the case, transecting the vas higher in the inguinal region, risking devascularization of the segment between the vasography site and the inguinal obstruction. If exploration at the site of previous inguinal hernia surgery fails to clearly reveal a site of obstruction the testis can be delivered and vasography performed through the inguinal incision.

If the site of obstruction is unknown and no previous inguinal incision is present, the testis is delivered through a high vertical scrotal incision. The vas deferens is identified and isolated at the junction of the straight and convoluted portions of the vas deferens. While employing an operating microscope and 10-power magnification, the vasal sheath is vertically incised and the vasal vessels carefully preserved. If vasovasostomy is subsequently necessary in the inguinal region of the vas, destruction of the vasal blood supply at the site of vasography may result in ischemia and necrosis of the intervening segment of vas.

A clean segment of bare vas is delivered, and a straight clamp is placed beneath the vas to act as a platform. Under 15-power magnification, a microknife is used to hemitransect the vas until the lumen is revealed (Fig. 87–2). Any fluid exuding from the lumen is placed on a slide, mixed with a drop of saline, and

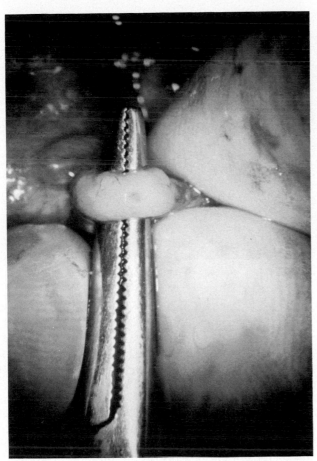

Figure 87–2. Hemitransected vas. Vasal vessels are excluded and preserved.

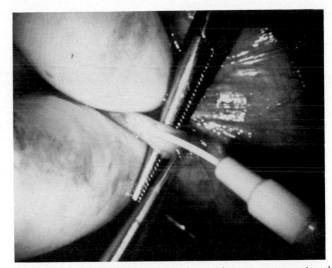

Figure 87–3. Cannulation of vasal lumen with a 24-gauge angiocath sheath. (From Goldstein, M.: Vasography and technique of testis biopsy. *In* Rajfer, J. (Ed.): Common Problems in Infertility and Impotence. New York, Mosby-Year Book, 1990.)

the first place. If the ureteral catheter passes to the internal inguinal ring without resistance, it is left in place, and an identical procedure is performed on the opposite side. After both vasa have been cannulated with ureteral catheters, simultaneous vasograms are performed with the injection of 50 per cent water-soluble contrast medium into both vasa (Fig. 87–4). Before

sealed with a coverslip for microscopic examination. If the vasal fluid is devoid of sperm, epididymal obstruction is present. If no fluid is found in the lumen, a 24-gauge angiocath sheath is passed into the testicular end of the vas and, while the epididymis and convoluted vas are milked, barbitage with 0.1 to 0.2 ml of saline or Ringer's solution is performed. If there is no sperm in this fluid, obstruction of the epididymis is confirmed. The seminal vesicle end of the vas is then cannulated with the 24-gauge antiocath sheath and is injected with saline to confirm its patency (Fig. 87–3). If the saline passes, formal vasography is not necessary. If proof of patency of the vas deferens is desired, dilute methylene blue may be injected and the bladder catheterized. The presence of blue dye in the urine confirms patency of the vas.

If a large amound of fluid is found in the vasal lumen and microscopic examination reveals the presence of sperm, obstruction toward the seminal vesicle end of the vas is suspected. In this case, the vas is usually markedly dilated and a No. 3 whistle-tip ureteral catheter can be gently passed toward the seminal vesicle end of the vas. If the obstruction is in the inguinal region, the calibrated catheter markings can be utilized to determine the exact site of obstruction. This circumstance is unusual because inguinal obstruction is invariably due to previous surgery. The exploration would have been carried out through an inguinal incision in

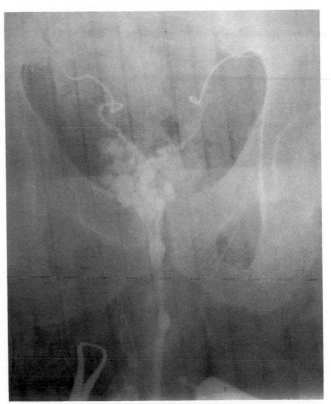

Figure 87–4. Normal vasogram with Foley catheter occluding bladder neck. (From Goldstein, M.: Vasography and technique of testis biopsy. *In* Rajfer, J. (Ed.): Common Problems in Infertility and Impotence. New York, Mosby-Year Book, 1990.)

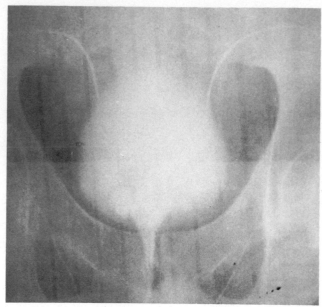

Figure 87–5. Vasogram without occlusion of bladder neck. Contrast material refluxing into the bladder obscures detail. (From Goldstein, M.: Vasography and technique of testis biopsy. *In* Rajfer, J. (Ed.): Common Problems in Infertility and Impotence. New York, Mosby-Year Book, 1990.)

vasography is performed, a Foley catheter should be placed in the bladder and pulled tightly against the bladder neck to prevent reflux of contrast material into the bladder, obscuring fine detail (Fig. 87–5). If vasography reveals obstruction at the site of the ejaculatory ducts (Fig. 87–6), a transurethral resection (TUR) of the ejaculatory ducts (described later in this chapter) is performed (Fig. 87–7). Opening of the ejaculatory ducts can be confirmed by injecting methylene blue through these ureteral catheters and by visualizing the dye through the resectoscope.

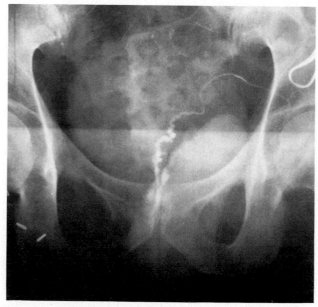

Figure 87–6. Ejaculatory duct obstruction. (From Goldstein, M.: Vasography and technique of testis biopsy. *In* Rajfer, J. (Ed.): Common Problems in Infertility and Impotence. New York, Mosby-Year Book, 1990.)

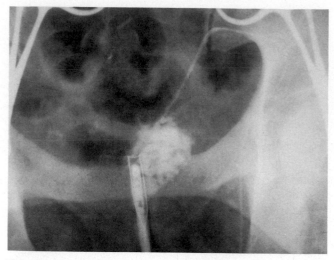

Figure 87–7. Vasography with resectoscope at verumontanum facilitates transurethral resection of ejaculatory ducts. (From Goldstein, M.: Vasography and technique of testis biopsy. *In* Rajfer, J. (Ed.): Common Problems in Infertility and Impotence. New York, Mosby-Year Book, 1990.)

Vasography may reveal the vas deferens blindly ending far away from the ejaculatory ducts (Fig. 87–8). If this finding is bilateral (Fig. 87–9), no further surgery is indicated. However, the patient is a good candidate for microsurgical aspiration of vasal or epididymal sperm for IVF. If vasography reveals obstruction in the inguinal region (Fig. 87–10), either inguinal vasovasostomy or crossed transseptal vasovasostomy may be performed. Vasography sites are carefully closed with microsurgical

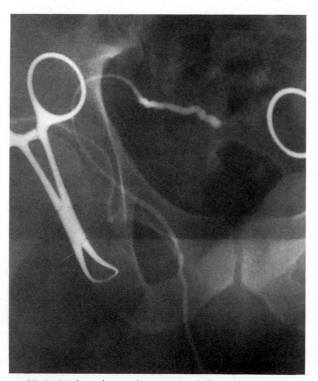

Figure 87–8. Unilateral partial agenesis of the vas deferens. (From Goldstein, M.: Vasography and technique of testis biopsy. *In* Rajfer, J. (Ed.): Common Problems in Infertility and Impotence. New York, Mosby-Year Book, 1990.)

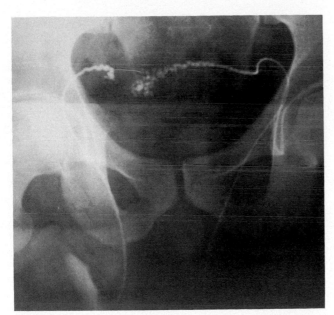

Figure 87–9. Bilateral partial agenesis of vas deferens. (From Goldstein, M.: Vasography and technique of testis biopsy. *In* Rajfer, J. (Ed.): Common Problems in Infertility and Impotence. New York, Mosby-Year Book, 1990.)

technique using 10–0 monofilament nylon for the mucosa and 9–0 for the muscularis and adventitia.

If the vasal fluid reveals no sperm and injection of the seminal vesicle end of the vas confirms its patency, the vas is completely transected and the end prepared for vasoepididymostomy. If the vasal fluid reveals many sperm and vasography is normal (see Fig. 87–4), retrograde ejaculation, lack of emission, or vas aperistalsis is the cause of azoospermia (Tiffany and Goldstein, 1985).

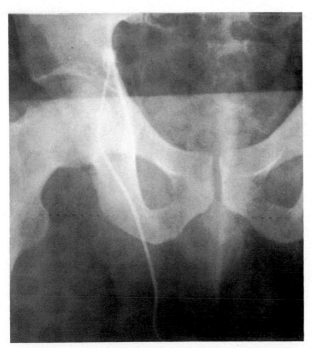

Figure 87–10. Inguinal obstruction of vas deferens. (From Goldstein, M.: Vasography and technique of testis biopsy. *In* Rajfer, J. (Ed.): Common Problems in Infertility and Impotence. New York, Mosby-Year Book, 1990.)

Contrast Agents for Vasography

Ringer's lactate or normal saline should be selected first. If the fluid injects toward the seminal vesicle end of the vas without difficulty, contrast vasography is unnecessary. When the vas is strictured and injection requires undue pressure, methylene blue can be injected and the bladder catheterized. The presence of dye in the bladder indicates a partial obstruction. Formal vasography may be performed with 50 per cent dilute water-soluble contrast material.

Complications of Vasography

Stricture

Multiple attempts at percutaneous vasography with sharp needles can result in stricture or obstruction at the site. Careless or crude closure of a vasotomy can also cause stricture and obstruction. Nonwater-soluble contrast agents may also produce stricture and should not be employed for vasography.

Injury to the Vasal Blood Supply

If the vasal blood supply is injured at the site of vasography, vasovasostomy proximal to the site may result in ischemia, necrosis, and obstruction of the intervening segment of vas.

Hematoma

A bipolar cautery should be employed for meticulous hemostasis at the time of vasotomy to prevent hematoma in the perivasal sheath.

Sperm Granuloma

Leaky closure of a vasography site may lead to the development of a sperm granuloma, which can result in stricture or vas obstruction. The microsurgical technique for closure of vasography sites is identical to that for vasovasostomy described later in this chapter.

VASECTOMY

Vasectomy is a safe and effective method of permanent contraception. In 1983, approximately 412,000 vasectomies were performed in the United States, more than any other urologic procedure (Kendrick et al., 1985). Impressive as these numbers may seem, far fewer vasectomies are performed than female sterilizations worldwide. Vasectomy is less expensive and associated much lower morbidity and mortality than tubal ligation. Some men will not consider vasectomy because they fear the trauma, pain, and possible complications associated with scrotal surgery. For other men, vasectomy may be equated with castration or loss of masculinity. Although vasectomy is conceptually a very simple procedure, its technical difficulty is reflected in the markedly increased incidence of postoperative complications in the hands of surgeons who perform relatively few vasectomies per year (Kendrick et al., 1987). Efforts to enhance the popularity of vasectomy have led Chinese physicians to develop refined methods of vasectomy that minimize trauma, pain, and complications. Their success in attaining these goals is evidenced by a complete reversal of the ratio of male to female sterilizations to 3:1 in favor of vasectomy in the Szechuan province. In this region, where the no-scalpel and percutaneous vasectomy methods were developed and popularized, 10 million men have undergone voluntary sterilization.

Local Anesthesia for Vasectomy

Vasectomy can safely be performed as an outpatient procedure employing local anesthetics. Poor local anesthetic technique results in pain and hematoma formation. The inadequacy of local anesthetic technique in the hands of many surgeons is partly responsible for the poor "word of mouth" about vasectomy revealed by focus group interviews in which men who had undergone vasectomies reported experiencing more pain and discomfort than they had been led to expect by their surgeons (Li et al., 1991).

With the surgeon standing on the patient's right side, the vas deferens is separated from the spermatic cord vessels and manipulated to a superficial position under the scrotal skin. The right vas is firmly trapped over the middle finger of the left hand and under the index finger and thumb (Fig. 87–11). A 1-cm diameter superficial skin wheal is raised utilizing a 1.5-inch, 25-gauge needle and 2 per cent plain lidocaine. The needle is advanced within the perivasal sheath toward the external inguinal ring, and 2 to 5 ml of lidocaine is injected around the vas without moving the needle in and out (Fig. 87–12).

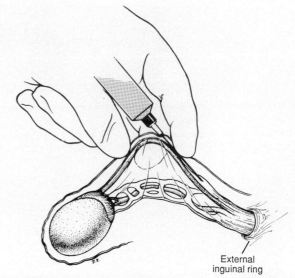

Figure 87–12. Vasal nerve block away from the vasectomy site.

This maneuver produces a vasal nerve block and minimizes edema at the actual vasectomy site. The left vas deferens is fixed and anesthetized employing the same three-finger technique (Fig. 87–13). The original skin wheal is pinched to reduce local edema. This anesthetic technique, when perfected, allows a virtually pain-free vasectomy to be performed, with minimal risk of hematoma. The relatively large amount of anesthetic ensures a complete block and is well below the limits of toxicity. Injection away from the vasectomy site prevents interference with exposure due to local edema. Avoidance of multiple punctures and needle movement minimizes the risk of hematoma.

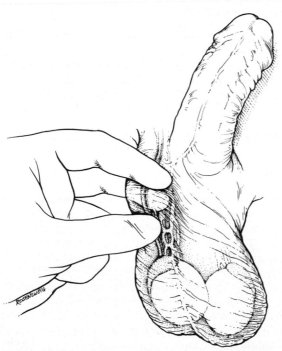

Figure 87–11. The three-finger technique of fixing the right vas deferens with the left hand. Surgeon is standing on the patient's right side.

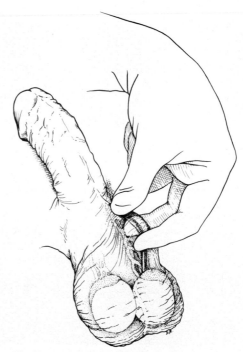

Figure 87–13. The three-finger technique of fixing the left vas with the left hand. Surgeon remains on the patient's right side. (From Li, S., Goldstein, M., Zhu, J., and Huber, D.: The no-scalpel vasectomy. J. Urol., 145:341–344, 1991. © By Williams & Wilkins, 1991.)

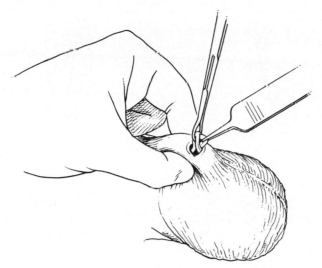

Figure 87–14. Incisional technique of accessing the vas.

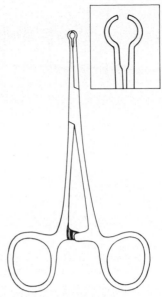

Figure 87–15. Ring-tipped vas deferens fixation clamp. Cantilever design prevents injury to the scrotal skin. (From Li, S., Goldstein, M., Zhu, J., and Huber, D.: The no-scalpel vasectomy. J. Urol., 145:341–344, 1991. © By Williams & Wilkins, 1991.)

Conventional Incisional Techniques of Vasectomy

Through 1-cm bilateral transverse incisions or a single medium raphe incision, the vas deferens is exposed high in the scrotum where it is more superficial and straight. The vas is mobilized to the most superficial position possible under the scrotal skin and is fixed with the fingers, a towel clip, or a needle. The incision is carried down through the vas sheath until bare vas is exposed (Fig. 87–14). The vas is delivered. The deferential artery and veins, with accompanying nerves, are dissected free of the vas and spared. Preservation of these structures minimizes bleeding complications and may enhance the success of subsequent attempts at reversal by preserving the innervation and blood supply necessary for normal vas function. After a 1- to 2-cm segment of vas has been delivered and cleaned, a segment may be removed and the ends occluded, employing one of the techniques described later in this chapter. Suture closure of the scrotal wounds is optional. Leaving the small incisions open helps prevent hematoma formation. The wound heals itself in 24 hours. Plain gauze dressings are held in place by a snug-fitting athletic supporter.

No-Scalpel Vasectomy

An elegant method for gaining access to the vas deferens through a single tiny puncture hole was developed in China by Li (1976). This method eliminates the scalpel, results in fewer hematomas and infections, and leaves a much smaller wound than conventional methods of accessing the vas deferens for vasectomy. The procedure is performed with the patient supine. The penis is retracted cephalad onto the abdomen using a rubber band secured to the patient's gown. The procedure should be performed in a warm room, and warm preparation solutions employed in order to relax the scrotum. The surgeon stands on the patient's right side.

The right vas deferens is fixed under the median raphe by the surgeon's left hand with the three-finger tech-

nique (see Fig. 87–11). After a skin wheal is raised, vasal nerve block is performed as described previously. After both vasa have been anesthetized, the right vas is again fixed under the skin wheal with the left hand by the three-finger method. The ring-tipped fixation clamp is grasped with the right hand and opened while pressing downward (Fig. 87–15), stretching the scrotal skin tightly over the vas and locking the vas within the clamp. The ring clamp is placed in the left hand and the trapped vas elevated with the left index finger, tightening the scrotal skin over the vas (Fig. 87–16).

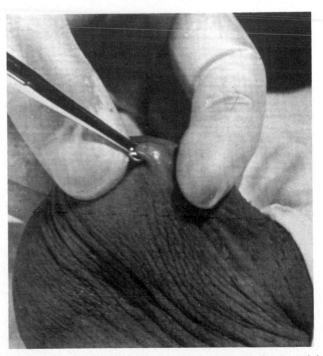

Figure 87–16. Vas fixed in the ring clamp. Scrotal skin is tightly stretched over the most prominent portion of the vas. (From Li, S., Goldstein, M., Zhu, J., and Huber, D.: The no-scalpel vasectomy. J. Urol., 145:341–344, 1991. © By Williams & Wilkins, 1991.)

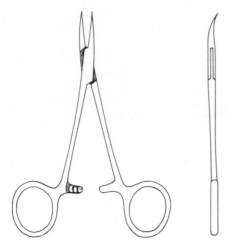

Figure 87–17. Sharp, curved mosquito hemostat. (From Li, S., Goldstein, M., Zhu, J., and Huber, D.: The no-scalpel vasectomy. J. Urol., 145:341–344, 1991. © By Williams & Wilkins, 1991.)

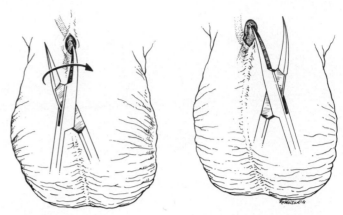

Figure 87–19. Vas wall is skewered with one blade of the clamp and delivered. (From Li, S., Goldstein, M., Zhu, J., and Huber, D.: The no-scalpel vasectomy. J. Urol., 145:341–344, 1991. © By Williams & Wilkins, 1991.)

A sharp pointed and curved mosquito hemostat punctures the scrotal skin, vas sheath, and vas wall (Fig. 87–17), with one blade of the clamp (Fig. 87–18).

The single blade of the hemostat is withdrawn, and the closed tip of the instrument introduced through the same puncture hole. The blades of the clamp are gently opened, spreading all layers until the bare vas wall can be visualized. With the right blade of the hemostat, the vas wall is skewered at a 45 degree angle and the dissecting clamp is rotated laterally 180 degrees (Fig. 87–18). The vas is delivered through the puncture hole while the ringed fixation clamp is released (Fig. 87–19). The ring clamp secures the delivered vas (Fig. 87–20). The sharp hemostat is used to clean the vasal vessels

away from the vas, yielding a clean segment at least 2 cm in length (Fig. 87–21). At this point, the vas is divided. Occlusion is effected utilizing one of the techniques described later in this chapter.

The ends of the right vas are returned to the scrotum. The left vas is fixed directly under the same puncture hole with the three-finger technique (see Fig. 87–13). On the left side, the ring clamp can first be introduced through the puncture hole, encircling the vas without the overlying skin. The remainder of the procedure is identical to that described for the right side. After both vasa are returned to the scrotum, the puncture hole is pinched for a minute and inspected for bleeding. The puncture hole contracts and is virtually invisible. Antibiotic ointment is applied to the site and sterile dressing held in place with snug-fitting athletic supporter.

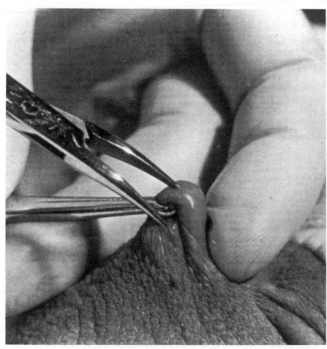

Figure 87–18. Puncture of the skin, vas sheath, and adventitia. (From Li, S., Goldstein, M., Zhu, J., and Huber, D.: The no-scalpel vasectomy. J. Urol., 145:341–344, 1991. © By Williams & Wilkins, 1991.)

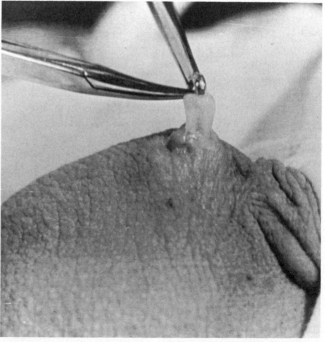

Figure 87–20. Delivery of clean vas. (From Li, S., Goldstein, M., Zhu, J., and Huber, D.: The no-scalpel vasectomy. J. Urol., 145:341–344, 1991. © By Williams & Wilkins, 1991.)

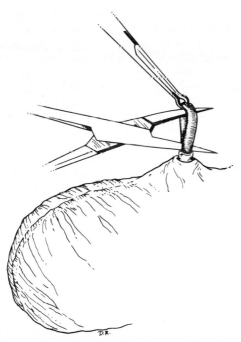

Figure 87–21. Segment cleaned. (From Li, S., Goldstein, M., Zhu, J., and Huber, D.: The no-scalpel vasectomy. J. Urol., 145:341–344, 1991. © By Williams & Wilkins, 1991.)

Studies in the United States and in China (Li et al., 1991), as well as a large controlled study carried out in Thailand comparing no-scalpel with conventional vasectomy (Nirapathpongporn et al., 1990), have clearly shown that the no-scalpel technique results in a markedly reduced incidence of hematoma, infection, and pain. In addition, the no-scalpel vasectomy is performed in about 40 per cent less time. In some ways, the no-scalpel technique may be compared with a percutaneous endoscopic technique, in which a small tract is dilated and blood vessels are pushed aside rather than cut.

Although this method of vasectomy appears deceptively simple, it is more difficult to learn than conventional vasectomy and requires intensive hands-on training. No-scalpel vasectomy promises to enhance the popularity of vasectomy and to make it a more significant part of the urologist's practice.

Percutaneous Vasectomy

The Chinese have performed over 500,000 truly percutaneous vasectomies utilizing chemical occlusion with a combination of cyanoacrylate and phenol (Ban, 1980; Li, 1980; Tao, 1980). After fixation of the vas with the same ring clamp as previously described, the scrotal skin and vas wall are punctured with a 22-gauge needle. The lumen is cannulated with a 24-gauge blunt needle. The needle's position within the vas lumen is confirmed by a series of ingenious tests with final confirmation obtained by injection of Congo red into the abdominal side of the right vas deferens and methylene blue into the left. Injection of 20 μL of two parts phenol mixed with one part n-butyl 2-cyanoacrylate mixture via the 24-gauge blunt-tipped needle occludes the lumen. The

patient voids at the termination of the procedure. Excretion of red urine means the left side was missed—blue urine means the right side was missed. Excretion of brown urine, however, means both sides were successfully cannulated. In China, pharmacologic tests of the cyanoacrylate and phenol mixture have demonstrated no toxicity or carcinogenesis. However, these chemicals are not approved by the Food and Drug Administration for use in the human vas deferens. Furthermore, gaining percutaneous access to the 300-μ diameter lumen of the vas is a procedure that requires great skill and considerable training.

Experimental work is currently in progress directed toward conversion of this percutaneous chemical method to a percutaneous electrical or laser method. Other research has been completed demonstrating the efficacy of a percutaneous clip occlusion device in dogs (Goldstein et al., 1992). Clinical trials with this device have not yet been completed.

Methods of Vasal Occlusion and Vasectomy Failure

The technique employed for occlusion of the vasal lumina, as well as the length of vas removed, determines the incidence of recanalization. Suture ligature, still the most common method employed worldwide, may result in necrosis and sloughing of the cut end distal to the ligature. On the testicular end of the cut vas, a sperm granuloma will result. If both ends slough, recanalization is more likely. Vasectomy failure due to recanalization has a frequency ranging from 1 to 5 per cent when ligatures alone are selected for occlusion.

When the vasa are sealed with two medium hemoclips on each end, failure rates are reduced to less than 1 per cent (Bennett, 1976; Moss, 1974). The wide diameter of hemoclips compared with sutures more evenly distributes pressure on the vasal wall, resulting in less necrosis and sloughing.

Intraluminal occlusion with a needle electrocautery, set at a power sufficient to destroy mucosa, but not sufficient to cause transmural destruction of the vas, further reduces recanalization rates to less than 0.5 per cent (Schmidt, 1987). At least 1 cm of lumen should be cauterized in each direction. Battery-driven thermal cautery devices can also be utilized intraluminally but are somewhat less effective.

Interposition of fascia between the cut ends, folding back of the vasal ends, and securing one end within the dartos muscle are all techniques that have been advocated with the intent of reducing vasectomy failure rates (Esho and Cass, 1978). However, no controlled studies have been performed documenting the efficacy of any of these methods in reducing failure rates. Moreover, these techniques complicate vasectomy and increase the time required to perform the procedure.

The length of vas removed undoubtedly influences the rate of vasectomy failure. Removing very long segments lessens the possibility of recanalization. Such destructive procedures are more likely to be associated with post-operative hematomas and decrease the possibility of vasectomy reversal in the future. Most urologists insist on removal of a segment of vas for pathologic verification, primarily for medicolegal reasons. Because the majority of vasectomy failures are due to recanalization, rather than failure to ligate or occlude the proper structure, there is little justification for this policy. Even from a legal point of view, a pathologist's report confirming the presence of vas in the vasectomy specimen offers no protection from litigation. Documented counseling, diligent follow-up to obtain at least two azoospermic semen specimens postoperatively, and careful selection of appropriate candidates for vasectomy in the first place provide the best protection from a medicolegal standpoint.

Preferred Methods of Occlusion

Occlusion techniques that result in very low rates of recanalization, without destruction of excessively long segments of vas and without complicated time-consuming strategies, include the following:

1. Intraluminal electrocautery of each end for a distance of 1 to 2 cm in each direction after removal of a 1-cm segment of vas
2. Intraluminal thermal cautery with a battery-driven device for a distance of 1 to 2 cm in each direction plus application of a medium hemoclip on the vasal end distal to the cauterized segment, also after removal of a 1 to 2-cm segment
3. Intraluminal cautery as previously described plus separation of the vasal ends into different tissue planes with or without removal of a segment
4. Double medium hemoclips on each end 1 cm apart after removal of a 1 to 2-cm segment with or without separation into different tissue planes.

No technique of vasal occlusion, short of removing the entire scrotal vas, is 100 per cent effective. Follow-up semen analysis with the goal of obtaining two absolutely azoospermic specimens 4 to 6 weeks apart is essential. If sperm are found in the ejaculate 3 months after vasectomy, the procedure should be repeated.

Open-Ended Vasectomy

For over 20 years, attempts have been made to develop reversible methods of vasectomy. Most of these efforts have been focused on mechanical valves that could be opened and closed. Unfortunately, these attempts have not been successful because of the damage to the epididymis that occurs after long-term obstruction. Evidence is now good that leakage of sperm at the vasectomy site prevents this pressure-induced damage and may increase the chances of successful reversal when accurate microsurgical vasovasostomy is performed (Silber, 1977). If the testicular end of the vas deferens is not sealed (open-ended technique), a sperm granuloma forms at the vasectomy site and damage to the epididymis is reduced. Early experience with this technique resulted in an unacceptably high incidence of vasectomy failure varying from 7 to 50 per cent (Goldstein, 1983;

Shapiro and Silber, 1979). Better methods of sealing and burying the abdominal end of the vas reduce the failure rate of open-ended vasectomy to about 4 per cent. This is still a substantially higher incidence of failure than that obtained with the closed occlusion techniques previously described. Because recanalization after vasectomy is invariably associated with sperm granuloma formation, it is likely that open-ended vasectomy will always be associated with higher failure rates unless extraordinary efforts are made to widely separate the vasal ends or unless very long lengths of vas are destroyed on the seminal vesicle side. These measures, however, would unduly complicate the performance of vasectomy or, paradoxically, make it less reversible.

Complications of Vasectomy

Hematoma and Infection

Hematoma is the most common complication of vasectomy, with an average incidence of 2 per cent but a range of 0.09 to 29 per cent (Kendrick et al., 1987). Infection is surprisingly common with an average rate of 3.4 per cent, but several series report rates from 12 to 38 per cent (Appell and Evans, 1980; Randall et al., 1983 and 1985). The experience of the surgeon is the single most important factor in regard to complication rates (Kendrick et al., 1987). The hematoma rate was significantly higher among surgeons performing one to ten vasectomies (4.6 per cent), than among those performing 11 to 50 vasectomies (2.4 per cent) or more than 50 vasectomies per year (1.6 per cent). A similar relationship was reported for hospitalization rate. Surprisingly, 22 per cent of physicians surveyed reported using general anesthesia for vasectomy.

Sperm Granuloma

Sperm granuloma associated with pain is reported after 0.1 to 3 per cent of vasectomies. The presence or absence of a sperm granuloma at the vasectomy site seems to be of importance in modulating the local effects of chronic obstruction on the male reproductive tract. The sperm granuloma's complex network of epithelialized channels provides additional absorptive surfaces that help vent the high intraluminal pressure in the obstructed excurrent ducts. Numerous animal studies have correlated the presence or absence of sperm granuloma at the vasectomy site with the degree of epididymal and testicular damage. Species that always develop granulomas after vasectomy have minimal damage to the seminiferous tubules. Studies of men undergoing vasectomy reversal have revealed somewhat higher success rates in men who have sperm granuloma at the vasectomy sites (Belker et al., 1983; Silber, 1977). Because sperm granulomas represent a violation of the blood-testis barrier, it was thought that they might increase the stimulation of antisperm antibody formation after vasectomy. Studies attempting to address this issue, however, have yielded conflicting results.

Although sperm granulomas at the vasectomy site are present microscopically in 10 to 30 per cent of men undergoing reversals, it is likely that, given enough time, virtually all men will develop sperm granulomas at the vasectomy site, epididymis, or rete testis.

When sperm granuloma results in chronic postvasectomy pain, excision and occlusion of the vasa with intraluminal cautery usually relieve the pain and prevent recurrence (Schmidt, 1979). Alternatively, men with postvasectomy congestive epididymitis may be relieved of pain by open-ended vasectomy designed to purposefully produce a pressure-relieving sperm granuloma.

Long-Term Complications

Long-term effects of vasectomy include vasitis nodosa, chronic testicular pain, testicular function alterations, and epididymal obstruction, and the postulated effect of vasectomy on the cardiovascular system. Although vasitis nodosa has been reported in up to 66 per cent of vasectomy specimens in men undergoing vasectomy reversals (Freund et al., 1989), this entity does not appear to be associated with pain or significant medical sequelae.

In humans, micropuncture studies have revealed that the markedly increased pressures that occur on the testicular side of the vas as well as the epididymis after vasectomy are not transmitted to the seminiferous tubules (Johnson and Howards, 1975). Therefore, little disruption of spermatogenesis is expected. Biopsy specimens up to 15 years after vasectomy show the testes to be essentially normal by light microscopy. Electron microscopic studies, however, have revealed thickening of the basal lamina and scattered areas of disrupted spermatogenesis in portions of the biopsy specimens (Jarow et al., 1985). Chronic orchialgia after vasectomy has been reported in approximately one in 10,000 patients. In some cases, a vasectomy reversal or an open-ended vasectomy as described previously might be considered. The brunt of pressure-induced damage after vasectomy falls on the epididymis and efferent ductules. These structures become markedly distended and then adapt to reabsorb large volumes of testicular fluid and sperm products. It is likely that, in time, all vasectomized men develop "blowouts" in either the epididymis or efferent ducts. Sperm granulomas may form at the site of rupture, and secondary epididymal or efferent duct obstruction may result. For this reason, reversal surgery is less successful as the time interval from the original vasectomy increases. The presence of a sperm granuloma at the vasectomy site may vent some of the high pressure ordinarily transmitted to the epididymis and, therefore, may confer some protection against damage to these structures.

Systemic effects of vasectomy have been postulated. Vasectomy results in violation of the blood-testis barrier producing detectable levels of serum antisperm antibodies in 60 to 80 per cent of men after vasectomy (Fuchs and Alexander, 1983; Lepow and Crozier, 1979). Some studies suggest that the antibody titers diminish 2 or more years after vasectomy; others suggest that these antibody titers persist. However, neither circulating immune complexes nor deposits are higher after vasectomy in men (Witkin et al., 1982). Studies in animals and men have failed to find any association between antisperm antibodies and immune complex–mediated diseases, such as lupus erythermatosus, scleroderma, rheumatoid arthritis, and myasthenia gravis (Massey, 1984). Although one study in cynomolgus monkeys found more frequent and extensive atherosclerosis of the major vessels in previously vasectomized monkeys fed a high cholesterol diet (Alexander and Clarkson, 1978), no evidence of excess cardiovascular disease (Walker et al., 1981a), illness requiring hospitalization (Petitti et al., 1982; Walker et al., 1981b), or biochemical alterations (Smith and Paulson, 1980) have been found in more than 12 reports on vasectomized men. Nine of these studies employed matched controls and the largest examined over 6000 men vasectomized 3 to 25 years previously (Goldacre et al., 1983). These reports indicate that the risk of any serious systemic long-term effects from vasectomy is very small.

VASOVASOSTOMY

Although the number of men in the United States who undergo vasectomy has remained stable at about 500,000 per year, the number who request surgical reversal of vasectomy has grown. Surveys suggest that 2 to 6 per cent of vasectomized men will ultimately seek reversal (Derrick et al., 1973). Prior to the refinement of microsurgical techniques, results of vasectomy reversal were relatively poor, with pregnancy rates of 15 to 50 per cent. Creating an accurate leak proof anastomosis of structures with a luminal diameter of only 0.3 to 0.4 mm is a formidable technical challenge.

Anesthesia

Light general or regional anesthesia is preferred. In cooperative patients, local anesthesia with sedation can be employed if the time interval since vasectomy is short, the vasal ends are palpable, and a sperm granuloma is present, decreasing the likelihood of secondary epididymal obstruction. Slight movements are greatly magnified by the operating microscope and disturb performance of the anastomosis. When large vasal gaps are present, extensions of the incisions high into the inguinal canal may be necessary. Furthermore, if vasoepididymostomy is necessary, the operating time could exceed 3 hours. Local anesthesia limits the options available to the surgeon. Hypobaric spinal anesthesia with long-acting agents, such as bupivacaine (Marcaine), can provide 4 to 5 hours of anesthesia and has the advantage of eliminating lower body motion. Epidural anesthesia with an indwelling catheter can be equally effective.

With local anesthesia and cord block, there is a small risk of inadvertent injury to the testicular artery (Goldstein et al., 1983). If the vasal artery has been disrupted by previous vasectomy, testicular artery injury could result in testicular atrophy.

Surgical Approaches

Scrotal

Bilateral high vertical scrotal incisions provide the most direct access to the obstructed site in cases of vasectomy reversal. If the vasal gap is large, this incision can be extended inguinally without difficulty. If the vasectomy site is low, it is simple to pull up the testicular end. This incision should be made at least 1 cm lateral to the base of the penis. A 2- to 3-cm incision can be made directly over the vasectomy site if both vasal ends are palpated. The testis should be delivered, with the tunica vaginalis intact, when the site of obstruction cannot be determined or when large vasal gaps are present. This approach provides excellent exposure of the entire scrotal vas deferens and, if necessary, the epididymis.

Infrapubic Incision

This approach has the advantage of exposing both vasa through a single incision. Because the incision is high, obtaining adequate length on the abdominal side vas is simplified. The disadvantage of this incision is that the skin and the subcutaneous tissue at this level are fairly thick—it also results in a thick scar.

Inguinal Incision

This is the preferred approach in a man with a suspected obstruction of the inguinal vas deferens from prior herniorrhaphy or orchiopexy. Incision through the previous scar usually leads directly to the site of obstruction. If the obstruction is scrotal or epididymal, it is a simple matter to deliver the testis through the inguinal incision.

Preparation of the Vasa

The vas is grasped with Babcock clamps above and below the vasectomy site. Penrose drains replace the Babcock clamps to facilitate dissection. Include the vasal vessels and periadventitial tissue. The vas is mobilized for a distance of 2 to 3 cm on either side of the vasectomy site. The vas should not be stripped of its sheath. The obstructed segment and, if present, sperm granuloma at the vasectomy site is removed. Granulomas can invade the adjacent vasovasostomy and cause reobstruction.

When large vasal gaps are present, a gauze-wrapped index finger separates the cord structures from the vas. Blunt finger dissection through the external ring will free the vas to the internal inguinal ring, if additional abdominal length is necessary. These maneuvers will leave all the vasal vessels intact. When the vasal gap is extremely large, additional length can be achieved by dissecting the entire convoluted vas free of its attachments to the epididymal tunic, allowing the testis to drop upside down. These maneuvers can provide an additional 4 to 6 cm length (Fig. 87–22). In order to maintain the integrity of the vasal vessels, this dissection is best performed while employing magnifying loupes or

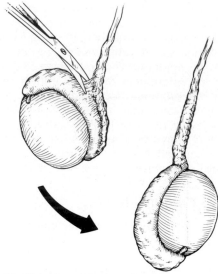

Figure 87–22. Dissection of the convoluted vas free of its attachments to the epididymal tunic allows the testis to drop down and provides 4 to 6 cm of additional length.

the operating microscope. If the amount of vas removed is so large that even these measures fail to allow a tension-free anastomosis, the incision can be extended to the internal inguinal ring. The floor of the inguinal canal is cut and the vas rerouted under the floor, as in a difficult orchiopexy. With this combination of maneuvers, 12-cm gaps can be bridged.

After the vasa have been freed, the testicular end of the vas is sharply cut. An ultrasharp knife drawn through a slotted 2- or 2.5-mm diameter nerve clamp yields a perfect 90 degree cut (Fig. 87–23). The cut surface of the testicular end of the vas deferens is inspected using

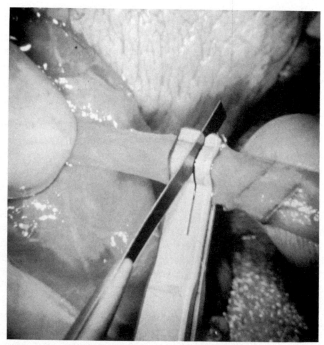

Figure 87–23. Ultrasharp knife drawn through a 1- to 3-mm diameter slotted nerve holder yields a perfect 90-degree cut.

8- to 15-power magnification. A healthy white mucosal ring should be seen, which springs back immediately after gentle dilation. The muscularis should be smooth and soft, not gritty. Healthy bleeding should be noted from both the cut edge of the mucosa as well as the surface of the muscularis. If the blood supply is poor or the muscularis is gritty, the vas is recut until healthy tissue is found. The vasal artery and vein are clamped and ligated with 4–0 plain catgut suture. Small bleeders are controlled with microbipolar forceps. Once a patent lumen has been established on the testicular end, the vas is milked and a clean glass slide is touched to its surface. The vasal fluid is immediately mixed with a drop or two of saline and preserved under a coverslip for microscope examination. The abdominal end of the vas deferens is prepared in a similar manner and the lumen gently cannulated with a 24-gauge angiocath sheath (see Fig. 87–3). Injection of saline or Ringer's lactate solution confirms its patency. A minimum of instrumentation of the mucosa should be performed.

After preparation, the ends of the vasa can be stabilized with an approximating clamp (Goldstein, 1985) or with sutures placed through the periadventitia to remove all tension prior to performing the anastomosis. A sterile tongue blade covered with a Penrose drain placed beneath the ends of the vasa provides an excellent platform on which to perform the anastomosis. Isolating the field through a slit in a rubber dam prevents microsutures from sticking to the surrounding tissue.

The decision when to perform vasoepididymostomy is made based on the evaluation of the vasal fluid and the examination of the epididymis. If microscopic examination of the vasal fluid reveals the presence of sperm with tails, vasovasostomy is performed. If no fluid is found, a 24-gauge angiocath sheath is inserted into the lumen and barbitage with 0.1 ml of saline performed, while the convoluted vas is vigorously milked. Men with large sperm granulomas often have virtually no dilation of the testicular end of the vas, and little or no fluid may be noticed initially. The barbitage fluid is expressed onto a slide and examined. Invariably, when granulomas are present, sperm is always found in this scant fluid. If the vas is absolutely dry and spermless after multiple samples are examined, vasoepididymostomy should be performed. If the fluid expressed from the vas is found to be thick, white, and water insoluble, and toothpaste-like in quality, examination rarely reveals sperm. Under these circumstances, the tunica vaginalis is opened and the epididymis inspected. If clear evidence of obstruction is found, i.e., an epididymal sperm granuloma with dilated tubules above and collapsed tubules below, vasoepididymostomy is performed. When in doubt, and when the vasal fluid contains no sperm or sperm heads only, vasovasostomy should be performed. Up to 60 per cent of men with bilateral absence of sperm in the vasal fluid will have sperm return to the ejaculate and 31 per cent will ultimately impregnate their partners (Belker et al., 1990).

When copious, crystal-clear, water-like fluid squirts out from the vas and no sperm is found in this fluid, a vasovasostomy is performed because the prognosis is good that sperm will return to the ejaculate.

Multiple Vasal Obstructions

If saline injection reveals that the abdominal end of the vas deferens is not patent, a 0.18-mm blunt-tipped guide wire is gently passed to determine the site of obstruction. If the obstruction is within 5 cm of the original vasectomy site the abdominal end of the vas deferens may be dissected to this site and excised. The incision should be extended inguinally to free the vas extensively toward the internal inguinal ring. The testicular end should also be freed to the vasoepididymal junction. If the site of the second obstruction is so far from the vasectomy site that two vasovasostomies are necessary, the distance to the inguinal obstruction is measured and recorded for future reference. A vasovasostomy is then performed at the vasectomy site. Re-exploration is scheduled for a later date for an inguinal vasovasostomy, after allowing the vasal segment beyond the original vasovasostomy site to become well vascularized. Performance of simultaneous vasovasostomies at two separate sites is risky and may lead to devascularization of the intervening segment.

Anastomotic Techniques

All successful vasovasostomy techniques depend on adherence to surgical principles that are universally applicable to anastomoses of all tubular structures. These include accurate mucosa-to-mucosa approximation, leak proof anastomosis, tension-free anastomosis, good blood supply, healthy mucosa and muscularis, and good atraumatic anastomotic technique.

ACCURATE MUCOSA-TO-MUCOSA APPROXIMATION. In human vasovasostomy, the testicular-side lumen is often dilated to diameters 3 or 4 times that of the abdominal-side lumen. Techniques that work well with lumens of equal diameters may be less successful with lumens of markedly discrepant diameters.

LEAK PROOF ANASTOMOSIS. Sperm are highly antigenic and provoke an inflammatory reaction when they escape from the normally intact lining of the excurrent ducts of the male reproductive tract. Extravasated sperm adversely influences the success of vasovasostomy (Hagan and Coffey, 1977; Silber, 1979).

TENSION-FREE ANASTOMOSIS. When an anastomosis is performed under tension, sperm may appear in the ejaculate for several months after surgery. Ultimately, sperm counts and motility decrease and azoospermia may ensue. At re-exploration, only a thin fibrotic band is found at the anastomotic site. This can be prevented by adequately freeing the ends of the vasa and by placing reinforcing sutures in the periadventitia of the vas.

GOOD BLOOD SUPPLY. If the cut vas exhibits poor blood supply it should be cut again until healthy bleeding is encountered. When extensive resection is necessary, additional length should be obtained utilizing the techniques previously described.

HEALTHY MUCOSA AND MUSCULARIS. If the mucosa or cut surface of the vas exhibits poor distensibility after dilation, peels away from the underlying muscularis, or shreds easily, the vas should be cut back until healthy mucosa is found. When the muscularis is fibrotic or gritty, the vas must be cut again until healthy tissue is found.

GOOD ATRAUMATIC ANASTOMOTIC TECHNIQUE. If multiple surgical errors occur during the procedure, such as cutting of the mucosa with needles, tearing through sutures, or backwalling of mucosa, the anastomosis should be immediately resected and redone.

Macroscopic Techniques

The diameter of the undilated abdominal end of the vas deferens is approximately 300 μ. Furthermore, one cannot predict the necessity for vasoepididymostomy until the time of surgery. For these reasons, macroscopic techniques are no longer appropriate for this type of surgery. Comparison of pregnancy and patency rates after macroscopic surgery and those after microscopic surgery in over a dozen studies have clearly shown that better results are obtained when magnification is used in the procedure. In a report from China, excellent results were achieved utilizing a needle-stented macroscopic technique of vasovasostomy (Xie-Yang and Yong-Xiong, 1988). However, in this study, the average time from vasectomy to reversal was only 1 year. Therefore, the vasal lumens were of equal diameter. Under these circumstances, most techniques of vasovasostomy yield fairly good results. Furthermore, this technique cannot be employed in the convoluted vas. In our experience, half of all vasovasostomies will be performed in the convoluted portion of the vas.

Loupe Magnification

Loupes are now available that can provide 6- to 8-power magnification—the minimum necessary for accurate vasovasostomy. The heavy weight of high-power loupes can make them uncomfortable after 1 or 2 hours. Surgeons who are experienced and comfortable with such loupes can obtain satisfactory results, however.

Microsurgical Techniques

These methods employ an operating microscope that provides variable magnification from 6 to 32 power. A diploscope providing identical fields for both surgeon and assistant, is preferred. Additionally, foot pedal controls for a motorized zoom and focus leave the hands free.

ONE-LAYER TECHNIQUE. Although we prefer the multilayer technique described next, a modified one-layer anastomosis (Sharlip, 1981) is satisfactory when the abdominal and testicular-end lumens have similar diameters and the anastomosis is performed in the straight portion of the vas. A single layer of four to eight interrupted 9–0 or 10–0 monofilament nylon sutures are placed through all layers. A second layer of 8–0 or 9–0 sutures is placed in the adventitia and muscularis (Fig. 87–24). A periadventitial layer of heavier sutures removes all tension from the anastomosis.

MULTILAYER TECHNIQUE. This method of vasovasostomy can handle lumens of markedly discrep-

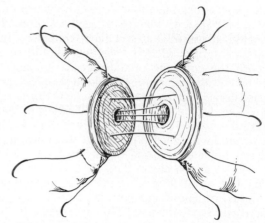

Figure 87–24. Modified one layer vasovasostomy.

ant diameters in the straight or convoluted vas (Owen, 1977; Silber, 1977b). Monofilament 10–0 nylon sutures, double-armed with 70-μ diameter taper-point needles bent into a fishhook configuration, are utilized. The anastomosis begins with the placement of three 10–0 monofilament nylon mucosal sutures (Fig. 87–25). The double-armed sutures allow inside-out placement, eliminating the need for manipulation or dilation of the mucosa and the possibility of backwalling. After these three mucosal sutures are tied, two 9–0 monofilament nylon deep muscularis sutures are placed exactly in between the previously placed mucosal sutures, just above, but not through the mucosa (Fig. 87–26). These sutures seal the gap between the two mucosal sutures without trauma to the mucosa from the larger 100-μ diameter cutting needle required to penetrate the tough vas muscularis and adventitia. A superficial adventitial 9–0 suture is placed between these two muscularis sutures to provide additional strength (Fig. 87–27). The vas is then rotated 180 degrees, and three to five additional 10–0 sutures are placed to complete the mucosal portion of the anastomosis (Fig. 87–28).

Just before tying the last mucosal suture, the lumen is irrigated with heparinized Ringer's solution to prevent the formation of clot. After completion of the mucosal layer, 9–0 deep muscularis sutures are placed exactly in between each mucosal suture, just above, but not penetrating the mucosa (Fig. 87–29). This step provides a

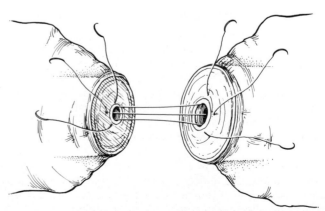

Figure 87–25. Three mucosal sutures are placed, inside out, and tied.

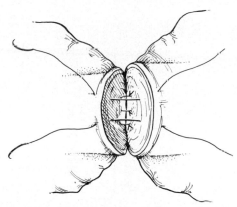

Figure 87–26. Deep submucosal sutures of 9–0 nylon, including all the muscularis and adventitia, are placed exactly in between each pair of mucosal sutures.

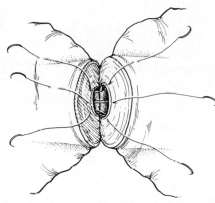

Figure 87–28. The vas is rotated 180 degrees, and an additional three or four 10–0 nylon sutures complete the mucosal portion of the anastomosis.

watertight anastomosis. Superficial adventitial 9–0 sutures are then placed exactly in between each of the previously placed deep muscularis sutures (Fig. 87–30). This placement closes the muscularis and adventitia over the underlying mucosal sutures and provides additional strength. The anastomosis is finished by approximating the vasal sheath with six to eight sutures of 6–0 Prolene (see Fig. 87–29). This layer completely covers the anastomosis and relieves it of all tension.

Anastomoses in the Convoluted Vas

Vasovasostomy performed in the convoluted portion of the vas deferens is technically more demanding than anastomoses in the straight portion. Fear of cutting back into the convoluted vas in order to obtain healthy tissues may lead surgeons to complete an anastomosis in the straight portion where the testicular end of the vas has poor blood supply, unhealthy or friable mucosa, or gritty fibrotic muscularis. Adherence to the following principles will ensure that anastomoses in the convoluted vas will succeed equally as often as those in the straight portion.

1. A perfect transverse cut yielding a round ring of mucosa and a lumen directed straight down is essential

(Fig. 87–31A). A very oblique lumen with a thin flap of muscle and mucosa on one side is not acceptable (Fig. 87–31B). The vas should be cut again at 0.5-mm intervals, until a perfect cut with good blood and healthy tissue is obtained. A slotted nerve clamp 2.5 or 3 mm in diameter and an ultrasharp knife facilitate this part of the procedure (see Fig. 87–23). Often, the vas must be cut 5 or 6 times until the correct cut is obtained.

2. The convoluted vas should not be unraveled—this disturbs the blood supply at the anastomotic line.

3. The sheath of convoluted vas may be carefully dissected free of its attachments to the epididymal tunic (see Fig. 87–22). This maneuver will minimize disturbance of its blood supply and will provide the necessary length to perform a tension-free anastomosis.

4. Care must be taken to avoid taking large bites of the muscularis and adventitial layers to prevent inadvertent perforation of adjacent convolutions.

5. Reinforce the anastomosis by approximating the vasal sheath of the straight portion to the sheath of the convoluted portion with multiple 6–0 sutures (see Fig. 87–30). This procedure will remove all tension from the anastomosis.

Crossed Vasovasostomy

This is a useful procedure (Fig. 87–32) that often provides a simple solution to an otherwise difficult

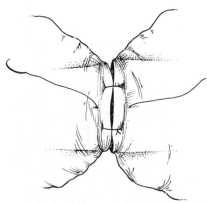

Figure 87–27. Adventitial sutures of 9–0 nylon are placed superficial to each mucosal suture and, therefore, in between each deep muscularis suture.

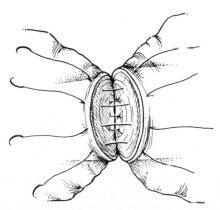

Figure 87–29. Remaining deep submucosal sutures are placed.

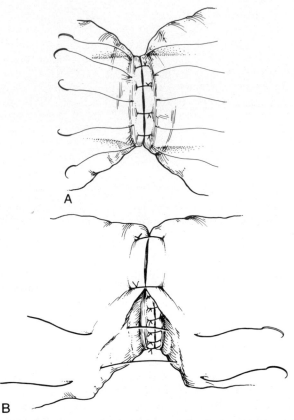

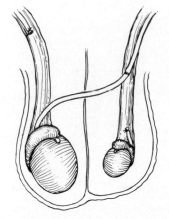

Figure 87–32. Crossed vasovasostomy.

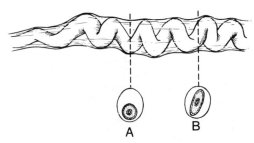

Figure 87–30. After completion of the superficial adventitial layer *(A)* the vasal sheath is approximated with 6–0 Prolene *(B)*. This step removes all tension from the anastomosis.

problem (Hamidinia, 1988; Lizza et al., 1985). Crossover is indicated in the following circumstances:

UNILATERAL INGUINAL OBSTRUCTION OF THE VAS DEFERENS ASSOCIATED WITH AN ATROPHIC TESTIS ON THE CONTRALATERAL SIDE. Transect the vas attached to the atrophic testis at the junction of its straight and convoluted portion and confirm its patency with a saline vasogram (see Fig. 87–3). Dissect the contralateral vas toward the inguinal obstruction. Transect it and cross it through a capacious opening made in the scrotal septum and proceed with vasovasostomy as previously described. This procedure is much less difficult than trying to find both ends of the vas within the dense scar of a previous inguinal operation.

UNILATERAL OBSTRUCTION OR APLASIA OF THE INGUINAL VAS OR EJACULATORY DUCT AND CONTRALATERAL OBSTRUCTION OF THE EPIDIDYMIS. It is preferable to perform one procedure with a high probability of success (vasovasostomy) than two procedures with a much lower probability of success, e.g., unilateral vasovasoepididymostomy and contralateral TUR of the ejaculatory ducts.

ONE OR TWO ANASTOMOSES. In general, opt for one good anastomosis instead of two mediocre ones; opt for one good vasovasostomy rather than a unilateral vasoepididymostomy and contralateral mediocre vasovasostomy.

Transposition of the Testis

Occasionally, when vasal length is critically short, a tension-free crossed anastomosis can best be accomplished by testicular transposition (Fig. 87–33).

Wound Closure

If extensive dissection and delivery of the testis were performed, Penrose drains are brought out the depen-

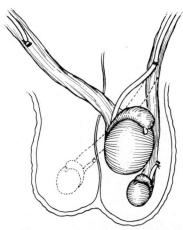

Figure 87–33. Transposition of testis for crossed vasovasostomy when vasal length is severely compromised.

Figure 87–31. *A,* The ideal cut for a convoluted vas anastomosis—round mucosal edge with lumen directed perpendicular to the cut. *B,* Unsatisfactory cut in the convoluted vas—eccentric mucosal ring with lumen directed obliquely.

dent portion of the right and left hemiscrota and fixed in place with sutures and safety pins. The dartos is loosely approximated with interrupted absorbable sutures and the skin with interrupted subcuticular sutures of 4–0 Vicryl. This closure promotes drainage from the wound, thereby minimizing hematoma formation. The wound heals with a fine scar and none of the "railroad tracks" associated with through-and-through skin closures. A majority of our procedures are not drained and are performed on an ambulatory basis.

Long-Term Follow-Up Evaluation

When sperm is found in the vasal fluid on at least one side at the time of surgery, carefully done microscopic anastomoses will result in the appearance of sperm in the ejaculate in 90 to 98 per cent of men. Late obstruction, after initial patency, occurs in 5 to 10 per cent of men followed for at least 2 years. Pregnancy occurs in 50 to 60 per cent of couples followed for at least 2 years when female factors are excluded and sperm was found in the vas on at least one side at the time of vasovasostomy. The role of antisperm antibodies, drug treatment, and assisted reproductive procedures in enhancing the chances of pregnancy after vasovasostomy is discussed in Chapter 15.

SURGERY OF THE EPIDIDYMIS

Detailed knowledge of epididymal anatomy and physiology (presented in Chapter 6) is essential prior to undertaking surgery of this delicate and important structure. Sperm motility and fertilizing capacity progressively increase during passage through the 200-µ diameter, 9- to 12-foot long, tightly coiled single tubule. When the epididymis is obstructed, or functionally shortened after vasoepididymostomy, even very short lengths of epididymis adapt and allow some sperm to acquire motility and fertilizing capacity (Silber, 1989). Adaptation may gradually continue up to 2 years after surgical reconstruction, with progressive improvement in the fertility and motility of sperm. Nevertheless, preservation of the greatest possible length of functional epididymis is most likely to result in the best sperm quality after vasoepididymostomy (Schoysman and Bedford, 1986). Furthermore, because the wall of the epididymis is thinnest in the caput region and gradually thickens, owing to the increasing numbers of smooth muscle cells in its more distal (inferior) end, anastomoses are technically simpler to perform and more likely to succeed in its distal regions. Because the epididymis is a single tubule with a very small diameter, injury or occlusion of a tubule, anywhere along its length, leads to total obstruction of output from that epididymis. For these reasons, magnification with loupes, or preferably the operating microscope, is essential for performing virtually all epididymal surgery.

Fortunately, the epididymis has a rich blood supply derived from the testicular vessels superiorly and the deferential vessels inferiorly. Because of the extensive interconnections between these branches, either the testicular or deferential branches to the epididymis may be divided without compromising epididymal viability.

Conversely, because the epididymal branches of the testicular artery are medial to and separate from the main testicular artery and veins, surgical procedures may be performed on the epididymis without compromise to testicular blood supply.

Epididymectomy

Epididymectomy may be indicated in men with chronic infections or abscesses of the epididymis that are unresponsive to antibiotic therapy. Men with acquired immune deficiency syndrome (AIDS) may develop cytomegalovirus infections of the epididymis and may require epididymectomy for treatment (Randazzo et al., 1986). Chronic unremitting pain after vasectomy may be relieved by total epididymectomy (Selikowitz and Schned, 1985). All patients should be counseled preoperatively that the procedure may impair fertility or render them sterile if bilateral epididymectomy is performed.

Surgical Technique

Through a vertical medium raphe or transverse scrotal incision, the vas deferens is isolated at the junction of its straight and convoluted regions and doubly ligated and divided including the deferential vessels. The convoluted vas is dissected free of its attachments to the epididymal tunic and traced to the vasoepididymal junction (see Fig. 87–22). The tunica vaginalis is opened, and dissection is continued in the plane between the epididymis and the testis. Optical loupe magnification (2.5×) and elevation of the epididymis with an encircling Penrose drain, with transillumination of the mesentery between the testis and epididymis, allow for better visualization of the epididymal blood supply and for avoidance of injury to the spermatic cord vessels. These are encountered at the junction of the middle and upper thirds of the testis, entering medial to the epididymis (Fig. 87–34). Care should be taken to preserve the testicular vessels. The efferent ducts, located superior to the testicular vascular pedicle, are ligated. The epi-

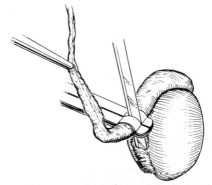

Figure 87–34. Preparation for end-to-end vasoepididymostomy.

didymectomy specimen may then be removed. For hemostasis, the edges of the tunica vaginalis along the base of the resected epididymis should be oversewn with a continuous catgut suture. The dartos and skin are loosely closed with interrupted absorbable sutures.

Spermatocelectomy

A spermatocele is the epididymal equivalent of a berry aneurysm; they may occur anywhere in the epididymis but are more common in the caput region. They are exceedingly common, increasing in frequency with age, and identified incidentally in upward of 70 per cent of men who are undergoing high resolution scrotal ultrasonography. Intervention for spermatocele is rarely indicated. Spermatoceles are usually painless and do not obstruct the epididymal tubule from which they arise. Resection of the spermatocele, however, may cause epididymal obstruction. Spermatocelectomy is only indicated when the spermatocele is associated with unremitting pain or when the spermatocele has grown to a large size.

Surgical Technique

The testis is delivered through a median raphe or transverse scrotal incision and the tunica vaginalis opened. The spermatocele is dissected free of the epididymis utilizing the operating microscope, to avoid inadvertent injury to the epididymal tubules. The attachment of the spermatocele to the epididymis is ligated to prevent extravasation of sperm and granuloma formation. The tunica vaginalis is reapproximated with continuous absorbable sutures, and the dartos and skin are closed in two layers.

Excision of Epididymal Tumors and Cysts

Most nontransilluminable epididymal masses are benign adenomatoid tumors. Malignant epididymal tumors are exceedingly rare. Like any potentially malignant testicular mass, tumors should be managed by inguinal exploration, clamping of the cord and delivery of the testis. If the diagnosis of malignancy is uncertain, the field should be isolated and cooled prior to opening the tunica vaginalis for direct inspection and biopsy. This modification of Chevassu's maneuver is particularly helpful for exploration of epididymal tumors (Goldstein and Waterhouse, 1983). These are usually benign, and needless orchiectomy is prevented. If the diagnosis of malignancy has been excluded, the epididymal tumor or cyst is excised in a fashion identical to that for a spermatocele.

Vasoepididymostomy

The indications for vasoepididymostomy are discussed in Chapter 15. The indications for vasoepididymostomy in men undergoing vasectomy reversals are discussed earlier in this chapter in the section on vasovasostomy.

Prior to the development of microsurgical techniques, accurate approximation of the vasal lumen to that of a specific epididymal tubule was not possible. Vasoepididymostomy was performed by aligning the vas deferens adjacent to a slash made in multiple epididymal tubules, while the surgeon anticipated that a fistula would form. Results with this primitive technique were poor. Microsurgical approaches allow an accurate approximation of the vasal mucosa to that of a single epididymal tubule (Silber, 1978), resulting in a marked improvement in the patency and pregnancy rates. Microsurgical vasoepididymostomy, however, is the most technically demanding procedure described in this chapter, and, probably, one of the most difficult procedures to perform in microsurgery. In virtually no other operation are results so dependent on technical perfection. Microsurgical vasoepididymostomy should be attempted only by the most experienced microsurgeons who perform the procedure frequently.

Microsurgical Vasoepididymostomy

END-TO-END ANASTOMOSIS. End-to-end vasoepididymostomy is a useful technique when the epididymal tubules are not dilated, which is often the situation in epididymides obstructed by sperm granulomas. The multiple epithelialized channels within the granuloma increase the surface area available for the absorption of sperm and testicular fluid. The granuloma, therefore, relieves pressure proximally resulting in minimal dilation of epididymal tubules above the site of obstruction. This situation is identical to the phenomena in vasovasostomy, whereby minimal dilation of the testicular end of the vas deferens occurs when a sperm granuloma is present at the vasectomy site. When the epididymal tubules are not dilated, a transverse cut across the epididymis allows the clearest visualization of the cut edges of the tubule.

An end-to-end operation is indicated in distal obstructions near the vasoepididymal junction. At this point, the epididymis is narrower and its outer diameter more closely matches that of the vas deferens. Furthermore, it is possible to perform a more distal anastomosis when the epididymis is dissected completely to the vasoepididymal junction and transversely sectioned. An end-to-side operation cannot be performed in the cauda of the epididymis unless the epididymis is dissected distally off the testis. If this maneuver is done, the additional dissection obviates the benefits of an end-to-side operation.

An end-to-end anastomosis is preferred when vasal length is compromised—a situation commonly encountered during vasectomy reversal. If the epididymis is obstructed distally, it can be dissected off the testis right up to the efferent ductules, if necessary, and flipped up to provide up to 5 cm of additional length (see Fig. 87–34). The superior epididymal branches of the testicular artery are preserved and provide excellent blood supply to the distal epididymis.

Surgical Technique

The testis is delivered through a 3- to 4-cm high vertical scrotal incision. The vas deferens is identified, isolated with a Babcock clamp, and surrounded with a Penrose drain at the junction of the straight and convoluted portions of the vas deferens. With 8- to 15-power magnification provided by the operating microscope, the vasal sheath is vertically incised with a microknife. A bare segment of vas, stripped of its carefully preserved vessels, is delivered. The vas is hemitransected with the knife until the lumen is entered (see Fig. 87–2). The vasal fluid is sampled. If microscopic examination of this fluid reveals the absence of sperm, the diagnosis of epididymal obstruction is confirmed. Saline vasography is performed as described earlier in this chapter to confirm patency of the abdominal side of the vas deferens (see Fig. 87–3). The vas is completely transected utilizing a 2.5-mm slotted nerve clamp, and the vas is prepared as described earlier for vasovasostomy (see Fig. 87–23). When an end-to-end vasoepididymostomy is performed, it is particularly important to avoid stripping the vas of its sheath. The vas should be sectioned with as much sheath and periadventitial tissue left attached to the vas as possible. This maneuver is critical for completing the outer layer of the anastomosis, especially in the proximal epididymis where the diameter of its tunic is much larger than that of the stripped vas.

After the vas has been prepared, the tunica vaginalis is opened and the testis delivered. Inspection of the epididymis under the operating microscope may reveal a clearly delineated site of obstruction. Often, a discrete yellow sperm granuloma is noted, above which the epididymis is indurated and the tubules dilated and below which the epididymis is soft and the tubules collapsed. Under these circumstances, the epididymis is encircled with a small Penrose drain at the level of obstruction and, with 2.5-power loupe magnification, dissected proximally 1 to 2 cm off the testis, yielding sufficient length to perform the anastomosis (see Fig. 87–34). Usually, a plane can be found between the epididymis and testis. Injury to the epididymal blood supply can be avoided by staying right on the tunica albuginia of the testis. The medial and inferior epididymal branches of the testicular artery are doubly ligated and divided, only if required to free an adequate length of epididymis. The superior epididymal branches entering the epididymis at the caput are always preserved. They can provide an adequate blood supply to the entire epididymis.

When the site of obstruction is not obvious, or the epididymis is indurated and dilated throughout its length, the epididymis is dissected to the vasoepididymal (VE) junction. This dissection is often facilitated by first dissecting the convoluted vas to the VE junction from below. After encircling the epididymis with a Penrose drain, one dissects the epididymis to the VE junction from above. In this way, the entire VE junction can be freed. This allows preservation of maximal epididymal length in the cases of distal obstruction or in the very rare cases of proximal obstruction of the convoluted vas near the VE junction.

When the dissection has been completed, the operating microscope is brought into the field. At the VE junction, or if clearly delineated, at the site of obstruction, the epididymis is encircled with a slotted nerve

clamp of appropriate diameter (4 to 6 mm) and transversely sectioned with an ultrasharp knife (see Fig. 87–34). The distal epididymal stump is ligated, and the proximal cut surface of the epididymis inspected under high-power magnification.

The epididymis is serially sectioned until a gush of cloudy fluid is seen effluxing from a single epididymal tubule. After hemostasis has been obtained with a bipolar cautery, a touch preparation of epididymal fluid is made, a drop of saline or Ringer's solution is added, and a careful microscopic examination of the slide performed. If many sperms are present, the single tubule continually effluxing fluid must be identified. Rubbing a fresh surgical marking pen on the cut surface of the epididymis helps clearly outline the cut edges of the epididymal tubules. Defunctionalized tubules empty in seconds and no longer have efflux of fluid. The tubule with efflux of fluid is gently probed with a microvessel dilator to identify the direction of its lumen. If no sperm are found or if the cut tubule is obliquely sectioned, the epididymis is cut again until sperm-bearing fluid is found in continual efflux from a round clearly visualized tubule. If fluid is in continuous efflux from more than one site, a tubule or tubules have been tangentially cut. The epididymis is sectioned again a few millimeters proximally until efflux is noted from only one round tubule. Painstakingly meticulous attention is paid to the attainment of absolutely perfect hemostasis with bipolar coagulation forceps with very fine tips.

The epididymis and vas deferens are stabilized with an approximating clamp so that the mucosa of the vas and a single epididymal tubule are adjacent to each other. The anastomosis begins with the placement of two posterior mucosal sutures of 10–0 monofilament nylon double-armed with 70-μ fishhook-shaped, taper-pointed needles. Inside-out placement of these sutures helps to prevent backwalling of the mucosa. Two to three additional anterior mucosal sutures are placed and tied (Fig. 87–35).

It is important to avoid taking wide bites during placement of mucosal sutures, to prevent inadvertent occlusion of an adjacent convolution of the epididymal tubule. After tying of the anterior mucosal sutures, interrupted 9–0 nylon sutures are utilized to approxi-

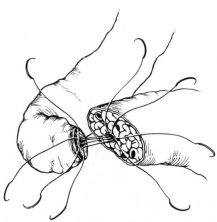

Figure 87–35. Placement of 10–0 mucosal sutures for end-to-end vasoepididymostomy.

mate the anterior outer muscularis and adventitial layers of the vas deferens to the epididymal tunic. These sutures are placed in such a way as to keep the mucosal anastomosis exactly aligned. Creativity is often required on the part of the surgeon, and 12 to 20 sutures may be necessary to secure a watertight anastomosis. It is hoped that this procedure will create a situation in which the path of least resistance for epididymal fluid is through the vasal lumen. As during vasovasostomy, persistent leakage of sperm with subsequent granuloma formation is likely to compromise the results of vasoepididymostomy. Avoid deep bites on the epididymal tunic side to prevent occlusion of a proximal epididymal tubule.

The anastomosis is now turned over, and the posterior epididymal sutures are tied. Additional 9–0 sutures are placed to complete the second layer of the anastomosis (Fig. 87–36). Two or three reinforcing sutures of 6–0 nylon or Prolene will bring the periadventitial tissue of the vas deferens and epididymis together and relieve all tension on the anastomosis. Hemostasis is obtained, and a Penrose drain is brought out in a dependent position of the hemiscrotum. The testis is replaced in the scrotum in a natural position, without torsion, that allows a tension-free anastomosis. The scrotum is closed as described for vasovasostomy. The drains are removed the day after surgery.

END-TO-SIDE ANASTOMOSIS. End-to-side vaso-epididymostomy has the advantage of being less traumatic to the epididymis and can often be performed in less time than an end-to-end anastomosis (Krylov and Borovikov, 1984; Wagenknecht et al., 1980). Because this procedure does not require extensive dissection of the epididymis or partial epididymectomy, it is less disruptive of the epididymal blood supply and associated with less bleeding. End-to-side anastomosis is most useful when marked dilation of the epididymal tubule is present, enabling clear visualization of the edges of the cut tubule. This method also obviates the necessity for identifying the single tubule effluxing sperm among the many tubules cut when the epididymis is sectioned transversely. The end-to-side approach also has the advantage of allowing accurate approximation of the muscularis and adventitia of the vas deferens to a precisely tailored opening in the tunic of the epididymis. This is the preferred technique when vasoepididymostomy is performed simultaneously with inguinal vaso-vasostomy or varicocelectomy, because it allows the vasal blood supply, deriving from epididymal branches

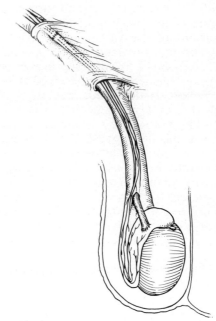

Figure 87–37. Simultaneous inguinal vasovasostomy and scrotal vaso-epididymostomy with preservation of the vasal branches of the epididymal artery.

of the testicular artery, to remain intact (Fig. 87–37). This maneuver preserves blood supply to the segment of vas intervening between the two anastomoses. In the case of simultaneous varicocelectomy, the technique maintains the integrity of the vasal veins for venous return after ligation of the internal and external spermatic veins. Maintenance of the deferential artery's contribution to the testicular blood supply is also important when the integrity of the testicular artery is in doubt because of prior surgery, such as orchiopexy, varicocelectomy, or hernia repair.

Vasotomy, preparation of the vas, and opening of the tunica vaginalis are performed as described for end-to-end anastomosis. The epididymis is inspected under the operating microscope. At a convenient point above the site of the suspected obstruction, a longitudinal 3- to 4-mm incision is made in the epididymal tunic over dilated tubules, with an ultrasharp microknife. The tunic is trimmed with microscissors to create a round opening that matches the diameter of the previously prepared vas deferens. The tubules are bluntly dissected with a microneedle holder and sharply dissected with microscissors, until a dilated loop of tubule is clearly exposed. The posterior edge of the epididymal tunic is approximated to the posterior edge of muscularis and adventitia, with three interrupted 9–0 nylon sutures (Fig. 87–38). This maneuver is done in such a way as to bring the vasal lumen in close approximation to the epididymal tubule selected for anastomosis. With 25- to 32-power magnification, employing an ultrasharp microknife, a longitudinal incision of about 0.5 mm is made in the selected tubule. Epididymal fluid is touched to a slide, diluted with saline, and inspected under the microscope for sperm. If no sperms are found, the opening in the tubule is closed with 10–0 sutures, the vas detached, and the tunic incision closed with 9–0 nylon. The procedure is repeated more proximally in the epididymis.

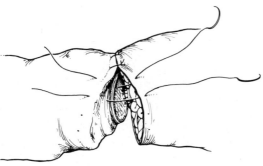

Figure 87–36. Second layer of 9–0 nylon sutures approximating vasal adventitia and perivasal sheath to the cut edge of the epididymal tunic.

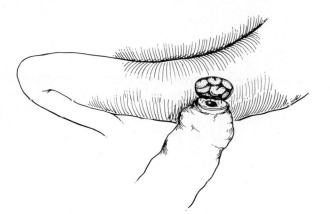

Figure 87–38. Preparation for end-to-side vasoepididymostomy. The 9–0 sutures approximate the posterior lip of the vasal adventitia to the lower edge of the opening tailored in the epididymal tunic.

Once sperm is identified, 1:1 methylene blue:lactated Ringer's solution is dripped onto the cut tubule to outline the mucosa. The posterior mucosal edge of the epididymal tubule is approximated to the posterior edge of the vasal mucosa with three interrupted 10–0 monofilament nylon double-armed sutures with fishhook-shaped 70-μ diameter tapered needles (Fig. 87–39). The lumen is irrigated with Ringer's lactate prior to placement of the sutures to keep the epididymal lumen open. After these mucosal sutures are tied, the anterior mucosal anastomosis is completed with three additional 10–0 sutures. Approximation of the outer muscularis and adventitia of the vas to the cut edge of the epididymal tunic is completed with six to ten additional interrupted sutures of 9–0 nylon (Fig. 87–40). Closure of the tunica vaginalis is optional. The scrotum is closed as previously described. Penrose drains are usually not necessary.

Long-Term Follow-Up Evaluation and Results

Microsurgical vasoepididymostomy in the hands of experienced and skilled microsurgeons results in the appearance of sperm in the ejaculate in 50 to 70 per cent of patients. In our experience, the transient appearance of sperm followed by azoospermia occurs in up to 25 per cent of initially patent anastomoses. In the approximately 50 per cent of all men operated on with long-term patency, about 60 per cent will impregnate their partners after a minimum follow-up of 2 years (Goldstein et al., 1991). Bottom line, overall pregnancy rates after vasoepididymostomy range from 15 to 30 per cent. Pregnancy rates are higher the more distal the anastomosis is performed. Additional pregnancies may be possible by further operations in men who remain azoospermic, by IVF in men with very low counts but fairly good sperm quality, and by IVF combined with the micromanipulation techniques of partial zona dissection or subzonal insertion (described later in this chapter) in men with poor sperm motility. In the individuals who remain azoospermic despite repeated attempts at surgical reconstruction, microscopic epididymal sperm aspiration combined with IVF and oocyte micromanipulation offers hope of pregnancy in the partner.

TRANSURETHRAL RESECTION (TUR) OF THE EJACULATORY DUCTS

The work-up leading to the diagnosis of probable ejaculatory duct obstruction is reviewed in Chapter 15. Briefly, ejaculatory duct obstruction is suspected in azoospermic or severely oligospermic men with at least one palpable vas deferens, low semen volume, and negative or low semen fructose level. If these men have normal serum levels of FSH and if the testis biopsy findings reveal normal spermatogenesis, the diagnosis of ejaculatory duct obstruction is entertained.

Confirmation of the diagnosis is made by vasography, described earlier in this chapter. If vasography reveals obstruction near the ejaculatory ducts (see Fig. 87–6), the catheters are left in the vasa. The patient is placed in the lithotomy position. The Foley catheter, occluding the bladder neck at the time of vasography, is removed. Cystoscopy is performed. Dilute methylene blue is injected into the vasography catheters. This maneuver will occasionally result in the appearance of a submucosal blue spot between the verumontanum and the bladder neck, signaling the location of the ejaculatory ducts. A urethrotome cold knife is selected to incise into the obstructed duct. The appearance of blue dye gushing

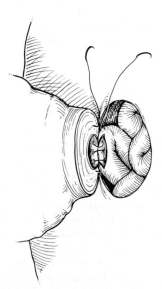

Figure 87–39. Posterior row of 10–0 mucosal sutures placed inside out.

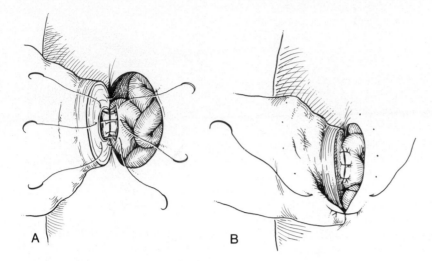

Figure 87–40. After completion of the anterior mucosal portion of the anastomosis *(A)*, the second layer of 9–0 nylon sutures is placed to provide a watertight seal *(B)*.

from the incision at the time of methylene blue injection into the vas will confirm the successful incision into the duct. The contralateral duct is incised in a similar fashion. A resectoscope is introduced (see Fig. 87–7). With a finger in the rectum elevating the urethra, the ducts on both sides are opened widely by resecting from just distal to the bladder neck to the verumontanum, immediately to the right and left of the midline (Fig. 87–41). The bladder neck should remain intact to prevent retrograde ejaculation. Resection is continued until a pair of round dilated ducts are clearly seen with efflux of methylene blue after injection in each vas. Cold knife incision may lead only to a higher incidence of reobstruction. If one ejaculatory duct is obstructed, resection need be done only to the immediate right or left of midline.

At the completion of the resection, a Foley catheter is left in the bladder. After flushing with saline or Ringer's solution, the vasotomy sites are carefully closed with microsurgical technique. If the initial vasotomy revealed no sperm in the vasal fluid and repeat sampling results after the TUR is completed are still negative for sperm, vasoepididymostomy may be performed during the same operation. If vasoepididymostomy is not performed and follow-up semen analysis reveals azoosper-

mia, but an increased semen volume and a return of seminal fructose, indicating patency of the ejaculatory ducts, vasoepididymostomy will have to be done subsequently.

When the ejaculatory ducts are markedly dilated, high resolution transrectal sonography will enable a diagnosis of ejaculatory duct obstruction to be made with a fair degree of reliability prior to vasography. A TUR of the ducts can be performed without violating the scrotum. The primary disadvantage of this approach is that epididymal obstruction cannot be diagnosed and repaired at the same time. Furthermore, methylene blue injection into the vas cannot be employed to facilitate the resection. The incidence of secondary epididymal obstruction in men with ejaculatory duct obstruction is unknown. As described earlier, if the patient remains azoospermic in spite of increased semen volume and a positive fructose test postresection conversion, a vasoepididymostomy will have to be performed.

The few scattered case reports and small published series (Goldwasser et al., 1985), as well as our own experience, suggest that ejaculatory duct resection will result in the appearance of sperm in the semen about 50 per cent of the time. Reports of pregnancy, however, are rare. IVF with aspirated vasal or epididymal sperm may achieve pregnancies in previously failed cases.

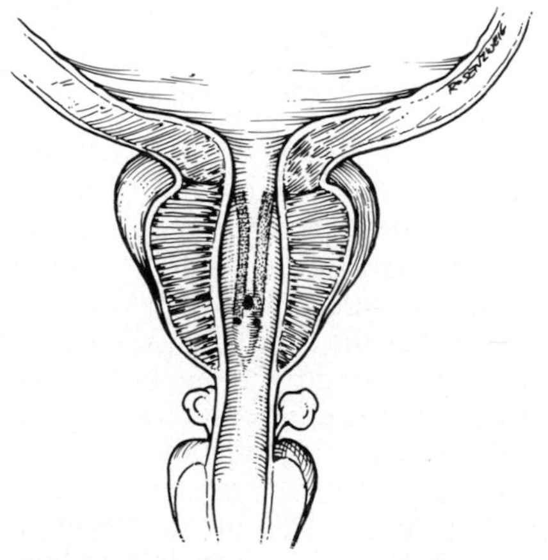

ALLOPLASTIC SPERMATOCELES

Prior to the development of IVF techniques, attempts to treat men with surgically unreconstructable obstructive azoospermia involved the creation or implantation of an artificial sperm reservoir—an alloplastic spermatocele. The reservoir would be percutaneously aspirated to obtain spermatozoa for artificial insemination. These attempts have been largely unsuccessful. A review by Turner in 1988 revealed only three term pregnancies in over 200 attempted implantations of alloplastic spermatoceles by different workers. Until an alloplastic spermatocele can be designed that remains patent and maintains sperm viability and fertilizing capacity, further implantations of alloplastic spermatoceles should not be attempted. Currently, microsurgical epididymal sperm

Figure 87–41. Transurethral resection of the ejaculatory ducts showing the location of resection.

aspiration combined with IVF techniques, described next, is the preferred approach to surgically unreconstructable obstructive azoospermia.

IN VITRO FERTILIZATION WITH MICROSURGICALLY ASPIRATED EPIDIDYMAL SPERM

Men with congenital absence or bilateral partial aplasia of vas deferens, or those with failed or surgically unreconstructable obstructions can now be treated by using microsurgically aspirated epididymal sperm in conjunction with IVF techniques. Sperm obtained from chronically obstructed systems usually has exceeding poor motility and markedly decreased fertilizing capacity. These effects are probably caused by a combination of factors including the following:

1. The adverse affects of chronic obstruction on epididymal function
2. The adverse effects on sperm function of breakdown products as well as leukocytes and macrophages migrating into the obstructed epididymal lumen
3. The partial absence of the epididymis in men with the congenital absence of the vas deferens.

For these reasons, the number of motile sperm with fertilizing capacity among the millions residing in the obstructed epididymis is exceedingly small. Therefore, IVF techniques are essential to achieve pregnancies with aspirated epididymal sperm. Even with IVF, oocyte fertilization rates with epididymal sperm are low. Oocyte micromanipulation techniques to facilitate fertilization, described later in this chapter, have now resulted in pregnancies with the sperm that had failed to fertilize with more conventional IVF methods.

Microsurgical Epididymal Sperm Aspiration Technique

The technique described here is that employed for previously reported epididymal sperm aspirations (Pryor et al., 1984; Silber et al., 1987; Temple-Smith et al., 1985). A median raphe approach allows delivery of both testes through a single incision. The tunica vaginalis is opened and the epididymis inspected under 16- to 25-power magnification utilizing the operating microscope. The epididymal tunic is incised as described previously for vasoepididymostomy. Meticulous hemostasis is obtained with the bipolar cautery. A dilated tubule is isolated and incised with a fine point knife. A 24-gauge angiocatheter attached to a 1-cc tuberculin syringe is employed to gently aspirate fluid while an assistant squeezes the testis and caput epididymis (Fig. 87–42). If no sperm is obtained, the epididymal tubule and tunic are closed with 10–0 and 9–0 nylon sutures. An incision is made more proximally in the epididymis or even the efferent ductules until motile sperms are obtained. The sperms are then processed for IVF. Standard swim-up techniques are usually unsatisfactory because of the low initial sperm motility (1 to 20 per cent). Mini-percoll methods and/or incubation with activating agents increases the yield of motile sperm.

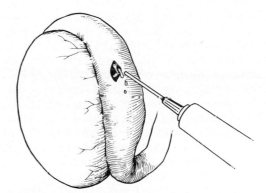

Figure 87–42. Microsurgical aspiration of epididymal sperm from an incision in the epididymal tubule.

The first reports of this technique describe very disappointing results with fertilization rates of 5 per cent and a rare pregnancy. Later experience, combining hyperstimulation and retrieval of 15 to 40 eggs per couple and better sperm processing, have resulted in a significant improvement in fertilization and pregnancy rates. A pregnancy rate of 20 per cent is reported in couples in whom more than ten eggs can be retrieved and in whom initial sperm motility is greater than 10 per cent (Silber et al., 1987 and 1990).

Experience with the technique has revealed that, paradoxically, in obstructed systems, sperm motility is better more proximally in the epididymis. The most motile sperms are often found in the efferent ductules. The environment in the obstructed epididymis appears to promote a natural swim-up. Initial motility and, consequently, fertilization rates are highest in men who have the longest epididymal tubule. Even when obstructed with debris distally, the epididymal tubule may be capable of secreting substances that can diffuse proximally and beneficially influence sperm motility and fertilizing capacity.

Blood has an extremely detrimental effect on the sperm's fertilizing capacity. The difficulty lies in maintaining absolute hemostasis when squeezing on the testis and aspirating the sperm that is leaking from an incision in the epididymal tubule. These lead to inevitable contamination of the aspirated sperm with blood and tissue fluids. We believe that this problem contributed to the poor results obtained at New York Hospital (Cornell Medical Center), in our initial attempts with this technique. In spite of retrieving over 40 mature eggs and between 500,000 and 550 million sperm from the epididymis of men with absent vasa, none of the eggs fertilized. Our embryologist thought that even the slightest contamination of the aspirated sperm with blood and/or tissue fluids inhibited fertilization, leading to the development of the technique described next.

Micropuncture of the Human Epididymal Tubule For Sperm Retrieval

Micropuncture of the epididymal tubule in laboratory animals has been employed for studies of epididymal function (Howards et al., 1975). When epididymal sperm is collected by incision into an epididymal tubule and aspiration of the effluxing fluid, contamination with some blood and tissue fluid is inevitable, regardless of meticulous attempts at hemostasis with a microbipolar cautery. Even microscopic quantities of such contaminants have an adverse effect on sperm motility and fertilizing capacity. Processing of human epididymal sperm by swim-up techniques, which ordinarily eliminate such contaminants, is usually not possible because of the low motility and poor progression of aspirated sperm. To circumvent this problem, we have adapted the micropuncture techniques perfected in animals to aspiration of human epididymal sperm.

Glass capillary tubes, 0.9 mm (outside diameter) × 0.6 mm (inside diameter) are washed and pulled to a tip width of 250 to 350 μ. The tips are sharpened on a fine grinding wheel. The micropuncture pipettes are again washed, siliconized, and attached to silicone tubing. A collecting system, similar to that used for epididymal micropuncture in animals, is employed (Fig. 87–43).

The epididymis is exposed and prepared as described previously, utilizing an operating microscope. Under 15- to 32-power magnification, with an assistant stabilizing the epididymis and squeezing the testis and epididymis, the epididymal tubule is punctured in an area devoid of blood vessels. Successful puncture is heralded by free flow of epididymal sperm and fluid up the pipette (Fig. 87–44). The pipette tip is gently advanced 0.5 to 1 mm into the lumen and adjusted for maximum flow. When no further fluid can be collected, the pipette is removed from the tubule and the collected fluid is flushed out

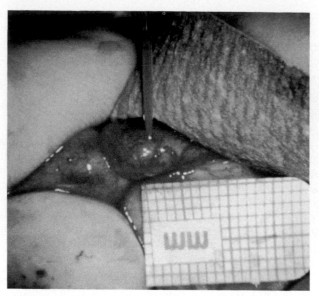

Figure 87–44. Successful micropuncture of the epididymal tubule.

with the medium being used for examination and processing. The puncture hole is sealed with a single stitch of 10–0 monofilament nylon. Repetitive punctures progressively more proximal can be made until motile sperm are retrieved. The efferent ductules can be punctured with equal success.

We have employed this technique in 15 men with congenital absence of the vas deferens or multiple failed vasoepididymostomy procedures (Schlegel et al., 1991). Oocyte retrieval was performed transvaginally with ultrasound guidance. From one to 15 embryos were obtained in each of 6 couples. Embryos were transferred transcervically by standard IVF techniques. Four pregnancies with confirmed heartbeats resulted. One of the pregnancies subsequently aborted. The three ongoing pregnancies resulted in delivery of six healthy infants (one single, one set of twins, and one set of triplets).

The micropuncture technique for human epididymal sperm aspiration yields sperm free of contaminants. The puncture is minimally traumatic and simply sealed, preserving the potential for repeated punctures. In the series described, the oocyte micromanipulation techniques described next were employed to facilitate fertilization.

OOCYTE MICROMANIPULATION TECHNIQUES FOR FACILITATED FERTILIZATION

The role of IVF and related technologies for the treatment of nonobstructive male factor infertility is discussed in Chapter 15. In men with critically low sperm counts and poor motility in whom conventional IVF attempts have resulted in no fertilizations, oocyte micromanipulation techniques can produce fertilizations and pregnancies. Poor progressive motility is also characteristic of microsurgically aspirated epididymal sperm. Oocyte micromanipulation techniques may improve the results of IVF with such sperm.

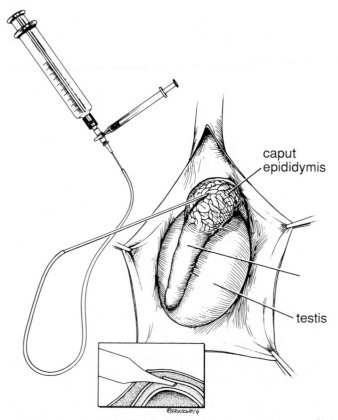

caput epididymis

testis

Figure 87–43. Micropuncture of the human epididymal tubule. Collection system.

Partial Zona Dissection (PZD)

Initial attempts at facilitating sperm penetration of the zona pellucida utilized the application of acid to dissolve a small hole in the zona. Although fertilization and cleavage of human oocytes were achieved with this technique (Gordon et al., 1988), no pregnancies resulted. Currently, mechanical dissection of the zona pellucida employing a micromanipulator and glass sliver to create a tangential rent has successfully achieved fertilizations, pregnancies, and live births in couples in whom initial IVF attempts failed owing to lack of fertilizations (Cohen et al., 1988 and 1989). At the Cornell IVF program a 12 per cent pregnancy rate has been achieved when PZD techniques have been applied in couples who have experienced previous IVF fertilization failures.

Sub-Zonal Insertion (SZI)

When sperm are viable but lack progressive motility, even PZD will not facilitate fertilization. Under these circumstances, four or five of the best sperms are collected with a 5-μm diameter glass pipette and injected into the perivitelline space with the aid of a micromanipulator (Cohen et al., 1988; Laws-King et al., 1987). At Cornell, a 25-per cent ongoing pregnancy rate has been achieved with this technique. Two of these pregnancies were in the partners of men with bilateral congenital absence of the vas deferens from whom sperm were retrieved with the micropuncture technique described previously. SZI produced the only fertilized eggs in these two couples.

Microinjection

Microinjection of a single sperm through the zona pellucida directly into the ooplasm has been attempted in humans but with little success. Fertilization has been achieved, but cleavage and embryo formation have not.

VARICOCELECTOMY

Varicocelectomy is the most commonly performed operation for the treatment of male infertility. Animal and human studies have demonstrated that varicocele is associated with a progressive and duration-dependent decline in testicular function (Gorelick and Goldstein, 1989; Hadziselimovic et al., 1989; Harrison et al., 1986; Kass et al., 1987; Lipshultz and Corriere, 1977; Nagler et al., 1985; Russell, 1957).

Repair of varicocele will halt any further damage to testicular function (Kass and Belman, 1987) and, in a large percentage of men, will result in improved spermatogenesis. The potentially important new role of urologists in preventing future infertility underscores the importance of developing techniques of varicocelectomy that minimize the risk of complications and failure.

Surgical Repair

A variety of surgical approaches have been advocated for varicocelectomy. The earliest recorded attempts at repair of varicocele date to antiquity and involved external clamping of the scrotal skin, including the enlarged veins. In the early 1900s, an open scrotal approach was employed, involving the mass ligation and excision of the varicosed plexus of veins. At the level of the scrotum, however, the complex of veins are intimately entwined with the coiled testicular artery. Therefore, scrotal operations are to be avoided, because damage to the arterial supply of the testis frequently results in testicular atrophy and further impairment of spermatogenesis and fertility.

Retroperitoneal Operations

Retroperitoneal repair of varicocele involves incision at the level of the internal inguinal ring, splitting of the external and internal oblique muscles, and exposure of the internal spermatic artery and vein retroperitoneally near the ureter (Fig. 87–45). This approach has the advantage of isolating the internal spermatic veins proximally, near the point of drainage into the left renal vein. At this level, only one or two large veins are present and, in addition, the testicular artery has not yet branched and is often distinctly separate from the internal spermatic veins. Retroperitoneal approaches involve ligation of the fewest number of veins and are relatively fast. This approach is still one of the most popular methods employed for the repair of varicocele.

A disadvantage of a retroperitoneal approach, however, is the high incidence of varicocele recurrence. Recurrence rates after retroperitoneal varicocelectomy are in the range of 15 per cent (Homonnai et al., 1980; Rothman et al., 1981). Failure is usually due to the presence of parallel inguinal and retroperitoneal collaterals, which may exit the testis and bypass the retroperitoneal area of ligation, rejoining the internal spermatic vein proximal to the site of ligation (Murray et al., 1986; Sayfan et al., 1981). Dilated cremasteric veins, another cause of varicocele recurrence (Sayfan et al., 1980), cannot be identified with a retroperitoneal approach. Furthermore, positive identification and preservation of the testicular artery via the retroperitoneal approach are difficult. The operation involves working in a "deep hole." Because, at this level, the internal spermatic vessels cannot be delivered into the wound, they must be dissected and ligated in situ in the retroperitoneum. The diameter of the testicular artery ranges from 0.5 to 0.8 mm; therefore, positive identification and preservation of the artery with this approach are uncertain. In addition, the difficulty in positively identifying and preserving lymphatics with this approach results in postoperative hydrocele formation after 7 to 33 per cent of retroperitoneal operations (Szabo and Kessler, 1984). The incidence of recurrence appears to be higher in children, with rates reported between 15 and 45 per cent in adolescents (Gorenstein et al., 1986; Levitt et al., 1987; Reitelman et al., 1987).

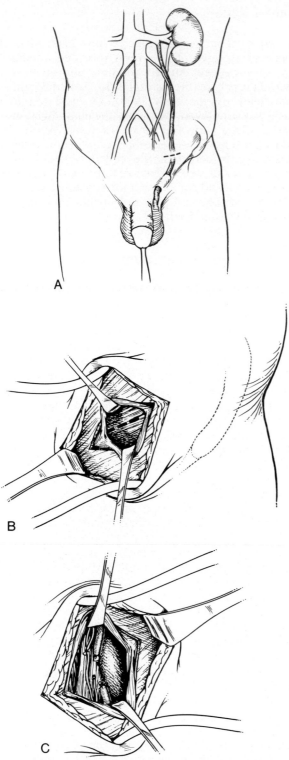

Figure 87–45. Retroperitoneal varicocelectomy.

Inguinal Operations

Inguinal varicocelectomy is currently the most popular approach. It has the advantage of allowing delivery of the spermatic cord structures near the internal inguinal ring where the testicular artery may be more easily identified, separated from the spermatic veins, and preserved. Although more veins will need to be ligated than in a retroperitoneal approach, with inguinal exposure the spermatic cord may be externalized, facilitating dissection of cord structures. An inguinal approach allows access to external spermatic and even gubernacular veins, which may bypass the spermatic cord and result in recurrence if not ligated.

Traditional approaches to inguinal varicocelectomy involve a 5- to 10-cm incision made over the inguinal canal, an opening of the external oblique aponeurosis, and an encirclement with delivery of the spermatic cord. The cord is dissected, and all internal spermatic veins are ligated. The vas deferens and its vessels are preserved (Dubin and Amelar, 1977). An attempt is made to identify and preserve the testicular artery and, if possible, the lymphatics. In addition, the cord is elevated, and any external spermatic veins that are running parallel to the spermatic cord or perforating the floor of the inguinal canal are identified and ligated. Compared with retroperitoneal operations, inguinal approaches lower the incidence of varicocele recurrence but do not alter the incidence of either hydrocele formation or testicular artery injury. Conventional inguinal operations are associated with an incidence of postoperative hydrocele formation varying from 3 to 15 per cent, with an average incidence of 7 per cent. Analysis of the hydrocele fluid has clearly indicated that hydrocele formation following varicocelectomy is due to ligation of the lymphatics (Szabo and Kessler, 1984). The incidence of testicular artery injury after inguinal varicocelectomy is unknown. Case reports, however, suggest that this complication may be more common than realized. It can result in testicular atrophy and, if the operation is performed bilaterally, azoospermia may ensue in a previously oligospermic man (Silber, 1979).

Microsurgical Techniques

The introduction of microsurgical techniques to varicocelectomy has resulted in a substantial reduction in the incidence of hydrocele formation, because the lymphatics can be more easily identified and preserved. Furthermore, magnification enhances the ability to identify and preserve the testicular artery, thus avoiding the complications of atrophy or azoospermia. Marmar and colleagues (1985) described a microscopic subinguinal approach, just below the external inguinal ring. This approach obviates the necessity for opening any fascial layer. The operating microscope enables the identification and preservation of the lymphatics and testicular artery. At the subinguinal level, however, a much larger number of veins are encountered. To deal with the profusion of veins at this level, a sclerosing agent is injected to occlude small unligated venous channels. At the subinguinal level, the testicular artery has often divided and several branches will need to be identified and preserved. An advantage of this approach is access to cremasteric veins and collaterals that perforate the floor of the canal. Results with this technique are good— no reported hydroceles or testicular atrophy and a recurrence rate of 6 per cent. The incision is small and recovery relatively painless and rapid.

Microsurgical High Inguinal Varicocelectomy With Delivery of the Testis

We have developed and refined an inguinal, microsurgical approach to varicocelectomy that combines the advantages of the previously described techniques and eliminates many of the disadvantages (Gilbert and Goldstein, 1988; Goldstein et al., 1990). An operating microscope allows preservation of the testicular artery and lymphatics, eliminating postoperative hydrocele formation and minimizing the risk of testicular atrophy or injury. Compared with a subinguinal operation, the high inguinal approach reduces the number of veins encountered and obviates the necessity for injection of sclerosing agents (Kaye, 1988). Delivery of the testis provides access to parallel inguinal, cremasteric, and even gubernacular collaterals, markedly reducing the incidence of recurrence.

A 2- to 3-cm inguinal incision is made, beginning at the external inguinal ring, and is extended within Langer's lines toward the internal inguinal ring (Fig. 87–46). After retraction of Camper's and Scarpa's fascia, the external oblique aponeurosis is opened in the direction of its fibers through the external inguinal ring. A 3–0 Vicryl suture is placed at the apex to facilitate closure after the repair. At this point, the ileoinguinal nerve is identified and preserved. The spermatic cord is encircled with a Babcock clamp and delivered through the incision. The genital branch of the genitofemoral nerve can often be identified on the posterior surface of the cord and excluded. The cord is freed with finger dissection into the scrotum and the testis delivered through the incision. Delivery of the testis allows positive identification of all external spermatic and cremasteric veins, which are doubly clamped and ligated with

4–0 silk (Fig. 87–47). The gubernaculum is inspected and any transscrotal collaterals are identified. They are either ligated or electrocoagulated.

After these preliminary procedures are completed, all venous drainage from the testis must be within the encircled spermatic cord. The testis is returned to the scrotum and the spermatic cord elevated by a platform made from a tongue blade covered with a Penrose drain (Fig. 87–48). The operating microscope is brought into the field, and under 8-power magnification the external and internal spermatic fasciae are opened (Fig. 87–49). A 1 per cent papavarine solution, is sprinkled on the cord to facilitate identification of the testicular artery. If the artery is immediately identified, it is dissected free of all surrounding veins and encircled with a 0 silk suture (Fig. 87–50). With a nonlocking curved microneedle-holder and fine smooth forceps, the cord is meticulously dissected transversally under the operating microscope; all internal spermatic veins are cleaned, doubly ligated with 4–0 silk or small hemoclips, and divided (Fig. 87–51). The lymphatics may be identified without difficulty and preserved (Fig. 87–52). The vas deferens and its vessels are preserved. The two sets of veins associated with the vas deferens provide collateral venous return. A markedly dilated vasal vein is rare, but if encountered is ligated. At the completion of the dissection, the spermatic cord is carefully run over the index finger to assure that all internal spermatic and cremasteric veins, however small, have been identified and ligated.

At the termination of the procedure, the testicular artery, the vas deferens and its vessels, and the lymphatics remain undisturbed. The testis is redelivered. Bleeders on the surface of the tunica vaginalis or cord are identified and cauterized. The testis is returned to the scrotum and the external oblique aponeurosis reapproximated with continuous sutures utilizing the previ-

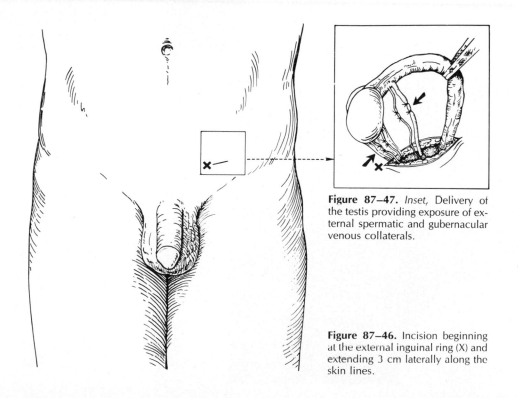

Figure 87–47. *Inset,* Delivery of the testis providing exposure of external spermatic and gubernacular venous collaterals.

Figure 87–46. Incision beginning at the external inguinal ring (X) and extending 3 cm laterally along the skin lines.

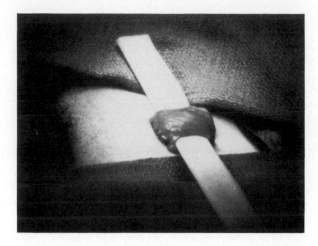

Figure 87–48. The testis has been returned to the scrotum and the spermatic cord elevated over a tongue blade covered with a Penrose drain.

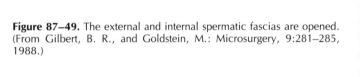

Figure 87–49. The external and internal spermatic fascias are opened. (From Gilbert, B. R., and Goldstein, M.: Microsurgery, 9:281–285, 1988.)

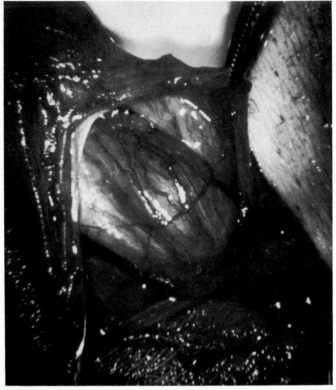

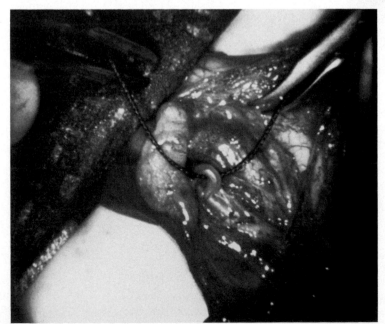

Figure 87–50. The testicular artery is identified and tagged with a 0 silk suture. (From Gilbert, B. R., and Goldstein, M.: Microsurgery, 9:281–285, 1988.)

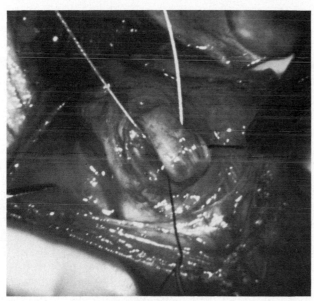

Figure 87–51. Internal spermatic veins are cleaned and double 4–0 silks, one black and one white, passed beneath them prior to ligation and division. (From Gilbert, B. R., and Goldstein, M.: Microsurgery, 9:281–285, 1988.)

ously placed 3–0 Vicryl. Scarpa's and Camper's fasciae are reapproximated with a continuous suture of 3–0 plain catgut. The wound is infiltrated with bupivacaine (Marcaine) and the skin closed with Steri-Strips (Fig. 87–53).

With experience, this procedure can be performed in less than 30 minutes per side. This varicocelectomy is done as an ambulatory procedure. We have compared the results of 710 operations performed in this way with an initial series of conventional inguinal varicocelectomies all done by the same surgeon (Goldstein et al., 1990). Using the conventional inguinal approach, the

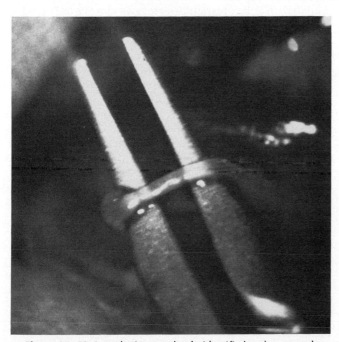

Figure 87–52. Lymphatics are clearly identified and preserved.

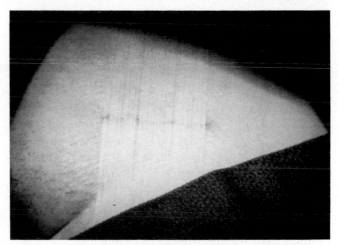

Figure 87–53. Steri-Strip closure of the skin.

incidence of hydrocele formation was 9 per cent and the incidence of varicocele recurrence was 9 per cent. In the microsurgical high inguinal approach with delivery of testis, there were no hydroceles and four recurrences (0.6 per cent). We have positively identified and preserved the testicular artery in all but six patients. Four hematomas have occurred, one requiring surgical drainage.

Radiographic Occlusion Techniques

Intraoperative venography has been employed to visualize the venous collaterals, that if left unligated, may result in varicocele recurrence (Belgrano et al., 1984; Levitt et al., 1987; Sayfan et al., 1981; Zaontz and Firlit, 1987). Intraoperative venography reduces the incidence of varicocele recurrence, but the two-dimensional view afforded often does not enable the surgeon to identify the location of all collaterals.

Radiographic balloon or coil occlusion of the internal spermatic veins has been successfully employed for varicocelectomy (Lima et al., 1978; Weissbach et al., 1981; Walsh and White, 1981). These techniques allow the procedure to be performed using a local anesthetic through a small cutdown incision over the femoral vein. The method eliminates the risk of hydrocele formation after varicocelectomy and poses virtually no risk of injury to the internal spermatic artery. The recurrence rate after balloon occlusion was originally 11 per cent and is now as low as 4 per cent (Kaufman et al., 1983; Mitchell et al., 1985; Murray et al., 1986). Recurrence results from failure to successfully cannulate small collaterals and external spermatic veins. Venographic placement of a balloon or coil in the internal spermatic vein is successfully accomplished in 75 to 90 per cent of attempts (Morag et al., 1984; White et al., 1981); therefore, a significant number of men undergoing attempted radiographic occlusion will ultimately require a surgical approach.

The radiographic techniques take between 1 and 3 hours to perform compared with 25 to 45 minutes in surgical repair. Although rare, serious complications of occlusion during radiography have included migration of the balloon or coil into the renal vein, resulting in loss of a kidney, or, more rarely, pulmonary embolization of the balloon or coil, femoral vein perforation, or thrombosis and anaphylactic reactions to the contrast medium.

Laparoscopic Varicocelectomy

Laparoscopic techniques have been employed by urologists for localization of intra-abdominal testes (Cortesi et al., 1976; Elder, 1989; Lowe et al., 1984) and for retroperitoneal lymph node sampling and dissection (Winfield and Ryan, 1990). Clearly, laparoscopic techniques are significantly less invasive alternatives to traditional open transperitoneal procedures.

The internal spermatic vessels and vas deferens can be visualized through the laparoscope, as they come through the internal inguinal ring. The magnification provided by the laparoscope allows visualization of the testicular artery. With experience, it is possible that lymphatics may be visualized and preserved as well. Laparoscopic varicocelectomy will allow internal spermatic vein ligation at the same level as the retroperitoneal approach described previously.

Although laparoscopic varicocelectomy should allow preservation of the testicular artery in a majority of cases, and possibly preservation of lymphatics as well, the incidence of varicocele recurrence would be expected to be the same as that of open retroperitoneal operations. These recurrences would be due to collaterals joining the internal spermatic vein, near its entrance to the renal vein, or entering the renal vein separately. Laparoscopic localization of these collaterals will require dissection of the renal vein, significantly increasing the potential morbidity of the procedure. Three video presentations of laparoscopic varicocelectomy demonstrate a procedure utilizing two 11-mm ports and one or two 5-mm ports (Donovan and Winfield, 1991; Hagood, 1991; Stone et al., 1991). The artery is visualized in half the cases presented, the lymphatics in none. All of these series are short-term studies of less than 25 patients. A 10 per cent incidence of hydrocele formation has been reported.

Varicocelectomy can be performed laparoscopically. The incidence of recurrence and complications has not yet been determined. The potential complications of laparoscopic varicocelectomy (e.g., injury to bowel, vessels, or viscera; air embolism; peritonitis) are significantly more serious than those associated with the open techniques previously described. The microsurgical techniques described in this chapter employ incisions of 2.5 to 3 cm, the same as the sum of incisions employed for a laparoscopic approach. Furthermore, laparoscopic varicocelectomy takes at least twice as long to perform (about 1 hour) as open varicocelectomy. Postoperative pain and recovery time for laparoscopic technique are probably similar to those for microsurgical varicocelectomy.

Laparoscopic techniques offer minimally invasive alternatives to many major urologic procedures. In the case of varicocelectomy, however, the laparoscopic technique is probably a more invasive alternative to current open microsurgical methods.

Complications of Varicocelectomy

Hydrocele

Hydrocele formation after nonmicroscopic varicocelectomy is the most common complication reported. The incidence of this complication varies from 3 to 33 per cent, with an average incidence of about 7 per cent. Analysis of the protein concentration of hydrocele fluid indicates that hydrocele formation after varicocelectomy is due to lymphatic obstruction (Szabo and Kessler, 1984). At least half of postvaricocelectomy hydroceles become large enough to warrant surgical excision because of the discomfort. The effect of hydrocele formation on sperm function and fertility is uncertain. It is known that men with varicoceles have significantly elevated intratesticular temperatures (Goldstein and Eid, 1989; Zorgniotti and MacLeod, 1979). This appears to be an important pathophysiologic phenomenon mediating the adverse effects of varicocele on fertility (Saypol et al., 1981). The development of a large hydrocele surrounds the testis with an abnormal insulating layer that may impair the efficiency of the countercurrent heat exchange mechanism and therefore may obviate some of the benefits of varicocelectomy.

Magnification to identify and preserve lymphatics can eliminate the development of hydrocele after varicocelectomy. In addition, radiographic balloon or coil occlusion techniques also prevent hydrocele formation.

Testicular Artery Injury

The diameter of the testicular artery in humans is 0.5 to 0.8 mm. Microdissections of the spermatic cord have revealed that the testicular artery is closely adherent to a large internal spermatic vein in 40 per cent of men. In another 20 per cent, the testicular artery is surrounded by a network of tiny veins (Beck and Goldstein, 1991). During the course of cord dissection for varicocelectomy, the artery may be in spasm. Even in its unconstricted state, this artery is often very difficult to positively identify and preserve. Injury or ligation of the testicular artery carries with it the risk of testicular atrophy. The actual incidence of testicular artery ligation during varicocelectomy is unknown, but some studies suggest it is common (Silber, 1979; Wosnitzer and Roth, 1983). Animal studies indicate that the risk of testicular atrophy after testicular artery ligation varies from 20 to 100 per cent (Goldstein et al., 1983; MacMahon et al., 1976). In humans, atrophy after artery ligation is probably less likely because of the contribution of the cremasteric as well as the vasal arterial supply. Magnifying loupes or an operating microscope or a fine-tipped Doppler probe facilitates identification and preservation of the testicular artery and, therefore, minimizes the risk of testicular injury. Radiographic balloon or coil occlusion techniques also eliminate this risk.

Varicocele Recurrence

The incidence of varicocele recurrence following surgical repair varies from 0.6 to 45 per cent. Recurrence is more common after repair of pediatric varicoceles. Radiographic studies of recurrent varicoceles demonstrate parallel inguinal or mid-retroperitoneal collaterals or, more rarely, transcrotal collaterals. Retroperitoneal operations will miss parallel inguinal collaterals. Inguinal operations have a lower incidence of varicocele recurrence but fail to address the issue of scrotal collaterals or small collaterals surrounding the testicular artery. The microsurgical approach lowers the incidence of varicocele recurrence to 0.4 per cent compared with 9 per cent with conventional inguinal techniques. Intraoperative venography or percutaneous balloon or coil occlusion techniques also significantly lower the incidence of recurrence, if the balloon or coil can be successfully placed.

Results

Varicocelectomy produces a significant improvement in semen analysis in 60 to 80 per cent of men. Reported pregnancy rates after varicocelectomy vary from 20 to 60 per cent, with most series averaging about 35 per cent. It seems likely that varicocelectomy will at least halt the progressive duration-dependent testicular injury associated with varicocele.

The results of varicocelectomy are also related to the size of the varicocele and the age of the patient at the time of repair. Repair of large varicoceles results in a significantly greater improvement in semen quality than repair of small varicoceles (Steckel et al., 1990). In addition, large varicoceles are associated with greater preoperative impairment in semen quality than small varicoceles; consequently, overall pregnancy rates are similar regardless of varicocele size. Evidence is also accumulating that the younger the patient is at the time of varicocele repair, the more likely the testis is to recover from varicocele-induced injury (Kass and Belman, 1987). Varicocele recurrence or postvaricocelectomy hydrocele formation are often associated with poor postoperative results.

Summary

Varicocele is an extremely common entity, present in 15 per cent of the male population. Varicoceles are found in approximately 35 per cent of men with primary infertility but up to 85 per cent of men with secondary infertility. Evidence is clearly accumulating that varicocele causes progressive duration-dependent injury to the seminiferous epithelium. Larger varicoceles appear to cause more damage than smaller varicoceles, and conversely repair of larger varicoceles results in greater improvement of semen quality. Varicocelectomy can almost certainly halt the progressive duration-dependent decline in semen quality found in men with varicoceles. The younger the age when varicocele is repaired, the more likely is recovery of spermatogenic function.

The most common complications after varicocelectomy are hydrocele formation, testicular artery injury, and varicocele persistence or recurrence. The incidence of these complications can be reduced by employing microsurgical techniques, inguinal operations, exposure of external spermatic and scrotal veins, and radiographic occlusion. Employment of these advanced techniques of varicocelectomy provides a safe, effective approach to the elimination of varicocele; the preservation of testicular function; and, in a substantial number of men, the improvement in semen quality and likelihood of a partner's pregnancy.

HYDROCELECTOMY

Inguinal Approach

High resolution scrotal ultrasound should be performed in all men with hydroceles. An inguinal approach to hydrocelectomy is indicated when sonography or palpation reveals any suspicion of intratesticular mass. The surgical approach is identical to that for radical orchiectomy. A modification of Chevassu's maneuver is employed (Goldstein et al., 1983). The cord is doubly occluded with rubber-shod clamps and the hydrocele delivered, and the gubernaculum is ligated and divided prior to opening the sac. The field is isolated and testis cooled after the sac is opened. This technique allows inspection of the testis and epididymis and biopsy of suspicious-looking areas without compromising an operation for cancer. If no malignancy is found, needless orchiectomy is avoided. Hydrocelectomy is performed utilizing one of the techniques subsequently described.

Scrotal Approach

Scrotal hydrocelectomy may be performed in older men beyond the age group in which cancer is more prevalent in whom sonography reveals normal testes. Scrotal hydrocelectomy may also be safely performed when sonographic examination findings are normal in a younger man with a clear etiology for hydrocele (e.g., postvaricocelectomy and postepididymitis). Under these circumstances a transverse incision within the scrotal folds and between the scrotal vessels or a median raphe incision results in minimal bleeding and a virtually invisible scar.

Methods of Repair

After the hydrocele sac has been exposed and, if excision techniques of repair are employed, delivered intact, it is opened anteriorly away from testis, epididymis, vas deferens, and cord structures in an avascular area. Samples of hydrocele fluid are collected for culture and cytology. Large hydroceles can severely distort the normal anatomic relationships. The internal spermatic vessels and vas deferens are encircled with Penrose drains for positive identification. Their courses are traced to avoid injury to these structures. The opening in the sac is enlarged, utilizing a Bovie cautery in a direction away from the testis, epididymis, vessels, and vas. The testis and epididymis are inspected for masses and for evidence of epididymitis or dilated epididymal tubules suggestive of obstruction. The margins of the epididymis may be difficult to clearly identify. In large long-standing hydroceles, the epididymis may be splayed out far from the testis. The convoluted portion of the vas deferens may be distorted and splayed out within the layers of the hydrocele sac. Loupe magnification is sometimes of assistance in positively identifying the margins of the epididymis.

After inspection and identification of all the key structures within and adjacent to the hydrocele sac, repair is accomplished, employing one of the techniques subsequently described.

Excisional Techniques

Excisional techniques are most certain to result in permanent elimination of the hydrocele. Excision is performed for long-standing hydroceles with thick-walled sacs and multiloculated hydroceles. After simple excision, leaving a good one fingerbreadth margin to avoid injury to the epididymis, the edges are oversewn with a 4–0 catgut suture baseball stitch (Fig. 87–54). When thin floppy sacs are excised, the bottleneck operation, in which the sac edges are sewn together behind the cord (Fig. 87–55), reduces the chance of recurrence caused by reapposition of the edges of the hydrocele sac. When the bottleneck operation is employed, the sac margins should be left 1 cm wider to prevent constriction of the cord. If necessary, a Penrose drain is

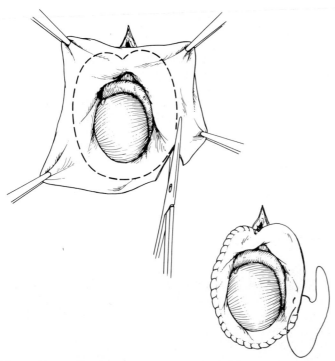

Figure 87–54. Simple excision of thick-walled hydrocele sac and oversewn edges.

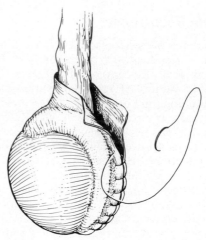

Figure 87–55. Bottleneck technique for excision of thin floppy sacs.

brought out the dependent portion of the hemiscrotum. The dartos is closed with a continuous catgut suture and the skin with a subcuticular absorbable suture. Fluff dressings are stuffed inside a snug-fitting scrotal supporter.

Plication Techniques

Plication operations can be employed for thin sacs (Lord, 1964) but are not suitable for multiloculated hydroceles or long-standing thick-walled hydroceles. Plication will leave a large bundle of residual tissue within the scrotum. Because the sac is not dissected, plication is quick and relatively bloodless.

The sac is opened and the cut edges are cauterized or oversewn for hemostasis. The testis is delivered, and the sac is inverted. Beginning one fingerbreadth away from the testis and epididymis, 8 to 12 catgut sutures are placed radially to plicate the sac (Fig. 87–56). Drains are not necessary. Closure is performed as previously described.

Window Operations

This is the quickest method of repair but associated with a high recurrence rate. After the sac is exposed an x-shaped incision is made into the sac, and the four resulting flaps are sewn back to produce a square window at least 5 cm on each edge. Drains are not necessary; closure is as previously described.

Dartos Pouch Technique

This method is suitable for thin-walled sacs. As in the plication and window techniques, sac dissection is not required and bleeding is minimal. After delivery of the testis, the cut edges of the sac opening are cauterized or oversewn with catgut suture for hemostasis and a Dartos pouch is created exactly as for orchiopexy. The testis is fixed in the pouch with three nonabsorbable (4–0 silk) sutures and the skin closed with interrupted 4–0 chromic catgut suture.

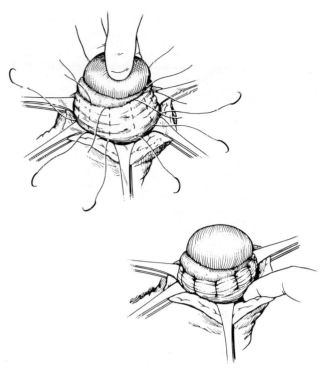

Figure 87–56. Lord's plication technique.

Sclerotherapy

Sclerotherapy with tetracycline or other irritating agents may result in epididymal obstruction. This sometimes is associated with substantial postoperative pain and is often followed by hydrocele recurrence (Odell, 1979). When recurrent hydrocele forms after sclerotherapy, it usually multiloculated and more difficult to repair.

Complications

Hematoma is the most common complication of hydrocelectomy. When excision techniques are completed, the incidence of hematoma can be minimized by meticulously oversewing all raw edges of sac and draining the scrotum when necessary.

In men desiring future fertility, the primary dangers associated with hydrocelectomy operations are injury to the epididymis or the vas deferens. In some large hydroceles, the anatomy can be extremely distorted. The epididymis may not be identifiable. The vas deferens, especially in its convoluted portion, may be splayed out within the hydrocele layers. Regardless of the approach to hydrocelectomy, the vas deferens and the epididymis should be positively identified and care taken to avoid injury to these structures. The internal spermatic vessels should also be positively identified and encircled with a Penrose drain to prevent injury during excision of the hydrocele sac.

SCROTAL ORCHIOPEXY FOR ADULT RETRACTABLE TESTIS

Spermatogenesis is exquisitely temperature sensitive. Varicocele is associated with elevated testicular temper-

ature, and this finding is thought to be the primary pathophysiologic feature of that disorder (Goldstein and Eid, 1989; Saypol et al., 1981; Zorgniotti and MacLeod, 1979). Cryptorchidism is associated with a high incidence of infertility even when unilateral. Both animal and human studies have shown that artificial elevation of testicular temperature results in impaired spermatogenesis. In pigs, testes that are pushed into the abdomen and pexed will stop making sperm (Wensing, 1986). Orchiopexy restores spermatogenesis. In pigs with surgically created cryptorchid testis, cooling of the testis with an intra-abdominal device restores spermatogenesis (Frankenhuis and Wensing, 1979). Long hot baths and saunas in men, on a regular basis, have been shown to impair spermatogenesis.

Retractile testes in boys are usually not surgically repaired if the testes can be manipulated down manually into the scrotum by the physician either in the office or using anesthesia. The fate of persistently retractile testis in adults is unknown. We have found a subset of infertile men who have retractile testes. The semen analysis characteristics of these men are similar to those of men with varicoceles. These men, however, do not have palpable varicoceles. They all have at least one testis and frequently both that retract out of the scrotum and into the abdomen and remain there for an hour or more a day. In some men, these testes remain in the abdomen virtually all the time, except when they are in a warm shower and when they are under anesthesia. It is likely that these testes will suffer from impaired temperature regulation and impaired spermatogenesis. Scrotal orchiopexy can improve the semen quality and fertility of some of these individuals.

When scrotal orchiopexy is performed for retractile testis, a dartos pouch operation should be performed. Simple suture orchiopexy of the tunica albuginea of the testis to the dartos, such as is performed for torsion, will not prevent retraction of these testes into the groin. Creation of a dartos pouch and fixation of the tunica albuginea to the dartos with at least three nonabsorbable sutures will hold the testis well down into the scrotum and permanently prevent retraction.

Jean Schweis and the administrative staff of the Population Council provided invaluable assistance in the preparation of this manuscript.

REFERENCES

Alexander, N. J., and Clarkson, T. B.: Vasectomy increases the severity of diet-induced atherosclerosis in *Macaca fasciculoris*. Science, 201:538, 1978.

Appell, R., and Evans, P.: Vasectomy: Etiology of infectious complications. Fertil. Steril., 33:52–53, 1980.

Ban, S. L.: Sterility by vas injection method. Hu Nan Med. J., 5:49–50, 1980.

Beck, E. M., and Goldstein, M.: Varicocele anatomy: A macro- and microscopic study. American Urological Association Annual Meeting, Toronto, 1991. [Abstract.]

Belgrano, E., Puppo, P., Quattrini, S., Trombetta, C., and Guiliana, L.: The role of venography and sclerotherapy in the management of varicocele. Eur. Urol., 10:124–129, 1984.

Belker, A. M., Fuchs, E. F., Konnak, J. W., Sharlip, I. D., and Thomas, A. J.: Results of 1247 first vasectomy reversals by the vasovasostomy study group. J. Urol., 143:383A, 1990. [Abstract.]

Belker, A. M., Konnak, J. W., Sharlip, I. D., and Thomas, Jr., A. J.: Intraoperative observations during vasovasostomy in 334 patients. J. Urol., 129:524–527, 1983.

Bennett, A. H.: Vasectomy without complication. Urology 7:184, 1976.

Chan, S. L., Lipshultz, L. I., and Schwartzendruber, D.: Deoxyribonucleic acid (DNA) flow cytometry: A new modality for quantitative analysis of testicular biopsies. Fertil. Steril., 41:485–487, 1984.

Cohen, J., Malter, H., and Fehilly, C.: Implantation of embryos after partial opening of oocyte zona pellucida to facilitate sperm penetration. Lancet, 1:162, 1988.

Cohen, J., Malter, H., Wright, G., Kort, H., Massey, J., and Mitchell, D.: Partial zona dissection of human oocytes when failure of zona pellucida penetration is anticipated. Human Reprod., 4:435–442, 1989.

Cortesi, N., Ferrari, P., Zambarda, E., et al.: Diagnosis of bilateral abdominal cryptorchidism by laparoscopy. Endoscopy, 8:33–34, 1976.

Derrick, F. C., Yarbrough, W., and D'Agostino, J.: Vasovasostomy: results of questionnaire of members of the American Urological Association. J. Urol., 110:556, 1973.

Donovan, J. F., and Winfield, H. M.: Laparoscopic varix ligation. Annual Meeting American Urological Association, Toronto, 1991. [Video.]

Dubin, L., and Amelar, R.: Varicocelectomy: 986 cases in a 12-year study. Urology, 10:446, 1977.

Elder, J. S.: Laparoscopy and Fowler-Stephens orchiopexy in the management of the impalpable testis. Urol. Clin. North Am., 16:399–411, 1989.

Esho, J. O., and Cass, A. S.: Recanalization rate following methods of vasectomy using interposition of fascial sheath of vas deferens. J. Urol., 120:178–179, 1978.

Frankenhuis, M. T., and Wensing, C. J. G.: Induction of spermatogenesis in the naturally cryptorchid pig. Fertil. Steril., 31:428, 1979.

Freund, M. J., Weidmann, J. E., Goldstein, M., Marmar, J., Santulli, R., and Oliveira, N.: Microrecanalization after vasectomy in man. J. Androl., 10:120–132, 1989.

Fuchs, E. F., and Alexander, N.: Immunologic considerations before and after vasovasostomy. Fertil. Steril., 40:497, 1983.

Gilbert, B. R., and Goldstein, M.: New directions in male reproductive microsurgery. Microsurgery, 9:281–285, 1988.

Goldacre, M. J., Holford, T. R., and Vessey, M. P.: Cardiovascular disease and vasectomy: findings from two epidemiologic studies. N. Engl. J. Med., 308:805–808, 1983.

Goldstein, M.: Vasectomy failure using an open-ended technique. Fertil. Steril., 40:699–700, 1983.

Goldstein, M.: Microspike approximator for vasovasostomy. J. Urol., 134:74, 1985.

Goldstein, M., and Eid, J. F.: Elevation of intratesticular and scrotal skin surface temperature in men with variocele. J. Urol., 142:743–745, 1989.

Goldstein, M., Gilbert, B. R., Dicker, A., Dwosh, J., and Gnecco, C.: Microsurgical varicocelectomy: An artery and lymphatic sparing technique. American Fertility Society, Annual Meeting, 1990. [Abstract.]

Goldstein, M., Li, P. S., Sandhaus, J. J., and Bardin, C. W.: Percutaneous clip vasectomy in dogs. (Abstract.) Annual Meeting, American Society of Andrology. Washington, D.C., 1992.

Goldstein, M., Schlegel, P. N., and Morrison, G. P.: Microsurgical vasoepididymostomy. American Urological Association, Annual Meeting, Toronto, 1991. [Abstract.]

Goldstein, M., and Schlossberg, S.: Men with congenital absence of the vas deferens often have seminal vesicles. J. Urol., 140:85–86, 1988.

Goldstein, M., and Waterhouse, K.: When to use the Chevassu maneuver during exploration of intrascrotal masses. J. Urol., 130:1199–1200, 1983.

Goldstein, M., Young, G. P. H., and Einer-Jensen, N.: Testicular artery damage due to infiltration with a fine gauge needle: Experimental evidence suggesting that blind cord block should be abandoned. Surgical Forum, 24:653–656, 1983.

Goldwasser, B. Z., Weinerth, J. L., and Carson, C. F.: Ejaculatory duct obstruction: the case for aggressive diagnosis and treatment. J. Urol., 134:964, 1985.

Gordon, J. W., Grunfeld, L., Garrisi, G. J., Talansky, B. E., Richards, C., and Laufer, N.: Fertilization of human oocytes by sperm from infertile males after zona pellucida drilling. Fertil. Steril. 50:68, 1988.

Gorelick, J., and Goldstein, M.: Loss of fertility in men with varicocele: concept of duration-dependent injury. Am. Fertil. Soc. Annual Meeting, San Francisco. Abstract:S48, 1989.

Gorenstein, A., Katz, S., and Schiller, M.: Varicocele in children: "To treat or not to treat"—venographic and manometric studies. J. Pediatr. Surg., 21:1046–1050, 1986.

Hadziselimovic, F., Herzog, B., Liebundgut, B., Jenny, P., and Buser, M.: Testicular and vascular changes in children and adults with varicocele. J. Urol., 142:583–585, 1989.

Hagan, K. F., and Coffey, D. S.: The adverse effects of sperm during vasovasostomy. J. Urol., 118:269–273, 1977.

Hagood, P. G.: Laparoscopic varicocelectomy. Annual Meeting American Urological Association, Toronto, 1991. [Video.]

Hamidinia, A.: Transvasovasostomy—an alternative operation for obstructive azoospermia. J. Urol., 140:1545–1548, 1988.

Harrison, R. M., Lewis, R. W., and Roberts, J. A.: Pathophysiology of varicocele in nonhuman primates: long-term seminal and testicular changes. Fertil. Steril., 46:500, 1986.

Homonnai, Z. T., Fainman, N., Engelhard, Y., Rudberg, Z., David, M. P., and Paz, G.: Varicocelectomy and male fertility: Comparison of semen quality and recurrence of varicocele following varicocelectomy by two techniques. Int. J. Androl., 3:447–456, 1980.

Howards, S. S., Jesse, S., and Johnson, A.: Micropuncture and microanalytic studies of the effect of vasectomy on the rat testis and epididymis. Fertil. Steril., 26:20, 1975.

Jarow, J. P.: Intratesticular arterial anatomy. J. Androl., 11:255–259, 1990.

Jarow, J. P., Budin, R. E., Dym, M., Zirkin, B. R., Noren, S., and Marshall, F. F.: Quantitative pathological changes in the human testis after vasectomy. N. Engl. J. Med., 313:1252, 1985.

Johnson, A. L., and Howards, S. S.: Intratubular hydrostatic pressure in testis and epididymis before and after vasectomy. Am. J. Physiol., 228:556, 1975.

Kass, E. J., Chandra, R. S., and Belman, A. B.: Testicular histology in the adolescent with a varicocele. Pediatrics, 79:996–998, 1987.

Kass, E. J., and Belman, A. B.: Reversal of testicular growth failure by varicocele ligation. J. Urol., 137:475, 1987.

Kaufman, S. L., Kadir, S., Barth, K. H., Smyth, J. W., Walsh, P. C., and White, R. I.: Mechanisms of recurrent varicocele after balloon occlusion or surgical ligation of the internal spermatic vein. Radiolog·, 147:435, 1983.

Kaye, K. W.: Modified high varicocelectomy: outpatient microsurgical procedure. Urology, 32:13–16, 1988.

Kendrick, J., Gonzales, B., Huber, D., Grubb, G., and Rubin, G.: Complications of vasectomies in the United States. J. Fam. Prac., 25:245–248, 1987.

Kendrick, J. S., Rhodenhiser, E. P., Rubin, G. L., and Greenspan, J. R.: Characteristics of vasectomies performed in selected outpatient facilities in the United States. J. Reprod. Med., 30:936, 1985.

Krylov, V. S., and Borovikov, A. M.: Microsurgical method of reuniting ductus epididymis. Fertil. Steril., 41:418–423, 1984.

Laws-King, A. O., Sathananthan, A. O., and Kola, H. I.: Fertilization of human oocytes by microinjection of a single spermatozoon under the zona pellucida. Fertil. Steril., 48:637–642, 1987.

Lepow, I. H., and Crozier, R.: Vasectomy: Immunologic and Pathophysiologic Effects in Animals and Man. New York, Academic Press, 1979.

Levitt, S., Gill, B., Katlowitz, N., Kogan, S. J., and Reda, E.: Routine intraoperative post-ligation venography in the treatment of the pediatric varicocele. J. Urol., 137:716–718, 1987.

Li, S.: Ligation of vas deferens by clamping method under direct vision. Chin. Med. J., 4:213–214, 1976.

Li, S.: Percutaneous injection of vas deferens. Chin. J. Urol., 1:193–198, 1980.

Li, S., Goldstein, M., Zhu, U., and Huber, D.: The no-scalpel vasectomy. J. Urol., 145:341–344, 1991.

Lima, S. S., Castro, M. P., and Costa, O. F.: A new method for the treatment of varicocele. Andrologia, 10:103, 1978.

Lipshultz, L. I., and Corriere, J. N.: Progressive testicular atrophy in the varicocele patient. J. Urol., 117:175, 1977.

Lizza, E. F., Marmar, J. L., Schmidt, S. S., Lanasa, J. A., Sharlip, I. D., Thomas, A. J., Belker, A. M., and Nagler, H. M.: Transseptal crossed vasovasostomy. J. Urol., 134:1131, 1985.

Lord, P. H.: A bloodless operation for the radical cure of idiopathic hydrocele. Br. J. Surg., 51:914, 1964.

Lowe, D. H., Brock, W. A., and Kaplan, G. W.: Laparoscopy for localization of nonpalpable testes. J. Urol., 131:728–729, 1984.

MacMahon, R. A., O'Brien, B. McG., and Cussen, L. J.: The use of microsurgery in the treatment of the undescended testis. J. Pediatr. Surg., 11:521, 1976.

Marmar, J. L., DeBenedictis, T. J., and Praiss, D.: The management of varicoceles by microdissection of the spermatic cord at the external inguinal ring. Fertil. Steril., 43:583–588, 1985.

Massey, F. J.: Vasectomy and health: Results from a large cohort study. JAMA, 252:1023, 1984.

Mitchell, S. E., White, R. I., Chang, R., et al.: Long-term results of outpatient balloon embolotherapy in 300 varicoceles. Radiology, 157:90, 1985.

Morag, B., Rubinstein, Z. J., Goldwasser, B., Yerushalmi, A., and Lunnenfeld, B.: Percutaneous venography and occlusion in the management of spermatic varicoceles. Am. J. Roentgen., 143:635–640, 1984.

Moss, W. M.: Sutureless vasectomy, an improved technique: 1300 cases performed without failure. Fertil. Steril., 27:1040–1045, 1974.

Murray, R. R., Mitchell, S. E., Kadir, S., Kaufman, S. L., Chang, R., Kinnison, M. L., Smyth, J. W., and White, R. I.: Comparison of recurrent varicocele anatomy following surgery and percutaneous balloon occlusion. J. Urol., 135:286–289, 1986.

Nagler, H. M., Li, X. -Z., Lizza, E. F., Deitch, A., and White, R. D.: Varicocele: Temporal considerations. J. Urol., 134:411–413, 1985.

Nirapathpongporn, A., Huber, D. H., and Krieger, J. N.: No-scalpel vasectomy at the King's birthday vasectomy festival. Lancet, 335:894–895, 1990.

Odell, T. H.: Sclerosant treatment for hydroceles and epididymal cysts. Br. Med. J., 2:704, 1979.

Owen, E. R.: Microsurgical vasovasostomy: a reliable vasectomy reversal. Aust. N. Z. J. Surg., 47:305, 1977.

Petitti, D. B., Klein, R., Kipp, H., and Friedman, G. D.: Vasectomy and the incidence of hospitalized illness. J. Urol., 129:760–762, 1982.

Pryor, J., Parsons, J., Goswamy, R., Matson, P., Vaid, P., Wilson, L., and Whitehead, M.: In vitro fertilization for men with obstructive azoospermia. Lancet, 2:762, 1984.

Randall, P. E., Ganguli, L. A., Keaney, M. G. L., and Marcuson, R. W.: Prevention of wound infection following vasectomy. Br. J. Urol., 57:227–229, 1985.

Randall, P. E., Ganguli, L., and Marcuson, R. W.: Wound infection following vasectomy. Br. J. Urol., 55:564–567, 1983.

Randazzo, R. F., Hulette, C. M., Gottlieb, M. S., and Rajfer, J.: Cytomegalovirus epididymitis in a patient with the acquired immune deficiency syndrome. J. Urol., 136:1095–1096, 1986.

Reitelman, C., Burbige, K. A., Sawczuk, I. S., and Hensle, T. W.: Diagnosis and surgical correction of the pediatric varicocele. J. Urol., 138:1038–1040, 1987.

Rothman, L. P., Newmark, M., and Karson, R.: The recurrent varicocele. A poorly recognized problem. Fertil. Steril., 35:552, 1981.

Russell, J. K.: Varicocele, age, and fertility. Lancet, 2:222, 1957.

Sayfan, J., Adam, Y. G., and Soffer, Y.: A new entity in varicocele subfertility: The "cremasteric reflux." Fertil. Steril., 33:88, 1980.

Sayfan, J., Adam, Y. G., and Soffer, Y.: A natural "venous bypass" causing postoperative recurrence of a varicocele. J. Androl., 2:108–110, 1981.

Saypol, D. C., Howards, S. S., and Turner, T. T.: Influence of surgically induced varicocele on testicular blood flow, temperature, and histology in adult rats and dogs. J. Clin. Invest., 68:39, 1981.

Schlegel, P., Gilbert, B., Alikani, M., Malther, H., Talansky, B., and Goldstein, M.: Micropuncture of the human epididymis: therapeutic applications for infertile men. American Urological Association Annual Meeting, Toronto, 1991. [Abstract.]

Schmidt, S. S.: Spermatic granuloma: an often painful lesion. Fertil. Steril., 31:178–181, 1979.

Schmidt, S. S.: Vasectomy. Urol. Clin. North Am., 14:149, 1987.

Schoysman, R. J., and Bedford, J. M.: The role of the human epididymis in sperm maturation and sperm storage as reflected in the consequences of epididymovasostomy. Fertil. Steril., 46:292–299, 1986.

Selikowitz, A. M., and Schned, A. R.: A late postvasectomy syndrome. J. Urol., 134:494–497, 1985.

Shapiro, E. I., and Silber, S. J.: Open-ended vasectomy, sperm granuloma, and postvasectomy orchialgia. Fertil. Steril., 32:546–550, 1979.

Sharlip, I. D.: Vasovasostomy: Comparison of two microsurgical techniques. Urology, 17:347, 1981.

Silber, S.: Microsurgical aspects of varicocele. Fertil. Steril., 31:230, 1979.

Silber, S., Ord, T., Borrero, C., Balmaceda, J., and Asch, R.: New treatment for infertility due to congenital absence of vas deferens. Lancet, 10:850–851, 1987.

Silber, S. J.: Sperm granulomas and reversibility of vasectomy. Lancet, 2:588–589, 1977.

Silber, S. J.: Microscopic vasectomy reversal. Fertil. Steril., 28:1191, 1977.

Silber, S. J.: Microscopic vasoepididymostomy. Specific microanastomosis to the epididymal tubule. Fertil. Steril., 30:565, 1978.

Silber, S. J.: Role of epididymis in sperm maturation. Fertil. Steril., 33:47–51, 1989.

Silber, S. J., Ord, T., Balmaceda, J., Patrizio, P., and Asch, R. H.: Congenital absence of the vas deferens: The fertilizing capacity of human epididymal sperm. N. Engl. J. Med., 323:1788–1792, 1990.

Smith, M. S., and Paulson, D. F.: The physiologic consequences of vas ligation. Urol. Surv., 30:31–33, 1980.

Steckel, J., Dicker, A. P., and Goldstein, M.: Influence of varicocele size on response to surgical ligation. American Urological Association Annual Meeting, New Orleans, 1990. [Abstract.]

Stone, H. N., Schlussel, R. M., Newman, L. H., and Leventhal, I.: Laparoscopic varicocelectomy. Annual Meeting American Urological Association, Toronto, 1991. [Video.]

Szabo, R., and Kessler, R.: Hydrocele following internal spermatic vein ligation: A retrospective study and review of the literature. J. Urol., 132:924–925, 1984.

Tao, T.: Vas deferens sterility by injection method. Qeng Dao Med. J., 5:65–68, 1980.

Temple-Smith, P. D., Southwick, G. J., Yates, C. A., Trounson, A. O., and DeKretser, D. M.: Human pregnancy by in vitro fertilization (IVF) using sperm aspirated from the epididymis. J. In Vitro Fertil. Embryo Transfer, 2:119, 1985.

Tiffany, P., and Goldstein, M.: Aperistalsis of the vas deferens corrected with administration of ephedrine. J. Urol., 133:1060–1061, 1985.

Turner, T. T.: On the development and use of alloplastic spermatoceles. Fertil. Steril., 49:387–394, 1988.

Wagenknecht, L. V., Klosterhalfen, H., and Schirren, C.: Microsurgery in andrologic urology: Refertilization. J. Microsurg., 1:370, 1980.

Walker, A. M., Hunter, J. R., Watkins, R. N., Jick, H., Danford, A., Alhadeff, L., and Rothman, K. J.: Vasectomy and non-fatal myocardial infarction. Lancet, 1:13–15, 1981a.

Walker, A. M., Jick, H., Hunter, J. R., Danford, A., and Rothman, K. J.: Hospitalization rates in vasectomized men. JAMA, 245:2315–2317, 1981b.

Walsh, P. C., and White, R. I.: Balloon occlusion of the internal spermatic vein for the treatment of varicoceles. JAMA, 246:1701, 1981.

Weissbach, L., Thelen, M., and Adolphs, H. -D.: Treatment of idiopathic varicoceles by transfemoral testicular vein occlusion. J. Urol., 126:354–356, 1981.

Wensing, C. J. G.: Testicular descent in the rat and a comparison of this process with that in the pig. Anat. Rec., 214:154, 1986.

White, R. I., Kaufman, S. L., Barth, K. H., Kadir, S., Smyth, J. W., and Walsh, P. C.: Occlusion of varicoceles with detachable balloons. Radiology, 139:327, 1981.

Winfield, H. N., and Ryan, K. J.: Experimental laparoscopic surgery: potential clinical applications in urology. J. Endourol., 4:37–47, 1990.

Witkin, S. S., Zelikovsky, G., and Bongiovanni, A. M.: Sperm-related antigens, antibodies, and circulating immune complexes in sera of recently vasectomized men. J. Clin. Invest., 70:33–40, 1982.

Wosnitzer, M., and Roth, J. A.: Optical magnification and Doppler ultrasound probe for varicocelectomy. Urology, 22:24–26, 1983.

Xie-Yang, Z., and Yong-Xiong, S.: Vasovasostomy with use of medical needle as a support. J. Urol., 139:53, 1988.

Zaontz, M. R., and Firlit, C. F.: Use of venography as an aid in varicocelectomy. J. Urol., 138:1041–1042, 1987.

Zorgniotti, A. W., and MacLeod, J.: Studies in temperature, human semen quality, and varicocele. Fertil. Steril., 24:40, 1979.

INDEX

Note: Page numbers in *italics* refer to illustrations; page numbers followed by t refer to tables.

A

Abdomen, computed tomography of, attenuation values in, 482, 483t
plain film radiographs of, in cloacal malformation, 1826, *1827*
in excretory urography, 412–413, *413*, 442, *442*
in neonatal abdominal mass evaluation, 1596, *1600*
in unilateral renal agenesis, 1363, *1363*
in urinary lithiasis, 2103, *2103*
in urinary schistosomiasis, 895, *896*
in urinary tract infection, 749
stab wounds to, during pregnancy, 2593, *2593*
Abdominal incision(s), in renal surgery, 2423, *2425–2428*, 2427
in renovascular surgery, 2528, *2529*
Abdominal mass, neonatal, 1595–1599
bilateral, 1596, *1597*
excretory urography in, 1596, *1600*
frequency of causes of, 1596, 1596t
midline, 1596, *1598–1599*
physical examination in, 1596
plain abdominal radiography in, 1596
radionuclide renal scan in, 1597
solid or mixed density, 1598–1599
transillumination in, 1596
ultrasonography in, 1596t, 1596–1597, 1598t
Abdominal musculature, congenital hypoplasia of, 1593, *1593*, 1605. See also *Prune-belly syndrome*
Abdominal paravertebral sympathetic ganglion, neuroblastoma of, 1989
Abdominal quadrant, upper, auscultation of, 312
Abdominal stoma(s), 2608–2610
circular incision for, 2609
flush stoma, 2609
loop end ileostomy, 2609–2610, *2610*
nipple stoma ("rosebud"), 2609, *2609*

Abdominal stoma(s) *(Continued)*
site of, 2608–2609
Abdominal wall, anterolateral, anatomy of, 3, *10–13*, 12
in prune-belly syndrome, 1852, *1852*, *1867–1868*, 1868–1869
posterior, anatomy of, 3, *10–13*, 12
Abscess. See also individual types
of appendix ureteral obstruction due to, 549
of kidney. See *Renal abscess*
of prostate, 819–820
of psoas muscle, ureteral obstruction due to, 557, *557*
of retroperitoneum, ureteral obstruction due to, 557
of Skene's gland, vs. urethral diverticula, 2816
of tubo-ovarian structures, ureteral obstruction due to, 543–544
of urethral diverticula, 2820
perinephric. See *Perinephric abscess*
renal. See *Renal abscess*
Absent testes syndrome, 1518–1519
Absorbent products, for detrusor overactivity, 654–655
for neuromuscular voiding dysfunction, 628
for stress incontinence, 655
Acetazolamide, for uric acid lithiasis, 2116
Acetrizoate, chemical structure of, *402*
Acetylcholine, as neurotransmitter, 166
for bladder emptying, 629
in erection, 715
ureteral effects of, 133
Acid-base balance, 79–80, *81*
in neonate, 1346
in renal insufficiency, 2332
net acid excretion in, 80
proximal bicarbonate reabsorption in, 80
Acidosis, in acute renal failure, 2053
metabolic. See *Metabolic acidosis*

Acquired immunodeficiency syndrome (AIDS), 846–859. See also *Human immunodeficiency virus (HIV); Human immunodeficiency virus infection*
as epidemic, 853–854
bacille Calmette-Guérin immunization and, 954
deficient cell-mediated immunity in, 851–852
definition of, 852t
nephropathy in, 857
progression in, 852
prostate in transmission of, 222, 222t
seminal vesicles in transmission of, 222, 222t
Acrosome, of spermatozoon, male infertility and, 670, 685–686
ACTH. See *Adrenocorticotropic hormone (ACTH)*
Actin, in smooth muscle contractility, 116–117, *116–117*, 145–146
Actinomycin D, in Wilms' tumor, 1983t
Action potentials, 113–114, *113–114*
motor unit, 591
Activity product ratio (APR), in estimation of calcium stone-forming activity, 2131
Acupuncture, for bladder contractility inhibition, 620–621
Addison's disease, due to histoplasmosis, 932
signs and symptoms of, 2381t, 2381–2382
test for, 2382–2383
treatment of, 2383
Adenocarcinoma, of bladder. See *Bladder cancer, adenocarcinoma*
of cervix, DES-related, 2002
of exstrophied bladder, 2002
of prostate, 1159–1214. See also *Prostatic cancer, adenocarcinoma*
of rete testis, 1253–1254
of seminal vesicles, characteristics of, 2948
management of, 2948–2949
of upper urinary tract, 1139
of vagina, DES-related, 2002
in infant, 2002
Adenofibroma, of testis, 1254

Infertility (Continued)
  due to congenital adrenal hyperplasia, 665, 679
  due to cryptorchidism, 681–682, 1552
  due to diethylstilbestrol, 685
  due to ductal obstruction, 691–692
  due to dyskinetic cilia syndrome, 662, 685
  due to ejaculatory problems, 692–693
  due to endocrine abnormalities, 677–680
  due to epididymal obstruction, 692
  due to estrogen excess, 679
  due to febrile illness, 685
  due to fertile eunuch syndrome, 678
  due to genetic abnormalities, 680–681
  due to glucocorticoid excess, 680
  due to gonadotoxic agents, 684
  due to hyperprolactinemia, 664, 679–680
  due to hyperthyroidism, 680
  due to hypogonadotropic hypogonadism, 676, 677–678
  due to isolated FSH deficiency, 679
  due to Kallmann's syndrome, 662, 677–678
  due to Kartagener's syndrome, 662, 685
  due to Klinefelter's syndrome, 680
  due to Laurence-Moon-Bardet-Biedl syndrome, 679
  due to marijuana use, 685
  due to myotonic dystrophy, 683
  due to nitrofurantoin, 685
  due to Noonan's syndrome, 681
  due to orchitis, 686
  due to pituitary disease, 677
  due to pituitary macroadenoma, 679–680
  due to Prader-Willi syndrome, 679
  due to primary testicular failure, endocrine evaluation in, 664, 664t
  due to prolactin excess, 679–680
  due to prolactin-secreting tumor, 664, 679–680
  due to prolonged storage of sperm, 208
  due to prostatitis, 820
  due to radiation therapy, 684
  due to Sertoli cell-only syndrome, 675, 675–676, 683
  due to sickle cell disease, 685
  due to systemic illness, 685
  due to ultrastructural sperm abnormalities, 685–686, 686
  due to uremia, 685
  due to vanishing testis syndrome, 681
  due to varicocele, 663–664, 682–683
  due to vasectomy, 692
  due to XX disorder, 681
  due to XYY syndrome, 680–681
  endocrine evaluation in, 664t, 664–665
    FSH levels in, 664
    GnRH stimulation test in, 664–665
    prolactin levels in, 664
  etiologic categories of, frequencies of, 678t
  genital examination in, 663t, 663–664
  genital tract culture in, 670–671
  hemizona assay in, 673–674
  history in, 661–663, 662t
    developmental, 662
    infections and, 662
    intercourse frequency and, 661
    lubricants and, 661–662
    surgical, 662
    syndromes associated with, 662
    toxic exposures and, 662–663
  hypoosmotic sperm membrane swelling assay in, 670
  idiopathic, 687–691

Infertility (Continued)
  androgens for, 688, 689t, 690
  aromatase inhibitor for, 688, 690t
  clomiphene for, 688, 689t
  gonadotropin-releasing hormone for, 689t, 690–691
  gonadotropins for, 689t, 690
  hCG for, 689t, 690
  hMG for, 689t, 690
  kallikreins for, 691
  nonsteroidal anti-inflammatory agents for, 691
  pentoxifylline for, 691
  prevalence of, 687
  tamoxifen for, 688, 689t–690t
  testolactone for, 688, 690t
  in vitro fertilization for, 694
  intrauterine insemination for, 693–694
  laboratory evaluation in, 664–677
  Mycoplasma hominis infection and, 670–671
  physical examination in, 663–664
  postcoital test in, 671
  radiologic evaluation in, 674, 674
  rectal examination in, 664
  semen analysis in, 665–670, 676t, 676–677. See also Semen analysis
  semen processing for, 693
  seminal plasma analysis in, 257
  sperm-cervical mucus interaction assay in, 671
  sperm-oocyte interaction assay in, 673–674
  surgical anatomy in, 3114–3115
  surgical management of, 3114–3147
  testicular biopsy in, 674–676, 675, 3115–3116. See also Testis(es), biopsy of
  testicular fine needle aspiration cytology in, 676
  tubal gamete placement for, 694
  ultrasonography in, 373, 373, 674, 674
  Ureaplasma urealyticum infection and, 670–671
  vasography in, 3116–3119, 3117–3119
  zona pellucida micromanipulation for, 694
Infrapubectomy, for displaced prostatic urethra, 3004–3005, 3005
Infravesical obstruction, urethral catheterization in, 331
Infrequent voider, 1659, 1659–1660
Infundibulopelvic dysgenesis, 1392–1393, 1393
Infundibulopelvic stenosis, hydrocalycosis due to, 1388, 1389
Infundibuloplasty, for infundibular stenosis, 2463, 2463, 2465
Infundibulorrhaphy, for infundibular stenosis, 2464, 2465
Infundibulotomy incision(s), longitudinal, in stone disease, 2460, 2460–2461
Infundibulum, 34. See also under Calyx(ces); Renal collecting system
  anatomic anomalies of, 37
  stenosis of, endoinfundibulotomy for, 2270–2272
    results of, 2272, 2273t
    technique of, 2271, 2271–2272
    management of, 2463, 2463–2464, 2465
Inguinal canal, male, embryology of, 1501
  physical examination of, 314, 314
Inguinal hernia, 1554–1555
  bilateral, 1554–1555
  cryptorchidism and, 1551
  diagnosis of, 1555
  hypospadias and, 1895

Inguinal hernia (Continued)
  in girls, 1555
  incarcerated, neonatal, 1602
  incidence of, 1554
  surgical management of, 1946, 1947
  testicular feminization syndrome and, 1555
Inguinal metastasis, in squamous cell carcinoma of penis, 1282–1290. See also under Penis, squamous cell carcinoma of
Inguinal node(s), surgical anatomy of, 3077–3078
Inguinal node dissection, reconstruction after, 1291, 1292
Inguinal ring, deep, embryology of, 1501
  superficial, embryology of, 1501
Inhibin, properties of, 248
  testicular, chemical structure of, 183
    in FSH feedback control, 183
Injury, associated with Peyronie's disease, 3011–3012
  causing renal artery thrombosis, 2526, 2526
  during pregnancy, 2593, 2593
  genitourinary, 2571–2593. See also at specific site
  to intestinal organs, as complication of percutaneous nephrostomy, 2245
Inositol triphosphate (IP3), in signal transduction, 276, 277
Insemination, intrauterine, for male infertility, 693–694
Insulin, for diabetic surgical patient, 2341–2342, 2342t
  for hyperkalemia, 2333t
  male, prostatic effects of, 236
  renal metabolism of, 101, 101–102
  renal physiologic effects of, 88
Insulin-like growth factor I, 97–98
  properties of, 249, 249t
  renal synthesis of, 97–98
Insulin-like growth factor II, properties of, 249, 249t
int-2 oncogene, prostatic epithelial hyperplasia due to, 247–248
Integrins, 245
Interaortocaval lymph nodes, anatomy of, 17
Intercostal blockade, in perioperative care, 2327
Interferon, for metastatic renal cell carcinoma, 1080–1081
  intravesical, for superficial bladder cancer, 1124
Interlabial mass, 1930–1931, 1930–1932
Interleukin, in immune response, 2513–2514, 2514t
Interleukin-2, for metastatic renal cell carcinoma, 1081–1082, 1082
Interleukin-2 receptor antibodies, 2516t, 2516–2517
Intermittency, definition of, 310
Intermittent catheterization. See Urethral catheterization, intermittent
Intermittent mandatory ventilation (IMV), postoperative use of, 2325
Intermittent positive-pressure breathing devices, in perioperative pulmonary care, 2324
Intersex states. See individual types; Sexual differentiation, disorders of
Interstitial cystitis. See Cystitis, interstitial
Interstitial nephritis. See also Pyelonephritis
  acute, drugs causing, 2048, 2048t
    eosinophilia in, 2048
    urine studies in, 2050
Interstitial radiation pneumonitis, due to Wilms' tumor therapy, 1984
Intertrigo, 863

Neurovascular bundle, in retropubic prostatectomy, clinical stage of excision of, 2878t
excision of, 2876, 2878, *2878–2879*
identification and preservation of, 2875–2876, *2875–2877*
Nevoid basal-cell carcinoma syndrome, renal cysts in, 1465
Nevus, *867*, 878–879
compound, *867*, 879
intradermal, 879
junctional, 879
of penis, 1264, *1265*
Newborn. See *Infant(s), newborn*
Nicotinic acid, for hyperchloremic metabolic acidosis, 2621
Nicotinic agonists, ureteral effects of, 133
Nifedipine, for bladder contractility inhibition, 616
Nil (minimal change) disease, chronic renal failure due to, 2055
Nipple stoma, 2609, *2609*
Nipple ureterointestinal anastomosis, split, 2615–2616, *2616*
complications of, 2613t
Nipple valve(s), antireflux, 2618, *2618*
in self-catheterizing pouches, construction of, 2700
with intussuscepted terminal ileum, 2707, 2709–2711, *2709–2711*
Nitrites, in urine, dipstick test for, 319–320
Nitrofurantoin, contraindicated in pregnancy, 794
for urinary tract infection prophylaxis, 787
for vesicoureteral reflux in children, 1681
male infertility due to, 685
plasma vs. prostatic fluid levels of, 813t
serum vs. urinary levels of, 743t
Nitrogen mustard, male infertility due to, 684
Nitroglycerin paste, for impotence, 3053
Nitroprusside, for pheochromocytoma patient, 2398
Nitrous oxide, avoidance of, in urinary undiversion operations, 2724
Nocturia, 649
aging and, 644
causes of, 649, 649t
definition of, 309
in neurourologic evaluation, 577
orthotopic voiding procedures and, 2685
voiding/incontinence record in, 649, 649t, 653–654, 654t
Nocturnal penile tumescence (NPT) testing, 3036–3037, *3037*
No-incision (Gittes) transvaginal bladder neck suspension, for stress incontinence, *2797*, 2797–2798
Noncalculous disease, diagnosis and treatment of, endosurgical techniques in, 2231–2306. See also specific procedure
instruments of change in, 2231–2233, *2233–2234*
"magic bullets" and surgery in, 2231, *2232*
urologic surgery in, metamorphosis in, 2233–2235
diagnostic endourology in, 2245–2255
laparoscopy in, 2303–2306
therapeutic endourology in, 2255–2303
Nonelemental diets, 2345
Nongonococcal urethritis, 826–829. See also *Urethritis, nongonococcal*
Non-Hodgkin's lymphoma. See *Lymphoma*

Nonhormonal medical therapy, for erectile dysfunction, 3053
Non-neurogenic/neurogenic bladder, 612–613
Non-neuropathic psychologic bladder, 1661t, 1661–1664, *1662–1663*, 1664t
Nonradiated complex vesicovaginal fistula, 2824
Nonseminoma, 1239–1248
clinical staging of, 1239
histologic findings in, 3093–3094
histology in, 1239–1240
natural history of, 1239
pathologic staging in, 1245t
primary tumor in, pathologic extent of, 3093
treatment of, 1240–1248
in disseminated disease, 1248, 1249t
in stage I disease, 1240–1244
historical, 1240–1241
limited retroperitoneal node dissection in, 3096–3097, *3097–3098*
orchiectomy in, 1240, 1241t
radiation therapy in, 1243, 1244t
retroperitoneal lymph node dissection in, 1241–1243, *1242–1243*. See also *Retroperitoneal lymph node dissection*
surveillance in, 1243–1244, 1245t, 3095t, 3095–3096
in stage II disease, 1244–1246, 3097–3100
adjuvant chemotherapy after node dissection in, 3099–3100
chemotherapy in, *1245*, 1245–1246
extension to full bilateral dissection in, 3097
primary surgery vs. chemotherapy in, 3097, 3099
radiation therapy in, 1246
surgical, 1244–1245
in stage III disease, 1246–1248
adjuvant chemotherapy in, 1248
PVB studies in, 1247–1248
salvage chemotherapy in, 1248
timing of surgery for, 3108–3111, *3109–3110*
VAB protocols in, 1247
Nonsteroidal anti-inflammatory drugs (NSAIDs), for male infertility, 691
nephrotoxicity of, 2077–2078, 2078t
Noonan syndrome, 1513
cryptorchidism in, 1552
male infertility due to, 681
Norepinephrine, as neurotransmitter, 165
for bacteremic shock, 772t
ureteral effects of, 134
Norfloxacin, serum vs. urinary levels of, 743t
Northern blots, *274*, 275
NSAIDs (nonsteroidal anti-inflammatory drugs), for male infertility, 691
nephrotoxicity of, 2077–2078, 2078t
Nuclear matrix, 243–244, 244t
biologic function(s) of, 244, 244t
DNA organization as, 244, 244t
DNA replication as, 244, 244t
nuclear regulation as, 244, 244t
RNA synthesis as, 244, 244t
constituents of, 243
definition of, 243
Nucleation, of crystals, 2094–2095, *2095*
Nucleic acid, historical, 267
Nutrients, malabsorption of, following urinary intestinal diversion, 2623
Nutrition, for surgical patients, 2343–2347
assessing response to, 2345
caloric requirement in, 2343–2344

Nutrition (Continued)
enteral, 2345
fat requirement in, 2344
hyperosmotic intravenous, 2346
intravenous, renal failure and, 2346–2347
isosmotic intravenous, 2346
protein requirement in, 2344
vitamin and mineral requirement in, 2344
poor, as risk factor, in perioperative pulmonary care, 2322
total parenteral, priapism due to, 724
Nutritional index, prognostic, in surgical patient, 2344–2345
Nutritional planning, goals of, 2344
Nutritional status, preoperative evaluation of, 2344–2345

O

Obesity, as risk factor, in perioperative pulmonary care, 2322
Oblique muscle, external, anatomy of, 3, *10*
internal, anatomy of, *10*, 12
Obstructive uropathy. See *Hydronephrosis; Ureteral obstruction; Ureteropelvic junction obstruction*
in schistosomiasis. See *Schistosomiasis, obstructive uropathy in*
Obturator fascia, anatomic relationships of, 64, *65*
Obturator nerve, anatomic distribution of, 63
anatomy of, 18, *19*
injury to, as complication of prostatectomy, 2883
Occupation, role of, in bladder cancer, 1096
in urinary lithiasis, 2092
Ogilvie's syndrome, 2352
following urinary intestinal diversion, 2607, 2608
OKT3 (muromonab CD3), 2502, 2515t
Oleandomycin, plasma vs. prostatic fluid levels of, 813t
Olfactory bulb, neuroblastoma of, 1989
Oligohydramnios, definition of, 1564
in bilateral renal agenesis, 1358–1359, 1360
in posterior urethral valve(s), 1885, 1885t
Oligomeganephronia, 1446
clinical features of, 1446
evaluation in, 1446
histopathology in, 1446, *1447*
treatment in, 1446
Oligospermia. See also *Infertility, male*
causes of, 676t, 676–677
Oliguria, cause of, sodium excretion in, 78
neonatal, 1601–1602
Omentum sleeves, wrapping ureters with, 2557, *2557*
Onchocerca volvulus, 907, 916
Onchocerciasis, 916
Oncocytoma, renal, 1056–1058, *1057*
Oncofetal protein expression, in bladder cancer prognosis, 1112
Oncogene(s), 1037–1040
assay technique for, 1037–1038
historical discovery of, 290
in bladder cancer, 1096
in malignant transformation, 276, 290–293
in renal cell carcinoma, 1062
nuclear transcriptional, 1039–1040
proto-oncogene conversion to, 290–292, *291*
receptors for, increased, 291

Pulmonary hypoplasia *(Continued)*
  in posterior urethral valve(s), 1876–1877, 1885–1886
  in prune-belly syndrome, 1857
Pulmonary patient, perioperative care of, 2321–2326. See also *Perioperative care, of pulmonary patient*
Pulse oximetry, in perioperative cardiac care, 2321
Pulsed-dye laser, 2924
  stone disruption with, 2939
Purine diet, low, for urinary lithiasis, 2146
Purinergic neurotransmitters, 152t, 154
Pyelogenic cyst(s), 1482–1485, *1483–1484*
Pyelography, in acute renal failure, 2050–2051
  in blind-ending ureteral duplication, 1410, *1410*
  in genitourinary tuberculosis, 963, 967
  in neuroblastoma, 1992, *1992–1993*
  in renal pelvis tumors, *1140,* 1140–1141
  in upper urinary tract urothelial tumors, 1141
  in urinary lithiasis, *2106,* 2106–2107
  retrograde, 337–338
    allergic reactions in, 337
    indications for, 337
    patient preparation in, 337
    technique in, 337–338, *338*
    ureteral catheters in, 337, *337*
    urinary sepsis due to, 337
Pyelolithotomy, coagulum, 2468–2469, *2469–2470*
  constituents for, preparation of, 2468t
  indications for, 2468
  extended, 2465–2466, *2467, 2468*
  for stone disease, 2465, *2466*
  standard, 2465, *2466*
Pyelolysis, 2272
Pyelonephritis, 758–771
  abacterial, 761
  acute, 758–760
    bacteriology in, 759
    clinical presentation in, 758–759
    computed tomography in, 759
    intravenous urography in, 759
    laboratory findings in, 759
    pathologic findings in, 760
    perinephric abscess vs., 764–765
    radiographic findings in, 759–760
    renal angiography in, 760
    renal ultrasonography in, 759
    treatment of, 760
  as complication of ureterointestinal anastomosis, 2619
  atrophic, definition of, 732
  bacteriuria due to, 737–740
    antibody-coated bacteria for, 739
    C-reactive protein for, 739–740
    Fairley bladder washout test for, 738–739
    fever and flank pain and, 740
    ureteral catheterization for, 737–738, 738t–739t
  calculous, associated with urinary lithiasis, 2112
  chronic, 760–763
    bacterial access in, 761
    clinical presentation in, 760
    due to immunologic responses, 761–762
    intravenous urography in, 760–761
    laboratory findings in, 760
    pathogenesis of, 761–762
    pathologic findings in, 761
    radiographic findings in, 760–761
    reflux nephropathy and, 762

Pyelonephritis *(Continued)*
    sequelae of, 762–763
    voiding cystourethrography in, 761
  definition of, 732
  due to candidal infection, 939
  due to obstructive uropathy, in schistosomiasis, 905
  emphysematous, diabetes mellitus and, 757–758, *758*
  excretory urography in, *432*
  hemorrhagic, ultrasonography in, 462, *466*
  immunoglobulin response in, 751
  in children, 1672. See also *Urinary tract infection, in children*
  in pregnancy, 1677–1678
    bacteriuria and, 791–792
    prematurity and perinatal mortality in, 792–793
    radiographic studies in, 793
    treatment of, 794
  radiographic imaging in, indications for, 749, 749t
  ureteral functional effects of, 128–129
  xanthogranulomatous, 765–767
    associated with urinary lithiasis, 2113
    bacteriology and laboratory findings in, 766
    clinical presentation in, 766
    due to obstructive uropathy, in schistosomiasis, 905–906
    pathologic findings in, 766–767
    radiologic findings in, 766
    treatment of, 767
Pyeloplasty, failed, management of, 2488–2489, *2488–2490*
  for ureteropelvic junction repair, dismembered, 2482–2483, *2483–2484*
    surgical principles of, *2481,* 2481–2482
  preoperative renal drainage and, 2481
  stents or nephrostomy tubes in, intraoperative placement of, 2481–2482
Pyelotomy, and tumor excision, for noninvasive transitional cell carcinoma, of renal pelvis, *2496,* 2496–2497
  "slash," for ureteropelvic junction repair, 2482
Pyloric stenosis, hypertrophic, in autosomal dominant (adult) polycystic kidney disease, 1456
Pyogenic reactions, to blood transfusion, 2337
Pyonephrosis, 763
  diagnosis in, 763
  ultrasonography in, 763
Pyrazinamide, challenge dose for hypersensitivity to, 973t
  for tuberculosis, 969
  in renal failure, 974t
Pyuria, dipstick test for, 320
  in diagnosis of urinary tract infection, 736–737
  in urinary lithiasis, 2103
  leukocyte esterase testing for, 320

Q

Q-switched neodymium:YAG laser, stone disruption with, 2939
Q-Tip test, for incontinence, 651, 2790
Quadratus lumborum muscle, anatomy of, 12
Quantitative fluorescent image analysis, in bladder cancer, 1114
Quartey flap, for urethral reconstruction, 2991, *2993*

R

RAAS. See *Renin-angiotensin-aldosterone system*
Radiation, 395–401. See also individual procedures; *Contrast media*
  definitions in, 395–397
  exposure to, as complication of shock wave lithotripsy, 2170
  half-value layer in, 396
Radiation dose (rad), 396
  exposure patterns in, *400,* 400t, *400*
  in computed tomography, 399
  in extracorporeal shock wave lithotripsy, 398
  in percutaneous nephrostolithotomy, 398–399
  NCRP maximal permissible dose equivalent for occupational exposure to, 400t
  organ dose tables for, 398, 398t–399t
  personnel monitoring and, 400–401
  regulatory guides for, 399–400, 400t
  typical examination data for, 396t–397t, 397–398
Radiation dose equivalent (H), 397
Radiation enteritis, due to Wilms' tumor therapy, 1984
Radiation exposure, 395
Radiation pneumonitis, interstitial, due to Wilms' tumor therapy, 1984
Radiation therapy, bladder cancer due to, 1097
  for bladder cancer, invasive, 1125–1129
    metastatic, 1133
    results of, 2751t
    superficial, 1120
  for Cushing's disease, 2374
  for inguinal metastasis, in squamous cell carcinoma of penis, 1288–1289
  for nonseminoma (stage I), 1243, 1244t
  for nonseminoma (stage II), 1246
  for Peyronie's disease, 3013
  for prostatic cancer, 1201–1203
  for seminoma, 1237–1239, 1238t
  for squamous cell carcinoma of penis, 1280–1282
  for upper urinary tract urothelial tumors, 1146
  for Wilms' tumor, 1982
  in squamous cell carcinoma of penis, 1280–1282, 3074
  male infertility due to, 662, 684
  penile injury due to, 2981
  ureteral obstruction due to, 555–557
  vesicovaginal fistula due to, 2824–2825
Radiculitis, renal pain vs., 312
Radiocontrast media. See *Contrast media*
Radiography. See also individual disorders; individual imaging techniques, e.g., *Computed tomography (CT)*
  chest, in bladder cancer staging, 1118
    in germ cell tumors of testis, 1231
    in neuroblastoma, 1993
    in perioperative cardiac care, 2316
  for bladder neck position, in relation to symphysis pubis, 2834–2838, *2835–2838*
  in neurourologic evaluation, 579–580, *581–583*
  in Peyronie's disease, 3013
  in upper urinary tract defect, 2251, 2253
  plain abdominal, in cloacal malformation, 1826, *1827*
    in excretory urography, 412–413, *413,* 442, *442*

Vesical artery(ies) *(Continued)*
identification of, in radical cystectomy, 2755
Vesical calculus(i), 2140–2142
age and sex as factors in, 2140, *2140*
as complication of cystoplasty, 2645
composition of, 2140–2141
diagnosis of, 2141, *2141*
electrohydraulic lithotripsy for, 2919
in children, 2135
mechanical litholapaxy for, 2918–2919, *2919*
pathologic changes due to, 2141
size of, 2097, *2097*
symptoms of, 2141
treatment of, 2141–2142
ultrasonography of, 470, *470*
Vesical dysfunction, neurogenic. See *Bladder, neurogenic*
Vesical fascia, anatomic relationships of, 65
Vesical leukoplakia, 1101, *1102*
Vesical pain, in medical history, 308
Vesical plexus, anatomic distribution of, 63
Vesicocutaneous fistula, endosurgical management of, 2293–2295
results of, 2294–2295, 2295t
technique for, 2293–2294, *2294*
Vesico-deferential artery(ies), 2942
Vesico-deferential vein(s), 2942
Vesicopsoas hitch, use of, 2569, *2569*
Vesicorenal reflex, 48
Vesicostomy, for urethral rupture, 2585, *2586*
for vesicoureteral reflux in meningocele, 1642–1643
Vesicoumbilical fistula, 1816, *1816*
Vesicoureteral reflux, 1689–1708
antireflux surgery indications in, 1696
associated anomalies in, 1703–1704
bladder diverticulum as, 1704
neuropathic bladder as, 1703
ureteral duplication as, 1703–1704
ureteropelvic junction obstruction as, 1703
causes of, 1690, 1692t
classification and grading of, 1694–1696, *1695–1696*
clinical correlations of intrarenal reflux in, 1702–1703
"big bang" theory of, 1702
embryonic renal dysgenesis and, 1703
lifelong renal reflux and, 1703
radiography in, 1702
renal scarring and, 1702–1703
congenital, 1418
congenital hydronephrosis due to, 1607
diagnosis of, 1693–1696
cystography in, 1693
radionuclide scan in, 1694, *1694*
embryology of, 1402, *1403*
experimental studies on, 1701–1702, *1702*
genetics in, 1692–1693
historical, 1689
HLA type in, 1692
hypertension in, 1706–1707
in children, 1672–1674, *1673*
management of, 1680–1681
antimicrobial prophylaxis in, 1680–1681
antireflux procedures in, 1681, 1681t
cephalexin in, 1681
nalidixic acid in, 1681
nitrofurantoin in, 1681
trimethoprim in, 1681
trimethoprim-sulfamethoxazole in, 1681

Vesicoureteral reflux *(Continued)*
reflux nephropathy and, 1674–1675
in hyperactive bladder and detrusor-sphincter dyssynergia, 1698–1699
in meningocele, 1642–1644, *1644*
in non-neurogenic/neurogenic bladder, 1698–1699
in peripubertal girls, renal damage due to, 1677–1678
in posterior urethral valve(s), 1880–1882
in prune-belly syndrome, 1854, *1854*
in siblings, 1691–1692
in spinal cord injury, 608–609
in ureteropelvic junction obstruction, 2475–2476
in urinary tract infection, 1691, 1699–1701, *1700*
incidence of, 1699
kidney growth and, 1699–1700
kidney scarring and, *1700*, 1700–1701
in utero, 1324–1325
incidence and epidemiology of, 1691–1693
lateral ectopic ureter in, 1696, *1697*
management of, 1704–1706
antireflux surgery in, 1705–1706
cystoscopy in, 1705
endoscopic correction in, 1733–1734
Polytef injection in, 1734
Teflon injection in, 1734
measurement of intravesical ureter in, 1705, *1705*
sequential intravenous pyelograms in, 1705
spontaneous resolution and, 1705
ureteral reimplantation for, 1718–1733. See also *Ureter(s), reimplantation of*
medical vs. surgical treatment of, clinical trials of, 1707
pregnancy and, 1707
primary, 1696–1697, *1697*
abnormal renal morphology and, 1697–1698, *1698*
prognostic factors in, 1695
renal function in, 1704
ureteral factors in, 128, 1689–1691, *1691–1692*, 1692t
ureteral orifice morphology in, 1690, *1692*, 1695–1696, *1696*
ureterovesical junction–bladder pressure gradient in, 128, *128*
Vesicoureteroplasty, Licht's, 1719, *1720*
Vesicourethral suspension, for bladder outlet resistance increase, 624
Vesicovaginal fistula, 2820–2825
complex, nonradiated, 2824
diagnosis of, 2821
etiology of, 2821
giant, 2824
radiation related, 2824–2825
surgical repair of, abdominal approach in, 2822, 2825
adjuvant measures in, 2822–2823
excision of fistulous tract in, 2822
postoperative care following, 2825
principles of, 2821–2822
results of, 2824
timing of, 2822
use of estrogens and antibiotics in, 2822
vaginal approach in, 2822, 2823–2824, *2823–2824*
symptoms and presentation of, 2821
V-flap skin inserts, in cutaneous ureterostomy, 2659, *2660–2661*, 2661
Video-urodynamic studies, incontinence evaluation with, 2793
voiding cystometry and, 588–589, *590–593*

Vinca alkaloids, male infertility due to, 684
Vincristine, in Wilms' tumor, 1983t
VIP pouch, 2686, 2689, *2689*
Visual sexual stimulation, in diagnosis of erectile dysfunction, 3037
Vitamin(s), daily requirement of, 2344
Vitamin B, for Peyronie's disease, 3021
Vitamin B_{12}, deficiency of, 2336–2337
for pernicious anemia, 2337
malabsorption of, following urinary intestinal diversion, 2623
Vitamin C, for Peyronie's disease, 3021
Vitamin D, 95
excess, hypercalcemia and hypercalciuria in, 2127t, 2128
Vitamin D_2, 95, *95*
Vitamin D_3, 95, *95*, 2125
metabolism of, 95, *95*
Vitamin D sterols, renal physiologic effects of, 88
Vitamin E, for Peyronie's disease, 3013, 3021
Vitamin K deficiency, 2340
Vitiligo, *868*, 879
lichen sclerosus vs., 879
Voided volume, in child, 1621–1622
in fetus, 1314t, 1327
in neonate, preterm, 1601
term, 1601, 1621
in stress incontinence, 2831
Voider, infrequent, 1659, *1659–1660*
Voiding, neonatal, abnormal, 1601t, 1601–1602
first, 1601t
neural reflex mechanisms of, 160–163, *160–163*, 575–576
lesioning studies of, 160–162, *161*
pathways of, 160, *160–161*
spinal cord tracts in, 161, *162*
normal, requirements for, 574
observed, in incontinence, 651–652
pressure flow studies of, 2838–2842, 2839t, 2841t
problems in, following perineal prostatectomy, 2898
prompted, for detrusor overactivity, 652–653
spontaneous, by Valsalva's maneuver, 2645, *2646*
staccato, in recurrent urinary tract infection, 1656, *1656*
trigger, for neuromuscular voiding dysfunction, 628–629
vaginal, 650
Voiding dysfunction. See also *Bladder, neurogenic; Enuresis; Incontinence*
classification of, 595–601
Bors-Comarr, 596t, 596–597
Bradley loop system, 597–598
functional, 600t, 600–601
Hald-Bradley, 597, 597t
International Continence Society, 599t, 599–600
Lapides, 598, 598t
urodynamic, 598–599, 599t
due to adult enuresis, 612
due to benign prostatic hyperplasia, 1021
due to bladder neck dysfunction, 612
due to brain tumor, 602
due to cerebellar ataxia, 602
due to cerebral palsy, 602–603, 1652–1654
due to cerebrovascular disease, 601–602
due to concussion, 602
due to dementia, 602
due to diabetes mellitus, 611
due to herpes zoster virus infection, 611